Murray & Nadel's Textbook of Respiratory Medicine

Murray & Nadel's Textbook of Respiratory Medicine

SEVENTH EDITION

Editor-in-Chief

V. Courtney Broaddus, MD
Professor Emeritus of Medicine
University of California San Francisco
Division of Pulmonary and Critical Care Medicine
Zuckerberg San Francisco General Hospital
San Francisco, California

Editors

Joel D. Ernst, MD
Professor of Medicine
Chief, Division of Experimental Medicine
University of California San Francisco School of Medicine
San Francisco, California

Talmadge E. King Jr, MD
Dean, UCSF School of Medicine
Vice Chancellor for Medical Affairs
University of California San Francisco
San Francisco, California

Stephen C. Lazarus, MD, FCCP, FERS
Professor of Medicine
Division of Pulmonary and Critical Care Medicine
Senior Investigator, Cardiovascular Research Institute
University of California San Francisco
San Francisco, California

Kathleen F. Sarmiento, MD, MPH
Associate Professor of Medicine
Division of Pulmonary, Critical Care, and Sleep Medicine
University of California San Francisco;
San Francisco VA Healthcare System
San Francisco, California

Lynn M. Schnapp, MD
George R. and Elaine Love Professor
Chair, Department of Medicine
School of Medicine and Public Health
University of Wisconsin-Madison
Madison, Wisconsin

Renee D. Stapleton, MD, PhD
Professor of Medicine
Division of Pulmonary and Critical Care Medicine
University of Vermont Larner College of Medicine
Burlington, Vermont

Thoracic Imaging Editor

Michael B. Gotway, MD
Professor of Radiology
Department of Diagnostic Imaging
Mayo Clinic
Scottsdale, Arizona;
Clinical Associate Professor
Departments of Diagnostic Radiology and Biomedical
    Imaging, and Pulmonary and Critical Care Medicine
University of California San Francisco
San Francisco, California;
Clinical Professor
University of Arizona College of Medicine
Phoenix, Arizona;
Adjunct Professor
Department of Biomedical Informatics
Arizona State University
Tempe, Arizona

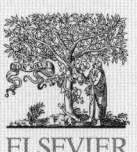

ELSEVIER

Elsevier
1600 John F. Kennedy Blvd.
Ste 1600
Philadelphia, PA 19103-2899

MURRAY & NADEL'S TEXTBOOK OF RESPIRATORY MEDICINE, ED 7   ISBN: 978-0-323-65587-3

Cover images courtesy Michael B. Gotway, MD (images 1 and 4), and U.S. Centers for Disease Control and Prevention/Alissa Eckert, MSMI; Dan Higgins, MAMS (image 2); https://phil.cdc.gov/Details.aspx?pid=23311.

Executive Content Strategist: Robin Carter
Senior Content Development Specialist: Jennifer Shreiner
Publishing Services Manager: Catherine Jackson
Senior Project Manager/Specialist: Carrie Stetz
Design Direction: Brian Salisbury

Printed in Canada

Last digit is the print number: 9   8   7   6   5   4   3   2   1

Working together
to grow libraries in
developing countries

www.elsevier.com • www.bookaid.org

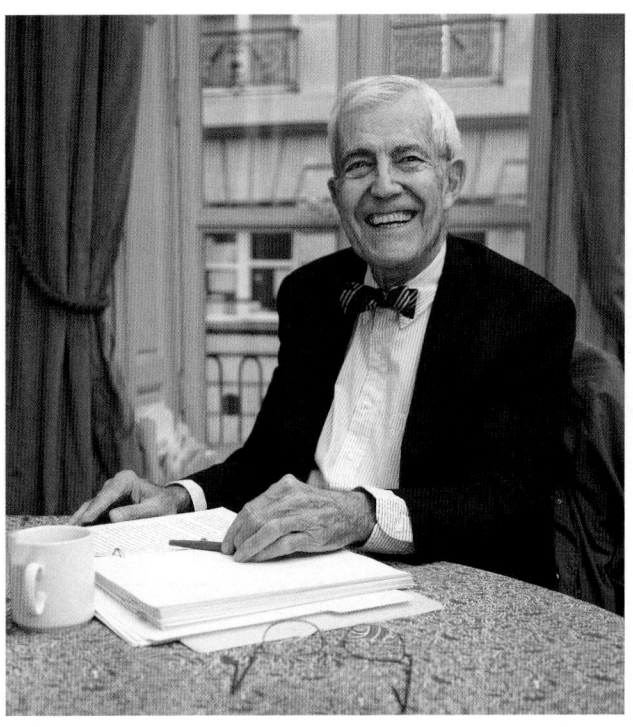

We dedicate this Textbook to Dr. John F. Murray. In 1988, Dr. Murray, together with Dr. Jay A. Nadel, published the first edition of this Textbook. Motivated by his love of teaching, he aimed to create a comprehensive, clear, authoritative, thoroughly annotated compendium of respiratory medicine, always integrated with scientific principles. Over the subsequent years and six more editions, he inspired us to continue his work and to maintain his high standards.

Of all his contributions to respiratory medicine, he was perhaps most proud of the Textbook.

John F. Murray, MD
(1927-2020)

Dedication

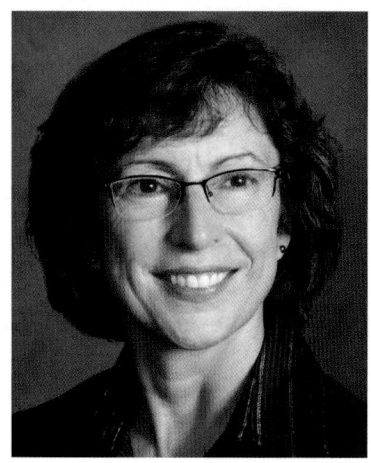

To my husband, Chuck, who has been the bedrock.

To the rest of our wonderful family, Chris and Clay, Mary and Lydia, and the grandboys Charlie and Rory.

To my mentors, colleagues and fellow editors for their inspiration and support of my career and of this project.
V. Courtney Broaddus, MD

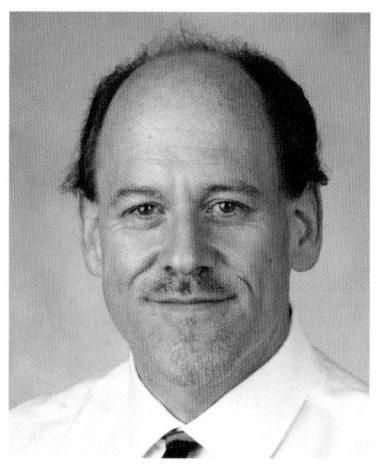

For my parents, to whom I owe all I have, and to my loving wife and daughter, Mary Pat and Allison, for all the support and inspiration they provide.
Michael B. Gotway, MD

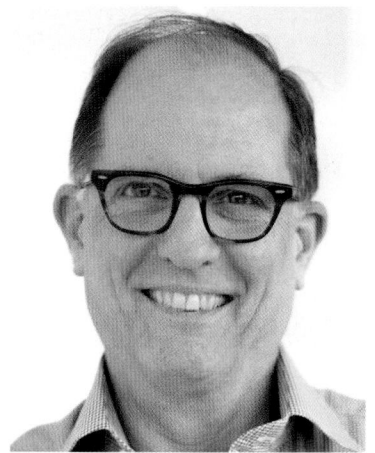

To Vicki, Kristina, and Genevieve, who make everything worthwhile.
Joel Ernst, MD

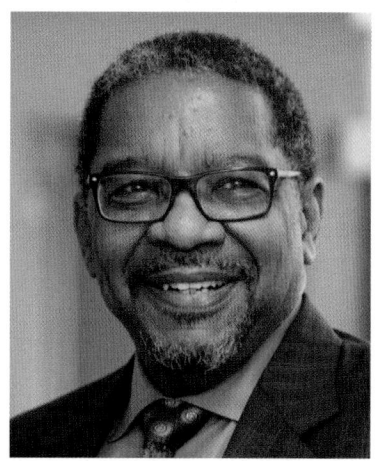

To my wife, Mozelle D. King

To my children, Consuelo King and Malaika King Kattke

To my grandchildren, Madison and Siena Kattke

To the memories of my mother and father, Almetta and Talmadge King
Talmadge E. King Jr, MD

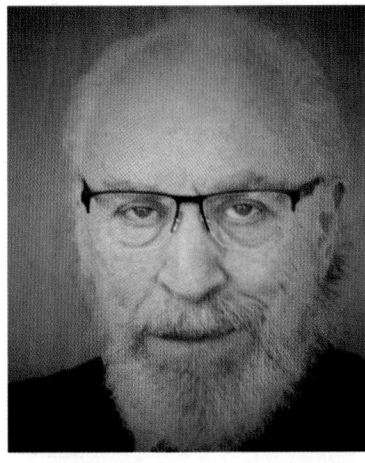

To my wife, Gail, who makes everything possible, and better; to my daughter, Hillary, and her husband, Andrew, who continue to ask about what I do, and encourage it; to my grandchildren Lola and Axel, who give me hope for the future and joy in the present; and to the many colleagues, students, and trainees, who made my first 49 years at UCSF so enjoyable.
Stephen C. Lazarus, MD, FCCP, FERS

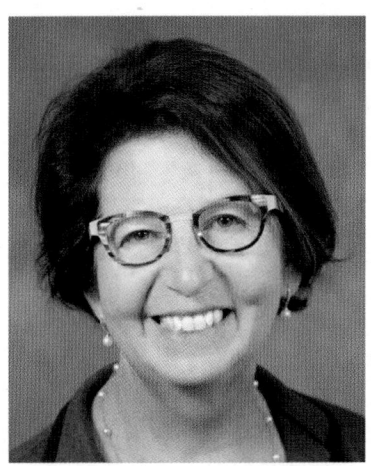

In loving memory of my parents, who were an unwavering source of support and encouragement for everything that I did. They may not have understood why I ran, but they were always at the finish line to cheer me on.
Lynn M. Schnapp, MD

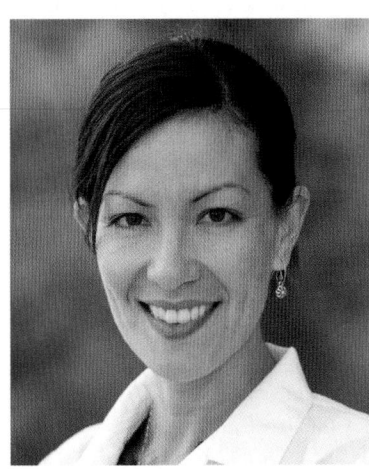

To my parents, Barbara and Barry Brennan, who taught by example the value of hard work, perseverance, and compassion.
Kathleen F. Sarmiento, MD, MPH

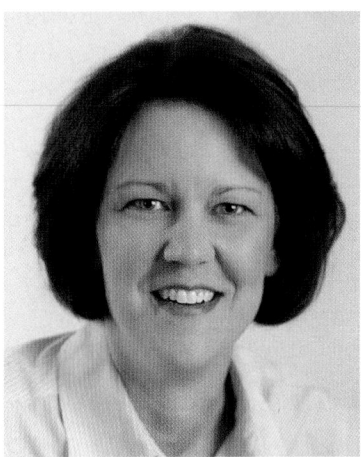

To my husband Jonathan; our children Walker, Emmerson, and Orion; my parents Myrna and Ted; and my mentors, colleagues, patients, and trainees for a lifetime of pushing me to learn, grow, and change.
Renee D. Stapleton, MD, PhD

Contributors

Lewis Adams, PhD
Professor of Physiology
School of Allied Health Sciences
Griffith University
Gold Coast, Queensland, Australia
Chapter 36: Dyspnea

Rosemary Adamson, MB, BS
Associate Professor of Medicine
Division of Pulmonary, Critical Care, and Sleep Medicine
University of Washington School of Medicine
Veterans Affairs Puget Sound Healthcare System
Seattle, Washington
Chapter 23: Ultrasonography: Principles and Basic Thoracic and Vascular Imaging

Dan E. Adler, MD
Professor of Pulmonary Medicine
Division of Pneumology
University Hospital of Geneva
Geneva, Switzerland
Chapter 136: Noninvasive Support of Ventilation

Evangelia Akoumianaki, MD, PhD
Consultant
Intensive Care Unit
University Hospital of Heraklion
Heraklion, Crete, Greece
Chapter 136: Noninvasive Support of Ventilation

Tyler J. Albert, MD
Assistant Professor of Medicine
Department of Medicine
Division of General Internal Medicine
University of Washington School of Medicine
Veterans Affairs Puget Sound Health Care System
Seattle, Washington
Chapter 12: Acid-Base Balance

Kurt H. Albertine, PhD, FAAAS, FAAA
Edward B. Clark Endowed Chair IV in Pediatrics
Adjunct Professor of Medicine and Neurobiology and Anatomy
University of Utah School of Medicine
Editor-in-Chief, *The Anatomical Record*
Salt Lake City, Utah
Chapter 1: Anatomy

Barbara D. Alexander, MD, MHS
Professor of Medicine and Pathology
Division of Infectious Diseases
Duke University Medical Center
Durham, North Carolina
Chapter 57: Fungal Infections: Opportunistic

Christopher I. Amos, PhD
Professor of Medicine
Director, Institute for Clinical and Translational Research Medicine
Associate Director of Quantitative Science
Dan L. Duncan Comprehensive Cancer Center
Baylor College of Medicine
Houston, Texas
Chapter 74: Lung Cancer: Epidemiology

Douglas A. Arenberg, MD, FACCP
Professor of Medicine
Division of Pulmonary and Critical Care Medicine
University of Michigan Medical School
Ann Arbor, Michigan
Chapter 79: Metastatic Malignant Tumors
Chapter 80: Benign Lung Tumors

A. Christine Argento, MD, FCCP
Assistant Professor of Medicine
Division of Pulmonary and Critical Care Medicine
Northwestern University Feinberg School of Medicine
Chicago, Illinois;
Professor of Medicine
Division of Pulmonary and Critical Care Medicine
Johns Hopkins University School of Medicine
Baltimore, Maryland
Chapter 27: Diagnostic Bronchoscopy: Advanced Techniques (EBUS and Navigational)

Shaikh M. Atif, PhD
Instructor of Medicine
Division of Clinical Immunology
University of Colorado Anschutz Medical Campus
Aurora, Colorado
Chapter 16: Adaptive Immunity

Najib T. Ayas, MD, MPH
Associate Professor of Medicine
University of British Columbia Faculty of Medicine
Vancouver, British Columbia, Canada
Chapter 11: Respiratory System Mechanics and Energetics

Jennifer M. Babik, MD, PhD
Associate Clinical Professor of Medicine
Division of Infectious Diseases
University of California San Francisco School of Medicine
San Francisco, California
Chapter 46a: COVID-19

Jessica B. Badlam, MD
Assistant Professor of Medicine
Division of Pulmonary Disease and Critical Care Medicine
University of Vermont Larner College of Medicine
Burlington, Vermont
Chapter 39: Wheezing and Stridor

John Randolph Balmes, MD
Professor of Medicine
Division of Occupational and Environmental Medicine
University of California San Francisco
Division of Pulmonary and Critical Care Medicine
Zuckerberg San Francisco General Hospital
San Francisco, California;
Professor of Environmental Health Sciences
University of California Berkeley School of Public Health
Berkeley, California
Chapter 102: Indoor and Outdoor Air Pollution

Niaz Banaei, MD
Professor
Departments of Pathology and Medicine (Infectious
    Diseases)
Stanford University School of Medicine
Stanford, California;
Medical Director, Clinical Microbiology Laboratory
Stanford University Medical Center
Palo Alto, California
Chapter 19: Microbiologic Diagnosis of Lung Infection

Christopher F. Barnett, MD, MPH
Director, Pulmonary Hypertension Program
Director, Medical Cardiovascular Intensive Care Unit
Department of Cardiology
Medstar Washington Hospital Center
Washington, DC
*Chapter 24: Ultrasonography: Advanced Applications and
Procedures*
*Chapter 85: Pulmonary Hypertension Due to Lung
Disease: Group 3*

Sonja D. Bartolome, MD
Professor of Medicine
Division of Pulmonary and Critical Care Medicine
University of Texas Southwestern Medical Center
Dallas, Texas
*Chapter 84: Pulmonary Arterial Hypertension:
Group 1*

Robert P. Baughman, MD
Professor of Medicine
Department of Internal Medicine
University of Cincinnati College of Medicine
Cincinnati, Ohio
Chapter 93: Sarcoidosis

Michael F. Beers, MD
Robert L. Mayock and David A. Cooper Professor of
    Medicine
Department of Medicine
Division of Pulmonary and Critical Care
Perelman School of Medicine at the University of
    Pennsylvania
Philadelphia, Pennsylvania
Chapter 3: Alveolar Compartment

Joshua O. Benditt, MD
Professor of Medicine
Division of Pulmonary and Critical Care Medicine
University of Washington School of Medicine
Director, Respiratory Care Services
University of Washington Medical Center
Seattle, Washington
*Chapter 130: The Respiratory System and Neuromuscu-
lar Diseases*

Neal L. Benowitz, MD
Emeritus Professor of Medicine
University of California San Francisco;
Attending Physician
Departments of Medicine and Biopharmaceutical Sciences
Program in Clinical Pharmacology
Division of Cardiology
Zuckerberg San Francisco General Hospital
San Francisco, California
Chapter 65: Smoking Hazards: Cigarettes, Vaping, Marijuana

Nirav R. Bhakta, MD, PhD
Associate Professor of Medicine
Division of Pulmonary, Critical Care, Allergy, and Sleep
    Medicine
Director of Education and Associate Director, Adult Pulmo-
    nary Function Laboratory
University of California San Francisco
San Francisco, California
*Chapter 31: Pulmonary Function Testing: Physiologic
and Technical Principles*
*Chapter 32: Pulmonary Function Testing: Interpretation
and Applications*
Chapter 60: Asthma: Pathogenesis and Phenotypes

Rahul Bhatnagar, MBChB, PhD
Honorary Lecturer
Academic Respiratory Unit
University of Bristol
Bristol, United Kingdom
Chapter 112: Pleural Fibrosis and Unexpandable Lung

Surya P. Bhatt, MD, MSPH
Associate Professor of Medicine
Division of Pulmonary, Allergy, and Critical Care Medicine
Medical Director, Pulmonary Function and Exercise
    Physiology Laboratory
University of Alabama at Birmingham
Birmingham, Alabama
*Chapter 32: Pulmonary Function Testing: Interpretation
and Applications*

Anna C. Bibby, MBChB, BSC, MRCP
Academic Respiratory Unit
Translational Health Sciences
University of Bristol Medical School;
Respiratory Department
North Bristol NHS Trust
Bristol, United Kingdom
Chapter 109: Pleural Infections

Alexandra Binnie, MD, DPhil, FRCP(C)
Invited Assistant Professor
University of Algarve
Faro, Portugal;
Critical Care Physician
William Osler Health System
Toronto, Canada
Chapter 134: Acute Respiratory Distress Syndrome

Paul D. Blanc, MD, MSPH
Professor of Medicine
Endowed Chair in Occupational and Environmental
    Medicine
University of California San Francisco
Chief, Division of Occupational and Environmental
    Medicine
UCSF Medical Center
San Francisco, California
Chapter 103: Acute Responses to Toxic Exposures

Zea Borok, MB, ChB
Professor of Medicine and Biochemistry and Molecular
    Medicine
Division of Pulmonary, Critical Care, and Sleep Medicine
Keck School of Medicine
University of Southern California
Los Angeles, California
Chapter 3: Alveolar Compartment

T. Douglas Bradley, MD, FRCPC
Professor of Medicine
Director, Division of Respirology
Centre for Sleep Medicine and Circadian Biology
University of Toronto Faculty of Medicine;
Director, Sleep Medicine Laboratory
University Health Network
Toronto Rehabilitation Institute
Toronto General Hospital
Toronto, Ontario, Canada
Chapter 121: Central Sleep Apnea

V. Courtney Broaddus, MD
Professor Emeritus of Medicine
University of California San Francisco
Division of Pulmonary and Critical Care Medicine
Zuckerberg San Francisco General Hospital
San Francisco, California
Chapter 14: Pleural Physiology and Pathophysiology
Chapter 44: Hypoxemia
Chapter 108: Pleural Effusion

Laurent J. Brochard, MD
Interdepartmental Division Director for Critical Care
University of Toronto Faculty of Medicine
Full Professor and Clinician Scientist
Department of Medicine
Division of Critical Care
Saint Michael's Hospital
Keenan Research Center for Biomedical Science
Toronto, Ontario, Canada
Chapter 136: Noninvasive Support of Ventilation

Steven L. Brody, MD
Dorothy R. and Hubert C. Moog Professor of Pulmonary
    Medicine
Washington University School of Medicine in St. Louis
St. Louis, Missouri
Chapter 4: Airway Biology

Kevin K. Brown, MD
Professor and Chair
Department of Medicine
National Jewish Health
Denver, Colorado;
Professor of Medicine
Division of Pulmonary Sciences and Critical Care Medicine
University of Colorado School of Medicine
Aurora, Colorado
Chapter 87: Pulmonary Vasculitis

Paul G. Brunetta, MD
Adjunct Associate Professor of Medicine
Division of Pulmonary and Critical Care Medicine
University of California San Francisco;
Fontana Tobacco Treatment Center
Mt. Zion Medical Center
San Francisco, California
Chapter 66: Smoking Cessation

Jacques Cadranel, MD, PhD
Professor of Respiratory Medicine
Service de Pneumologie
Hôpital Tenon, Assistance Publique Hôpitaux de Paris
Paris, France
Chapter 78: Rare Primary Lung Tumors

Shamus R. Carr, MD
Associate Research Physician
Thoracic Surgery Branch
Center for Cancer Research
National Cancer Institute
Bethesda, Maryland
Chapter 30: Thoracic Surgery

Tara F. Carr, MD
Associate Professor of Medicine
College of Medicine, Tucson
Asthma and Airway Disease Research Center
University of Arizona Health Sciences
Tucson, Arizona
Chapter 62: Asthma: Diagnosis and Management

Adithya Cattamanchi, MD, MAS
Professor of Medicine and Epidemiology
Division of Pulmonary and Critical Care Medicine
University of California San Francisco Center for
    Tuberculosis
University of California San Francisco School of Medicine
San Francisco, California
*Chapter 53: Tuberculosis: Clinical Manifestations and
Diagnosis*

Lara Chalabreysse, MD
Département de Pathologie
Groupement Hospitalier Est Hospices Civils de Lyon
Lyon, France
Chapter 78: Rare Primary Lung Tumors

Edward D. Chan, MD
Professor of Medicine
University of Colorado Anschutz Medical Campus
Staff Physician
Department of Medicine
Rocky Mountain Regional Veterans Affairs Medical Center
Aurora, Colorado;
Staff Physician
Department of Academic Affairs
National Jewish Health
Denver, Colorado
Chapter 69: Bronchiectasis

Ken K.P. Chan, MBChB, MRCP (UK), FHKCP, FHKAM
Clinical Assistant Professor (Honorary)
Department of Medicine & Therapeutics
Chinese University of Hong Kong;
Associate Consultant
Department of Medicine & Therapeutics
Prince of Wales Hospital
Hong Kong
Chapter 111: Chylothorax

Jean Chastre, MD
Professor
Service de Réanimation Médicale
Institut de Cardiologie, Groupe Hospitalier Pitié-Salpêtrière
Paris, France
Chapter 49: Ventilator-Associated Pneumonia

Guang-Shing Cheng, MD
Associate Professor, Clinical Research Division
Fred Hutchinson Cancer Research Center;
Associate Professor of Medicine
Division of Pulmonary, Critical Care, and Sleep Medicine
University of Washington School of Medicine
Seattle, Washington
Chapter 115: Mediastinal Tumors and Cysts
Chapter 125: Pulmonary Complications of Stem Cell and Solid Organ Transplantation

Kelly M. Chin, MD, MSCS
Associate Professor of Medicine
Division of Pulmonary and Critical Care Medicine
Director, Pulmonary Hypertension Program
University of Texas Southwestern Medical Center
Dallas, Texas
Chapter 84: Pulmonary Arterial Hypertension: Group 1

Michael H. Cho, MD, MPH
Associate Professor of Medicine
Channing Division of Network Medicine and Division of Pulmonary and Critical Care Medicine
Brigham and Women's Hospital
Harvard Medical School
Boston, Massachusetts
Chapter 9: Genetics of Lung Disease
Chapter 63: COPD: Pathogenesis and Natural History

David C. Christiani, MD
Professor of Medicine
Harvard Medical School
Elkan Blout Professor of Environmental Genetics
Department of Environmental Health
Harvard School of Public Health;
Physician
Division of Pulmonary and Critical Care
Massachusetts General Hospital
Boston, Massachusetts
Chapter 74: Lung Cancer: Epidemiology

Kian Fan Chung, MD, DSc, FRCP
Professor of Respiratory Medicine
Head of Experimental Studies
National Heart & Lung Institute
Imperial College London;
Consultant Physician
Royal Brompton and Harefield NHS Trust
London, United Kingdom
Chapter 37: Cough

Amelia O. Clive, MBBS, PhD
Consultant in Thoracic Medicine
North Bristol Lung Centre
Southmead Hospital
Bristol, United Kingdom
Chapter 112: Pleural Fibrosis and Unexpandable Lung

Robert A. Cohen, MD
Professor of Medicine
Northwestern University Feinberg School of Medicine
Clinical Professor of Environmental and Occupational Health Sciences
University of Illinois at Chicago School of Public Health
Chicago, Illinois
Chapter 101: Pneumoconioses

Thomas V. Colby, MD
Professor Emeritus
Department of Laboratory Medicine and Pathology
Mayo Clinic Alix College of Medicine
Scottsdale, Arizona
Chapter 89: Idiopathic Pulmonary Fibrosis

Carlyne D. Cool, MD
Clinical Professor of Pathology
University of Colorado School of Medicine
Aurora, Colorado;
Adjunct Professor
National Jewish Health
Denver, Colorado
Chapter 87: Pulmonary Vasculitis

Ricardo Luiz Cordioli, MD, PhD
Medical Staff
Division of Intensive Care
Albert Einstein Hospital
Oswaldo Cruz Hospital
São Paulo, Brazil;
Intensive Care Unit
University Hospital of Geneva
Geneva, Switzerland
Chapter 136: Noninvasive Support of Ventilation

Tamera J. Corte, MBBS, PhD, FRACP
Associate Professor of Medicine
University of Sydney Medical School
Consultant Respiratory Physician
Director of Interstitial Lung Disease Service
Royal Prince Alfred Hospital
Sydney, Australia
Chapter 92: Connective Tissue Diseases

Vincent Cottin, MD, PhD
Professor of Respiratory Medicine
Claude Bernard University
University of Lyon;
Head, Coordinating Reference Center for Rare Pulmonary
    Diseases, Hospices Civils de Lyon
Louis Pradel Hospital
Lyon, France
Chapter 96: Eosinophilic Lung Diseases

Kristina Crothers, MD
Professor of Medicine
University of Washington School of Medicine
Chief, Section of Pulmonary, Critical Care, and Sleep
    Medicine
Veterans Affairs Puget Sound Health Care System
Seattle, Washington
Chapter 123: Pulmonary Complications of HIV Infection

Jeffrey L. Curtis, MD
Professor of Internal Medicine
University of Michigan Medical School
Staff Physician, Medicine Service
VA Ann Arbor Healthcare System
Ann Arbor, Michigan
Chapter 63: COPD: Pathogenesis and Natural History

Charles L. Daley, MD
Professor and Chief
Division of Mycobacterial and Respiratory Infections
National Jewish Health
Denver, Colorado;
Professor of Medicine
Division of Pulmonary and Critical Care Medicine and
    Infectious Diseases
University of Colorado School of Medicine
Aurora, Colorado;
Professor of Medicine
Division of Pulmonary and Critical Care Medicine
Icahn School of Medicine at Mt Sinai
New York, New York
Chapter 55: Nontuberculous Mycobacterial Infections

Bruce L. Davidson, MD, MPH
Former Clinical Professor of Medicine
Division of Pulmonary and Critical Care Medicine
University of Washington School of Medicine
Seattle, Washington
*Chapter 82: Pulmonary Thromboembolism: Prophylaxis
and Treatment*

Helen E. Davies, MD, FRCP
Consultant Respiratory Physician
Department of Respiratory Medicine
University Hospital of Wales
Cardiff, United Kingdom
Chapter 114: Pleural Malignancy

J. Lucian Davis, MD
Associate Professor of Epidemiology
Department of Epidemiology of Microbial Diseases
Yale School of Public Health;
Associate Professor of Medicine
Pulmonary, Critical Care, and Sleep Medicine Section
Yale School of Medicine
New Haven, Connecticut
Chapter 18: History and Physical Examination

Teresa De Marco, MD
Professor of Medicine
RH and Jane G. Logan Endowed Chair in Cardiology
Chief, Advanced Heart Failure and Pulmonary
    Hypertension
Medical Director, Heart Transplantation
University of California San Francisco
San Francisco, California
*Chapter 85: Pulmonary Hypertension Due to Lung
Disease: Group 3*

Stanley C. Deresinski, MD
Clinical Professor of Medicine
Division of Infectious Diseases and Geographic Medicine
Stanford University School of Medicine
Stanford, California
Chapter 19: Microbiologic Diagnosis of Lung Infection

Christophe M. Deroose, MD, PhD
Associate Professor of Nuclear Medicine and Molecular
    Imaging
Katholieke Universiteit Leuven;
Deputy Head of Clinic
Nuclear Medicine
University Hospitals Leuven
Leuven, Belgium
Chapter 25: Positron Emission Tomography

Anne E. Dixon, MA, BM, BCh
Professor of Medicine
Chief, Division of Pulmonary Disease and Critical Care
    Medicine
Director, Vermont Lung Center
University of Vermont Larner College of Medicine
Burlington, Vermont
Chapter 61: Asthma and Obesity

David H. Dockrell, MD, FRCPI, FRCP(Glas), FACP
Professor of Infection Medicine
University of Edinburgh
Edinburgh, United Kingdom
Chapter 46: Community-Acquired Pneumonia

Christophe Dooms, MD, PhD
Assistant Professor of Pneumology
Katholieke Universiteit Leuven;
Deputy Head of Clinic
Pneumonology
University Hospitals Leuven
Leuven, Belgium
Chapter 25: Positron Emission Tomography

Gregory P. Downey, MD
Executive Vice President, Academic Affairs
Department of Medicine
National Jewish Health;
Professor
Departments of Medicine and Immunology and
    Microbiology
Associate Dean
University of Colorado Denver School of Medicine
Denver, Colorado
Chapter 8: Regeneration and Repair

Hilary DuBrock, MD, MMSc
Assistant Professor of Medicine
Mayo Clinic
Rochester, Minnesota
*Chapter 126: Pulmonary Complications of Abdominal
Diseases*

Souheil El-Chemaly, MD, MPH
Assistant Professor of Medicine
Division of Pulmonary and Critical Care Medicine
Harvard Medical School
Brigham and Women's Hospital
Boston, Massachusetts
Chapter 7: Lymphatic Biology

C. Gregory Elliott, MD
Professor of Internal Medicine
University of Utah School of Medicine
Salt Lake City, Utah;
Chairman, Department of Medicine
Intermountain Medical Center
Murray, Utah
*Chapter 82: Pulmonary Thromboembolism: Prophylaxis
and Treatment*

Joel D. Ernst, MD
Professor of Medicine
Chief, Division of Experimental Medicine
University of California San Francisco School of Medicine
San Francisco, California
Chapter 52: Tuberculosis: Pathogenesis and Immunity

Christopher M. Evans, PhD
Professor of Medicine
Division of Pulmonary Sciences and Critical Care
University of Colorado School of Medicine
Aurora, Colorado
Chapter 4: Airway Biology

John V. Fahy, MD, MSc
Professor of Medicine
Division of Pulmonary, Critical Care, Allergy, and Sleep
    Medicine
Cardiovascular Research Institute
University of California San Francisco
San Francisco, California
Chapter 60: Asthma: Pathogenesis and Phenotypes

Elaine Fajardo, MD
Assistant Professor of Medicine
Pulmonary, Critical Care, and Sleep Medicine Section
Yale School of Medicine
New Haven, Connecticut
Chapter 18: History and Physical Examination

Eddy Fan, MD, PhD
Associate Professor of Medicine
Interdepartmental Division of Critical Care Medicine
University of Toronto Faculty of Medicine
Toronto, Ontario, Canada
Chapter 135: Mechanical Ventilation

Marie E. Faughnan, MD, MSc
Professor of Medicine
Division of Respirology
University of Toronto Faculty of Medicine
Toronto, Ontario, Canada
Chapter 88: Pulmonary Vascular Anomalies

David Feller-Kopman, MD, FCCP
Professor of Medicine, Anesthesiology, and Otolaryngology–
 Head and Neck Surgery
Director, Bronchoscopy and Interventional Pulmonology
Department of Pulmonary and Critical Care Medicine
Johns Hopkins Medical Institutions
Baltimore, Maryland
*Chapter 27: Diagnostic Bronchoscopy: Advanced
Techniques (EBUS and Navigational)*
*Chapter 28: Therapeutic Bronchoscopy: Interventional
Techniques*

Brett E. Fenster, MD
Cardiologist
Kaiser Permanente
Denver, Colorado
Chapter 38: Chest Pain

Timothy M. Fernandes, MD, MPH
Associate Clinical Professor of Medicine
Division of Pulmonary, Critical Care, and Sleep Medicine
University of California San Diego School of Medicine
San Diego, California
*Chapter 86: Pulmonary Hypertension Due to Chronic
Thromboembolic Disease: Group 4*

Evans R. Fernández Pérez, MD, MS
Associate Professor of Medicine
Division of Pulmonary, Critical Care, and Sleep Medicine
National Jewish Health
Denver, Colorado
Chapter 91: Hypersensitivity Pneumonitis

William A. Fischer II, MD
Assistant Professor of Medicine
Institute of Global Health and Infectious Diseases
Division of Pulmonary and Critical Care Medicine
The University of North Carolina School of Medicine
Chapel Hill, North Carolina
Chapter 59: Outbreaks, Pandemics, and Bioterrorism

Andrew P. Fontenot, MD
Henry N. Claman Professor of Medicine
Division of Clinical Immunology
University of Colorado Anschutz Medical Campus
Aurora, Colorado
Chapter 16: Adaptive Immunity

James Frank, MD, MA
Professor of Clinical Medicine
Division of Pulmonary, Critical Care, Allergy, and Sleep
 Medicine
University of California San Francisco School of Medicine
San Francisco, California
*Chapter 23: Ultrasonography: Principles and Basic
Thoracic and Vascular Imaging*

Stephen K. Frankel, MD, FCCM, FCCP
Executive Vice President, Clinical Affairs
Professor of Medicine
National Jewish Health
Denver, Colorado;
Professor of Medicine
Division of Pulmonary Sciences and Critical Care Medicine
University of Colorado School of Medicine
Aurora, Colorado
Chapter 87: Pulmonary Vasculitis

Joseph Friedberg, MD
Charles Reid Edwards Professor of Surgery
Head, Division of Thoracic Surgery
Director, Pleural Mesothelioma Program
University of Maryland School of Medicine
Baltimore, Maryland
Chapter 30: Thoracic Surgery
Chapter 113: Hemothorax

Monica Fung, MD
Assistant Professor of Medicine
Division of Infectious Diseases
University of California San Francisco School of Medicine
San Francisco, California
Chapter 46a: COVID-19

Yuansheng Gao, PhD
Professor of Physiology and Pathophysiology
Peking University Health Science Center
Beijing, China
Chapter 6: Vascular Biology

Erik Garpestad, MD
Associate Professor of Medicine
Division of Pulmonary, Critical Care, and Sleep Medicine
Director, Medical ICU
Tufts Medical Center
Boston, Massachusetts
Chapter 132: Acute Ventilatory Failure

Eric J. Gartman, MD
Associate Professor of Medicine
Division of Pulmonary, Critical Care, and Sleep Medicine
Alpert Medical School of Brown University;
Staff Physician
Division of Pulmonary, Critical Care, and Sleep Medicine
Providence VA Medical Center
Providence, Rhode Island
*Chapter 131: The Respiratory System and Chest Wall
Diseases*

G.F. Gebhart, PhD
Professor of Anesthesiology, Medicine, Neurobiology, and
 Pharmacology
Director, Center for Pain Research
University of Pittsburgh School of Medicine
Pittsburgh, Pennsylvania
Chapter 38: Chest Pain

Gautam George, MD
Assistant Professor of Medicine
Division of Pulmonary, Allergy, and Critical Care Medicine
Jane and Leonard Korman Respiratory Institute
Sidney Kimmel Medical College
Thomas Jefferson University
Philadelphia, Pennsylvania
Chapter 5: Lung Mesenchyme

Yaron B. Gesthalter, MD
Assistant Professor of Medicine
Division of Pulmonary and Critical Care
Section of Interventional Pulmonology
University of California San Francisco School of Medicine
San Francisco, California
Chapter 40: Hemoptysis

Mark T. Gladwin, MD
Jack D. Myers Professor and Chair
Department of Medicine
University of Pittsburgh School of Medicine
Director, Pittsburgh Heart, Lung, Blood, and Vascular
    Medicine Institute
University of Pittsburgh Medical Center
Pittsburgh, Pennsylvania
*Chapter 127: Pulmonary Complications of Hematologic
Diseases*

Leonard H.T. Go, MD
Research Assistant Professor of Environmental and
    Occupational Health Sciences
University of Illinois at Chicago School of Public Health;
Department of Medicine
Stroger Hospital of Cook County;
Department of Medicine
Northwestern University Feinberg School of Medicine
Chicago, Illinois
Chapter 101: Pneumoconioses

Nisha H. Gidwani, MD
Associate Professor of Clinical Medicine
Division of Pulmonary, Critical Care, Allergy, and Sleep
    Medicine
University of California San Francisco
San Francisco, California
Chapter 50: Lung Abscess

Nicolas Girard, MD, PhD
Professor of Respiratory Medicine
Institut du Thorax Curie Montsouris
Institut Curie
Paris, France
Chapter 78: Rare Primary Lung Tumors

Robb W. Glenny, MD
Professor of Medicine and of Physiology and Biophysics
Division of Pulmonary and Critical Care Medicine
University of Washington School of Medicine
Seattle, Washington
Chapter 33: Exercise Testing

Ewan C. Goligher, MD, PhD
Assistant Professor of Medicine
Interdepartmental Division of Critical Care Medicine
University of Toronto Faculty of Medicine;
Scientist
Toronto General Hospital Research Institute;
Attending Physician
Department of Medicine, Division of Respirology
University Health Network
Toronto, Ontario, Canada
Chapter 135: Mechanical Ventilation

Antonio Gomez, MD
Associate Professor of Medicine
University of California San Francisco
Medical Director, Critical Care Services
Zuckerberg San Francisco General Hospital
San Francisco, California
Chapter 44: Hypoxemia

Anne V. Gonzalez, MD, MSc
Associate Professor of Medicine
McGill University Faculty of Medicine
Montreal, Quebec, Canada
Chapter 76: Lung Cancer: Diagnosis and Staging

Stephen B. Gordon, MD, MA, FRCP, DTM&H
Director, Malawi Liverpool Wellcome Programme
University of Malawi College of Medicine
Blantyre, Malawi;
Professor of Clinical Sciences
Liverpool School of Tropical Medicine
Liverpool, United Kingdom
Chapter 46: Community-Acquired Pneumonia

Dominique Gossot, MD
Institut du Thorax Curie Montsouris
Institut Mutualiste Montsouris
Paris, France
Chapter 78: Rare Primary Lung Tumors

Jeffrey E. Gotts, MD, PhD
Assistant Professor of Medicine
Division of Pulmonary and Critical Care Medicine
University of California San Francisco
San Francisco, California
Chapter 65: Smoking Hazards: Cigarettes, Vaping, Marijuana

Michael B. Gotway, MD
Professor of Radiology
Department of Diagnostic Imaging
Mayo Clinic
Scottsdale, Arizona;
Clinical Associate Professor
Departments of Diagnostic Radiology and Biomedical
    Imaging, and Pulmonary and Critical Care Medicine
University of California San Francisco
San Francisco, California;
Clinical Professor
University of Arizona College of Medicine
Phoenix, Arizona;
Adjunct Professor
Department of Biomedical Informatics
Arizona State University
Tempe, Arizona
*Chapter 20: Thoracic Radiology: Noninvasive Diagnostic
Imaging*

Michael Gould, MD, MS
Director for Health Services Research
Department of Research and Evaluation
Kaiser Permanente Southern California
Pasadena, California
Chapter 41: Pulmonary Nodule

Bridget A. Graney, MD
Instructor in Medicine
Division of Pulmonary Sciences and Critical Care
University of Colorado School of Medicine
Aurora, Colorado
*Chapter 90: Nonspecific Interstitital Pneumonitis and
Other Idiopathic Interstitital Pneumonias*

Giacomo Grasselli, MD
Associate Professor
Department of Pathophysiology and Transplantation
University of Milan
Dipartimento di Anestesia-Rianimazione e Emergenza
    Urgenza
Fondazione IRCCS Ca' Granda Ospedale Maggiore Policlinico
Milan, Italy
Chapter 138: Extracorporeal Support of Gas Exchange

John R. Greenland, MD, PhD
Associate Professor of Medicine
University of California San Francisco School of Medicine;
Staff Physician
Medical Service
San Francisco Veterans Administration Health Care
    System
San Francisco, California
Chapter 72: Bronchiolitis

David E. Griffith, MD
Professor of Medicine
Division of Mycobacterial and Respiratory Infections
National Jewish Health
Denver, Colorado
Chapter 55: Nontuberculous Mycobacterial Infections

Nishant Gupta, MD, MS
Associate Professor of Internal Medicine
Division of Pulmonary, Critical Care, and Sleep Medicine
University of Cincinnati College of Medicine
Cincinnati, Ohio
Chapter 97: Lymphangioleiomyomatosis

Rob Hallifax, DPhil, BMCh, MSc, MRCP
Academic Clinical Lecturer
Respiratory Trials Unit
Oxford Centre for Respiratory Medicine
Churchill Hospital NHS Trust
Oxford, United Kingdom
Chapter 110: Pneumothorax

Meilan K. Han, MD, MS
Professor of Medicine
Division of Pulmonary and Critical Care Medicine
University of Michigan School of Medicine
Ann Arbor, Michigan
Chapter 64: COPD: Diagnosis and Management

Nadia N. Hansel, MD, MPH
Professor of Medicine
Division of Pulmonary and Critical Care Medicine
Johns Hopkins University School of Medicine
Baltimore, Maryland
Chapter 63: COPD: Pathogenesis and Natural History

Umur Hatipoğlu, MD, MBA
Associate Professor of Medicine
Cleveland Clinic Lerner College of Medicine of Case
    Western Reserve University
Director, COPD Center
Respiratory Institute, Cleveland Clinic Foundation
Cleveland, Ohio
Chapter 106: Air Travel

William R. Henderson, MD, PhD
Clinical Professor of Critical Care Medicine
University of British Columbia Faculty of Medicine
Staff Intensivist
Division of Critical Care Medicine
Vancouver General Hospital
Vancouver, British Columbia, Canada
Chapter 11: Respiratory System Mechanics and Energetics

Susanne Herold, MD, PhD
Professor of Medicine
Universities of Giessen and Marburg Lung Center
Giessen, Germany
Chapter 8: Regeneration and Repair

Margaret S. Herridge, MSc, MD, MPH, FRCP(C)
Professor of Medicine
University of Toronto Faculty of Medicine;
Attending Physician
Division of Respirology and Critical Care
University Health Network
Toronto, Canada
Chapter 134: Acute Respiratory Distress Syndrome

Robert Hiensch, MD
Assistant Professor of Medicine
Division of Pulmonary, Critical Care, and Sleep Medicine
Icahn School of Medicine at Mount Sinai
New York, New York
Chapter 119: Sleep-Disordered Breathing: A General Approach

Janet Hilbert, MD
Assistant Professor of Clinical Medicine
Division of Pulmonary, Critical Care, and Sleep Medicine
Yale School of Medicine
New Haven, Connecticut
Chapter 130: The Respiratory System and Neuromuscular Diseases

Nicholas S. Hill, MD, FPVRI
Professor of Medicine
Chief, Division of Pulmonary, Critical Care, and Sleep Medicine
Tufts University Medical Center
Boston, Massachusetts
Chapter 132: Acute Ventilatory Failure

Antonia Ho, MBChB, PhD
Clinical Senior Lecturer
MRC-University of Glasgow Centre for Virus Research
Institute of Infection, Immunity & Inflammation
Glasgow, United Kingdom
Chapter 46: Community-Acquired Pneumonia

Stephanie M. Holm, MD, MPH
Assistant Clinical Professor of Medicine
Division of Occupational and Environmental Medicine
University of California San Francisco;
Co-Director
Western States Pediatric Environmental Health Specialty Units (WSPEHSU)
San Francisco, California;
Doctoral Student in Public Health
Division of Epidemiology
University of California Berkeley School of Public Health
Berkeley, California
Chapter 102: Indoor and Outdoor Air Pollution

Wynton Hoover, MD
Professor of Pediatrics
Division of Pulmonary and Sleep Medicine
University of Alabama at Birmingham
Birmingham, Alabama
Chapter 68: Cystic Fibrosis: Diagnosis and Management

Philip C. Hopewell, MD
Professor of Medicine
Director, Curry International TB Center
University of California San Francisco
San Francisco, California
Chapter 51: Tuberculosis Epidemiology and Prevention

David J. Horne, MD, MPH
Associate Professor of Medicine
Division of Pulmonary, Critical Care, and Sleep Medicine
Adjunct Associate Professor of Global Health
Harborview Medical Center
University of Washington
Seattle, Washington
Chapter 54: Tuberculosis: Treatment of Drug-Susceptible and Drug-Resistant

Richard L. Horner, PhD, FCAHS
Professor of Medicine and Physiology
Faculty of Medicine, University of Toronto;
Canada Research Chair in Sleep and Respiratory Neurobiology
Fellow, Canadian Academy of Health Sciences
Toronto, Ontario, Canada
Chapter 117: Control of Breathing and Upper Airways During Sleep

Connie C.W. Hsia, MD
Professor of Internal Medicine
Division of Pulmonary and Critical Care Medicine
University of Texas Southwestern Medical Center
Dallas, Texas
Chapter 128: Pulmonary Complications of Endocrine Diseases

Laurence Huang, MD
Professor of Medicine
University of California San Francisco School of Medicine
Chief, HIV/AIDS Chest Clinic
Zuckerberg San Francisco General Hospital
San Francisco, California
Chapter 123: Pulmonary Complications of HIV Infection

Lindsey L. Huddleston, MD
Assistant Clinical Professor of Anesthesia
University of California San Francisco School of Medicine
San Francisco, California
Chapter 24: Ultrasonography: Advanced Applications and Procedures

Robert C. Hyzy, MD
Professor of Medicine
Division of Pulmonary & Critical Care Medicine
University of Michigan Medical School
Director, Critical Care Medicine Unit
University of Michigan Hospital
Ann Arbor, Michigan
Chapter 137: Noninvasive Support of Oxygenation

Yoshikazu Inoue, MD, PhD
Executive Director, Clinical Research Center
National Hospital Organization Kinki-Chuo Chest Medical Center
Sakai, Osaka, Japan
Chapter 97: Lymphangioleiomyomatosis

Claudia V. Jakubzick, PhD
Associate Professor of Microbiology and Immunology
Dartmouth College
Hanover, New Hampshire
Chapter 15: Innate Immunity

Shijing Jia, MD
Assistant Professor of Medicine
Division of Pulmonary & Critical Care Medicine
University of Michigan Medical School
Ann Arbor, Michigan
Chapter 137: Noninvasive Support of Oxygenation

Kerri A. Johannson, MD, MPH
Assistant Professor of Medicine
University of Calgary Cumming School of Medicine
Calgary, Alberta, Canada
Chapter 91: Hypersensitivity Pneumonitis

Meshell Johnson, MD
Professor of Medicine
University of California San Francisco
Chief, Division of Pulmonary, Critical Care, and Sleep
    Medicine
San Francisco VA Health Care System
San Francisco, California
Chapter 71: Large Airway Disorders

Clinton E. Jokerst, MD
Assistant Professor of Radiology
Department of Diagnostic Imaging
Mayo Clinic
Scottsdale, Arizona
*Chapter 20: Thoracic Radiology: Noninvasive
Diagnostic Imaging*

Kirk D. Jones, MD
Professor of Pathology
University of California San Francisco School of Medicine
San Francisco, California
*Chapter 22: Pathology: Neoplastic and Non-neoplastic
Lung Disease*
Chapter 72: Bronchiolitis

Marc A. Judson, MD
Chief, Division of Pulmonary and Critical Care Medicine
Albany Medical Center
Albany, New York
Chapter 93: Sarcoidosis

Andre C. Kalil, MD, MPH
Professor of Internal Medicine
Division of Infectious Diseases
University of Nebraska Medical Center
Omaha, Nebraska
Chapter 48: Hospital-Acquired Pneumonia

Marta Kaminska, MD, MSc
Associate Professor of Medicine
Division of Respiratory Medicine
McGill University Faculty of Medicine
Sleep Laboratory
McGill University Health Centre
Montreal, Quebec, Canada
Chapter 120: Obstructive Sleep Apnea

David A. Kaminsky, MD
Professor of Medicine
Division of Pulmonary and Critical Care Medicine
University of Vermont Larner College of Medicine;
Attending Physician
Division of Pulmonary and Critical Care Medicine
University of Vermont Medical Center
Burlington, Vermont
*Chapter 31: Pulmonary Function Testing: Physiologic
and Technical Principles*
Chapter 39: Wheezing and Stridor

Midori Kato-Maeda, MD, MS
Associate Professor of Medicine
University of California San Francisco
Zuckerberg San Francisco General Hospital
San Francisco, California
Chapter 51: Tuberculosis Epidemiology and Prevention

David A. Kaufman, MD
Assistant Professor of Medicine
NYU Grossman School of Medicine
New York, New York
Chapter 46a: COVID-19

Kim M. Kerr, MD
Clinical Professor of Medicine
Division of Pulmonary, Critical Care, and Sleep Medicine
University of California San Diego School of Medicine
San Diego, California
*Chapter 86: Pulmonary Hypertension Due to Chronic
Thromboembolic Disease: Group 4*

Shaf Keshavjee, MD, MSc, FRCSC, FACS
Professor of Surgery
Division of Thoracic Surgery
University of Toronto Faculty of Medicine
Surgeon-in-Chief
Sprott Department of Surgery
Director, Toronto Lung Transplant Program
Director, Latner Thoracic Research Laboratories
University Health Network
Toronto, Ontario, Canada
Chapter 140: Lung Transplantation

Fayez Kheir, MD, MSCR
Assistant Professor of Medicine
Division of Pulmonary, Critical Care, and Environmental
    Medicine
Tulane University School of Medicine
New Orleans, Louisiana
Chapter 40: Hemoptysis

Kristen M. Kidson, MD
Clinical Instructor
Department of Anesthesiology, Pharmacology, and
Therapeutics
University of British Columbia Faculty of Medicine
Vancouver, British Columbia, Canada
Chapter 11: Respiratory System Mechanics and Energetics

Kami Kim, MD
Andor Szentivanyi Professor of Medicine
Director, Division of Infectious Disease & International
Medicine
University of South Florida Morsani College of Medicine
Global Health Infectious Disease Research Program
University of South Florida College of Public Health
Tampa, Florida
Chapter 58: Parasitic Infections

Suil Kim, MD, PhD
Assistant Professor
Departments of Medicine, Physiology, and Pharmacology
Oregon Health & Science University
Director, Pulmonary Function Laboratory
VA Portland Health Care System
Portland, Oregon
Chapter 71: Large Airway Disorders

R. John Kimoff, MD, FRCP(C)
Professor of Medicine
Division of Respiratory Medicine
McGill University Faculty of Medicine
Director, Sleep Laboratory
McGill University Health Centre
Montreal, Quebec, Canada
Chapter 120: Obstructive Sleep Apnea

Talmadge E. King Jr, MD
Dean, UCSF School of Medicine
Vice Chancellor for Medical Affairs
University of California San Francisco
San Francisco, California
Chapter 89: Idiopathic Pulmonary Fibrosis
*Chapter 90: Nonspecific Interstitial Pneumonitis and
Other Idiopathic Interstitial Pneumonias*

Georgios Kitsios, MD, PhD
Assistant Professor of Medicine
Division of Pulmonary, Allergy, and Critical Care
Medicine
University of Pittsburgh School of Medicine
Pittsburgh, Pennsylvania
Chapter 17: Microbiome

Jeffrey S. Klein, MD
A. Bradley Soule and John P. Tampas Green and Gold
Professor of Radiology
University of Vermont College of Medicine
Burlington, Vermont
*Chapter 21: Thoracic Radiology: Invasive Diagnostic
Imaging and Image-Guided Interventions*

Kristine Konopka, MD
Assistant Professor of Pathology
University of Michigan Medical School
Ann Arbor, Michigan
Chapter 80: Benign Lung Tumors

Laura L. Koth, MD
Professor of Medicine
Division of Pulmonary and Critical Care Medicine
University of California San Francisco
San Francisco, California
Chapter 93: Sarcoidosis

Robert M. Kotloff, MD
Professor of Clinical Medicine
Pulmonary, Allergy, and Critical Care Division
The Perelman School of Medicine at the University of
Pennsylvania
Philadelphia, Pennsylvania
Chapter 140: Lung Transplantation

Monica Kraft, MD
Robert and Irene Flinn Professor and Chair
Department of Medicine
College of Medicine, Tucson;
Deputy Director, Asthma and Airway Disease Research Center
University of Arizona Health Sciences
Tucson, Arizona
Chapter 62: Asthma: Diagnosis and Management

Vidya Krishnan, MD, MHS
Associate Professor of Medicine
Case Western Reserve University School of Medicine
Associate Director, Center for Sleep Medicine
Division of Pulmonary, Critical Care, and Sleep Medicine
The MetroHealth System
Cleveland, Ohio
Chapter 118: Consequences of Sleep Disruption

Lisa Kroon, PharmD
Professor and Chair
Department of Clinical Pharmacy
University of California San Francisco School of Pharmacy
San Francisco, California
Chapter 66: Smoking Cessation

Wolfgang M. Kuebler, MD, FERS, FAPS
Professor of Physiology
Institute of Physiology
Charite–Universitatsmedizin Berlin
Berlin, Germany
Chapter 6: Vascular Biology

Elif Küpeli, MD, FCCP
Professor of Medicine
Pulmonary Department
Baskent Üniversitesi Hastanesi Göğüs Hastalıkları AD
Ankara, Turkey
*Chapter 26: Diagnostic Bronchoscopy: Basic
Techniques*

Ware G. Kuschner, MD
Chief, Pulmonary Section
VA Palo Alto Health Care System;
Professor of Medicine
Stanford University School of Medicine
Palo Alto, California
Chapter 103: Acute Responses to Toxic Exposures

Bart N. Lambrecht, MD, PhD
Department Director
Center for Inflammation Research (IRC)
Vlaams Instituut voor Biotechnologie
Zwijnaarde, Belgium;
Professor of Pulmonary Medicine
Ghent University
Ghent, Belgium
Chapter 60: Asthma: Pathogenesis and Phenotypes

Matthew R. Lammi, MD, MSCR
Associate Professor of Medicine
Division of Pulmonary/Critical Care and Allergy/
    Immunology
Louisiana State University Health Sciences Center
New Orleans, Louisiana
Chapter 83: Pulmonary Hypertension: General Approach

Stephen E. Lapinsky, MBBCh, MSc, FRCPC
Professor of Medicine
University of Toronto Faculty of Medicine
Director, Intensive Care Unit
Mount Sinai Hospital
Toronto, Ontario, Canada
*Chapter 129: The Lungs in Obstetric and Gynecologic
Diseases*

Stephen C. Lazarus, MD, FCCP, FERS
Professor of Medicine
Division of Pulmonary and Critical Care Medicine
Senior Investigator, Cardiovascular Research Institute
University of California San Francisco
San Francisco, California
Chapter 64: COPD: Diagnosis and Management

Jarone Lee, MD, MPH, FCCM
Associate Professor of Surgery and Emergency Medicine
Harvard Medical School
Medical Director, Blake 12 ICU
Trauma, Emergency Surgery, Surgical Critical Care
Department of Emergency Medicine
Massachusetts General Hospital
Boston, Massachusetts
Chapter 104: Trauma and Blast Injuries

Joyce S. Lee, MD
Associate Professor of Medicine
Division of Pulmonary Sciences and Critical Care
University of Colorado School of Medicine
Aurora, Colorado
Chapter 89: Idiopathic Pulmonary Fibrosis
*Chapter 90: Nonspecific Interstitial Pneumonitis and
Other Idiopathic Interstitial Pneumonias*

Warren L. Lee, MD, PhD, FRCP(C)
Associate Professor of Medicine
University of Toronto Faculty of Medicine;
Attending Physician
Medical-Surgical Intensive Care Unit
Canada Research Chair, Mechanisms of Endothelial
    Permeability
Staff Scientist, Keenan Research Center
St. Michael's Hospital, Unity Health Network
Toronto, Canada
Chapter 134: Acute Respiratory Distress Syndrome

Won Y. Lee, MD
Associate Professor of Internal Medicine
Division of Pulmonary and Critical Care Medicine
University of Texas Southwestern Medical Center
Dallas, Texas
*Chapter 128: Pulmonary Complications of Endocrine
Diseases*

Y.C. Gary Lee, MBChB, PhD, FRACP, FCCP
Professor of Respiratory Medicine
Centre for Respiratory Health
University of Western Australia;
Consultant, Department of Respiratory Medicine
Director of Pleural Services
Sir Charles Gairdner Hospital
Perth, Australia
Chapter 111: Chylothorax
Chapter 114: Pleural Malignancy

Teofilo L. Lee-Chiong Jr, MD
Professor of Medicine
University of Colorado School of Medicine
National Jewish Health
Denver, Colorado
Chapter 38: Chest Pain

Jonathan M. Lehman, MD, PhD
Instructor in Medicine
Division of Hematology and Oncology
Vanderbilt University Medical Center
Nashville, Tennessee
Chapter 73: Lung Cancer: Molecular Biology and Targets

Catherine Lemière, MD, MSc
Professor of Medicine
University of Montréal Faculty of Medicine
Chest Physician
Department of Medicine
Sacré-Coeur de Montréal Hospital
Montréal, Canada
Chapter 100: Asthma in the Workplace

Robert J. Lentz, MD
Assistant Professor of Medicine and Thoracic Surgery
Vanderbilt University Medical Center
Nashville, Tennessee
Chapter 116: Mediastinitis and Fibrosing Mediastinitis

Richard W. Light, MD
Professor of Medicine
Division of Allergy, Pulmonary, and Critical Care Medicine
Vanderbilt University School of Medicine
Nashville, Tennessee
Chapter 108: Pleural Effusion

Andrew H. Limper, MD
Associate Dean for Practice Transformation
Annenberg Professor of Pulmonary Research
Department of Internal Medicine
Director, Thoracic Diseases Research Unit
Mayo Clinic College of Medicine
Rochester, Minnesota
Chapter 99: Drug-Induced Pulmonary Disease

Michael S. Lipnick, MD
Associate Professor of Anesthesia and Perioperative Care
University of California San Francisco School of Medicine
Dive Medical Officer
California Academy of Sciences
San Francisco, California
Chapter 107: Diving Medicine

Stanley Yung-Chuan Liu, MD, DDS, FACS
Assistant Professor of Otolaryngology
Assistant Professor of Plastic and Reconstructive Surgery, by Courtesy
Co-director, Sleep Surgery Fellowship
Department of Otolaryngology
Stanford University School of Medicine;
Chief, Maxillofacial Surgery
Stanford Health Care
Stanford, California
Chapter 122: Sleep-Disordered Breathing: Treatment

James E. Loyd, MD
Professor of Medicine
Rudy W. Jacobson Chair in Pulmonary Medicine
Division of Allergy, Pulmonary, and Critical Care Medicine
Vanderbilt University Medical Center
Nashville, Tennessee
Chapter 116: Mediastinitis and Fibrosing Mediastinitis

Njira Lugogo, MD
Associate Professor of Medicine
Division of Pulmonary, Critical Care Medicine
University of Michigan Medical School
Ann Arbor, Michigan
Chapter 62: Asthma: Diagnosis and Management

Andrew M. Luks, MD
Professor of Medicine
Division of Pulmonary, Critical Care, and Sleep Medicine
University of Washington School of Medicine
Seattle, Washington
Chapter 33: Exercise Testing
Chapter 105: High Altitude

Nicole Lurie, MD, MSPH
Strategic Advisor to the CEO
Coalition for Epidemic Preparedness Innovations (CEPI)
Oslo, Norway
Chapter 59: Outbreaks, Pandemics, and Bioterrorism

Charles-Edouard Luyt, MD, PhD
Professor
Medical Intensive Care Unit
Pitié-Salpêtrière Hospital
Paris, France
Chapter 49: Ventilator-Associated Pneumonia

Stuart M. Lyon, MBBS, FRANZCR, EBIR
Associate Professor of Radiology
Monash University
Melbourne, Australia;
Associate Professor of Radiology
Monash Health
Ormond, Australia
Chapter 111: Chylothorax

Roberto F. Machado, MD
Dr. Calvin H. English Professor of Medicine
Chief, Division of Pulmonary, Critical Care, Sleep, and Occupational Medicine
Indiana University School of Medicine
Indianapolis, Indiana
Chapter 127: Pulmonary Complications of Hematologic Diseases

Lisa A. Maier, MD, MSPH, FCCP
Professor of Medicine
Chief, Division of Environmental and Occupational Health
National Jewish Health
University of Colorado, Colorado School of Public Health
Denver, Colorado
Chapter 35: Evaluation of Respiratory Impairment and Disability

Atul Malhotra, MD
Peter C. Farrell Presidential Chair in Respiratory Medicine
Research Chief of Pulmonary and Critical Care Medicine
Director of Sleep Medicine
University of California San Diego School of Medicine
San Diego, California
Chapter 117: Control of Breathing and Upper Airways During Sleep

Thomas R. Martin, MD
Emeritus Professor of Medicine
University of Washington School of Medicine
Seattle, Washington;
Global Head, Respiratory Therapeutic Area
Global Drug Development
Novartis Pharmaceuticals
East Hanover, New Jersey
Chapter 15: Innate Immunity

Nick A. Maskell, DM, FRCP
Academic Respiratory Unit
Translational Health Sciences
University of Bristol Medical School;
Respiratory Department
North Bristol NHS Trust
Bristol, United Kingdom
Chapter 109: Pleural Infections

Pierre P. Massion, MD
Professor of Medicine, Cancer Biology, Radiology, and
    Radiological Sciences
Division of Allergy, Pulmonary, and Critical Care
    Medicine
Vanderbilt University School of Medicine
Director, Cancer Early Detection and Prevention Initiative
Co-leader, Cancer Health Outcomes and Control Research
    Program
Vanderbilt Ingream Cancer Center
Nashville, Tennessee
*Chapter 73: Lung Cancer: Molecular Biology and
Targets*

Stephen C. Mathai, MD, MHS
Associate Professor of Medicine
Division of Pulmonary and Critical Care Medicine
Johns Hopkins University School of Medicine
Baltimore, Maryland
*Chapter 83: Pulmonary Hypertension: General
Approach*

Scott M. Matson, MD
Assistant Professor of Medicine
Division of Pulmonary, Critical Care, and Sleep Medicine
University of Kansas School of Medicine
Kansas City, Kansas
Chapter 94: Diffuse Alveolar Hemorrhage

Michael A. Matthay, MD
Professor of Medicine and Anesthesia
Cardiovascular Research Institute
University of California San Francisco
San Francisco, California
Chapter 133: Pulmonary Edema

Richard A. Matthay, MD
Professor Emeritus and Senior Research Scientist in
    Medicine
Yale School of Medicine
New Haven, Connecticut
Chapter 38: Chest Pain

Anna M. May, MD, MS
Assistant Professor
Staff, Sleep Medicine Division
Staff, Pulmonary and Critical Care Division
Staff, Research Division
VA Northeast Ohio Healthcare System;
Staff, Division of Pulmonary, Critical Care, and Sleep
    Medicine
University Hospitals Cleveland Medical Center
Staff, School of Medicine
Case Western Reserve University
Cleveland, Ohio
Chapter 122: Sleep-Disordered Breathing: Treatment

Annyce S. Mayer, MD, MSPH
Associate Professor of Medicine
Division of Environmental and Occupational Health
National Jewish Health
University of Colorado, Colorado School of Public Health
Denver, Colorado
*Chapter 35: Evaluation of Respiratory Impairment and
Disability*

Peter J. Mazzone, MD, MPH, FCCP
Clinical Assistant Professor of Medicine
Case Western Reserve University School of Medicine;
Director, Lung Cancer Program
Respiratory Institute
Cleveland Clinic
Cleveland, Ohio
Chapter 75: Lung Cancer: Screening

Stuart B. Mazzone, PhD
Professor of Neuroscience
Department of Anatomy and Neuroscience
University of Melbourne
Parkville, Victoria, Australia
Chapter 37: Cough

Cormac McCarthy, MD, PhD
Associate Professor of Medicine
University College Dublin
Consultant Respiratory Physician
St. Vincent's Hospital Group
Dublin, Ireland
Chapter 98: Pulmonary Alveolar Proteinosis Syndrome

F. Dennis McCool, MD
Professor of Medicine
Division of Pulmonary and Critical Care Medicine
Alpert Medical School of Brown University
Providence, Rhode Island
Chapter 130: The Respiratory System and Neuromuscular Diseases
*Chapter 131: The Respiratory System and Chest Wall
Diseases*

Francis X. McCormack, MD
Taylor Professor and Director
Division of Pulmonary, Critical Care, and Sleep Medicine
University of Cincinnati College of Medicine
Cincinnati, Ohio
Chapter 97: Lymphangioleiomyomatosis

Meredith C. McCormack, MD, MHS
Associate Professor of Medicine
Division of Pulmonary and Critical Care Medicine
Johns Hopkins University School of Medicine
Baltimore, Maryland
Chapter 10: Ventilation, Blood Flow, and Gas Exchange

David McCulley, MD
Assistant Professor of Pediatrics
University of Wisconsin School of Medicine
Madison, Wisconsin
Chapter 2: Lung Growth and Development

Bryan J. McVerry, MD
Associate Professor of Medicine, Environmental and Occupational Health, and Clinical and Translational Science
Division of Pulmonary, Allergy, and Critical Care Medicine
University of Pittsburgh School of Medicine
Pittsburgh, Pennsylvania
Chapter 17: Microbiome

Reena Mehra, MD, MS, FCCP, FAASM, FAHA
Professor of Medicine
Cleveland Clinic Lerner College of Medicine of Case Western Reserve University
Director, Sleep Disorders Research, Neurologic Institute
Staff, Respiratory Institute
Staff, Heart and Vascular Institute
Staff, Department of Molecular Cardiology, Lerner Research Institute
Cleveland Clinic
Cleveland, Ohio
Chapter 122: Sleep-Disordered Breathing: Treatment

Atul C. Mehta, MBBS, FACP, FCCP
Buoncore Family Endowed Chair in Lung Transplantation
Professor of Medicine
Lerner College of Medicine
Staff Physician
Respiratory Institute
Cleveland Clinic
Cleveland, Ohio
Chapter 26: Diagnostic Bronchoscopy: Basic Techniques

Mark L. Metersky, MD
Professor of Medicine
Division of Pulmonary, Critical Care, and Sleep Medicine
University of Connecticut School of Medicine
Farmington, Connecticut
Chapter 48: Hospital-Acquired Pneumonia

Nuala J. Meyer, MD, MS
Associate Professor of Medicine
Division of Pulmonary, Allergy, and Critical Care Medicine
Perelman School of Medicine at the University of Pennsylvania
Philadelphia, Pennsylvania
Chapter 133: Pulmonary Edema

Isabel C. Mira-Avendano, MD
Assistant Professor of Medicine
Mayo Clinic Florida
Jacksonville, Florida
Chapter 95: Pulmonary Langerhans Cell Histiocytosis and Other Rare Diffuse Infiltrative Lung Diseases

Gita N. Mody, MD, MPH
Assistant Professor of Surgery
Division of Cardiothoracic Surgery
University of North Carolina School of Medicine
Chapel Hill, North Carolina
Chapter 77: Lung Cancer: Treatment

Babak Mokhlesi, MD, MSc
Professor of Medicine
Section of Pulmonary and Critical Care
Director, Sleep Disorders Center
Director, Sleep Medicine Fellowship Program
The University of Chicago Pritzker School of Medicine
Chicago, Illinois
Chapter 45: Hypercapnia

Alison Morris, MD, MS
Professor of Medicine
Division Chief, Pulmonary, Allergy, and Critical Care Medicine
Director, Center for Medicine and the Microbiome
University of Pittsburgh School of Medicine
Pittsburgh, Pennsylvania
Chapter 17: Microbiome

Amy E. Morris, MD
Associate Professor of Medicine
Division of Pulmonary, Critical Care, and Sleep Medicine
University of Washington School of Medicine
Seattle, Washington
Chapter 23: Ultrasonography: Principles and Basic Thoracic and Vascular Imaging

Timothy A. Morris, MD
Professor of Medicine
Division of Pulmonary and Critical Care Medicine
University of California San Diego School of Medicine
Clinical Service Chief
University of California San Diego Medical Center
San Diego, California
Chapter 81: Pulmonary Thromboembolism: Presentation and Diagnosis

Rory E. Morty, PhD
Department of Translational Pulmonology
University Hospital Heidelberg
Heidelberg, Germany
Chapter 1: Anatomy

Lakshmi Mudambi, MBBS
Assistant Professor of Medicine
Oregon Health & Science University
Director, Interventional Pulmonology
VA Portland Health Care System
Portland, Oregon
Chapter 71: Large Airway Disorders

John S. Munger, MD
Associate Professor of Medicine and Cell Biology
New York University Grossman School of Medicine
New York, New York
Chapter 46a: COVID-19

**Mohammed Munavvar, MD, DNB, FRCP(Lon),
FRCP(Edin)**
Consultant Chest Physician
Department of Respiratory Medicine
Lancashire Teaching Hospitals
Preston, United Kingdom
Chapter 29: Thoracoscopy

Payam Nahid, MD, MPH
Professor of Medicine
Division of Pulmonary and Critical Care Medicine
University of California San Francisco Center for
 Tuberculosis
University of California San Francisco School of Medicine
Zuckerberg San Francisco General Hospital
San Francisco, California
*Chapter 54: Tuberculosis: Treatment of Drug-Susceptible
and Drug-Resistant*

Catherine Nelson-Piercy, MBBS, MA, FRCP, FRCOG
Professor of Obstetric Medicine
Women's Health Academic Centre
King's Health Partners
Consultant Obstetric Physician
Women's Health Service
Guy's & St Thomas' Foundation Trust
Consultant Obstetric Physician
Queen Charlotte's and Chelsea Hospital
Imperial College Healthcare Trust
London, United Kingdom
*Chapter 129: The Lungs in Obstetric and Gynecologic
Diseases*

Linda Nici, MD
Professor of Medicine
The Warren Alpert Medical School of Brown University
Chief, Pulmonary and Critical Care Medicine
Providence Veterans Affairs Medical Center
Providence, Rhode Island
Chapter 139: Pulmonary Rehabilitation

Stephen L. Nishimura, MD
Professor of Pathology
University of California San Francisco School of Medicine
San Francisco, California
*Chapter 22: Pathology: Neoplastic and Non-neoplastic
Lung Disease*

Joshua D. Nosanchuk, MD
Senior Associate Dean
Professor of Medicine and Microbiology & Immunology
Albert Einstein College of Medicine
New York, New York
Chapter 56: Endemic Fungal Infections

Thomas G. O'Riordan, MD, MPH
Vice President US Medical Affairs
Respiratory Therapeutic Area Head
GlaxoSmithKline
Philadelphia, Pennsylvania
Chapter 13: Aerosols and Drug Delivery

Victor Enrique Ortega, MD, PhD
Associate Professor of Medicine
Center for Precision Medicine
Wake Forest School of Medicine
Winston-Salem, North Carolina
Chapter 60: Asthma: Pathogenesis and Phenotypes

Justin R. Ortiz, MD, MS, FCCP
Associate Professor of Medicine
Center for Vaccine Development and Global Health
Department of Medicine
University of Maryland School of Medicine
Baltimore, Maryland
Chapter 47: Influenza

Sushmita Pamidi, MD, MSc
Assistant Professor of Medicine
Division of Respiratory Medicine
McGill University Faculty of Medicine
Sleep Laboratory
McGill University Health Centre
Montreal, Quebec, Canada
Chapter 120: Obstructive Sleep Apnea

Nicholas J. Pastis, MD, FCCP
Professor of Medicine
Division of Pulmonary and Critical Care
Medical University of South Carolina
Section Chief, Pulmonary and Critical Care
Ralph H. Johnson Veterans Administration Medical Center
Charleston, South Carolina
Chapter 76: Lung Cancer: Diagnosis and Staging

Sanjay R. Patel, MD, MS
Professor of Medicine, Epidemiology, and Clinical and
  Translational Science
Division of Pulmonary Allergy and Critical Care Medicine
University of Pittsburgh School of Medicine
Pittsburgh, Pennsylvania
Chapter 118: Consequences of Sleep Disruption

Nicolò Patroniti, MD
Professor
Anesthesia and Intensive Care
Ospedale Policlinico San Martino
IRCCS
Department of Surgical Sciences and Integrated
  Diagnostics (DISC)
University of Genoa
Genoa, Italy
Chapter 138: Extracorporeal Support of Gas Exchange

Steven A. Pergam, MD, MPH
Associate Professor
Vaccine and Infectious Disease Division
Fred Hutchinson Cancer Research Center;
Associate Professor of Medicine
University of Washington School of Medicine;
Director, Infection Prevention
Seattle Cancer Care Alliance
Seattle, Washington
*Chapter 125: Pulmonary Complications of Stem Cell and
Solid Organ Transplantation*

Antonio Pesenti, MD
Professor of Anesthesia and Critical Care
Department of Pathophysiology and Transplantation
University of Milan
Director, Dipartimento di Anestesia–Rianimazione e Emer-
  genza Urgenza
Fondazione IRCCS Ca' Granda–Ospedale Maggiore Policlinico
Milan, Italy
Chapter 138: Extracorporeal Support of Gas Exchange

Michael C. Peters, MD, MAS
Assistant Professor of Medicine
Division of Pulmonary and Critical Care Medicine
University of California San Francisco
San Francisco, California
Chapter 61: Asthma and Obesity

Kurt Pfeifer, MD, FACP, SFHM
Professor of Medicine
Division of General Internal Medicine
Medical College of Wisconsin
Milwaukee, Wisconsin
Chapter 34: Preoperative Evaluation

Jennifer A. Philips, MD, PhD
Associate Professor of Medicine
Co-director, Division of Infectious Diseases
Washington University in St. Louis
St. Louis, Missouri
Chapter 52: Tuberculosis: Pathogenesis and Immunity

Benjamin A. Pinsky, MD, PhD
Associate Professor
Departments of Pathology and Medicine (Infectious
  Diseases)
Stanford University School of Medicine
Medical Director, Clinical Virology Laboratory
Stanford Health Care and Stanford Children's Health
Stanford, California
Chapter 19: Microbiologic Diagnosis of Lung Infection

Steven D. Pletcher, MD
Professor and Director, Residency Training Program
Department of Otolaryngology–Head and Neck Surgery
University of California San Francisco
San Francisco, California
Chapter 70: Upper Airway Disorders

Vikramaditya Prabhudesai, MBBS, MS, FRCR
Assistant Professor of Medicine
University of Toronto Faculty of Medicine;
Interventional Radiologist
Department of Medical Imaging
St. Michael's Hospital
Toronto, Ontario, Canada
Chapter 88: Pulmonary Vascular Anomalies

Loretta G. Que, MD
Professor of Medicine
Division of Pulmonary, Allergy, and Critical Care Medicine
Duke University Health System
Durham, North Carolina
Chapter 62: Asthma: Diagnosis and Management

Bryon D. Quick, MD
Chair, Department of Pulmonary and Sleep Medicine
Kaiser Permanente Oakland Medical Center
Oakland, California
*Chapter 126: Pulmonary Complications of Abdominal
Diseases*

**Najib M. Rahman, BM, BCh, MA(Oxon), MSc, FRCP,
DPhil**
Professor of Respiratory Medicine
Head, Oxford Pleural Unit
Director of Oxford Respiratory Trials Unit (ORTU)
Nuffield Department of Medicine
University of Oxford
Oxford, United Kingdom
Chapter 29: Thoracoscopy
Chapter 110: Pneumothorax

J. Usha Raj, MD, MHA
Anjuli S. Nayak Professor of Pediatrics
University of Illinois College of Medicine at Chicago
Chicago, Illinois
Chapter 6: Vascular Biology

Maria I. Ramirez, PhD
Associate Professor of Medicine
Division of Pulmonary, Allergy, and Critical Care Medicine
Center for Translational Medicine
Jane and Leonard Korman Respiratory Institute
Sidney Kimmel Medical College at Thomas Jefferson
    University
Philadelphia, Pennsylvania
Chapter 1: Anatomy
Chapter 5: Lung Mesenchyme

Rishindra M. Reddy, MD
Associate Professor of Surgery
Section of Thoracic Surgery
University of Michigan Medical School
Ann Arbor, Michigan
Chapter 79: Metastatic Malignant Tumors

Elizabeth F. Redente, PhD
Associate Professor of Pediatrics
Division of Cell Biology
National Jewish Health
Denver, Colorado
Chapter 15: Innate Immunity

Hasina Outtz Reed, MD, PhD
Assistant Professor of Medicine
Division of Pulmonary and Critical Care Medicine
Weill Cornell Medicine
New York, New York
Chapter 7: Lymphatic Biology

R. Lee Reinhardt, PhD
Associate Professor of Biomedical Research
National Jewish Health
Department of Immunology and Microbiology
University of Colorado Anschutz Medical Campus
Aurora, Colorado
Chapter 16: Adaptive Immunity

David W.H. Riches, PhD
Professor of Medicine and Immunology
Division of Pulmonary Sciences and Critical Care Medicine
University of Colorado Anschutz Medical Campus
Aurora, Colorado;
Professor and Division Head
Program in Cell Biology
National Jewish Health
Denver, Colorado
Chapter 15: Innate Immunity

M. Patricia Rivera, MD
Professor of Medicine
Division of Pulmonary and Critical Care Medicine
University of North Carolina School of Medicine
Chapel Hill, North Carolina
Chapter 77: Lung Cancer: Treatment

Carolyn L. Rochester, MD
Professor of Medicine
Section of Pulmonary, Critical Care, and Sleep Medicine
Yale University School of Medicine
Director, Yale COPD Program
Director, Pulmonary Rehabilitation
VA Connecticut Healthcare System
New Haven, Connecticut
Chapter 139: Pulmonary Rehabilitation

Jesse Roman, MD
Professor of Medicine
Division of Pulmonary, Allergy, and Critical Care Medicine
Center for Translational Medicine
Jane and Leonard Korman Respiratory Institute
Sidney Kimmel Medical College at Thomas Jefferson
    University
Philadelphia, Pennsylvania
Chapter 5: Lung Mesenchyme

Alexandra Rose, MD
Assistant Clinical Professor of Medicine
Division of Pulmonary and Critical Care Medicine
University of California San Diego School of Medicine
San Diego, California
*Chapter 81: Pulmonary Thromboembolism: Presentation
and Diagnosis*

Clark A. Rosen, MD
Lewis Francis Morrison, MD, Endowed Chair in
    Laryngology
Professor, Department of Otolaryngology–Head and Neck
    Surgery
Chief, Division of Laryngology
Co-Director, UCSF Voice and Swallowing Center
University of California San Francisco
San Francisco, California
Chapter 70: Upper Airway Disorders

John M. Routes, MD
Professor of Pediatrics, Medicine, and Microbiology and
    Immunology
Medical College of Wisconsin
Milwaukee, Wisconsin
*Chapter 124: Pulmonary Complications of Primary
Immunodeficiencies*

Steven M. Rowe, MD, MSPH
Professor of Medicine
University of Alabama at Birmingham School of Medicine
Birmingham, Alabama
Chapter 67: Cystic Fibrosis: Pathogenesis and Epidemiology
Chapter 68: Cystic Fibrosis: Diagnosis and Management

Clodagh M. Ryan, MBBCh, BAO, MD, FRCPC
Assistant Professor of Medicine
Centre for Sleep Medicine and Circadian Biology
University of Toronto Faculty of Medicine;
Division of Respirology
University Health Network
Toronto Rehabilitation Institute
Toronto General Hospital
Toronto, Ontario, Canada
Chapter 121: Central Sleep Apnea

Jay H. Ryu, MD
Professor of Medicine
Division of Pulmonary and Critical Care Medicine
Mayo Clinic Alix College of Medicine
Rochester, Minnesota
Chapter 89: Idiopathic Pulmonary Fibrosis

Sarah Sanghavi, MD
Clinical Assistant Professor of Medicine
Department of Medicine
Division of Nephrology
University of Washington School of Medicine
Veterans Affairs Puget Sound Health Care System
Seattle, Washington
Chapter 12: Acid-Base Balance

Kathleen F. Sarmiento, MD, MPH
Associate Professor of Medicine
Division of Pulmonary, Critical Care, and Sleep Medicine
University of California San Francisco
San Francisco VA Healthcare System
San Francisco, California
Chapter 119: Sleep-Disordered Breathing: A General Approach

Jennifer L. Saullo, MD, PharmD
Assistant Professor of Medicine
Division of Infectious Diseases
Duke University Medical Center
Durham, North Carolina
Chapter 57: Fungal Infections: Opportunistic

Robert B. Schoene, MD
Sound Physicians
Division of Pulmonary and Critical Care Medicine
St Mary's Medical Center
San Francisco, California
Chapter 105: High Altitude

Gregory L. Schumaker, MD
Assistant Professor of Medicine
Division of Pulmonary, Critical Care, and Sleep Medicine
Tufts University School of Medicine;
Director, Medical ICU
Chief, Critical Care Section
Lowell General Hospital
Boston, Massachusetts
Chapter 132: Acute Ventilatory Failure

David A. Schwartz, MD
Chair and Professor
Department of Medicine
Professor of Immunology
University of Colorado Anschutz Medical Campus
Aurora, Colorado
Chapter 9: Genetics of Lung Disease

Richard M. Schwartzstein, MD
Ellen and Melvin Gordon Professor of Medicine and Medical Education
Harvard Medical School
Executive Director, Carl J. Shapiro Institute for Education and Research
Chief, Division of Pulmonary, Critical Care, and Sleep Medicine
Vice President for Education
Beth Israel Deaconess Medical Center
Boston, Massachusetts
Chapter 36: Dyspnea

Marvin I. Schwarz, MD
Professor of Medicine
Pulmonary Sciences and Critical Care Medicine
University of Colorado School of Medicine
Aurora, Colorado
Chapter 94: Diffuse Alveolar Hemorrhage

Moisés Selman, MD
Distinguished Investigator
Research Unit
Instituto Nacional de Enfermedades Respiratorias
Mexico City, Mexico
Chapter 89: Idiopathic Pulmonary Fibrosis

Neomi Shah, MD, MPH
Associate Professor of Medicine
Division of Pulmonary, Critical Care, and Sleep Medicine
Icahn School of Medicine at Mount Sinai
New York, New York
Chapter 119: Sleep-Disordered Breathing: A General Approach

Rupal J. Shah, MD, MSCE
Assistant Professor of Medicine
Division of Pulmonary, Allergy, and Critical Care Medicine
University of California San Francisco School of Medicine
San Francisco, California
Chapter 43: Aspiration

Priya B. Shete, MD, MPH
Assistant Professor of Medicine
Division of Pulmonary and Critical Care Medicine
University of California San Francisco Center for Tuberculosis
University of California San Francisco School of Medicine
San Francisco, California
Chapter 53: Tuberculosis: Clinical Manifestations and Diagnosis

Samira Shojaee, MD, MPH
Associate Professor of Medicine
Fellowship Director, Interventional Pulmonology Program
Division of Pulmonary and Critical Care Medicine
Virginia Commonwealth University
Richmond, Virginia
Chapter 28: Therapeutic Bronchoscopy: Interventional Techniques

Gerard A. Silvestri, MD, MS, FCCP
Professor of Medicine
Division of Pulmonary and Critical Care Medicine
Medical University of South Carolina
Charleston, South Carolina
Chapter 76: Lung Cancer: Diagnosis and Staging

Jonathan P. Singer, MD, MS
Associate Professor of Medicine
Division of Pulmonary, Critical Care, Allergy, and Sleep Medicine
University of California San Francisco School of Medicine
San Francisco, California
Chapter 72: Bronchiolitis

Christopher G. Slatore, MD, MS
Investigator
Center to Improve Veteran Involvement in Care
VA Portland Health Care System
Associate Professor of Medicine
Division of Pulmonary and Critical Care Medicine
Oregon Health & Science University
Portland, Oregon
Chapter 41: Pulmonary Nodule

Gerald C. Smaldone, MD, PhD
Professor of Medicine, Physiology, and Biophysics
State University of New York at Stony Brook
Chief, Division of Pulmonary, Critical Care, and Sleep Medicine
Stony Brook University Medical Center
Stony Brook, New York
Chapter 13: Aerosols and Drug Delivery

Gerald W. Smetana, MD, MACP
Professor of Medicine
Harvard Medical School
Attending Physician
Division of General Medicine and Primary Care
Beth Israel Deaconess Medical Center
Boston, Massachusetts
Chapter 34: Preoperative Evaluation

George M. Solomon, MD
Associate Professor of Medicine
Division of Pulmonary, Allergy, and Critical Care
University of Alabama at Birmingham School of Medicine
Birmingham, Alabama
Chapter 67: Cystic Fibrosis: Pathogenesis and Epidemiology
Chapter 68: Cystic Fibrosis: Diagnosis and Management
Chapter 69: Bronchiectasis

Eric J. Sorscher, MD
Professor of Pediatrics
Emory University School of Medicine
Atlanta, Georgia
Chapter 67: Cystic Fibrosis: Pathogenesis and Epidemiology
Chapter 68: Cystic Fibrosis: Diagnosis and Management

Renee D. Stapleton, MD, PhD
Professor of Medicine
Division of Pulmonary and Critical Care Medicine
University of Vermont Larner College of Medicine
Burlington, Vermont
Chapter 141: End-of-Life Care in Respiratory Failure

Daniel Sterman, MD
Professor of Medicine and Cardiothoracic Surgery
New York University Grossman School of Medicine
New York, New York
Chapter 114: Pleural Malignancy

Shelby J. Stewart, MD
Assistant Professor of Thoracic Surgery
University of Maryland School of Medicine
Baltimore, Maryland
Chapter 113: Hemothorax

James K. Stoller, MD, MS
Jean Wall Bennett Professor of Medicine
Samson Global Leadership Academy Endowed Chair
Cleveland Clinic Lerner College of Medicine of Case Western Reserve University
Staff, Respiratory Institute
Cleveland Clinic
Cleveland, Ohio
Chapter 106: Air Travel

Xin Sun, PhD
Professor of Pediatrics
University of California San Diego School of Medicine
San Diego, California
Chapter 2: Lung Growth and Development

Bernie Y. Sunwoo, MBBS
Associate Professor of Medicine
Division of Pulmonary, Critical Care, and Sleep Medicine
University of California San Diego School of Medicine
San Diego, California
Chapter 45: Hypercapnia

Daniel A. Sweeney, MD
Associate Professor of Medicine
University of California San Diego School of Medicine
San Diego, California
Chapter 24: Ultrasonography: Advanced Applications and Procedures

Erik R. Swenson, MD
Professor of Medicine, Physiology, and Biophysics
Department of Medicine
Division of Pulmonary Medicine and Critical Care
University of Washington School of Medicine
Veterans Affairs Puget Sound Health Care System
Seattle, Washington
Chapter 12: Acid-Base Balance
Chapter 105: High Altitude

Nichole T. Tanner, MD, MSCR, FCCP
Associate Professor of Medicine
Division of Pulmonary and Critical Care Medicine
Medical University of South Carolina;
Staff Pulmonologist
Ralph H. Johnson Veteran Affairs Hospital
Charleston, South Carolina
Chapter 41: Pulmonary Nodule
Chapter 75: Lung Cancer: Screening

Lynn Tanoue, MD
Professor and Vice Chair for Clinical Affairs
Department of Internal Medicine
Section of Pulmonary, Critical Care, and Sleep Medicine
Yale School of Medicine
New Haven, Connecticut
Chapter 75: Lung Cancer: Screening

George R. Thompson III, MD
Associate Professor of Clinical Medicine
Division of Infectious Diseases
University of California Davis School of Medicine
Davis, California
Chapter 56: Endemic Fungal Infections

Bruce C. Trapnell, MD
Professor of Medicine and Pediatrics
University of Cincinnati College of Medicine
Director, Translational Pulmonary Science Center
Cincinnati Children's Hospital Medical Center
Cincinnati, Ohio
Chapter 98: Pulmonary Alveolar Proteinosis Syndrome

Matthew Triplette, MD, MPH
Assistant Professor of Medicine
Division of Pulmonary, Critical Care, and Sleep Medicine
University of Washington School of Medicine;
Assistant Professor, Clinical Research Division
Fred Hutchinson Cancer Research Center
Seattle, Washington
Chapter 115: Mediastinal Tumors and Cysts

Melissa H. Tukey, MD, MSc
Department of Pulmonary and Critical Care
Kaiser Permanente Oakland Medical Center
Oakland, California
Chapter 126: Pulmonary Complications of Abdominal Diseases

George E. Tzelepis, MD
Professor of Medicine
National and Kapodistrian University of Athens Medical School
Athens, Greece
Chapter 131: The Respiratory System and Chest Wall Diseases

Anatoly Urisman, MD, PhD
Assistant Professor of Pathology
University of California San Francisco School of Medicine
San Francisco, California
Chapter 22: Pathology: Neoplastic and Non-neoplastic Lung Disease

Olivier Vandenplas, MD, PhD
Professor of Medicine
Department of Chest Medicine
Mont-Godinne University Hospital Center
Catholic University of Louvain
Yvoir, Belgium
Chapter 100: Asthma in the Workplace

Karen B. Van Hoesen, MD
Clinical Professor of Emergency Medicine
Associate Dean for Health Sciences Faculty Affairs
University of California San Diego School of Medicine
Co-Director, San Diego Center of Excellence in Diving
San Diego, California
Chapter 107: Diving Medicine

Thomas K. Varghese Jr, MD, MS
Associate Professor of Surgery
Head, Section of General Thoracic Surgery
Co-Director, Thoracic Oncology Program
Program Director, Cardiothoracic Surgery Residency
University of Utah School of Medicine
Salt Lake City, Utah
Chapter 115: Mediastinal Tumors and Cysts

Robert Vassallo, MD
Professor of Medicine
Mayo Clinic
Rochester, Minnesota
Chapter 95: Pulmonary Langerhans Cell Histiocytosis and Other Rare Diffuse Infiltrative Lung Diseases

James W. Verbsky, MD, PhD
Associate Professor of Pediatrics and Microbiology and Immunology
Medical College of Wisconsin
Milwaukee, Wisconsin
Chapter 124: Pulmonary Complications of Primary Immunodeficiencies

Ajay Wagh, MD, MS, FCCP
Interventional Pulmonology Fellow
Division of Pulmonary and Critical Care Medicine
Northwestern Memorial Hospital
Chicago, Illinois
Chapter 27: Diagnostic Bronchoscopy: Advanced Techniques (EBUS and Navigational)

Ryan Walsh, MD
Associate Professor of Radiology
University of Vermont Medical Center
Shelburne, Vermont
Chapter 21: Thoracic Radiology: Invasive Diagnostic Imaging and Image-Guided Interventions

David J. Weber, MD, MPH
Professor of Medicine, Pediatrics, and Epidemiology
University of North Carolina School of Medicine
Medical Director
Hospital Epidemiology and Occupational Health
Associate Chief Medical Officer
Department of Epidemiology
University of North Carolina Health Care
Chapel Hill, North Carolina
Chapter 59: Outbreaks, Pandemics, and Bioterrorism

Ashley A. Weiner, MD, PhD
Assistant Professor of Radiation Oncology
University of North Carolina School of Medicine
Chapel Hill, North Carolina
Chapter 77: Lung Cancer: Treatment

Louis M. Weiss, MD, MPH
Professor of Pathology
Division of Parasitology and Tropical Medicine
Professor of Medicine
Division of Infectious Diseases
Albert Einstein College of Medicine
New York, New York
Chapter 58: Parasitic Infections

Athol U. Wells, MBChB, MD, FRCR, FRCP
Professor of Respiratory Medicine
Faculty of Medicine, National Heart & Lung Institute
Imperial College London;
Consultant Physician
Interstitial Lung Disease Unit
Royal Brompton Hospital
London, United Kingdom
Chapter 92: Connective Tissue Diseases

John B. West, MD, PhD, DSc
Professor of Medicine and Physiology
University of California San Diego School of Medicine
San Diego, California
Chapter 10: Ventilation, Blood Flow, and Gas Exchange

T. Eoin West, MD, MPH, FCCP
Associate Professor of Medicine
Division of Pulmonary, Critical Care, and Sleep Medicine
University of Washington School of Medicine
Adjunct Associate Professor of Global Health
University of Washington Schools of Medicine and Public Health
Seattle, Washington
Chapter 47: Influenza

Douglas B. White, MD, MAS
UPMC Endowed Chair of Ethics in Critical Care Medicine
Department of Critical Care Medicine
University of Pittsburgh School of Medicine
Director, Program on Ethics and Decision Making in Critical Illness
University of Pittsburgh Medical Center
Pittsburgh, Pennsylvania
Chapter 141: End-of-Life Care in Respiratory Failure

Kevin L. Winthrop, MD, MPH
Professor of Infectious Diseases and Public Health
Department of Medicine
Oregon Health & Science University–Portland State University School of Public Health
Portland, Oregon
Chapter 55: Nontuberculous Mycobacterial Infections

David A. Wohl, MD
Professor of Medicine
Division of Infectious Diseases
Institute of Global Health and Infectious Diseases
University of North Carolina School of Medicine
Chapel Hill, North Carolina
Chapter 59: Outbreaks, Pandemics, and Bioterrorism

Lisa F. Wolfe, MD
Associate Professor of Medicine
Division of Pulmonary, Critical Care, and Sleep Medicine
Northwestern University Feinberg School of Medicine
Chicago, Illinois
Chapter 130: The Respiratory System and Neuromuscular Diseases

Prescott G. Woodruff, MD, MPH
Professor of Medicine
Division of Pulmonary, Critical Care, Allergy, and Sleep Medicine
Cardiovascular Research Institute
University of California San Francisco
San Francisco, California
Chapter 60: Asthma: Pathogenesis and Phenotypes

William Worodria, MBChB, MMed, PhD, MSc
Staff Physician
Department of Medicine
Mulago Hospital
Kampala, Uganda
Chapter 123: Pulmonary Complications of HIV Infection

D. Dante Yeh, MD, MHPE, FACS, FCCM
Associate Professor of Surgery
Department of Surgery
University of Miami Miller School of Medicine
Acute Care Surgeon
Jackson Memorial Hospital
Miami, Florida
Chapter 104: Trauma and Blast Injuries

Christina Yoon, MD, MPH, MAS
Assistant Professor of Medicine
Division of Pulmonary and Critical Care Medicine
University of California San Francisco Center for
  Tuberculosis
University of California San Francisco School of Medicine
San Francisco, California
Chapter 42: Positive Screening Test for Tuberculosis
*Chapter 53: Tuberculosis: Clinical Manifestations and
Diagnosis*

VyVy N. Young, MD
Associate Professor of Clinical Otolaryngology
Department of Otolaryngology–Head and Neck Surgery
University of California San Francisco School of Medicine
San Francisco, California
Chapter 43: Aspiration

William J. Zacharias, MD, PhD
Assistant Professor of Pediatrics and Internal Medicine
Divisions of Pulmonary Biology, Developmental Biology,
  and Pulmonary and Critical Care Medicine
University of Cincinnati School of Medicine
Cincinnati, Ohio
Chapter 3: Alveolar Compartment

Alberto Zanella, MD
Department of Pathophysiology and Transplantation
University of Milan
Dipartimento di Anestesia-Rianimazione e Emergenza
  Urgenza
Fondazione IRCCS Ca' Granda–Ospedale Maggiore
  Policlinico
Milan, Italy
Chapter 138: Extracorporeal Support of Gas Exchange

Preface to the Seventh Edition

This seventh edition of the Textbook represents the first major reorganization since the first edition in 1988. You will notice many changes in structure and content, all aimed to enhance its readability and educational value.

There are two major changes. The first is that the number of chapters has been increased from 106 in the sixth edition to the current 142. This strategic change enabled us to create more focused shorter chapters, which we hope are easier to find and to read. We were able to bring new chapters out of their hiding places under other headings (e.g., Influenza, Idiopathic Pulmonary Fibrosis, and Pneumothorax), to create new chapters on topics not directly covered before (e.g., Hypoxemia, Aspiration, and Air Travel), and to cover entirely new topics (e.g., Microbiome and COVID-19). The second major change was the creation of a new section particularly with our trainees in mind, "The Evaluation of Common Presentations in Respiratory Disease," built on the classic triad of Dyspnea, Cough, and Chest Pain. Seven new chapters were added on topics ranging from Hypercarbia to Hemoptysis to Pulmonary Nodule, which we hope will be a valuable resource for our readers. Other changes to the Textbook are noteworthy: in particular, the sections on Basic Science and on Sleep have been revamped, reflecting the major rethinking of those topics in the last decade.

These changes were spearheaded by our exceptional editorial board, with three new members. The makeup of our editors is now equally women and men, a remarkable change from the time in 2005 when I (V.C.B.) joined as the inaugural woman. Our new editors have brought a fresh outlook and diverse areas of expertise that helped chart this new course. With these new editors have come a slew of new authors. Of our 317 authors, we welcome almost 180 new authors, either to take on new chapters or to take the place of authors who have rotated off. Overall, our authors come from 33 states of the United States and from 18 countries. Here, too, we have increased the participation of women; women now make up 32% of our authors, almost double that in the previous edition (17%).

The printed textbook is a gateway to rich resources online. While there are a whopping 900 figures in the printed text, they are joined by others to make a total of 1650 figures online, all available for download. The text is expanded by an additional 25% online. A total of 190 videos and audio clips are accessible online, popping up with just a click to the link in the text. All the references are online, and each one links to the actual publication. Most importantly, the online textbook will feature regular updates from our editors and authors, with the aim of realizing a "living textbook."

We wish to thank our valuable and skilled colleagues at Elsevier, who made this herculean work possible. In particular, our thanks go to Jennifer Shreiner, who has remained dedicated to the Textbook over the last three editions and made this task a pleasure. In addition, Carrie Stetz had the attention to detail and the high standards necessary to produce a lovely book. Thanks go also to Dolores Meloni and Robin Carter. We also wish to thank the authors and editors who contributed to the past editions.

The COVID-19 pandemic has loomed over us during this project. Much of the book was written and edited during lockdowns and hospital surges, with many of our authors simultaneously juggling heavy frontline clinical and family responsibilities with chapter deadlines. In recognition of this momentous experience, we have added a chapter (46a) devoted to the topic—a chapter that has been updated up to the last moment and will continue to be updated frequently online—and placed an image of the novel coronavirus on our cover. The impact of the pandemic on our lives has made the successful outcome of this project all the more remarkable. A special thanks again to our authors and staff for their outstanding efforts during this particularly difficult time.

Sadly, Dr. Murray, who started this Textbook together with Dr. Jay Nadel and guided it up to this point, died of COVID-19 in March 2020. He remained committed to the textbook until his last days. Over his illustrious career, he taught many of us and inspired all of us to the highest callings of teaching and caring for patients. This Textbook is dedicated to him.

V. Courtney Broaddus, MD

Joel D. Ernst, MD

Talmadge E. King Jr, MD

Stephen C. Lazarus, MD, FCCP, FERS

Kathleen F. Sarmiento, MD, MPH

Lynn M. Schnapp, MD

Renee D. Stapleton, MD, PhD

Michael B. Gotway, MD

Contents

Video Contents

PART 1

SCIENTIFIC PRINCIPLES OF RESPIRATORY MEDICINE

ANATOMY AND DEVELOPMENT OF THE RESPIRATORY TRACT
Anatomy
Lung Growth and Development
Alveolar Compartment
Airway Biology
Lung Mesenchyme

Vascular Biology
Lymphatic Biology
Regeneration and Repair
Genetics of Lung Disease
RESPIRATORY PHYSIOLOGY
Ventilation, Blood Flow, and Gas Exchange
Respiratory System Mechanics and Energetics

Acid-Base Balance
Aerosol and Drug Delivery
Pleural Physiology and Pathophysiology
DEFENSE MECHANISMS AND IMMUNOLOGY
Innate Immunity
Adaptive Immunity
Microbiome

ANATOMY AND DEVELOPMENT OF THE RESPIRATORY TRACT

1 *ANATOMY*

KURT H. ALBERTINE, PHD, FAAAS, FAAA • MARIA I. RAMIREZ, PHD • RORY E. MORTY, PHD

INTRODUCTION

The lung has two essential, interdependent functions. One essential function is ventilation-perfusion matching to deliver *oxygen* (O_2) to the body and to remove the *carbon dioxide* (CO_2) produced by the body (Fig. 1.1). The second essential function is host defense against the onslaught of airborne pathogens, chemicals, and particulates. These essential functions are emphasized through the gross, subgross, histologic, cellular, and molecular determinants of the respiratory gas-exchange process in the normal human lung.[1] Other secondary functions of the lung, which support the essential functions, are important, such as cellular functions of surfactant synthesis, secretion and recycling, mucociliary clearance, neuroendocrine signaling, and synthesis and secretion of myriad molecules by the epithelial and endothelial cells of the lung. The diversity of secondary functions emphasizes the importance of the lung in homeostasis. Finally, the widespread use of murine models in lung research as surrogates for the human lung highlights the need to understand the similarities and differences of the lung between these species. The anatomic features that support the essential and secondary functions and comparative anatomy topics are the focus of this chapter. In addition, online supplemental digital videos linked to this chapter provide views of lung movements related to changes in tidal volume, airway pressures, and respiratory rate. (Videos 1.1 to 1.5).

GROSS AND SUBGROSS ORGANIZATION

The position of the lungs in the chest and in relationship to the heart is shown in Fig. 1.2. Fig. 1.2A shows a midfrontal section through the thorax of a frozen human cadaver. Fig. 1.2B shows a posterior-anterior chest radiograph of a normal human at *functional residual capacity* (FRC). The two illustrations represent the extremes of the approaches to study lung anatomy. On one hand, the cadaver lung (see Fig. 1.2A) shows the gross anatomic arrangements and relationships. The main distortion is that the lungs are at low volume. The height of the lungs is only about 18 cm, which is well below FRC height (see Fig. 1.2A). The diaphragm is markedly elevated in Fig. 1.2A, probably about 5 cm relative to its end-expiratory position in life. Another distortion is the abnormally wide pleural space. However, that fixation shrinkage artifact serves as a useful reminder that the lung is not normally attached to the chest wall. In life, the separation between the parietal and visceral pleurae is only several micrometers.[2,3] On the other hand, the chest radiograph (see Fig. 1.2B) shows that the height of

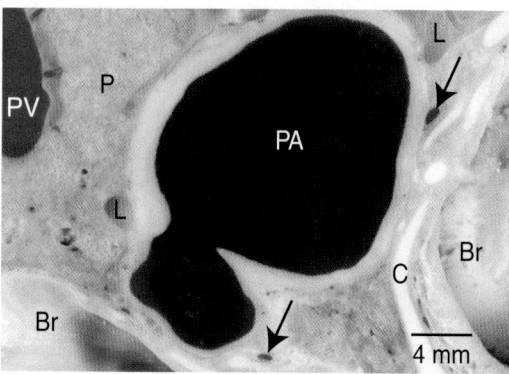

Figure 1.1 Levels of oxygenation of blood in a frozen block of lung tissue. Air is brought into the lung via the bronchus (Br). Pulmonary arterial (PA) blood is dark purple because it is poorly oxygenated. Gas exchange across the lung's parenchyma (P) results in oxygenated pulmonary venous (PV) blood, which is crimson. Also present in the peribronchovascular connective tissue are bronchial arteries *(arrows)*, cartilage (C), and lymphatics (L). (Frozen sheep lung, unstained.)

the lung at FRC is approximately 24 cm, with the level of the bifurcation of the pulmonary artery about halfway up the lungs. The diaphragm is lower and flatter than in the cadaver. However, the radiographic image is only a shadow of dense structures.

In life, the human lungs weigh 900 to 1000 g, of which nearly 40–50% is blood.[4,5] At end-expiration, the gas volume is about 2.5 L, whereas, at maximal inspiration, the gas volume may be 6 L. Thus, overall lung density varies from 0.30 g/mL at FRC to 0.14 g/mL at *total lung capacity* (TLC). However, the density of the lung is not distributed uniformly, being about 1 g/mL near the hilum and 0.1 g/mL peripherally. If one likens each lung to a half cylinder, more than 50% of all the lung's alveoli are located in the outer 30% of the lung radius (hilum to chest wall). This is why the peripheral portion of the lung appears relatively empty in the chest radiograph (see Fig. 1.2). Variability in density also exists from top to bottom. In Fig. 1.2, the blood vessels are more distended in the lower lung fields. The increasing distention of vessels from apex to base also illustrates the increase in vascular distending pressures at the rate of 1 cm H_2O/cm height down the lung.

The composition of the various tissues that comprise the lung is summarized in Table 1.1. An amazing point is how little tissue is involved in the architecture of the alveolar walls.[6,7] However, this is as it should be because the major physical obstacle to gas exchange is the slowness of O_2 diffusion through water.[8,9] Thus, the alveolar walls must be extremely thin. In fact, the thickness of the *red blood cell* (RBC) forms a substantial portion of the air-blood diffusion pathway. Advantage was taken of this fact to separate the carbon monoxide diffusing capacity measurement into two components: the capillary blood volume and the membrane diffusing capacity.[10] (For a discussion of diffusing capacity, see Chapter 31.)

The lung has two well-defined interstitial connective tissue compartments arranged in series, as described by Hayek[11] (Fig. 1.3). These are the parenchymal (alveolar wall) interstitium and the loose binding (extra-alveolar) connective tissue (peribronchovascular sheaths, interlobular septa, and visceral pleura). The connective

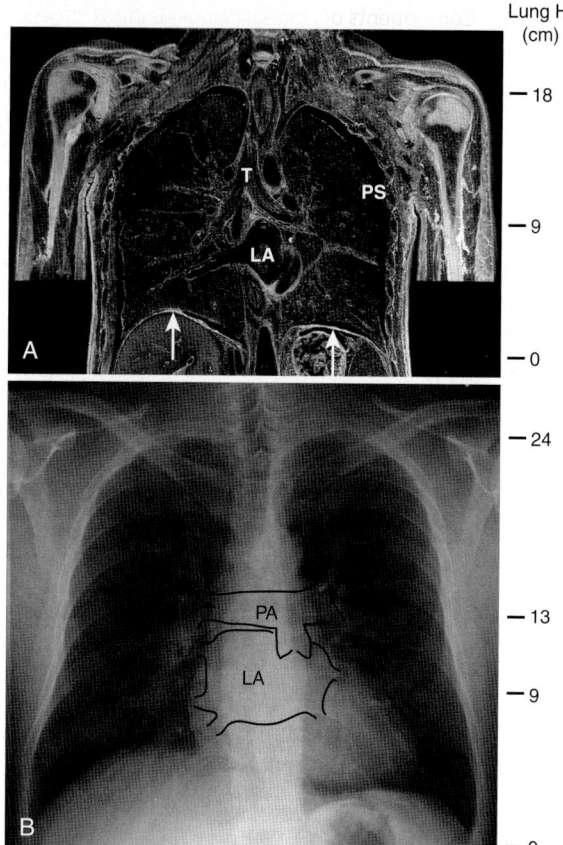

Figure 1.2 Comparison views of the position of the lungs in the chest and their relationship to the heart. (A) Midfrontal section through the thorax of a frozen cadaver of a 35-year-old human. The cadaver was prepared by routine embalming procedures, stored horizontally for 3 months in 30% alcohol, and frozen in the horizontal position for 1 week at −20°C. Frontal sections were cut with a band saw. Because the cadaver was preserved in the horizontal position, the weight of the abdominal organs compressed the contents of the thoracic cavity. The domes of the diaphragm *(arrows)* are elevated about 5 cm relative to their end-expiratory position in life. Pleural space (PS) width is artifactually enlarged; normally, in life it is several micrometers in width. The trachea (T) is flanked on its left by the aortic arch and on its right by the azygos vein. The left pulmonary artery lies on the superior aspect of the left mainstem bronchus. Pulmonary veins from the right lung enter the left atrium (LA), which is located about 7 cm above the lung's base. These structures at the root of the lungs caused the esophagus to be cut twice as it follows a curved path behind them to reach the stomach. (B) Chest radiograph of a normal human adult taken in the upright position at functional residual capacity. The lung height (cm) was measured from the costodiaphragmatic angle to the tubercle of the first rib. The main pulmonary artery (PA) and LA are outlined. The vascular structures, especially the pulmonary veins, are more easily seen near the base of the lung. This is partly because vascular distending pressures are greater near the bottom. The density of the lung is also graded, being higher at the bottom than the top and higher near the hilum than peripherally. (From Koritké JG, Sick H. *Atlas of Sectional Human Anatomy.* vol. 1: *Head, Neck, Thorax.* Baltimore: Urban and Schwarzenberg; 1983:83.)

tissue fibrils (collagen, elastin, and reticulin) form a three-dimensional basket-like structure around the alveoli and airways (Fig. 1.4).[12] This basket-like arrangement allows the lung to expand in all directions without developing excessive tissue recoil. Because the connective tissue fibrils in the parenchymal interstitium are extensions of the coarser fibers in the loose-binding connective tissue, stresses imposed at the alveolar wall level during lung

Table 1.1 Components of Normal Human Lung

Component	Volume or Mass (mL)	Thickness (μm)	Reference
Gas	2400		9
Tissue	900		4, 5
Blood	400		5
Lung	500		9
Support structures	225		6
Alveolar walls	275		6, 7
Epithelium	60	0.18	6, 7
Endothelium	50	0.10	6, 7
Interstitium	110	0.22	6, 7
Alveolar macrophages	55		7

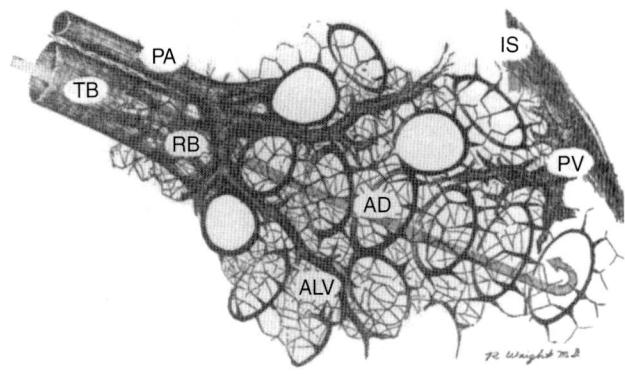

Figure 1.4 Illustration of the connective tissue support of the normal human adult lung lobule. The weave of fibers composing the "elastic continuum" is demonstrated. AD, alveolar duct; ALV, alveolus; IS, interstitial space; PA, pulmonary artery; PV, pulmonary vein; RB, respiratory bronchiole; TB, terminal bronchiole. (From Wright RR. Elastic tissue of normal and emphysematous lungs. *Am J Pathol.* 1961;39:355–363.)

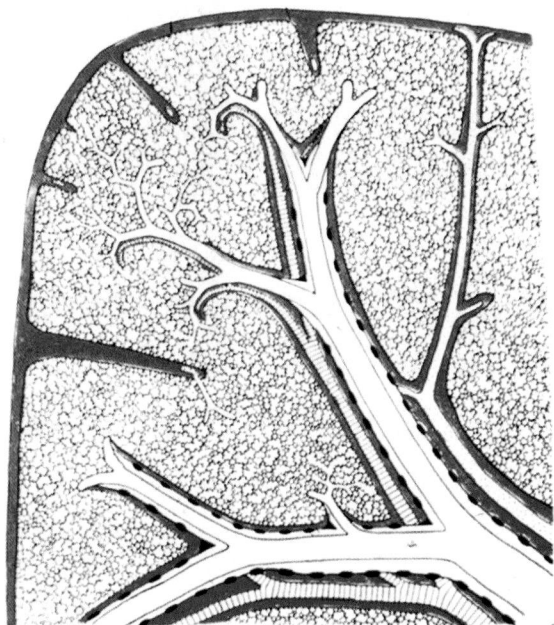

Figure 1.3 General plan depicting the interstitial connective tissue compartments of the lung. All of the extra-alveolar support structures (airways, blood vessels, interlobular septa, visceral pleura) are subsumed under the term, loose-binding connective tissue. The alveolar walls' interstitium comprises the parenchymal interstitium. This organizational plan of the lung follows the general organization of all organs. (From Hayek H. *The Human Lung.* New York: Hafner; 1960:298–314.)

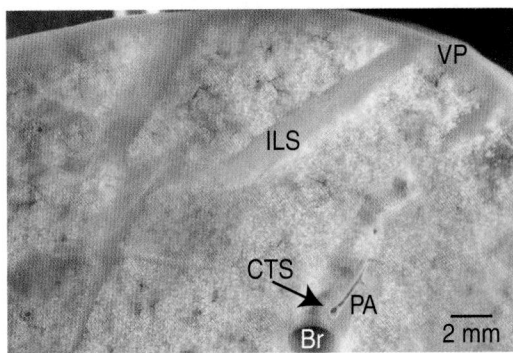

Figure 1.5 Accumulation of interstitial pulmonary edema in the loose-binding interstitial spaces. The edema fluid accentuates the loose-binding (peribronchovascular) connective tissue spaces (CTS) that surround the bronchi (Br) and pulmonary arteries (PA). Interstitial edema also expanded the interlobular septa (ILS) that are contiguous with the connective tissue of the visceral pleura (VP). (Frozen sheep lung, unstained.)

inflation are transmitted not only to adjacent alveoli, which abut each other, but also to surrounding alveolar ducts and bronchioles, and then to the loose-binding connective tissue supporting the whole lobule, and ultimately to the visceral pleural surface (see Fig. 1.3). These relations become more apparent in certain pathologic conditions. For example, in interstitial emphysema,[13] air enters the loose-binding connective tissue and dissects along the peribronchovascular sheaths to the hilum and along the lobular septa to the visceral pleura. Interstitial pulmonary edema fluid enters and moves along the same interstitial pathways (Fig. 1.5).[14]

The bulk of the interstitium is occupied by a matrix of proteoglycans (Fig. 1.6).[15,16] Proteoglycans constitute a complex group of gigantic polysaccharide molecules (≈30

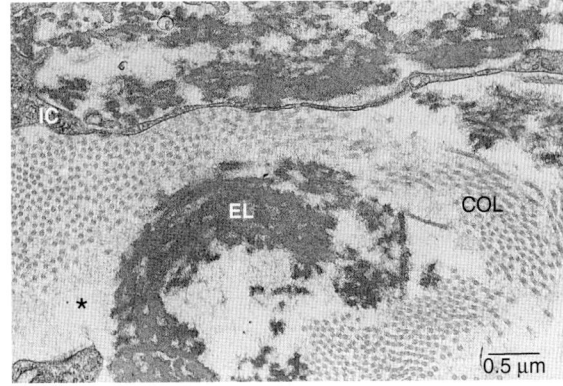

Figure 1.6 Structure of the interstitial compartment. The connective tissue compartment of the lung contains interstitial cells (IC; fibroblasts), fibrils of collagen (COL), and bundles of elastin (EL). The bulk of the interstitium, however, is occupied by matrix constituents (asterisk), such as glycosaminoglycans. (Human lung surgical specimen, transmission electron microscopy.)

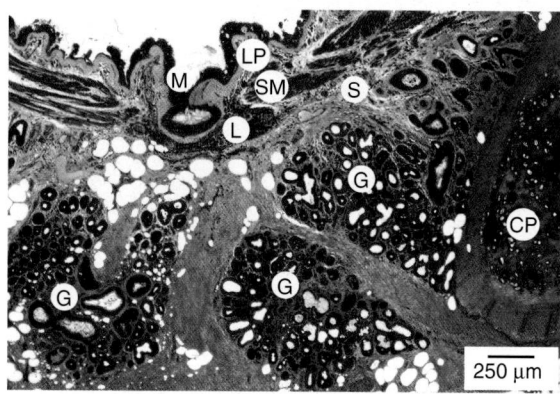

Figure 1.7 Wall structure of a bronchus. The bronchial wall is composed of mucosa (M), lamina propria (LP), smooth muscle (SM), and submucosa (S). Seromucous glands (G) are located between the spiral bands of SM and cartilaginous plates (CP). Diffuse lymphoid tissue (L) has infiltrated the lamina propria and submucosa. (Human lung surgical specimen, right middle lobar bronchus, 2-μm–thick glycol methacrylate section, light microscopy.)

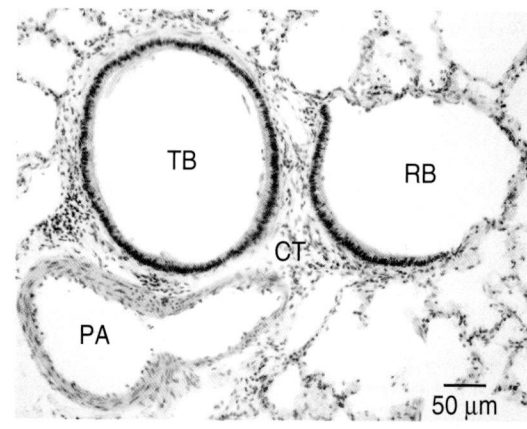

Figure 1.8 Differences in wall structure of terminal bronchioles and respiratory bronchioles. The wall of the terminal bronchiole (TB) is constructed of a single layer of ciliated, cuboidal epithelium that rests over thin, discontinuous bands of smooth muscle and loose areolar connective tissue (CT). In contrast, the wall of the respiratory bronchiole (RB) is only partially lined by ciliated cuboidal epithelium *(lower left).* The remainder of its wall is lined by squamous epithelium *(upper right).* The connective tissue also surrounds the adjacent pulmonary arteriole (PA). (Human lung surgical specimen, 10-μm–thick paraffin section, light microscopy.)

different core proteins, with great diversity of glycosaminoglycan side chains) whose entanglements impart a gel-like structure to the interstitium. That structural role, although essential, is not the sole role of these important molecules. A growing view is emerging of the lung's extracellular matrix components as regulators of lung physiology, such as determining epithelial cell phenotype; binding of and subsequent signaling by cytokines; chemokines and growth factors; and cell proliferation, migration, differentiation, and apoptosis.[17–24] In disease states, degradation products of extracellular matrix components may activate the Toll-like receptor pathways (see discussion later), thus the degradation products may serve as endogenous sentinels of tissue damage and initiators of innate immune responses.[19,23–25] Within this gel-like interstitium reside several varieties of interstitial cells (contractile and noncontractile interstitial cells,[26,27] mast cells, plasma cells, and occasional leukocytes). The remainder of the interstitium is composed of laminin, collagens, elastin and reticulin fibrils, fibronectin, and tenascin (see Fig. 1.6). (For more details on the lung mesenchyme see Chapter 5.)

AIRWAYS

The airways, forming the connection between the outside world and the *terminal respiratory units* (TRUs), are of central importance to lung function in health and disease.[28,29] Intrapulmonary airways are divided into three major groups: bronchi (conducting airways with cartilage) (Fig. 1.7), membranous bronchioles (distal conducting airways without cartilage) (Fig. 1.8), and respiratory bronchioles (distal airways participating to some extent in gas exchange) (Fig. 1.9; Table 1.2). Bronchi, by definition, have cartilage in their wall. The trachea, bronchi, and membranous bronchioles peripherally to and including terminal bronchioles (together the *conducting airways*) do not participate in respiratory gas exchange. Respiratory bronchioles serve a dual function as airways and as part of the alveolar volume that participates in respiratory gas exchange.[29]

The anatomic dead space, as measured by the single-breath nitrogen dilution technique, is approximately 30% of each tidal volume. Anatomically, this dead space

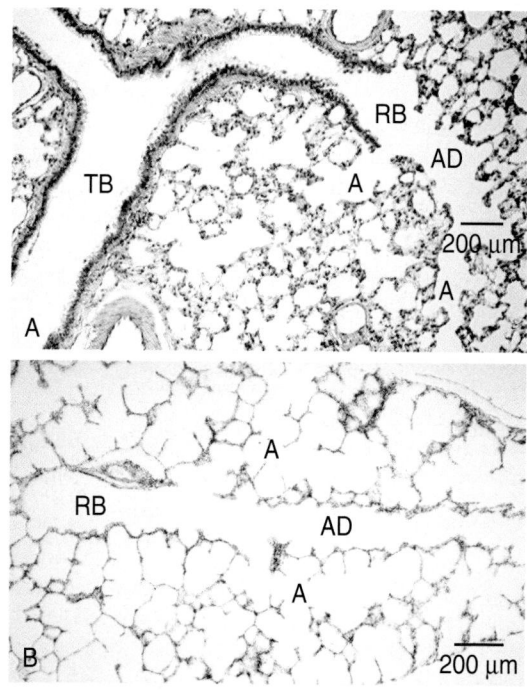

Figure 1.9 Longitudinal sections along membranous bronchioles. (A) Diameter remains relatively constant along the terminal bronchiole (TB), respiratory bronchiole (RB), and alveolar duct (AD). Alveoli (A) communicate with the gas-exchange duct. (B) This longitudinal section along an RB and AD shows that their diameter is relatively constant and that both gas-exchange ducts communicate with clusters of alveoli (A). (Human lung surgical specimen, 10-μm–thick paraffin section, light microscopy.)

is accounted for principally by the volume of the extrapulmonary (upper) airways, including the nasopharynx, trachea, and the intrapulmonary bronchi.[30] The trachea and bronchi are cartilaginous and do not change shape substantially with ventilation. The membranous bronchioles (noncartilaginous airways of ≈1-mm diameter or less), although exceedingly numerous, are short. They

Table 1.2 Characteristics of Airway Generations in Humans

Airway Generation	Generations	Characteristic	Role	TRU	Reference
Trachea	0	Cartilaginous	Conducting		28, 29
Bronchi	1–3	Cartilaginous	Conducting		28, 29
Bronchioles	4–13	Membranous	Conducting		28, 29
Terminal bronchioles	14	Membranous	Conducting		96
Respiratory bronchioles	16–18	Partially membranous	Partially conducting and gas exchange	Yes	96
Alveolar ducts	19–22		Gas exchange	Yes	96
Alveoli	23		Gas exchange	Yes	96

TRU, terminal respiratory unit.

consist of about five branching generations and end at the terminal bronchioles. In contrast to the bronchi, the membranous bronchioles are tightly embedded in the connective tissue framework of the lung and therefore enlarge passively as lung volume increases.[31] Histologically, the bronchioles down to and including the terminal bronchioles ought to contribute about 25% to the anatomic dead space. In life, however, they contribute little because of gas-phase diffusion and mechanical mixing along the distal airways, resulting from the cardiac impulse (refer to the supplemental videos on lung movements). By definition, the respiratory bronchioles and alveolar ducts participate in gas exchange and thus do not contribute to the anatomic dead space. The volume of the respiratory bronchiole-alveolar duct system is approximately one-third of the total alveolar volume, and it is into this space that the fresh-air ventilation enters during inspiration.

Most airway resistance arises from the upper airways and bronchi. Normally, the large airways are partially constricted. The minimum airway diameter in the human lung, about 0.5 mm, is reached at the level of the terminal bronchioles; succeeding generations of exchange ducts (respiratory bronchioles and alveolar ducts) are of constant diameter (see Fig. 1.9).[29,32] The functional significance of centralized resistance is that the TRUs are regionally ventilated chiefly in proportion to their individual distensibilities (compliances) because most of their airway resistance is common. This is demonstrated normally by the finding that regional lung ventilation is dependent primarily upon the initial volumes of the alveoli. TRUs toward the top of the lung, which are more expanded at FRC, do not receive as great a share of the inspiratory volume as do the TRUs near the bottom of the lung.

Airway diameter represents a balance between anatomic dead space volume and airflow resistance. Airway diameter ought to be as small as possible to minimize anatomic dead space and maximize efficient alveolar ventilation by reducing the dead space–to–tidal volume ratio, whereas airway diameter ought to be as large as possible to minimize airway resistance and the work of breathing. In disease, airways are often narrowed (Fig. 1.10), which increases resistance and the work of breathing.

The presence of apical junctional complexes between airway epithelial cells (Fig. 1.11) has important functional implications for metabolically regulated secretion into and absorption of electrolytes and water from the lining liquid.

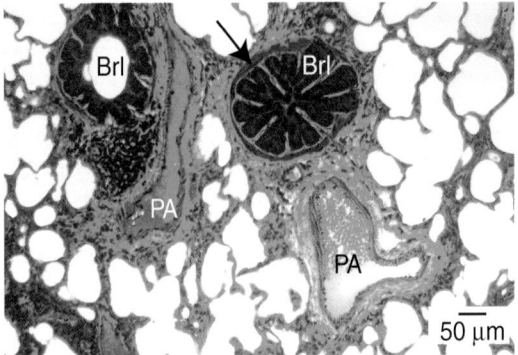

Figure 1.10 Cross-sections of two bronchioles that would contribute to increased airway resistance. On the left is a bronchiole (Brl) that is partially narrowed, evident by the folded and thick epithelium. The bronchiole to the right is completely narrowed. Its lumen is obliterated by the infolded epithelium. This bronchiole's smooth muscle is thick *(arrow)*, suggesting that the narrowing is related to constriction of the smooth muscle. Each bronchiole is flanked by a pulmonary arteriole (PA). (Sheep lung, 5-μm–thick paraffin section, light microscopy.)

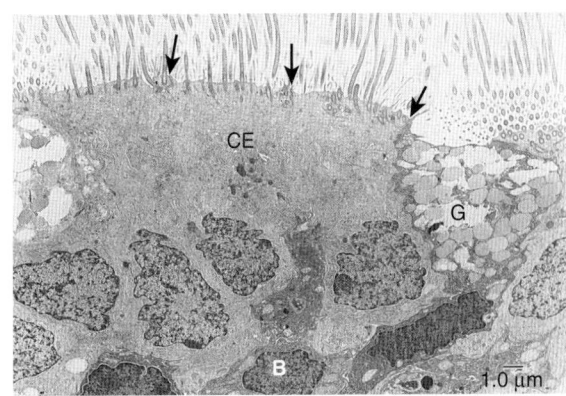

Figure 1.11 Cells constituting the bronchial epithelium. The *arrows* at the apical surface of the airway cells indicate the location of junctional complexes between contiguous epithelial cells. The bronchial epithelium has ciliated epithelial cells (CE), goblet cells (G), and basal cells (B). Goblet cells have abundant mucous granules in the cytoplasm, and their apical surface is devoid of cilia. Basal cells, as their name indicates, are located along the abluminal portion of the lining epithelium, adjacent to the basal lamina. (Human lung surgical specimen, transmission electron microscopy.)

Apical junctional complexes consist of three elements: *zonula occludens* (tight junction), *zonula adherens*, and *macula adherens* (desmosome).[33] Tight junctions serve two important functions: (1) restriction of passive diffusion by blocking the lateral intercellular space and (2) polarization of cellular functions (ion and water transport) between the apical and basolateral membranes.[34] Polarization of chloride and sodium transport allows the airway epithelium either to secrete or absorb ions, with associated passive water movement (see Chapter 3).

Trapping of foreign material, such as particulates or bacteria, is accomplished by mucins. Mucins are complex glycoproteins that form gels. MUC5AC and MUC5B are the main gel-forming mucins in human airways.[35,36] MUC5AC is produced by surface epithelia in proximal cartilaginous airways.[37] Normally, MUC5B is produced by airway glandular cells[37,38] but, in a variety of pulmonary diseases, its cell source is expanded. Other mucins (e.g., MUC5B, MUC7)[38,39] become expressed by airway epithelial cells in diseases, such as cystic fibrosis. In that disease, MUC5B is produced by airway epithelial cells.[40]

Glands are limited to the submucosa of the bronchi. Airway glands secrete water, electrolytes, and mucins into the lumen. Studies of regulation of secretion in vivo and by explant culture systems in vitro show that secretion can be modulated by neurotransmitters, including cholinergic, adrenergic, and peptidergic transmitters,[41,42] and by inflammatory mediators, such as histamine,[43] platelet-activating factor,[44] and eicosanoids.[45] The absence of airway glands and goblet cells distal to ciliated epithelial cells makes teleologic sense because that arrangement should minimize the flow of mucus backward into alveolar ducts and alveoli.

Although most foreign material and immunologic stimuli are carried up the airways by mucociliary action, some are cleared by the lymphatics. In addition, lymphoid tissue is found within the lungs and referred to as *inducible bronchus-associated lymphoid tissue* (iBALT).[46] These lymphoid aggregates are distributed along the tracheobronchial tree (see Fig. 1.7) and, to a lesser extent, along the blood vessels.[46–48] BALT in the human lung is called inducible because it is not present at birth in humans or in germ-free animals but develops after antigenic stimulation.[47,48] Lymphocytes in these structures are principally B cells, which often form follicles.[49] The presence of lymphocytes along the airways provides a reminder that the respiratory system is constantly challenged by airborne immunologic stimuli. The tracheobronchial lymphoid tissue appears to provide an important locus for both antibody-mediated and cell-mediated immune responses.[50] Another important locus of immune response is provided by the epithelial cells that line the airways and comprise the airway glands. The importance of epithelial cells arises from their expression of *Toll-like receptors* (TLRs), whose role is identification of pathogen-associated molecular patterns.[51] Activation of TLRs leads to downstream signaling cascades involved in mucin production, leukocyte recruitment, antimicrobial peptide production, and wound repair[52–57] (see also Chapter 15).

BRONCHIAL CIRCULATION

The trachea (and esophagus), mainstem bronchi, and pulmonary vessels entering the lung (see Fig. 1.1), as well as the visceral pleura in humans (see "Pleural Space and

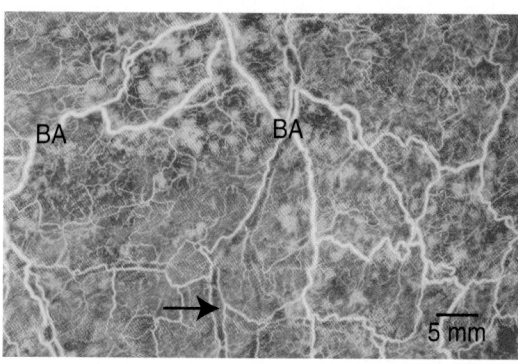

Figure 1.12 Surface view of the visceral pleura. Yellow latex polymer fills the rich network of the bronchial arteries (BA) and subsequent microvascular network. Some bronchial arterioles flank lymphatics *(arrow)* that comprise the superficial lymphatic plexus of the lung. (Sheep lung visceral pleural surface.)

Pleural Membranes" toward the end of this chapter), are supplied by the bronchial (systemic) blood circulation.[58–60] Measurements of bronchial circulation, by microsphere studies in animals, indicate that flow is 0.5–1.5% of cardiac output and is predominantly to the large airways.[58,59,61–64] The bronchial arteries arborize into bronchial capillaries that form a network in the lamina propria (the underlying connective tissue), in the submucosa, and in the region external to the cartilage of bronchi, as well as in the lamina propria of neighboring pulmonary arteries.[65] Venous blood from the trachea and large airways enters bronchial venules, which converge to form bronchial veins that drain into the azygos or hemiazygos veins. Thus, most bronchial blood flow returns to the right side of the heart. Deeper in the lung, however, bronchial blood passes via short anastomotic vessels into the pulmonary venules, thus reaching the left side of the heart to contribute to the venous admixture. The relationships among the bronchial, pulmonary, and systemic arterial and venous circulations are diagrammed in eFig. 1.1.

The bronchial circulation has enormous growth potential in contrast to the pulmonary circulation, which, after childhood, is unresponsive to growth signals. As a result, the bronchial circulation is the primary source of new vessels for repair of tissue after lung injury. In long-standing inflammatory and proliferative diseases, such as bronchiectasis or carcinoma, bronchial blood flow may be greatly increased.[59,66] Scar tissue and tumors greater than 1 mm in diameter receive their blood supply via the bronchial circulation.[67,68] As will be discussed near the end of this chapter, the bronchial circulation also supplies the visceral pleura of species that have thick visceral pleura (Fig. 1.12), which includes humans.

PULMONARY CIRCULATION

In humans, the pulmonary artery enters each lung at the hilum in a loose connective tissue sheath adjacent to the main bronchus (see Fig. 1.1). The pulmonary artery travels adjacent to and branches with each airway generation (Fig. 1.13) down to the level of the respiratory bronchiole (see Fig. 1.8). The anatomic arrangements of the pulmonary arteries and the airways are a continual reminder of the relationship between perfusion and ventilation

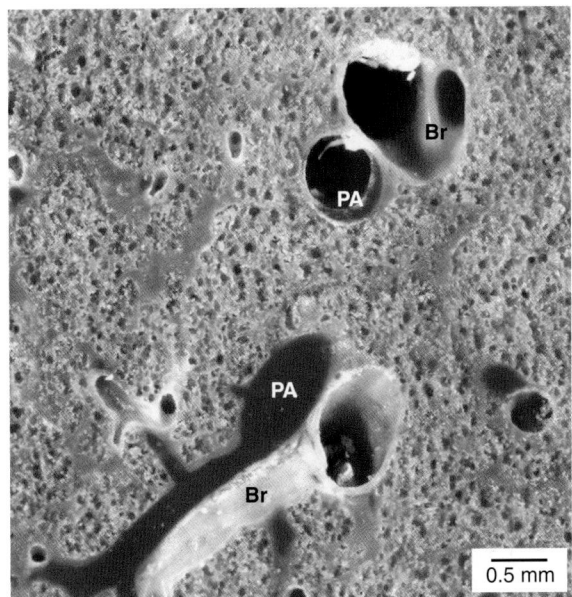

Figure 1.13 Divisions of the pulmonary artery (PA) within the lung. The PA divides and travels beside the bronchi and bronchioles (Br) out to the respiratory bronchioles. Thus, at all airway generations, an intimate relationship exists with pulmonary arterial generations. Note that the loose-binding (peribronchovascular) connective tissue sheaths are not distended, compared to the interstitial edema cuffs in Fig. 1.5. (Frozen normal sheep lung, unstained.)

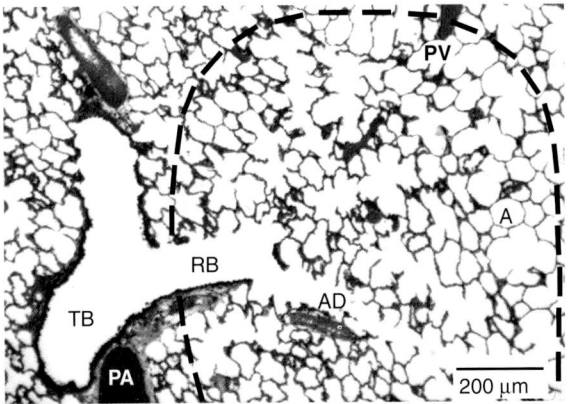

Figure 1.14 Anatomy of terminal respiratory units. Terminal respiratory units (the physiologist's alveolus) consist of the alveoli (A) and alveolar ducts (AD) arising from a respiratory bronchiole (RB). Each unit is roughly spherical, as suggested by the *dashed outline*. Pulmonary venous vessels (PV) are peripherally located. PA, pulmonary artery; TB, terminal bronchiole. (Normal sheep lung, somewhat underinflated, 2-μm–thick glycol methacrylate section, light microscopy.)

that determines the efficiency of normal lung function. Although the pulmonary veins also lie in loose connective tissue sheaths adjacent to the main-stem bronchus and pulmonary artery at the hilum, once inside the lung they follow Miller's dictum that the veins will generally be found as far away from the airways as possible.[58] Peripherally, the pulmonary arteries branch out into the TRU, whereas the veins occupy the surrounding connective tissue envelope (Fig. 1.14). Each small muscular pulmonary artery supplies a specific volume of respiratory tissue, whereas each vein drains portions of several such zones.

Table 1.3 Quantitative Data on Intrapulmonary Blood Vessels in Humans

Vessel Class (With Diameter)	Volume (mL)	Surface Area (m²)	Reference
Arteries (>500 μm)	68	0.4	69
Arterioles (13–500 μm)	18	1.0	69
Capillaries (10 μm)	60–200	50–70	70
Venules (13–500 μm)	13	1.2	71
Veins (>500 μm)	58	0.1	71

Considerable quantitative data about the pulmonary circulation are available for the human lung (Table 1.3).[69-71] Although most of the intrapulmonary blood volume is in the larger vessels down to approximately 500 μm diameter, nearly all of the surface area is in the smaller vessels. For example, the surface area of arterioles 20 to 500 μm in diameter exceeds that of the larger vessels by a factor of two, and the maximal capillary surface area is 20 times that of all other vessels. Such impressive expansion of surface area maximizes the area for respiratory gas exchange.

Because the vertical height of the lung at FRC is about 24 cm (see Fig. 1.2), the pressure within the pulmonary blood vessels varies by approximately 24 cm H_2O over the full height of the lung. Thus, if pulmonary arterial pressure is taken as 20 cm H_2O (15 mm Hg, 1.9 kPA)* at the level of the main pulmonary artery, which is about halfway up the height of the lung, pressure in the pulmonary arteries near the top of the lung will be about 12 cm H_2O, whereas pressure in pulmonary arteries near the bottom will be about 36 cm H_2O. Pulmonary venous pressure, which is about 8 cm H_2O at the level of the pulmonary artery in midchest (left atrial pressure), would be −4 cm H_2O near the top of the lung and +20 cm H_2O at the bottom. In the normal lung, the blood volume is greater at the bottom because of increased luminal pressure, which expands those vessels and increases their volume. This effect of distention also decreases the contribution of the blood vessels at the bottom of the lung to total pulmonary vascular resistance.

From birth through adulthood, the normal pulmonary circulation is a low-resistance circuit. The resistance is distributed somewhat differently than in the systemic circulation, where the major drop in resistance is across the arterioles. In the pulmonary circulation, although the pressure drop along the pulmonary capillaries is only a few centimeters of water (similar to the pressure drop in systemic capillaries), the pulmonary arterial and venous resistances are low, so a relatively larger fraction of the total pulmonary vascular resistance (35–45%) resides in the alveolar capillaries at FRC.[72,73] (For further information about pulmonary circulation in health and disease see Chapters 6 and 83.)

Vasoactivity plays an important part in the local regulation of blood flow in relation to ventilation.[74,75] Because smooth muscle surrounds the pulmonary vessels on both

---

*To convert from kPA to cm H_2O, multiply by 10.3; to mm Hg, multiply by 7.5.

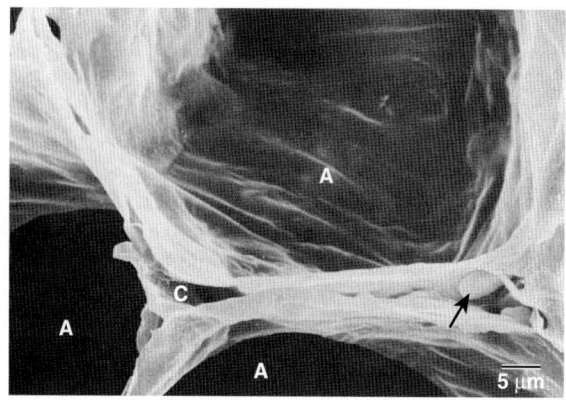

Figure 1.15 Alveolar capillaries are long. An alveolar capillary (C) is shared longitudinally along its path across three alveoli (A). The alveolar walls are flattened, and the wall junctions are sharply curved because the lung is fixed in zone 1 conditions. Some red blood cells remain in the capillary at an alveolar corner *(arrow)*. (Perfusion-fixed normal rat lung; airway pressure = 30 cm H_2O, pulmonary artery pressure = 25 cm H_2O, left atrial pressure = 6 cm H_2O, scanning electron microscopy.)

the arterial and the venous side down to precapillary and postcapillary vessels,[76,77] any segment can contribute to active vasomotion.[78] In pathologic conditions, vascular smooth muscle may extend down to the capillary level.[79,80]

Theoretically, gas exchange may take place through the thin wall of almost any pulmonary vessel. At normal alveolar O_2 tensions, however, little O_2 and CO_2 is exchanged before the blood reaches the true capillaries.[81] In the pulmonary arterioles, because of their small volume (see Table 1.3), blood flow is rapid. As blood enters the vast alveolar wall capillary network, its velocity slows, averaging about 1000 μm/s (or 1 mm/s). Flow in the microcirculation is pulsatile because of the low arterial resistance.[82] Pulsations reach the microvascular bed from both the arterial and the venous sides. In fact, one sign of severe pulmonary hypertension is the disappearance of capillary pulsations.[83]

The capillary network is long and crosses several alveoli (Fig. 1.15) before coalescing into venules. The vast extent of the capillary bed together with the length of the individual paths allows a transit time for RBCs sufficient for gas exchange to take place. The estimate based on anatomy of approximately 0.5- to 1-second average transit time is essentially the same as that found using the carbon monoxide diffusing capacity method, in which one divides capillary blood volume by cardiac output to obtain mean capillary transit time.[84] In the normal lung, there is sufficient time for equilibrium between the O_2 and CO_2 tensions in the alveoli and the erythrocytes in the pulmonary capillaries. Only under extreme stress (heavy exercise at low inspired O_2 tensions) or in severe restrictive lung disease are the RBCs predicted to pass through the microcirculation without enough time to reach diffusion equilibrium.[85]

Normally, capillary blood volume is equal to or greater than stroke volume. Under normal resting conditions, the volume of blood in the pulmonary capillaries is well below its maximal capacity, however. Recruitment can increase this volume by a factor of about three. Thus, the normal capillary blood volume of 60 to 75 mL is one-third of the capacity (200 mL) measured by quantitative histology.[6] This reserve capacity of the capillaries allows them

to accommodate rapid increases in cardiac output during times of high demand.

Anatomically, the pulmonary blood vessels can be divided into two groups: extra-alveolar and alveolar. *Extra-alveolar vessels* lie in the loose-binding connective tissue (peribronchovascular sheaths, interlobular septa). Extra-alveolar vessels extend into the TRUs. *Alveolar vessels* lie within the alveolar walls and are embedded in the parenchymal connective tissue. They are subject to whatever forces operate at the alveolar level. They are referred to as alveolar vessels in the sense that the effective hydrostatic pressure external to them is alveolar pressure. Not all of the alveolar vessels are capillaries, however. Small arterioles and venules, which bulge into the air spaces, may also be affected by changes in alveolar pressure. Likewise, not all of the capillary bed is subjected to alveolar pressure under all conditions.[86] The corner capillaries in the alveolar wall junctions are protected from the full effects of alveolar pressure by the curvature and alveolar air-liquid surface tension.[87] This may account for the fact that, even under conditions in which alveolar pressure exceeds both arterial and venous pressure ("zone 1"),[88] some blood continues to flow through the lung.[89] One has to go several centimeters up into zone 1 before blood flow stops completely. (For a discussion of distribution of pulmonary blood flow and lung zones, see Chapter 10.)

An important question is whether the normal human lung contains connections between the pulmonary arteries and veins that permit some portion of pulmonary blood flow to bypass the capillary network. Whereas such vessels may develop congenitally or pathologically,[90] functioning short circuits probably do not exist in the normal lung. (Pathologic arteriovenous communications are discussed in Chapter 88.)

In addition to its function in gas exchange, the pulmonary circulation is involved in a number of other functions important to homeostasis. The pulmonary vascular bed serves as a capacitance reservoir between the right and left sides of the heart. Consequently, the reservoir of blood in the pulmonary circulation is sufficient to buffer changes in right ventricular output for two to three heartbeats. The pulmonary vascular bed also serves as a filter, trapping embolic material and preventing it from reaching systemic vascular beds. For example, during intravascular coagulation or in processes involving platelet or neutrophil aggregation, the predominant site of sequestration is the lung. The main anatomic reason for this is that 75% of the total circulating blood volume is in the venous circuit, and the lung's microvascular bed is the first set of small vessels through which the blood flows. Moderate numbers of microemboli generally produce no detectable dysfunction in the lung because of the huge array of parallel pathways in the pulmonary microcirculation. At most, microemboli temporarily block flow to a portion of or to an entire TRU. The fate of such emboli is not clear. Some are phagocytosed and removed into the lung tissue.[91] Some emboli can be degraded to a small size, pass through into the systemic circulation, and be removed by the reticuloendothelial system. The filtering function of the lung enables such clinical studies as the perfusion scan, in which macroaggregated albumin is trapped by the lung vessels as a measure of perfusion. (Further information about the pathophysiology of thromboembolic disorders is presented in Chapter 81.)

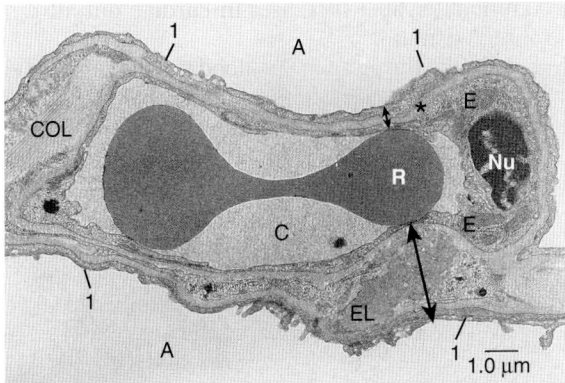

Figure 1.16 Cross-section of an alveolar wall showing the path for oxygen and carbon dioxide diffusion. The thin side of the alveolar wall barrier *(short double-headed arrow)* consists of type 1 epithelium (1), interstitium (asterisk) formed by the fused basal laminae of the epithelial and endothelial cells, capillary endothelium (E), plasma in the alveolar capillary (C), and finally the cytoplasm of the red blood cell (R). The thick side of the gas-exchange barrier *(long double-headed arrow)* has an accumulation of elastin (EL), collagen (COL), and matrix that jointly separate the alveolar epithelium from the alveolar capillary endothelium. As long as the red blood cells are flowing, oxygen and carbon dioxide probably diffuse across both sides of the air-blood barrier. (See also Video 3.1 for a three-dimensional ultrastructural view of alveolar walls.) A, alveolus; Nu, nucleus of the capillary endothelial cell. (Human lung surgical specimen, transmission electron microscopy.)

TERMINAL RESPIRATORY UNITS

The TRU consists of a respiratory bronchiole and all the alveolar ducts together with their accompanying alveolar ducts and alveoli (see Fig. 1.14; see Table 1.2). The TRU has both a structural and a functional existence and was first described in the human lung by Hayek.[11] In the human lung, this unit contains approximately 100 alveolar ducts and 2000 alveoli. At FRC, the unit is approximately 5 mm in diameter, with a volume of 0.02 mL. There are about 150,000 such units in the lungs of normal adult humans.[6]

The functional definition of the TRU is physiologic; namely, gas-phase diffusion is so rapid along patent airways that the partial pressures of O_2 and CO_2 are uniform throughout the unit.[28] Therefore, physiologically, O_2 in the gas phase anywhere along the TRU will diffuse along its concentration gradient across the extremely thin walls into RBCs flowing in the capillaries (Fig. 1.16), where O_2 combines with hemoglobin. CO_2 diffuses in the opposite direction along its concentration gradient. A key point about diffusion is that the process is much faster in the gas phase than in the liquid phase. Thus, the TRU size is defined in part by the fact that gas molecules can diffuse and equilibrate anywhere within the unit more rapidly than they can diffuse across the air-blood barrier into the blood. Of note, the solubility of O_2 in water is low relative to its concentration in gas. CO_2 is much more soluble in water (20 times the solubility of O_2 in water), and therefore CO_2 diffuses rapidly into the gas phase, even though the driving pressure for CO_2 diffusion is only one-tenth that for O_2 entering the blood.

A source of confusion is the term *acinus* in the context of the lung. Historically, the term acinus has been defined differently by different fields. In pathology, the acinus is bigger than a TRU. The pathologists' *acinus* consists of a terminal bronchiole and all of the subsequent respiratory bronchioles

together with their accompanying alveolar ducts and alveoli.[92–95] Alas, the term *acinus* also has been used to describe the TRU unit.[96] This chapter uses the physiologists' *alveolus*: the TRU. The physiologists' *alveolus* is the TRU because the unit's definition is functional.

In general, O_2 diffusion is not limiting in the normal lung, except during heavy exercise while breathing gas containing very low O_2 concentrations (e.g., at high altitudes).[85] Even at that, it is not so much diffusion that is limiting, but the fact that the transit time of the RBCs is reduced due to increased cardiac output. However, most disorders of oxygenation are due to ventilation-perfusion inequalities[97] (see also Chapter 44).

All portions of the TRU participate in volume changes with breathing.[98,99] When a unit increases its volume from FRC, the alveolar gas that had been in the alveolar duct system enters the expanding alveoli, together with a small portion of the fresh air. Most of the fresh air remains in the alveolar duct system. This does not lead to any significant gradient of alveolar O_2 and CO_2 partial pressures because diffusion in the gas phase is so rapid that there is equilibrium within a few milliseconds. However, nondiffusible (suspended or particulate) matter remains away from the alveolar walls and is expelled in the subsequent expiration.[100] This explains why it is difficult to deposit aerosols on the alveolar walls and why large inspired volumes and breath-holding are needed for efficient alveolar deposition.

The anatomic alveolus is not spherical (Fig. 1.17, see Fig. 1.15). It is a complex geometric structure with flat walls and sharp curvature at the junctions between adjacent walls. The most stable configuration is for three alveolar walls to join together, as in foams.[6] The resting volume of an alveolus is at 10–14% of TLC. When alveoli go below their resting volume, they must fold up because their walls have a finite mass (see Fig. 1.17). Most of the work required to inflate the normal lung is expended across the air-liquid interface to overcome surface tension; the importance of the air-liquid interface is demonstrated by the low pressure required to "inflate" a liquid-filled lung with more liquid[101] (see Fig. 3.5 and Chapter 3).

The phenomenon of TRU, or alveolar, stability is complex because not only is air-liquid interfacial tension involved but each flat alveolar wall is part of two alveoli, and both must participate in any volume change. Therefore atelectasis does not usually involve individual alveoli but rather relatively large units (Fig. 1.18).[102]

The alveolar walls are composed predominantly of pulmonary capillaries. In the congested alveolar wall the blood volume may be greater than 75% of the total wall volume. Alveoli near the top of the lung show less filling of the capillaries than those at the bottom.[103,104] This affects regional diffusing capacity, which is dependent on the volume of RBCs in the capillaries.

The transition from a cuboidal epithelium of the respiratory bronchiole to the squamous epithelium of the alveolus is abrupt (Fig. 1.19). Little is known about the function, if any, of this transitional junction. Although Macklin[105] speculated that the permeability of the bronchiole-alveolar epithelial junctions might be unique, no definitive difference has been demonstrated.[106] The controversy continues as to whether this region shows unique permeability features that might participate in clearance of particles or leakage of edema.[107–109]

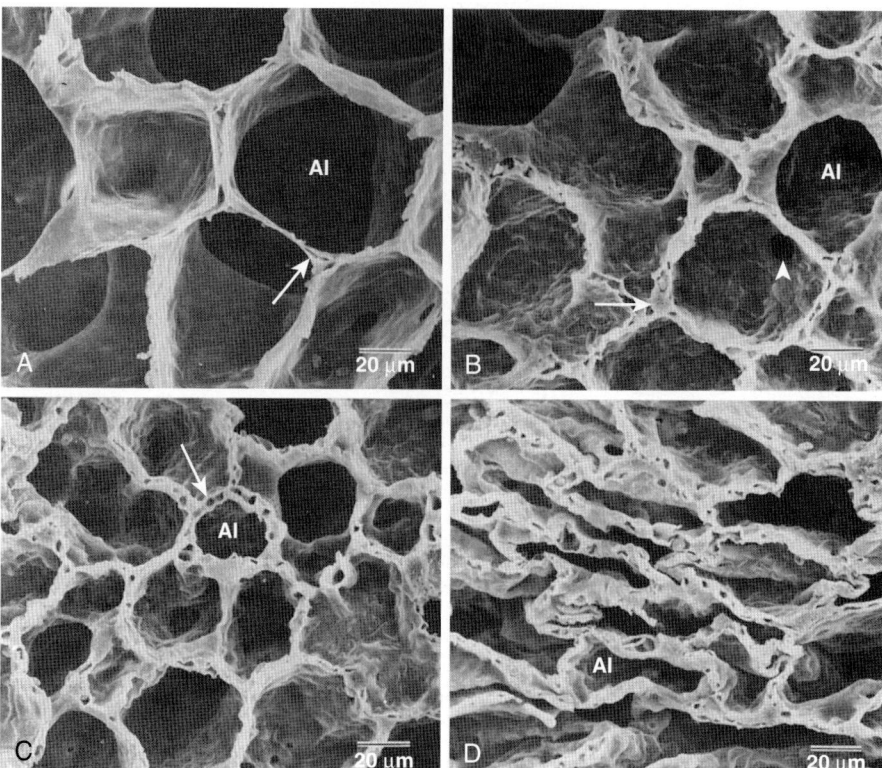

Figure 1.17 Alveolar shape changes at representative points along the air deflation pressure-volume curve of the lung. The four micrographs are at the same magnification. The air deflation pressure points are as follows: (A) airway pressure = 30 cm H$_2$O (total lung capacity [TLC]); (B) 8 cm H$_2$O (≈50% TLC); (C) 4 cm H$_2$O (near functional residual capacity [FRC]); and (D) 0 cm H$_2$O (minimal volume). Vascular pressures are constant (pulmonary artery pressure = 25 cm H$_2$O and left atrial pressure = 6 cm H$_2$O). Intrinsic alveolar shape (AI) is maintained from TLC to FRC (A–C). The alveolar walls are flat, and there is sharp curvature at the junctions between adjacent walls. Note the flat shape of the alveolar capillaries *(arrow)* at TLC ([A] lung zone 1 conditions) compared to their round shape *(arrow)* at FRC ([C] lung zone 3 conditions). The alveolar walls are folded and alveolar shape is distorted at minimal lung volume (D). The *arrow* in (B) identifies an alveolar type 2 cell at an alveolar corner. The *arrowhead* in (B) identifies a pore of Kohn. (Perfusion-fixed normal rat lungs, scanning electron microscopy.)

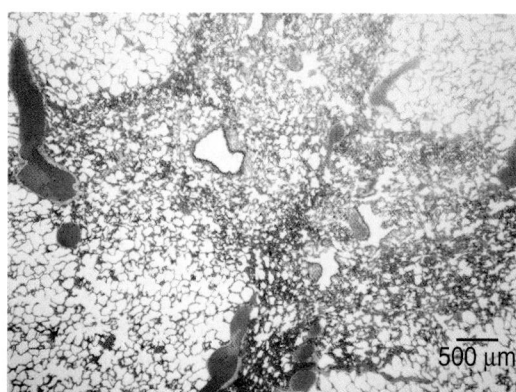

Figure 1.18 Histologic appearance of atelectasis. Atelectasis usually involves relatively large units of lung parenchyma, rather than individual alveoli. Alveolar walls in the atelectatic units are folded, distorting alveolar air space and capillary shape, as shown in Fig. 1.17D. (Sheep lung injured by air emboli, 2 μm–thick glycol methacrylate section, light microscopy.)

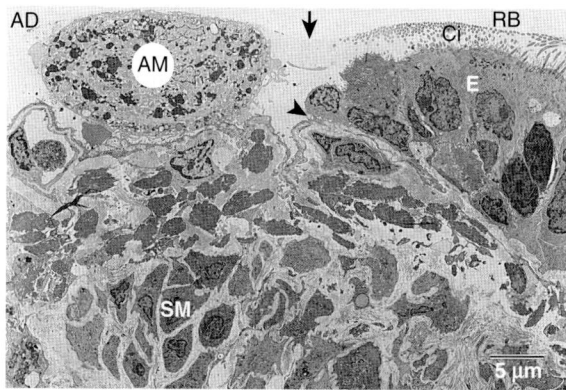

Figure 1.19 The respiratory bronchiole (RB)–alveolar duct (AD) junction is abrupt. The junction is demarcated by an abrupt transition *(arrowhead)* from low cuboidal epithelial cells (E) with cilia to squamous epithelial cells. Submerged in the lining liquid *(arrow)* are an alveolar macrophage (AM) and cilia (Ci). Airway smooth muscle cells (SM) extend to this level of the airway tree. (Human lung surgical specimen, transmission electron microscopy.)

Trapping and clearance of particulate matter impinging on the alveolar surfaces is vital and takes place in the alveolar surface liquid. Within this liquid are suspended alveolar macrophages (see Fig. 1.19).[110] The majority of alveolar macrophages that reach the terminal airways via the slow, upward flow of alveolar lining liquid are expelled with the surface film as it is pulled up onto the mucociliary escalator.[111,112]

LYMPHATICS

Another route for clearance of particulate matter and fluid from the lung is the pulmonary lymphatic system (see Chapter 7). Lymphatics of the lung are subdivided into two principal groups based on their location: a deep plexus and a superficial plexus.[11,58,113,114] Both plexuses are made up of initial and collecting lymphatics, with communications between the two.[11,58,108,113] The *deep plexus* is situated in the peribronchovascular connective tissue sheaths of the lung (see Fig. 1.1).[11,58,108,113] Lymphatics in the deep plexus are distributed around the airways, extending peripherally to the respiratory bronchioles and next to branches of the pulmonary arteries and veins.[11,58,108,113] Lymphatics are not found in the alveolar walls. The *superficial plexus* is located in the connective tissue of the visceral pleura. This plexus is

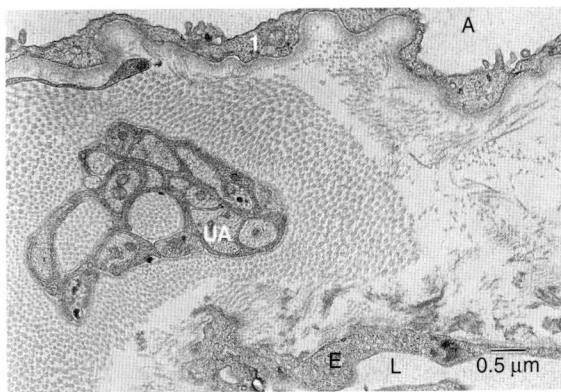

Figure 1.20 Ultrastructure of unmyelinated axons in the lung parenchyma. Unmyelinated axons (UA), known as C fibers, are shown situated in the interstitium of a respiratory bronchiole, between an alveolar type 1 cell (*white 1*) lining an alveolus (A) and an initial lymphatic (L). Although the presence of small clear vesicles is suggestive of cholinergic (autonomic) axons, unequivocal identification as either motor or sensory fibers is not possible in random thin sections. E, lymphatic endothelial cell. (Human lung surgical specimen, transmission electron microscopy.)

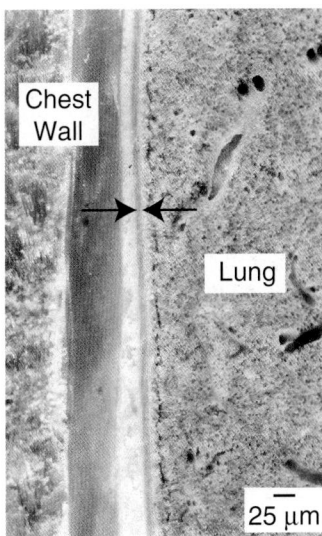

Figure 1.21 The pleural space is a real space. The dark band delimited by the *opposed arrows* is the pleural space, which is located between the chest wall and lung. (Frozen sheep chest wall and lung, unstained.)

prominent in the lung of species with thick visceral pleura, including human lung (see the section "Pleural Space and Pleural Membranes").[11,58,113] Collecting lymphatics have one-way valves and in large species, such as humans and sheep, a discontinuous, thin layer of smooth muscle. Of note, the visceral pleural lymphatics do not open into the pleural space and do not participate in pleural liquid clearance.

Lymph is propelled centripetally toward the lung's hilum or pulmonary ligament by movements of the lungs through the respiratory cycle and by heart pulsations, to reach regional lymph nodes. In the human, pulmonary lymph flows to extrapulmonary lymph nodes located around the primary bronchi and trachea.[11,58,113]

INNERVATION

Innervation of the human lung consists of sensory (afferent) and motor (efferent) pathways.[92,113,115,116] Fibers of the sensory pathway include myelinated, slowly adapting stretch receptors (Hering-Breuer reflex) and irritant receptors, but most sensory fibers are unmyelinated, slow-conducting C fibers located in the TRUs, either along the bronchioles or within the alveolar walls (Fig. 1.20). Investigators have speculated about the function of C fibers since Paintal first suggested that they played a role in sensing parenchymal connective tissue distortion, as during pulmonary vascular congestion and interstitial edema.[117–120] The speculation has neither been proven nor disproven.

The motor pathways reach the lung through the sympathetic and parasympathetic nervous systems. Preganglionic contributions to the sympathetic nerves arise from the upper four or five thoracic paravertebral ganglia, whereas the preganglionic parasympathetic nerves originate in the brainstem motor nuclei associated with the vagus nerves. Postganglionic sympathetic nerve fibers terminate near airways, vascular smooth muscle cells, or submucosal glands. Postganglionic parasympathetic fibers extend from ganglia mainly located external to the smooth muscle and cartilage.

Some submucosal ganglia exist, but they are generally smaller and have fewer neurons.

PLEURAL SPACE AND PLEURAL MEMBRANES

As stated earlier, the primary function of the lung is ensuring efficient gas exchange between alveolar air and alveolar capillary blood. This vital function is met, in part, by extensive and rapid movement of the lung within the pleural space and its pleural liquid.[121,122] Online supplemental digital videos linked to this chapter provide a glimpse of the view that surgeons have during dissection through the intercostal muscles: The lungs glide along the deep surface of the translucent endothoracic fascia and parietal pleura (see Videos 1.1 to 1.5). The pleural space also serves as an outlet into which pulmonary edema liquid can escape.[123,124] The pleural liquid also serves to couple the lung to the chest wall.[125] What are the anatomic features of the pleural space and pleurae that contribute to these functions?

An important anatomic fact is that the pleural space is a real space (Fig. 1.21); it is not a potential space.[3,125] The pleural space surrounds the lung, except at its hilum, where the parietal pleura and visceral pleura join.[11,91] Separations are present between the parietal and visceral pleurae along the interlobar fissures and costodiaphragmatic recesses. The normal volume of pleural liquid is 0.1 to 0.2 mL/kg body weight in most mammals.[125,126] This volume is distributed across a pleural surface area of approximately 1000 cm^2/lung and pleural space width of 10 to 20 μm (see Fig. 1.21).[3,125] Normally, there is little or no contact across the pleural space because the microvilli that extend from the parietal and visceral mesothelial cells are only 3 to 5 μm long.[2,3,127,128]

The unique anatomic features of the parietal pleura are the lymphatic stomata.[128–133] The lymphatic stomata are openings (≈1–12 μm in diameter) between parietal and mesothelial cells (Fig. 1.22), which are continuous with

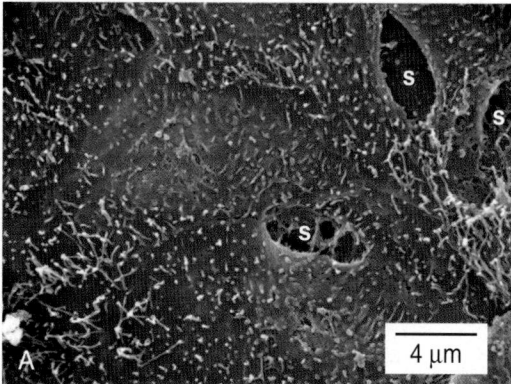

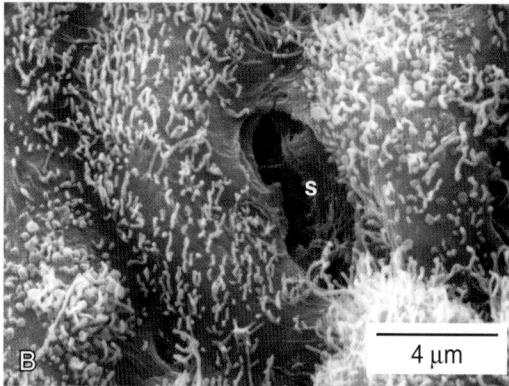

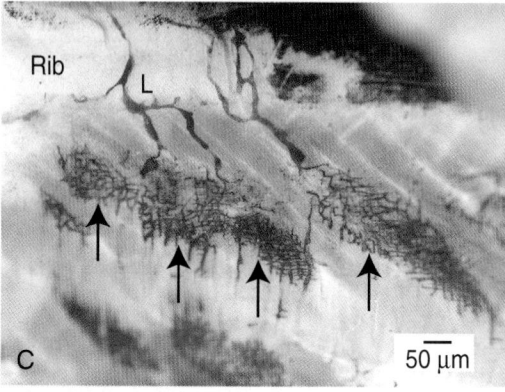

Figure 1.22 Surface view of lymphatics stomata, initial lymphatics, and collecting lymphatics of the parietal pleura. (A–B) Scanning electron micrographs that show the unique structure of lymphatic stomata (S). Stomata are apertures between the pleural space and the initial lymphatics in the parietal pleura. Three stomata are visible in a low-magnification field of view in (A). Stomata are located over intercostal muscles. (B) shows a different stoma at a higher magnification. Microvilli are not present at the aperture of the stomata, which are lined by mesothelial cells. (Sheep parietal pleura, scanning electron microscopy.) (C) shows a portion of the parietal pleura, where colloidal carbon is seen in four beds of initial lymphatics *(arrows)* located over an intercostal space. Colloidal carbon is also in collecting lymphatics (L) that cross a rib, where the collecting lymphatics drain into lymphatic vessels that accompany the intercostal vessels. (Rabbit, macroscopic view of the parietal pleural after colloidal carbon was placed in the pleural space in situ.)

the lumen of lymphatic capillaries. The size likely varies as the chest moves with ventilation. Tracer studies reveal that India ink and chicken RBCs (which are nucleated and therefore easily identifiable) are cleared almost exclusively from the pleural space by the stomata, which are located over the intercostal spaces in the distal half of the thorax, and along the sternum and pericardium of experimental

animals that have been studied.[128,134] Physiologic studies showed that protein and particulate matter in the pleural space are cleared almost entirely by the parietal pleural system of stomata and lymphatics.[129,135] The lymphatics transport the cleared pleural liquid (lymph) to regional lymph nodes along the sternum and vertebral column and then, to the thoracic duct and right lymphatic duct. In these regards, normal pleural liquid is cleared by mechanisms consistent with normal interstitial liquid turnover in the peritoneum.

CELLULAR ANATOMY OF THE LUNG

AIRWAY LINING CELLS

The airway epithelium of the human proximal conducting airways contains different types of epithelial cells with specific functions. These cells include basal cells, ciliated cells, and goblet cells, as well as some club cells and a small number of brush cells, single neuroendocrine cells,[136–139] and ionocytes.[140,141] Submucosal gland epithelium, contiguous to the airway surface epithelium, contains serous and goblet secretory cells.[142] The proportion of the different epithelial cell types that form the healthy adult human airways varies along the proximal-to-distal axis, with a decreasing number of submucosal glands and an increasing number of club secretory cells.[137,143]

Basal cells function as progenitor cells within the airway epithelium because these cells are able to self-renew or differentiate into secretory, goblet, and ciliated cells in homeostasis and during injury repair[144,145] (see Chapter 8). In humans, basal cells cover most of the airway basement membrane[146]; however, they do not reach the airway lumen and thereby contribute to the pseudostratified appearance of the airway epithelium. These cells interact with columnar epithelium, basement membrane, and underlying mesenchymal cells, inflammatory cells, lymphocytes, and dendritic cells.[147,148]

Ciliated cells protect the TRUs by filtering the inhaled air for solid particles and removing them by mucociliary clearance. Nearly half of the epithelial cells in the normal human airway are ciliated at all airway generations (Fig. 1.23), down to bronchioles (see Fig. 1.19).[149] Each ciliated cell has multiple cilia (≈200 cilia) that have a specialized capping clawlike structure called a ciliary crown, to make the distal portion stiff to propel the liquid lining layer along the airways and to promote debris clearance from the airways. The cilia have structural and motor proteins that produce coordinated and directional beating at 8 to 15 Hz, which is critical for mucociliary clearance.[136–138,150] As the airway superficial lining liquid moves centripetally, it encounters larger and fewer airways, which have a smaller *total* perimeter. For example, the total perimeter of approximately 150,000 terminal bronchioles is much greater than the total perimeter of the five lobar bronchi.[6] If the lining liquid volume remained constant, the liquid layer ought to grow in thickness, but this does not happen, suggesting that much of the liquid is reabsorbed during its ascent along the airways.

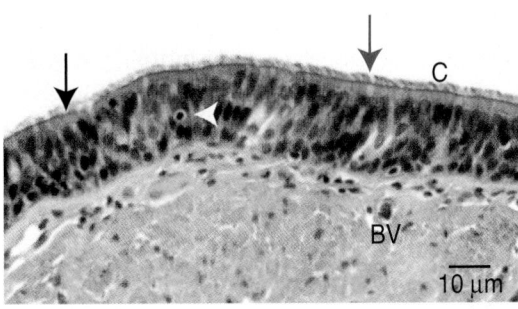

Figure 1.23 Structure of bronchial mucosa. The bronchial mucosa consists of pseudostratified, columnar epithelium with cilia (C) and goblet cells *(red arrow)*. The cilia, which form a thick carpet, move rhythmically and thereby propel liquid, mucus, cells, and debris centrally toward the pharynx. The dark band immediately beneath the cilia *(black arrow)* is produced by the basal bodies. By transmission electron microscopy, basal bodies are recognized as modified centrioles. A lymphocyte *(white arrowhead)* is intercalated among the epithelial cells. A bronchial blood vessel (BV) is located beneath the mucosal layer. (Human lung surgical specimen, 10 μm–thick paraffin section, light microscopy.)

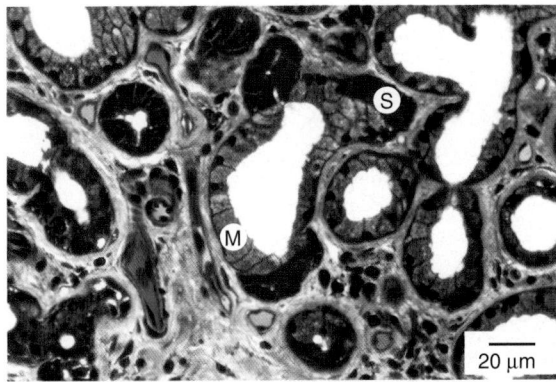

Figure 1.25 Structure of submucosal glands. This figure provides a higher magnification view of a region shown in Fig. 1.7. The mixed, compound tubuloacinar glands contain mucus-secreting cells (M) and serous-secreting cells (S). The latter type form crescentic caps, or demilunes, over the ends of the acini, the rounded secretory units of the gland. Mucous cells are the predominant glandular cell type. (Human lung surgical specimen, right middle lobar bronchus, 2 μm–thick glycol methacrylate section, light microscopy.)

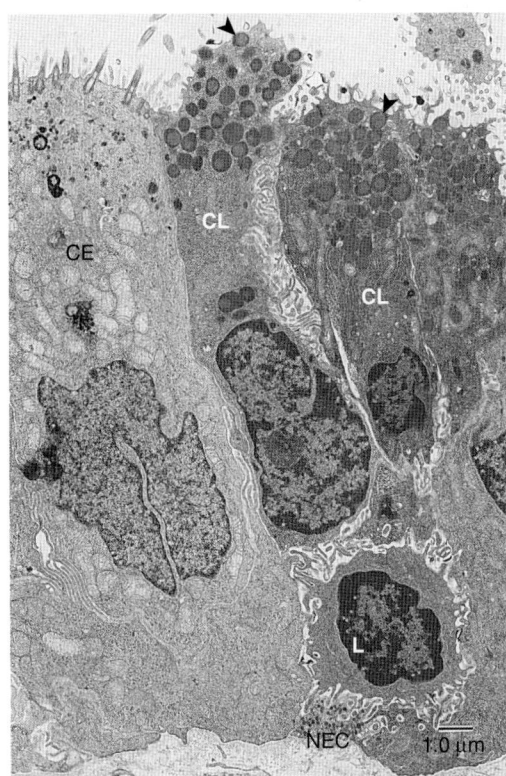

Figure 1.24 Cellular structure of terminal airway epithelium. The epithelium consists mainly of ciliated epithelium (CE) and nonciliated club cells (CL). Club cells have the ultrastructural features of secretory cells; namely, they possess basally located rough endoplasmic reticulum, perinuclear Golgi apparatus, apically located smooth endoplasmic reticulum, and prominent membrane-bound granules *(arrowheads)*. A lymphocyte (L) is intercalated among the epithelial cells. A small portion of a neuroendocrine cell (NEC) containing characteristic dense-cored vesicles is also visible at the base of the epithelial cells. (Human lung surgical specimen, transmission electron microscopy.)

Goblet cells are secretory cells that produce and store mucus in granules of about 800 nm diameter. Secretion of the correct amount of mucus with an optimum viscoelastic profile is essential for maintenance of normal mucociliary clearance.[137,151] Goblet cells also secrete inflammatory mediators that participate in the recruitment and activation of immune cells. Goblet cells are found on the airway surface and in the submucosal glands.[11,58] Furthermore, goblet cells are capable of division and may show stem cell multipotency.[152]

Club cells[153] are dome-shaped cells with dense cytoplasmic granules and microvilli that, in humans, are restricted to terminal and respiratory bronchioles,[154,155] where club cells serve as facultative progenitors for themselves and for ciliated epithelial cells, and they maintain the normal epithelium of the distal conducting airways (see Fig. 1.24).[154,156] Single-cell transcriptome analyses have suggested novel roles for club cells in host defense, antiprotease activity, and physical barrier function.[157] Club cells also secrete secretoglobin 1A1; surfactant proteins A, B, and D; and lipids.[156,158,159]

Submucosal gland epithelial cells line the submucosal glands (Fig. 1.25), which are continuous with the airway epithelium and are located below the airway luminal surface of all of the cartilaginous proximal airways. Submucosal gland epithelial cells secrete mucins, water and electrolytes, and other substances that help protect the lungs from particles and infectious agents. Studies of the regulation of secretion in vivo and in vitro show that secretion is modulated by neurotransmitters, including cholinergic, adrenergic, and peptidergic transmitters,[42] and by inflammatory mediators, such as histamine,[43] platelet-activating factor,[44] and eicosanoids.[45] Submucosal glands are connected to the airway surface by a duct lined by epithelial cells identified as ductal cells.[160] The submucosal gland epithelium contains goblet cells (described earlier) and serous cells. *Serous cells* are the defensive cells of the mucosa because they secrete innate immunity proteins, such as lysozyme, SPLUNC1, β-defensins,[161] mucins, and electrolytes, including chloride and bicarbonate, to control the fluidity of the mucus. These cells, in contrast to goblet cells, have discrete electron-dense granules of about 600 nm diameter. A few serous cells are also present in the surface epithelium of the human bronchioles.[162]

Rare lung epithelial cell types include pulmonary neuroendocrine cells, ionocytes, and brush (tuft) cells. These cell

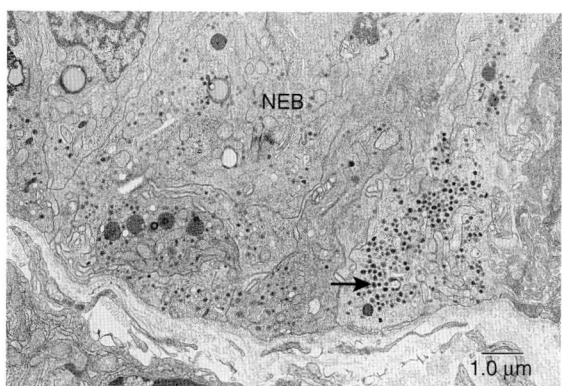

Figure 1.26 Neuroepithelial body (NEB) located in a peripheral airway. Neuroepithelial bodies contain aggregates of neuroendocrine cells. A characteristic ultrastructural feature of neuroendocrine cells is the presence of small (0.1–0.3 μm in diameter) dense-cored vesicles in their cytoplasm *(arrow)*. Each dense-cored vesicle is bounded by a unit membrane. (Human lung surgical specimen, transmission electron microscopy.)

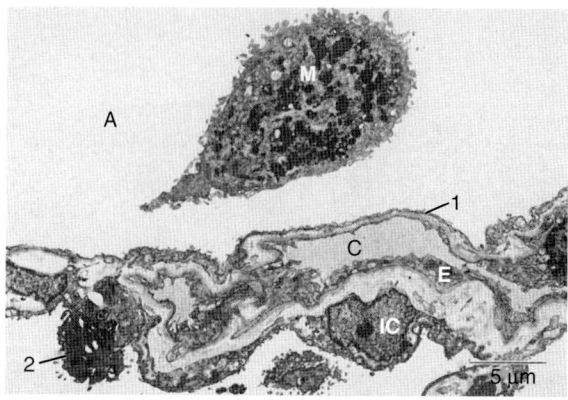

Figure 1.27 Cells of the terminal respiratory unit. An alveolar macrophage (M) is located in an alveolus (A). Alveolar macrophages are the air space scavengers that are cleared either up the mucociliary escalator or into the interstitium. These cells can be activated to express and secrete cytokines, which may interact with other cells. Cells of the alveolar wall are the lining alveolar type 1 and 2 cells (1 and 2, respectively) and the enclosed capillary (C), endothelial cells (E), and interstitial cells (IC; fibroblasts). (Human lung surgical specimen, transmission electron microscopy.)

types are continually and directly replenished by basal progenitor cells.

Pulmonary neuroendocrine cells serve as O_2 sensors[163,164] and release hormones that affect smooth muscle (e.g., vasoactive intestinal peptide[165,166] and substance P).[167–170] Pulmonary neuroendocrine cells represent less than 1% of airway epithelial cells and are a component of the diffuse neuroendocrine system called the amine uptake and decarboxylation system.[171,172] This system is composed of single neuroendocrine cells and clusters of such cells, known as neuroepithelial bodies,[173] distributed along the airway epithelium down to the region of alveolar ducts.[174–177] The neuroepithelial bodies are preferentially located at airway bifurcations. Pulmonary neuroendocrine cells are ultrastructurally characterized by dense-cored vesicles in their cytoplasm (Fig. 1.26). The dense-cored vesicles are the storage sites of amine hormones (serotonin, dopamine, norepinephrine) and peptide hormones (bombesin, calcitonin, leu-enkephalin).[166] Neurons are also associated with neuroendocrine cells.

Ionocytes are a recently identified and rare cell population that serves as the primary source of cystic fibrosis transmembrane conductance regulator activity in the conducting airway epithelium in mice and humans.[140,141] The cystic fibrosis transmembrane conductance regulator is a membrane protein that conducts chloride ions and water across epithelial cell membranes. Mutations in this gene cause cystic fibrosis (see Chapters 67 and 68).

Brush (tuft) cells are pear-shaped cells, with a narrow apex from which extend a tuft of blunt, squat microvilli that stretch their filaments into the underlying cytoplasm. Brush cells also contain numerous intracytoplasmic membrane-bound inclusions and seem to have a chemosensory role, although their function has not been clearly defined.[178]

The complex and diverse cellular composition of the airway epithelium in mammalian organisms has evolved to support the main functions of the airways, namely to connect the outside world to the TRUs, to maintain a balanced secretion and absorption of electrolytes and water from the lining liquid, and to facilitate mucociliary clearance.

ALVEOLAR LINING CELLS

The alveolar epithelial cells that line the anatomic alveoli include *alveolar type 1* (AT1) and *alveolar type 2* (AT2) cells and a minor subpopulation of *alveolar epithelial progenitors* (AEPs), all supported by a shared basal membrane and the subjacent capillaries and fibroblasts.[179,180] AT2 cells outnumber AT1 cells (≈15% vs. 8–10% of total peripheral lung cells, respectively). However, AT1 cells account for approximately 90–95% of the alveolar surface area of the peripheral lung.[181] (See also Video 3.1 for a three-dimensional ultrastructural view of AT1 cells.)

AT1 cells have extensive, attenuated cytoplasmic processes that form a large, thin surface area for gas exchange (Figs. 1.27 and 1.28). AT1 cells express water channels[182] and also epithelial sodium channels and membrane sodium-potassium–adenosine triphosphatase,[183,184] which play a role in pulmonary water flux.[185] Adult rodent and human AT1 cells have a limited proliferative capacity and are sensitive to injury. Under normal conditions, AT1 cells attach via tight junctions to neighboring AT2 cells to form a relatively impermeable seal between alveolar air and alveolar wall interstitial spaces. AT1 cells contain many small, non–clathrin-coated vesicles, or caveolae, that are open either to the alveolar lumen or interstitium or are detached from the surface as free vesicles in the cytoplasm.[186] The vesicles contain caveolin-1 protein, a scaffolding protein that organizes specialized membrane phospholipids and proteins into vesicles. Caveolin-1 can bind free cholesterol and modulate the efflux of cholesterol from the cell when intracellular concentrations rise.[187,188] Caveolae appear to sequester various proteins into the vesicles, such proteins that include growth factor receptors, signaling molecules such as G proteins, calcium ion receptors, and pumps.

AT2 cells are small (≈300 μm³) cuboidal cells with short stubby apical microvilli (see Figs. 1.27 and 1.29). AT2 cells are specialized in the production and recycling of proteins and phospholipids that form surfactant. Surfactant is stored in cytoplasmic lamellar bodies, which are membrane-bound inclusions (diameter from <0.1–2.5 μm) that are stacked layers of cell membrane-like material (Fig. 1.29) composed

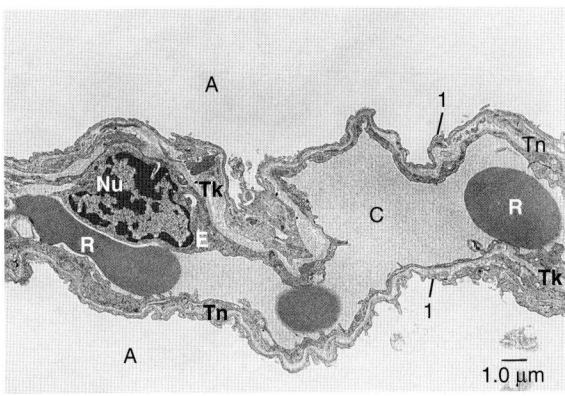

Figure 1.28 Ultrastructure of alveolar walls. The thick (Tk) and thin (Tn) sides of an alveolar capillary (C) change as the capillary crosses between alveoli (A). The basal laminae of the capillary endothelium and alveolar epithelium fuse in the thin regions. The nucleus (Nu) of an endothelial cell (E) is visible above a red blood cell (R). (See also Video 3.1 for a three-dimensional ultrastructural view of alveolar walls.) 1, alveolar type 1 cell. (Human lung surgical specimen, transmission electron microscopy.)

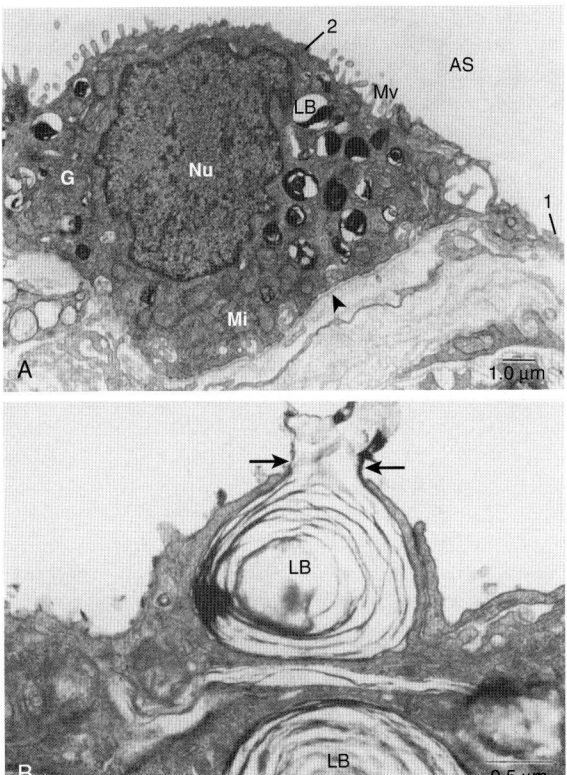

Figure 1.29 Cellular structure of alveolar type 2 cells. (A) Alveolar type 2 (or granular) cells (2) are cuboidal epithelial cells that contain characteristic lamellar bodies (LB) in their cytoplasm and have stubby microvilli (Mv) that extend from the apical surface into the alveolar air space (AS). Other prominent cytoplasmic organelles in alveolar type 2 cells are mitochondria (Mi) and Golgi apparatus (G). Adjacent to the alveolar type 2 cell is a process of an alveolar type 1 cell (1). The abluminal surface of the epithelial cells rests on a continuous basal lamina (*arrowhead*). Nu, nucleus of an alveolar type 2 cell. (B) The apical region of an alveolar type 2 cell contains two LB, one of which has been fixed in the process of secretion by exocytosis (*arrows*). The lamellar osmiophilic bodies are the source of surface-active material (surfactant). Alveolar type 2 cells are usually located in the alveolar corners (see Fig. 1.17B). (Human lung surgical specimen, transmission electron microscopy.)

of phospholipids[189] and various proteins, including surfactant proteins A, B, C, and D; lysosomal enzymes; and other molecules.[190,191] Surfactant is secreted to the alveolar space where it decreases the alveolar surface tension.[181] AT2 cells also have immunomodulatory functions. The presence of various ion channels and transporters supports earlier evidence that AT2 cells are actively involved in liquid resorption and transepithelial water fluxes.[192] Studies in mice support a role for AT2 cells as the facultative stem cells of the alveolar epithelium because AT2 cells can both self-renew and differentiate into AT1 cells.[193–195] AEP cells are a subpopulation of AT2 cells that can serve as alveolar epithelial progenitors. AEPs have been identified in adult mouse and human alveoli.[194,195] Human AEPs can be directly isolated by virtue of their expression of the conserved cell surface marker TM4SF1.[194] AEPs are a stable lineage during steady-state turnover in homeostasis but rapidly expand to regenerate the alveolar epithelium after acute lung injury.

The above epithelial cells that line the alveoli are critical for the ultimate function of the lung, which is the gas-exchange process. These cells are shaped and arranged in a way that allows the formation of very thin alveolar septa, where the epithelial cells are in close contact with the capillaries to support the diffusion of gases between air and blood. AT2 cuboidal epithelial cells maintain the integrity of the respiratory units and produce surfactant to control the surface tension of the alveoli.

MESENCHYMAL CELLS

Vascular endothelial cells of both pulmonary and bronchial vessels are continuous (nonfenestrated) endothelial cells (see Fig. 1.16). These flattened cells have an individual area of 1000 to 3000 μm^2 and an average volume of 600 μm^3.[196] The pulmonary capillary bed covers a total surface area of approximately 130 m^2, or the equivalent of one side of a doubles tennis court (260 m^2). Other structural features of capillary endothelial cells are the large number of plasmalemmal vesicles and small number of organelles. Despite having relatively few organelles, capillary endothelial cells have organelles involved in protein synthesis, such as endoplasmic reticulum, ribosomes, and Golgi apparatus, and vesicles, such as caveolae, multivesicular bodies, and lysosomes.[197] The endocytic apparatus participates in receptor-mediated uptake and transport (transcytosis) of albumin, low-density lipoproteins, and thyroxine.[198–202] Vascular endothelial cell functions include O_2 and nutrient transport, control of blood coagulation, interaction with inflammatory cells, and maintenance of epithelial homeostasis.[203] Although all vascular endothelial cells share core properties, there are differences among the endothelial cells in large blood vessels versus capillaries.[204] The large artery endothelium, for example, has a lower barrier strength and angiogenic potential than the capillary endothelium.

Lymphatic endothelial cells share many of the structural and functional characteristics of vascular endothelial cells. The ultrastructural distinction of initial lymphatics (lymphatic capillaries) is that their basement membrane is discontinuous, whereas that of pulmonary and bronchial capillaries is continuous.[205,206]

Fibroblasts are located subjacent to epithelial cell layers of airways or in the interstitium, between the epithelial and endothelial layers of alveolar walls.[207,208] Fibroblasts produce extracellular matrix components and direct cell growth and differentiation of neighboring cells by cell-cell and cell-matrix interactions. Lung fibroblast populations are highly heterogeneous.[209] For instance, human lung fibroblasts derived from the airway or alveolar regions differ in their gene expression patterns and their phenotype. *Airway fibroblasts* are morphologically and functionally distinct from alveolar fibroblasts, with differences in contractile forces and in gene expression.[210,211] Genes highly expressed in airway fibroblasts are involved in extracellular matrix deposition and organization, whereas genes highly expressed in alveolar fibroblasts participate in actin binding and cytoskeletal organization. Airway fibroblasts synthesize more collagen and eotaxin-1 than alveolar fibroblasts. Also, airway fibroblasts proliferate faster and are more myofibroblast-like, expressing higher levels of α-smooth muscle actin than alveolar fibroblasts. *Alveolar fibroblasts* play an important role during alveologenesis. During lung alveologenesis, two distinct subpopulations of fibroblasts are located in the growing secondary septa: alveolar myofibroblasts and lipofibroblasts.[212] *Myofibroblasts* are considered to be the cell type responsible for secondary septa formation. These cells are located at the tip of growing secondary septa, where they deposit elastin in the apical tip. Myofibroblasts express α-smooth muscle actin and high levels of platelet-derived growth factor receptor-β and contain myofibrils oriented parallel to the alveolar walls. Myofibroblasts differentiate from different precursor cells in disease, being the principal cell in the fibrotic foci.[213,214] *Lipofibroblasts* are characterized by the presence of lipid droplets and specific molecular markers and are located close to AT2 epithelial cells, which is consistent with lipofibroblast support of growth and differentiation of AT2 cells by providing the lipids for surfactant production. Lipofibroblasts are abundant in the late stages of lung development and postnatally. The expression of lipofibroblast marker genes, such as adipose differentiation-related protein, is reduced in the lungs of individuals with interstitial pulmonary fibrosis.[213,215] However, the existence of lipofibroblasts in human lung is still controversial because some electron microscopy studies have not detected lipofibroblasts in developing human lung.[216,217]

Smooth muscle cells in the lung are of two major subtypes[218,219] that differ in their origin and function. *Airway smooth muscle* cells form circular bands around the airway epithelium (see Figs. 1.7 and 1.10) and extend from the trachea throughout the bronchial tree to the terminal bronchioles. Airway smooth muscle cells derive from undifferentiated mesenchymal cells in closest proximity to prodifferentiation signals released from the lung epithelial layer. Newly differentiated airway smooth muscle cells in the embryonic lung are proliferative, but their proliferative capacity decreases with maturation in the fetal and postnatal stages of lung development. The spontaneous phasic contraction of fetal airway smooth muscle cells is important for normal lung development by regulating intraluminal fluid movement. In the adult lung, this phasic contraction is absent and regulation of tonic contraction and airflow is under neuronal and humoral control. Airway smooth muscle responsiveness contributes to the pathophysiology of lung diseases such as asthma.[220]

Airway smooth muscle expresses heavy chain α-smooth muscle actin arranged in contractile filaments, along with other contractile proteins.[221,222] *Vascular smooth muscle cells* play an essential physiologic role in regulation of blood flow through the pulmonary and bronchial vasculature. Smooth muscle forming around these vessels derives partly through proliferation/migration of the neighboring airway smooth muscle cell population and de novo differentiation of mesenchymal cells. Airway and vascular smooth muscle cells have differences in phenotype and gene expression that support their distinct structure and function within the lung.[222]

Pericytes are another mesenchymal cell type located along capillary basement membranes in close contact with the endothelial cells.[208,223,224] Pericytes are contractile, sharing characteristics of vascular smooth muscle cells and myofibroblasts. Lung pericytes might serve as myofibroblast progenitors and amplify inflammatory responses by expressing cytokines and adhesion molecules.[225,226]

Chondrocytes are embedded in a collagenous extracellular matrix rich in proteoglycan and elastin fibers that form the C-shaped cartilaginous rings around bronchi.[227,228]

Mesenchymal cells as a group provide the lungs with the structural support, elasticity, and blood supply necessary for sustaining respiratory movements, oxygenation of the lung tissue, and gas exchange at the capillary level in the alveoli.

NEURAL CELLS

Innervation of the lung is mediated by intrinsic neurons, whose cell bodies reside within the lung, and extrinsic neurons, whose cell bodies are located elsewhere. Intrinsic neurons originate in the neural crest and are located asymmetrically around the trachea and primary bronchi.[229] These intrinsic neurons are located close to innervated tissues, including smooth muscle cells in the trachea, airways, and neuroendocrine cells, and their numbers decrease along the proximal-distal axis of the lung.[229]

Extrinsic neuron axons, when found, resemble known sensory endings in other organs (<1 μm in diameter, electron-lucent, and containing microtubules and smooth endoplasmic reticulum).[230] The terminal processes of sympathetic efferent fibers and parasympathetic efferent fibers pierce the epithelial basement membrane, where they initiate airway reflexes, such as bronchoconstriction and cough.[231,232]

HEMATOPOIETIC AND LYMPHOID CELLS

Resident immune cells, including peribronchial and perivascular interstitial macrophages and alveolar macrophages (see Figs. 1.19 and 1.27), control the immune response during homeostasis and disease. Interstitial macrophages and alveolar macrophages, however, have different functional properties. *Interstitial macrophages* are involved in homeostasis and protection against continuous pathogen exposure from the environment. Interstitial macrophages have a high turnover rate and a short life span in the steady state. Interstitial macrophages have been proved to derive from blood monocytes and serve as intermediates for differentiation into alveolar macrophages in primates and in mice.[233]

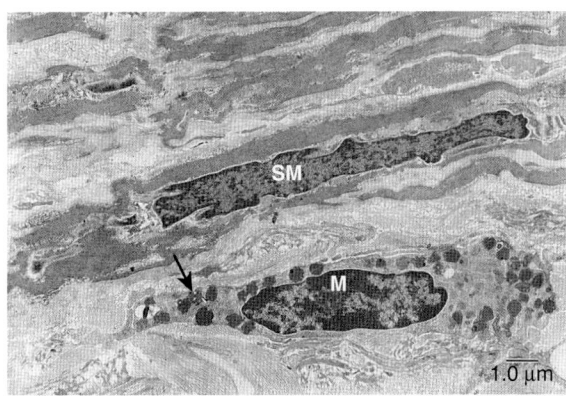

Figure 1.30 Mast cell (M) located adjacent to an airway. The mast cell flanks airway smooth muscle cells (SM). Granules in mast cells demonstrate heterogeneous morphology, including whorled and scrolled contents *(arrow).* (Human lung surgical specimen, transmission electron microscopy.)

Alveolar macrophages, by comparison, are relatively static under normal conditions, but undergo apoptosis and replacement by interstitial macrophages after exposure to bacterial endotoxin or *Streptococcus* pneumonia.[234,235] Alveolar macrophages actively express and secrete cytokines, such as tumor necrosis factor-α and transforming growth factor-α, and function in surfactant homeostasis and innate immunity.[236] Alveolar macrophages are weak antigen-presenting cells but are active in phagocytosis and production of host defense molecules, such as nitric oxide and cytokines.[237]

Immune response cells, including monocyte-derived macrophages, recruited to the lung during inflammation or infections, migrate through the epithelial basement membrane and pass through to the luminal surface, where some remain intercalated within the surface epithelium. Other immune cells that can be found in the lung, particularly in disease, are mast cells, lymphocytes, eosinophils, neutrophils, basophils, and megakaryocytes.[238] Mast cells in the human lung contain membrane-bound secretory granules (Fig. 1.30) that contain a host of inflammatory mediators, including histamine, proteoglycans, lysosomal enzymes, and metabolites of arachidonic acid.[239] Not only can these mediators induce bronchoconstriction, they can also stimulate mucus production and induce mucosal edema by increasing permeability of bronchial vessels. Lymphocytes are frequently seen intercalated between airway epithelial cells (see Figs. 1.23 and 1.24). These cytotoxic T lymphocytes undergo immunoglobulin A–class antibody responses.[240] T and B lymphocytes also accumulate in the lamina propria beneath the airway epithelium.[240]

The lung is one of the organs in the body in direct contact with the environment. The presence or recruitment of immune cells to the lung is of high importance as a first-line protective mechanism to fight infections, control inflammatory responses, and provide innate immunity.

PLEURAL CELLS

Two types of pleurae exist in the chest: the visceral pleura, which covers the lungs and other chest structures, and the parietal pleura, which is attached to the chest wall.[241] Both visceral and parietal pleurae have a superficial layer of

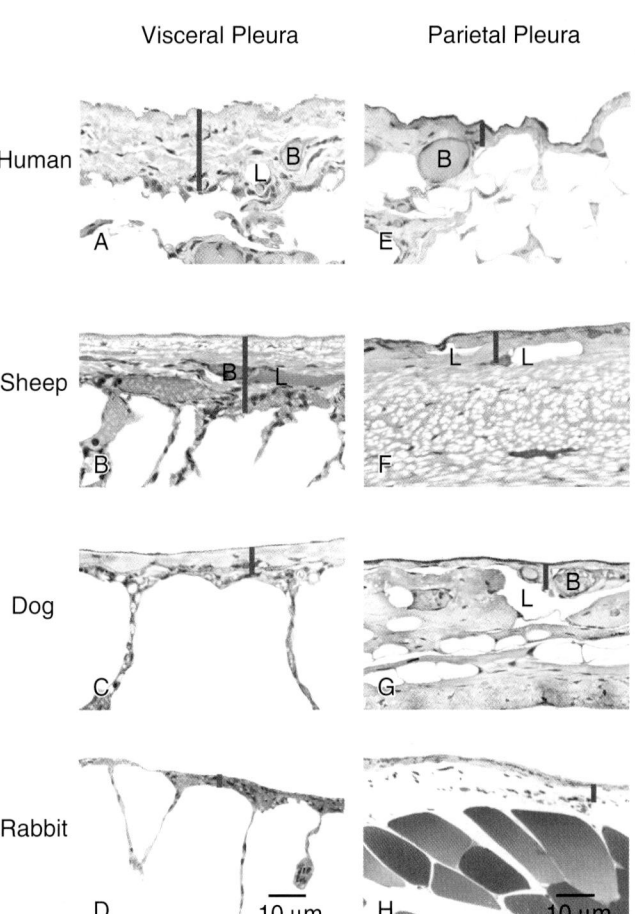

Figure 1.31 Comparative histologic features of the visceral and parietal pleurae among humans, sheep, dogs, and rabbits. The eight panels are shown at the same magnifications. (A–D) Visceral pleura. (E–H) Parietal pleura. The most obvious feature of the visceral pleura is its greater thickness *(longer red vertical bars)* among humans and sheep compared to thinner visceral pleura of dogs and rabbits *(shorter red vertical bars).* The parietal pleura is thinner and consistently so among species. Both the visceral and parietal pleurae are lined by a single layer of mesothelial cells that have microvilli extending from their surface into the pleural space. Subjacent to the mesothelial cell lining layer is loose areolar connective tissue. Among species with "thick" visceral pleura, the loose areolar connective tissue is traversed by bronchial microvessels (B), lymphatics (L), and nerves. By comparison, among species with "thin" visceral pleura, the loose areolar connective tissue is devoid of microvessels, other than the subjacent pulmonary microvessels at the perimeter of the most superficial alveoli. Lymphatics and nerves are infrequent. In the parietal pleura's loose areolar connective tissue are systemic blood microvessels (B), lymphatics (L), and nerves. This histologic organization is consistent among species. (Human, sheep, dog, and rabbit lung, 2 μm–thick glycol methacrylate sections, light microscopy.)

simple, cuboidal or flattened, mesothelial cells, with various amounts of microvilli on the luminal surface[128,131,132,134] (Fig. 1.31). This mesothelial cell layer is supported by a thin submesothelial connective tissue layer, which includes a basal lamina. Subjacent to this layer is a thin superficial elastic layer, a loose connective tissue layer containing vessels and lymphatics, and a deep fibroelastic layer. Among these layers, thickness of the loose connective tissue layer of the visceral pleura is different across species. For species with thick visceral pleura (human, sheep; see Fig. 1.31), the loose connective tissue layer is much thicker compared to species with thin visceral pleura (dog, rabbit; see Fig. 1.31; rat and mouse; Albertine, unpublished results).

Table 1.4 Comparative Anatomy of Human and Mouse Lungs

Anatomic Feature of the Lung	Human	Mouse
Visceral pleura thickness	25–100 μm	5–20 μm
Visceral pleura arterial supply	Systemic (bronchial)	Pulmonary
Lobes	3 right; 2 left	4 right; 1 left
Airway generations	17–21	13–17
Airway branching pattern	Dichotomous	Monopodial
Main bronchus diameter	≈10–15 mm	≈1 mm
Intrapulmonary airway cartilage	Yes	No
Tracheal epithelium thickness	50–100 μm	11–14 μm
Tracheal club cells	None	≈50%
Tracheal goblet cells	Present	Absent
Tracheal cartilaginous rings	15–20	15–18
Tracheal submucosal glands	Present	Absent
Proximal intrapulmonary airway thickness	40–50 μm	8–17 μm
Proximal intrapulmonary airway club cells	None	≈60%
Proximal intrapulmonary airway goblet cells	Present	Absent
Proximal intrapulmonary airway submucosal glands	Present	Absent
Terminal bronchiole diameter	≈600 μm	≈10 μm
Terminal bronchiole thickness	Not determined	≈8 μm
Terminal bronchiole club cells	≈11%	≈70%
Respiratory bronchioles	Present (≈150,000)	Absent (or 1)
Respiratory bronchiole club cells	≈20%	Absent
Lung parenchyma/total lung volume ratio	≈12%	≈18%
Alveolar diameter	100–200 μm	30–80 μm
Number of alveoli	≈500 million	≈15 million
Alveolar lipofibroblasts	Absent	Present
Blood-air barrier thickness	≈0.68 μm	≈0.32 μm
Pulmonary venule location	Along interlobular septa	Next to bronchioles
Developmental stage at full term	Alveolar	Saccular

Modified from references 154, 155, and 247–249.

The pleural cells provide a smooth tissue surface on the lung and the chest wall. The normal amount of fluid in the pleural cavity facilitates the movement of the lung during breathing.

MOLECULAR ANATOMY OF THE LUNG

Advances in cell isolation and molecular methodologies during the past 3 decades are allowing identification of genes uniquely expressed in the different cell types that form the lung, thus serving as markers to recognize the distinct populations and study their function in health and disease (eTable 1.1). Most markers were first identified in rodents because these models allow genetic manipulation to perform cell lineage tracing to establish lineage and location, as well as cell-specific mutations to study cell-specific function. However, although many markers are common among rodents and humans (see eTable 1.1, uppercase genes), others have been identified only in rodents (see eTable 1.1, lowercase genes) or only in humans (see eTable 1.1, asterisk).

Remarkable technologic advances in the last few years in high-throughput methods for single-cell genomic and transcriptomic analyses and in bioinformatics methodologies have revolutionized the field of lung cell biology. These methods allow studying individual cells within a tissue to classify their cell types, identify new cell types, and characterize variations in their molecular profiles in health and disease.[242] The Human Lung Atlas project[243] is working toward mapping the different structures of the human lung and identifying their cellular and molecular composition. Initial studies show high diversity within each cell population of the lung and emphasize that our knowledge about the number and type of cells that form the human lung in health and disease is incomplete. These single-cell approaches will soon provide a comprehensive cellular composition of the healthy lung[244] and allow dissecting the alterations in cell composition and function associated with the initiation, progression, and resolution of human lung diseases.[245,246]

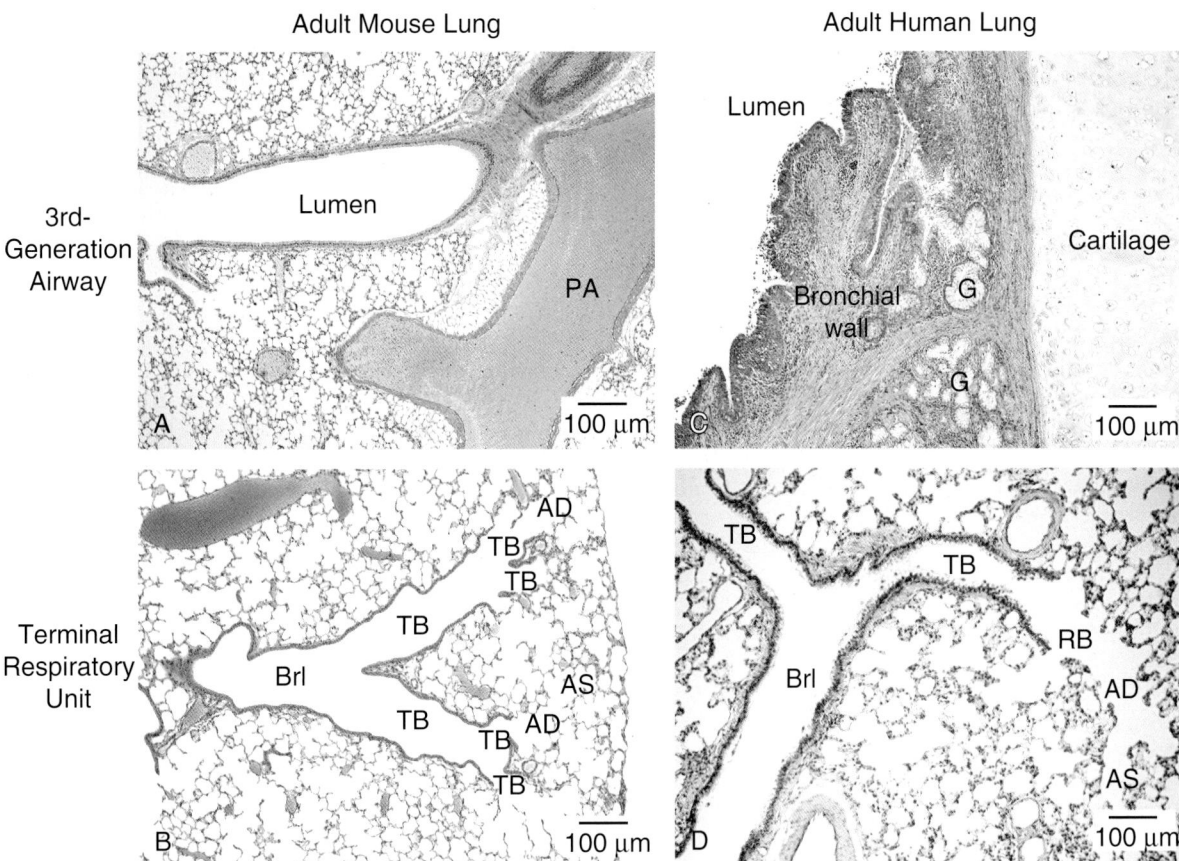

Adult Mouse Lung

3rd-Generation Airway

Lumen

PA

A   100 μm

Terminal Respiratory Unit

AD
TB
TB
TB
Brl
AS
TB   AD
TB
TB

B   100 μm

Adult Human Lung

Lumen

Cartilage

Bronchial wall   G

G

C   100 μm

TB

TB

Brl   RB

AD

AS

D   100 μm

Figure 1.32 Comparison of lung morphology between adult mice *(left column)* and humans *(right column)*. The four panels are the same magnification, as shown by the scale bar in each panel. The upper row compares third-generation, intrapulmonary airways between mouse (A) and human (C). The mouse's airway lumen is narrower than the same generation airway (bronchus) in the human. Absent from the wall of the mouse's airway wall are cartilage and submucosal glands (G), both of which are obvious in the wall of the bronchus of the human airway. The lower row compares terminal respiratory units between mouse (B) and human (D). The mouse's terminal respiratory units do not have respiratory bronchioles; therefore terminal bronchioles (TB) open directly into alveolar ducts (AD). By comparison, the human's terminal respiratory units have respiratory bronchioles, which open into ADs. AS, air space; Brl, bronchiole; PA, pulmonary artery. (Mouse and human lung tissue, 5 μm–thick paraffin-embedded sections, light microscopy.)

COMPARISON OF THE LUNG OF HUMANS AND MICE

A point made in the previous section is that species variations are significant in the visceral pleural structure (see Fig. 1.31) and the blood supply to the lung. This point raises the question of what other species variations are found in the lung. For the purpose of this chapter, comparison is made between human and mouse, owing to the fantastic discoveries about genetic and molecular regulation of lung biology by making mouse constructs to identify normal lung structure and function, as well as to study the impact of disease on lung structure and function. For this discussion, the lung will be divided into the conducting airways (bronchi through terminal bronchioles), which do not participate in respiratory gas exchange, and the lung parenchyma (respiratory bronchioles, alveolar ducts, and alveoli), which do participate in respiratory gas exchange.

Key structural features of human and mouse pulmonary morphology are summarized in Table 1.4.[247-249] This table reveals that many anatomic and developmental differences are present in both the conducting airways and lung parenchyma of the human and mouse lower respiratory systems.

Although the general anatomic organization of the human and mouse lower respiratory system is largely similar, important differences also exist, at both the gross anatomy level and in the cellular composition of the lower respiratory system.

Human and mouse lungs have different lobe structures. The human lung has five lobes, with the right lung divided into three lobes by the oblique and horizontal interlobar fissures, whereas the left lung is divided into two lobes by the oblique fissure. The lobe structure of the mouse lung is markedly different, with the right lung divided into four lobes and the left lung consisting of a single lobe. The upper airways in the human lung include the trachea and bronchi, whereas the upper airway in the mouse lung is the trachea alone.[250] In the human lung, airway branching is dichotomous, where the parent airway divides at an approximately 45-degree angle into two daughter segments, generating 17 to 21 generations of branches between the trachea and the lung parenchyma, at which point terminal bronchioles transition into up to three generations of respiratory bronchioles, which are part of the lung parenchyma in humans. In contrast, branching in the mouse lung is monopodial (asynchronous), yielding 13 to 17 generations of airways, with a single axial airway (the central bronchiole) running the entire length of its associated lobe, with lateral branches forming irregularly along the length of the central bronchiole. The lateral branches (lateral bronchioles) bifurcate repeatedly before terminating into short terminal bronchioles that abruptly give rise to alveolar ducts at the bronchoalveolar duct junctions, which are part of the lung parenchyma in mice. Furthermore, in contrast to the human lung, the walls of intrapulmonary conducting airways in mice do not have cartilage, which may impact the distribution of airway resistance compared to the human lung (Fig. 1.32). A potential impact of the fewer airway generations, as well as narrower conducting airways, in the mouse lung is that the deposition of inhaled particulates may have a different distribution in the lungs of mice compared to those of humans. Also, because the mouse lung has fewer airway generations, the parenchyma makes up a larger proportion of total lung volume ($\approx18\%$) compared to humans ($\approx12\%$). Furthermore, the different lobar structure of the mouse lung has implications for studies on compensatory lung regrowth after unilateral pneumonectomy. For example, left pneumonectomy in mice allows prominent expansion of the right lung, predominantly of the cardiac (often called the accessory) lobe. Thus, the lobar structure of the mouse lungs facilitates studies on lung regeneration, which may be more difficult in lungs from species with a different lobar structure.

The lung parenchyma of human and mouse lungs also has important differences. In the human lung, the terminal bronchioles transition into respiratory bronchioles, of which the human lung has about 150,000 (see Fig. 1.32). These respiratory bronchioles transition into as many as 11 alveolar ducts, which then subsequently transition into up to six alveolar sacs, which are lined by, in total, approximately 500 million alveoli in the adult human lung.[251] In contrast, in the mouse lung, respiratory bronchioles are essentially absent, and the lung parenchyma encompasses exclusively alveolar ducts and alveoli, with the approximately 15 million alveoli in the adult mouse lung constituting the terminus of the lung parenchyma.[252] Thus, the mouse lung has fewer airway generations than the human lung. In both human and mouse lungs, adjacent alveoli are physically connected through pores of Kohn, which facilitate the maintenance of similar pressures across the alveoli by allowing collateral ventilation. Although these pores are similar in human and mouse lungs, the number of pores increase with age in human lungs, whereas in the mouse the number of pores does not change with age.[253,254]

The cellular structure of human and mouse lungs also has marked contrasts. In the conducting airways, the inner surface of both the human and the mouse trachea is lined by a pseudostratified columnar epithelial layer. In humans, the bulk of the cells lining the trachea are ciliated cells, including columnar, basal, and goblet cells; whereas the mouse trachea is lined largely with nonciliated cells. Indeed, in the upper airways of the human lung, the principal secretory cells are goblet cells (see Fig. 1.32), whereas, in the upper airways of the mouse lung, the principal secretory epithelial cells are club cells. Club cells in the human lung are found in the terminal airways. In addition, in the upper airways of the human lung, additional secretory cells are mucous and serous epithelial cells in submucosal glands, which

extend along the trachea and bronchi, whereas in the mouse lung, submucosal glands are limited to the proximal aspect of the trachea. Thus, different cell types contribute to airway secretions, and hence airway defense in the two species. Likewise, the distribution of BALT is different between the two species. In the human lung, BALT is located along bronchi. In the mouse lung, BALT is limited to bronchioles.[255]

Differences in the cellular composition of human *versus* mouse lungs have also been noted in the lung parenchyma, taking the example of the lipofibroblast, a lipid-laden fibroblast subset that has been credited with a key role in lung development and repair. To date, lipofibroblasts remain elusive in human lungs. Lipofibroblasts are present in abundance in mouse lungs.[217] The cellular composition of the conducting vessels of the pulmonary circulation in human *versus* mouse lungs also exhibits differences, notably, cardiomyocytes. In humans, cardiomyocytes are not typically detected in intrapulmonary veins in healthy individuals.[256] Cardiomyocytes are present as part of the pulmonary vein structure in mice, extending along the pulmonary vein beyond the hilum, and surrounding individual intrapulmonary veins, even those of small ($<100\ \mu m$) diameter. Their presence may lead to misidentification of intrapulmonary veins in mice as intrapulmonary arteries, if the cardiomyocyte layer, which may be substantial, is mistaken for vascular smooth muscle. These differences in cellular composition present some challenges for the extrapolation of experimental studies in mice to human pulmonary physiology. For example, the critical role ascribed to lipofibroblasts during distal lung development cannot be generalized to all mammalian lung development if lipofibroblasts are not present in human lungs.

The lung's developmental stage at full term is different between humans and mice. In humans, lung development at full term is at the beginning of the alveolar stage. In mice, lung development at full term is the saccular stage. This timing difference is helpful to keep in mind when developmental comparisons are made and is particularly relevant to studies addressing lung maturation in preterm-born infants; preterm infants born between the 27th and 36th week of gestational age and mouse pups are both delivered in the saccular stage of lung development. Despite being born at a comparatively earlier stage in terms of lung development, term-born mouse pups in the saccular stage of lung development are fully competent for gas exchange, whereas preterm-born infants in the same stage of lung development may require respiratory and supplemental O_2 support due to a limited capacity for gas exchange. This phenomenon highlights important developmental differences between humans and mice during late lung maturation.[257]

Differences in the structure and cellular composition of lungs are not only evident between species but also between strains of the same species. For example, the apparent size of the alveolar unit in the C3H/He mouse strains is appreciably larger than in four other mouse strains—C57BL/6, BALB/c, FVB/N, and DBA/2—by visual inspection of lung sections, a phenomenon confirmed by the determination of the mean linear intercept, a very rough surrogate for the distance between adjacent alveolar walls.[258,259] This is important in experimental studies that assess the impact of an intervention (such as genetic interference) on alveolar development or alveolar structure, because mice on a complete or partial C3H/He strain background will have intrinsic differences in the dimensions of their alveoli compared with other mouse strains.

- Genes uniquely expressed in the different cell types that form the lung are serving as markers to recognize the distinct populations and study their function in health and disease.
- Although mouse and human lung share many common characteristics, there are a number of differences in structure, cell composition, and development that need to be considered when using mouse models to study human lung function and structure.

Key Points

- The primary function of the lung is gas exchange, achieved by ventilation-perfusion matching between alveolar air and alveolar capillary blood.
- The anatomic arrangements of the pulmonary arteries beside the airways are a reminder that the relationship between perfusion and ventilation determines the efficiency of normal lung function.
- The major obstacle for gas exchange is the slow rate of oxygen diffusion through water. Thus, the alveolar walls must be extremely thin. Because of that thinness, the thickness of the red blood cell forms a substantial portion of the air-blood diffusion pathway.
- The airways form the connection between the outside world and the terminal respiratory units.
- Smooth muscle cells form circular bands around the airway epithelium as far peripherally as the respiratory bronchioles. Tone in the smooth muscle is altered by the autonomic nervous system and by mediators released from mast cells, inflammatory cells, and neuroendocrine cells.
- Normally, capillary blood volume is equal to or greater than stroke volume and, under normal resting conditions, the volume of blood in the pulmonary capillaries is well below its maximal capacity. Recruitment can increase capillary blood volume threefold.
- The alveolar type 2 cell is the major synthesizing and secreting factory of the alveolar epithelium and implements epithelial repair via its ability to proliferate.
- The terminal respiratory unit consists of all the alveolar ducts together with their accompanying alveoli that stem from the most proximal (first) respiratory bronchiole, and contains approximately 100 alveolar ducts and 2000 alveoli. The functional definition of the terminal respiratory unit is that, because gas phase diffusion is so rapid, the partial pressures of oxygen and carbon dioxide are uniform throughout the unit.

Key Readings

Bienenstock J. The lung as an immunologic organ. *Annu Rev Med.* 1984;35:49–62.

Clements JA. Surface phenomena in relation to pulmonary function. *Physiologist.* 1962;5:11–28.

Coleridge JC, Coleridge HM. Afferent vagal C fibre innervation of the lungs and airways and its functional significance. *Rev Physiol Biochem Pharmacol.* 1984;99:1–110.

Comroe Jr JH. *Physiology of Respiration.* 2nd ed. Chicago: Yearbook; 1974.

Cutz E. Neuroendocrine cells of the lung. an overview of morphologic characteristics and development. *Exp Lung Res.* 1982;3:185–208.

Dawson CA. Role of pulmonary vasomotion in physiology of the lung. *Physiol Rev.* 1984;64:544–616.

Forster RE. Exchange of gases between alveolar air and pulmonary capillary blood: pulmonary diffusing capacity. *Physiol Rev.* 1957;37:391–452.

Fung YC. Stress, deformation, and atelectasis of the lung. *Circ Res.* 1975;37:481–496.

Horsfield K, Cumming G. Morphology of the bronchial tree in man. *J Appl Physiol.* 1968;24:373–383.

Johnson MD, Widdicombe JH, Allen L, Barbry P, Dobbs LG. Alveolar epithelial type I cells contain transport proteins and transport sodium, supporting an active role for type I cells in regulation of lung liquid homeostasis. *Proc Natl Acad Sci USA.* 2002;99(4):1966–1971.

Lai-Fook SJ. Pleural mechanics and fluid exchange. *Physiol Rev.* 2004;84:358–410.

Mason RJ, Dobbs LG, Greenleaf RD, Williams MC. Alveolar type II cells. *Fed Proc.* 1977;36:2697–2702.

Murray JF. *The Normal Lung: The Basis for Diagnosis and Treatment of Pulmonary Disease.* Philadelphia: Saunders; 1986.

Plasschaert LW, Zilionis R, Choo-Wing R, et al. A single-cell atlas of the airway epithelium reveals the CFTR-rich pulmonary ionocyte. *Nature.* 2018;560(7718):377–381.

Schiller HB, Montoro DT, Simon LM, et al. The human lung cell atlas: a high-resolution reference map of the human lung in health and disease. *Am J Respir Cell Mol Biol.* 2019;61(1):31–41.

Staub NC, Albertine KH. Biology of lung lymphatics. In: Johnston M, ed. *Experimental Biology of the Lymphatic Circulation.* Amsterdam: Elsevier Science; 1985:305–325.

Staub NC. Pulmonary edema. *Physiol Rev.* 1974;54:678–811.

Weibel ER. It takes more than cells to make a good lung. *Am J Respir Crit Care Med.* 2013;187:342–346.

Complete reference list available at ExpertConsult.com.

2 LUNG GROWTH AND DEVELOPMENT

XIN SUN, PHD • DAVID MCCULLEY, MD

INTRODUCTION

The human lungs, serving as the primary respiratory organ, have an estimated surface area of approximately 130 m.[1,2] The gas-exchange function is carried out by approximately 480 million respiratory units called alveoli.[2] Gas is transported to and from alveoli through an elaborate branched network of conducting airways. Forming in parallel is a network of blood vessels, the pulmonary vasculature, which carries deoxygenated blood to the lungs and oxygenated blood from the lungs, a partnership opposite to other tissues in the body. Because gas exchange is required immediately after birth, developmental patterns leading to a functional lung are key to survival at first breath.

Defects in lung development not only cause mortality and morbidity in the neonatal and pediatric period, they often lead to respiratory deficiency later in life. For example, *bronchopulmonary dysplasia* (BPD), a common consequence of preterm birth, results in poor gas exchange in infancy. This deficiency in respiratory function frequently persists into adulthood and is complicated by increased susceptibility to respiratory infections.[3] It is well established that reduced lung capacity due to abnormalities in early lung growth can lead to premature decline of respiratory function during aging or in chronic conditions such as COPD.[4] Thus understanding and supporting a healthy course of lung development will have long-term benefits.

Human lung development is visible starting at approximately 4 *postconceptual weeks* (PCW 4) of gestation with the appearance of the trachea and paired lung buds. This is followed by an elaborate program of branching morphogenesis. The formation of conducting airways is completed well before birth. In comparison, the gas-exchange regions of the lungs, composed of alveoli, begin to develop relatively late in gestation. It is estimated that 95% of the surface area is added after birth. Although the conventional view suggests that elaboration of gas-exchange surface area is complete by 6 to 7 years of age, a more recent study shows that addition of new alveoli continues into the 20s in humans.[5]

Based on classical morphologic categorization, there are more than 40 resident cell types in a mature lung.[6] An even greater number of cell types is becoming evident from the use of newer technologies, including single-cell RNA sequencing.[7–9] During development, the epithelial cells arise from the endoderm, whereas the mesenchymal or endothelial cells arise from the mesoderm. Lung epithelial cells can be broadly categorized into airway versus alveolar. In the airway epithelium, goblet and club cells are secretory, whereas ciliated cells sport motile cilia that clear inhaled particles and pathogens. Rare airway cells, including pulmonary neuroendocrine cells, ionocytes, and tuft cells, have also been investigated.[10–12] These luminal cells are underlined by basal cells that serve as progenitors and can replace damaged luminal cells after airway injury. Invaginating from the surface airway, submucosal glands are a prevalent and regular feature in the human lung. These glands are lined by serous cells and goblet cells, with myoepithelial cells in the basal layer. In the alveolar epithelium, *alveolar type 2* (AT2) cells produce surfactant and can give rise to *alveolar type 1* (AT1) cells that cover approximately 95% of the surface area and serve as both a barrier and interface for gas exchange. Airway epithelial cells begin to differentiate at midgestation, whereas alveolar epithelial cells begin to differentiate near the end of gestation, in time to support lung expansion and gas exchange at birth.

The lung epithelium is underlined by lung mesenchyme and endothelium. Although both are derived from the mesoderm, the mesenchymal and endothelial lineages become distinct from each other early in lung development. Pulmonary endothelial cells give rise to three distinct vascular networks.

MAJOR STAGES OF LUNG DEVELOPMENT

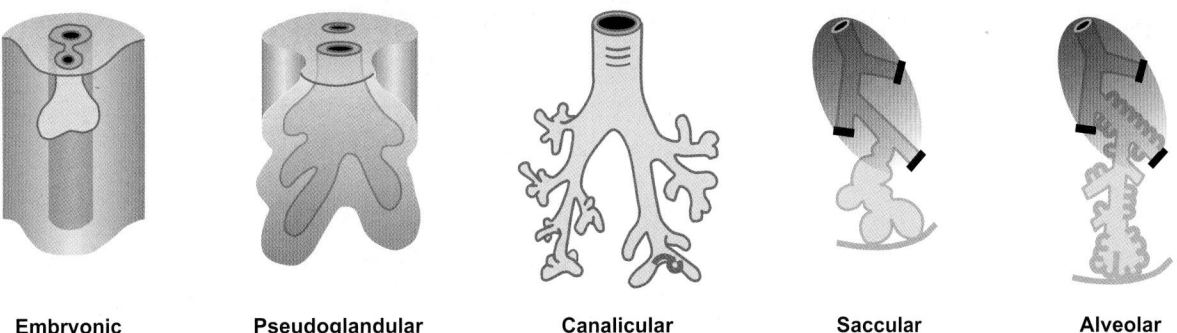

| Embryonic | Pseudoglandular | Canalicular | Saccular | Alveolar |

Figure 2.1 Diagrams of key features of the lung at progressive developmental stages, from the embryonic, pseudoglandular, canalicular, saccular, to alveolar stages. See text for stages and details of these events of lung development. (Modified from Swarr DT, Wert SE, Whitsett JA. Molecular determinants of lung morphogenesis. In Wilmott RW, Deterding R, Li A, et al, editors. *Kendig's Disorders of the Respiratory Tract in Children*, ed 9. Philadelphia: Elsevier; 2019.)

The pulmonary vascular network brings deoxygenated blood, via the pulmonary artery, into the lungs for gas exchange before returning oxygenated blood to the heart via the pulmonary veins. In parallel, the bronchial vasculature brings oxygenated blood from the systemic circulation to sustain the survival of lung cell types. Complementing these blood vascular networks, the lymphatic vascular network maintains fluid homeostasis in the lungs and serves as a conduit for antigens and antigen-presenting cells.[13,14] Compared to the epithelium and endothelium, the distinction among lung mesenchymal cell types is more poorly defined. Nevertheless, it is generally agreed that the human lung mesenchyme contains airway smooth muscle, vascular smooth muscle, myofibroblasts, matrix fibroblasts, pericytes, and chondrocytes.

Much of the current knowledge of cellular and molecular control of lung development is gained from animal studies. Among all animal models, mouse models are the most frequently used. Mouse lung development follows a progression that shares many of the same cellular and molecular characteristics as human lung development. With access to tissues with defined genetic backgrounds at any desired stage, the process of mouse lung development has been extensively characterized. Using sophisticated genetic tools in mice, gene networks that control lung development have been elucidated, and progenitor-progeny relationships have been defined in vivo. Furthermore, with CRISPR/Cas9-based genome editing, patient-specific mutations have been engineered into homologous mouse genes, providing patient-specific platforms to study disease etiology and test therapy. Despite the enormous contribution of mouse models to lung development, it should be noted that there are key distinctions between the mouse lung and the human lung, including their size, airway cell type composition, and physiology (reviewed in Chapter 1).[2,15,16] Validation in human cell–based settings is essential and will become more mainstream as new technologies, such as induced pluripotent stem cell–derived lung cell differentiation and single-cell sequencing, are implemented.

In addition to premature birth leading to lung diseases such as BPD, disruptions of lung development can be caused by genetic mutations, early respiratory infections, or exposure to toxic agents, such as pollutants, cigarette smoke, and e-cigarette vapor. With increasing understanding of the normal process of lung growth and development, more avenues are opened for early prevention, treatment, and reversal of developmental defects responsible for pediatric and adult respiratory conditions.

STAGES OF LUNG DEVELOPMENT WITH CELLULAR AND MOLECULAR MECHANISMS

Mammalian lung development can be broadly divided into two major sets of processes: budding and branching morphogenesis responsible for generating the conducting airways, and septation and alveologenesis responsible for generating the surface area in the distal lung for gas exchange.[17] The morphologic changes of lung development have classically been subdivided into five stages: embryonic, pseudoglandular, canalicular, saccular, and alveolar (Fig. 2.1). Although each stage is defined by a distinct period of time, the cellular and molecular processes that direct lung development transition smoothly from one stage to the next.

EMBRYONIC STAGE

The embryonic stage of lung development takes place between PCW 4 and 7 in humans and between embryonic day 8.5 and 11.5 (E8.5–11.5) in mice (Fig. 2.2A–B).[17] At the beginning of this stage, a small number of endoderm-derived ventral foregut epithelial cells become specified to take on the respiratory fate, as demonstrated by their expression of *Nkx2-1*, the earliest known marker of the respiratory epithelium.[18,19] After specification of these respiratory progenitor cells, the first morphologic change is budding of the posterior portion of the nascent respiratory primordium into the surrounding mesenchyme to generate the left and right lung buds.[20] Concurrent with budding, the common foregut tube, anterior to the lung buds, divides into the trachea ventrally and the esophagus dorsally. At the time of budding, the left-right asymmetry of the lung buds is already specified, as part of left-right determination of all visceral organs. After establishment of the respiratory primordium, the lung buds rapidly elongate into the surrounding mesenchyme and initiate branching morphogenesis as they transition into the pseudoglandular stage.

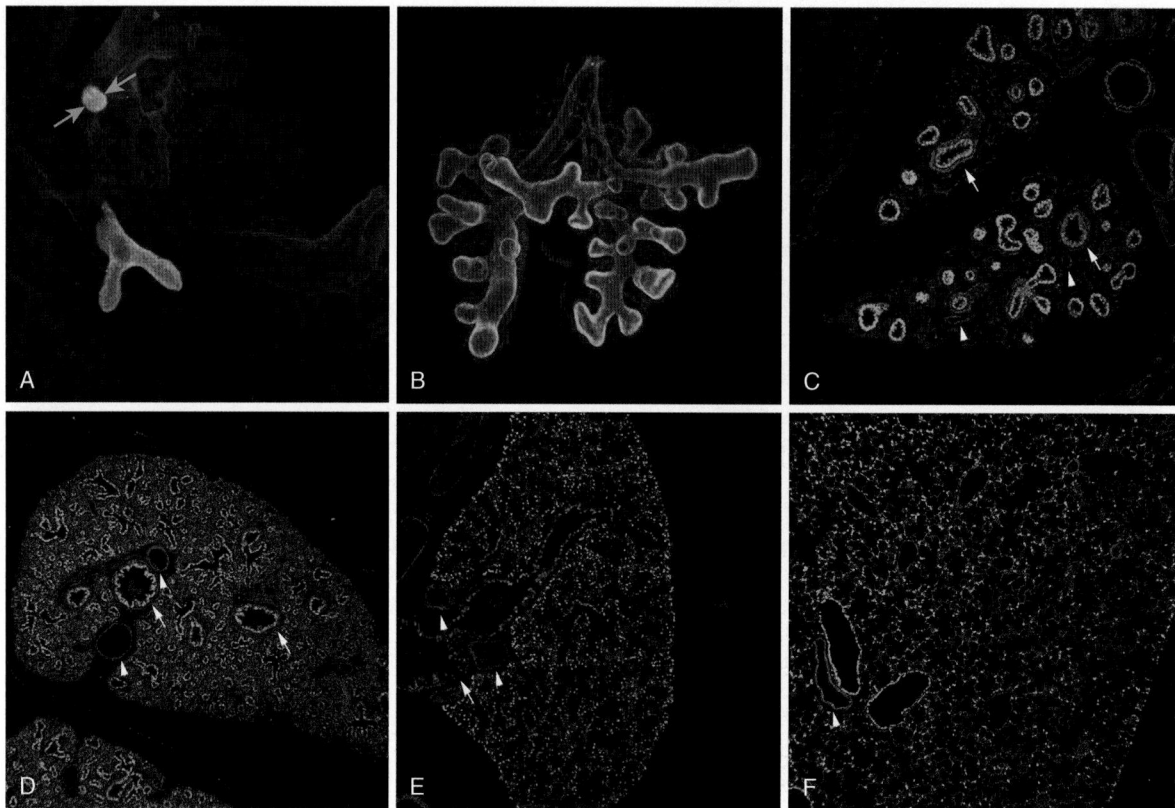

Figure 2.2 Morphology of the stages of lung development. Mouse lungs from the indicated developmental stages were stained with an antibody against Nkx2-1 to identify epithelial cells in the respiratory lineage *(green)*, an antibody against endomucin to identify vascular cells *(red)*, and an antibody against α-smooth muscle actin to identify smooth muscle cells *(magenta)*. An antibody against E-cadherin identifies the foregut endodermal epithelium *(blue)*. (A) Lung buds originate as a pair of outpocketings from the ventral foregut endoderm on day E9.5 in the mouse; the lung endoderm stains positive for Nkx2-1, as does the primitive thyroid rudiment *(double arrow)*. (B) During the embryonic stage, dichotomous and lateral branching of the lung epithelium continues. Vascular precursors are already present and form a plexus surrounding the epithelium. (C) During the pseudoglandular stage, the lung primarily consists of epithelial tubules surrounded by a relatively thick mesenchyme. Proximal epithelial cells show tall columnar morphologic characteristics, whereas more distal epithelial cells are cuboidal. The vasculature branches in parallel with the epithelium, and smooth muscle cells surrounding airways *(white arrows in all panels)* and vessels *(white arrowheads in all panels)* are evident. (D) During the canalicular stage, epithelial acini appear, and the vasculature becomes more abundant and closely apposed to the epithelium. (E) During the saccular stage, alveolar type 1 cell differentiation increases air space size. The vasculature has continued to expand, fully investing the lung parenchyma. Fusion of the epithelial and endothelial basal laminae brings alveolar type 1 cells and capillaries into close association. (F) During the alveolar stage, the formation, lengthening, and thinning of secondary septa markedly increase the epithelial surface area. All images of sectioned lungs (C–F) are at the same magnification. *Arrows,* airways; *arrowheads,* vessels; *green,* respiratory lineage; *red,* vascular; *magenta,* smooth muscle. (Confocal images generated by Jamie Havrilak, Graduate Program in Molecular and Developmental Biology, Cincinnati Children's Hospital Medical Center.)

All lung lobes are enclosed in pleura, also termed mesothelium, a thin layer of squamous epithelial cells that provide protection and lubrication to allow sliding of lung lobes against the chest wall.[21] By 3 weeks of gestational age, the pleural, pericardial, and peritoneal spaces begin to form from the mesoderm. By 9 weeks, the pleural cavity has become separated from both the pericardial and peritoneal spaces. After lung specification, the lung buds invaginate into the visceral mesoderm, which is covered by pleura. Thus the lungs retain a pleural covering starting at budding.

Findings from mouse models indicate that the site of lung initiation is specified by signaling molecules, including *wingless types* (WNTs). *Wnt2* and *Wnt2b*, two canonical Wnt pathway genes, are both required for lung specification.[18] They act through β-catenin, a downstream nuclear effector, to maintain the expression of *Nkx2-1*, the earliest known marker of respiratory fate.[18,19] In mice, inactivation of Wnts or β-catenin leads to complete failure of trachea and lung development.[18,19] After specification of respiratory

progenitor cells, *fibroblast growth factor 10* (FGF10) signaling is essential for lung budding. Inactivation of *Fgf10* leads to lung agenesis, while development of the trachea is maintained.[22,23] Furthermore, retinoic acid signaling has been shown to control budding via regulation of WNT, *transforming growth factor-β* (TGF-β), and FGF10 signaling.[24] In humans, mutations in the WNT pathway gene *RSPO2*, the retinoic acid downstream gene *STRA6*, the FGF pathway gene *FGF10*, and the transcription factor gene *TBX4* have all been tied to lung agenesis or severe hypoplasia.[25–27]

PSEUDOGLANDULAR STAGE

The pseudoglandular stage of lung development takes place during PCW 5 to 17 in humans and E11.5 to E15.5 in mice (see Fig. 2.2C).[17] The primary cellular event in this stage is branching morphogenesis.[28] After lung bud elongation, the epithelial tubules and tips initiate branching with the support and guidance of the mesenchyme. Mapping of lung branching has revealed a largely stereotypic program composed of three subroutines: domain branching, where side branches emerge from bronchi in proximal-to-distal sequence with regular spacing; planar bifurcation, where distal tips engage in repeated rounds of bifurcation in the same two-dimensional plane; and orthogonal bifurcation, where distal tips bifurcate and then bifurcate again in a plane 90 degrees to the former.[29] In mice, these three subroutines are programmed in a stereotypic sequence, suggesting that they are tightly controlled by genetic circuits.[29,30] In humans, this process is believed to be more variable.[31] Regardless, by the end of the pseudoglandular stage, the majority of proximal airways are formed, and the distal tips are poised to form gas-exchange units in the following stages.

Based on mouse mutants that exhibit lung branching defects and aided by mathematical and computational modeling, the genetic circuits that control branching morphogenesis are beginning to be elucidated.[32] Elegant studies have demonstrated that the mesenchyme provides instructive cues to the airway epithelium to direct the branching pattern.[33] Key among these signals is again *Fgf10*, which is expressed in the lung mesenchyme and concentrated at future sites toward where the epithelial tips grow.[34] FGF10 acts to promote regional proliferation and chemotaxis of the distal tip epithelium toward the signaling source.[35] Bypassing its requirement for earlier budding, conditional inactivation of *Fgf10* in mice during the pseudoglandular stage disrupts branching morphogenesis.[36,37] These data support the notion that the site-specific expression of *Fgf10* establishes the subsequent branching pattern. However, a more recent study showed that lungs with indiscriminate overexpression of *Fgf10* in the mesenchyme still underwent branching morphogenesis. These data suggest that other regulators, including heparin sulfate proteoglycans, may coordinate with FGF activity to coordinate branching.[38]

Multiple models suggest that reciprocal interactions between the mesenchyme and epithelium are required for branching morphogenesis. FGF10 cooperates with other signaling factors in feedback regulatory loops across the epithelium/mesenchyme boundary. For example, FGF10 from the mesenchyme acts through FGF receptor 2 and downstream transcription factors ETV4/5 in the epithelium to promote the expression of sonic hedgehog *(Shh)*.[39] SHH in turn signals to the mesenchyme to inhibit the expression of *Fgf10*. Evidence from genetic, pharmacologic, and mathematical modeling suggests that this feedback regulation may contribute to the repeated bifurcation program.[36,37,39–41]

Concurrent with branching morphogenesis, the overall pattern of the lungs, namely proximal airway versus distal alveolar region, becomes established in the pseudoglandular stage. During this stage, distal tips continue to elongate while undergoing repetitive branching to form the future airways. Molecularly, this distinction between the airways and future air spaces for gas exchange is marked by proximal expression of *Sox2* and distal expression of *Sox9*, two transcription factor genes.[37,42] In mice, *Sox2* and *Sox9* domains are distinct starting from early branching morphogenesis. However, in human lungs, *SOX2* continues to be expressed distally, overlapping with *SOX9* until approximately 20 weeks of gestation, when the *SOX2* expression becomes more restricted to the proximal airway domain.[43–45]

At the end of branching morphogenesis, airway epithelial cells begin to differentiate. Pulmonary neuroendocrine cells, a rare airway cell type with sensory function, are the first cells known to differentiate in the airway epithelium.[46–48] This is followed by basal cells that serve as a prominent source of airway progenitor cells required for airway epithelial cell regeneration in the adult.[49] Concurrently, the adjacent mesenchymal cells differentiate into cartilage and smooth muscle. Elaboration of the pulmonary vascular network continues in parallel to the airway with an increasing number of vessel branches leading into the elaborate capillary network.

CANALICULAR STAGE

The canalicular stage of lung development takes place between PCW 16 and 26 in humans and E15.5 and E16.5 in mice (see Fig. 2.2D).[17] During this stage, there is a transition from the genetic program that directs branching morphogenesis to the program that directs septation of the distal air spaces in preparation for gas exchange. Although the majority of branching morphogenesis happens during the pseudoglandular stage, the distal epithelium undergoes three final rounds of branching during the canalicular stage.[28] In distal tips, canalization of the parenchyma happens as the respiratory air spaces increase in length and width and the capillaries grow in size and complexity.[17] Thinning of the mesenchyme allows a close juxtaposition of the alveolar epithelium and capillaries, establishing the alveolar-blood interface essential for gas exchange. The epithelial cells in the distal lung also begin to differentiate into AT1 and AT2 cells. Production of surfactant by AT2 cells is first detected between PCW 22 and 24.[50] Surfactant production is a key developmental milestone that impacts the survival of premature infants and can be enhanced in utero by the administration of steroids.

SACCULAR STAGE

The saccular stage of lung development happens between PCW 24 and 38 in humans and E16.5 and postnatal day 3 (P3) in mice (see Fig. 2.2E).[17] By this stage, branching morphogenesis is complete and the airways are laid out. During the saccular stage, the major morphologic changes take place in the terminal air spaces that continue to increase in volume, resulting in further compression and thinning of the adjacent mesenchyme.[17] The primary septa that separate the air spaces are covered by an alveolar barrier composed of AT1 cells with interspersed AT2 cells. The alveolar epithelial barrier is underlined by a basket of capillaries. In the thin walls are also fibroblasts and extracellular matrix, which are positioned to support but not to interfere with gas exchange across the epithelium-capillary juxtaposition. During this stage, AT2 cells increase their production of surfactant stored in lamellar bodies.

The timing of sacculation coincides with an increase of amniotic fluid in the fetus that peaks at approximately PCW 34. Experimental evidence in mice suggests that mechanical pressure from the increasing amniotic fluid plays a role in alveolar epithelial cell differentiation during sacculation.[51] Both AT1 and AT2 cells arise from the columnar distal tip epithelial cells and are present in a near 1:1 ratio by birth. Reduction of amniotic fluid volume in mice led to a decrease in the AT1:AT2 ratio, whereas an increase in the amniotic fluid led to an increase in the AT1:AT2 ratio.[51] These findings suggest that the volume of amniotic fluid and the pressure it exerts on the developing respiratory air space epithelium plays an important role in the differentiation and balance of AT1 and AT2 cell fate. These findings raised the possibility that a similar mechanism may be at play in AT1/AT2 differentiation in humans.

Relatively little is known of the specific genetic control of sacculation due to the paucity of genes specifically required for this process and the lack of genetic tools to target this stage. It is possible that many of the same signaling pathways involved in earlier stages of lung development, such as FGF, *bone morphogenetic protein* (BMP), WNT, SHH, and WNT pathways also function in sacculation. If so, it will be interesting to determine how the same signaling pathway can execute distinct cell morphogenesis programs, such as those that direct branching versus sacculation. Immune regulators, such as nuclear factor kappa B, play a role in the proliferation and thinning of the epithelium and mesenchyme.[52] Hippo signaling, in particular its downstream effector Yap, is central to mechanical force-induced gene expression and cell fate changes.[53–56]

ALVEOLAR STAGE

The final stage of lung development, the alveolar stage, happens between PCW 36 and young adulthood in humans and between P3 and P39 in mice[17,57] (see Fig. 2.2F). The primary goal of alveologenesis (also termed alveolarization) is to expand the surface area for gas exchange. The exact age at which alveologenesis, and thereby lung maturation, ends in humans is debated. As mentioned, although the conventional view suggests that alveologenesis is complete by 6 to 7 years of age, advanced imaging experiments indicate that new septa continue to be added in lungs of early 20-year-olds.[5] Because lung development continues postnatally, exposure of young lung to pollution, secondary smoke, and e-cigarette vapor not only damages existing alveoli but also truncates the program to form new alveoli. This explains why early exposure to toxic aerosols leads to more profound damage than does late exposure, leading to predisposition of adult-onset diseases, such as COPD.

At the beginning of the alveolar stage, each alveolus is a simple balloon-shaped gas-exchange unit extending from an alveolar duct and separated from each other by primary septa. The primary septa remain relatively thick and contain a double-layered capillary network capable of gas exchange, albeit not optimized for efficiency. During alveologenesis, new septa rise from the alveolar wall into the lumen. Each nascent septum is a delicate new gas-exchange surface, with flat AT1 cells and interspersed AT2 cells, overlying a dense capillary network. As mentioned, in humans, an estimated 95% of the final alveolar surface area is constructed by alveologenesis after birth.

The mechanisms that direct alveologenesis are poorly understood. Multiple lines of evidence suggest that smooth muscle actin-positive myofibroblasts are required for septum formation; however, their precise role is debated.[58–60] Conventional studies of alveologenesis relied

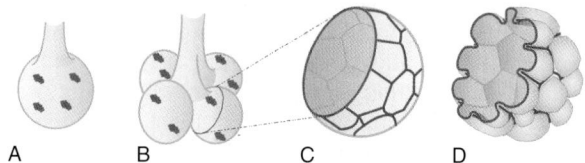

Figure 2.3 Three-dimensional model of septum formation. (A–B) During sacculation, myofibroblast precursors *(red)* proliferate and are evenly spaced in the alveolar mesenchyme. (C–D) During alveologenesis, myofibroblasts differentiate into contractile cells *(red strings)*, connect into a network and constrict (D), leading to coordinated rise of septal ridges into the lumen.

on two-dimensional sections and depict nascent septa as finger-like protrusions into the lumen, with myofibroblasts frequently found at the tips.[61] These observations led to the hypotheses that septa arise from either repulsion of the myofibroblasts from the alveolar wall into the lumen or growth of the septa along a signaling gradient with FGF at the tip and retinoic acid at the base.[61,62] More recent experiments using confocal microscopy and three-dimensional reconstructions of the alveoli have led to a different view. Instead of the finger-like protrusions, a nascent septum forms a ridge that arises from the walls of the alveolus.[63] Instead of a single point at the tip of a finger-like protrusion, each smooth muscle actin-positive myofibroblast is instead a long, stringlike cell that interconnects with other myofibroblasts, forming a network. This fishnet-like pattern was first described in 1970 by Dr. Embry after analysis of human alveoli.[64] Rather than repulsion or growth to form new septa, the myofibroblasts may guide contraction of this fishnet-like network to form novel septa (Fig. 2.3).[63] Myofibroblasts also produce elastin and elastin cross-linking enzymes to generate the extracellular matrix essential for formation of the septa. In addition to myofibroblasts, other cells within the septa, including alveolar endothelial cells, are required for the formation of this structure. Inactivation of *Vegf-a* and simplification of the capillary network led to alveolar simplification.[65] It remains to be determined how myofibroblasts and the endothelial cells collaborate to establish and maintain the septa.[66]

DEVELOPMENTAL INSIGHTS INTO LUNG REPAIR AND REGROWTH

Continuing into adulthood, the lung maintains a certain degree of repair and regenerative capacity following injury.[67] For example, upon exposure to pollution or toxic injury, the remaining airway and/or alveolar epithelial cells proliferate and differentiate to replace lost cells (see Chapter 8). Beyond this type of epithelial cell–based repair, the adult lungs are also capable of growing en masse. For example, upon lung resection, also termed pneumonectomy, even though there is no regeneration at the site of the resection, the remaining lobes grow to fill the open space.[68–70] This type of compensatory regrowth is achieved through proliferation and morphogenesis of the alveolar epithelium, mesenchyme, and endothelium, coming together to make new septa.

Growing evidence suggests that after injury there is a general reactivation of the dormant developmental program, leading to repair and regrowth.[67] For example, bleomycin-induced alveolar injury leads to AT2 proliferation and differentiation into AT1 cells to regenerate gas-exchange capacity.[71] This mimics AT2 behavior during development. Similar AT2 activation is also induced after pneumonectomy. During postpneumonectomy compensatory regrowth, there is also reactivation of secondary crest myofibroblasts, which likely drives the reseptation of enlarged lung lobes.[72]

On the molecular level, there is also reactivation of developmental signals in repair and regrowth. For example, FGFs, WNTs, and TGF-β pathways are reactivated during naphthalene-induced airway repair.[38,73] The Hippo/YAP pathway controls AT2 proliferation and differentiation, similar to its role in alveolar development.[51,53] These findings open the possibility of manipulating these developmental programs to stimulate proper and efficient repair and regrowth.

EMERGING TECHNOLOGIES TO STUDY LUNG DEVELOPMENT

INDUCED PLURIPOTENT STEM CELL–DERIVED LUNG CELLS

An adult skin fibroblast can be erased of its differentiation program and reversed into a pluripotent cell, called an *induced pluripotent stem cell* (iPSC), when it is engineered to express just four transcription factor genes: *OCT4*, *SOX2*, *KLF4*, and *cMYC* (OSKM or Yamanaka factors named after Dr. Shinya Yamanaka's seminal work).[74] The fibroblast-derived iPSCs can then be used to generate individual differentiated cell types. Since the first publication in 2006, iPSCs have been manipulated to generate a kaleidoscope of differentiated cell types, including neurons, cardiomyocytes, intestinal epithelial cells, skeletal myocytes, immune cells, and lung epithelial cells.[75–77] During iPSC differentiation into lung cells, the cells follow a similar sequence as during lung development, that is, transitioning first into endoderm, then foregut endoderm, followed by NKX2-1–positive lung progenitors, and finally into either airway or alveolar lineages.[78–81] Thus this technology can be used to study human lung cell specification and differentiation. Furthermore, it holds tremendous promise for studying disease mechanisms in a human cell context and for generating a sufficient number of corrected, healthy, and mature lung cells for autologous transplantation back into a patient from whom iPSCs are generated.

LUNG ORGANOIDS

Emerging from studies of lung progenitor cells, it was found that adult progenitors, such as airway basal cells and AT2 cells, are capable of forming organoids if given the proper nutrient and extracellular matrix support.[71,82] In the organoids, the progenitors can proliferate and differentiate, often from the origin of an individual cell. Analysis of colony number, size, and proportion of differentiated progeny offers a quantitative measure of progenitor potential. Change of growth factors, addition of agonists and antagonists, and introduction of small interfering RNA agents for gene knockdown have allowed interrogation of the molecular mechanisms that control progenitor cell maintenance and activation. Other cell types, such as mesenchymal cells, have been incorporated into organoid assays to establish tissue niches.[83,84] The prototype of lung-on-a-chip may allow the use of increasingly sophisticated combinations of cells and environmental cues to capture and manipulate the in vivo microenvironment in a dish.[85,86]

CRISPR/CAS9 GENOME EDITING

CRISPR/Cas9-based genome editing technology is a simple yet powerful tool that can target specific stretches of genetic code to edit, allowing investigators to make precise deletions, insertions, nucleotide changes, and other genomic or epigenomic changes in cells.[87–89] These technologies have led to remarkable advances in generating animal models for lung diseases and to investigations of the effects of mutations in human iPSC-derived lung cells.[89,90] Teams are working with the approach to correct disease mutations in patient-derived iPSCs, differentiate them into lung cell types, and engraft these into the same patient from where the cells were derived. In a parallel approach, a recent study succeeded with in utero CRISPR editing of lung cells in animal models, opening the door for in vivo editing of disease mutation somatically in cells in a formed organ.[91] A combination of these technologies holds promise toward bringing cures to patients with congenital diseases such as cystic fibrosis.

SINGLE-CELL SEQUENCING

In 2015, a pair of studies were published on a new, microfluidics-based technology that interrogated the transcriptome at single-cell resolution, at a capacity of thousands of cells at a time.[92,93] This technology, widely known as Drop-seq, has since exploded in its usage and spin-off improvements. Among these, bead-based chemistry improved cell capture efficiency, leading to *single-cell RNA sequencing* (scRNA-seq). More recently, the technology was applied to analyze chromatin accessibility in *single-cell Assay for Transposase-Accessible Chromatin by sequencing* (scATAC-seq), one indicator of the epigenomic state. Several consortia in the lung biology field, including efforts from the *National Heart, Lung, and Blood Institute*–funded LungMAP consortium, have taken advantage of these technologies to reveal the exciting new molecular properties of the lung at single-cell resolution (Fig. 2.4).

Among the explosion of publications with scRNA-seq data are studies of the developing lung[8,9,94–96] The data confirmed all known cell types and added much needed markers for some of these cell types. More important, the data solidified long-suspected heterogeneity within morphologically similar cell types. For example, in published studies and in the LungMAP-generated publicly available datasets, single-cell analysis defined complexity within alveolar mesenchyme with signatures for myofibroblasts, matrix fibroblasts 1 (also known as lipofibroblasts), matrix fibroblasts 2, and pericytes.[8,83,84,97] Single-cell analysis of the trachea uncovered heterogeneity within the basal cell population.[10] A population along the differentiation path of AT2-to-AT1 transition was captured in early postnatal samples.[8] Furthermore, single-cell technology provided the resolution needed to detect rare cell populations, including pulmonary neuroendocrine cells, ionocytes, and tuft cells.[10,98] The importance of these rare cell populations in lung function is just starting to be appreciated.[10,11,46,98] Studies

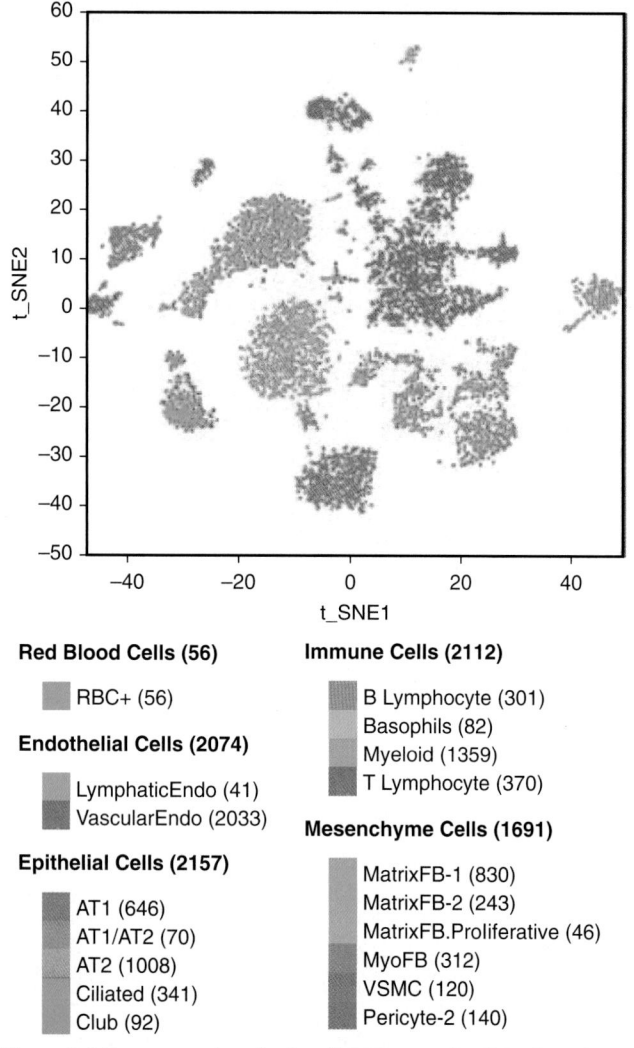

Red Blood Cells (56)

RBC+ (56)

Endothelial Cells (2074)

LymphaticEndo (41)
VascularEndo (2033)

Epithelial Cells (2157)

AT1 (646)
AT1/AT2 (70)
AT2 (1008)
Ciliated (341)
Club (92)

Immune Cells (2112)

B Lymphocyte (301)
Basophils (82)
Myeloid (1359)
T Lymphocyte (370)

Mesenchyme Cells (1691)

MatrixFB-1 (830)
MatrixFB-2 (243)
MatrixFB.Proliferative (46)
MyoFB (312)
VSMC (120)
Pericyte-2 (140)

Figure 2.4 Representative single-cell RNAseq *t-distributed stochastic neighbor embedding* (tSNE) plot to demonstrate cell-type–based clustering. Data from single-cell analysis of whole mouse normal lung at postnatal day 3 (beginning of alveologenesis phase). On the tSNE plot, each dot represents a cell placed in in silico space based on its RNA transcript profile. Cells with similar transcriptional profiles are placed near each other. Hence each cluster displayed here represents a cell type, with annotations below. Numbers in the bracket indicate the number of cells captured on this tSNE plot. AT1/AT2, alveolar epithelial type 1/2 cell; MyoFB, myofibroblast; VSMC, vascular smooth muscle cell. (Data from Lung Gene Expression Analysis Web portal, courtesy Dr. Yan Xu, Dr. Jeffery Whitsett, and *National Heart, Lung, and Blood Institute*–funded LungMAP team of the Cincinnati Children's Hospital Medical School. https://research.cchmc.org/pbge/lunggens/mainportal.html.)

of single-cell analysis of the diseased lung are expanding. Examples are emerging on how single-cell resolution analysis has revealed variations in cell populations among patients that may improve the precision of diagnosis of lung diseases.[99,100]

REPRESENTATIVE DEVELOPMENTAL LUNG DISEASES

Developmental defects of the lungs can arise at any stage during their formation. They include abnormalities of the airways, the gas-exchange components of the lungs, and the pulmonary vasculature. Although major structural abnormalities of the lungs are often not compatible with life, many congenital malformations can be detected by prenatal ultrasound and addressed by specialized neonatal care, including surgical treatment in the newborn period. Aside from congenital malformations, preterm birth itself is a significant contributor to lung disease and impacts survival and long-term health outcomes. Although many diseases with disruption of lung development manifest with symptoms soon after birth, there are also many categories of disease that do not become apparent until childhood or even adulthood. Below are described some of the common congenital diseases of the lungs and pulmonary vasculature, organized by the time they arise during development.

DEFECTS IN TRACHEA/ESOPHAGUS SPECIFICATION AND SEPARATION

An abnormal or persistent connection between the airway and the digestive tract, as in tracheoesophageal fistula, develops in approximately 1 in 3500 live births and is frequently accompanied by atresia of the esophagus.[101,102] The fistula can be ligated surgically after birth; however, repair of the esophagus may be complicated depending on the distance between the disconnected proximal and distal esophageal segments. Furthermore, many patients have a spectrum of associated malformations of the *vertebral bodies* (V), *gastrointestinal tract atresia* (A), *cardiac defects* (C), *tracheoesophageal* defects (TE), *renal* and distal urinary defects (R), and *limb* malformations (L) that all make up the VACTERL syndrome.[101] Even more rare, and frequently lethal, is atresia of the trachea.[103] Tracheal atresia may be survivable only if identified before birth or if there is a fistula connecting the lower airways to the esophagus. Tracheal reconstruction using synthetic and stem cell–based approaches is an area that continues to be investigated for these infants and for patients who have tracheal injury or cancer in later life.

DEFECTS IN BRANCHING MORPHOGENESIS

Abnormalities of lung initiation and branching morphogenesis can lead to a variety of congenital lung masses, seen in 1 in 10,000 to 35,000 live births, which include bronchogenic cysts, *congenital pulmonary airway malformation* (CPAM), and pulmonary sequestration.[104,105] Bronchogenic cysts, the result of abnormal budding of the ventral foregut, result in cystic duplications of the proximal airway that frequently do not communicate with the tracheobronchial tree and have a blood supply from either the pulmonary or systemic circulation.[106] Bronchogenic cysts are often not identified until later in life due to recurrent infection; however, they can result in respiratory distress during the newborn period if they rapidly enlarge or cause compression of the normal lungs or heart.[106,107] CPAMs are the most common type of congenital lung mass and are the result of abnormal branching morphogenesis.[108,109] They connect to the normal tracheobronchial tree and have a blood supply derived from the pulmonary circulation. CPAMs are classified according to a variety of approaches; the most widely adopted scheme includes clinical, macroscopic, and microscopic information.[110] More recently, classification of CPAMs has been based on the size of the abnormal cystic structures as either macrocystic or microcystic. Their treatment includes a wide variety of fetal interventions when the mass impairs development of the normal lungs or the function of the heart.[109,111,112] Due to concern for malignant transformation, CPAMs are typically removed after birth even if they do not cause respiratory distress. This practice is gradually changing, with some practitioners opting to observe patients with CPAMs using serial imaging.[113,114] In contrast, bronchopulmonary sequestrations are another, but rarer, type of congenital lung mass; they do not connect to the tracheobronchial tree and have a blood supply derived from the systemic circulation.[115–117] Sequestrations are subdivided based on their position and characteristics as intralobar, within a normal lobe of the lung; extralobar, outside of the normal lung and separated by an independent layer of visceral pleura; or hybrid, where there are histologic characteristics typical of a CPAM, but blood supply is derived from the systemic circulation. Intralobar sequestrations account for the majority of sequestrations and typically present with infections.

LUNG HYPOPLASIA

Hypoplasia of the lungs and pulmonary vasculature can happen for a variety of reasons. One of the major causes of lung hypoplasia is *congenital diaphragmatic hernia* (CDH), affecting in 1 in 3500 live births.[118,119] Patients with CDH have an opening in the diaphragm allowing the abdominal organs to herniate into the chest. The lungs and pulmonary vasculature are underdeveloped in patients with CDH due to a combination of mechanical compression and intrinsic defects in branching morphogenesis, septation, and vascular development.[120,121] Extrinsic compression of the developing fetal lungs can also result from skeletal dysplasias, pleural effusions, or other structure birth defects such as omphalocele, causing life-limiting lung hypoplasia.[122] Low amniotic fluid levels caused by premature rupture of membranes or bladder outlet obstruction in the fetus, also result in lung hypoplasia.[122] Lack of sufficient amniotic fluid decreases the intrauterine space for lung growth and the volume and pressure of amniotic fluid itself appears to be required for normal lung development and postnatal lung function.[123]

SURFACTANT PROTEIN DEFICIENCIES

In addition to structural lung defects, loss of function of individual molecules can also lead to significant respiratory distress and life-threatening lung disease in the newborn period. Mutations in the genes that encode surfactant proteins B and C (*SFTPB* and *SFTPC*) or in the phospholipid transport protein *ABCA3* gene are among the most common genetic causes of surfactant dysfunction.[124] Surfactant metabolism and function is discussed in Chapter 3. Inadequate pulmonary surfactant production due to preterm birth, gene mutations, or increased surfactant inactivation results in impaired gas exchange in the newborn period with diffuse collapse of the alveoli.

PRETERM BIRTH AND BRONCHOPULMONARY DYSPLASIA

Perhaps the most significant cause of impaired lung development is preterm birth, or birth before 37 weeks of gestation, which complicates 10% of all pregnancies.[125] Infants who are born prematurely are exposed to multiple treatments, including steroids, positive-pressure ventilation, and supplemental oxygen, treatments that improve survival but come at the cost of limiting normal development during the saccular and alveolar stages. The infants who are most commonly and severely affected are those born extremely preterm, or before 28 weeks of gestation. These infants have a high incidence of persistent respiratory distress throughout the newborn period. Preterm infants who require treatment with supplemental oxygen and/or positive-pressure ventilation beyond 36 weeks corrected gestational age are given the diagnosis of BPD.[126] Premature arrest of lung development in these infants is often made worse by inadequate nutrition, recurrent lung infection, and other cardiovascular and inflammatory insults.[126] Despite the association between preterm birth and BPD, the disease itself is very heterogeneous, and it is unclear what treatments improve the outcome. What is clear is that as more and more preterm infants are surviving and technical advances, such as surfactant therapy and better controlled ventilation, have permitted improved survival for infants born at even earlier gestational ages (<24 weeks), care for this group of patients will require specialized management throughout their lifetime.

CHILDHOOD INTERSTITIAL LUNG DISEASES

In addition to preterm birth, there are many other diseases that result from developmental defects arising during the later stages of lung development. Defects in alveolar septation cause a wide variety of interstitial lung diseases presenting in the newborn period or in later life.[127,128] One of the most severe forms of this category of disease is *alveolar capillary dysplasia with misalignment of the pulmonary veins* (ACD/MPV). Infants with ACD/MPV present with respiratory distress, hypoxemia, and pulmonary hypertension during the newborn period.[129,130] Histologic samples from lung biopsies and autopsy specimens show decreased density of pulmonary capillaries, thickening of the alveolar septal walls, hypertrophy of the pulmonary artery smooth muscle, and abnormal positioning of the pulmonary veins. ACD/MPV has been associated with mutations and deletions in the *FOXF1* gene in 40% of patients; however, there are other chromosome and single-gene defects that result in a similar phenotype.[131,132] Historically, the majority of patients with the ACD/MPV did not survive; however, there are increasing reports of patients being identified later in life or of infants who survive despite the disease.[133]

One rare childhood interstitial lung disease whose etiology remains unclear is pulmonary *neuroendocrine cell hyperplasia of infancy* (NEHI), with a frequency of 1 in 10,000 live births.[134] Patients with NEHI are often asymptomatic after birth but develop respiratory deficiency around 6 months of life accompanied by failure to thrive.[135] It has remained an intriguing disease because biopsies show normal alveolar density, unlike many other diseases with gas-exchange defects. Furthermore, computed tomography scans show ground-glass opacities that are not explained by any histologic defects found in biopsies.[136] The only consistent histologic feature is an increase in the number of pulmonary neuroendocrine cells, thus explaining the name of the disease.[137] However, it remains debated whether changes in an airway cell type can cause the gas-exchange abnormalities manifested in the alveolar region. The first NEHI mutation was identified as a point mutation in *NKX2-1*, the quintessential lung transcription factor gene.[138] These genetic changes provide an entry point to uncovering the mechanism underlying NEHI.

PULMONARY VASCULAR DISEASE

Abnormal development and function of the vasculature in the lungs can result in pulmonary hypertension independent of defects in airway development. The primary mechanisms that contribute to pulmonary hypertension include abnormal or insufficient vascular development causing a decrease in the number of proximal pulmonary arteries, capillaries in the alveolar region, or pulmonary veins. Pulmonary hypertension can also result from hypertrophy or persistent contraction of the pulmonary vascular smooth muscle causing a reduction in the size of vessels in the lungs. Many lung diseases resulting in pulmonary hypertension do so because a combination of these mechanisms causes failure of normal pulmonary vascular smooth muscle relaxation after birth. Mutations in *BMPR2* account for the majority of heritable forms of pulmonary hypertension; however, many other genetic variants have been identified in pediatric and adult patients with pulmonary hypertension, including genes that encode transcription factors, receptor and signaling molecules, and channel proteins.[139,140] In addition, pulmonary hypertension complicates many developmental defects of the airways, including congenital diaphragmatic hernia, alveolar capillary dysplasia, and preterm birth with or without BPD.[141,142]

CONGENITAL OR LUNG DEVELOPMENTAL DEFECTS THAT MANIFEST LATER IN LIFE

Although many congenital lung diseases result in respiratory distress in the newborn period, there are many genetic and developmental diseases that do not become apparent until later life. Among this list are several important diseases that affect large groups of individuals, including cystic fibrosis, primary ciliary dyskinesia, and childhood asthma. These diseases will be discussed in later chapters.

Key Points

- Normal development of the lungs requires complex interactions among cell types across the epithelium, mesenchyme, and endothelium.
- Deviations from normal lung development contribute not only to pediatric lung diseases but also to adult respiratory conditions and the premature decline of respiratory function with aging.
- Lung development is characterized by highly stereotypical programs of branching, sacculation, and alveolar formation.
- Many signaling pathways, involving fibroblast growth factor, wingless type, hedgehog, retinoic acid, bone morphogenic protein, and transforming growth factor-β pathways, play important roles in lung development.
- Airway formation is completed before birth, whereas alveolar development continues after birth.
- There are many contributors to developmental origins of lung diseases, including mutations, premature birth, infections, and early exposures to toxins, such as cigarette smoke and e-cigarette vapor.

Key Readings

Kurland G, Deterding RR, Hagood JS, et al. American Thoracic Society Committee on Childhood Interstitial Lung Disease (chILD) and the chILD Research Network. An official American Thoracic Society clinical practice guideline: classification, evaluation, and management of childhood interstitial lung disease in infancy. *Am J Respir Crit Care Med.* 2013;188(3):376–394.

Morrisey EE, Hogan BLM. Preparing for the first breath: genetic and cellular mechanisms in lung development. *Cell.* 2010;18(1):8–23.

Nikolić MZ, Sun D, Rawlins EL. Human lung development: recent progress and new challenges. *Development.* 2018;145(16).

Schittny JC. Development of the lung. *Cell Tissue Res.* 2017;367(3):427–444.

Swarr DT, Morrisey EE. Lung endoderm morphogenesis: gasping for form and function. *Annu Rev Cell Dev Biol.* 2015;31:553–573.

Whitsett JA, Kalin TV, Xu Y, Kalinichenko VV. Building and regenerating the lung cell by cell. *Physiol Rev.* 2019;99(1):513–554.

Complete reference list available at ExpertConsult.com.

3

ALVEOLAR COMPARTMENT

WILLIAM J. ZACHARIAS, MD, PHD • MICHAEL F. BEERS, MD •
ZEA BOROK, MB, CHB

INTRODUCTION

The major function of the lung is to facilitate gas exchange, a process that takes place in the distal alveolar region. The alveolar compartment comprises greater than 99.5% of the large surface area of the lung,[1,2] estimated in the adult human to be approximately 100 to 150 m^2. The adult human lung contains approximately 480 million alveoli, each about 4.2×10^6 μm^3 in size.[3] In these alveoli, an intricate mixture of epithelial, mesenchymal, and endothelial lineages combine to form a thin air-blood interface for efficient gas exchange[4] (Fig. 3.1), and maintenance of this structure is required to maintain tissue oxygenation.[5] The epithelial cells of the distal lung include *alveolar type 1* (AT1) cells, which share a common fused basement membrane with capillary endothelial cells to facilitate gas exchange, and *alveolar type 2* (AT2) cells, which synthesize pulmonary surfactant components and act as progenitor cells for repair and regeneration of the alveolus (Fig. 3.2). In the mesenchyme, multiple supportive fibroblast lineages participate in alveolar homeostasis, forming niches for both epithelial and endothelial cells. This alveolar unit regulates fluid homeostasis and ion transport; provides protection against inhaled toxins, pathogens, and irritants; and via the biophysical properties of surfactant, prevents atelectasis, alveolar flooding, and severe hypoxemia. The alveolus maintains efficient gas exchange across a large variety of organism sizes, physiologic stresses, and pathologic processes.

This chapter reviews key features of alveolar structure and function, with an emphasis on the functions of alveolar epithelial cells, the physiologic properties and pathophysiologic roles of pulmonary surfactant, and management of ion and fluid homeostasis in the alveolar epithelium. The chapter ends with a brief discussion of diseases of the lung with a primary pathology centered in the alveolus. The topics presented here complement additional discussions found elsewhere focused on the structure of the alveolus (see Chapter 1), lung development (see Chapter 2), and lung mesenchyme (see Chapter 5). The reader is also directed to Chapter 8 for a detailed discussion focused on regeneration of the alveolus. A comprehensive review of *acute respiratory distress syndrome* (ARDS) can be found in Chapter 134.

CELLULAR COMPOSITION OF THE ALVEOLAR EPITHELIUM

ALVEOLAR TYPE 1 CELLS

AT1 cells comprise approximately 10% of the cells in the alveolar region but cover approximately 95% of the internal alveolar surface area,[6] with remarkable conservation of size and function across species.[2] AT1 cells are large squamous cells with a mean volume of 2000 μm^3, whereas AT2 cells are much smaller with a mean volume of 850 μm^3 in the human lung.[6] The average area covered by one AT1 cell is remarkably independent of species and body size, with an estimated area of 5100 mm^2 in humans (76 kg), 4000 mm^2 in the baboon (29 kg), 5300 mm^2 in the rat (0.36 kg), and 5200 mm^2 in the shrew (2.5 g).[2,6–8] Increases in lung size with increased body size thus result from increases in alveolar cell number. Electron microscopy studies demonstrate that the alveolar surface is lined by a continuous epithelium and highlight the complexity of AT1 cell structure.[9,10] AT1 cells contain eccentric nuclei surrounded by perinuclear cytoplasm and attenuated cytoplasmic extensions that come into close contact with the capillaries to form the epithelial component of the air-blood barrier.[10–12] A complex internal structure includes microvilli, mitochondria, Golgi, rough and smooth *endoplasmic reticulum* (ER), small intracellular vesicles, and caveolae,[13,14] suggesting subcellular domains for both metabolic and endocytic functions.[15]

An expanded discussion of the structure and modeling of AT1 cells can be found at ExpertConsult.com.

The basal surface of the AT1 cell is attached to the basement membrane, whereas the apical surface comes into contact with air. Where the epithelium lies directly over the capillary endothelial cells, their two basement membranes can fuse (Fig. 3.3 A–B). AT1 cells are not confined to one alveolus; their cytoplasmic extensions penetrate across several alveolar septa or cross interalveolar pores to

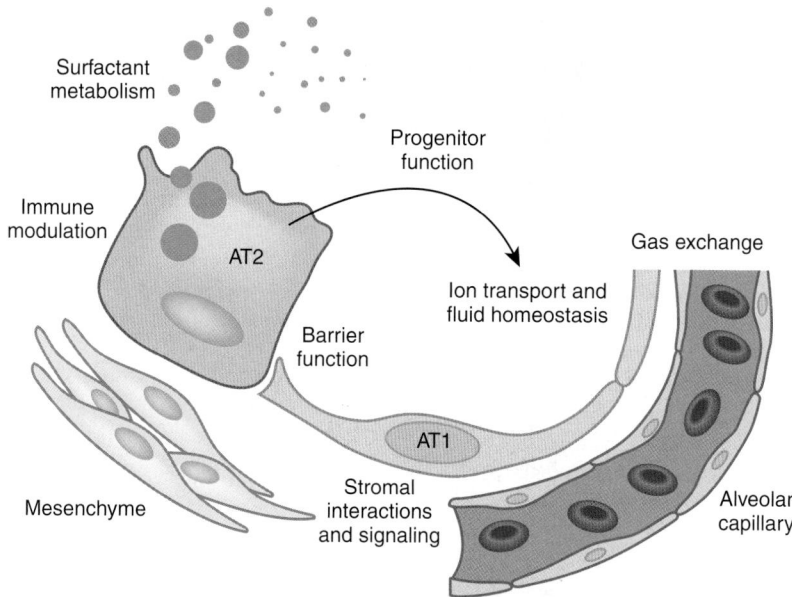

Figure 3.1 **The cellular components and functional roles of the lung alveolus.** The alveolus is made up of alveolar type 1 (AT1) and alveolar type 2 (AT2) cells that associate closely with supportive mesenchymal lineages and the alveolar capillary endothelium to coordinate major alveolar functions, including gas exchange, surfactant metabolism, ion transport and fluid homeostasis, barrier function, immune modulation, and regeneration.

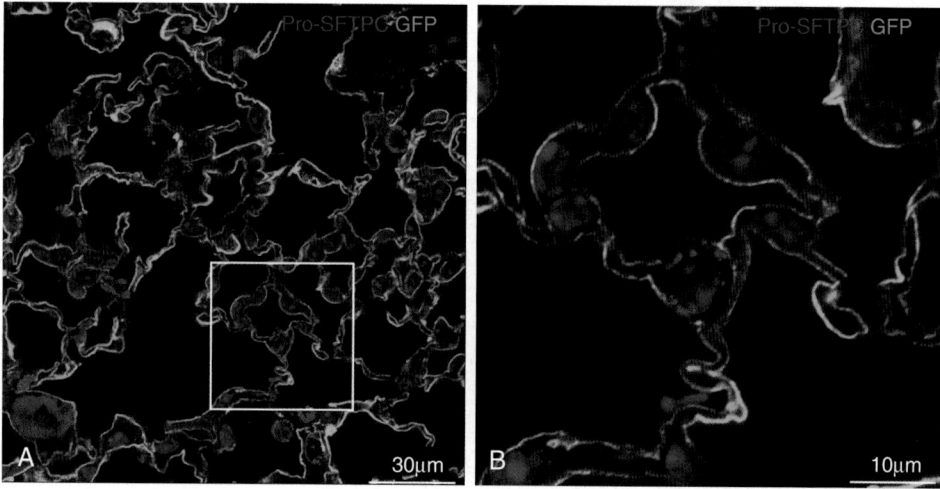

Figure 3.2 **Immunofluorescence microscopy of *alveolar type 1* (AT1) and *alveolar type 2* (AT2) cells in adult mouse lung.** (A) The majority of the alveolar epithelial surface is lined by AT1 cells. In reporter mice, labeled AT1 cells express green fluorescent protein (GFP, *green*), whereas immunofluorescent staining shows that AT2 cells express prosurfactant protein C (pro-SFTPC, *red*). Panel B shows higher magnification images for the boxed area in panel A. (Courtesy Y. Liu, B. Zhou, and Z. Borok.)

bridge two or three different alveoli.[10,11] AT1 cells also form close contacts with surrounding mesenchymal and inflammatory cells. New volume techniques, such as serial bloc face scanning electron microscopy, which allows for three-dimensional reconstruction, have revealed the morphologic diversity of AT1 cells and their ability to make cell junctions with each other, and have confirmed that entire AT1 cell bodies can cross the alveolar wall, where their cytoplasmic extensions can line both sides of the alveolar septum[20] (Video 3.1). These complex three-dimensional morphologic relationships may complicate simple interpretations of cellular function that assume distinct apical, basal, and lateral membrane domains.

Classically, AT1 cells were thought to play a largely passive role in alveolar homeostasis, serving as an impermeable lining of the alveolar surface and providing the surface area for gas exchange. Although AT1 cells do function in these roles, recent improvements in techniques, including identification of AT1 cell markers,[21–25] methods for AT1 cell isolation and enrichment,[26–32] and generation of novel transgenic mouse models for genetic labeling of AT1 cells,[33–36] have provided new insights (see Fig. 3.2). In vitro and in vivo studies and gene expression profiling[59–67] support an active, important role for AT1 cells in numerous alveolar functions, including ion transport,[26,27,68–70] barrier formation and function,[59-67,71–75] and immunomodulation[30,76] (reviewed in individual sections later).

A number of classical genes and their protein products are enriched in AT1 cells, including *aquaporin-5* (AQP5),[23,77] T1α/podoplanin/*RT140*,[21,78,79] receptor for advance glycation end products,[16,36,61,80,81] caveolin-1,[13,82] and homeodomain-only protein,[35] have been used to identify AT1 cells, facilitate AT1 cell isolation,[28–30,32] and generate AT1 cell–specific lineage tracing and deletion mouse models. However, all have some limitations with regard to cell specificity, and identification of a gene with comparable AT1 cell specificity to that of *surfactant protein C* (*SFTPC* gene) in AT2 cells remains elusive. Although functional or intact AT1 cells are still not highly represented in isolated mixed lung cell populations, recent advances in *fluorescence activated cell sorting* (FACS) and lineage tracing[35,65,83–85] have led to improved yields and purity of sorted AT1 cells.[26,28,29,79,86]

RNA-sequencing analysis[63–67] of these isolated cells has identified novel AT1 cell–enriched proteins[25] and emphasized the role of AT1 cells in fluid handling and signaling interactions in the alveolus. Comparison of AT1 cells from mouse[30] and human lungs[32] demonstrates both

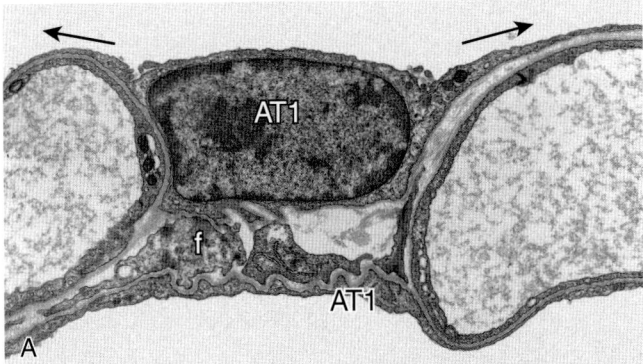

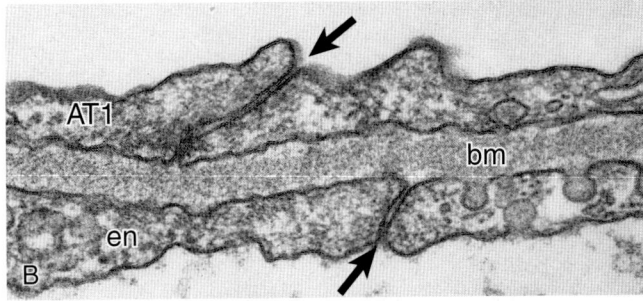

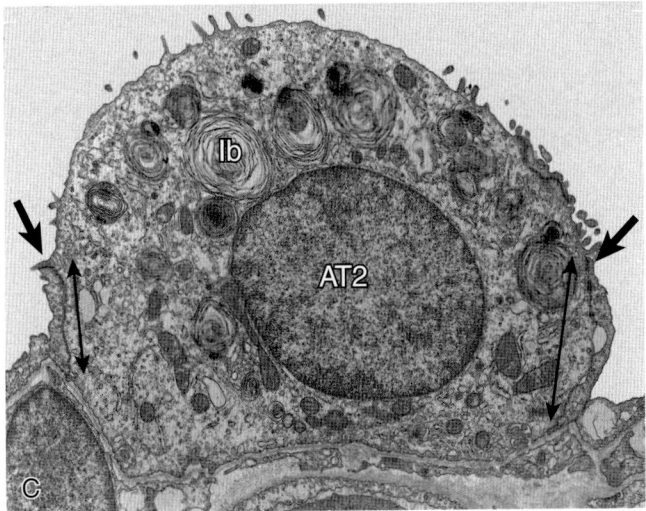

Figure 3.3 Basic features of alveolar epithelial cells. (A) Alveolar type 1 cell (AT1) sitting in a niche of a capillary mesh and extending a thin cytoplasmic leaflet to form the air-blood barrier *(long arrows)*. Interstitial space with fibroblast (f) separates this cell from type 1 cells lining the lower surface. (B) Higher-power view of the cytoplasmic leaflets of type 1 epithelial and endothelial cells (en) separated by fused basement membranes (bm) in thin part of barrier. *Arrows* point to intercellular junctions with tight junction in both cell layers. (C) Alveolar type 2 (AT2) epithelial cell is a cuboidal cell with a cytoplasm rich in organelles related to the production of surfactant elements, such as phospholipids in lamellar bodies (lb) and apoproteins. Note extended lateral membrane *(double-headed arrows)* with junctional complex between AT1 and AT2 cells *(heavy single-headed arrows)*. (A, From Weibel ER, Claassen H, Gehr P, et al. The respiratory system of the smallest mammal. In: Schmidt-Nielsen K, Bolis L, Taylor CR, eds. *Comparative Physiology: Primitive Mammals.* Cambridge, UK: Cambridge University Press; 1980:181–191; B–C, From Weibel ER. On the tricks alveolar epithelial cells play to make a good lung. *Am J Respir Crit Care Med.* 2015;191:504–513.)

conservation[25] and divergence[62] of gene expression in AT1 cells from different organisms and between freshly isolated AT1 cells and cultured AT1-like cells, suggesting both a core AT1 cell gene signature and plasticity of AT1 cells under different conditions. Recent methods allowing isolation and propagation of AT1 cells from three-dimensional

lung organoid cultures[35] will likely provide new insights to refine the properties of individual AT1 cells. Advanced techniques, including single cell and single nuclear RNA sequencing, continue to provide new insight into AT1 biology and hold promise to advance our understanding of alveolar biology.

ALVEOLAR TYPE 2 CELLS

AT2 cells (see Fig. 3.3C) are the second major epithelial lineage of the lung alveolus.[88] Although AT2 cells comprise only 3–5% of the alveolar surface area, they constitute 60% of all alveolar epithelial cells and 10–15% of all lung cells. AT2 cells were first comprehensively described by Macklin in 1954[89] before the advent of the electron microscope, and subsequent findings have validated many of the initial predictions about the function of these cells. Starting in 1974 with the seminal report of Kikkawa and Yoneda[90] and continuing over the past 5 decades with pioneering efforts of Dobbs, Williams, Mason, and others,[91–95] a wealth of data from multiple species have been generated implicating AT2 cells in important biosynthetic, secretory, metabolic, host defense, and repair/regenerative functions.[96,97] A combination of robust animal studies and isolation of primary human AT2 cells from both adult and fetal samples[86,98–101] has demonstrated the importance of AT2 cells in the maintenance of alveolar homeostasis and frequently in driving the pathogenesis of parenchymal lung diseases.[85,99,102,103]

The primary role of the AT2 cell is to produce surfactant lipids and proteins and transport them into the alveolar space. AT2 cells of all mammalian species contain specialized cytoplasmic, osmiophilic, lamellated organelles termed *lamellar bodies* (LBs), the storage organelle from which surfactant is released into the alveolar lumen[104] (Fig. 3.4). Biochemically, LBs resemble other lysosomal-related organelles in that they are acidic and express lysosomal markers (CD63, LAMP-1), but LBs also contain surfactant components (phospholipids, surfactant proteins) required for their specialized function. The apparatus for biosynthesis, processing, and exocytosis of surfactant protein is unique to AT2 cells.[88,97,105] AT2 cells are also unique in their exclusive expression and complete processing of one of the *surfactant proteins* (SPs), SP-C (SFTPC)[106,107] (see Fig. 3.2). Both human (*SFTPC*) or murine SP-C (*Sftpc*) promoter elements have been extremely useful for expressing or deleting genes in murine AT2 cells.[108] Of importance, whereas AT2 cells express the surfactant proteins SP-A, SP-B, and SP-D, these proteins are expressed in nonciliated bronchiolar cells, such as club cells, and at low levels in some extrapulmonary tissues.[109–112]

To support the synthesis and secretion of surfactant, which is rich in phospholipids, the lipid metabolism and energy capacity of AT2 cells are highly specialized: (1) the AT2 cell transcriptome is highly enriched in genes involved in lipid metabolism; (2) AT2 cell metabolism is geared toward high glucose and *oxygen* (O_2) consumption; and (3) AT2 cells contain a high density of mitochondria to support lipid biosynthesis, processing of surfactant, and the uptake and reutilization of surfactant.[7,113] Lipogenesis in AT2 cells is up-regulated at the end of gestation and, similar to other lipogenic cells, is regulated by the transcription factors sterol regulatory element binding protein-1c and CCAAT/enhancer-binding protein alpha, as well as dexamethasone, *keratinocyte growth factor* (KGF/FGF7),

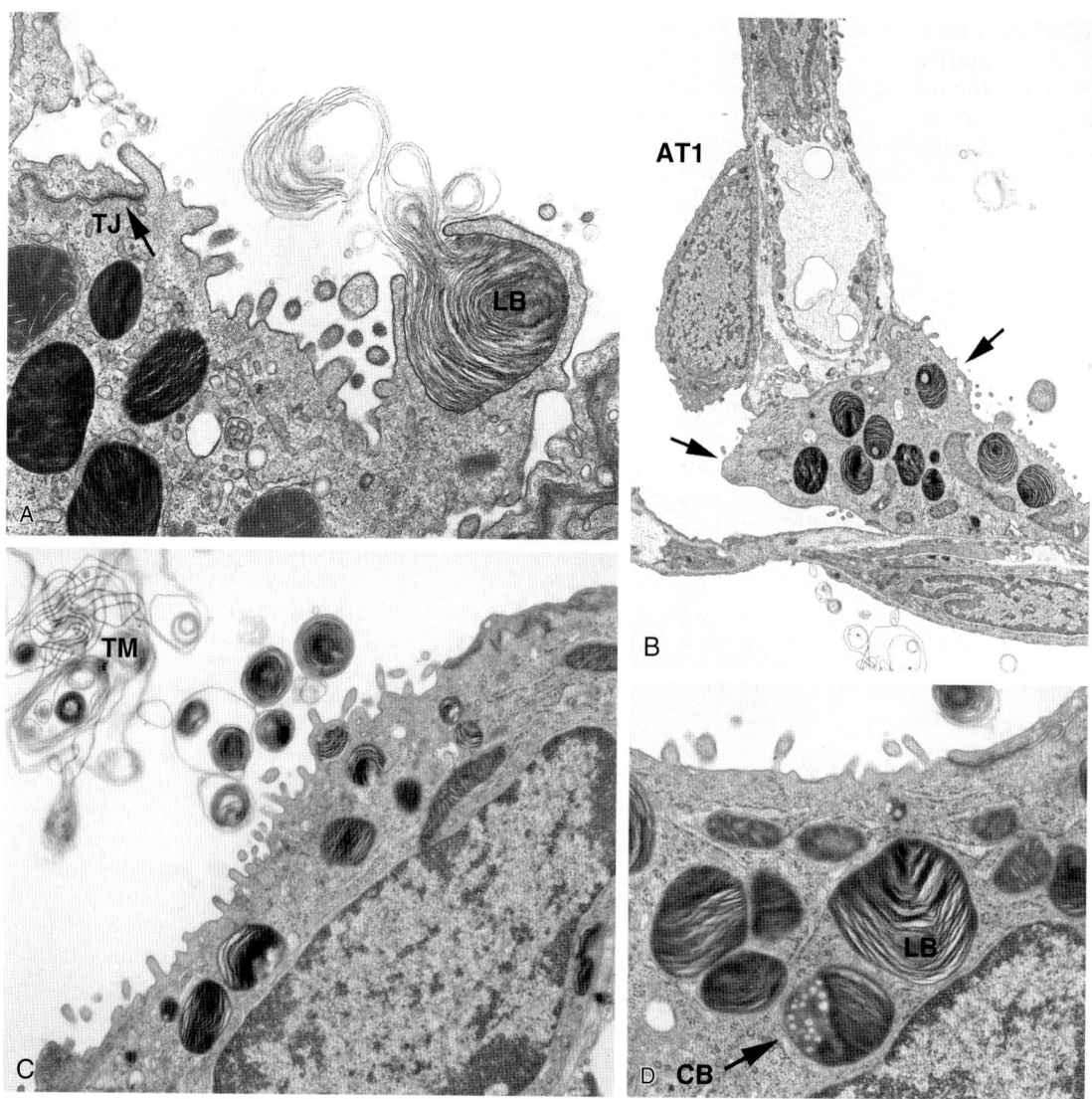

Figure 3.4 *Alveolar epithelial type 2* **(AT2) cells.** (A) A portion of an AT2 cell, showing lamellar bodies (LBs), a portion of a tight junction (TJ, *arrow*) between AT1 and AT2 cells, and an LB undergoing exocytosis. (B) Alveolar epithelium showing an AT2 cell bridging two different alveolar surfaces *(arrows)* adjacent to the nucleus of an AT1 cell. (C) A portion of an AT2 cell and secreted LBs and tubular myelin (TM) in the alveolar space. (D) A portion of an AT2 cell with an LB and a composite body (CB), which serves as an intermediate endosomal compartment between the multivesicular body and the LB. (Courtesy Lennell Allen and L. Dobbs.)

and *cyclic adenosine monophosphate* (cAMP).[100,114,115] Lipogenesis is crucial in preparing the alveolus for the first breath of air after birth. AT2 cells are therefore responsible for the biosynthesis, assembly, and complex intracellular trafficking of a diverse and challenging set of cargo. This trafficking requires activation of overlapping processes in multiple subcellular compartments, including the secretory, endocytic, and degradative (lysosomal) pathways.[105] The complexity of this cargo renders AT2 cells highly susceptible to cellular stress, and multiple studies indicate AT2 cell dysfunction is driven by activation of the unfolded protein and impaired cellular quality control pathways[105] (Table 3.1).

In addition to surfactant metabolism, AT2 cells perform critical roles in transporting fluid to prevent the alveoli from flooding and are important participants in innate lung immunity. Finally, AT2 cells function as a progenitor cell during regeneration of the lung alveolus, as discussed in detail later. This extensive secretory burden, other critical roles in the response to and repair from injury, and intrinsic susceptibility to injury highlight AT2 cells as an important participant in lung injury and aberrant repair. Failure of these systems in AT2 cells has been causally associated with a variety of lung diseases and syndromes in both pediatric and adult populations (Table 3.1).

FUNCTIONAL ROLES OF THE ALVEOLAR UNIT

PULMONARY SURFACTANT AND ALVEOLAR SURFACE TENSION

The requirement for an extensive, hydrated, and patent surface for gas exchange presents a challenging bioengineering problem because the surface tension at air-liquid interfaces creates forces promoting alveolar collapse at low lung volumes. Alveolar collapse then results in ventilation-perfusion mismatch that impairs normal gas exchange. In 1929, von Neergaard[116] discovered that there was a difference in the mechanics and elastic recoil properties of the respiratory system depending on whether the lung was inflated with air or saline (Fig. 3.5). More pressure was required to inflate the lungs with air than with saline, but once inflated, alveoli remained open even at low lung volumes, leading to the hypothesis that the surface tension in the distal lung was lower than predicted for a simple air-water interface due to an "antiatelectasis factor." In the 1950s, Clements[117] and Pattle[118] used lung extracts to demonstrate that surfactant, specifically its phospholipid components, was responsible for lowering alveolar surface tension, decreasing the work of breathing, preventing alveolar collapse, and promoting stability of alveoli of different sizes with different radii of curvature. Soon after these discoveries, Avery and Mead[119] causally demonstrated a deficiency in surface-active material in the lungs of premature infants with neonatal respiratory distress syndrome. This led to the current understanding that the alveolar gas exchange surface is coated with a thin film of *surface active agent* (surfactant), a biochemically heterogeneous complex composed of primarily lipids and protein, that functions to reduce surface tension at the air-liquid interface along the distal lung epithelial lining.

Surfactant Composition

Surfactant is a mixture of lipids and proteins secreted into the alveolar space by AT2 cells. These lipids play a key role in modulating surface tension. The critical lipid component of surfactant is *dipalmitoylphosphatidylcholine* (DPPC), an atypical phospholipid species of phosphatidylcholine in that both fatty acid side chains are saturated. DPPC, along with unsaturated phosphatidylcholine, phosphatidylglycerol, and four surfactant-associated proteins (reviewed later) represent the bulk of the secreted AT2 cell surfactant (Table 3.2). Approximately 50–60% of surfactant lipid is DPPC, which distinguishes it from the composite of phosphatidylcholine species found in cellular membranes. Pulmonary phospholipids are amphophilic (i.e., contain both hydrophilic and hydrophobic parts) and therefore can spontaneously form a monolayer film at air-liquid interfaces to stabilize the surface film at low alveolar volumes.[120] Of note, the

TABLE 3.1 Diseases of the Distal Lung Epithelium

Category	Clinical Diagnosis	Lung Phenotype	Molecular and Cellular Mechanism(s)
SURFACTANT SYSTEM DISORDERS			
Surfactant Deficiencies			
Developmental	Neonatal RDS	Immature lung hyaline membranes Respiratory failure	Decreased surfactant system components Increased surface tension
Inherited	SP-B deficiency	Respiratory failure Alveolar proteinosis PAS-positive staining	Absent SP-B in BAL Dysfunctional surfactant Misprocessed SP-C Increased BAL phospholipids
	ABCA3 mutations (null)	Respiratory failure	Absent lamellar bodies Decreased BAL and AT2 phospholipids Dysfunctional surfactant
Surfactant Dysfunction Syndromes			
Acquired/intrinsic	ARDS	Hyaline membranes Respiratory failure/shunt	Epithelial cell death, barrier dysfunction Surfactant inactivation Inflammatory cell recruitment
	Primary graft dysfunction	Focal pulmonary infiltrates Hypoxic respiratory failure	Epithelial cell death, barrier dysfunction Surfactant inactivation Inflammatory cell recruitment
Extrinsic toxins	Hyperoxic lung injury Nitrogen mustard	Hypoxic respiratory failure	AT2/AT1 cell death Inflammatory cell recruitment Surfactant inactivation
Infectious	*Pneumocystis jirovecii*	Hypoxic respiratory failure Alveolar proteinosis	Defective AT2 surfactant secretion Surfactant inactivation
Altered Surfactant Metabolism			
Pulmonary Alveolar Proteinosis (PAP)			
Autoimmune	iPAP	Alveolar proteinosis PAS (+) alveolar material "Crazy paving" CT scan	GM-CSF autoantibodies
Hereditary	hPAP	Alveolar proteinosis	Recessive variants in GM-CSF receptor common beta chain or alpha chains
Acquired	Secondary PAP	Alveolar proteinosis	Dust exposure: silica, aluminum, titanium Hematologic malignancy Post-allogenic BMT *Pneumocystis jirovecii*

Continued

TABLE 3.1   Diseases of the Distal Lung Epithelium—cont'd

Category	Clinical Diagnosis	Lung Phenotype	Molecular and Cellular Mechanism(s)
INTRINSIC EPITHELIAL CELL DYSFUNCTION			
Mutations in AT2 Cell or Surfactant Component Genes			
SFTPC mutations	Child (children) IPF (adult)	NSIP ± PAP UIP	Epithelial cytotoxicity from protein aggregation or mistrafficking including ER stress. apoptosis, impaired autophagy Cytokine/TGF-β generation
SFTPA mutations	chILD IPF (adult) Lung cancer	NSIP/PAP UIP pathology Adenocarcinoma	Epithelial dysfunction ER stress Cytokine generation
ABCA3 mutations	chILD (children) IPF (adult)	NSIP/PAP UIP (adult)	ER stress Impaired autophagy
Short telomere syndrome	Interstitial lung diseases ± dyskeratosis congenita	IPF/UIP NSIP	Short telomeres Genetic variants: *RTEL1, TERT, PARN, TERC DKC1, NAF1, TINF2*
Organellar Homeostasis			
Hermansky-Pudlak syndrome	Interstitial lung disease	Early-onset UIP	Genetic variants in *HPS1, HPS2,* or *HPS4* Abnormal (giant) lamellar bodies Macrophage-dominant alveolitis
Birt-Hogg-Dubé syndrome	Parenchymal cystic lung disease	Bilateral basolateral lung cysts Pneumothoraces Skin fibrofolliculomas Renal tumors	Variants in *FLCN* (folliculin)
Disorders of AT2 Cell Metabolism			
Macromolecule metabolism	Niemann-Pick disease	Interstitial lung disease Alveolar proteinosis	Mutation in *NPD-A, SMPD1, NPC1, NPC2* Altered LDL cholesterol, sphingomyelin
Ion homeostasis	Pulmonary microlithiasis	CT scan: micronodular "sandstorm" calcifications ± crazy paving pattern	Mutation in *SLC34A2* (Na-PO$_4$ transporter) Air space accumulation of CaPO$_4$ microliths
BARRIER DYSFUNCTION			
Altered Barrier Integrity			
Genetic	None		
Acquired	Sepsis ARDS	Diffuse alveolar damage Alveolar edema Respiratory failure	Barrier disruption
Transport Dysfunction			
Acquired lower respiratory tract infections	ARDS		Decrease expression of ion transport proteins Proinflammatory cytokines Reactive oxygen and nitrogen species Extracellular nucleotides
Genetic	Multisystem pseudohypoaldosteronism	Recurrent lower respiratory tract infections	Homozygous or compound heterozygous mutations of α-, β-, γ-ENaC subunits

ARDS, acute respiratory distress syndrome; AT1, AT2, alveolar type 1 and 2, respectively; BAL, bronchoalveolar lavage; BMT, bone marrow transplant; chILD, interstitial lung disease of childhood; CT, computed tomography; ENaC, epithelial sodium channel; ER, endoplasmic reticulum; GM-CSF, granulocyte-macrophage–colony-stimulating; hPAP, hereditary pulmonary alveolar proteinosis; iPAP, inspiratory positive airway pressure; IPF, idiopathic pulmonary fibrosis; LDL, low-density lipoprotein; NSIP, nonspecific interstitial pneumonitis; PAP, pulmonary alveolar proteinosis; PAS, periodic acid–Schiff; RDS, respiratory distress syndrome of the newborn; SP-B, -C, surfactant protein B and C, respectively; TGF-β, transforming growth factor-beta; UIP, usual interstitial pneumonitis.

composition of surfactant lipid is important for optimal lung function, and changes are associated with disease; for instance, during ARDS, a reduction in the percentage of phosphatidylglycerol is the earliest alteration detected in the composition of surfactant.[121]

See ExpertConsult.com for more information on the study of composition and measurement of surfactant.

DPPC-enriched phospholipid films reduce surface tension at the air-liquid interface, but these lipids alone demonstrate slow film formation and cannot provide optimal surfactant function. Surfactant proteins play a key supportive role in stabilizing and supporting the lipid monolayer and participate in innate immune functions. Although united by a common nomenclature defined by order of discovery as SP-A, SP-B, SP-C, and SP-D,[131] these surfactant components have both overlapping and distinct functions. The two smaller hydrophobic proteins, SP-B and SP-C, can each improve the rate of delivery (adsorption and spreading) of DPPC and other phospholipids at the air-liquid interface.[132] Of importance, either protein alone or a mixture of the two improves the surfactant-like properties of the phospholipids present in the alveolus and are

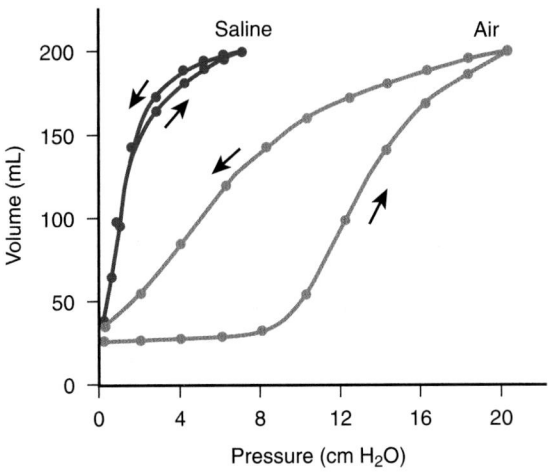

Figure 3.5 **Air and saline volume-pressure curves.** The classic physiologic observation that led to the discovery of surfactant. It takes more pressure to inflate the lung with air than with saline. However, the pressure difference is much less than would be expected if the alveolar lining had the same surface tension as other biologic fluids, which indicates the presence of a surface-active material. The descending limb of the air volume-pressure curve is highly reproducible and is used to estimate the surface tension of the lung and static compliance. (Modified from Radford EP Jr. Recent studies of mechanical properties of mammalian lungs. In: Remington JW, ed. *Tissue Elasticity.* Washington, DC: American Physiological Society; 1957:177–190.)

TABLE 3.2 Composition of Pulmonary Surfactant

Phospholipids: 85%	% of Phospholipids
Phosphatidylcholine	76.3
Dipalmitoylphosphatidylcholine	47.0
Unsaturated phosphatidylcholine	29.3
Phosphatidylglycerol	11.6
Phosphatidylinositol	3.9
Phosphatidylethanolamine	3.3
Sphingomyelin	1.5
Other	3.4
Neutral Lipids: 5%	
Cholesterol free fatty acids	
Proteins 10%	
SP-A	++++
SP-B	+
SP-C	+
SP-D	++
Other	

SP-A, SP-B, SP-C, and SP-D, surfactant protein A, B, C, and D, respectively.
+, relative abundance.

the major protein components in the current surfactant replacement therapies used to treat neonatal respiratory distress syndrome.[133] The other two surfactant proteins, SP-A and SP-D, are hydrophilic and do not appear to have a primary role in modulating surfactant biophysics.[134] They are members of the collectin family of C-type lectins with known host defense functions. Although SP-A coisolates with surfactant phospholipids and can recapitulate some of the biophysical properties of SP-B and SP-C in vitro, its main functions are in innate immunity and homeostasis of surfactant (see also Chapter 15).

After secretion into the alveolus, surfactant can be found in several forms that can be visualized in transmission electron microscopy and freeze fracture images. These include LBs, highly organized structures termed tubular myelin, and phospholipid-rich sheets and vesicles.[135,136] Tubular myelin is a unique extracellular form of surfactant that sediments rapidly on centrifugation and is surface active. Tubular myelin appears as an organized lattice of surfactant bilayers formed at right angles and represents a surfactant intermediate between the LB and the surface monolayer. SP-A, in combination with SP-B, is necessary for the formation of tubular myelin in vitro.[137] However, because SP-A–deficient mice lack tubular myelin but have normal respiratory mechanics at rest, the formation of tubular myelin is not considered absolutely necessary for surfactant function.[138] Overall, this multistage surfactant system promotes a low surface tension in the alveoli and small airways but not in the large airways or trachea.[126–130]

Surfactant Protein A

SP-A was the first surfactant protein identified[139] and is the most abundant of the surfactant proteins. In contrast to SP-B and SP-C, the main role of SP-A in the lung is related to host defense. SP-A is a secreted octadecameric collagenous glycoprotein with a complex tertiary structure similar to serum mannose-binding lectin and the complement component C1q.[134,140] SP-A forms a polarized bouquet-like structure composed of 18 monomers organized as six trimeric units. The SP-A monomer contains a COOH-terminal C-type lectin motif, a triple helical collagen domain, and *carbohydrate recognition domain* (CRD) (Fig. 3.6). The CRD is essential for SP-A host defense function and consists of a globular domain that binds carbohydrate and other ligands recognized by SP-A. In humans, there are two SP-A genes, *SFTPA1* and *SFTPA2*, 4.5 kb each, located on chromosome 10 near the closely related genes SP-D and mannose-binding lectin. The amino acid differences that distinguish SP-A1 from SP-A2 are in general conservative and located mainly in the collagen-like domain, with only one shown to affect protein structure.[141–143]

Greater than 99% of secreted SP-A in lavage fluid is bound to phospholipid.[144] SP-A is localized primarily in the gas exchange units of the lung and small airways.[145] In rodents, SP-A is found in AT2 cells and in nonciliated bronchiolar cells (club cells) lining the conducting airways. In humans, most SP-A is found in the alveoli, with less prominent expression in human tracheal submucosal glands.[146] SP-A is also expressed in extrapulmonary sites, including salivary glands, lacrimal glands, and the female urogenital tract,[147] although the exact physiologic relevance of SP-A in other organs is unknown. At the ultrastructural level, immunogold electron microscopy has detected SP-A in both AT2 cell organelles and intra-alveolar surfactant.[148] A number of factors can increase the synthesis of SP-A, including cAMP, KGF/FGF7, and *interleukin* (IL)-1.[149]

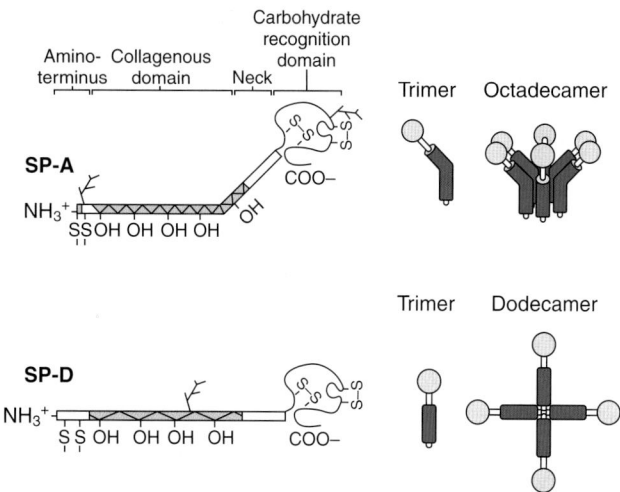

Figure 3.6 Structural organization of *surfactant proteins A and D* (SP-A and SP-D). SP-A *(top)* and SP-D *(bottom)* are collagenous glycoproteins with four important domains. The amino-terminal region contains cysteines for intermolecular disulfide bonding to form covalent oligomeric units. The collagen-like domain imparts structural rigidity and elongated molecular structure to both proteins. In SP-A, the collagen region has a kink, which accounts for the bend in the collagen region and the bouquet-like structure of the octadecamer. In SP-D, the collagen domain is straight and allows formation of a cross-shaped dodecamer. The neck contributes to the trimeric assembly of polypeptide subunits and spacing for the terminal carbohydrate recognition domain (CRD). The CRD is a globular region of the molecule that plays a major role in the recognition of multiple ligands. In SP-A, the CRD accounts for most of the binding to dipalmitoylphosphatidylcholine vesicles, alveolar type 2 cells, macrophages, and inhaled organisms. In SP-D, the CRD unit is responsible for all the reported interactions with viruses and bacteria. (Modified from Kuroki Y, Voelker DR. Pulmonary surfactant proteins. *J Biol Chem.* 1994;269:25943–25946.)

The intracellular trafficking and secretion of nascent SP-A involves both LB-dependent (regulated)[150] and LB-independent (constitutive) pathways.[151] Directly secreted SP-A is newly synthesized, whereas the SP-A found in LBs is likely derived from SP-A recycled via endocytosis and via reincorporation into LBs, which may play an important role in regulation of reuptake of other lipids.[152–154] Beyond the presence of a signal peptide and N-linked glycosylation, structural motifs and signals regulating trafficking of SP-A remain incompletely defined.

The major function of extracellular SP-A appears to be in innate immunity. SP-A binds to a variety of microorganisms and particles, promotes their clearance by phagocytic cells, and directly alters the function of immune effector cells.[155–159] Because SP-A binding is somewhat promiscuous with a low affinity, the physiologic effects of SP-A are likely due to its polyvalent structure and multiple binding sites on cells and organisms. SP-A is capable of binding both the surfactant lipid in alveolar fluid and inhaled organisms or particles. SP-A binds gram-negative bacteria with the rough form of lipopolysaccharide, aggregates these bacteria, and increases their phagocytosis and killing. In contrast, SP-A binds poorly to smooth variant forms of lipopolysaccharide; gram-negative bacteria that colonize the respiratory tract usually express smooth variants that avoid detection.

SP-A enhances the adherence and subsequent clearance of mycobacteria,[160] certain fungal pathogens, and the opportunistic pathogen *Pneumocystis jirovecii*.[161] SP-A also binds to a variety of viruses, including influenza and respiratory syncytial virus, and likely aggregates the virus, which may inhibit infection.[162–165]

SP-A suppresses the secretion of inflammatory cytokines by macrophages in the normal lung but enhances cytokine production during infection or lung injury, a duality referred to as the inflammatory paradox of SP-A. The precise receptors on target immune cells mediating this function are unknown. Identifying functional cell receptors for SP-A and SP-D has been challenging because both are polyvalent lectins and can bind to a variety of glycoproteins and glycolipids.[140] Receptors for SP-A exist on AT2 cells[166–168] for surfactant recycling and on macrophages for clearance of apoptotic cells,[169,170] surfactant clearance, and modulation of the innate immune response.[171,172] Currently, the precise role of individual SP-A receptors in normal surfactant metabolism or in disease is unknown.

Surfactant Protein B

SP-B is one of two extremely hydrophobic surfactant proteins (with SP-C) crucial for the biophysical activity of surfactant preparations. As a member of the saposin-like family of peptides that interact with lipids, SP-B avidly associates with phospholipids in surfactant and facilitates their adsorption and surface spreading.[132,173–176] SP-B protein found in lung lavage is a homodimer composed of two 79–amino acid polypeptide chains linked by disulfide bonds. Each monomer has five amphipathic helices that interact with the surface of the surfactant monolayer but do not span the entire monolayer.[177] After a process of posttranslational modification, the mature peptide is secreted into the alveolar space exclusively via regulated LB exocytosis as an 18-kDa disulfide-linked homodimer that is exceptionally hydrophobic due to residues comprised predominantly of valine and leucine.

See ExpertConsult.com for a more detailed discussion of SP-B genetics and processing.

In addition to its role in formation of tubular myelin and generation of a surface film, SP-B is necessary for formation of AT2 cell LBs.[184] Both SP-B–deficient patients with homozygous loss of function mutations and SP-B knockout mice lack LBs.[185–187] In vitro, the interaction of SP-B with lipid vesicles causes lysis and fusion, resulting in the formation of phospholipid sheets,[188,189] a process believed to facilitate transformation of multivesicular bodies into the densely packed lamellae characteristic of the LB. Importantly, SP-B deficiency is uniformly fatal (or requires lung transplantation) due to a lack of both mature SP-B and SP-C. The molecular basis for this double deficiency lies in the critical role of the LB in posttranslational processing of the SP-C propeptide.[105,190,191] Therefore, in contrast to SP-C deficiency (discussed later), loss of functional SP-B protein results in complete loss of all hydrophobic surfactant protein function and very high alveolar surface tension.

Surfactant Protein C

Of all surfactant proteins, only SP-C is made exclusively by AT2 cells; SP-C cooperates with SP-B to enhance the surfactant properties of the lipid monolayer. The mature SP-C protein is an extremely hydrophobic peptide composed of 33 to 35 highly conserved amino acids containing a high content of valine, isoleucine, and leucine ($\approx$60–65% of the primary sequence).[192] The segment between residues 13 and 28 forms a hydrophobic α-helix, which is the membrane-spanning portion of SP-C and is extremely stable in lipids or organic solvents. However, in aqueous solutions, SP-C self-aggregates, adopting a β-sheet conformation and forming amyloid fibrils.[193–195] SP-C is thought to stabilize the surface film and minimize film collapse via insertion into the surface monolayer to organize surfactant phospholipids during the respiratory cycle. Unlike SP-B, SP-C does not appear to interact with SP-A and is not needed for the formation of tubular myelin. SP-C is found in all preparations of natural surfactant, and a recombinant form of SP-C has been used in one version of a surfactant replacement therapy. Both normal posttranslational processing events and the processing of disease-causing *SFTPC* mutants are influenced by four main functional domains and structural motifs contained within proSP-C. Extensive work has led to a detailed understanding of these domains and their relative function in SP-C activity.

More information on these domains can be found at ExpertConsult.com.

Although SP-C is dispensable for surfactant biophysical activity, both loss of function and toxic gain of function mutations in the *SFTPC* gene are implicated in chronic parenchymal lung disease in humans. While autosomal recessive *SFTPC* null mutations have not yet been described in humans, SP-C null mice appear normal at birth but eventually develop a strain-dependent chronic pneumonitis and air space enlargement in adulthood and are more sensitive to bleomycin injury.[209–211] Since 2001, heterozygous expression of more than 60 inherited and sporadic *SFTPC* mutations have been linked with interstitial lung disease in both children and adults.[212–215] Mutations in the COOH-terminus domain produce a misfolded proSP-C protein that accumulates in the ER, self-aggregates, and causes AT2 cell ER stress. Mutations in other regions appear to disrupt other AT2 cell quality control pathways, such as macroautophagy.[105] In familial forms of *SFTPC*-related interstitial lung disease, the age of onset of interstitial lung disease varies from the early perinatal period through older adulthood, indicating that genetic background and other disease-modifying genes contribute to fibrotic pathophysiology in these patients.[215] Recently, expression of either of two clinical *Sftpc* mutations in mice induced a fibrotic lung phenotype, providing proof of concept that *SFTPC* mutations and AT2 cell dysfunction are likely drivers of interstitial lung disease.[216,217] Additional disease associations of alveolar cells and proteins are summarized in Table 3.1.

Surfactant Protein D

Like SP-A, SP-D is a multimeric, calcium-dependent lectin that functions primarily as an important component of innate lung immunity.[155,218,219] SP-D binds the phospholipids of surface-active material weakly and is mostly soluble in alveolar fluid. SP-D is found in ER of AT2 cells and in the secretory granules of club cells, but not in LB of AT2 cells or in tubular myelin, and only sparsely in major conducting airways.[110,145] These characteristics emphasize the immune function of SP-D, a collagenous glycoprotein with a complex but highly ordered tertiary structure (see Fig 3.6). The C-terminal CRD domain contains calcium and carbohydrate binding sites[140,220] and is primarily responsible for multivalent binding to surface ligands on microorganisms. Like SP-A, SP-D binds to a variety of microorganisms to promote clearance from the alveolar space. Full oligomerization of both SP-D and SP-A causes amplification of relatively weak interactions across multiple pathogen binding sites, improving clearance.

In addition to its interactions with microbes, SP-D has both pro-inflammatory and anti-inflammatory signaling functions, which involve posttranslational modifications of the protein. The lectin-like CRD head of SP-D inhibits inflammation, whereas the collagenous tail domain stimulates inflammation.[221,222] S-Nitrosylation results in a disruption of SP-D multimers so that monomers predominate, exposing collagenous tail domains,[223] leading to chemoattraction of macrophages. SP-D is up-regulated in a variety of infectious and inflammatory disease states, including allergic asthma, hyperoxic lung injury, bleomycin injury, and *Pneumocystis* pneumonia.[58,224–230] Up-regulation of SP-D has also been observed in hyperplastic AT2 cells present in interstitial lung diseases. SP-D can be detected in normal serum, and elevation of serum SP-D has been proposed as a diagnostic and/or predictive biomarker in a variety of lung diseases, including idiopathic pulmonary fibrosis, COPD, and post–lung transplant recipients.[231–233]

Surfactant Secretion and Turnover

AT2 cells can synthesize, secrete, and recycle all components of pulmonary surfactant, directing the process of surfactant production and turnover. From 10–20% of the surfactant pool is secreted hourly from AT2 cells.[234] Secretion requires active extrusion of the lamellar body contents,[235] which involves fusion of the lamellar body with the plasma membrane.[236,237] Secretion is highly regulated, and multiple checks and balances likely balance surfactant turnover. In vivo, secretion is stimulated by hyperventilation or even a single deep breath or sigh.[238] Secretion is also stimulated by stretch, an important physiologic stimulus leading to an elevation of intracellular calcium in AT1 cells, which is then propagated to adjacent AT1 and AT2 cells via gap junctions,[239,240] potentiating prosecretory signaling[241] and increasing surfactant secretion. In vitro, secretion is greatly stimulated by tetradecanoyl acetate and *adenosine triphosphate* (ATP)[242–245] and is more modestly increased by other agents, including β-agonists and cholera toxin.

After exocytosis by AT2 cells, the secreted LBs undergo physical rearrangements extracellularly (Fig. 3.7). The initial change is the conversion from the multilamellar state to tubular myelin, which as noted earlier requires SP-A, SP-B, and calcium. In lavage samples, surfactant can be segregated by its sedimentation properties into large and small aggregates. Large-aggregate surfactant contains SP-A and SP-B and is composed of tubular myelin, multilamellar structures, and other loose lipid arrays, which are forms of secreted and unraveling LBs.[246] Large aggregates adsorb rapidly to the air-liquid interface and can be considered

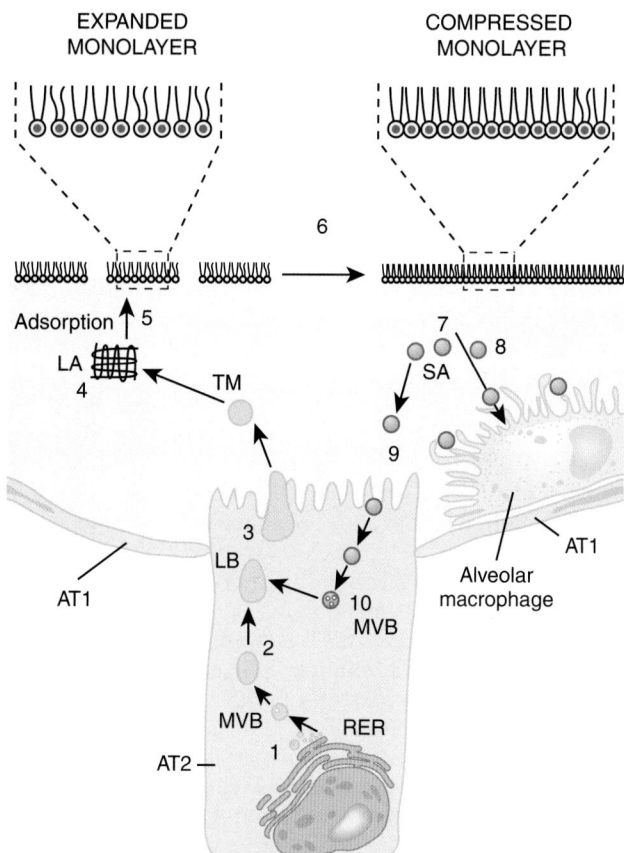

EXPANDED MONOLAYER

COMPRESSED MONOLAYER

Figure 3.7 Metabolic trafficking of surfactant phospholipids. The phospholipids are synthesized in the rough endoplasmic reticulum (RER) of the alveolar type 2 (AT2) cell (1). They are transported to the multivesicular bodies (MVB) (2), where the first lamellae are formed. These lamellae increase to form lamellar bodies (LB), which are subsequently secreted by exocytosis (3). The secreted LB unfolds to form tubular myelin (TM) (4) and other large aggregates (LA). These forms adsorb into the expanded surface monolayer (5). This is a critical step for producing a low surface tension in the alveolus. During the respiratory cycle, as the film is compressed during exhalation, the film pressure rises, and a compressed, closely packed monolayer of nearly pure dipalmitoylphosphatidylcholine is formed (6). Material is excluded from the monolayer (7) and forms small aggregates (SA). Some of these aggregates are ingested by macrophages (8), but most are endocytosed for reprocessing by AT2 cells (9 and 10). AT1, alveolar type 1 (cell).

an extracellular reservoir of surfactant. Small aggregates, which are much less surface active,[247] are thought to represent surfactant that has left the air-liquid interface and is available to be cleared from the alveolar space.

To maintain steady-state pool sizes of extracellular surfactant, secretion needs to be counterbalanced by surfactant removal. The two dominant routes for the clearance of surface-active material are reuptake by AT2 cells for reprocessing (≈50–85%) and phagocytosis by alveolar macrophages for catabolism.[236,237] Reuptake of extracellular surfactant by AT2 cells can be increased in response to surfactant secretagogues, such as ATP and phorbol myristate acetate.[248] Catabolism of extracellular surfactant is regulated by *granulocyte-macrophage–colony-stimulating factor* (GM-CSF) and its ability to activate macrophages (more details of this pathway can be found in Chapter 98).[249–253] Taken together, these data emphasize that the full complement of surfactant components, the appropriate management of cellular secretion, and regulated surfactant reuptake and removal from the alveolar space are all

collectively required to maintain alveolar homeostasis and promote gas exchange.

ALVEOLAR IMMUNE DEFENSE AND INFLAMMATORY MODULATION

The alveolar epithelium forms a thin, single cell surface separating the outside world from the pulmonary circulation. Due to the large amounts of air exchanged during breathing, the distal lung is bombarded with environmental pathogens, particulates, and toxins. To maintain immune quiescence, pulmonary epithelial cells partner with professional immune cells in both the alveolar space and the interstitium to activate adaptive immunity appropriately in the event of barrier breach or infection, while at the same time preventing aberrant inflammatory responses to limit damage. There are three major components of the alveolar immune defense: (1) the surfactant system (reviewed earlier), (2) alveolar epithelial barrier function (reviewed later), and (3) innate host defense in coordination with alveolar cells. This section focuses on the role of the alveolar epithelium in directing immune defense in the alveolus.

Alveolar epithelial cells are constantly exposed to both commensal and pathogenic microorganisms throughout life. Traditional teaching that the alveolus is a sterile space has been supplanted by an understanding, based on modern molecular techniques, that healthy patients harbor a microbiome in the distal lung similar to that in the more proximal airways[254] (see Chapter 17). The resident microbes differ between smokers and healthy patients and vary in multiple lung diseases, including cystic fibrosis and COPD. Antibiotic treatment during late gestation, which limits acquisition of these commensal bacteria, alters the development of pulmonary innate immunity and worsens outcomes of experimental pneumonia, emphasizing the instructive role of commensal bacteria in priming the alveolar immune system.[255]

Alveolar epithelial cells also directly participate in immune defense. AT2 cells express cell surface receptors, including *toll-like receptor* (TLR) family molecules, which allow direct recognition of both commensal and pathogenic bacteria in the alveolar space. TLR2 and TLR4 on AT2 cells are activated in response to viral infections, cigarette smoke, and multiple inflammatory cytokines.[256] Epithelial cells then coordinate with innate immune lineages, especially alveolar macrophages, to balance the immune response. AT2 cells, for example, produce the macrophage growth factor GM-CSF,[257] which is required for proper differentiation of alveolar macrophages in the alveolar space; abnormalities in alveolar macrophage maturation can lead to pulmonary alveolar proteinosis (reviewed in Chapter 98). AT1 cells express high amounts of *receptor for advanced glycation end products* (RAGE),[61] a protein associated with modulation of inflammation in both inflammatory and stromal cells in the lung[258] and a major danger-associated molecular pattern receptor in multiple tissues, including the lung. Finally, as reviewed in detail later, multiple inflammatory stimuli modify the secretion and absorption of fluid in the alveolus during pathologic conditions, directly impacting gas exchange by modifying airway surface-liquid properties. These findings implicate alveolar epithelial cells as direct participants in lung inflammation and immune defense and emphasize the coordinated activity required to maintain functional surface area for gas exchange.

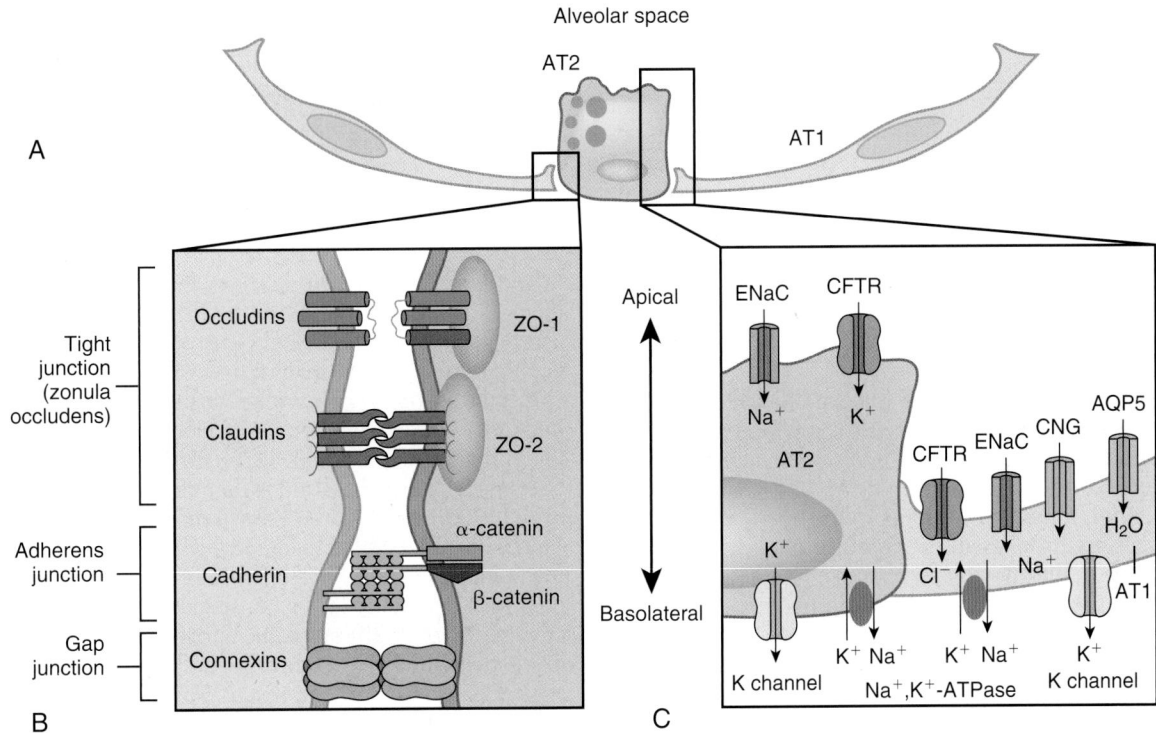

Figure 3.8 Schematic representation of junctions and ion transporters critical to lung epithelial barrier function and fluid handling. (A) Overall schematic showing *alveolar type 1* (AT1) and *alveolar type 2* (AT2) cells in the alveolus. Cell-cell junctions are important to maintain the alveolar epithelial barrier. (B) Schematic of junctional complexes and proteins in the alveolus. Alveolar epithelial cells are connected by tight, adherens, and gap junctions with differential localization of claudins, occludins, cadherins, and connexins. See text for details. (C) Schematic of key apical and basal transporters regulating ion and fluid flow in the alveolar epithelium. See text for detailed discussion of the role of each transporter in alveolar physiology. AT2 cell has been reduced in size to simplify representation. AQP5, aquaporin 5; ATPase, adenosine triphosphatase; CFTR, cystic fibrosis transmembrane regulator; Cl^-, chloride ion; CNG, cyclic nucleotide–gated sodium channels; ENaC, epithelial Na^+ channel; K^+, potassium ion; Na^+, sodium ion; ZO-1, ZO-2, zonula occludens–1 and –2, respectively.

ALVEOLAR EPITHELIAL INTEGRITY AND BARRIER FUNCTION

Alveolar epithelial cells form a barrier separating "external" environmental hazards from the inside of the body. This barrier is constantly challenged. Therefore multiple cellular and extracellular components form a multilayered barrier designed to maintain epithelial integrity without impairing gas exchange. As noted earlier, the first barrier encountered by environmental pathogens is the surfactant system, where SP-A and SP-D bind particulates and pathogens in a pattern-specific manner, augmenting alveolar macrophage function in clearing the alveolar space. Alveolar fluid also contains other defense molecules, including lysozyme, an enzyme that catalyzes the destruction of bacterial cell walls, providing a further barrier above the epithelial surface.

If pathogens and environmental particulates circumvent these barriers, they then reach the epithelial layer. Alveolar epithelial cells are connected by a series of cell-cell junctions that function to coordinate cell behavior and prevent passage of solutes and deleterious molecules between cells (Fig. 3.8). Proper gas exchange is predicated on minimization of fluid in the air space, and the alveolar epithelium contains a host of junctional connections to create one of the tightest epithelial barriers in the human body. The homeostatic function of this barrier is to prevent passive leak of fluid into the air spaces. Thus injury to the junctional proteins and complex leads to alveolar edema and hypoxemia. Barrier damage is a major part of the pathophysiology of ARDS (see Chapter 134), and fluid management in the alveolus is reviewed in detail later.

Tight junctions (also called *zonula occludens* [ZO]) connect adjacent alveolar epithelial cells, where claudins, including Cld3, Cld4, and Cld18,[73] form close connections between AT2 and AT1 cells. Although each of these claudins is expressed in both AT1 and AT2 cells, levels of expression differ between cell types, and AT1-AT1, AT2-AT1, and AT2-AT2 tight junctions have different stoichiometry of these components, as well as other core tight junction proteins, including occludin, tricellulin, junctional adhesion molecule, and ZO-1 and ZO-2.[11] Mouse knockout studies[72,74,239,259] have demonstrated key roles for claudins in both tight junction function and fluid clearance, and injury studies have implicated claudins as key regulators of severity of injury in several human disease and animal models. Within the tight junction, claudins form selective pores allowing regulation of passage of ions and molecules between adjacent epithelial cells.[260] Regulation of formation and degradation of these tight junctions impact both the integrity of the epithelial barrier and the management of fluid and ion transport in the alveolus. Permeability of the alveolar epithelial barrier to ions and solutes is regulated by the precise distribution and interactions of claudins, which are expressed in a cell-specific manner. Recent studies also implicate claudins in regulation of other cellular functions, such as cell proliferation.[261]

Below the tight junction, the adherens junctions, formed of E-cadherin and β-catenin, connect alveolar epithelial cells under homeostatic conditions.[262] Disruption of adherens junctions can potentiate injury to tight junctions after inflammatory injury to the lung,[263] and breakdown in the adherens junctions is also associated with increased neutrophil infiltration. Both AT1 and AT2 cells also express connexins, form gap junctions, and coordinate cellular signaling in response to stretch and other stimuli. Below the epithelial cell, endothelial cells also form both tight and adherens junctions, forming an additional barrier to passage of fluid, ions, and pathogens.[264] This combination of cellular and extracellular barriers forms a multilayered, resilient, and coordinated system protecting the integrity of the lung.

ALVEOLAR FLUID CLEARANCE AND ION TRANSPORT

An intact barrier is also required to keep the alveolus free of fluid. The close apposition between the alveolar epithelium and the vascular endothelium, in addition to facilitating gas exchange, creates a tight barrier restricting passive movement of liquid, ions, and proteins from the interstitial and vascular spaces, thus assisting in maintaining the relatively dry condition of the alveolar air spaces.[265] Of note, the alveolar epithelium, rather than the endothelium, is believed to be the chief permeability barrier to small, water-soluble molecules.[266,267] Therefore, directed transport of ions, fluid, and proteins across this epithelial layer is essential for maintenance of normal gas exchange and for resolution of both cardiogenic and noncardiogenic pulmonary edema. This transport is made possible via a combination of active and passive transport, mediated by both ion channels and ion pumps.[268] Channels, when open, allow the passive diffusion of ions rapidly down electrical and concentration gradients, which results in the generation of transmembrane electric currents. In contrast, pumps actively transport ions against the electrochemical gradient in an energy-dependent fashion. Ion transporters and other membrane proteins asymmetrically distributed on apical and basolateral surfaces coordinately regulate the directional transport properties of the alveolar epithelium (see Fig. 3.8).[269,270]

For many years, differences in hydrostatic and protein osmotic pressures (Starling forces) were thought to account for the removal of excess fluid from the air spaces of the lung.[270,271] Evidence for the contribution of active ion transport to *alveolar fluid clearance* (AFC) came from extensive in vivo and in vitro experimental studies.[270,272–274] Intratracheally administered fluid is cleared from the alveolus into the interstitium,[275–277] and lymphatic drainage subsequently removes the fluid from the interstitium.[278,279] Clearance is inhibited by amiloride and ouabain, pharmacologic inhibitors of *sodium* (Na^+) channels and Na^+ pumps, respectively,[280,281] emphasizing the importance of Na^+ movement in alveolar fluid clearance. Of interest, there are major species differences in both basal and stimulated rates of AFC, although mechanisms responsible for these differences are not entirely clear.[275,277,281–290]

It is now accepted that the asymmetrical distribution of ion transporters and other membrane proteins on opposing cell surfaces confer directional transport properties to the polarized alveolar epithelium.[270,276] Furthermore, whereas active ion transport was initially thought to be primarily a function of AT2 cells, it is now appreciated that both AT1 and AT2 cells contribute,[26,27,68,70] and it is likely that AT1 cells make a larger contribution to ion transport and fluid clearance than AT2 cells[15,26] due to their extensive surface area. AT1 and AT2 cells express a partially overlapping set of membrane ion channels and pumps, including the *epithelial sodium channel* (ENaC),[270,272,291] *cyclic nucleotide-gated* (CNG) cation channels,[292] *cystic fibrosis transmembrane regulator* (CFTR),[68,293,294] *potassium* (K^+) channels,[295] β-aminobutyric acid type A (GABA$_A$) channels, and voltage-gated *chloride channels* (CLC2 and CLC5) (see Fig. 3.8).[68]

These transporters coordinate to maintain appropriate fluid clearance. Na^+ ions enter *alveolar epithelial cells* (AECs) at the apical membrane and are pumped out at the basolateral membrane by Na^+,K^+-*adenosine triphosphatase* (ATPase).[38,270,276,296] The apical entry step is passive, and Na^+ flows down a chemical potential gradient, whereas basolateral transport requires energy to move ions against the gradient. Because of pump activity, the K^+ electrochemical potential is larger inside the cell, and K^+ leaks through K^+ channels at the basolateral membrane and is then actively transported back into the cell by Na^+,K^+-ATPase to maintain the Na^+ gradient. Mechanisms for Na^+ transport are better understood than are mechanisms for chloride (Cl^-) and K^+ transport.[297] Water channels, including AQPs, participate in passive movement of water through the epithelial barrier, driven by the osmotic gradient created by ion movement. The water channel AQP5, which is localized in the apical plasma membrane of AT1 cells, is thought to be responsible for their extremely high osmotic water permeability,[23,298,299] although, surprisingly, *Aqp5* knockout mice show reduced osmotic water permeability but intact fluid clearance, suggesting that other water channels also participate in fluid clearance by AT1 cells. The molecular basis for water transport across the basal surface of the alveolar epithelium remains unknown.[300,301]

Developmental Ion and Fluid Management

During in utero gestation in mammals (reviewed in Chapter 2), the alveolus is suffused in amniotic fluid and is primarily secretory.[300] During gestation the lung epithelium actively secretes Cl^-, although the precise channel responsible for this activity is unknown. Na^+ is driven across the membrane passively, secondary to high intracellular concentrations and Cl^- flux, and the combined activity of Na^+ and Cl^- provide an osmotic gradient driving water into the alveolar lumen. Absence of appropriate secretion of fluid can lead to development of hypoplastic lungs, a process likely mediated primarily by physical forces, including stretch.[302] At birth, the lung must transition from fluid secretion to fluid absorption.[300,303] Whereas some fluid is mechanically expelled due to compression of the chest wall during labor, the majority of fluid clearance is driven by ENaC; up-regulation of ENaC expression in alveolar epithelium is dependent on the combination of glucocorticoid and thyroid hormone signaling.[304] ENaC activity leads to Na^+ absorption, reversing the gradient for osmotic water flow and helping remove fluid from the alveolus. After this transition, the alveolar surface in the postnatal lung is lined by a thin (average, 0.2 µm) layer of *alveolar lining fluid* (ALF).[305–307] ALF is thought to prevent cells from drying out by preventing direct contact between alveolar epithelial cells and air.[307] The volume, depth, and pH of this fluid are tightly regulated, in part through management of Na^+ flux. Inhibition of ENaC or Na^+,K^+-ATPase reduces fluid clearance in adult lungs by as much as 80%, depending on the species,[270,287,308] and inhibition of either is associated with increased depth of alveolar

TABLE 3.3 Impact of Signaling Pathway Modulation on Alveolar Fluid Clearance

Ion Transport Modulator	Effect on Alveolar Fluid Clearance	Proposed Mechanisms	References
Glucocorticoids	Increased	Up-regulates ENaC expression	370, 409, 410
Thyroid hormone	Increased	Increases Na^+,K^+-ATPase translocation to cell surface	411
Insulin	Increased	Up-regulates ENaC expression	412
Estradiol	Increased	Increases α-ENaC at cell surface	413
Dopamine	Increased	Increases activity of Na^+,K^+-ATPase	414
Leukotriene D4	Increased	Increases activity of Na^+,K^+-ATPase by recruitment of α subunit to membrane	415
Serine proteases	Increased	Activates ENaC	416–418
KGF/FGF7	Increased	Stimulates AT2 cell proliferation and activates ENaC	47, 419–421
EGF	Increased	Increases expression of α and β subunits of Na^+,K^+-ATPase	355, 356
TGF-β	Mixed	Decreases ENaC at membrane and increases Na^+,K^+-ATPase activity	422–424
Purine nucleotides (e.g., adenosine)	Mixed	Regulates ENaC and CFTR activity	374, 425–427
Angiotensin II	Decreased	Decreases cAMP	428
IL-8	Decreased	Decreases cAMP	429
IL-1β	Decreased	Decreases α-ENaC expression and barrier dysfunction	430
TNF-α	Mixed	Mediates barrier dysfunction, but activates ENaC	431–439
Maresins/resolvins	Increased	Stimulates Na^+ channels and Na^+,K^+-ATPase activity	440–442

AT2, alveolar type 2 (cell); ATPase, adenosine triphosphatase; cAMP, cyclic adenosine monophosphate; CFTR, cystic fibrosis transmembrane regulator; EGF, epithelial growth factor; ENaC, epithelial sodium channel; FGF, fibroblast growth factor; IL, interleukin; K^+, potassium ion; KGF, keratinocyte growth factor; Na^+, sodium ion; TGF-β, transforming growth factor-β; TNF-α, tumor necrosis factor-α.

surface fluid. ALF depth influences the diffusion rate for O_2 and carbon dioxide, implying that substantial increases may be deleterious for gas exchange, but limited evidence is available to determine the consequences of changes in ALF volume or composition during more normal conditions.

Roles of Individual Ion Transporters

Epithelial Na^+ channels. The primary pathway for Na^+ entry is via apical amiloride-sensitive ENaC, with basolateral Na^+,K^+-ATPase driving Na^+ into the interstitium to maintain intracellular Na^+ at low levels to allow passive apical transport.[309,310] ENaC channels comprise both *highly selective cation* (HSC) and *nonselective cation* (NSC) channels, with differing cation and amiloride sensitivity. Both AT1 and AT2 cells express the two types of ENaC channels, with HSC exceeding NSC by 10- to 15-fold.[68,311–313] HSC channels have a selectivity for Na^+ over K^+ and are inhibited by amiloride.[68,272] NSC channels are equally selective for Na^+ and K^+ and are inhibited by higher concentrations of amiloride. HSC channels have been proposed to constitute the rate-limiting step for amiloride-sensitive Na^+ absorption.[314] HSC channels are composed of three homologous α, β, and γ subunits.[315–317] A fourth novel δ subunit has been identified in human lungs and most closely resembles the α subunit, but its expression level is low,[318] and its functional role is unclear. The four ENaC subunits have distinct patterns of tissue distribution,[319] and AT1 and AT2 cells express α, β, and γ ENaC subunits.[26,27,68] The composition of NSC channels is less clear; these have been suggested to consist of α-ENaC alone[320] or a combination of α-ENaC with acid-sensing ion channel 1a proteins.[321] ENaC can be regulated

at transcriptional and posttranscriptional levels, including by changes in membrane trafficking and altered stability in the apical membrane. Alterations in activity after physiologic and pathologic factors may contribute to impairment of alveolar fluid clearance (Table 3.3).[309,311,319] α-ENaC knockout mice die at birth due to inability to clear fluid from their lungs,[314,322] and α-ENAC knockdown decreases basal AFC and response to β-agonists.[323] The β and γ subunits appear less important.[324–327]

Cyclic nucleotide-gated channels. Apically located amiloride-insensitive CNG channels provide another Na^+ entry pathway in the alveolar epithelium. CNG channels have been observed in cultured, but not freshly isolated, AT2 cells[328] and in both freshly isolated AT1 cells[68] and AT1 cells in lung slices.[292] CNG channels have equal selectivity for Na^+ and K^+, are inhibited by *guanosine monophosphate* (GMP) inhibitors, stimulated by GMP analogues, and variably blocked by pimozide and L-*cis*-diltiazem.[329] Other Na^+ channels implicated in amiloride-insensitive transport in AECs include the sodium-glucose transporter[330,331] and the Na^+-coupled neutral transporter.[332,333] The exact role of these channels is unclear.[334]

Chloride channels. Both AT1 and AT2 cells express a number of Cl^- transport proteins, including CFTR, the CLC2 and CLC5 channels of the CLC family of voltage-gated Cl^- channels, and the $GABA_A$ channel of the ionotropic receptor family of Cl^- channels[68,69,335,336]; however, consensus is lacking as to their role in adult Cl^- absorption versus secretion in the alveolar epithelium. CFTR allows bidirectional transport of Cl⁻, depending on the electrochemical gradient. Activation of CFTR is dependent on intracellular cAMP or GMP.[337] The role of CFTR in Cl⁻ transport under basal conditions in the adult alveolus is controversial, with some studies demonstrating that CFTR is responsible for Cl⁻ absorption[293,294,337] and other studies demonstrating that CFTR is responsible for Cl⁻ secretion.[335,338,339] Under conditions of β-agonist stimulation, Cl⁻ absorption appears to be important for AFC in whole mouse lungs and human lungs ex vivo. CFTR function in the alveolus is not associated with regulation of lung mucocilliary clearance, an important consequence of CFTR function in the airway epithelium. As noted later, the precise role of Cl⁻ balance remains unclear to date.

Na⁺,K⁺-ATPase. The activity of the Na⁺,K⁺-ATPase pump provides the driving force for Na⁺ resorption by maintaining low intracellular levels of Na⁺. The Na⁺ pump exchanges cytoplasmic Na⁺ for extracellular K⁺ at the basolateral membrane[310] and is inhibited by ouabain. Na⁺,K⁺-ATPase is a heterodimer composed of two subunits, α and β, and small accessory transmembrane proteins that modulate pump activity.[269,340–342] The existence of four α, three β, and up to seven accessory subunit isoforms leads to extensive isozyme diversity.[343] The specific subunit expression pattern of a cell is a major determinant of overall Na⁺ pump activity, based on the differing enzymatic properties of the various isozymes.[344] The α subunit harbors the catalytic domain of the Na⁺ pump, is phosphorylated by ATP, and binds ouabain, whereas the β subunit regulates pump activity and localization at the cell membrane.[340,345,346] Na⁺ pumps comprised of α_1 and β_1 subunits are the predominant isozymes expressed in freshly isolated AT2 and AT1 cells,[26,27,47,347] although the α_2 isoform was also expressed in AT1 cells in whole lung and in cultured AT2 cells.[348] Activity of Na⁺,K⁺-ATPase can be regulated by changes in ion affinity and/or abundance.[349] Na⁺ pumps are also regulated either indirectly in response to increases in intracellular Na⁺[350] or directly by several mechanisms, including β-adrenergic agonists,[351,352] dopamine,[353] corticosteroids,[354] and growth factors,[355,356] among others[343] (see Table 3.3).

Potassium channels. A number of K⁺ channels are present on AECs and are important for maintaining membrane potential and the electrochemical gradient required for ion and fluid transport.[295,297,357] It has been suggested that K⁺ channels modulate fluid clearance through effects of Na⁺ and Cl⁻ transport.[358] Maintenance of high extracellular K⁺ helps maintain Na⁺ gradients through the activity of Na⁺,K⁺-ATPase as noted earlier, and K⁺ (ATP) channels have been functionally identified in freshly isolated and cultured AECs.[358] Potassium channels also have been shown to play a role in O₂ sensing. The precise nature of how these channels function and coordinate with other currents is an area of active investigation.

Physiologic Regulation of Ion and Fluid Transport

Directional fluid transport across the distal pulmonary epithelium is regulated by catecholamine-responsive effects on Na⁺ channels, Na⁺ pumps, and CFTR. Elevated levels of endogenous catecholamines or exogenous administration of β₂-adrenergic receptors can each increase alveolar fluid clearance. Endogenous catecholamines (e.g., epinephrine) stimulate fluid reabsorption from fetal lung at birth[359,360] and increase fluid clearance in conditions such as septic shock[361] and neurogenic pulmonary edema.[362] In most adult mammalian species, stimulation of β₂-adrenergic receptors increases fluid clearance.[284,363–366] Increased fluid clearance in response to β₂-agonists can be inhibited by amiloride or by RNA interference against α-ENaC, indicating that stimulation is related to increased transepithelial Na⁺ transport.[323,364] Both AT2[367,368] and AT1 cells express β₁- and β₂-adrenergic receptors, and increased fluid clearance in response to β₂-agonists can also be inhibited by β₂-adrenergic receptor antagonists.

Chloride transport cooperates with Na⁺ transport during periods of adrenergic stimulation, with in vitro studies suggesting that CFTR-mediated Cl⁻ transport[294] is required for cAMP-stimulated fluid Na⁺ absorption.[337,369–371] Furthermore, β-agonist stimulation does not increase fluid clearance in Δ508 CFTR mice.[366,372] These results contrast with other studies suggesting Cl⁻ secretory pathways are active at baseline in rats,[336] mice,[373] and human AT2 cells,[374] and after terbutaline stimulation in rats[375] and rabbits.[376] Furthermore, in hydrostatic pulmonary edema, reversal of transepithelial Cl⁻ flux via CFTR has been shown to drive alveolar fluid secretion accompanied by inhibition of amiloride-sensitive Na⁺ uptake.[339] Therefore the precise role of Cl⁻ absorption versus secretion during alveolar fluid clearance remains controversial and may depend on the experimental model and specific conditions tested.

Catecholamine-independent mechanisms have also been identified that regulate ion and fluid transport across the distal air spaces of the lung. A number of such pathways are listed in Table 3.3. Effects of many of these modulators, especially growth factors and inflammatory cytokines, are complex because they also affect cell proliferation, barrier function, and resolution of injury independent of effects on ion transport. Several of these modulators provide effects that could potentially be harnessed therapeutically in the future to improve fluid clearance under conditions of alveolar flooding, potentially with additional regenerative effects.

Impaired Fluid Clearance and Resolution of Alveolar Edema Under Pathologic Conditions

Accumulation of fluid in the alveolar air spaces is a common cause of clinically relevant hypoxemia, common to cardiogenic pulmonary edema, usually caused by increases in hydrostatic pressure and conditions of increased vascular and epithelial permeability, such as ARDS. An intact epithelial barrier is crucial for the resolution of alveolar edema in humans.[377] Patients with severe hydrostatic edema generally demonstrate intact fluid clearance.[378] In contrast, most patients with ARDS have markedly impaired fluid clearance, which is associated with worse clinical outcomes.[379] Consistent with the notion that the degree of epithelial injury is an important determinant of outcome in patients with ARDS, elevated levels of RAGE, a marker of AT1 cell injury, correlate with impaired AFC in isolated perfused lungs.[380]

Several conditions coexisting with ARDS also adversely impact fluid clearance and worsen alveolar edema.

Exposure of human AT2 cells to edema fluid from ARDS patients decreased expression of ENaC, Na$^+$,K$^+$-ATPase, and CFTR with reduction in net vectorial fluid transport. Respiratory pathogens, including influenza virus, can impair epithelial fluid transport via direct and indirect effects on ENaC, Na$^+$,K$^+$-ATPase, and CFTR,[381] thus promoting edema accumulation. Chronic alcohol ingestion exacerbates alveolar edema during ARDS due to inhibitory effects on ion transport. Both hypoxemia and hypercapnia can inhibit transepithelial Na$^+$ transport through acute and chronic effects on both ENaC and Na$^+$,K$^+$-ATPase, further limiting fluid clearance and exacerbating alveolar edema.[382,383] Finally, the overall inflammatory milieu during ARDS includes a number of soluble mediators that also impair AFC, including classical proinflammatory cytokines (e.g., TNF-α and L-1β), reactive O$_2$ species and reactive O$_2$-nitrogen species,[384,385] and extracellular nucleotides (see Table 3.3).

Given the impact of decreased fluid clearance on outcomes in ARDS, strategies to increase AFC have been an important focus both experimentally and therapeutically. Although β-adrenergic agonists effectively up-regulate AFC in hydrostatic pulmonary edema and experimental lung injury models,[386–389] two randomized clinical trials of either aerosolized (albuterol) or intravenous selective β$_2$-agonists (salbutamol) failed to show improved clinical outcomes in patients with ARDS, perhaps because the injury to the alveolar epithelium was too severe[390,391] or because of the challenges in delivering the drug to injured alveoli. Similarly, prophylactic use of corticosteroids and β-agonists in patients at risk of developing ARDS was not effective.[392] Other approaches being explored therapeutically include mesenchymal cells, which, among a variety of effects, improve ion transport in experimental models, with conditioned medium from mesenchymal stem cells restoring Na$^+$ transport in primary rat AECs.[393] Further studies will be needed to identify patients who may benefit from tailored strategies to improve AFC and to identify the ideal time to provide such therapy to patients with ARDS.

ALVEOLAR EPITHELIAL REPAIR

After acute injury to the alveolar epithelium, restoration of the cellular components, barrier function, and fluid transport are required to restore gas exchange. Under homeostatic conditions, the alveolar epithelium is relatively quiescent, with limited cell renewal.[44,99,394,395] After injury, AT2 cells proliferate rapidly and differentiate to regenerate the epithelial surface. Landmark studies demonstrating the differentiation of AT2 to AT1 cells were performed in rodents using radiolabeling with tritiated thymidine to identify the proliferating cells after oxidant injury; these studies showed labeling first in AT2 cells and later in AT1 cells.[41–43,396] More recent studies of primary AT2 cells in two-dimensional and three-dimensional culture conditions confirm that AT2 cells serve as a progenitor cell for AT1 cells, whereas genetic lineage tracing experiments in mouse models confirm the progenitor role of AT2 cells for repair of the alveolar epithelium—capable of both self-renewal and differentiation into AT1 cells.[41–44,99,397]

A number of signaling pathways and transcription factors have been implicated in the regulation of AT2 to AT1 cell differentiation, including Wnt/β-catenin,[99,398–401] TGF-β,[48,49,66] Hippo (both YAP and TAZ),[402,403] retinoid X receptor,[63] and Notch.[404] There is also evidence of heterogeneity among AT2 cells, with subsets of cells having greater proliferative capacity[99,405] and ability to give rise to AT1 cells.[99,397,406] Furthermore, single-cell RNA sequencing of AT2 cells during regeneration after lipopolysaccharide-induced lung injury has identified distinct populations of AT2 cells in different states, including proliferating, cell cycle–arrested, and transdifferentiating.[66]

In contrast, AT1 cells have been regarded as terminally differentiated cells without significant proliferative potential, although recent data have shown that a small number of AT1 cells exhibit increased plasticity in mouse models[35] or in culture,[46,57,86,407,408] raising the possibility that at least some AT1 cells are not terminally differentiated. Heterogeneity among AT1 cells was further interrogated by single-cell RNA sequence analysis of postnatal AT1 cells,[65] which demonstrated that 95% of AT1 cells did not proliferate after pneumonectomy or form organoids in culture, suggesting these cells were terminally differentiated. Together, these findings indicate that AT2 cells are the predominant progenitor during alveolar repair and highlight the complexity of the regenerative process. Ongoing work continues to identify the factors needed to balance proliferation and differentiation for effective epithelial repair. For a discussion of additional potential progenitor relationships in the lung and their possible contributions to alveolar repair, see Chapter 8.

DISEASES OF THE DISTAL LUNG EPITHELIUM

Consistent with the central role of the alveolus in the maintenance of functional gas exchange and the complex roles reviewed earlier, numerous disease entities have been identified involving alveolar structure and function. Many of the subsequent chapters in this text contain detailed descriptions of lung diseases with a primary or secondary pathogenesis in alveolar injury. A number of diseases, however, specifically relate to dysfunction of the lung epithelium in one of the key roles reviewed earlier. Table 3.1 lists many of the key clinical entities associated with distal epithelial dysfunction. Of note, these diseases present throughout the human life span, with both congenital and acquired alveolar dysfunction often presenting both in childhood and adulthood. Surfactant mutations, for example, are associated with interstitial lung disease in both children and adults and share some common pathophysiology, while also exhibiting distinct characteristics depending on age of presentation. Alveolar proteinosis (reviewed in Chapter 98) can be acquired, hereditary, or autoimmune. Dysfunctional transport of ions and fluids across the alveolar surface is a prominent feature of ARDS (see Chapter 134) but is also present in rare genetic disorders, such as multisystem pseudohypoaldosteronism. This range and spectrum of disorders associated with alveolar function emphasize the important physiologic roles of the alveolar epithelium and provide a number of opportunities to learn more about alveolar function for a better understanding of dysfunction in disease.

Key Points

- The lung alveolus is the primary site of gas exchange.
- Normal function of the alveolar unit requires the combined function of epithelial, mesenchymal, and endothelial cells.
- Alveolar type 1 cells provide the surface for gas exchange and are active participants in maintenance of alveolar fluid homeostasis.
- Alveolar type 2 cells produce, process, and regulate surfactant components; function in ion transport; participate in immune surveillance; and serve as alveolar progenitor cells during regeneration.
- Surfactant lipids and proteins function to maintain appropriate surface tension to prevent alveolar collapse and function as integral members of the alveolar innate immune system.
- Surfactant processing and pool management are crucial for maintenance of alveolar function.
- Epithelial cells lining the alveolus provide a tight barrier to protect the distal air spaces for gas exchange.
- Resolution of alveolar edema requires an intact epithelial barrier and is driven by active ion transport.
- The primary mechanism for reabsorption of excess alveolar fluid is active Na^+ and Cl^- transport driven by basolaterally located Na^+,K^+-ATPase.
- Alveolar fluid transport is impaired in patients with various forms of lung injury, including acute respiratory distress syndrome.
- Many lung diseases originate from disruption of alveolar structure and function.

Key Readings

Barkauskas CE, et al. Lung organoids: current uses and future promise. *Development.* 2017;144:986–997.

Beers MF, Moodley Y. When is an alveolar type 2 cell an alveolar type 2 cell? A conundrum for lung stem cell biology and regenerative medicine. *Am J Respir Cell Mol Biol.* 2017;57:18–27.

Borok Z. Alveolar epithelium: beyond the barrier. *Am J Respir Cell Mol Biol.* 2014;50:853–856.

Dobbs LG, et al. Highly water-permeable type I alveolar epithelial cells confer high water permeability between the airspace and vasculature in rat lung. *Proc Natl Acad Sci U S A.* 1998;95:2991–2996.

Gadsby DC. Ion channels versus ion pumps: the principal difference, in principle. *Nat Rev Mol Cell Biol.* 2009;10:344–352.

Hanukoglu I, Hanukoglu A. Epithelial sodium channel (ENaC) family: phylogeny, structure-function, tissue distribution, and associated inherited diseases. *Gene.* 2016;579:95–132.

Hogan BLM, et al. Repair and regeneration of the respiratory system: complexity, plasticity, and mechanisms of lung stem cell function. *Cell Stem Cell.* 2014;15(2):123–138.

Koval M. Claudin heterogeneity and control of lung tight junctions. *Annu Rev Physiol.* 2013;75:551–567.

Marconett CN, et al. Cross-species transcriptome profiling identifies new alveolar epithelial type I cell-specific genes. *Am J Respir Cell Mol Biol.* 2017;56:310–321.

Pattle RE. Properties, function, and origin of the alveolar lining layer. *Nature.* 1955;175:1125–1126.

Reyfman PA, et al. Single-cell transcriptomic analysis of human lung provides insights into the pathobiology of pulmonary fibrosis. *Am J Respir Crit Care Med.* 2019;199:1517–1536.

Weibel ER. On the tricks alveolar epithelial cells play to make a good lung. *Am J Respir Crit Care Med.* 2015;191:504–513.

Whitsett JA, Weaver TE. Hydrophobic surfactant proteins in lung function and disease. *N Engl J Med.* 2002;347:2141–2148.

Wilson SM, Olver RE, Walters DV. Developmental regulation of lumenal lung fluid and electrolyte transport. *Respir Physiol Neurobiol.* 2007;159:247–255.

Complete reference list available at ExpertConsult.com.

4 *AIRWAY BIOLOGY*

STEVEN L. BRODY, MD • CHRISTOPHER M. EVANS, PhD

INTRODUCTION

The primary function of the airways is to allow airflow while protecting the alveolar compartment from the hazards in environmental air. The airway is constantly exposed to pathogens, particles, allergens, and toxic pollutants (Fig. 4.1). It is not surprising that airway responses to acute and chronic environmental exposure directly account for a significant proportion of the burden of lung disease in respiratory virus infections, asthma, COPD, bronchiectasis, and *cystic fibrosis* (CF). Airway structure, cellular functions, host response, genetic variants, and the nature of exposure are important factors in pathologic responses. As a platform for understanding the biologic basis of disease, normal human airway structure and function, cellular components, physiologic functions, and the cellular and molecular control of airway functions are described in this chapter. Chapters 70 to 72 cover diseases of the airways, in particular upper airway disorders, large airway disorders, and bronchiolitis.

OVERVIEW

AIRWAY STRUCTURE AND CELLULAR COMPONENTS

Airways are divided anatomically into upper and lower divisions, which can be conceptually separated at the level of the vocal cords (see Fig. 4.1). Airway surfaces possess a continuous layer of epithelial cells with regional differences in morphology, function, and gene expression patterns.

UPPER AIRWAY STRUCTURE AND FUNCTION

The upper airway consists of the nose, paranasal sinuses, posterior pharynx, and larynx, although some sources consider the trachea as part of the upper airway.[1,2]

Paranasal sinuses are highly vascularized to provide warming and humidification of air. The nasal mucosa covers 160 cm^2 and secretes 20 to 40 mL/day of mucus.[3] Foreign particles impact on nasal and oropharyngeal surfaces, where they become trapped in mucus or saliva for elimination by expectoration or swallowing. Thus, the upper airway epithelium defends the lung from particles, allergens, and pathogens by mucociliary clearance, swallowing, coughing, and innate barrier function.[4] Particles cleared by the upper airways are typically large (≥10 μm diameter). Smaller particles (particularly <0.5 μm diameter) bypass the mouth and sinuses to deposit in the lower airways[5,6] (see also Chapter 70).

LOWER AIRWAY STRUCTURE AND FUNCTION

The general structure of the lower airway allows movement of inspired gas from the trachea to large airways, then to a very large number of smaller airways, which create a huge cross-sectional surface area. The continuous branching of the airways limits access of particles and pathogens by impaction in large airways and by deposition in smaller airways.[7]

Airway components and cell populations vary with airway generation, from the upper airway to the conducting zone and finally the respiratory zone (Table 4.1) (see also Chapter 1). The large tracheobronchial portion of the airway has greater amounts of airway wall collagen, smooth muscle, and autonomic innervation relative to bronchiolar portions. Within the first 10 to 12 airway generations, smooth muscle, cartilage plates or plaques, and *submucosal glands* (SMGs) are abundant (Fig. 4.2).[8–10] A surrounding structure of incomplete cartilaginous rings and plates, together with smooth muscle, allows airways to remain pliable during breathing while preventing airway collapse.[11] Distal to the

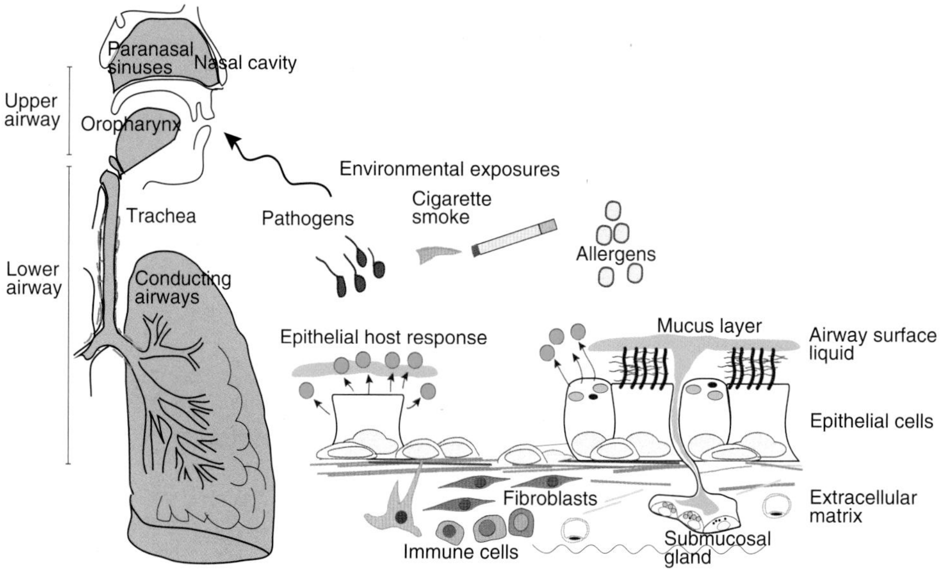

Figure 4.1 Cellular responses of airways to injury. Upper and lower airways are subject to environmental exposures that lead to defensive epithelial responses provided by secreted mucus (*green*) and secreted peptides (*blue*). Upper airway includes the nasal cavity and paranasal sinuses; the lower airway includes the trachea and conducting airways of the lung. Injury and epithelial cell responses are coordinated with responses of the submucosal glands, extracellular matrix, and immune cells.

Table 4.1 Airway Structures

Airway Component (Approximate Generation)	Cartilage	Smooth Muscle	Major Epithelial Cell Types
UPPER AIRWAY			
Nasal and paranasal sinuses	+++	+	Squamous, ciliated and mucous cells; olfactory epithelial cells, SMG
CONDUCTING ZONE			
Trachea (0)	+++	++	Tall columnar ciliated and mucous/goblet cells; SMG
Bronchi (1–3)	++	++	
Small bronchi (4–10)	+	+++	Columnar ciliated and secretory; SMG
Bronchioles (11–14)	0	+	Cuboidal ciliated and secretory cells
RESPIRATORY ZONE			
Respiratory bronchioles (16–18)	0	0	Cuboidal secretory cells
Alveolar ducts (19–22)	0	0	Squamous-like secretory cells
Alveolar sacs (23)	0	0	Alveolar epithelial type 1 and 2 cells

Abundance scored 0 to +++.
SMG, submucosal glands.
Data from Hayward J, Reid LM. Observations on the anatomy of the intrasegmental bronchial tree. *Thorax.* 1952;7(1):89-97.

trachea and mainstem bronchi, airways are embedded within and attached to the lung parenchyma. This "tethering" provides structural and functional interdependence of airways and alveoli during lung inflation and deflation.[12]

Bronchi are primarily lined by ciliated cells and mucin-secreting cells that contribute to the mucociliary escalator for clearance. Mucin refers to the glycoproteins forming a viscoelastic mucus hydrogel for maintaining tissue hydration and supporting host defense (see later). SMG ducts are found along large airway surfaces at a frequency of 0.5 to 1 gland opening/mm².[13] Lymph nodes on the outer surface of the trachea and bronchi provide antigen processing for defense in infection, but they may also contribute to metastases in cancer and immune hyperreactivity in asthma.[14]

Bronchioles are lined with ciliated cells and secretory club cells, but they contain few mucin-secreting cells,

lack cartilage and submucosal glands, and show progressive decreases in smooth muscle (see Fig. 4.2D). Bronchioles have diameters of less than 2 mm, compared to the 2 mm or greater size of bronchi. Whereas airway diameters provide practical means for identifying "small" and "large" airways, the specific distinction between bronchioles and bronchi are defined by their histologic composition.

See ExpertConsult.com for a discussion of airflow principles.

MICROVASCULATURE

Airway Microvasculature

Airway tissues are supplied with blood by the systemic bronchial circulation.[20] Bronchial arteries branch off from the aorta and extend longitudinally along bronchi to the terminal bronchioles.[21] A plexus of bronchial microvessels in airway walls perfuse tissues while also warming and

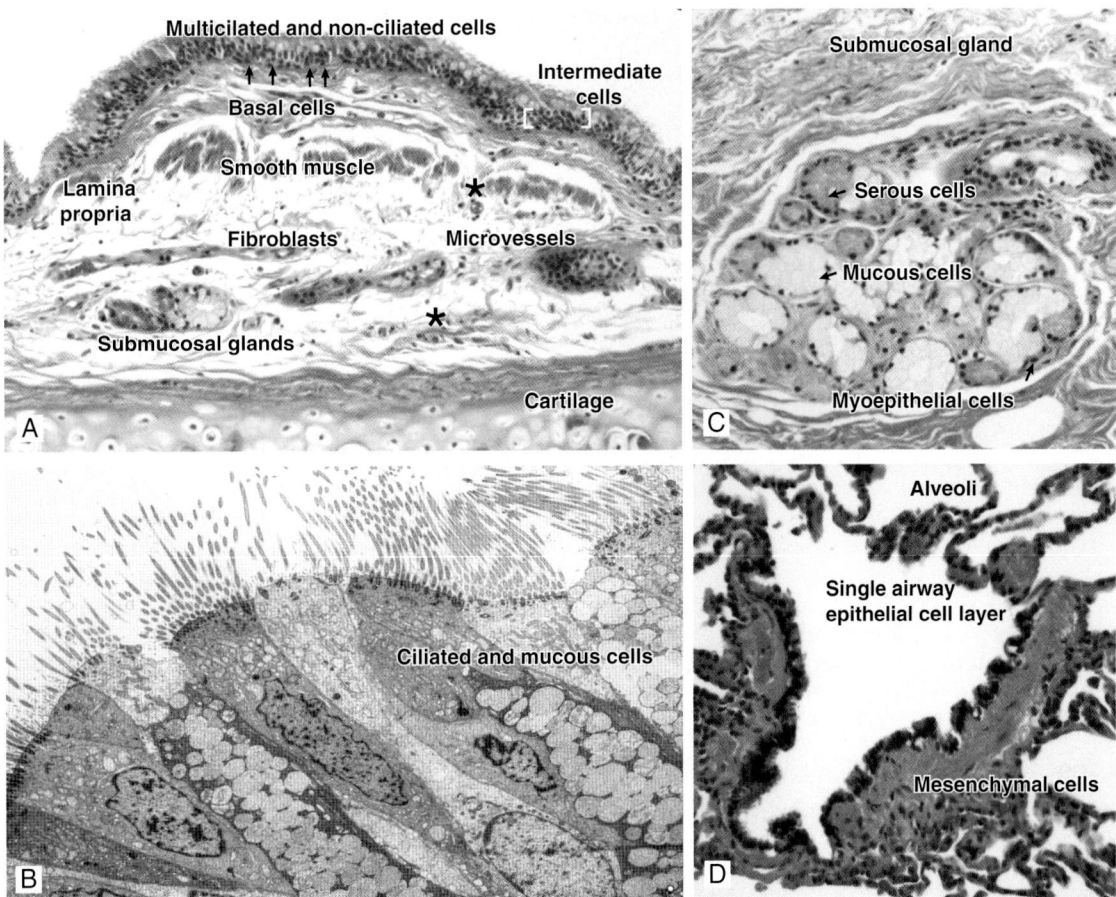

Figure 4.2 Airway structures and cell types. (A) Cellular components and epithelial architecture of bronchi demonstrating a pseudostratified layer. Basal cells are indicated by *arrows*, intermediate cells by *white brackets*, and microvasculature by *asterisks* above vessels. (B) Ultrastructure of bronchial multiciliated and mucous cells by transmission electron microscopy. (C) Epithelial cell types in submucosal glands. (D) Epithelial architecture of terminal bronchiole, demonstrating a single layer of epithelial cells and absence of mucosal glands and smooth muscle. (Hematoxylin and eosin stain.) (Courtesy Dr. Steven L. Brody.)

humidifying large airways.[22] The bronchial arteries drain either to the azygous vein or into the pulmonary veins; the latter route constitutes a small right-to-left shunt as deoxygenated bronchial venous flow enters the oxygenated postcapillary blood.

The airway microvasculature is embedded within the subepithelial matrix and supported by collagen IV in the epithelial lamina propria (see Fig. 4.2). Pericytes that wrap around the capillary and postcapillary venules help maintain endothelial integrity in health. Signals from the endothelium, such as nitric oxide, control vascular tone, while the surrounding extracellular matrix–endothelial interactions maintain normal levels of angiogenesis. Following airway injury, proteolytic extracellular matrix fragments and activated pericytes emit inflammatory signals that can alter endothelial cell function and lead to angiogenesis and remodeling.[23,24]

Mechanisms that regulate flow in the bronchial circulation are extrapolated from animal studies to humans.[22] Bronchial microvessels express α- and β-adrenergic receptors that respond to sympathetic neurotransmission.[25] Adrenergic control of airway vascular tone is dependent on nitric oxide and is sensitive to endothelium-mediated dilation, which, along with histamine, prostaglandin F2α, prostacyclin, and bradykinin, likely play roles in vascular leak and remodeling in airway diseases.

Airway Lymphatic Vessels

Airways also incorporate an extensive network of lymphatic vessels.[26] The importance of lymphatics in fluid homeostasis is especially evident in preterm infants, whose poorly developed lymph networks may contribute to bronchopulmonary dysplasia. Lymph vessels are lined internally by endothelial cells, which, like blood vessels, express the surface protein CD31, but lymphatic endothelial cells also express Prox1 and vascular endothelial growth factor receptor. These and other lymphatic endothelial markers are being used to understand the importance of lung lymphatics in health and disease[27] (see Chapter 7).

Microvascular-Related Inflammation

The airway microvasculature is an important regulator of airway inflammatory responses.[25,28,29] Endothelial cells express cell adhesion proteins, in particular E-selectin, intracellular adhesion molecule-1, and endothelial leukocyte adhesion molecule-1, that facilitate leukocyte attachment. Stimuli such as cigarette smoke, allergens, and viruses cause endothelial cell production of inflammatory mediators. Proinflammatory factors contribute to the disassembly of tight junctions between endothelial cells, allowing leukocytes to migrate into tissues and air spaces. Endothelial cells produce angiogenic growth factors that induce vascular remodeling in airways disease such as asthma, COPD, and bronchiectasis,[29] potentially through the recruitment of bone marrow–derived endothelial progenitors.[25,30,31]

EXTRACELLULAR MATRIX AND FIBROBLASTS

Structural support and biomechanical properties of lung tissues, including recoil of the airways, is provided by *extracellular matrix* (ECM), consisting of proteins, proteoglycans, and glycosaminoglycans. ECM makes up the thin basal lamina (basement membrane) firmly linked to airway epithelial cells by fibronectin and integrin proteins and also fills the interstitial space (lamina propria) to provide structure and organization to the airway. ECM is produced mainly by the resident fibroblasts, although many other cell types can contribute. (See also Chapter 5.)

ECM is composed of over 300 proteins (collectively called the matrisome), including collagens, elastin, fibrous glycoproteins, fibronectin, laminin, and heparan sulfate proteoglycans.[32] In addition to structural support, integrins relay signals between mucosal epithelia and submucosal microcirculation, lymphatics, fibroblasts, cartilage, and smooth muscle.[32–34] ECM serves as a storage depot for growth factors such as transforming growth factor-β and cytokines, which regulate cell growth, inflammation, repair, and remodeling.[32]

Anatomic Specificity of Extracellular Matrix

ECM composition differs in tracheobronchial, bronchiolar, and alveolar compartments. Across the lung, collagen is the major structural component providing airway elasticity. However, among compartments, the subtypes of collagen, the fibrous nature of collagen structure, and the composition of noncollagen ECM components differ greatly (eTable 4.1).

A discussion of additional protein components is available at ExpertConsult.com.

ECM Alterations in Airway Disease. Remodeling of the ECM is a characteristic of diseases of the airways, including asthma and chronic bronchitis,[45–52] as well as diseases of the lung parenchyma, such as emphysema, pulmonary hypertension, pulmonary fibrosis, and lung cancer,[53–58] that can have etiologic relationships to airway diseases.[32,44,59] Changes in ECM with diseased lungs are related to changes in the production and cross-linking of collagen (eFig. 4.1, and see eTable 4.1), and also to changes in elastin, and other proteins and proteoglycans. Persistent activity of proteases such as *matrix metalloproteinases* (MMPs) and leukocyte-derived elastases further contributes to matrix remodeling and pathology.[32]

SMOOTH MUSCLE

Airway smooth muscle (ASM) surrounds the large airways. In health, the role of ASM contraction is debated.[60] ASM may limit airway distension during normal breathing and cough. ASM may also sequester damaged or infected lung regions to promote ventilation of healthy tissues, and it may compress SMGs to facilitate mucus secretion. Although these homeostatic functions of ASM are unclear, it is well known that ASM contraction causes airway obstruction in asthma and COPD.[61] Accordingly, for maintaining healthy airflow steady state, ASM relaxation is crucial.

ASM normally exists in a relaxed state due to low-level contractile stimulation and to tonic activation of bronchodilatory signals.[62] Contraction is caused by Ca^{2+}-dependent activation of myosin light chain kinase, which stimulates formation of actin-myosin cross-bridges that shorten myocytes. Reversal of myosin light chain kinase phosphorylation and sequestration of intracellular Ca^{2+} are drivers of smooth muscle relaxation.[63]

The main ASM relaxant signal originates from interaction of circulating epinephrine with β_2-adrenergic receptors on ASM.[62,64–67] β_2-receptors stimulate dilation by increasing intracellular cyclic adenosine monophosphate and decreasing intracellular calcium levels (eFig. 4.2). ASM relaxation is also induced by non-adrenergic noncholinergic neurons using *nitric oxide* (NO) and vasoactive intestinal peptide as neurotransmitters[62,68–70] (eTable 4.2).

Steady-state bronchodilation can be overridden by stimuli such as airway surface irritants, chemicals, and inflammatory mediators, leading to ASM contraction and bronchoconstriction. Bronchoconstriction may also be activated by ASM mechanosensory and neural reflex responses[71–73] (eTable 4.2).

INNERVATION

Airway neural control derives from *central nervous system* (CNS) and peripheral nervous system pathways that coordinate breathing,[74–76] airflow, and host defense.[77,78] CNS centers regulate breathing rate and depth by integrating voluntary and involuntary (sensory) inputs from the peripheral nervous system. Efferent signals from the medulla and pons transmit signals that stimulate contraction and relaxation of diaphragm and intercostal muscles during breathing. Additional innervation and muscle contractions control the glottis and larynx during consciously controlled breathing, sneezing, or coughing.[74,75]

To regulate airflow and host defense, CNS and peripheral nervous system pathways exert autonomic control over airway structures (Fig. 4.3). The predominant autonomic control is supplied by the vagus nerves.[72] Neurally mediated bronchoconstriction is mediated by parasympathetic vagal fibers that impinge upon ganglia embedded in tracheobronchial airway submucosal tissues.[72] Inflammatory signals can activate sensory nerves and evoke reflex-mediated bronchoconstriction.

Afferent Autonomic Control of Airway Smooth Muscle

Trachea, bronchi, and bronchioles contain vagal sensory nerve termini.[74,79–81] These nerves have cell bodies in the jugular and nodose ganglia and transmit mechanoreceptive and chemoreceptive signals to synapses in the medulla. The main vagal sensory neurotransmitters in the CNS are gamma-aminobutyric acid and glutamate, and their signals can be potentiated or suppressed by peptide neurotransmitters called tachykinins.[74,76]

Local sensory nerves also terminate in the airway, where the tachykinins, substance P, neurokinin A, and neurokinin B amplify parasympathetic neurotransmission[82,83] independent of CNS-mediated reflexes.[84,85]

However, M_2 receptors on prejunctional nerve terminals can mediate bronchodilation by suppressing vagally induced acetylcholine release by 80–90%[100,101]; absence of neuronal M_2 inhibitory function causes excessive ASM contraction in animal models of airway obstruction.[102–107] Given the pleiotropic effects of M_2 receptor functions, highly selective M_3 receptor antagonists such as tiotropium have been developed for clinical use as bronchodilators.[95–99]

Other Neural Controls

Additional nonvagal inputs from nerves originating in cervical and thoracic vertebrae and in dorsal root ganglia affect the lower airways (see Fig. 4.3). These include sensory signals involved in airway tone and cough via substance P and efferent signals mediated by norepinephrine and neuropeptide Y that affect SMG secretion.[75,108] Additional sympathetic fibers also regulate vascular flow.

AIRWAY EPITHELIUM

MORPHOLOGY

The tracheobronchial epithelium is pseudostratified, meaning it appears as a multilayered sheet even though it is actually a single layer of cells (see Fig. 4.2). Each cell is firmly attached to the basal lamina, thereby establishing basal-to-apical polarity.[109] From the trachea to the bronchioles, epithelia progressively transition from pseudostratified columnar to simple cuboidal morphologies. Throughout this proximal-distal axis, the heights of individual epithelial cells and thickness of mucosal sheets and submucosal layers also decrease.[17,109,110] Along the distal respiratory bronchioles, the cuboidal epithelial layer becomes discontinuous as conducting airways transition to alveoli.

CELL-CELL JUNCTIONS

Airway Barrier Function

Airway epithelial cells have specialized structures mediating attachment to the ECM and to neighboring cells. In both upper and lower airways, physical barrier function is provided by adhesion of epithelial cells to basal lamina through hemidesmosomes,[111] which are rich in proteins called integrins. The integrin α6β4 facilitates communication between the epithelial cell cytoskeleton and the ECM to provide structural integrity, mechano-coupling, and host defense.[112] The basolateral attachments are also selectively permeable to regulate ion and water flux.

Types of lateral attachments include desmosomes, tight junctions, and adherens junctions (eFig. 4.3).[113–123] These junction complexes provide basolateral barrier strength, cell-cell communication, and control of the selective movements of molecules across cells. Lateral junctions may be disrupted by injury and inflammatory responses following exposure to toxicants, particulates, or pathogens, leading to paracellular leak.[114,120,124,125] In addition, disruption of epithelial junctions triggers epidermal growth factor receptor–mediated repair programs.[125]

Additional junctions are discussed at ExpertConsult.com.

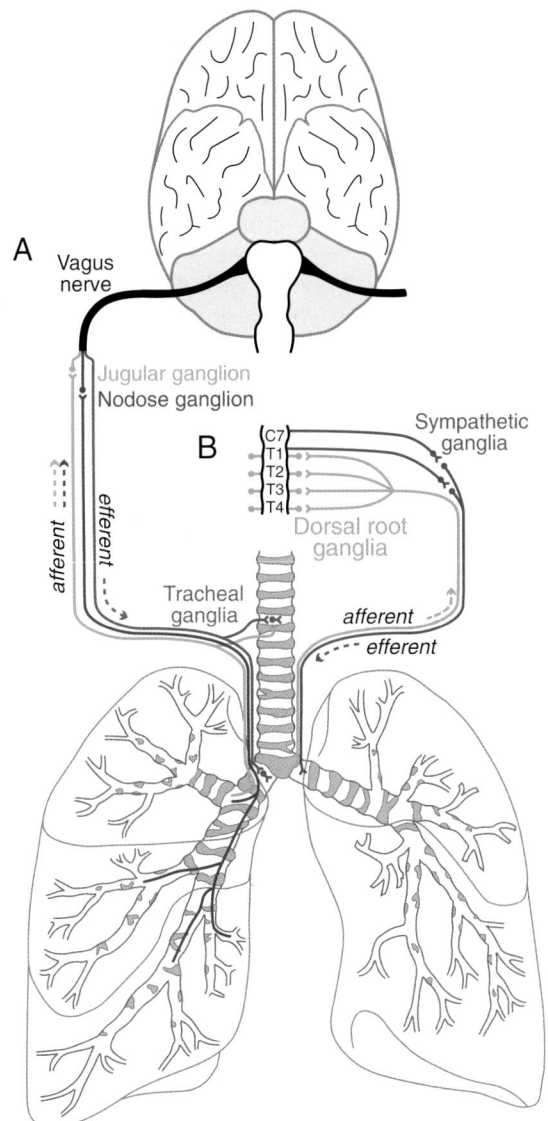

Figure 4.3 Autonomic innervation of the lung. (A) Cranial innervation from the vagus nerve (*black*) includes afferent sensory nerves with cell bodies in jugular (*green*) and nodose (*blue*) ganglia and efferent fibers with cell bodies in tracheal ganglia (*violet*). Postganglionic cholinergic fibers extend into the airways (*violet*). (B) Spinal innervation from afferent fibers (*orange*) with cell bodies in dorsal root ganglia transmit signals to the central nervous system, and efferent fibers (*red*) with cell bodies in the sympathetic ganglia transmit adrenergic signals to the pulmonary vasculature (not shown).

Efferent Autonomic Control of Airway Smooth Muscle

The dominant neural control of ASM contraction is provided by parasympathetic fibers within the vagi.[86–91] Acetylcholine released by parasympathetic nerves stimulates contraction by activating M_3 muscarinic receptors on ASM.[92] In contrast to M_3 receptors, M_2 receptors found on the ASM or on the nerve terminals can have pleiotropic effects. For example, M_2 muscarinic receptor subtypes on ASM facilitate contraction by suppressing β_2-adrenergic receptor signaling.[93,94] Thus, antagonism of the muscarinic receptors on ASM dilates human airways, which can be useful for treating obstructive lung diseases.[95–99]

CELL POPULATIONS

Upper Airway Epithelial Cells

The majority of the nasal airway epithelium is lined by ciliated respiratory epithelium with numerous interspersed mucous cells. In humans, olfactory cells cover only a small percentage of the epithelium (<5%). Squamous epithelial cells dominate the posterior pharynx, with the exception of specialized cells in the adenoids and tonsils. The luminal aspect of the adenoids is comprised of multiciliated and secretory cells, whereas surfaces of the tonsils have secretory cells.[126]

Lower Airway Epithelial Cell Populations and Frequencies

Major epithelial cell types present within the conducting airway epithelium are basal, intermediate, multiciliated, mucous, club, and pulmonary neuroendocrine cells[127,128]

(Fig. 4.4). At the epithelial-lumen surface, approximately equal proportions of ciliated and nonciliated cells can be identified based on morphologies.[129]

In addition to cell appearances, the use of molecular markers and single-cell RNA sequencing reveals a more nuanced and complex view of the lung epithelium in health and disease.[4,130–134] At least a dozen well-defined epithelial cell populations can be found in the upper and lower airways (Table 4.2).[127,128,132–134] Mouse studies have laid the groundwork for understanding each epithelial cell type at molecular and functional levels.

Basal Cells

Airway basal cells are small round cells located on the basal epithelial layer, adherent to the basement membrane throughout the airway, and function as stem cells and barrier components.[110,135] The essential markers of the basal

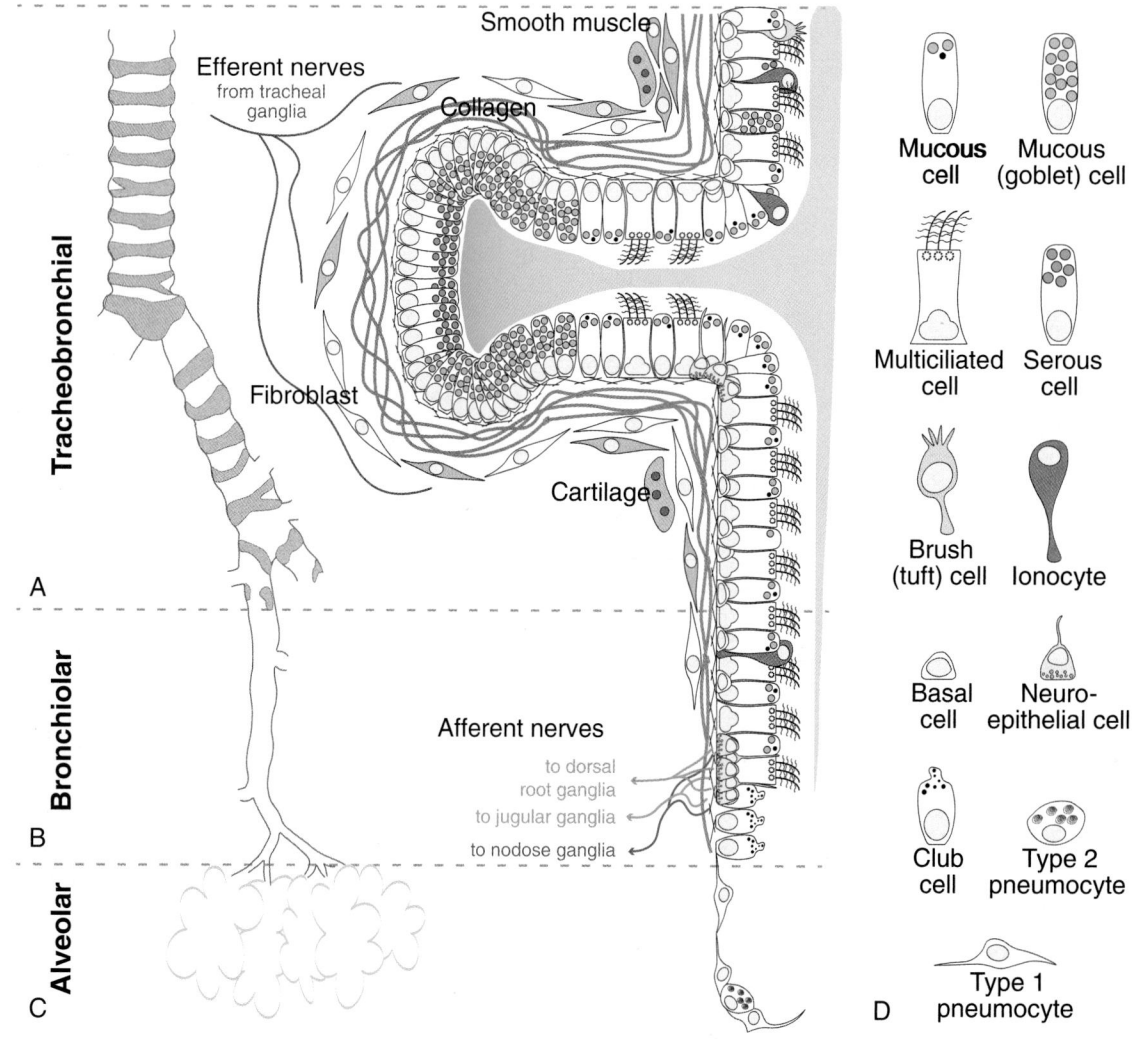

Figure 4.4 Airway cell types. (A) Tracheobronchial airway walls have abundant cartilage, extracellular matrix, and smooth muscle, as well as submucosal glands. Epithelial cells at tracheobronchial surfaces include mucous cells, mucin-packed goblet-shaped mucous cells, serous cells, and multiciliated cells that all contribute to airway surface liquid hydration and mucociliary defense. Hydration and defense properties are strongly enhanced locally by neurally regulated secretions from serous and mucous cells within submucosal glands. Brush cells and ionocytes are rare epithelial types that sense and control the chemical and ionic environments at airway surfaces. (B) Bronchioles have progressively thinner airway walls, with many of the same epithelial cell types found in the tracheobronchial airways, including basal cells. Neuroepithelial cells and club cells are enriched in bronchioles, where they have progenitor, chemosensory, and detoxification functions. Neuroepithelial cells found in clusters called neuroepithelial bodies are innervated by sensory fibers. (C) Distal airways include club cell–lined respiratory bronchioles that terminate at type 1 and type 2 pneumocyte-lined alveoli. (D) Figure key identifying distal airway cell types depicted in A–C.

Table 4.2 Epithelial Cell Types and Features

Cell Type	Morphology and Markers	Major Functions	Location
Basal cells	Small Round Attached to lamina propria *Markers:* TRP63, KRT5	Stem/progenitor	Trachea, bronchi, bronchioles ≈5% in terminal bronchioles
Ciliated cells	Columnar Multiple apical motile cilia *Markers:* Acetylated α-tubulin, FOXJ1	Airway clearance Osmoregulation	Lumen interface in large and small airways
Club cells	Columnar Secretory vesicles Head of cell may protrude into lumen (bronchioles) *Markers:* SCGB1A1, MUC5B	Xenobiotic metabolism Host defense Progenitor Osmoregulation	Bronchioles Absent in trachea and bronchi
Mucous cells	Columnar Large cytoplasmic vesicles varying in numbers and contents Small base (goblet) *Markers:* MUC5AC, MUC5B, CLCA1, SCGB1A1	Host defense Hydration Stem/progenitor Mucin secretion	Submucosal glands Lumen interface in large and small airways <3% in terminal bronchioles
Intermediate cells	Positioned between basal and well-differentiated ciliated, club, and mucous cells. *Markers:* none specific, MYB	Pre-specialized or progenitor	Variable in large airways with multilayered epithelium
Pulmonary neuroendocrine cells	Irregular shaped Dendrites Found in insolation or in clusters (NE bodies) Basolaterally secreted vesicles *Markers:* CGRP, CGA	Chemosensory Stem/progenitor	Rare in all levels Enriched at airway branch points
Ionocytes	Small cells *Marker:* FOXI1, CFTR	Osmoregulation	Very rare Present in bronchi Not well described in humans
Brush (or tuft) cells	Pear-shaped Short apical microvilli *Markers:* ACh-containing vesicles, bitter-taste receptors	Chemosensory Secrete IL-25 postinjury	Very rare Present throughout airways Not well described in humans

ACh, acetylcholine; CFTR, cystic fibrosis transmembrane conductance regulator; CGA, chromogranin A; CGRP, calcitonin gene–related peptide; CLCA1, calcium-activated chloride channel regulation 1; Il-25, interleukin-25; MUC, mucin; NE, neuroepithelial; SCGB1A1, secretoglobin 1A1.
Data from references 132, 133, 135, 161, 177, 423, 424.

cell are the transcriptional regulator transformation protein 63 (p63) and the intermediate filament cytokeratin keratin 5, with its heterodimeric partner keratin 14.[136] In the human airway, basal cells are found in the nasal sinuses and throughout the large and small airways, including the most distal regions. Basal cells are occasionally noted in the bronchoalveolar ducts, the site of transition to the alveoli.[135] The wide distribution of basal cells in human airways is in marked contrast to the mouse, where basal cells are rarely observed distal to the large bronchi.

Intermediate Cells

During repair and regeneration, proliferating basal cells move from the basal lamina toward the lumen, to an intermediate position beneath the well-differentiated luminal cells[135–137] (see Fig. 4.2). These intermediate cells lose typical basal cell markers through down-regulation of p63[136] and lack histologic features of specialized cells, so they are also referred to as parabasal or indeterminant cells. Analysis by single-cell RNA sequencing during differentiation reveals transcriptional features of preciliated or presecretory cells. Specific molecular markers are not known, but transcription factor MYB is expressed in a subpopulation of intermediate cells.[138] Though still poorly understood functionally, intermediate cells may serve as reserve

populations for mature types while also serving structural and host defense roles.

Multiciliated Cells. Ciliated cells are the most common type of differentiated cells lining the airway lumen of the bronchi and are present in high proportions in the bronchi and in SMG ducts. The major function of multiciliated cells is airway clearance, which is driven by movements of motile cilia that project apically into air spaces. These cells are referred to as multiciliated cells to avoid confusion with cells that have a single, sensory (nonmotile) cilium.[139] Multiciliated cells are terminally differentiated[140] and have 200 to 300 motile cilia, each 5 to 8 μm in length, that extend into the lumen (Fig. 4.5).[141] Multiciliated cell height and cilia length decrease along the proximal-distal axis of the airways.

In addition to the presence of apical cilia that may be identified by the presence of acetylated α-tubulin, other features of multiciliated cells include the expression of transcription factor FOXJ1, which regulates the assembly of motile cilia.[142,143] The cells also contain hundreds of basal bodies docked in an actin mesh at the apical membrane.[144] Cilia arise from each basal body.

The ultrastructure of the ciliary cytoskeleton or *axoneme* is a circular 9 + 2 arrangement of paired microtubules

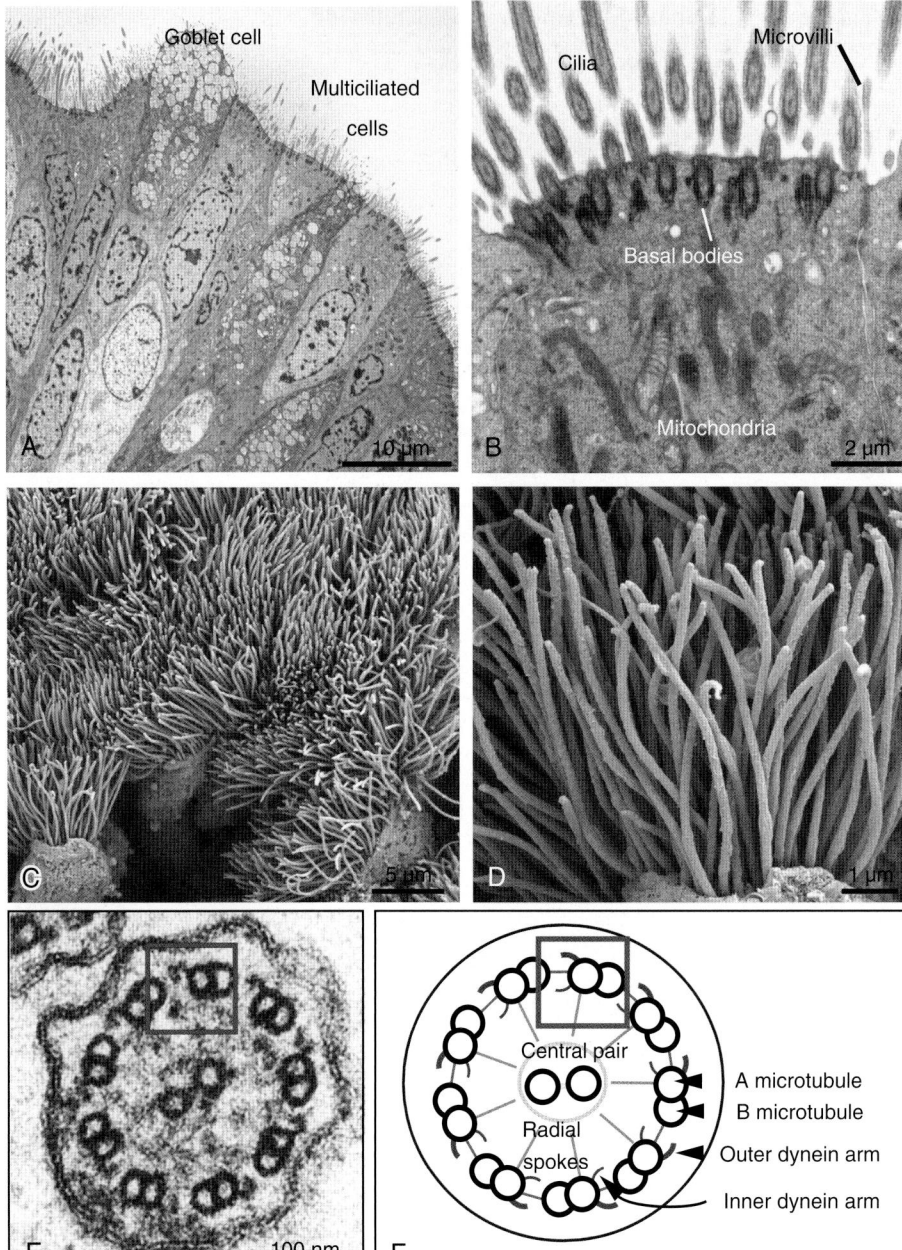

Figure 4.5 Multiciliated airway epithelial cells. (A) Ultrastructure of multiciliated and goblet cells in human bronchi by transmission electron microscopy. (B) Detail of the apical region of a multiciliated cell showing basal bodies with rootlets securing the cilia and relative to the mitochondria. (C) *Scanning electron micrograph* (SEM) of cilia on the surface of a human bronchus. (D) SEM of a single ciliated cell. (E) SEM of transverse section of ciliary axoneme (i.e., cytoskeleton of the cilia). (F) Diagram of part E indicating microtubule organization and the location of dynein motor complexes. Outer doublet A and B microtubules, inner pair, and connecting spokes are shown. Dynein motor complexes appear as arms on the inner and outer portion of the A microtubule. The box shows the same structures in the SEM image and the diagram. (A–E, Courtesy Dr. Steven L. Brody.)

composed of nine outer doublets and a central pair organization (see Fig. 4.5).[141,145] The outer doublets hold dynein motor complexes that power the cilia beating.[146–148] Cilia beat at a frequency of 8 to 15 Hz (8-15 beats/second), as measured ex vivo[149,150] (Video 4.1). Mutations in the genes coding for the motor proteins and ciliary assembly machinery result in abnormal ciliary motility, defining the autosomal recessive disease, primary ciliary dyskinesia[151] (see also Chapter 69).

Secretory Cells

Lumen-facing secretory cells are identified by the presence of cytoplasmic secretory vesicles (or granules) classified based on their numbers, subcellular localization, morphology, and cargo. Secretory cells include mucous cells, serous cells, and club cells. These determinations can be made morphologically by electron microscopy or histochemically by light microscopy and the use of dyes, antibodies, or lectins to identify their secreted products.[152,153] Secretory cells are less numerous than either the ciliated or basal cells.[129] Secretory cells are also present in SMGs.

There is some overlap in secretory cell types depending on whether they are defined by morphologic versus molecular criteria. There is also considerable interspecies heterogeneity in the abundance, distribution, and ultrastructure of secretory cell types in the airways, so experimental studies in nonhuman species must be considered carefully for their relevance to humans.

Mucous Cells

Cells containing abundant granules filled with secreted gel-forming mucin glycoproteins are called mucous cells. Mucous cells can be identified by electron microscopy with dyes such as Alcian blue and periodic acid–Schiff stain,[154] or with molecular markers for airway mucins such as *mucin 5B* (MUC5B) and MUC5AC.[154–157] Throughout the airways, MUC5B and MUC5AC are the most abundant gel-forming mucins produced in the airways of healthy individuals.[154] In general, MUC5B is the predominant mucin produced in health, and MUC5AC is increased during inflammation.[132–134,154,158–160]

Goblet cells are recognized by their characteristic morphology. When mucous cells accumulate large numbers of granules at their apices, they have a disproportionately small basal lamina attachment site and assume a swollen cuplike morphology or goblet-like appearance (see Fig. 4.5A). Thus goblet cells are a subclass of mucous cells. Historically, "goblet" and "mucous" were terms used to distinguish cells at airway surfaces and at SMGs, respectively. However, these morphologic appraisals are not accurate descriptors of molecular identity. In fact, cells with goblet-shaped morphologies account for the majority of mucous cells in the SMG and also along the surfaces of the large airways.

Although goblet-shaped cells are undetectable in bronchioles by electron microscopy,[129] Alcian blue and periodic acid–Schiff staining, RNA in situ hybridization, and anti-MUC5B antibody labeling reveal that mucin-producing cells are indeed present in bronchioles. These mucous cells account for up to 50% of the luminal epithelia in proximal bronchioles, become less prevalent in terminal bronchioles, and are absent from respiratory bronchioles.[154,161]

Serous cells are secretory cells with electron-dense apical secretory granules that do not stain positively with Alcian blue or periodic acid–Schiff stain. Serous cells are present along large surfaces, but they are most abundant in SMGs. Within the SMGs, serous cells are sources of water and defensive proteins such as lactoferrin, lysozyme, and defensins.[162–164]

Club cells are a subclass of secretory cells with a morphologically distinct clublike or dome-shaped head that may extend into the lumen, a particularly prominent feature in rodent lungs.[152,165] Club cells are defined by the expression of *secretoglobin1A1* (SCGB1A1, also called club cell secretory protein, CC-10, CC16, or uteroglobin), a distinctive secretory protein present only in granules of epithelial cells of the airway and uterus.[152,161,166,167]

In human nonterminal bronchioles, nearly all club cells express both MUC5B and SCGB1A1.[154] In contrast, terminal and respiratory bronchiolar club cells do not express MUC5B. A similar distribution of these club and mucous cell markers is seen in mouse airways.[168–170]

Club cells also produce essential host defense factors, including *surfactant proteins* (SPs) A, B, and D, complement factor C3, and cytochrome P450 enzymes.[171,172] In mouse airways, the P450 enzyme Cyp2f2 is a reliable club cell marker,[173,174] but it is not conserved in human lungs. Club cells are shown experimentally to be highly plastic and capable of differentiating into different types, thus providing progenitor function.[134,168,175,176]

Pulmonary Neuroendocrine Cells

Pulmonary neuroendocrine cells (PNECs) are rare (<1%) airway cells that may be found alone or as clusters of up to 25 cells called *neuroepithelial bodies* (NEBs). PNECs and NEBs are located throughout the entire upper respiratory tract, including the nasal epithelium and lower tract from trachea to the terminal airways. NEBs are frequently present at airway bifurcations and bronchioloalveolar duct junctions.[177]

PNECs and NEBs form contacts with subepithelial nerve terminals.[177,178] The PNEC basal aspect broadly attaches to the basement membrane while the cell has thin apical dendritic-like projections extending across cell layers to the lumen.[179] PNECs contain cytoplasmic secretory granules in the basolateral region for release of contents towards the submucosa, likely signaling to nerves.

PNECs and NEBs are thought to have sensory functions, including detection of environmental hypoxia and allergens.[180,181] PNEC secretory products vary but include combinations of serotonin, calcitonin, calcitonin gene–related peptide, chromogranin A, gastrin-releasing peptide, and cholecystokinin.[179,182] It is suspected that these secreted peptides act as signaling molecules from PNECs and NEBs to sensory nerves.

In mouse models, PNECs proliferate in response to injury, and they have the capacity to differentiate to other cell types.[183–185] Neuroendocrine cell hyperplasia of infancy is a rare pediatric lung disease syndrome in which PNEC numbers are increased, but their role in the etiology of the disease is unclear; increased PNECs are also observed in other pediatric lung diseases.[186] PNECs are considered the cell of origin for malignant neuroendocrine cells, including those of small cell lung cancer.[185,187]

Ionocytes

Although well known for osmoregulation in fish and amphibians,[188,189] ionocytes are a rare epithelial cell recently identified in human airways by single-cell RNA sequencing. Ionocytes are specialized for ion transport, and they have molecular features similar to cells in the kidney collecting duct. Ionocytes are identified by expression of the transcription factor FOXI1. The function of ionocytes in humans is incompletely understood. An intriguing feature of this cell type is its high expression of *cystic fibrosis transmembrane conductance regulator* (CFTR), suggesting that ionocytes may play a role in the pathogenesis of CF[132,133] (see also Chapter 67).

Respiratory Brush (Tuft) Cells

Brush cells, also called tuft cells, are chemosensory cells that express elements of the bitter taste transduction system.[190] In health, they are found in nasal, laryngeal, and tracheobronchial airways, often intertwined with nerve fibers.[190–193] In mice, stimulation of taste receptors results in reduced respiratory rate.[194] Markers that identify brush cells include taste receptors and the signaling molecule α-gustducin. Brush cells may share some chemosensory functions of PNECs.[195] In models of allergic asthma, brush cells secrete the type 2 cytokine *interleukin* (IL)-25,[196] suggesting a role in type 2 inflammation.

Bronchoalveolar Stem Cells

A minute population of cells called *bronchoalveolar stem cells* (BASCs) resides at the bronchoalveolar duct junction in mice. BASCs are marked by dual expression of the club cell protein SCGB1A1 and the alveolar epithelial type 2 cell protein SP-C.[197] It is not clear whether this is a unique cell population or a variant population of SCGB1A1- and SP-C-expressing cells. A proposed function of these cells is to repopulate airway and alveolar cells following severe injury[198,199]; this feature may promote tumorigenesis in lung adenocarcinoma models.[197] Similar cells have not yet been identified in humans.

SUBMUCOSAL GLANDS

Submucosal glands are invaginations of the airway that are buried within the ECM among the layers of smooth muscle (see Figs. 4.2 and 4.4). SMGs are continuous with the airway epithelium, connected by a ciliated cell–lined duct that terminates in grapelike structures called acini that are lined by mucous and serous cells. SMGs are the major source of airway surface liquid.[108]

SMGs are present in the nasal passages, sinus cavities, trachea, and cartilaginous bronchi. In the nose, SMGs humidify air, provide hydration, and are an important source of airway mucus. Individual glands have volumes of approximately 100 to 150 nL.[200] In the lower airways, SMG ducts can be found at a frequency of 0.5 to 1 gland openings/mm². [13] Owing to their multi-acinar structures and frequency across airway surfaces, SMGs support ample fluid production for maintaining airway health.[108] Gland size and duct diameter are increased in cigarette smoking and inflammatory airway diseases, notably chronic bronchitis, COPD, bronchiectasis, asthma, and CF.[13,108,201–204] When ducts are dilated, SMG openings appear as pits that can be easily observed during bronchoscopy.[13,204]

In SMGs, mucous cells produce MUC5B, and serous cells produce peptides that mediate microbial killing and regulate water and ion transport through ion channels to hydrate secretions. SMG secretions pass through ducts to the airway surface.[162–164] SMGs are a major source of mucus supporting hydration of airway surfaces and participating in host defense.[108,162–164] SMGs are embryonically derived from myoepithelial cells,[205,206] and a small population of myoepithelial cells in adult SMGs may serve as progenitor cells during injury repair.[205,207,208]

PROGENITOR CELLS

Airway Epithelial Cell Life Span

Cells within the airway have a very low turnover. Animal studies show that the half-life of ciliated airway epithelial cells is about 6 months in the trachea and 17 months in the bronchioles.[209,210] In the absence of lung disease, about 1% of cells are actively proliferating,[209,211,212] which increases with lung injury.[213–216]

Tissue-Specific Stem Cells of the Airway

Airway epithelial cell proliferation, repair, and regeneration are primarily dependent on basal cells.[136,209,211,212,217–219] The basal cell is considered the major stem cell of the airway and is distinct from a stem cell type in the alveolar epithelial compartment.[128,220–222]

Facultative Progenitor Epithelial Cells

Regionally specific differentiated cells provide a niche for facultative progenitor function through multipotent responses to injury.[175,184,222,223] In fact, nearly all airway epithelial cell types are shown to be highly plastic, so that, in response to injury, differentiated airway epithelial cells may acquire specialized functions of another cell type

without proliferation.[134,168,175,224] At least four distinct cell types may have progenitor capacity:

- Club cells. These secretory cells can self-renew and differentiate into multiciliated cells. Club cells may serve as the major progenitor in mice because basal cells, the major progenitor in human airways, are exceedingly rare in mouse bronchioles.[215,225]
- Bronchoalveolar stem cells. The mouse bronchoalveolar duct junction lies where the bronchiole transitions to the alveoli. Within this zone, small numbers of *bronchoalveolar stem cells* (BASCs) are found with the capacity to repair both the airway and alveolar epithelial cells in experimental severe lung injury.[197–199] An analogous BASC population in humans has not yet been identified.
- Cells of SMG ducts and acini. These cells may also function as a rescue progenitor cell population.[207,208] Following severe lung injury, the myoepithelial cells and duct cells proliferate and then migrate to serve as progenitors in the mouse airway surface epithelium.[206,226,227] Evidence for proliferative SMG populations in human glands suggests this is a clinically relevant niche in humans.[206,228]
- Pulmonary neuroendocrine cells. These cells are present as solitary or small clusters throughout the upper and lower airway and can proliferate in human tissues.[177] During severe lung injury, PNECs proliferate and perform progenitor functions to generate differentiated secretory and multiciliated cells.[185]

AIRWAY EPITHELIAL CELL DIFFERENTIATION

Notch Signaling

Notch is the primary signal transduction mechanism that determines whether a basal cell differentiates into a secretory cell or a nonsecretory cell (eFig. 4.4).[137,220,229–231] In the presence of Notch signaling (by engagement of a jagged/delta-like ligand to a Notch receptor), basal cells differentiate into secretory cells. In the absence of Notch signaling and in the presence of other transcription factors, cells differentiate into multiciliated cells,[137,229–234] ionocytes,[133] or PNECs.[230,235,236]

Through this coordinated approach, a balance of secretory and multiciliated, nonsecretory cells is maintained.[230,237,238] In adult cells, interruption of active Notch signaling results in transdifferentiation of secretory to multiciliated cells.[231] Because inhibition of Notch directs mucous cells to multiciliated cells, such an approach could serve as a therapy for COPD.[137]

Differentiation Pathways for Secretory and Ciliated Cells

Following Notch-mediated fate determination, daughter cells undergo secretory cell differentiation and form club cells, serous cells, and mucous cells.[132,133,137,220,230,231,233] Multiciliated cell specification is a default cell fate in the absence of Notch signaling in transgenic animal models.[137,229–234] The transcriptional landscape of multiciliated cells includes the transcription factor MCIDAS early in specification, followed by FOXJ1 later in ciliogenesis.[143,145,239–245] Despite programmatic lineage determinations and defined differentiation pathways, airway epithelial cells are highly plastic, leading cells to assume different fates and functions, through the influence of multiple other factors, particularly in the setting of injury.[224]

AIRWAY SURFACE LIQUID

The surface of the respiratory system is lined by a thin layer of liquid. This layer differs in thickness in airway and alveolar compartments. Alveolar lining fluid is essential for preventing desiccation, but it is extremely thin (<0.1 μm) to maximize gas-exchange efficiency. The fluid lining the nose, trachea, bronchi, and bronchioles is called *airway surface liquid* (ASL). ASL is essential for maintaining surface hydration throughout the conducting airways. ASL is also crucial for defense and, although thicker than alveolar lining fluid, is ordinarily still thin enough (<10 μm) to permit gas diffusion into underlying epithelia.[108,154]

In tracheobronchial airways, serous and mucous cells in SMGs and on airway surfaces are sources of ASL and macromolecules. The overall volume of ASL is related to numbers of SMGs present (1 to 2 SMGs per mm^2) and stimulation of ASL secretion by homeostatic or neural inputs described above. In bronchioles, which lack SMGs, club cells are the main sources of both mucous and serous components. These secretory cells, along with other surface cells such as ciliated cells and ionocytes, also contribute to ion and water transport.[108]

COMPOSITION

Airway Surface Liquid Layers

ASL comprises a mucus gel, approximately 2 to 5 μm thick, atop a *periciliary layer* (PCL) in which the motile cilia beat.[246,247] Traditionally, mucus was illustrated as a gel-on-liquid model, with mucus above a PCL that was watery and diluted and hence referred to as a "sol" phase. However, microscopic, biochemical, and biophysical measurements show that the PCL is itself a gel.[248] Accordingly, the contemporary view of ASL is a gel-on-gel arrangement, with a mucus gel atop a mesh-like mucin layer in which the cilia beat.

To maintain ASL homeostasis, water is drawn from mucosal and submucosal compartments in a steady-state equilibrium. Along airway surfaces, osmotic pressures across the PCL and mucus layer are driving forces controlled by water diffusion, ion transport, and macromolecule secretions (Fig. 4.6).

Water

Water moves across airway epithelial cells via diffusion between cells and through aquaporin channels located on plasma membranes of basal, ciliated, serous, and club cells. The aquaporins involved in airway epithelial fluid movement are aquaporin 3 on basolateral surfaces and aquaporin 5 on apical membranes.[249–251]

Ions

Cation and anion transporters control fluxes of Na^+, K^+, Cl^-, and HCO_3^- across basolateral and apical surfaces.[252–259] Basolateral transporters maintain the balance of electrolytes supplied from tissues. Apical cation channels also mediate K^+ and Na^+ conductance, with the *epithelial sodium channel* (ENaC) playing a predominant role in Na^+ absorption.[259–261] ENaC is normally inhibited by the anion channel CFTR; however, if CFTR is mutated as in CF, ENaC is unregulated.[259] ENaC overactivity drives CF-like ASL depletion in mice.[262]

Mucins and Other Macromolecules

Proteins and carbohydrates are abundant macromolecules crucial for ASL homeostasis. There are over 130 proteins present in ASL, including mucin glycoproteins that play critical roles in ASL in both the mucus and PCL gel phases.[267]

Mucins are grouped as gel-forming or membrane-associated. Both groups are rich in the amino acids serine and threonine, which are sites of the heavy glycosylation that is a defining characteristic of mucins. In mature mucins, glycans comprise 50–80% of their dry mass and yield strong osmotic potentials.[268]

- *Gel-forming mucins.* MUC5B and MUC5AC are the predominant gel-forming mucins in airway mucus, accounting for approximately one-third of all proteins present. Individually, MUC5AC and MUC5B monomers are very large (>3000 amino acids in length). During synthesis, they multimerize via disulfide bonds formed in the endoplasmic reticuli and the Golgi, resulting in polymers that are tens to hundreds of microns long. MUC5AC and MUC5B are even more massive due to their extensive glycosylation.[268] To fit into secretory granules, mucin glycopolymers form non-covalent interactions with Ca^{2+} and become dehydrated.[266] When secreted into the airway, mucins can hydrate and expand up to 500-fold.[269,270]
- *Membrane-associated mucins.* The surfaces of cilia are coated with three membrane-associated mucins, MUC1, MUC4, and MUC16, which have transmembrane spanning C-terminal domains and extracellular glycosylated domains. Their presence along the apical surfaces of cilia suggests that these mucins play roles in motile cilia structure and function. MUC1, MUC4, and MUC16, also regulate ASL hydration by maintaining osmotic equilibrium between the PCL and mucus gel layer.[248]

Periciliary Layer Contribution to Airway Surface Liquid Hydration

On the extracellular surfaces of multiciliated cells, MUC1, MUC4, and MUC16 absorb water and extend into hydrated brushlike extensions occupying much of the space between individual cilia (see Fig. 4.6). In addition, their glycosylation domains vary in size and carbohydrate mass (MUC16 > MUC4 > MUC1), which causes them to form a mass density gradient from the bases to the tips of cilia.

The smallest of these mucins, MUC1, aggregates against cell surfaces at the bases of cilia projections. The largest, MUC16, concentrates along distal regions of cilia. The intermediate size mucin, MUC4 distributes between cilia bases and tips.[248] This continuum imparts an osmotic force gradient directed towards cilia bases, thereby preventing airway surface desiccation and promoting cilia stability.

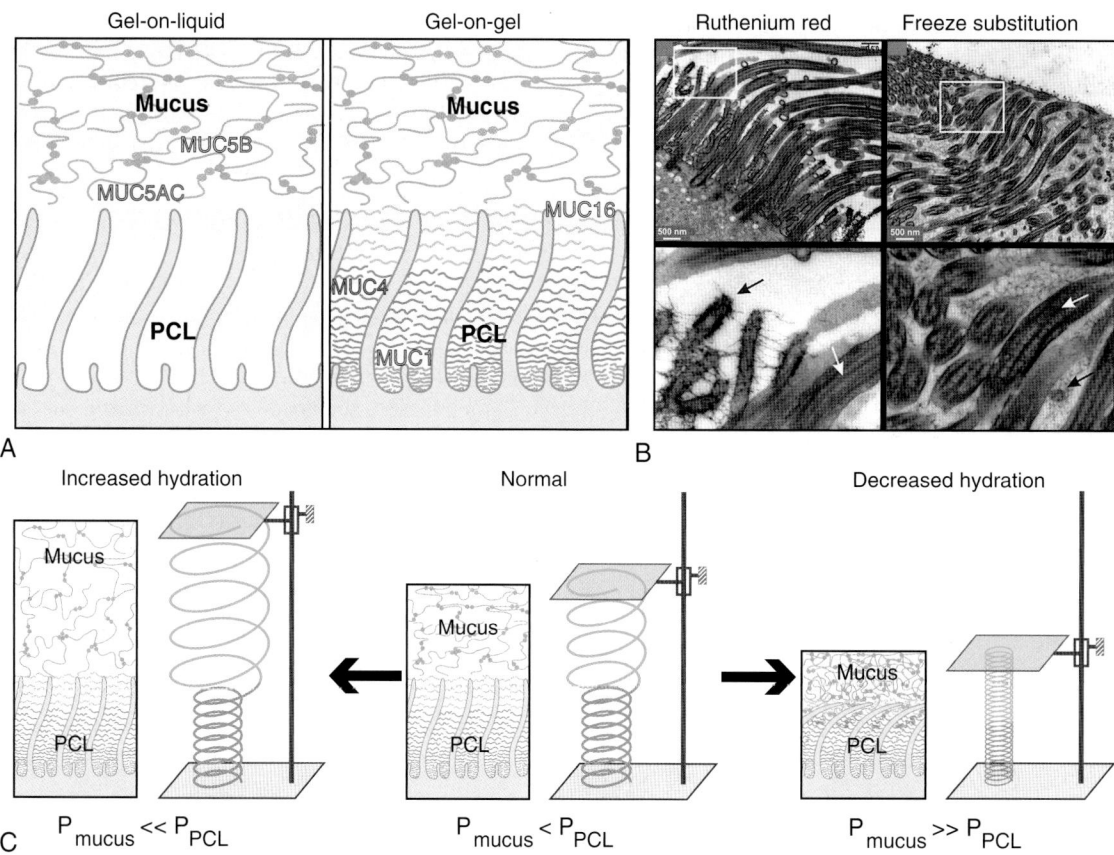

Figure 4.6 Airway surface liquid. (A) Classic gel-on-liquid mucus layer model (*left*) with MUC5AC (*green*) and MUC5B (*blue*) lying on a watery "sol" layer. The revised gel-on-gel model (*right*) shows mucus lying on a periciliary gel comprising hydrated MUC1 (*purple*), MUC4 (*red*), and MUC16 (*orange*) transmembrane mucins. (B) Transmission electron micrographs with cilia (*white arrows*) and periciliary glycans (*black arrows*) shown by ruthenium red staining (*left*) and freeze substitution (*right*). (C) Diagram illustrating mucus and periciliary layer (PCL) osmotic pressure (P) at equilibrium and when concentrations of macromolecules and water change. When P_{mucus} is less than P_{PCL}, mucus is loose and easily cleared. When macromolecules increase or when water decreases in concentration, as in COPD or cystic fibrosis, P_{mucus} exceeds P_{PCL}, and P_{mucus} draws water away from cilia resulting in PCL collapse. (A and C, Modified from Button B, Cai LH, Ehre C, Kesimer M, Hill DB, Sheehan JK, Boucher RC, Rubinstein M. A periciliary brush promotes lung health by separating the mucus layer from airway epithelia. *Science.* 2012;337[6097]:937-941. B, Modified from Kesimer M, Ehre C, Burns KA, Davis CW, Sheehan JK, Pickles RJ. Molecular organization of the mucins and glycocalyx underlying mucus transport over mucosal surfaces of the airways. *Mucosal Immunol.* 2013;6[2]:379-392.)

Mucus Gel Layer

Mucus gels also exert substantial osmotic forces on the ASL. Under healthy conditions, mucus gels contain solid materials at concentrations of approximately 2% weight per ASL volume and, when the percent of solid mass increases, a greater osmotic potential is generated that favors hydration of the mucus gel and drawing of water from the PCL.[248,271] Accordingly, even small increases in the amounts of MUC5AC or MUC5B in the mucus gel can result in strong osmotic forces drawing water away from airway surfaces, resulting in cilia collapse and mucus adhesion (see Fig. 4.6C). In fact, the concentrations of MUC5B and MUC5AC in individuals with cigarette smoke–induced COPD are up to 10 times those of nonsmokers, contributing to reduced airway clearance.[272]

Integrated Effects of PCL and Mucus Gels on ASL Hydration

To explain how mucus and PCL gels regulate airway surface hydration, the ASL can be considered a gel composed of competing osmotic force centers between the mucus and periciliary layers.[248,271,273] A healthy 2% solids mucus gel exerts an osmotic potential of approximately 100 to 200

Pa. At the same time, the graded packing of membrane mucins in the PCL creates an osmotic potential gradient of 300 to 500 Pa that draws water towards epithelial plasma membrane surfaces (see Fig. 4.6).[273]

In equilibrium, sufficient PCL hydration keeps membrane mucins in extended brushlike structures on the apical surface.[248] Small changes can cause water to flow out of the PCL, resulting in cilia collapse and impaired motility. As noted, decreased hydration of the PCL due to excessive mucin polymer concentrations in the mucus gel is one mechanism of impaired clearance in the dehydrated ASL of CF, COPD, and other airway diseases.[248,271,273]

SECRETION

ASL secretion depends on neural mechanisms that regulate bulk release of water and solids from SMGs and on local signaling mechanisms that induce MUC5B and MUC5AC mucin granule exocytosis in airway surface cells (see eFig. 4.2). Water flux is primarily controlled by diffusion. Airway epithelial cells maintain ASL homeostasis by regulating transepithelial ion and water fluxes in large part through extracellular purinergic signaling pathways. *Adenosine triphosphate* (ATP) and adenosine are released into the ASL as a function of cilia-mucus interactions that result in G protein–coupled receptor activation in SMG and surface mucous cells.

Submucosal Gland Secretion

SMG content release is caused by neuronal inputs, including cholinergic, adrenergic, and neuropeptide-mediated signals such as vasoactive intestinal peptide.[274-278] Additional stimuli include eicosanoids and leukocyte products, as well as NO, nucleotides, and nucleosides, although these latter mediators may have both neuronal and non-neuronal origins.[108] Collectively, these mediators affect mucin exocytosis, fluid flow, and myoepithelial cell contraction during acute secretion.[108,279]

During exit from SMG ducts, bundled strands of mucus become coated and mix with materials from airway surfaces.[280-283] A single SMG can increase mucous secretion 10-fold (from <1 to ≥10 nL/min per gland) within seconds.[275-278] With approximately 100 SMGs per cm^2 of airway surface in bronchi,[108] the rapid release of large amounts of mucus underscores the importance of SMG secretions in acute ASL control and subsequent particle clearance by bulk ASL secretions.

Surface Mucous Cell Secretion

Under healthy homeostatic conditions, mucin is secreted at a low steady-state rate in equilibrium with mucin production. This phenomenon accounts for the apparent paucity of mucous cells in healthy airways.[155,284] Low baseline rate secretion is adequate to support defense against inhaled particles and pathogens while facilitating the elimination of shed epithelial cells or resident leukocytes during normal turnover.[285]

In response to irritant triggers, inflammatory mediators, and pharmacologic or neural stimuli,[286] an exocytic burst results in over a thousand-fold increase in mucin release for brief periods of time (10 to 120 seconds)[284,287-289] (Video 4.2). This allows for localized thickening of mucus to trap particles, which are then transported out of the airways. Steady-state and stimulated secretion are both regulated processes and utilize similar but distinct extracellular ligands, signal transduction pathways, and exocytic machinery.

In the steady state, small deformations in the mucosa can cause shear and compressive stress-triggered ATP release from epithelia. ATP acts on P2Y2 purinergic receptors to cause mucin secretion, and the ATP catabolite adenosine acts on A2b adenosine receptors to control changes in ion and water flux.[247,290-294] ATP is also released during cell injury, inflammation, and in response to neural activation. The precise mechanisms of mucin granule exocytosis in respiratory SMG mucous cells have not been elucidated at a molecular level.

MUCUS AND MUCOCILIARY INTERACTIONS

Mucus is the vehicle used by cilia to transport inhaled particles to the mouth, where they are eliminated by expectoration or swallowing. Mucociliary function requires regulation of cilia and mucus components, including water, ions, and macromolecules, to achieve a composition that falls within biophysical constraints for barrier and transport activities.

MUCOCILIARY CLEARANCE

Establishment of Directional Mucociliary Clearance

Effective *mucociliary clearance* (MCC) is defined by the movement of materials from peripheral air spaces towards the mouth.[271,295] At the tissue level, MCC is controlled by the anatomic distributions of mucous and ciliated cells and the coordinated regulation of mucociliary functions.[129]

Multiciliated cells use highly conserved mechanisms to organize across a directional gradient on tissue surfaces resulting in planar cell polarity.[296,297] In establishing planar cell polarity, signaling along a proximal-to-distal axis results in asymmetric orientation of cytoskeletal cadherins, junction proteins, and cilia basal bodies in sheets of multiciliated cells.[298]

Specific cues for planar cell polarity are being studied, and Wnt signaling pathways are involved in airway surface flow sensing.[297] Planar cell polarity appears to be developmentally programmed and autonomous because surgical removal and reversal of tracheal segments of rabbits or rats does not reverse the direction of cilia beating or mucus transport.[299,300]

Regulation of Cilia Beat Frequency and Motility

Ciliary beating and waveforms are generated by coordinated enzymatic activity. In each cilium, thousands of dynein ATPase motors walk back and forth along the microtubules of the ciliary axoneme (see Fig. 4.5).[147,148,301,302] Rapid, coordinated, asymmetric dynein activity results in ciliary bending.[147,148,303] ATP/adenosine diphosphate–generating enzymes are maintained within the cilia for dynein activity.[304-306]

Several other molecules also control ciliary motility. Intracellular calcium concentration increases cilia motility as regulated by adenosine nucleotide phosphorylation.[149,150,307,308] Increased NO also increases ciliary beat frequency, while imbalanced cell redox state can depress ciliary motility.[309-311] In bronchi, in which multiciliated cell populations are dense, mucociliary transport takes place on coordinated *metachronal* waves, a result of sequential (not synchronized) action of the cilia (Video 4.3). As a result of friction at the margin of the mucus gel layer and the cilia in the PCL, mucus is transported distal to proximal.

Periciliary Layer and Ciliary Beating

In addition to osmoregulation, the gel-on-gel nature of the ASL also optimizes motile cilia function. In health, hydrated membrane mucin extensions from cilia form "grafted brushes" that create lubricative electro-repulsion between cilia.[248] Increased osmotic pressures of mucus gels that draw water away from the PCL cause cilia to collapse, increase friction between cilia, and thereby impair mucociliary transport.[248] It is therefore essential to maintain homeostatic balance among aqueous, ionic, and macromolecular components.[271]

Purinergic Signals Integrate Mucociliary Functions

Adenosine nucleotide and nucleoside signaling mechanisms have well-described roles in mucociliary functions. ATP is released into extracellular spaces in response to tonic or inflammatory signals. ATP activates P2Y2 receptors and drives mucin secretion, ion channel opening, and increased cilia beat frequency.[271,284] Subsequent ATP dephosphorylation activates A2b-dependent hydration signals along with sustained potentiation of cilia beating.[304] Collectively, the physiologic and stimulated release of mucin granule contents in response to ATP-mediated activation of P2Y2 receptors is matched by parallel P2Y2-dependent ion and water fluxes and by potentiated motile cilia functions.

Mucociliary Transport

With gel structure and cilia function in equilibrium in healthy human airways, clearance is approximately 3 to 11 mm/min.[246,312,313] This is validated by measurements of inhaled tracer compounds that are cleared from the human lung in 1 to 2 hours.[312,314,315] Impaired MCC is a primary defect in primary ciliary dyskinesia and CF, and it is a contributing pathophysiologic factor in asthma and COPD.[271,316,317]

MCC does not account for the removal of all particles. Very small particles (<1 μm diameter) can bypass areas of the most efficient MCC.[312] These particles deposit in distal air spaces (including alveoli), where they are ingested by macrophages and may persist for extended periods of time (days to weeks). Because of the anatomic distribution of SMGs in tracheobronchial airways, there are strong correlations between SMG secretion rates, volumes, hydration, and MCC. The absence of SMGs in bronchioles, along with the presence of fewer ciliated cells, likely restrains MCC velocity in small airways.

Cough Clearance of Mucus

In settings of accumulated mucus or overwhelming exposure to particles or irritants, cough becomes another significant means for clearance. Cough efficiency depends on airflows that, in large airways, can reach velocities of 100 to 300 m/sec (approximately 200 mph).[318] If shear forces can overcome adhesive and cohesive forces of mucus, cough can peel mucus from airway surfaces or break the mucus layer, allowing parts of mucus to be cleared. Thus, the efficacy of cough clearance also depends on mucus composition and biophysical properties.[318]

Studies have identified that mucus adhesion and cohesion are key properties determining the effectiveness of cough; both depend on the concentration of mucins in the mucus gel. Efforts to decrease the concentration of mucins by hydration and to decrease the cohesive strength of the long mucin strands with mucolytics may provide additive benefit by improving mucus biophysical properties.[338]

In addition, cough is more effective in clearing thicker mucus gels.[271,318] In large bronchi, high-velocity airflow disrupts thick accumulations of mucus while preserving the thin protective ASL coat. However, in small airways (e.g., 1-mm diameter bronchioles), mucus is less likely to become thick; that fact, coupled with much lower forced airflow velocities, can result in the inability to clear mucus with coughing and, ultimately, small airway obstruction.

Airway mucus gels also function as semi-porous barriers to pathogens and particles. In health, airway mucus has a mean porosity of 100 to 1000 nm, which is sufficient for blocking penetration by most microbes.[319–321] Although mucus may be present as a continuous blanket, there are often insoluble mucin rafts (or "flakes") dispersed across heterogenous mucus strands.[322] In the PCL, the mucins tightly packed along the cilia create a mesh-like region with openings of less than 40 nm diameter, which keeps the mucus gel from penetrating the PCL and maintains the two layers as separate entities.[248] As with ASL hydration, the control of the porosity of mucus gel also requires equilibrium between its aqueous, ionic, and macromolecular components.

MUCOUS CELL METAPLASIA AND HYPERPLASIA

Baseline Mucin Expression

In health, mucous differentiation is controlled by cues that specify secretory lineages (see eFig. 4.4). Signals that promote mucous cell differentiation include Notch, SPDEF, β-catenin, epidermal growth factor, and retinoid receptor pathways.[323–327] Conversely, some factors inhibit mucous differentiation, including NKX2-1, FOXA2, and epigenetic regulation.[328–333] Collectively, these signals determine spatial and temporal patterns that regulate mucous cell differentiation.

Injurious, infectious, or inflammatory responses increase the number of mucous cells and the amounts of MUC5AC and MUC5B they produce. Epithelial cell remodeling leads to excessive mucin production and secretion, which are prominent features in CF, idiopathic pulmonary fibrosis, asthma, and lung adenocarcinoma.[170,330,334–337] The potential importance of MUC5AC and MUC5B in human lung diseases is supported by findings in mouse models.[170,285,338–341]

Mucous Cell Metaplasia

If resident cells transition to a mucous phenotype (i.e., without proliferation), the process is termed *metaplasia*. Metaplasia takes place when mucin is induced in cells, such as serous or club cells, that already possess secretory phenotypes.[168,169] In fact, many of these cells are already "mucous" when defined at the molecular level based on expression of MUC5B.[154–156] In the setting of mild injury or inflammation, metaplastic changes may be transient, resolving within days or weeks.[168,169] Resolution of metaplasia involves down-regulation of *MUC5AC* and *MUC5B* gene expression, coupled with emptying of their contents through secretion, autophagy, or potentially apoptosis.[168,169,342–344]

Mucous Cell Hyperplasia

In contrast to metaplasia, *hyperplasia* involves cell proliferation. In severe or chronic situations, mucous cells arise during proliferation-dependent replacement of epithelia.[168,345] Club cells, serous cells, and basal cells are capable of proliferating, increasing in numbers, and differentiating into secretory cells that synthesize MUC5AC and MUC5B.[132,134,221,346] Resolution of mucous cell hyperplasia may involve secretion, autophagy, and apoptosis.[344,347–349]

Mechanisms of Mucin Overproduction

MUC5AC and *MUC5B* gene expression is regulated by conserved regulatory elements that control baseline and inducible expression.[329,334,350,351] Triggers for mucin gene expression include pathways with proinflammatory, allergic, and innate immune signatures, as well as pathways related to baseline differentiation signals.[352,353] In allergic asthma, type 2 cytokine pathways are major drivers of the transition from normal to pathologic mucin production via signal transducer and activator of transcription 6.[346,354–359]

In addition to allergic stimuli, innate cytokines such as tumor necrosis factor, IL-1β, and IL-17A induce mucin production.[360–362] Inflammatory signals are transmitted by mitogen-activated protein kinases,[363,364] and inducible transcription factors that have been implicated in mucous cell differentiation include CREB, STAT1, STAT3, MyD88, NF-kB, HIF-1, FOXM1, FOXA2, and FOXA3.[324,346,362,365–371] These diverse signals ultimately lead to activation of transcription factor SPDEF, which mediates mucous cell differentiation and induced production of MUC5AC.[372–374]

Current evidence suggests that epidermal growth factor receptor signaling is a parallel pathway involved in mucin overproduction. Epidermal growth factor receptor signaling is necessary for MUC5AC induction in a wide range of settings, including cigarette smoke exposure, viral infection, bacterial infection, and both innate and adaptive immune response signals.[326,354,362,364,375,376]

Mechanisms of Regulated Mucin Secretion

The biosynthesis and secretion of mucins are independent steps. As MUC5AC and MUC5B are synthesized, they are packaged into secretory vesicles that are stored in apical cytoplasmic compartments while they await secretory triggers. Stimuli, such as ATP acting via P2Y2 receptors, result in rapid docking of mucin granules with exocytic machinery present on the inner leaflets of apical plasma membranes[284] (eFig. 4.5).

Mucin granule docking and fusion involve proteins such as vesicle-associated membrane proteins and plasma membrane-associated proteins called syntaxins and SNAPs.[377] Exocytic core complex formation is aided by Munc13 and Munc18 family syntaxin binding proteins.[377–379] In rapid succession, increased cytoplasmic Ca²⁺ levels drive tightening of SNAP receptor complexes, followed by fusion of mucin granule membranes with the plasma membrane mediated by synaptotagmin.[284] After secretory granule fusion, mucin contents become hydrated and expand to form strands that organize into mucus gel layers in the lumen.

INNATE DEFENSE MOLECULES AND MICROBIOTA

INTEGRATION OF BARRIER FUNCTION AND AIRWAY DEFENSE

Components of innate defense include physical, structural, biochemical, and immune factors. As noted, airway branching leads to pathogen impaction and, at the cellular level, an epithelial barrier is provided by the integrity of tight cell–cell junctions. Airway mucus gels are a first-line, essential barrier to pathogens within the lumen.[319–321]

ASL contains many antimicrobial and immunomodulatory proteins secreted by epithelial cells that have broad, nonspecific activity or act as soluble pattern recognition receptors. Important soluble pattern recognition receptors are surfactants and complement.[353,380]

In addition to surfactant proteins and complement, the airways contain many additional antimicrobial factors, including lactoferrin, the bactericidal permeability-increasing protein family, human β-defensins, and cathelicidin (LL37). These members of the innate immune response are produced by airway secretory epithelia and recognize bacteria, viruses, and environmental particles.[381] Resident airway immune cells, including dendritic cells, resident lymphocytes, and interstitial macrophages, are essential participants in airway host defense.

See also Chapter 15 and ExpertConsult.com for a discussion of innate immunity.

SOLUBLE PATTERN RECOGNITION RECEPTOR PROTEINS

Multiple epithelial cell secretory products perform antimicrobial activities, participate in responses to allergens, and clear airway pollutants.

- *Airway complement.* Complements C3 and C5 are broadly expressed in airway epithelial cells, and C3 is particularly high in club cells.[172] Complement cascades activate antibody binding to antigen (classical pathway), mannose-binding lectin binding to bacterial carbohydrates (lectin pathway), and alternative pathways.[392] The active form of complement C3 is cleaved to bind and opsonize bacteria and mediate local inflammation through phagocyte recruitment and bacterial killing.[380] Activated complement can be identified in the airway epithelial cells of individuals with asthma, CF, and obliterative bronchiolitis.[172]
- *Surfactant protein (SP)-A, SP-D, and mannose-binding lectin* are large, hydrophilic glycoproteins categorized as collectins.[393] Collectins can bind to microorganisms and eliminate them by aggregation, complement activation, and activation of phagocytosis, or by inhibiting their growth. SP-A and SP-D are secreted by the nonciliated cells of the bronchioles.[353,380,391] Specific collectins, including mannose-binding lectin on the airway surface or in the serum, bind to oligosaccharides or lipids of bacteria, fungi, and viruses.[380] SP-A and SP-D can effectively inhibit the invasion of respiratory syncytial virus, adenovirus, and influenza A virus and promote neutrophil-mediated phagocytosis. These proteins can also modulate other inflammatory responses.[394,395]
- *Human β-defensins* (hβD-1, -2, -3, and -4) are among the most abundant of antimicrobial factors produced by large airway epithelial cells. These are cationic peptides that bind bacteria and virus, form pores in bacterial membranes, suppress pathogen replication, and induce cytokine expression.[396]
- *Bacterial binding proteins* are another superfamily of epithelial cell defense proteins called the lipid transfer/lipopolysaccharide binding proteins. The proteins share the ability to bind lipid substrates. They can bind lipid A, the lipopolysaccharide region of gram-negative

bacteria, to facilitate killing. The *bactericidal/permeability increasing* (BPI) family of antibacterial proteins are enriched in the upper airway epithelial cells. *BPI fold-containing family A1* (BPIFA1; also called SPLUNC1) and *BPI fold-containing family B member 1* (BPIFB1; also called LPLUNC1) are expressed at high levels in epithelia of the nasopharynx, oral cavity, and large airways with high levels in the nasal and respiratory lining fluids.[397,398] These proteins recognize and coat bacteria, while some members also kill. BPIFA1 is reported to regulate ASL hydration through the epithelial sodium channel ENaC.[399]

- *Lactoferrin* is a cationic lipoprotein produced by SMG epithelial cells. A member of the transferrin family, it contains ferrins that chelate iron essential for bacterial function.[400] Lactoferrin also has a broad ability to interfere with both RNA and DNA virus infections by binding virus or receptors.[401,402]
- *Lysozyme* is secreted in abundant amounts by serous cells in the upper airway and in submucosal glands. Lysozyme degrades the polysaccharide capsules of multiple species of bacteria.[403,404]

AIRWAY IMMUNOGLOBULIN A

Dimeric *immunoglobulin A* (IgA) is released by subepithelial B cells and binds the poly Ig receptor on the basal airway epithelial cell surface.[405] The complex of poly Ig receptor and dimeric IgA is transported across the cell in secretory vesicles for apical secretion into the lumen. Secreted IgA then targets and binds viral pathogens or allergens for entrapment in mucus. Evidence suggests a beneficial role of IgA in chronic airway diseases. Patients with COPD, asthma, and chronic rhinosinusitis have impaired poly Ig receptor expression and reduced secretory IgA levels in airway epithelial secretions.[406–409]

NITRIC OXIDE

NO is produced by airway epithelial cells as a stress response through the induction of NO synthases 1, 2, or 3.[410,411] NO acts as an antimicrobial agent by directly causing nitrosative and oxidative damage to pathogens. NO also increases cilia beat frequency.[309,310] Multiple sensors are capable of inducing NO. NO synthase 2 is highly induced in response to infections with respiratory viruses and other pathogens.[412] In the sinuses, *Pseudomonas* can activate the bitter-taste receptors to release NO, increasing cilia beat frequency and airway clearance.[413] Whereas exhaled NO is increased with exacerbations of asthma, nasal NO is decreased in CF, and low levels may support the diagnosis of primary ciliary dyskinesia.[414,415]

AIRWAY MICROBIOTA

The upper and lower airways harbor a microbiome of diverse communities of bacteria, viruses, and fungi that are a component of normal health of the respiratory tract[416,417] (see also Chapter 17). It is proposed that microbes within the respiratory tract prevent invasion and colonization of pathogenic organisms.[416] Acquisition of an upper airway microbiome begins with delivery at birth[416,418] and increases in complexity from birth until stable communities are developed at approximately age 3 years.[416] Bacteria from the upper tract and airway normally enter the lower tract by breathing and micro-aspiration. A hallmark of the airway diseases asthma, CF, non-cystic fibrosis bronchiectasis, and COPD is a change in the microbial diversity or abundance.[419,420]

Key Points

- The major function of the airways is to conduct airflow while also protecting the alveoli from environmental insults. Inspired air is hydrated and diverted into trachea, bronchi, and bronchioles.
- Airways are composed of a mucosal layer lined by epithelium, and a submucosal layer containing smooth muscle, autonomic nerves, and extracellular matrix. Mucosal and submucosal tissues are in constant communication and dynamically respond to environmental challenges.
- Airway structure and function are maintained in part by interactions among matrix, nerves, and smooth muscle. Extracellular matrix provides a rigid support for maintaining airway patency and tissue tensile strength. Smooth muscle provides dynamic changes in airway tone in response to autonomic neural inputs and immune mediators.
- Airway epithelial cells maintain airway barrier function. Basal cells are tightly adherent to the basal lamina by connections between cell cytoskeleton and extracellular matrix by hemidesmosomes and integrins. Cell-cell tight and adherens junctions impart selective movement of paracellular water, proteins, and ions between cells. Specialized epithelial cells lining the lumen provide mucociliary clearance and host defense.
- Airway epithelial cells are a diverse population with specific roles and locations. Multiciliated and mucous cells are the major cell types of the upper tract and large airways. Basal cell populations have progenitor functions. Rarer epithelial cell types include ionocytes, neuroendocrine cells, and tuft cells.
- Airway epithelial cells all survive many months. The basal cell is the major stem cell for maintenance of differentiated epithelial cell types. The dominant pathway for airway epithelial cell differentiation of basal cells is Notch signaling, which generates secretory cells, while an absence of Notch signaling generates multiciliated cells.
- Lumen surfaces are protected by airway surface liquid comprising a gel-on-gel structure, with a mucus gel overlying a periciliary gel layer. Submucosal glands are the major source of airway surface liquid in the healthy lung.
- Mucociliary clearance is the first line of airway host defense. Effective clearance depends on both the mucus gel and the underlying periciliary gel in which the cilia move. Mucus and periciliary layers are in osmotic equilibrium. The mucus gel is composed of roughly 98% water and 2% solid materials, including gel-forming mucins MUC5AC and MUC5B. This composition creates an efficiently transported gel while also imparting homeostatic osmotic forces that support periciliary layer hydration and cilia motility.

Key Readings

Asosingh K, Weiss K, Queisser K, et al. Endothelial cells in the innate response to allergens and initiation of atopic asthma. *J Clin Invest.* 2018;128(7):3116–3128.

Boucher RC. Muco-obstructive lung diseases. *N Engl J Med.* 2019;380(20):1941–1953.

Burgstaller G, Oehrle B, Gerckens M, White ES, Schiller HB, Eickelberg O. The instructive extracellular matrix of the lung: basic composition and alterations in chronic lung disease. *Eur Respir J.* 2017;50(1).

Bustamante-Marin XM, Ostrowski LE. Cilia and mucociliary clearance. *Cold Spring Harb Perspect Biol.* 2017;9(4).

Button B, Cai LH, Ehre C, Kesimer M, et al. A periciliary brush promotes the lung health by separating the mucus layer from airway epithelia. *Science.* 2012;337(6097):937–941.

Fahy JV, Dickey BF. Airway mucus function and dysfunction. *N Engl J Med.* 2010;363(23):2233–2247.

Fischer AJ, Pino-Argumedo MI, Hilkin BM, et al. Mucus strands from submucosal glands initiate mucociliary transport of large particles. *JCI Insight.* 2019;4(1).

Hogan BL, Barkauskas CE, Chapman HA, et al. Repair and regeneration of the respiratory system: complexity, plasticity, and mechanisms of lung stem cell function. *Cell Stem Cell.* 2014;15(2):123–138.

Montoro DT, Haber AL, Biton M, et al. A revised airway epithelial hierarchy includes CFTR-expressing ionocytes. *Nature.* 2018;560(7718):319–324.

Okuda K, Chen G, Subramani DB, et al. Localization of Secretory Mucins MUC5AC and MUC5B in Normal/Healthy Human Airways. *Am J Respir Crit Care Med.* 2019;199(6):715–727.

Plasschaert LW, Zilionis R, Choo-Wing R, et al. A single-cell atlas of the airway epithelium reveals the CFTR-rich pulmonary ionocyte. *Nature.* 2018;560(7718):377–381.

Rock JR, Gao X, Xue Y, Randell SH, Kong YY, Hogan BL. Notch-dependent differentiation of adult airway basal stem cells. *Cell Stem Cell.* 2011;8(6):639–648.

Tata PR, Rajagopal J. Plasticity in the lung: making and breaking cell identity. *Development.* 2017;144(5):755–766.

Whitsett JA, Alenghat T. Respiratory epithelial cells orchestrate pulmonary innate immunity. *Nat Immunol.* 2015;16(1):27–35.

Widdicombe JH, Wine JJ. Airway gland structure and function. *Physiol Rev.* 2015;95(4):1241–1319.

Complete reference list available at ExpertConsult.com.

5 | *LUNG MESENCHYME*

GAUTAM GEORGE, MD • MARIA I. RAMIREZ, PHD • JESSE ROMAN, MD

INTRODUCTION

The lung mesenchyme is a loosely organized mesodermal tissue composed of the cells and connective tissue matrices within the lung interstitium. It includes a few different cell types, including smooth muscle cells, fibroblasts, and pericytes, and contains *extracellular matrices* (ECMs) that occupy the acellular spaces of the lung. Initially considered a compartment containing an inert ground substance solely responsible for providing structural support, the lung mesenchyme is now known to provide key spatial and contextual cues to surrounding cells, thereby exerting roles in physiologic and pathologic processes.[1,2] Proteoglycans, glycoproteins, and collagens make up the lung ECM and, through disulfide bonds and other interactions, connect with each other and with adjacent cells, thereby establishing a vast acellular network of multifunctional molecules that provide support, drive cell behavior, and influence responses to injury.

Pulmonary cells submerged within the lung mesenchyme recognize and interact with individual ECM components through cell surface signaling receptors called *integrins*.[3] Thus the impact of cell-ECM interactions is determined by the relative amount and composition of the ECM in any given compartment and the cellular repertoire of integrins and other matrix binding molecules. Cell-ECM binding allows the transfer of tensile strength, which affects cell phenotypes through mechanotransduction.[4] Embedded within this entangled ECM framework are growth factors and other cell-derived bioactive molecules that lay dormant until the ECM is disturbed (e.g., during lung injury), at which time they are released and activated in the microenvironment, where they interact with adjacent cells.[5]

Considering its distinct ECM components, its ability to influence cell behavior, and its function as a reservoir for extracellular bioactive molecules, the lung mesenchyme is recognized as a dynamic and complex structure necessary to maintain homeostasis during health, while driving repair or disrepair after injury. Most, if not all, pulmonary disorders are associated with alterations in ECM expression, degradation, and turnover. Although it has been difficult to ascertain the exact role of individual ECMs and their cellular receptors in the lung due to the lack of appropriate tools or models, research generated over the past 3 decades has unveiled roles for the mesenchyme in lung morphogenesis and in human disorders, characterized by aberrant tissue remodeling ranging from emphysema and asthma to pulmonary vascular disease, fibrosis, and cancer.[6–10]

This chapter discusses these subjects with a focus on the ECM and emphasizes its roles in the control of cell functions during physiologic processes and lung disease.

THE LUNG EXTRACELLULAR MATRIX

In healthy states, the lung mesenchyme contains few mesenchymal cells (e.g., fibroblasts) surrounded by a vast network of intertwined ECMs. These ECMs are arranged into two types of compartments: *interstitial matrix* and *basement membranes*.[11] The interstitial matrix is a loose meshwork that interconnects cellular structures and maintains the *three-dimensional* (3D) organization and biochemical characteristics of the lung. Even though interstitial matrices represent the main parenchyma of the lung, basement membranes are arranged in thin specialized ECM layers located beneath epithelial and endothelial cell sheets, where they separate distinct cellular structures, thereby allowing the development of specialized and functional pulmonary structures, such as the airways and alveoli.[12]

The composition of the ECM in mouse and human lung has been characterized by isolating the matrix after removing all cellular material (decellularized scaffold), followed by proteinase digestion of the matrix, and analysis of its components by mass spectrometry. The collection of proteins, glycoproteins, proteoglycans, and associated modifying proteins identified by this type of analysis has been termed the *matrisome*. This approach allowed the identification of at least 150 different ECM proteins and modifying enzymes, including some previously unknown, in addition to collagens, elastin, glycosaminoglycans, and laminin.[13,14] The number of core structural components of the entire mammalian ECM is approximately 300 proteins (also termed the *core matrisome*).[15] The ECM serves as a reservoir for many secreted proteins, including growth factors, ECM-modifying enzymes, and other ECM-associated proteins, together known as the *ECM-associated matrisome*.

The composition and properties of the ECM are heterogeneous among the different regions within the lung (i.e., bronchi, bronchioles, alveoli, vasculature) and among physiologic states (i.e., fetal, adult, aged, injured).[14,16] Each type of ECM component (e.g., proteins, glycoproteins, and proteoglycans) has subcomponents with different physical and biochemical properties. For example, collagen and elastin proteins form fibrils from protein monomers and contribute to the tensile strength and viscoelasticity of the lung.[17] Other proteins, such as *fibronectin* (FN) and laminin, participate in building the matrix network as connectors or linking proteins (Fig. 5.1).[18,19] Individual ECM components might be cross-linked and organized via covalent modifications or undergo further modifications, including glycosylation, that influence cell-ECM interactions and change overall ECM properties, such as stiffness or fiber orientation.[20]

The most abundant proteins in the lung ECM are *collagens*. They provide tensile strength but also regulate cellular communication and developmental functions.[21] Collagen molecules form triple-stranded helices that assemble into complexes called fibrillar (types I, II, III, V, and XI) and nonfibrillar (IV, VI, VIII, and X) forms of collagen (Fig. 5.1B). Fibrillar collagen subtypes I and III predominate in the interstitial matrix and are integral to maintaining the architecture of the lung.[22] Fibrillar collagens are resistant to enzymatic degradation, which is important for limiting the turnover and remodeling of the interstitium during injury. The nonfibrillar form collagen IV is a major constituent of basement membranes.[23] For the most part, collagens are increased in restrictive disorders associated with pulmonary fibrosis.[24]

Another component of the lung ECM is *elastin*, a constituent formed by tropoelastin coalescing to form large polymers[25] (see Fig. 5.1C). Lung compliance and elastic recoil are dependent on the appropriate deposition and alignment of elastin fibers. The production of elastin ceases in the human lung after birth, and elastin has an extremely long half-life under normal conditions. Significant elastin turnover is seen only in pathologic states such as emphysema.[26]

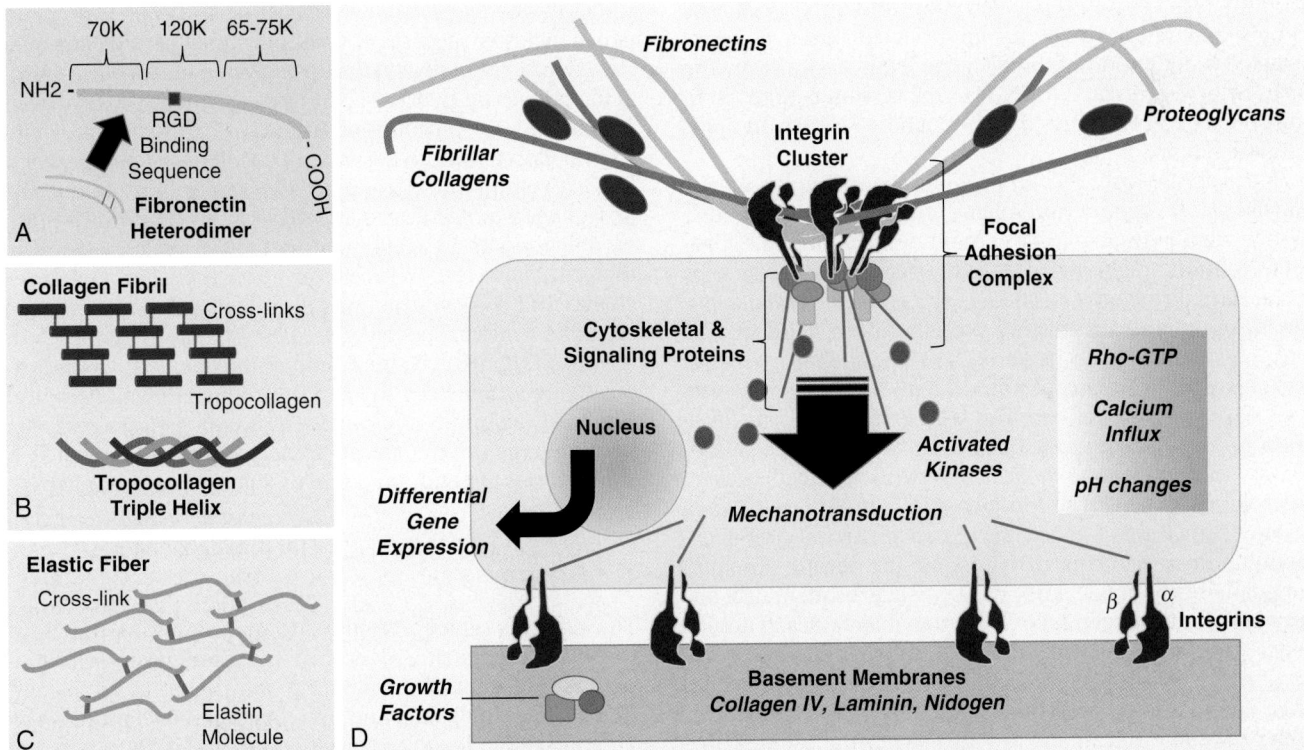

Figure 5.1 Cell–extracellular matrix (ECM) interactions via integrins. (A) ECMs assemble and organize into distinct structures that provide support to cells within the mesenchyme. Fibronectin, for example, is expressed as a heterodimer linked at its carboxy terminal end by disulfide bonds and is secreted into the extracellular environment, where it interacts with other ECMs and with cells through its *arginine-glycine-aspartic acid* (RGD) site located in its midsection (the 120K cellular domain), among others, that binds to cell surface integrins. (B) Collagen is initially produced as procollagen, followed by the assembly of a triple helix by three procollagen chains. Once outside, the procollagen ends are cleaved, and tropocollagen molecules form collagen fibrils deposited around cells, where they provide tensile strength. (C) The elastin fiber is formed by microfibrils, along with central cross-linked elastin, and its alignment contributes to lung compliance and elastic recoil. (D) Mesenchymal cells are submerged within a complex mesh of ECM with which they interact through cell surface integrin receptors. Cells interact with ECMs organized within basement membranes (e.g., collagen IV, laminin, nidogen; see *bottom of figure*) or ECMs within the interstitium (e.g., fibrillary collagens, fibronectin, proteoglycans; see *top of figure*). Upon ligand binding, integrin receptors cluster in focal adhesion complexes, where they "integrate" the ECM with cytoskeletal molecules and activate signaling pathways that ultimately impact protein kinase activation, Rho-GTP, calcium influx, and intracellular pH, among other signals. Tension generated through these interactions promotes mechanotransduction, which also stimulates signals that affect differential gene transcription. These interactions can be disrupted by affecting the relative composition of the ECM, disrupting basement membranes (with the release of active growth factors), and impairing integrin signaling. GTP, guanosine triphosphate.

Small peripheral glycoproteins called microfibrils, along with central cross-linked elastin, form the lung's elastic fibers. The glycoproteins fibrillin-1, -2, and -3 represent the major structural components of microfibrils.[27] Elastin–cross-linking *lysyl oxidase* (LOX), elastin microfibril interface-located proteins, and fibulins are associated with microfibrils and elastin.[28]

Laminins are composed of α, β, and γ chains that assemble into approximately 20 distinct cross-shaped high-molecular-weight proteins found in basement membranes. There they serve as bridging molecules with collagen type IV and nidogen (a glycoprotein formerly known as entactin), thereby enabling communication between cells and other ECM proteins, and promoting cell adhesion, migration, and differentiation, which are necessary for appropriate organogenesis.[29–31]

FNs are glycoproteins involved in the organization of the interstitial matrix where they mediate a host of cellular interactions[32] (see Fig. 5.1A and D). A single FN gene results in multiple splicing variants, of which the best studied is the FN *extracellular domain A* (EDA).[32,33] These multifunctional domain molecules have significant roles in matrix assembly, cell adhesion, migration, growth, and differentiation and are increased in embryonic tissues. FN is highly expressed in the developing lung and is assumed to play an important role in lung development. In mice, targeted inactivation of the FN gene leads to death during early embryogenesis.[34,35] FN-EDA expression is reduced in adulthood except in injured tissues, where FNs are involved in tissue repair.

Proteoglycans are the other main constituents of the matrisome. In general, proteoglycans are hydrophilic due to their high polysaccharide content, which enables hydrogel formation and contributes to the viscoelastic properties of the lung. Proteoglycans are composed of *glycosaminoglycan* (GAG) chains linked to a protein core.[36] GAG chains may be sulfated, such as keratin sulfate, heparin sulfate, and chondroitin sulfate, or nonsulfated, such as hyaluronic acid. Based on the GAG chain and the protein core, the three main groups of proteoglycans are *small leucine-rich proteoglycans* (SLRPs), modular proteoglycans, and cell surface proteoglycans. SLRPs are involved in signaling pathways and the activation of *transforming growth factor-β* (TGF-β).[37] Modular proteoglycans in basement membranes include perlecans, agrin, hyalectans, versican, aggrecan, neurocan, brevican, and collagen type XVIII; they have roles in angiogenesis and influence cell adhesion, migration, and proliferation.[38] Cell surface proteoglycans, such as syndecans, have ligand and receptor functions.[39] The SLRPs, decorin, biglycan, and lumican, are among the most abundant proteoglycans found in a matrisome dataset from healthy adult murine lungs and differentially affect TGF-β activation.[40]

DYNAMIC REGULATION OF THE EXTRACELLULAR MATRIX

Throughout the human life span, the lung ECM is remodeled to adapt to mechanical, biochemical, and structural changes that take place during lung morphogenesis, the onset of breathing at birth, injury, repair, aging, and disease.[41] ECM remodeling helps drive lung cell differentiation and tissue organization.[42,43] The remodeling of the ECM is regulated through various mechanisms, including ECM rate of synthesis, deposition, degradation, and posttranslational modifications. These mechanisms control the composition of the ECM, its dynamic organization into 3D structures, and its biomechanical properties.

The main cell type in the interstitial spaces of the lung is the resident fibroblast, which is mainly responsible for the production of the ECM core components (e.g., FN, collagen). Other ECM components (e.g., laminins, thrombospondin-1) are also produced by other mesenchymal cells, such as airway smooth muscle cells, or by endothelial and epithelial cells in close contact to the mesenchyme.[44] The synthesis of collagen, elastin, laminin, FN, proteoglycans, and other ECMs involves multistep mechanisms that are tightly regulated. As an example, there are approximately 30 types of collagen in the human body, which are coded by different collagen genes, with types I, III, IV, and V being the most common.[45] Collagen genes are transcribed in the cell nucleus, where transcription factors and chromatin modifications control the rate of transcription of each collagen gene into pre-RNA. After splicing of the pre-RNA, procollagen *messenger RNAs* (mRNAs) are translated into protein in the cytoplasm. The resulting pre–propolypeptide chains travel to the endoplasmic reticulum, where they undergo posttranslational processing to become procollagen. The latter requires N-terminal signal peptide removal, the addition of hydroxyl groups to lysine and proline amino acid residues by hydroxylase enzymes, and glycosylation of selected hydroxyl groups on lysines. Afterward, three of the hydroxylated and glycosylated procollagen chains assemble by twisting into a triple helix by zipper-like folding. This procollagen molecule moves to the Golgi apparatus for final modification and assembly into secretory vesicles. Once the molecule is in the extracellular space, collagen peptidases cleave and remove the ends of procollagen, and the molecule becomes tropocollagen. Lysyl oxidases then act on lysine and hydroxylysine residues and covalently bond tropocollagen molecules to form the collagen fibril. Although this is an example of a particularly complex process, it is by no means unique, because the production of most ECM components depends on complex synthetic mechanisms.

EXTRACELLULAR MATRIX DEGRADATION AND TURNOVER

The proteins, glycoproteins, and proteoglycans that form the ECM are mostly degraded by proteinases belonging to different families, including *matrix metalloproteinases* (MMPs), adamalysins, and cysteine and serine proteases.[46] The most significant proteinases are the MMPs, a family of more than 30 zinc-dependent endopeptidases expressed in a cell type–specific manner,[47–49] which degrade ECMs and other substrates. MMPs influence several cellular functions, including cell migration, and modulate the activity of molecules by cleavage or release from a storage state. Macrophages, fibroblasts, bronchiolar and alveolar epithelial cells, and other cells express MMPs as well as their inhibitors, the *tissue inhibitors of metalloproteinases* (TIMPs). MMPs are secreted along with their inhibitors in a 1:1 ratio; in consequence, the bioactivity of any given MMP depends on the relative concentration and spatial colocalization of its inhibitor. TIMPs appear to be dysregulated in distinct lung disorders, such as *idiopathic pulmonary fibrosis* (IPF) and lung cancer.[50,51]

Several MMPs are essential in lung remodeling before and after birth; others are reactivated in response to environmental factors, infection, and injury. Studies performed in null mutant mice indicate that complete absence of MMP2 or MMP14[52] alters lung development, yet mutations of other MMPs do not impair normal lung development. Only after a stimulus or "second hit" do notable differences appear. For example, the absence of MMP9 results in enhanced allergen-induced lung inflammation, whereas the loss of MMP7 and MMP10 results in differential response to *Pseudomonas* infection.[53,54] Like ECMs, MMP expression levels are regulated at the transcriptional, translational, and epigenetic levels.[55] Meanwhile, MMP activity is regulated by vesicle trafficking and secretion, activation of latent pro-forms, deactivation by other proteinases, and complexing with specific TIMPs.

Adamalysins, such as *a disintegrin and metalloproteinases* (ADAMs), and *ADAMs with a thrombospondin motif* (ADAMTs),[56,57] are expressed by many cell types and cleave membrane-bound growth factors, cytokines, proteoglycans, and Fas ligand, leading to the detachment or shedding of mature soluble forms implicated in distinct physiologic and pathologic processes.[58,59] The *serine proteases* include several subfamilies, such as the coagulation proteases, neutrophil serine proteases, and *type II transmembrane serine proteases* (TTSPs), among others. The coagulation proteases play pivotal roles in tissue repair by generating fibrin.[51] However, the coagulation proteinases have functions independent of fibrin formation because they exert profibrotic effects by inducing the expression of potent fibrogenic factors, including platelet-derived growth factors and connective tissue growth factor. The TTSPs are the newest subfamily identified and comprise a large number of proteinases, such as matriptases, hepsin, corin, and human airway trypsin-like protease, which have distinct roles in the lung. The neutrophil serine proteases, such as neutrophil elastase, are found in various chronic inflammatory lung diseases. *Cysteine proteases* degrade ECMs and limit the release of newly synthesized ECM from fibroblasts. Within this subfamily, the cathepsins (i.e., cathepsin K, L, and S)[60] are expressed by epithelial cells and fibroblasts and show elastase and collagenase activities.[61–63]

EXTRACELLULAR MATRIX MODIFICATION AND CROSS-LINKING

ECM components (i.e., collagen and elastin) are cross-linked to form and maintain the 3D structure of the mesenchyme. There are two major groups of cross-links: those initiated by the enzyme LOX and those derived from nonenzymatically glycated lysine and hydroxylysine residues. In contrast, *lysyl hydroxylases* (LHs) reduce the levels of cross-linking between ECMs.[64–66] Thus the balance between LOX and LH regulates the level of cross-linking between collagen and elastin, thereby controlling their biomechanical properties.

Modification and cross-linking enzymes that remodel the ECM (i.e., MMPs, TIMPs, LOX, LHs) are regulated by targeting them to different subcellular locations, by secreting them to the extracellular milieu, or by keeping them tethered to the cell membrane of epithelial and endothelial cells. Furthermore, some ECM modification enzymes exist as inactive precursors, in which their catalytic domain is masked and rendered inactive. Specific proteinases cleave and remove masking peptides, thus activating the modifying enzyme. Posttranslational modifications can further modify the physical properties of the ECM, including glycation and glycosylation, transglutamination, oxidation, carbamylation, and citrullination.[67,68]

CELL–EXTRACELLULAR MATRIX INTERACTIONS VIA INTEGRINS

Integrins are heterodimeric cell surface proteins, members of a large multigene family of receptors involved in cell-cell and cell-ECM interactions. They are characterized by a large α-subunit that noncovalently partners with a smaller β-subunit; both subunits contain large extracellular domains and small intracellular domains[69–71] (see Fig. 5.1D). Mammals express 18 α-subunits and 8 β-subunits capable of forming at least 24 receptors with distinct ligand specificities. The β-subunits can be shared by more than one integrin, whereas the α-subunits typically provide ligand-binding specificity.

The extracellular domain of integrins interacts with ECMs, whereas the intracellular domain interacts with the cytoskeleton. Many ECMs contain an evolutionarily conserved *arginine-glycine-aspartic acid* (RGD) amino acid sequence that mediates binding with specific integrins. Such RGD motifs are found in FN, vitronectin, osteopontin, collagens, thrombospondins, fibrinogen, fibulin-5, and von Willebrand factor, among others.[72] Upon encountering a ligand, integrins cluster at the cell surface, which promotes conformational changes in their cytoplasmic domain that attract cytoskeletal and signaling components. In consequence, ECM ligands, integrins, and cytoskeletal components come together in what has been termed *focal adhesion complexes* (FACs)[73] (see Fig. 5.1D). Signaling molecules assemble within the intracellular aspect of FACs and activate signal transduction through intracellular calcium fluxes, pH changes, and activation of protein kinases, including focal adhesion kinase, integrin-linked kinase, and mitogen-activated protein kinases, among others. These signals, in addition to signals transmitted from cytoskeletal-associated signaling proteins, promote differential gene expression in what is termed *outside-in* signaling. However, intracellular signals may affect integrin activation and ligand binding through *inside-out* signaling. In this fashion integrins bidirectionally "integrate" the extracellular ECM with the intracellular signaling machinery.

By mediating cell-ECM interactions, integrins allow the transfer of tensile strength into cells. The integrin signaling is dependent on ECM composition, its biochemical properties, ligand density, and the way the ligands are spatially displayed.[74] The influence of ECM on cell behavior is demonstrated by in vitro studies showing that fibroblasts align and migrate along ECM fibers and invade areas of reduced matrix rigidity.[75] Aided by the use of atomic force microscopy, matrix stiffening has been confirmed in ECM from human IPF lungs and from animals with experimental lung fibrosis.[76] These studies showed that the normal lung stiffness or Young's modulus (measured in Pascals [Pa]) is about 0.4 to 7.5 kPa, whereas it is on average 16.5 kPa in idiopathic pulmonary fibrosis. These values are dramatically less than the stiffness of plastic dishes used for in vitro studies, which ranges from 2 to 4×10^6 kPa, which may limit the in vivo relevance of these studies.

GROWTH FACTORS WITHIN THE LUNG MESENCHYME

The lung ECM serves as a reservoir for growth factors and other mediators. Insulin-like growth factor, *fibroblast growth factors* (FGFs), *vascular endothelial growth factor* (VEGF), and hepatocyte growth factor, among others, have been found embedded in the lung mesenchyme, where they may associate with ECM proteins or with heparin sulfate.[77] During ECM remodeling observed during lung injury, these growth factors are released and activated and can gain access to cells. TGF-β1, for example, is secreted as a homodimer together with its *latency associated propeptide* (LAP) and binds *latent TGF-β–binding proteins* (LTBPs) that secure it to the ECM. The LAP portion of latent TGF-β1 contains an RGD consensus site for binding of αv integrins. These integrins may bind latent TGF-β1 and activate it through the release of the LTBP via mechanical strain.[78] Newly released TGF-β can also be activated through oxidative stress or via MMP cleavage. In this fashion growth factor activity can be controlled and made available during tissue remodeling or during organ development.[79]

THE LUNG MESENCHYME IN DEVELOPMENT

The lung mesenchyme is mostly derived from the embryonic splanchnic mesenchyme, which provides crucial signals for the progenitor cells that form stromal cells, smooth muscle, cartilage, and ECM-supporting structures. The importance of the mesenchyme in lung development was highlighted in early experiments showing that the transplantation of the lung mesenchyme from one area of the embryonic lung to another led to alterations in morphogenesis with changes consistent with the origin of the transplanted mesenchyme.[80] For example, mesenchyme obtained from distal lung buds induced branching when inserted next to the more proximal tracheal epithelium, whereas branching was prevented when tracheal mesenchyme was inserted in the distal lung bud. Further work revealed that the composition and structure of the ECM within the lung mesenchyme changed during different stages of lung development and served not only as structural support but also as a biomechanical and signaling hub.[81] Reciprocal biochemical and biomechanical signals elicited during epithelial-mesenchymal, endothelial-mesenchymal, and mesenchymal-mesenchymal interactions drive morphogenesis of the distinct structures of the lung. The most studied and critical processes of lung development, which show rapid and precise changes in the composition and organization of the ECM, are branching morphogenesis, vascularization, and alveolarization.

BRANCHING MORPHOGENESIS

Once the lung bud emerges from the foregut during the initial stages of lung development, the organ grows and undergoes branching to form the primitive airway tree through lung *branching morphogenesis*, which consists of iterative rounds of bud formation, extension, and dichotomous bifurcation; this takes place during the pseudoglandular stage of lung development (7–16 weeks of gestation in humans and from embryonic day 9.5–16.5 in mice).[82,83] At the interface of the epithelium and the mesenchyme is the basement membrane, which coordinates branching morphogenesis. Basement membrane components, such as collagen IV, laminin, FN, nidogen, *heparan sulfate proteoglycans* (HSPGs), and netrin, are expressed in a spatially and temporally regulated manner by mesenchymal and epithelial cells.[84–86] Specific signaling molecules, such as FGFs secreted by fibroblasts, induce cell differentiation and budding of the epithelium; conversely, the epithelium expresses the FGF receptors to establish epithelial-mesenchymal communication[87,88]; FGF-10 is considered the main morphogen driving lung branching morphogenesis in mice. During bud bifurcation, FN is found at the site where the epithelium will invaginate to split the epithelial tip. The thinning of the basement membrane at the tip of the buds and the presence of low-sulfated HSPG at the adjacent mesenchyme facilitates branching by allowing the diffusion of FGF-10, whereas highly-sulfated HSPG, with higher affinity for FGF-10, and netrin around the neck, prevents branching by reducing diffusion of FGF-10 and blocking FGF-10 signaling, respectively.[82,89–96] A role for cell-ECM interactions in lung branching morphogenesis is also demonstrated in studies showing that RGD-containing peptides and interventions targeting laminins and other ECMs inhibit this process in embryonic lung explants.[97,98] It must be noted that most of the studies about mesenchymal factors that regulate branching morphogenesis have been performed in mouse models.[94,95] In humans, the importance of the mesenchyme in branching morphogenesis is best demonstrated by the congenital malformations caused by mutations of two transcription factors central to mesenchymal cell functions, FOXF1[99] and TBX4,[100] which result in alveolar capillary dysplasia and acinar hypoplasia, respectively, in newborn infants.

VASCULARIZATION

Overlapping with lung branching morphogenesis is the emergence of vascular structures, which signals the start of the *canalicular stage* of lung development, spanning from 16 to 24 weeks of gestation in humans and embryonic days 16.5 to 17.5 in mice. Mesenchymal cells in the distal parts of the lung coalesce to form vascular structures through the process of vasculogenesis and connect with more proximal vessels through the process of angiogenesis. The distal vascular structures align with alveolar spaces to form the alveolar-capillary unit. Elegant studies in vitro have demonstrated that both vasculogenesis and angiogenesis are driven by ECM composition. Endothelial cells cultured on two-dimensional scaffolds containing basement membrane components, such as laminin, type IV collagen, and nidogen (e.g., Matrigel), undergo vasculogenesis; similar observations were made in collagen-fibrin matrices.[101] FGF and VEGF are required for blood vessel formation. VEGF produced by the airway epithelium is stored within the mesenchyme and released by MMP-mediated cleavage. In turn, FGFs and VEGFs are capable of increasing the expression of MMPs, which are important in vascular biology.[102] Thus the ECM is essential for driving vasculogenesis in the developing lung.

ALVEOLARIZATION

Lung alveolarization spans from 36 weeks of gestation through 3 years of age in humans and from postnatal day 5 to approximately day 30 in mice.[103] During this period, the epithelium, the endothelial capillary network, and the mesenchyme undergo coordinated remodeling to form functional gas exchange units. Early in development, epithelial cells and endothelial cells are separated from each other by two basement membranes and a thick interstitium. During alveolarization, this structure becomes simplified with a reduction in the amount of mesenchymal ECM and focal deposition of elastin, mainly along the sites of the future alveolar septae.[41] The terminal respiratory units are supported by an extensive network of flexible collagen and elastin fibers produced by fibroblasts that support the expansion and recoil mechanisms in each inhaling-exhaling respiratory cycle. Lipofibroblasts store neutral lipids and retinoids to support alveolar epithelial type 2 cell growth, whereas interstitial myofibroblasts confer flexibility to the alveolar septum.[104] Together, these observations suggest that mesenchymal ECMs and cells regulate alveolar septation and, ultimately, the formation of functional alveoli.

THE LUNG MESENCHYME IN AGING

Aging is associated with a number of changes, ranging from mitochondrial dysfunction and oxidative stress to chronic inflammation and stem cell exhaustion.[105] This is also true for the aging lung, where these changes are thought to render the host susceptible to infection and to disrepair after injury in both rodents and humans.[106–114] Although the exact mechanisms responsible for these events remain incompletely elucidated, increasing attention is being paid to the role of the ECM.

Lung aging is associated with physiologic enlargement of air spaces, resulting in the so-called *emphysema of aging*.[115,116] This is thought to be caused by an increased expression and unopposed activity of proteases, leading to the destruction of elastin fibers. Consistent with this idea, a decrease in the number of elastin fibers has been detected via immunohistochemistry within the alveolar walls of aging lungs. These studies also showed increased collagen type III deposition.[117] In other studies, however, decreased collagen and limited changes in elastin were detected in postmortem examinations.[118] Changes in proteoglycans have also been demonstrated with age.[118,119] Although these changes can be measured, their magnitude is typically small, and their clinical significance is unclear.

Early observations made in animal studies, especially rodents, were somewhat inconsistent.[120,121] In more recent studies performed in lungs harvested from young (2-month-old) and aged (24-month-old) mice, increased mRNAs encoding for FN-EDA, collagen type I, and plasminogen activator-1 were detected,[122,123] as were mRNAs and gelatinolytic activity related to MMP-2 and MMP-9. TGF-β1 and its receptor TGF-βRI were also elevated as was the intracellular TGF-β1–dependent transcription factor SMAD3. Primary lung fibroblasts isolated from senescent murine lungs showed decreased expression of Thy-1, a surface protein that regulates TGF-β1 activation and FN expression; animals deficient in Thy-1 show increased fibrosis when exposed to bleomycin.[124]

In addition to increased accumulation of certain ECMs, aging is associated with ECM protein modifications induced by their reaction with reducing sugars; this results in the production of advanced glycation end products.[125,126] Together, these studies suggest that the senescent lung has a "profibrotic" phenotype, resulting in alterations in ECM production and turnover, perhaps driven by altered fibroblasts.

It is well known that the proliferative and migratory capabilities of human lung and skin fibroblasts decrease with age.[127] Loss of fibroblast clonogenicity and progressive myofibroblastic differentiation have been observed in murine lungs and are implicated in the changes described.[128] Oxidative stress has also been proposed as a mechanism responsible for ECM remodeling in the aging lung.[129] Exactly how oxidant stress is generated during aging is not clear, but aging lung fibroblasts are deficient in controlling their redox state; this deficiency is associated with decreased expression of the cystine transporter Slc7a11/xCT, which regulates redox potential for the cysteine/cystine thiol disulfide couple.[130,131]

It should be highlighted that the changes in ECM content and composition noted in aging uninjured lungs are not typically associated with major changes in lung architecture. In fact, except for rare changes suggestive of the so-called emphysema of aging described earlier, senescent lungs appear normal under microscopic examination. It is only under biochemical scrutiny that alterations in ECM, MMPs, and profibrotic growth factors are detected. This "transitional" state between normal and remodeled lung, as traditionally considered, has been termed *transitional remodeling* to denote its transitory state and potential for reversal with appropriate interventions, although the latter requires confirmation.[116] In mice, chronic exposure to nicotine and alcohol also leads to alterations in the expression and relative composition of the lung ECM without causing overt architectural changes.[116,132–134] The role of transitional remodeling in the lung is unclear, but considering the ability of lung cells to recognize specific ECM components that trigger differential intracellular signaling, it is likely that these changes impact the phenotype of resident cells. Furthermore, injuries to the aging lung with transitional remodeling could potentially lead to the rapid upregulation of "maladaptive" pathways resulting in tissue disrepair and loss of organ function, but this requires further exploration.

THE LUNG MESENCHYME IN DISEASE

Essentially every form of lung disease is characterized by alterations in ECM synthesis, deposition, and turnover. In emphysema, destruction of elastin within the alveolar septae leads to enlarged air spaces and fewer gas exchange units. In IPF, the original architecture of the lung is replaced by excessive deposition of collagens and other ECMs, leading to stiffness and inadequate oxygen transfer. In pulmonary vascular disease, the hypertrophy of vascular smooth muscle cells and excess deposition of ECM leads to pulmonary hypertension. In asthma, chronic inflammation and airway wall remodeling are associated with airways hyperreactivity and airflow limitation. In infection, alterations in ECMs may result in fibrosis, bronchiectasis, and cavitation, such as seen in *Mycobacterium tuberculosis* infection.

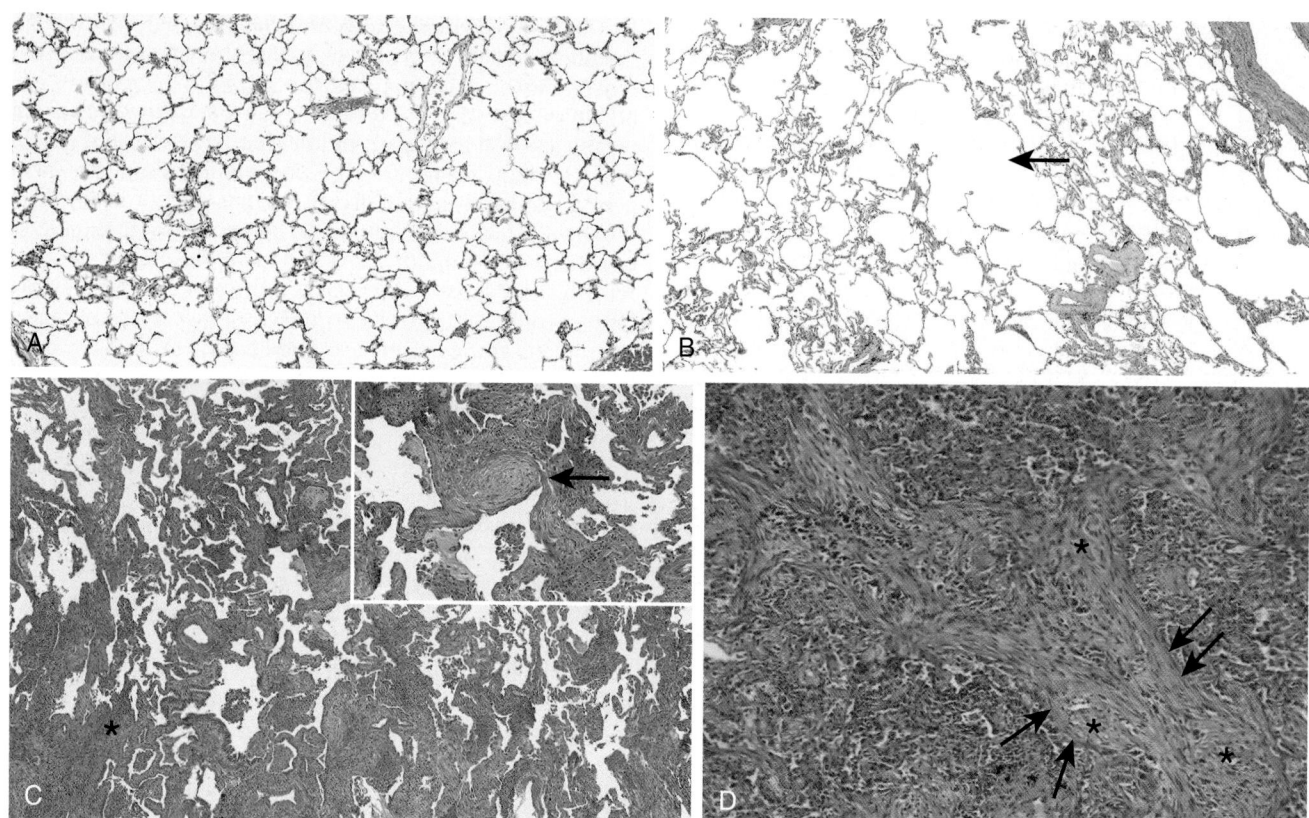

Figure 5.2 *Extracellular matrix* **(ECM) deposition in chronic lung disease.** Essentially all forms of chronic lung disease are associated with alterations in ECM expression and turnover resulting in architectural derangements that affect lung function. (A) Normal lung. (B) In emphysema, there is degradation of the ECM resulting in destruction of the alveolar septae leading to enlarged air spaces *(arrow)*. (C) In idiopathic pulmonary fibrosis, there is excessive fibro-proliferation and excessive deposition of ECM. These changes result in a heterogeneous pattern with abnormal areas of fibrosis *(asterisk)* located adjacent to normal lung tissue. Fibroblasts organize into fibroblastic foci (insert, *arrow*), which are thought to represent the leading edge of the fibrotic process. In this and related conditions, the basement membranes are disrupted. The disruption of basement membranes is thought to eradicate the original "map" of the tissue, thereby impairing restoration of the original lung architecture after the insult (A–C shown at 40× original magnification; C and inset shown at 200× original magnification). (D) In other conditions, such as in organizing pneumonia, tissue injury leads to the excessive accumulation of ECMs within the air spaces *(asterisk)* without greatly altering basement membranes *(arrows)*, which permits adequate tissue repair after the elimination of the initiating injury or by other interventions (D shown at 40× original magnification). (Courtesy Dr. Jeffrey Baliff, Department of Pathology, Thomas Jefferson University.)

Even in cancer, either primary or metastatic to the lung, tumor cell–stromal interactions are believed to influence cancer progression. If uncontrolled, alterations in ECM composition and content in disease states lead to enhanced inflammation, induction of oxidative stress, and phenotypic cellular changes, ultimately resulting in a progressively remodeled structure with impaired organ function.

OBSTRUCTIVE AIRWAY DISEASES

Most components of the lung ECM can be potentially altered in COPD and asthma. In the normal lung, the ECM supports the delicate structure of the lung (Fig. 5.2A). In emphysema, however, inflammation caused by the excess influx of neutrophils leads to the destruction of elastin in alveolar walls[135] (Fig. 5.2B). Early studies pointed to deficiency in alpha$_1$-antitrypsin in the development of the disease.[136] These and other early observations led to the development of the "protease-antiprotease" hypothesis, the idea that imbalances in the production and activity of proteases and antiproteases are responsible for the development of emphysema. This hypothesis is being challenged by new information regarding the immunologic functions of alpha$_1$-antitrypsin and other proteases.[137] In addition, the fact that alpha$_1$-antitrypsin deficiency is uncommon

(with <1% of the population affected) suggests that other protease-antiprotease pairs are important, such as MMPs considered pathogenic in COPD.[138]

In one study that compared COPD and IPF, COPD lungs were characterized by increased ECM regulators TIMP 3 and MMP-28, whereas IPF lungs were characterized by impaired expression of proteins, such as collagen VI and laminins, involved in cell adhesion.[139] Proteins involved in regulation of endopeptidase activity and serpins were increased in both COPD and IPF. However, the tissues examined included end-stage COPD, which may not be representative of all stages of the condition. In studies using samples harvested from moderate COPD subjects, alterations were noted in elastin, FN, collagens, tenascin-C, and versican.[140] Taken together, these studies demonstrate that COPD is accompanied by substantial changes in ECM composition.

Thickening of collagen fibrils and remodeling also take place in the alveolar walls of emphysematous lungs.[141] A tripeptide fragment containing three to five *proline, glycine, and proline* (PGP) repeats is derived from collagen degradation and induces neutrophil chemotaxis.[142] PGP levels, osteopontin, and FN are elevated in COPD, and PGP levels are highest during COPD exacerbations, indicating increased ECM turnover during periods of increased inflammation.[142–144]

Oxidants produced during the combustion of tobacco not only induce the expression and oxidation of ECMs but may also cleave and inactivate protective molecules, such as alpha$_1$-antitrypsin.[145] Cigarette extract stimulates airway smooth muscle cells harvested from patients with COPD to produce exaggerated amounts of collagen VIII alpha 1 and MMP-1, MMP-3, and MMP-10.[146] Nicotine promotes the expression of FN and collagen type I through induction of protein kinase C and activation of mitogen-activated protein kinases.[134]

In asthma, ECMs accumulate in the submucosal and adventitial areas of large and small airways, with changes in collagens I, III, and V and in FN.[147,148] Decorin and hyaluronan deposition are increased,[149] as are the protease activities of MMP-9 and MMP-12, especially in severe fatal asthma.[150] In long-standing uncontrolled asthma, levels of collagen deposition were found to be increased in the alveolar parenchyma, versican was increased in the central airways, and decorin and biglycan were increased in both.[151]

LUNG FIBROSIS

In IPF and other types of interstitial lung disease, there is an increase in the formation of fibrous tissue, leading to changes in compliance of the lungs. Collagen production, proteoglycans, and glycosaminoglycans are upregulated. Genetic factors and recurrent environmental injuries to the lung epithelium are believed to cause the release of proinflammatory cytokines, proteases, and growth factors. These mediators can activate TGF-β1, which has a central role in fibrosis along with alterations in fibroblast signaling and increased epithelial-mesenchymal transformation and myofibroblast transdifferentiation.[152,153]

Proteomic analysis revealed that the expression of 662 proteins was altered in lung tissue from patients with IPF when compared to controls.[154] Pathway enrichment analysis revealed that these proteins mainly belonged to pathways related to PI3K-Akt signaling, focal adhesion, ECM-receptor interactions, and carbon metabolism. About 229 matrisome proteins were identified: 104 core matrisome proteins and 125 matrisome-associated proteins. Of these, 56 proteins were differentially expressed, including many well-known ECM proteins (e.g., COL1A1) and novel ECM proteins of unknown function. These results illustrate the profound changes in the matrisome found in IPF, which are distinct from those detected in other conditions.

Increased deposition of fibrillar collagen in the ECM around fibroblastic foci and an increase in the expression of cross-linking enzyme LOXL2 are observed in IPF.[155,156] In contrast to emphysema, where elastin levels are reduced by protease enzymes, increased elastin has been seen in mouse models of pulmonary fibrosis, which increases TGF-β1–induced myofibroblast differentiation.[157] FN-EDA and tenascin-C are high, and these molecules promote inflammation and fibrosis.[158] The absence of FN-EDA is protective in the bleomycin model of pulmonary fibrosis in mice,[158] further emphasizing the importance of the ECM.

There is also a significant increase in the turnover and deposition of proteoglycans and glycosaminoglycans. Versican, for example, is increased in concert with collagen in fibroblastic foci.[159] Decorin, which downregulates TGF-β1

and has antifibrotic effects, is decreased in IPF.[91] Membrane-bound hyaluronan synthases accumulate in areas of tissue injury, and these molecules increase ECM production and myofibroblast differentiation. In contrast, low-molecular-weight hyaluronan is also increased, which promotes the release of cytokines and stimulates chemotaxis.[160]

Studies using decellularized normal lungs (declined for lung transplantation) and IPF lungs (explants from patients undergoing transplantation) have allowed the study of the impact of these ECM changes on cellular function. Naive fibroblasts cultured atop fibrotic decellularized lungs show increased expression of α-smooth muscle actin, denoting myofibroblastic differentiation; these changes were not detected when cells were cultured on normal decellularized lungs.[13] Further studies evaluating the transcriptional and translational programs expressed by fibroblasts harvested from normal or IPF-derived lungs or normal fibroblasts cultured atop normal or IPF-derived ECMs show dramatic responses driven by the ECM. In other words, changes in fibroblast gene transcription and translation were primarily driven by the ECM environment rather than being autonomous.[161] Taken in total, the changes in ECM in IPF not only affect the architecture of the lung but also affect cells in ways that promote a profibrotic environment.

OTHER LUNG DISORDERS

Altered ECM structure and function have been demonstrated in bronchopulmonary dysplasia where MMPs have been implicated.[162] Pulmonary hypertension is associated with vasoconstriction and vascular remodeling of the three layers of the pulmonary vasculature (i.e., the intima, media, and adventitia). Increased synthesis of elastin and collagen have been identified in hypoxia-induced pulmonary hypertension.[163] During acute lung injury, a syndrome characterized by noncardiogenic pulmonary edema and refractory hypoxemic respiratory failure,[164] injury to the basement membrane results in increased deposition of FNs, fibrin, collagens, and other ECM proteins within the affected alveolar spaces and interstitium. Newly released fibronectin and collagen fragments promote chemotaxis via integrin-dependent signals, thereby enhancing inflammation.[165] Fibronectin promotes fibroblast proliferation, whereas β$_6$ integrins serve to activate TGF-β1 after its latent form is released, which further promotes remodeling.[166] The N-terminal peptide of type III procollagen is elevated in acute lung injury, and the excess presence of this peptide is associated with poor outcomes.[167] Chronic alcohol abuse increases susceptibility to acute lung injury in both rodents and humans, perhaps by promoting oxidative stress, epithelial cell dysfunction with increased expression of TGF-β, impairments in macrophage phagocytosis, and surfactant abnormalities. These abnormalities are also associated with increased FN and MMP expression, perhaps highlighting another example of transitional remodeling. Together, these changes result in the "alcoholic phenotype," which is associated with increased incidence of and enhanced mortality from acute lung injury in at-risk individuals (e.g., sepsis).[133,168,169] Chronic tissue rejection is a major cause of limited survival after lung transplantation. Among other things, this process is characterized by the exaggerated deposition of connective tissue matrices, such as collagens and FN, within the bronchioles resulting in obliterative bronchiolitis. Lack of TGF-β1 and MMP-9 is protective in animal models of tracheal transplantation.[170,171] Thus the matrisome is impacted in essentially every pulmonary disorder studied, and these changes are likely to impact disease development and progression.

In cancer, the role of the lung mesenchyme remains controversial, but most lung cancers emerge in patients with an abnormal lung structure, such as emphysema and pulmonary fibrosis, thereby implicating the ECM. In vitro studies have shown that ECMs influence the proliferation, migration, and invasion of tumor cells.[172] In rodents, the subcutaneous injection of tumor cells silenced for the FN-binding integrin subunit α5 resulted in reduced lung metastasis.[10] Further studies dissecting the role of the lung mesenchyme in lung cancer are needed.

CURRENT UNDERSTANDING AND GAPS IN KNOWLEDGE

In summary, the lung mesenchyme contains distinct cell types submerged in a mesh of multifunctional ECMs interwoven together to provide structure to the lung, while influencing cellular functions in ways that sustain homeostasis. When disrupted, however, alterations in ECM expression, the release of latent and subsequently activated growth factors, and the generation of ECM fragments by newly released proteases, among other events, promote inflammation, oxidative stress, cell apoptosis, and other actions to rid the lung of the injurious agent, while promoting adaptive tissue repair. Under most circumstances, these events are tightly controlled and lead to the recovery and maintenance of organ function. However, host factors, as well as the type, duration, and severity of the insult, may trigger self-perpetuating mechanisms that drive the aberrant deposition and/or destruction of ECMs, upregulate inflammation, and promote cell death and dysfunction, thereby leading to organ destruction during maladaptive repair or disrepair. In doing so, the distorted ECM does not represent the final stage of injury but contributes to it and becomes an important driver of organ destruction. This nuanced understanding of the complex nature and roles of ECMs in lung health and disease guides current research efforts in this area.

Over the past 2 decades, it has become clear that, although individual ECMs play distinct roles that can be investigated in vitro, the relative concentration, spatial presentation, and physical properties of a combination of ECMs is more likely to be determinant of outcomes in vivo. Technological advances have allowed the identification of the matrisome, but there is still much to be learned about how patterns of ECM expression and turnover exert their influence on cellular functions.

One of the key requirements for tissue healing is the delivery of appropriate physical and biochemical cues for adequate cell reorganization into functional structures. This is mostly driven by ECMs in basement membranes, which provide a map for the reorganization and polarization of epithelial cells into functional units aligned with vascular structures. Diseases characterized by severe basement membrane disruption (e.g., IPF) are typically associated with irreversible organ damage, whereas disorders characterized by the relative maintenance of basement membranes may show recovery of organ function with appropriate interventions (e.g., acute lung injury, organizing pneumonia) (Fig. 5.2C–D).[173,174] This leads to the following obvious question: How can we possibly repair a lung with disrupted basement membranes? Currently, there are very few clues as to how to accomplish this.

Host factors, such as age, genetics, and environmental and occupational factors are undoubtedly important in orchestrating the repair response to injury. How these factors influence inflammation, autophagy, redox stress, mitochondrial function, and other cellular events needs to be defined. In particular, how these events converge with, and are influenced by, signals transmitted from ECMs needs to be elucidated. Lipopolysaccharide, cigarette smoke, and other exposures also have an effect, either through actions on gene transcription or epigenetic control of ECM expression, but the implications of these events to the response to injury remain uncertain. By the same logic, it is likely that medications (e.g., corticosteroids, bronchodilators) also affect ECM composition or integrin signaling in ways that might promote detrimental long-term consequences, such as activation of tissue remodeling.[175] It is also important to understand how such exposures during the perinatal period and childhood affect ECMs in ways that might promote disease susceptibility in the adult.[176]

A major hindrance to advancements in understanding the role of the lung mesenchyme in disease and the impact of interventions is the lack of adequate and sensitive markers of activation of tissue remodeling, which should provide valuable information about disease initiation and progression and about early response to interventions.

Ultimately, it is anticipated that new knowledge in understanding the lung mesenchyme will lead to safer and more efficient therapeutics. Current efforts in lung regeneration focus on the delivery of multipotential cells (e.g., stem cells) capable of differentiating into distinct cells or inducing anti-inflammatory responses.[177] However, emerging data suggest that this approach alone may not succeed in generating a fully functional organ. Because the ECM provides cellular cues that alter cell behavior, aberrant ECMs newly generated and cursorily deposited after injury may not adequately assist in stem cell–induced healing. A better understanding of the mechanisms responsible for these events and the development of interventions that take into consideration both cells and their surrounding ECM are necessary to advance this field.

Finally, it is important to emphasize that, although the complex regulation of the expression, deposition, and turnover of distinct ECMs in diseased states makes it difficult to define effective therapeutic strategies, the complexity also provides diverse opportunities for intervention. Simultaneous multipronged approaches, rather than single specific interventions, are more likely to succeed in halting, and perhaps reversing, the many maladaptive mechanisms triggered during injury. Studies evaluating such approaches targeting ECM and fibroblasts in well-defined experimental models are needed to determine the usefulness of new interventions.

Key Points

- The lung mesenchyme is formed by different cell types, including smooth muscle cells, fibroblasts, and pericytes, and contains *extracellular matrices* (ECMs), including proteoglycans, glycoproteins, and collagens.
- Pulmonary cells submerged within the lung mesenchyme interact with individual ECMs through cell surface signaling receptors called *integrins*. In this fashion the lung mesenchyme provides spatial, contextual, and mechanical cues to surrounding cells, thereby exerting roles in physiologic and pathologic processes.
- Embedded within the ECM framework are growth factors and other cell-derived bioactive molecules that lay dormant until the ECM is disturbed (e.g., during lung injury), at which time they are released and activated in the microenvironment, where they interact with adjacent cells.
- ECM expression, turnover, and distribution are altered in lung development and aging, as well as in pathologic processes related to obstructive airways disease and lung fibrosis, among others. Although the exact role that ECMs play under these circumstances remains incompletely elucidated, information generated over the past 2 decades suggest that they play prominent roles.

Key Readings

Aschner Y, Downey GP. Transforming growth factor-β: master regulator of the respiratory system in heath and disease. *Am J Respir Cell Mol Biol.* 2016;54:647–655.

Barnes PJ. Pulmonary diseases and ageing. *Subcell Biochem.* 2019;91:45–74.

Bonnans C, Chou J, Werb Z. Remodeling the extracellular matrix in development and disease. *Nat Rev Mol Cell Biol.* 2014;15:786–801.

Booth AJ, Hadley R, Cornett AM, et al. Acellular normal and fibrotic human lung matrices as a culture system for in vitro investigation. *Am J Respir Crit Care Med.* 2012;186:866–876.

Budinger GRS, Kohanski RA, Gan W, Kobor MS, et al. The intersection of aging biology and the pathobiology of lung diseases: a joint NHLBI/NIA workshop. *J Gerontol A Bio Sci Med Sci.* 2017;72:1492–1500.

Burgstaller G, Oehrle B, Gerckens M, White ES, Schiller HB, Eickelberg O. The instructive extracellular matrix of the lung: basic composition and alterations in chronic lung disease. *Eur Respir J.* 2017;50(1).

Daley WP, Peters SB, Larsen M. Extracellular matrix dynamics in development and regenerative medicine. *J Cell Sci.* 2008;121(Pt 3):255–264.

Duijits L, Reiss IK, Brusselle G, de Jonqste JC. Early origins of chronic obstructive lung diseases across the life course. *Eur J Epidemiol.* 2014;29:871–885.

Gharib SA, Manicone AM, Park WC. Matrix metalloproteinases in emphysema. *Matrix Biol.* 2018;73:34–51.

Gotte M, Kovalszky I. Extracellular matrix functions in lung cancer. *Matrix Biol.* 2018;73:105–121.

Hendrix AY, Kheradmand J. The role of matrix metalloproteinases in development, repair, and destruction of the lungs. *Prog Mol Biol Transl Sci.* 2017;148:1–29.

Hynes RO, Naba A. Overview of the matrisome—an inventory of extracellular matrix constituents and functions. *Cold Spring Harb Perspect Biol.* 2012;4:a004903.

Iozzo RV. Matrix proteoglycans: from molecular design to cellular function. *Annu Rev Biochem.* 1998;67:609–652.

Kechagia JZ, Ivaska J, Roca-Cusachs P. Integrins as biomechanical sensors of the microenvironment. *Nature Rev Mol Cell Biol.* 2019;20:457–473.

Matthes SA, Hadley R, Roman J, White ES. Comparative biology of the normal lung extracellular matrix. In: Parent RA, ed. *Comparative Biology of the Normal Lung.* Cambridge, MA: Elsevier; 2015:387–402.

Muro AF, Moretti FA, Moore BB, Yan M, Atrasz RG, et al. An essential role for fibronectin extra type III domain a in pulmonary fibrosis. *Am J Respir Crit Care Med.* 208;177:638-645

Parker MW, Rossi E, Peterson M, Smith K, et al. Fibrotic extracellular matrix activates a profibrotic positive feedback loop. *J Clin Invest.* 2014;124:1622–1635.

Postma DS, Timens W. Remodeling in asthma and chronic obstructive pulmonary disease. *Proc Am Thorac Soc.* 2006;3:434–439.

Pozzi A, Yurchenco PD, Iozzo RV. The nature and biology of basement membranes. *Matrix Biol.* 2017:1–11. 57-58.

Roman J. Remodeling of the extracellular matrix in the aging lung. In: Rojas M, Meiners S, Le Saux CJ, eds. *Molecular Aspects of Aging.* Hoboken, NJ: Wiley Blackwell; 2014:145–157.

Shiller HB, Fernandez IE, Burgstaller G, Schaab C, Scheltema RA, et al. Time- and compartment-resolved proteome profiling of the extracellular matrix niche in lung injury and repair. *Mol Syst Biol.* 2015;11:819.

Strieter RM. What differentiates normal lung repair and fibrosis? Inflammation, resolution of repair, and fibrosis. *Proc Am Thorac Soc.* 2008;5:305–310.

Suki B, Sato S, Parameswaran H, et al. Emphysema and mechanical stress-induced lung remodeling. *Physiology (Bethesda).* 2013;28:404–413.

Tschumperlin DJ. Matrix, mesenchyme, and mechanotransduction. *Ann Am Thorac Soc.* 2015;(12 suppl 1):S24–S29.

Zhou Y, Horowitz JC, Naba A, et al. Extracellular matrix in lung development, homeostasis and disease. *Matrix Biol.* 2018;73:77–104.

Complete reference list available at ExpertConsult.com.

6 VASCULAR BIOLOGY

YUANSHENG GAO, PHD • WOLFGANG M. KUEBLER, MD, FERS, FAPS • J. USHA RAJ, MD, MHA

INTRODUCTION

The lung is supplied by two different circulations: the pulmonary and the bronchial. The pulmonary circulation is a unique low-pressure, low-resistance circuit that receives the entire cardiac output for gas exchange and yet maintains low perfusion pressures so that fluid filtration is kept low and pulmonary edema does not develop. It is made up of three vascular networks arranged in series: the arterial, capillary, and venous networks. The resistance of each of these networks can change independent of each other, and total *pulmonary vascular resistance* (PVR) is the sum of these three resistances.[1-3] Control of the pulmonary circulation is achieved by complex interactions between endothelial and smooth muscle cells, which include elaboration of vasoactive substances and propagation of signals through direct communications.[4-6] In addition to the key roles of facilitating gas exchange and maintaining barrier function, pulmonary endothelial cells have other functions, including some metabolic functions.[7] The bronchial circulation, which arises from the systemic circulation, supplies nutrients and oxygen to the airways and pulmonary vessel walls.[8,9]

OVERVIEW OF DEVELOPMENT OF THE PULMONARY CIRCULATION

From the earliest stage of development, the lung circulation develops in parallel with the lung parenchyma and airways.[4,10-13] A continuous circulation between the heart and lungs with a pulmonary capillary plexus is formed by the 34th day of gestation in the human fetus, with the artery arising from the outflow tract of the heart and the veins draining into the future left atrium. During the canalicular stage (16–26 weeks of gestation), the number of capillaries increases greatly, and the capillaries grow in close apposition to the epithelium to form the first air-blood barrier. This phase contains the first primitive air sacs. During the saccular stage (24–38 weeks), the terminal air sacs are lined by primary septa that have a capillary on either side separated by mesenchymal tissue. Very premature babies are born with air sacs with this double capillary structure. In the alveolar stage (36 weeks onward), the endothelial layers of the two capillaries fuse to form a single capillary, and the septa become thin and attain the adult form with a single capillary layer.[14] After birth, the arterial walls continue to remodel and thin out with a continued fall in PVR.[15]

In human fetuses at term gestation, pulmonary blood flow is only 11–21% of the combined ventricular output because PVR is very high, and blood is shunted away from the lungs through the foramen ovale and the ductus arteriosus.[16-18] At birth, there is a dramatic fall in PVR. With the first breath and inflation of the lung, the outward tension of the lung parenchyma on the walls of the extra-alveolar vessels leads to a fall in perivascular interstitial pressure, increase in transmural pressure, distention of the vessels, and an immediate fall in PVR.[19] This passive vasodilation increases pulmonary blood flow and increases shear stress on the endothelium, which results in the release of vasodilators from the endothelium, such as *nitric oxide* (NO)[20] and *prostaglandin* I_2 (PGI$_2$),[21] mediating active vasodilation. In addition, in response to an increase in oxygen tension with breathing, the endothelium releases more vasodilators and inhibits the release of vasoconstrictors, such as platelet activating factor.[4] Thus, during resuscitation of the newborn, it is critically important to inflate and aerate the lungs first, which will immediately lead to an increase in pulmonary blood flow and oxygenation.[19,22] Closure of the foramen ovale and ductus arteriosus after birth directs the entire cardiac output to flow through the lungs. Remodeling of the pulmonary vasculature after birth enables the cardiac output to be accommodated at low perfusion pressures and low PVR, making the lungs ideal organs for gas exchange.[4,10]

PHYSIOLOGIC CONTROL OF THE PULMONARY CIRCULATION

Pulmonary artery pressure in adults is typically one-fifth to one-sixth that in the aorta of the systemic circulation.

PVR in adults is also substantially lower than systemic vascular resistance. A comparison of the characteristics of the pulmonary and systemic circulations is shown in eTable 6.1.[1,6,23–30] PVR can be affected by many passive and active factors. The pulmonary vasculature is highly distensible and not fully recruited and perfused at rest; therefore, various mechanical factors can affect PVR by changing the degree of distension and recruitment of the blood vessels in the lung.[1,6,9,31–33] The pulmonary vasculature is also actively regulated by oxygen tension and various vasoactive factors, in particular those released from the endothelial cells, such as NO, prostacyclin, and *endothelin-1* (ET-1).[4,6,9,34] The current understanding of the influence of mechanical or passive factors on PVR, the active regulation of pulmonary vasomotor tone via various mediators and neural factors, and the important contribution of the veins to total PVR are discussed in this section.

MECHANICAL FACTORS OR PASSIVE REGULATION

The pulmonary vasculature, unlike that in other organs, is unique because it is subject to many mechanical forces that affect the resistances of its three vascular networks.[35] Lung volume increases by approximately 500% when going from residual volume to total lung capacity, which differentially affects the resistances of the three vascular networks within it.[32] Changes in alveolar pressure affect the resistances of the capillaries and corner vessels, vessels that are exposed to alveolar pressure.[35] In addition, other mechanical forces generated by alveolar surfactant and surface tension affect capillary resistance,[36] and the interdependence between parenchymal structures can significantly affect local and total vascular resistance in the lungs. The height of the lungs enables gravity to influence regional pressures and flow within the lungs (see Chapter 10).[31]

Gravity

In the upright position, the pressure in pulmonary vessels increases with increasing distance down the lungs from the hilum due to gravity. Based on the relationship among *pulmonary artery pressure* (PPA), *pulmonary venous pressure* (PPV), and *alveolar air pressure* (PA), the lungs are divided into three zones (eFig. 6.1).[31] In zone 1 (apex), where PA > PPA > PPV, there is no blood flow. In most adult humans at physiologic conditions, zone 1 does not exist. In zone 2 (middle), where PPA > PA > PPV, there is blood flow only when the pressure of PPA exceeds PA, which may happen only in systole. The increase in blood flow in zone 2 results largely from recruitment of vessels that were previously closed. In zone 3 (bottom), where PPA > PPV > PA, the lungs are continuously perfused, and the amount of blood flow is determined by the pressure gradient between PPA and PPV independent of PA. The increase in blood flow in zone 3 results predominantly from distension of patent capillaries (see Chapter 10 for additional details). It should be noted that the zone concept is functional, not anatomic. The borders between zones are fluid and are altered by changes in PPA, PPV, and PA under various physiologic and pathophysiologic conditions, including changes in body position, lung volume, and changes in right ventricular output and left atrial pressure.[1,31,37] In the clinical setting,

the measurement of *pulmonary capillary wedge pressure* (PCWP) is only accurate when done in lungs in zone 3, where flow is continuous. In a supine patient, the dorsal, dependent portions of the lungs are in zone 3 but, if the patient is sitting upright or is under high airway pressures on a ventilator, the placement of the Swan-Ganz catheter to measure PCWP correctly becomes very important.[38]

Lung Volume

Changes in lung volume exert opposite effects on the resistance of alveolar (capillary network) and extra-alveolar (arterial and venous networks) vessels. For alveolar vessels, the perivascular pressure is generally slightly lower than alveolar pressure as a result of the elastic recoil of alveolar walls, reflecting both surface tension created by the layer of liquid at the air-liquid interface[39] and traction on membranes surrounding the interstitial space produced by alveolar wall attachments.[40] In effect, surface tension forces tend to collapse alveoli, thereby decreasing perivascular pressure relative to alveolar pressure. During lung inflation, alveolar vessels are compressed and elongated.[41] Therefore, as the lung volume increases from residual volume to total lung capacity, resistance of alveolar vessels progressively increases. In contrast, extra-alveolar vessels are subjected to different stresses. The interstitial pressure surrounding extra-alveolar vessels decreases with lung inflation; the resulting increased transmural pressure causes a decrease in resistance of these vessels. Any increase in perivascular pressure of alveolar vessels or extra-alveolar vessels increases the resistance of these vessels.[9,42] Because the resistances of alveolar and extra-alveolar vessels are in series, their resistances are additive, and the change in PVR forms a U-shaped curve, with the nadir of the curve at approximately functional residual capacity, the end-expiratory lung volume (see Fig. 10.10). Hence, measurement of PVR in patients should be made when lung volume is close to functional residual capacity and the lungs are neither severely underinflated or overinflated.

Shear Stress

In the vasculature, shear stress is defined as the tangential force of blood flow that acts on the endothelium. The magnitude of shear stress (τ) in a straight tube is calculated by the formula: $\tau = 4\mu Q/\pi r^3$, where μ is the blood viscosity, Q the blood flow, π is the ratio of a circle's circumference to its diameter, and r is the radius of the circle. Normally, the shear stress in human blood vessels is approximately 10 to 50 dyne/cm^2 in highly pulsatile arteries and about 10-fold less in the minimally pulsatile veins.[43–45] Pulsatility of flow affects segmental vascular resistances in the lungs, independent of active vasomotion,[46] and abnormalities in flow and shear stress in disease affect local vascular resistances in the lungs.[44,47] Shear stress induces the release of NO and PGI$_2$ from the endothelium,[48,49] which plays a role in the fall in PVR at birth,[50,51] in the maintenance of a low baseline vasomotor tone, and in the accommodation of the increased cardiac output during exercise.[52] Patients with *pulmonary artery hypertension* (PAH) have been noted to have significantly larger proximal pulmonary arteries than normal, which results in a significant reduction in shear stress in these vessels compared with healthy subjects.[53] In addition, the large pulmonary arteries are stiffer in *pulmonary hypertension* (PH) patients, and hence wall shear stress is lower.[54] This reduced shear stress may contribute to reduced NO production and thus compromised protection and/or enhanced vascular remodeling and vasoconstriction.

ACTIVE REGULATION

Hypoxic Pulmonary Vasoconstriction

A pulmonary vasoconstrictor response is evoked when alveolar oxygen tension falls below 60 mm Hg, and the response increases proportional to the degree of hypoxia. *Hypoxic pulmonary vasoconstriction* (HPV) is a unique feature of the pulmonary vasculature because systemic vessels generally *dilate* in response to hypoxia. Both pulmonary arteries and veins, but predominantly small arteries and arterioles, constrict in response to hypoxia. Most studies in a variety of species, including humans, indicate that the greatest and most consistent HPV response takes place in small pulmonary arteries.[30]

Underventilation in small defined regions of the lungs, such as develops in patchy pneumonia or segmental atelectasis, results in local HPV due to local alveolar hypoxia.[30,55] The blood is diverted to better ventilated areas of the lungs, and perfusion is matched better with ventilation. However, under conditions of global hypoxia, such as at high altitude, HPV is generalized. With sustained exposure to global hypoxia, there is suppression of HPV.[56]

Perfusion of isolated cat lungs with partially deoxygenated blood increases pulmonary arterial pressure only when the lungs are ventilated with hypoxic gas mixtures and not with atmospheric air, indicating that HPV is driven by alveolar hypoxia.[57] When isolated rat lungs were perfused under alveolar hypoxic conditions, the pulmonary arterial pressure increased only when perfusion was forward (through the pulmonary artery) and not during retrograde perfusion (through the left atrium), indicating that the oxygen sensor for HPV is likely situated at a precapillary site. Both alveolar and perfusate oxygen tensions determine the magnitude of HPV.[58]

It is generally recognized that HPV is an intrinsic property of pulmonary *vascular smooth muscle cells* (VSMCs). Currently there are two major hypotheses regarding the mechanisms underlying HPV: the *redox hypothesis* and the *reactive oxygen species* (ROS) *hypothesis*.[30,55] Both hypotheses propose that the oxygen sensor is located in the mitochondrial electron transport chain in pulmonary VSMCs. The *redox hypothesis* proposes that hypoxia causes decreased generation of ROS by mitochondria, which results in a less oxidized intracellular redox environment. In consequence, the sulfhydryl groups on the voltage-dependent potassium ion (K^+) channel $K_V1.5$ are reduced, causing K^+ channels to close, followed by membrane potential depolarization, opening of voltage-dependent calcium ion (Ca^{2+}), and activation of the contractile apparatus in VSMCs.[56] The *ROS hypothesis* proposes that hypoxia stimulates mitochondrial electron transport chain complex III to generate ROS, which, when released into the cytosol, stimulate Ca^{2+} influx from the extracellular space through nonselective cation channels and promote Ca^{2+} release from the sarcoplasmic reticulum. These events lead to increased intracellular levels of Ca^{2+} ions and vasoconstriction. ROS also activates *Rho kinase* (ROCK), leading to sensitization of myofilaments

to Ca^{2+}, and thus augments the contractile response.[59,60] There is experimental evidence in support of both hypotheses, and different methodologies used in the experiments may explain some of the controversy.[61,62]

HPV is modulated by many physiologic variables and by neuronal and humoral factors.[30,55] In anesthetized dogs, HPV is enhanced by metabolic acidosis but attenuated by metabolic alkalosis. HPV is not affected by respiratory acidosis but is blunted by respiratory alkalosis, suggesting that the effect of carbon dioxide is pH independent.[63] Zucker rats have increased sympathetic nerve activity associated with obesity,[64] and they have an enhanced HPV response that may be the result of increased pulmonary sympathetic nerve activity and decreased expression of lung *β2-adrenergic receptors* (β2-ARs).[65] Obese humans also have increased sympathetic nerve activity.[66,67] Although hypoxia-induced pulmonary hypertension is enhanced in diabetic mice,[68] and patients with diabetes mellitus exhibit a high prevalence of PH,[69,70] a potential role of an elevated sympathetic activity in the pathophysiologic process of PH in patients with diabetes mellitus remains to be determined. HPV is profoundly affected by a variety of vasoactive substances, in particular those released from endothelial cells such as NO, prostacyclin, and ET-1. Under pathophysiologic conditions, the production and activity of these molecules are often altered, resulting in an exaggerated HPV response.[30,71,72] For example, acute alveolar hypoxia stimulates the production of ET-1,[73,74] which can augment pulmonary vasomotor tone and thus the HPV response. However, ET-1 acts via two receptors: ET_A, with mainly vasoconstrictor activities, and ET_B, with more vasodilatory activities. ET-1 can inhibit HPV by stimulating ET_B receptors on endothelial cells leading to the release of NO and PGI_2.[75] ET-1 can also stimulate the aldosterone system, and hyperaldosteronism can inactivate ET_B receptors on *pulmonary artery endothelial cells* (PAECs) by oxidative modification of cysteinyl thiols, in which case the ET_A-mediated vasoconstrictor effect of ET-1 can prevail, leading to an exaggerated HPV response.[76]

Endothelium-Derived Vasoactive Agents

The endothelium, which is strategically located at the interface between the flowing blood and the vascular smooth muscle of the vessel wall, plays a pivotal role in regulating the pulmonary VSMCs, mainly by the release of a variety of vasoactive agents, specifically NO, PGI_2, and ET-1[34,72,77] (Fig. 6.1).

Nitric Oxide Signaling. Although minor roles for the gaseous molecules carbon monoxide and hydrogen sulfide have been shown in the modulation of HPV[78] and in pulmonary vascular homeostasis,[79-81] NO is the gaseous molecule with the primary role in the regulation of pulmonary vasomotor tone. Endothelial cells synthesize NO from L-arginine by using *endothelial nitric oxide synthase* (eNOS). NO is a highly lipophilic gas that readily diffuses into the underlying VSMCs to exert its vasodilator and antiproliferative actions, primarily by elevating *cyclic 3′,5′-guanosine monophosphate* (cGMP) through activation of *soluble guanylyl cyclase* (sGC) and cGMP-mediated activation of cGMP-dependent protein kinase.[82,83]

In animal models and in humans, inhibition of endogenous endothelial NO production leads to an increase in PVR, suggesting a tonic level of vasodilation induced by

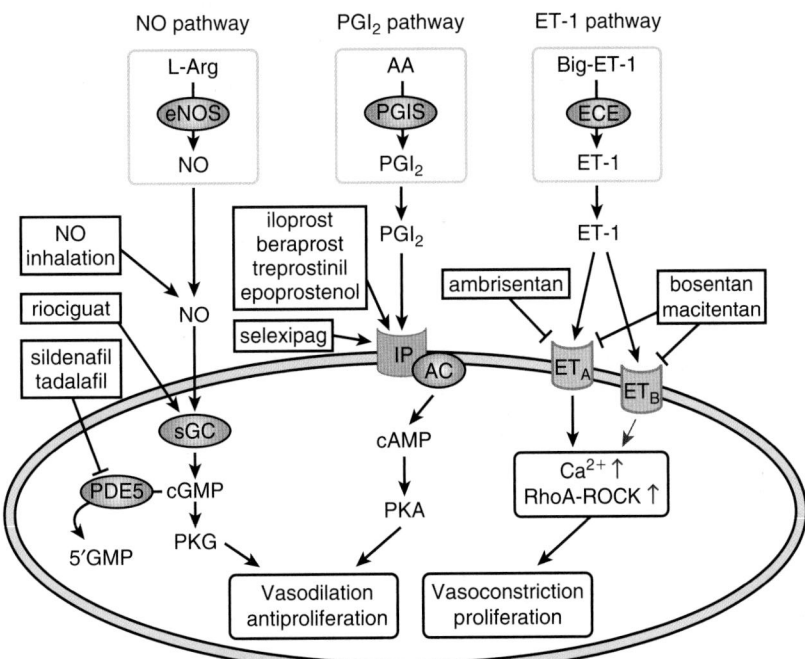

ENDOTHELIAL CELL

Figure 6.1 Signaling pathways of pulmonary endothelial cells. Shown are the endothelium-derived vasoactive agents *nitric oxide* (NO), *prostacyclin* (PGI₂), and *endothelin-1* (ET-1), which regulate pulmonary *vascular smooth muscle cell* (VSMC) tone and proliferation and the relevant pharmacologic agents used in the treatment of *pulmonary hypertension* (PH). NO is synthesized in *endothelial cells* (ECs) from *L-arginine* (L-arg) by *endothelial NO synthase* (eNOS). It diffuses easily into the underlying VSMCs and stimulates *soluble guanylyl cyclase* (sGC), resulting in increased *cyclic guanosine monophosphate* (cGMP) levels. cGMP then activates *cGMP-dependent protein kinase* (PKG), which leads to relaxation of VSMCs and inhibition of VSMC proliferation. cGMP is degraded by *type 5 phosphodiesterase* (PDE5) into a biologic inactive compound, 3′,5′-GMP. To counteract the impaired NO signaling in PH, NO inhalation, riociguat, an sGC stimulator, and PDE5 inhibitors, sildenafil, and tadalafil, are used clinically. PGI₂ is synthesized in EC from *arachidonic acid* (AA) by cyclooxygenase and *PGI₂ synthase* (PGIS) sequentially. Upon release, it binds to *PGI₂ receptors* (IP), which results in activation of *adenylyl cyclase* (AC), increased *cyclic adenosine monophosphate* (cAMP) levels and activation of *cAMP-dependent protein kinase* (PKA). This results in relaxation of VSMCs and inhibition of their proliferation. Clinically, several synthetic analogs of PGI₂ (iloprost, beraprost, treprostinil, and epoprostenol) and a synthetic IP receptor agonist, selexipag, are in use in the treatment of PH. ET-1 is synthesized in EC by translation from preproendothelin messenger RNA, followed by cleavage to Big–ET-1, which is then converted to ET-1 by *endothelin-converting enzyme* (ECE). ET-1 stimulates VSMC constriction and proliferation via ET$_A$ or ET$_B$ receptors, predominantly the former. ET-1 acts by elevating intracellular Ca^{2+} levels and stimulating *RhoA–RhoA kinase* (RhoA-ROCK) signaling. ET-1 can also stimulate the production of NO and PGI₂ via ET$_B$ receptors present on EC (not shown). Currently, there are three ET-1 receptor antagonists available for the treatment of PH. Ambrisentan is a selective ET$_A$ receptor antagonist, whereas bosentan and macitentan are dual endothelin receptor antagonists (ET$_A$ and ET$_B$). The *arrow* and T-end lines denote stimulatory and inhibitory effects, respectively.

endothelial-derived NO.[24,26,84] In patients with PAH and other forms of PH, the expression of eNOS, endothelial NO production, and their bioavailability are decreased.[85–88] The expression and activity of sGC is also compromised in PAH, likely due to oxidative stress.[89–91] Net intracellular levels of cGMP are determined by its production via sGC and by its degradation by *phosphodiesterases* (PDEs), in particular the *type 5 PDE* (PDE5).[82,92] In animal models of PH, the expression and/or activity of PDE5 is increased, which leads to augmented cGMP degradation and thus impaired NO-mediated vasodilation.[93–95] PDE5 is highly expressed in lungs, allowing for the use of selective PDE5 inhibitors in the treatment of pulmonary hypertension.[96] Currently, two PDE5 inhibitors, sildenafil and tadalafil, are approved by the *U.S. Food and Drug Administration* (FDA) for the treatment of PAH.[97] In addition to PDE5 inhibitors, inhaled NO is commonly used as first-line vasodilator therapy in persistent PH of the newborn.[98,99] Riociguat, an sGC stimulator, has also been approved by the FDA for the treatment of PAH and chronic thromboembolic pulmonary hypertension.[97]

Prostaglandin I₂/Prostacyclin. Prostaglandin is a potent vasodilator and antiproliferative agent in the pulmonary

circulation. PGI₂ is primarily synthesized in endothelial cells by prostacyclin synthase from arachidonic acid. Upon release, PGI₂ binds to *I-prostanoid* (IP) receptors on VSMCs. The IP receptor is coupled to G proteins, which activate adenylate cyclase. This leads to increased generation of *cyclic adenosine monophosphate* (cAMP). cAMP causes pulmonary vasodilation and inhibits vascular proliferation through the activation of protein kinase A.[100,101]

In patients with PAH, the expression of prostacyclin synthase and IP receptors is down-regulated, which contributes to the exaggerated pulmonary vasoconstriction and vascular remodeling seen in this disease.[102,103] Clinically, several synthetic analogs of PGI₂ (epoprostenol, treprostinil, iloprost, and beraprost) have been approved by the FDA for the treatment of PAH and PH related to scleroderma, congenital heart disease, and other causes. Selexipag, a synthetic IP receptor agonist, has been shown to be of therapeutic benefit in PAH.[97,104]

Endothelin-1. ET-1, a 21–amino acid peptide, is a vasoactive agent capable of vasoconstriction and vasodilation and is a pro-proliferation agent of VSMCs. It is synthesized predominantly in endothelial cells, initially as a

212–amino acid precursor prepro–ET-1. It is then cleaved sequentially by a signal peptidase and furin enzymes to generate pro–ET-1 and Big–ET-1, respectively. Big–ET-1 is converted to ET-1 by endothelin-converting enzyme. ET-1 exerts its effect by binding to its receptors—ET_A, which mediates vasoconstriction, and ET_B, which mediates vasodilation. Both receptor types are present in pulmonary VSMCs, with ET_A being dominant. The binding of ET-1 to its receptor ET_A in VSMCs causes vasoconstriction by stimulating the influx of extracellular Ca^{2+} and the release of Ca^{2+} from the sarcoplasmic reticulum into the cytosol. ET-1 also enhances vasoconstriction by increasing the sensitivity of myofilaments to Ca^{2+} through RhoA-ROCK signaling. ET_B receptors are mainly located in pulmonary endothelial cells. Activation of ET_B receptors stimulates the production and release of NO and PGI_2 from the endothelium, resulting in vasodilation. ET-1 has a weak mitogenic effect on VSMCs, which is enhanced by other growth factors, such as transforming growth factor-β1. Under normal conditions, the vasoconstrictive effect of ET-1 via ET_A is balanced by its vasodilatory effect via ET_B. However, when the integrity of the endothelium is compromised, the vasoconstrictive effect of ET-1 prevails.[105–107]

Patients with PH have both increased circulating levels of ET-1 and increased expression of ET-1 in the pulmonary vasculature, which are closely associated with increased PVR and the severity of structural abnormalities in the distal pulmonary arteries.[108–111] Elevated intracellular Ca^{2+} levels and enhanced Ca^{2+} sensitivity of myofilaments induced by ET-1 are implicated in the exaggerated contractility of pulmonary vessels in PAH.[112] Moreover, ET_B-mediated production of endothelial-derived NO is diminished in PAH. NO normally exerts an inhibitory effect on the synthesis and release of ET-1.[113] Decreased NO production would increase the release of ET-1 from the endothelium, thus leading to further vasoconstriction and vascular remodeling.[114] The role of ET-1 signaling in vascular tone has been successfully translated into new therapeutic agents for PAH. Currently, three FDA-approved ET-1 receptor antagonists are available for the treatment of PH. Bosentan and macitentan are dual endothelin receptor antagonists (ET_A and ET_B), whereas ambrisentan is a selective ET_A receptor antagonist.[115,116] In an event-driven study, macitentan significantly reduced morbidity and mortality among patients with PAH.[117] The combination therapy with ambrisentan and PDE5 inhibitor tadalafil was found to have a significantly lower risk of clinical failure events than with ambrisentan or tadalafil monotherapy[118] (see Fig. 6.1).

NEURAL CONTROL

The pulmonary vasculature is innervated by sympathetic, parasympathetic, and sensory-motor nerve fibers but is typically less richly innervated than the systemic vessels. The density of the nerve fibers is greatest in large vessels and at branch points. Sympathetic activation increases PVR via the release of norepinephrine, which causes vasoconstriction via *α-adrenergic receptors* (α-ARs) and vasodilation via β-ARs, with the vasoconstrictive effect being more dominant.[9,34] Under basal conditions, there is limited sympathetic influence on pulmonary vasomotor tone, but sympathetic

activation happens during exercise and hypoxia.[119,120] In PH patients, the sympathetic nervous system is activated and may contribute to increased vasomotor tone.[121] In an animal model of PH, denervation of the large pulmonary arteries significantly reduced pulmonary artery pressure and PVR.[122] Parasympathetic stimulation induces the release of *acetylcholine* (ACh). ACh induces relaxation of isolated human pulmonary arteries through release of endothelial-derived NO, whereas its direct effect on denuded vessels is contraction.[123] Under basal conditions, there is limited parasympathetic influence on pulmonary vasomotor tone.[34,124] In addition to the classic neurotransmitters, a number of neuropeptides and bioactive agents can be co-released from the nerve terminals in the pulmonary vessel wall, such as neuropeptide Y, vasoactive intestinal peptide, calcitonin gene–related peptide, substance P, adenosine triphosphate, and NO. Their roles in regulation of pulmonary vasomotor tone remain to be fully elucidated.[125–127]

ROLE OF PULMONARY VEINS

In the lungs, venous differentiation and patterning are genetically controlled through the coordinated actions of specific transcription factors.[13] In most developing organs, including the lungs, arterial and venous identity is also modulated by hemodynamic forces.[128–131] Arterial fate is acquired by the combined effect of transcription factors FOXC1 and FOXC2 and vascular endothelial growth factor signaling, whereas venous identity is regulated by the orphan nuclear receptor *chicken ovalbumin upstream promoter transcriptional factor-II* (COUP-TFII) through the repression of Notch1.

In the lung, there is now a large body of evidence indicating that the veins are not simple conduits that return blood to the left atrium. Unlike the systemic veins, pulmonary veins play an active role in the regulation of lung blood flow, capillary filtration pressures, and PVR.[4,132,133] Significant vasoreactivity has been described in pulmonary veins in the fetus and newborn[134–139] and in the adult.[140–144] Data from many animal species indicate that, similar to pulmonary arteries, pulmonary veins are reactive to a broad range of vasoconstrictors, such as platelet activating factor, thromboxane and leukotrienes, and vasodilators, such as NO and PGI_2.[4,130,133] Pulmonary veins in the fetus and newborn are exquisitely sensitive to NO and cGMP.[145,146] In the hypoxic environment of the fetus, both pulmonary arteries and veins are constricted. The enhanced responsiveness of veins and arteries in the perinatal period to NO facilitates their relaxation at birth as NO is released from the endothelium with the initiation of respiration.[4]

Although the primary site of resistance to flow in the pulmonary circulation under both normal and hypoxic conditions is the precapillary pulmonary arterioles,[34] numerous studies have shown that hypoxia causes vigorous constriction of pulmonary veins in a variety of species, including rat,[147] guinea pig,[148] ferret,[149] dog,[150] sheep,[132,151] and pig.[152] In dog lungs, acute alveolar hypoxia predominantly constricts pulmonary arteries. However, when the lungs are perfused with histamine, the vasoconstrictor response to acute alveolar hypoxia is in veins.[153] By increasing microvascular pressures, venous constriction can cause distention and recruitment of capillaries with the possibility of better ventilation-perfusion matching; however, venous constriction can also increase capillary filtration pressures and the likelihood of edema formation.[133,154]

Postcapillary pathology with venous abnormalities as a cause of PH is now recognized in the updated Classification of Pulmonary Hypertension and listed as group 1.6. This group has venous pathology in addition to arterial pathology and therefore is included in group 1. Also, for group 2 patients with PH due to left heart disease, a subcategory of group 2.4 was added to distinguish congenital and acquired pulmonary venous lesions that lead to PH.[155,156] To distinguish patients with both precapillary and postcapillary lesions with venous pathology from those who have isolated postcapillary PH with left heart failure, the hemodynamic definition of PH was updated. Isolated precapillary PH is associated with *mean pulmonary arterial pressure* (mPAP) greater than 20 mm Hg, PCWP less than 15 mm Hg, and PVR greater than 3 Wood units. Isolated postcapillary PH is associated with mPAP greater than 20 mm Hg, PCWP greater than 15 mm Hg, and PVR less than 3 Wood units, and combined precapillary and postcapillary PH is associated with mPAP greater than 20 mm Hg, PCWP greater than 15 mm Hg, and PVR greater than 3 Wood units.[157]

In chronic pulmonary hypertensive disorders, there is vascular remodeling of pulmonary arteries as well as veins[158,159] in a number of species, including rat,[160,161] sheep,[162] and humans.[163–167] In humans, the changes in veins consist of medial hypertrophy and arterialization of bundles of smooth muscle cells within the venous intima.[164] In one study of 19 patients with PAH, intimal and adventitial thickening of pulmonary veins less than 250 μm in diameter was observed in approximately one-half of the subjects studied, suggesting that venous pathology in PAH is underdiagnosed.[165]

COMMUNICATION BETWEEN ENDOTHELIAL AND SMOOTH MUSCLE CELLS

Endothelial cells have an important role in the regulation of pulmonary vasoreactivity, primarily via the release of various diffusible molecules, such as NO, prostacyclin, and ET-1. Increasing evidence indicates that the relationship between the endothelial cells and the underlying VSMCs is bidirectional rather than unidirectional. Paracrine signaling is the primary mechanism by which the endothelium modulates the activity of VSMCs.[168] However, vasoactive agents released from the endothelium can induce the underlying VSMCs to generate diffusible molecules that in turn affect endothelial function. For example, ET-1 can increase VSMC production of hydrogen peroxide, which can then suppress eNOS expression in endothelial cells.[114] In addition to paracrine signaling, additional cross-talk mechanisms exist, including communications via *myoendothelial junctions* (MEJs)[169] and *extracellular vesicles* (EVs).[170] All these mechanisms are crucial to the homeostasis of the pulmonary circulation. Under pathophysiologic conditions, the altered interactions between endothelial cells and VSMCs may promote increased vasoconstriction and hyperproliferation of endothelial cells and VSMCs, the development of pulmonary vascular remodeling, increased PVR, and eventual right ventricular failure.[5,72,169–171]

MYOENDOTHELIAL JUNCTIONS

Functional MEJs are emerging as an important mechanism for communication between vascular endothelial and VSMCs.[172] Abnormal communication via MEJs is implicated in pulmonary vascular disease.[173,174] Located at the boundary between the endothelium and smooth muscle, the MEJs form gap junctions that allow fine tuning of vascular function. MEJs enable the direct transfer of current and small molecules (<1.2 kDa) between the cytoplasm of the adjacent cells. MEJs also provide a microdomain to localize other signaling pathways and proteins involved in intercellular communication and paracrine-based signaling. MEJs are more numerous in small resistance arteries than in larger elastic arteries, which enables a faster endothelial response to signaling from the smooth muscle in these vessels.[172]

The MEJ is composed of two hemichannels termed *connexons*, each composed of six *connexin* proteins. Of the connexin family, only Cx37, Cx40, and Cx43 are found in MEJs.[175] Although ultrastructural localization of MEJs was first described in 1957,[176] functional confirmation of MEJs has lagged behind. Dye transfer studies and comparison of membrane potentials between endothelial cells and VSMCs have provided evidence of functional MEJs. For example, green fluorescent dye loaded in PAECs can diffuse into the underlying *pulmonary arterial smooth muscle cells* (PASMCs). This effect is inhibited by small interfering RNA knockdown of the connexin Cx43, indicating the existence of functional MEJs.[174] There is also evidence that superoxide anion production originating from the VSMCs can diffuse into the endothelial cells to react with NO, leading to inactivation of NO.[5,169] MEJs may facilitate transfer of neurotransmitters between endothelial cells and VSMCs. In pulmonary blood vessels, serotonin is released by endothelial cells and causes pulmonary vasoconstriction by elevating intracellular Ca^{2+} levels and activating ROCK in VSMCs. Serotonin also promotes vascular proliferation via the activation of mitogen-activated protein kinase, Akt, and ROCK.[177–180] Although serotonin acts on VSMC via its cell surface receptors and serotonin transporter, emerging evidence suggests that it can also diffuse from endothelial cells into VSMCs through the MEJs.[177,181,182] For instance, serotonin synthesized in rat PAECs is transferred to PASMCs in a co-culture system when the cells are in contact, but not without contact. The transfer of serotonin between these cell types is suppressed by blockade of the MEJ.[174,177]

EXTRACELLULAR VESICLES

EVs are cell-derived membrane-bound structures that originate from different subcellular membrane compartments. EVs contain *micro-RNAs* (miRNAs), proteins, lipids, and so forth, and they can transmit information to their target cells by delivering their cargo by membrane fusion, endocytosis, or receptor-mediated binding. EVs represent an important mechanism for cell-cell communication. They have been shown to transfer information from one cell to another under physiologic conditions and in disease.[170] However, more is known now about their pathophysiologic role in disease than under normal conditions.[183,184] EVs are classified into three main populations: exosomes, microvesicles, and apoptotic bodies. *Exosomes* are approximately 40 to 100 nm membrane vesicles of endocytic origin released into the extracellular space after fusion of multivesicular bodies with the plasma membrane. Exosomes contain endosome-specific proteins, such as ALIX and TSG101; components of microdomains in the plasma membrane, such as cholesterol, ceramide, integrins, and tetraspanins; messenger RNA; miRNA; and other noncoding RNAs. The larger *microvesicles* (MVs), sometimes referred to as microparticles, are approximately 100 to 1000 nm in size. They are formed by the outward budding and separation of the plasma membrane and therefore retain surface molecules from parent cells and part of their cytosolic content (proteins, RNA, miRNA). *Apoptotic bodies* are the largest EV (>1 μm). They are formed by outward blebbing of the cell membrane during the late steps of apoptosis and contain cellular organelles, proteins, DNA, RNA, and miRNA. EVs are released from most cell types, including endothelial cells and VSMCs.[5,171,185]

Under physiologic conditions, EVs are actively involved in the maintenance of the hemostasis in various organs, including the lungs.[183,184] Human PAECs can take up PASMC-derived EVs containing *zinc finger E-box–binding homeobox 1* (ZEB1, a well-known gatekeeper for endothelial-to-mesenchymal transition) and transforming growth factor-β superfamily ligands, which may facilitate endothelial-to-mesenchymal transition during normal angiogenesis[186] or during the development of PH[187] and other vascular diseases.[188,189] Pericytes, which are mural cells that wrap around and support the endothelial cells, may be recruited by Wnt5a-containing exosomes released from pulmonary venous endothelial cells, thereby preserving the number of functional vessels within the microcirculation. A lack of Wnt5a production impairs the interaction between endothelium and pericytes, resulting in loss of small vessels and the development of PAH.[190]

The cargo content of EVs has the distinct characteristics of the parental cells. Hence, EVs have a great potential for use as biomarkers in the diagnosis and/or prognosis of various diseases.[191–193] Circulating endothelial MVs are shed from activated or injured endothelial cells. In patients with PAH, the plasma levels of endothelial MVs, as identified by the endothelial markers CD31+ (platelet endothelial cell adhesion molecule) or CD144+ (vascular endothelial cadherin), are significantly increased compared with controls. Moreover, the CD31+ and CD144+ MV levels correlate with mean pulmonary artery pressure, PVR, and mean right atrial pressure in patients with PAH.[194] Endothelial MVs may serve as biomarkers of PAH and be involved in the pathogenesis of PAH.[195–197] Endothelium-dependent relaxation of rat pulmonary arteries is diminished after incubation with MVs obtained from rats exposed to chronic hypoxia, compared to control animals, and is accompanied by decreased eNOS activity and increased production of ROS.[195] Cell migration is an important step in the development of pulmonary vascular remodeling and PAH. The migration of PAECs can be induced by *micro-RNA-143* (miR-143) generated in PASMCs via exosomes. The miR-143–enriched exosomes derived from PASMCs are internalized by PAECs, leading to increased EC migration and angiogenesis.[198] Thus MVs may serve to amplify the pathologic response in PAH.

NONRESPIRATORY FUNCTIONS OF THE PULMONARY CIRCULATION

Although the primary purpose of the pulmonary circulation is gas exchange, it has other functions, such as metabolism.[199] The vast vascular surface area of the lungs and the fact that they receive the entire cardiac output, make them uniquely suited to metabolize and modify blood-borne compounds. Compounds can be either activated or inactivated within the pulmonary circulation.

The relatively inactive polypeptide angiotensin I is converted to the potent vasoconstrictor angiotensin II within the pulmonary circulation by an enzyme, *angiotensin I–converting enzyme* (ACE), located in small pits (caveolae intracellulares) on the surface of the capillary endothelial cells.[200,201] After being converted to angiotensin II by ACE, this potent vasoconstrictor can be converted to a vasodilator, *angiotensin 1-7* (Ang 1-7), by *angiotensin-converting enzyme II* (ACE2),[202] an enzyme abundantly expressed in various organs and tissues.[203,204] Of interest, ACE2 is the key cell receptor for *severe acute respiratory syndrome coronavirus 2* (SARS-CoV-2) to enter human cells and replicate, ultimately leading to the global pandemic of *coronavirus disease 2019* (COVID-19).[205] After binding of SARS-CoV-2 to ACE2, both the virus and ACE2 are internalized, which leads to reduced expression of ACE2 and thus reduced conversion of angiotensin II to Ang 1-7. This results in increased ROS production, increased inflammatory response, vasoconstriction, vascular leakage, a profibrotic response, and eventually severe lung injury.[206] Although COVID-19 is primarily considered a lung parenchymal disease, ACE2 is expressed on both endothelial cells and VSMCs, and the pulmonary vascular system can be infected by the virus.[203,204] The relative resistance of young people to this virus is thought to be in part due to a lower expression of ACE2 because it is developmentally regulated, and its expression is lower the younger the age.[207] In SARS-CoV-2 infection, there is an increased release of von Willebrand factor from the endothelial cells, which may contribute to the hypercoagulable state in COVID-19.[208,209] Currently, there are only a few reported cases of COVID-19 disease in patients with PH. Considering the limited numbers of patients with PH, the relationship between these diseases remains to be explored.[210] Currently there is also no evidence to suggest that PH per se is an independent risk factor for COVID-19.[206]

A number of vasoactive substances are completely or partially inactivated during passage through the lung. Bradykinin is largely inactivated (up to 80%) by ACE. The lung is the major site of inactivation of serotonin (5-hydroxytryptamine), not by enzymatic degradation but by an uptake and storage process. Some of the serotonin is transferred to platelets in the lung or stored and released during anaphylaxis.[199,211] Endothelin, although it is stable in plasma and whole blood, undergoes extensive pulmonary removal after binding to ET$_B$ on the endothelial cells during its passage through the pulmonary circulation.[106,107] Prostaglandins E$_1$, E$_2$, and F$_{2\alpha}$ are inactivated in the lung. Norepinephrine is also taken up by the lung to some extent (up to 30%). Histamine appears not to be inactivated by the intact lung but is stored there.[199]

Several vasoactive substances are normally synthesized or stored within the lung but are released into the circulation under pathologic conditions. For example, in anaphylaxis or during an asthmatic attack, histamine, bradykinin, prostaglandins, and leukotrienes are discharged into the circulation. Other conditions in which the lung may release potent chemicals include pulmonary embolism and alveolar hypoxia.[7,199] There is evidence that the lung plays a role in blood clotting under normal and abnormal conditions. There are large numbers of mast cells containing heparin in the interstitium that participate in health and disease.[212] The pulmonary circulation also acts as a filter of blood. Small intravascular thrombi are removed from the circulation before they can reach the brain or other vital organs, in part due to a high fibrinolytic activity expressed in the endothelial cells of pulmonary arteries compared with that of systemic vessels.[213] Abnormal vascular connections in pulmonary arteriovenous malformations bypass the filtering effect of pulmonary capillaries, which may lead to paradoxical septic or nonseptic embolization. In particular, the brain is usually the most frequent target, and any right-to-left shunts would render patients vulnerable to cerebral abscesses or stroke.[214]

Compared with a majority of other organs, there is a higher concentration of neutrophils sequestrated in pulmonary capillaries, which are readily recruitable to serve as important host defense agents.[215,216] In the lung, neutrophils emigrate primarily through capillaries, with about 70% of migrating neutrophils leaving the capillaries at tricellular corners where the margins of three endothelial cells converge (eFig. 6.2).[217]

PERICYTES, ADVENTITIAL CELLS, AND OTHER CELLS

In the pulmonary vessel wall, in addition to endothelial cells and VSMCs, other structures exist, such as the vasa vasorum (the vessels that feed the blood vessel walls), lymphatic vessels, and nerves, as well as fibroblasts, immunomodulatory cells (dendritic cells and macrophages), adipocytes, and vascular progenitor cells.[218]

Pericytes are contractile cells that surround the endothelial cells and are embedded within the basement membrane of the microvasculature, particularly in precapillary arterioles, capillaries, and postcapillary venules.[219] In the process of new vessel formation, although the endothelial cells can form tubelike structures independently, a close interplay between the endothelial cells and pericytes is indispensable for the formation of functional vasculature capable of conducting blood flow.[220–222] For example, when primary human lung pericytes are added to endothelial cells during in vitro microfluidics experiments, the microvessels formed are narrower, less tortuous, and significantly less leaky than vessels formed with endothelial cells alone.[223] The pericytes in microvessels constrict in response to phenylephrine, indicating an active role for pericytes in the regulation of the microcirculation. Pericytes may also act as sentries of the immune system. In response to inflammatory mediators, such as necrotic cell lysates or *tumor necrosis factor-α* (TNF-α), pericytes along arterioles and capillaries up-regulate the expression of adhesion molecule intercellular adhesion molecule-1 and release chemoattractant macrophage migration-inhibitory factor. These pericytes can attract and greatly augment leukocyte extravasation and can "instruct" extravasated leukocytes by increasing the expression of toll-like receptors and enhancing the ability of innate immune cells to detect and migrate to their final destination.[224] Increased numbers of pericytes have been observed around lung blood vessels in chronic lung diseases and are thought to be involved in vascular remodeling through pericyte-to-myofibroblast transformation in both humans and rodents.[225] The underlying mechanisms and their role in the development of PH remain to be elucidated.

Fibroblasts are the most abundant cell type in the adventitia of the blood vessel wall. They are the main cell type that synthesizes extracellular matrix to provide structural and biochemical support to the vessel wall. When exposed to hypoxia, ischemia, abnormal mechanical forces, or certain biochemical stimuli, fibroblasts can release a mixture of cytokines, chemokines, adhesion molecules, growth factors, and ROS, which initiate and perpetuate an inflammatory response. The adventitia of the pulmonary vasculature contains innate immune cells, particularly macrophages and *dendritic cells* (DCs). Under various pathophysiologic conditions, macrophages can fight pathogens, promote and restrict T cell responses, promote or resolve fibrosis, regulate angiogenesis, and control homeostasis in local immune networks. The principal role of pulmonary DCs is to encounter putative self and nonself environmental antigens and coordinate appropriate innate and acquired immunity responses. The coordinated actions of fibroblasts, macrophages, DCs, and other resident and recruited cells are essential for initiation, propagation, and resolution of local immune responses. When the response becomes chronic, the dysregulated activities of these cells contribute to the immunopathology of PH.[226–228]

Stem and progenitor cells, both resident and circulating, are present in pulmonary vessels, being most abundant in the adventitia. These cells have the potential to differentiate into various cell types, including endothelial cells, VSMCs, pericytes, fibroblasts, myofibroblasts, and macrophages. Under physiologic conditions, they are inactive and reside in stem cell niches of the vessel wall. When activated, they can be mobilized and migrate to the areas where the stimuli originated. Within the microenvironments surrounding these cells, in addition to soluble factors, the mechanical characteristics of the extracellular matrix exert profound influences on the lineage specification of stem and progenitor cells.[226,229,230]

PULMONARY VASCULAR ENDOTHELIUM AND CONTROL OF ENDOTHELIAL PERMEABILITY

The pulmonary circulation should be viewed as a series of networks from arteries to capillaries and veins. The endothelium in each of these vessels displays unique characteristics, and endothelial phenotypes vary distinctly in terms of origin, morphology, and function along the length of the pulmonary circulation.[231] Whereas pulmonary artery endothelial cells are derived from the pulmonary truncus through angiogenesis, lung capillary endothelial cells are derived from blood islands via vasculogenesis.[6] Pulmonary artery, capillary, and venous endothelial cells differ in their staining properties, with lectins suggesting differences in glycan composition of their respective glycocalyces. They also differ in their intracellular organelle content (e.g., Weibel-Palade bodies are present only in endothelial cells lining pulmonary arteries and veins, but not in lung capillaries) and in their function because precapillary endothelial cells produce more NO and do not form as tight a barrier as capillary endothelial cells.[6,232] Recent single-cell analytics and cloning identified additional lung endothelial subsets with specific proliferative, angiogenic, and bioenergetic profiles[233] and unique functions specifically in alveolar revascularization after injury.[234] A newly discovered population of pulmonary endothelial cells, called *Car4-high EC*, express a unique gene signature, and ligand-receptor analysis shows that they are primed to receive reparative signals from alveolar type 1 cells. After acute lung injury, they preferentially localize in regenerating regions of the alveolus and contribute to recovery and repair of the lung.[234]

To subserve the function of gas exchange, the overall capillary surface area is extensive (≈ 60 m^2), and the alveolar-capillary membrane at the gas-exchanging site is only approximately 200 nm thick. On the vascular side, this barrier is composed of approximately 68×10^9 endothelial cells[235] covering roughly 300×10^9 alveolar capillaries[236,237] (Fig 6.2). Hence each endothelial cell spans an average of four adjoining alveolar capillary segments. On the alveolar epithelial side of the membrane, the alveolar type 1 cell is extremely thin to facilitate gas exchange. At the blood-gas barrier, the endothelial and alveolar epithelial basement membranes fuse into a single one, a phenomenon that is unique to the alveolar-capillary membrane, with the single exception of the similarly fused basement membrane between capillary endothelial cells and podocytes in the kidney glomerulus. At the alveolar-capillary membrane, this results in a thin, yet particularly resilient, basement membrane considered as the major component responsible for the surprising strength of the blood-gas barrier[238,239] (Fig 6.3). This strong fused basement membrane facilitates diffusive gas exchange, while it also provides the tensile strength for this extremely thin membrane to resist rupture, even though it is exposed to constant mechanical stresses from both the vascular and the airspace side, demonstrating the remarkable engineering of the lung[240] (see Video 3.1).

In the intact lung, endothelial barrier function is maintained via restrictive interendothelial junctions composed of *tight junctions* and *adherens junctions*, as well as focal adhesions anchoring the endothelium to the underlying extracellular matrix (Fig. 6.4). For the tight junction, the predominant molecules in the lung endothelium are occludin, zonula occludens-1, and claudin-5, which form band-like structures around the endothelial cells in lung capillaries to ensure intact barrier function.[241,242] Claudin-5 expression is inversely correlated with lung endothelial leak,[243] with various pathogenic stimuli that cause loss of claudin-5.[244] If claudin-5 is silenced, the ability of simvastatin to stabilize the endothelial barrier, either in cultured endothelial cells or in a mouse model of acute lung injury, is decreased, indicating the important role of claudin-5 in maintaining endothelial barrier integrity.[245] For the

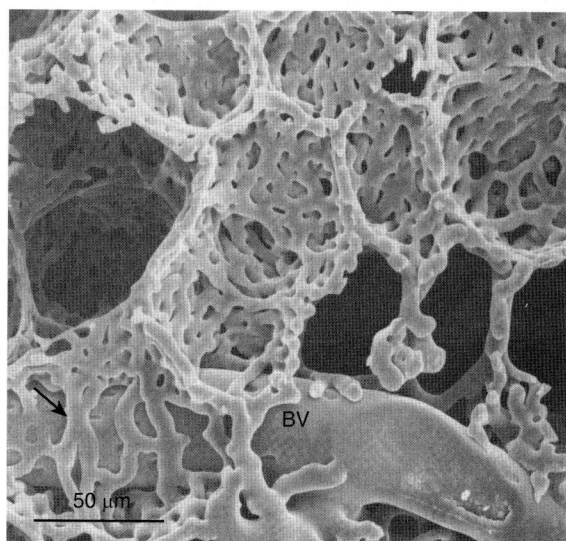

Figure 6.2 A scanning electron micrograph showing alveolar capillaries in a rat lung. Alveolar capillaries are seen as densely matted and intersecting tubules surrounding alveolar spaces. Other less numerous vessels are seen. At the bottom of the micrograph is a large *blood vessel* (BV), and running across this vessel is a nonalveolar capillary (*arrow*). (From Guntheroth WG, Luchtel DL, Kawabori I. Pulmonary microcirculation: tubules rather than sheet and post. *J Appl Physiol Respir Environ Exerc Physiol.* 1982;53[2]:510–515.)

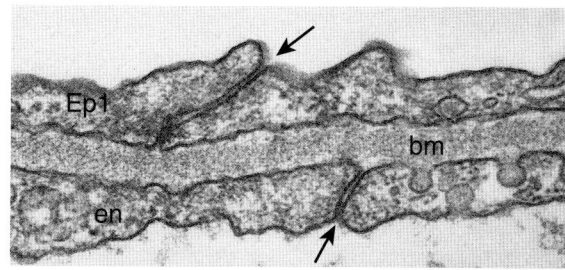

Figure 6.3 The alveolar-capillary barrier. A scanning electron micrograph of diffusion membrane shows the alveolar type 1 cells (Ep1) and *endothelial cells* (en) separated by fused *basement membrane* (bm) in the thin part of barrier. *Arrows* point to intercellular junctions with tight junctions in both cell layers. (From Weibel ER. On the tricks alveolar epithelial cells play to make a good lung. *Am J Respir Crit Care Med.* 2015;191[5]:504–513.)

adherens junctions, the major protein in the vasculature is vascular endothelial–cadherin, which forms homomeric intercellular adhesions linked to the endothelial cytoskeleton at its cytoplasmic tail via β-catenin, p120-catenin, and α-catenin.[246] Disassembly of vascular endothelial–cadherin junctions causes loss of lung endothelial barrier function.[247,248] In lung microvascular endothelial cells, which line alveolar capillaries as well as small nonmuscularized precapillary arterioles and postcapillary venules of up to 18 μm in size,[249] but not in pulmonary artery endothelial cells, expression of activated leukocyte cell adhesion molecules is highly correlated with N-cadherin expression.[250] Our understanding of the individual contribution of various cell adhesion molecules to the maintenance of an intact endothelial barrier in the lung is far from complete and may ultimately be crucial for the development of barrier-stabilizing interventions that can specifically target endothelial barrier function in individual vascular subcompartments (e.g., capillaries vs. arteries).

Endothelial Barrier

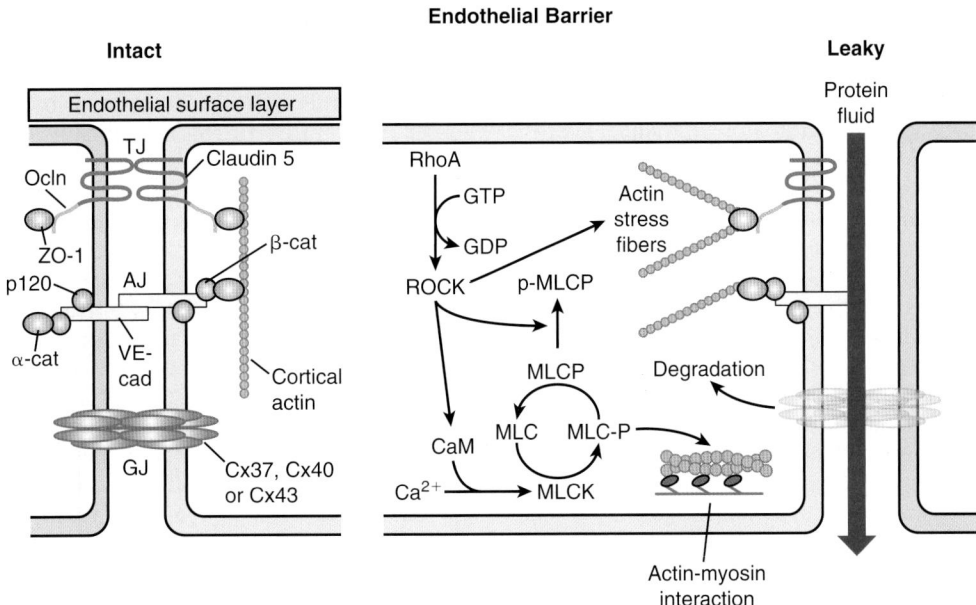

Figure 6.4 Regulation of lung endothelial barrier function. Under normal conditions (at *left*), the intact endothelial barrier restricts fluid and solute exchange due to the presence of an endothelial surface layer hydrogel and intact interendothelial junctions. The latter consist of *tight junctions* (TJs) composed of claudin, which is anchored to the cortical actin cytoskeleton via *occludin* (Ocln) and *zonula occludens* (ZO)-1, and of *adherens junctions* (AJ), which contain *VE-cadherin* (VE-cad) and p120, and α-catenin and *β-catenin* (cat). *Gap junctions* (GJs) composed of *connexins* (Cx) 37, 40, and 43 mediate interendothelial communication. Upon exposure to barrier-disruptive agonists (at *right*), the endothelial barrier can become leaky. The endothelial surface layer is shed and interendothelial gap junctions are degraded. Activation of *RhoA kinase* (RhoA-ROCK) signaling leads to phosphorylation and inhibition of *myosin light chain phosphatase* (MLCP). RhoA-ROCK activation increases Ca²⁺ signaling and by binding to *calmodulin* (CaM) activates *myosin light chain kinase* (MLCK), which leads to myosin light chain phosphorylation and enhanced and prolonged actin-interactions. In parallel, RhoA-ROCK signaling promotes the formation of actin stress fibers in lieu of the cortical actin cytoskeleton. In combination, these effects result in endothelial contraction and disruption of interendothelial junctions, resulting in unrestricted fluid and protein flux across a leaky endothelium.

Gap junctions situated between endothelial cells do not physically stabilize the endothelial barrier but regulate its permeability, in part by creating intercellular communication pathways by the assembly of two juxtaposed hemichannels and in part by direct protein-protein interactions.[251] Analogous to MEJs discussed earlier, interendothelial gap junctions in the lung are composed of connexins, with lung microvascular endothelial cells expressing Cx37, Cx40, and Cx43. There is evidence that connexins play an important role in the regulation of endothelial permeability. Inhibition or genetic deficiency of both Cx40 and Cx43 protects against the increase in endothelial permeability in various lung injury models, which suggests that gap junctions spread local increases in permeability along the pulmonary endothelium.[252,253] A recent study showed that when thrombin or lipopolysaccharide was applied locally to the endothelium of lungs with inhibition or deficiency of connexins, not only was there no spread of increased endothelial permeability, but there was also protection from injury at the site of application of the injurious agent. This finding cannot be explained by intercellular propagation of a permeability signal via gap junctions but, rather, points to additional functions of connexins in barrier regulation at the level of the individual endothelial cell. Of note, connexins seem to up-regulate expression of ROCK and stimulation of its downstream signaling pathway, which plays an important role in endothelial barrier failure.[253,254]

The luminal side of the microvascular endothelium is covered with a two-tiered hydrogel surface layer forming an additional physical barrier for transendothelial fluid and solute flux.[255–258] The lower tier, referred to as the glycocalyx, is approximately 70 nm thick and is anchored firmly in the cell membrane. It consists of proteoglycans with long unbranched *glycosaminoglycan* (GAG) side chains and glycoproteins with short-chain branched carbohydrate side chains. The upper tier, which can exceed 1000 nm in thickness, is formed by a thick layer of GAGs, predominantly hyaluronan, heparan sulfate, and chondroitin sulfate.[216] Degradation of this endothelial surface layer by invading pathogens or inflammatory responses markedly increases endothelial permeability[259,260]; hence, strategies for preservation or reconstitution of the surface layer, such as by GAG fragments[261] or growth factor signaling,[262] may present promising strategies to prevent or limit lung endothelial leak.

The pulmonary endothelium is not impermeable under normal conditions, and there is a constant basal exchange of fluid, electrolytes, and solutes between the vascular lumen and the lung interstitium. This exchange takes place via two main routes: a paracellular and a transcellular route.

The *paracellular* pathway of fluid and solute exchange is via interendothelial junctions and is governed by the variables in the Starling equation:

$$J_v = L_p \times S \left[(P_c - P_i) - \sigma(\pi_c - \pi_i) \right]$$

where J_v is fluid flux rate, L_p is hydraulic conductivity, S is the vessel surface area, σ is the reflection coefficient for plasma proteins, P is hydrostatic pressure, and π is oncotic pressure. The subscripts c and i refer to the capillary and interstitial compartments, respectively. The product of L_p and S is referred to as the endothelial *filtration coefficient* (K_f). Because K_f can be quantified in isolated perfused lungs, it remains the gold standard parameter for assessing endothelial permeability in the intact lung.[6] Under basal conditions, this fluid flux is largely driven by the hydrostatic pressure difference. Fluid filtered into the interstitium is rapidly cleared by passive movement of liquid from the filtration site to the initial lymphatics along a hydraulic pressure gradient of approximately 3 cm H_2O.[263] Along with fluid flux, small solutes and particles can extravasate by solvent drag along the paracellular route, yet their ability to permeate across the endothelial barrier decreases exponentially with molecular size. Alveolar epithelial cells also actively secrete solutes and, via the generated osmotic pressure, maintain a fluid layer in the alveolar space.[264] Under normal conditions at rest, the rate of basal paracellular fluid flux across the intact lung microvascular endothelium is relatively low.

Transcellular transport or endothelial transcytosis is the preferred pathway for macromolecules to move across the barrier because they are too big to pass through the paracellular route. Macromolecules move in a receptor-mediated manner via caveolae, clathrin-coated pits, or via clathrin- and caveolin-independent mechanisms, as well as in a receptor-independent manner via fluid-phase uptake. The best studied of these pathways in the lung is caveolar transport. Caveolae are abundant in the lung vasculature and comprise approximately 15–20% of the total endothelial volume.[265] In caveolar transcytosis, macromolecules such as albumin bind to their receptor on the apical endothelial membrane, resulting in activation of downstream kinases, in particular Src. Src phosphorylates both caveolin-1, the structural protein of caveolae, and the small guanosine triphosphatase, dynamin, resulting in "pinching off" of the caveolar vesicle from the cell membrane. Once caveolae reach the abluminal side of the endothelium, they fuse with the plasma membrane, releasing their cargo into the subendothelial space.[266] However, the physiologic significance of endothelial transcytosis across the pulmonary microvascular wall is not certain, and many questions regarding the dynamics and regulation of endothelial transcytosis remain unclear, such as whether caveolar trafficking within endothelial cells is directed or random, or how receptors change their affinity to bind cargo on the luminal side and release it again on the abluminal side. Mice with a genetic knockout of caveolin-1 (Cav1$^{-/-}$) lack endothelial caveolae and develop endothelial hypercellularity and pulmonary hypertension.[267] The Cav1$^{-/-}$ phenotype has fueled the notion that caveolar transport is essential for lung homeostasis, yet the multiple signaling functions of caveolin-1 make it impossible to attribute this phenotype to changes in endothelial transcytosis alone.

A myriad of pathologic and proinflammatory stimuli can impair lung endothelial barrier function and result in an increased permeability-type lung edema, rich in protein and inflammatory cells.[268] Well-established mediators that cause lung endothelial barrier failure are proteins such as thrombin or angiopoietin-2, cytokines such as TNF-α, peptides such as bradykinin, or bioactive lipids such as platelet-activating factor or ceramide.[269] Mediators generally act via two main signaling pathways, namely the RhoA-ROCK pathway and endothelial Ca^{2+} signaling (Fig. 6.4). The downstream effector ROCK is activated by the monomeric Rho guanosine triphosphatase as a result of ligand binding to Gα12/13-coupled receptors. ROCK phosphorylates and

inhibits myosin light chain phosphatase, the enzyme that dephosphorylates myosin light chain and thus terminates its interaction with F-actin filaments. ROCK activation enhances and prolongs actin-myosin–driven contractile forces transmitted to the endothelial adherens junctions complex, resulting in disruption of interendothelial junctions and gap formation.[246] With in vitro experiments, barrier-disrupting stimuli, such as TNF-α, cause characteristic ROCK-mediated cytoskeletal remodeling and actin stress fiber formation,[270] which further increases the contractile forces in the endothelium and, in parallel, leads to microtubule dissolution and loss of the cortical actin ring, which anchors interendothelial junction molecules under baseline junctions.[271] The Ca^{2+} pathway represents the other major barrier modification pathway. Barrier-disrupting stimuli, such as thrombin or platelet-activating factor, can increase endothelial Ca^{2+} signaling either by increasing Ca^{2+} release from intracellular stores, typically mediated by Gα12/13-coupled receptors and phospholipase C–dependent formation of inositol trisphosphate, and subsequent activation of store-operated Ca^{2+} channels, or by direct or indirect (e.g., via phospholipase C–derived diacyl glycerol) activation of transmembrane Ca^{2+} channels. The resulting increase in cytosolic Ca^{2+} concentration causes Ca^{2+}/calmodulin-dependent activation of myosin light chain kinase and phosphorylation of myosin light chain, which again increases contractile forces in the endothelium, promoting interendothelial gap formation. Of note, Ca^{2+}-dependent increases in lung endothelial permeability are not restricted to permeability-type lung edema but can also contribute, albeit to a lesser extent, to hydrostatic lung edema formation, which has traditionally been viewed as increased fluid filtration across an intact endothelial barrier with no change in permeability. This paradigm has, however, been revised by the finding that increased vascular pressures stimulate mechanosensitive cation channels, such as transient receptor potential vanilloid 4 on the endothelial plasma membrane, thereby increasing endothelial permeability and contributing to the formation of hydrostatic lung edema.[272]

Whether endothelial barrier disruption is primarily mediated via RhoA-ROCK or via Ca^{2+} signaling depends on the triggering stimulus and its respective receptor on the endothelial cell membrane, and whether the studies have been done under in vitro or in vivo conditions. RhoA-ROCK signaling and stress fiber formation play a key role in virtually all endothelial permeability assays in vitro; in contrast, Ca^{2+} signaling seems to be the dominant regulator in intact lungs, where endothelial stress fiber formation is less prominent or totally absent and inhibition of ROCK signaling does not prevent endothelial hyperpermeability.[269] The reasons for these differences in experimental findings are not fully understood but may relate to the fact that ROCK-dependent formation of stress fibers in endothelial cells becomes more prominent when the cells are on a stiff substrate; the stiffness of plastic or glass used in culture dishes is in the range of 2 to 4 *gigapascals* (GPa) but is a million times less (below 1 kPa) in the intact lung.[273]

Other factors also play a role in barrier function. Paracellular leak of plasma proteins in response to barrier-disruptive stimuli can be amplified by stimulation of protein transcytosis, by mediators such as endotoxin[274] or thrombin.[266] Finally, a variety of mediators and second messengers can help to reconstitute or preserve endothelial barrier function by attenuating activation of RhoA-ROCK and Ca^{2+} signaling pathways with their effects on cytoskeletal remodeling and contraction. Barrier-protective mediators such as sphingosine-1-phosphate or angiopoietin-1 are potential therapeutic molecules for lung endothelial barrier preservation and repair, but their clinical use awaits definitive clinical trials.

BRONCHIAL CIRCULATION

The bronchial circulation supplies nutrition and oxygenated blood to the conducting airways, walls of the pulmonary arteries and veins, regional lymph nodes, nerves, and the visceral pleura. The bronchial circulation is a high-pressure, low-volume system supplied by the bronchial arteries, which arise directly from the thoracic aorta or one of its branches, although there is significant anatomic variability. Upon entering the lung, the intrapulmonary bronchial arteries travel and branch within the bronchi down to the terminal bronchioles, forming a vast network of capillaries and establishing extensive anastomoses with other bronchial arteries and the pulmonary vasculature. Bronchial blood flow to the lung is estimated to be less than 3% of the cardiac output. A small portion ($\approx$25–33%) of the bronchial arterial supply returns to the right atrium via bronchial veins, and approximately 67–75% flows into the left atrium via pulmonary veins, constituting an intrinsic right-to-left shunt. In consequence, blood in the left atrium is slightly less oxygenated than in the pulmonary capillaries[9,275–277] (eFig. 6.3).

Although often overlooked because of its relatively low blood flow compared to that in the pulmonary circulation, the bronchial circulation is an important contributor to lung homeostasis. For example, although most particulate matter in the airways is cleared by the mucociliary machinery, soluble particles can also be removed by direct uptake into the bronchial vessels.[278,279] Absorption of inhaled drugs by the submucosal bronchial venous system in airways may provide inhaled drugs direct access to the systemic circulation, bypassing hepatic degradation. Such a possibility and its clinical relevance, however, have not yet been evaluated.[280] Compared to the pulmonary circulation, the bronchial circulation also has a much greater capacity to expand and proliferate in response to chronic inflammation. Because the bronchial circulation is a high-pressure system, disruption of the vessels leads to significant bleeding. Indeed, the vast majority of massive and submassive hemoptysis episodes arise from the bronchial circulation.[280,281]

Key Points

- The pulmonary circulation is a low-pressure, low–vascular-resistance circulation functionally different from the systemic circulation.
- Gravity and changes in lung volume during breathing profoundly affect the distribution of blood flow within the lung.

- Pulmonary vessels constrict in response to hypoxia, which leads to improved matching of perfusion to ventilation. However, chronic and global hypoxic vasoconstriction may lead to pulmonary hypertension.
- The pulmonary veins also play an important role in the regulation of pulmonary microvascular filtration pressures and segmental and total pulmonary vascular resistances.
- Endothelial cells play a pivotal role in the regulation of pulmonary vascular contractility and remodeling through the release of nitric oxide, prostacyclin, and endothelin-1.
- Endothelial cells communicate with the underlying vascular smooth muscle cells via paracrine signaling, myoendothelial gap junctions, and extracellular vesicles.
- Pericytes, fibroblast, immune cells, and other cells in the pulmonary vasculature contribute to its vasoreactivity.
- The pulmonary circulation also possesses certain nonrespiratory functions, including activation/inactivation and clearance of various vasoactive agents, anticoagulation and fibrinolytic activity, clearance of particles, and host defense.
- Endothelial cells demonstrate heterogeneity across the arteries, capillaries, and veins.
- Endothelial barrier integrity is maintained by intact interendothelial junctions and an endothelial surface layer hydrogel; barrier-disruptive agents cause shedding of the surface layer, endothelial contraction, and loss of interendothelial junctions, allowing protein and fluid leak into the interstitial space.
- The bronchial circulation is a part of the systemic circulation and is required for the metabolic needs of the lungs. Because it is a high-pressure system, disruption of these vessels can lead to massive hemoptysis.

Key Readings

Dhaun N, Webb DJ. Endothelins in cardiovascular biology and therapeutics. *Nat Rev Cardiol.* 2019;16(8):491–502.

Gao Y, Chen T, Raj JU. Endothelial and smooth muscle cell interactions in the pathobiology of pulmonary hypertension. *Am J Respir Cell Mol Biol.* 2016;54(4):451–460.

Klinger JR, Kadowitz PJ. The nitric oxide pathway in pulmonary vascular disease. *Am J Cardiol.* 2017;120(8S):S71–S79.

Lan NSH, Massam BD, Kulkarni SS, Lang CC. Pulmonary arterial hypertension: pathophysiology and treatment. *Diseases.* 2018;6(2):E38. pii.

Lanyu Z, Feilong H. Emerging role of extracellular vesicles in lung injury and inflammation. *Biomed Pharmacother.* 2019;113:108748.

Stenmark KR, Frid MG, Graham BB, Tuder RM. Dynamic and diverse changes in the functional properties of vascular smooth muscle cells in pulmonary hypertension. *Cardiovasc Res.* 2018;114(4):551–564.

Suresh K, et al. Lung circulation. *Compr Physiol.* 2016;6(2):897–943.

Sylvester JT, Shimoda LA, Aaronson PI, Ward JP. Hypoxic pulmonary vasoconstriction. *Physiol Rev.* 2012;92(1):367–520.

Thind GS, Zanders S, Baker JK. Recent advances in the understanding of endothelial barrier function and fluid therapy. *Postgrad Med J.* 2018;94(1111):289–295.

Wettschureck N, Strilic B, Offermanns S. Passing the vascular barrier: endothelial signaling processes controlling extravasation. *Physiol Rev.* 2019;99(3):1467–1525.

Complete reference list available at ExpertConsult.com.

7 LYMPHATIC BIOLOGY

SOUHEIL EL-CHEMALY, MD, MPH • HASINA OUTTZ REED, MD, PHD

INTRODUCTION

The lymphatic vasculature has long been poorly studied. Over the past 2 decades, the advent of markers that could reliably differentiate *lymphatic endothelial cells* (LECs) from vascular endothelial cells led to important progress in the understanding of lymphatic biology. Lung lymphatics play important roles in lung homeostasis, particularly in the drainage of fluid and macromolecules and immune cell trafficking. The role(s) of lymphatic vessels in lung disease is poorly understood. Most lung diseases are associated with changes in lymphatic distribution and/or density. It is unclear, however, if these changes are secondary to the remodeling process or directly contribute to disease pathogenesis. This chapter focuses on current knowledge regarding the distribution and function of lymphatics in the normal lung and highlights new evidence demonstrating that changes in the lymphatic vasculature play a critical role in lung disease initiation and progression.

ANATOMY OF THE PULMONARY LYMPHATICS

The pulmonary lymphatics drain fluid and traffic leukocytes from the distal lung parenchyma to the mediastinal and hilar lymph nodes. Anatomic studies have defined the relationship of the lymphatics to the other structures in the lung, but historically this was challenging given the lack of specific markers for pulmonary lymphatic endothelium and the fact that, in a normal lung, the lymphatics are thin, collapsed vessels that are difficult to detect. Some of the most detailed early descriptions of the pulmonary lymphatics resulted from casting procedures using resins in rodents in which pulmonary edema was induced to expand and visualize these vessels.[1–3]

These studies described lymphatic structures on the pleural surface (the superficial lymphatic plexus) and within the lung itself (the deep lymphatic plexus); in both cases a network of smaller initial lymphatic capillaries drain into larger conduit or collecting lymphatic vessels.[4] Whole mount imaging techniques using reporter mice in which all LECs are labeled with *green fluorescent protein* (GFP) (Prox1-GFP) have allowed for in-depth imaging of these vessels in the lungs and elsewhere.[5]

Initial lymphatic capillaries are small, thin-walled, blind-ended structures (Fig. 7.1C–D). Initial lymphatics feed into the larger collecting lymphatics containing a series of valves (Fig. 7.1A, B, D). LECs in lymphatic vessels have unique junctions specialized for the uptake of fluid and cells. Initial lymphatic capillaries have discontinuous junctions that form flaps between adjacent areas (called "buttons") and allow cells to enter the lumen of the lymphatic capillary[6,7] (Fig. 7.2). These junctions differ greatly from those of the collecting lymphatics, which have continuous zipper-like junctions that resemble those found between blood endothelial cells in both structure and function (see Fig. 7.2).[8] Collecting lymphatics in the periphery of the lung drain toward the visceral pleura but do not connect to the pleural space, whereas more centrally located lymphatics drain to the mediastinum.

The collecting lymphatics in tissues outside of the lung contain functional subunits known as lymphangions that consist of smooth muscle cell–lined segments of lymphatic vessel separated by valves, which actively pump lymph.[9–11] However, collecting pulmonary lymphatics in humans have only sporadic smooth muscle cell coverage, and collecting pulmonary lymphatics in rodents lack any smooth muscle cell coverage.[12–14] Therefore, collecting pulmonary lymphatics cannot contract robustly,[15] suggesting that extrinsic forces such as changes in thoracic pressure associated with ventilation may play a more central role in driving lung lymph flow.[16–18]

Within the human lung, the vast majority of lymphatic vessels are located either in the interlobular septa or subpleural space rather than within the lobule.[18] Among intralobular lymphatics, nearly all are associated with a blood vessel or in a bronchovascular bundle (Fig. 7.3).[4,19] Casting studies as well as conventional and whole mount immunohistochemistry of lung tissue have failed to identify a significant component of lymphatics in close association with alveoli in humans or rodents.[1–3,20,21]

PULMONARY LYMPHATIC MARKERS

Over the past 2 decades, major advances in the study of lymphangiogenesis were made possible by the identification of

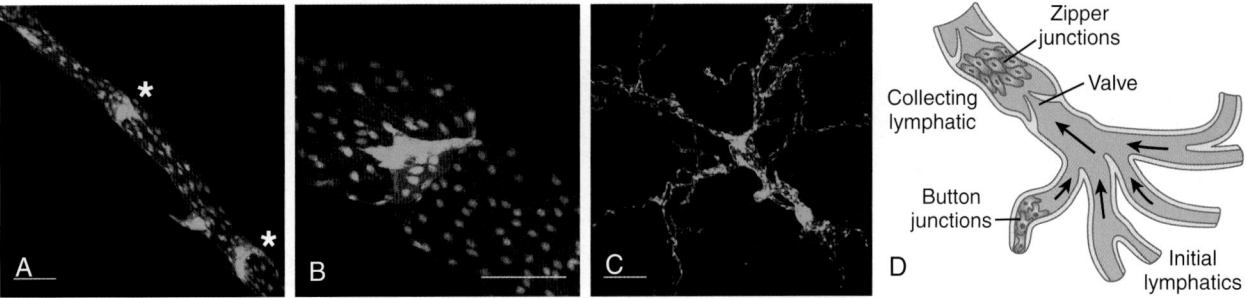

Figure 7.1 **Pulmonary lymphatic vessel structure.** (A–B) Whole mount imaging of lungs from adult *Prox1-GFP* lymphatic reporter mice shows pulmonary lymphatic vessels in green. (A) Collecting lymphatic vessel, with asterisks indicating areas of Prox1^{hi} endothelial cells that mark lymphatic valves. (B) High-magnification image of collecting pulmonary lymphatic vessel with Prox1^{hi} area demonstrating valve leaflet. (C) Smaller initial lymphatic vessels are blind-ended vessels without valves. (D) Illustration of pulmonary lymphatic vessels. Initial lymphatics begin as blind ends with button junctions. These initial lymphatics drain into larger collecting lymphatics characterized by zipper junctions and a series of valves. Scale bars = 25 μM.

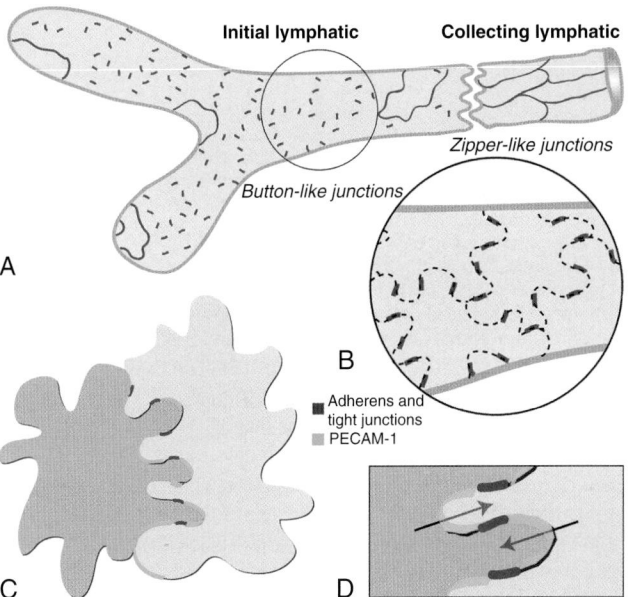

Figure 7.2 **Specialized lymphatic junctions.** (A) Schematic diagram showing distinctive, discontinuous buttons in endothelium of initial lymphatics and continuous zippers in collecting lymphatics. Both types of junctions consist of proteins typical of adherens junctions and tight junctions. (B) More detailed view showing the oak-leaf shape of endothelial cells (*dashed lines*) of initial lymphatics. Buttons (*red*) appear to be oriented perpendicular to the cell border but are in fact parallel to the sides of flaps. In contrast, most PECAM-1 expression is at the tips of flaps. (C and D) Enlarged views of buttons show that flaps of adjacent oak leaf–shaped endothelial cells have complementary shapes with overlapping edges. Adherens junctions and tight junctions at the sides of flaps direct fluid entry (*arrows*) to the junction-free region at the tip without repetitive disruption and re-formation of junctions. (From Baluk P, Fuxe J, Hashizume H, et al. Functionally specialized junctions between endothelial cells of lymphatic vessels. *J Exp Med.* 2007;204[10]:2349–2362.)

many lymphangiogenic growth factors, including *vascular endothelial growth factor* (VEGF)-C and VEGF-D, which signal through their canonical receptor *VEGF receptor 3* (VEGFR3) present on the surface of LECs.[22] Importantly, the identification of markers of pulmonary lymphatics allows the pulmonary lymphatics to be distinguished from the blood vasculature and capillary network in the lung. While many of these markers are also expressed by LECs in other organs, the repertoire of markers expressed by LECs varies according to the organ in which they are located. Therefore, careful analysis is required

to ensure that pulmonary lymphatics are properly identified. In the mouse lung, two commonly used markers of lymphatic endothelium, lymphatic vessel endothelial hyaluronan receptor and podoplanin, are not specific for pulmonary lymphatics because they are highly expressed by blood endothelial cells and the epithelium, respectively.[23,24] Combination of these markers with other more specific lymphatic markers such as PROX1, a transcription factor and master regulator of lymphatic lineage, increase their utility. Expression of VEGFR3 can be used to identify lymphatics in the mouse lung whereas, in the human lung and in other mouse organs, this marker lacks specificity for the lymphatic endothelium. In humans, podoplanin (D2-40 epitope) has good specificity for identifying lymphatic vessels by immunohistochemistry staining.[25] Further complicating the identification of pulmonary lymphatic vessels is the finding that expression of lymphatic markers may change in the setting of lung injury.[26,27] Whenever possible, co-staining using two markers of the lymphatic endothelium should be used to ensure proper distinction of these vessels from the blood endothelium. Commonly used markers of the lymphatic endothelium are detailed in Table 7.1.

ROLE OF LYMPHATICS IN THE LUNG

FLUID UPTAKE AND PREVENTION OF PULMONARY EDEMA

An established role of lymphatic vessels in all organs is uptake of interstitial fluid; therefore, the consequence of a loss of lymphatic function is tissue edema.[28] In the lung, the role of lymphatics for drainage of interstitial fluid and prevention of alveolar edema is essential, because the lungs are exquisitely sensitive to alveolar pulmonary edema, which would negatively affect gas exchange. Accordingly, normal lymphatic function during lung development is required to drain fluid and increase the compliance necessary for neonatal lung inflation.[29,30] However, despite the importance of normal lymphatic development in the clearance of lung fluid immediately after birth, studies in adult large animals have shown that pulmonary lymph flow is relatively minimal even in the presence of lung edema.[16,31,32] In the traditional model by Ernest Starling, fluid balance in the lung

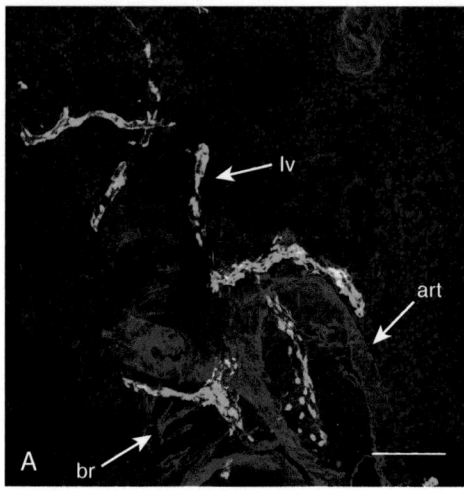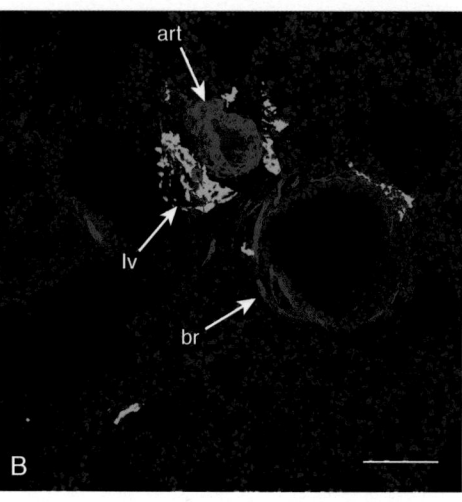

Figure 7.3 **Pulmonary lymphatics are closely associated with bronchovascular bundles.** (A–B) Immunohistochemistry of thick lung sections from *Prox1-GFP* mice with smooth muscle actin staining (*red*) shows lymphatic vessels (lv, *green*), in close association with arteries (art) and bronchi (br) in bronchovascular bundles. Nuclei stained with DAPI shown in blue. Scale bars = 25 μM.

Table 7.1   Lung Lymphatic Markers

Marker	Species	Comments
VEGFR3	Mouse	Unlike in other tissues, this is a specific marker for pulmonary lymphatics in the mouse lung. Use caution when using this marker in lung injury models because there can be increased VEGFR3 staining of pulmonary capillaries in this setting.
GFP (in *Prox1-GFP* mice)	Mouse	This lymphatic reporter mouse is the best and most specific way to visualize the pulmonary lymphatics in mice. In these mice, the GFP signal expressed from the Prox1 promoter can be detected in fresh or frozen sections, or immunohistochemistry can be used to detect GFP. The Prox1-GFP transgene can be crossed into other backgrounds for use in multiple mouse models. In the mouse lung, Prox1-GFP transgene expression is specific for lymphatic endothelial cells.
tdTomato (in *Prox1-tdTomato* mice)	Mouse	The tdTomato signal can be visualized in fresh or frozen sections, or immunohistochemistry can be used to detect tdTomato. Difficulty breeding these mice and issues with sterility limit their usefulness.
Prox1	Mouse	Nuclear stain labels lymphatic endothelial cells, but also labels other cell types in the lung, limiting its usefulness as a lymphatic marker on its own.
Lymphatic vessel endothelial hyaluronan receptor	Mouse	As opposed to other tissues in mice, this is not a specific marker of lymphatics in the lungs, because it strongly stains much of the blood vascular endothelium. Though it cannot be used on its own, when combined with Prox1 for double staining, it can be used to identify pulmonary lymphatic vessels.
CCL21	Mouse	Provides specific staining of lymphatic endothelial cells in the lungs.
Podoplanin	Mouse/human	Not a specific marker of pulmonary lymphatics in the mouse lung. However, staining for podoplanin (D2-40 clone) in human lungs does provide specific staining and is the best pulmonary lymphatic marker for human tissue.

CCL21, C-C motif chemokine ligand 21; GFP, green fluorescent protein; VEGFR, vascular endothelial growth factor receptor.

is maintained by a balance of hydrostatic forces moving fluid from the blood into the lung interstitium with oncotic forces moving fluid back into the blood capillary system. In this model, lung edema can be considered primarily a consequence of imbalanced Starling forces rather than inadequate pulmonary lymphatic function.[32–34] Nonetheless, lymphatics clearly have a role in the drainage of lung fluid, and pulmonary lymph flow increases in settings of injury and inflammation.[35,36] Genetic mouse models of impaired pulmonary lymphatic flow have been lacking until recently, making testing the role of these vessels in lung biology challenging. Recent work examining a mouse model of impaired lymph flow (from defects in lymphatic-venous separation) has demonstrated that these mice are susceptible to pulmonary edema in the setting of lung injury despite intact lymphatic vessels,[15] though notably these mice did not

have evidence of pulmonary edema at baseline. Thus, the role of the pulmonary lymphatics in lung fluid drainage is likely most important in settings of injury and pulmonary edema. These observations are analogous to those of the parietal pleural lymphatics, which drain the pleural fluid (see Chapter 14). At baseline with a normal slow entry rate of pleural fluid, impairment of lymphatic drainage of the pleural space may have little consequence whereas, when entry of fluid into the pleural space increases, the limitation of lymphatic drainage contributes to formation of pleural effusions.

IMMUNE CELL TRAFFICKING

The role of the pulmonary lymphatics goes beyond providing a conduit for excess edema. An additional well-studied role of the pulmonary lymphatics is regulating the immune response. The lung is constantly exposed to the outside environment and must maintain a quiescent immune state as well as be able to mount a robust immune response to pathogens. Immune cell trafficking to draining lymph nodes via the pulmonary lymphatics plays a central role in coordinating the adaptive immune response.[37,38] At steady state in healthy animals, the migration of antigen-presenting cells from the airways to the mediastinal lymph nodes via the lymphatics takes 1 to 2 days.[39,40] Some studies have shown similar kinetics of the migration of these cells in the setting of infection, while others have shown that the migration of these cells increases in the first few days after infection.[41–44] Of note, the kinetics for upper airway antigen-presenting cells is much faster than for their counterparts in the lung parenchyma, where the migration rate is greater than 7 days in some models.[40,43] Immune cell trafficking via the lymphatics is dependent on signaling between the lymphatic endothelium and antigen-presenting cells, which coordinates their migration. In particular, *C-C motif chemokine ligand* (CCL)21 expressed on the lymphatic endothelium and its receptor CCR7 expressed on T cells and dendritic cells appears to be essential for uptake and migration of these immune cells in pulmonary lymphatic vessels.[45] Immobilized CCL21 on the lymphatic endothelium is also important in directing the leukocytes moving within lymphatic vessels.[46–48] Other factors expressed by the lymphatic endothelium, including S1P, intercellular adhesion molecule-1, and vascular cell adhesion molecule-1, are also important for leukocyte trafficking via lymphatics, particularly in response to inflammation.[26,49,50] Migration of immune cells to draining lymph nodes ensures antigen presentation resulting in either an adaptive immune response or tolerance.

LOCAL IMMUNITY AND INDUCIBLE BRONCHUS-ASSOCIATED LYMPHOID TISSUE

Migration of antigen-presenting cells to the draining lymph node via the lymphatics is essential for proper immune responses. In response to inflammation, the pulmonary lymphatics proliferate and play a role in the local inflammatory environment.[20,51] Lymphatics contribute to the development of *bronchus-associated lymphoid tissue* (BALT), which is a tertiary lymphoid organ not present in normal lung. Because BALT is induced only in response to a stimulus, the term *inducible bronchus-associated lymphoid tissue* (iBALT) is preferred.[52,53] iBALTs are accumulations of lymphoid cells that resemble lymph nodes in cellular content, organization, and the presence of lymphatic vessels. Chronic inflammation is often associated with the development of iBALT, where antigen presentation and lymphocyte priming can take place in close proximity to the area of inflammation, bypassing the need for antigen-presenting cells to traffic to the draining lymph nodes. However, this can have both favorable and unfavorable consequences. For example, in the setting of infection, iBALT allows for more rapid pathogen clearance and is protective.[54–57] However, in response to cigarette smoke exposure, iBALT may be a source of autoantibodies and destructive inflammatory mediators.[58–61] In mouse models of lung transplantation, iBALT can contribute to rejection through local immune activity,[60] though iBALT may also be a source of regulatory T cells that promote tolerance and acceptance

of the graft.[61,62] Although tertiary lymphoid organs are a hallmark of chronic lung disease,[63] the reason they form from such widely differing insults and the role they play in different settings is unclear. Lymphatics are likely to be important in this process, because lymphatic vessels are key features of iBALT[20,52] and, in the setting of inflammation, active lymphangiogenesis is observed in association with these structures.[20] In addition, lymphatic dysfunction can contribute to iBALT formation and alveolar damage, even in the absence of inflammation or insult,[15] suggesting that lymphatic impairment may play a role in the pathogenesis of lung diseases in which iBALT is prominent.

PULMONARY LYMPHATICS IN LUNG INJURY

Apart from iBALT, pulmonary lymphatic function (and dysfunction) likely plays an important role in a variety of lung diseases (Table 7.2). Though lymphangiogenesis is often seen in response to lung inflammation, chronic inflammation leads to impaired lymphatic function,[64–67] perhaps in part due to a change in the LEC junctions that makes them less conducive to leukocyte entry.[6] When lymphatic function is impaired, accumulation of fluid, immune cells, proteins, and hyaluronan leads to inflammation, fibrosis, and changes in immune function.[67–69] However, the precise mechanism of how pulmonary lymphatics play a role in the pathogenesis of lung injury remains elusive. Abnormal lymphatics have been described in association with a variety of lung diseases,[70] but whether they are simply a consequence of the disease or whether lymphatic dysfunction actively contributes to lung injury is not always clear. The current state of knowledge of the role of lymphatics in lung disease is discussed further later.

LYMPHATIC DISORDERS DURING LUNG DEVELOPMENT

The lymphatic vasculature arises mainly from the venous endothelial cells driven by a combination of the expression of lymphatic-specific transcription factors (e.g., Prox1) and response to growth factors such as VEGF-C via VEGFR3 signaling in LECs.[71] LECs undergo a complex maturation program in preparation for birth,[72] which is critically important for the first breath.[32] Thus, disorders of lung lymphatics may be an underrecognized cause of early respiratory failure in preterm infants.[73] Experimental data in genetically engineered mice have shown that VEGF-C overexpression in utero leads to dilated lymphatics, chylous effusions, and respiratory failure, all features of human lymphangiectasia.[74] Importantly, there was a time-dependent response to exposure to VEGF-C overexpression, with worse outcomes with earlier exposures in utero, which was not reversed by stopping VEGF-C overexpression or blocking its receptors (VEGFR2 and VEGFR3) after the development of lymphangiectasia.[74] However, treatment with rapamycin, an inhibitor of the *mammalian target of rapamycin* (mTOR), reversed the aberrant lymphatics without affecting existing normal lymphatics.[75] Even though the mouse phenotype resembled human pulmonary lymphangiectasia, the role of VEGF-C in human disease is unclear.

Table 7.2   Evidence of Lymphatic Involvement in Lung Disease

	Clinical Findings	Experimental Findings
Asthma	Decreased airway lymphatics associated with edema and fibrosis in fatal asthma	Chronic airway inflammation results in lymphangiogenesis in rat and mouse models. Blocking lymphatic vessel formation results in airway edema.
COPD	Increased lymphatic vessel density especially associated with alveolar spaces and in advanced stage COPD	Lymphatic dysfunction alone leads to BALT formation and air space enlargement.
Interstitial lung disease	Increased lymphatic vessel density especially associated with alveolar spaces. Fragmented lymphatic vessels. Diffuse lymphatic anomalies can manifest as ILD	A decrease in lymphatic vessels after ionizing radiation precedes development of fibrosis. After bleomycin injury, mural cells lining lymphatic lumens result in lymphatic dysfunction.
Lung transplantation	Acute rejection is associated with increased lymphatic vessel density. No change in lymphatic vessel density in chronic allograft dysfunction	Stimulation of lymphangiogenesis decreased acute allograft rejection.
Tuberculosis	Elevated serum VEGF-C levels correlate with disease burden	VEGF-C induces lymphangiogenesis. *Mycobacterium tuberculosis* grows in lymphatic endothelial cells.
Sarcoidosis	Elevated VEGF and VEGF-C levels in bronchoalveolar lavage and serum. Atypical lymphatics around sarcoid granulomas	

BALT, bronchus-associated lymphoid tissue; ILD, interstitial lung disease; VEGF, vascular endothelial growth factor.

Other diseases characterized by systemic lymphatic malformations such as *Gorham-Stout disease* (GSD) and generalized lymphatic anomaly can affect the lung, causing chylous effusions and respiratory failure.[76] Bone-specific overexpression of VEGF-C in mice results in the bone lymphatic malformations observed in GSD and in the development of chylous effusions, thought to be due to the chyle leakage from aberrant lymphatics in the periosseous chest wall muscles.[77] In GSD, there is an increase in lung lymphatic surface area and in the proliferative capacity of lung LECs.[78] While rapamycin has been shown to be effective in the management of vascular and lymphatic anomalies,[79] precision medicine approaches have recently led to the identification of novel somatic mutations in pathways involved in lymphatic homeostasis leading to rational selection of therapy with either mTOR inhibitors[80] or MEK inhibitors.[81] Additional lymphatic diseases with pulmonary manifestations are listed in Table 7.3.

ASTHMA

Asthma is characterized by airway inflammation leading to mostly reversible airways obstruction. Chronic inflammation, angiogenesis, subepithelial fibrosis, and extracellular matrix deposition are often features of the disease.[82]

There is a paucity of data regarding the fate of the lymphatic vasculature in human asthma. One study showed that, in fatal asthma, there is decreased lymphatic vessel density associated with airway edema and fibrotic changes, despite an increase in VEGF-C and VEGF-D levels,[82] suggesting a link between lymphatics and outcome in severe asthma.[82]

The role of the lymphatic vasculature in chronic airway inflammation has been studied in a mouse model using *Mycoplasma pulmonis*[51,83,84] and in a rat model using house dust mites.[85] Both of these models have yielded important

new knowledge in the understanding of chronic airway inflammation. These models showed that inflammation resulted in an increase in lymphatic vessels in the airways. Chronic airway inflammation using *Mycoplasma pulmonis*[51,83,84] in a mouse model resulted in a significant increase in number of lymphatic and blood vessels. VEGF-C/D signaling through VEGFR 3 was partially driving the de novo lymphangiogenesis, but not angiogenesis.[51] Critically, blocking lymphangiogenesis resulted in an increase in airway edema,[51] potentially linking lymphatics to the development of airways obstruction. Moreover, while angiogenesis regressed with anti-inflammatory and antibiotic therapy, these treatments did not result in involution of the newly formed lymphatics.

Importantly, LECs isolated from house dust mite–sensitized rats showed increased proliferative, chemotactic, and tubulation properties, which persisted over multiple passages.[85] Although these models have yielded important insights into chronic airway inflammation, the role and contribution of lymphatics to human asthma pathogenesis remains to be elucidated.

CHRONIC OBSTRUCTIVE PULMONARY DISEASE

COPD is characterized by fixed airway obstruction, excess mucus production, and enlarged alveolar spaces, most commonly due to cigarette smoke exposure.[86] The role and fate of the lymphatic vessels in animal models of emphysema and cigarette smoke exposure has not been studied, and the effects of cigarette smoke exposure on LECs are unknown. Lymphoid follicles are increasingly recognized as central to the pathogenesis of COPD.[87] Furthermore, in lung tissues of patients with COPD, there is an increase in lymphatic vessel density, particularly in association with the alveolar spaces, which is associated with worse disease severity.[88,89] These findings are associated with a dysregulation of CCL21 and

Table 7.3 Miscellaneous Lymphatic Diseases With Pulmonary Manifestations

Disorder	Pulmonary Manifestations	Comments
Congenital pulmonary lymphangiectasias[124]	Severe neonatal respiratory distress	▪ Dilated saccular lung lymphatics ▪ Presumed impaired development of the fetal central lymphatic conduction system ▪ Can be associated with other congenital disorders
Diffuse pulmonary lymphangiomatosis[125]	Interstitial infiltrates, chylous effusions	▪ Lymphangiomas within normal lymphatic pathways ▪ Positive staining for endothelial markers such as CD31, factor VIII-related antigen, and D2-40 ▪ Absence of HMB45-positive LAM cells
Gorham-Stout disease[126]	Chylous effusions due to thoracic cage involvement	▪ Primary systemic manifestation is osteolysis ▪ Increased lymphatic and proliferative properties of lung LEC
Lymphangioleiomyomatosis	Pneumothorax, chylous effusions, thin-walled pulmonary cysts	▪ Elevated serum VEGF-D levels ▪ Presence of HMB-45 cells
Yellow nail syndrome[127]	Exudative pleural effusions, bronchiectasis	▪ Impaired lymph transport by lymphoscintigraphy ▪ Possible microvasculopathy

HMB, human melanoma black; LAM, lymphangioleiomyomatosis; LEC, lymphatic endothelial cells; VEGF, vascular endothelial growth factor.

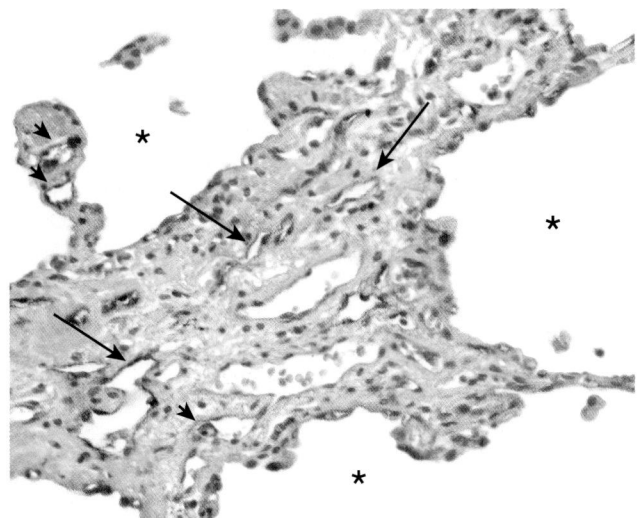

Figure 7.4 Alveolar lymphangiogenesis in *idiopathic pulmonary fibrosis* (IPF). IPF lung tissue section was stained with anti-CD34 (*red*) and anti-D2-40 (*brown*) antibodies. There is an increase in both blood capillary (*red, arrowheads*) and lymphatics (*brown, arrows*), with lymphatic vessels in proximity to alveolar spaces (*asterisks*). In the normal lung, there is a paucity of lymphatics associated with the alveoli.

chemokine scavenger receptor D6, which may alter transit of immune cells through the lymphatics in COPD.[89] Further evidence of lymphatic involvement in the pathogenesis of COPD is suggested by models of lymphatic impairment in mice that demonstrate that lymphatic dysfunction alone results in development of iBALT and air space enlargement that resembles emphysema.[15] Additional studies are needed to identify the effects of cigarette smoke on LECs, the effects of modulation of lymphangiogenesis on air space enlargement due to cigarette smoke, and whether these newly formed lymphatic vessels are functional.

INTERSTITIAL LUNG DISEASE

Interstitial lung diseases are a heterogenous group of disorders characterized by diffuse parenchymal involvement, with the potential development of fibrosis. Multiple studies have shown an increase in lymphatic vessel density and altered lymphatic distribution in *idiopathic pulmonary fibrosis* (IPF) and other forms of interstitial lung disease[25,90] (Fig. 7.4). These studies have also shown that increased alveolar lymphangiogenesis is associated with worsening fibrosis.[25,90] What remains unclear is the role of these vessels in fibrotic lung disease and whether these newly formed lymphatic vessels are functional or, as one study suggests, whether they are fragmented, and therefore nonfunctional.[91] Intriguingly, diffuse lung lymphatic anomalies can manifest as interstitial lung disease, with pathologic evidence of fibrosis.[92] In a description of three patients with lung lymphatic abnormalities (two cases of pulmonary lymphangiectasia and one case of lymphangiomatosis), CT scan of the chest at the time of presentation showed thickened interlobular septa, and other features of parenchymal lung involvement. However, the main histologic feature was dilated and abnormal lymphatic structures. This report demonstrates that primary lymphatic anomalies may present as interstitial lung disease.

In a mouse model of radiation-induced fibrosis, lung lymphatic vessel density decreased prior to the development of fibrosis,[93] suggesting that these changes are not simply in response to fibrosis. In the bleomycin mouse model of fibrosis, although there were no differences in lymphatic vessel density at day 28, lymphatic vessels were lined with *platelet-derived growth factor receptor* (PDGFR)-β mural cells that blocked the ability of lymphatics to drain hyaluronan, a key regulator of lung injury.[94] Although no preclinical or clinical studies have been undertaken to modulate lymphangiogenesis in fibrotic lung disease, it is important to note that a clinical trial using a PDGFR inhibitor did not improve outcome in IPF, although it is unclear in this study if the target was engaged and whether PDGFR was adequately inhibited.[95] Conversely, nintedanib, a pan–tyrosine kinase inhibitor, has been shown to decrease lung function decline in IPF, and it is tempting to hypothesize that some of the activity of nintedanib is derived from its targeting of LECs.[96]

LYMPHANGIOLEIOMYOMATOSIS

Lymphangioleiomyomatosis (LAM), a rare cystic lung disease that primarily affects women, is characterized by the proliferation of cells carrying inactivating mutations in the tuberous sclerosis complex gene (see Chapter 97). LAM can be sporadic or in association with the tuberous sclerosis complex. Chylothorax can develop in about 10–30% of patients with LAM.[97] The presence of chylous effusions or ascites in combination with cystic lung disease is diagnostic of LAM.[98]

The origin of LAM cells remains unknown, but some evidence suggests that these cells could be of lymphatic endothelial lineage.[99,100] Further, lymphatic vessels are thought to be the conduit of LAM cell metastasis.[101] VEGF-D, elevated in approximately 70% of women with LAM, is a biomarker used for diagnosis and response to rapamycin, the FDA-approved treatment for LAM.[102]

LUNG TRANSPLANTATION

Lung transplantation carries the worst outcome of any solid organ transplant, with a 60% 5-year survival.[103,104] Acute rejection, which happens in about 30% of recipients,[105] is a major risk factor for the development of chronic lung allograft dysfunction, a driver of poor long-term outcomes.[106,107]

Human studies of transbronchial lung biopsies have shown that acute allograft rejection is associated with an increase in lymphatic vessel density.[108] However chronic lung allograft dysfunction, whether bronchiolitis obliterans syndrome or restrictive allograft syndrome, was not associated with changes in lymphatic vessel density.[109]

Because lymphatic vessels act as a major conduit for immune cell trafficking, they may contribute to graft rejection.[110] In rat models of cardiac transplantation[111] or the orthotopic tracheal transplant model[112] blocking lymphangiogenesis resulted in improved graft survival. However, in a mouse model of orthotopic lung transplantation, enhancing lymphangiogenesis by exogenous administration of VEGF-C decreased acute allograft rejection by increasing the clearance of excess short-fragment hyaluronan, a known alloimmune agonist.[113,114] During lung transplant surgery, lymphatics are severed and not reconnected.[115] This impaired lymphatic drainage has the potential to promote acute allograft rejection by impeding the clearance of proinflammatory molecules. These seemingly contradictory findings may be explained by the different models used.[112] In the mouse orthotopic lung transplant model, recent evidence demonstrates that posttransplant, there is a reestablishment of a functional lymphatic bed, as a result of donor lymphatics sprouting towards the host.[116] Understanding mechanisms of lymphatic regeneration as well as modalities that could enhance lymphangiogenesis posttransplant could result in novel therapies for acute allograft rejection.

TUBERCULOSIS

Mycobacterium tuberculosis (MTB) infection leads to the development of caseating granulomas in the lungs and other infected tissues.[117] Granulomas are composed of a large percentage of CD11b[+] macrophages, which produce VEGF-C leading to de novo lymphangiogenesis.[118] The newly formed lymphatic vessels in the granulomatous tissue facilitate the egress of CD11c[+] macrophages from the granulomas into the lymph nodes to prime T cells. Blocking lymphangiogenesis in animal models of tuberculosis infection resulted in decreased T cell activation. Although this did not translate to decreased bacterial burden in granulomas in the acute phase, the effects

of long-term blockade of lymphangiogenesis in MTB infection are unknown.[118] Moreover, an additional role of lymphatics has recently been identified with the demonstration that lymph node LECs harbor replicating MTB.[119] Interferon-γ is a critical mediator of the interaction between MTB, macrophages, and granuloma formation. LEC stimulation with IFN-γ leads to induction of autophagy and nitric oxide production, which in turn restricts intracellular MTB proliferation.[116] In patients with TB infection, serum levels of VEGF-A, VEGF-C, and VEGFR2 positively correlated with pulmonary involvement and disease burden,[120] suggesting that lymphangiogenesis may be involved in the pathogenesis of human disease, consistent with preclinical model findings. Taken together, these data suggest the importance of lymphatics and LECs in the response to MTB and the persistence of infection.

SARCOIDOSIS

Sarcoidosis is a systemic granulomatous disease with noncaseating granulomas as a hallmark for diagnosis. Sarcoidosis can lead to parenchymal lung involvement as well as hilar lymphadenopathy.[121] The sarcoid granuloma is a source of VEGF and VEGF-C, which are elevated in sera and bronchoalveolar lavage fluid of patients with sarcoidosis.[122] Sarcoid granulomas are surrounded by tubular structures thought to be lymphatics but, in one study, these structures weakly expressed the LEC markers podoplanin and VEGFR2 but not VEGFR3, and were in part connected to afferent lymphatics, suggesting that these structures were likely atypical lymphatic vessels.[122] Evidence shows that mTORC1 signaling in macrophages leads to granuloma formation.[123] Whether these macrophages result in excess production of lymphangiogenic growth factors is unknown. The exact mechanisms driving lymphangiogenesis in sarcoidosis and the contribution of lymphatics to the development of lung granulomas remains unclear.

Key Points

- Lymphatic vessels run along the major airways and the blood vessels. There are very few lymphatics alongside the alveoli in the normal lung.
- Lymphatics are important for fluid homeostasis, macromolecule drainage including hyaluronan, and immune cell trafficking.
- Lymphatic endothelial cells can be identified using a panel of markers, including podoplanin, VEGFR3, and CCL21. Specificity and sensitivity depends on animal species and organ location.
- A functioning lung lymphatic system is essential for proper lung development and for the first breath at birth.
- Lymphatic changes have been observed in almost every lung disease including asthma, COPD, and interstitial lung disease.
- The exact contribution of the lymphatic system to lung disease pathogenesis remains unclear. However, dysfunctional lymphatics are sufficient for the development of air space enlargement mimicking emphysema, blocking lymphatic vessels results in airway edema, and stimulating lymphatic vessel formation leads to decreased transplant rejection.

Key Readings

Alitalo K. The lymphatic vasculature in disease. *Nat Med.* 2011;17(11):1371–1380.

Baluk P, Tammela T, Ator E, et al. Pathogenesis of persistent lymphatic vessel hyperplasia in chronic airway inflammation. *J Clin Invest.* 2005;115(2):247–257.

Baluk P, Yao LC, Flores JC, Choi D, Hong YK, McDonald DM. Rapamycin reversal of VEGF-C-driven lymphatic anomalies in the respiratory tract. *JCI Insight.* 2017;2(16).

Baluk P, McDonald DM. Imaging lymphatics in mouse lungs. *Methods Mol Biol.* 2018;1846:161–180.

Cui Y, Liu K, Monzon-Medina ME, et al. Therapeutic lymphangiogenesis ameliorates established acute lung allograft rejection. *J Clin Invest.*125(11):4255–4268.

El-Chemaly S, Malide D, Zudaire E, et al. Abnormal lymphangiogenesis in idiopathic pulmonary fibrosis with insights into cellular and molecular mechanisms. *Proc Natl Acad Sci U S A.* 2009;106(10):3958–3963.

Jakus Z, Gleghorn JP, Enis DR, et al. Lymphatic function is required prenatally for lung inflation at birth. *J Exp Med.* 2014;211(5):815–826.

Lara AR, Cosgrove GP, Janssen WJ, et al. Increased lymphatic vessel length is associated with the fibroblast reticulum and disease severity in usual interstitial pneumonia and nonspecific interstitial pneumonia. *Chest.* 2012;142(6):1569–1576.

Outtz Reed H, Wang L, Sonett J, et al. Lymphatic impairment leads to pulmonary tertiary lymphoid organ formation and alveolar damage. *J Clin Invest.* 2019.

Schraufnagel DE. Forms of lung lymphatics: a scanning electron microscopic study of casts. *Anat Rec.* 1992;233(4):547–554.

Yao LC, Baluk P, Srinivasan RS, Oliver G, McDonald DM. Plasticity of button-like junctions in the endothelium of airway lymphatics in development and inflammation. *Am J Pathol.* 2012;180(6):2561–2575.

Complete reference list available at ExpertConsult.com.

REGENERATION AND REPAIR

SUSANNE HEROLD, MD, PHD • GREGORY P. DOWNEY, MD

INTRODUCTION

The pathobiology of many pulmonary diseases involves injury to the lung, followed by delayed, incomplete, or dysfunctional repair. Injury can be viewed at different levels, including at the level of the whole organ or of individual cells or molecules. Repair can be also be viewed at many levels, including restoration of the function of an injured organ (e.g., improvement in the gas exchange function of the lung), of cells (e.g., replacement of terminally injured cells or repair of defects in plasma membranes), or of molecules (e.g., damaged molecules can be degraded in the proteasome and replaced by de novo synthesis). We will emphasize the cellular injury resulting in the dysfunction or death of cells that underlies the pathogenesis of diverse pulmonary diseases. Injury to any of the different cell types residing in the lung can ultimately lead to organ dysfunction (for a review of lung structure, see Chapter 1). A broad concept of lung repair encompasses processes resulting in restoration of the function of the injured lung and in the return to a homeostatic state. This chapter focuses on the cellular and molecular aspects of repair, including replacement of irreversibly damaged cells from endogenous progenitor cells residing in specified niches and restoration of normal cellular function.

The lung is continuously exposed to a diverse array of chemical and biologic agents that are potentially toxic and can cause cellular dysfunction or even death if a threshold is exceeded. The lung frequently undergoes minor damage as a result of viral or bacterial infection or chemical exposures, leading to transient alterations in lung function. *Repair* can be defined as restitution of the cells, and thus the lung, to the preinjury level of structure and function. Normal repair returns the lung to a healthy state capable of responding to subsequent injuries. Aging is manifest by steady and progressive declines in cell number and/or function and decline in overall lung function. The declines are in part due to episodes of recurrent microinjury from environmental toxicants (e.g., pollutants) and decreased capacity of the epithelium or endothelium to heal itself, related to senescence of the lung cells and waning of the ability of the immune system to combat pathogenic microorganisms. Mutations in the genes controlling senescence (e.g., telomerase genes) may impede the ability of lung cells to repair themselves after injury, resulting in prolonged cellular and organ dysfunction. Defective repair leads to episodic decrements in pulmonary function that may ultimately lead to respiratory failure (Fig. 8.1).

LUNG INJURY

LUNG INJURY IN DISEASE PATHOGENESIS

Many pulmonary disorders, such as asthma, COPD, pneumonia, *interstitial lung disease* (ILD), cystic fibrosis, and *acute respiratory distress syndrome* (ARDS), are characterized by cellular injury and faulty repair, resulting in physiologic dysfunction of the lung. The intensity and duration of the insult contribute to the rapidity of onset of symptoms and the chronicity of disease. In ARDS, a severe insult causes widespread lung injury and respiratory failure in hours to days. By contrast, in COPD, years of exposure to the offending agent (usually cigarette smoke in the developed world and smoke from biomass fuels in developing countries) results in slowly progressive loss of respiratory function. Patients with ILD often have a stuttering course with periods of rapidly declining lung function. Dysfunctional repair and "remodeling" contribute to the pathogenesis and clinical course of these and other lung diseases.

The pathogenesis of many lung diseases involves exposure to exogenous toxic agents (e.g., inhaled toxins, allergens, or microbial pathogens) triggering host responses (inflammation or autoimmune responses) that may cause cellular dysfunction or death. In COPD, inhaled toxins, such as those that comprise cigarette smoke, initiate pathologic processes, including inflammation and infection, which culminate in epithelial and endothelial cell death[1–5] and destruction of the scaffolding of the lung.[6] In asthma, allergens, environmental pollutants, pathogens, and the inflammatory response to these agents induce injury to the bronchial epithelium.[7–9] Pulmonary fibrosis/ILD is thought to reflect repetitive injury to the distal lung epithelium interspersed with periods of relative quiescence.[10]

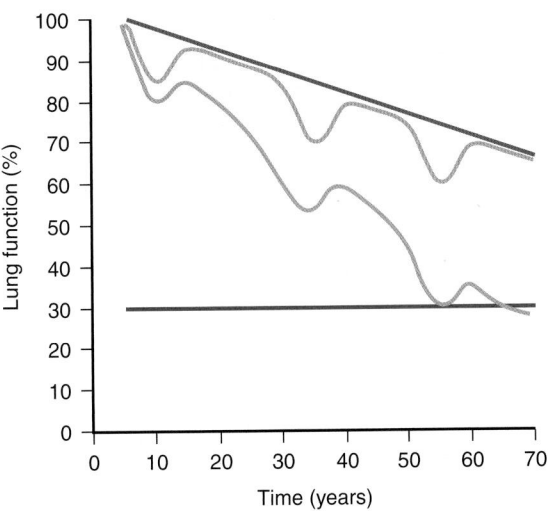

Figure 8.1 Conceptual relationship between lung function and time. Normal aging can be viewed as a process in which steady and progressive declines in cell number and/or function reflect parallel decrements in the capacity of the epithelium or endothelium to heal itself *(straight blue line)*. Acute episodes of injury to the lung and its cellular and structural components, such as viral infection or chemical exposures, result in temporary fluctuations in lung function *(fluctuating blue line)*. Chronic lung disease is associated with a progressive loss of lung function that is exacerbated by environmental exposures. Individuals affected by chronic lung disease may be predisposed to repeated episodes of lung injury and may undergo cycles of injury that result in an accelerated decline in lung function *(orange line)*. Once a hypothetical functional threshold is reached *(red line)*, the lung may no longer have the capacity to repair itself and functionality is irreversibly lost. (Modified from Lazaar AL, Panettieri RA Jr. Is airway remodeling clinically relevant in asthma? *Am J Med.* 115:652–659, 2003.)

FACTORS MEDIATING ACUTE EPITHELIAL AND ENDOTHELIAL CELL INJURY

To illustrate the processes involved in lung injury, we will focus on the clinical problem of ARDS, a process that involves inflammatory injury to the lung. An extensive review of the causes, pathogenesis, clinical manifestations, and treatment of ARDS is included in Chapter 134. ARDS is a heterogeneous syndrome rather than a single disease, and predisposing causes include pneumonia, sepsis, inhalational injury, aspiration, injurious (high tidal volume) mechanical ventilation, pancreatitis, trauma, and blood transfusion.[11]

Epithelial and endothelial cells form selective barriers separating the vascular and air space compartments in the lung; the respiratory epithelium also provides a barrier from the environment. This barrier function depends on the presence of an intact layer of viable cells and the intercellular junctions that link adjacent cells, thus restricting the movement of fluid, ions, and macromolecules. In the healthy lung, the epithelium, due to its tight intercellular junctions, prevents fluid from leaking into the alveolar spaces. In addition, there is active removal of fluid, ions, and protein from the alveolar space via the action of channels, ionic pumps, and transporters in the epithelial cells. In ARDS, compromise of the endothelial and/or epithelial barriers, either via disruption of intercellular junctions or via death and sloughing of cells, results in an increase in lung permeability and the influx of protein-rich edema fluid,[12,13] which leads to refractory hypoxemia and bilateral opacities on chest radiographs.[14–17] Impaired fluid, ion, and protein

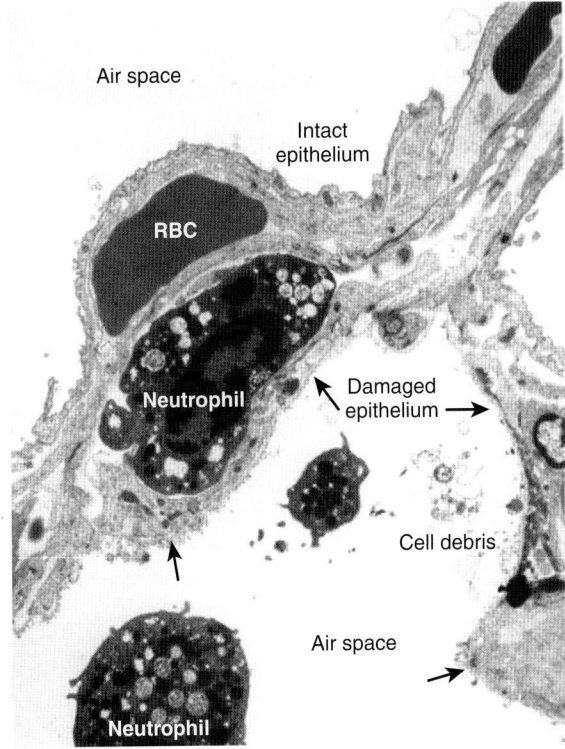

Figure 8.2 Electron micrograph of inflammatory injury in the murine lung. A key contributor to lung injury, from either the vascular or epithelial surface, is the inflammatory process, including the effects of inflammatory mediators and the accumulation and activation of inflammatory cells. This electron micrograph depicts damage to endothelial and alveolar epithelial cells *(arrows)* accompanying sequestration and activation of neutrophils in an acute inflammatory response. The process is usually associated with increased vascular and alveolar permeability, sometimes with sufficient damage to the alveolar wall to result in coagulation (fibrin) and erythrocyte accumulation in the air spaces. RBC, red blood cell.

transport[18,19] and decreased surfactant production and function[20,21] further contribute to the impaired lung compliance and gas exchange abnormalities.

In ARDS, structural and functional epithelial and endothelial injury is largely attributable to excessive and dysregulated inflammation[16,22] (Fig. 8.2; see also Chapter 134). During pneumonia, the most common cause of ARDS, microbial products are recognized by resident lung cells, which in turn secrete chemoattractants that recruit inflammatory cells, initially neutrophils, into the lungs.[23–27] During immune surveillance or a normal immune response, neutrophils ingest (phagocytose) microorganisms and release potent antimicrobial compounds, including oxidants, proteinases, and cationic peptides into the phagosome.[28] Thus neutrophil influx into the lungs under most circumstances does not result in tissue injury.[29,30] However, during excessive and dysregulated inflammation in ARDS, large numbers of activated neutrophils release these microbicidal compounds into the extracellular space, causing tissue injury.[31–33] For example, neutrophil elastase, although inherently antimicrobial and critical for host defense,[34,35] can also cause injury to the extracellular matrix in COPD[36,37] and also to the alveolar capillary membrane in ARDS.[38–45] Of importance, neutrophil elastase can cause both a disruption of intercellular junctions[46,47] and death of endothelial[48–50] and epithelial[51,52] cells. ARDS patients have elevated levels of elastase in the bronchoalveolar lavage fluid and plasma, and these levels correlate with the severity of lung injury.[53–56] Unfortunately, pharmacologic agents that inhibit neutrophil elastase have not proven to be effective in the treatment of ARDS.[57,58] In addition to neutrophil elastase, other serine proteases—*matrix metalloproteinases* (MMPs) and cysteine proteinases—are released by inflammatory cells and contribute to tissue destruction during lung injury.[38] Increased levels of MMPs, derived from both neutrophils and macrophages, are present in patients with ARDS[59–63] and contribute to lung injury.[64–69] The mechanisms by which MMPs cause lung injury have not been fully elucidated. MMPs are able to degrade junctional proteins in both epithelia[70–72] and endothelia[73,74] and induce cell death,[72] although the latter is dependent on the cell type and the specific MMP. Conversely, some MMPs promote survival of the lung epithelium,[75] and others may attenuate injury[76] or even promote repair.[77,78]

In addition to proteinases and antimicrobial peptides such as defensins,[79–86] oxidants, including reactive oxygen and nitrogen species, are released by inflammatory cells during ARDS[87–89] and contribute to tissue injury,[90–98] including epithelial[99–107] and endothelial[108,109] cell death and disruption of tight junctions.[110–112] Although the lung possesses potent endogenous antioxidant mechanisms, which serve to limit injury,[113–121] in ARDS these mechanisms are overwhelmed by the large amount of reactive oxygen and nitrogen species generated. In addition, oxidants can potentiate proteinase-induced lung injury, in part by inactivating antiproteinases.[122] Finally, oxidized phospholipids[98] and another antimicrobial weapon, neutrophil extracellular traps, can cause epithelial and endothelial injury.[123–126]

Although neutrophils and their mediators cause much of the early injury to the alveolar capillary membrane,[31,127–129] they are not the only perpetrators of lung injury, because ARDS can develop even in neutropenic patients.[130] Recruitment of monocytes to the lungs follows the initial neutrophilic response in ARDS.[131] Recruited monocytes gradually acquire the phenotype of macrophages and secrete proinflammatory mediators, including cytokines, chemokines, and lipids, that propagate the inflammatory response. Recruited macrophages also release endogenous toxic and proapoptotic mediators, including reactive oxygen and nitrogen species,[132,133] MMPs,[62,67,68,134] *tumor necrosis factor-α* (TNF-α),[135] vascular endothelial growth factor,[136] *TNF-related apoptosis-inducing ligand* (TRAIL),[135,137] and interferon-β,[138] which may enhance host defense but also induce tissue injury.[139,140] In addition, macrophages also play a critical role in both tissue repair[141–143] and the resolution of inflammation[144,145] (also see later). The role of macrophages in lung inflammation, injury, and repair is further reviewed in Chapter 15. In addition to neutrophils and macrophages, platelets (mostly observed as neutrophil-platelet aggregates) have recently been identified as crucial drivers of the increase in vascular permeability.[146,147] Furthermore, free hemoglobin from red blood cells,[148] angiopoietin-2 released from the pulmonary endothelium,[149] coagulation factors,[150,151] products of infectious agents that directly injure lung cells,[152] inhaled toxins,[153] oxygen,[154] and mechanical forces[155,156] can all contribute to injury to the alveolar capillary membrane. Indeed, a diverse array of mechanisms, mediators, and signaling pathways has been implicated in lung injury.[11,63,157–165] Because the spectrum

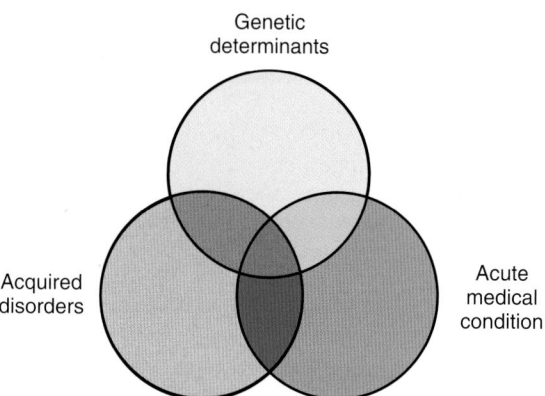

Figure 8.3 Acute lung injury: clinical risk factors. Based on the results of several epidemiologic studies published over the last 2 decades, a variety of factors have been identified that can alter the susceptibility of an individual patient to the development of acute lung injury. These factors can be separated into three general categories: genetic determinants, preexisting acquired disorders, and the acute medical condition. The identification of such patient-specific characteristics could significantly improve both our understanding of the pathogenesis of acute lung injury and our ability to care for these critically ill patients.

of injurious agents in ARDS is so broad, and their effects can be modified by preexisting lung disorders and genetic predispositions (Fig. 8.3), it is not surprising that pharmacologic strategies to block a single pathway or class of mediators have been ineffective.

HISTOPATHOLOGY AND MECHANISMS THAT CONSTITUTE ALVEOLAR CELL INJURY

Having reviewed the pathogenic agents that induce lung injury, we will now focus on exploring what constitutes lung injury. As mentioned earlier, we define injury as cellular dysfunction or death. Although cellular dysfunction in ARDS includes impaired production of surfactant,[166] which is essential for lung compliance and important in host defense,[167] we focus on the cellular dysfunction and death that contribute to increased lung permeability. In inflammatory lung injury, this includes (1) disruption of intercellular junctions responsible for maintaining the barrier function of the endothelium and epithelium and (2) impaired active ion and fluid transport responsible for fluid reabsorption and maintenance of dry air spaces. Although transient opening and closing of intercellular junctions is necessary for the transmigration of immune cells during immune surveillance or a normal immune response[168] and can take place without compromising barrier function,[30] during ARDS, intercellular junctions of the endothelium[110,169–172] and epithelium[46,112] are disrupted, resulting in enhanced paracellular permeability, which contributes to the flooding of the alveolar spaces with edema fluid. This alveolar flooding is exacerbated by impaired function of the epithelial Na^+/K^+ pumps and epithelial sodium channels responsible for fluid reabsorption.[137,173–179] It should be noted, however, that attempts at stimulating fluid clearance with β-agonists did not improve outcomes in ARDS.[180]

In addition to the disruption of intercellular junctions, severe lung injury in ARDS and other lung diseases[3,181–183] is characterized by cell death. In ARDS, inflammatory mediators induce death of endothelial cells[184] and *type 1 alveolar epithelial* (AT1) cells, leaving surviving *type 2 alveolar epithelial* (AT2) cells, which are more, but not fully, resistant to injury, for repopulating a largely denuded basement membrane.[13,185–188] This dramatic injury to the alveolar epithelium, together with hyaline membrane formation, protein-rich edema, and hemorrhage, engendered the pathologic term *diffuse alveolar damage* (DAD),[189] which describes the histologic appearance of lungs from patients who died of ARDS. More recent evidence revealed that DAD was only found in some patients with the clinical diagnosis of ARDS, and the pathologic findings were relatively heterogeneous.[190] A study that analyzed postmortem samples reported that 45% of patients who were diagnosed with ARDS according to the Berlin definition revealed DAD, whereas 55% showed an inflammatory pattern consistent with acute pneumonia, and the frequency of the DAD pattern declined in the decade after lung protective ventilation was implemented, suggesting a substantial contribution of ventilator-induced injurious mechanical forces to the DAD pattern.[11,191]

Endothelial Damage

Even in severe DAD, in contrast to epithelial cells, alveolar endothelial cells are often morphologically preserved and, although the endothelial lining remains continuous, there is significant impairment of endothelial function rather than frank cell death and denudation. Homophilic vascular endothelial cadherin bonds between adjacent endothelial cells are crucial for maintaining lung microvascular integrity; loss of these bonds results in functional impairment of the endothelial barrier and increased alveolar-capillary permeability.[11,192]

Epithelial Damage

The extent of epithelial cell loss determines the severity of ARDS. The loss of endothelial and epithelial cells can result from necrotic cell death or programmed cell death, the latter termed *apoptosis*. Originally a morphologic definition, apoptosis might best be defined on the basis of nuclear condensation and characteristic DNA fragmentation and other morphologic alterations; biochemically, it is based on its induction mechanisms and requirement for the action of a series of intracellular proteases termed caspases.[193,194] There are two major pathways leading to apoptosis: the intrinsic pathway, involving signaling from the mitochondria, and the extrinsic pathway, deriving from signals generated from external stimulation of "death" receptors. Mitochondrial regulation of alveolar epithelial apoptosis may be induced by p53[195] or by the proapoptotic Bcl-2 family members BAX or BAK.[99,196] In the extrinsic pathway, death receptors of the TNF receptor family, such as Fas, mediate apoptosis. In animal models of lung injury, Fas[197] and TRAIL[135] induce epithelial cell apoptosis, and inhibition of apoptosis improves survival.[198,199] Apoptotic epithelial cells are engulfed by both professional phagocytes (macrophages) and other epithelial cells.[200,201] Both Fas and Fas ligand levels are elevated in the edema fluid of ARDS patients, induce epithelial cell apoptosis in a manner dependent on their modulation by oxidants and proteases, and predict worse clinical outcomes.[202–204]

In ARDS, cells can also die by necroptosis (programmed cell death leading to necrosis), or direct necrosis, a form of cell death that does not require active participation of cellular processes and generally leads to disruption of the cell membrane with subsequent release of cellular contents that may be additionally injurious. Causes of epithelial necrosis in ARDS include physical effects of acid from inspiration of stomach contents, inhalation of toxic materials or fumes, infection with lytic viruses or bacterial products, hyperoxia,[205] mechanical disruption of cell membranes during mechanical ventilation, and other effects. In summary, cell death is a major mechanism of lung injury, resulting in epithelial denudation and contributing to increased lung permeability and the massive influx of edema fluid into the alveolar space, despite the existence of endogenous protective mechanisms.

LUNG REGENERATION AND REPAIR

The ability of the lung to withstand considerable damage and repair itself enables recovery and survival from a variety of noxious stimuli, independent of containment of pathogens by host defense systems.[206] We define repair broadly as *processes by which the function of the injured lung is restored to normal*. Repair of the lung after acute injury requires coordinated processes to reconstitute the endothelial and epithelial barriers, clear edema fluid,[207–212] and resolve inflammation.[213] In the case of ARDS, survival depends on repair of the injured lung, although some survivors do not completely regain normal lung function.[214]

RESOLUTION OF INFLAMMATION

Inflammation resolution and tissue repair are processes that usually happen in parallel and are closely interrelated: The inflammatory response must resolve to halt ongoing injury to the lung and, vice versa, persistent cell damage will trigger ongoing inflammation due to presence of danger-associated molecular patterns from dead cells and matrix components.

Neutrophils undergo apoptosis as a noninflammatory, nonimmunogenic form of cell death, during which they retain and sequester toxic mediators within their plasma membrane. This is in contrast to a necrotic neutrophil death, in which neutrophils disintegrate and release their intracellular constituents, including toxic and proinflammatory mediators, resulting in prolongation of the inflammatory response. Apoptotic neutrophils are engulfed by macrophages in a phagocytic process termed *efferocytosis* without release of toxic intracellular contents.[144,145] Efferocytosis depends on the recognition by a variety of receptors of "eat me" signals, including phosphatidylserine[215] and calreticulin,[216] displayed on the apoptotic cell surface.[217,218] This is followed by activation of Rho *guanosine triphosphatases* (GTPases), leading to engulfment, which is regulated by the mitochondrial membrane protein Ucp2,[219] as well as high mobility group box-1[220] and urokinase-type plasminogen activator.[221] Efferocytosis results in the release of anti-inflammatory mediators that further promote the resolution of inflammation.[222] In particular, efferocytosis induces an anti-inflammatory, previously termed *M2*, or alternatively activated phenotype of macrophages that will trigger further resolution and repair processes.[223] Apoptotic neutrophils can also be efferocytosed by myeloid-derived suppressor cells in an *interleukin-10* (IL-10)-dependent manner.[224] Whereas clearance of apoptotic neutrophils is usually highly efficient, yielding a low number of observable apoptotic cells at any given time,[225] if defective or overloaded, apoptotic neutrophils can undergo secondary necrosis or postapoptotic cytolysis.[226] Thus impaired neutrophil apoptosis and efferocytosis prolongs the duration of the inflammatory response, resulting in a chronic inflammatory state.[227] Lipid mediators such as resolvins promote the resolution of inflammation by enhancing neutrophil apoptosis[228] and efferocytosis,[229–231] as well as through other mechanisms.[232–236] In addition to neutrophils, recruited inflammatory macrophages may also be cleared during the resolution of lung injury,[237] or they may replace alveolar macrophages lost during the inflammatory process to regenerate the local tissue-resident pool.[238] Anti-inflammatory, tissue-reparative subsets of T cells (*T regulatory cells* [T_{Regs}]) are additional important cellular players in lung injury resolution, involving *transforming growth factor-β* (TGF-β) and IL-10.[239]

RESORPTION OF EDEMA FLUID

The primary force driving fluid reabsorption from the alveolar space into the interstitium and the pulmonary circulation is active Na^+ transport. Sodium is taken up on the apical surface of the alveolar epithelium by amiloride-sensitive and -insensitive Na^+ channels and is subsequently pumped out of the cell by the *Na^+,K^+-adenosine triphosphatase* (Na^+,K^+-ATPase) on the basolateral side. This process generates an osmotic gradient, which drives passive movement of water from the apical side of the epithelium (the alveolar space) to the basolateral side (the interstitium), mainly paracellularly. Fluid reabsorption requires a widely intact alveolar epithelium and resolution of inflammation.[240] Excess alveolar protein, a hallmark of ARDS, is cleared by active albumin transport via a glycoprotein called megalin.[241–243]

ENDOTHELIAL REPAIR

Given that endothelial cell injury involves disruption of intercellular junctions and, to a lesser extent, cell death, endothelial repair mainly requires reassembly of these junctions. Primary barrier-stabilizing and reparative mechanisms involve adrenomedullin, angiopoietin-1, and sphingosine-1-phosphate, the latter released from activated platelets to stimulate reassembly of endothelial intercellular junctions via Rho- and Rac-dependent cytoskeletal rearrangement.[244–248] This process is dependent on $\alpha_v\beta_3$ integrin.[249] In addition, Slit/Robo stabilizes the endothelial adherens junctions by promoting p120-catenin/E-cadherin association,[250,251] and Rho GTPases stabilize the actin cytoskeleton, thereby enhancing endothelial barrier integrity.[252]

EPITHELIAL REPAIR

The following sections describe basic principles in lung epithelial repair and provide an overview on the current view of epithelial stem cell hierarchies, stem/progenitor cells involved in lung epithelial repair, and the cellular cross-talk and molecular mechanisms involved. To illustrate the underlying basic mechanisms, we will first focus on re-epithelialization of the denuded epithelium by general mechanisms of cell spreading and migration, cell proliferation, and junctional (re)sealing. Re-epithelialization of airways or of the denuded alveolar basement membrane involves different subsets of stem cells, including basal cells, specialized club/secretory cells, and alveolar progenitors, such as specialized AT2 cells, the "defender of the alveolus."[253] Alveolar repair involves AT2 cell proliferation and differentiation into AT1 cells to restore a normal alveolar epithelium. Of note, if the injury is extensive, *bronchioalveolar stem cells* (BASCs) migrate and proliferate to repopulate the injured alveolus (Fig. 8.4; Video 8.1). If these stem/progenitor cell niches are depleted due to extensive injuries, further stem cell niches might be recruited for repair; however, such responses frequently result in aberrant remodeling processes with nonresolving injury or tissue fibrosis. Epithelial injury and repair promotes the activation of resident fibroblast subsets,[254,255] which, although important for physiologic wound repair, can result in fibrotic lung disease. Each of these phenomena is discussed in more detail later.

Basic Principles in Epithelial Repair: Cell Spreading and Migration, Cell Proliferation, and Junctional Resealing

Repair of the epithelium is crucial for clinical recovery, including reestablishment of AT1 cells and resolution of alveolar edema fluid. AT1 cells are flat cells that normally cover the majority of the gas exchange surface and exhibit active ion and fluid transport properties, whereas AT2 cells are cuboidal and synthesize surfactants to prevent the alveoli from collapsing.[256,257] After death of AT1 cells, surviving AT2 cells supposedly spread and migrate onto the denuded basement membrane as an immediate process to reestablish the cellular barrier. Although this has not been directly observed in the lung in vivo, cell spreading and migration is likely to be the initial mechanism for resealing the leaky epithelium[189] based on in vitro observations[258–260] and on the importance of these phenomena in wound repair of other organs.[261] Cell migration depends on a tightly regulated assembly of the cytoskeleton leading to protrusion of "lamellipodia" and "filopodia" from the leading edge, followed by contractile forces that drive release of the rear edge from the extracellular matrix, processes that depend on the Rho GTPases.[262,263] In the lung epithelium, cell spreading and migration after injury are triggered by soluble factors such as *keratinocyte growth factor* (KGF), also known as *fibroblast growth factor 7* (FGF7),[260] TGF-α,[259] TGF-β,[264] *interleukin-1β* (IL-1β),[265,266] and CXC motif chemokine 3.[267] Cell migration is controlled by signaling pathways involving Rac1/Tiam1,[268] *phosphatase and tensin homolog* (PTEN),[269] β-catenin,[270–273] syndecan-1,[274,275] *adenosine triphosphate* (ATP) and dual oxidase 1,[276,277] and vimentin,[264] as reviewed elsewhere.[278] Integrins, which are up-regulated in the alveolar epithelium after injury,[279] contribute to cell migration via interactions with both the actin cytoskeleton[280] and the *extracellular matrix* (ECM).[258,281–283] The production of ECM and MMPs is essential for cell migration.[141,275] MMPs enhance wound healing by cleavage of

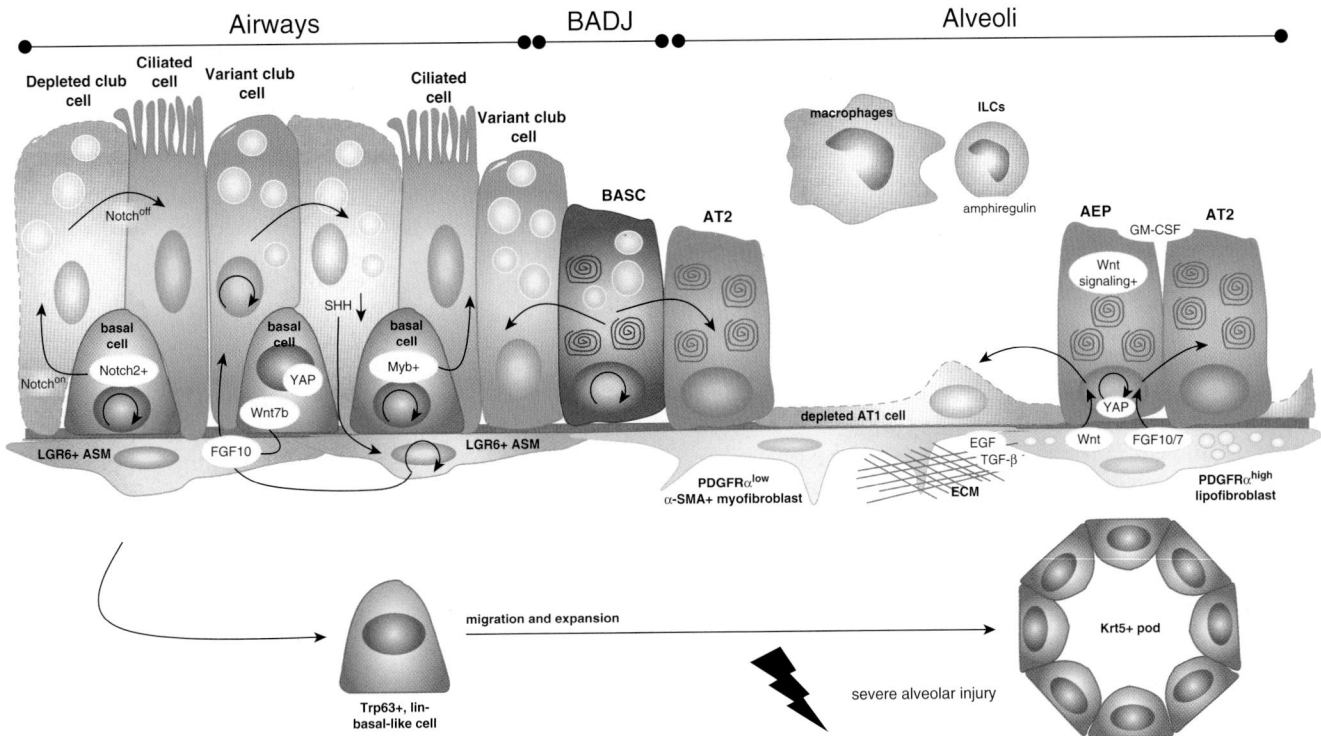

Figure 8.4 Cell types and signaling pathways involved in airway, bronchioalveolar duct, and alveolar epithelial cell repair. In response to *airway injury*, Notch 2–expressing basal cells give rise to club/secretory cells and Myb-expressing basal cells give rise to ciliated cells. Loss of *sonic hedgehog* (SHH) signaling between the airway epithelium and *airway smooth muscle* (ASM) induces ASM cell proliferation as part of the wound healing response. Upon selected loss of secretory/club cells, remaining "variant club/secretory cells" proliferate and repopulate the lost secretory/club cells. Airway injury causes YAP-mediated epithelial Wnt7b expression, which promotes FGF10 expression in the nearby niche ASM cells, in turn stimulating secretory/club cell proliferation and differentiation. In response to *alveolar injury*, the Wnt-responsive, bipotent *alveolar epithelial progenitor* (AEP) subset of *type 2 alveolar epithelial cells* (AT2) proliferates and differentiates into *type 1 alveolar epithelial cells* (AT1) and AT2 cells, responses driven by YAP/TAZ and the release of Wnt ligands and FGFs, respectively, from lipofibroblast niche cells. Myofibroblasts are activated to secrete ECM during wound healing. Additional growth factors are released from the matrix (e.g., EGF, TGF-β), by the inflamed AT2 cell pool (e.g., GM-CSF), and by immune cells such as macrophages, *innate lymphocyte cells* (ILC; amphiregulin) and T regulatory cells (TGF-β), and contribute to wound healing. CCSP + SFTPC + BASC residing at the *bronchoalveolar duct junctions* (BADJ) proliferate upon airway and alveolar injury and give rise to both differentiated airway and AT2 cells.[319] Very severe alveolar injury with substantial depletion of endogenous stem cells and facultative progenitors (e.g., after influenza virus infection) can result in a dysplastic (keratinization) wound healing response with generation of abnormal cell clusters ("pods") from basal-like, Trp63+ lineage-negative cells that maintains the tissue barrier but does not result in reestablishment of functional alveolar epithelium. *Arrows* indicate differentiation into or action upon; *circular arrows* indicate proliferation. *Dashed lines* indicate dead cells to be replaced. BASC, bronchioalveolar stem cell; CCSP, club cell secretory protein; ECM, extracellular matrix; EGF, epidermal growth factor; FGF, fibroblast growth factor; GM-CSF, granulocyte-macrophage colony stimulating factor; lin-, lineage negative; Krt5, keratin 5; PDGFRα, platelet-derived growth factor receptor α; SFTPC, surfactant protein C; SMA, smooth muscle actin; TGF, transforming growth factor; Trp63, transformation-related protein 63; YAP, Hippo–yes-associated protein. (Modified from Zepp JA, Morrisey EE. Cellular crosstalk in the development and regeneration of the respiratory system. *Nat Rev Mol Cell Biol.* 2019;20:551–566.)

cell-cell and cell-ECM adhesion molecules, proteolytic activation of chemokines and growth factors, and degradation of the provisional matrix.[142] Of note, cyclic stretch, imposed by mechanical ventilation during the acute and the recovery phase in ARDS, impedes cytoskeletal reorganization during cell spreading.[284]

In addition to cell spreading and migration, the denuded epithelial basement membrane is repopulated through the proliferation of surviving AT2 cells with progenitor cell potential (outlined in more detail later), which accounts for the epithelial cell hyperplasia observed on histologic samples from ARDS patients.[13,188,253,285] In animal models, significant acute lung injury resulting in cell death triggers alveolar epithelial cell proliferation.[286] Factors that promote AT2 cell proliferation after injury include the growth factors KGF, FGF10, *hepatocyte growth factor* (HGF), and *epidermal growth factor* (EGF).[287–294] In animal models of lung injury, exogenous administration of KGF resulted in decreased mortality,[295] although the protective role of KGF may in part be attributable to enhanced epithelial

cell survival.[296] Of note, a recently completed phase II trial revealed no improvement when KGF was administered to ARDS patients.[297] Other factors and pathways implicated in AT2 cell proliferation after injury include *granulocyte-macrophage colony stimulating factor* (GM-CSF),[298,299] which is also protective against injury in animal models,[300–302] β-catenin signaling,[303,304] Hippo–*yes-associated protein* (YAP)/*transcriptional coactivator with PDZ-binding motif* (TAZ) signaling,[305] macrophage migration inhibitory factor,[306] and the transcription factor FoxM1.[307]

Although the alveolar epithelial junctions seem more resistant to injury than the endothelial junctions,[308] increased epithelial permeability is a prerequisite for the development of air space edema. Conversely, repair of the alveolar epithelium is critically important for the resolution of edema, restoration of critical lung functions, including surfactant production and ion and fluid transport, and ultimately clinical outcomes.[173,309] In the epithelium, KGF,[112] interferon-γ,[310] PTEN,[311] EGF,[211] and the tyrosine kinase c-Met[312] are protective of tight junctional integrity during lung injury by a mechanism that involves cytoskeletal reorganization and possibly enhanced expression of junctional proteins,[313] including claudin-4.[314,315]

Stem and Progenitor Cells in the Lung

Replenishment of destroyed lung cells is a key element in repair of the injured lung. A *stem cell* is defined as a reparative cell with the capacity for unlimited self-renewal and with the greatest differentiation potential. A *progenitor cell* is defined as an early descendant of stem cells that can differentiate to form one or more kinds of cells but cannot divide and reproduce indefinitely. In addition, a progenitor cell is often more limited than a stem cell in the kinds of cells it can become. Thus the stem and progenitor cells can be distinguished by the capacity to reproduce (unlimited ability of stem cells vs. limited ability of progenitor cells) and the ability to differentiate into any cell of the body (stem cell) compared to relatively few cell types (progenitor cell).

For the stem cell, the attributes of "stemness" are controlled by interaction with the stem cell microenvironment or niche. The niche serves to protect or sequester stem cells from factors that promote their differentiation. Many of the current concepts about the function of stem and progenitor cells in the lung derive from studies of airway epithelial cells. Comparatively less is known regarding the identity of stem cells in the alveolar region, and even less is known about stem and progenitor cells for the diverse lung mesenchymal cell populations. In addition, most of the studies have been performed in murine models, and it is unknown whether similar progenitor cell populations exist in humans.

Stem Cell Division. Stem cell division produces two daughter cells whose fate is determined by interactions with the stem cell niche. *Symmetrical cell division* results in both daughter cells retaining contact with the niche and maintenance of these nascent cells as stem cells. This mechanism, which results in amplification of stem cell number, takes place in tissues with rapid cell turnover, such as the bone marrow and gut. In contrast, *asymmetrical cell division* results in generation of one daughter cell that maintains contact with the niche and is retained as the stem cell. The second daughter cell is the founding cell for the transit-amplifying cell population. Transit-amplifying cells are temporary constituents of the niche. They proliferate repeatedly over a short time period and then withdraw from the cell cycle as they commit to a differentiation pathway. Thus transit-amplifying cells serve to increase cell number and are destined to produce terminally differentiated cells. Within any organ or tissue the majority of cells are terminally differentiated cells. Terminally differentiated cells are postmitotic. In accordance, turnover of the terminally differentiated cell population acts as a stimulus for differentiation of transit-amplifying cells that resupply this population.

Progenitor Cell. As mentioned earlier, the term *progenitor cell* is a collective term used to describe any cell that has the capacity to proliferate and generate daughter cells, whereas the term *stem/progenitor cells* includes all cells with stem and/or progenitor potential. It is commonly used to indicate a cell in the process of cell division or with the potential to enter the cell cycle. The functional distinctions among lung progenitor cells are defined later.

Tissue-Specific Stem Cells. A tissue-specific stem cell is a rare cell type that is undifferentiated and has the potential to repopulate all of the cell types in their resident tissue,[316] as opposed to embryonic or pluripotent stem cells, which can generate any cell in the body. Due to the relatively quiescent state of the pulmonary epithelium, lung stem cells are mainly identified in various studies as cells activated in response to severe cell depletion.

Tracheobronchial tissue-specific stem cells exhibit a low cuboidal to pyramidal morphology and are termed *basal cells* (Trp63/Krt5-positive) and reside within specialized microenvironments located at the submucosal gland duct junction and in intercartilagenous regions of the trachea and bronchial epithelium.[317] In bronchioles and alveoli, additional tissue-specific stem cells include the BASC, the variant secretory/club cell,[318,319] and the *alveolar epithelial progenitor* (AEP) in the alveoli[320,321] (discussed further later).

Facultative Progenitor Cell Pools. A facultative progenitor cell exhibits defined differentiated features in the quiescent state, yet has the capacity to proliferate for maintenance of normal tissue and in response to injury. Facultative progenitor cells exist in two states: quiescent and reparative. In the quiescent state, facultative progenitor cells are nonmitotic and carry out differentiated functions necessary for tissue homeostasis. In response to injury, facultative progenitor cells dedifferentiate, enter the cell cycle, self-renew, and can differentiate into regionally specific differentiated cell types (e.g., ciliated epithelial cells).[322–325] Examples of facultative progenitor cells in the lung include the club cells in the airway and subsets of AT2 cells in the alveolus.[318,326] In contrast to the bone marrow and gut, the lung epithelium is maintained and repaired under most conditions by an abundant, broadly distributed facultative progenitor cell pool.

Stem/Progenitor Cells Involved in Lung Repair

Airway Repair. In contrast to other mucosal surfaces constantly exposed to external stimuli, such as the gut, the cells of the lung airways and alveoli are relatively quiescent, with a low turnover rate under homeostatic conditions. However, upon injury, several stem and progenitor cells and their niche cells (i.e., adjacent cells that communicate directly or via soluble mediators with stem and progenitor cells) are engaged to repopulate the injured area immediately. In the upper and lower airways, basal cells are located in the basal regions of the pseudostratified epithelium and are considered to be stem cells for the pseudostratified epithelial cells (ciliated cells, secretory cells, club cells) under homeostasis and after injury. As opposed to mice, where basal cells are located in the large conducting airways and the trachea, basal cells in humans are found throughout the proximal and distal airways, suggesting a key role in airway epithelial maintenance and repair.[327] In mice, basal cells preferentially give rise to secretory cells rather than ciliated cells, and this fate decision is regulated by Notch signaling. Secretory cells can then transdifferentiate into ciliated cells upon Notch inhibition.[328,329] However, upon injury, basal cells are capable of immediately generating both secretory and ciliated cells, with Notch 2–expressing basal cells giving rise to secretory cells, and Myb-expressing basal cells giving rise to ciliated cells.[330] Pathways involved in basal cell-mediated airway repair include FGF10-*FGF receptor 2b* (FGFR2b), bone morphogenic protein, p53, and the Hippo-YAP/TAZ pathway.[327] In addition, so-called "variant" secretory or club cells can repopulate secretory airway cells in mouse models in which secretory cells are depleted by naphthalene.[331] Whether these findings translate to humans remains unclear. A related stem cell population, the BASC, is characterized by coexpression of the AT2 cell marker *surfactant protein C* (SFTPC) and the club cell marker *club cell secretory protein* (CCSP) and is located at the bronchioalveolar duct junctions. The BASC is the only cell that can give rise to both airway and alveolar epithelial cells under homeostasis and after injury in mice[319,332] (see Fig. 8.4).

Alveolar Repair. AT1 and AT2 cells represent the two major epithelial cell types lining the alveoli that function as the gas-exchanging respiratory units of the lung. Alveolar epithelial cells are in close contact with underlying capillary endothelial cells and fibroblasts, and bidirectional communication exists between these cell types that is essential for repair of the injured lung.[257,333,334] Until recently, AT1 cells were considered to be fragile and susceptible to cell death in the setting of acute lung injury. By contrast, AT2 cells were considered to be more resistant to injury, and the surviving AT2 cells were thought to function as alveolar facultative stem or progenitor cells that would proliferate and transdifferentiate to AT1 cells, thus repopulating the alveoli. Recent studies have demonstrated the presence of bipotent alveolar progenitors that can give rise to both AT2 and AT1 cells during development,[321] whereas after birth new AT1 cells derive from rare, self-renewing, long-lived, mature AT2 cells. In this regard a population of AEPs[320,321] that rely on Wnt signaling, a crucial pathway regulating cell fate, was recently described that functions as a major facultative progenitor cell in the distal lung.[320]

During acute lung injury, AEPs express autocrine Wnts that recruit and expand the pool of facultative progenitor AT2 cells to repair the gas exchange surface of the lung.[320,327,335,336] TGF-β is a key regulator of AT2 cell expansion: it halts AT2 cell proliferation and is then inactivated to allow differentiation into AT1 cells during the repair process.[337] Additional important growth factors are released by the alveolar epithelium itself (e.g., GM-CSF)[298,299] or by invading and tissue-resident leukocytes (e.g., amphiregulin by *innate lymphocyte cells* [ILC]; TGF-β by T_Regs) (see Fig. 8.4).[239,336] An additional source of alveolar cells is the population of BASC located in the bronchioalveolar duct junctions.[319,332] BASC can give rise to the majority of distal lung epithelial cells after damage but only moderately contribute to homeostatic turnover. Of importance, ablation of BASC impairs regeneration of distal lung epithelia, identifying BASC as crucial components of the lung repair machinery, particularly after severe injury involving the bronchiolar and alveolar compartment[319] (see Fig. 8.4). To date it remains unclear whether an equivalent of the murine BASC exists in the human distal lung.

Loss of Regenerative Potential: Depletion of the Facultative Progenitor Cell Pool

Repeated epithelial injury and repair may deplete the mitotic potential of the facultative progenitor cell pool. Depletion of the facultative progenitor cell pool would leave the epithelium deficient in both regenerative and differentiation functions and contribute to epithelial fragility through loss of cellular autocrine/paracrine protective mechanisms, epithelial hypoplasia, and dysregulation of interactions between the epithelial, mesenchymal, and vascular compartments. In addition, specific properties of pulmonary facultative progenitor cells may limit their ability to repair the injured epithelium. For example, the metabolic pathways that allow the club cell to eliminate lipophilic agents also sensitize it to the toxic effects of excessive amounts of these compounds, leading to depletion of the progenitor pool.[338–340] In addition, the phenotypic plasticity essential to the club cell's ability to detect and eliminate pathogens and toxic agents may compromise the reparative functions of this cell type.[341–343] Thus, even though the progenitor cells are more resistant to injury in most settings, they are also particularly fragile to certain stresses or severe injuries.

In patients with acute lung injury and in chronic lung diseases, there are decreased numbers of club cells, as measured by expression of the club cell marker CCSP. Within small airways of those with COPD and asthma, club cells undergo a metaplastic transition to a mucosecretory phenotype,[344] which removes these cells from the progenitor pool. In addition, a reduction in the number of club cells is associated with tissue remodeling characterized by an increase in the number of an alternative progenitor, the basal cell, and consequent squamous metaplasia.[345–347] Furthermore, increased epithelial proliferation in the lungs of smokers suggests an ongoing injury process and the potential for the facultative progenitor cell pool to undergo replicative senescence, characterized by irreversible arrest of cell proliferation and altered cell functions.[348] Senescent cells persist and consequently inhibit activation of the remaining reparative cells by several mechanisms. Thus senescent cells could compromise differentiated functions while also acting to block cell replacement.

Defects in cellular maturation may also contribute to a failure to establish the facultative progenitor cell pool or to the depletion of the facultative progenitor cell pool after injury. The lung undergoes rapid and extensive maturation during the postnatal period. However, the maturation process can be interrupted by preterm birth and associated oxygen treatment, resulting in bronchopulmonary dysplasia, and can be impaired by postnatal exposure to environmental harms, including ozone and side-stream tobacco smoke in term infants.[349–351] These exposures are associated with depressed protective and reparative functions and morphologic and functional alterations to airway and alveolar facultative progenitor cells. These observations suggest that irritant exposure impairs lung maturation, leading to dysregulation of airway reparative processes. These studies support the concept that failure to establish or maintain an appropriately sized pool of facultative progenitor cells during lung development limits the repair potential after future injury and fosters chronic injury and dysfunctional repair cycles characteristic of chronic lung disease.

Another important aspect to consider is that the extent and severity of lung injury may determine whether the appropriate stem/progenitor cell type repopulates the lung. In a mouse model of severe influenza lung injury, an alveolar epithelial cell expressing $\alpha_6\beta_4$ integrin and basal cell markers, but not prosurfactant protein C, functioned as alternative AEP cells when local facultative progenitors such as AEP cells (and likely the BASC) were depleted.[352,353] This regenerative response was associated with aberrant remodeling and sustained Notch activation. Likewise, in the same model of severe lung injury, cells expressing basal cell makers migrated to alveolar regions in an attempt to repair the alveolar tissue devoid of facultative progenitor cells and resulted in abnormal repair, forming clusters ("pods") with tissue keratinization (see Fig. 8.4).[353–356] Thus the lung is capable of initiating repair even in settings where the primary progenitor cells are destroyed; however, repair by these "back-up" progenitor cells generally does not restore normal lung architecture. Thus significant depletion or changes in function of the facultative progenitor pool may contribute to the complex pathophysiologic alterations characteristic of acute and chronic lung diseases.

The Mesenchymal Niche in Epithelial Repair

The local microenvironment of a stem or progenitor cell (termed *niche*) is crucial in maintaining or activating repair processes in these cells by direct and indirect crosstalk mechanisms between different cell types. Mesenchymal cells play an important role in this niche, both during normal and abnormal repair. As such, the mesenchyme, comprised of populations of fibroblasts embedded within the extracellular matrix in the interstitium of the lung, represents another area important for consideration of normal and abnormal repair. Normal repair depends on epithelial-mesenchymal interactions, including the proliferation of subepithelial fibroblasts with focal deposition of ECM forming new connective (granulation) tissue that serves to fill in the "wound." We are just beginning to understand the functional heterogeneity of mesenchymal lung cells during these processes. In the airways, smooth muscle cells constitute a niche that harbors *leucine-rich repeat-containing G-protein–coupled receptor 6* (LGR6)-positive *airway smooth muscle* (ASM) cells that surround airway epithelia and drive their repair, involving the Wnt-FGF10 and Hippo pathways.[357,358] Loss of sonic hedgehog signaling between the airway epithelium and ASM induces ASM cell proliferation, thus triggering the wound healing response. During alveolar repair, distinct *platelet-derived growth factor receptor-α*

(PDGFRα)-positive mesenchymal cell populations have defined roles in development and regeneration. Lipid droplet-containing "lipofibroblasts" are Wnt-responsive, PDGFRα-high cells that release factors such as HGF and FGFs to drive proliferation and differentiation of AEP cells.[294] In addition, the mesenchyme contains a PDGFRα-low, α-smooth muscle actin–positive profibrotic myofibroblast that releases ECM during the repair process and constitutes a source of growth factors[359,360] (see Fig. 8.4). A leucine-rich repeat-containing G-protein–coupled receptor 5–positive alveolar mesenchymal cell was identified that supports alveolar cell proliferation; however, the lineage relation to the previously mentioned mesenchymal cells remains elusive.[357] Repetitive and/or nonresolving injury can result in fibroblast migration, proliferation, and differentiation into myofibroblasts, with deposition of excessive ECM comprised of collagen and other matrix components.[254,255,273,285,361–363] This is observed in idiopathic pulmonary fibrosis[360,364–367] and many other lung diseases, including ARDS,[13,15,368–370] asthma,[7,8] and COPD.[371–373] Although cytokines and growth factors that induce physiologic repair can prevent fibrosis,[271,273,304,374,375] under other circumstances these same factors, such as TGF-β, may actually promote fibrosis,[303,376–378] underscoring the importance of context in lung repair.

Does Lung Repair Recapitulate Mechanisms of Lung Development?

One of the proposed strategies to assist lung repair is to engage the normal pathways of lung development, at which time the entire lung is generated by the integration of developmental programs. Normal lung development involves the integration of numerous signaling pathways, including Wnt/β-catenin, Notch-delta, sonic hedgehog-patched, Hippo-YAP/TAZ, FGF-FGFR, and bone morphogenetic protein/TGF-β pathways.[305,379,380] These pathways interact to direct the appropriate differentiation of the epithelium, mesenchyme, and vasculature during lung development. During lung injury and repair, many of these pathways are reactivated to drive tissue regeneration and resolution of inflammation.[327] It is unclear, however, how these various signaling pathways are integrated during repair and whether they can be therapeutically exploited to drive productive cell replacement without causing aberrant remodeling or malignant proliferation. Key potential differences between lung development and lung repair include the presence of immune cells and other mediators during injury that might interfere with the normal response to developmental signals and the increased age of the lung, which might not respond the same as a developing lung to the same signals. Hence it is not known if the key regulatory pathways that are dominant during development can ultimately be targeted to improve repair in the adult.

Key Points

- The mechanisms of injury involve changes at the cellular and molecular level that initiate structural alterations and lead to compromised lung function. At the tissue and cellular level, exogenous insults and/or inflammatory stimuli result in increased vascular permeability and loss of alveolar epithelial barrier function due to disruption of intercellular junctions and cell death.
- Susceptibility to lung injury is determined by previous exposures, the level of stem/progenitor cells and their depletion after injury, and the individual's genetic constitution. This "gene-environment interaction" is the cornerstone of research initiatives directed at identification of susceptibility genes and those that modify the response to treatment.
- The pathways leading to injury involve so many mediators and cell types that it is not surprising that pharmacologic strategies to block a single pathway or class of mediators have so far been ineffective.
- Lung repair involves restoration of normal cellular composition, lung architecture, barrier function, and gas exchange.
- The inflammatory response must resolve to halt ongoing injury to the lung and allow reparative processes to proceed. Inflammatory cells undergo apoptosis and are cleared by macrophages in a phagocytic process termed *efferocytosis*, and lung edema fluid and protein are actively cleared from the air spaces.
- In response to cellular injury by noxious stimuli, such as infection and toxic compounds, endogenous stem and progenitor cells undergo rapid proliferation and differentiation to repair and regenerate the injured lung. Under normal circumstances, repair of the alveolar epithelium after injury relies on cell spreading, migration, and proliferation of surviving type 2 alveolar cells, followed by differentiation of specified type 2 cell subsets (or common alveolar progenitor cells) into alveolar type 1 cells. More upstream progenitors, such as the bronchioalveolar stem cells, give rise to both bronchiolar and alveolar cells, depending on the type and extent of injury.
- Repetitive epithelial injury or severe depletion of local stem/progenitor cells can lead to aberrant healing involving basal-like cells and to fibroproliferative responses in the airways and parenchyma, processes which are critically important for the pathogenesis of diseases, including pulmonary fibrosis, COPD, and asthma.

Key Readings

Bachofen M, Weibel ER. Structural alterations of lung parenchyma in the adult respiratory distress syndrome. *Clin Chest Med.* 1982;3(1):35–56.

Beers MF, Morrisey EE. The three R's of lung health and disease: repair, remodeling, and regeneration. *J Clin Invest.* 2011;121(6):2065–2073.

Jamieson AM, Pasman L, Yu S, Gamradt P, Homer RJ, Decker T, et al. Role of tissue protection in lethal respiratory viral-bacterial coinfection. *Science.* 2013;340(6137):1230–1234.

Kumar PA. Distal airway stem cells yield alveoli in vitro and during lung regeneration following H1N1 influenza infection. *Cell.* 2011:525–538.

Leach JP, Morrisey EE. Repairing the lungs one breath at a time: how dedicated or facultative are you? *Genes Dev.* 2018;32(23-24):1461–1471.

Mason RJ, Williams MC. Type II alveolar cell. Defender of the alveolus. *Am Rev Respir Dis.* 1977;115(6 Pt 2):81–91.

Matthay MA, Zemans RL, Zimmerman GA, Arabi YM, et al. Acute respiratory distress syndrome. *Nat Rev Dis Primers.* 2019;14(1):18. 5.

Ranieri VM, Rubenfeld GD, Thompson BT, Ferguson ND, Caldwell E, Fan E, et al. Acute respiratory distress syndrome: the Berlin definition. *JAMA.* 2012;307(23):2526–2533.

Serhan CN, Savill J. Resolution of inflammation: the beginning programs the end. *Nat Immunol.* 2005;6(12):1191–1197.

Vaughan AE, et al. Lineage-negative progenitors mobilize to regenerate lung epithelium after major injury. *Nature.* 2015;517(7536):621–625.

Zepp JA, Morrisey EE. Cellular crosstalk in the development and regeneration of the respiratory system. *Nat Rev Mol Cell Biol.* 2019; 20(9):551–566.

Zuo W, et al. p63(+)Krt5(+) distal airway stem cells are essential for lung regeneration. *Nature.* 2015;517(7536):616–620.

Complete reference list available at ExpertConsult.com.

9 GENETICS OF LUNG DISEASE

MICHAEL H. CHO, MD, MPH • DAVID A. SCHWARTZ, MD

INTRODUCTION

Our genome is a complete set of genetic code. Each genome is unique to an individual; on average, any two people will have approximately 4 to 5 million differences among their 3 billion letters of DNA sequence. Genetics is the study of this inherited variation. One of the first steps in investigating genetics of a trait or disease is to determine whether there is, in fact, a genetic contribution. The relative contribution of genetic factors to disease is called heritability. Formally, it is the fraction of variation of a phenotype—broadly defined as an observable characteristic of an individual, such as lung function—that can be attributed to genetic factors. This measure depends on the population studied and the relative contribution of the environment.[1] Although heritability has traditionally been measured using family studies, more recent methods allow estimation of heritability in unrelated individuals. These studies broadly confirm a significant genetic contribution to most traits and diseases.[2,3]

The field of human genetics has experienced tremendous growth over the last few decades. Technological advances in microarrays and in next-generation sequencing have driven the cost of genome-wide genotyping to less than $50 and whole-genome sequencing to less than $1000. In parallel, bioinformatic platforms and statistical methods have advanced to allow the rapid, efficient, and accurate measurement of this human genetic variation and its association to disease. Large epidemiologic efforts, including recruitment of large populations and biobanks, have enabled larger and better phenotyped samples.

The genome encodes all cellular processes, and genetic variants are assigned at birth. This essentially random assignment has the potential to reveal novel and causal mechanisms of disease pathobiology and confirm existing or uncover new targets for therapeutics. Human genetic evidence for a drug target significantly increases the likelihood of success of a drug trial.[4] Genetic variants also have the ability to identify disease subgroups or subtypes.[5] Complex and polygenic diseases may also be amenable to genetic risk prediction. For example, polygenic risk scores developed using *genome-wide association studies* (GWASs) for obesity and cardiovascular disease have been shown to identify subsets of individuals at a similar risk of disease as those who harbor mendelian variants.[6] These persons may be targets for preventive therapy, including specific pharmacologic treatments or lifestyle modification. The progress made in cystic fibrosis, from the discovery of the causal gene to the development of novel and mutation-specific therapies,[7] serves as a model for precision medicine in other diseases.

HUMAN GENETICS

CHARACTERIZATION OF GENETIC VARIATION

Molecular genetics is elegant in its simplicity. Just four base pairs (two purines [adenine and guanine] and two pyrimidines [thymine and cytosine]) code for 20 amino acids that form the molecular building blocks of complex proteins. However, the assemblage of inherited genes (genotypes), control mechanisms, resultant proteins, and posttranslational modifications have the capacity to create a complex panoply of unique biologic, physiologic, or visible traits of an organism called a *phenotype*. The relationship between these rather simple molecular characteristics and the vast array of complex phenotypes is, in part, explained by a number of seminal discoveries. Gregor Mendel[8] was the first to demonstrate that discrete traits could be inherited as separable factors (genes) in a predictable manner. Mendel's laws established the concept that each gene has alternative forms (alleles). Darwin[9] made the observation that evolution represents a series of environmentally responsive "genomic" upgrades. Thomas Morgan[10] established the concept of linkage to discover that genes were organized (and inherited) on individual chromosomes, and that genetic material was recombined or exchanged between maternal and paternal chromosomes during meiosis and that the frequency of recombination could be used to establish the relative genomic distance between genes. However, it was not until 1944 that Avery, MacLeod, and McCarty, while working with *Pneumococcus*, discovered that DNA was the essential molecule that transmitted the genetic code.[11] The double-helix structure of DNA was discovered by Watson, Crick, Chargaff, Franklin, and Wilkins in 1953[12] and, since then, genetics assumed a central role in understanding the biologic and physiologic differences between and among species and between states of health and states of disease.

LINKAGE DISEQUILIBRIUM

Over the past several decades, genomic maps have evolved from karyotypes (i.e., microscopic images of chromosomes during metaphase) to maps with specific base-pair sequences. Two major breakthroughs at the end of the 20th and beginning of the 21st centuries changed human genetics forever—the sequencing of the human genome[13,14] and the creation of the International HapMap Project to identify the common sequence differences and similarities between individuals.[15] With the sequencing of the human genome, investigators for the first time had a detailed road map of the human genome that identified the genes, regulatory units, and noncoding sequences with a high degree of resolution. Of the 3.2 billion base pairs in the human genome, fewer than 1% uniquely identify each human being.[16] Although there are several types of variation in the human genome (Table 9.1), the most common types of variation are *single nucleotide variants* (SNVs), which result from the substitution of a single base (e.g., A to G). Common SNVs are referred to as *single nucleotide polymorphisms* (SNPs). To date, more than 450 million SNVs and small insertions or deletions (i.e., indels) have been identified in the human genome. These variants provide much of the genetic diversity that underlies the variable susceptibility to disease development and progression.[16] The 1000 Genomes Project[17] and, more recently, the Trans-Omics in Precision Medicine program,[18] have been developed to expand the catalog of uncommon and rare variation among diverse human populations.

Genetic maps are based on the frequency of recombination events, defined as a specific form of exchange of genetic material between the maternal and paternal chromosomes during meiosis. Genes on the same chromosome that are closer together are more likely to be inherited together (i.e., linked) than genes that are farther apart, which may demonstrate more random and independent assortment. In general, the greater the distance is between genes, the higher the recombination frequency (eFig. 9.1A). A *haplotype* (i.e., haploid genotype) is a set of linked, contiguous genetic variants that are inherited together. The Haplotype Map (HapMap) project leveraged this key concept called *linkage disequilibrium* (see eFig. 9.1B). Linkage disequilibrium exists when two markers in close physical proximity are correlated in a population, when they are in association more than would be expected with random assortment. This "blocky" nature of the genome facilitates genetic discovery because instead of having to interrogate and test all variants in the genome, one achieves nearly the same power by testing a smaller set of variants that are correlated with or "tag" other variants.

PUBLIC DATABASES

Online resources are a major source of information about genetics, such as the Online Mendelian Inheritance in Man (https://www.omim.org) and the Human Gene Mutation Database (http://www.hgmd.cf.ac.uk/ac/index.php).[19] Up-to-date genetic sequence, variant, and other annotation information can be obtained from Ensembl (www.ensembl.org). The University of California at Santa Cruz Genome Browser (genome.ucsc.edu), Ensembl and LDLink (https://ldlink.nci.nih.gov/) provide linkage disequilibrium information across a range of populations, whereas the Genome Aggregation Database (gnomAD; gnomad.broadinstitute.org) and BRAVO (https://bravo.sph.umich.edu) provide resources for interrogating variation across large-scale whole-genome sequencing studies. Resources such the GWAS catalog (https://www.ebi.ac.uk/gwas/) store genome-wide association information.

GENETIC EPIDEMIOLOGY

LINKAGE STUDIES

Genetic epidemiology is the study of genetic factors in families and in populations. Historically, identifying disease regions involved linkage. Linkage analyses use family data, which can be made up by a wide range of pedigree structures from extended pedigrees to affected sibling pairs. There are two broad types of linkage analysis: parametric and nonparametric. Both types of linkage analysis rely on the coinheritance of disease alleles with genetic markers used in the analysis. When a mutation arises on a particular chromosome, initially there is a large shared segment of DNA and hence linkage disequilibrium around it. With each subsequent generation, this region of linkage disequilibrium becomes smaller as a result of meiotic recombination. *Parametric* linkage analysis aims to determine if alleles at a genotyped marker segregate together with the alleles at a putative disease locus more often than one would expect by random assortment, or chance. *Nonparametric* linkage analysis refers to a group of analysis methods that, in contrast to parametric linkage analysis, does not require

---

Table 9.1 Commonly Used DNA Markers

Single nucleotide variant (SNV)—Individual point substitutions of a single nucleotide that do not change the length of the DNA sequence and are present throughout the genome. Common variants are often referred to as single nucleotide polymorphisms.

Indel—Insertion/deletion variant, leading either to inserted or deleted base pairs. When present in coding regions and not a multiple of three, indels can result in frameshift mutations. Usually short (a few base pairs in length, although can be up to 1000 base pairs in length), and together with SNVs, indels make up the majority of cataloged human variation.

Copy number variant (CNV)—A duplication or deletion of a region of a genome that is 1000 to 5 megabases in length.

assumptions about a particular form of inheritance. This nonparametric approach has been combined with genetic association within the linked region to identify disease susceptibility genes for asthma, Crohn disease, and pulmonary fibrosis.[20–25]

ASSOCIATION STUDIES

Association studies that test for the relationship of a marker to a phenotype are not limited to families and can be an order of magnitude more powerful than linkage analyses.[26] Today genetic association studies are the most commonly used study designs to find disease genes in complex traits and can test for quantitative, binary, or other (e.g., survival) outcomes; contain varying degrees of unrelated and related individuals; and use population-based, case-control, or family studies. Genetic association studies are similar to other epidemiologic study designs and involve identifying genetic markers with significant genotype frequency differences between individuals with the phenotype of interest (cases) and a set of unrelated control individuals.[27] One problem with association studies is that, although genetic data are generally less subject to confounding, differences in genetic background between cases and controls can cause spurious results,[28] termed *population stratification.* Genotyping and adjusting for the effects of a set of randomly distributed markers can address this problem.[29–33] A second problem with early case-control studies has been that often the sample size was too small to allow robust evaluation of the evidence for association. Because of the small genetic effect sizes seen and expected for complex traits, sample sizes at least in the thousands are generally required in addition to replication to generate rigorously validated association results. Thus key considerations when evaluating genetic association studies[34] include (1) accounting for population stratification, (2) assessing nonrandom and evolutionary forces on allele frequencies (i.e., Hardy-Weinberg equilibrium), (3) replicating results, and (4) adjusting for multiple comparisons.

Genetic association tests can also include related subjects. Two main types of models can be used. The first type of statistical model incorporates correlation between samples, such as linear mixed models. Advances in statistical methods have led to faster and more convenient implementations[35,36] that can incorporate sample correlation between family members and correlation due to population substructure (i.e., they can be used to adjust for population stratification). The second type of family-based statistical model is based on the transmission disequilibrium test.[37,38] The test is predicated on the assumption that, if a genetic locus is uninvolved (neither linked nor associated) in the phenotype of interest, one would expect each of the two parental alleles at that locus to be transmitted equally to an affected child (i.e., transmitted 50% of the time). However, if the locus is actually linked and associated with disease, there will be overtransmission (or undertransmission) of one allele at that locus, and its transmission will differ significantly from the expected 50%. These types of tests need to recruit both affected individuals and their parents, which often limits diseases studied and sample size but is immune to population stratification and can be used to identify de novo mutations.

GENOME-WIDE ASSOCIATION STUDIES

GWASs have arguably revolutionized the field of complex trait genetics. In GWASs, single nucleotide variants are selected using linkage disequilibrium information from the population to cover the entire genome; approximately 500,000 variants result in greater than 90–95% coverage of common variants. GWAS have well-accepted approaches to the design, data collection, data cleaning, and data analysis required for these large complex studies. These include proper attention to technical artifacts and batch effects,[39,40] population stratification,[28] and statistical significance, usually a P value of less than 5×10^{-8},[41] although more recent studies may require a more stringent cutoff,[42] ideally with replication in a second study. The number of robustly associated genetic loci for complex diseases has increased dramatically since 2000.[43]

Several important lessons have been learned from the GWAS era. Perhaps the most important lesson is that very few of the candidate genes from previously hypothesized genes have been replicated in large GWASs; nearly all the findings are for genes that have not been studied in the disease of interest. A second is the extensive degree of overlap between genetic association findings among different diseases. This setting, in which a genetic variant has many phenotypic effects, is called *pleiotropy.* Pleiotropy can be horizontal, affecting traits in different causal pathways, or vertical, with different traits mediated by the same pathway. Pleiotropy can lead to insights into gene function or prioritize regions for follow-up.[44] Third is the recognition that the heritability of many traits and diseases appears to be accounted for by common variants, with a smaller proportion of heritability due to rare variants.[45,46] However, these findings do not imply that finding rare variants is unimportant, particularly for understanding disease pathobiology.

GENETIC ARCHITECTURE AND RARE VARIANTS

The specific genetic variants responsible for phenotype exist along a spectrum (Fig. 9.1). This relationship can be illustrated by examining the relationship between two factors. The first, *allele frequency,* represents how common a genetic factor or "version" of a gene (allele) is in the population. The second factor is *penetrance,* or the chance that someone who has the risk allele has disease, and corresponds to *effect size.* For decades, the primary application of human genetics focused on disorders due to these high penetrance, rare variants, and rare diseases, also termed *mendelian.* Examples of these types of diseases include cystic fibrosis and Huntington disease.

At the opposite end of this spectrum are complex, or polygenic diseases. In this setting, no single variant leads to disease; instead, many genetic variants each modestly increase risk. A typical variant in this scenario more commonly lies in the 99% of the genome that is noncoding (does not change a protein amino acid) and has a modest odds ratio in the range of 1.1 to 1.4. Due to these small effect sizes, studying these diseases usually relies on large sample sizes.

These two examples represent opposite ends of what is increasingly being recognized as a spectrum. For mendelian diseases, studies have found that some variants

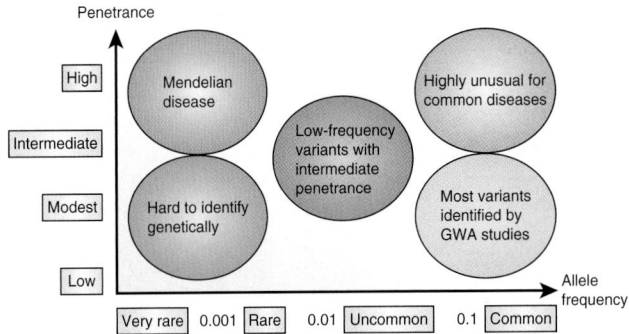

Figure 9.1 The relationship of allele frequency to penetrance. Traditional mendelian diseases harbor very rare genetic variants that have very high penetrance (e.g., large effect sizes); in contrast, most genome-wide association studies identify common variants of weak effect. However, these two contrasting study designs exist on a spectrum, and rare variants can contribute to common disease, whereas common variants can also modify mendelian disease. (From McCarthy MI, Abecasis GR, Cardon LR, et al. Genome-wide association studies for complex traits: consensus, uncertainty and challenges. *Nat Rev Genet.* 2008;9:356–369.)

previously considered fully penetrant do not result in disease,[47] and common genetic variants can also contribute to mendelian disease, as in genetic modifiers of cystic fibrosis.[48] In common diseases, some of the contributing variants are rare coding variants of large effect.[49,50]

Identification of rare variants often requires sequencing. In contrast to genotyping studies—where an individual DNA base pair known to vary in the population is tested—sequencing studies assay all variants in a given region. The advent of *next-generation sequencing* has dropped the cost of sequencing more than a millionfold. This technological advance has led to a revolution in analyzing rare diseases, which formerly required slow and painstaking linkage and mapping. Due to these advances over the past decade,[51] sequencing studies of affected subjects can directly identify the causal gene and variant by screening for very rare, predicted deleterious mutations. Genome centers now routinely perform exome or whole-genome sequencing on patients with rare genetic disorders, with an appreciable rate of success in identifying the likely causal gene.[52]

Sequencing studies are not just limited to very rare diseases. Rare variants can also contribute to the burden of more common diseases. Sequencing studies have identified rare variants in lipid disorders, diabetes, and inflammatory bowel disease.[46,50,53] In pulmonary disease, rare variants are responsible for cases of pulmonary hypertension, allergic diseases, and pulmonary fibrosis, all of which are also due to common variants.[54–57]

Just as there is no true dichotomy between common and rare variant studies, the differences between genotyping and sequencing studies are also less clear. As sequencing studies get larger and more diverse, these data can be used to reconstruct the haplotypes in a population. These population-based "reference panels" allow increasingly accurate genotype *imputation* from genetic microarray data[58] (Fig. 9.2). Imputation refers to a statistical technique of "filling in" variants not covered by genotyping, using sequencing data as a reference. Although imputation is more challenging for rare than

for common variants, with the most recent large imputation panels, some rare variants, for example, *BRCA1*, can also be imputed.[18] The decision to perform more economical but less accurate genotyping and imputation, versus more expensive but comprehensive sequencing, depends on the disease and types of analysis to be done. For most complex polygenic diseases, most genetic associations will be identified through genotyping with imputation.[45]

GENE BY ENVIRONMENT INTERACTION

Because both genes and environmental exposures are known to be related to complex traits, performing studies to test both factors in one study design is of great value. The two major challenges for these studies are statistical power and accurate measurement of exposure. Tests for gene-environment interaction require larger sample sizes than tests for the genetic effect alone. Alternative approaches may address some of these limitations. For example, a gene by environment interaction study on lung function and smoking did not find convincing evidence of interaction, but a study using genetic variants in aggregate did find an association.[59,60] Although some environmental factors, such as diet, are hard to measure accurately and require complex techniques, other exposures, such as lifetime cigarette smoking, can be measured with relatively high precision. Accurate and consistent measures of exposure will greatly enhance the ability of these studies to provide new insights into disease pathogenesis.

EPIGENETICS

Epigenetics is the study of changes in gene transcription that are dependent on the molecules that bind to DNA, rather than on the base-pair sequence of DNA.[61,62] This includes both heritable changes in gene expression in the progeny of cells or of individuals and stable, long-term alterations in the transcriptional potential of a cell or tissue that are not necessarily heritable. Because epigenetic processes are highly interdependent and regulate gene expression in an age-, state-, cell-, and tissue-dependent manner, collectively these mechanisms constitute a complex system of molecular controls that affects biologic processes and human diseases.

Although our understanding of the fundamental mechanisms of epigenetics continues to evolve, it is recognized that epigenetic regulation of the genome results in a hierarchy of transcriptional switches that facilitate development and differentiation, normal tissue function, and the ability of the host to respond to stress.[61,62] There are three primary mechanisms that govern gene expression—DNA methylation, histone modifications, and noncoding RNAs—that may be inherited, independent of the sequence of DNA (Table 9.2 and eFig. 9.2). Hypermethylation of cytosine-guanosine motifs, particularly at promoter and enhancer sites, silences gene transcription. Conversely, hypomethylation of these motifs enhances gene transcription. Histones, the building blocks of nucleosomes, undergo numerous posttranslational modifications (methylation, acetylation, or phosphorylation with more than 100 conserved, covalent modifications) that affect chromatin structure and alter gene expression. Noncoding RNAs bind to DNA and interfere with transcription and posttranscriptional regulation

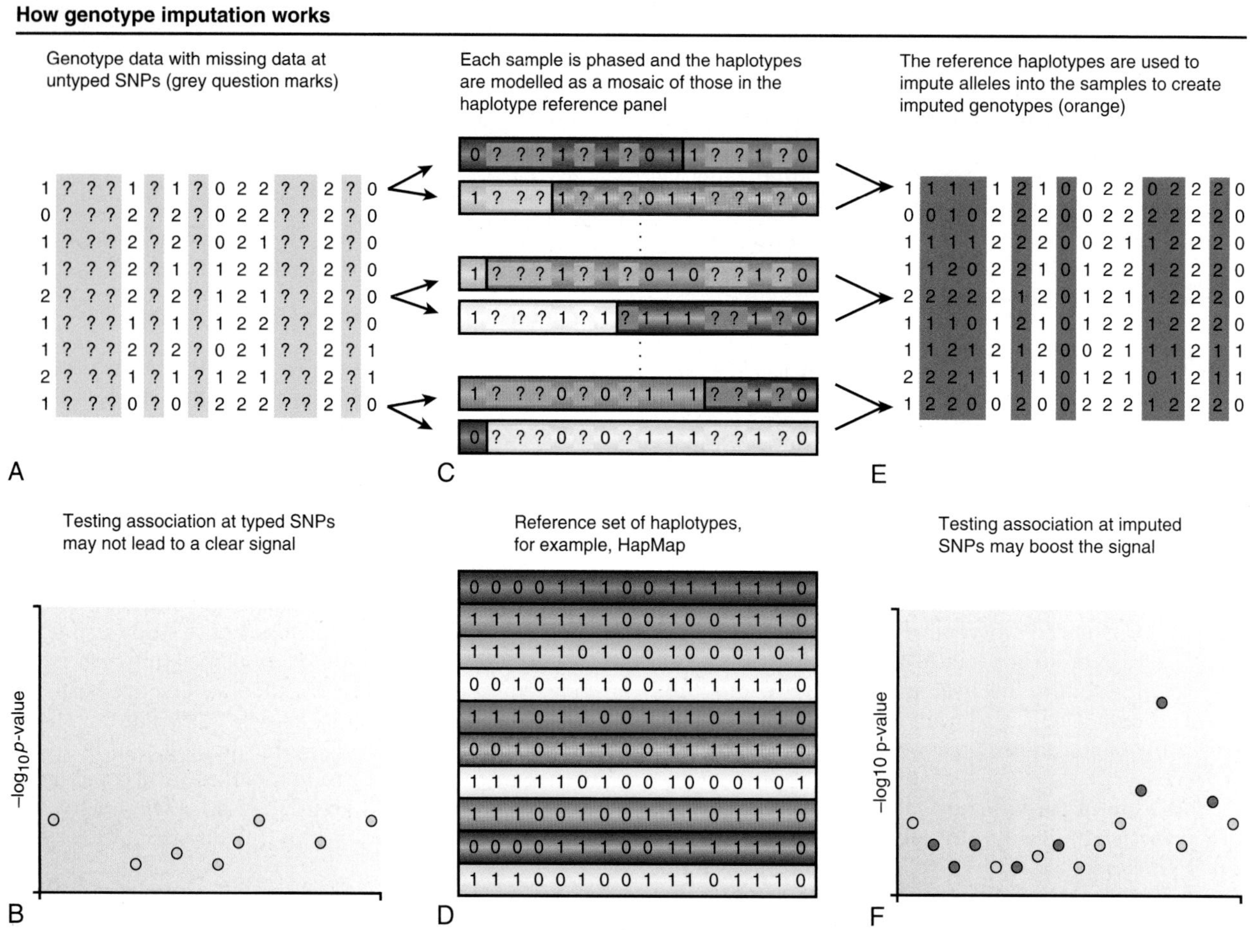

How genotype imputation works

Figure 9.2 **The process of genotype imputation.** Genotype imputation is a technique by which a reference panel with detailed genetic variation information from a sequencing-based study is used to provide additional information for a study using genotyping arrays. This method increases power of genome-wide association studies and blurs the distinction between rare variant, sequencing-based studies and genome-wide association studies. (A) Genotyping arrays only cover a select set of single nucleotide polymorphisms. (B) Association testing may not show a signal. By computational approaches to phase the data (C) and matching to a reference set (D), these missing values can be filled in (E), leading to a new signal (F). (From Marchini J, Howie B. Genotype imputation for genome-wide association studies. *Nat Rev Genet*. 2010;11:499–511.)

Table 9.2   Known Epigenetic Mechanisms

DNA methylation—The methyl group is transferred from *S*-adenosylmethionine to the C-5 position of cytosine by a cytosine-methyltransferase. Hypermethylation of CpG motifs, particularly at promoter and enhancer sites, silences gene transcription. Alternatively, hypomethylation of these motifs enhances gene transcription.

Histone modification—Histones, the building blocks of nucleosomes, undergo numerous posttranslational modifications (methylation, acetylation, or phosphorylation with >100 conserved, covalent modifications) that regulate chromatin structure and gene expression.

Noncoding RNAs—These RNAs bind to DNA and interfere with transcription and posttranscriptional regulation of gene expression (e.g., miRNA).

CpG, cytosine-guanosine; miRNA, micro-RNA.

---

of gene expression. In aggregate, these mechanisms serve to regulate the transcriptional activity of specific genes, at specific stages of development, and in response to specific forms of endogenous and exogenous stress. Of importance, these mechanisms are conserved in eukaryotic organisms, from yeast to humans.

Epigenetic mechanisms can have profound effects on cellular, tissue, and whole-organism phenotype, including fundamental mechanisms such as stem cell differentiation[63]

and inactivation of the X chromosome.[64] Although epigenetic marks can be inherited, these potent regulators of transcription can also be modified throughout development[65] and by environmental exposures.[66] For instance, although monozygotic twins are genetically identical, as they age, twin pairs develop divergent epigenetic marks associated with differences in gene expression.[65] Environmental endocrine disruptors have been shown to induce transgenerational effects on male fertility as a result of DNA methylation.[66] These findings suggest that the epigenome can be reprogrammed, potentially affecting the risk, cause, and treatment of various disease states.

The technology to measure epigenetic changes is continuing to evolve and, with the advent of methylation sequencing, it will soon be feasible to detect the epigenetic modifications of the entire genome during states of stress and disease. High-quality antibodies have been used to detect known modifications in the amino acid residues of histones. Chromatin immunoprecipitation can be used in conjunction with either microarrays (chromatin immunoprecipitation chip) or next-generation sequencing (ChIP-seq, FAIRE-seq, and ATAC-seq) to evaluate global changes in histone modifications. As the cost of sequencing decreases, these assays will become increasingly accessible.

Considering the importance of the environment in the development of lung disease, it is somewhat surprising that more attention has not been devoted to epigenetic mechanisms that lead to acute and chronic forms of lung disease. Epigenetic mechanisms have been associated with a number of tumors, and the methylation pattern of six genes is associated with the development of lung cancer.[67] However, research is just beginning to demonstrate the relevance of epigenetic changes to nonmalignant forms of lung disease. In patients with *idiopathic pulmonary fibrosis* (IPF), DNA methylation is markedly altered in their lung tissue.[68] In airway diseases such as asthma and COPD, bronchial biopsy specimens and alveolar macrophages have increased histone acetyltransferase activity and reduced histone deacetylase activity,[69–71] thought to be important in the transcriptional regulation of inflammatory mediators.[71] Because cigarette smoke, vitamin supplementation, and other environmental exposures can alter the epigenetic marks along the human genome, studying the importance of changes in DNA methylation, structural changes in amino acid residues of histones, and expression of noncoding RNAs should help us to understand the fundamental mechanisms associated with the etiology and progression of several types of lung disease. Moreover, the epigenome can be modified by a variety of drugs. Of interest, in a murine model of asthma, trichostatin A, a histone deacetylase inhibitor, can decrease ovalbumin-induced allergic airway disease.[72] As we begin to understand the role of epigenetic mechanisms in the development of lung disease, it will become much more obvious how we can modify these mechanisms therapeutically to reduce the burden of lung disease among our patients.

FINE MAPPING AND FUNCTIONAL GENETICS

Genetic association studies, with few exceptions, identify an associated locus, not a causal variant or gene. This result is due to linkage disequilibrium, which, although facilitating discovery, impairs identification of the specific causal variant, a process requiring "fine mapping." Similarly, although an association is often denoted by the closest gene, for instance, *FAM13A*, in most cases the nearest gene is not actually the causal gene,[43,73] nor is the cell or tissue type, the timing of action, or environmental conditions known. This issue is exemplified by one of the strongest genetic associations for obesity, where the most significant variant is located within the *FTO* gene. *FTO* as the causal gene was supported by early studies.[74] However, subsequent work identified a mechanism that did not involve *FTO*; instead, the causal variant disrupted a motif for the *ARID5B* repressor, affecting *IRX3* and *IRX5* expression in preadipocytes and leading to a shift in lipid storage.[75]

Despite hundreds of replicated loci for respiratory disease, the underlying biologic mechanisms are completely unknown for most. In a minority of loci, the associated variant is *nonsynonymous*, which means it results in an amino acid change that can directly affect the function or expression of the encoded protein (e.g., *AGER*, *SFTPD*, or *TERT* variants in COPD and pulmonary fibrosis). However, in most cases, the causal variant is likely regulatory.

Although identifying an effect of the identified variant on gene expression can help narrow down the gene of interest, gene expression is pervasive, expression may be condition specific, and directionality may not be consistent.[76,77] To date, most loci have required careful and customized approaches. These examples include *MUC5B*, *ORMDL3*, and *HHIP* in studies of IPF, asthma, and COPD, respectively.[78–80] Methods to perform fine mapping and functional assessment are improving, through increased availability of open chromatin profiling, three-dimensional genome maps, high-throughput functional assays, gene editing, and other methods.[81–84]

INTEGRATIVE GENOMICS AND SYSTEMS GENETICS

The discovery of large numbers of genetic risk factors, most affecting novel genes with unknown mechanisms of action, makes it clear that consideration of single genes in isolation is insufficient. The field of integrative genomics aims to relate genetic variants to other omics. Systems genetics is an approach to understand mechanisms, beginning from genetic variants through intermediate phenotypes, such as transcripts, proteins, and metabolites, and then to determine how these converge on pathways and networks[85] (Fig. 9.3). Network medicine, in turn, is the related concept that diseases arise from perturbations and interactions in a complex intra- and intracellular network, linking tissues and organ systems, and that these processes can be studied using principles of network science.[86]

Although these fields are still emerging, they are already influencing discovery. For example, identification of expression quantitative trait loci—genetic loci that affect gene expression—is a key tool in identifying gene function, as exemplified by *ORMDL3* in asthma (see later). In COPD, specific pathways have been implicated by leveraging gene or protein expression from individual associations.[87]

APPLICATION TO PULMONARY DISEASES

ASTHMA

Asthma has long been known to have a significant genetic component. Although there have been hundreds of reports of associations, many of the studies from the candidate gene era for asthma suffer from the methodologic problems discussed earlier. The first asthma GWAS identified a genome-wide significant locus at 17q21[88] and also was one of the first to integrate gene expression, demonstrating differential expression of *ORMDL3*, a gene involved in the endoplasmic reticulum found to regulate sphingolipid synthesis. The most recent large GWAS include multi-ethnic studies, and studies of adult and childhood asthma,[89–91] the latter of which appears to harbor more genetic susceptibility than adult asthma.[92] Some of the major findings include associations near *interleukin-1 receptor-like 1 (IL1RL1), thymic stromal*

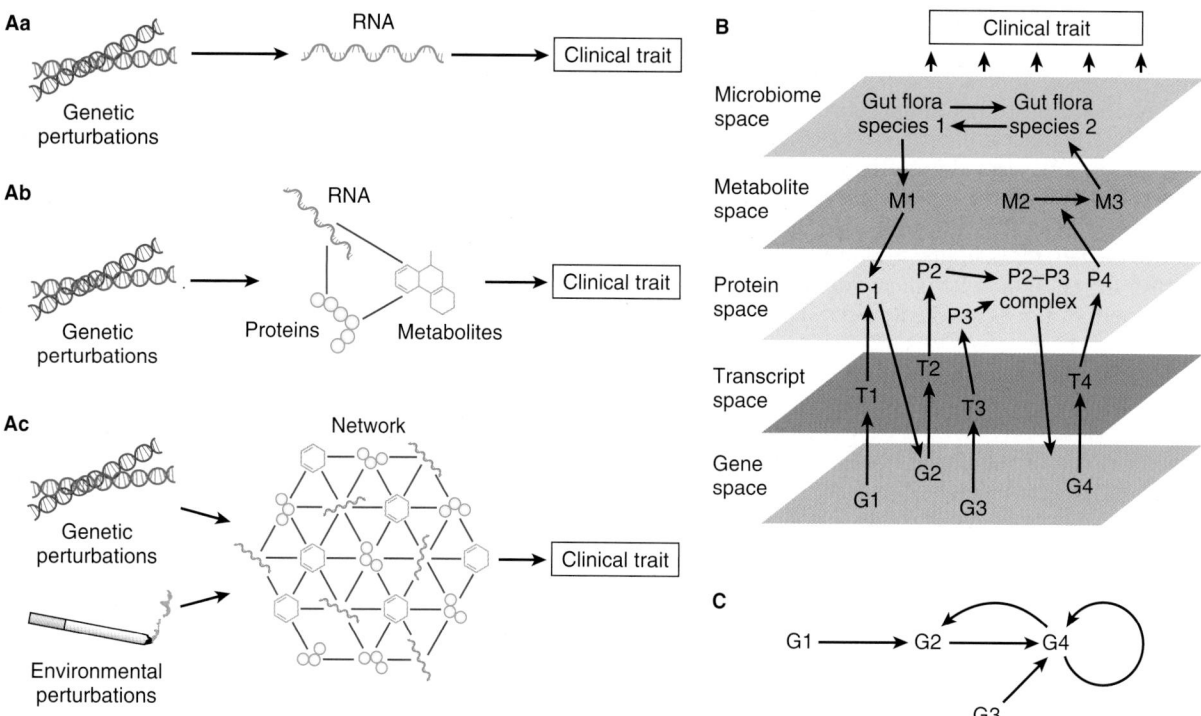

Figure 9.3 Systems genetics. (Aa) A genetic perturbation can have an effect on transcription and a resulting clinical trait; (Ab) or can affect proteins or metabolites; (Ac) or, in conjunction with an environmental perturbation, can affect a network. (B) These interactions can involve multiple genes and molecular phenotypes and (C) result in specifically derived models. (From Civelek M, Lusis AJ. Systems genetics approaches to understand complex traits. *Nat Rev Genet.* 2014;15:34–48; A, Modified from Schadt EE. Molecular networks as sensors and drivers of common human diseases. *Nature.* 2009;461:218–223.)

lymphopoietin (TSLP), and *IL-33 (IL33)*, all genes implicated in type 2 T helper cell–mediated immune responses and genes related to allergy and dysregulated epithelial barrier function. Additional investigations into related traits, such as immunoglobulin E levels and other allergic diseases, have also identified loci that have an influence on asthma.[93,94]

COPD AND LUNG FUNCTION

One of the first genetic causes of COPD was identified more than 50 years ago with the discovery of *alpha₁-antitrypsin deficiency* (AATD). However, even after controlling for cigarette smoking exposure and excluding AATD patients, studies in families, twins, and unrelated individuals have found clear evidence of additional genetic contributions. Despite years of candidate gene studies, it has only been with the advance of GWASs that clear, reproducible genetic signals have been identified. The first GWAS for COPD[95] identified a region on chromosome 15q25, and additional studies identified the *hedgehog-interacting protein gene (HHIP)*[96-98] and a *family with sequence similarity 13, member A*[96] *(FAM13A)*. Pulmonary function is also highly heritable. As COPD is defined using lung function, perhaps it is not surprising that GWASs of *forced expiratory volume in 1 second* (FEV₁) and the *FEV₁ to forced vital capacity* (FEV₁/FVC) ratio have a high degree of overlap. Most lung function loci and COPD loci are shared with a consistent direction of effect, and a genetic risk score comprising lung function loci strongly predicts COPD.[99,100] The most recent large studies have identified dozens of loci for COPD[87] and hundreds for lung function.[99,100]

ACUTE RESPIRATORY DISTRESS SYNDROME

Genetic analysis of inbred mouse strains first revealed that acute lung injury susceptibility was strain dependent and therefore may, in part, be genetically determined.[101] Although no studies to date have identified and replicated variants of genome-wide significance,[102] several suggestive associations have emerged. For example, a variant in the *IL-1 receptor antagonist (IL1RN)* reached a predetermined level of significance for coding variants, was replicated, and was associated with an increased IL-1 receptor antagonist response in plasma.[103] Additional bioinformatic analysis in 232 African Americans and 162 control subjects identified a nonsynonymous variant in *selectin P ligand (SELPLG)* as a risk factor for *acute respiratory distress syndrome* (ARDS), with support from preclinical models, including knockout mice.[104] Genetic studies in ARDS still are limited by sample size and heterogeneity; integration of additional omics data, including biomarkers, and identification of more homogeneous phenotypes will likely be helpful.[102]

LUNG CANCER

In a recent pooled analysis from the International Lung Cancer Consortium, first-degree relatives had a 1.5-fold increase in the risk of lung cancer after adjustment for smoking and other confounders, and this relationship seemed to be consistent across histologic subtypes.[105] GWAS have identified several susceptibility loci, including the *CHRNA3/5* and *CYP2A6* loci, both of which are also associated with COPD and cigarette smoking, as well as loci at genes related to telomere maintenance, such as

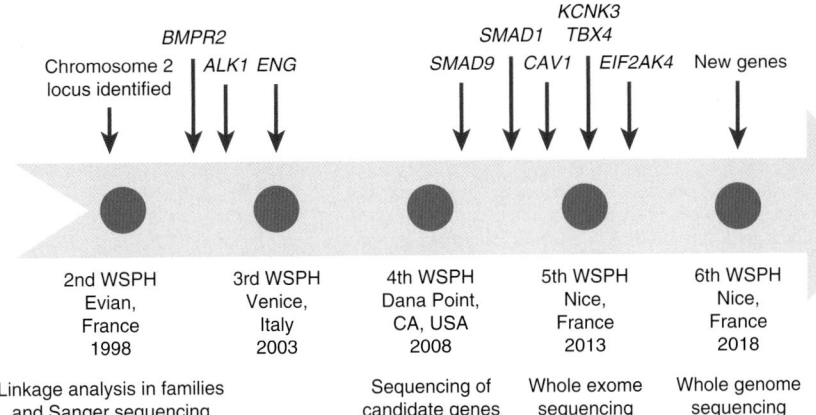

Figure 9.4 **Genetics of pulmonary hypertension.** The discovery of genes in pulmonary hypertension also traces the development of genetic technology for rare variants to increasingly powerful and unbiased approaches, from linkage analysis and Sanger sequencing, to candidate gene, exome, and whole-genome sequencing studies. WSPH, World Symposium on Pulmonary Hypertension; Sanger sequencing, the standard method of sequencing from 1977 for the next 40 years. (From Morrell NW, Aldred MA, Chung WK, et al. Genetics and genomics of pulmonary arterial hypertension. *Eur Respir J.* 2019;53:1801899.)

TERT, OBFC1, and *RTEL1,* and other genes, such as *HLA, BRCA2, CHEK2, RNASET2, SECISBP2L,* and *NRG1.* This most recent study also identified subtypes as an important consideration in lung cancer association studies; of the 10 novel loci, six appeared to be specific for adenocarcinoma.[106,107] In addition to inherited, germline variation—present in all cells in an individual's genome—another type of genetic variation is important in cancer. Somatic mutations are those that develop in specific tissues during the course of cell division and drive much of lung cancer pathogenesis. These have led to tumor-specific targets,[108–110] an impressive accomplishment of genomic medicine that provided a seamless link between the pathogenesis, prediction of treatment effect, and successful application of treatment (see Chapters 73 and 74).

FIBROSING IDIOPATHIC INTERSTITIAL PNEUMONIA

Fibrosing *idiopathic interstitial pneumonia* (IIP) refers to a group of lung diseases that are characterized by progressive scarring of the alveolar interstitium that leads to significant morbidity and mortality. IPF is the most common and severe form of fibrosing IIP. There is substantial evidence for a genetic basis for IPF.[111–113] Although rare mutations in the *TERT, TERC, SFTPC,* and *SFTPA2* genes have been associated with familial interstitial pneumonia and IPF,[114–119] in aggregate these mutations account for a small proportion of the population attributable risk. One of the most striking findings in respiratory genetics is the identification of a promoter variant in the *MUC5B* gene (rs35705950), found to be present in approximately 50% to 60% of individuals with familial or sporadic forms of IPF. In contrast to most other common variants that are of modest (odds ratio <1.5) effect, the *MUC5B* variant is estimated to increase the risk 6-fold for heterozygotes and 20-fold for homozygotes (eFig. 9.3).[25,120] Of importance, the *MUC5B* promoter SNP also appears to be predictive of early disease; in the Framingham population, the SNP is associated with a threefold to sixfold excess risk per allele for interstitial lung abnormalities that likely represent early radiographic evidence of interstitial lung disease,[121] suggesting that the *MUC5B* promoter SNP could be used to identify individuals with preclinical

forms of IPF. Additional loci revealed by GWAS include *TERT/TERC, FAM13A, DSP, OBFC1, ATP11A, DPP9,* and *AKAP13.*[122] Recently, targeted sequencing across the original 10 GWAS loci[123] identified 10 common variants that, in aggregate, account for at least 35% of the risk of IPF.[124] Further characterizing these IIP-associated loci will provide important targets for functional studies that will ultimately allow the development of new prevention and treatment strategies.[113]

PULMONARY HYPERTENSION

In contrast to asthma, COPD, and IPF, where susceptibility appears to be driven primarily by common variants, the genetic susceptibility of pulmonary arterial hypertension (World Health Organization Group 1) appears to be due frequently to rare variants.[125] An overview of discoveries in the genetics of pulmonary hypertension is shown in Fig. 9.4. *Bone morphogenetic protein type II receptor (BMPR2)* variants may account for as many as 80% of familial cases and up to 10–20% of cases without a family history,[126] although only about 25% of carriers actually develop disease. Additional studies have identified *ALK1, ACVRL1,* and *ENG* as associated with hereditary hemorrhagic telangectasia; BMPR pathway genes, including *SMAD1, SMAD4,* and *SMAD9,*[127] and *EIF2AK4,* appear to be relatively specific to pulmonary capillary hemangiomatosis and pulmonary veno-occlusive disease.[128,129] Recent exome sequencing identified rare variants in *ATP13A3, AQP1, SOX17,* and *GDF2* and found approximately 15% also had *BMPR2* mutations. Common variants, identified by GWAS, have loci near *SOX17* and *HLA-DPA1/DPB1.* The identification of causative mutations in pulmonary hypertension has focused research efforts on developing strategies that restore the function and expression of defective pathways.

SARCOIDOSIS

Siblings of those with sarcoidosis are at a relative risk of disease of approximately four- to fivefold.[130,131] Early studies identified a strong association signal in a region of the genome responsible for immune function, the *major histocompatibility complex* (MHC) locus[132]; subsequent studies identified associations at *ANXA11, CCDC88B, RAB23,* and

Table 9.3   Selected Mendelian Syndromes Associated With Pulmonary Disorders

Disorder	Description	Example Gene(s)
Primary ciliary dyskinesia	Also known as *immotile-cilia syndrome;* defect in the cilia resulting in impaired mucociliary clearance, recurrent respiratory tract infections and bronchiectasis, infertility, and situs inversus	*CCDC39, CCDC40, DNAAF1, DNAAF2, DNAH11, DNAH5, DNAI1, DNAI2, DNAL1, NME8*
Neurofibromatosis	Systemic manifestations include café au lait macules, Lisch nodules, neurofibromas, bone abnormalities, cognitive defects, and other tumors. Lung manifestations include pulmonary hypertension, pulmonary artery stenosis, interstitial lung disease, and bullous lung disease	*NF1*
Cutis laxa	Abnormality in elastic fiber resulting in loose, redundant skin, vascular abnormalities, and pulmonary emphysema	*ELN, EFEMP2, FBLN5, LTBP4*
Hermansky-Pudlak syndrome	Lysosomal-related disorder resulting in oculocutaneous albinism, bleeding diathesis, and pulmonary fibrosis	*AP3B1, BLOC1S3, BLOC1S6, DTNBP1, HPS1-6*
Marfan syndrome	Connective tissue disorder resulting in aortic root dilation, arachnodactyly, ectopia lentis, and emphysematous/bullous changes and pneumothorax	*FBN1*
Birt-Hogg-Dubé syndrome	Hamartoma syndrome with skin fibrofolliculomas, renal cancers, and cystic lung disease/pneumothorax	*FLCN*
Familial pulmonary alveolar proteinosis	Diffuse lung disease characterized by lipoproteinaceous material in distal air spaces (*SLC7A7*, in setting of lysinuric protein intolerance)	*ABCA3, CSF2RA, CSF2RB, SFTPB, STPBC, SLC7A7*

IL23R.[133–135] The most recent large association study identified novel associations, but also three independent signals in the MHC,[136] and confirmed and extended the role of IL23/T helper cell type 17 signaling.

RARE DISEASES

In addition to these and other common diseases, many other diseases or syndromes with a primary or a major pulmonary manifestation have been described (Table 9.3). Several panels exist that test for different genes, including the PulmoGene panel that tests for 64 different genes related to cystic lung disease, bronchiectasis (including primary ciliary dyskinesia), fibrosis (including Hermansky-Pudlak syndrome), pulmonary hypertension, and central hyperventilation syndrome (see https://personalizedmedicine.partners.org/Assets/documents/Laboratory-For-Molecular-Medicine/Gene_Disease_Association/PulmoGene_Gene_Assoc_Table.pdf).

THE PATH FORWARD

In the approximately 2 decades since the initial draft of the Human Genome Project was completed, there has been tremendous progress in human genetics, with the development of genotyping and next-generation sequencing, characterization and cataloging of human genetic variation, identification of genes for mendelian diseases and genetic loci for complex diseases, and elucidation of mechanisms of gene regulation.[43,137] Despite tremendous progress, however, less than 10% of the genetic regions responsible for the observed heritability have been identified in most diseases and, of these identified genetic factors, the specific causal variant, gene, cell type, and mechanism are nearly all unknown.[43] Thus, continued investigation is clearly needed. Attention to phenotypic heterogeneity and other ethnicities is important not only to confirm variant effects but can also lead to novel genetic discoveries and elucidate causal variants due to differences in variant allele frequencies.[138–142]

Translating these discoveries into clinical medicine and public health remains challenging. The magnitude of the task of converting a genetic association to functional studies for the correct variant, gene, cell type, and ultimately translational mechanistic insight is only beginning to be realized. The advent of tools such as high-throughput functional studies[84] will help advance what is currently a process that requires bespoke experimental design. Many of these limitations arise from the fact that human diseases are a result of extraordinary complex gene-gene and gene-environment interactions, where exposures affect those that are vulnerable temporally (age), spatially (geographically), and by unique circumstance (comorbid disease, nutritional status, economic status, and ethnicity). Environmental health research and genomic research are logical, even necessary, partners. These concepts are essential to understanding the network relationship of genetics to epigenetics, gene expression, proteomics, metabolomics, and eventually disease phenotypes, all of which reflect a combination of genetics and environment, from the organism down to the single-cell level. The next decade of discoveries that are made in human genetics—incorporating new associations, identification of causal genes and cell types, and environmental genomics—will lead to better diagnosis, treatment, and prevention of these common, complex human diseases.

Key Points

- Heritability is a measure of the contribution of genetic variation to variation in a phenotype.
- Complex genetic disorders account for the majority of lung diseases and are caused by multiple genetic variants and environmental factors.
- The human genome comprises approximately three billion base pairs. There are more than 450 million single nucleotide polymorphisms in the human genome, although the majority of these are rare.
- Genome-wide association studies have emerged as the most commonly used study design to find disease genes in complex disorders. Sequencing provides more detailed characterization of variation and is useful for rare variant studies and enhancing the power of these studies.
- Epigenetics is the study of changes in gene transcription that are dependent on the molecules that bind to DNA, rather than on the base pair sequence of DNA. This includes both heritable changes in gene expression and stable long-term alterations in the transcriptional potential of a cell or tissue that are not necessarily heritable.
- Asthma genetic studies have identified immune cell, epithelial, allergic response genes, and differences between heritability of childhood- and adult-onset disease. As in most complex diseases, only a small portion of the heritability of this disease has been explained.
- COPD risk is largely related to genetic factors independent of smoking, and most of the currently described variants are also determinants of lung function in the population.
- Lung cancer develops in only a minority of smokers, and thus genetic and epigenetic mechanisms need to be considered. Epidemiologic studies have identified germline, inherited risk variants, but somatic mutations, such as those in the *EGFR* and *ALK* families, predict prognosis and response to therapy.
- Interstitial lung disease is caused by environmental and genetic factors. Mutations in surfactant protein C and the telomerase genes enhance the risk for developing this disorder. A common polymorphism in the promoter of the *MUC5B* gene is strongly associated with the development of familial and sporadic forms of idiopathic pulmonary fibrosis. Recently additional novel loci have been found to be associated with the development of pulmonary fibrosis.
- Most familial pulmonary hypertension cases are caused by mutations in *BMPR2*, but other rare variants, including some indicative of specific forms of pulmonary hypertension, and common variants have been identified.
- Sarcoidosis susceptibility is due in part to variants in the human leukocyte antigen A region and other immune-related pathways.
- Rare variants underlie several mendelian syndromes, with pulmonary disease as the primary or commonly associated manifestation, including pulmonary ciliary dyskinesia, cutis laxa, and pulmonary alveolar proteinosis.

Key Readings

Bush WS, Moore JH. Genome-wide association studies. *PLoS Comput Biol.* 2012;8(12):e1002822.

Demenais F, Margaritte-Jeannin P, Barnes KC, et al. Multiancestry association study identifies new asthma risk loci that colocalize with immune-cell enhancer marks. *Nat Genet.* 2018;50(1):42–53.

Feinberg AP, Tycko B. The history of cancer epigenetics. *Nat Rev Cancer.* 2004;4:143–153.

Fingerlin TE, Murphy E, Zhang W, et al. Genome-wide association study identifies multiple susceptibility loci for pulmonary fibrosis. *Nat Genet.* 2013;45:613–620.

Kwak EL, Bang YJ, Camidge DR, et al. Anaplastic lymphoma kinase inhibition in non-small-cell lung cancer. *N Engl J Med.* 2010;363:1693–1703.

Reich DE, Cargill M, Bolk S, et al. Linkage disequilibrium in the human genome. *Nature.* 2001;411:199–204.

Reilly JP, Christie JD, Meyer NJ. Fifty years of research in ARDS. Genomic contributions and opportunities. *Am J Respir Crit Care Med.* 2017;196(9):1113–1121.

Sakornsakolpat P, Prokopenko D, Lamontagne M, et al. Genetic landscape of chronic obstructive pulmonary disease identifies heterogeneous cell-type and phenotype associations. *Nat Genet.* 2019;51(3):494–505.

Shrine N, Guyatt AL, Erzurumluoglu AM, et al. New genetic signals for lung function highlight pathways and chronic obstructive pulmonary disease associations across multiple ancestries. *Nat Genet.* 2019;51(3):481–493.

Silverman EK, Palmer LJ. Case-control association studies for the genetics of complex respiratory diseases. *Am J Respir Cell Mol Biol.* 2000;22:645–648.

Timpson NJ, Greenwood CMT, Soranzo N, et al. Genetic architecture: the shape of the genetic contribution to human traits and disease. *Nat Rev Genet.* 2018;19(2):110–124.

Visscher PM, Wray NR, Zhang Q, et al. 10 years of GWAS discovery: biology, function, and translation. *Am J Hum Genet.* 2017;101(1):5–22.

Complete reference list available at ExpertConsult.com.

RESPIRATORY PHYSIOLOGY

10 *VENTILATION, BLOOD FLOW, AND GAS EXCHANGE*

MEREDITH C. MCCORMACK, MD, MHS • JOHN B. WEST, MD, PHD, DSC

INTRODUCTION

This first chapter in the section on respiratory physiology is devoted to the primary function of the lung: gas exchange. Herein, the principles of ventilation and blood flow that underlie gas exchange are reviewed. Although the lung has other functions, such as metabolizing some compounds, filtering unwanted materials from the circulation, and acting as a reservoir for blood, gas exchange is its chief function. Respiratory diseases frequently interfere with ventilation, blood flow, and gas exchange and may ultimately lead to respiratory failure and death.

VENTILATION

The anatomy of the airways and the alveolar region of the lung is discussed in Chapter 1. There we saw that the airways consist of a series of branching tubes that become narrower, shorter, and more numerous as they penetrate deeper into the lung. This process continues down to the terminal bronchioles, which are the smallest airways

without alveoli. All these bronchi make up the conducting airways. Their function is to channel inspired gas to the gas-exchanging regions of the lung. Because the conducting airways contain no alveoli and therefore take no part in gas exchange, they constitute the anatomic dead space.

Each terminal bronchiole conducts air to a respiratory unit, or acinus. The acinus is where alveolization, and therefore gas exchange, begins. The acinus can also be termed the terminal respiratory unit, indicating its chief role in gas exchange. The terminal bronchioles divide into respiratory bronchioles that have occasional alveoli budding from their wall, which then transition to the alveolar ducts, structures that are completely lined with alveoli. This alveolated region of the lung where gas exchange takes place is known as the respiratory zone. The distance from the terminal bronchiole to the most distal alveolus is only approximately 5 mm, but the respiratory zone makes up most of the lung in terms of gas volume (some 2–3 L).

The morphologic characteristics of the human airways were greatly clarified by Weibel.[1] He measured the number, length, width, and branching angles of the airways, and he

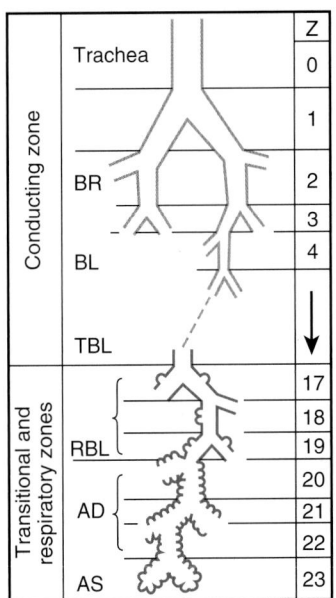

Figure 10.1 Idealization of the human airways according to Weibel's model A. The first 16 generations of airways constitute the conducting zone, the next three generations are the respiratory bronchioles constituting the transitional zone, and the final three generations are the alveolar ducts and alveolar sacs constituting the respiratory zone. Note that the RBL, AD, and AS make up the transitional and respiratory zones. AD, alveolar duct; AS, alveolar sac; BL, bronchiole; BR, bronchus; RBL, respiratory bronchiole; TBL, terminal bronchiole; Z, airway generation. (Modified from Weibel ER. *Morphometry of the Human Lung.* Berlin: Springer-Verlag; 1963.)

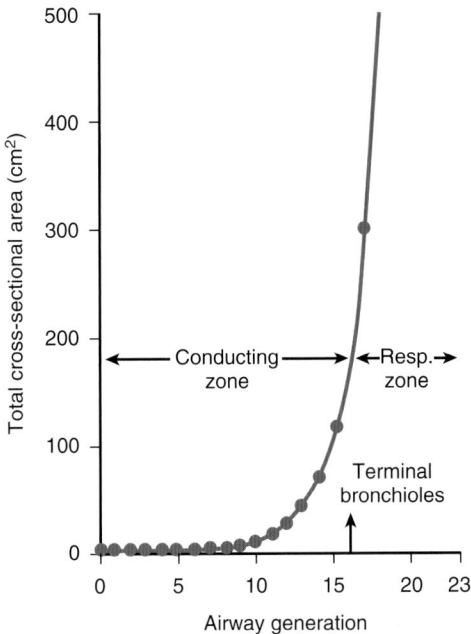

Figure 10.2 Cross-sectional area of the different zones. Diagram showing the extremely rapid increase in total cross-sectional area of the airways in the respiratory (Resp.) zone as predicted from the Weibel model in Fig. 10.1. (Modified from West JB. *Respiratory Physiology: The Essentials.* 9th ed. Baltimore: Lippincott Williams & Wilkins; 2012.)

proposed models that, although they are idealized, make pressure flow and other analyses much more tractable.

The most commonly used Weibel model is the so-called model A, shown in Figure 10.1. Note that the first 16 generations (Z) make up the conducting airways ending in the terminal bronchioles. The next three generations constitute the respiratory bronchioles, in which the degree of alveolation steadily increases. This is called the transitional zone because the nonalveolated regions of the respiratory bronchioles do not have a respiratory function. Finally, there are three generations of alveolar ducts and one generation of alveolar sacs. These last four generations constitute the true respiratory zone.

Other models of the airways have been proposed.[2] However, the Weibel model has been of great value to respiratory physiology, and an example of its use is shown in Figure 10.2. Here the model clarifies the nature of gas flow in all generations of the airways in the lung. Figure 10.2 shows that, if the total cross-sectional area of the airways of each generation is calculated, there is relatively little change in area until we approach generation 16, that is, the terminal bronchioles. Near this level, the cross-sectional area increases very rapidly. This has led some physiologists to suggest that the shape of the combined airways is similar to a trumpet or even a thumbtack.

The result of this rapid change in area is that the mode of gas flow changes in the region of the terminal bronchioles. Proximal to this point, flow is convective, or "bulk," that is, similar to the sort of flow that results when beer is poured out of a pitcher. However, when the gas reaches the region approximating the level of the terminal bronchioles, its forward velocity decreases dramatically because of the very

sudden increase in cross-sectional area. As a consequence, diffusion begins to take over as the dominant mode of gas transport. Naturally, there is no sharp transition; flow changes gradually from primarily convective to primarily diffusive in the general vicinity of generation 16.

One implication of this change in mode of flow is that many aerosol particles penetrate to the region of the terminal bronchioles by convective flow, but they do not penetrate further because of their large mass and resulting low diffusion rate. Thus, sedimentation of these particles is heavy in the region of the terminal respiratory bronchioles. This is one reason why this region of the lung is particularly vulnerable to the effects of particulate air pollutants (see Chapters 72 and 102).

Another implication of this dichotomously branching airway tree is that the greater the number of branch points, the greater the potential for nonuniform distribution of airflow among the distal airways and alveoli. In addition, repeated, possibly minor, differences in flow distribution at each branch point will give rise to spatial correlation of flow; in other words, neighboring regions will tend to have more similar flows than regions located far apart, other factors being equal.

Figure 10.3 shows the major divisions of lung volume. Total lung capacity is the volume of gas contained in the lungs at maximal inspiration. The vital capacity is the volume of gas that can be exhaled by a maximal expiration from total lung capacity. The volume remaining in the lung after maximal expiration is the *residual volume* (RV). Tidal volume refers to the normal respiratory volume excursion. The lung volume at the end of a normal expiration is the *functional residual capacity* (FRC). Figure 10.3 also indicates the inspiratory reserve volume and the expiratory reserve volume. These volumes change in characteristic directions with different respiratory diseases, such as COPD and lung

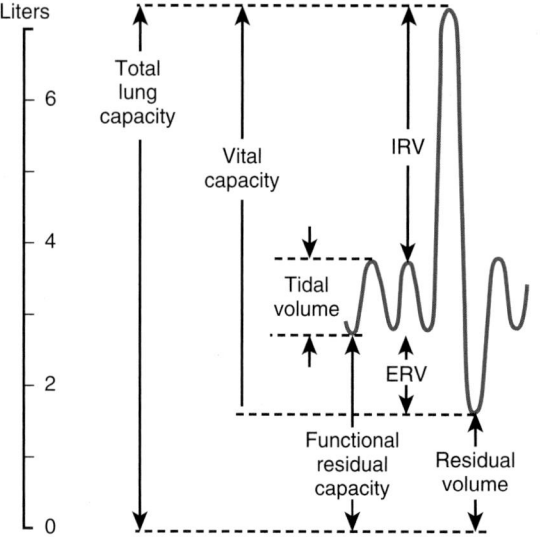

Figure 10.3 Major divisions of lung volumes. Values are illustrative only; there is considerable normal variation. ERV, expiratory reserve volume; IRV, inspiratory reserve volume. (Modified from West JB. *Respiratory Physiology: The Essentials*. 9th ed. Baltimore: Lippincott Williams & Wilkins; 2012.)

fibrosis, so their measurement becomes important (see Chapters 31 and 32).

TOTAL AND ALVEOLAR VENTILATION

Total Ventilation

Total ventilation, also called minute ventilation, is the total volume of gas exhaled per minute. It is equal to the tidal volume times the respiratory frequency. (The volume of inhaled air is slightly greater than the exhaled volume because more oxygen is inhaled than carbon dioxide is exhaled, but the difference is usually less than 1%.) Alveolar ventilation is the amount of fresh inspired air (non–dead-space gas) that enters the alveoli per minute and is therefore available for gas exchange.

Alveolar Ventilation

Because the *tidal volume* (V_T) is made up of the *dead-space volume* (V_D) and the *volume of gas entering (or coming from) the alveoli* (V_A), the alveolar ventilation can be measured from the following equations:

$$V_T = V_D + V_A \qquad \text{Eq. 1}$$

Multiplying by respiratory frequency gives

$$\dot{V}_E = \dot{V}_D + \dot{V}_A \qquad \text{Eq. 2}$$

where $\dot{V}_A$ is the alveolar ventilation, and $\dot{V}_E$ and $\dot{V}_D$ are the expired total ventilation and dead-space ventilation, respectively.
Therefore,

$$\dot{V}_A = \dot{V}_E - \dot{V}_D \qquad \text{Eq. 3}$$

A difficulty with this method is that the anatomic dead space is not easy to measure, although a value for it can be assumed with little error. One milliliter per pound of body weight is a common assumption. This approximation will overestimate dead space in obese subjects and so should be applied using ideal body weight for height.

Another way of measuring alveolar ventilation in normal subjects is to use the alveolar ventilation equation, which expresses mass conservation of carbon dioxide by defining *carbon dioxide production* ($\dot{V}_{CO_2}$), which in a steady state is equal to the amount of CO_2 exhaled in a given time, as the product of *alveolar ventilation* ($\dot{V}_A$) and *fractional alveolar concentration of carbon dioxide* (F_{ACO_2}). Because concentration is proportional to partial pressure, the relationship can be written as:

$$\dot{V}_{CO_2} = \dot{V}_A \times F_{ACO_2} = \dot{V}_A \times P_{ACO_2}/K \qquad \text{Eq. 4}$$

This can then be rearranged as follows:

$$\dot{V}_A = \frac{\dot{V}_{CO_2}}{P_{ACO_2}} \times K \qquad \text{Eq. 5}$$

where $\dot{V}_{CO_2}$ is the volume of carbon dioxide exhaled per unit time, P_{ACO_2} is the alveolar P_{CO_2}, and K is a constant (0.863 when $\dot{V}_A$ is expressed in L/min, $\dot{V}_{CO_2}$ in mL/min, and P_{ACO_2} in mm Hg). In patients with normal lungs, the P_{CO_2} of alveolar gas and that of arterial blood are virtually identical. Therefore, the arterial P_{CO_2} can be used to determine alveolar ventilation from Eq. 5. The equation then becomes

$$\dot{V}_A = \frac{\dot{V}_{CO_2}}{P_{aCO_2}} \times K \qquad \text{Eq. 6}$$

This equation is often used in patients with lung disease, but the value then obtained is the *effective* alveolar ventilation. This is not the same as the alveolar ventilation as defined in Eq. 3. Because patients with lung disease must increase their total ventilation to overcome the inefficiency of gas exchange caused by ventilation-perfusion inequality just to keep arterial P_{CO_2} normal, $\dot{V}_A$ from Eq. 6 will be less than that from Eq. 3.

Anatomic Dead Space

The anatomic dead space is the gas volume contained within the conducting airways. The normal value is in the range of 130 to 180 mL and depends on the size and posture of the subject. It can be estimated, as described earlier, as 1 mL per pound of ideal body weight. The value increases slightly with large inspirations because the radial traction exerted on the bronchi by the surrounding lung parenchyma increases their size. Anatomic dead space can be measured by Fowler's method,[3] in which a single breath of oxygen is inhaled and the concentration of nitrogen in the subsequent expiration is analyzed, as shown in Figure 10.4.

Physiologic Dead Space

Unlike anatomic dead space, which is determined by the anatomy of the airways, physiologic dead space is a functional measurement based on the ability of the lungs to eliminate carbon dioxide. It is defined by the Bohr equation:

$$\frac{V_D}{V_T} = \frac{P_{ACO_2} - P_{ECO_2}}{P_{ACO_2}} \qquad \text{Eq. 7}$$

where A and E refer to alveolar and mixed expired gas, respectively. In subjects with normal lungs, the P_{CO_2} of alveolar gas and that of arterial blood are virtually the same, so that the equation is often written as

$$\frac{V_D}{V_T} = \frac{P_{aCO_2} - P_{ECO_2}}{P_{aCO_2}} \qquad \text{Eq. 8}$$

INEQUALITY OF VENTILATION

Not all the alveoli are equally ventilated, even in the normal lung. There are several reasons for this, related both to gravitational and to nongravitational influences on gas distribution.

Gravitational Influences on Inequality

Hyperpolarized helium and xenon magnetic resonance imaging have been used to measure regional ventilation,[4,5]

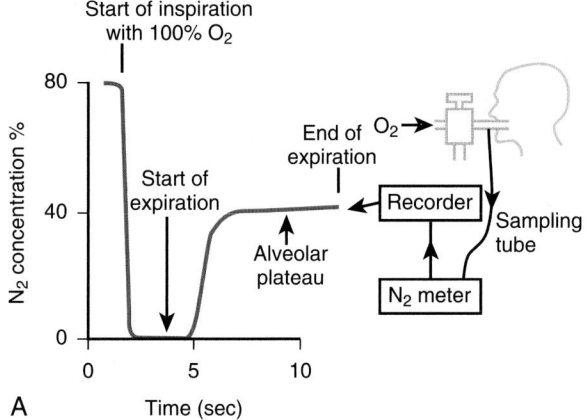

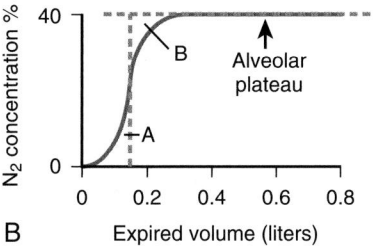

Figure 10.4 **Fowler's method of measuring the anatomic dead space with a rapid N$_2$ analyzer.** (A) After a test inspiration of 100% O$_2$, the N$_2$ concentration rises during expiration to an almost level plateau representing pure alveolar gas. (B) N$_2$ concentration is plotted against expired volume, and the dead space is the volume at the vertical dashed line that makes the areas to the left and to the right of the dashed vertical lines (*A* and *B*) equal. In this example, the dead space is ≈150 mL (or 0.15 L). (Modified from West JB. *Respiratory Physiology: The Essentials.* 9th ed. Baltimore: Lippincott Williams & Wilkins; 2012.)

and more recent studies have used ventilation single-photon emission computed tomography and positron emission tomography scanning techniques.[6–8]

Measurements in upright normal subjects show that the ventilation per unit volume of the lung is greatest near the base of the lung and becomes progressively smaller toward the apex. When the subject lies supine, this difference becomes much less, but the ventilation of the dependent (posterior) lung exceeds that of the uppermost (anterior). In the lateral decubitus position, again, the dependent lung is better ventilated. (These results refer to an inspiration from FRC.)

An explanation of this gravitational inequality of ventilation is shown in Figure 10.5A, which depicts conditions at FRC.[9] The intrapleural pressure is less negative at the bottom than at the top of the lung. This pattern can be attributed to the weight of the lung, which requires a larger pressure below the lung than above it to balance the downward-acting weight forces.[10] There are two consequences of this lower expanding pressure on the base of the lung. First, the resting volume of the basal alveoli is smaller, as shown by the pressure-volume curve. Second, the change in volume for a given change in intrapleural pressure is greater because the alveoli are operating on a steeper part of the pressure-volume curve. Thus, the ventilation (change in volume per unit resting volume) is greater at the base than the apex. However, if a normal subject makes a small inspiration from RV (rather than from FRC), an interesting change in the distribution of ventilation is seen. The major share of the ventilation now goes to the apex of the upright lung, whereas the base becomes very poorly ventilated. Figure 10.5B shows why a different pattern is seen in this case. Now the intrapleural pressures are less negative, and the intrapleural pressure at the base of the lung actually exceeds atmospheric pressure. For a small fall in intrapleural pressure, no gas will enter the extreme base of the lung, and only the apex will be ventilated. Thus, the normal pattern of ventilation is reversed in this early phase of inhalation.

In this way, obesity may change the distribution of ventilation; for example, obesity-associated factors may alter the gravitational distribution of inhaled methacholine, and thus methacholine-induced bronchoconstriction. Findings from studies using two-dimensional and three-dimensional imaging modalities suggest diversion of

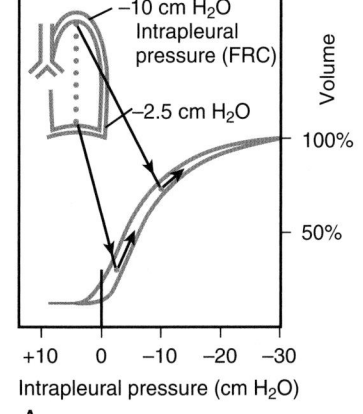

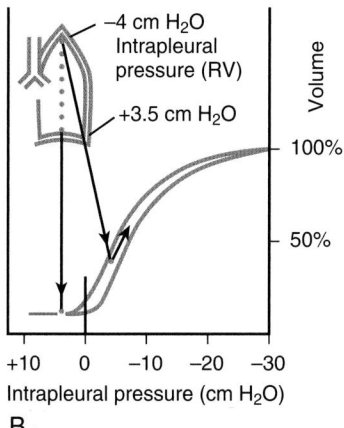

Figure 10.5 **The inequality of ventilation down the lung due to gravity.** (A) An inspiration from functional residual capacity. (B) The situation at very low lung volumes (see text for details). FRC, functional residual capacity; RV, residual volume. (Modified from West JB. *Respiratory Physiology: The Essentials.* 9th ed. Baltimore: Lippincott Williams & Wilkins; 2012.)

ventilation from the base into the upper lung zone among obese individuals.[6]

Airway Closure

At RV, the compressed region of the lung at the base in Figure 10.5B does not have all its gas squeezed out because small airways, probably in the region of the respiratory bronchioles, close first and trap gas in the distal alveoli. This is known as *airway closure.* In young normal subjects, airways close only at lung volumes below FRC. However, in older normal subjects, the volume at which the basal airways close (closing volume) increases with age and may encroach on the FRC. The reason for this increase is that, with aging, the lung loses some of its elastic recoil, and the intrapleural pressures therefore become less negative, thus approaching the situation shown in Figure 10.5B. Under these conditions, basal regions of the lung may be ventilated only intermittently, with resulting defective gas exchange. A similar situation frequently develops in patients with COPD in whom lung elastic recoil decreases. Airway closure promotes air trapping and hyperinflation characteristic of poorly controlled asthma. Exaggerated airway closure may be a feature of airway hyperresponsiveness in asthma,[11] particularly among obese individuals with asthma.[12,13]

Nongravitational Influences on Inequality

In addition to the inequality of ventilation caused by gravitational factors (Fig. 10.5), nongravitational mechanisms also exist. This is proved by the fact that even astronauts in space, in microgravity, show uneven ventilation.[14,15] This has been confirmed by studies in which labeled small particles in inspired gas demonstrate variability in ventilation at a given horizontal level at which gravitational forces are equal.[4] At least three factors have been proposed to explain the uneven ventilation in the distal, smaller regions of the lung.

One of these factors is the existence of uneven time constants.[16] The time constant of a region of lung is given by the product of its resistance and compliance (analogous to the time constant in electrical circuits, which is the product of electrical resistance and capacitance). Lung units with different time constants inflate and deflate at different flow rates. Depending on the breathing frequency, a unit with a large time constant does not complete its filling before expiration begins and therefore is poorly ventilated; the faster the frequency, the less time for ventilation. In contrast, a unit with a small time constant, which fills rapidly, may receive a high proportion of gas from the anatomic dead space, reducing its effective alveolar ventilation.

Another cause of uneven ventilation in small lung units is the asymmetry of their structure, which can result in a greater penetration of gas by diffusion into the smaller units than into the larger.[17] The resulting somewhat complex behavior is known as diffusion- and convection-dependent inhomogeneity and may play an important role in lung disease.

A third possible reason for uneven ventilation is the presence of concentration gradients along the small airways. This is known as series inequality. Recall that inspired gas reaches approximately the region of the distal terminal or proximal respiratory bronchioles by convective flow, but gas flow over the rest of the distance to the alveoli is accomplished principally by diffusion within the airways. If there is abnormal dilation of an airway, the diffusion process may not be complete within the breathing cycle, and the distal alveoli will be less well ventilated than the proximal alveoli.

Heterogeneity in ventilation can be assessed by single-breath and *multibreath nitrogen washout* (MBNW) methods, which are described in Chapters 31 and 32. Three major indices are derived from the MBNW.[18,19] The *lung clearance index* is a global measure of ventilation heterogeneity but does not allow any specific anatomic localization of the site of heterogeneity. The more uneven the ventilation, the higher the lung clearance index, and abnormalities are apparent in obstructive airways disease, such as asthma, COPD, and cystic fibrosis. Two other indexes, *Scond* and *Sacin*, describe the contribution of convection (driven by pressure gradients, which take place in the conducting airways) and diffusion (driven by concentration gradients, which take place in the extreme periphery of the lung, likely beginning at the entrance to the lung acinus) to overall heterogeneity of ventilation.

BLOOD FLOW

Blood flow is as important for gas exchange as is ventilation. This has not always been appreciated, partly because the process of ventilation is more obvious, especially in the dyspneic patient, and is more accessible to measurement. Much has been learned about the pulmonary circulation in the past few years, especially about its metabolic functions. The anatomy and function of the pulmonary circulation are described in Chapters 1 and 6.

PRESSURES OF THE PULMONARY CIRCULATION

The pressures in the pulmonary circulation are very low compared with those in the systemic circulation, and this feature is responsible for much of its special behavior. The normal pressures in the human pulmonary artery are typically approximately 25 mm Hg systolic, 8 mm Hg diastolic, and 15 mm Hg mean. Normal mean pulmonary arterial pressure is thus six times lower than that in the systemic arterial circulation, which is approximately 100 mm Hg. The evolutionary force keeping the pressures in the pulmonary circulation low is the mechanical vulnerability of the extremely thin blood-gas barrier; higher pressures in the pulmonary capillaries would cause stress failure of the capillary wall.[20]

Pressure Inside Blood Vessels

Because the pulmonary arterial pressure is so low, hydrostatic effects due to gravity within the pulmonary circulation become very important. The adult upright human lung is some 30 cm high, giving a hydrostatic difference in pressure of 30 cm blood between the extreme apex and the base, which is equivalent to approximately 23 mm Hg. As a result, there are very substantial differences in flow within the small pulmonary arteries and the capillaries between the top and bottom of the upright lung. This topic is discussed further in the section "Distribution of Pulmonary Blood Flow."

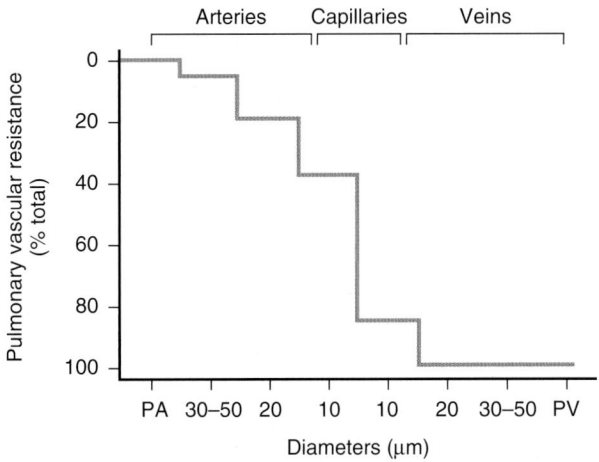

Figure 10.6 Pressure drop along the pulmonary circulation as determined by direct puncture of vessels. The normal pressure drop is greatest at the capillaries, and its mean pressure is approximately halfway between pulmonary artery (PA) pressure and pulmonary vein (PV) pressure. (Modified from Bhattacharya J, Nanjo S, Staub NC. Factors affecting lung microvascular pressure. *Ann N Y Acad Sci.* 1982;384:107–114.)

Various techniques have been used to determine the pattern of pressure drop along the pulmonary blood vessels. These include measurement of the transudation pressure on the pleural surface of isolated lung, measurement of the pressure transient resulting from the injection of a slug of low- or high-viscosity blood into the pulmonary artery,[21] and direct puncture of different-sized vessels along with direct measurement of hydrostatic pressure.[22] The direct puncture measurements indicate that much of the normal pressure drop in the pulmonary circulation probably takes place in the pulmonary capillaries (alveolar vessels), and that the mean capillary pressure is approximately halfway between that in the pulmonary artery and that in the pulmonary vein (Fig. 10.6). The distribution of pressure along the pulmonary blood vessels depends on lung volume. At low states of lung inflation, the resistance of the extra-alveolar vessels (see next section) increases and more pressure drop then takes place across the pulmonary arteries and veins instead of the capillaries. By contrast, there is evidence that, at very high states of lung inflation, the resistance of the capillary bed is increased, and therefore there will be an additional pressure drop in the capillaries.

Of interest, the pressures in the pulmonary circulation are highly pulsatile; indeed, if the normal systolic and diastolic pressures in the main pulmonary artery are 25 and 8 mm Hg, respectively, this is a much greater proportional change than the systolic-diastolic difference in systemic arteries (120 and 80 mm Hg, respectively). There is good evidence that the pulsatility of pressure, and therefore flow, extends to the pulmonary capillaries.[23]

Pressures Outside Blood Vessels

Some pulmonary blood vessels are exposed to alveolar pressure (or very nearly), whereas others are outside the influence of alveolar pressure but are very sensitive to the state of lung inflation. These two types of vessels are known as *alveolar* and *extra-alveolar*, respectively (Fig. 10.7).

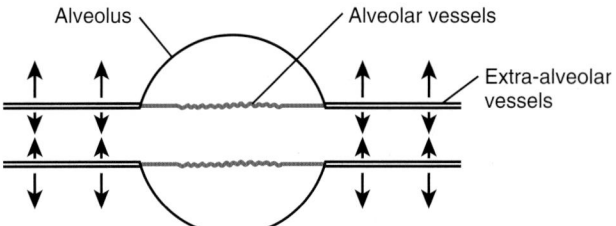

Figure 10.7 Diagram of alveolar and extra-alveolar vessels. The alveolar vessels are mainly the capillaries and are exposed to alveolar pressure. The extra-alveolar vessels have their lumina enlarged by the pull of radial traction (*outward-oriented arrows*) of the surrounding parenchyma. (Modified from West JB. *Respiratory Physiology: The Essentials.* 9th ed. Baltimore: Lippincott Williams & Wilkins; 2012.)

The alveolar vessels are largely capillaries that course through the alveolar walls. The pressure to which they are exposed is very nearly alveolar pressure. However, it can be shown that, when the lung is expanded from a very low lung volume, this pericapillary pressure falls below alveolar pressure because of surface tension effects in the alveolar lining layer.[24] By contrast, during deflation from high lung volumes, surface tension effects are much reduced and the pericapillary pressure is very close to alveolar pressure.

The extra-alveolar vessels are not exposed to alveolar pressure. The caliber of these vessels is determined by the radial traction of the surrounding alveolar walls and therefore depends on lung volume. When the lung inflates, the caliber of these vessels increases; when the lung deflates, their caliber decreases because of the elastic tissue in their walls and also because of a small amount of smooth muscle tone. The important point is that extra-alveolar vessel resistance falls with lung inflation, whereas alveolar vessel (capillary) resistance rises with lung inflation.

The small vessels (≈30 μm diameter) in the corners of the alveolar walls behave in a manner that is intermediate between that of the alveolar capillaries and the extra-alveolar vessels. These corner vessels can remain open when the capillaries are closed. Indeed, this is the normal appearance in zone 1 lung[25] (see later section on the distribution of blood flow). However, the shape and attachments of the corner vessels are very different from those of the larger extra-alveolar vessels, and it is unlikely that the pressure outside them varies in the same way when the lung expands.

The extra-alveolar vessels are surrounded by an interstitial perivascular space, which has an important role in the passive movement of extravascular fluid in the lung. The lymph vessels run in this space, although these lymph vessels do not open into this space or drain this fluid. One of the earliest histologic signs of interstitial pulmonary edema is "cuffing" of the interstitial perivascular space around the extra-alveolar vessels (see Figs. 14.4 and 14.5).[26,27] There is evidence that the perivascular pressure is very low compared with the hydrostatic pressure in the interstitium of the alveolar wall. As a consequence, fluid that moves from the capillaries into the interstitial space of the alveolar wall eventually flows to the perivascular low-pressure region by virtue of the hydrostatic pressure gradient.[28] The interstitial edema fluid then moves toward the hilum or toward the pleural space (see Chapter 14).

PULMONARY VASCULAR RESISTANCE

Pulmonary vascular resistance is given by the following relationship:

$$PVR = \frac{\text{Pulmonary arterial pressure} - \text{Pulmonary venous pressure}}{\text{Pulmonary blood flow}} \quad \text{Eq. 9}$$

Because all three variables vary between systole and diastole, mean values are generally used. This definition is similar to that used for electrical resistance, which is the difference of voltage across a resistor divided by the current. However, whereas the resistance of an electrical resistor is independent of the voltage at both ends and the current, this is not the case for pulmonary vascular resistance. For example, an increase in either pulmonary arterial pressure or pulmonary venous pressure generally results in a decrease in pulmonary vascular resistance because, as capillary pressure rises, there is both capillary recruitment and distention (see later). Similarly, if pulmonary blood flow is increased (e.g., by raising pulmonary arterial pressure), pulmonary vascular resistance usually decreases.

It is important to appreciate that a single number for pulmonary vascular resistance is an incomplete description of the pressure-flow properties of the pulmonary circulation. However, in practice, pulmonary vascular resistance is often a useful measurement because, although the normal value varies considerably, we often wish to compare the value in a normal lung with the higher values in abnormal ones.

Pressure-Flow Relations

If pulmonary blood flow is measured in an isolated, perfused lung, when pulmonary arterial pressure is raised (while pulmonary venous pressure, alveolar pressure, and lung volume are held constant), then flow increases relatively more than pressure. Figure 10.8 shows that pulmonary vascular resistance decreases both when pulmonary arterial pressure is raised and when pulmonary venous pressure is raised (other pressures held constant). The unifying explanation for reduced resistance in both cases is that the increases in intravascular pressure induce vascular recruitment and distension.

The decreases in pulmonary vascular resistance shown in Figure 10.8 help to limit the work of the right heart under conditions of high pulmonary blood flow. For example, during exercise, both pulmonary arterial and venous pressures rise. Although the normal pulmonary vascular resistance is remarkably low (the normal 5 L/min pulmonary blood flow is associated with an arterial-venous pressure difference of only approximately 10 mm Hg), the resistance falls to even lower values when the pulmonary arterial and venous pressures rise, as during exercise.

Two mechanisms responsible for the fall in pulmonary vascular resistance are *recruitment*, the opening up of previously closed blood vessels, and *distention*, the increase in caliber of vessels. Figure 10.9A shows experimental data from rapidly frozen dog lung preparations, indicating the importance of recruitment as the pulmonary arterial pressure is raised from low values.[29] Note that the number of open capillaries per millimeter of length of alveolar wall increased from approximately 25 to more than 50 as pulmonary arterial pressure was raised from zero to almost

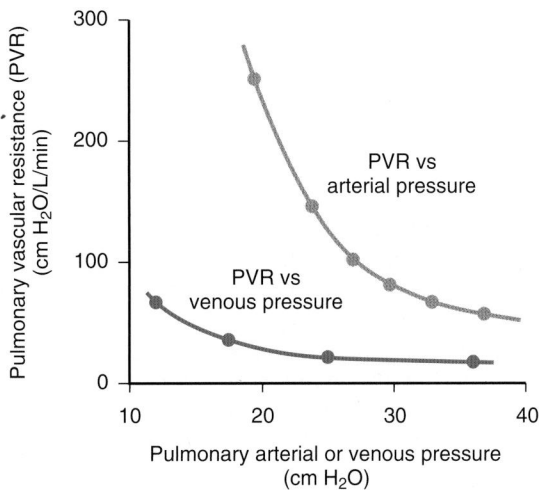

Figure 10.8 The drop in pulmonary vascular resistance seen when the pulmonary arterial or venous pressure is raised in a canine lung preparation. When one pressure was changed, the other was held constant. (Modified from West JB. *Respiratory Physiology: The Essentials.* 9th ed. Baltimore: Lippincott Williams & Wilkins; 2012.)

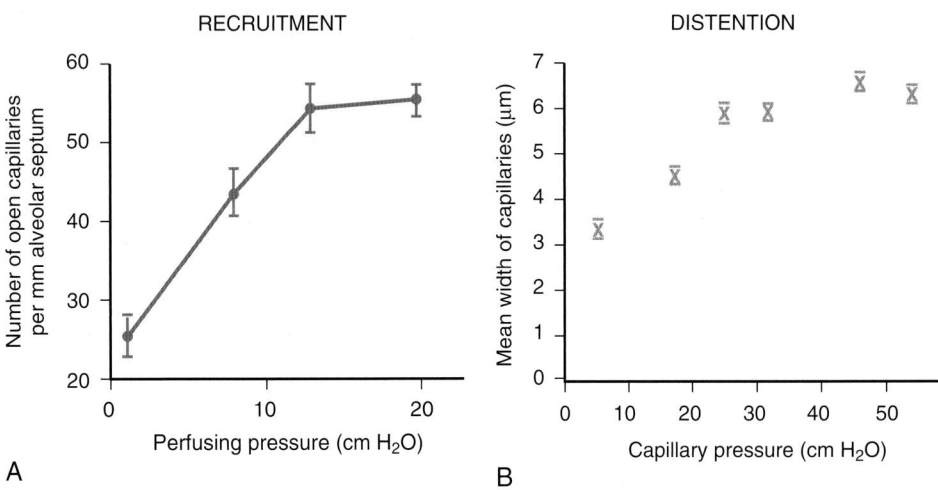

Figure 10.9 Mechanisms responsible for the fall in pulmonary vascular resistance with increases in vascular pressures. (A) Recruitment of pulmonary capillaries as the pulmonary arterial pressure, the perfusing pressure, is raised. (B) Distention of pulmonary capillaries as their pressure is increased. (A, Modified from Warrell DA, Evans JW, Clarke RO, et al. Pattern of filling in the pulmonary capillary bed. *J Appl Physiol.* 1972;32:346–356. B, Modified from Glazier JB, Hughes JMB, Maloney JE, West JB. Measurements of capillary dimensions and blood volume in rapidly frozen lungs. *J Appl Physiol.* 1969;26:65–76.)

15 cm H$_2$O. Figure 10.9B shows data on the importance of distention of pulmonary capillaries.[25] Note that the mean width of the capillaries increased from approximately 3.5 to nearly 7 µm as the capillary pressure was increased to approximately 50 cm H$_2$O. Beyond that, there was very little change.

The mechanism of recruitment of pulmonary capillaries is not fully understood. It has been suggested that, as the pulmonary arterial pressure is increased, the critical opening pressures of various arterioles are successively overcome. However, it has been shown that the red blood cell concentration, used as a measure of perfusion, varied within areas supplied by single arterioles, indicating that capillaries, not arterioles, probably accounted for the heterogenous perfusion.[29] This suggests that vessels are recruited at the capillary rather than the arterial level.

The mechanism of distention of pulmonary capillaries is apparently simply the bulging of the capillary wall as the transmural pressure of the capillaries is raised. This behavior is likely caused by a change in shape of the capillaries rather than actual stretching of the capillary wall. Surface tension forces and also longitudinal tension in the alveolar wall associated with lung inflation tend to flatten the capillaries at low capillary transmural pressures; this means that their diameter can then increase when capillary pressure rises. In photomicrographs of rapidly frozen lung preparations, pulmonary capillaries with very high intracapillary pressures show remarkable bulging.[25]

Recruitment and distention also provide mechanisms for increasing both the surface area of the lung microvasculature in contact with alveolar gas and the red cell transit time through the microvasculature, which may facilitate gas exchange.

Effect of Lung Volume

Lung volume has an important influence on pulmonary vascular resistance. Figure 10.10 shows that, as lung

volume is increased from very low values, vascular resistance first decreases and then increases. The lung normally operates near the minimal value of vascular resistance, that is, FRC coincides with a low vascular resistance.

At very low lung volume, the increase in pulmonary vascular resistance is caused by the decrease in caliber of the extra-alveolar vessels. Because these vessels are normally held open by the radial traction of the surrounding parenchyma, their caliber is least in the collapsed lung.[30] Another factor that may contribute to the high pulmonary vascular resistance at low states of lung inflation is folding and distortion of pulmonary capillaries.[31,32]

At high lung volume, the increase in pulmonary vascular resistance is probably caused by narrowing of the pulmonary capillaries. An analogy is a piece of thin rubber tubing that narrows considerably when it is stretched sideways, across its diameter. This distortion increases the resistance to fluid moving through it. Direct measurements on rapidly frozen dog lungs show that the mean width of the capillaries is greatly decreased at high states of lung inflation.[25]

In considering the effects of lung inflation, a distinction should be made between "positive" and "negative" pressure inflation. The results shown in Figure 10.10 were found with negative-pressure inflation, that is, when the lung was expanded by reducing pleural pressure and the relationship between pulmonary arterial and alveolar pressures was held constant. If positive-pressure inflation is used (i.e., alveolar pressure is increased with respect to pulmonary arterial pressure), pulmonary vascular resistance increases even more at high states of lung inflation. The reason is that lung inflation is then associated with a decrease in the transmural pressure of the capillaries and they are, in effect, squashed by the increased alveolar pressure.

Other Factors Affecting Pulmonary Vascular Resistance

Various drugs affect pulmonary vascular resistance. In some instances, the effects depend on the species of animal. However, in general, serotonin, histamine, and norepinephrine cause contraction of pulmonary vascular smooth muscle and increase vascular resistance. These drugs are particularly effective as vasoconstrictors when the lung volume is small and the radial traction of surrounding parenchyma on the extra-alveolar vessels is weak. Drugs that often relax smooth muscle in the pulmonary circulation include acetylcholine and isoproterenol. However, normal pulmonary blood vessels have little resting tone, so the degree of potential relaxation is small.

The autonomic nervous system exercises a weak control on the pulmonary circulation. There is evidence that increased sympathetic tone can cause vasoconstriction and stiffening of the walls of the larger pulmonary arteries. Both α- and β-adrenergic receptors are present.[33] Increased parasympathetic activity has a weak vasodilator action. As already indicated, any changes of vascular smooth muscle tone are much more effective at low states of lung inflation, when the extra-alveolar vessels are narrowed or, in the fetal state, when the amount of smooth muscle present is much greater than in the adult.

Pulmonary edema increases vascular resistance by poorly understood mechanisms. It may be that mechanisms

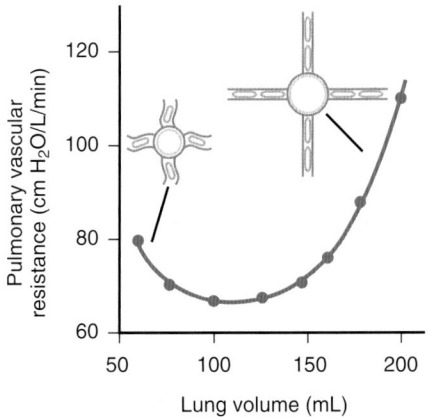

Figure 10.10 Effect of changing lung volume on pulmonary vascular resistance. At low lung volumes, resistance is high because the extra-alveolar vessels are narrowed (central circle) and because pulmonary capillaries become folded and distorted (vessels radiating from central circle). At high lung volumes, capillaries are stretched and their caliber reduced; this is probably the major contributor to increased vascular resistance at high lung volumes. (Data from a canine lung preparation.) (Modified from West JB. *Respiratory Physiology: The Essentials.* 9th ed. Baltimore: Lippincott Williams & Wilkins; 2012.)

differ depending on the type and stage of edema. Interstitial pulmonary edema causes marked cuffing of the perivascular spaces of the extra-alveolar vessels. Presumably, the edema increases their vascular resistance[34] because the edema widens the perivascular space and thereby reduces the radial traction of the surrounding parenchyma that normally holds the vessels expanded. In addition, however, edema in the interstitium of the alveolar wall may encroach on the pulmonary capillaries to some extent, thus increasing their vascular resistance.[35] Pulmonary edema may also increase pulmonary vascular resistance by reducing ventilation to the most affected regions, thereby reducing the local alveolar P_{O_2} and stimulating hypoxic pulmonary vasoconstriction.

DISTRIBUTION OF PULMONARY BLOOD FLOW

Just as for ventilation, blood flow is not partitioned equally to all alveoli, even in the normal lung. Both gravitational and nongravitational factors affect the distribution of blood flow.

Normal Distribution

The distribution of pulmonary blood flow can conveniently be measured using radioactive materials. In one technique, radioactive xenon is dissolved in saline and injected into a peripheral vein. When the xenon reaches the pulmonary capillaries, it diffuses into the alveolar gas because of its low blood solubility. The resulting distribution of radioactivity within the lung can be measured using a gamma camera and reflects the regional distribution of blood flow. Subsequently, the distribution of alveolar volume is obtained by having the subject rebreathe radioactive xenon to equilibrium. By combining the two measurements, the blood flow per unit alveolar volume of the lung can be obtained. In another technique, the distribution of blood flow can be measured with radioactive albumin macroaggregates and with a variety of radioactive gases, such as ^{15}O-labeled carbon dioxide and ^{13}N. Finally, functional magnetic resonance imaging of the lung can be used to assess distribution of pulmonary blood flow.[36] This noninvasive technique does not expose subjects to radioactivity; therefore, it can be used repetitively and shows great promise for the future.

In the normal upright human lung, pulmonary blood flow decreases approximately linearly with distance up the lung, reaching very low values at the apex.[37] However, if the subject lies supine, apical and basal blood flow become the same, and now blood flow is less in the anterior (uppermost) than posterior (lowermost) regions of the lung. Thus, blood flow distribution is highly dependent on gravitational effects. During exercise in the upright position, both apical and basal blood flow rates increase, and the relative differences are reduced.

The factors responsible for the uneven distribution of blood flow due to gravitational influences can be studied conveniently in isolated lung preparations. These studies show that, in the presence of normal vascular pressures, blood flow decreases approximately linearly up the lung[38] as it does in intact humans. However, if the pulmonary arterial pressure is reduced, blood flows only up to the level at which pulmonary arterial equals alveolar pressures; above

this point, no flow can be detected. These observations and others have led to the following model of blood flow.

Three-Zone Model for the Distribution of Blood Flow

Figure 10.11 shows a simple model for understanding the factors responsible for the inequality of blood flow in the lung.[38] The lung is divided into three zones according to the relative magnitudes of the pulmonary arterial, alveolar, and venous pressures.

Zone 1 is that region of the lung above the level at which pulmonary arterial equals alveolar pressures; in other words, in this region, alveolar pressure exceeds arterial pressure. Measurements in isolated lungs show that there is no blood flow in zone 1, the explanation being that the collapsible capillaries close because the pressure outside exceeds the pressure inside. Micrographs of rapidly frozen lung from zone 1 show that the capillaries have collapsed, although occasionally trapped red blood cells can be seen within them.[25] The vertical level of blood flow can also be influenced by the surface tension of the alveolar lining layer, as discussed earlier. If measurements are made on a lung immediately after it is inflated from a near-collapsed state, blood flow reaches 3 or 4 cm above the level at which pulmonary arterial and alveolar pressures are equal.[24] This can be explained by the surface tension, which lowers the pericapillary hydrostatic pressure to below the alveolar pressure and permits flow.

Zone 2 is the part of the lung in which pulmonary arterial pressure exceeds alveolar pressure, but alveolar pressure exceeds venous pressure. Here the vessels behave like Starling resistors,[39] that is, as collapsible tubes surrounded by a pressure chamber. Under these conditions, flow is determined by the difference between arterial and alveolar pressures, rather than by the difference between arterial and venous pressures. One way of looking at this is that the thin wall of the vessel offers no resistance to the collapsing pressure, so the pressure inside the vessel at some point

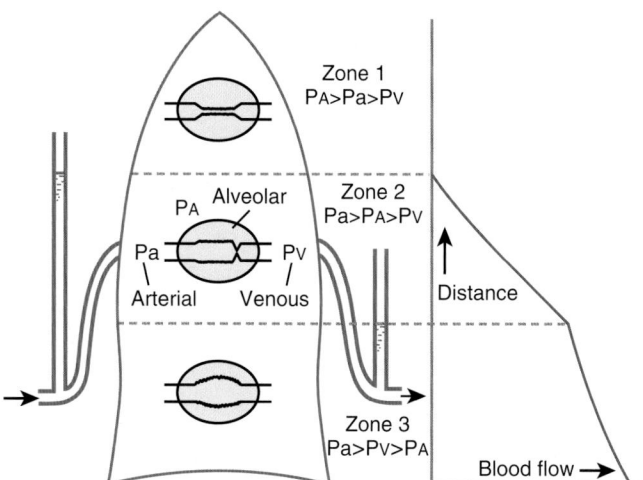

Figure 10.11 Three-zone model designed to account for the uneven gravitational distribution of blood flow in the lung. Pa, pulmonary arterial pressure; PA, pulmonary alveolar pressure; Pv, pulmonary venous pressure. (Modified from West JB, Dollery CT, Naimark A. Distribution of blood flow in isolated lung: relation to vascular and alveolar pressures. *J Appl Physiol.* 1964;19:713–724.)

along its length becomes equal to chamber pressure, and the flow is determined by arterial minus chamber pressure. This behavior has been variously referred to as the waterfall[39] or sluice[40] effect and can be demonstrated in rubber-tube models on the laboratory bench. The increase in blood flow down zone 2 can be explained by the increase in hydrostatic pulmonary arterial pressure down the zone, whereas the alveolar pressure remains constant. Thus, the pressure difference determining flow increases linearly with distance down the lung.

Zone 3 is that part of the lung in which venous pressure exceeds alveolar pressure. Radioactive gas measurements show that blood flow also increases as one measures vertically down this zone, although, in some preparations at least, the rate of increase appears less than found in zone 2. Because the pressure difference responsible for flow is arterial minus venous pressure and because these two pressures increase similarly with distance down the zone, the increase in blood flow is not explained by changes in perfusing pressure. Instead, blood flow increases down this zone because vascular resistance falls with distance down the zone, likely because of progressive distention (confirmed histologically[25]) from the increasing transmural pressure (intravascular pressure increasing down the zone while alveolar pressure is constant). However, resistance may also be reduced by recruitment of capillaries.

The Effect of Lung Volume on the Distribution of Blood Flow—Zone 4

The three-zone model of Figure 10.11, based on the effects of pulmonary arterial, alveolar, and venous pressures, accounts for many of the distributions seen in the normal lung. However, other factors play a role; one of these is lung volume. For example, under most circumstances, a zone of reduced blood flow, known as zone 4, is seen in the lowermost region of the upright human lung.[41] This zone becomes smaller as lung volume is increased, but careful measurements indicate that a small area of reduced blood flow is still present at the lung base at total lung capacity. As lung volume is reduced, this region of reduced blood flow extends further and further up the lung so that, at FRC, blood flow decreases in the bottom half of the lung.

These patterns cannot be explained by the interactions of the pulmonary arterial, venous, and alveolar pressures at the alveolar vessels as in Figure 10.11. Instead, we have to take into account the contribution of the extra-alveolar vessels. As pointed out previously (see Fig. 10.10), the caliber of these vessels is determined by the degree of lung inflation; as lung volume is reduced, the vessels narrow. In the upright human lung, the alveoli are less well expanded at the base than at the apex because of distortion of the elastic lung caused by its weight (see Fig. 10.5). As a result, the extra-alveolar vessels are relatively narrow at the base, and their increased contribution to pulmonary vascular resistance results in the presence of a zone of reduced blood flow in that region. As lung volume is reduced, the contribution of the extra-alveolar vessels to the distribution of blood flow increases, and zone 4 extends further up the lung.

Vasoactive drugs and interstitial edema can also modify the contribution of extra-alveolar vessels to pulmonary vascular resistance. With injection of vasoconstrictor drugs such as serotonin, the role of the extra-alveolar vessels can be exaggerated[42] and, under these conditions, zone 4 extends further up the lung. The opposite effect is seen if a vasodilator drug such as isoproterenol is infused into the pulmonary circulation. With interstitial edema, the contribution of the extra-alveolar vessels increases because the edema creates a cuff of fluid around the vessels and the vessels narrow. This is thought to be the cause of the increased pulmonary vascular resistance seen at the base of the human lung in conditions of interstitial pulmonary edema,[34] in which the distribution of blood flow often becomes inverted (e.g., in chronic mitral stenosis).[43] Under these conditions, the blood flow to the apex of the upright lung consistently exceeds the flow to the basal regions. However, the effects of interstitial edema on blood flow distribution are still not fully understood.

Other Factors Affecting the Distribution of Blood Flow

Because the influence of gravity on the distribution of blood flow in the normal lung is so important, it is not surprising that, during acceleration of the body in an upward direction, the distribution of blood flow becomes more uneven.[44] For example, during exposure to $+3g$ acceleration, that is, three times the normal acceleration experienced by someone in the upright posture, the upper half of the lung is completely unperfused.

By contrast, in astronauts at weightlessness in space, the distribution of blood flow becomes more uniform.[45] Because it is not possible to use radioactive gases in this environment, the inequality of blood flow has been determined indirectly from the size of the cardiogenic oscillations for P_{CO_2}. Cardiogenic oscillations are fluctuations in the concentrations of gases such as oxygen, carbon dioxide, and nitrogen during a single expiration. They have the same frequency as the heart rate and are considered to be caused by differential rates of emptying of different parts of the lung due to contraction and dilation of the heart exerting direct pressure on nearby lung parenchyma. For oscillations to be detected, these differentially emptying regions must also have different alveolar P_{O_2} and P_{CO_2} values; this happens when blood flow and ventilation are not uniformly distributed throughout the lung. Weightlessness almost abolishes cardiogenic oscillations, implying greater uniformity in the distribution of blood flow and/or ventilation. Of interest, because these oscillations can still be seen, albeit to a much smaller extent than on Earth, some inequality remains, indicating an effect of nongravitational factors.

Several nongravitational factors may account for an uneven distribution of blood flow. One is that there may be regional differences of vascular resistance, with some regions of the pulmonary vasculature having an intrinsically higher vascular resistance than others. This has been shown to be the case in isolated dog lungs,[46] and there is some evidence for higher blood flows in the dorsal than the ventral regions of the lung in both intact dogs and horses. Another possible factor is a difference in blood flow between the central and peripheral regions of the lung,[47] although this finding is controversial. Some measurements show differences in blood flow along the acinus, with the more distal regions of the acinus being less well perfused than the proximal regions.[48,49] Also, as pointed out earlier, because of the complexity of the pulmonary circulation at the alveolar level, including the very large number of capillary segments, it is likely that there is inequality of blood flow at this level.[50] There is also work suggesting that the distribution of pulmonary blood flow in small vessels may follow a fractal pattern.[51] The term *fractal* describes a branching pattern of both structure (blood vessels) and function (blood flow) that repeats itself with each generation. This means that any subsection of the vascular tree exhibits the same branching pattern as the entire tree. Were a picture of such a subsection to be enlarged, it would overlie and match the pattern of the whole tree. The repeated branching of blood vessels has implications for how blood flow is distributed independently of gravitational influences. The greater the number of branch points, the greater the likely inequality of perfusion among alveoli. This implies that the finer the spatial resolution of the method used to assess flow distribution, the greater the amount of inequality likely to be detected.

Abnormal Patterns of Blood Flow

The normal distribution of pulmonary blood flow is frequently altered by lung and heart disease. Localized lung disease, such as fibrosis and cyst formation, usually causes a local reduction of flow. The same is true of pulmonary embolism, in which the local reduction in blood flow, as determined from a perfusion scan, is usually coupled with normal ventilation, and this pattern provides important diagnostic information. Lung cancer may reduce regional blood flow, and occasionally a small hilar lesion can cause a marked reduction of blood flow to one lung, presumably through compression of the main pulmonary artery. Generalized lung diseases, such as COPD and asthma, also frequently cause patchy inequality of blood flow.[52,53]

Heart disease frequently alters the distribution of blood flow, as might be expected from the factors responsible for the normal distribution (see Fig. 10.11). For example, patients with increased blood flow through left-to-right shunts or with pulmonary hypertension usually show a more uniform distribution of blood flow because of their higher pulmonary artery pressure.[54] Diseases in which pulmonary arterial pressure is reduced, such as tetralogy of Fallot with oligemic lungs, are associated with reduced perfusion of the lung apices. Increased pulmonary venous pressure, as in mitral stenosis, initially causes a more uniform distribution than normal. However, in advanced disease, an inversion of the normal distribution of blood flow is frequently seen, with more perfusion to the upper than to the lower zones. The mechanism for this shift is not fully understood, but, as indicated earlier, perivascular edema causing an increased vascular resistance of the extra-alveolar vessels is thought to be a factor.

ACTIVE CONTROL OF THE PULMONARY CIRCULATION

The distribution of pulmonary blood flow and the pressure-flow relations of the pulmonary circulation are normally dominated by the passive effects of the hydrostatic pressure gradient described earlier. Thus, the roles of gravity, of variation in vascular lengths and diameters, and of recruitment and distention can account for much of the behavior of the normal circulation. The normal adult pulmonary

circulation has a limited amount of smooth muscle in the walls of the vessels, and active control of vascular tone is weak. However, in some conditions there is an increase in the amount of smooth muscle. This is the case in the fetal lung, in long-term residence at high altitude, and in prolonged pulmonary hypertension. In these situations, the tone of the vascular smooth muscle plays a more significant role. However, even in the normal lung, some active control of the circulation is seen.

Hypoxic Pulmonary Vasoconstriction

In a region of a lung with alveolar hypoxia, vascular smooth muscle contracts and raises local vascular resistance, which may reduce blood flow. The precise mechanism of such hypoxic pulmonary vasoconstriction is still not known but, because it can be observed in excised isolated lungs, it clearly does not depend on central nervous system connections. Studies indicate that voltage-gated potassium channels in the vascular smooth muscle cells are involved, leading to increased intracellular calcium ion concentrations.[57–60] Furthermore, excised segments of pulmonary artery can constrict if their environment is made hypoxic, so there appears to be a local action of hypoxia on the artery itself.[55] It is also known that it is P_{O_2} of the *alveolar* gas, not of the pulmonary arterial blood, that chiefly determines the response.[56] This can be proved by perfusing a lung with blood with a high P_{O_2} while keeping the alveolar P_{O_2} low; under these conditions the vasoconstrictive response is still seen. The importance of local factors is supported by observations that hypoxic pulmonary vasoconstriction exists in transplanted lungs, despite the absence of autonomic neural innervation.[55]

For further discussion of the mechanisms of hypoxic pulmonary vasoconstriction, see ExpertConsult.com and Chapter 6.

The major site of vasoconstriction is in the small pulmonary arteries.[67] In the normal human lung, the small arteries have a meager amount of smooth muscle, which may be uneven in its distribution. This may explain why, even in global alveolar hypoxia (e.g., at high altitude), vasoconstriction is uneven. For example, during alveolar hypoxia, the variation in transit times through the pulmonary circulation of a lobe of a dog lung nearly doubles,[68] and the distribution of India ink particles injected into the pulmonary circulation becomes more uneven.[69] This uneven vasoconstriction probably plays a role in the mechanism of high-altitude pulmonary edema[70] (see later).

Hypoxic pulmonary vasoconstriction has the effect of directing blood flow away from hypoxic regions of lung, a redistribution that is beneficial to gas exchange. Other things being equal, this effect reduces the amount of ventilation-perfusion inequality in a diseased lung and limits the depression of the arterial P_{O_2}. An example of this is seen in patients with asthma treated with certain bronchodilators, which can decrease hypoxic pulmonary vasoconstriction. These sometimes reduce arterial P_{O_2} by increasing blood flow to poorly ventilated areas.[71,72]

Probably the most important role for hypoxic pulmonary vasoconstriction is in the fetal period. During fetal life, when the lungs do not undertake gas exchange, pulmonary vascular resistance is very high, partly because of hypoxic vasoconstriction, and only some 15% of the cardiac output flows through the lungs. The rest bypasses the lungs via the ductus arteriosus. The vasoconstriction is particularly effective because of the abundance of smooth muscle in the pulmonary arteries. At birth, when the first few breaths oxygenate the alveoli, the vascular resistance falls dramatically because of relaxation of vascular smooth muscle, and pulmonary blood flow increases enormously. In this situation, the release of hypoxic vasoconstriction is essential for the transition to air breathing.

DAMAGE TO PULMONARY CAPILLARIES BY HIGH WALL STRESSES

The blood-gas barrier has a basic dilemma. On one hand, the barrier has to be extremely thin to allow efficient gas exchange by passive diffusion. On the other hand, the blood-gas barrier must be strong because of the large mechanical stresses that develop in the capillary wall when the pressure in the capillaries rises or when the wall is stretched by inflating the lung to high volumes. There is evidence that the blood-gas barrier is just strong enough to withstand the highest stresses to which it is normally subjected. Unusually high capillary pressures or lung volumes can result in ultrastructural damage or stress failure of the capillary wall, leading to a high-permeability type of pulmonary edema, or even pulmonary hemorrhage.

When the capillary transmural pressure is raised in animal preparations, disruption of the capillary endothelium, alveolar epithelium, or sometimes all layers of the capillary wall is seen. In the rabbit lung, the first changes are seen at a transmural pressure of approximately 24 mm Hg, and the frequency of breaks increases as the pressure is raised.[73] Although these capillary pressures seem very high, there is now good evidence that the capillary pressure rises to the mid-30s (mm Hg) in the normal lung during heavy exercise.[74] This is largely secondary to the increase in left ventricular filling pressure.[75]

At these increased capillary transmural pressures, the "hoop" or circumferential stresses in the capillary wall become extremely high. The main reason for the very high stresses is the extreme thinness of the wall which, in the human lung, is less than 0.3 μm in some places. It is now believed that the strength of the blood-gas barrier on the thin side comes from type IV collagen in the basement membranes. The thickness of the type IV collagen layer is only approximately 50 nm. The delicacy of the alveoli can be appreciated by scanning electron microscopy, which demonstrates the interface of the alveolar epithelial cells and the alveolar capillary network (see Video 3.1).

Stress failure is the likely mechanism of several clinical conditions characterized by high-permeability pulmonary edema or hemorrhage.[76] Neurogenic pulmonary edema is associated with very high capillary pressures, the edema is of the high-permeability type, and ultrastructural damage to the capillaries is consistent with stress failure. High-altitude pulmonary edema is apparently caused by uneven hypoxic pulmonary vasoconstriction (referred to earlier), which allows some of the capillaries to be exposed to high pressure.[77] Again, the edema is of the high-permeability type, and typical ultrastructural changes in the capillaries have been demonstrated in animal preparations.[78]

A particularly interesting condition is seen in racehorses, which can suffer bleeding into the lungs while galloping. This is a common problem caused by extremely high pulmonary capillary pressures, which approach 100 mm Hg. Direct evidence of stress failure of pulmonary capillaries has been shown in these animals.[79] In fact, there is evidence that elite human athletes develop some ultrastructural changes in their blood-gas barrier during extreme exercise because significantly higher concentrations of red blood cells, total protein, and leukotriene B_4 are seen in their bronchoalveolar lavage fluid compared with sedentary controls.[80] This leakage only happens at extremely high levels of exercise[81]; a similar group of athletes who exercised at submaximal levels for 1 hour showed no changes in the bronchoalveolar lavage fluid.[82]

Overinflation of the lung is also known to increase the permeability of pulmonary capillaries. Stress failure is apparently the mechanism because it has been shown that, for the same capillary transmural pressure, high lung volumes greatly increase the frequency of capillary wall damage.[83] This is because some of the increased tension in the alveolar wall associated with lung inflation affects the capillary wall. Damage to the capillaries by overinflation may be an important mechanism in ventilator-induced lung injury.

BLOOD-GAS TRANSPORT

The partial pressure of a gas is an important concept in any discussion of gas exchange, as described later in the section on gas exchange. The *partial pressure* (P) of a gas is found by multiplying its concentration by the total pressure. For example, the P_{O_2} in dry room air at sea level is 159 mm Hg (0.209×760 mm Hg), where oxygen is 20.9% of room air and barometric pressure is 760 mm Hg. However, the relationship between P_{O_2} and its concentration in blood is not linear and is commonly described by an oxygen dissociation curve. Similar considerations apply to carbon dioxide in blood. The physiologic factors that determine the oxygen and carbon dioxide dissociation curves are considered later.

OXYGEN

Oxygen is carried in the blood in two forms. By far the most important component is in combination with hemoglobin. In addition, a small amount of oxygen is dissolved in the blood.

Hemoglobin consists of heme, an iron-porphyrin compound, and a protein (globin) that has four polypeptide chains. There are two types of chains, α and β, and differences in their amino acid sequences give rise to different types of human hemoglobin. There are unique conditions in which alterations in hemoglobin have clinical consequences. Examples include the normal hemoglobin F (fetal), which has a high affinity for oxygen, and hemoglobin S (sickle), which has a reduced affinity for oxygen and, in the deoxygenated form, tends to aggregate and deform the red cell. Methemoglobin, formed as a result of exposure to various drugs or chemicals, is not useful for carrying oxygen and increases the oxygen affinity of the remaining hemoglobin, thus impairing unloading of oxygen in the tissues.

Blood is able to transport large amounts of oxygen because oxygen forms an easily reversible combination with *hemoglobin* (Hb) to give *oxyhemoglobin* (HbO$_2$):

$$O_2 + Hb \rightleftharpoons HbO_2 \qquad \text{Eq. 10}$$

The relationship between the partial pressure of oxygen and the number of binding sites of the hemoglobin with oxygen attached is known as the *oxygen dissociation curve* (Fig. 10.12). Each gram of pure hemoglobin can combine with 1.39 mL of oxygen and, in normal blood with 15 g Hb/100 mL, the oxygen capacity (reached when all the binding sites are full) is 1.39 × 15, or approximately 20.8 mL O$_2$/100 mL of blood. The total *oxygen content* of a sample of blood (expressed as mL O$_2$/100 mL of blood), which includes the oxygen combined with hemoglobin and the dissolved oxygen, is given by

$$O_2 \text{ content} = (1.39 \times Hb) \times \frac{\% \text{ saturation}}{100}$$
$$+ (0.003 \times P_{O_2}) \qquad \text{Eq. 11}$$

where *Hb* is the hemoglobin concentration and the final term is the oxygen dissolved in the blood (see later).

The characteristic shape of the oxygen dissociation curve has several physiologic advantages. The fact that the upper portion is almost flat means that a fall of 20 to 30 mm Hg in arterial P$_{O_2}$ in a healthy subject with an initially normal value (e.g., ≈100 mm Hg) causes only a minor reduction in arterial oxygen content. However, this also means that noninvasive monitoring of oxygen saturation by pulse oximetry will often fail to indicate substantial falls in arterial P$_{O_2}$ (see Chapter 44). Another consequence of the flat upper part of the curve is that the diffusive loading of oxygen in the pulmonary capillary is enhanced. This results from the large partial pressure difference between alveolar gas and capillary blood that is maintained even when most of the oxygen has been loaded. The steep lower part of the

oxygen dissociation curve means that a relatively small drop in capillary P$_{O_2}$ can lead to the unloading of considerable amounts of oxygen. This also maintains the blood P$_{O_2}$ and assists the diffusion of O$_2$ into the tissue. A useful measure of the position of the dissociation curve is the P$_{O_2}$ for 50% oxygen saturation, known as the P$_{50}$. The normal value for human blood is approximately 27 mm Hg.

Various factors affect the position of the oxygen dissociation curve (see Fig. 10.12). A rightward shift indicates a decrease in the affinity of hemoglobin for oxygen. The curve is shifted to the right by an increase of temperature, hydrogen ion concentration, the concentration of *2,3-diphosphoglycerate* (2,3-DPG) in the red cell, and the P$_{CO_2}$. Increased P$_{CO_2}$ reduces the oxygen affinity mainly by the increased H$^+$ concentration and increases oxygen unloading. The ability of carbon dioxide to reduce the affinity of hemoglobin for oxygen is called the *Bohr effect*. One consequence of the Bohr effect is that, as peripheral blood loads carbon dioxide, the unloading of oxygen is assisted. A rightward shift is also caused by 2,3-DPG, an end product of red cell metabolism.[84,85] The concentration of 2,3-DPG can be increased in the setting of chronic hypoxia.

Leftward shifts of the oxygen dissociation curve mean an increased affinity of hemoglobin for oxygen, as can be caused by a reduced concentration of 2,3-DPG or by the presence of carbon monoxide. The concentration of 2,3-DPG falls in stored blood, which can lead to blood with a high affinity for oxygen but with difficulty releasing oxygen to the tissues. Small amounts of carbon monoxide in the blood increase the affinity of the remaining oxygen for hemoglobin and therefore cause a leftward shift of the dissociation curve. As a result, the unloading of oxygen in the peripheral tissue is hampered. In addition, of course, the oxygen content of the blood is reduced at the same P$_{O_2}$ because some of the hemoglobin is bound to carbon monoxide. This is particularly dangerous because arterial chemoreceptors respond to decreases in P$_{O_2}$ and not to decreases in oxygen content, so the usual physiologic responses to hypoxemia may be absent.

Dissolved oxygen, when compared to oxygen carried by hemoglobin, plays a small role in oxygen transport because the solubility of oxygen is so low (0.003 mL O$_2$/100 mL blood/mm Hg). Thus, normal arterial blood with a P$_{O_2}$ of approximately 100 mm Hg contains only 0.3 mL of dissolved oxygen per 100 mL, whereas approximately 20 mL is combined with hemoglobin. However, dissolved oxygen can become important under some conditions. The most common is when a patient is given 100% oxygen to breathe. This typically raises the alveolar P$_{O_2}$ to greater than 600 mm Hg, with the result that, if the lungs are normal, the dissolved oxygen may increase from 0.3 to approximately 2 mL/100 mL blood. This dissolved oxygen then becomes a significant proportion of the normal arterial-venous oxygen content difference of approximately 5 mL O$_2$/100 mL blood.

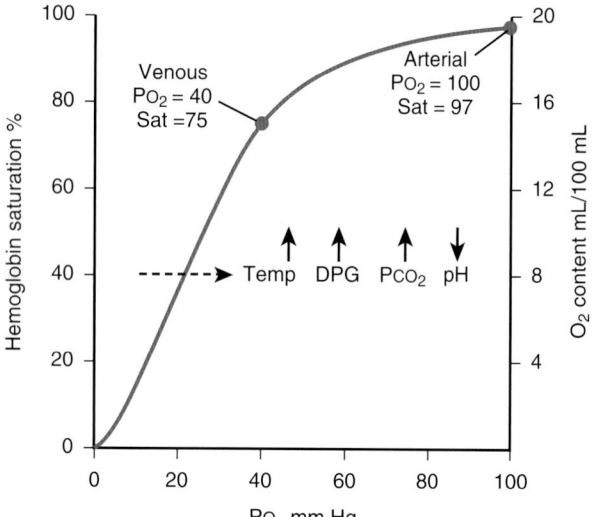

Figure 10.12 Oxygen dissociation curve showing typical values for arterial and mixed venous blood. The curve is shifted to the right by increases of temperature, 2,3-diphosphoglycerate (DPG), P$_{CO_2}$, and H$^+$ concentration. P$_{CO_2}$, partial pressure of carbon dioxide; P$_{O_2}$, partial pressure of oxygen; Sat, saturation; Temp, temperature. (Modified from West JB. *Respiratory Physiology: The Essentials.* 9th ed. Baltimore: Lippincott Williams & Wilkins; 2012.)

CARBON DIOXIDE

Carbon dioxide is transported in the blood in three forms: as bicarbonate (≈90%), as dissolved CO$_2$ (≈5% of the total), and in combination with proteins such as carbamino compounds (≈5%). Because carbon dioxide is some 24 times more soluble than oxygen in blood, dissolved carbon dioxide plays a more significant role in carbon dioxide transport than dissolved oxygen does in oxygen transport. For example, approximately 10% of the carbon dioxide that diffuses into the alveolar gas from the mixed venous blood comes from the dissolved form.

Bicarbonate is formed in blood by the following hydration reaction:

$$CO_2 + H_2O \xleftrightarrow{CA} H_2CO_3 \rightleftharpoons H^+ + HCO_3^- \qquad \text{Eq. 12}$$

The hydration of carbon dioxide to carbonic acid (and vice versa) is catalyzed by the enzyme *carbonic anhydrase* (CA), present in high concentrations in the red cells but absent from the plasma; some CA is apparently located on the surface of the endothelial cells of the pulmonary capillaries. Because the majority of the CA is in the red cell, carbon dioxide is mostly hydrated there, and bicarbonate ion moves out of the red cell to be replaced by chloride ions to maintain electrical neutrality (the chloride shift). Some of the hydrogen ions formed in the red cell are bound to hemoglobin and, because deoxygenated hemoglobin is a better proton acceptor than the oxygenated form, deoxygenated blood can carry more carbon dioxide for a given P_{CO_2} than can oxygenated blood (Fig. 10.13). In this way, oxygen decreases the affinity of hemoglobin for carbon dioxide, thereby increasing carbon dioxide delivery at the lung. This is known as the *Haldane effect*.

The carbon dioxide dissociation curve describing the relationship between P_{CO_2} and total carbon dioxide concentration is shown in Figure 10.13. Note that the curve is much more linear in its working range than the oxygen dissociation curve (see Fig. 10.12) and that, as we have seen, the lower the saturation of hemoglobin with oxygen, the larger the carbon dioxide concentration for a given P_{CO_2}.

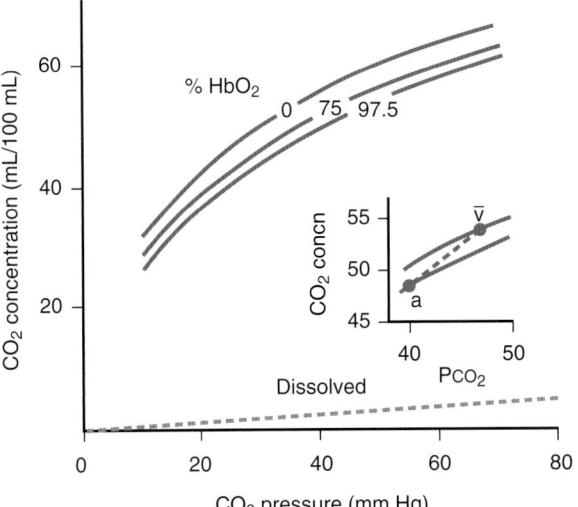

Figure 10.13 Carbon dioxide dissociation curves for blood of different oxygen saturations (oxyhemoglobin [HbO₂]). *Inset*, The physiologic curve between arterial (a) and mixed venous (v̄) blood, shown with two dissociation curves representing the %HbO₂ for venous blood (*top*) and for arterial blood (*bottom*). concn, concentration; Pco₂, partial pressure of carbon dioxide. (Modified from West JB. *Respiratory Physiology: The Essentials*. 9th ed. Baltimore: Lippincott Williams & Wilkins; 2012.)

The transport of carbon dioxide by the blood plays an important role in the acid-base status of the body. This topic is discussed at length in Chapter 12.

GAS EXCHANGE

The primary function of the lungs is gas exchange, that is, allowing oxygen to move from the air into the blood and allowing carbon dioxide to move out. It is now established that movement of gas across the blood-gas interface is by simple passive diffusion, that is, random (brownian) motion at a rate determined by temperature. Diffusion results in net transfer of molecules from an area of high to an area of low partial pressure, and active transport is not required. The structure of the lung is well suited to this mechanism of gas exchange. The blood-gas barrier is extremely thin (only 0.3 μm over much of its extent), and its area is between 50 and 100 m². Because Fick's law of diffusion states that the amount of gas that moves across a tissue sheet is proportional to its area and inversely proportional to its thickness, the blood-gas barrier is ideal for its gas-exchanging function.

An important concept in any discussion of gas exchange is partial pressure. As described earlier in "Blood-Gas Transport," the partial pressure of a gas is the product of its concentration and the total pressure. For example, $P_{O_2} = 0.209 \times 760$ mm Hg = 159 mm Hg in dry air with 20.9% oxygen at sea level, where the barometric pressure is 760 mm Hg. When air is inhaled into the upper airway, it is warmed and saturated with water vapor. The water vapor pressure at 37°C is 47 mm Hg. Under these conditions, the total dry gas pressure is only $760 - 47 = 713$ mm Hg. The P_{O_2} of moist inspired air is therefore $(20.9/100) \times 713 = 149$ mm Hg. In general, the relationship between the *partial pressure* (P) and *fractional concentration* (F) of a gas when water vapor is present is given by $Px = Fx (Pb - P_{H_2O})$, where *Pb* is barometric pressure and *x* is the species of gas.

Figure 10.14 shows an overview of the oxygen cascade from the air that we breathe to the tissues where it is used. The line represents an ideal situation that does not actually exist but does make a useful backdrop for purposes of discussion. One of the first surprises is that, by the time the oxygen has reached the alveoli, its partial pressure has fallen from approximately 150 to 100 mm Hg. The reason for this decline is that the P_{O_2} in the alveolar gas is determined by a balance between two factors. On the one hand, there is the essentially continuous addition of oxygen by the process of alveolar ventilation and, on the other hand, there is the continuous removal of oxygen by the pulmonary blood flow. The net result is that the alveolar P_{O_2} settles out at approximately 100 mm Hg.

It is true that the process of ventilation is intermittent with each breath and not continuous. By the same token, pulmonary capillary blood flow is known to be pulsatile. However, the volume of gas in the lung at FRC is sufficient to dampen both of these oscillations, with the result that the alveolar P_{O_2} varies by only 3 or 4 mm Hg with each breath and by less than that with each heartbeat. Thus, alveolar ventilation and capillary blood flow can be regarded as continuous processes from the point of view of gas exchange. This greatly simplifies consideration of gas exchange.

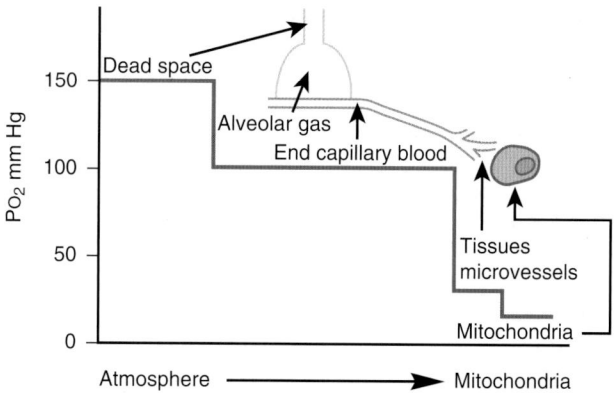

Figure 10.14 Scheme of the oxygen partial pressures from air to tissues. A hypothetically perfect situation. Po$_2$, partial pressure of oxygen. (Modified from West JB. *Ventilation/Blood Flow and Gas Exchange.* 5th ed. Oxford: Blackwell Scientific; 1990.)

In an ideal lung (see Fig. 10.14), the effluent pulmonary venous blood, which becomes the systemic arterial blood, would have the same Po$_2$ as that of the alveolar gas, namely, approximately 100 mm Hg. This is very nearly the case in the normal lung. However, when the arterial blood reaches the peripheral tissues, Po$_2$ falls substantially en route to the mitochondria. The movement of oxygen in the peripheral tissues is also essentially by passive diffusion, and the mitochondrial Po$_2$ is considerably lower than that in either the arterial or mixed venous blood. Indeed, the Po$_2$ in the mitochondria may vary considerably throughout the body, depending on the type of tissue and its oxygen uptake. Nevertheless, it is useful to bear in mind that the mitochondria are the targets for the oxygen transport system and that any fall in the arterial Po$_2$ caused, for example, by inefficient pulmonary gas exchange must be reflected in a reduced tissue Po$_2$, other factors being equal.

For carbon dioxide, the process is reversed. There is essentially no carbon dioxide in the inspired air, and the alveolar Pco$_2$ is approximately 40 mm Hg. Under normal conditions, arterial and alveolar Pco$_2$ values are the same, whereas the Pco$_2$ of mixed venous blood is in the range of 45 to 47 mm Hg. The Pco$_2$ of the tissues is probably quite variable, depending, for example, on the state of metabolism. Nevertheless, any inefficiency of the lung for carbon dioxide removal tends to raise the Pco$_2$ of the tissues, other factors being equal.

CAUSES OF HYPOXEMIA (See Chapter 44)

Hypoxemia refers to a reduction in arterial Po$_2$ to below normal values. There are five causes of hypoxemia. Four processes from within the body can impair pulmonary gas exchange and cause hypoxemia when breathing room air at sea level: hypoventilation, diffusion limitation, shunt, and ventilation-perfusion inequality. There is an additional cause from outside the body, namely from a decrease in inspired oxygen concentration. Such a decrease in fractional concentration of oxygen in inspired gas may be found at high altitude or with accidents in which oxygen is consumed or displaced in inspired air.

Hypoventilation

Hypoventilation is used here to refer to conditions in which alveolar ventilation is abnormally low in relation to oxygen uptake or carbon dioxide output (see also Chapter 45). Alveolar ventilation is the volume of fresh inspired gas going to the alveoli (i.e., non–dead-space ventilation), as mentioned earlier. As we shall see, hypoventilation always causes a raised arterial Pco$_2$ and also arterial hypoxemia (unless the patient is breathing an enriched oxygen mixture). It should be noted that other conditions (e.g., ventilation-perfusion inequality) can also result in carbon dioxide retention, and some use the terms *hypoventilation* and *carbon dioxide retention* interchangeably. However, this can be confusing because carbon dioxide can be retained even when a patient is breathing more than normal, so we do not use the terms interchangeably.

As previously mentioned, the Po$_2$ of alveolar gas is determined by a balance between the rate of addition of oxygen by alveolar ventilation and the rate of removal by the pulmonary blood flow to satisfy the oxygen demands of the tissues. Hypoventilation results when the alveolar ventilation is reduced and the alveolar Po$_2$ therefore settles out at a lower level than normal. For the same reason, the alveolar Pco$_2$, and therefore also arterial Pco$_2$, are also raised.

Causes of hypoventilation include depression of the respiratory center by drugs, such as opiates, or diseases of the brainstem, such as encephalitis; abnormalities of the spinal cord–conducting pathways, such as high cervical dislocation; anterior horn cell diseases, including poliomyelitis, affecting the phrenic nerves or supplying the intercostal muscles; diseases of nerves to respiratory muscles (e.g., Guillain-Barré syndrome); diseases of the myoneural junction, such as myasthenia gravis; diseases of the respiratory muscles themselves, such as progressive muscular dystrophy; thoracic cage abnormalities (e.g., crushed chest); upper airway obstruction (e.g., thymoma); hypoventilation associated with extreme obesity (obesity hypoventilation syndrome); and other causes, such as metabolic alkalosis and idiopathic states.

Note that, in all these conditions, the lungs are normal. Thus, this group can be clearly distinguished from those diseases in which the carbon dioxide retention is associated with chronic lung disease. In the latter conditions, the lungs are abnormal, and a major factor in the raised Pco$_2$ is the ventilation-perfusion inequality that causes gross inefficiency of pulmonary gas exchange (see later).

The rise in alveolar Pco$_2$ as a result of hypoventilation can be calculated using the alveolar ventilation equation (see earlier section "Total and Alveolar Ventilation" for derivation):

$$\dot{V}_A = \frac{\dot{V}_{CO_2}}{P_{ACO_2}} \times K \qquad \text{Eq. 5}$$

where *K* is a constant. This can be rearranged as follows:

$$P_{ACO_2} = \frac{\dot{V}_{CO_2}}{\dot{V}_A} \times K \qquad \text{Eq. 13}$$

Because, in normal lungs, the alveolar (P$_{ACO_2}$) and arterial (Pa$_{CO_2}$) Pco$_2$ are almost identical, we can write:

$$Pa_{CO_2} = \frac{\dot{V}_{CO_2}}{\dot{V}_A} \times K \qquad \text{Eq. 14}$$

This very important equation indicates that the level of P_{CO_2} in alveolar gas or arterial blood is inversely related to the alveolar ventilation. For example, if the alveolar ventilation is halved, the P_{CO_2} doubles. Note, however, that this is true only after a steady state has been reestablished and the carbon dioxide production rate is the same as before. In practice, if the alveolar ventilation of a patient is suddenly decreased (e.g., by changing the setting on a ventilator), the P_{CO_2} rises over a period of 10 to 20 minutes. The rise is rapid at first and then is more gradual as the body stores of carbon dioxide are gradually filled.[86]

The same principles used for carbon dioxide can be applied to oxygen to understand the effect of hypoventilation on alveolar, and thus arterial, P_{O_2}. The corresponding mass conservation equation for oxygen is as follows, where $\dot{V}_{O_2}$ is the oxygen uptake:

$$\dot{V}_{O_2} = (\dot{V}_I \times F_{IO_2}) - (\dot{V}_A \times F_{AO_2}) \qquad \text{Eq. 15}$$

Here $\dot{V}_I$ is inspired alveolar ventilation, whereas $\dot{V}_A$ is expired alveolar ventilation. Eq. 15 expresses oxygen uptake as the difference between the oxygen inhaled (volume per minute of inspired gas [$\dot{V}_I$] × *fractional concentration of oxygen* [F_{IO_2}]) and that exhaled (volume per minute of alveolar ventilation [$\dot{V}_A$] × *fractional concentration of oxygen in alveolar gas* [F_{AO_2}]). Normally, because a little more oxygen is taken up per minute than carbon dioxide exhaled, $\dot{V}_I$ exceeds $\dot{V}_A$. However, this difference is usually no more than 1% of the ventilation, and clinically it can most often be ignored. If this is done, $\dot{V}_I$ may then be replaced by $\dot{V}_A$, and Eq. 15 simplifies to

$$\dot{V}_{O_2} = \dot{V}_A \times (F_{IO_2} - F_{AO_2}), \; or$$

$$\dot{V}_{O_2} = \dot{V}_A \times \frac{(P_{IO_2} - P_{AO_2})}{K} \qquad \text{Eq. 16}$$

where P_{IO_2} is the partial pressure of oxygen in the inspired gas. Thus, as ventilation falls, P_{AO_2} must fall as well to maintain the rate of oxygen uptake necessary for metabolic function.

Eq. 13 (reexpressed as $\dot{V}_{CO_2} = \dot{V}_A \times P_{ACO_2}/K$) and Eq. 16 can be usefully combined. If Eq. 13 is divided by Eq. 16, we get

$$\frac{\dot{V}_{CO_2}}{\dot{V}_{O_2}} = R = \frac{P_{ACO_2}}{(P_{IO_2} - P_{AO_2})} \qquad \text{Eq. 17}$$

Here R is the respiratory exchange ratio (volume of carbon dioxide exhaled/oxygen taken up in the same time). Both K and $\dot{V}_A$ cancel out when the division is performed. Rearranging this equation yields

$$P_{AO_2} = P_{IO_2} - \frac{P_{ACO_2}}{R} \qquad \text{Eq. 18}$$

This is called the *alveolar gas equation*, and it uniquely relates alveolar P_{O_2} to P_{CO_2} for given values of inspired P_{O_2} and R. It is the basis of calculations of the *alveolar-to-arterial P_{O_2} difference*, a commonly used index of efficiency of pulmonary gas exchange. Because we assumed that $\dot{V}_I = \dot{V}_A$ in deriving this equation, it is an approximation. It is possible to account for the difference between $\dot{V}_I$ and $\dot{V}_A$, and, when this is done, the alveolar gas equation contains an additional term:

$$P_{AO_2} = P_{IO_2} - \frac{P_{ACO_2}}{R} + \left[P_{ACO_2} \times F_{IO_2} \times \frac{(1-R)}{R} \right] \qquad \text{Eq. 19}$$

The term in brackets is the correction factor for the difference between inspired and expired volumes. It is generally small during air breathing (1 to 3 mm Hg) and can be ignored in most clinical settings if the patient is breathing air. However, if the patient is being given an enriched oxygen mixture, the correction factor increases. In someone with normal lungs breathing pure oxygen, the factor is approximately 10 mm Hg.

As an example of the use of the alveolar gas equation, suppose that a patient with normal lungs takes an overdose of a barbiturate drug that depresses alveolar ventilation. The patient's alveolar P_{CO_2} might rise from 40 to 60 mm Hg (the actual value is determined by the alveolar ventilation equation). Before the drug, the patient's alveolar P_{O_2} can be calculated assuming R = 1.0, and the small correction factor is neglected:

$$P_{AO_2} = P_{IO_2} - (P_{ACO_2}/R)$$
$$= 149 - (40/1)$$
$$= 109 \text{ mm Hg}$$

After the drug, and making the same assumptions, with an increase of P_{CO_2} by 20 mm Hg, the alveolar P_{O_2} will fall by 20 mm Hg:

$$P_{AO_2} = P_{IO_2} - (P_{ACO_2}/R)$$
$$= 149 - (60/1)$$
$$= 89 \text{ mm Hg}$$

Hence, when R = 1.0, alveolar P_{O_2} falls by 20 mm Hg, which is the same amount by which the P_{CO_2} rises. If R = 0.8, which is a more typical resting value, and we ignore the small correction factor in Eq. 19, then, when alveolar P_{CO_2} increases by 20 mm Hg, alveolar P_{O_2} decreases by 25 mm Hg, from 99 mm Hg (the P_{AO_2} when the CO_2 is 40 mm Hg and R 0.8) to 74 mm Hg.

Both examples emphasize that, in practical terms, the hypoxemia is generally of minor importance compared with the carbon dioxide retention and consequent respiratory acidosis. This is further illustrated in Figure 10.15, which shows calculated changes in gas exchange as a result of hypoventilation. Note that severe hypoventilation sufficient to double the P_{CO_2} from 40 to 80 mm Hg decreases the alveolar P_{O_2} from only, say, 100 to 50 or 60 mm Hg. Although the arterial P_{O_2} is likely to be a few millimeters of mercury lower than the alveolar value, the arterial oxygen saturation is still approximately 80%. However, at that level of P_{CO_2}, there is substantial respiratory acidosis, with an arterial pH of approximately 7.2. This fact emphasizes that, in pure hypoventilation, the hypoxemia is usually not as important as the carbon dioxide retention and respiratory acidosis.

An important feature of alveolar hypoventilation is that, although the arterial P_{CO_2} is always elevated, the arterial P_{O_2} may be returned to normal very easily by giving supplementary oxygen. Suppose that the patient with barbiturate intoxication just discussed is given 30% oxygen to breathe. If we assume that the ventilation remains unchanged, it can be shown (from Eq. 19) that the alveolar P_{O_2} increases from 74 to approximately 140 mm Hg. Thus, a relatively small increase in inspired P_{O_2} is very effective in eliminating the arterial hypoxemia of hypoventilation.

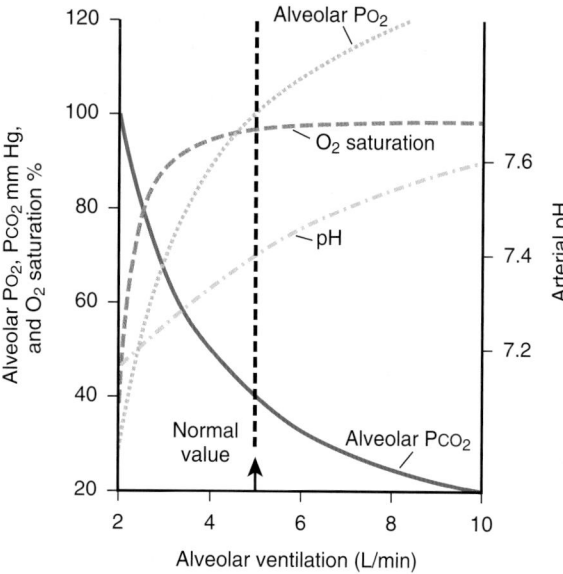

Figure 10.15 Gas exchange during changes in ventilation. With hypoventilation, note the relatively large rise in P_{CO_2} and consequent fall in pH compared with the modest fall in arterial oxygen saturation. P_{CO_2}, partial pressure of carbon dioxide; P_{O_2}, partial pressure of oxygen. (Modified from West JB. *Respiratory Physiology: The Essentials.* 9th ed. Baltimore: Lippincott Williams & Wilkins; 2012.)

Diffusion Limitation

Oxygen, carbon dioxide, and all other gases cross the blood-gas barrier by simple passive diffusion. Fick's law of diffusion states that the rate of transfer of a gas through a sheet of tissue is proportional to the tissue *area* (A) and the difference in partial pressure ($P_1 - P_2$) between the two sides, and it is inversely proportional to the *thickness* (T):

$$\dot{V}gas = \frac{A}{T} \times D \times (P_1 - P_2) \qquad \text{Eq. 20}$$

As we have seen already, the area of the blood-gas barrier in the lung is enormous (50–100 m²), and the thickness is less than 0.3 µm in some places, so the dimensions of the barrier are ideal for diffusion.

The rate of diffusion is also proportional to a *constant* (D), which depends on the properties of the tissue and the particular gas. The constant is proportional to the *solubility* (Sol) of the gas and inversely proportional to the square root of the *molecular weight* (MW):

$$D \propto \frac{Sol}{\sqrt{MW}} \qquad \text{Eq. 21}$$

This equation can be used to compare the difference of rate of diffusion of oxygen and carbon dioxide. For each millimeter of mercury difference between capillary and alveolar partial pressures, carbon dioxide diffuses approximately 20 times more rapidly than oxygen through tissue sheets because carbon dioxide has a much higher solubility (24:1 at 37°C), whereas the square roots of the molecular weights are not very different (1.17:1). Note that this calculation applies only to tissue sheets and does not fully account for the uptake of oxygen or output of carbon dioxide by the lung because the chemical reactions between these gases and components of blood also play a role (see later discussion).

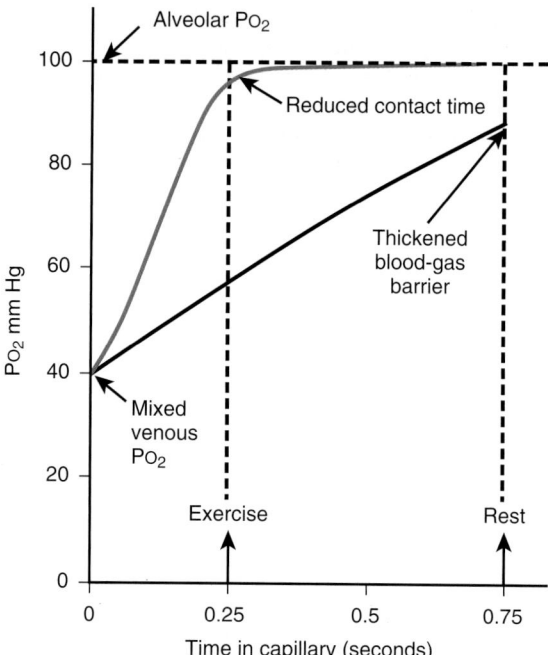

Figure 10.16 Oxygen uptake along the pulmonary capillary. Typical time courses for the change in P_{O_2} in the pulmonary capillary when diffusion is normal (*green line*), when the contact time is reduced as during exercise (*arrow at green line*), and when the blood-gas barrier is abnormally thick (*black line*). P_{O_2}, partial pressure of oxygen. (Modified from West JB. *Respiratory Physiology: The Essentials.* 9th ed. Baltimore: Lippincott Williams & Wilkins; 2012.)

Oxygen Uptake Along the Pulmonary Capillary.

Figure 10.16 shows calculated changes in the P_{O_2} of the blood along the pulmonary capillary as oxygen is taken up under normal conditions. The calculation is based on Fick's law of diffusion (see Eq. 20). One of the several assumptions is that the diffusion characteristics of the blood-gas barrier are uniform along the length of the capillary. The calculation is complicated by the fact that the change in the P_{O_2} of the capillary blood depends on the oxygen dissociation curve. This is not only nonlinear, but it is also influenced by the simultaneous elimination of carbon dioxide. The calculation describing this is often known as the Bohr integration because it was first carried out in a simplified form by Christian Bohr.[87] Modern computations take into account reaction times of oxygen with hemoglobin and also reaction rates associated with carbon dioxide elimination (see later discussion).[88]

Figure 10.16 shows that the time spent by the blood in the pulmonary capillary under normal resting conditions is approximately 0.75 second. This number is obtained by dividing the volume of blood calculated to be in the pulmonary capillaries (75 mL) by the cardiac output (6 L/min).[89] The figure shows that the P_{O_2} of pulmonary capillary blood very nearly reaches that of alveolar gas after approximately one-third of the available time in the capillary. This means that there is normally ample time for essentially complete oxygenation of the blood or, as it is sometimes said, the normal lung has substantial diffusion reserves.

If the blood-gas barrier is thickened, the rate of transfer of oxygen across the barrier is reduced in accordance with Fick's law, and the rate of rise of P_{O_2} is slower, as shown in Figure 10.16. Under these circumstances, diffusion may not be sufficient, and a P_{O_2} difference may develop between alveolar gas and end-capillary blood. This means that there is some diffusion limitation of oxygen transfer. It is important to appreciate that, under most conditions at sea level, oxygen transfer is perfusion limited, meaning that oxygen uptake is entirely dependent on blood flow. Only under unusual conditions, such as severe interstitial lung disease, is there some diffusion limitation. However, at high altitude, diffusion limitation during exercise is universal, even in health. In well-trained athletes with very rapid transit time through the capillaries, diffusion may be limiting during exercise even at sea level.

For further discussion of diffusion and perfusion limitation and diffusion capacity measurements, see ExpertConsult.com and Chapter 31.

Shunt

Shunt refers to the entry of blood into the systemic arterial system without going through ventilated areas of lung. Even the normal cardiopulmonary system shows some depression of the arterial P_{O_2} as a result of this factor. For example, in the normal lung, some of the bronchial artery blood is collected by the pulmonary veins after it has perfused the bronchi. Because the oxygen content of this blood has been reduced, its addition to the normal end-capillary blood results in a reduction of arterial P_{O_2}. Another source of normal shunting is the small amount of coronary venous blood that drains directly into the cavity of the left ventricle through the thebesian veins. Of course, most of the coronary venous blood ends up in the coronary sinus, and only a minute fraction reaches the left ventricle directly. Such shunts depress arterial P_{O_2} only by approximately 1 to 2 mm Hg.

In patients with congenital heart disease, there may be a direct addition of venous blood to arterial blood across a defect between the right and left sides of the heart. In general, this needs an increase in pressure on the right side; otherwise, the shunt would only take place from left to right. In lung disease, there may be gas-exchanging units that are completely unventilated because of airway obstruction, atelectasis, or alveolar filling with fluid or cells. The unoxygenated blood draining from these constitutes a shunt. It could be argued that such units are simply at the extreme end of the spectrum of ventilation-perfusion inequality (see next section), but the gas exchange properties of unventilated units are so different (e.g., in their response to supplemental oxygen) that it is convenient to separate them.

When the shunt is caused by the addition of mixed venous blood (pulmonary arterial) to blood draining from the capillaries (pulmonary venous), it is possible to calculate the amount of shunt flow. This is done using a mixing equation. The total amount of oxygen delivered into the systemic circulation per minute is the *total blood flow* ($\dot{Q}T$), that is, cardiac output, multiplied by the *oxygen content in the systemic arterial blood* (CaO_2), or $\dot{Q}T \times CaO_2$. This must equal the sum of the amounts of oxygen in the shunted blood ($\dot{Q}s \times C\overline{v}O_2$) and the nonshunted or end-capillary blood [$(\dot{Q}T - \dot{Q}s) \times Cc'O_2$]. Also, it is assumed that all regions of lung not subject to shunt are normal. Thus,

$$\dot{Q}T \times CaO_2 = (\dot{Q}s \times C\overline{v}O_2) + (\dot{Q}T - \dot{Q}s) \times Cc'O_2 \qquad \text{Eq. 26}$$

where $\dot{Q}s$ is pulmonary physiologic shunt (in mL/min), QT is cardiac output (in mL/min), $Cc'O_2$ is end-pulmonary capillary oxygen content, CaO_2 is arterial oxygen content, and $C\overline{v}O_2$ is mixed venous oxygen content.

Rearranging, this gives

$$\frac{\dot{Q}s}{\dot{Q}T} = \frac{(Cc'O_2 - CaO_2)}{(Cc'O_2 - C\overline{v}O_2)} \qquad \text{Eq. 27}$$

The oxygen content of end-capillary blood is usually calculated from the alveolar P_{O_2} and the hemoglobin concentration, assuming 100% oxyhemoglobin saturation (Eq. 11), hence the assumption of normalcy of all regions not subject to shunt.

When the shunt is caused by blood that does not have the same oxygen content as mixed venous blood (e.g., bronchial venous blood), it is generally not possible to calculate its true magnitude. However, it is often useful to calculate an "as if" shunt, that is, what the shunt would be if the observed depression of arterial oxygen content were caused by the addition of mixed venous blood.

An important diagnostic feature of a shunt is that the arterial P_{O_2} does not rise to the normal level, which in theory should be 670 mm Hg, when the patient is given 100% oxygen to breathe. The reason for this is that the shunted blood that bypasses ventilated alveoli is never exposed to the higher alveolar P_{O_2}. Its addition to end-capillary blood therefore continues to depress the arterial P_{O_2}. Nevertheless, the arterial P_{O_2} is elevated somewhat because of the oxygen added to the capillary blood of the ventilated lung. Most of this added oxygen is in the dissolved form rather than attached to hemoglobin because the blood that is perfusing lung regions with normal ventilation-perfusion ratios is normally nearly fully saturated.

The administration of 100% oxygen to a patient with a shunt is a very sensitive method of detecting small amounts of shunting. This is because when the arterial P_{O_2} is very high, a very small reduction of arterial oxygen content (or hemoglobin saturation) caused by the addition of the shunted blood causes a relatively large fall in P_{O_2}. This is directly attributable to the almost flat slope of the oxygen dissociation curve in this region.

A patient with a shunt usually does not have an increased P_{CO_2} in the arterial blood in spite of the fact that the shunted blood is rich in carbon dioxide. The reason is that the chemoreceptors sense any elevation of arterial P_{CO_2} and respond by increasing the ventilation. As a consequence, the P_{CO_2} of the unshunted blood is reduced by the hyperventilation until the arterial P_{CO_2} is back to normal. Indeed, in some patients with large shunts caused, for example, by cyanotic congenital heart disease, the arterial P_{CO_2} is low because the arterial hypoxemia increases the respiratory drive.

Ventilation-Perfusion Relationships

The mismatching of ventilation and blood flow is the most common cause of hypoxemia in lung disease. Uneven ventilation and blood flow are also a cause of carbon dioxide retention. Early intimations of the importance of the subject go back to Krogh and Lindhard[94] and Haldane.[95] However, in the late 1940s, our understanding advanced when Fenn and colleagues[96] and Riley and Cournand[97] introduced graphic analysis of gas exchange. This was an important advance because the interrelationships of ventilation, blood flow, and gas exchange depend on the oxygen and carbon dioxide dissociation curves, which are not only nonlinear but interdependent, and direct solutions to the gas exchange equations that relate the ventilation-perfusion ratio to gas exchange (see later, Eqs. 29 and 30) are not possible.

Later, computers were used to describe the oxygen and carbon dioxide dissociation curves.[98,99] These procedures enabled investigators to answer questions about gas exchange that had been impossibly difficult before that time. The behavior of distributions of ventilation-perfusion ratios was analyzed,[100] and Wagner and colleagues[101] introduced the multiple inert gas elimination technique, which allowed, for the first time, information about the dispersion, number of modes, and shape of the distributions of ventilation, of perfusion, and of their ratio to be obtained.

Gas Exchange in a Single Lung Unit. The P_{O_2}, P_{CO_2}, and P_{N_2} in any gas-exchanging unit of the lung are uniquely determined by three major factors: (1) the ventilation-perfusion ratio, (2) the composition of the inspired gas and the composition of the mixed venous blood, and (3) the slopes and positions of the relevant blood-gas dissociation curves.

Formally, the key role of the ventilation-perfusion ratio can be derived as follows. The amount of carbon dioxide exhaled into the air from alveolar gas per minute is given by Eq. 4:

$$\dot{V}_{CO_2} = \dot{V}_A \times P_{A_{CO_2}}/K$$

where $\dot{V}_{CO_2}$ is the carbon dioxide production, $\dot{V}_A$ is the alveolar ventilation, K is a constant, and there is no carbon dioxide in the inspired gas.

The amount of carbon dioxide that diffuses into alveolar gas from capillary blood per minute is given by:

$$\dot{V}_{CO_2} = \dot{Q}(C\bar{v}_{CO_2} - Cc'_{CO_2}) \qquad \text{Eq. 28}$$

where $\dot{Q}$ is blood flow, and $C\bar{v}_{CO_2}$ and Cc'_{CO_2} are the concentrations of carbon dioxide in mixed venous and end-capillary blood, respectively. Now, in a steady state, the amount of carbon dioxide lost from the alveoli and from the capillary blood must be the same. Therefore,

$$\dot{V}_A \times P_{A_{CO_2}}/K = \dot{Q}(C\bar{v}_{CO_2} - Cc'_{CO_2}), \ or$$

$$\frac{\dot{V}_A}{\dot{Q}} = K \times \frac{(C\bar{v}_{CO_2} - Cc'_{CO_2})}{P_{A_{CO_2}}} \qquad \text{Eq. 29}$$

Thus, the alveolar P_{CO_2} and the corresponding end-capillary carbon dioxide concentration (assuming end-capillary and alveolar P_{CO_2} are identical) are determined by (1) the ventilation-perfusion ratio, (2) the mixed venous carbon dioxide concentration, and (3) the carbon dioxide dissociation curve relating P_{CO_2} to carbon dioxide concentration.

Although this equation looks simple, its appearance is deceiving because, when the ventilation-perfusion ratio, for example, increases, the alveolar P_{O_2} rises. This means that the oxygen saturation of the blood increases, and the relationship between P_{CO_2} and carbon dioxide concentration is altered. Thus, the alveolar P_{O_2} is an implicit variable in the

equation. In addition, the relationship between P_{CO_2} and carbon dioxide concentration in blood is nonlinear.

Just as in the context of the alveolar ventilation equation (see "Hypoventilation" earlier), it is possible to write an equation similar to Eq. 29 for oxygen exchange based on the same principles as applied for carbon dioxide. Again, the approximation is made that $\dot{V}_I = \dot{V}_A$ to keep the equation simple but, as for the alveolar gas equation, the fact that $\dot{V}_I$ slightly exceeds $\dot{V}_A$ can formally be taken into account. Using this approximation, the equation for oxygen is

$$\frac{\dot{V}_A}{\dot{Q}} = K \times \frac{(Cc'_{O_2} - C\bar{v}_{O_2})}{(P_{I_{O_2}} - P_{A_{O_2}})} \qquad \text{Eq. 30}$$

Just as for carbon dioxide, the alveolar and end-capillary P_{O_2} values are taken to be identical, implying diffusion equilibrium across the blood-gas barrier. It is seen that the determinants of alveolar P_{O_2}, as for carbon dioxide, are threefold: (1) the ventilation-perfusion ratio, (2) inspired and mixed venous oxygen levels, and (3) the relationship between P_{O_2} and oxygen content in blood (i.e., the oxygen dissociation curve).

Graphic analysis of these relationships is assisted by the use of the oxygen–carbon dioxide diagram, in which P_{O_2} is on the horizontal axis and P_{CO_2} is on the vertical axis. Figure 10.17 is an example of the use of the oxygen–carbon dioxide diagram to show how the P_{O_2} and P_{CO_2} of a lung unit change as the ventilation-perfusion ratio is either decreased below or increased above the normal value. Note that for a given composition of inspired gas (I) and mixed venous blood ($\bar{v}$), the possible combinations of P_{O_2} and P_{CO_2} are constrained to a single line known as the ventilation-perfusion ratio line. Each point on that line uniquely corresponds to a value of the ventilation-perfusion ratio. Note also that, when the ventilation-perfusion ratio is zero, the P_{O_2} and P_{CO_2} of end-capillary blood are those of mixed venous blood and, when the ventilation-perfusion ratio is infinity, the P_{O_2} and P_{CO_2} of alveolar gas are the same as those of inspired gas. In this diagram and in the rest of this section, we assume that there is complete diffusion equilibration between the P_{O_2} and P_{CO_2} of alveolar gas and end-capillary blood. This is a reasonable assumption unless

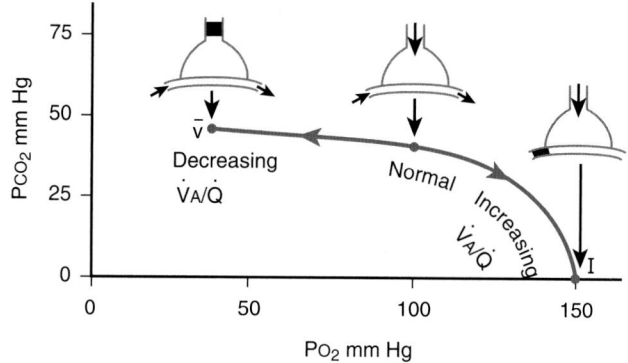

Figure 10.17 Oxygen–carbon dioxide diagram shows how the P_{O_2} and P_{CO_2} of a lung unit change as the ventilation-perfusion ratio ($\dot{V}_A/\dot{Q}$) is changed. I, inspired gas; P_{CO_2}, partial pressure of carbon dioxide; P_{O_2}, partial pressure of oxygen; $\bar{v}$, mixed venous blood. (Modified from West JB. *Respiratory Physiology: The Essentials.* 9th ed. Baltimore: Lippincott Williams & Wilkins; 2012.)

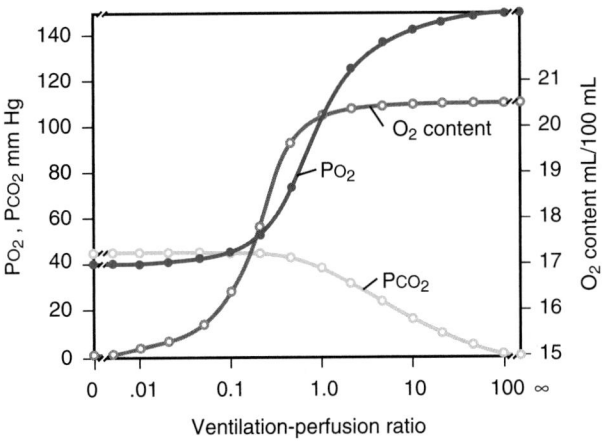

Figure 10.18 **Changes in P_{O_2}, P_{CO_2}, and end-capillary oxygen content in a lung unit are shown as its ventilation-perfusion ratio is altered.** See text for assumptions. P_{CO_2}, partial pressure of carbon dioxide; P_{O_2}, partial pressure of oxygen. (Modified from West JB. State of the art: ventilation-perfusion relationships. *Am Rev Respir Dis.* 1977;116:919–943.)

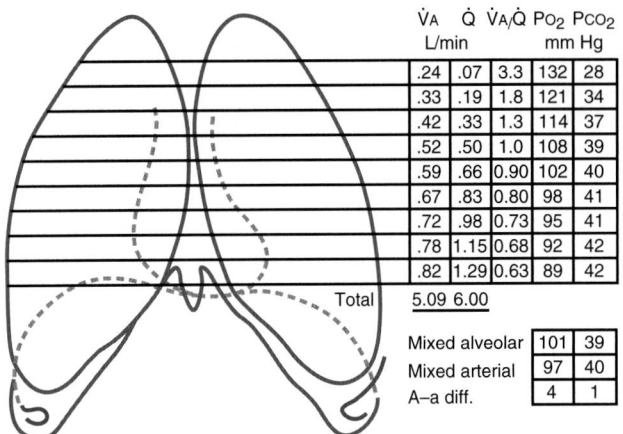

$\dot{V}_A$	$\dot{Q}$	$\dot{V}_A/\dot{Q}$	P_{O_2}	P_{CO_2}
L/min			mm Hg	
.24	.07	3.3	132	28
.33	.19	1.8	121	34
.42	.33	1.3	114	37
.52	.50	1.0	108	39
.59	.66	0.90	102	40
.67	.83	0.80	98	41
.72	.98	0.73	95	41
.78	1.15	0.68	92	42
.82	1.29	0.63	89	42

Total 5.09 6.00

Mixed alveolar	101	39
Mixed arterial	97	40
A–a diff.	4	1

Figure 10.19 **Regional differences of gas exchange down the upright normal lung.** The lung is divided into nine imaginary slices. $\dot{Q}$, blood flow; $\dot{V}_A$, alveolar ventilation. A–a diff, alveolar-arterial difference. (Modified from West JB. *Respiratory Physiology: The Essentials.* 9th ed. Baltimore: Lippincott Williams & Wilkins; 2012.)

there is marked thickening of the blood-gas barrier or one is considering a subject exercising in hypoxia.

Figure 10.18 shows the P_{O_2}, P_{CO_2}, and oxygen content of end-capillary blood of a lung unit as its ventilation-perfusion ratio is increased from extremely low to extremely high values. The inspired gas is assumed to be air, the P_{O_2} and P_{CO_2} of mixed venous blood are normal (40 and 45 mm Hg, respectively), and the hemoglobin concentration is 14.8 g/100 mL. The normal value of the ventilation-perfusion ratio is in the range of 0.8 to 1. Note that as the ratio is altered either above or below that value, the P_{O_2} changes considerably. By contrast, the oxygen content increases little as the ventilation-perfusion ratio is raised above the normal value because the hemoglobin is normally almost fully saturated. The P_{CO_2} falls considerably as the ventilation-perfusion ratio is raised but rises relatively little at lower ventilation-perfusion ratio values. The quantitative information in this figure is consistent with the graphic analysis of Figure 10.17.

Pattern in the Normal Lung. Both ventilation and perfusion vary throughout the lung. It is thus instructive to look at the inequality of gas exchange in different regions due to gravitational influences in the normal upright lung. As previously stated, both ventilation and blood flow per unit volume decrease from the bottom to the top of the upright lung. However, the changes for blood flow are more marked than those for ventilation. As a consequence, the ventilation-perfusion ratio increases from low values at the base to high values at the apex of the normal upright lung (Fig. 10.19).

Because the ventilation-perfusion ratio determines the gas exchange in any region (see Eqs. 29 and 30), the variation in P_{O_2} and P_{CO_2} in the lung can be calculated. Normal composition of mixed venous blood is assumed. Note that the P_{O_2} increases by some 40 mm Hg from base to apex, whereas the P_{CO_2} falls by 14 mm Hg. The pH is high at the apex because the P_{CO_2} there is low (the base excess is the same throughout the lung). Very little of the total oxygen uptake takes place at the apex, principally because the blood flow there is very low.

Figure 10.19 also helps to explain why ventilation-perfusion inequality interferes with overall gas exchange. Note that the base of the lung has most of the blood flow, but the P_{O_2} of the end-capillary blood is lowest there. As a result, the effluent pulmonary venous blood, which becomes the systemic arterial blood, is loaded with moderately oxygenated blood from the base. The net result is a depression of the arterial P_{O_2} below that which would be seen if ventilation and blood flow were uniformly distributed.

The same argument applies to carbon dioxide. In this case, the P_{CO_2} of the end-capillary blood is highest at the base, where the blood flow is greatest. As a result, the P_{CO_2} of arterial blood is elevated above that which would be seen if there was ventilation-perfusion equality. In other words, a lung with mismatched ventilation and blood flow is less efficient at exchanging gas, be it oxygen or carbon dioxide. In fact, the inefficiency applies to any gas that is being transferred by the lung. The extent of the impairment of gas exchange caused by any given amount of ventilation-perfusion inequality depends mostly on the solubility, or slope of the blood dissociation curve, of the gas. For example, in a lognormal distribution of ventilation-perfusion ratios, gases with medium solubility experience the greatest interference with pulmonary transfer.[104] In the normal lung, the effect of inequality due to gravity on arterial P_{O_2} can be modeled, as shown in Figure 10.19. Of interest, the overall effect of the normal inherent ventilation-perfusion inequality on gas exchange turns out to be very small, reducing arterial P_{O_2} by only approximately 4 mm Hg from that in a homogeneous lung.

Traditional Assessment of Ventilation-Perfusion Inequality. A central question that has engaged the attention of physiologists and physicians for many years has been how best to assess the amount of ventilation-perfusion inequality. Ideally, we would like to know the actual distribution of ventilation-perfusion ratios (see next section), but the procedure required for this is too complicated for many clinical situations. Traditionally, we rely on measurements of P_{O_2} and P_{CO_2} in arterial blood and expired gas.

The arterial P_{O_2} certainly gives some information about the degree of ventilation-perfusion inequality. In general, the lower the P_{O_2}, the more marked is the mismatching of ventilation and blood flow. The chief merit of this measurement is its simplicity, but a disadvantage is that its value is sensitive to the overall ventilation and pulmonary blood flow, to inspired P_{O_2}, and to other potential causes of hypoxemia already discussed.

Arterial P_{CO_2} is so sensitive to the level of ventilation that it gives little information about the extent of the ventilation-perfusion inequality. However, the most common cause of an increased P_{CO_2} in chronic lung disease is mismatching of ventilation and blood flow, as explained later in the section on ventilation-perfusion inequality and carbon dioxide retention.

Because of these limitations, the alveolar-arterial P_{O_2} difference is frequently measured and is more informative than the arterial P_{O_2} alone because it is less sensitive to the level of overall ventilation. To understand the significance of this measurement, we need to look in more detail at how gas exchange is altered by the imposition of ventilation-perfusion inequality.

Figure 10.20 shows an oxygen–carbon dioxide diagram with the same ventilation-perfusion line as that in Figure 10.17. Suppose initially that this lung has no ventilation-perfusion inequality. The P_{O_2} and P_{CO_2} of the alveolar gas and arterial blood would then be represented by point i, known as the ideal point. This is at the intersection of the gas and blood respiratory exchange ratio (R) lines; these lines indicate the possible compositions of alveolar gas and arterial blood consistent with the overall respiratory exchange ratio (carbon dioxide output/oxygen uptake) of the whole lung. In other words, a lung in which R = 0.8 would have to have its mixed alveolar gas point (A) located somewhere on the line joining points i and I. A similar statement can be made for the arterial gas point (a).

What happens to the composition of mixed alveolar gas and arterial blood as ventilation-perfusion inequality

is imposed on the lung? The answer is that both points diverge away from the ideal point (i) along the gas and blood R lines. The more extreme the degree of ventilation-perfusion inequality, the further the divergence. Moreover, the type of ventilation-perfusion inequality determines how much each point will move. For example, a distribution containing a large amount of ventilation to units with high ventilation-perfusion ratio especially moves point A down and to the right, away from point i. By the same token, a distribution containing large amounts of blood flow to units with low ventilation-perfusion ratios predominantly moves point a leftward along the blood R line.

It is clear that the horizontal distance between points A and a (i.e., the mixed alveolar-arterial P_{O_2} difference) would be a useful measure of the degree of ventilation-perfusion inequality. Unfortunately, this index is impossible to obtain in most patients because A denotes the composition of mixed expired gas, excluding the anatomic dead-space gas. In most diseased lungs the alveoli empty sequentially, with poorly ventilated alveoli emptying last, so that a post–dead-space sample is not representative of all mixed expired alveolar gas. In a few patients who have essentially uniform ventilation but uneven blood flow, this index can be used, and it is occasionally reported in patients with pulmonary embolism. In this instance, the P_{O_2} of end-tidal gas is taken to represent mixed expired alveolar gas.

Because the mixed expired alveolar P_{O_2} is usually impossible to obtain, a more useful index is the P_{O_2} difference between ideal alveolar gas and arterial blood, that is, the horizontal distance between points i and a. The ideal alveolar P_{O_2} is calculated from the full alveolar gas equation:

$$P_{AO_2} = P_{IO_2} - \frac{P_{ACO_2}}{R} + \left[P_{ACO_2} \times F_{IO_2} \times \frac{(1-R)}{R} \right] \quad \text{Eq. 19}$$

To use this equation, we assume that the P_{CO_2} of ideal alveolar gas is the same as the P_{CO_2} of arterial blood. The rationale for this is that the line along which point a moves (in Fig. 10.20) is so nearly horizontal that the value is close enough for clinical purposes. It is important to note that this ideal alveolar-arterial P_{O_2} difference is caused by units situated on the ventilation-perfusion ratio line between points i and $\bar{V}$, that is, units with abnormally low ventilation-perfusion ratios. This means that a diseased lung may have substantial ventilation-perfusion inequality but a nearly normal ideal alveolar-arterial P_{O_2} difference if most of the inequality is caused by units with abnormally high ventilation-perfusion ratios.

Physiologic shunt is another useful index of ventilation-perfusion inequality. It measures that movement of the arterial point away from the ideal point along the blood R line (see Fig. 10.20). It is therefore caused by blood flow to lung units with abnormally low ventilation-perfusion ratios. To calculate physiologic shunt, we pretend that all of the leftward movement of the arterial point a is caused by the addition of mixed venous blood $\bar{V}$ to ideal blood i. This is not so unreasonable as it might at first seem because units with very low ventilation-perfusion ratios put out blood that has essentially the same composition as that of mixed venous blood (see Figs. 10.17 and 10.18). The shunt equation is used in the following form:

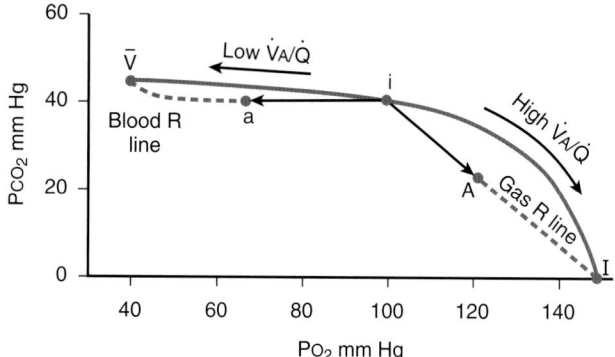

Figure 10.20 Effect of ventilation-perfusion inequality on gas exchange. Oxygen–carbon dioxide diagram showing the ideal point (i) and the points for arterial blood (a) and alveolar gas (A) (see text for details). I, inspired gas; P_{CO_2}, partial pressure of carbon dioxide; P_{O_2}, partial pressure of oxygen; Q, blood flow; R, respiratory exchange ratio; $\bar{V}$, mixed venous blood; $\dot{V}_A$, alveolar ventilation. (Modified from West JB. *Respiratory Physiology: The Essentials*. 9th ed. Baltimore: Lippincott Williams & Wilkins; 2012.)

$$\frac{\dot{Q}_{PS}}{\dot{Q}_T} = \frac{(C_{IO_2} - Ca_{O_2})}{(C_{IO_2} - C\bar{v}_{O_2})} \qquad \text{Eq. 31}$$

where $\dot{Q}_{PS}$ refers to physiologic shunt, $\dot{Q}_T$ refers to total blood flow through the lung, and C_{IO_2}, Ca_{O_2}, and $C\bar{v}_{O_2}$ refer to the oxygen content of ideal, arterial, and mixed venous blood, respectively. The oxygen content of ideal blood is calculated from the ideal P_{O_2} and the oxygen dissociation curve. The normal value for physiologic shunt as a ratio of total blood flow is less than 0.05.

The last traditional index to be discussed is physiologic dead space (also known as wasted ventilation). Whereas physiologic shunt reflects the amount of blood flow going to lung units with abnormally low ventilation-perfusion ratios, physiologic dead space is a measure of the amount of ventilation going to units with abnormally high ventilation-perfusion ratios. Thus, the two indices provide measurements of both ends of the spectrum of ventilation-perfusion ratios.

To calculate physiologic dead space, we pretend that all the movement of the alveolar point A away from the ideal point i (Fig. 10.20) is caused by the addition of inspired gas I to ideal gas. Again, this is not so unreasonable as it may first appear because units with very high ventilation-perfusion ratios behave very much like point I (see Fig. 10.20). Because, as indicated earlier, it is usually impossible to obtain a pure sample of mixed expired gas, we generally collect mixed expired gas and measure its composition, E. The mixed expired gas contains a component from anatomic dead space, which therefore moves its composition further toward point I. The Bohr equation (see Eq. 8) is then used in the form

$$\frac{V_{D_{phys}}}{V_T} = \frac{(Pa_{CO_2} - P_{ECO_2})}{Pa_{CO_2}} \qquad \text{Eq. 32}$$

where $V_{D_{phys}}$ is physiologic dead space, V_T is tidal volume, and P_{ECO_2} is mixed expired P_{CO_2}, and again we exploit the fact that the P_{CO_2} of ideal gas and that of arterial blood are virtually the same. The normal value for physiologic dead space as a ratio of total ventilation is less than 0.3. (For applications of these principles in pulmonary function testing, see Chapter 31.)

Distributions of Ventilation-Perfusion Ratios. The analysis of ventilation-perfusion inequality briefly described in the last section is sometimes known as the three-compartment model because the lung is conceptually divided into an unventilated compartment (shunt), an unperfused compartment (dead space), and a compartment that is normally ventilated and perfused (ideal). This way of looking at the diseased lung, which was introduced by Riley and Cournand,[97] has proved to be of great clinical usefulness in assessing the effects of mismatching of ventilation and blood flow.

However, it was recognized many years ago that real lungs must contain some sort of distribution of ventilation-perfusion ratios and that a three-compartment model is therefore remote from reality. Computer analysis facilitated considerable advances in the understanding of the behavior of distributions of ventilation-perfusion ratios.[100] This allowed the multiple inert gas elimination technique to become the standard research technique for measuring patterns of ventilation-perfusion distributions in normal subjects and patients with lung disease.[101]

For further discussion of measuring the distribution of ventilation-perfusion ratios by the multiple inert gas technique, see ExpertConsult.com.

DISTRIBUTION IN THE NORMAL LUNG. Figure 10.21A shows the distribution of ventilation-perfusion ratios in a 22-year-old normal volunteer derived from the multiple inert gas technique.[108] The distribution shows that the plots of both ventilation and blood flow are narrow, spanning only one decade of ventilation-perfusion ratios (i.e., from a ventilation-perfusion ratio of 0.3 to one 10 times higher, of 3). As expected, this range of ventilation-perfusion ratios is slightly greater than the regional differences, which mainly depend on gravity alone (see Fig. 10.19). However, there was essentially no ventilation or blood flow outside this range on the ventilation-perfusion ratio scale. Note also that there was no shunt, that is, blood flow to unventilated alveoli. The absence of shunt was a consistent finding in all the normal subjects studied and was initially surprising. It should be pointed out that this technique is very sensitive, in that a shunt of only 0.5% of the cardiac output approximately doubles the arterial concentration of sulfur hexafluoride. Apparently, young normal subjects are able to ventilate essentially all of their alveoli. One can conclude that bronchial and thebesian shunts are not detected by the method.

In normal subjects, the measured arterial P_{O_2} value is consistent with that modeled for a given ventilation-perfusion distribution and assuming diffusion equilibrium for oxygen. This means that ventilation-perfusion heterogeneity explains all of the difference between ideal alveolar P_{O_2} and arterial P_{O_2} in normal lungs. For example, in older normal subjects the variation of the ventilation-perfusion distribution increases, which explains the gradual fall in arterial P_{O_2} observed with aging. Ventilation-perfusion mismatching must take place between lung units perfused by vessels 150 μm in diameter or larger to have a significant effect on arterial P_{O_2}.[109] This means the functional unit of oxygen exchange in terms of ventilation-perfusion matching is the acinus, or lung units distal to a terminal bronchiole.

DISTRIBUTIONS IN LUNG DISEASE. Ventilation-perfusion relationships vary by disease state. Figure 10.21B–C and eFigure 10.5 show typical distributions of ventilation-perfusion ratios from patients with COPD, contrasting a patient with an emphysematous phenotype with a patient with a chronic bronchitis phenotype. The distribution typical of the pattern seen in patients with predominantly emphysema shows a broad bimodal distribution, with large amounts of ventilation to lung units with extremely high ventilation-perfusion ratios (alveolar dead space)[110] (see Fig. 10.21B). Note the small shunt of 0.7%. Mild hypoxemia in this patient would be explained mostly by the slight displacement of the main mode of blood flow to the left of normal. Presumably, the high ventilation-perfusion ratio mode reflects ventilation to lung units in which many capillaries have been destroyed by the emphysematous process, reducing their perfusion. Patients with COPD whose predominant lesion is severe bronchitis generally show a different pattern (see Fig. 10.21C). The main abnormality in the distribution

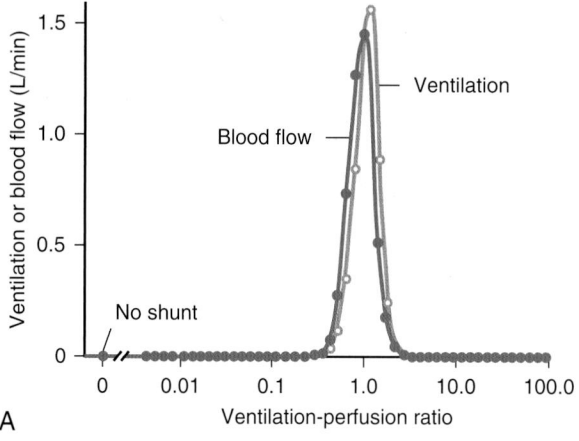

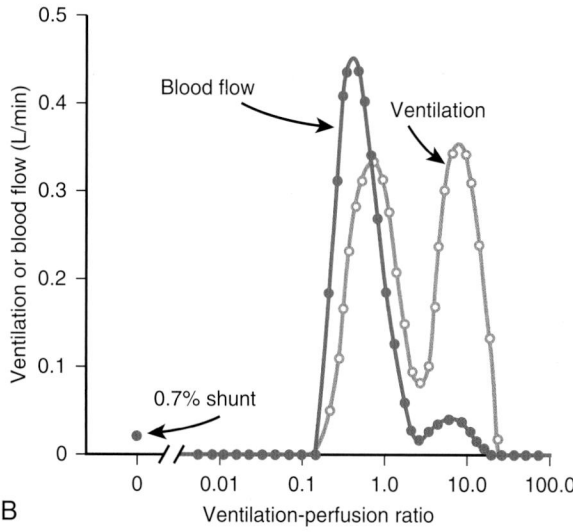

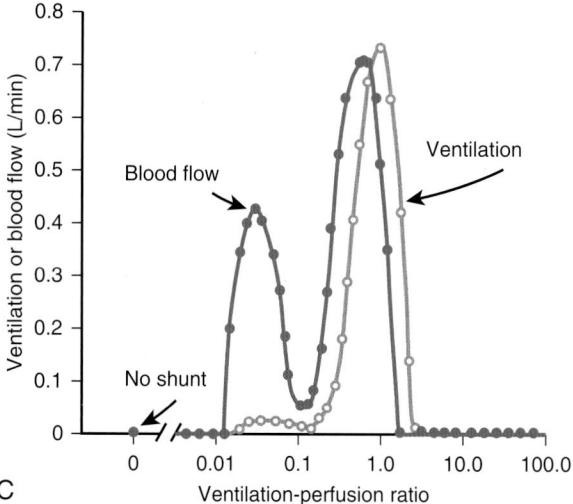

Figure 10.21 Ventilation-perfusion ratios in normal and in patients with COPD of different mechanisms. (A) In a healthy person, the distribution of ventilation (*open circles*) and perfusion (*closed circles*) is narrow, unimodal, and centered around a $\dot{V}_A/\dot{Q}$ of 1. (B) In a person with emphysema-type COPD, the ventilation distribution is bimodal, with areas of high $\dot{V}_A/\dot{Q}$ ratio. (C) In a person with bronchitis-type COPD, the perfusion distribution is bimodal, with areas of low $\dot{V}_A/\dot{Q}$. (From West JB. Causes of and compensations for hypoxemia and hypercapnia. *Compr. Physiol.* 2011;1:1541–1553.)

is a large amount of blood flow going to lung units with very low ventilation-perfusion ratios, between 0.005 and 0.1. This explains the more severe hypoxemia in this type of patient and is consistent with a large physiologic shunt. Presumably, the low ventilation-perfusion ratios in some lung units are the result of partially blocked airways due to retained secretions and airway disease that reduces airway diameter. It should be emphasized that the distributions found in severe chronic bronchitis show considerable variability.

Newer techniques are being developed to image and quantify ventilation-perfusion matching.[111–113] These have the advantage of being less invasive and may be more widely available in the future, providing the ability to detect pathologic changes earlier and to improve the understanding of subgroups of patients.

Ventilation-Perfusion Inequality and Carbon Dioxide Retention. It is important to remember that ventilation-perfusion inequality interferes with the uptake and elimination of all gases by the lung (oxygen, carbon dioxide, carbon monoxide, and anesthetic gases). In other words, mismatching of ventilation and blood flow reduces the overall gas exchange efficiency of the lung. There has been considerable confusion in this area, particularly about the role of ventilation-perfusion inequality in carbon dioxide retention.

Imagine a lung that is uniformly ventilated and perfused and that is transferring normal amounts of oxygen and carbon dioxide. Suppose that the matching of ventilation and blood flow is suddenly disturbed while everything else remains unchanged. What happens to gas exchange? It can be shown that the effect of this "pure" ventilation-perfusion inequality (i.e., with all other factors held constant) is to reduce both the oxygen uptake and carbon dioxide output of the lung.[100] The lung becomes less efficient as a gas exchanger for both gases, and therefore mismatching of ventilation and blood flow must cause hypoxemia and hypercapnia (carbon dioxide retention), other things being equal.

In practice, however, as mentioned earlier for shunt, patients with ventilation-perfusion inequality often have a normal arterial P_{CO_2}. The reason is that whenever the chemoreceptors sense a rising P_{CO_2}, there is an increase in ventilatory drive. The consequent increase in ventilation to the alveoli usually returns the arterial P_{CO_2} to normal. However, such patients can only maintain a normal P_{CO_2} at the expense of this increased ventilation to their alveoli. The ventilation in excess of what they would normally require is sometimes referred to as wasted ventilation and is necessary because the lung units with abnormally high ventilation-perfusion ratios contribute little to eliminating carbon dioxide. Such units are part of the alveolar (physiologic) dead space. Patients with ventilation-perfusion ratio inequality causing carbon dioxide retention are sometimes said to be "hypoventilating," but in fact they may actually be breathing more than normal.

Although patients with mismatched ventilation and blood flow can usually maintain a normal arterial P_{CO_2} by increasing the ventilation to the alveoli, this strategy is much less effective at increasing the arterial P_{O_2}. The reason for the different behavior of the two gases lies in the different shapes of the carbon dioxide and oxygen dissociation curves. The carbon dioxide dissociation curve is almost straight in the physiologic range, with the result that an increase in ventilation raises the carbon dioxide output of lung units with both high and low ventilation-perfusion ratios. By contrast, the nonlinearity of the oxygen dissociation curve means that not all lung units benefit from increased ventilation by increasing oxygen content in their effluent blood. Those units with high ventilation-perfusion ratios, which operate high on the flat portion of the dissociation curve, increase the oxygen content in blood very little despite large increases in PO_2. In units with a low ventilation-perfusion ratio, PO_2 in blood will increase more but some hypoxemia always remains.

In summary, carbon dioxide retention can result from two clearly distinct mechanisms: pure hypoventilation and ventilation-perfusion inequality. The latter is a common cause in clinical practice.

Effect of Changes in Cardiac Output on Gas Exchange in the Presence of Ventilation-Perfusion Inequality.

In a lung with no ventilation-perfusion inequality, the cardiac output has no effect on arterial PO_2 or PCO_2. This follows from Eqs. 4 and 16, the mass conservation equations for CO_2 and O_2, respectively, which do not contain cardiac output. By contrast, these equations show that the level of total ventilation is very important.

However, in a lung with ventilation-perfusion inequality, cardiac output can have a major effect on arterial PO_2 by altering the mixed venous PO_2, which affects the arterial PO_2 via shunts through the lung. A reduction in cardiac output reduces the PO_2 of mixed venous blood; when this venous blood transits low ventilation-perfusion regions, it exaggerates the hypoxemia. This is sometimes seen in patients with myocardial infarction, in whom the reduction in arterial PO_2 seems to be out of proportion to the degree of ventilation-perfusion inequality. The opposite is sometimes seen in patients with bronchial asthma, who may have unusually high cardiac outputs and a high mixed venous PO_2, especially when treated with some β-agonist drugs. The result is that the arterial PO_2 is higher than would be expected from the degree of ventilation-perfusion inequality. This important modulating effect of cardiac output on gas exchange is often overlooked in the clinical setting.

OXYGEN SENSING

The responses of the body to hypoxia have been greatly clarified by the discovery of *hypoxia inducible factors* (HIFs). The initial finding was of a protein that bound to the hypoxia response element of the erythropoietin gene under hypoxic conditions.[114] Later it became clear that HIFs are critically important in a large number of responses of cells to hypoxia.

More information on the physiology of hypoxia can be found at ExpertConsult.com.

Acknowledgment

We acknowledge the contributions of Frank L. Powell, PhD, and Peter D. Wagner, MD, who authored this chapter in the previous edition of this text and contributed substantially to the content.

Key Points

- The magnitudes of ventilation and perfusion, as well as their distribution, are key factors determining pulmonary gas exchange.
- Distribution of ventilation and perfusion is predominantly affected by gravity in the normal lung, but intrinsic lung structure also plays a role.
- Distribution of *ventilation-perfusion* ($\dot{V}A/\dot{Q}$) ratios is nonuniform, with the $\dot{V}A/\dot{Q}$ ratio being generally higher in nondependent lung regions and lower in dependent lung regions.
- Regional alveolar PO_2 and PCO_2 are determined principally by the $\dot{V}A/\dot{Q}$ ratio of each region. Secondary factors are the PO_2 and PCO_2 of inspired gas and of mixed venous blood and also the shape of the oxygen and carbon dioxide dissociation curves.
- There are five causes of hypoxemia: decreased inspired oxygen, hypoventilation, alveolar-capillary diffusion limitation, shunt, and $\dot{V}A/\dot{Q}$ inequality.
- There are two principal causes of hypercapnia: hypoventilation and $\dot{V}A/\dot{Q}$ inequality.
- $\dot{V}A/\dot{Q}$ inequality is the most important cause of gas exchange abnormalities in most lung diseases.

Key Readings

Barer GR, Howard P, Shaw JW. Stimulus-response curves for the pulmonary vascular bed to hypoxia and hypercapnia. *J Physiol (Lond).* 1970;211:139–155.
Frostell C, Fratacci M-D, Wain JC, et al. Inhaled nitric oxide: a selective pulmonary vasodilator reversing hypoxic pulmonary vasoconstriction. *Circulation.* 1991;83:2038–2047.
Glazier JB, Hughes JMB, Maloney JE, et al. Measurements of capillary dimensions and blood volume in rapidly frozen lungs. *J Appl Physiol.* 1969;26:65–76.
Milic-Emili J, Henderson JAM, Dolovich MB, et al. Regional distribution of inspired gas in the lungs. *J Appl Physiol.* 1966;21:749–759.
Petousi N, Talbot NP, Pavord I, Robbins PA. Measuring lung function in airways diseases: current and emerging techniques. *Thorax.* 2019;74(8):797–805.
Rahn H, Fenn WO. *A Graphical Analysis of the Respiratory Gas Exchange.* Washington, DC: American Physiological Society; 1955.
Riley RL, Cournand A. "Ideal" alveolar air and the analysis of ventilation/perfusion relationships in the lung. *J Appl Physiol.* 1949;1:825–847.
Wagner PD, Dantzker DR, Dueck R, et al. Ventilation-perfusion inequality in chronic obstructive pulmonary disease. *J Clin Invest.* 1977;59:203–216.
Wagner PD, Dantzker DR, Iacovoni VE, et al. Ventilation-perfusion inequality in asymptomatic asthma. *Am Rev Respir Dis.* 1978;118:511–524.
Wagner PD, Laravuso RB, Uhl RR, et al. Continuous distributions of ventilation-perfusion ratios in normal subjects breathing air and 100% O_2. *J Clin Invest.* 1974;54:54–68.
Wagner PD, West JB. Effects of diffusion impairment on O_2 and CO_2 time courses in pulmonary capillaries. *J Appl Physiol.* 1972;33:62–71.
West JB. *Ventilation/Blood Flow and Gas Exchange.* 5th ed. Oxford-Philadelphia:Blackwell Scientific Publications–Lippincott; 1990:1–120.
West JB. Ventilation/perfusion inequality and overall gas exchange in computer models of the lung. *Respir Physiol.* 1969;7:88–110.
West JB, Dollery CT. Distribution of blood flow in isolated lung: relation to vascular and alveolar pressures. *J Appl Physiol.* 1964;19:713–724.
West JB, Lahiri S, Gill MB, et al. Arterial oxygen saturation during exercise at high altitude. *J Appl Physiol.* 1962;17:617–621.
West JB, Mathieu-Costello O. Structure, strength, failure and remodeling of pulmonary capillaries. *Annu Rev Physiol.* 1999;61:543–572.

Complete reference list available at ExpertConsult.com.

11 RESPIRATORY SYSTEM MECHANICS AND ENERGETICS

KRISTEN M. KIDSON, MD • NAJIB T. AYAS, MD, MPH •
WILLIAM R. HENDERSON, MD, PHD

INTRODUCTION

The movement of gases in and out of the respiratory system may be described by the physical laws that govern pressure, volume, and flow of gas. The study of these relationships is called *respiratory mechanics*, and the study of the energy cost of gas movement is called *energetics*.

This chapter reviews basic terminology, respiratory mechanics under static and dynamic conditions, and energetics, including measurements of the work of breathing. The chapter also highlights how physiologic principles can be applied to specific clinical problems.

TERMINOLOGY

FLOW

Flow is defined as the volume of gas passing a fixed point per unit of time. Flow is usually measured with a pneumotachograph (flowmeter), which consists of a tube with a known fixed resistance. Flow can be calculated by measuring the pressure drop across the resistor.

Gas velocity is the distance moved by a gas molecule per unit of time and should not be confused with flow. At a constant flow, gas velocity will be greater in narrower tubes.

VOLUME

Volume is defined by the space occupied by a gas. The volume occupied by a fixed number of gas molecules is influenced by temperature and pressure.

The volume of gas entering and leaving the lung can be determined by a spirometer that measures volume displacement or by integrating the flow signal measured by a pneumotachograph. The subdivisions of lung volumes are shown in Figure 11.1 (see also Chapters 31 and 32). Some of these subdivisions can be measured by spirometry alone (vital capacity, *tidal volume* [VT]), whereas others require use of helium dilution or plethysmography. *Total lung capacity* (TLC) is the lung volume at the end of a maximal inspiration. *Residual volume* (RV) is the volume at the end of a maximal expiratory effort. *Functional residual capacity* (FRC) refers to the volume in the lung at the end of a normal tidal exhalation, where there is normally relaxation of both inspiratory and expiratory muscles.

Total gas volume in the lung is usually measured using plethysmographic methods or by inert gas dilution methods, and each of these techniques has advantages and disadvantages.[1] In body plethysmography, subjects are completely enclosed in a gas-tight container. Lung volume can be calculated by comparing changes in *alveolar pressure* (Palv) (measured at the mouth while the patient pants against an occluded mouthpiece) with changes in pressure

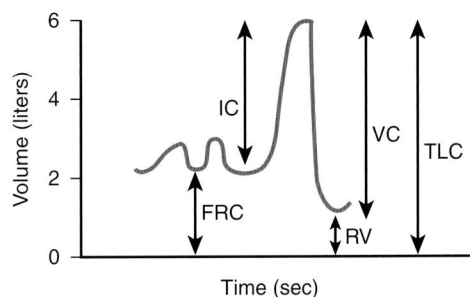

Figure 11.1 Subdivisions of lung volume. Volume-time tracing of a subject taking two normal tidal breaths, inhaling to *total lung capacity* (TLC), and exhaling to *residual volume* (RV). *Vital capacity* (VC) and *inspiratory capacity* (IC) may be measured with a spirometer. The measurement of *functional residual capacity* (FRC), RV, and TLC requires a determination of intrathoracic gas volume by helium dilution, nitrogen washout, or plethysmography.

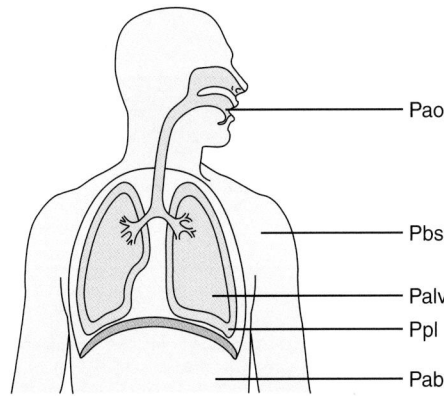

Figure 11.2 Respiratory system pressures. Pao, pressure at airway opening (mouth or nose) in spontaneously breathing patient; Pbs, pressure at body surface; Palv, pressure in alveolus; Ppl, pressure in pleural space; Pab, pressure in abdomen. Trans-pulmonary pressure: Pao − Ppl; trans-lung pressure: Palv − Ppl; trans-chest wall pressure: Ppl − Pbs; trans-respiratory system pressure: Pao − Pbs; trans-diaphragmatic pressure: Ppl − Pab. Under static conditions, when the subject is not on assisted ventilation, Pao = 0 (atmospheric pressure). However, Pao may be positive when the patient is receiving positive-pressure mechanical ventilation. Pbs is equivalent to atmospheric pressure unless the subject is in a negative-pressure device such as an iron lung.

in the container.[2] Body plethysmography is widely available and accurate but may overestimate lung volumes because it will include measurement of abdominal gas if that gas is compressed and decompressed during the panting maneuver. In addition to using body plethysmography to estimate FRC, inert gas dilution techniques or radiologic assessments can be used. Historically, inert gas methods have usually used helium. For this method, subjects at FRC inhale a known concentration and volume of helium from a bag. The helium mixes with and is diluted by gas already in the lung. A sample of exhaled gas is analyzed for helium concentration, allowing calculation of the FRC thus:

$$C_1 \times V_1 = C_2 \times (V_1 + FRC)$$

Where C_1 is the initial (known) helium concentration in the bag, C_2 is the final (measured) helium concentration, and V_1 is the initial volume of gas in the bag. Therefore:

$$FRC = [(C_1 \times V_1)/C_2] - V_1$$

By the same principle other nonrespiratory gases, such as sulfur hexafluoride, can be used to calculate FRC. In general, inert gas dilution measurements tend to underestimate total lung volume, especially in patients with substantial airway obstruction who may have gas trapped in lung units that do not mix with inspired gas.

Respiratory gases naturally present in a subject's lungs (such as nitrogen) can also be used for FRC determination. Multiple techniques have been described that rely on using nitrogen dilution or "washout." In this test, the subject breathes 100% oxygen, allowing the nitrogen in the respiratory system to "wash out." During this maneuver, the volume of expired nitrogen is calculated and is used to estimate FRC.[3] Similar to inert gas dilution measurements, the nitrogen washout technique may underestimate the lung volume in patients with obstructive lung disease.

Imaging modalities such as chest radiography, computed tomography, and magnetic resonance imaging can provide accurate assessment of FRC.[3-7] Computed tomography may overestimate the volume of alveolar gas available for gas exchange because it measures the entire volume of gas in the lung, whether or not that gas participates in gas exchange.[8] In summary, understanding the

advantages and limitations with each method is essential for appropriate interpretation of values.

PRESSURE

The pressure of a gas is generated from the momentum of molecules colliding against a surface and is expressed as the force per unit area. Pressure, as opposed to force, is the same in all directions. Respiratory system pressures are usually reported relative to atmospheric pressure.

The pressures relevant to the respiratory system are shown in Figure 11.2. Although it is possible to measure *pleural pressure* (Ppl) directly, esophageal pressure is a less invasive surrogate. Esophageal pressure may be measured using an air-filled balloon inserted into the middle third of the esophagus, approximately 35 to 45 cm from the nares.[9-11] Values obtained by esophageal balloon only reflect the pressure at one level of the lung, adjacent to the esophagus, and can be affected by movement of the neck, weight of the mediastinum from patient positioning, esophageal elastance, and the volume of air in the balloon.[12-14]

Boyle's Law

For an ideal gas at a constant temperature, the relationship between volume and pressure is described by Boyle's law:

$$P_1 \times V_1 = P_2 \times V_2$$

where P_1 is the absolute pressure of the gas and V_1 is the volume. Because the number of particles in an ideal gas remains constant, P_2 and V_2 are the resulting pressure and volume if any parameter is modified. The combined gas law describes how changes in volume of the lung alveoli (through contraction of the respiratory muscles) cause a change in pressure and thus drive ventilation. Although this equation theoretically applies only to an ideal or perfect gas, it is an adequate approximation for clinical purposes.

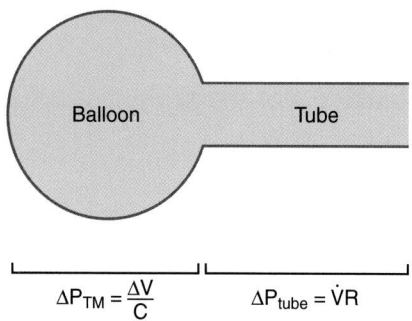

Figure 11.3 Balloon-and-tube analogy of the respiratory system. ΔP_{TM}, change in transmural pressure (inside − outside) of balloon; ΔV, change in volume; C, compliance; $\dot{V}$, flow; R, resistance; and ΔP_{tube}, pressure difference from one end of the tube to the other.

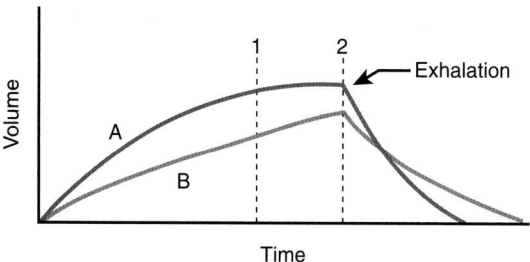

Figure 11.4 Time constants. Shown are two lung units of equal volume, one with a short time constant (A) and one with a long time constant (B). Each is inflated under a constant pressure until point 2 and then exhalation is passive. At point 2, unit A is completely filled but unit B is not. Of note, when time constants are uneven, decreasing inspiration time to point 1 will worsen heterogeneity in ventilation.

COMPLIANCE, RESISTANCE, AND TIME CONSTANTS

The respiratory system can be thought of as a combination of balloons and tubes (Fig. 11.3). As the pressure across the wall of a balloon increases (called transmural pressure, or pressure inside minus pressure outside), the volume inside the balloon increases. The ratio between the change in volume and the change in transmural pressure is the compliance of the balloon. The units of compliance are volume/pressure. A larger compliance indicates that volume changes more for every change in pressure. The inverse of compliance is elastance, with a larger elastance indicating a stiffer system.

Resistance is a measure of the pressure required to generate flow through a tube. The narrower the tube, the greater the pressure needed and the higher the resistance. The units of resistance are pressure/flow. Airway conductance, the inverse of resistance, represents the flow per unit of pressure. Assuming that all other factors are constant, a greater conductance indicates a more dilated airway.

When a pressure is applied to a lung unit (Fig. 11.4), the time required to fill the unit is dependent on its compliance and resistance. That is, it will take longer to fill if resistance is high because the flow will be low. Similarly, it will take longer to fill the unit if compliance is high because it will require more volume to reach the applied pressure. The product of the resistance and compliance of a lung unit is the time constant and represents the time required for the lung unit to fill to 63% of the final volume if a constant

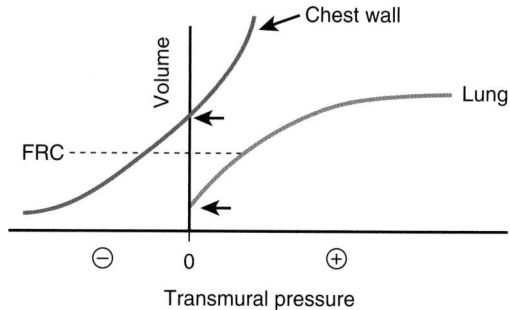

Figure 11.5 Volume-pressure curves of lung and chest wall. The relationship between transmural (inside − outside) pressure of lung and relaxed chest wall volume are shown. At *functional residual capacity* (FRC), outward chest wall recoil is balanced by inward lung recoil. At FRC, transmural pressure for the lung = Pao − Ppl; because Ppl is negative, this yields a positive value. For the chest wall, transmural pressure = Ppl − Pbs, which yields a negative value. The static equilibrium (resting volume) of the chest wall is above FRC whereas that for the lung is below FRC (*arrows*). Pbs, pressure at body surface; Pao, pressure at airway opening; Ppl, pleural pressure.

pressure is applied. Areas of the lung with small time constants (i.e., low resistance and/or low compliance) will fill more rapidly than areas with larger time constants.

This concept has clinical implications when there are heterogeneous time constants between parallel lung units, as in patients with chronic airflow obstruction or patchy alveolar edema/atelectasis as is found in *acute respiratory distress syndrome* (ARDS). As long as the respiratory rate is low, all units will fill fully. However, if the respiratory rate increases so that the inspiratory time becomes less than the time constant of some units, these units will receive less ventilation and contribute to ventilation-perfusion mismatch.

RESPIRATORY MECHANICS IN STATIC CONDITIONS

We first consider the lung during static conditions, when the respiratory system is maintained at a fixed volume with no gas flow. Even under static or no-flow conditions, pressure gradients are still required to distend the respiratory system. The energy used to distend the respiratory system during inhalation (elastic work) is stored as potential energy. Because of this stored energy, normal exhalation does not require work and is a passive process. The elastic work used to inflate the respiratory system has both lung and chest wall components.

ELASTIC RECOIL OF THE LUNGS

If removed from the body, an isolated lung will deflate to a minimal volume containing only trapped gas, due to its elastic recoil. Because airways close before complete alveolar emptying, application of a negative pressure to the airway opening will not remove the trapped gas. The relationship between lung volume and transpulmonary pressure during inflation is shown in Figure 11.5. Lung compliance is fairly high at the lung volumes associated with normal breathing, but then decreases markedly near TLC. At this volume, very large increases in transmural pressure result in small changes in volume.

Two major factors are responsible for the elastic recoil of the lung: (1) lung connective tissue and (2) surface tension related to the air-liquid interface of the alveolar surface.

Lung Connective Tissue

A network of connective tissue fibers, composed primarily of collagen and elastin, provide the framework for the alveoli and structural integrity for the lung (see also Chapter 5). Collagen fibers exhibit high tensile strength but are relatively noncompliant, whereas elastin, which has a lower tensile strength, is more compliant.[15]

At low lung volumes, elastin fibers are the major contributor to the volume-pressure relationship, facilitating lung inflation and stability, whereas collagen fibers remain curled and unstressed.[16,17] At high lung volumes, collagen fibers uncurl and straighten to have a stiffening effect on the lung. Destruction of lung connective tissue, such as from smoking-induced emphysema, can substantially increase lung compliance.[18]

Alveolar Surface Forces and Surfactant

When a lung is completely filled with water, compliance is much greater than when it is filled with air.[19] This suggests that lung elastic recoil is mostly due to surface tension at the air-liquid interface lining the alveoli rather than from elastin and collagen connective tissue fibers.

Because there are intermolecular forces of attraction between molecules of liquids, the surface of an air-liquid interface is under tension. Whereas molecules in the interior of a liquid are subjected to equal forces in all directions, molecules at the surface are pulled toward each other and pulled down by molecules below the surface. These forces, referred to as surface tension, cause a gas-filled bubble to collapse.

Because of surface tension, a positive pressure must be present to prevent the collapse of a gas-filled bubble of liquid. The pressure of gas within a bubble is related to the *surface tension* (T) and the *radius of curvature* (r) of the bubble by Laplace's law (P = 2T/r). The alveolus can be likened to a bubble with a radius of approximately 0.1 mm at FRC. If the surface tension were similar to that of water (72 mN/m), the lungs would be very noncompliant, and ventilation with transpulmonary pressures in the physiologic range (3 to 5 cm H_2O) would be impossible. Furthermore, the high surface tension would lead to alveolar instability. Smaller alveoli with smaller radii of curvature, by the nature of Laplace's law, would generate higher alveolar pressures than larger alveoli. Because gas travels from an area of higher pressure to one of lower pressure, smaller alveoli would tend to empty into larger alveoli, eventually resulting in one large air-filled alveolus.

Many factors contribute to alveolar stability in normal lungs. First, pulmonary surfactant, a mixture of lipids and proteins secreted by type 2 alveolar epithelial cells, reduces surface tension (see Chapter 3).[20] The lipid component of surfactant is amphiphilic, containing both hydrophobic and hydrophilic groups. At an air-liquid interface, the amphiphilic nature of the phospholipids creates a monolayer and displaces water molecules. The saturation of the acyl group allows the phospholipids in surfactant to form ordered monolayers and confers the ability to be compressed (during expiration), which is essential to decreasing surface tension at low lung volumes.[21] Second, alveoli

are interconnected (alveolar interdependence) by common walls and structures. Therefore, if one alveolus began to collapse, it would stretch adjacent alveolar walls, creating a tethering effect on the collapsing unit. Third, the connective tissue scaffolding limits overdistention of alveoli.

Hysteresis and Stress Adaptation

During inflation of the lung, the pressure required at any given lung volume is greater than that during deflation (Fig. 11.6). The difference between the inflation and the deflation curves is due to hysteresis and stress adaptation.

Hysteresis refers to changes in mechanical properties due to the volume history of the lung and is caused by several factors. First, the effect of surfactant on surface tension is dependent on volume history, with surfactant less effective at reducing surface tension during inspiration than during expiration. This is due to movement of surfactant molecules from below the surface of the fluid to the liquid surface during inhalation. Second, much higher pressures are required to open collapsed airways or alveoli than are required to keep them open. In disease states characterized by collapse of alveoli (e.g., ARDS), significant hysteresis of the pressure-volume curve can be seen (see Fig. 11.6) and higher inflation pressures are often required for ventilation.[22]

In contrast, *stress adaptation* refers to changes in mechanical properties over time. When lung tissue is stretched to a particular length, the tension required to maintain the length gradually diminishes due to time-dependent properties of surfactant and deformation of viscoelastic tissues of the lung. Therefore, after a sustained lung inflation, the pressure required to keep the lung at that volume will decrease.

ELASTIC RECOIL OF THE CHEST WALL

Movement of the chest wall by the muscles of ventilation generates pressure gradients between the alveoli and the surrounding air, enabling gas to be moved in and out of the lungs.

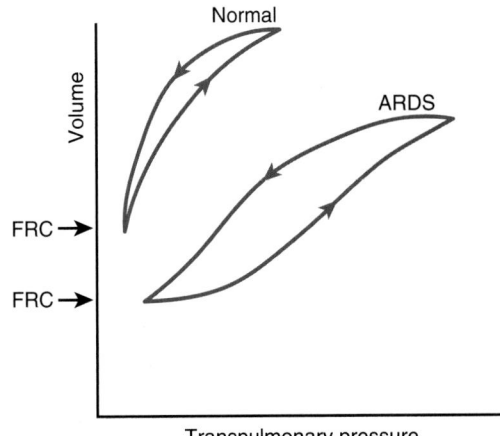

Figure 11.6 Hysteresis in a normal lung and an acutely injured lung. In *acute respiratory distress syndrome* (ARDS) the lung is stiffer than the normal lung and greater inflation pressure is required at any given lung volume. Furthermore, the degree of hysteresis is much greater in ARDS lungs, with a greater separation of the volume-pressure curves on inspiration (*upward arrow*) and exhalation (*downward arrow*). FRC, functional residual capacity.

Chest Wall Compliance

The compliance of the chest wall can be determined by measuring changes in the transmural pressure across the thorax (trans-chest wall pressure, Ppl – Pbs) relative to change in volume (see Fig. 11.5). (Body surface pressure is the pressure acting on the surface of the body, normally atmospheric pressure.) The resting volume of the relaxed chest wall is approximately 1 L above FRC. The difference between the resting volume of the chest wall and that of the lung can be appreciated in patients with a pneumothorax or pleural effusion, when the chest wall recoils outward and the lung recoils inward. When the chest wall is distended to a volume above its resting volume, the chest wall recoils inward; when it is pulled in to a volume below its resting volume, it recoils outward. The compliance of the normal chest wall is approximately 200 mL/cm H_2O, but it becomes progressively stiffer at lower lung volumes. This stiffness predominantly determines RV in normal young subjects.[23]

Factors such as severe kyphoscoliosis, skin eschars from burns, and abdominal distention may reduce chest wall compliance. Chest wall compliance is higher in the sitting position than in the supine position, but the overall effect is usually modest.[24]

INTEGRATION OF LUNG AND CHEST WALL MECHANICS

The chest wall and lung are juxtaposed and, in the absence of pleural disease (e.g., pneumothorax or pleural effusion), changes in chest wall volume are essentially identical to changes in lung volume (Fig. 11.7). An integration of lung and chest wall mechanics can be represented graphically by plotting Ppl against the relaxed volumes of the lung and chest wall (Campbell diagram) (Fig. 11.8A). These plots help to explain the determinants of the commonly measured static lung volumes. At FRC (relaxation volume), the outward recoil pressure of the chest wall is balanced by the inward recoil of the lung. The Ppl at which the recoil pressures are balanced is negative (approximately −3 to −4 cm H_2O) in

normal subjects. Changes in the compliance of the lung or chest wall may change the relaxation volume (see Fig. 11.8A).

Increases in lung compliance (e.g., due to emphysema) will tend to shift the volume-pressure curve of the lung upward and to the left. If chest wall compliance remains constant, FRC will increase. In contrast, if lung compliance is reduced (e.g., pulmonary fibrosis), the volume-pressure curve of the lung will shift downward and to the right, leading to a reduction in FRC. Similarly, changes in chest wall compliance can lead to increases or decreases in FRC. FRC is believed to represent the balance of forces in a relaxed state with no muscle activation. However, there is a reduction in FRC with paralysis compared to the relaxed state. This suggests that inspiratory muscle tone of the rib cage muscles and diaphragm may contribute to a "passive" decrease in chest wall compliance and thus to an increase in FRC.[25]

With activation of inspiratory and expiratory muscles, the configuration of the chest wall changes (Fig. 11.8B). Activation of inspiratory muscles effectively shifts the volume-pressure curve of the chest wall, so that at any given Ppl, the volume of the chest wall is increased relative to the relaxed state. The horizontal difference between the relaxed curve and the curve with inspiratory muscle activation represents the net pressure generated by the inspiratory muscles.

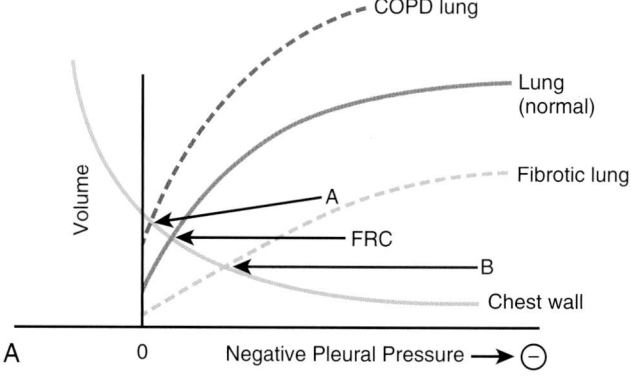

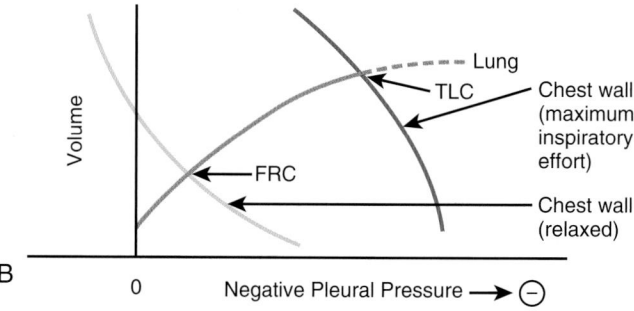

Figure 11.8 Integration of lung and chest wall mechanics. (A) Changes in lung and relaxed chest wall volumes as a function of pleural pressure (Campbell diagram). This is basically the same plot as in Figure 11.5 except that the x-axis is pleural pressure rather than transmural pressure for the lung and chest wall. The point at which the two curves meet is the *functional residual capacity* (FRC) (lung recoil balanced by chest wall recoil). If lung compliance is increased (e.g., in COPD), the point at which the two curves meet (FRC) is greater (point A). In contrast, if lung compliance is reduced (e.g., in pulmonary fibrosis), the point at which the two curves meet is less (point B). (B) Maximal inspiratory effort (Campbell diagram). With maximal inspiratory effort, the volume-pressure curve of the chest wall moves to the right. The point at which there is intersection of this curve and the lung volume-pressure curve is the *total lung capacity* (TLC).

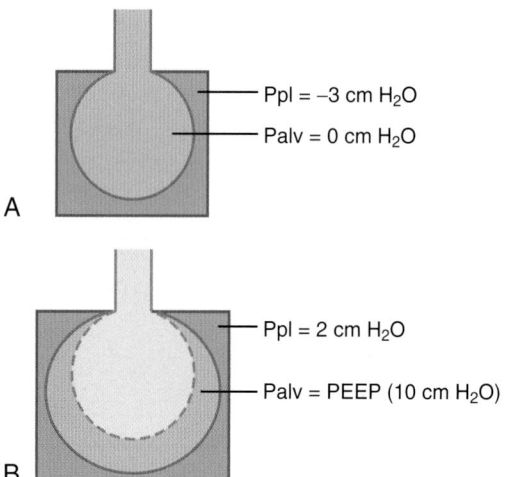

Figure 11.7 Changes in *pleural pressure* (Ppl) with applied *positive end-expiratory pressure* (PEEP). (A) Shown is a lung at end-exhalation with no PEEP. (B) With the application of PEEP, there is an increase in the volume of the respiratory system (lung and chest wall) and an increase in Ppl. The magnitude of the increase in Ppl is dependent on the relative compliances of the lung and chest wall. Palv, pressure in alveolus.

TLC is determined by the balance between inward lung recoil plus the inward chest wall recoil and the strength of the inspiratory muscles. However, in normal subjects, TLC is predominantly determined by the increased stiffness of the lung at high lung volume, rather than the recoil of the chest wall or respiratory muscle strength.[26] In support of this concept, inspiratory muscle training in normal subjects increases strength substantially (55% increase in maximal inspiratory pressure) but results in a very modest change in TLC and vital capacity (about 4%).[27] The situation in patients with neuromuscular disease is very different; in such individuals, reduced TLC is largely due to respiratory muscle weakness and can be improved to some extent by inspiratory muscle training.[28]

Activation of expiratory muscles shifts the volume-pressure curve of the chest wall in the other direction, and the degree of shift is a measure of the net pressure exerted by the expiratory muscles. In young subjects, RV is determined by the balance of static forces among the outward recoil of the chest wall, inward lung recoil (small component), and expiratory muscle strength.[26] In older subjects or patients with obstructive lung disease, RV is determined by gas trapping during airway closure upon exhalation before a static balance is achieved.[26]

Calculation of Total Respiratory System Compliance from Lung and Chest Wall Compliance

Mechanical properties of the lungs can be compared to a Newtonian model, which consists of a resistor and capacitor. Airway resistance acts as the resistor and respiratory compliance acts as the capacitor. Because the two components of the respiratory compliance, the chest wall and lung, are arranged in series, the relationship between total *respiratory system compliance* (C_{RS}), *lung compliance* (C_L), and *chest wall compliance* (C_W) is:

$$1/C_{RS} = 1/C_L + 1/C_W$$

Alternatively, because elastance = 1/compliance,

$$Elastance_{RS} = Elastance_L + Elastance_W$$

For example, in a supine paralyzed subject, lung compliance is approximately 150 mL/cm H_2O pressure and chest wall compliance is approximately 200 mL/cm H_2O pressure[29]; the calculated compliance of the respiratory system would thus be approximately:

$$1/(1/150 + 1/200) = 85.7 \text{ mL/cmH}_2O$$

CLINICAL APPLICATIONS

Positive End-Expiratory Pressure and its Impact on Pleural Pressure

Patients with diseases that decrease lung compliance receive positive-pressure mechanical ventilation to maintain positive pressure at the end of exhalation to prevent alveolar collapse.[30] Some—but not all—of this *positive end-expiratory pressure* (PEEP) is transmitted from the alveolar space to the pleural space (see Fig. 11.7B). During mechanical ventilation, changes in both Ppl and transpulmonary pressure depend on the relationships between the *elastance*

of the chest wall (E_W), *elastance of the lung* (E_L) and *elastance of the total respiratory system* (E_{RS}, the sum of E_W and E_L), a relationship that can be described by the equation:

$$\Delta Ppl = \Delta Paw \times E_W / E_{RS}$$

where *Paw* represents the airway pressure at the end of the endotracheal tube in a mechanically ventilated patient. In healthy individuals, E_W and E_L are approximately equal, and E_W/E_{RS} has a value of approximately 0.5, within the range of normal ventilation.[31] In this situation, it is reasonable to infer the value of Ppl from Paw. However, in disease, both E_W and E_L demonstrate great variability, so that the ratio of E_W to E_{RS} is unpredictable.[32] In this situation, Ppl cannot be assumed to be directly related to Paw.[33] If lung compliance is much greater than chest wall compliance (e.g., in a patient with emphysema and kyphoscoliosis), a greater proportion of PEEP will be transmitted to the pleural space. In healthy individuals, as described, the chest wall and lung compliances are equal and thus the increase in Ppl is roughly equal to one-half of the applied PEEP (e.g., 5 cm H_2O pressure if the PEEP is 10 H_2O pressure). In contrast, if lung compliance is low and chest wall compliance is high (as in thin patient with severe ARDS), very little of the Palv will be transmitted to the pleural space, and thus Ppl will change minimally with PEEP.

PEEP has two major benefits. PEEP helps to recruit alveolar units and thereby improves ventilation-perfusion mismatch and gas exchange by reducing atelectasis. PEEP also helps reduce the shear stress of repeated alveolar opening and closing (atelectrauma), which can contribute to lung injury.[34] While the addition of PEEP may be beneficial to alveolar recruitment, the amount of PEEP transmitted to each alveolar unit may not be homogenous in disease states (see "PEEP Optimization and Recruitment Maneuvers" later).

PEEP has a number of adverse consequences. First, if PEEP increases Ppl, that can lead to an increase in pericardial pressure and reduce venous return and cardiac output.[35] Second, if PEEP increases Ppl, this will increase central venous pressure and pulmonary artery occlusion pressure to a similar magnitude, which, if not taken into account, may result in errors when using these parameters to asses intravascular volume status. Finally, PEEP acts as an inspiratory threshold load requiring inspiratory muscles to counteract this intrinsic PEEP (see later) to generate airflow.

Plateau Pressures in Patients Receiving Positive-Pressure Mechanical Ventilation

In patients receiving positive-pressure mechanical ventilation, the *plateau pressure* (Pplat) is the distending pressure of the respiratory system at end inspiration when there is no flow. When possible, Pplat should be limited to a maximum of 30 to 35 cm H_2O because higher pressures can damage the lung through overdistention. At TLC in a normal subject, the distending pressure across the lung (Palv − Ppl) is approximately 35 cm H_2O.[36] Therefore, limiting Pplat to less than 35 cm H_2O should limit lung expansion to below TLC and avoid overdistention. Avoiding high Pplat may be even more important in settings where the lung parenchyma is not homogenous because highly compliant lung units may be more at risk of overdistension than less compliant lung units. The use of low V_T during mechanical ventilation for ARDS has led to improved clinical outcomes, presumably due to decreased alveolar distension and volutrauma, the term referring to injury caused by overdistention of alveoli.[37,38]

During mechanical ventilation, Pplat is often used as a surrogate for transpulmonary pressure (pressure used to distend the lung), when it is actually a measure of transrespiratory system pressure (pressure used to distend both the lung and chest wall). When lung compliance is much less than chest wall compliance (i.e., the lung is quite stiff), this is a reasonable assumption, because during mechanical ventilation most of the pressure will be used to distend the lung, not the chest wall. However, in conditions in which the chest wall is stiff (e.g., obesity, ascites, kyphoscoliosis), Pplat may substantially overestimate the distending pressure of the lung.[39]

Esophageal manometry can be used to separate the contributions of airway pressure into the components that distend the lung (transpulmonary pressure = Paw – Ppl) or chest wall (Ppl). A small air-filled balloon is placed in the midesophagus and attached to a pressure transducer. Assuming that the pressure surrounding the esophagus is properly transmitted, the *esophageal balloon pressure* (Pes) can be used as a surrogate to estimate Ppl at end inspiration.[12] In a mechanically ventilated patient on volume-control mode, Paw is equal to Pplat at end-inspiration. Consider a ventilated patient who develops ascites. In order to maintain the transpulmonary pressure, the increase in Ppl (as measured by Pes) would be matched by an increase in Pplat. In this example, the increase in Pplat is related to reduced chest wall compliance from ascites. An increase in Pplat as in this example may be less injurious to the lung than in a patient with the same Pplat but low Ppl (see later discussion on driving pressure). Thus, the esophageal balloon can provide clinically useful measurements. However, there are limitations to the use of esophageal balloons, including movement of the balloon, inadequate inflation, and patient positioning.[12–14]

STRESS AND STRAIN

A discussion of the mechanics of stress and strain is available at ExpertConsult.com.

THE RESPIRATORY SYSTEM IN DYNAMIC CONDITIONS

The work to distend the chest wall and lung during inhalation is stored as potential energy (elastic work). Work also must be done to overcome the inertia of the gas (which is negligible when breathing air at normal breathing frequency and atmospheric pressures) and nonelastic resistance (resistive work), which cannot be stored but is dissipated as heat. Resistive work has two components that must be considered.

RESISTIVE WORK DUE TO GAS FLOW THROUGH AIRWAYS

When gas flows through an airway, frictional and viscous forces cause energy loss and a pressure drop along the airway. The extent of this pressure drop is dependent on the resistance to gas flow, physical properties of the gas (e.g., density and viscosity), and the nature of flow (laminar versus turbulent).

Laminar versus Turbulent Flow

The pressure drop due to friction is lowest with pure laminar flow, in which gas molecules travel in a straight line. The velocity profile of the gas is parabolic, with the molecules closer to the wall traveling slower than molecules in the center of the airway. When gas flow is laminar, the flow is proportional to the pressure gradient (ΔP) along the airway and inversely proportional to resistance (R).

$$\text{Flow} = \Delta P / R$$

For a straight airway under conditions of laminar flow, resistance of a tube is related to viscosity, length, and radius of the tube by the Poiseuille equation:

$$\text{Flow} = \frac{\pi \times \text{radius}^4 \times \Delta P}{8 \times \text{length} \times \text{viscosity}}$$

Because of this relationship, flow through a tube is dramatically affected by even small changes in tube diameter (i.e., reducing the radius by half causes a 16-fold decrease in gas flow). If the dimensions of a tube are held constant, the most important variable in determining laminar gas flow is viscosity.

In turbulent flow, the orderly movement of gas molecules becomes haphazard. When gas flow is turbulent, the flow is proportional to the square root of the pressure gradient (as opposed to a linear relationship seen with laminar flow)[43]:

$$\text{Flow} = \text{constant} \times (\Delta P)^{1/2}$$

Because resistance is defined as the pressure gradient divided by the flow rate, the "resistance" for turbulent flow is not constant but increases in proportion to flow. In contrast to laminar flow, turbulent flow differs in that (1) a higher ΔP is required for gas flow, (2) gas flow depends on gas density, not viscosity, and (3) ΔP is proportional to the fifth power of the radius of the airway.

Reynolds Number

The Reynolds number is a dimensionless coefficient that predicts whether flow through an unbranched tube will be predominantly laminar, turbulent, or mixed. The equation is as follows:

$$Re = \rho DV / \mu$$

where ρ is the gas density, D is the diameter of the airway, V is the mean gas velocity, and μ is the viscosity. In general, a Reynolds number of less than 2000 is associated with laminar flow, whereas a value greater than 4000 is associated with predominantly turbulent flow. Intermediate values are associated with mixed flow patterns. Increased gas density, increased gas velocity, and increased tube diameter predispose to turbulent flow.[43]

Air flow through the airways of the lung is more complex than flow through theoretical tubes. The cross-sectional diameter of a small peripheral airway (e.g., bronchiole) is much smaller than that of a central airway (e.g., trachea). However, because of the greater number of peripheral airways, the sum of the entire cross-sectional area of the peripheral airways greatly exceeds that of the central airways. Therefore, as gas moves from the peripheral to the central airways during exhalation, the gas velocity increases. The different flow rates along the airways results in predominantly laminar flow in the periphery and turbulent flow in the larger central airways (except at very low flow rates).

Clinical Effects of Heliox

Heliox is a mixture of oxygen and helium. Heliox has a density less than air because helium has a lower density than the nitrogen it replaces. For instance, a mixture of 20% oxygen and 80% helium has a density of 0.33 relative to air.[44] In patients who have upper airway narrowing (e.g., partial tracheal obstruction),[45] substituting heliox for air reduces gas density, lowers the Reynolds number, and helps to convert turbulent to laminar flow. This reduces the pressure required to move gas and diminishes the work of breathing, unloading the respiratory muscles. Heliox may be useful in patients with asthma or COPD, although this is controversial due to mixed clinical results.[46–48] The clinical benefit of heliox is lost when the gas mixture contains less than 70% helium; thus heliox is not a good option for patients who require more than 30% oxygen supplementation.

Flow Limitation

In a normal subject, increasing expiratory effort will increase air flow until a threshold is reached. Once this effort threshold is exceeded, expiratory flow will not increase with a further increase in effort, resulting in flow limitation (Fig. 11.9).[49] In contrast, patients with very poor effort or marked expiratory muscle weakness may be unable to generate sufficient expiratory pressures to reach flow limitation. If maximum flow was not relatively effort independent, measures such as forced expiratory volume in 1 second would have little utility in monitoring patients because variable effort would result in poorly reproducible results.

The concept of expiratory flow limitation is important and relates to the properties of the airways. For simplicity, the airways are often likened to a rigid tube but, in reality,

the airways are partially collapsible. During inhalation, Ppl is negative, and the intrathoracic airways tend to be pulled open. During forced exhalation, Ppl becomes positive, increasing pressure around the intrathoracic airways and predisposing to their collapse.

Several theories have been developed to explain the limitation of flow on expiration, by which a maximal flow cannot be increased even with increasing effort. These theories include the equal pressure point theory, the Bernoulli effect, and the wave speed theory.

Equal Pressure Point Theory. Consider the respiratory system depicted as a balloon (lung) inside a box (chest wall) connected by a tube that extends through the box (intrathoracic airway) (Fig. 11.10). The pressure inside the lung is equal to the Ppl (created by expiratory muscle activation) plus the recoil pressure of the lung. As air travels down the airway, pressure in the airway decreases, predominantly due to frictional losses. A point is eventually reached where the Ppl in the box is equivalent to the pressure inside the tube, termed the *equal pressure point* (EPP).[50,51] Downstream (mouthward) of this EPP, the pressure outside the airway exceeds the pressure within the airway, and the airway tends to collapse. Further increases in effort increase Ppl, but this simply causes greater narrowing of the airway downstream of the EPP so that flow remains constant. Under these conditions, the airway acts as a Starling resistor; flow is now not proportional to the difference between Palv and mouth pressure, but rather is proportional to the difference between Palv and pressure at the EPP. In this case, the pressures downstream from the EPP have no effect on expiratory flow.

This concept can be mathematically expressed as follows:

Because

$$Palv = Ppl + Lung\ recoil\ pressure$$

and

$$Pressure\ at\ EPP = Ppl$$

and

$$Driving\ pressure = Palv - Pressure\ at\ EPP$$

therefore

$$Driving\ pressure = Lung\ recoil\ pressure$$

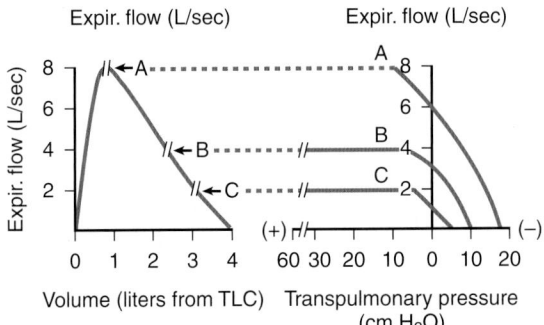

Figure 11.9 Expiratory flow limitation. *Left,* The expiratory flow volume curve for a normal subject. Maximal flow rates are plotted against their corresponding volumes at A, B, and C and define the maximal expiratory flow-volume curve. *Right,* Three isovolume pressure-flow curves for the same subject. Once a threshold transpulmonary pressure is achieved, no increase in flow is seen. (From Hyatt RE. Forced expiration. In: Macklem PT, Mead J, eds. *Handbook of Physiology. Section 3. The Respiratory System. Vol III: Mechanics of Breathing [part 1].* Bethesda, MD: American Physiological Society; 1986:295–314.)

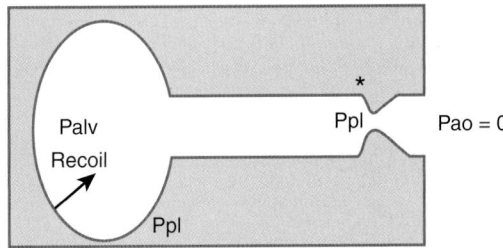

Figure 11.10 Equal pressure point theory. At the *equal pressure point* (EPP; asterisk), pressure inside the tube is equal to the pressure outside the tube (pleural pressure, Ppl) due to pressure drop related to flow-resistive losses from alveolus to the asterisk. Downstream (mouthward) from the EPP, the airway is compressed. Once an EPP develops, increasing expiratory effort, although increasing the *alveolar pressure* (Palv), also increases the downstream compression and causes no increase in flow. Pao, airway opening pressure.

Therefore, further increases in effort will increase both Palv and pressure at the EPP equally, resulting in no difference in driving pressure and airflow.

The Bernoulli Effect and Wave Speed Theory. The Bernoulli effect provides an alternative explanation for flow limitation.[52] As gas flows through a tube, the intraluminal pressure decreases, and the lateral pressure exerted by the gas is less than the pressure driving flow by an amount proportional to the velocity of the gas. If the tube is collapsible, as gas velocity increases, there is a tendency for the tube to collapse, leading to a reduction in airflow.

The wave speed theory is yet another explanation for expiratory flow limitation.[53] When fluid is pushed through a collapsible tube, a pressure wave is propagated along the wall of the tube. The speed of this pressure wave is dependent on the characteristics of the tube and the density of the gas rather than the driving pressure. The velocity of the gas in the tube cannot exceed the velocity of the pressure wave; thus the velocity of this wave represents a "speed limit" for the gas in the tube.

Interestingly, the maximal flow of gas derived using the Bernoulli effect and wave speed theory are identical, as shown by the following formula:

$$\text{Maximal flow} = A \sqrt{\left(\frac{A}{\text{gas density}}\right) \times \frac{dP}{dA}}$$

where A represents the cross-sectional area of the airway wall and dP/dA represents the slope of the relationship between changes in transmural pressure of the tube and changes in tube area. Therefore, maximal flow should increase if the tube area increases, gas density decreases, or tube stiffness increases.

Different mechanisms for flow limitation may predominate at different lung volumes. As lung volume increases, there is a proportional decrease in airway resistance and an increase in volume of the airways. Air flow in larger airways is often turbulent and is affected by changes in gas density, not viscosity (see earlier discussion of laminar versus turbulent flow). At high lung volumes, the Bernoulli effect may be more important in flow limitation because it is also related to gas density. Conversely, flow in smaller airways is laminar and influenced by gas viscosity, not density. Thus at low lung volumes, the wave speed effect may be less significant, whereas the EPP mechanism may be more important in determining flow limitation.[54]

OTHER RESISTIVE WORK

Besides the elastic work done by the respiratory muscles on the lung and chest wall, an additional component of work is expended to overcome what is sometimes called "tissue resistance." This is energy required to distort the lung and chest wall during inhalation and is dissipated as heat.

Equation of Motion

During ventilation, gas moves down a pressure gradient (ΔP). This pressure difference must be created by either the patient's own muscular efforts (Pmus) or a mechanical ventilator (Paw). The energy loss represented by this pressure drop is used to overcome resistance to airflow and tissue deformation, to expand the lungs and chest wall, and to

overcome gas inertance (resistance to changes in velocity or direction of gas flow). The first-order linear equation of motion describes the relationship between these variables as:

$$\Delta P = Paw + Pmus = \left(\dot{V} \times R\right) + V_T/C + \left(I \times \ddot{V}\right) + \left(PEEPi + PEEPset\right)$$

The work done to overcome airflow and tissue resistance is represented by $\left(\dot{V} \times R\right)$, where $\dot{V}$ is gas flow and R is resistance; the work done to expand the respiratory system is represented by V_T/C, where V_T is tidal volume and C is compliance; and the work done to overcome gas inertance is represented by $\left(I \times \ddot{V}\right)$ where I represents inertance and $\ddot{V}$ represents acceleration of gas flow. *PEEPi* represents intrinsic PEEP above PEEPset, and *PEEPset* represents PEEP provided by the ventilator. In most practical situations involving adults, inertance is ignored because it makes such a small contribution to work.

INTRINSIC PEEP DURING POSITIVE-PRESSURE VENTILATION OF COPD

An appreciation of the dynamics of the respiratory system aids in understanding clinical scenarios, such as for patients with COPD who are treated with positive-pressure ventilation for respiratory failure. Because lung resistance and compliance are variable in these patients, heterogeneity of time constants will result in variable emptying times. If insufficient time is allowed for complete emptying of lung units, the result will be a positive mean Palv in the alveoli at the end of exhalation or *intrinsic PEEP* (PEEPi; also known as auto-PEEP). High end-expiratory Palv acts as an inspiratory threshold load. In order to generate a negative pressure great enough to trigger the ventilator and initiate inspiratory flow, the inspiratory respiratory muscles must exert adequate pressure to counteract the PEEPi and reduce Palv to a subatmospheric value before inspiratory flow can be initiated.[55] PEEPi can also develop in the absence of airflow obstruction if the expiratory time is too short (e.g., in the setting of high minute ventilation).

As mentioned, high PEEPi may lead to inspiratory efforts that are ineffective in triggering the ventilator if the respiratory muscles cannot reduce Palv to less than the applied PEEP (Fig. 11.11).[56] This may lead to patient

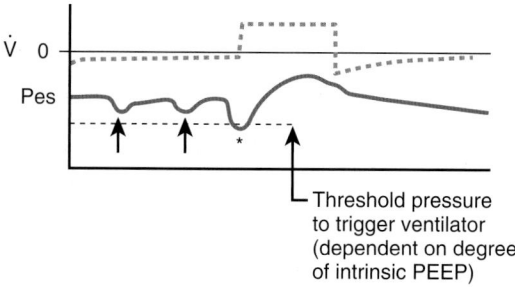

Figure 11.11 Failure to trigger the ventilator in a COPD patient. Graph of flow (V̇) and esophageal pressure (Pes) over time in a patient with COPD and intrinsic positive end-expiratory pressure receiving positive-pressure mechanical ventilation. The patient has made two attempts (*up arrows*) at triggering inspiration but could not due to the positive end-expiratory alveolar pressure. When pleural pressure is sufficiently negative to exceed the ventilator's threshold (*dotted line*), this triggers the ventilator (asterisk) and a breath is provided. Note the failure of expiratory flow to reach 0 prior to a triggered breath.

ventilator dysynchrony and places the inspiratory muscles at a mechanical disadvantage,[57] which can lead to failure of weaning from mechanical ventilation.

Management of PEEPi should include treatment of the underlying contributing disorder, such as an acute COPD or asthma exacerbation, as well as efforts to decrease minute ventilation and ventilator maneuvers to increase expiratory time. In patients with expiratory flow limitation, dynamic airway collapse acts as an equal pressure point causing flow limitation and an inability to increase expiratory flow at end-expiration (see earlier discussion on flow limitation). Increasing expiratory effort raises pleural and alveolar pressure but does not improve expiratory air flow. If a patient is unable to expire to FRC because of flow limitation, end-expiratory lung volume increases and leads to dynamic hyperinflation, or PEEPi.

If expiratory flow limitation results in the development of PEEPi, then increasing PEEPset to match the PEEPi should decrease the gradient between the mouth and alveoli at end-expiration (i.e., the inspiratory threshold load). This may improve ventilator synchrony.[58] Pressures downstream from the equal pressure point will not have any effect on expiratory flow, thus the application of PEEPset will not produce further hyperinflation or reduce the expiratory flow if the PEEPset is less than or equal to the PEEPi.[59]

Conversely, PEEPi may not be due to expiratory flow limitation, for example at very high respiratory rates, if the lungs simply do not have enough time to empty to FRC. In this instance, there is still a pressure difference between the mouth and alveoli to allow for expiratory flow. If PEEPi is present, without evidence of expiratory flow limitation, additional application of PEEP will worsen respiratory mechanics.[60]

The end-expiratory occlusion method is commonly used to measure static PEEPi (Fig. 11.12A). The expiratory line in the ventilator is occluded at the end of an exhalation; with flow now at zero, the pressure can be measured.[60] If PEEPi is present, Paw will increase until a plateau is reached, usually in 2 to 4 seconds. Given sufficient time for lung units to equilibrate, this represents the "average" measure of PEEPi because volume will redistribute from some alveoli to others depending on regional compliance.

Alternatively, PEEPi can be measured under dynamic conditions. This can be done by determining the change in pressure required to initiate lung inflation, or the difference between Paw at zero flow and at end-expiratory pressure. Dynamic PEEPi, which is measured just prior to the initiation of inspiratory flow, is usually less than that measured under static conditions, that is, at end-expiration. Inspiratory flow starts when airway pressure exceeds end-expiratory alveolar pressure; air flows first to the lung regions with the shortest time constants. Dynamic PEEPi therefore corresponds to the lowest PEEPi in regional lung tissue with the shortest time constants as opposed to the average amount of PEEPi.[60]

PEEPi is not limited to patients on mechanical ventilation. Spontaneously breathing patients who have COPD can develop PEEPi, especially when they increase their inspiratory rate during exertion, a phenomenon that has been termed dynamic hyperinflation. PEEPi and hyperinflation increases the work of breathing (see later) and contributes to exercise limitation in these patients.

MEASUREMENT OF STATIC COMPLIANCE AND RESISTANCE DURING MECHANICAL VENTILATION

In the intensive care unit, measurement of respiratory system compliance and resistance can be helpful in assessing weaning from mechanical ventilation. Normal C_{RS} in a supine subject is approximately 100 mL/cm H_2O. A markedly decreased compliance should prompt a search for causes of reduced C_L (e.g., edema) and/or Cw (e.g., abdominal distention) that might be potentially reversible. Similarly, a markedly increased resistance should prompt a search for reversible causes, including bronchospasm, or partial obstruction of the endotracheal tube from kinking or secretions.

Calculation of compliance and resistance should be performed with a square wave flow pattern after an inspiratory pause. Patients need to be relaxed or paralyzed to obtain accurate measurements. If respiratory efforts are present, Paw may not reflect transmural pressures across the respiratory system.

Consider a paralyzed sedated patient treated with positive-pressure mechanical ventilation in the assist-control mode. The changes in flow, volume, and pressure over time are shown in Figure 11.12B. Assume a constant inspiratory flow rate (1 L/sec) and a VT of 500 mL (0.5 sec inspiratory time). Because flow is constant, volume increases linearly over time. Peak pressure is 40 cm H_2O, Pplat is 35 cm H_2O, and PEEP is set at 5 cm H_2O.

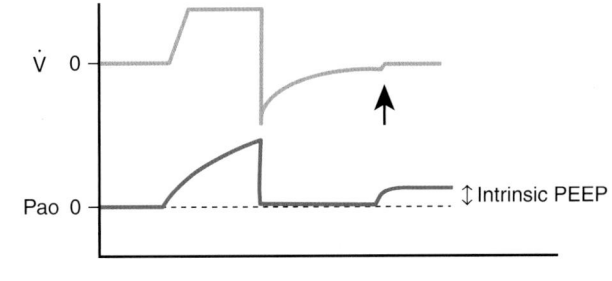

A

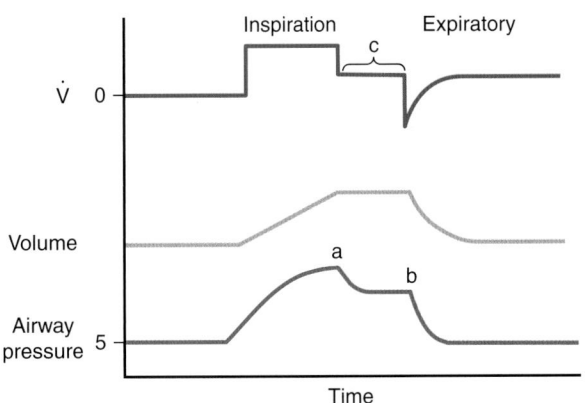

B

Figure 11.12 Pressures measured in a patient on mechanical ventilation. (A) Measurement of intrinsic *positive end-expiratory pressure* (PEEP), flow (V) and airway pressure over time. *Arrow* represents the point at which the expiratory line is occluded, leading to an increase in measured pressure that represents the degree of intrinsic PEEP. (B) Ventilator mechanics. Point a is the peak pressure (40 cm H_2O). Point b is the plateau pressure (35 cm H_2O). The bracket at *c* indicates the inspiratory pause.

Using the balloon and tube analogy of the respiratory system (see Fig. 11.3), the components of pressure required to ventilate are as follows:

$$\text{Total pressure} = \text{Pressure to distend respiratory system} \\ + \text{Pressure to maintain gas flow} \\ + \text{Inertial pressure losses}$$

Because the inertial component can be ignored at the respiratory rates commonly used:

$$\text{Total pressure} = \text{Pressure to distend respiratory system} \\ + \text{Pressure to maintain gas flow} \\ = \Delta\,\text{Volume/compliance} \\ + \text{Flow} \times \text{resistance}$$

The difference between Pplat (measured during an inspiratory hold) and PEEP represents the pressure required to distend the respiratory system at 0 flow.

Therefore,

$$\text{Pplat} - \text{PEEP} = \Delta\text{Volume/Compliance} + \text{Flow} \times \text{Resistance}$$

Because flow = 0, rearranging the equation yields:

$$\text{Compliance} = \Delta\text{Volume/(Pplat} - \text{PEEP)} \qquad [1]$$

The difference between peak pressure (a) and Pplat (b) represents the pressure required to overcome resistance of the respiratory system. This predominantly represents flow resistance, but also includes contributions from tissue resistance, stress relaxation, and time constant heterogeneity within the lung (i.e., pendelluft). Therefore,

$$\text{Peak pressure} - \text{PEEP} = \Delta\text{Volume/Compliance} \\ + \text{Flow} \times \text{Resistance} \qquad [2]$$

Rearranging Equations 1 and 2:

$$\text{Peak pressure} - \text{Pplat} = \text{Flow} \times \text{Resistance}$$

Because flow is known:

$$\text{Resistance} = (\text{Peak pressure} - \text{Pplat})/\text{Flow}$$

Going back to the patient:

$$\text{Compliance} = 500\text{ mL}/(30\text{ cm H}_2\text{O}) = 16.7\text{ mL/cmH}_2\text{O}$$

$$\text{Resistance} = \frac{40 - 35\text{ cm H}_2\text{O}}{1\text{ L/sec}} = 5\text{ cm H}_2\text{O/L/sec}$$

In other words, the patient's resistance is relatively low but the compliance is severely reduced, suggesting an extremely stiff respiratory system (as mentioned above, normal respiratory system compliance in a supine subject is approximately 100 mL/cm H$_2$O).

RESPIRATORY MECHANICS IN ARDS

ARDS is an inflammatory disease state resulting in heterogenous parenchymal changes, poorly compliant lung units, a reduction in FRC from atelectasis, and shunting from airspace filling resulting in profound hypoxemia.[61] In order to maintain viable gas exchange, mechanical ventilation is required, but it is associated with potential for *ventilator-induced lung injury* (VILI).[62]

Conceptually, the term *baby lung* has been coined to reflect the small volume of lung parenchyma relatively spared from disease which demonstrates relatively normal mechanics.[63] Although the mechanics of this small lung may be normal, the potential for VILI is possible if it is inadvertently ventilated with high volumes (see later). Lung injury is also possible because aerated lung in ARDS demonstrates altered permeability and susceptibility to inflammation. The use of lung protective ventilation in ARDS is predominantly to spare the baby lung from additional injury while maintaining adequate gas exchange (see Chapter 135 for more details).

PEEP OPTIMIZATION AND RECRUITMENT MANEUVERS

At low lung volumes, atelectrauma and repetitive sheer forces from recruitment-derecruitment likely contribute to VILI.[64] In patients with recruitable lung, PEEP can improve oxygenation and promote homogenous ventilation by preventing alveolar collapse.[65] Esophageal pressure is a surrogate for Ppl and has been used to separate contributions of the lung and chest wall to the reduced respiratory system compliance in ARDS patients.[66] While PEEP titrated by use of an esophageal balloon has been shown to improve oxygenation, a recent study found no difference in death or ventilator-free days in ARDS patients when esophageal balloon-titrated PEEP was compared to PEEP titrated according to FiO$_2$.[67]

Trials examining low versus high levels of PEEP in ARDS have failed to show improvements in mortality, possibly due to unrecognized variation in the amount of recruitable lung.[30,68–70] Previously collapsed alveoli may become newly recruited, whereas PEEP applied to previously functional alveoli may cause added stress and strain.[65] The degree of recruitment or overdistention could be assessed by the stress index.

STRESS INDEX

A discussion of the stress index is available at ExpertConsult.com.

RECRUITMENT MANEUVERS IN ARDS

ARDS is also thought to lead to surfactant dysfunction. The dysfunction of surfactant increases surface tension at the air-liquid interface of the alveoli, leading to collapse, intrapulmonary shunting, and hypoxemia.[74]

Recruitment maneuvers with high pressure to open alveoli have been used in ventilated patients with ARDS who remain hypoxemic despite moderate levels of PEEP.[75–79] A recruitment maneuver consists of a sustained inflation at a constant high pressure, which opens collapsed alveoli. Because closing pressures are much less than opening pressures, the alveoli stay open (at least temporarily) after the sustained inflation is ended as long as the lung is not allowed to return to a low volume. Although recruitment maneuvers may be useful at treating hypoxemia, frequent and aggressive recruitment with high PEEP has led to respiratory and hemodynamic complications.[80]

VENTILATING ARDS USING PLATEAU PRESSURE, TIDAL VOLUME, AND DRIVING PRESSURE

A landmark study in ARDS concluded that lung protective ventilation using small V_T (6 mL/kg predicted body weight) and minimizing Pplat (<30 cm H_2O) improved clinical outcomes, presumably due to decreased alveolar distention and volutrauma of the more normal areas of lung (see Chapter 135 for further discussion).[37,38,81] Although limiting Pplat and V_T during mechanical ventilation has demonstrated benefit in decreasing ventilator-associated lung injury, it is not known whether additional reduction will improve outcomes even further.[82] There may not be a safe level of pressures or tidal volume in patients with ARDS.

Driving Pressure

Driving pressure (DP) is the difference between Pplat and PEEP following a mechanically delivered V_T. It reflects the distending pressure of the lung. In mechanically ventilated patients, C_{RS} is a ratio between V_T/(Pplat – PEEP) or, alternatively, DP = V_T/C_{RS}. DP thus describes the relationship between V_T and functional lung available for ventilation. An excessive Pplat, and thus excessive DP, increases the risk of lung injury whereas potential benefits of high levels of PEEP depend on lung recruitability and resulting change in compliance.[83] Reexamination of randomized clinical trials of ARDS patients demonstrated that DP was the pulmonary mechanical variable most predictive of 60-day mortality.[84] Limiting DP to 14 cm H_2O or less may reduce lung injury.[85]

It is important to recall that C_{RS} reflects the distending pressure of the lung but does not represent the true stress on the lung, which is represented by the transpulmonary pressure. Transpulmonary pressure represents Paw – Ppl. Remembering that esophageal balloons can be used to measure pleural pressure, then *transpulmonary driving pressure* (TPDP) equals

(Pplat − PEEP) − (Esophageal plateau pressure

− End-expiratory esophageal pressure)

Unlike DP, TPDP considers the effect of chest wall elastance.[86] A patient with high chest wall elastance and normal pulmonary elastance (as in chest wall edema) will have a large DP and low TPDP with minimal stress across lung parenchyma. This patient may be less susceptible to lung injury than a patient with a large DP and high TPDP who has high lung and chest wall elastance (e.g., ARDS with chest wall edema). This may explain why DP was not associated with mortality reduction in obese ARDS patients.[87] Other limitations of DP include the underestimation in spontaneously breathing patients, overestimation in prone patients, and the lack of randomized control trials supporting the benefit of DP to guide ventilator strategies.[88–89]

ENERGETICS AND WORK OF BREATHING

When a force is applied to an object over a distance, energy is required; the work done is equal to:

$$Work = Force \times Distance$$

Similarly, because pressure is force over an area and volume is an area multiplied by a distance, work in a fluid system may be defined as the integral of applied pressure over a change in volume:

$$Work = \int PdV$$

During inspiration, work must be performed to distend the respiratory system (elastic work), which is stored as potential energy. Also, nonelastic work must be done to generate flow through the airways (to overcome resistance to gas flow), to overcome lung and chest wall tissue resistance, and to accelerate gas (to generate the inertial component). This work cannot be stored as potential energy and is dissipated as heat. The inertial component is minimal and is usually ignored in measuring total work.

MEASURING WORK OF BREATHING DONE BY A POSITIVE-PRESSURE VENTILATOR IN A PARALYZED PATIENT

Consider a paralyzed patient receiving positive-pressure mechanical ventilation, for whom the entire work of breathing is performed by the ventilator (Fig. 11.13A). On a volume-pressure plot, pressure applied to the airway will track to the right of the static volume-pressure curve of the respiratory system because additional pressure is required to overcome resistive forces. In Figure 11.13A, the blue shaded area represents the elastic work done by the ventilator during one inhalation, whereas the gray shaded area represents the resistive work expended to generate flow and overcome tissue resistance. With exhalation, the stored elastic energy can be used to deflate the lungs so that exhalation is normally a passive process. Increases in resistance or decreases in compliance can increase the work of breathing significantly.

MEASURING WORK OF BREATHING IN A SPONTANEOUSLY BREATHING PATIENT

In a spontaneously breathing patient, work is performed by the inspiratory muscles rather than by a ventilator. Graphing the pressure-volume characteristics of the lung and chest wall against Ppl illustrates the work performed by inspiratory muscles (Fig. 11.13B). During inspiration, Ppl decreases to expand the lungs (see Fig. 11.13B). The distance between the two curves at any given lung volume represents the pressure the inspiratory muscles must exert to overcome elastic forces of the lung and chest wall. In Figure 11.13B, the blue shaded area thus represents the elastic work of breathing against the lung and chest wall. To overcome the resistive forces, additional pressure and work are required, as indicated by the gray shaded area.

Under normal conditions, exhalation is passive, because the stored potential energy from elastic work is more than sufficient to overcome resistive work. However, in the presence of severe airflow obstruction (e.g., an asthma attack), the necessary resistive work may exceed this stored energy, requiring active generation of force by expiratory muscles and additional work for exhalation.

OXYGEN COST OF BREATHING

The oxygen cost of breathing is an indicator of the total amount of energy required by the respiratory muscles for ventilation. At rest, the oxygen cost of breathing is low at 0.25 to 0.5 mL/L of ventilation, or 1–2% of total body oxygen consumption. However, at maximal exercise in normal subjects, the oxygen cost of breathing represents approximately 10–15% of total oxygen consumption.[90] The oxygen cost of breathing can increase markedly as minute ventilation increases (eFig. 11.2).

Patients with COPD have an increased oxygen cost of breathing as a function of ventilation (see eFig. 11.2). This may be related to a combination of increased work of breathing and decreased efficiency of the respiratory muscles due to dynamic hyperinflation. Dynamic hyperinflation is an increase in end-expiratory lung volume seen when patients with airflow obstruction develop PEEPi. PEEPi is caused when there is incomplete expiration of air from the lungs due to long time constants for gas distribution and an increased respiratory rate.[91] Dynamic hyperinflation can be exacerbated by tonic inspiratory muscle activity at end-expiration.

Although the dynamic increase in lung volume can have a beneficial effect by dilating intraparenchymal airways to decrease the resistive work, the end-expiratory alveolar pressure acts as an inspiratory threshold load, which increases the work of breathing. Furthermore, the mechanical efficiency of the inspiratory muscles is compromised by hyperinflation because the zone of diaphragmatic apposition is reduced and the inspiratory muscles are shorter than the optimal length for force generation. The efficiency of breathing (defined as the ratio between the rate of mechanical work accomplished and the rate of energy consumed) may be further diminished if postural or other stabilizing muscles (trunk, neck, shoulder) need to be recruited.

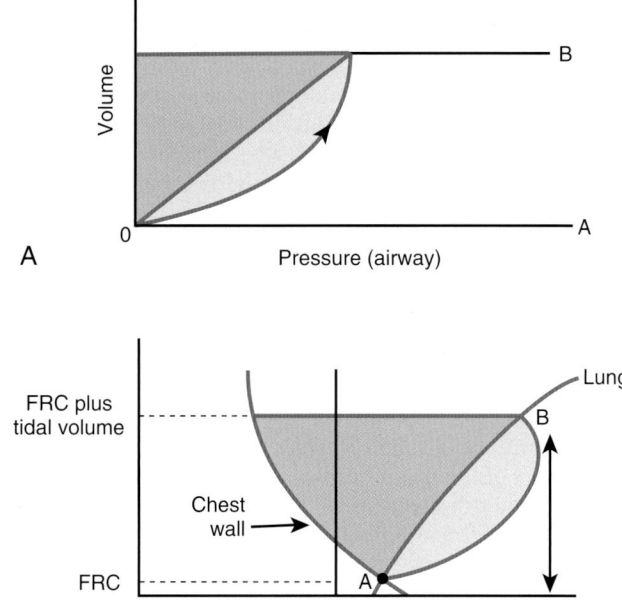

Figure 11.13 The work of breathing. (A) Work of breathing during mechanical ventilation. Consider a paralyzed patient receiving one tidal breath while on positive-pressure mechanical ventilation (point A to point B). The *diagonal blue line* represents the volume-pressure curve of the static respiratory system; the *shaded dark blue area* to the left of this line thus represents the elastic work done during the inflation. This work can be stored as potential energy and can be used during exhalation. The *gray shaded area* to the right of the line represents the resistive work done. (B) Work of breathing during spontaneous breathing (Campbell diagram). Consider a patient taking a spontaneous breath from *fuctional residual capacity* (FRC; point A) with a volume equal to the height of the *double-headed arrow* (point B). In order to overcome elastic forces of the lung and chest wall, the inspiratory muscles must exert a force equal to the horizontal distance between the chest wall and lung volume pleural pressure curves. Thus, the entire elastic work done will be equal to the *blue shaded area*. Resistive work must also be done, requiring the inspiratory muscles to generate an even greater negative pleural pressure. This is indicated by the *gray shaded area*. The total work done will be the sum of both areas.

Key Points

- Under conditions of laminar flow, flow is directly proportional to the pressure difference along the path of flow. Under conditions of turbulent flow, flow is directly proportional to the square root of the pressure difference. Turbulent flow, such as with partial upper airway obstruction, can be reduced by using a less dense gas mixture like heliox.
- The majority of the elastic recoil of the lung is due to surface forces generated by fluid lining the alveoli. The unique properties of surfactant help to reduce surface tension and stabilize alveoli at low lung volumes, preventing their collapse.
- At functional residual capacity (relaxation volume), the outward recoil pressure of the chest wall is balanced by the inward recoil of the lung. Total lung capacity is determined by the balance between the maximal inspiratory pressure generated by the respiratory muscles and the opposing pressure generated by the inward recoil of the lungs and chest wall.

- Measuring respiratory system resistance and compliance can be easily accomplished in ventilated patients and is useful for assessing reasons for difficulty weaning from the ventilator.
- In ventilated patients, the proportion of the applied airway pressure transmitted to the pleural space is dependent on the ratio of lung and chest wall compliance.
- In patients with airflow obstruction who are treated with positive-pressure ventilation, intrinsic positive end-expiratory pressure can lead to hemodynamic compromise, increased work of breathing, an inspiratory threshold load, mechanical inefficiency of the diaphragm, and patient-ventilator asynchrony.
- Patients with acute respiratory distress syndrome benefit from a ventilation strategy using low tidal volume, low plateau pressures, low driving pressures and positive end-expiratory pressure.

Key Readings

Akoumianaki E, Maggiore SM, Valenza F, et al. The application of esophageal pressure measurement in patients with respiratory failure. *Am J Respir Crit Care Med.* 2014;189:520–531.

Amato MBP, Meade MO, Slutsky AS, et al. driving pressure and survival in the acute respiratory distress syndrome. *N Engl J Med.* 2015;372:747–755.

Bellani G, Laffey JG, Pham T, et al. Epidemiology, patterns of care, and mortality for patients with acute respiratory distress syndrome in intensive care units in 50 countries. *JAMA.* 2016;315:788–800.

Beitler JR, Sarge T, Banner-Goodspeed VM, et al. Effect of titrating positive end-expiratory pressure (PEEP) with an esophageal pressure–guided strategy vs an empirical high PEEP-FiO2 strategy on death and days free from mechanical ventilation among patients with acute respiratory distress syndrome. *JAMA.* 2019;321:846–857.

Blanch L, Bernabé F, Lucangelo U. Measurement of air trapping, intrinsic positive end-expiratory pressure, and dynamic hyperinflation in mechanically ventilated patients. *Respir Care.* 2005;50:110–123.

Colebourn CL, Barber V, Young JD. Use of helium-oxygen mixture in adult patients presenting with exacerbations of asthma and chronic obstructive pulmonary disease: a systematic review. *Anaesthesia.* 2007;62:34–42.

Frerking I, Günther A, Seeger W, Pison U. Pulmonary surfactant: functions, abnormalities and therapeutic options. *Intensive Care Med.* 2001;27:1699–1717.

Henderson WR, Chen L, Amato MBP, Brochard LJ. Fifty years of research in ARDS. Respiratory mechanics in acute respiratory distress syndrome. *Am J Respir Crit Care Med.* 2017;196:822–833.

Hoppin FG, Stothert Jr JS, Greaves IA, et al. Lung recoil: Elastic and rheologic properties. In: Macklem P, Mead J, eds. *Handbook of Physiology. Section 3. The Respiratory System. Mechanics of Breathing (Part 1).* Vol III. Bethesda, MD: American Physiological Society; 1986:195–216.

Leith DE, Brown R. Human lung volumes and the mechanisms that set them. *Eur Respir J.* 1999;13:468–472.

Lumb AB. Elastic forces and lung volumes. In: *Nunn's Applied Respiratory Physiology.* 8th ed. Italy: Elsevier; 2017:17–32.

Malhotra A. Low-tidal-volume ventilation in the acute respiratory distress syndrome. *N Engl J Med.* 2007;357:1113–1120.

Mead J, Takishima T, Leith D. Stress distribution in lungs: a model of pulmonary elasticity. *J Appl Physiol.* 1970;28:596–608.

Ranieri VM, Dambrosio M, Brienza N. Intrinsic PEEP and cardiopulmonary interaction in patients with COPD and acute ventilatory failure. *Eur Respir J.* 1996;9:1283–1292.

Sahetya SK, Goligher EC, Brower RG. Fifty years of research in ARDS. Setting positive end-expiratory pressure in acute respiratory distress syndrome. *Am J Respir Crit Care Med.* 2017;195:1429–1438.

Writing Group for the Alveolar Recruitment for Acute Respiratory Distress Syndrome Trial (ART) Investigators, Cavalcanti AB, Suzumura ÉA, et al. Effect of lung recruitment and titrated positive end-expiratory pressure (PEEP) vs low PEEP on mortality in patients with acute respiratory distress syndrome: a Randomized. *JAMA.* 2017;318:1335–1345.

Talmor D, Sarge T, Malhotra A, et al. Mechanical ventilation guided by esophageal pressure in acute lung injury. *N Engl J Med.* 2008;359:2095–2104.

Complete reference list available at ExpertConsult.com.

12 · ACID-BASE BALANCE

SARAH SANGHAVI, MD • TYLER J. ALBERT, MD • ERIK R. SWENSON, MD

In all things you shall find everywhere the Acid and Alcaly.
OTTO TACHENIUS, HIPPOCRATES CHEMICUS (1670)

FUNDAMENTAL CONCEPTS

The care of critically ill patients requires a thorough understanding of acid-base balance. Maintenance of normal arterial pH (7.35–7.45 in plasma) is a critical factor in maintaining stable extracellular fluid and intracellular acid-base homeostasis. Arterial pH is kept under tight control by both pulmonary and renal mechanisms, each of which also regulate other processes, such as gas exchange in the lungs and fluid and electrolyte balance by the kidneys. Although, in most cases of acid-base disorders, deviations of arterial pH are moderated by specific compensatory responses to maintain acid-base homeostasis, other physiologic priorities may intervene. For example, hypoxemia stimulates the carotid bodies, resulting in hyperventilation and respiratory alkalosis. In the case of metabolic alkalosis generated by severe vomiting, alkalosis will be maintained by the overriding need for the kidneys to maintain extracellular volume. What follows is a review of some of the more important concepts and disorders of acid-base balance.

ACID-BASE CHEMISTRY

pH, the logarithmic function of H^+ concentration ([H^+], normally 35–45 nanomole/L [nmol/L or nM] in plasma; Eq. 1), is used to represent a broad range of concentrations in body fluids from 1 in gastric acid to 8 in alkaline urine and pancreatic and biliary fluid.

$$pH = -\log_{10}[H^+] \qquad [1]$$

Using the Henderson-Hasselbalch equation (Eq. 2), pH can be calculated from two variables, *partial pressure of carbon dioxide* (P_{CO_2}) and *bicarbonate* (HCO_3^-), without consideration of other acid-base pairs in the plasma.

$$pH = pK_a + \log\left[\frac{[HCO_3^-]}{\alpha P_{CO_2}}\right] \qquad [2]$$

The Kassirer-Bleich approximation (Eq. 3) is a more practical tool that allows determination of pH when P_{CO_2} and HCO_3^- are known.

$$H^+ = 24\, P_{CO_2} / [HCO_3^-] \qquad [3]$$

In this equation, the units of H^+, P_{CO_2}, and HCO_3^- are nmol/L, mm Hg, and mEq/L, respectively. The calculated [H^+] can then be converted to pH, with [H^+] of 25, 40, and 63 roughly correlating to a pH of 7.6, 7.4, and 7.2, respectively. It is a useful check for internal consistency of laboratory-reported values.

CARBON DIOXIDE AND BICARBONATE

Buffer systems minimize changes in pH upon the addition of acid or alkali and are therefore paramount to normal enzymatic function and protein structure. The HCO_3^- buffer system is extremely important in maintaining arterial pH at approximately 7.4 (Eqs. 4 and 5).

$$CO_2 + H_2O \underset{CA}{\overset{CA}{\rightleftharpoons}} H_2CO_3 \rightleftharpoons H^+ + HCO_3^- \qquad [4]$$

$$CO_2 + OH^- \underset{CA}{\overset{CA}{\rightleftharpoons}} HCO_3^- \qquad [5]$$

Gas exchange by the lungs keeps HCO_3^- concentration 20 times greater than that of dissolved *carbon dioxide* (CO_2), favoring H^+ consumption and CO_2 production. A low P_{CO_2} is a prerequisite for optimal function of the HCO_3^- buffer system. The predominant pathway to form HCO_3^- from CO_2 is shown in Eq. 4, with an alternative pathway shown in Eq. 5. However, generation of HCO_3^- through either pathway is slow in the absence of the catalyst *carbonic anhydrase* (CA), which is present in erythrocytes, vascular endothelium, alveolar epithelium, and in most other organs, including the kidney.[1–3]

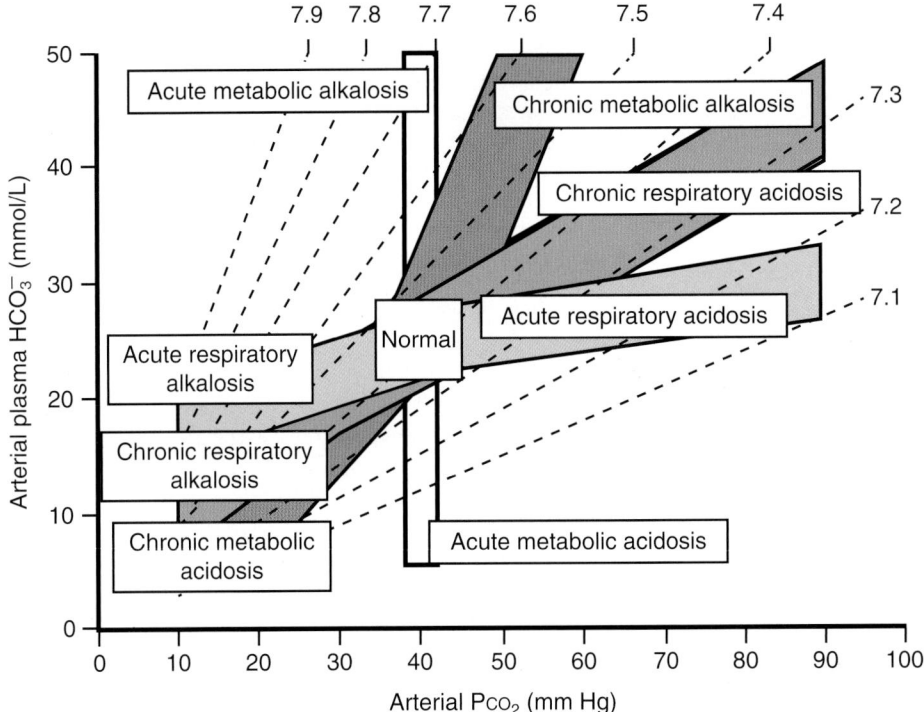

Figure 12.1 The relation between bicarbonate (HCO₃⁻) and Pco₂ in a variety of clinical disorders. For discussion, see text. The 95% confidence levels for acute and chronic respiratory and metabolic abnormalities are denoted by the colored boxes. The *vertical transparent bar* indicates the absence of any change in arterial Pco₂ with acute changes in HCO₃⁻. However, the respiratory response to the onset of metabolic acidosis and alkalosis is rapid, and the metabolic band rotates clockwise toward the chronic metabolic position within a matter of minutes to hours. Compensatory metabolic responses to respiratory changes in arterial Pco₂ are much slower, making it easier to observe the acute respiratory bands before metabolic compensation.

Base Excess

Although HCO_3^- is the most commonly used metabolic parameter in assessing acid/base status, it underestimates the amount of acid (or base) that must be used to titrate samples of blood, plasma, or the body as a whole to a pH of 7.4. This reflects the presence of other buffer pairs that are titrated by the addition of strong acids and bases. The second problem with using HCO_3^- as a metabolic parameter is that it is influenced by changes in arterial Pco_2.

The *base excess* (BE) is a complex equation developed in response to these limitations. It estimates how much strong acid or alkali must be added to titrate fully oxygenated blood to a pH of 7.4 at 37°C and at the hemoglobin concentration in that sample. The term *base deficit* is simply the negative of BE. Standard BE is provided by most *arterial blood gas* (ABG) machines and is commonly used as an indicator of metabolic acidosis in the setting of trauma.

ARTERIAL AND VENOUS BLOOD GAS ANALYSIS

Arterial blood gas (ABG) analysis is the standard for assessing oxygenation and the concentration of CO_2 in arterial blood. *Partial pressure of oxygen* (Po_2), Pco_2, and pH are directly measured with electrodes in blood and plasma samples, whereas HCO_3^- is calculated from pH and Pco_2 values. *Acidemia* and *alkalemia* refer to the deviations in arterial plasma pH from normal plasma pH. *Acidosis* and *alkalosis* refer to processes pushing the pH in the acid or alkaline direction but do not designate the actual pH.

The pH and Pco_2 of blood are prone to error if blood samples are exposed to air, inadvertently diluted, or measured without temperature correction for hypothermia or hyperthermia. Exposure to air decreases Pco_2, raises pH, and more gradually decreases CO_2 content. Dilution of samples by saline or other fluids in indwelling catheters causes both Pco_2 and HCO_3^- to fall equally. Failure to temperature correct for hypothermia leads to spuriously higher Pco_2, lower pH, and higher Po_2; the opposite is seen with hyperthermia.[4]

Venous blood gas (VBG) measurement is less invasive than ABG measurement and may be used in its place if the clinician does not require an arterial Po_2 measurement. On average, compared to arterial values, venous pH is lower by 0.05 units, and venous Pco_2 is higher by 5 mm Hg. In states of low cardiac output, high CO_2 production or inhibition of red cell carbonic anhydrase, the arteriovenous differences can increase by as much as 10-fold.[5]

Alternatively, $[HCO_3^-]$ can be estimated from the total CO_2 content measured as part of a basic metabolic profile in venous blood. It tends to run approximately 5% higher (2–3 mmol/L) than arterial HCO_3^- because venous blood includes CO_2 produced from cellular metabolic activity not yet excreted by the lung. It also includes carbonic acid (H_2CO_3), dissolved CO_2, carbonate, and CO_2 bound to amino acids (carbamates).

NOMENCLATURE OF ACID-BASE DISORDERS

Procedures for naming acid-base disorders become quite simple if CO_2 and HCO_3^- are used as the respiratory and metabolic parameters. An additional assumption is made that compensation is incomplete, especially with severe acid-base disturbances. If arterial pH is low, the primary disorder must be an acidosis and, if high, the primary disorder is an alkalosis. Based on this approach, abnormal combinations of pH, Pco_2, and HCO_3^- can be designated in terms of a primary disorder and any compensation that might be present.

Figure 12.1 indicates the ranges in which HCO_3^- and Pco_2 changes have been observed in normal persons subjected to acute or chronic respiratory or metabolic changes.

Figure 12.1 is based on the simple assumption that changes in P_{CO_2} reflect respiratory events, whereas changes in HCO_3^- reflect metabolic events. Note that if respiratory and metabolic parameters change proportionately, pH does not change. Baseline patient values for both P_{CO_2} and HCO_3^- are helpful in understanding compensatory responses. When no baseline values are available, a lack of appropriate compensation for a primary metabolic acidosis may suggest an underlying respiratory disorder; of note, these patients may appear to be breathing comfortably without tachypnea. Similarly, a lack of renal response after 48 to 72 hours may indicate a concurrent renal disorder. "Triple disorders" may also be encountered, involving an anion gap acidosis, non–anion gap acidosis or metabolic alkalosis, and a primary respiratory disorder.

Several caveats should be noted in the interpretation of acid-base status. The distinction between primary and compensatory disorders is based simply on which alteration is proportionately greater at the time the blood was drawn rather than on the sequence of events involved. For example, it is common for patients with COPD to be admitted to the hospital with compensated respiratory acidosis. With therapy, P_{CO_2} may decrease, revealing what might be interpreted as "a primary metabolic alkalosis with secondary respiratory compensation" if the clinical history is unknown.

ROLE OF VENTILATION: ARTERIAL P_{CO_2}

Arterial P_{CO_2} is determined by the rate of CO_2 production relative to the rate of alveolar ventilation. If arterial P_{CO_2} exceeds the normal range (35–45 mm Hg), then the patient is hypoventilating; conversely, if the arterial P_{CO_2} is lower, the patient is hyperventilating. These terms are distinct from hyperpnea and hypopnea, which refer to the increases or decreases of ventilation (high and low minute ventilation) to meet respiratory requirements, and from tachypnea and bradypnea, which indicate rapid and slow respiratory rates, respectively. Thus arterial P_{CO_2} can be interpreted as a "ventilatory" parameter that reflects the adequacy of ventilation relative to the rate of CO_2 production.

The utility of arterial P_{CO_2} as a ventilatory parameter is readily illustrated by a few brief examples. Arterial P_{CO_2} is usually normal during moderate exercise, and the subject is neither hyperventilating nor hypoventilating, despite obvious hyperpnea and tachypnea. Patients with severe lung disease frequently hypoventilate despite both hyperpnea and tachypnea at rest because much of the inhaled air is delivered to an enlarged physiologic dead space because of both shunting and regions of low $\dot{V}_A/\dot{Q}$ ratio. Regardless of the reason that ventilation fails to keep pace with CO_2 production, the concomitant increase in arterial P_{CO_2} is classified as hypoventilation.

ROLE OF THE KIDNEYS

The kidney is essential in maintaining acid-base balance under physiologic conditions and correcting deviations under pathologic conditions. In general, to maintain homeostasis, the kidney reclaims filtered HCO_3^- in the proximal tubule and excretes dietary acid in the cortical collecting tubule (Fig. 12.2).

Metabolic Alkalosis

As much as 80–90% of the filtered HCO_3^- is indirectly reclaimed in the proximal tubule by secretion of H^+ via the Na^+, H^+–exchanger 3 (NHE3) on the luminal membrane. The driving force for this exchanger is the low intracellular Na^+ concentration generated by the basolateral Na^+, K^+-adenosine triphosphatase (ATPase) pump. The distal nephron is responsible for the reabsorption of a small quantity of HCO_3^-. In states of alkalosis, the capacity of the proximal tubule to reclaim HCO_3^- is overwhelmed, and HCO_3^- is excreted in the urine, aiding in the resolution of the metabolic alkalosis.

Metabolic Acidosis

In conditions of acidosis, the increased acid load is excreted predominantly as *ammonium chloride* (NH_4Cl) in the collecting duct. NH_4^+ is produced from glutamine by the proximal tubular cells; this process can be stimulated by chronic acidosis and hypokalemia. Through a complex pathway of secretion and reabsorption, *ammonia* (NH_3) is present in the cortical collecting tubule, where it may accept protons secreted by the cortical collecting tubule cells. Because the collecting duct fluid tends to be very acidic, NH_3 becomes "trapped" as NH_4^+ and is excreted in the urine.[11,12] Distal tubular acid secretion is mediated by K^+, H^+-ATPase and H^+-ATPase on the luminal surface of cortical collecting tubule cells.

COMPENSATION

Respiratory Acidosis

Although the acute increase in HCO_3^- is relatively modest after onset of hypercapnia, HCO_3^- continues to rise if hypercapnia persists and reaches a peak value after approximately 5 days (Table 12.1). An increase in HCO_3^- of approximately 4 mEq/L may be expected when P_{CO_2} is increased in steps of 10 mm Hg. Increases in plasma HCO_3^- require an initial net loss of H^+, which is made possible by the loss of increased quantities of NH_4^+ in the urine. Mechanisms mirror those that arise with an increase in exogenous acids. Chronic respiratory acidosis may down-regulate activity of the apical HCO_3^-, Cl^--exchanger pendrin in the distal tubule.[13] Once plasma HCO_3^- has reached a new steady state, H^+ secretion need only be sufficient to reabsorb HCO_3^- from the tubular fluid, and NH_4^+ and H^+ excretion usually return to normal.

Respiratory Alkalosis

Hypocapnia results in a decrease in renal acid excretion and a fall in HCO_3^- that becomes fully evident within 2 to 3 days. As indicated in Table 12.1, HCO_3^- decreases by 2.5 mEq/L for each decrease of 10 mm Hg in P_{CO_2}[14] and does not generally fall much below 16 mEq/L in respiratory alkalosis unless there is an independent metabolic acidosis present. Confidence bands for chronic compensation are indicated in Figure 12.1.

Metabolic Acidosis

Respiratory compensation for metabolic disorders is quite fast (within minutes) and reaches maximal values within 24 hours. In metabolic acidosis, a decrease in P_{CO_2} of 1 to 1.5 mm Hg should be observed for each mEq/L decrease of HCO_3^-.[15] A simple rule for deciding whether the fall in P_{CO_2} is appropriate for the degree of metabolic acidosis is that the P_{CO_2} should be equal to the last two digits of the pH. For example, compensation is adequate if the P_{CO_2} decreases to

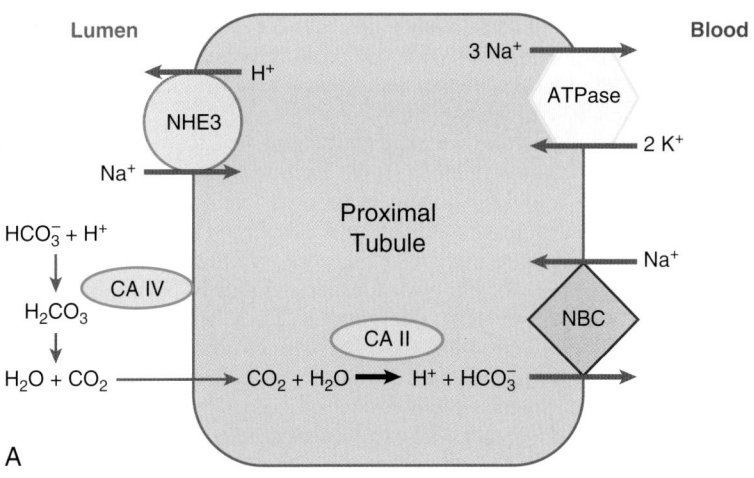

A

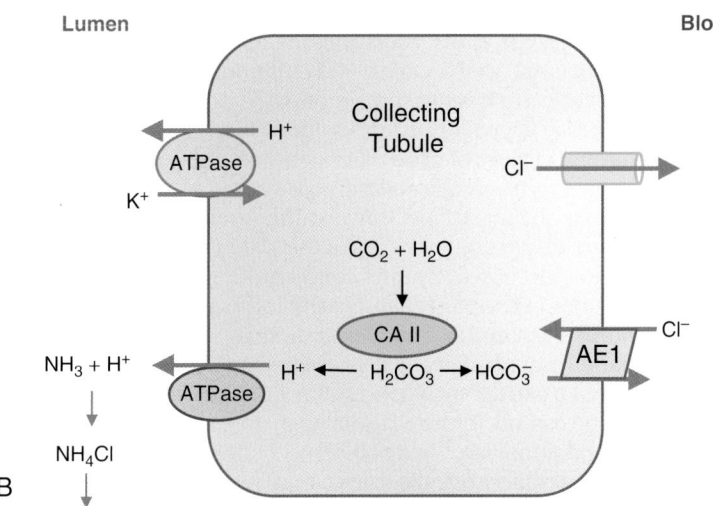

B

Figure 12.2 Acid-base handling by the kidney. (A) Reclamation of bicarbonate (HCO_3^-). In the proximal tubule, the Na^+, H^+–exchanger 3 (NHE3) secretes H^+ into the lumen. H^+ combines with filtered HCO_3^- producing carbonic acid (H_2CO_3), which is then catalyzed to H_2O and carbon dioxide (CO_2) by membrane-bound carbonic anhydrase (CA) type IV. CO_2 is recycled back into the proximal tubule cell, where it is hydrated to H_2CO_3 by carbonic anhydrase type II and subsequently dissociates into HCO_3^- and H^+. The HCO_3^- is reabsorbed into the blood via the sodium-bicarbonate cotransporter (NBC), and the H^+ enters the lumen to continue the cycle of HCO_3^- reclamation. No net acid is excreted in this process. (B) Acid excretion and generation of HCO_3^-. In acidosis, the acid load is excreted predominantly as ammonium chloride (NH_4Cl) in the collecting duct. Ammonia (NH_3) in the lumen combines with H^+ secreted by K^+, H^+–adenosine triphosphatase (ATPase) and H^+-ATPase on the luminal side of the collecting duct cells. NH_4Cl is excreted in the urine, and HCO_3^- is reabsorbed via a chloride-bicarbonate exchanger. AE1, anion exchanger 1.

Table 12.1 Rules of Chronic Compensation

		EXAMPLES	
Primary Disorder	**Secondary Compensation**	**Primary Change**	**Compensation**
↑Pco_2	↑HCO_3^-: 4 mEq/L for each 10 mm Hg increase in Pco_2 (±3 mEq/L)	Pco_2: 40 → 80	HCO_3^-: 24 → 40 pH: 7.1 → 7.32
↓Pco_2	↓HCO_3^-: 2.5 mEq/L for each 10 mm Hg decrease in Pco_2 (±3 mEq/L)*	Pco_2: 40 → 20	HCO_3^-: 24 → 19 pH: 7.70 → 7.60
↓HCO_3^-	↓Pco_2: 1–1.5 mm Hg for each mEq/L decrease in HCO_3^-	HCO_3^-: 24 → 9	Pco_2: 40 → 25 pH: 7.00 → 7.20
↑HCO_3^-	↑Pco_2: 0.5–1.0 mm Hg for each mEq/L increase in HCO_3^-	HCO_3^-: 24 → 34	Pco_2: 40 → 50 pH: 7.56 → 7.46

*HCO_3^- seldom falls below 18 mEq/L in acute and 16 mEq/L in chronic respiratory alkalosis.

28 when the pH is 7.28. Another helpful formula is Winter's formula (Eq. 6),[15] which can be used provided pH > 7.1.

$$\text{Expected } Pco_2 = 1.5 (HCO_3^-) + 8 \pm 2 \qquad [6]$$

Metabolic Alkalosis

Compensation for metabolic alkalosis results in a decrease in tidal volume, resulting in a rise of Pco_2 by approximately 0.6 to 0.7 mm Hg for each mEq/L increase in HCO_3^-. This compensatory hypoventilation generally does not exceed a Pco_2 of 55 mm Hg because the accompanying fall in arterial Po_2 evokes increased ventilation to defend body oxygenation. This general rule may not apply in severe metabolic alkalosis, where compensatory values of Pco_2 greater than 60 mm Hg have been documented.[16] Respiratory compensation for metabolic alkalosis, such as that for metabolic acidosis, can have a counterproductive effect on renal H^+ transport: increases in Pco_2 associated with metabolic alkalosis decrease intracellular pH in the kidney, thereby promoting acid secretion and further increasing serum HCO_3^- levels.[17]

METABOLIC ACIDOSIS

ANION GAP CONCEPT

The most useful classification of metabolic acidosis is based on the concept of the anion gap, which is calculated by subtracting the sum of plasma concentrations of Cl^- and HCO_3^- from that of Na^+ (eFig. 12.1). This difference provides a convenient index of the relative concentrations of plasma anions other than Cl^- and HCO_3^-. Normally the anion gap is between 8 and 16 mEq/L, although somewhat lower values (5–11 mEq/L) have been observed when newer techniques for measuring ion activities rather than total concentrations are used.[6,18] The anion gap accounts for anions present in plasma that are not included in the equation, including albumin (which normally constitutes approximately half of the gap), lactate, pyruvate, sulfate, and phosphate.

Elevations of the anion gap are generally accompanied by a similar decrease in HCO_3^- ("anion gap acidosis"). In contrast, loss of *sodium bicarbonate* ($NaHCO_3$) results in acidosis without a rise in the anion gap (hyperchloremic acidosis). The mnemonic GOLDMARK may be used to remember many of the causes for an anion gap acidosis: *g*lycols including ethylene glycol and propylene glycol, 5-*o*xoproline [pyroglutamic acid], *l*actic acidosis, *D*-lactic acidosis, *m*ethanol, *a*spirin, *r*enal failure, and *k*etoacidosis.[7]

Once the presence of an anion gap has been established, the next step is to assess for other metabolic disturbances. This is achieved by calculating the delta gap, which is the difference in the anion gap from the patient's baseline value or from a normal value of 12. In a pure anion gap acidosis, the delta gap should equal the deficit in HCO_3^-. Thus, when the delta gap is added to the total CO_2, the sum is 24. If the sum is much greater than 24, a concurrent metabolic alkalosis exists. If the sum is lower than 24, then a coexisting hyperchloremic acidosis exists. The actual value is approximate because either the H^+ or the conjugate base may leave the extracellular space, altering this 1:1 relationship. For example, in lactic acidosis, the delta gap often exceeds the decrease in HCO_3^-, whereas the opposite is true in diabetic ketoacidosis (see later sections).

A low anion gap reflects an increase in cations other than Na^+ (e.g., *calcium* [Ca^{2+}], *magnesium* [Mg^{2+}], *lithium* [Li^+], and abnormal cationic proteins, such as in multiple myeloma) or a decrease in unmeasured anions, typically albumin. Hypoalbuminemia decreases the anion gap by approximately 2.5 mEq/L for each decrease in albumin concentration of 1 g/dL.[18] Alkalemia tends to decrease H^+ binding to albumin, thereby increasing the number of negatively charged groups and the anion gap.

CAUSES OF ANION GAP ACIDOSIS

Lactic Acidosis

Approximately 1400 mEq of lactate are normally produced each day.[8] At rest, production is balanced by consumption and precisely regulated so that serum levels are kept at approximately 1 mEq/L. Most lactate is produced by skeletal muscle contraction but, with various stresses, such as ischemia, profound hypoxemia, sepsis, and high sympathetic tone, other tissues may also generate lactate due to anaerobic metabolism. In resting healthy individuals, the liver and, to a lesser extent, the kidneys are responsible for most of its consumption,[8] with oxidation in red skeletal muscle accounting for the remainder. In states of acidosis, renal lactate metabolism increases, and hepatic lactate metabolism decreases.[9]

As noted earlier, the delta gap in lactic acidosis may exceed the decrease in HCO_3^-. Lactate is poorly cleared by the kidney and tends to stay in the extracellular space, whereas H^+ moves intracellularly and is buffered by non-HCO_3^- buffers. This difference may be more profound in severe acidosis because the capacity for intracellular buffering increases as the serum HCO_3^- decreases.[10] Thus, when the delta gap is added to the total CO_2, the sum can be greater than 24. This is frequently seen in lactic acidosis and should not be misinterpreted as evidence for a coexisting metabolic alkalosis.[18] Also, lactic acidosis may cause hyperkalemia due to concomitant renal dysfunction and cellular ischemia.

Lactic acidosis can be divided into two types: type A, in which tissue hypoxia is evident, and type B, in which the tissue P_{O_2} appears to be adequate for aerobic metabolism.[19] Type A disorders include all forms of shock, acute hypoxemia, and a variety of conditions that impair oxygen delivery, such as carbon monoxide poisoning and severe anemia. Type B disorders include illnesses such as liver disease, a variety of drugs and poisons, and congenital metabolic enzyme deficiencies (Table 12.2).

In diabetic patients, low insulin levels reduce the metabolism of pyruvate by pyruvate dehydrogenase, resulting in an increased lactate concentration. Accumulation of ketones in the plasma may inhibit the monocarboxylic acid pump responsible for hepatic uptake of lactate.[20] In some patients with *diabetic ketoacidosis* (DKA), elevated lactate may be caused by extracellular fluid volume depletion due to the osmotic diuresis induced by hyperglycemia.

Malignancies, particularly lymphoproliferative and myeloproliferative disorders, may result in overproduction of lactic acid, which may impair normal immune tumor surveillance. This phenomenon results from the reliance of cancer cells on aerobic glycolysis as an ATP source rather than mitochondrial oxidative phosphorylation, the so-called Warburg effect, as a means to generate carbon intermediates necessary for rapid cell growth.[21] Renal or hepatic failure may impair metabolism of lactate, delaying its clearance once perfusion has been restored.

Although L-lactate is usually the cause of lactic acidosis, D-lactate accumulation due to intestinal bacterial metabolism has been documented in patients with short bowel syndrome, bowel ischemia, or obstruction. Bacteria in the colon metabolize carbohydrates to D-lactic acid, which is absorbed systemically. Because D-lactate cannot be converted into pyruvate by L-lactate dehydrogenase, it may accumulate. It may be treated by avoiding foods that contain lactobacilli (e.g., yogurt and sauerkraut), by decreasing dietary carbohydrates, and by the administration of oral antibiotics.

Of interest, lactic acidosis is not frequently observed in patients with severe respiratory insufficiency or cyanotic heart diseases. Lactic acidosis is much more likely to develop when tissue perfusion is impaired than when arterial blood oxygen content is moderately reduced. Several compensations for chronic arterial hypoxemia help minimize tissue hypoxia: cardiac output rises, the hematocrit rises and, if pH declines in those with CO_2 retention, hemoglobin oxygen affinity falls because of increased 2,3-diphosphoglycerate

Table 12.2 Causes of Anion Gap Acidosis

LACTIC ACIDOSIS

Type A: Tissue Hypoxia

Poor tissue perfusion: distributive shock, cardiogenic shock, obstructive shock
Severe hypoxemia: pulmonary disorders, acute respiratory distress syndrome, carbon monoxide poisoning
Exercise above anaerobic threshold, seizures, shivering
Rhabdomyolysis
Severe anemia

Type B: Altered Lactate Metabolism Without Hypoxia

Liver disease, renal failure, diabetes mellitus, malignancies (especially hematopoietic), SIRS, HIV
Drugs: acetaminophen, β-agonists, biguanides, cocaine, cyanide, ethanol, diethyl ether, fluorouracil, halothane, iron, methanol, salicylates, ethylene and propylene glycol, isoniazid toxicity, linezolid, nalidixic acid, niacin, zidovudine (azidothymidine [AZT]), metformin, chemotherapy, propofol, total parenteral nutrition, valproic acid
Hereditary: glucose-6-phosphatase deficiency, fructose-1,6-phosphatase deficiency
D-Lactic acidosis

KETOACIDOSIS

Diabetes mellitus
Starvation
Ethanol
Inherited errors of metabolism

UREMIA

TOXIC ANIONS

Salicylates
Ethylene glycol (glyceraldehyde, oxalate)
Methanol (formaldehyde, formate)
Paraldehyde (acetoacetate)
Aminocaproic acid

HIV, human immunodeficiency virus; SIRS, systemic inflammatory response syndrome.

production, permitting more oxygen to be released at the tissue level.

Diabetic Ketoacidosis

Ketoacidosis refers to the accumulation of acetoacetate, β-hydroxybutyrate, and acetone ("ketone bodies") in the body. Development of ketoacidosis requires both increased mobilization of free fatty acids from lipid stores and their excessive conversion within hepatocytes to ketone bodies (eFig. 12.3). Triglycerides within fat are normally broken down by lipase into free fatty acids and glycerol. Lipase activity is enhanced by low concentrations of insulin and increased concentrations of glucagon, catecholamines, and growth hormone. Free fatty acids released from adipocytes are taken up by the liver and linked to *coenzyme A* (CoA) to form acyl CoA. Acyl CoA is either transformed by esterification to triglycerides and lipoproteins or transferred into the mitochondria, degraded to form acetyl CoA, and then metabolized to CO_2 and water via the Krebs cycle or converted to ketone bodies. In DKA, the acetyl CoA produced exceeds the capacity of handling by the mitochondria and is converted to ketone bodies. Ketoacids are normally taken up and metabolized to CO_2 and water by muscle and kidney rather than by the liver, but this process may be reduced in DKA.[22]

In normal subjects, the ratio of β-hydroxybutyrate to acetoacetate is 2:1. With DKA, this ratio increases to 2.5:1 to 3:1 and, with poor tissue perfusion and associated lactic acidosis, it can exceed 8:1.[23] The urine nitroprusside test detects acetoacetate but not β-hydroxybutyrate. Therefore, as patients improve with appropriate therapy, conversion of β-hydroxybutyrate to acetoacetate may be misinterpreted as worsening of the ketoacidosis.[23] Serum and point-of-care capillary blood assays are now available that directly measure β-hydroxybutyrate levels.

The decrease in HCO_3^- may be lower than the delta gap during the treatment of DKA. During volume resuscitation, ketoacid anions are renally excreted with Na^+ and K^+. The excretion of ketoacids removes conjugate anions from the extracellular space, thereby decreasing the anion gap. Thus, when the delta gap is added to the total CO_2, the sum can be less than 24. As noted earlier, this should not be interpreted as an additional acid-base disorder.

The observed hyperkalemia in DKA is due to cellular insulin deficiency preventing cellular uptake of K^+. Hyperosmolarity also causes water efflux from cells, a process that moves K^+ extracellularly by solute drag. However, despite hyperkalemia at presentation, most patients with DKA have total body depletion of potassium and require potassium supplementation during treatment, as acidosis and hyperosmolarity resolve and potassium shifts intracellularly.

Starvation Ketoacidosis

Starvation often leads to ketoacidosis within 1 or 2 days, particularly after exercise, but HCO_3^- levels seldom decline below 18 mEq/L. Starvation ketoacidosis may decrease insulin concentrations, but the insulin does not fall to levels as low as those encountered in DKA. Furthermore, there is evidence that ketosis stimulates insulin secretion in those with normal pancreatic function. Alcoholics who binge and then abruptly stop drinking and eating may develop severe ketoacidosis,[24,25] which may be underestimated because of a disproportionate rise in β-hydroxybutyrate. They usually become dehydrated from vomiting before hospital admission, and they may develop severe acidosis, frequently with concomitant lactic acidosis. Glucose concentrations are frequently low, and glucose (given with thiamine to avoid the Wernicke-Korsakoff syndrome of cerebral beriberi) stimulates insulin secretion and corrects the ketoacidosis. Supplementation with K^+, phosphate, and Mg^{2+} is frequently required.

Uremic Acidosis

Acute kidney injury does not usually produce an anion gap acidosis until the *glomerular filtration rate* (GFR) falls below 20 mL/min. However, because of differences in diet and sites of renal damage, there is some variation in the filtration threshold at which anion gap acidosis develops.[23] The loss of nephrons is accompanied by a decrease in the ability to excrete both NH_4^+ and anions. Numerous anions normally kept low by renal clearance contribute to the anion gap, including sulfate, phosphate, and lactate.

Toxic Forms of Anion Gap Acidosis

Salicylates. Large ingestions of salicylates, such as aspirin, cause a mixed disorder with both an anion gap metabolic acidosis and a primary respiratory alkalosis due to *central nervous system* (CNS) stimulation. Although salicylates are themselves anions, most of the acidosis observed after an overdose is related to formation of organic acids, particularly lactic acid and ketones.[26] Associated symptoms include tinnitus, nausea/vomiting, and vertigo. The most severe consequence is neurotoxicity, which may manifest as altered mental status, seizures, and cerebral edema. Salicylates lower cerebral glucose concentrations, resulting in neuroglycopenia despite normal serum glucose concentrations.[27] Salicylate levels above 40 mg/dL are associated with increased toxicity, and levels above 100 mg/dL are associated with increased morbidity and mortality. First-line therapy is intravenous $NaHCO_3^-$, which promotes salicylic acid excretion in the urine and flux from the CNS into plasma by ionic trapping of salicylate anion.

Volatile Alcohols. Methanol, isopropyl ethanol, and ethylene glycol ingestions are frequent causes of anion gap metabolic acidoses. Methanol (rubbing alcohol) is converted to formic acid, and ethylene glycol (antifreeze, radiator fluid) is converted to glycoxalic acid and oxalic acid by alcohol dehydrogenase. Both methanol and ethylene glycol contribute to serum osmolarity but are not represented in the calculated osmolarity (Eq. 7):

$$\text{Serum osmolality} = 2 \times [Na^+] + BUN/2.8 + glucose/18 \quad [7]$$

In acute ingestions, the difference in measured serum osmolarity and calculated serum osmolarity (osmolar gap) is greater than 10. However, as these alcohols are metabolized to acids, the osmolar gap may decrease as the anion gap increases. Ethanol consumption will also increase the osmolar gap. In addition, any severe critical illness may raise the osmolar gap to greater than 10 due to increased membrane permeability and leakage of intracellular solutes.[31] Nonetheless, an unexplained, large osmolal gap is highly suggestive of toxic volatile alcohol ingestion.

Treatment with fomepizole,[28] an alcohol dehydrogenase inhibitor, prevents the accumulation of toxic metabolites, such as formic acid, glycoxalic acid, and oxalic acid. The parent drugs are ultimately cleared by the kidney. Hemodialysis is a very effective method to remove parent drug and toxic metabolites, particularly in the setting of end-organ damage.

HYPERCHLOREMIC ACIDOSIS

Metabolic acidosis in the absence of an elevated anion gap is usually associated with hyperchloremia. The first step in the workup of a hyperchloremic acidosis is determining if the kidneys are handling acid excretion appropriately. The normal response to a metabolic acidosis is increased excretion of urinary NH_4^+, which can be estimated using the urine anion gap (Eq. 8).

$$\text{Urine Anion Gap} = U_{NA^+} + U_{K^+} - U_{Cl^-} \quad [8]$$

The normal urine anion gap is greater than 20. When the kidneys are excreting more acid, because the majority of NH_4^+ is excreted with Cl^- as NH_4Cl, the U_{Cl^-} should increase and the urine anion gap should decrease. Therefore, in the setting of an acidosis, a urine anion gap greater than 20 suggests that the kidneys are not excreting the excess acid and thus a renal tubular acidosis is the cause of the hyperchloremic acidosis. The cardinal feature of all types of renal tubular acidosis is a low rate of NH_4^+ excretion in the setting of a chronic metabolic acidosis, out of proportion to the GFR.[29]

Type 1 Renal Tubular Acidosis

Type 1 (distal) *renal tubular acidosis* (RTA) involves defects in distal tubular acid secretion, resulting in a urine pH > 6.5. Hypokalemia is also a prominent feature of type 1 RTA. As indicated in Table 12.3, many disorders are associated with type 1 RTA, which most commonly affects the activity of carbonic anhydrase II or the proton pump (H^+-ATPase) of the renal cortical collecting duct. Amphotericin B may induce an RTA by making pores in luminal cell membranes allowing leak of H^+ from the tubular fluid back into the intercalated cells.

Chronic acidosis leads to osteopenia with Ca^{2+}, Mg^{2+}, and PO_4^{2-} loss in the urine. Decreased tubular citrate secretion promotes precipitation of Ca^{2+} and PO_4^{2-}, which contributes to the development of nephrolithiasis and nephrocalcinosis in patients with type 1 RTA.

If untreated, the acidosis progresses relentlessly because the normally generated acids cannot be excreted at their rate of production. Correction of hypokalemia and treatment with 1 mEq/kg $NaHCO_3^-$ daily (roughly the rate of bodily fixed acid generation) is usually sufficient to normalize acid-base status in adults.

Type 2 Renal Tubular Acidosis

In type 2 (proximal) RTA, HCO_3^- reabsorption is impaired because of a defect in the proximal tubule apical membrane NHE3. Normally, HCO_3^- is completely reabsorbed from glomerular filtrate, and maximal reabsorption rates are not observed until concentrations are approximately 28 mEq/L. In proximal RTA, maximal reabsorption values may top out at a serum concentration of approximately 18 mEq/L. The distal tubules cannot absorb more than 15–20% of the filtered load of HCO_3^-, so bicarbonaturia ensues. If the serum HCO_3^- level falls below the HCO_3^- recovery threshold, then urinary HCO_3^- loss ceases, urine pH falls, and the acidosis does not progress. A typical patient will have a steady-state serum HCO_3^- value in the range of 12 to 20 mEq/L. When serum HCO_3^- is normalized to 24 mmol/L by HCO_3^- infusion, more than 15% of the filtered HCO_3^- is lost in the urine in type 2 RTA, compared with less than 5% in normal subjects and in those with type 1 RTA. Therefore, patients with type 2 RTA tend to have a urine pH of 5 to 6 under chronic steady-state conditions, with a rise to close to 7 with $NaHCO_3$ infusion.

Table 12.3   Causes of Hyperchloremic Acidosis

RENAL TUBULAR ACIDOSIS

Type 1 (Distal) Hypokalemic

Congenital defects without systemic disease (anion exchanger, AE1 deficient) or with systemic disease (e.g., Ehlers-Danlos syndrome, sickle cell anemia, Southeast Asian ovalocytosis)

Autoimmune disorders (e.g., Sjögren syndrome, thyroiditis, systemic lupus erythematosus, autoimmune hepatitis/biliary cirrhosis, rheumatoid arthritis)

Drug toxicity (e.g., amphotericin B, analgesics, lithium, ifosfamide)

Nephrocalcinosis (e.g., primary hyperparathyroidism, vitamin D intoxication, hyperoxaluria, Fabry disease, Wilson disease)

Tubular and interstitial renal disease (e.g., pyelonephritis and obstructive renal disease, renal transplant rejection)

Type 2 (Proximal) Hypokalemic

Selective carbonic anhydrase inhibitors: topiramate, acetazolamide, methazolamide

Genetic (e.g., cystinosis, Wilson disease, tyrosinemia, galactosemia, Lowe syndrome)

Dysproteinemias (e.g., multiple myeloma, amyloidosis)

Drug or chemical toxicity (e.g., lead, cadmium, ifosfamide, tenofovir)

Secondary hyperparathyroidism with hypocalcemia (e.g., vitamin D deficiency or resistance)

Renal interstitial disease (e.g., medullary cystic disease, Sjögren syndrome, renal transplant)

Combined Type 1 and 2 RTA

Carbonic anhydrase II deficiency

Type 4 Hyperkalemic

Mineralocorticoid deficiency: Addison disease, tuberculosis, autoimmune, adrenal hemorrhage, AIDS, critically ill patients,

Hyporeninemic states: diabetes mellitus, AIDS

Mineralocorticoid resistance: pseudohypoaldosteronism (congenital, spironolactone)

Medications: potassium-sparing diuretics (amiloride, triamterene), angiotensin-converting enzyme inhibitors, trimethoprim, pentamidine, nonsteroidal anti-inflammatory drugs, cyclosporine A, β-adrenergic inhibitors, α-adrenergic agonists, heparin, digitalis overdose, lithium, insulin antagonists (diazoxide, somatostatin), succinylcholine drugs (ketoconazole, phenytoin, rifampin)

NONRENAL HYPERCHLOREMIC ACIDOSIS

Excessive intravenous saline administration

Diarrhea

Pancreatic drainage

Ureterosigmoidostomy

Cholestyramine (diarrhea)

Hyperalimentation with amino acid infusions

Administration of NH_4Cl or $CaCl_2$

Toluene exposure (hippurate production)

Loss of ketones with Na^+ or K^+

AE1, anion exchanger 1; AIDS, acquired immunodeficiency syndrome; RTA, renal tubular acidosis.

Type 2 (proximal) RTA may be an isolated tubular lesion, but it is more frequently associated with other proximal tubular defects that lead to loss of glucose, phosphate, amino acids, and low-molecular-weight proteins (Fanconi syndrome) (see Table 12.3). If the acidification defect is associated with calcium and phosphate loss, patients are susceptible to osteomalacia and rickets. In contrast to distal RTA, nephrolithiasis and nephrocalcinosis are not characteristic of proximal RTA. Treatment of proximal RTA requires much more $NaHCO_3$ (10–15 mEq/kg/day) to correct the acidosis than treatment of distal RTA. In addition, large amounts of $NaHCO_3$ exacerbate losses of K^+, and potassium supplements and/or potassium-sparing diuretics are commonly required.

Type 4 Renal Tubular Acidosis

Type 4 RTA is distinguished from other RTAs by the presence of hyperkalemia and a less severe acidosis. It is classically associated with hypoaldosteronism, but newer data suggest hyperkalemia-induced inhibition of ammoniagenesis may also be causative.[30] Aldosterone increases the number of open *epithelium sodium channels* (ENaCs) in the luminal membranes of cortical collecting tubule cells, which stimulates distal secretion of H^+ and K^+. Hyperkalemia itself also suppresses proximal NH_3 production, resulting in low NH_4^+ excretion. Because NH_3 cannot buffer H^+ secreted by H^+-ATPase, urine pH may still be less than 5.5. A wide variety of disorders lead to low aldosterone production (see Table 12.3) but, in clinical practice, it is most commonly seen in diabetic kidney disease due to hyporeninemic hypoaldosteronism. Potassium-sparing diuretics, angiotensin-converting enzyme inhibitors, and heparin, which can inhibit aldosterone production, may also cause hyperkalemia and type 4 RTA.

Acidosis of Progressive Renal Failure

Hyperchloremic RTA without hyperkalemia is characteristic of many chronic renal diseases associated with loss of renal tissue and a decrease in the GFR. Acid retention in these patients is attributable to a decrease in the ability of the kidneys to excrete NH_4^+. Although the decline in serum HCO_3^- is relatively modest, it is recommended that serum HCO_3^- concentrations should be maintained above 22 mEq/L, with $NaHCO_3$ supplementation to minimize bone reabsorption, protein catabolism, and progression of chronic kidney disease.[31]

Gastrointestinal Causes of Hyperchloremic Acidosis

Diarrhea is a common cause of hyperchloremic acidosis. In the bowel, Cl^- is selectively absorbed in exchange for HCO_3^-. In the setting of diarrhea, significant amounts of HCO_3^- can be lost: each liter of diarrheal fluid can result in the loss of 200 mEq of HCO_3^-. Acidosis is exacerbated by absorption of NH_4^+ generated by gut bacteria. Ureterosigmoidostomy or ureteroileostomy can also produce hyperchloremic acidosis because the Cl^- in the urine diverted to the bowel tends to be absorbed instead of the HCO_3^-. Severe losses of pancreatic or biliary fluids, which contain 50 to 100 mEq of HCO_3^- per liter, can cause a severe hyperchloremic acidosis. Finally, extracellular volume depletion promotes aldosterone secretion, which in turn enhances urinary K^+ loss. Chronic acidosis increases renal NH_4^+ secretion, distinguishing it from RTA. A nonrenal cause of acidosis may be inferred from a urinary anion gap less than 20.

Miscellaneous Causes of Hyperchloremic Acidosis

A common cause of hyperchloremia in hospitalized patients is the administration of large amounts of normal saline. Other causes of hyperchloremia causes include some hyperalimentation fluids and administration of NH_4Cl, or $CaCl_2$. Because chronic respiratory alkalosis is normally compensated by a decrease in proximal HCO_3^- reabsorption, the correction of an underlying respiratory alkalosis may transiently produce a hyperchloremic acidosis. Toluene inhalation can also cause hyperchloremic acidosis due to its conversion to benzoic acid and hippurate, which are rapidly excreted renally with cations.[32]

CLINICAL MANIFESTATIONS

A classic sign of metabolic acidosis is Kussmaul respiration, which consists of slow, deep breaths. Kussmaul respiration is particularly effective because the dead-space fraction and its contribution to ventilation is minimized. However, most patients with chronic metabolic acidosis are often asymptomatic, and their hyperventilation may not be clinically obvious. With more severe acidosis, patients may complain of dyspnea with exertion, along with headache, nausea, and vomiting. Although acidosis decreases myocardial contractility and inotropic responsiveness in vitro and in animal models,[33] there are no convincing data that acidosis decreases total peripheral resistance or vasoconstrictor response to vasopressors.

THERAPY

Treatment of metabolic acidosis should focus on correcting the underlying metabolic disorder responsible for its emergence and the hemodynamic, oxygenation, and electrolyte derangements that ensue, rather than the acidemia itself.

$NaHCO_3$ administration is indicated in patients with chronic metabolic acidosis, such as those with significant hyperchloremic acidosis (e.g., RTA) to prevent bone and muscle catabolism, relieve exertional dyspnea, and promote growth in children. In acute severe metabolic acidosis (especially the endogenous anion gap acidoses), HCO_3^- administration is not always helpful or effective. In severe DKA, even with an arterial pH as low as 6.8, HCO_3^- administration does not alter rates of glucose correction or ketoacid clearance when compared with equivalent NaCl administration. Likewise, there are no clear benefits of HCO_3^- administration for sepsis, severe hypoxemia, and cardiogenic shock, and even suggestions of worse outcomes in HCO_3^--treated patients (for review, see Swenson[35]). Although it is often claimed that when the pH is lower than 7.2, $NaHCO_3$ infusions may be lifesaving by enhancing cardiac contractility and response to vasopressors, the supporting data are unconvincing. Any transient hemodynamic benefits of HCO_3^- administration may simply be the result of volume expansion by any sodium-containing fluid. Potential downsides of serum alkalization in these conditions include a left-shift of the oxygen-hemoglobin dissociation curve that may impair oxygen delivery in already hypoxic tissues, a decrease in ionized calcium, and nonmetabolic generation of CO_2 from HCO_3^- with paradoxical intracellular acidosis.[36–38] As the underlying disorders improve, both ketone bodies and lactate may be metabolized to HCO_3^-, resulting in the development of posttherapeutic alkalosis.

Alkalinizing agents may be indicated to treat associated severe hyperkalemia or to enhance excretion of acid metabolites of certain toxins.[39] $NaHCO_3$ infusions should be kept as low as possible (usually <200 mmoL) to avoid volume overload, which may alternatively be managed by hemodialysis against a $NaHCO_3$ solution. If $NaHCO_3$ is indicated acutely, determinations of arterial blood PO_2, PCO_2, HCO_3^-, pH, glucose, and electrolytes must be repeated at frequent intervals to monitor the response to therapy.

METABOLIC ALKALOSIS

GENERAL CONSIDERATIONS

For both diagnostic and therapeutic reasons, it is helpful to divide the causes of metabolic alkalosis into those associated with a decrease in the extracellular volume or chloride (chloride-sensitive) and those associated with a normal or increased extracellular volume (chloride resistant)[40] (Table 12.4). In general, maintenance of a metabolic alkalosis requires the presence of increased aldosterone *and* distal Na^+ delivery. Severe chloride depletion and hypokalemia may also independently contribute to the maintenance of a metabolic alkalosis.[41] Urine chloride values less than 20 mEq/L suggest a chloride-responsive process, whereas levels greater than 40 mEq suggest a chloride-resistant process. Bicarbonaturia may be present in metabolic alkalosis, which can pull cations such as Na^+ in the urine, so urine Na^+ is not useful in determining volume status in this setting. Metabolic alkalosis may be associated with an elevated anion gap due to an increase in the negative anion charges on albumin, but the anion gap is not helpful in determination of the cause.

CHLORIDE-RESPONSIVE ALKALOSIS

Gastrointestinal Losses

Upper gastrointestinal tract acid losses generate an alkalosis that is initially associated with increased renal Na^+ excretion. *Extracellular fluid* (ECF) volume depletion causes the GFR to fall and is associated with increased aldosterone secretion. This enhances HCO_3^- reabsorption, and alkalosis persists even after all initiating factors (e.g., protracted vomiting and continuous nasogastric suction) have abated. In these patients, Cl^- is avidly reabsorbed from the tubules, and urine concentrations remain less than 10 mEq/L. Although diarrhea usually generates a hyperchloremic acidosis (see earlier discussion), alkalosis may rarely be seen with Cl^--HCO_3^- exchange across the ileal mucosa[42] and in a minority of patients with villous adenomas of the colon. In general, correction of the metabolic alkalosis depends on replacement of Cl^- losses, given as saline in the setting of volume depletion.

Diuretics

These agents are the most common cause of excessive renal fluid losses. When Na^+ delivery to the distal nephron persists despite ECF depletion (e.g., after diuretic therapy), H^+ secretion by this segment is enhanced. In these conditions, Cl^- concentrations in the urine may be appreciable. Both loop diuretics (furosemide, bumetanide, ethacrynic acid) and thiazides can promote H^+ and K^+ secretion from the more distal segments of the nephron. This frequently results in severe hypokalemic alkalosis.

Table 12.4 Causes of Metabolic Alkalosis

LOSS OF H+ FROM THE BODY

Chloride-Responsive With Urine Cl− < 20 mEq/L

Gastrointestinal losses of chloride: stomach (vomiting), some villous adenomas, congenital chloride-wasting diarrhea, high-volume ileostomy drainage
Renal losses of chloride with volume depletion: recent use of loop and thiazide diuretics
Sweat losses of chloride: cystic fibrosis
Posthypercapnia: elevated HCO_3^- after resolution of chronic respiratory acidosis

Chloride-Resistant With Urine Cl− > 40 mEq/L With Hypertension

Hyperaldosteronism: primary adrenal hyperplasia, aldosterone producing adenoma, Cushing syndrome, 11-β-hydroxysteroid dehydrogenase type 2 deficiency, glycyrrhetinic acid (licorice)
Liddle syndrome: increased epithelial sodium channel expression in collecting duct

Chloride-Resistant with Urine Cl− > 40 mEq/L Without Hypertension

Bartter syndrome: impaired reabsorption of sodium ions (Na^+) and chloride ions (Cl^-) in the thick ascending loop of Henle (variants)
Gitelman syndrome: impaired thiazide-sensitive Na^+/Cl^- transporter in the distal convoluted tubule
Administration of poorly absorbed anions (e.g., penicillin)

EXCESSIVE INTAKE OF HCO_3^-

Milk-alkali syndrome
Bicarbonate dialysis in end-stage renal disease
Recovery from ketoacidosis or lactic acidosis after bicarbonate administration
Massive blood transfusions (citrate)

EXTRACELLULAR FLUID VOLUME REDUCTION

Sweat

Metabolic alkalosis is reported in patients with cystic fibrosis, who lose proportionately more Cl^- than HCO_3^- in their sweat.

Mechanical Ventilation

In patients with chronic respiratory acidosis and chronic metabolic compensation, initiation of mechanical ventilation with an acute increase in minute ventilation to "normalize" the Pco_2 may result in life-threatening metabolic alkalosis. The arterial pH and plasma levels of HCO_3^- of these persons may remain high and inhibit spontaneous ventilation unless Cl^- is restored, generally in the form of KCl. An additional consideration is that normalizing the CO_2 while on mechanical ventilation can result in reversal of chronic metabolic compensation. Once patients are liberated from the ventilator and assume their baseline CO_2, the serum pH will be much lower than at their baseline.

CHLORIDE-RESISTANT ALKALOSIS

Metabolic alkalosis may be associated with either normal or increased ECF volume, particularly in the presence of excessive aldosterone secretion. Mineralocorticoids increase Na^+ retention by the distal nephron, resulting in H^+ and K^+ wasting. Unlike situations in which the ECF is decreased, Cl^- is lost in the urine with metabolic alkalosis caused by excessive mineralocorticoid secretion (urine Cl^- > 40 mEq/L). Maintenance of the metabolic alkalosis is a result of persistent excess mineralocorticoid secretion as well as hypokalemia.

Any alteration in the renin-angiotensin-aldosterone axis that promotes aldosterone secretion also causes a metabolic alkalosis (see Table 12.4). Patients with edema due to liver disease, nephrotic syndrome, or congestive heart failure may secrete excessive aldosterone because their effective arterial blood volume is reduced, even though their total ECF volume is increased. The development of hypokalemic alkalosis is particularly likely when they receive diuretics.

The pathogenesis of several forms of congenital hypokalemic, hypochloremic metabolic alkalosis not associated with hyperaldosteronism (Bartter and Gitelman syndromes) has been traced to abnormalities in renal tubular transporters.[43] In patients who are volume depleted, sodium salts of penicillin or other anions that cannot be reabsorbed by the renal tubules pulls sodium distally, which causes acid and K^+ losses and results in a metabolic acidosis.

EXCESSIVE INTAKE OF ALKALI

Although the kidneys normally can excrete large quantities of HCO_3^-, metabolic alkalosis may occasionally be generated by excessive intake of HCO_3^- or other anions metabolized to HCO_3^-, especially in patients with renal insufficiency. For example, metabolic alkalosis may be observed after ingestion of extremely large amounts of HCO_3^- and milk (milk-alkali syndrome, which is associated with renal calcification, reduced GFR, and reduced ability to filter HCO_3^- for excretion), after fasting (due to conversion of ketones to HCO_3^-),[44] and after transfusions of large amounts of blood (conversion of citrate to HCO_3^-).[45] In the absence of volume depletion or renal disease, alkalosis due to increased HCO_3^- intake rapidly resolves once intake is restricted.

Extracellular Fluid Contraction

Water loss from plasma may induce a modest alkalemia that is sometimes referred to as a "contraction" alkalosis and is related to the relatively greater increase of HCO_3^- compared with Pco_2. It would probably be more appropriate to designate this as a *concentration alkalosis* to distinguish it from the alkalosis of contraction caused by ECF fluid depletion, which promotes renal acid excretion and alkalemia.

CLINICAL MANIFESTATIONS

Metabolic alkalosis frequently remains asymptomatic and is often untreated even after discovery. Nevertheless, it may be associated with significant mortality, particularly when pH > 7.5 and $[HCO_3^-]$ > 45 mmol/L.[46-48] Alkalosis increases the affinity of hemoglobin for oxygen, thereby reducing oxygen delivery to the tissues. It also decreases ventilation by suppressing the carotid body and may constrict the peripheral vasculature, further limiting oxygen supply to tissues. Neuromuscular hyperirritability may be observed in alkalosis and has been attributed in part to increased calcium binding to albumin. Twitching and tetany may be preceded by the Chvostek and Trousseau signs, and seizures can ensue. The myocardium may also become irritable, leading to ventricular arrythmias.[47] Thus prompt recognition and treatment is important.

THERAPY

Treatment of metabolic alkalosis depends on the status of the ECF volume. Patients with ECF volume loss can be distinguished from those with excess volume on the basis of urine Cl^-. For patients who have sustained severe volume losses, fluids that contain Na^+, Cl^-, K^+, and Mg^{2+} are frequently indicated.

Fluid administration to edematous patients with alkalosis is usually inappropriate, and KCl may resolve the metabolic alkalosis without the administration of Na^+.[41] Spironolactone is useful in the presence of excessive mineralocorticoid secretion. The carbonic anhydrase inhibitor, acetazolamide, may be helpful in patients with post-hypercapnic alkalosis, although it may increase loss of K^+ and occasionally cause hepatic encephalopathy in those with cirrhosis by interfering with NH_4^+ detoxification to urea and CO_2 retention in patients with severe lung disease.

Infusions of HCl (at a concentration of 100–200 mEq/L) may be safer than NH_4Cl in patients with liver and kidney disease, but these infusions require central access confirmed radiologically by location of the catheter tip in the superior vena cava to minimize the likelihood of tissue necrosis and hemolysis caused by the acid infusion. Alternatively, intubation and intentional hypoventilation to increase the Pco_2, thereby reducing arterial pH, may be used.

RESPIRATORY ACIDOSIS

GENERAL CONSIDERATIONS

Respiratory acidosis is common in patients with severe respiratory insufficiency, generally when lung function falls below 25% of the predicted value. Chemoreceptors located in the medulla (central chemoreceptors) and in the carotid bodies (peripheral chemoreceptors) normally keep Pco_2 within narrow limits. Normally, arterial Pco_2 is controlled primarily by the central chemoreceptors, which may have increased sensitivity because of concomitant hypercapnic peripheral chemoreceptor input. However, central chemoreceptors may be suppressed by chronic hypercapnia because compensatory renal generation of HCO_3^- increases the cerebrospinal fluid pH and reduces the magnitude of a pH change with fluctuations in arterial Pco_2. This blunting of the central chemoreceptor response is seen mostly in patients with severe COPD. When this happens, ventilation is maintained by the carotid bodies responding to alterations in Po_2 and pH. In this setting, if Po_2 is raised excessively, carotid body output may be suppressed, leading to progressive hypercapnia and narcosis.

Acute increases in Pco_2 are buffered by non-HCO_3^- buffers to form HCO_3^-, but HCO_3^- concentrations seldom exceed 30 mEq/L during the first 24 hours of hypercapnia. Increases in Pco_2 also result in an intracellular acidosis within the renal tubular cells that favors acid excretion and, over the next few days, acid excretion is accelerated by a rise in NH_4^+ formation, as compensation for respiratory acidosis.

CAUSES

Any process interfering with ventilation can lead to respiratory acidosis (Table 12.5). COPD is the most frequent cause of this problem, related primarily to mechanical conditions that decrease alveolar ventilation and lead to respiratory muscle weakness, either from reduced intrinsic strength or effective weakness as hyperinflation puts the respiratory muscles at a disadvantageous position in their length-tension relationship. Interstitial lung disease is less likely to increase Pco_2 until it becomes severe and the increased work of breathing cannot be maintained. Extensive infiltrative processes, including pneumonias and all forms of pulmonary edema, and large pleural effusions can decrease alveolar ventilation. With significant acute pulmonary artery embolic obstruction, wasted ventilation due to increased alveolar dead space can explain sudden increases in ventilation; hypercapnia may ensue if ventilation cannot be increased sufficiently. In such situations, the dead-space ventilation to tidal volume ratio (V_D/V_T) may be measured by sampling both arterial blood and mixed expired gases. A paralyzed diaphragm or extensive rib fractures that lead to a unilateral flail chest can produce an inefficient mode of ventilation and lead to hypoventilation.

Hypoventilation is the most serious complication of a wide variety of neuromuscular disorders. The central respiratory centers may be depressed acutely or chronically by narcotics or by any process that injures the brainstem, including chronic hypoxemia and hypercapnia. A complex disturbance of the respiratory center may be encountered in patients with the obesity-hypoventilation syndrome. Apneic episodes during sleep are common in these persons and are related to airway obstruction or to a central failure to initiate ventilation, or both.

Rarely, if cardiac output is low, if anemia is severe, and/or if certain drugs are used that interfere with the normal high efficiency of red cell CO_2 transport and exchange, CO_2 retention in the tissues may develop and yet not be reflected in the arterial Pco_2.[49] In fact, as CO_2 rises in the vicinity of the central chemoreceptors, ventilation may be stimulated sufficiently to cause a paradoxical arterial hypocapnia that can be mistaken as evidence of a primary respiratory alkalosis. If Pco_2 is measured in the venous circulation (mixed venous Pco_2), one will find an elevated Pco_2 and lower pH, revealing the true state of CO_2 homeostasis.

CLINICAL MANIFESTATIONS

If hypoventilation is caused by neuromuscular or mechanical problems, the patient will be dyspneic and tachypneic. In contrast, if the respiratory center is impaired, ventilation may be reduced without any sensation of dyspnea.

Table 12.5 Causes of Respiratory Disorders

RESPIRATORY ACIDOSIS

Central Nervous System Depression

Drugs: opiates, sedatives, anesthetics
Excessive administration of oxygen in COPD
Obesity-hypoventilation syndrome
Central nervous system disorders

Neuromuscular Disorders

Neurologic: multiple sclerosis, poliomyelitis, phrenic nerve injuries, high spinal cord lesions, Guillain-Barré syndrome, botulism, tetanus, amyotrophic lateral sclerosis
End plate: myasthenia gravis, succinylcholine chloride, curare, aminoglycosides, organophosphorus
Muscle: hypokalemia, hypophosphatemia, muscular dystrophy, polio

Airway Obstruction

COPD
Acute aspiration, laryngospasm

Chest Wall Restriction

Pleural: effusions, empyema, pneumothorax, fibrothorax
Chest wall: kyphoscoliosis, scleroderma, ankylosing spondylitis, extreme obesity

Severe Pulmonary Restrictive Disorders

Pulmonary fibrosis
Parenchymal infiltration: pneumonia, edema

Abnormalities in Blood Carbon Dioxide Transport

Decreased perfusion: heart failure, cardiac arrest with cardiopulmonary resuscitation, extensive pulmonary embolism, severe anemia
Carbonic anhydrase inhibition—high-dose acetazolamide

RESPIRATORY ALKALOSIS

Central Nervous System Stimulation

Hyperventilation syndrome, anxiety
Pregnancy
Cerebrovascular disease, subarachnoid hemorrhage
Meningitis, encephalitis
Septicemia, hypotension
Hepatic failure
Drugs: salicylates, nicotine, xanthines, quetiapine, progestational hormones

Pulmonary Disease

Pneumonia, interstitial fibrosis, pulmonary fibrosis, embolism, edema
Right-to-left shunt

Hypoxia

High altitude
Severe anemia, hemoglobinopathy
Decreased cardiac output

Excess Carbon Dioxide Removal

Mechanical ventilation
Acetate hemodialysis, heart-lung machine, extracorporeal membrane oxygenation

Decreased Carbon Dioxide Production

Myxedema, hypothermia

The physiologic and clinical consequences of respiratory acidosis tend to be more serious in acute than in chronic states. Elevations in PCO_2 cause systemic vasodilation that is particularly evident in the cerebral circulation. Cerebral blood flow and intracerebral pressures increase and may lead to a picture of pseudotumor cerebri with papilledema, retinal venous distention, and retinal hemorrhages. The patient may complain of dyspnea and manifest myoclonic jerks, asterixis, tremor, restlessness, and confusion. Coma may be observed at PCO_2 values of 70 to 100 mm Hg when the onset of hypercapnia is abrupt. Significantly higher levels may be well tolerated in patients with chronic respiratory acidosis, who have much higher HCO_3^- concentrations from renal compensation. Peripheral vasodilation and increased cardiac output promote warm, flushed skin and a bounding pulse. Arrhythmias are observed occasionally. Mild increases in serum phosphate and K^+ and decreases in lactate and pyruvate have been described in acute respiratory acidosis, and serum Na^+ may increase modestly in both acute and chronic hypercapnia.

THERAPY

Treatment of respiratory acidosis depends on the restoration of adequate ventilation. In COPD, attention must be focused on bronchodilation, adequate oxygen supplementation, and relief of anxiety or other causes of an increased metabolic rate. Judicious use of supplemental oxygen to correct hypoxemia is warranted to avoid the phenomenon of oxygen-induced hypercapnia in these patients. Sudden correction of arterial hypoxemia causes further hypercapnia by a combination of three mechanisms: (1) by relief of hypoxic pulmonary vasoconstriction in poorly ventilated lung regions that further reduces the ability of the lung to eliminate CO_2 because local perfusion to poorly ventilated regions increases, (2) by saturation of hemoglobin with oxygen that causes previously buffered protons on deoxyhemoglobin to be released with subsequent generation of new CO_2 from HCO_3^- stores (Haldane effect) and from hemoglobin carbamate, and (3) by depression of the hypoxia-driven peripheral chemoreceptor drive that causes more hypoventilation. Low-flow oxygen generally suffices to increase PO_2 to satisfactory levels (60 mm Hg and arterial oxygen saturation [arterial SO_2] approximately 90%); greater elevations are neither needed nor advisable. If mechanical ventilation becomes necessary, care must be taken that PCO_2 is not decreased by more than 10 mm Hg each hour to avoid life-threatening metabolic alkalosis. If opiates are responsible for central respiratory depression, the respiratory acidosis may be relieved by naloxone. Aminophylline acts as a respiratory center stimulant, but blood levels must be monitored carefully. Bicarbonate is generally contraindicated because it tends to decrease respiratory drive and increases CO_2 levels in the tissues.

"Permissive hypercapnia" with gradual increases in PCO_2 of 10% per hour to levels as high as 100 mm Hg may help mitigate lung damage by barotrauma associated with mechanical ventilation. This approach is frequently used in patients with acute respiratory distress syndrome, neonatal respiratory failure, or asthma by hypoventilation with tidal volumes less than 7 mL/kg and plateau pressures less than 30 to 35 cm H_2O. The value of HCO_3^- infusions to reverse acidosis in these patients remains uncertain. Permissive hypercapnia should be avoided in those with head trauma, increased intracerebral pressure, acute renal insufficiency, or cardiac dysfunction.

RESPIRATORY ALKALOSIS

GENERAL CONSIDERATIONS

Respiratory alkalosis is a common disorder, but it seldom has a significant impact on the clinical status of patients. Changes in pH related to hyperventilation are quickly moderated by tissue buffering and, to a lesser extent, by generation of lactic acid, as described earlier. However, HCO_3^- concentrations do not usually fall below 18 mEq/L acutely and, even with renal compensation, a HCO_3^- concentration below 16 mEq/L should raise the possibility of an independent metabolic acidosis. Although respiratory alkalosis may have prognostic implications, it generally requires little in the way of specific therapy to reverse the hyperventilation directly.

CAUSES

It is convenient to divide the causes of respiratory alkalosis into three major categories: CNS stimulation, pulmonary diseases, and hypoxia (see Table 12.5).

CNS stimulation is among the most common cause of respiratory alkalosis. Anxiety can provoke hyperventilation (hyperventilation syndrome). Central stimulation of respiration is also common in a wide variety of intracerebral injuries. Many drugs and hormones (notably salicylates, theophylline, thyroxine, and progesterone) stimulate ventilation, and hyperventilation may be an early sign of both sepsis and hepatic insufficiency due to the accumulation of ammonia and amines known to be responsible for respiratory center stimulation.

Many pulmonary disorders are associated with hyperventilation. Hypoxia certainly plays a role but, in addition, receptors have been described in lung tissue that are activated by local irritant stimuli and fluid accumulation and remain activated even after hypoxemia has been corrected.

Both central (arterial) and peripheral (capillary) hypoxia are causes of hyperventilation. Decreases in arterial PO_2 stimulate the carotid bodies directly. In contrast, tissue hypoxia caused by decreased cardiac output, shock, severe anemia, or excessive hemoglobin oxygen affinity results in the production of lactic acid and other stimuli, which are sensed in blood by the carotid chemoreceptors and by other less well-defined chemoreception in the affected tissues themselves. Acute ascent to altitudes greater than 8000 feet predictably leads to hypocapnia as a result of hypoxic stimulation of breathing.

CLINICAL MANIFESTATIONS

Many manifestations of respiratory alkalosis may be related in part to a fall in free serum Ca^{2+} due to increased calcium binding to serum proteins. Phosphate may also decline slightly and sometimes fall to rather low concentrations in patients who have prolonged severe respiratory alkalosis. The decline in phosphate may be related to activation of glycolysis and phosphorylation of the produced glucose metabolites. Some of the CNS changes of acute respiratory alkalosis may be caused by hypocapnic cerebral vasoconstriction leading to reduced blood flow and tissue hypoxia.

Often, deliberate hyperventilation is used to reduce cerebral blood flow in states of impending brain herniation from high intracranial pressure, but evidence is mounting that it is useful only for a few hours as a temporizing measure to allow more definitive pressure relief by other means.

Panic, weakness, and a sense of impending doom are common, as are paresthesias and muscle weakness or cramping. As in metabolic alkalosis, Trousseau and Chvostek signs can often be elicited, and overt tetany or seizures may follow, particularly in patients with previous seizure diatheses. Vision and speech may become impaired, and syncope can follow. Transient electrocardiographic changes can resemble those of myocardial ischemia; this finding can be particularly misleading because it is not uncommon for hyperventilating patients to complain of chest discomfort. Indeed, acute hypocapnia, for example with mechanical ventilation, can induce coronary artery vasospasm, angina, ominous cardiac arrhythmias, and ST elevations in patients with coronary artery disease. Acute respiratory alkalosis can increase lactate and reduce serum K^+ concentrations.

THERAPY

Reassurance and rebreathing in a small paper bag are frequently all that is needed to control hyperventilation associated with anxiety attacks. In more severe cases, β-adrenergic inhibitors have proved useful, and specific therapy for anxiety may be indicated. Correction of respiratory alkalosis in other conditions, such as hepatic coma and pulmonary disorders, depends on treatment of the primary disorder. CO_2 inhalation by patients with hepatic coma has not been helpful.

Key Points

- Arterial PCO_2 provides a suitable criterion for determining whether alveolar ventilation is appropriate for the rate at which CO_2 is produced in the body. Abnormalities in arterial PCO_2 may be "primary" causes of abnormal pH or "secondary" responses, which act to compensate for pH disturbances.
- Changes in total CO_2 reflect net accumulation or loss of nonvolatile acids and bases from the body and can be primary or secondary. Both the kidneys and other organs, including the gastrointestinal tract and skin, may be involved.
- Incorporation of electrolyte concentrations into the analysis permits calculation of the anion "gap" and identification of various processes involved in both metabolic acidosis and alkalosis. However, these measurements must always be accompanied by measurement of conventional acid-base parameters (pH_a, arterial PCO_2, and HCO_3^-).
- Correction of the underlying metabolic or respiratory disorder represents the most effective way to treat any acid-base disorder but, in specific circumstances, judicious direct manipulation of PCO_2 and HCO_3^- may be considered.

Key Readings

Berend K. Diagnostic use of base excess in acid–base disorders. *N Engl J Med.* 2018;378:1419–1428.

Berend K, de Vries AP, Gans RO. Physiological approach to assessment of acid-base disturbances. *N Engl J Med.* 2014;371(15):1434–1445.

Buckley MS, Leblanc JM, Cawley MJ. Electrolyte disturbances associated with commonly prescribed medications in the intensive care unit. *Crit Care Med.* 2010;38(suppl 6):S253–S264.

Casey JR, Grinstein S, Orlowski J. Sensors and regulators of intracellular pH. *Nat Rev Mol Cell Biol.* 2010;11:50–61.

Gennari FJ. Pathophysiology of metabolic alkalosis: a new classification based on the centrality of stimulated collecting duct ion transport. *Am J Kidney Dis.* 2011;58(4):626–636.

Halperin M, Kamel K, Goldstein M. *Fluid, Electrolyte, and Acid-Base Physiology: A Problem- Based Approach.* Philadelphia: Elsevier; 2010.

Hamm L, Nakhoul N, Hering-Smith K. Acid-base homeostasis. *CJASN.* 2015;10:2232–2242.

Kraut JA, Madias NE. Differential diagnosis of nongap metabolic acidosis: value of a systematic approach. *Clin J Am Soc Nephrol.* 2012;7:671–679.

Kurtz I, Kraut J, Ornekian V, et al. Acid-base analysis: a critique of the stewart and bicarbonate-centered approaches. *Am J Physiol Renal Physiol.* 2008;294:F1009–F1031.

Nguyen MK, Kao L, Kurtz I. Calculation of the equilibrium pH in a multiple-buffered aqueous solution based on partitioning of proton buffering: a new predictive formula. *Am J Physiol Renal Physiol.* 2009;296:F1521–F1529.

Palmer BF. Evaluation and treatment of respiratory alkalosis. *Am J Kidney Dis.* 2012;60(5):834–838.

Palmer BF, Alpern RJ, Seldin DW. Normal acid-base balance, chapter 11, and metabolic acidosis, chapter 12. In: Floege J, Johnson RJ, Feehally J, eds. *Comprehensive Clinical Nephrology.* 4th ed. St. Louis: Saunders; 2011.

Rice M, Ismail B, Pillow MT. Approach to metabolic acidosis in the emergency department. *Emerg Med Clin N Am.* 2014;32:4403–4420.

Rogovik A, Goldman R. Permissive hypercapnia. *Emerg Med Clin N Am.* 2008;26:941–952.

Soifer JT, Kim HT. Approach to metabolic alkalosis. *Emerg Med Clin N Am.* 2014;32:453–463.

Vernon C, Letourneau JL. Lactic acidosis: recognition, kinetics, and associated prognosis. *Crit Care Clin.* 2010;26:255–283.

Complete reference list available at ExpertConsult.com.

13 AEROSOLS AND DRUG DELIVERY

THOMAS G. O'RIORDAN, MD, MPH • GERALD C. SMALDONE, MD, PHD

INTRODUCTION

The human lung has a large surface area, which for an average-size person approximates half a doubles tennis court, thus maximizing the approximation and apposition of capillaries to the epithelial surface. Although this design optimizes gas exchange, it also has the intrinsic risk of exposing the delicate alveolar tissues to potentially noxious particles present in the ambient air. There are various safeguards against the danger posed by inhaled particles. The first line of defense is the configuration of the nasopharynx and serial branching of the airways, which causes particles to deposit proximal to the more vulnerable alveolar structures.[1,2] Second, if an insoluble particle deposits in the lung, there are processes by which it can be cleared from the airways or alveoli. Clearance of insoluble particles that deposit in the ciliated airways is achieved by mucociliary clearance.[3] The particles are trapped in a mucus blanket, which is then transported proximally by beating cilia. If the cilia are not functioning optimally or if the quantity or quality of the airway mucus is abnormal, the mucus and its entrapped particulates can be cleared by cough. Particles that deposit distal to the ciliated airways are removed by alveolar clearance, mainly by macrophages ingesting the particles and transporting them to regional lymph nodes.

The branching structure of the airways is a barrier not only to noxious environmental aerosols but also to therapeutic aerosols. However, the application of the principles of deposition facilitates the design of therapeutic aerosols.[4] For the most part, therapeutic aerosols are "targeted" to the lungs; that is, they are designed to treat lung diseases directly and avoid systemic toxicity. Theoretically the large surface area of the lungs can facilitate the systemic delivery of nonrespiratory drugs via the lung as aerosols, usually proteins, such as insulin, that cannot be given by the oral route. However, to date the use of this pathway has not had a major impact on clinically successful systemic therapeutic drugs.

DEFINITION AND DESCRIPTION OF AN AEROSOL

An *aerosol* can be defined as a system of solid particles or liquid droplets that can remain dispersed in a gas, usually air. Naturally occurring aerosols and those emitted by clinical aerosol generators almost always contain a wide range of particle sizes. Because the aerodynamic behavior of an aerosolized particle is critically influenced by its mass, it is important to be able to describe precisely the size distribution of aerosolized particles. In clinical studies, the *mass median aerodynamic diameter* (MMAD) and the geometric standard deviation are often used to characterize the dimensions of an aerosol. When the mass distribution of particles in an aerosol is fractionated and the cumulative particle distribution plotted as a lognormal distribution, it often approximates a straight line. However, recent studies of clinical aerosols have indicated that nebulized particles are often not lognormal in distribution.[5] The MMAD represents the point in the distribution above which 50% of the mass resides, expressed as the diameter of a unit density (1 g/mL) sphere having the same terminal settling velocity as the aerosol particle in question, regardless of its shape and density.

The lognormal plot is convenient because, if linear, it defines a statistically "normal" distribution and the data can be described accurately by the MMAD and the standard deviation alone. For a lognormal distribution, one standard deviation is called the *geometric standard deviation* (σg). The σg is the ratio of the size at 84% (or 16%) to the MMAD and is an indicator of the variability in particle diameters. If the particle size varies over a wide range (σg > 1.2), it is described as having a *polydisperse* particle distribution; if the particles are of similar size (σg < 1.2), the particle distribution is described as *monodisperse*. Monodisperse aerosols are usually encountered only in research studies where specialized generators are used to create such an aerosol.[6] For clinical aerosols that are not lognormal and are widely polydisperse, it is best to relate deposition studies to the entire distribution of particles and avoid focusing on simple descriptive terms, such as the MMAD and σg.[5,7]

PRINCIPLES OF DEPOSITION

The fraction of inhaled particles that deposit (as opposed to being exhaled) is called the *deposition fraction*.[1,2] The likelihood that a particle will deposit in a particular airway depends on the interaction of three factors: the physical characteristics of the particle (e.g., mass, shape), the gas flow in which the particle is transported (the patient's breathing pattern[8] and any velocity provided to the particle by a propellant), and the airway anatomy (especially the presence of airway obstruction[9]). Particles deposit in the lung by three primary mechanisms: inertial impaction, gravitational sedimentation, and Brownian diffusion.

Inertial impaction is the dominant mechanism by which particles deposit in the nasopharynx and more proximal airways. In general, the greater the mass, the faster the velocity, and the narrower the airway, the greater the likelihood that the particle will deposit by impaction. Impaction describes the process by which a particle fails to follow the air stream in which it is suspended, thereby impacting on an obstacle instead of circumventing it. The probability of a particle undergoing inertial impaction can be estimated using Equation 1[1]:

$$I = \alpha\,(V_t V_a \sin\theta / gR) \qquad \text{[Eq. 1]}$$

where I is inertial impaction, V_t is the settling velocity of the entrained particle, V_a is the air stream velocity, θ is the angle required to circumvent the obstacle, g is the acceleration due to gravity, and R is the airway radius. The settling velocity (defined in Equation 2) increases as particle size increases. This equation applies to situations in which laminar flow predominates. The presence of turbulent nonlaminar flow will tend to increase impaction further. Particles that fail to deposit in proximal airways by inertial impaction can deposit in peripheral airways and alveoli by a process called gravitational sedimentation.

Gravitational sedimentation is the process by which a particle accelerates under gravity until it reaches a terminal settling velocity (V_t), which is determined by Equation 2[1]:

$$V_t = (\rho - \sigma)\,gd^2/18\gamma \qquad \text{[Eq. 2]}$$

where ρ is the density of the particle, σ is the density of air, g is the acceleration due to gravity, d is the diameter of the particle, and γ is the viscosity of air. Therefore, for a given velocity, the greater the aerodynamic mass of an aerosol, the shorter the time it will remain suspended in the air stream. Gravitational sedimentation is the main mechanism by which particles between 0.5 and 5.0 μm in diameter deposit in the peripheral regions of the lung. Sedimentation is critically dependent on the patient's breathing pattern.[8] If there is a breath-hold before exhalation, particles are more likely to sediment; without a breath-hold, particles are more likely to be exhaled rather than deposited. It has also been suggested that alveolar volume may affect deposition fraction (larger air spaces require more time for sedimentation).

Brownian diffusion describes how very small particles (<0.2 μm) can deposit. The diffusion coefficient of a particle (D) reflects the rate of diffusion of the particle in air and can be expressed as in Equation 3:

$$D = kT/3\pi\eta d \qquad \text{[Eq. 3]}$$

where k is the Boltzmann constant, T is the temperature in Kelvin, η is the gas viscosity, and d is particle diameter.[2] These tiny particles are rarely important in therapeutic aerosols but can be produced by combustion and may be clinically relevant, even though they tend to be transient because of the tendency to agglomeration. In addition, human-made nanoparticles, which are of increasing interest in electronics and biomedical research, would, if inadvertently inhaled, likely deposit by diffusion. Particles between 0.2 and 0.5 μm in diameter tend to be too small to deposit efficiently by sedimentation and yet too large to deposit efficiently by Brownian diffusion and tend to be exhaled rather than deposited in the lung.[1,2]

MEASUREMENTS AND APPLICATIONS OF AEROSOL PARTICLE SIZE

Particle size is an important factor in determining whether a particle will undergo nasopharyngeal deposition, airway deposition, or alveolar deposition.[10] Particle size is usually measured by light scattering or cascade impaction. Light scattering is based on the principle that there is differential scattering of polarized light by particles of different sizes; cascade impaction is based on a different trajectory of particles of different mass. In cascade impaction, particles at a set flow rate go through a series of apertures of decreasing diameter and impact on a series of plates if they fail to follow the air stream. Cascade impactors with high flow rates (e.g., 28 L/min) were originally designed for environmental sampling of ambient air to collect 100% of the emitted dose. They have been adopted as the method of choice for monitoring quality control in manufacturing plants for aerosol delivery. Cascade impaction has an advantage over light scattering in that it facilitates the correlation of different methods of quantifying the distribution of the active drug (e.g., chemical analysis of drug on each plate compared with radioactive label or weight). However, measuring the emitted dose of aerosol using a high-flow cascade impactor is not ideal for predicting how an aerosol will perform in clinical practice. Although low-flow cascade impactors sample only some of the output, they more closely duplicate in vivo conditions.[5,11–13]

Particle size measurements using different techniques are not necessarily interchangeable. Meaningful comparisons of the sizes of clinical aerosols, especially those produced by a pressurized *metered-dose inhaler* (MDI), can be made only if obtained with identical techniques. Nevertheless, despite the technical difficulties, some investigators have established that, when used with appropriate caution, data obtained by in vitro measurement of particle size provide useful predictive information for subsequent clinical studies.[5,7,11,13]

The classic studies of the influence of particle size on lung deposition were performed with monodisperse aerosols consisting of particles that would not absorb moisture from the air (nonhygroscopic).[6] In contrast, pharmaceutical aerosols tend to be polydisperse liquid droplets, with the active pharmaceutical ingredient and, in some cases, pharmaceutically inactive ingredients, such as preservatives and hydrofluoralkane, being either in solution or suspended as micronized particles. Droplets can change size by exchanging water with either the dry carrier gas or the humid environment of the upper airway.[2,14] In addition, some drug ingredients are hygroscopic, and some diluent solutions are hypertonic, both of which could lead to an increase in particle size due to an increase in aqueous content of the particle; the clinical significance of such changes is not clear.[15] Thus measuring the particle distribution of droplet aerosols is difficult because the particles can be affected by ambient humidity. The predictive value of cascade impaction data from droplet aerosols for in vivo deposition (e.g., for upper airway deposition as measured by gamma scintigraphy) is strongly dependent on the specific technique used for cascade impaction.[12]

GENERATION OF THERAPEUTIC AEROSOLS

Therapeutic aerosols can be generated in three ways. First, the patient's inspiratory airflow can aerosolize a micronized dry powder (*dry powder inhalers* [DPI]). Second, micronized particles can be suspended in a volatile pressurized liquid that vaporizes when at atmospheric pressure, thus imparting velocity to the emitted particles (MDIs). Third, a dispersal force can be applied to a liquid to generate droplets, which are then inhaled by tidal breathing. The generation of the dispersal force can be as simple as using a compressed air source attached to a narrow orifice to generate a Venturi effect (i.e., jet nebulizer) or by more complex vibrating membranes and meshes. In addition, a novel delivery system, Soft Mist, a metered liquid aerosol that does not use a propellant, is briefly described below.

DRY POWDER DEVICES

Because DPI aerosols are generated by the patient's inspiration, they are by definition coordinated with inspiration, a feature that enhances drug deposition (Fig. 13.1A).[4,16–19] The need to trigger the aerosol generation by an inspiratory effort makes them unsuitable for infants and for patients with severe cognitive impairment, who may be unable to comprehend the instructions. The design of DPI devices has evolved over several decades to meet the key objective that the emitted dose should not vary significantly within the clinically relevant range of inspiratory flow. By so doing, the DPI intersubject dosing remains consistent and meets stringent regulatory standards for the quality and reproducibility

of the emitted aerosol. For dry powder devices to maintain reproducible dosing over time, it is essential that the powder be protected from moisture. The design of DPIs has greatly improved, and the devices approved in major markets now perform at high levels of efficiency and reproducibility.[20] Devices can be single-dose devices in which a capsule of powder is perforated in the device (HandiHaler, Boehringer Ingelheim), a multidisk with individual doses wrapped in foil blisters[17] (Diskus and Ellipta, GlaxoSmithKline), or a multidose metered reservoir (Turbuhaler and Flexhaler, AstraZeneca).

A DPI device (Trelegy Ellipta, GlaxoSmithKline) has recently been developed that can deliver three medications simultaneously (an inhaled corticosteroid, a long-acting β_2-agonist, and a long-acting muscarinic antagonist) and is used once daily, making this a more convenient device for patients with COPD to use.[18] Clinical trials in patients with COPD demonstrate that the three-drug combination as a single inhaler was superior to a two-drug combination single-inhaler therapy and was noninferior to the three drugs being administered in two inhalers.[18,19]

PRESSURIZED METERED-DOSE INHALERS

Pressurized MDIs (pMDIs) using chlorofluorocarbon propellants were developed 60 years ago to treat obstructive lung disease. Chlorofluorocarbon-containing pMDI formulations have been replaced by formulations that use hydrofluoroalkane as a propellant.[21–23] pMDIs remain the most popular method of administering short-acting rescue inhalers and are an alternative to DPIs in delivering controller medications to patients with asthma and COPD. They are portable and discreet, but many patients have difficulty with inhaler technique, which can contribute to poor control of disease. For adequate lung deposition, there must be precise coordination with a patient's ventilation. Even with optimal technique, 80% of the emitted dose may deposit on the pharynx and cause local irritation (see Fig. 13.1B). In addition, some orally bioavailable medications cause significant systemic exposure from swallowed medication. Valved holding chambers ("spacers") reduce pharyngeal deposition because high-velocity particles impact on the inside of the chamber; use of these devices decreases the need for precise coordination with respiration.[21] For young children, a

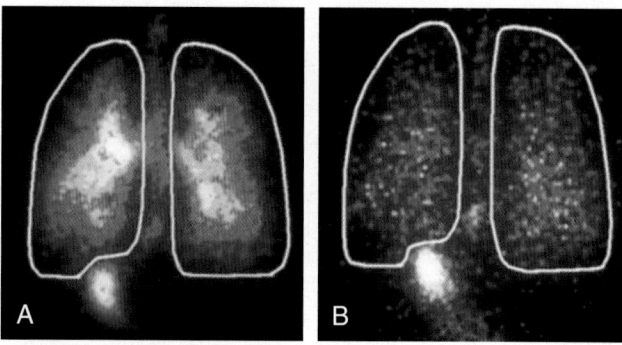

Figure 13.1 Comparison of drug deposition using common aerosol delivery systems. Deposition images after inhalation of radiolabeled aerosols using a dry powder inhaler (A) or a *metered-dose inhaler* (MDI) (B). The dry powder inhaler provided more lung deposition than the MDI. With the MDI, most of the inhaled dose was deposited in the oropharynx due to inertial impaction and detected in the stomach after being swallowed.

face mask can be used in conjunction with a valved holding chamber. Pivotal studies of novel MDI medications undertaken for regulatory approval are almost always performed without a holding chamber because manufacturers do not want their product's prescription tied to a specific holding chamber. To make the chambers more acceptable to patients, small-volume chambers (140 mL) and collapsible chambers have been developed.

As an alternative to using a holding chamber, pMDIs have been developed that are actuated during inspiration and have similar performance characteristics as an optimally used conventional pMDI (Qvar RediHaler, Teva Respiratory).[24]

Increasing frequency of rescue inhaler use may be a sign of worsening control of asthma. As a result, electronic monitoring devices have been attached to these devices to measure their use in real time. Electronic monitoring devices are also being developed for controller medications given via pMDI or DPI in efforts to encourage improved adherence and facilitate early intervention during exacerbations.[25,26]

JET NEBULIZERS

The ubiquitous small-volume jet nebulizer is the mainstay of bronchodilator delivery in hospitalized patients and patients at the extremes of age. These devices are inexpensive and require little patient cooperation. In addition, they are useful for delivering medications with a relatively large mass, such as antibiotics. Generation of the driving pressure requires either a tank of pressurized gas or an electric compressor. Although the manufacturers of compressors have made these devices more portable, they are far from convenient for ambulatory patients. In addition, conventional nebulizers take 10 to 20 minutes to deliver a single treatment, which may decrease adherence. Most generic nebulizers are inefficient and deliver less than 10% of the drug to the lung. The remainder is left in the nebulizer chamber as so-called dead volume (droplets and dried particles left on the nebulizer walls), lost through the expiratory port because the device generates aerosol throughout the respiratory cycle, or deposited in the extrapulmonary upper airway because most of the emitted dose is contained in large, poorly respirable particles. Recent enhancements of jet nebulizers include addition of internal recycling baffles to reduce emitted particle size and addition of expiratory filters to trap potentially hazardous aerosols and reduce collateral exposure.[27]

During the COVID-19 respiratory virus pandemic of 2020, concerns regarding exposure of health care workers to potentially contaminated aerosols during nebulization of bronchodilators led hospital clinicians to switch from using jet nebulizers to MDIs with spacers (https://www.cdc.gov/coronavirus/2019-ncov/hcp/infection-control-recommendations.html).

Increased drug delivery by nebulizers is possible by the use of breath actuation, which coordinates nebulization with inspiration and essentially turns the nebulizer off during expiration, or by the use of breath enhancement, which uses the patient's inspiratory flow through the nebulizer to increase drug delivery (e.g., LC Star, Pari; Medicaid Ventstream, Medicaid, Ltd.).[28]

VIBRATING MESH NEBULIZERS

These devices provide an alternative to jet nebulizers for delivery of larger quantities of drugs such as antibiotics or proteins. Instead of bulky compressors, the devices use either vibrating mesh or crystal, extrude the liquid through tiny holes (microextrusion), or use a combination of both vibration and microextrusion.[29] Vibrating mesh systems vary in durability, cost, and the relative ease with which they can be cleaned between treatments. They usually have a lower dead volume in the nebulizer chamber than the conventional jet nebulizers, resulting in increased efficiency and shorter treatment times.[30] The increased efficiency increases the risk of overdosage if a patient has previously been using a less-efficient device. Some aerosol devices are customized for specific drug approval; for example, different iterations of the eFlow device (Pari) deliver specific aerosolized antibiotics to *cystic fibrosis* (CF) patients more rapidly than conventional nebulizers. The Aerogen vibrating mesh nebulizers are used to deliver bronchodilators more rapidly than conventional nebulizers and to deliver novel medications (insulin, Dance Biopharm Holdings) now in clinical trials. Another vibrating mesh device (I-neb) has been adapted to administer inhaled prostacyclin (Ventavis, Actelion), a drug with a relatively narrow therapeutic index, to treat pulmonary hypertension. The I-neb device uses adaptive aerosol technology, monitors the breathing pattern of a patient, and provides feedback to the patient to facilitate a more consistent inhaled dose. As discussed earlier, a "slow" inspiration reduces inertial impaction and thus decreases oropharyngeal deposition, allowing distal delivery of particles that would otherwise deposit in the oropharynx during tidal breathing. "Smart" nebulizers that provide feedback to patients can help patients adjust their breathing pattern to achieve more consistent dosing.[30,31]

SOFT MIST AEROSOLS

The Respimat Soft Mist (Boehringer Ingelheim) device is approved for delivery of short-acting and long-acting bronchodilators. It is a small hand-held device significantly different in design from a conventional pMDI or DPI.[32] The drug is stored in a liquid reservoir, and an aerosol is generated when a precisely calibrated volume of liquid is forced through a nozzle to produce two jets of liquid that converge at a defined angle. The velocity of the resulting aerosol mist is much slower than that generated by a pMDI and is thus both less likely to impact on the upper airway and easier to coordinate with a patient's inspiration. The efficiency is higher than with a conventional DPI. For example, the nominal dose of tiotropium is 18 µg by DPI but only 5 µg with the Respimat.

The challenge of demonstrating clinical equivalence of the same drug from two devices is illustrated by a regulatory requirement to perform a 17,000-patient head-to-head safety study comparing the safety of DPI to Respimat in patients with COPD. No difference in mortality was observed in this large study, which was performed to evaluate a potential mortality signal with soft mist aerosols in earlier smaller studies.[33] Improved drug delivery by soft mist aerosols will decrease the amount of drug needed per dose. However, the small metered volume limits this device to high-potency drugs.

PRINCIPLES OF ASSESSMENT OF DELIVERY SYSTEMS

Assessing effects of an aerosolized drug requires the understanding of three major factors: the characteristics of the aerosol delivery system, the quality of the aerosol produced, and the quantification of deposition within the lungs.[34] Quantification of deposition is performed in vivo, is time consuming and costly, and involves some degree of risk and uncertainty to the patient. The other two components of the aerosol delivery process can be well characterized and studied in vitro. The field of aerosol delivery has advanced significantly in the last 10 years so that aerosol delivery characteristics and the quality of the aerosol can be significantly optimized on the bench before exposure to patients.

THE INHALED MASS

The term *inhaled mass* has been coined to represent the amount of drug that passes the lips of the patient, that is, *drug delivery* to the patient, to distinguish this quantity from drug *dose* or drug *deposition* (see later). Bench models are useful in identifying the parameters that define the inhaled mass for different devices and experimental conditions[11] (eFig. 13.1). A mouthpiece is replaced by a filter that captures the aerosolized particles, and a breathing device (piston ventilator) can duplicate conditions such as routine tidal breathing and mixing of ambient air with the nebulized particles. The quantity of drug captured on the inspiratory filter represents the inhaled mass. The setup can be modified to incorporate a ventilator circuit and endotracheal tube to duplicate aerosol delivery in the setting of mechanical ventilation and determine the impact of the brand of nebulizer, humidification, ventilator settings, and nebulizer fill volume on drug delivery before proceeding to clinical studies.[35,36]

DEPOSITION

The term *deposition* implies a "dose" to the patient. The term *deposition* needs to be further refined in a given situation (e.g., oropharyngeal vs. parenchymal deposition, or central vs. peripheral deposition within the lung). Each of these terms may be important depending upon the disease entity to be treated. Obviously, the measurement of the actual deposition requires an in vivo experiment. However, deposition can be estimated based on parameters measured in vitro as shown in Equation 4:

$$\text{Deposition} = \text{Inhaled mass} - \text{Exhaled mass} \quad \text{[Eq. 4]}$$

Clinical deposition studies using gamma scintigraphy can be used to assess the regional distribution of drug deposited in the patient.[37] Deposition can be divided into extrapulmonary deposition versus pulmonary deposition, whereas pulmonary deposition can be further subdivided into deposition in central airways versus in peripheral air spaces. A radiotracer (usually technetium) is mixed with the study drug and aerosolized and inhaled. It is important to confirm that the size distribution of the radiotracer and the drug are identical.[35] The drug deposition images on the gamma camera are superimposed on an outline of the patient's lung, obtained by a separate radioactive gas study,[38,39] or a transmission image from an external standardized radioactive source.[30,40] Quantification of lung deposition can be obtained by expressing the radioactivity detected in the lungs as a percentage of the radioactivity initially placed in the nebulizer (see Fig. 13.1).

Several other methods can be used to assess deposition. A mass balance technique uses filters placed near a patient's mouth to measure the amount inhaled and, in a separate experiment, the amount exhaled, with the difference being what was deposited in the patient.[38,39] However, this technique does not provide information on the specific compartment in which the material was deposited. Pharmacokinetic approaches include comparison of blood levels of aminoglycosides obtained after an intravenous calibration standard to blood levels obtained after inhalation[41] or the urinary concentrations of pentamidine after inhalation.[42,43] Oral charcoal can be used to block the absorption of swallowed pharyngeal deposited drug so that blood levels will be due entirely to drug absorbed through lung deposition and absorption.[16]

STRATEGIES TO OPTIMIZE DEPOSITION OF THERAPEUTIC AEROSOLS

The determinants of aerosol deposition apply to both therapeutic and environmental inhaled particles. To optimize deposition of therapeutic aerosols, a number of strategies have been developed.

GETTING PARTICLES PAST THE OROPHARYNX

In clinical studies, predicting penetration of aerosol beyond the oropharynx and subsequent lung deposition is a major criterion for device selection. Deposition estimations are often based on particle size measurements defined by in vitro characterization of the aerosol produced by a given device. During tidal breathing, most investigators would expect aerosols with particles smaller than 5 μm to be deposited primarily in the lungs (the fine particle fraction). Conventional aerosol delivery devices (DPI, pMDI, and jet nebulizer) emit particles with a wide range of sizes and velocities (i.e., polydisperse particles). It is estimated that the combined effect of particle size, particle inertia, and the geometry of the oropharynx result in upper airway deposition ranging from 30–90% of the total deposition in the patient. Only nebulizers producing particles with particularly small MMAD (e.g., AeroTech II, Biodex; MMAD, 1.0 μm) bypass the upper airways (5% oropharyngeal deposition in adults).[44] In children, the smaller oropharyngeal airways make the task more difficult.[45] In children, compared to adults, significantly more drug may be deposited in the oropharynx and less in the lung (Fig. 13.2).

CONTROL OF BREATHING PATTERN AND AEROSOL DEPOSITION

In normal subjects, the pattern of breathing is the most important factor affecting aerosol delivery and deposition.

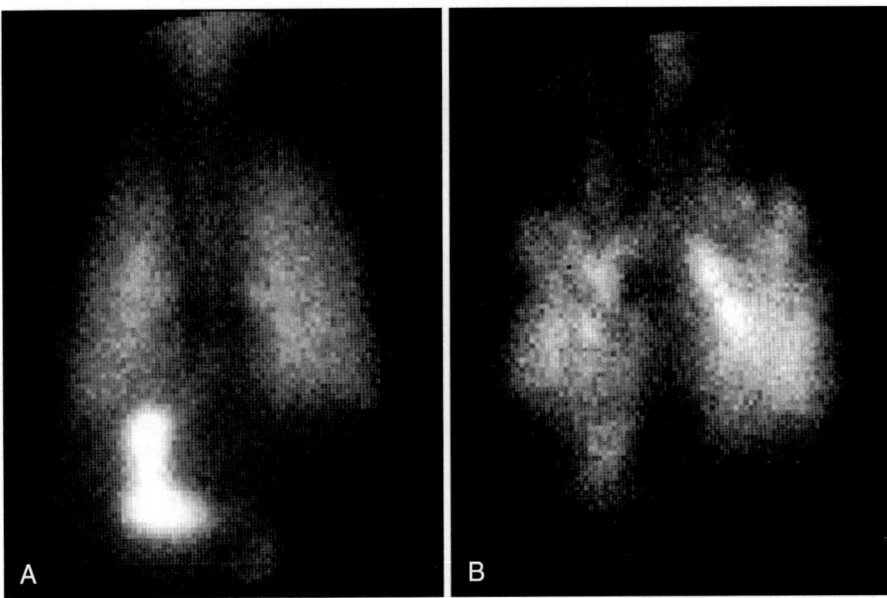

Figure 13.2 Differences in aerosol deposition between adults and children illustrated by deposition scans from patients with cystic fibrosis breathing the same aerosol. (A) A 9-year-old boy with 48% upper airway deposition, which appears in the stomach after a drink of water. (B) A 31-year-old woman demonstrating a more peripheral but patchy distribution but minimal activity in stomach. Aerosols that can readily bypass the upper airways of an adult frequently deposit in the oropharynx of a child. (From Diot P, Palmer LB, Smaldone A, et al. RhDNase I aerosol deposition and related factors in cystic fibrosis. *Am J Respir Crit Care Med.* 1997;156:1662–1668.)

How the patient breathes can affect the performance of the device, the particle distribution, the penetration of particles past the oropharynx, and the deposition within the parenchyma. Earlier studies suggested that much of the variation in parenchymal deposition was related to differences in airway geometry among subjects. However, variability in deposition among subjects appears well controlled if the pattern of breathing is controlled. As tidal volume increases and breathing frequency decreases, the time of inspiration is prolonged (e.g., slow and deep inspiration). As demonstrated in Figure 13.3, changes in the deposition fraction can largely be accounted for by changes in the tidal volume and breathing frequency.

EXPIRATION AND PROBLEMS WITH AEROSOL DEPOSITION

Particles that pass through the oropharynx during inspiration enter the central airways and traverse them without difficulty because lobar and segmental bronchi are generally widely patent during inspiration. Then the particles enter alveoli, with a few depositing by sedimentation and, like cigarette smoke, the bulk of the aerosol is exhaled. Deposition is controlled by sedimentation in small airways and is influenced by local geometry and, to a strong degree, by the residence time (period of breathing). In normal subjects the particles that do not deposit during inspiration are largely exhaled completely.

In obstructive lung disease, maximal expiratory flows are diminished. With moderate disease, maximal flows can be superimposed on tidal breathing; as the disease progresses, maximal flows can be reduced even further. Therefore, it is common to observe that patients are often breathing on their maximal expiratory flow-volume curves even during quiet, tidal breathing[46] (eFig. 13.2). In these patients, the flow-limiting segments exist in the

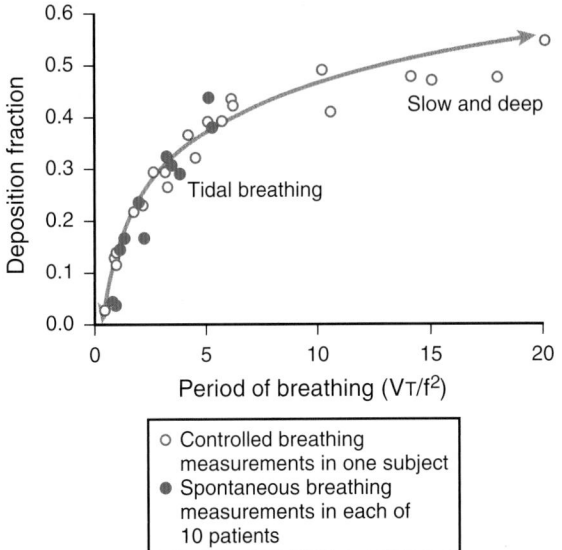

Figure 13.3 Deposition in the lungs is primarily determined by the pattern of breathing. Deposition fraction of 2.6-μm monodisperse particles from one subject during controlled breathing (*open circles*) and from 10 patients during spontaneous breathing (*solid circles*). The deposition fraction is the fraction of inhaled particles that deposited in the subject; breathing pattern is illustrated by the period of breathing (tidal volume divided by breathing frequency squared [V_T/f^2]). Typical tidal breathing is found near the origin; slow and deep inspirations appear away from the origin. The deposition fraction varied over a wide range, but changes in the deposition fraction were accounted for by changes in the breathing parameter. (Modified from Bennet WD, Smaldone GC. Human variation in the peripheral airspace deposition of inhaled particles. *J Appl Physiol.* 1987;62:1603–1610.)

same airways as in normal subjects during forced expiration but, in patients with obstructive lung disease, they form during every tidal breath. Therefore, in patients with obstructive lung disease, deposition in the peripheral

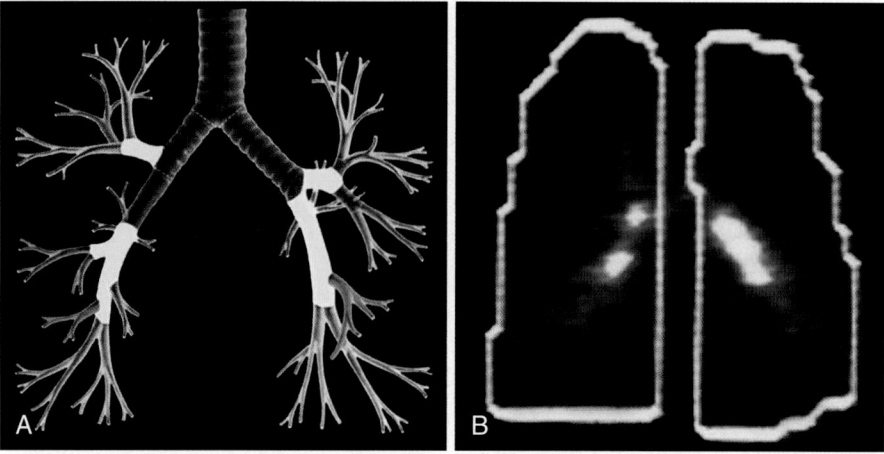

Figure 13.4 Particles are deposited preferentially at sites of flow-limiting segments in patients with COPD. Sites of flow-limiting segments (A, *yellow*) and the corresponding deposition image (B) in a patient with severe COPD (*posterior view*). (Modified from Smaldone GC. Advances in aerosols: adult respiratory disease. *J Aerosol Med.* 2006;19:36–46.)

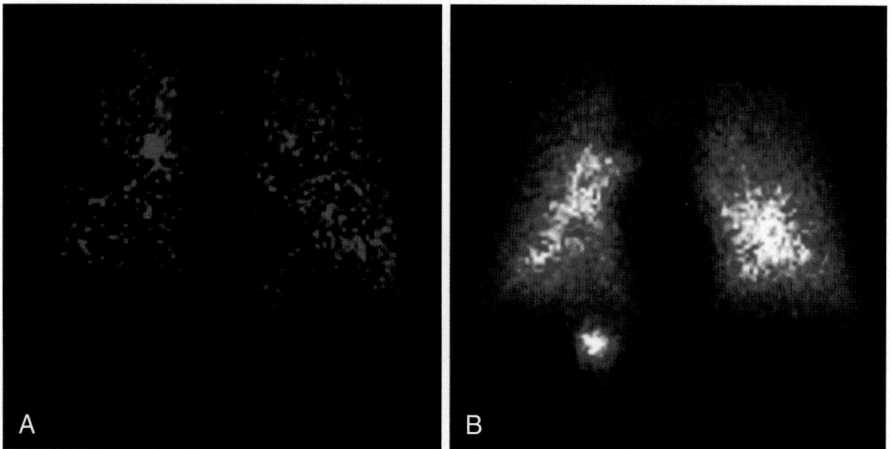

Figure 13.5 Slow and deep breathing improves aerosol delivery and deposition. Deposition scans from a normal subject after breathing from I-neb, a breath-actuated vibrating mesh nebulizer in which particles are generated only during inspiration. (A) After 20 breaths of normal tidal breathing. (B) Scan repeated after 3 breaths of very slow and deep inspiration (~7 sec/breath). For slow and deep breathing, deposition was 50 times more efficient per breath, a combination of enhanced delivery and more efficient deposition. (Courtesy G.C. Smaldone, unpublished data.)

lung poses a significant challenge because deposition of aerosol is enhanced during expiration at sites of flow limitation (Fig. 13.4). Based on these physiologic considerations, peripheral deposition of aerosol in these subjects would be favored by a slow prolonged inspiration with a breath of sufficiently long duration to promote deposition by settling and to minimize the particles available to the airways during expiration.

For many aerosol applications, inhaling particles slowly and deeply solves the problems outlined previously. A slow inhalation will minimize oropharyngeal deposition. Slow inspiration reduces particle inertia and allows inhalation of larger particles that would have deposited in the oropharynx during tidal breathing. Subsequently, commercial applications of these principles have combined slow and deep inspiration with direct mechanical feedback to the patient for particles of relatively large MMAD, resulting in more efficient delivery to the more distal airways (Fig. 13.5).[47]

ADDITIONAL FACTORS INFLUENCING DEVELOPMENT OF THERAPEUTIC AEROSOLS

In addition to efforts to bypass the oropharynx and optimize lung deposition, other factors influence the design of therapeutic aerosols. Some of these factors are disease related and others relate to specific patient populations.

INHALED PROTEINS

Most approved inhaled products are small molecular chemical entities. Larger molecules can also be inhaled, such as proteins,[48] including inhaled recombinant DNase for CF, *granulocyte-macrophage colony-stimulating factor* (GM-CSF) for alveolar proteinosis,[49] interferon-γ for pulmonary fibrosis,[50] and recombinant alpha$_1$-antitrypsin for emphysema.[51] Development programs of inhaled proteins face additional challenges. Preclinical evaluation is important to ensure that the nebulization process does not denature these agents. In addition, the structure of these proteins may be modified to decrease risk of being denatured by the proteolytic enzymes present in airway secretions. In addition to their use as therapeutic agents for pulmonary disease, the inhaled route of administration can be used to take advantage of the large alveolar surface area of the lung to facilitate systemic absorption. To date, the most extensively studied class of inhaled protein has been inhaled insulin,[52,53] based on the rationale that patients may prefer the inhaled administration to subcutaneous injection. Despite two products achieving U.S. regulatory approval, inhaled insulin has not been widely adopted by prescribers or patients. Some patients, especially those with preexisting airways disease, complained of cough after inhalation. Hypoglycemia was observed particularly in smokers in whom systemic absorption appeared to be accelerated. In rare cases, there was evidence of a decline in diffusion capacity, an observation that may result in requirements for extensive testing of future inhaled proteins. There are also theoretical concerns that exposure to insulin could accelerate the growth of lung cancer in populations at increased risk for cancer.

Despite these concerns, with the rapid progress in development of new biologic treatment modalities (fusion proteins, RNA silencing, gene therapy, etc.), it is likely that many of these agents will be evaluated for their potential to be delivered by inhalation.

ASTHMA

It is important that commercial formulations of inhaled corticosteroids, the mainstay of maintenance therapy for asthma, have a low oral bioavailability.[54–56] Because many delivery systems for inhaled corticosteroids have high levels of oropharyngeal deposition (up to 80% with pMDIs and DPIs), it is crucial that, when this oropharyngeal-deposited drug is subsequently swallowed, its systemic exposure be kept as low as possible. The oral bioavailability of beclomethasone, one of the oldest of the inhaled corticosteroids, is approximately 20%, fluticasone is approximately 1%, and mometasone less than 1%, whereas ciclesonide does not become activated until it deposits in lung tissue.[56] However, even if there is no oral bioavailability, there can still be systemic exposure when inhaled corticosteroids are absorbed from the lung itself, either from the alveoli or airways. Alveolar deposition may give rise to more systemic exposure than airway deposition because particles depositing in the alveoli are not removed by mucociliary clearance and because the alveoli may be more permeable to diffusion than the airway. There are some pharmacodynamic data that, when fluticasone is administered to both normal subjects and asthmatics, the asthmatic subjects have less systemic absorption, likely due to the more proximal deposition in the asthmatic subjects because of reduced airway caliber.[57] Most pharmaceutical manufacturers have therefore tried to target airway deposition while avoiding alveolar deposition. This appears reasonable because asthma is thought to be an airways disease. Some investigators, however, have suggested that there may be an alveolar inflammatory component in asthma, thus suggesting that alveolar deposition

may be beneficial.[58] Nonetheless, this remains a minority viewpoint.

Targeting the airways in asthma is complicated by the polydisperse nature of therapeutic aerosols. Making the average aerosol diameter smaller reduces oropharyngeal deposition but increases the amount of alveolar deposition. A low oral bioavailability is more important for polydisperse aerosols with larger MMADs to minimize systemic exposure from swallowed drug. Systemic exposure to inhaled corticosteroids can lead to short-term growth suppression in children, decreases in bone mineral density, and possibly an increase in cataracts.[54–56] The potential role of inhaled corticosteroids in cataract development is confounded by concomitant use of intermittent systemic corticosteroids, smoking, and ultraviolet light exposure.[58,59] However, an epidemiologic study from Australia that controlled for use of systemic and ocular steroid use found an association between inhaled steroids and the prevalence of cataracts.[60] Theoretically, cataracts could also be due to inadvertent spraying of aerosol into the eyes in addition to systemic exposure.

Although the search continues for the ideal method of delivery for inhaled steroids to patients with asthma, advances in drug design, formulation, and delivery now provide a wider array of options to the clinician. However, no delivery system can be considered to be intrinsically superior to all others. The delivery system should be judged instead by its ability to optimize the pharmacokinetic properties of the drug, most notably oral bioavailability, and by its suitability for the target subpopulation of asthmatics.[4]

CYSTIC FIBROSIS AND NON–CYSTIC FIBROSIS BRONCHIECTASIS

CF, the most common fatal single-gene genetic disease in Europe and North America, is associated with severe bronchiectasis.[61,62] Antibiotics such as tobramycin, aztreonam, and polymyxin are commonly inhaled for treatment. Antibiotics usually require the aerosolization of several hundred milligrams of medication. Jet nebulizers or vibrating mesh devices are usually needed to deliver such a large mass of drug. However, only approximately 10% of the dose is deposited in the lungs because of inefficiencies of the delivery systems. Nevertheless, inhalation can be effective at targeting the drug to the lung and avoiding systemic side effects and toxicity. For example, aminoglycosides, when given systemically, have poor airway penetration and are limited by renal and ototoxicity. Inhalation of tobramycin, on the other hand, can result in sputum levels two orders of magnitude higher than those associated with systemic delivery. For the purposes of inhalation, tobramycin was reformulated without the preservative present in the intravenous preparation.[63] Aztreonam was reformulated with a lysine side chain for inhalation instead of the methionine side chain found in the intravenous formulation, to reduce the risk for airway irritation.[64]

In addition to antibiotics, inhalation of mucolytics (recombinant DNase) and osmotic hydrating agents (hypertonic saline and mannitol) are of benefit in patients with CF.[65] The multiplicity of inhaled treatments, however, is likely to reduce patient adherence[66] and therefore creates the need to explore the use of devices with shorter treatment duration.

Because the key physiologic finding in the lungs of patients with CF is bronchiectasis with chronic bacterial infection, inhaled antibiotics effective in treating CF (tobramycin, aztreonam) were also evaluated in non-CF bronchiectasis. However, the antibiotics were much less effective in demonstrating efficacy, and the primary end points were not met in most trials. Recently, randomized trials evaluating a novel formulation of inhaled ciprofloxacin produced inconsistent evidence of efficacy.[67] The reasons for the disappointing outcomes in non-CF bronchiectasis are not understood but may include greater heterogeneity of disease severity, lower bacterial load, lower frequency of exacerbation, and more localized lobar distribution of disease in the non-CF patients.[68–72]

IDIOPATHIC PULMONARY FIBROSIS

Idiopathic pulmonary fibrosis (IPF) is a progressive interstitial lung disease with a peak incidence of onset in the sixth decade. Although there are two approved orally administered agents (pirfenidone and nintedanib) demonstrated to slow the rate of decline in lung function, there remains an unmet need for more effective and better tolerated medications.[73] There has been a recent increase in interest in exploring the inhaled route for IPF therapeutics.

In addition to the challenges facing all development programs in IPF (an incomplete understanding of the pathogenesis and requirement for relatively large and prolonged trials), an inhaled agent faces additional challenges: the need to target alveolar deposition rather than airway deposition, a requirement for a well-tolerated aerosolized drug in patients prone to debilitating cough, and a need to address marked regional variation in distribution, given that IPF is usually more severe in the lower lobes. Current inhalational strategies under development include an agent already approved through the systemic route (e.g., inhaled pirfenidone[74]), agents that were not effective by systemic administration (e.g., interferon-γ[50]), and agents not previously evaluated (e.g., galectin).[75]

PULMONARY MYCOBACTERIAL INFECTIONS

The emergence of resistance to first-line antibacterial agents has prompted a search for novel therapeutic approaches for pulmonary mycobacterial diseases, including tuberculosis and nontuberculous mycobacterial lung disease.

Several candidate aerosolized agents for treating multidrug-resistant tuberculosis have been formulated, with the majority of new formulations being dry powders.[76,77] Most antitubercular drugs require high doses (tens to hundreds of milligrams), rendering them unsuitable for many conventional DPIs, necessitating development of high-volume DPI systems.[77] Administration of aerosolized drugs to patients with multidrug-resistant tuberculosis may induce cough and increase risk of infecting other individuals in the vicinity of the treatment area. Several novel formulations have advanced to Phase I tolerability studies in healthy volunteers but, to date, none has advanced to registration trials of tuberculosis. In addition to development of direct antimicrobial agents, there was a preliminary evaluation of adding inhaled interferon-γ as adjunctive therapy with evidence of increased clearance of infection, but this has not been further advanced.

For treatment of nontuberculous mycobacterial infection, aerosolized amikacin as a liposomal formulation received preliminary approval from the U.S. Food and Drug Administration for treatment of *Mycobacterium avium* complex, to be used as an adjunct with standard oral combination therapy. The rationale for the use of a liposomal formulation is that airway macrophages are believed to ingest liposomes, which could potentially enhance intracellular killing of organisms.[77]

DELIVERY OF INHALED MEDICATIONS TO YOUNG CHILDREN

See ExpertConsult.com for a brief discussion of pediatric considerations.

DELIVERY OF THERAPEUTIC AEROSOLS TO THE NASAL MUCOSA

Diseases of the nasal mucosa are now being treated by an increasing list of aerosolized medications, including corticosteroids, anticholinergics (ipratropium bromide), antihistamines, cromoglycate, saline, and decongestants. In general, these formulations use large particle sizes to maximize nasal deposition. Manual pumps that produce large, relatively low-velocity particles are being used as an alternative to high-velocity pMDIs. There are isolated reports of nasal perforation with high-velocity inhalers,[86] and patients should be advised to direct the spray in the direction of the ipsilateral ear and away from the nasal septum. In addition, directing the inhaler against the lateral wall of the nares reduces the risk for epistaxis (caused by irritating the septum by delivery in a medial direction) or headache (caused by stimulating the olfactory nerve by delivery in a vertical direction). In severe allergic sinusitis, the mucosa may be so congested that a short course of systemic corticosteroids may be needed to allow penetration of aerosolized therapy. Prolonged use of topical decongestant sprays may lead to rebound hyperemia and intractable nasal congestion. In certain cases, systemic administration of decongestants may be preferable. For children who use inhaled corticosteroids for perennial rhinitis, formulations with low oral bioavailability, such as fluticasone, mometasone, and ciclesonide, are preferable and reduce the risk for growth suppression.[87,88]

Nasally inhaled mometasone is an effective topical treatment for chronic rhinosinusitis with nasal polyps.[89] However, obstruction of the nasal passages with large polyps can impair delivery, and surgical implants of topical corticosteroids have been developed as adjuncts to nasal inhalation.[90] In addition, a novel device for fluticasone (Xhance, Optinose) has been approved to treat chronic rhinosinusitis with nasal polyps. This device has a mouthpiece and a nasal piece for drug delivery. Delivery of corticosteroids to the nasal mucosa is achieved when the patient *exhales* through the device. Exhalation releases drug from the device and directs it to the nose. With exhalation, the soft palate also separates the nasal cavity from the mouth, and the drug is sent into one nostril, filling the nasal cavity and exiting via the other nostril.[91]

AEROSOL DELIVERY DURING MECHANICAL VENTILATION

Bronchodilators, either delivered by nebulizer or pMDI, are commonly used to treat patients with airway obstruction while they undergo mechanical ventilation.[92] The use of a pMDI is feasible provided certain conditions are met.[93] For example, delivery during mechanical ventilation must be synchronized with inspiration, and a spacer/holding chamber must be used with a pMDI. Not all holding chambers are equivalent in efficiency, and different brands are not necessarily interchangeable. For a therapeutic effect, it is essential that a dose-escalation protocol be used because it may be necessary to use doses far in excess of those used in ambulatory patients. Hence, objective evidence on response to treatment (e.g., peak airway pressure, dynamic compliance) and toxicity (tachycardia, arrhythmias) should be sought. In endeavoring to maximize delivered doses, however, it must be remembered that the efficiency of pMDI delivery decreases significantly if there is no pause between serial actuations and if the synchronization with inspiration is suboptimal.[94] Nebulizers are less dependent on timing or technique; modeling has shown similar delivery from nebulizers or pMDIs when both are optimally used.[94] Despite limitations, delivery of bronchodilators through ventilator circuitry is a mainstay of treatment of patients with obstructive diseases.

There is also interest in delivering aerosolized antimicrobial therapy via nebulizers in patients with purulent tracheobronchitis and ventilator-associated pneumonia.[92,95,96] The dose delivered in this setting can be highly variable, and delivery can be subtherapeutic if certain factors are not optimized. Similar to drug delivery in spontaneously breathing patients, drug delivery in intubated patients is highly dependent on the breathing pattern.[92] Delivery can be improved by reduced humidification (temporary discontinuation of humidification doubles the delivered dose by reduced rainout of medication), coordination with inspiration, and the appropriate selection of delivery system. If these factors are optimized, delivery can be consistently achieved at doses that approximate those delivered in spontaneously breathing subjects.[35,36] Single-center studies suggested that use of aerosolized antibiotics decreased rate of ventilator-associated pneumonia and other signs and symptoms of respiratory infection, facilitated weaning, reduced bacterial resistance, and decreased use of systemic antibiotics.[92,95–97] However, recent large-scale clinical trials of aerosolized antibiotics in the intubated critically ill patient have failed to reach clinical end points. These trials did not disclose how the delivery of the test drugs was ensured. Controlling drug delivery during mechanical ventilation is a requirement for the success of any future studies.

In conclusion, once technical factors have been identified and optimized, efficient delivery of aerosolized medications to patients undergoing mechanical ventilation is readily attainable.[36]

DIAGNOSTIC RADIOAEROSOLS

The radiolabeled ventilation-perfusion scan is an important clinical tool for detection of pulmonary emboli. Perfusion is measured by injecting radiolabeled macroaggregates of protein that impact in capillaries, whereas ventilation is evaluated by inhalation of a radioactive gas or aerosol. Discrepancies between perfusion abnormalities and ventilation abnormalities are used to assess the probability of pulmonary emboli. The measurement of ventilation should ideally be performed by using a radioactive gas (e.g., xenon-133). However, xenon-133 has a relatively long half-life and needs to be trapped after exhalation. In response to these concerns, aerosols labeled with technetium were developed on the assumption that aerosols would distribute similarly to the gas. In general, that assumption is true if submicron aerosols are inhaled, but it must be remembered that aerosol behavior is not identical to that of a gas.[98] For example, patients who are tachypneic with high inspiratory flows and who have airway obstruction will have central "hot spots" (see Fig. 13.5). This limits the use of the aerosol techniques in certain patient groups.

MUCOCILIARY CLEARANCE AND DISEASE

Mucociliary clearance is the primary mechanism to remove inhaled insoluble particles in the normal host. Inhaled particles that deposit in the ciliated airways are trapped in a blanket of mucus. This free-floating mucus gel overlies the respiratory epithelium. The equilibrium between the osmotic modulus of the gel and brush layers maintains an adequate periciliary depth to facilitate optimal movement of cilia. Mucus is transported proximally by the rhythmic beating of the cilia (a fast, forward-power stroke and slower, backward-recovery stroke) to the pharynx, where it is swallowed, a process called mucociliary clearance.[3] Mucociliary clearance in healthy subjects is usually completed within 24 hours of deposition.[3] The mucus path can be followed using radiolabeled aerosols (Video 13.3).

Ciliated respiratory epithelial cells are most numerous in the tracheal and lobar bronchi and decrease progressively in more distal airways. Secretory cells are also more numerous in proximal airways; goblet cells produce thick carbohydrate-rich secretions, whereas other cells produce more serous secretions. In diseases such as chronic bronchitis and bronchiectasis, the number of goblet cells increases in more distal airways. Airway secretions are also produced by submucosal glands. The latter are lined by mucinous and serous epithelial cells and become hypertrophic and hyperplastic in chronic bronchitis and other types of chronic airway inflammation.

Mucociliary clearance can be impaired by intrinsic defects in ciliary function, which can be congenital (primary ciliary dyskinesias[99]) or acquired (tobacco smoking, influenza).[3] Mucociliary clearance impairment can also be due to changes in the quantity and composition of airway secretions (chronic bronchitis, CF).[3] If the mucociliary apparatus is significantly impaired, secretions are cleared predominantly by coughing. If both mucociliary clearance and cough clearance become ineffective, retained secretions produce both physical obstruction of the airway lumen and amplification of the underlying inflammatory processes.

Primary ciliary dyskinesia is a genetically heterogeneous disorder of the dynein arms or other components of the cilia, resulting in loss of ciliary movement[99] (see Chapter 69).

In the absence of ciliary movement, these patients will have mucus stasis and develop bronchiectasis and sinusitis. In males, ciliary dyskinesia is also associated with infertility due to immotile spermatozoa. Patients may also have abnormalities of visceral organs, such as situs inversus and dextrocardia due to the role of monociliated cells during embryogenesis.[99]

CF management is complicated by impaired mucociliary clearance.[61,62] The mucus becomes dehydrated and less easy to clear because of an impaired chloride channel (*cystic fibrosis transmembrane conductance regulator* [CFTR]), which leads to reduced secretion of chloride into the airway lumen.[62] In addition, an increase in epithelial sodium channel activation due to inflammatory proteases promotes absorption of sodium from the lumen, further exacerbating the dehydration of mucus. Adequate hydration of airway secretions is essential for optimal mucociliary clearance. Hypertonic saline, when administered to the airways of patients with CF, creates an osmotic gradient that draws water into the airway lumen; this treatment is associated with decreased rates of acute exacerbation.[100] Inhaled mannitol is another inhaled osmolyte for patients with CF and has been approved by some regulatory authorities.[101] The airway secretions in CF not only contain mucus secreted by the airway but also consist of DNA and actin from dead neutrophils. Inhaled recombinant DNase can facilitate clearance of secretions and destroy neutrophil extracellular traps, the extracellular DNA released by neutrophils at sites of infection.[102] The development of drugs that modulate CFTR receptor function has significantly improved the clinical course of CF.[103] In addition to demonstrating improvements in standard clinical end points, such as lung function and exacerbation frequency, modulation of CFTR function improves the homogeneity of aerosol deposition and increases clearance of radiolabeled mucus[104,105] (see also Chapter 68).

In chronic bronchitis, there is hypertrophy and hyperplasia of the submucosal glands as well as an increase in the number of goblet cells and the presence of goblet cells in more distal airways, compared to normal. The resultant mucus has an increase in the mucous component relative to the serous component, which means that the mucus layer is relatively dehydrated.[106] In addition, chronic airway inflammation is associated with an increase in secretion of the mucin MUC5AC, which may have proinflammatory properties promoting a positive feedback cycle of inflammation and hypersecretion.[107] Both of these mechanisms contribute to impaired mucociliary clearance in chronic bronchitis.

In patients who die of status asthmaticus, the airways at autopsy are filled with inspissated mucus.[3] The mucus in patients with status asthmaticus has abnormal viscoelastic static properties that may be due in part to excessive cross-linking of mucus glycoproteins.[108,109] In addition, increases in the type 2 cytokine interleukin-13 in asthma promotes a hypersecretory phenotype and impairment of mucus transport.[110,111] Mucociliary clearance is severely impaired acutely in patients with status asthmaticus but can recover within weeks.[112]

In conclusion, mucociliary clearance is impaired in asthma, chronic bronchitis/COPD, CF, bronchiectasis, and primary ciliary dyskinesia and may be an index of disease severity.[113–115] Serial measurements of mucociliary clearance by tracking radiolabeled particles can be useful in measuring pharmaceutical enhancement of mucociliary clearance as, for example, in the sustained effects of hypertonic saline in CF[100] and CFTR modulation.[104] In addition to addressing the primary pathophysiologic defect, such as inflammation, CFTR dysfunction, or dehydration, efforts are being undertaken to develop novel inhaled agents to optimize rheologic properties of airway mucus and improve clearance.[116]

ALVEOLAR CLEARANCE

Particles deposited in the alveoli are cleared by alveolar rather than mucociliary clearance.[117,118] Particle solubility affects clearance in alveoli. Soluble particulates may be absorbed through the thin membrane of the peripheral air spaces. Insoluble particulates, however, tend to be phagocytosed by alveolar macrophages. Their metal content influences the free radical–generating properties of the particle and can promote inflammation, especially when the particle is delivered to the lysosomes. Lysosomes have a very low pH designed to kill microorganisms, but the low pH may promote solubility of transition metals, such as ferrous iron, and therefore be proinflammatory.[119]

Cells primed by one type of inflammation (e.g., by tobacco smoke or endotoxin) may be more reactive to a second stimulus from an inhaled particulate. Excessive particulate exposure can lead to overloading of alveolar macrophages, which can be proinflammatory even with relatively nonreactive particulates. Macrophages migrate to regional lymph nodes, and inhalational exposure to certain particles can be characterized by a distinctive adenopathy (e.g., silicosis and its eggshell calcifications).

The alveolar deposition and clearance of nanoparticles (<100 nm diameter) differ from the clearance of larger but fine particles that deposit in alveoli.[120,121] Nanoparticles are more likely to be absorbed through the alveolar epithelium, resulting in systemic exposure. Environmental nanoparticles arising from combustion tend to be unstable and aggregate into larger particles. However, engineered nanoparticles may be less likely to aggregate and may pose an increased risk of systemic exposure and potential health hazards.

Key Points

- The likelihood that a particle will deposit in an airway depends on the physical characteristics of the particle, the gas flow transporting the particle, and the airway anatomy. The greater the mass, the faster the flow, and the more narrow the airway, the greater is the potential for inertial impaction. For the clinician, forces that define inertial impaction are most important in determining upper airway deposition and the passage of aerosol into the lungs.
- Once particles pass through the upper airways, deposition in the lungs is largely defined by sedimentation. This process is dependent on a subject's breathing pattern, both the depth and the duration of the breath.
- Holding chambers ("spacers") reduce pharyngeal deposition and reduce the need for precise coordination to get the full dose.
- Face mask seal and design can be important factors in the delivery of clinical aerosols in pediatric populations.
- The design of dry powder inhaler devices has evolved to meet the key objective that emitted dose should not vary significantly within a clinically relevant range of inspiratory flow so that intersubject delivery remains consistent and thereby meets stringent regulatory standards for the quality and reproducibility of the emitted aerosol.
- Compared to systemic therapy, medicines can be delivered by aerosol in greater concentration to the target organ, the lung, with fewer side effects, but most traditional jet nebulizers are inefficient and deliver less than 10% of the drug to the lung.
- Directing the jet of high-velocity nasal sprays laterally avoids the side effects of epistaxis when directed medially, and headache when directed vertically.
- Serial measurements of mucociliary clearance may be of value in evaluating novel medications.

Key Readings

de Boer AH, Hagedoorn P, Hoppentocht M, Buttini F, Grasmeijer F, Frijlink HW. Dry powder inhalation: past, present and future. *Expert Opin Drug Deliv.* 2017;14(4):499–512.

Diaz KT, Smaldone GC. Quantifying exposure risk: surgical masks and respirators. *Am J Infect Control.* 2010;38(7):501–508.

Easa N, Alany RG, Carew M, Vangala A. A review of non-invasive insulin delivery systems for diabetes therapy in clinical trials over the past decade. *Drug Discov Today.* 2019;24(2):440–451.

Messina MS, O'Riordan TG, Smaldone GC. Changes in mucociliary clearance during acute exacerbations of asthma. *Am Rev Respir Dis.* 1991;143:993–997.

Palmer LB, Smaldone GC, Chen JJ, et al. Aerosolized antibiotics and ventilator-associated tracheobronchitis in the intensive care unit. *Crit Care Med.* 2008;36:2008–2013.

Shine KI, Rogers B, Goldfrank LR. Novel H1N1 influenza and respiratory protection for health care workers. *N Engl J Med.* 2009;361:1823–1825.

Stuart BO. Deposition and clearance of inhaled particles. *Environ Health Perspect.* 1984;55:369–390.

Torres A, Motos A, Battaglini D, Li Bassi G. Inhaled amikacin for severe gram-negative pulmonary infections in the intensive care unit: current status and future prospects. *Crit Care.* 2018;22(1):343.

Complete reference list available at ExpertConsult.com.

PLEURAL PHYSIOLOGY AND PATHOPHYSIOLOGY

V. COURTNEY BROADDUS, MD

INTRODUCTION

The pleural space is bounded by two membranes, the visceral pleura covering the lung and the parietal pleura covering the chest wall and diaphragm. Pleural pressure is subatmospheric and ensures inflation of the lung. In the normal state, it is now believed that liquid moves into the pleural space along the pressure gradient and across a leaky mesothelium; the low protein concentration suggests that the liquid originates as a filtrate from a systemic circulation, as opposed to a pulmonary filtrate which has a higher protein concentration. The liquid normally exits via the parietal pleural lymphatics, which open directly onto the pleural space. These lymphatics can increase their rate of liquid clearance approximately 30-fold and thus can accommodate large variations in the entry of pleural liquid without allowing accumulation. Therefore, the most likely explanation for the accumulation of an abnormal volume of pleural liquid (i.e., a pleural effusion) is if *both* the pleural liquid entry rate increases and the pleural liquid exit rate decreases. The pleural liquid may originate from a wide variety of sources and reach the pleural space because of (1) the subatmospheric pleural pressure, (2) the leaky pleural membranes, and (3) the high capacitance of the pleural space. Depending on the protein and *lactate dehydrogenase* (LDH) concentrations of the liquid, these effusions can be categorized initially as transudates or exudates. This chapter covers these points in more detail, focusing on how liquid normally moves into and out of the pleural space and how disturbances of the normal pattern allow the accumulation of a pleural effusion.

Other related chapters cover the anatomy of the pleural membranes (see Chapter 1) and the embryology of the pleural space (see Chapter 2) and the clinical information about pleural effusions in general (see Chapter 108), pleural infections (Chapter 109), and pleural malignancy (Chapter 114). In addition, pneumothorax, chylothorax, pleural fibrosis, and hemothorax are covered in Chapters 110 through 113.

FUNCTION

The visceral and parietal pleural membranes cover the lung and the chest wall, respectively, and meet at the hilar root of the lung. In the sheep, an animal with a pleural anatomy similar to humans, the surface area of the visceral pleura of one lung, including that invaginating into the lung fissures, is similar to that of the parietal pleura of one hemithorax, approximately 1000 cm^2.[1] The normal pleural space is approximately 10 to 30 μm in width, although it widens more at its most dependent areas.[1] It has been shown that the pleural membranes do not touch each other and that the pleural space is a real, not a potential, space (see Fig. 1.21).[1]

It is likely that the primary function of the pleural membranes is to allow extensive movement of the lung relative to the chest wall. If the lung adhered directly to the chest wall, its expansion and deflation would be more limited. Encased in its slippery coat, the lung, although still coupled mechanically to the chest wall, is able to expand across a breadth of several intercostal spaces. Nonetheless, in clinical and experimental studies, obliteration of the pleural space by pleurodesis via talc or surgical procedures has not been associated with abnormalities in overall lung function,[2–4] although there may be minor differences in regional lung function with changes in the distribution of air flow.[5] When there is pleural thickening, there may be measurable decreases in lung ventilation or blood flow to the affected lung and also, to some degree, to the opposite lung as well.[6] Thus, abnormalities of lung function may result more from pleural fibrosis than from obliteration of the pleural space alone (see Chapter 112).

The visceral pleura may also provide mechanical support for the lung: contributing to the shape of the lung, providing a limit to expansion, and contributing to the work of deflation. Because the submesothelial connective tissue is continuous with the connective tissue of the lung parenchyma, the visceral pleura may help to distribute the forces produced by negative inflation pressures evenly over the lung. In this way, overdistention of alveoli at the pleural

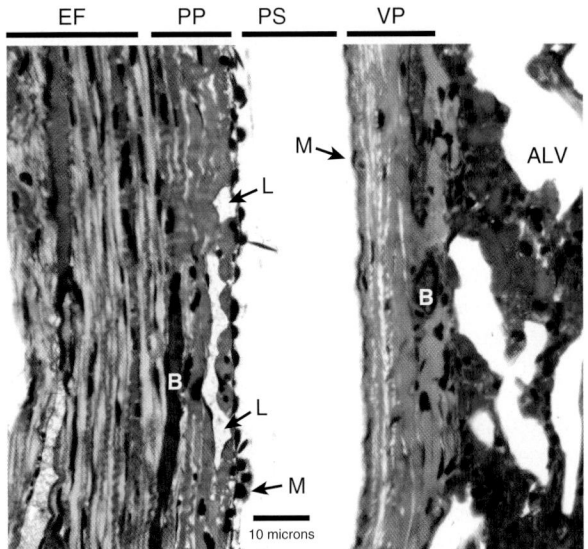

Figure 14.1 **Light micrograph showing the parietal and visceral pleurae of the sheep, an animal with a pleural anatomy similar to that of humans.** The two pleural membranes are positioned side by side at a distance of 20 μm, which represents an average width of the pleural space (PS).[1] On the left, the parietal pleura (PP) lies between the pleural space and the endothoracic fascia (EF). Within the loose connective tissue of the parietal pleura are blood microvessels (B) from the intercostal arteries and lymphatic lacunae (L), which open into the pleural space via stomata. On the right, the visceral pleura (VP) lies between the pleural space and the alveoli (ALV). The blood supply is via the bronchial arteries (B), which drain into pulmonary veins. (From Staub NC, Wiener-Kronish JP, Albertine KH. Transport through the pleura: physiology of normal liquid and solute exchange in the pleural space. In: Chrétien J, Bignon J, Hirsch A, eds. *The Pleura in Health and Disease.* New York: Marcel Dekker; 1985:174-175.)

surface may be avoided, lessening the chance of rupture and pneumothorax.

Another function of the pleural space may be to provide a route by which edema can escape the lung.[7] As has been shown in several experimental studies of either hydrostatic or increased-permeability lung edema[8,9] and summarized in this review,[10] edema fluid can and does move from the lung into the pleural space. In this way, the pleural space can function as an additional safety factor protecting against the development of alveolar edema. Seen in this way, the formation of transudative effusions in patients with *congestive heart failure* (CHF) reflects the movement of edema from the lung to a space where its effects on lung function are relatively small (see discussion of effusions from CHF later).

ANATOMY

PLEURAL MEMBRANES

The pleural membranes are smooth glistening coverings for the constantly moving lung. Overlying each pleural membrane is a single cell layer of mesothelial cells. These cells, the most numerous cell of the pleural space, have a variety of functions important to pleural biology.[11] Mesothelial cells can secrete and organize extracellular matrix proteins, phagocytose particles, produce fibrinolytic and procoagulant factors, and secrete neutrophil and monocyte chemotactic factors that may be important for inflammatory cell recruitment into the pleural spaces. The mesothelial cells also produce cytokines such as transforming growth

factor-β, epidermal growth factor, and platelet-derived growth factor, cytokines important in pleural inflammation and fibrosis.

On the mesothelial cell surface are microvilli. Although microvilli presumably exist to increase surface area for metabolic activity, the function of these prominent features is unknown. Mesothelial cells produce hyaluronan but not mucin, express keratin microfilaments, stain positively for calretinin and mesothelin, and fail to stain with epithelial-specific antibodies (Ber-EP4, B72.3, Leu.M1, and CEA), all features important for histochemical and immunohistochemical identification of the cells in pleural effusions.[12,13]

The mesothelial cells lie on a thin basement membrane overlying a region of connective tissue containing mostly collagen and elastin. The parietal pleural thickness is relatively constant in an individual and among species, whereas the visceral pleural thickness varies greatly. In a single individual, the visceral pleura varies from a thinner layer at the cranial region to a thicker layer at the caudal region.[14] Among mammalian species, the visceral pleura thickness also varies, from a "thin" pleura without a separate blood supply, as seen in small mammals, to the "thick" pleura with a bronchial arterial circulation, as seen in humans (see Fig. 1.31). Analysis of the constituents of the visceral pleura has shown that there is more collagen relative to elastin than is found in the lung parenchyma, a finding consistent with a structural role for the pleura.[15] This connective tissue layer contains blood vessels and lymphatics and joins with the connective tissue of the lung. The submesothelial tissue has been shown to have mechanical strength and to contain various growth factors supporting cell growth, suggesting that mesothelium could function as a repair and regeneration platform.[16] There is also evidence that mesothelial cells floating freely in the pleural liquid are viable and can adhere to denuded areas of the pleura to contribute to repair.[17]

BLOOD SUPPLY

The parietal pleura is supplied by intercostal arteries (Fig. 14.1).[18] In humans as well as in other large mammals with a "thick" visceral pleura, the visceral pleura is supplied by the bronchial circulation, which drains, not into systemic veins, but into pulmonary veins (Fig. 14.1).[14] The drainage route via pulmonary veins may have contributed to earlier confusion about whether the visceral pleural blood supply was from a systemic (bronchial) or pulmonary circulation. Thus, both pleuras in humans have a systemic circulation, although the visceral pleural circulation may have a slightly lower perfusion pressure than the parietal pleural intercostal circulation because of its drainage into a lower pressure venous system.

LYMPHATICS

If one injects carbon particles into the pleural space as a visible tracer of lymphatic drainage pathways, one later finds that the carbon has been taken up into lymphatics on the parietal side, not the visceral side (Fig. 14.2; also see Fig. 1.22C). The visceral pleura has extensive lymphatics, but they do not connect to the pleural space.[14] The parietal

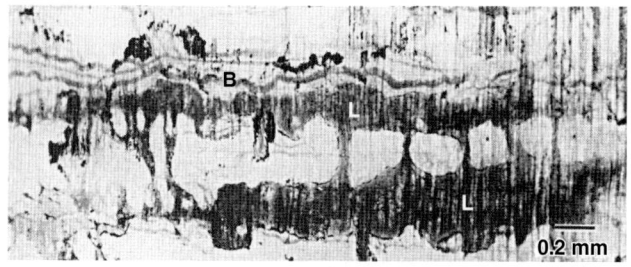

Figure 14.2 Macroscopic photograph of lymphatic lacunae in the parietal pleura over an intercostal space. Carbon particles were instilled into the pleural space to label the draining lymphatics. When looking down on the pleura, the lymphatic lacunae (L) appear as broad cisterns. (Original magnification ×39.) B, blood vessel. (From Albertine KH, Wiener-Kronish JP, Staub NC. The structure of the parietal pleura and its relationship to pleural liquid dynamics in sheep. *Anat Rec.* 1984;208:406.)

pleural lymphatics connect to the pleural space via stomata, openings of 2 to 12 µm in diameter formed by discontinuities in the mesothelial layer where mesothelium joins to the underlying lymphatic endothelium (see Fig. 1.22A–B).[19–21] Although lymphatics were known for some time to be important in drainage of liquid, protein, and cells from the pleural space,[22] the connection between the pleural space and the lymphatics could not be identified until the advent of scanning electron microscopy, at which time the existence of stomata was confirmed in rabbits and mice.[19] Lymphatic stomata have since been demonstrated in many other species, including monkeys[23] and humans.[24] Although their size has been reported to vary from 1 to 6 µm in rabbits, mice,[19] and sheep[18] to 3 to 12.5 µm in monkeys[23] and humans,[24,20] the reported size is probably a minimum and likely increases with expansion of the chest with ventilation. From the stomata, which can accommodate particles as large as erythrocytes, liquid drains to lacunae (spider-like submesothelial collecting lymphatics) and then to infracostal lymphatics, to parasternal and periaortic nodes,[25,26] to the right lymphatic duct and thoracic duct,[27] and into the central veins. The right lymphatic duct empties near the junction of the right internal jugular and right subclavian veins; the thoracic duct empties near the junction of the left internal jugular and left subclavian veins. The right lymphatic and the thoracic ducts likely drain all the lymph from the two hemithoraces. In animal studies, Courtice and Simmons showed that all the labeled protein introduced into the pleural space was drained by these ducts.[27] Interference with the drainage of lymph at these sites can be important clinically, as when large persistent transudative effusions arise when the brachiocephalic veins are thrombosed, stenosed, or otherwise compressed.[28–30]

NERVE SUPPLY

The parietal pleura contains sensory nerve fibers, supplied by the intercostal and phrenic nerves, and has long been thought to be the major site of pain sensation in the pleura. The costal and peripheral diaphragmatic regions are innervated by the intercostal nerves, and pain from these regions is referred to the adjacent chest wall. The central diaphragmatic region is innervated by the phrenic nerve, and pain from this region is referred to the ipsilateral shoulder. The visceral pleura has more recently been shown to have

sensory nerve fibers that may participate in pain or other sensations such as dyspnea.[31] In addition, pleural adhesions may become innervated with pain fibers and contribute to postthoracotomy or postpleurodesis pain[32] (see also Chapter 38).

PLEURAL PRESSURE

The pleural pressure in humans is approximately −5 cm H_2O at midchest at functional residual capacity and −30 cm H_2O at total lung capacity.[33] If the compliance of the lung were to decrease, pleural pressures at the same lung volume would be more negative. In one study of patients undergoing thoracentesis, those with more negative pleural pressures had a smaller improvement in lung volume than those with less negative pressures, presumably reflecting the presence of underlying noncompliant lung.[34]

The pleural pressure is the lowest pressure of the body and can explain how liquids accumulating elsewhere can move along pressure gradients toward the pleural space. Combined with a leaky mesothelium (see later), this pressure gradient can pull liquid into the pleural space. The pressure can become more negative if the lung collapses or can become more positive if liquid or air enters the pleural space. However, as long as the lung is inflated, even partially, the pleural pressure must be subatmospheric. A corollary to that is, as long as the aerated lung is partially inflated, a large pneumothorax even with some mediastinal shift cannot be a tension pneumothorax.[35]

Although the pleural space pressure is subatmospheric, gases do not normally accumulate there. The sum of all partial pressures of gases in capillary blood is approximately 700 mm Hg, or 60 mm Hg below atmospheric ($P_{H_2O} = 47$, $P_{CO_2} = 46$, $P_{N_2} = 570$, and $P_{O_2} = 40$ mm Hg). The subatmospheric pressure of dissolved gases in capillary blood helps to maintain the pleural space free of gas and facilitates absorption of any gas that does enter the pleural space. Of note, to increase the gradient favoring absorption of gas from the pleural space (e.g., pneumothorax), the partial pressure of nitrogen in the blood can be lowered by having a patient breathe higher concentrations of inspired oxygen. The oxygen displaces alveolar nitrogen, thereby lowering the partial pressure of nitrogen in capillary blood; at the same time, the increased inspired oxygen does not increase the oxygen tension in capillary blood due to the threshold of absorption demonstrated by the plateau of the oxygen-hemoglobin dissociation curve. The net result is a decrease in the partial pressure of gases in capillary blood and an accelerated absorption of pleural gas.

PHYSIOLOGY OF THE PLEURAL SPACE

A consensus currently exists that the normal pleural liquid arises from the systemic pleural vessels in both pleurae, flows across the leaky pleural membranes into the pleural space, and exits the pleural space via the parietal pleural lymphatics[36,37] (Fig. 14.3). In this way, the pleural space is analogous to other interstitial tissues of the body, such as muscle or subcutaneous tissue.[22,36] Knowing how the

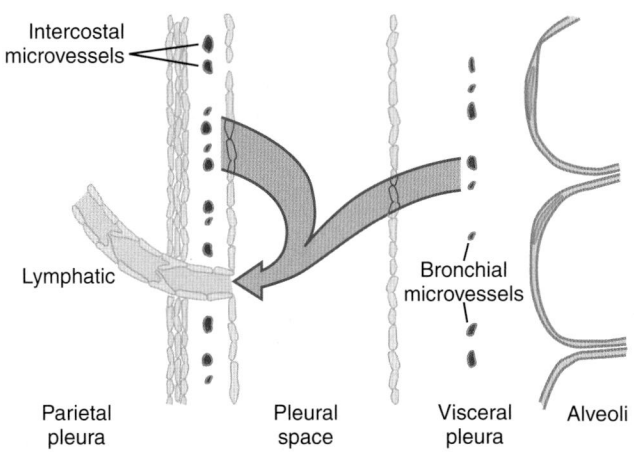

Figure 14.3   Schema showing normal pleural liquid entry and exit. The microvascular filtrate from the systemic microvessels in the parietal and visceral pleura flows across the leaky pleural mesothelial layers into the pleural space. The pleural liquid exits the pleural space via the parietal pleural lymphatic stomata. (From Staub NC, Wiener-Kronish JP, Albertine KH. Transport through the pleura: physiology of normal liquid and solute exchange in the pleural space. In: Chrétien J, Bignon J, Hirsch A, eds. *The Pleura in Health and Disease*. New York: Marcel Dekker; 1985:182.)

pleural liquid enters and exits is helpful in understanding how things go awry to allow effusions to form. This understanding also removes some of the mystery about how the pleural space functions, a mystery that arose in large part because of the difficulty of studying the narrow space without introducing inflammation or injury.

ENTRY OF NORMAL PLEURAL LIQUID

A Systemic Microvascular Source

There are two main lines of evidence that normal pleural liquid originates from the systemic circulation of the pleural membranes. For one, the low protein concentration of pleural liquid is more in keeping with systemic filtrate and is quite unlike pulmonary filtrates. For another, the protein concentration changes in concert with changes in systemic pressures, not pulmonic pressures.

Protein Concentration is Similar to Systemic Filtrates. The protein concentration of normal pleural liquid is low in sheep[38] and probably in humans, which implies sieving of the protein across a high-pressure, low-permeability microvascular barrier, as would be expected in systemic capillaries.[36] The protein concentration of sheep pleural liquid (1.0 g/dL) and pleural-to-plasma protein concentration ratio (0.15) is also much lower than found in filtrates from the low-pressure pulmonary vessels (protein concentration [4.5 g/dL] and ratio [lymph-to-plasma protein concentration ratio 0.69]).[39]

Protein Concentration Changes With Changes in Systemic Hydrostatic Pressures. With increases in filtration rates across a semipermeable membrane, proteins are retarded relative to liquid and electrolytes, and the protein concentration of the filtrate decreases. Therefore, if the systemic circulation is the source of pleural liquid, an increase in filtration pressure in the systemic circulation should manifest as a decrease in protein concentration

of pleural liquid. Two studies demonstrate this concept. In the first study, spontaneously hypertensive rats were found to have pleural liquid with lower total protein and albumin concentration ratios (pleural/serum) than in the control, normotensive rats.[40] In the second study, sheep were studied at different stages of development. As mammals grow from fetuses to newborns to adults, systemic arterial pressure increases while pulmonary arterial pressure decreases. Thus, if pleural liquid arose from the systemic circulation, pleural liquid protein concentrations would be expected to decrease; if they arose from the pulmonary circulation, it would be the opposite. Indeed, pleural liquid protein concentration ratios decreased from fetuses (ratio 0.50) to newborns (ratio 0.27) to adults (ratio 0.15).[41] These physiologic observations support the concept that the systemic circulation is the source of normal pleural liquid.

The Parietal Pleura Is the Major Source

The pleural space is sandwiched between two adjacent systemic circulations: the intercostal arterial circulation of the parietal pleural and the bronchial arterial circulation of the visceral pleura. Although both likely contribute to normal pleural liquid, the major source is likely the parietal pleura, for the following reasons:

1. The parietal pleural circulation is constant among species, with an anatomy nearly interchangeable from small mammals to humans. However, the visceral pleura changes dramatically depending on whether the visceral pleura is "thick" as in humans, sheep, and most large animals or is "thin" as in smaller mammals like dogs, rabbits, and mice (see Fig. 1.31).[14] Thick visceral pleura has a systemic bronchial blood supply, whereas the thin visceral pleura has no circulation of its own and is fed by the underlying pulmonary circulation. Interestingly, the measured rates of pleural entry are similar among different species, even when their visceral pleurae are strikingly different.[53] Thus, the parietal pleura is the likely constant and major source of normal pleural liquid.

2. The parietal pleura microvessels are closer and have a higher microvascular pressure. Although both pleurae have a systemic circulation, as in sheep and humans, the systemic arteries of the parietal pleura are closer to the pleural space (10–12 μm) than are the systemic arteries of the visceral pleura (20–50 μm).[14,18,36] The parietal pleural vessels also likely have a higher microvascular pressure due to their drainage into systemic venules, whereas the visceral bronchial vessels drain into lower resistance pulmonary venules.[36]

Pleural Membranes Are Leaky

The pleural membranes are leaky, at least compared with the very tight membranes of the alveolar epithelium. Whether tested in vitro[42,43] or in situ,[44,45] the pleura offers little resistance to liquid or protein movement. Indeed, the peritoneal membrane, a closely related mesothelial structure, is leaky enough to permit peritoneal dialysis, with a relatively free movement of solutes and water. Studies of peritoneal transport have concluded that the barrier to flow into the peritoneal space is primarily the vascular endothelium; the peritoneal mesothelial surface is not a significant barrier.[46]

In addition, the mesothelium, although it may exhibit microvilli and express various transporters and aquaporins, has not been shown to participate in active fluid transport.[47,48] Such a function would not be expected in a cell without tight cell-cell junctions providing a barrier to the movement of ions. Nonetheless, one argument for active transport has been that the pleural liquid contains more bicarbonate than does the plasma.[49,50] However, this bicarbonate difference is likely explained by a passive phenomenon called the Donnan equilibrium, which describes how ions move to achieve electroneutrality. In a Donnan equilibrium, differences in protein concentrations (and their negative charges) alter ionic balances passively between two electrolytic solutions separated by a semipermeable membrane. With the lower protein concentration in pleural liquid than in plasma, there is less of a negative charge; the distribution of bicarbonate allows for a balance of negative charge across the pleural membrane.[51]

Entry From the Interstitium into the Pleural Space

Once the liquid filters across the systemic microvessels, it can then flow along the pressure gradient toward the pleural space and across the mesothelial layer into the pleural space. The pressure gradient exists from the high-pressure pleural systemic microvessels into the surrounding interstitial tissue and from there into the subatmospheric pleural space.[52]

The entry of pleural liquid is slow, as shown by radiolabeled albumin studies in which the equilibration into the pleural space of mammals was calculated without instrumenting the pleural space. As mentioned, the rates were surprisingly similar among different species, at approximately 0.01 mL/kg/hr. Such a rate would be equivalent to an entry of 0.5 mL/hr, or 12 mL/day in a 50-kg person.[38,53] Much higher rates previously reported were most likely due to the disturbance of the pleural space by the placement of catheters that led to inflammation and injury, thereby increasing the entry of liquid.

The Pleural Space Is Vulnerable to Liquid Entry

The pleural space is susceptible to the entry of liquid from any source of excess liquid in the body. The subatmospheric pressure in the space establishes a gradient for liquid entry. The leaky mesothelium allows the entry of the liquid and protein into the pleural space. The large surface area of the pleural space provides a large area for liquid flow. Finally, the space itself can accommodate a large amount of liquid without a rapid elevation in pressure (i.e., the space is compliant). Thus, perhaps the interesting question is why there are not more effusions. The key must lie in the mechanisms that remove liquid from the pleural space.

EXIT OF NORMAL PLEURAL LIQUID

Lymphatics Are the Major Exit Route

The majority of liquid exits the pleural space by bulk flow, not by diffusion or active transport. This is evident because the protein concentration of pleural effusions remains constant as the effusion is absorbed, as is expected with bulk flow.[54] If liquid were absorbed by diffusion or active transport, proteins would diffuse at a slower rate, and the protein

concentration would progressively increase. (In fact, in *alveolar* liquid, protein concentration does increase as ions and water are actively absorbed across the alveolar epithelium, with protein absorbed more slowly by other routes.[55])

As a demonstration of the route of exit, sheep erythrocytes instilled into the sheep pleural space are absorbed intact and in almost the same proportion as the liquid and protein.[54] This indicates that the major route of exit is via holes large enough to accommodate sheep erythrocytes (~4.5 μm diameter). In addition, when chicken erythrocytes (identifiable because avian erythrocytes contain a nucleus) were instilled into a sheep pleural space, they could later be seen intact in the parietal pleural lymphatics.[18] The only possible exit for these particles is via the parietal pleural stomata into the pleural lymphatics. To visualize the lymphatic route of exit, ink, which consists of tiny particles of carbon, can be instilled into the pleural space, allowed to dwell for several hours, and then washed out. The absorbed carbon can be seen within the parietal pleural lymphatics, outlining them (see Fig. 14.2). Thus, a lymphatic route of clearance explains how protein can be absorbed without a change in concentration and how erythrocytes can be removed intact.

Lymphatics Have a Large Reserve Capacity

Importantly, the pleural lymphatics have a large reserve capacity for absorption. When artificial effusions were instilled into the pleural space of awake sheep, the measured exit rate (0.28 mL/kg/hr) was nearly 30 times the baseline exit rate (0.01 mL/kg/hr).[54] A reserve capacity of lymphatic absorption is a feature of lymphatics throughout the body; baseline lymphatic flow is slow, handling the normal low filtrate from microvessels, but increases briskly when faced with a higher filtration load.[56] Pleural lymphatics likely increase their flow for at least two reasons: because more liquid reaches them and because the pleural pressure rises slightly with the presence of more liquid. The ability of lymphatics to increase their rate of absorption and their large reserve capacity is probably a key feature in limiting the accumulation of excess liquid in the pleural space and anywhere in the body.

In earlier theories of pleural liquid absorption, it was postulated that the liquid diffused into the lung. However, as discussed earlier, diffusion cannot play a major role in absorption given the unchanging protein concentration of pleural effusions as they are absorbed. In addition, the pleural space has a pressure less than that of the lung, thereby inflating the lung. Thus, for liquid to enter the lung, the liquid would be moving against the pressure gradient, in effect flowing "uphill." Lymphatics, by virtue of their active pumping and one-way valves, perform the function of returning extravascular, interstitial liquid and protein to the venous system, for pleural liquid and also for interstitial liquids throughout the body. Both the intrinsic pumping of the collecting lymphatics and the extrinsic contractions of the chest wall muscles with ventilation can propel the lymph[27,57]; certain studies have attempted to distinguish the intrinsic and extrinsic mechanisms.[58]

Despite the large reserve capacity of lymphatic clearance, there is ultimately a maximum rate that limits absorption. Perhaps over time, when faced with increased loads, the lymphatics can increase their maximum absorption rate, as by increases in the number of lymphatics or in their contractility. However, the maximal lymphatic capacity will establish an upper limit to the exit rate of pleural liquid.

PATHOPHYSIOLOGY OF THE PLEURAL SPACE

WHAT IS REQUIRED TO PRODUCE A PLEURAL EFFUSION?

Based on the understanding of the normal turnover of pleural liquid, we can consider what is required to create a pleural effusion. For sufficient pleural liquid to accumulate to form an effusion, it is most likely that both the entry rate of liquid must increase and the exit rate must decrease. If only the entry rate increased and the exit rate could increase normally, it would require a sustained entry rate more than 30 times normal to exceed the reserve lymphatic absorptive capacity and allow excess liquid to accumulate.[54] Alternatively, if the exit rate was completely stopped and the entry rate did not change, it would take more than a month at the normal entry rate of 12 mL/day to accumulate an effusion detectable by chest radiograph.[37] Thus, for the creation of persistent and clinically relevant pleural effusions, it is most likely that changes in both the entry and exit rates are required.

WHAT DISEASES COULD ACCOUNT FOR THIS?

Of course, one disease can simultaneously increase the entry rate of liquid and decrease the exit rate. For example, a pleural infection could increase liquid entry from leaky pleural vessels and could also interfere with the exit of liquid by obstructing the parietal pleural lymphatics with fibrin. As another example, central venous obstruction could increase liquid entry by increasing parietal systemic capillary pressures and also decrease the exit of liquid by increasing the downstream venous pressure into which the parietal pleural lymphatics must drain.

But then, one could imagine that two different disease processes might cooperate to form an effusion; these disease processes could also take place at different times. For example, one disease might first interfere with lymphatic function, thereby decreasing the lymphatic reserve. This could happen gradually without notice because there would still be enough reserve to handle the slow entry rate. Then, if a second disease led to an increase in the liquid entry rate, the increased liquid could then exceed the reduced lymphatic capacity and accumulate as an effusion. The concept that different diseases can cooperate to form an effusion has some clinical support; in a prospective study, as many as 30% of effusions could be shown to have more than one etiology.[59] The concept can also explain how one pleural effusion could have multiple etiologies,[60] especially if one condition renders the pleural space more susceptible to liquid accumulation from other causes. For example, the interaction of different disease entities may account for the presence of transudates in the setting of pleural malignancy, especially when another transudative process like CHF coexists with malignancy.[61–63]

MECHANISMS OF INCREASED ENTRY OF LIQUID

Liquid is constantly filtered out of the microvessels, entering the interstitial (i.e., the peri-microvascular) space and then being returned to the vascular space by lymphatics. There are three mechanisms by which flow of liquid out of microvessels is governed: the hydrostatic pressure gradient, the osmotic pressure gradient, and the permeability or leakiness of the microvascular barrier. These forces are classically described by the Starling equation:

$$\dot{Q} = Kf\left[(P_{mv} - P_{pmv}) - \sigma(\pi_{mv} - \pi_{pmv})\right]$$

where $\dot{Q}$ is the net liquid filtration rate, Kf is the filtration coefficient or the leakiness of the barrier to water and electrolytes, P_{mv} is microvascular hydrostatic pressure, P_{pmv} is peri-microvascular hydrostatic pressure, σ is the protein reflection coefficient describing the leakiness of the barrier to protein, π_{mv} is microvascular osmotic pressure, and π_{pmv} is peri-microvascular osmotic pressure. Mechanisms of increased liquid entry due to changes in these Starling forces and other mechanisms are shown in Table 14.1. Relevant clinical examples including hypothetical ones are listed.

Increased Filtration Pressure

Hydrostatic Pressures. An increase in microvascular pressure (i.e., capillary pressure) will increase the filtration

Table 14.1 Mechanisms of Increased Liquid Entry Into the Pleural Space

Mechanism	Starling Symbol	Relevant Clinical Examples
Increased filtration pressure	↑ P_{mv}	Increased systemic venous pressure, increased pulmonary venous pressure
	↓ P_{pmv}	Atelectasis, trapped lung, (chest tube suction)
	↓ π_{mv}	Hypoalbuminemia, plasmapheresis
	(↑ π_{pmv})	(Hemothorax, iatrogenic tube feeding instillation)
Increased microvascular permeability	↑ Kf, ↓ σ	Inflammation, injury, malignancy
Entry of other biologic liquids		Chyle, bile, urine, pancreatic secretions, cerebrospinal fluid, hemothorax
Entry of nonbiologic liquids		Intravenous fluids, tube feedings, peritoneal dialysis fluids

Hypothetical examples are shown in parentheses.
Kf, filtration coefficient or the leakiness of the barrier to water and electrolytes; P_{mv}, microvascular hydrostatic pressure; P_{pmv}, peri-microvascular hydrostatic pressure; σ, protein reflection coefficient describing leakiness of the barrier to protein; π_{mv}, microvascular osmotic pressure; π_{pmv}, peri-microvascular osmotic pressure.

across the microvascular barrier. The microvascular pressure is particularly sensitive to elevations of venous pressure and is less likely to increase with elevations of arterial pressure because of the regulation of precapillary resistance. (Note: actual precapillary sphincters have been described only in the mesentery.[64])

A decrease in the peri-microvascular pressure (i.e., the pressure around the capillaries) also increases the hydrostatic gradient for liquid filtration. In the case of pleural microvessels, the peri-microvascular pressure of pleural microvessels is influenced by the nearby pleural pressure. Thus, a decrease in pleural pressure decreases peri-microvascular pressure and increases filtration.

Osmotic Pressures. A decrease in the osmotic pressure of the blood within microvessels would be expected to increase filtration. The osmotic pressure of blood is driven mostly by serum protein, comprised primarily of albumin. However, the effects of hypoalbuminemia are likely minimal, because hypoalbuminemia usually develops gradually and is accompanied by a decrease in the peri-microvascular osmotic pressure and the osmotic gradient as filtration of low-protein liquid dilutes the interstitial protein concentration. Nonetheless, a low serum osmotic pressure likely decreases the threshold for other factors, such as the hydrostatic forces, to increase filtration. Lowering the threshold for filtration may explain why, although it is not commonly a sole cause for effusions,[65] hypoalbuminemia is commonly found in patients with effusions of all causes; it may increase the likelihood of effusions[66,67] and increase their size.[68]

In comparison to the gradual scenario just described, a rapid decrease in microvascular osmotic pressure could be expected to swing the balance quickly toward increased filtration and the formation of pleural effusions. Such a picture has been described in an interesting case in which plasmapheresis of a patient with Waldenstrom macroglobulinemia dropped the serum osmotic pressure rapidly and was quickly followed by the appearance of large bilateral pleural effusions.[69] Again, the effusions would be expected to be transient until a new osmotic balance reestablished itself.

An increase in peri-microvascular osmotic pressure would also be expected to increase filtration, although this phenomenon has not been described in the clinical setting. One could speculate that pleural and secondarily peri-microvascular osmotic pressure could increase following a hemothorax or the intrapleural instillation of a hyperosmolar or high-protein liquid such as a tube feeding solution. Of note, there has been a modification of the Starling equation in recent years, which has deemphasized the role of the peri-microvascular osmotic force.[70]

Increased Microvascular Permeability

Filtration Coefficient (Kf) and Reflection Coefficient (σ). When the permeability of the microvascular barrier increases due to inflammation, infection, or malignancy, the resistance to the filtration of liquid and electrolytes and to protein is lowered (i.e., there is an increase in Kf and a decrease in σ). With an increase in microvascular permeability, the rate of filtration of liquid, electrolytes, and protein increases even without any change in hydrostatic pressures. However, in addition to the change in permeability, inflammation may also increase the hydrostatic pressure by relaxing the precapillary resistance.[71] The combination of an increase in hydrostatic pressure in the setting of a leakier barrier greatly enhances filtration.

Other Biologic Liquids and Iatrogenic Sources. As mentioned, the Starling factors discussed above are relevant to all the circulations of the body, systemic and pulmonary, and increases in filtration anywhere can lead to increased interstitial liquid that can then migrate to the pleural space. In addition, pleural effusions can be composed of other biologic liquids, such as blood, urine, chyle, pancreatic secretions from a pseudocyst, bile, and cerebrospinal fluid. In addition, pleural effusions can be composed of nonbiologic liquids such as intravenous fluids or tube feedings (see Table 14.1).

MECHANISMS OF DECREASED EXIT OF LIQUID

As postulated earlier, the accumulation of an effusion likely requires not only an increase in the entry of liquid, but also a decrease in the exit rate by interference with lymphatic function. Otherwise, if lymphatic function was normal, the exit rate could increase approximately 30-fold rapidly and, in most cases, handle the increased entry of liquid.[54]

Lymphatic function may become impaired in many ways. There may be reduced patency of the parietal pleural stomata, inhibition of lymphatic contractility,[56] infiltration of the lymphatics or their draining parasternal lymph nodes, an increase in the downstream central venous pressure, a complete obstruction of the central vein into which they drain, a decrease in the pleural pressure against which they must pump, or primary lymphatic disorders (Table 14.2).[37] There are few studies on the rate of removal of liquid in humans; however, decreases in lymphatic clearance have been confirmed in patients with tuberculous and malignant effusions,[72] and in those with the yellow-nail syndrome, a disease of lymphatic function.[73]

As previously stated, for either transudates or exudates, interference with lymphatic function may contribute to the accumulation of the effusion. Nonetheless, because the exit of pleural liquid via lymphatics does not alter the

Table 14.2 Mechanisms of Decreased Liquid Exit via Parietal Pleural Lymphatics From the Pleural Space

Mechanism	Examples*
Decreased lymphatic stomata patency	Inflammation (granulomas, empyema, fibrin), malignancy
Decreased lymphatic contractility	Hypothyroidism, drug effect
Infiltration of lymphatics or lymph nodes	Malignancy
Increased venous (downstream) pressure	Central venous pressure elevation
Blocked lymphatic drainage	Central venous thrombosis
Reduced pleural (upstream) pressure	Atelectasis, trapped lung
Lymphatic disorders	Yellow nail syndrome

*Many of these examples also increase entry; see Table 14.1.

pleural liquid protein concentration, the protein concentration gives insight into the *formation* of the liquid, not its *removal*.[37]

CATEGORIES OF PLEURAL EFFUSIONS

Effusions can be categorized based on their protein concentration. Because the protein concentration is not altered by its removal by the lymphatics, the protein concentration of pleural effusions stays relatively constant during the life of the effusion. This feature allows protein concentration to be a useful biomarker; the protein concentration and its ratio with that of serum give information about the formation of the liquid. It is for this reason that effusions can be divided into transudates (protein concentration ratio (pleural/serum) < 0.5) and exudates (protein ratios > 0.5), which constitute part of Light's criteria.[74] Of course, LDH is also used as a biomarker for effusions but, because LDH is at high levels intracellularly, this marker is more useful as a marker of cell turnover and inflammation (see Chapter 108).[74]

Transudates

Transudates form by filtration of liquid across an intact microvascular barrier owing to increases in hydrostatic pressures or decreases in osmotic pressures across that barrier. Transudates generally indicate that the pleural membranes and their microvessels are not themselves diseased. Transudates may form from increased filtration across either the systemic or the pulmonary circulations. However, if the protein concentration is very low (pleural/serum ratio <0.1–0.2), the effusion is likely caused by either (1) liquids formed from CSF or urine that normally have very low protein and have migrated to the pleural space or (2) nonbiologic liquids such as intravenous fluids.

Exudates

Exudates arise from inflamed or injured microvessels in the pleura, the lung, or other tissues. Many exudates arise from direct pleural injury due to inflammation, infection, or malignancy. Other exudates, such as those associated with pneumonia, may arise from inflammation or injury to the lung, creating a high-protein lung edema that leaks into the pleural space. Exudates can also form when exudative liquid in the mediastinum (esophageal rupture or chylothorax), retroperitoneum (pancreatic pseudocyst), or peritoneum (ascites with spontaneous bacterial peritonitis or Meigs syndrome) enters the pleural space.

Pseudoexudates

Pseudoexudate refers to an effusion that presumably starts as a transudate and develops exudative characteristics following diuresis. Although a common concern, the creation of a pseudoexudate is likely uncommon.[75] By removing protein-free liquid, diuresis will increase the concentration of protein in all liquids of the body. However, that does not mean that the *ratio* of pleural protein to serum will necessarily increase. Studies of this phenomenon show that only a few effusions move from a transudative to an exudative category,[75] and these studies did not always control for the effect of multiple thoracenteses that themselves might have increased pleural protein concentrations.[76]

An effusion may be considered a possible pseudoexudate if the diuresis has been effective in removing salt and water, particularly if it has reduced the size of the effusion. Even then, diuresis should only account for a small change in protein ratio (pleural/serum). In other words, pleural effusions with clearly exudative pleural characteristics should be considered exudative and not readily labeled pseudoexudative. Dismissing a true exudate as a pseudoexudate might lead to missing diagnoses such as cancer, pulmonary embolism, and other serious clinical conditions. When there is doubt, these effusions should undergo a thorough workup for underlying causes of exudates.

Indeterminate Effusions

Indeterminate is an acceptable term to use when the protein ratio and/or LDH ratios are near their cutoff values, making it difficult to determine if the effusion is clearly a transudate or an exudate. In such a case, which can arise frequently, it is better to avoid categorizing the effusion, especially if it would be categorized as a transudate and falsely reassure the clinician about the absence of serious exudative conditions. It is worth remembering that protein concentration ratios described in Light's criteria are most accurate at the extremes, when they are clearly high or low. Ratios in the middle are less helpful.

One possible reason for ambiguity is worth keeping in mind—there may be more than one thing going on. In fact, there could be an underlying transudative process (e.g., CHF, hypoproteinemia) and a secondary exudative process (e.g., pneumonia, viral pleuritis). One could imagine then that the protein values could reflect contributions from both processes.[59]

MECHANISMS BY WHICH SPECIFIC DISEASES CAUSE PLEURAL EFFUSIONS

Congestive Heart Failure

The cause of most transudates, and likely the cause of most effusions, is CHF.[77] Thus it is particularly important to understand how these effusions develop.

These transudates now are thought to form from leakage of interstitial edema across the leaky visceral pleura into the pleural space.[8,10] It is worth noting that once interstitial edema reaches the interstitial spaces of the lung, collecting around the bronchovascular bundles to form what are called "cuffs," the edema is not in contact with the pulmonary lymphatics and is not cleared by them (Fig. 14.4).[78] This extravascular interstitial edema flows along the interstitial spaces to the mediastinum, where lymphatics are available, or to the pleural space.[52] In edematous lungs, subpleural interstitial pressure rises steeply, enhancing the gradient for edema flow into the pleural space.[79] Once at the visceral pleura (Fig. 14.5), the edema can cross a leaky mesothelium to enter the pleural space. Such flow from the edematous lung into the pleural space has been described in a variety of animal models of lung injury,[9,10] showing that this route of movement of edema is not specific to any particular type of edema.

The protein concentration of pleural effusions in the setting of CHF is around 3 gm/dL with a ratio of 0.3 to 0.4 to that of serum. Such a protein concentration is higher than the normal pleural liquid (ratio 0.15) and is more consistent with a pulmonary filtrate than a systemic filtrate.[8] The movement of edema from the lung has been estimated in sheep experiments to account for up to 30% of the edema formed.[8] The pleural space may thus serve as a "safety factor" for clearance of interstitial edema from the lung, reducing the risk of alveolar edema.

When there are bilateral effusions, the right-sided effusion is often larger than the left. Given that the origin of the effusion is the edematous lung, a possible explanation may be that the right lung is larger and has more surface area for edema to move across than the left. In support of this idea, in studies in sheep, the lymphatic exit rate for pleural liquid was the same from the two hemothoraces[54]; however, the entry of liquid from the edematous lungs was greater on the right.[8]

By itself, central venous pressure elevation due to pulmonary hypertension may be associated with either no effusions[80] or with small effusions.[81,82] However, elevated central venous pressure may act cooperatively with CHF in the formation of effusions, although this has not been confirmed.

Malignancy

Malignancy can cause effusions by its effects either outside the pleural space or inside the pleural space. Outside the pleural space, malignancy can infiltrate lymphatics and lymph nodes and interfere with lymphatic absorption; it can obstruct a lung leading to collapse and to a decrease in pleural pressure. These mechanisms could explain the formation of transudative effusions. Inside the pleural space, the malignancy increases the permeability of the pleural microvasculature by cytokine production[83,84]; less commonly, it can invade vessels leading to a hemothorax. In their studies of liquid and protein turnover in pleural effusions of patients with different diseases, Leckie and Tothill reported that malignant effusions had an elevated entry of protein and a slow exit, suggesting both an increased permeability and decreased lymphatic flow.[72] In one interesting case, a young patient without other illnesses developed a transudate with negative cytology; within a short time, this effusion changed to an exudate with positive cytology and a biopsy showing malignant infiltration of the subpleural lymphatics. One interpretation of this case is that the malignancy induced a transudate by lymphatic obstruction outside the pleural space and then induced an exudate when the malignant cells invaded the pleural space.[62] Although one cannot be certain, this case illustrates what might be found if one is alert to the different ways malignancy may cause effusions. In addition, malignancy can induce many abnormalities

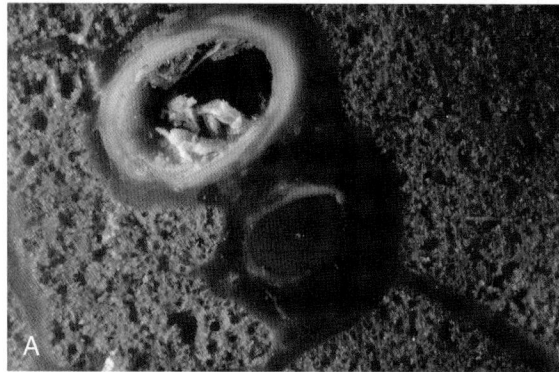
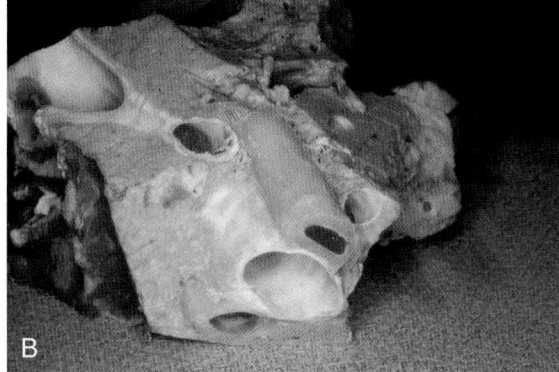

Figure 14.4 A frozen edematous sheep lung cut in cross section and dissected to show bronchovascular cuffs. Interstitial edema in the lung first collects in interstitial spaces around the bronchi and vessels. (A) A cross section showing a bronchovascular "cuff" of interstitial edema. Note the surrounding alveoli are air-filled, showing that there is no alveolar edema. (B) A dissection of a cuff showing its extent along the bronchovascular bundle. Interstitial edema in this location is not accessible to pulmonary lymphatics and flows either to the mediastinum or to the pleural space. When these "cuffs" are sampled, the protein concentration matches that of the pleural effusion.[8] (Courtesy V. Courtney Broaddus, MD.)

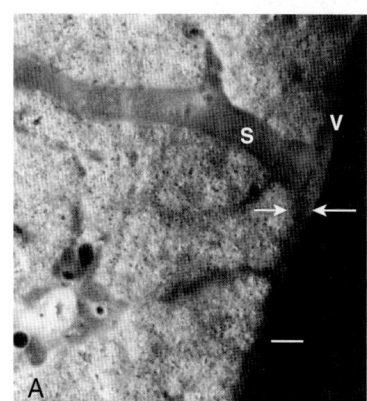
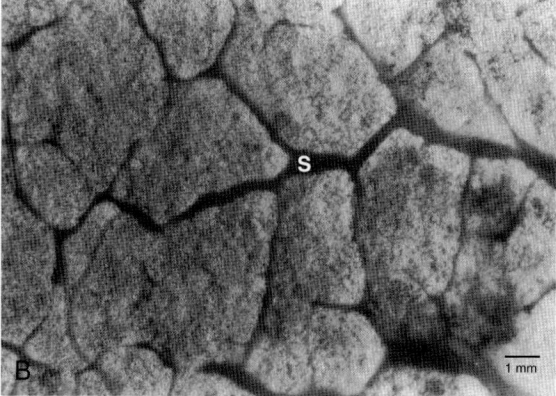

Figure 14.5 The interstitial edema seen at the visceral pleural surface. (A) A frozen edematous sheep lung cut to show the edema in the interlobular septum (S) and the subpleural space (V, visceral). The arrows indicate the width of the edema. (B) En face view of the lung showing interlobular septae (S) expanded by interstitial edema. The edema is only separated from the pleural space by a leaky visceral pleura. (A, From Broaddus VC, et al. Clearance of lung edema into the pleural space of volume-loaded anesthetized sheep. *J Appl Physiol.* 1990;68[6]:2627. B, From Wiener-Kronish JP, Broaddus VC, Albertine KH, et al. Relationship of pleural effusions to increased permeability pulmonary edema in anesthetized sheep. *J Clin Invest.* 1988;82[4]:1422-1429.)

that can lead to effusions, such as central venous thrombosis[61] or pulmonary embolism, among others.

Pulmonary Embolism

Pulmonary embolism (PE) is associated with exudative effusions.[85] PE may increase liquid entry in several ways: by increasing pulmonary and pleural vascular permeability (via bradykinin or VEGF), increasing central venous pressures thereby increasing pleural microvascular hydrostatic pressures, and creating atelectasis thereby decreasing pleural pressure. All these changes would tilt the balance toward increased entry of liquid into the pleural space. PE could also decrease liquid exit by increasing central venous pressure. Interestingly, it is not entirely clear that PE is the direct cause of effusions or whether it is merely associated with them. In three *computed tomography* (CT) studies, patients presenting with symptoms and signs suggestive of PE were studied by CT pulmonary angiography; effusions were common in all patients but not different in those found to have PE or not.[86–88] In the three studies, effusions were found in 50% to 58% of patients, without regard to the presence of PE. Thus, it appears that patients suspected of PE are highly likely to have effusions, although the exact cause of these effusions is not clear.

Tuberculosis

Tuberculosis is discussed here as representative of an infection targeted to the pleural membranes. In pleural tuberculosis, the intense granulomatous infiltration of the pleural membranes both increases the entry of a high-protein liquid into the pleural space and interferes with the exit of the liquid from the pleural space by lymphatics in the infiltrated parietal pleura. The study of effusions by Leckie and Tothill found that lymphatic flow from patients with TB was low, about 50% of that in patients with CHF.[72]

PLEURAL EFFUSION EFFECTS ON LUNG AND CARDIAC FUNCTION

In the presence of space-occupying liquid in the pleural space, the lung recoils inward, the chest wall expands outward, and the diaphragm is depressed inferiorly and is sometimes inverted.[89] If the lung and chest wall have normal compliances, the decrease in lung volume accounts for approximately one-third of the volume of the pleural effusion, and the increase in the size of the hemithorax accounts for the remaining two-thirds. As a result, lung volumes are reduced by less than the pleural effusion volume.

These mechanical abnormalities may explain dyspnea, exercise intolerance, and diaphragm dysfunction. All may be improved with thoracentesis. Dyspnea is most likely caused by the mechanical inefficiency of the respiratory muscles stretched by the outward displacement of the chest wall and the downward displacement of the diaphragm.[89] After the removal of large amounts of pleural liquid, dyspnea is generally relieved promptly, although the reduction in pleural liquid volume is associated with only small increases in lung volume. In one study, nine patients underwent removal of over 1800 mL of pleural liquid and, despite increases in vital capacity of only 300 mL, all patients experienced immediate relief of dyspnea.[90] Although the vital capacity changed little, patients could generate a more negative pleural pressure at the same lung volume after thoracentesis than before, indicating an improved efficiency of the respiratory muscles following the return of the chest wall and diaphragm to a more normal position after thoracentesis. A related explanation is that dyspnea is due to the inversion of the diaphragm caused by the weight of the pleural effusion, and that dyspnea is promptly relieved when thoracentesis allows the restoration of a dome-shaped diaphragm.[91] A mechanical explanation for the relief of dyspnea is supported by a case of a man with chronic absent lung perfusion on the side of a large effusion who nonetheless experienced significant relief of dyspnea with thoracentesis.[91a] Thoracentesis of a unilateral effusion (mean value 1.5 L) has also been shown to improve exercise tolerance.[92] Thoracentesis of an effusion in a ventilated patient has been shown to improve diaphragmatic function.[93] It appears that mechanical effects of a pleural effusion account for dyspnea and related symptoms.

If the lung is otherwise normal, there is no evidence that an effusion causes significant hypoxemia, presumably because ventilation and perfusion decrease similarly and remain reasonably matched. In fact, in one study, mild hypoxemia present before thoracentesis worsened *after* thoracentesis,[94] when perfusion presumably was restored while ventilation lagged behind. In another study using multiple inert gas techniques to quantify ventilation-perfusion distributions, pleural effusion was associated with a small intrapulmonary perfusion shunt (6.9%) that did not change significantly when measured again 30 minutes after thoracentesis of approximately 700 mL (6.1%).[95] Draining pleural effusions in patients with refractory hypoxemia on mechanical ventilation may improve oxygenation,[96] although there is no consensus on the indications for thoracentesis in this setting.[97] It appears therefore that the effects of pleural effusion and thoracentesis on oxygenation are variable and may depend on the underlying lung function.

Less well appreciated is the fact that large pleural effusions may impair cardiac function, most likely by decreasing the distending pressures of the cardiac chambers and thereby reducing cardiac filling. In a study of 27 patients with large effusions occupying more than half the hemithorax, clinical and echocardiographic findings of cardiac tamponade were identified in most patients. These findings, including elevated jugular venous pressure, pulsus paradoxus, right ventricular diastolic collapse, or flow velocity paradoxus, resolved in all patients when studied again 24 hours after thoracentesis of more than 1.0 L.[98] Large pleural effusions should be considered as potentially reversible causes of cardiac dysfunction.[99]

Understanding the physiology of the pleural space, liquid and protein turnover and the mechanics of pleural pressure lend themselves to understanding the abnormalities that commonly arise.

Key Points

- At baseline, pleural liquid entry is slow and balanced by an equal rate of pleural absorption (0.01 mL/kg/hr, or 12 mL/day in a 50-kg person).
- Normal pleural liquid enters from the pleural systemic microvessels and represents a filtrate from these high-pressure, low-permeability vessels, explaining the low protein concentration (1 gm/dL or ≈15% of serum protein).
- Normal pleural liquid exits via bulk flow through lymphatics which open directly onto the pleural space at the parietal pleura. This explains why pleural liquid protein concentration remains relatively constant even as liquid is absorbed.
- Lymphatics have a large reserve capacity and can normally accommodate increases in liquid entry into the pleural space without the development of an effusion.
- Pleural effusions develop when a disease or a combination of diseases increases liquid entry into the pleural space and decreases its exit from the pleural space; both changes are likely necessary for formation of a clinically relevant effusion.
- Because the protein concentration does not change with absorption via bulk flow through lymphatics, the protein concentration of pleural effusions gives information about the formation of the pleural liquid, not its removal.
- Transudates usually result from changes in hydrostatic and/or osmotic pressures that lead to increased filtration and accumulation of a protein concentration (pleural/serum protein ratio <0.5) lower than that of exudates.
- Transudates with a very low protein concentration (protein ratio <0.1–0.2) are most likely caused by entry of cerebrospinal liquid, urine, or intravenous fluids into the pleural space.
- Exudates result from pleural or extrapleural injury that can be due to a multitude of inflammatory, infectious or malignant diseases, leading to an effusion with a relatively high protein concentration.
- Excess liquid anywhere in the body can move to and enter the pleural space due to (1) its subatmospheric pleural pressure (−5 to −30 cm H_2O), (2) the leaky mesothelial layer, and (3) the high capacitance of the pleural space.

Key Readings

Bintcliffe OJ, Hooper CE, Rider IJ, et al. Unilateral pleural effusions with more than one apparent etiology. *Annals ATS*. 2016;13:1050–1056.

Broaddus VC, Wiener-Kronish JP, Staub NC. Clearance of lung edema into the pleural space of volume-loaded anesthetized sheep. *J Appl Physiol*. 1990;68:2623–2630.

Broaddus VC, Wiener-Kronish JP, Berthiaume Y, et al. Removal of pleural liquid and protein by lymphatics in awake sheep. *J Appl Physiol*. 1988;64:384–390.

Estenne M, Yernault J-C, de Troyer A. Mechanism of relief of dyspnea after thoracocentesis in patients with large pleural effusions. *Am J Med*. 1983;74:813–819.

Leckie WJH, Tothill P. Albumin turnover in pleural effusions. *Clin Sci*. 1965;29:339–352.

Light RW. *Pleural Diseases*. 6th ed. Philadelphia: Lippincott, Williams & Wilkins; 2013.

Romero-Candeira S, Fernandez C, Martin C, et al. Influence of diuretics on the concentration of proteins and other components of pleural transudates in patients with heart failure. *Am J Med*. 2001;110:681–686.

Wiener-Kronish JP, Broaddus VC. Interrelationship of pleural and pulmonary interstitial liquid. *Annu Rev Physiol*. 1993;55:209–226.

Complete reference list available at ExpertConsult.com.

DEFENSE MECHANISMS AND IMMUNOLOGY

15 *INNATE IMMUNITY*

CLAUDIA V. JAKUBZICK, PHD • ELIZABETH F. REDENTE, PHD •
DAVID W.H. RICHES, PHD • THOMAS R. MARTIN, MD

INTRODUCTION

The immune system is broadly conceptualized as having two separate but interconnected arms. In evolutionary terms, the innate immune arm is an older and more primitive system that has developed to provide early host defense against viruses, fungi, and bacteria. The fundamental basis of innate immunity is a system for pathogen detection that relies on the recognition of *pathogen-associated molecular patterns* (PAMPs), which include complex lipids, carbohydrates, unmethylated cytosine-guanosine DNA sequences, and double-stranded RNAs. PAMPs are recognized by a series of secreted, cell surface, and intracellular *pattern recognition receptors* (PRRs). These PRRs promote the recognition, phagocytosis, antigen presentation, and killing of microbial invaders. In addition, recognition of PAMPs by PRRs initiates inflammation, which in turn leads to the recruitment of phagocytes that kill and degrade microbes, promote the repair of damaged tissues, and assist in the restoration of tissue function. Although some organisms, such as sea urchins, have evolved a system of host defense based exclusively on the innate immune system,[1] mammals and higher animals have evolved an adaptive immune system

that differs from the innate immune system in its exquisite antigenic specificity and the ability to develop immunologic memory, allowing a more rapid response to previously encountered microbes and antigens. Both the innate and adaptive immune systems operate together and exist in a classic symbiotic relationship to provide optimal defense of the lung and other organs and tissues (see Chapter 16).

The broad concepts of innate and adaptive immunity outlined previously have evolved to protect most organs and tissues from microbes, a term that includes bacteria, yeasts, fungi, protozoa, multicellular parasites, and viruses. However, most organs and tissues, including the lung, have evolved additional mechanisms to tailor the immune system to their own specific needs. The lung epithelium has a surface area approximately the size of one side of a doubles tennis court and represents the largest epithelial surface in the body (see Chapter 1). With an average respiratory rate of 10 to 12 breaths/min and an average tidal volume of 600 mL, the lungs are exposed to more than 10,000 L of ambient air per day. The air we breathe is a complex mixture of gases and particulates containing pollutants, oxidants, inorganic and organic dusts, pollens, toxins, bacteria and their constituents (e.g., bacterial endotoxin, *lipopolysaccharides* [LPSs]), and viruses. In addition, the airways and gas-exchange surfaces of the lung can be exposed by aspiration to acidic gastric contents and to infected mucus from the nasal sinuses. Thus, all surfaces of the respiratory tract from the nasal passages to the alveoli are constantly exposed to a spectrum of harmless and harmful agents, raising the key question of how the lung differentiates between what is harmful and what is essentially harmless.

Like the gut, the lung has evolved discriminative mechanisms both to suppress unwanted and potentially harmful responses to harmless materials and to retain the ability to activate a vigorous innate and adaptive immune response when encountering harmful microbes and stressors. The overall goal of this chapter is to review current concepts of lung innate immunity and its fundamental underlying mechanisms. Multiple cell lineages participate in innate protection of the lung, and many share similarities in the way they recognize and respond to microbes and other harmful agents. Therefore, this chapter is organized into four broad sections: (1) an overview of lung innate immunity and its fundamental components, (2) a general mechanism of innate immune recognition, (3) a review of innate lung cells and their effector mechanisms, and (4) an outline of how these systems and mechanisms are integrated. Throughout the chapter we also discuss how the innate immune system primes the adaptive immune system as a prelude to the chapter on adaptive immunity (Chapter 16).

OVERVIEW OF THE COMPONENTS OF LUNG INNATE IMMUNITY

The long-held view that the lower respiratory tract of healthy individuals is sterile has now been invalidated through the application of culture-independent methodologies, especially bacterial 16S ribosomal RNA sequencing. Based initially on a single-center study with a modest number of subjects,[2] the National Heart, Lung, and Blood Institute–sponsored multicenter Lung HIV Microbiome Project analyzed bronchoalveolar lavage fluid and provided indisputable data that bacterial DNA is present in the lower respiratory tract of healthy subjects. Furthermore, the bacterial sequences found in bronchoalveolar lavage closely resembled the diversity seen in the mouth,[3,4] although the bacterial load was estimated to be approximately 0.1% of that found in oral washes.[5] Whether the DNA found in the lower respiratory tract was derived from reproducing bacterial colonies or represented bacteria that may have been inhaled or aspirated remains to be determined. These groundbreaking studies have ignited interest into how dysbiosis of the lung microbiome may contribute to susceptibility or to the pathogenesis of multiple lung diseases. Thus, as knowledge of the lung microbiome continues to grow, it will become increasingly important to integrate emerging information into our understanding of how the innate immune system interfaces with these potentially commensal bacteria.[6–8] For more information, see Chapter 17.

The innate immune system provides protection against a diverse spectrum of resident microbes, in addition to inhaled particles and antigens, ranging from harmless nonmicrobial particles (e.g., dusts and pollens) to harmful pathogenic microbes (e.g., *Mycobacterium tuberculosis*). To accomplish this range of protection, the lungs have evolved multiple mechanisms to survey and respond to inhaled particles based on their size, physicochemical properties, and especially the presence or absence of PAMPs. As illustrated in Figure 15.1, innate immune protection in the lung can be broadly divided into considerations of the conducting airways and the alveoli. At the cellular level, innate protection is afforded by the coordinated functions of airway and alveolar epithelial cells, *innate lymphoid cells* (ILCs),[9,10] resident macrophages (alveolar and interstitial macrophages), monocytes, *dendritic cells* (DCs), and recruited neutrophils (*polymorphonuclear leukocytes* [PMNs]).

Although often underestimated, an important component of airway host defense resides in the anatomic structure and epithelial cell lineages of the tracheobronchial tree. Air turbulence created by the nasal passages and the cartilaginous segmentation of the trachea and large airways ensures that particles in excess of 10 μm in diameter are deposited on the mucus-coated surfaces of the nose, pharynx, trachea, and descending airways. In turn, mucus, with its ensnared particulates and dissolved solutes, is constantly wafted toward the pharynx by the coordinated beating of ciliated airway epithelial cells, where its removal is aided by coughing, sneezing, and swallowing. In addition to the biophysical properties of mucus in innate host defense of the airways, the gel and pericellular liquid phases also contain an array of antimicrobial peptides, proteins, antioxidants, antiproteases, and specific *immunoglobulin* (Ig) A antibodies, all of which are maintained at a modestly acidic pH (pH 6.6).[11] Principal among airway antimicrobial peptides in humans are salt-sensitive cysteine-rich cationic β-defensins and the cathelicidin LL37/hCAP18.[12–16] β-Defensin-1 is constitutively secreted by airway epithelia and accumulates in airway surface liquid at μg/mL concentrations.[17] Expression of other β-defensins and LL37/hCAP18 is induced after exposure to LPS and other proinflammatory mediators.[18–20] Antimicrobial proteins, including lactoferrin and lysozyme, are also present in airway epithelial secretions.[21,22]

The conducting airways are lined with ciliated and secretory epithelial cells that serve a key role in the initial evaluation of large particles with which they come into contact. In addition, a network of DCs resides throughout the airway epithelium and continuously samples the airway lumen (see Fig. 15.1). DCs are particularly abundant in the trachea and large conducting airways, where most large particulates are deposited. In the absence of PAMPs, DCs and trafficking monocytes capture airway antigens and migrate to regional lymph nodes, where they process and present foreign and self-antigens to cognate T cells.

In contrast to large particles, particles smaller than 5 μm in diameter are able to descend the entire tracheobronchial tree and lodge at bronchiolar-respiratory duct junctions or deposit onto the surfactant-rich surfaces of the alveoli. Although sharing many similarities with innate protection of the airways—for example, the presence of antioxidants, antiproteases, and antimicrobial enzymes—additional innate protection of the alveoli is afforded by the presence of alveolar macrophages and the lung-specific collectins *surfactant protein A* (SP-A) and *surfactant protein D* (SP-D) (see Fig. 15.1). In addition to expressing *toll-like receptors* (TLRs), alveolar macrophages express *scavenger receptors* (SRs) that participate in the phagocytosis of microbial and

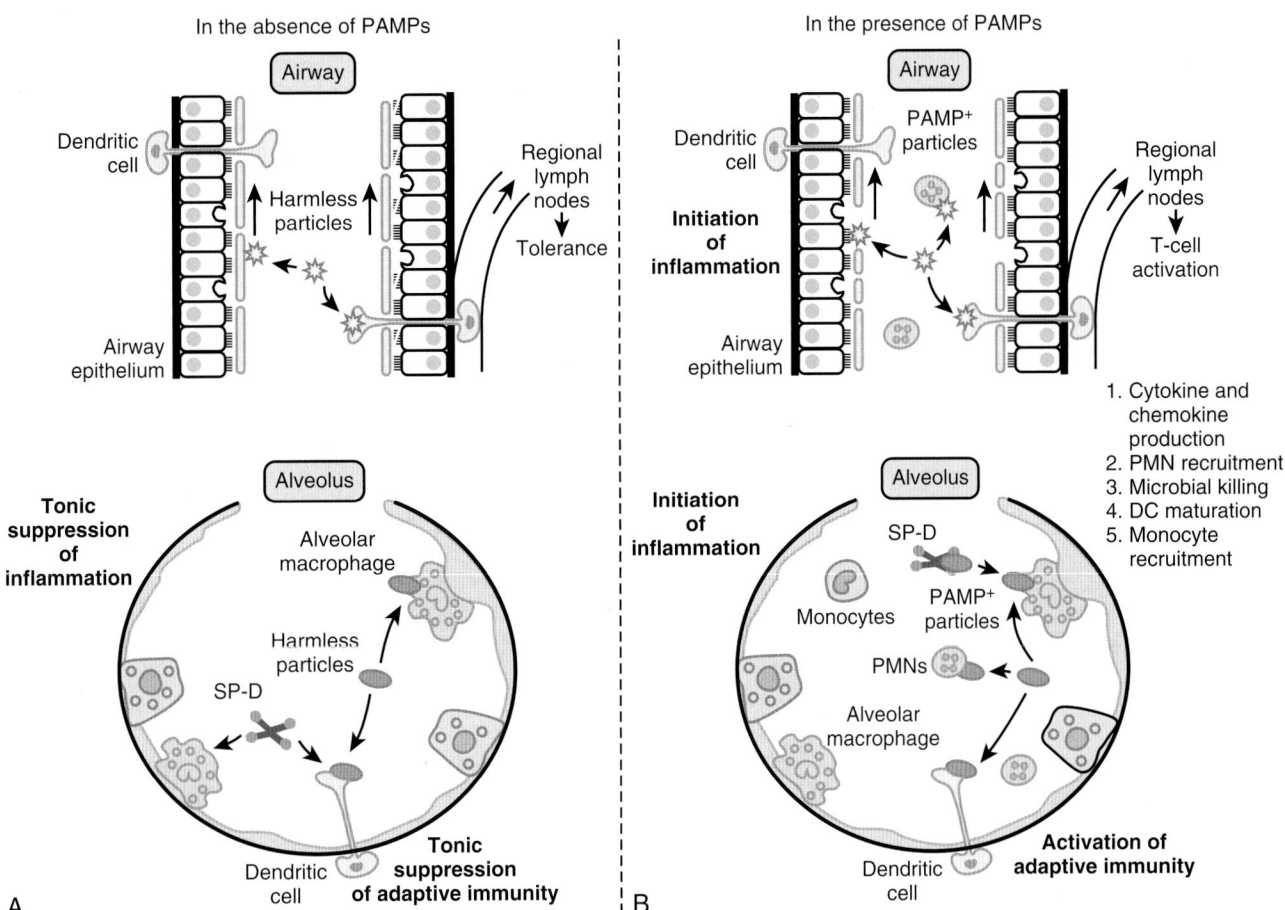

Figure 15.1 Overview of innate immune protection in the conducting airways (*upper*) and alveoli (*lower*) of the lung. (A) In the absence of *pathogen-associated molecular patterns* (PAMPs), that is, in the steady state, the airways are protected by mucus that captures harmless particulates and transports them along the mucociliary escalator. *Dendritic cells* (DCs) also capture particles, traffic to regional lymph nodes, and promote tolerance to commonly inhaled antigens. Also, in the absence of PAMPs, the alveoli are maintained in an anti-inflammatory and immunosuppressed state to prevent unwanted inflammation and immune activation toward commonly inhaled particles and antigens. (B) In the presence of PAMPs, innate immunity is activated. PAMPs stimulate airway epithelial cells to express chemokines, cytokines, and lipid mediators that attract neutrophils (polymorphonuclear leukocytes), which in turn kill PAMP-expressing microbes. Airway DCs respond to PAMPs by maturing, migrating to regional lymph nodes, and stimulating T cell proliferation. A similar program is activated in the alveoli upon PAMP detection by alveolar macrophages, alveolar epithelial cells, and DCs, resulting in the initiation of inflammation and activation of adaptive immunity. PMN, polymorphonuclear leukocytes; SP-D, surfactant protein D.

nonmicrobial particles, such as *macrophage receptor with collagenous structure* (MARCO). SP-A and SP-D are secreted PRRs and are capable of binding to microbial PAMPs, leading to opsonization and phagocytosis by alveolar macrophages and by intraseptal DCs, which then crawl into the airways and move up the mucociliary escalator or migrate to regional lymph nodes, respectively. In the absence of PAMPs, alveolar macrophages also play an important role in suppressing inflammation and adaptive immunity, thereby protecting the alveoli from unwanted responses to harmless inhaled particulates. SP-A and SP-D have a key role in suppressing inflammation through tonic signaling effects on alveolar macrophages. Thus, the innate immune system not only protects the lungs from harmful microbes but also prevents inflammation, injury, and activation of the adaptive immune system in the steady state and in response to harmless inhaled particulates.

How, then, do the airways and alveoli respond to the presence of potentially harmful microbes? As illustrated in Figure 15.1, resident airway and alveolar macrophages,

DCs, and airway and alveolar epithelial cells are capable of recognizing different PAMPs through their repertoires of cell surface and intracellular PRRs and by the interaction of PAMP-bound secreted PRRs with specific receptors on epithelial cells, macrophages, and DCs. In turn, these interactions induce signaling responses that promote the expression of an array of innate response genes (Table 15.1). These gene products collectively promote the migration of PMNs and monocytes from the pulmonary circulation into the air spaces, facilitate changes in endothelial and epithelial permeability to enhance inflammatory cell transmigration into the air spaces, and initiate the expression of specific genes involved in microbial killing. In addition, DCs and monocytes phagocytose PAMP-expressing microbes, mature, and migrate to regional lymph nodes (see Fig. 15.1).[23] During this process, ingested microbial products are digested, captured by *major histocompatibility complex* (MHC) class II and I molecules, and displayed on the plasma membrane together with co-stimulatory molecules, such as CD40, CD80, and CD86, for effective presentation to naive CD4[+] and CD8[+] T cells. After activation

Table 15.1   Representative Genes Activated by Pattern Recognition Receptors

CXCL CHEMOKINES

CXCL1, CXCL2, CXCL4, CXCL9, CXCL10, CXCL11

CCL CHEMOKINES

CCL1, CCL2, CCL7

CYTOKINES

TNF-α, IL-1β, TGF-β, IL-10

TOLL-LIKE RECEPTORS

TLR2, TLR4, TLR9

PROSURVIVAL

BCL2, cIAP1, cIAP2, BCL10

ANTIMICROBIAL

β-Defensins, cathelicidins

DC MATURATION

CD40, CD80, CD86, MHC class II, class II

Transcription of most of these genes is initiated by the activation of NF-κB and/or AP1. NF-κB activation is initiated by most PRRs.
AP1, activator protein-1; BCL, B-cell lymphoma; CCL, CC chemokine ligand; CD, cluster of differentiation; cIAP, cellular inhibitor of apoptosis; CXCL, CXC chemokine ligand; DC, dendritic cell; IL, interleukin; MHC, major histocompatibility complex; NF-κB, nuclear factor-κB; PRR, pattern recognition receptor; TGF, transforming growth factor; TLR, Toll-like receptor; TNF, tumor necrosis factor.

and expansion in regional lymph nodes, effector CD4⁺ and CD8⁺ T cells then migrate back to the site of microbial infection to augment specific host defense through their ability to activate macrophages and other effector cells. In addition, long-term central and resident memory T cells become resident in the lung and lymph nodes for future pathogen encounters.[24,25]

In summary, innate immune mechanisms involving the airway and alveolar epithelium, secreted antimicrobial enzymes, PRRs and peptides, mucus and mucociliary transport, and resident macrophages and DCs protect the lung against inhaled microbial and nonmicrobial particulates to maintain lung homeostasis. During steady-state conditions, the innate immune system actively suppresses inflammation and promotes tolerance to commonly inhaled harmless particulates. However, above a certain threshold and/or upon sensing the presence of PAMPs, additional mechanisms are activated to protect the lungs by promoting inflammation and adaptive immunity and by establishing communication and cooperation between these systems. Although it is convenient to think of these events separately, innate host responses both to harmless nonmicrobial particulates and to harmful microbes take place simultaneously and silently to maximize lung health and protection.

INNATE RECOGNITION IN THE LUNG

With this broad overview of the key elements in innate host defense of the lung and their connections to adaptive immunity, we now consider how microbes are recognized by resident and recruited lung cells. For this purpose, we specifically focus on the mechanisms of recognition by PRRs

expressed by epithelial cells, macrophages, and DCs or that are present in airway or alveolar surface liquids.

SECRETED PATTERN RECOGNITION RECEPTORS

Secreted PRRs have evolved to serve as bridges between certain PAMPs and specific receptors for these molecules. In the lung, secreted PRRs have particularly important roles in innate protection of the alveolar surfaces.

Collectins

The collectins are a family of secreted PRRs; SP-A and SP-D are collectins uniquely expressed in the distal lung.[26] All members of the collectin family are characterized by the presence of a cysteine-rich N-terminal noncollagenous domain, a collagen-like domain, an α-helical coiled-coil neck domain, and a globular C-type lectin domain, also called the carbohydrate recognition 2 domain, that interacts with microbial PAMPs (Fig. 15.2A). At baseline, SP-A and SP-D suppress inflammation (see later; shown for SP-D in Fig. 15.2B); in the presence of a variety of PAMPs, SP-A and SP-D stimulate microbial phagocytosis, the production of reactive oxidant species, and the expression of proinflammatory cytokines (see Fig. 15.2C).[27,28] A proinflammatory response is activated when PAMP-bound SP-A and SP-D interact with macrophages via their collagenous tails through a multifunctional protein made of calreticulin bound to CD91[29–31] (see Fig. 15.2C). Consistent with these findings, SP-A–deficient and SP-D–deficient mice have increased susceptibility to pulmonary infection with *Pseudomonas aeruginosa* and *Staphylococcus aureus*,[32,33] emphasizing the important contribution of these lung-specific collectins to innate lung host defense. Additional information on SP-A and SP-D can be found in Chapter 3.

The lung is remarkable in that it is capable of eliminating harmful pathogens from the alveolar surfaces while actively suppressing unwanted and potentially harmful inflammatory responses to harmless inhaled materials. Several studies have shed new light on this dichotomy by revealing an additional role for SP-A and SP-D in the tonic suppression of lung inflammation. When initially created, SP-D–deficient mice were found to have increased numbers of foamy, activated alveolar macrophages, suggesting that SP-D may somehow tonically suppress lung macrophage activation and lung inflammation (see Fig. 15.2B).[34] As illustrated in Figure 15.2C, in the steady state (i.e., in the absence of PAMPs), SP-D and SP-A interact with alveolar macrophages via their globular head groups and signal via *signal-inhibitory regulatory protein-α* (SIRPA) to suppress proinflammatory responses.[29] Thus, SP-A and SP-D, through their ability to interact under different circumstances with SIRPA and with calreticulin/CD91, play a pivotal role in the maintenance of the anti-inflammatory environment of the alveoli under steady-state conditions, while promoting an inflammatory and innate response when microbes are sensed. Other studies suggest that lipid and phospholipid constituents of surfactant also contribute to maintenance of the anti-inflammatory environment of the alveoli.[35]

Complement

The complement system functions as a pattern recognition system and a bridge to adaptive immunity through its ability to recognize repetitive structures on some microbes and

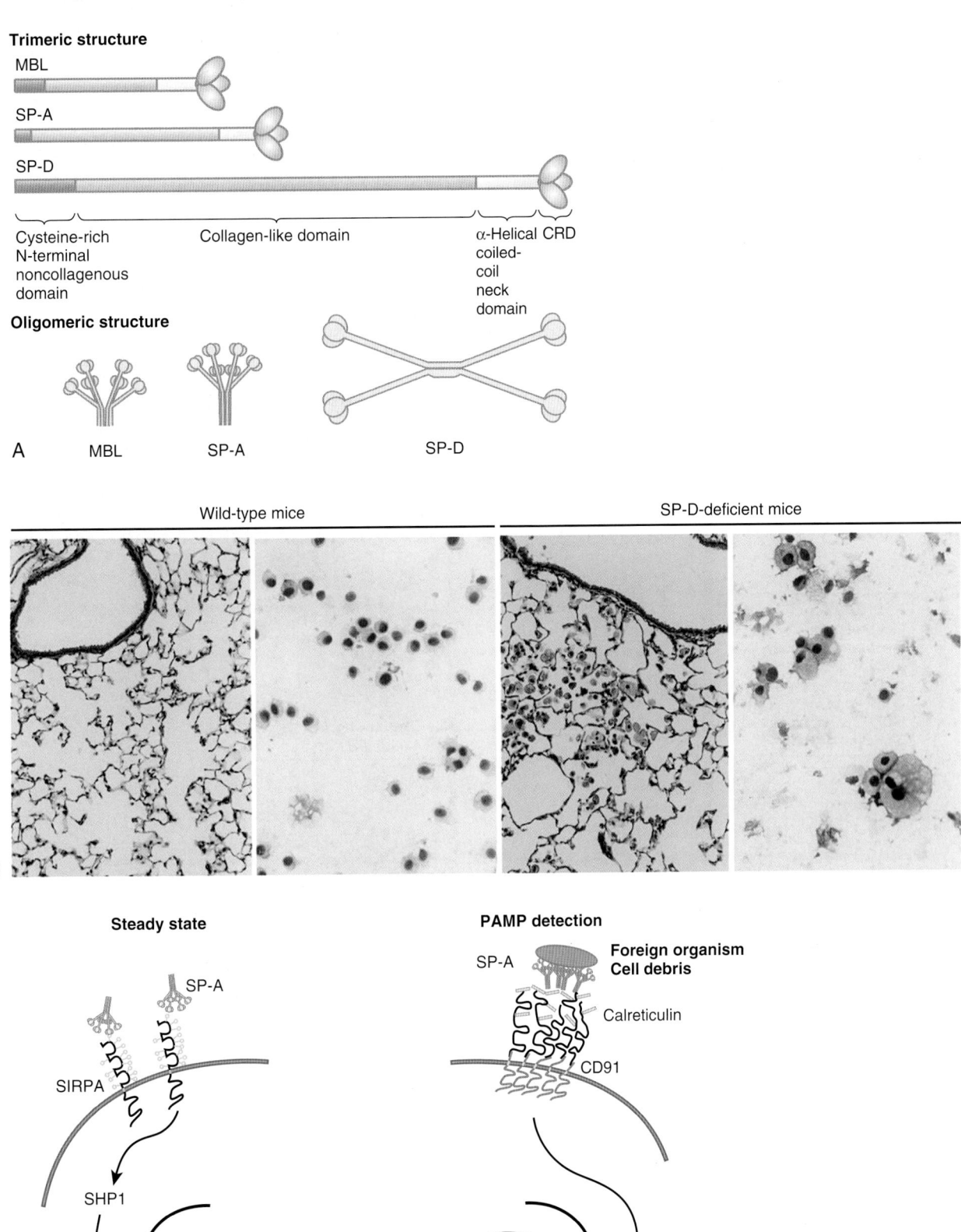

Figure 15.2 Pulmonary collectins, especially *surfactant protein A* (SP-A) and *surfactant protein D* (SP-D), play a key role in suppressing inflammation in the absence of *pathogen-associated molecular patterns* (PAMPs) while stimulating inflammation in the presence of PAMPs. (A) Structure of pulmonary collectins. (B) The importance of SP-D in tonic suppression of lung inflammation is illustrated by the spontaneous proinflammatory phenotype of SP-D–deficient mice. (C) Tonic suppression of inflammation is mediated by the binding of collectins to signal-inhibitory regulatory protein α (SIRPA) via their head groups, whereas activation of inflammation is mediated when PAMP-bound collectins interact with calreticulin/CD91 via their collagenous tail regions. CRD, carbohydrate recognition domain (C-type lectin domain); MBL, mannose-binding lectin; NFκB, nuclear factor-κB; SHP1, Src homology 2 domain-containing protein tyrosine phosphatase-1. (A, Modified from Wright JR. Immunoregulatory functions of surfactant proteins. *Nat Rev Immunol.* 2005;5:58–68. B, Modified from Fisher JH, Sheftelyevich V, Ho YS, et al. Pulmonary-specific expression of SP-D corrects pulmonary lipid accumulation in SP-D gene-targeted mice. *Am J Physiol Lung Cell Mol Physiol.* 2000;278:L365–L373. C, Modified from Gardai SJ, Xiao YQ, Dickinson M, et al. By binding SIRPalpha or calreticulin/CD91, lung collectins act as dual function surveillance molecules to suppress or enhance inflammation. *Cell.* 2003;115:13–23.)

on the Fc region of IgG and IgM antibodies. Complement activation is important in lung innate immunity because it promotes the opsonization of microbes and the generation of the potent chemotactic factor C5a, which in turn assists in the recruitment of phagocytic cells. Complement components of the classical, alternative, and mannose-binding lectin activation pathways are present in the lung airway and alveolar fluids[36–38] and are synthesized by alveolar epithelial type 2 cells, macrophages, and DCs.[22,39–41] Many microbes can directly activate the alternative complement pathway, resulting in the covalent attachment of C3b to the microbial cell wall. Microbes expressing cell wall–associated mannose-rich polysaccharides can also bind mannose-binding lectin and activate the mannose-binding lectin pathway to promote C3b attachment to the microbial cell wall. Phagocytic cells, especially macrophages, PMNs, and DCs, express various receptors for C3b and C3bi and, together with other receptors, phagocytose and kill complement-opsonized microbes. Moreover, the top genes expressed by three recently identified interstitial macrophages are *C1qa, C1qb,*

and *C1qc,* which form the C1q complex required to initiate the classical complement pathway.[42]

Pentraxins and Other Secreted Pattern Recognition Receptors

The pentraxins, including C-reactive protein, serum amyloid P, and pentraxin 3, also recognize PAMPs on microbes and activate the complement system to assist in microbial removal by phagocytic cells.[43,44] Similarly, ficolins promote phagocytosis and complement activation by binding to the gram-positive bacterial cell wall components N-acetylglucosamine and lipoteichoic acid.[45]

CELLULAR PATTERN RECOGNITION RECEPTORS

Different families of PRRs have evolved to enable the host to sense the presence of PAMPs in extracellular, endosomal, and cytoplasmic compartments in each of the lineages involved in lung innate immunity (Fig. 15.3). Transmembrane cell surface and endosome-associated PRRs include the TLRs widely

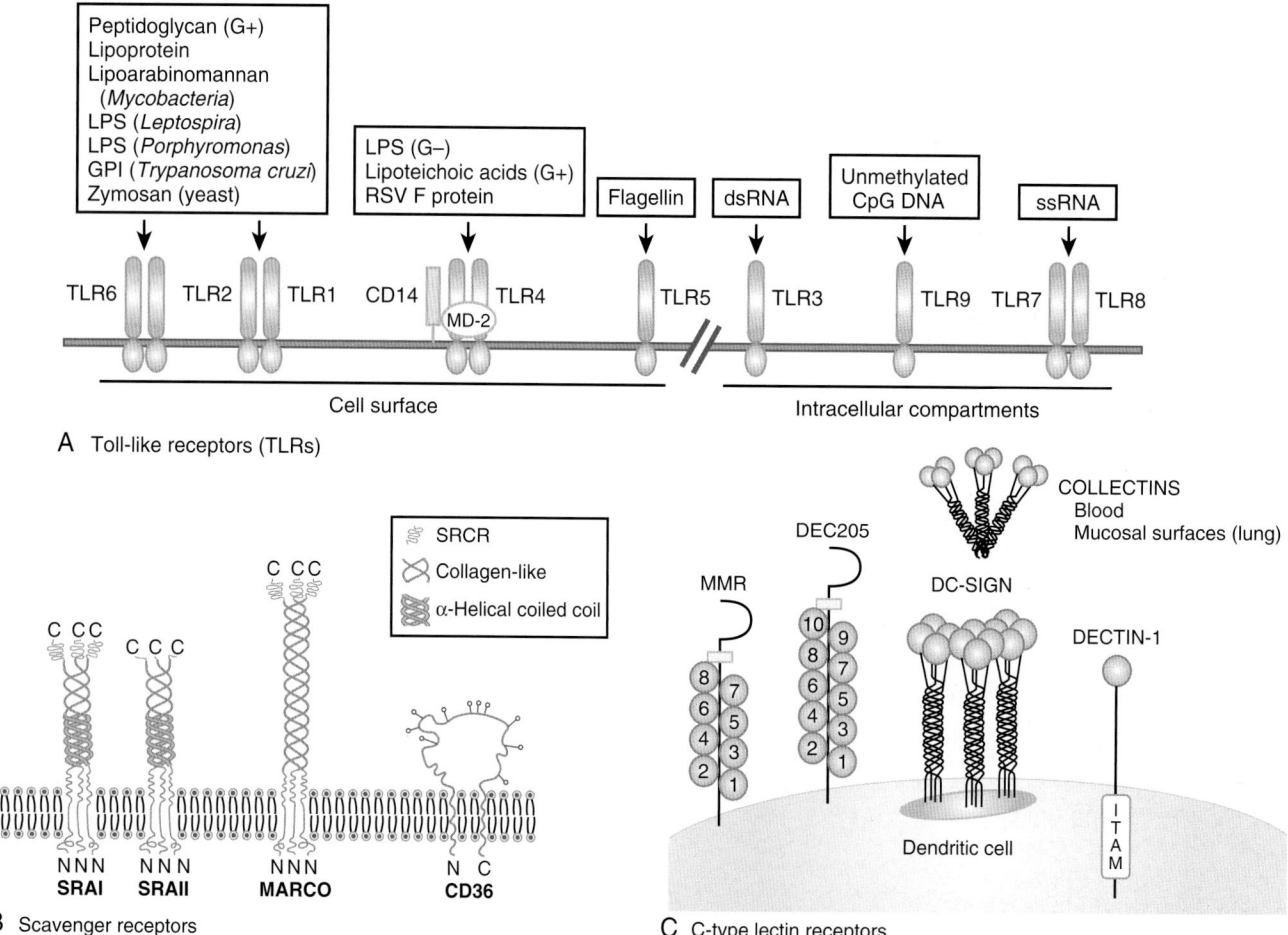

Figure 15.3 Major classes of transmembrane cell surface pattern recognition receptors expressed by lung cells. (A) Toll-like receptors. (B) Scavenger receptors. (C) C-type lectin receptors. CpG, cytosine-guanosine; DC-SIGN, dendritic cell–specific intercellular adhesion molecule–grabbing nonintegrin; DEC205, dendritic and thymic epithelial cell-205; dsRNA, double-stranded RNA; GPI, glycosylphosphatidylinositol; ITAM, immunoreceptor tyrosine-based activation motif; LPS, lipopolysaccharide; MARCO, macrophage receptor with collagenous structure; MD2, myeloid differentiation protein-2; MMR, macrophage mannose receptor; RSV, respiratory syncytial virus; SRAI, scavenger receptor AI; SRAII, scavenger receptor AII; SRCR, scavenger receptor cysteine-rich domain; ssRNA, single-stranded RNA. (A, Modified from Medzhitov R. Toll-like receptors and innate immunity. *Nat Rev Immunol.* 2001;1:135–145. B, Modified from Taylor PR, Martinez-Pomares L, Stacey M, et al. Macrophage receptors and immune recognition. *Annu Rev Immunol.* 2005;23:901–944. C, Modified from Gijzen K, Cambi A, Torensma R, Figdor CG. C-type lectins on dendritic cells and their interaction with pathogen-derived and endogenous glycoconjugates. *Curr Protein Pept Sci.* 2006;7:283–294. D, Modified from Geddes K, Magalhães JG, Girardin SE. Unleashing the therapeutic potential of NOD-like receptors. *Nat Rev Drug Discov.* 2009;8:465–479.)

expressed on epithelial cells, macrophages, PMNs, and DCs (see Fig. 15.3A); SRs primarily expressed on macrophages (see Fig. 15.3B); and C-type lectin receptors mainly expressed on DCs (see Fig. 15.3C). Cytoplasmic PRRs are composed of *nucleotide-binding and oligomerization domain (NOD)-like receptors* (NLRs) and RNA helicases of the *retinoic acid–inducible gene* (RIG) family. Each of the cytoplasmic PRRs has evolved as a strategy to alert the host to the presence of PAMPs within the cytoplasm, as often happens during the intracellular replication of facultative bacteria and viruses.

Plasma Membrane and Endosomal Pattern Recognition Receptors

Toll-like Receptors. TLRs are expressed on airway and alveolar epithelial cells, macrophages, PMNs, and DCs.[46–49] There are 10 TLRs in humans (TLR 1–10) and 12 TLRs in mice (TLR 1–9, 11–13).[50] TLR2, TLR4, TLR5, TLR7, TLR8, and TLR13 are expressed by most macrophages, with TLR4 being part of a core macrophage signature gene,[51] and TLR1 and TLR5 are highly expressed by interstitial macrophages.[42] Significant progress has been made in understanding the functions and downstream signal transduction pathways of TLRs.[52–55] TLRs can be divided into those expressed on the cell surface (TLR1, TLR2, TLR4, TLR5, TLR6, and TLR12) and those expressed in intracellular compartments (TLR3, TLR7, TLR8, TLR9, and TLR13) (see Fig. 15.3A).[50] TLRs also recognize endogenous ligands called *danger-associated molecular patterns* (DAMPs), including heat shock proteins, low-molecular-weight hyaluronan, heparin sulfate, fibronectin, high-mobility-group box-1 protein, and low-density lipoproteins. Recognition of DAMPs by TLRs and other PRRs is usually associated with the initiation of sterile inflammation. Surface TLRs recognize a wide variety of PAMPs, whereas intracellular TLRs mainly recognize nucleic acid–based PAMPs. TLRs not only recognize their individual cognate PAMPs but also combine with other TLRs to form heteromeric complexes that recognize a broader range of PAMPs.[55–58] For example, TLR1 associates with TLR2 to recognize microbial lipopeptides,[58] TLR2 and TLR4 recognize the LPS-binding protein/myeloid differentiation protein-2 complex when presented by CD14, and TLR2 recognizes broad patterns of lipoproteins in concert with either TLR1 or TLR6.[59] CD14 is a PRR that exists in membrane and soluble forms and recognizes both PAMPs and DAMPs and greatly amplifies signaling through TLR2, TLR3, and TLR4.[60] Of importance, soluble CD14 can present PAMPs to cells that do not respond to direct stimulation, such as endothelial and epithelial cells, thereby broadening inflammatory responses.[61] TLR5 recognizes flagellin and is particularly important in the response of airway epithelial cells to *P. aeruginosa* infection. Similarly, TLR6 can functionally associate with TLR2 to recognize a variety of microbial lipopeptides and peptidoglycans from gram-positive bacterial cell walls.[62] TLR3, TLR7, TLR8, and TLR9 are expressed intracellularly in endosomal and endoplasmic reticulum membranes, where they sense nucleic acids released from ingested and digested microbes.[52–55] TLR3 recognizes viral double-stranded RNA and induces the production of type I *interferons* (IFNs; IFN-α/IFN-β),[63] which in turn play a vital role in antiviral immunity and in the maturation of the cross-presenting Batf3+ DC, also known as DC1.[64–66] TLR7 recognizes single-stranded RNA

from viruses and is highly expressed by DC2, monocytes, and *plasmacytoid DCs* (pDCs),[67] whereas TLR9, which recognizes unmethylated cytosine-guanosine motifs in microbial DNA, is highly expressed by pDCs.[68,69] Of note, pDCs were previously thought to be myeloid derived. However, recent findings have shown them to be derived from lymphoid progenitors.[70]

Scavenger Receptors. The first macrophage SR was described by Goldstein and colleagues and Brown and associates[71,72] and was shown to bind and internalize acetylated low-density lipoprotein. Since then, multiple SRs have been identified and shown to play diverse roles in the phagocytosis of a variety of particles and molecules ranging from bacteria to lipids (see Fig. 15.3B). The SR family comprises eight classes (A–H), of which class A (SR-A) and class B (SR-B) are primarily involved in innate immunity through their ability to recognize and promote phagocytosis of a wide range of bacteria. Members of the SR-A and SR-B subfamilies are abundantly expressed on macrophages but do not appear to be expressed by airway or alveolar epithelial cells. The lack of expression on epithelial cells is in keeping with the notion that, during exposure to inhaled microbes and particles, the lung epithelium has evolved mechanisms to respond to PAMPs by promoting inflammation but not to engage in phagocytosis, leaving this activity to professional phagocytes.

Class A SRs are homotrimeric type II transmembrane proteins (extracellular C-terminal). SRA exists as two splice variants (SRAI and SRAII) of a single gene whose primary function is to promote the phagocytosis of a range of non-opsonized bacteria, including *S. aureus*, *Streptococcus pneumoniae*, and *Escherichia coli*.[73] SRA-deficient mice have increased susceptibility to systemic infections with *S. aureus* and *Listeria monocytogenes*[74,75] and to pulmonary infections with *S. pneumoniae*.[76] MARCO is an additional SRA involved in innate pulmonary host defense against *S. pneumoniae*.[77] Down-regulation of MARCO by IFN-γ increases susceptibility to *S. pneumoniae* in mice and may contribute to the development of pulmonary bacterial pneumonias after influenza infections.[78] MARCO may also play a role in dampening pulmonary inflammation because MARCO-deficient mice exhibit increased lung inflammation in response to inhaled silica and oxidants.[79,80] There is a notable difference in MARCO expression when alveolar macrophages are derived from embryonic monocytes compared to monocytes replenished postnatally. (Alveolar macrophages only replenish after birth if there is a significant loss of alveolar macrophages, such as by experimental depletion after intranasal delivery of liposome-encapsulated clodronate.) Postnatal-derived alveolar macrophages express significantly less MARCO than embryonic-derived alveolar macrophages,[81] and the lack of MARCO expression could be disadvantageous during certain infections, as described earlier.

Class B SRs are primarily represented in the lung by CD36. CD36 is expressed on monocytes, macrophages, DCs, and vascular endothelium.[82–84] Like class A SRs, CD36 has been implicated in PAMP recognition[85] and in the phagocytosis of *S. aureus*.[86,87] However, whereas CD36 deficiency in mice results in impaired host defense against *S. aureus*,[85] the absence of CD36 in humans, via a natural genetic deficiency, is not associated with a pulmonary phenotype.[88]

C-Type Lectin Receptors. *C-type lectin receptor* (CLR) domains are also present in a family of cell surface receptors that plays an important role in the function of DCs and macrophages (see Fig. 15.3C). CLRs recognize high-density carbohydrate-based PAMPs on microbial cell walls and viral coats. Carbohydrate binding can be divided into mannose and galactose specificity.[89] Type I CLRs include macrophage mannose receptor and *dendritic and thymic epithelial cell-205* (DEC205), and type II CLRs include DC-specific *intracellular adhesion molecule 3* (ICAM3), *DC–specific intercellular adhesion molecule–grabbing nonintegrin* (DC-SIGN), and *DC-specific receptor-1* (DECTIN1). As will be discussed later, studies in mice bearing targeted disruptions of CLR genes have emphasized their importance in innate host defense and particularly in DC maturation and antigen presentation.

DEC205 is a type 1 transmembrane receptor protein found on alveolar macrophages and the cross-presenting Batf3+ DC1 subset in humans and mice.[90,91] The natural carbohydrate ligands remain largely uncharacterized, although the receptor has been shown to induce the endocytosis of experimental antigen–anti-DEC205 receptor complexes and promote their delivery to endosomes before antigen processing and presentation. When DCs are treated with the antigen–anti-CD205 fusion protein alone, they induce tolerance to the antigen by deleting specific CD4+ and CD8+ T cells and by promoting the development of T regulatory cells.[92] In the presence of an inflammatory stimulus, DCs exposed to the antigen–anti-DEC205 fusion proteins promote long-lived immunity mediated by antigen-specific CD4+ and CD8+ T cells.[93,94] Antigens delivered by targeting DEC205 may be presented in association both with MHC class II molecules and by cross-presentation with MHC class I molecules.[95–98] Furthermore, a recent study showed that DEC205 mediates the uptake of self-antigens via the endocytosis of apoptotic cells, thereby providing a plausible mechanism for the cross-presentation of self-antigens, resulting in the induction of both central and peripheral tolerance.[99]

DECTIN1 is expressed on DCs, macrophages, monocytes, PMNs, and some T cell subsets.[91,100–102] DECTIN1 specifically recognizes β-(1,3)-linked glucans and β-(1,6)-linked glucans[103] and is thought to play a key role in the non-opsonic phagocytosis of a number of pathogenic yeasts, fungi, and bacteria by macrophages and DCs.[104] Ligation of DECTIN1 also stimulates the production of an array of proinflammatory cytokines, oxidants, and lipid mediators.[105–109]

DC-SIGN is also a type II CLR[110,111] but differs from DECTIN1 by its specificity for microbial mannose-rich carbohydrates.[110,112–114] DC-SIGN is important in DC trafficking and DC–T cell interactions through its ability to interact with ICAM3 and ICAM2, respectively.[102] DC-SIGN is also expressed on the surface of a subset of peripheral blood and lung BDCA-2+ pDCs and alveolar macrophages.[115] Of interest, increased expression of DC-SIGN by alveolar macrophages has been reported in response to stimulation with *interleukin-13* (IL-13), suggesting a possible role for DC-SIGN+ cells in the pathogenesis of *type 2 T helper* (Th2)–mediated lung diseases.[115]

Cytoplasmic Pattern Recognition Receptors

Nucleotide-Binding and Oligomerization Domain–like Receptors (NLRs). In humans, NLRs are a family of intracellular PRRs that have evolved to sense PAMPs in the cytoplasm of most cells. Cytoplasmic PAMPs recognized by NLRs include bacterial peptidoglycans and flagellin from gram-positive and gram-negative bacteria, as well as microbial toxins, such as *Bacillus anthracis* lethal factor.[116–118] Earlier, we briefly introduced DAMPs as a collection of nuclear and cytoplasmic molecules, including high-mobility-group box-1 protein, adenosine triphosphate, *nicotinamide adenine dinucleotide* (NAD+), and adenosine, which are released after tissue injury.[119] Studies have also shown that, although not technically DAMPs, uric acid and crystalline silica are also sensed by NLRs and, like PAMPs, initiate sterile inflammatory responses.[120–122] In turn, the recognition of cytoplasmic PAMPs and DAMPs by NLRs activates an array of signal transduction pathways that lead to the production of proinflammatory cytokines. Inflammasomes,[123–126] which are large protein-protein complexes comprising an NLR, an *apoptosis-associated speck-like protein containing a caspase activation and recruitment domain* ([CARD], ASC) adaptor protein, and procaspase-1, are important in the development of the inflammatory response. *Nucleotide-binding oligomerization domain, leucine-rich repeat and pyrin domain–containing protein 3* (NLRP3) is particularly relevant because it promotes the cleavage of pro–IL-1β and pro–IL-18 and the subsequent release of mature IL-1β and IL-18.[127] Inflammasomes also initiate several different forms of programmed cell death, including apoptosis, necrosis, pyroptosis, and pyronecrosis.[128] NLRs may also play a role in the maturation of immature DCs after exposure to PAMPs or cytokines.[125] The precise mechanisms by which NLRs signal is an area of intense investigation, but studies show that NLRs participate in the formation of three distinct inflammasomes, including the NLRP1 and NLRP3 inflammasomes and interleukin-1β–converting enzyme protease–activating factor–containing inflammasomes.[116,124] Although the role of NLRs in a variety of human disorders has been characterized, the complete role of these molecules in lung homeostasis and defense is not yet fully understood. More information about NLR structure and function is available in several reviews.[116,118,124,128–134]

Retinoic Acid–Inducible Gene-1–like Receptors. The last group of cytoplasmic PAMP sensors is the RIG-I–like receptors that have evolved to detect the presence of RNA from RNA viruses (as recently reviewed[135]). Recent studies have also revealed that host-derived RNA can trigger these sensors in herpesvirus (a double-stranded DNA virus) infected cells.[136] Three family members—RIG-I, myeloma-differentiation–associated gene 5, and laboratory of genetics and physiology 2—have been identified. RIG-I has been shown to recognize viral RNA sequences from several viruses and is involved in the response of lung epithelial cells to influenza virus.[137,138] In contrast, myeloma-differentiation–associated gene 5 has been shown to respond to polyriboinosinic-polyribocytidylic acid and picornoviruses.[139] Upon sensing viral RNA sequences, RIG-like family members promote the expression of type I IFNs and proinflammatory cytokines,[140] thereby inducing and augmenting host and lung innate immunity.

SUMMARY

Secreted, plasma membrane, endosomal, and cytosolic PRRs provide remarkable flexibility in innate protection of the lung. In the descending airways, plasma membrane PRRs, especially TLRs, are poised to sense PAMPs but are generally unable to phagocytose PAMP-containing microbes. However, TLR signaling in airway epithelial cells results in the production of proinflammatory mediators, especially chemokines and cytokines, which call in PMNs and macrophages to the site of PAMP detection to enable microbial clearance. In addition, intraepithelial DCs constantly sample the airway lumen to maintain immunologic tolerance to commonly encountered antigens that do not express PAMPs, while remaining poised to activate the adaptive immune system once PAMPs are sensed. The alveoli are also protected by epithelial cells, DCs, resident memory T cells, ILCs, and alveolar macrophages that also sense PAMPs via alveolar PRRs. However, in the alveoli, two additional levels of protection exist. First, secreted PRRs, especially SP-A and SP-D, protect the alveolar surfaces by tonically suppressing unwanted inflammation in the steady state, while remaining poised to stimulate innate responses in the presence of PAMPs. Second, alveolar macrophages express an additional array of PRRs, especially SRs that promote the phagocytosis of microbes and other particulates. It seems reasonable to suggest that, in the steady state, the innate immune system responds to inhaled particulates and microbes continuously, but silently. In the next section we discuss how ligation of these various PRRs activates and regulates innate host defense responses in lung cells.

EFFECTOR MECHANISMS

The cell types primarily responsible for innate protection of the lung in the steady state are airway and alveolar epithelial cells, macrophages, monocytes, and DCs and ILCs. In addition, in response to the initial activation of these cells, PMNs, although not an abundant cell type in the steady state, are rapidly recruited to augment lung phagocyte numbers once the presence of PAMPs is detected. In the following section, we review the origin and functions of these resident and recruited cells in innate protection of the lung.

EPITHELIUM

The lung epithelium has an important role in host defense against microbes that pass through the glottis and reach the conducting airways and gas-exchange parenchyma. The conducting airways of the lower respiratory tract are lined by ciliated columnar epithelial cells down to the terminal airways; these cells become nonciliated in the respiratory bronchioles. In contrast, the alveolar epithelium consists of flattened type 1 epithelial cells forming most of the alveolar surface and type 2 cuboidal epithelial cells that project into the subepithelial structures of the lungs, produce surfactant and surfactant-related proteins, and serve as both self-renewing stem cells and progenitors of type 1 epithelial cells. The classic antimicrobial defense mechanism in the conducting airways is the mucociliary system, which moves microbes deposited on the airway epithelial surface upward and out of the lungs. In addition to this physical removal system, the airway and alveolar epithelium participate actively in the innate defense of the

lungs, with the major goal of protecting the critical gas-exchange surface from microbial invasion.[141] The mucociliary system provides for the removal of all particles that deposit on the airway epithelium, and the clearance times in the trachea and proximal airways are measured in minutes (see Video 13.3). The cilia on the epithelial surface beat in coordinated waves, directing the movement of particles upward toward the larynx. Epithelial cell activation is not required for optimal ciliary beating, although beat frequency can be increased by β-agonists and slowed by opiates and other drugs.[142] Additional information on mucociliary clearance can be found in Chapter 13.

The mucociliary system and antimicrobial constituents of airway epithelial fluid discussed in the "Overview of the Components of Lung Innate Immunity" section (see Table 15.1) can be thought of as constitutive host defenses because they do not depend on specific microbial recognition mechanisms and do not need activation. However, the airway and alveolar epithelium also participate in innate immune mechanisms in that they express bacterial recognition molecules (PRRs) common to innate immune cells and can produce an array of proinflammatory mediators that recruit leukocytes into the airways directly through the airway and alveolar epithelial walls. Bacterial products stimulate the airway epithelium to produce chemotactic signals that recruit inflammatory cells into the airways. Endogenous cytokines also stimulate airway and alveolar epithelial cells to amplify leukocyte migration. Bacterial LPS stimulates ciliated airway epithelial cells to produce CXC and CC chemokines, which recruit PMNs and monocytes, respectively, into the airway lumen.[143] Airway epithelial cells also produce IL-1β, IL-6, IL-8, *regulated on activation, normal T cell expressed and secreted* (RANTES), *granulocyte-macrophage colony-stimulating factor* (GM-CSF), and *transforming growth factor-β* (TGF-β).[141] As with other cells involved in innate immunity, airway epithelial cells produce cytokines via the activation of transcription factors, including *nuclear factor-κB* (NF-κB), activator protein-1, and nuclear factor IL-6.[144] Of interest, noninfectious environmental agents, such as ozone,[145] asbestos,[146] diesel exhaust particles,[147] and air pollution particles,[148] all lead to NF-κB activation in airway epithelial cells under experimental conditions, which is typically followed by IL-8 production and release. Airway epithelial cells also recognize unmethylated bacterial DNA via TLR9, leading to NF-κB activation and production of IL-6, IL-8, and $β_2$-defensin in the airways.[149] Unlike airway epithelial cells, alveolar epithelial cells do not respond directly to LPS but do produce chemokines in response to the *tumor necrosis factor-α* (TNF-α) and IL-1β produced by alveolar macrophages in response to PAMPs.

The critical role of the lung epithelium in innate immunity and microbial defense has been supported by studies using transgenic mice. When a dominant negative IκB construct was expressed in the distal airway epithelial cells of mice, thereby preventing NF-κB activation, airway PMN recruitment in response to inhaled LPS was impaired.[150] This finding supports the importance of bacterial recognition by distal airway epithelial cells in vivo and shows that epithelium-derived cytokines produced by the NF-κB pathway probably are just as important as macrophage-derived cytokines in driving innate inflammatory responses in the airways and alveolar spaces. Hajjar and colleagues[151] created bone marrow chimeras in which either myeloid (leukocytes) or nonmyeloid (epithelial) cells lacked Myd88, a key adapter molecule required for signaling via all TLRs except TLR3. Unexpectedly, nonmyeloid deficiency of Myd88 impaired bacterial clearance more than myeloid deficiency. Specifically, mice lacking Myd88 (and therefore lacking TLR signaling) in nonmyeloid cells, including the airway and alveolar epithelium, had markedly impaired clearance of *P. aeruginosa*, whereas mice with or without Myd88 in myeloid cells had normal bacterial clearance. This surprising result further supports the important role of the airway and alveolar epithelium in bacterial recognition and clearance from the lungs, a role perhaps equivalent to that of resident and recruited leukocytes.

Innate immune responses in the airway epithelium can generate or influence adaptive responses. For example, recognition of β-(1,3)-glucan in house dust mites stimulates the production of CCL20, a chemokine that recruits immature DCs into the airways.[152] The airway epithelium can directly influence the function of lung DCs, inducing adaptive Th2 responses thought to be important in the pathogenesis of asthma, and LPS responses in the airway epithelium involved in some DC-driven Th2-cell responses.[153] Airway epithelial cells produce thymic stromal lymphopoietin, GM-CSF, IL-1β, IL-25, IL-33, and osteopontin, all of which activate DCs.[154]

An emerging concept is that deliberate stimulation of innate immunity in the airways and air spaces produces broad enhancement of antimicrobial defenses. Exposure of mice to a crude extract of nontypeable *Haemophilus influenzae* bacteria via aerosol initially stimulated innate immunity and then protected the mice from lethal infection with *S. pneumoniae*.[155] This was associated with enhanced production of lysozyme, lactoferrin, and defensins in the lungs. Similarly, exposure to this crude bacterial extract protected mice from *S. aureus*, *P. aeruginosa*, and the fungus *Aspergillus fumigatus*.[156] Thus, prestimulation of innate immune mechanisms in the airway and perhaps alveolar epithelium enhances antimicrobial activity and host defense of the lungs against a broad array of bacteria and fungi. The implication is that deliberate low-level stimulation of innate immunity in the lungs could be used as a protective strategy; however, the recognition of the important role of lung epithelial innate immunity in stimulating and regulating adaptive immune mechanisms raises the possibility that

such a strategy might have unexpected effects, such as promoting a hyperinflammatory state.

Thus, innate immune mechanisms in the airways stimulate endogenous defenses by enhancing production of airway defensins and other antimicrobial products, by stimulating PMN and monocyte recruitment into the airways to augment antimicrobial defenses, and by setting the stage for DCs and Th2-mediated adaptive immune responses that could be important in the pathogenesis of allergic lung diseases.

POLYMORPHONUCLEAR LEUKOCYTES

PMNs serve as the immediate effector arm of the innate immune system.[157,158] PMNs are produced from progenitor cells in the bone marrow, circulate for a short time in the bloodstream, and migrate to sites of tissue inflammation in response to signals produced by local innate immune mechanisms. Mature PMNs are released from the marrow in response to granulocyte colony–stimulating factor and other stimuli and circulate for up to 6 to 8 hours.[159] The bone marrow releases between 10^9 and 10^{10} PMNs each day, and marrow release can increase several fold in response to acute signals from the lungs and other tissues. PMNs contain several different kinds of cytoplasmic granules, containing an array of proteins (Fig. 15.4). Small specific granules serve as a source of new membrane during cell migration. Primary (azurophilic) granules contain myeloperoxidase, which accounts for the green color of pus, bacterial permeability–increasing protein, neutrophil elastase, matrix metalloproteinases, other proteinases, and defensins.

Circulating PMNs are spherical, with a diameter of approximately 8 μm, and must deform to make their way through the capillary microcirculation in the lungs and other organs.[160] Under normal circumstances, this migration is not associated with injury to the endothelial or epithelial barriers. PMNs bear surface adhesion molecules that recognize carbohydrate and protein moieties expressed on activated endothelial cells. In the systemic circulation, PMNs migrate into tissue through postcapillary venules in a four-step process by (1) weakly adhering to the venular endothelium, (2) rolling along the endothelial surface, (3) arresting on the endothelial surface, and (4) migrating between endothelial junctions into tissue in response to local chemotactic gradients.[160,161] In addition, the

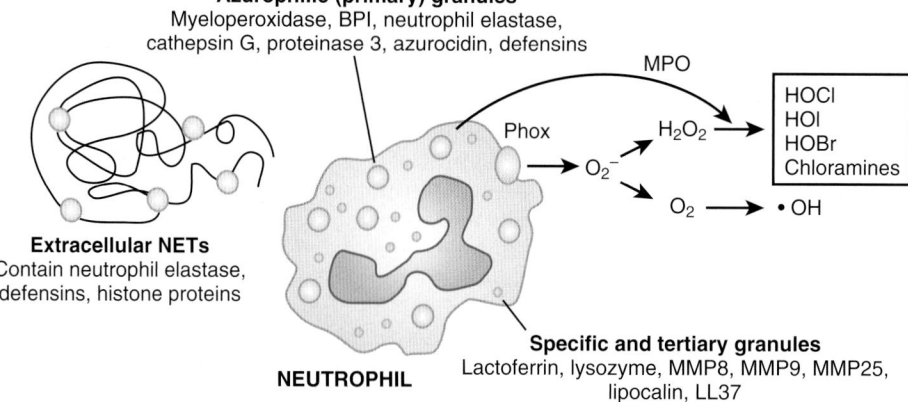

Figure 15.4 **Neutrophils use several mechanisms to kill microbes.** BPI, bacterial permeability–increasing protein; HOBr, hypobromous acid; HOCl, hypochlorous acid; HOI, hypoiodous acid; LL37, cathelicidin; MMP, matrix metalloproteinase; MPO, myeloperoxidase; NET, neutrophil extracellular trap; Phox, phagocyte oxidase. (Modified from Nathan C. Neutrophils and immunity: challenges and opportunities. *Nat Rev Immunol.* 2006;6:173–182.)

endothelial cells undergo reversible contraction in response to thrombin and other inflammatory stimuli, thereby opening endothelial junctions and allowing the passage of leukocytes. The alveolar barrier is much tighter, and yet PMNs reach the air spaces with only minor and transient changes in epithelial permeability.[162,163] Within the lungs, the small cross-sectional size of the pulmonary capillaries slow the transit of PMNs, producing a reservoir of capillary PMNs poised to respond directly to signals from the innate immune system in the air spaces.[164,165]

When bacteria or their products, such as gram-negative LPS, circulate in the bloodstream, PMNs undergo activation with cytoskeletal rearrangements that cause stiffening,[166] promoting increased entrapment of PMNs in the pulmonary capillaries. During migration, specific granules fuse with the leading edge of the cell membrane, providing new membrane material bearing specific adhesion molecules initiating the migratory process. Metabolic studies of PMNs in rabbits with pneumococcal pneumonia and humans with bronchiectasis have shown that most PMNs become fully activated in the air spaces and not during their migration into the lung.[162,167,168] However, when endothelial activation is intense or when PMN activation signals are present within the circulation, PMNs become preactivated, and migration can be associated with damage to the endothelial and epithelial barriers, with the development of increased-permeability pulmonary edema.[169]

When innate immunity is activated in the lungs, chemotactic factors are produced by alveolar macrophages and activated epithelium, which create complex, combinatorial, soluble, and tissue-fixed gradients that recruit PMNs into the alveolar spaces.[170] Leukotriene B_4 is a product of arachidonic acid metabolism in alveolar macrophages that produces an immediate and short-lived soluble gradient that recruits PMNs into the air spaces but dissipates within minutes.[171,172] Release of leukotriene B_4 is closely followed by the release of IL-8, a chemokine that binds to heparin residues on tissue matrix, creating a tissue reservoir promoting long-lived gradients that guide PMNs sequestered in the pulmonary capillaries into the airspaces.[173,174] IL-8 is the dominant member of a group of CXC chemokines, which also include GRO-α, GRO-β, and GRO-γ, and ENA-78. The CXC chemokines have a C-X-C sequence at the N-terminus, which provides PMN specificity, and an N-terminal Glu-Leu-Arg peptide sequence, which is important in chemotactic receptor binding. The CXC chemokines recruit PMN to sites of inflammation, whereas chemokines with the CC N-terminal sequence recruit monocytes. Whereas PMNs bear a single receptor for leukotriene B_4, they express two different receptors with differing affinity for IL-8. The low-affinity receptor (CXCR2) is thought to recruit PMNs to sites of inflammation, whereas the high-affinity receptor (CXCR1) is thought to guide PMN migration into the tissues. The low-affinity receptor is shed from the surface of circulating PMNs in sepsis, leaving the high-affinity CXCR1 receptor as the dominant IL-8 receptor.[175] This suggests that a CXCR1 receptor–targeted strategy could be effective in limiting PMN inflammation in patients with sepsis. PMNs also have receptors for the complement component C5a and for formylated peptides produced by bacteria in the air spaces so that endogenous and exogenous signals attract PMNs to sites of inflammation.

PMN migration into most tissues depends on the integrin CD11/CD18 on the PMN surface recognizing the counterligand ICAM1 on the endothelial surface. In the lungs, however, both CD18-dependent and CD18-independent mechanisms exist, and the signals that determine the dependence on CD18 are not clear.[176] For example, PMN migration into the lungs in response to *E. coli* and *P. aeruginosa* is CD18 dependent, whereas PMN migration in response to *S. pneumoniae* does not require CD18. TNF-α and IL-1β appear to direct CD18-dependent migration, whereas IFN-γ is more important for CD18-independent migration.

Once in the air spaces, PMNs ingest bacteria and fungi opsonized by complement and immunoglobulins that accumulate in the air spaces at sites of inflammation. PMNs contain a series of effector mechanisms to kill bacteria and fungi, including oxidant production, microbicidal proteins in primary azurophilic granules, and extracellular traps (see Fig. 15.4). As microbes are recognized, they are enveloped by plasma membrane to form the phagosomes. The phagosome is the intracellular compartment where digestion and killing of ingested particles takes place in a tightly regulated manner.[177] Within the phagosome, the subunits of a *nicotinamide adenine dinucleotide phosphate, reduced form* (NADPH) oxidase are assembled in the cell membrane, and the cell undergoes a respiratory burst; a superoxide anion is formed and reduced to form hydrogen peroxide. This happens on the invaginating phagosomal membrane. As the phagosome forms, the primary granules fuse with the phagosomal membrane, adding myeloperoxidase and cationic antimicrobial peptides to the phagolysosome. Myeloperoxidase catalyzes the formation of hypochlorous acid from hydrogen peroxide and a halide, typically *chloride* (Cl⁻), because of its high concentration in the cellular environment. Hypochlorous acid is a highly reactive oxidant that oxidizes methionines, tyrosines, and other amino acids on proteins, facilitating the killing of the microbes.

When α-defensins or human neutrophil protein 1, 2, and 3 (present in the primary azurophilic granules) are added to the phagolysosomal space, they attach to negatively charged microbial membranes via electrostatic interactions and are thought to form lytic pores in the microbial cell wall.[178,179] PMN defensins have antimicrobial activity for gram-positive and gram-negative organisms, fungi, and some viruses. Defensins are most active under conditions of low ionic strength and lose activity with increasing concentrations of salt or plasma proteins, which interfere with electrostatic interactions between the cationic defensins and the anionic microbial surface.[178] The loss of defensin activity in higher salt concentrations has been proposed as a contributing factor for the pathogenesis of chronic airway infection in cystic fibrosis.[180] In addition to their antimicrobial activity, defensins participate directly in innate and adaptive immunity because they stimulate IL-8 production by epithelial cells and modulate the responses of T cells and immature DCs.[179,181]

When phagocytosis is appropriately regulated, microbes are killed within the protected environment of the PMN phagolysosome. However, at sites of intense inflammation, PMNs release superoxide anions, hydrogen peroxide, and granular contents directly into the extracellular environment, leading to oxidant formation in the alveolar spaces with oxidation of structural proteins in the alveolar walls and intracellular proteins in leukocytes, and the accumulation of defensins and other granular contents in the alveolar spaces.[182] These extracellular products contribute to tissue injury by PMNs.

In addition to killing intracellular microbes using oxidants, chlorination, and antimicrobial peptides, as a final act, PMNs can project uncoiled nuclear DNA into the surrounding environment to form *neutrophil extracellular traps* (NETs) that ensnare and destroy bacteria.[183,184] NET formation depends on the initial respiratory burst of the PMN and leads to the death of the PMN in a process distinct from apoptosis and necrosis.[185] The PMNs of patients with chronic granulomatous disease, which lack a functional membrane NADPH oxidase, do not form NETs after appropriate stimulation.[185] A variety of proinflammatory stimuli activate NET formation, including LPS and IL-8. C5a triggers NET formation in PMNs after priming with IFNs or GM-CSF. Some microbes, including *S. aureus*, *E. coli*, *P. aeruginosa*, and *M. tuberculosis*, directly stimulate NET formation by PMNs.[186] The extracellular DNA mesh contains cationic proteins embedded in the negatively charged DNA net, including histones, defensins, and cathelicidin, which kill enmeshed bacteria. NET formation thickens secretions at sites of inflammation, creating a viscous pus with enmeshed microbes. As might be expected, some bacteria produce extracellular enzymes that degrade DNA NETs, including *S. pyogenes* (DNase Sda1/2) and *S. pneumoniae* (DNase EndA).[187,188] The mechanisms by which NETs are cleared from the air spaces during resolution of inflammation are not clear. Recent evidence suggests that NETs contribute to disease pathology in several immune-mediated diseases, including cystic fibrosis, where clinical isolates of *P. aeruginosa* are resistant to NET-mediated killing.[189–193]

PMNs have an important role in signaling the activation of adaptive immunity.[194] In rabbits with tuberculous pleurisy, PMNs are the first cells that migrate into the infected pleural space, where they produce chemotactic factors that direct the subsequent wave of monocyte recruitment, which characterizes the full inflammatory reaction to *M. tuberculosis*.[195] PMN granule proteins cathepsin G and azurocidin are chemoattractants for mononuclear cells, which mature into macrophages and DCs at sites of inflammation, and neutrophil-derived CC chemokines recruit DCs.[196,197] PMNs release limited amounts of TNF-α and IFN-γ, which regulate macrophage, T cell, and DC activation and maturation; however, the large numbers of PMNs at sites of inflammation can bring the concentrations of these PMN-derived cytokines into biologically relevant ranges. PMNs also produce CXC chemokine ligand 10 (IFN-γ inducible protein-10), which is a chemoattractant for natural killer cells and Th1 cells.[198] They also produce the lipid mediators prostaglandin E2 and leukotriene D4, which are potent activators of ILCs.[199,200]

At the same time that PMNs participate in and intensify inflammation in tissue, they also produce signals that control and begin the resolution of inflammation. PMNs, like macrophages and endothelial cells, release the secretory leukocyte protease inhibitor, which inhibits neutrophil elastase.[201] After migration into tissues, PMNs produce lipoxins from membrane arachidonic acid, which inhibit PMN recruitment, superoxide anion generation, and NF-κB activation, and enhance the uptake of apoptotic PMNs by macrophages.[202] PMN-derived oxidants inactivate proteases and other proteins at sites of inflammation.

PMNs and their products are cleared largely by macrophages during the resolution of inflammation. PMNs die primarily by apoptosis, necrosis, or NET formation. PMNs undergoing apoptosis express phosphatidylserine on the outer leaflet of the cell membrane and undergo nuclear chromatin condensation and cell shrinkage. Apoptotic PMNs are recognized by macrophages via the class B SR, CD36, and are rapidly ingested, so that large numbers of apoptotic PMNs are usually not seen. Macrophages that ingest apoptotic PMNs produce TGF-β and IL-10, which have anti-inflammatory effects. This process results in the clearance of PMNs and their residual intracellular contents and the dampening of inflammation.

However, in some cases inflammation may not be appropriately dampened. PMNs not ingested by macrophages undergo secondary necrosis with loss of membrane integrity, cytoplasmic swelling, and release of remaining intracellular contents into the inflammatory environment. Intracellular components are recognized as danger signals by macrophages, some of which function as "alarmins," or DAMPs.[203] DAMPs include the nuclear protein high-mobility-group box-1, granular antimicrobial peptides, and other intracellular products. Macrophages recognizing these danger signals produce IL-1β, TNF-α, IL-8, and other proinflammatory cytokines, initiating or perpetuating inflammatory responses. Some PMNs recovered from the lungs of patients with the acute respiratory distress syndrome have features of apoptosis, with small cytoplasmic features and nuclear pyknosis, whereas many have features of necrosis, including severe degranulation, membrane blebbing, and cytoplasmic swelling. The signals that govern the balance between apoptosis and necrosis, and therefore the balance between controlled or sustained inflammation, are incompletely understood.

Thus PMNs are important effector cells in innate immunity, ideally designed to circulate through the body and accumulate rapidly at tissue sites during acute inflammation. Under normal circumstances, they arrive in tissue ready to ingest and kill microbes, then quietly go away by programmed cell death. PMN-derived signals regulate local inflammation and stimulate adaptive immune responses, providing a broader role for PMNs in host defense.

INNATE LYMPHOID CELLS

ILCs are a newly identified class of lymphoid cells that are $CD45^+$ $Thy1^+$ but do not have antigen specificity, either through recombination of antigen receptors or through clonal selection.[204–206] ILCs are found within mucosal tissues, including the respiratory tract, and respond to pathogens through PRRs.[207] Once they are activated, they secrete immunoregulatory cytokines associated with Th1, Th2, or Th17 responses.[208] An important feature of IL-17–mediated diseases is the regulation of PMNs, both during homoeostasis and inflammation, thus making ILCs a potent influencer of neutrophil trafficking.[209] Additional information on ILCs can be found in Chapter 16.

MONONUCLEAR PHAGOCYTES

The concept of the mononuclear phagocyte system as a functionally and phenotypically heterogeneous system distributed throughout the body was developed in the 1960s and 1970s through a series of insightful studies pioneered by van Furth and Cohn[210] and Volkman and Gowans.[211] The central concept was that the resident macrophages of all organs and tissues were derived from progenitor cells in the bone marrow. In turn, the progenitor cells gave rise to circulating blood monocytes that were recruited into organs and tissues, where they differentiated into macrophages, to maintain macrophage homeostasis and to respond during inflammation or infection.[212–214] Fate-mapping studies involving lineage-tagged mice and other genetic models have refuted this notion by showing that there is a pool of "primitive" F4/80-high resident macrophages located within tissues derived from the yolk sac beginning on *embryonic day 8* (E8) (Fig. 15.5A).[215–217] In addition to expressing high levels of F4/80, these yolk sac–derived macrophages express CX3CR1, macrophage mannose receptor, and *colony-stimulating factor 1 receptor* (CSF1R; *c-fms* [gene]) and are dependent upon IL-34, CSF1, and the transcription factor PU.1 for their development (see Fig. 15.5A).[216,218–221] By E10.5, yolk sac–derived macrophages reside in most tissues, including the lung, and are able to undergo self-renewal.[212,214,216,222–230]

At E10.5, the fetal liver becomes the major site of hematopoiesis[231] and, with its development, a unique "definitive" macrophage population derived from the hematopoietic stem cell can also be found.[216,220] These cells express low levels of F4/80, high levels of CD11b, and, in contrast to the yolk sac–derived macrophages, are dependent on the transcription factor c-Myb for development.[216] During liver hematopoiesis, macrophages constitute up to 15% of the total cells in many organs,[220] and their importance in embryonic development has been definitively shown in studies using *c-fms*–, colony-stimulating factor 1–, CX3CR1-, c-Myb–, and PU.1-deficient mice.[216,232–235] These studies also showed that adult Langerhans cells, the prominent antigen-presenting cells of the skin, are produced by the fetal liver and that their development is dependent on IL-34 and CSF1. In studies using these and other models, macrophages have been shown to play important roles in bone morphogenesis, ductal branching in the mammary gland, neuronal patterning, angiogenesis, vascular remodeling, and kidney and endocrine development.[234,236,237] Analysis of embryonic tissue has shown that the lungs basally contain macrophages of fetal liver and hematopoietic stem cell origin.[216,238]

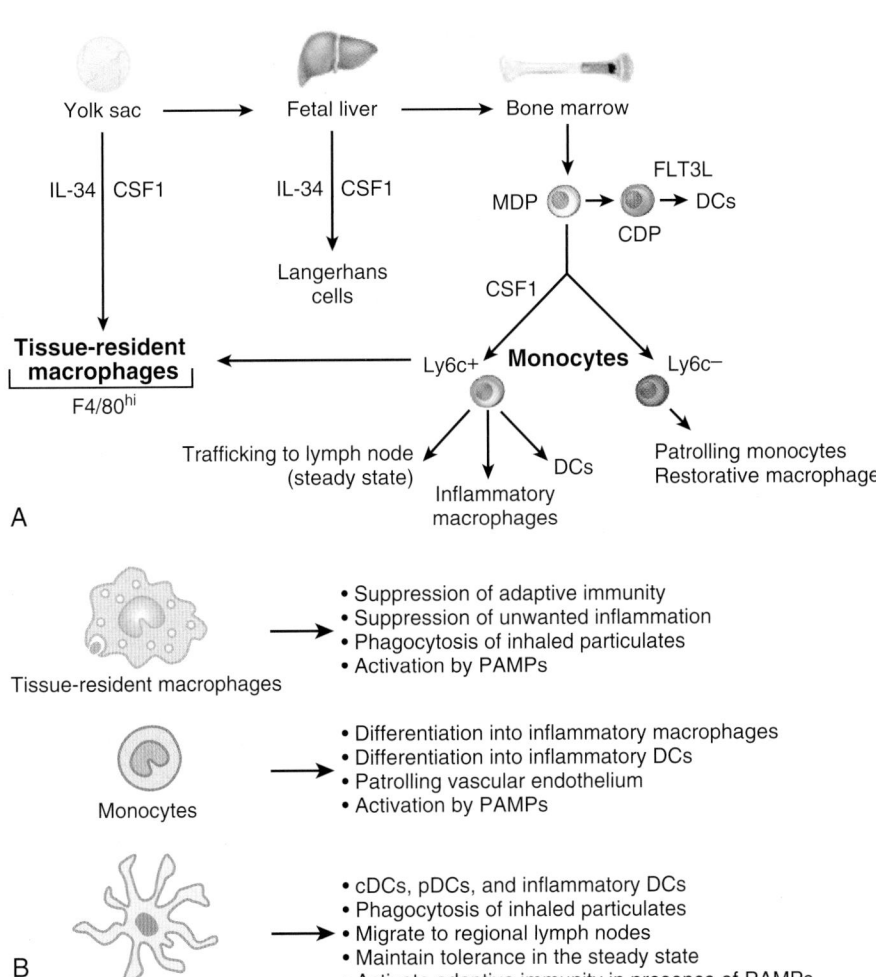

Figure 15.5 Pathways of development of tissue-resident macrophages and blood monocytes. (A) During embryogenesis, macrophages derived from the yolk sac populate most tissues, including the lung. Later, the fetal liver and the bone marrow become sites of hematopoiesis. (B) In the steady state, lung mononuclear phagocytes can be considered to include (1) tissue-resident macrophages of the alveoli and interstitium, (2) marginating monocytes of the lung microvasculature, and (3) resident DCs. Each of these subsets exhibits overlapping and unique functions. cDC, conventional DC; CDP, common DC precursor cell; CSF1, colony-stimulating factor 1; FLT3L, FMS-like tyrosine kinase 3 ligand; IL, interleukin; MDP, macrophage and DC precursor; PAMP; pathogen-associated molecular pattern; pDC, plasmacytoid DC. (A, Modified from Wynn TA, Chawla A, Pollard JW. Macrophage biology in development, homeostasis and disease. *Nature.* 2013;496:445–455.)

In addition to macrophages, DCs play a fundamental role in lung innate immunity. Steinman[239] published the first report on a population of antigen-presenting cells in mouse spleen and, based on their morphologic characteristics, coined the name dendritic cells. This work was recognized in 2011 with the posthumous award of the Nobel Prize in Physiology or Medicine. Since the late 1980s, a vast array of monoclonal antibodies against monocytes, macrophages, and DC cell surface antigens, together with lineage-tracing mice, have been developed and used to classify monocytes/macrophages and DCs.[42,240] With the onset of single-cell RNA sequencing technology, the ability to classify and define macrophages, monocytes, and DCs has been greatly expanded.[81,241–244] Cell surface molecules that help distinguish mononuclear phagocytes in humans and mice are FcgR1/CD64 and C5aR1/CD88, which are highly expressed on monocyte/macrophages and not DCs. F4/80 and CD11c, originally thought to distinguish monocytes/macrophage and DCs, are expressed on all mononuclear phagocyte classifications. In addition, much of our initial understanding of the functions of lung mononuclear phagocytes has come from studies conducted without the use of extensive cell surface marker panels or lineage-tracing technologies or using in vitro systems. Thus, although it is clear that the cells described in many studies are mononuclear phagocytes, it is sometimes difficult to classify them further without the use of multiple antibody markers combinations.[245] As illustrated in Figure 15.5B, pulmonary mononuclear phagocytes can be broadly thought of as three overlapping subpopulations: (1) *resident macrophages* of alveoli and interstitium; (2) *monocytes*, which marginate in the lung microvasculature, survey the lung environment, and can be recruited into the air spaces in response to innate activation; and (3) *resident and recruited DCs* of the airways and lung parenchyma. In this section, we discuss the localization and innate immune functions of each group of cells.[239,242,246]

Resident Macrophages

Tissues have two classes of resident macrophages: one that is *tissue specific*—in the lungs, the alveolar macrophage—and one that is *common* among all tissues—in the lungs, the interstitial macrophage.

Alveolar macrophages are distinguished from interstitial macrophages by several factors. The first is origin, with alveolar macrophages being derived from the yolk sac embryogenesis and interstitial macrophages derived from the fetal liver and circulating monocytes.[238] However, it is still unclear how origin dictates the functional outcome of a macrophage population.[247] The second is transcriptional signatures. There are major transcriptional differences between alveolar and interstitial macrophages.[51,248–251] All tissue-resident macrophages share core macrophage signature genes, but each tissue-specific macrophage displays their own unique transcriptional signature adapted to a given environment.[51] Tissue-specific macrophages also differ functionally, in parallel with the variation in their transcriptomes. By contrast, interstitial macrophages from the skin, heart, intestine, and lung have transcriptionally overlapping profiles independent of their local tissue environment.[248–251] The conserved transcriptional profile

across multiple organs, also observed in DCs,[42] suggest that interstitial macrophages may have a similar function in different organs.

ALVEOLAR MACROPHAGES

The primary functions of alveolar macrophages are to (1) dispose of inhaled microbes and particulates, (2) clear pulmonary surfactant, and (3) suppress the development of inappropriate inflammatory and immune responses. Alveolar macrophages are capable of phagocytosing a wide spectrum of harmless and harmful microbes and other particulates. Under basal conditions, most ingested phagocytosed particulates are enclosed within phagosomes, which ultimately fuse with lysosomes, leading to their degradation by an array of acid-pH optimum hydrolytic enzymes. Some inhaled microbes (e.g., *M. tuberculosis*) and some environmental particulates (e.g., crystalline silica) are resistant to this process and become sequestered in secondary lysosomes, where they remain for the life span of the macrophage. Most of these latter cells probably crawl into the airways and are cleared via the mucociliary escalator.[252,253] Some particle-laden macrophages may remain in the lung for extended periods of time before either dying and releasing their particle burden, thereby rendering it available for phagocytosis by other macrophages, or undergoing apoptosis and being cleared by other phagocytes.

Alveolar macrophages reside in the mixed environment of epithelial lining fluid and ambient inhaled air,[42,254–256] where they actively contribute to the normal homeostasis of pulmonary surfactant. This point is most clearly emphasized in patients with pulmonary alveolar proteinosis, a disorder characterized by the accumulation of proteinaceous and lipid-rich surfactant in the alveoli, leading to impaired gas exchange. A fundamental characteristic of the disorder is the finding that alveolar macrophage numbers are reduced, and those present are inefficient in clearing pulmonary surfactant.[257,258] Several studies have shown that pulmonary alveolar proteinosis can be associated with the development of autoantibodies against GM-CSF,[257–259] emphasizing the importance of GM-CSF in the activities of alveolar macrophages. Additional information about alveolar proteinosis syndromes can be found in Chapter 98.

Last, alveolar macrophages play a critically important role in tonic suppression of alveolar inflammation and adaptive immunity. Based in part on studies by MacLean and associates,[260] the concept has evolved that the lung can deal with inhaled microbes and particulates until a certain threshold burden is reached. The threshold is in part determined by the phagocytic capacity of alveolar macrophages. Once the threshold is exceeded, microbes and other particulates are phagocytosed by resident DCs that "snorkel" through tight junctions of the alveolar epithelium to sample the alveolar compartment. Consistent with this concept, studies have shown that depletion of alveolar macrophages with liposome-encapsulated clodronate augments antigen presentation by pulmonary DCs, which in turn augments adaptive immune responses to intranasal delivered antigens.[261,262]

INTERSTITIAL MACROPHAGES

There are three *interstitial macrophage* (IM) subtypes: Two IMs, IM1 (CD206^hiMHCII+) and IM2 (CD206^hiMHCII^lo), display classical macrophage characteristics, whereas the third IM, IM3 (CD206^loMHCII+), although containing macrophage properties, has a higher rate of turnover and expresses proinflammatory mediators, monocytic and DC genes.[42,248–251] Furthermore, all IMs express high levels of standard macrophage markers, such as MerTK, CD64, CD11b, and F4/80, while differing in their expression of CX3CR1, Lyve-1, CCR2, CD11c, and MHC class II.[42,248–251] Interstitial macrophages have been observed to interact with lymphatic vessels and sympathetic nerves in the bronchovascular bundle.[42,263,264] With the advent of single-cell RNA sequencing and identification of interstitial macrophage subtypes, new questions can now be addressed to determine their functional properties and relationship to cells in close proximity (i.e., blood vessels, lymphatic vessels, fibroblasts, nerves, and epithelial cells).

Monocytes

After birth and postnatal bone formation, liver hematopoiesis declines and is replaced by bone marrow hematopoiesis, which then becomes the exclusive source of circulating monocytes. Circulating monocytes have the potential to differentiate into macrophages or DC-like cells.[265–270] In 1989, Passlick and associates reported heterogeneity among human macrophages based on the differential expression of CD14 and CD16.[271] *Classical* CD14^hiCD16− monocytes make up approximately 95% of circulating monocytes in the steady state, and *nonclassical* CD14^loCD16+ monocytes constitute the remaining 5%.[272,273] Similar to human monocytes, mouse monocytes have been classified into *classical* (Ly6C^hi) and *nonclassical* (Ly6C^lo) monocyte subsets.[269,274,275] During steady state, Ly6C^lo monocytes patrol the lung vasculature; they express high levels of the fractalkine receptor CX$_3$CR1, which interacts with fractalkine CX$_3$CR1L, expressed on the luminal face of vascular endothelial cells, and promotes adherence.[274,276] The Ly6C^hi monocytes enter tissue in a CCR2-dependent manner in steady-state and inflammatory conditions. In the steady state, circulating Ly6C^hi monocytes continuously traffic into the lung and lymph nodes without differentiating into resident macrophages, unless there is a macrophage niche to fill.[277] Ly6C^hi monocytes survey the tissue environment and can acquire antigen and traffic to regional lymph nodes for antigen presentation (see Fig. 15.5A).[277,278] During inflammation, monocytes can differentiate into inflammatory and resolving macrophages, which display distinct properties from resident macrophages,[241,244,279,280] or monocyte-derived DCs. In lymphoid tissue, even though lymph node monocytes are highly present, their role in adaptive immunity is less defined than DCs. Last, Ly6C^hi monocytes are a short-lived obligatory precursor intermediate for Ly6C^lo monocytes under steady-state conditions.[223] Additional information about the mechanisms of monocyte, macrophage, and DC migration can be found in other reviews.[278,281,282]

Functions of Recruited Monocytes and Macrophages

In contrast to alveolar macrophages, recruited monocytes and macrophages have important proinflammatory and host-defense activities, including (1) microbial killing and (2) amplification of inflammation. Monocytes and macrophages kill microbes with *reactive oxygen species* (ROS) and reactive nitrogen species. *Superoxide anion* (O_2^-) is mainly produced by the phagocyte NADPH oxidase.[283] Like PMNs, monocytes subsequently convert O_2^- into additional ROS in a myeloperoxidase-dependent fashion[284] but, as they differentiate into macrophages, intracellular myeloperoxidase content declines, and additional ROS (e.g., hydroxyl radical [OH−]) are formed by the Fenton reaction.[285]

The generation of ROS is critical to host defense against commonly encountered and pathogenic bacteria. Patients with chronic granulomatous disease and mice bearing a targeted disruption of the p47^phox component of the NADPH oxidase[286,287] are deficient in their ability to control pulmonary and other infections.[286–289] Thus, whereas ROS play a vital role in the protection of the lung against microbes, inappropriate production in response to nonmicrobial particulates and pollutants, including cigarette smoke,[290] can result in a spectrum of injury to the airway and alveolar epithelium. *Nitric oxide* (NO) produced by *inducible nitric oxide synthase* (iNOS or NOS2) also contributes to macrophage-mediated microbial killing and epithelial injury after condensation with O_2^- to form peroxynitrite.[291,292] Whereas the importance of NO in microbial killing of *L. monocytogenes* and *M. tuberculosis* has been clearly demonstrated in mice,[293] the role of NO in host defense in humans is less clear.

Recruited monocytes that develop into macrophages are also capable of further differentiation. Based on earlier work in which different PAMPs were found to induce distinct patterns of macrophage gene expression,[39,294–296] the concept evolved that different patterns of gene expression could be induced in response to the conditions or stimuli prevailing at the sites to which macrophages have been recruited.[297–299] Much of the initial work describing macrophage programming subtypes was conducted using in vitro studies and macrophage cell lines. The diversity, complexity, and flexibility of macrophage programming in homeostasis and disease is now recognized, and the simple classification of macrophages into "classical" and "alternative" programming is being redefined because there are often overlapping patterns of gene expression in response to multiple stimuli.[300,301] Macrophages have the capacity to respond to a diverse range of environmental stimuli, and it may be more appropriate to think about these adaptive responses as points on a continuum in which the response generated is purely an adaptation to the microenvironment that macrophages encounter.[297,299,302,303]

In summary, macrophages play key roles in the maintenance of lung homeostasis through their abilities to suppress unwanted inflammation and immune responses to harmless, commonly encountered inhaled materials. However, they remain constantly poised to respond to harmful inhaled microbes and other substances. Part of this response involves calling in additional support through

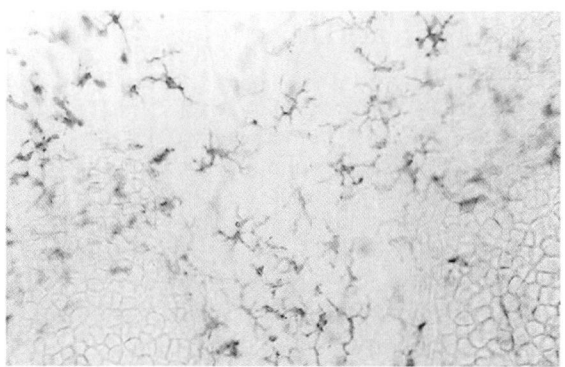

Figure 15.6 Airway dendritic cells exist as an interdigitating network within the epithelium and below the basement membrane. This population requires specific tissue preparation techniques for visualization. This whole-mount section of a mouse trachea was stained for major histocompatibility complex class II. (From Vermaelen K, Pauwels R. Pulmonary dendritic cells. *Am J Respir Crit Care Med.* 2005;172:530–551.)

the recruitment of circulating blood PMNs and monocytes. In turn, recruited monocytes can differentiate into macrophages or DCs, which can then express appropriate responses to microenvironmental cues at the site to which they have been attracted.

Resident and Recruited Dendritic Cells

DCs are the "professional" antigen-presenting cells of most tissues. DCs represent an important group of phagocytic and antigen-presenting cells acting as a bridge between the innate and the adaptive immune systems. In the lung, DCs have been shown to form an extensive intraepithelial and subepithelial network throughout the respiratory tract (Fig. 15.6).

DCs differ from alveolar macrophages in their (1) ontogeny, (2) antigen processing (macrophages rapidly degrade exogenous antigen), (3) expression of the receptor CCR7 mediating lymphatic migration, and (4) presentation of antigen to naive T lymphocytes in the lymph nodes and initiation of their maturation into effector cells. In the mouse, a division of labor by the two migratory DCs has been demonstrated in part on the basis of their transcription factors Batf3[+] versus Irf4[+] or integrins CD103[+] versus CD11b[+], respectively.[24,64,251,304–306] Both DCs migrate to the draining lymph node and present antigen to lymphocytes[307,308] but differ in a number of other important ways.[64,65,309–322] The *Batf3[+] CD103[+] DC* (DC1) selectively takes up apoptotic cells and cross presents cell-associated antigens on class 1 MHC to CD8 T cells in vivo, and mediates their subsequent differentiation to cytotoxic CD8[+] T cells, processes important for combating intracellular pathogens and cancer.[64,306,310,323] In fact, most studies have suggested that DC1s are the dominant cross-presenting DCs in the lung. On the other hand, the *Irf4[+] CD11b[+] DC* (DC2) cannot ingest apoptotic cells (i.e., is less likely involved in immune responses to cell-associated antigens), and is inefficient at cross-presentation to CD8 T cells but is highly efficient in presenting to CD4 T cells.[64,313]

Studies of human lung DC subsets are limited by difficulties in the availability of tissue samples, as is the case for interstitial macrophages. Human lung DCs are distinguished from alveolar macrophages by their expression of CD1c and CD1a.[324,325] Human lung DCs can be distinguished from other myeloid and lymphoid cells by the elimination of T cell, B cell, natural killer–cell, monocyte/macrophage, and granulocyte lineage markers. MHC class II[+] DCs are found in normal human airway epithelium, lung parenchyma, and visceral pleura,[326] and a langerin[+] DC subset is present in bronchioles.[327] Large numbers of DCs are present in alveolar septa.[328,329] Many subsets of DC have been identified in the lung.[330–333] As multiple unique DC subsets are identified and found to be associated with specific lung tissue structures, further studies can be conducted to understand the functional division of labor of DCs and how they contribute to the maintenance of lung homoeostasis and response to a harmful challenge.

SYSTEM INTEGRATION

The innate and adaptive immune systems have evolved to protect the lungs from harm by environmentally acquired microbes and other inhaled substances, as well as from host-derived harmful stressors, such as unwanted inflammation and inappropriate activation of adaptive immunity. Several core concepts emerge from considering innate immune mechanisms in the lungs. The first is that innate immune protection in the lungs is not a consequence of individualized responses of individual cells but represents coordinated responses and collective cooperation between many resident and recruited lung cell types. These coordinated events result in homeostasis of the airways and gas-exchange units, tolerance to harmless inhaled substances and self-antigens, and vigilance to respond to harmful microbes and substances. In addition, innate immune mechanisms assist in the rapid resolution of injury and restoration of lung function.

A second core concept is that from the nose to the alveolus, the respiratory epithelium, interdigitating DCs, and resident and recruited macrophages have evolved exquisite, diverse, and overlapping mechanisms to distinguish between the harmful and harmless. In its simplest form, this distinction is achieved by sensing the presence of microbial PAMPs. In the absence of PAMPs the epithelium remains largely ignorant of inhaled particulates, whereas "snorkeling" DCs continuously sample the airways and alveoli for particles, antigens, and apoptotic cells to phagocytose and to present antigen to lymph node resident naive CD4[+] and CD8[+] T cells, thereby maintaining tolerance to harmless commonly encountered antigens and self-antigens. Similarly, resident macrophages phagocytose and dispose of particulates that reach the alveoli, while tonically maintaining an anti-inflammatory and immunosuppressive environment through the production of anti-inflammatory cytokines, especially TGF-β and IL-10, and eicosanoids, such as prostaglandin E_2.

A third core concept is that integration of innate functions is dependent on cell-cell communication. In some settings, communication is fostered by proximity: DCs exist as a network within the airway epithelium and contact each other through tight junctions, whereas alveolar macrophages use integrins to communicate with alveolar epithelial cells. In other settings, cell-cell communication is mediated through the secretion of a vast array of cytokines and lipid mediators, which can act in autocrine or paracrine fashions. Thus, different cell lineages can communicate with each other and among themselves. Communication between different cell types also plays an important role in the coordination of innate immunity and in the activation of adaptive immunity. For example, depletion of alveolar macrophages reduces tolerance to inhaled antigens and induces alveolitis and lung injury, emphasizing the importance of alveolar macrophages for suppressing inflammation. Integration of innate immunity in the lung is also associated with "coordinated burden sharing." Airway goblet cells and submucosal glands produce mucus, whereas ciliated epithelial cells propel mucus and entrapped particulates toward the pharynx. Similar coordinated burden sharing is exhibited by airway epithelial cells, which are poorly phagocytic but are highly capable of sensing PAMPs and calling in PMNs and monocytes, which in turn are highly phagocytic, microbicidal, and able to eliminate an array of microbes.

A final core concept is that the clinical symptoms and consequences of innate immunity in the lungs depend on where in the respiratory system innate immunity is triggered—nasopharynx, airways, or alveoli. For example, streptococci that deposit on the posterior pharynx and stimulate innate immunity trigger acute tonsillitis, and rhinoviruses trigger initial symptoms in the nasopharynx. In contrast, adenoviruses, influenza viruses, and some bacteria, such as *Haemophilus* and *Moraxella* species, attach to cellular receptors in the ciliated airway epithelium and typically cause severe acute airway inflammation with cough, bronchospasm, and airway mucus production, leading to exacerbations of asthma or COPD in susceptible individuals. Yet other pyogenic bacteria, such as staphylococci, pneumococci, *E. coli*, *Klebsiella pneumoniae*, and others, reach distal airways and alveolar spaces and cause localized or severe lobar pneumonia. Viruses such as severe acute respiratory syndrome CoV-1 and -2 attach to alveolar epithelial and capillary endothelial cells via the angiotensin-converting enzyme-2 receptor, triggering an initial wave of innate immunity that leads to the acute respiratory distress syndrome with few if any upper respiratory symptoms (see Chapter 46a).

Taken together, innate immunity in the lungs involves a number of integrated systems that have evolved to provide the lungs with maximum protection against harmful microbes, while minimizing harmful responses against harmless inhaled substances. The net result is an exquisite system for protecting the delicate and critically important gas-exchanging parenchyma of the lungs from harm.

Key Points

- A primitive host defense system is broadly based on the recognition of repetitive structures on microbes called *pathogen-associated molecular patterns* (PAMPs) by pattern recognition receptors expressed on lung cells.

- Airway epithelium of the trachea and large airways is protected by (1) airway surface liquid, which contains antibacterial proteins; (2) mucus, which traps large inhaled particulates and transports them to the pharynx by mucociliary transport; and (3) immune cells, which produce chemokines, cytokines, and lipid mediators in response to PAMPs.
- Alveolar epithelium is protected by surfactant proteins A and D, which serve the dual purpose of (1) opsonizing microbes and (2) suppressing unwanted inflammation and adaptive immune responses to commonly encountered antigens.
- Polymorphonuclear leukocytes (i.e., neutrophils) are recruited to the airways and alveoli when airway and alveolar epithelial cells detect PAMPs. Neutrophils phagocytose and kill microbes by combined oxidative and nonoxidative mechanisms.
- Macrophages are resident phagocytic cells of the alveolar lumen involved in the removal of a wide range of microbial and nonmicrobial inhaled particulates. Macrophages also suppress unwanted alveolar inflammation and adaptive immunity in the steady state but can be activated by PAMPs to amplify inflammation.
- Dendritic cells are the primary antigen-sensing and -presenting cells of the innate immune system. In the absence of PAMPs, immature dendritic cells traffic to regional lymph nodes and promote tolerance to inhaled antigens. In the presence of PAMPs, dendritic cells mature, express co-stimulatory molecules, and promote T cell development into T helper cells type 1, 2 and 17, or T regulatory effector cells.
- The cell lineages of innate lung immunity collaborate to promote optimal responses to perceived danger signals (primarily PAMPs) while maintaining tolerance to inhaled antigens in the steady state.
- The clinical consequences of innate immune reactions in the lungs depend on where and how microbial pathogens deposit in the respiratory system.

Key Readings

Barlow JL, McKenzie ANJ. Innate lymphoid cells of the lung. *Annu Rev Physiol*. 2019;81:429–452.
Fitzgerald KA, Kagan JC. Toll-like receptors and the control of immunity. *Cell*. 2020;180(6):1044–1066.
Geissmann F, Manz MG, Jung S, et al. Development of monocytes, macrophages, and dendritic cells. *Science*. 2010;327(5966):656–661.
Hoffmann M, Kleine-Weber H, Schroeder S, Muller MA, Drosten C, Pohlmann S. SARS-CoV-2 cell entry depends on ACE2 and TMPRSS2 and is blocked by a clinically proven protease inhibitor. *Cell*. 2020;181:1–10.
Mould KJ, Jackson ND, Henson PM, Seibold M, Janssen WJ. Single cell RNA sequencing identifies unique inflammatory airspace macrophage subsets. *JCI Insight*. 2019;4(5):e126556.
Papayannopoulos V. Neutrophil extracellular traps in immunity and disease. *Nat Rev Immunol*. 2018;18(2):134–147.
Rehwinkel J, Gack MU. RIG-I-like receptors: their regulation and roles in RNA sensing. *Nat Rev Immunol*. 2020;20(9):537–551.
Wright JR. Immunoregulatory functions of surfactant proteins. *Nat Rev Immunol*. 2005;5(1):58–68.

Complete reference list available at ExpertConsult.com.

16 ADAPTIVE IMMUNITY

ANDREW P. FONTENOT, MD • SHAIKH M. ATIF, PHD •
R. LEE REINHARDT, PHD

INTRODUCTION

The human immune system consists of many cell types and organs that have evolved to destroy or control potentially harmful foreign substances. The immune response is essential for survival because it constitutes the principal means of defense against infection by pathogenic microorganisms, including those that enter and reside in the respiratory tract. The immune response is also critically involved in pathologic processes of the lung and upper respiratory tract. This chapter provides an understanding of the adaptive (or acquired) immune response, which depends on the specific recognition of antigens by T and B lymphocytes. Immune recognition is highly specific for a particular pathogen, and yet an individual's immune cells can collectively respond to an almost unlimited number of foreign antigens. The molecular mechanisms underlying this specificity and diversity are unique to the immune system. The adaptive immune response also changes after successive encounters with the same pathogen. For example, memory of an antigen allows the immune system to respond faster and in greater magnitude compared with the initial encounter. This chapter also describes how primary and secondary immune responses are regulated by complex cellular interactions and the release of particular types of soluble mediators. Antigen-specific immune responses are also regulated and augmented by nonspecific inflammatory cells of the immune system, such as dendritic cells, macrophages, monocytes, neutrophils, eosinophils, innate lymphoid cells, and mast cells. Defects in the development of adaptive immunity are discussed in Chapter 124. Innate immunity is covered in Chapter 15.

COMPONENTS OF THE IMMUNE SYSTEM: OVERVIEW

Cells of the immune system arise from pluripotent hematopoietic stem cells through two main lines of differentiation that give rise to the lymphoid lineage and the myeloid lineage.[1] Specificity within the immune system is primarily provided by lymphocytes. The two major categories of lymphocytes are T cells,[2] which are derived from bone marrow stem cells and primarily develop in the thymus, and B cells, which develop in the bone marrow in adult humans.

Lymphocytes and other cells of the immune system express a large number of different molecules on their surfaces. Some of these can be used as markers to separate cells with different functions or to distinguish cells at particular stages of differentiation. Monoclonal antibodies to many different cell surface markers have been produced, and a systematic nomenclature has been developed. The CD (cluster of differentiation, or cluster determinant) system provides a basis by which monoclonal antibodies that bind to the same surface molecule are grouped together, and the CD number is used to indicate the specific molecule recognized. Tables 16.1 to 16.3 provide a partial list of surface antigens, particularly those mentioned in this chapter. The markers are grouped based on the cell type expressing them. It may be necessary to refer to this list of molecules throughout this chapter.

T cells are distinguished by the presence of the *T cell receptor* (TCR).[3–5] Most T cells express a receptor composed of an α and a β chain, whereas a much smaller subset expresses a structurally similar receptor composed of a γ and a δ chain. Both receptors are associated with a complex of polypeptides, the CD3 complex, which provides a transmembrane signaling function and allows TCR engagement to be coupled to cellular activation. T cells expressing $\alpha\beta$ TCRs can be divided into CD4+ and CD8+ T cell subsets. CD4+ T cells primarily recognize antigens presented by *major histocompatibility complex* (MHC) class II molecules expressed on antigen-presenting cells. CD8+ T cells primarily recognize antigens presented by MHC class I molecules expressed by all nucleated cells.

Functionally, T cells can be divided into several major subsets. For example, T helper cells may interact with B cells and help them to survive and divide, make antibody, and become

Table 16.1 Selected Cell Surface Markers of Human T Cells

Cell Surface Markers	Identity/Function
TCR	Interacts with peptide/MHC complex on antigen-presenting cells
CD2	Binds to LFA-3; involved in co-stimulation and adhesion
CD3	T cell signaling complex
CD4	T cell subset with helper function; interacts with MHC class II molecule
CD8	T cell subset with cytotoxic function; interacts with MHC class I molecule
CD25	α chain of IL-2 receptor; expressed on activated T cells and on a subset of regulatory CD4+ T cells
CD28	Binds B7-1 (CD80) and B7-2 (CD86); co-stimulatory molecule involved in T cell activation
CD45	Phosphatase involved in cellular activation and differentiation; different isoforms (CD45RA, CD45RO) mark naive versus previously activated T cells and stages of activation
CD62L	L-selectin; involved in lymphocyte adhesion; levels mark naive versus memory cells
CD69	Activation marker
CD95 (FAS)	FAS; receptor involved in apoptosis
CD95L (FAS ligand)	Ligand for FAS; involved in T cell–mediated killing
CD152 (CTLA4)	Binds to B7-1 (CD80) and B7-2 (CD86); involved in down-regulation of TCR signaling
CD154 (CD40 ligand)	Ligand for CD40; important for T cell activation and T cell–dependent B cell activation
CD134 (OX40), CD137 (4-1BB), ICOS, PD1	Additional co-stimulatory molecules in the TNF or CD28 family; involved in T cell activation and regulation

CTLA4, cytotoxic T lymphocyte antigen-4; ICOS, inducible co-stimulator; IL-2, interleukin-2; LFA-3, lymphocyte function–associated antigen-3; MHC, major histocompatibility complex; PD1, programmed cell death-1; TCR, T cell receptor; TNF, tumor necrosis factor.

Table 16.2 Selected Cell Surface Markers of Human B Cells

Cell Surface Markers	Identity/Function
BCR	Immunoglobulin molecules; recognizes antigen
CD5	Binds to CD72; regulation of cell proliferation/activation; identifies B1a cell subset
CD19	B cell coreceptor subunit; involved in co-stimulation
CD20	B cell marker
CD21	Complement receptor type II; B cell coreceptor subunit; marks certain B cell subsets; EBV receptor
CD22	Adhesion molecule; involved in B cell activation
CD23	Identifies B cell subset; low-affinity receptor for IgE
CD40	Binds CD40L; involved in T cell–dependent B cell activation
CD79a (Ig-α)	Involved in B cell activation; signaling through BCR
CD79b (Ig-β)	Involved in B cell activation; signaling through BCR
CD80 (B7-1)	Binds CD28 and CD152 (CTLA4) on T cells
CD86 (B7-2)	Binds CD28 and CD152 (CTLA4) on T cells

BCR, B cell receptor; CD40L, CD40 ligand; CTLA4, cytotoxic T lymphocyte antigen-4; EBV, Epstein-Barr virus; Ig, immunoglobulin.

a large number of other surface markers that are critically involved in their function and interaction with T cells. For example, most B cells express MHC class II molecules that allow them to present antigen to T helper cells. Other B cell surface molecules are listed in Table 16.2.

A third population of lymphocytes recently classified as *innate lymphoid cells* (ILCs) seed the peripheral tissues early in life and modulate tissue-specific immunity and barrier homeostasis.[7] ILCs are characterized by expression of the interleukin-7 receptor but are devoid of other immune cell lineage markers.[8] They are grouped into three distinct subsets (ILC1, ILC2, and ILC3) and resemble different T helper cell subsets based on their differential expression of key transcription factors and cytokines.[9,10] However, unlike T helper cells, ILCs do not express a classical antigen receptor like TCR or Ig, and, as a result, ILCs do not undergo antigen-specific expansion upon activation. Instead, these innate lymphocytes sense alterations in the local tissue microenvironment caused by tissue damage. Because ILCs are tissue resident, they can rapidly respond to these tissue cues (often in the form of cytokines or alarmins) by proliferating as well as by secreting effector cytokines in much the same way that memory T cells quickly respond to reinfection.[11] In addition to their role as early tissue sentinels, ILCs help to educate adaptive immune responses via regulation of dendritic cells and B cells as well as to modulate CD4+ T cells through expression of MHC class II molecules.[12–16] In sum, ILCs serve three key functions: (1) modulate tissue homeostasis, (2) serve as an early line of innate defense against infection and promote tissue repair after sensing tissue damage, and (3) instruct the adaptive immune response after barrier insult.

The myeloid lineage consists primarily of monocytes, macrophages, dendritic cells, and neutrophils, which

memory B cells. T helper cells also may interact with cytotoxic T cells or with phagocytic cells and help them destroy intracellular pathogens. Different subsets of T helper cells can be distinguished by the presence of specific transcription factors and the pattern of cytokines that they secrete during an immune response. T helper cells are generally encompassed within the CD4+ T cell subset. Another subset of T cells is responsible for destruction of cells that have become infected by virus or other intracellular pathogens. These cells are called *cytotoxic T cells* and usually express the CD8 phenotypic marker. Although not clearly distinguished by phenotypic markers, separate subsets of T cells, within both the CD4 and CD8 subsets, have been termed *T regulatory (or suppressor) cells* because they down-regulate immune responses.

B cells are identified by the expression of surface *immunoglobulin* (Ig) or antibody molecules, which represent their specific *B cell receptor* (BCR) for antigen. Analogous to the CD3 complex on T cells, BCRs are also linked to accessory molecules, Ig-α (CD79a) and Ig-β (CD79b), which are required for cellular activation after antigen interaction.[6] After differentiation, B cells can develop the ability to produce high levels of antibody (soluble Ig). B cells also express

Table 16.3   Other Cell Surface Markers of General Interest

Cell Surface Markers	Distribution	Identity/Function
CD1	Thymocytes, subset of lymphocytes, antigen-presenting cells	MHC class I–like molecule; involved in presentation of nonpeptide antigens
CD11a	Leukocytes	α chain of LFA-1; associates with CD18; interacts with ICAM1; involved in adhesion and migration
CD11b	NK cells, monocytes, granulocytes	α chain of CR3; adhesion molecule
CD11c	Monocytes, granulocytes	α chain of CR4; adhesion molecule; identifies dendritic cells
CD14	Granulocytes, monocytes	Receptor for LPS/LPB complex; myeloid differentiation antigen; cell activation
CD16	NK cells, monocytes	Receptor for Fc domain of IgG, type 3 (FCGR3); low-affinity receptor for IgG; involved in ADCC
CD18	Leukocytes	β chain of $β_2$ integrin molecules, including LFA-1, CR3, and CR4
CD29	Leukocytes	β chain of $β_1$ integrin molecules, including VLA1-VLA6
CD32	B cells, monocytes, granulocytes	Receptor for Fc domain of IgG, type 2 (FCGR2)
CD35	B cells, subset of NK cells, monocytes, granulocytes	CR1
CD45	Leukocytes	Leukocyte common antigen; phosphatase; involved in cell signaling
CD46	Broad distribution	Membrane cofactor protein; regulates complement activation
CD54 (ICAM1)	Broad distribution	Binds LFA-1; adhesion molecule
CD56	NK cells	Neural cell adhesion molecule
CD58 (LFA-3)	Broad distribution	Binds CD2; adhesion molecule; involved in cell signaling

ADCC, antibody-dependent cellular cytotoxicity; CR, complement receptor; ICAM1, intercellular adhesion molecule-1; IgG, immunoglobulin G; LFA, lymphocyte function–associated antigen; LPB, LPB binding protein; LPS, lipopolysaccharide; MHC, major histocompatibility complex; NK, natural killer; VLA, vascular leukocyte adhesion molecule.

provide nonspecific inflammatory mediators and phagocytic function. These cells are critically involved in the nonspecific component of the inflammatory response (see Chapter 15). In addition, macrophages and dendritic cells are specialized to present antigens to T cells, thus contributing to specific immune responses.

The cells involved in the immune response are organized into tissues and organs. Primary lymphoid organs are the major sites of lymphopoiesis, in which stem cells and their committed precursor cells differentiate into lymphocytes and acquire specific functions. In humans, T lymphocytes mainly develop in the thymus, and B lymphocytes develop in the fetal liver and adult bone marrow. In the thymus, T cell differentiation also includes acquiring the ability to recognize foreign antigens in the context of self-MHC molecules and the elimination of self-reactive cells (self-tolerance). B cell acquisition of self-tolerance during development appears to take place in the bone marrow.

Differentiated lymphocytes migrate to secondary lymphoid organs, which include lymph nodes, spleen, and mucosa-associated lymphoid tissues, such as the tonsils, lymph nodes of the respiratory tract, and Peyer patches of the gut. These tissues provide an environment for lymphocytes to interact with each other, with antigen-presenting cells and other accessory cells, and with foreign antigens. The immune response is generated mostly within these secondary lymphoid organs, and lymphocytes migrate through the blood and lymph from one lymphoid organ to another and to nonlymphoid tissues. For example, foreign antigen exposure in the lung usually involves the movement of antigen to surrounding lymph nodes, where the specific immune response by T and B cells takes place. Generation

of a cell-mediated immune response or antibody response allows antigen-specific effector T cells or specific antibodies, respectively, to circulate to lung tissue for a direct assault on foreign antigens.

Under normal conditions, there is a continuous active flow of lymphocyte traffic through the lymph nodes. About 1–2% of the lymphocyte pool recirculates each hour, allowing a large number of antigen-specific lymphocytes to come into contact with their appropriate antigen. Recirculating lymphocytes leave the blood and enter the lymph node through specialized postcapillary venules, known as *high endothelial venules* (HEVs). Specific interacting receptors on lymphocytes and HEV cells facilitate this homing process. Lymphocytes return to the circulation by way of afferent lymphatics that pass via the thoracic duct into the left subclavian vein. Lymphocytes also enter mucosa-associated lymphoid tissues, such as the tonsils and Peyer patches, via HEVs. The recirculation and trafficking of memory and effector T and B cells is tightly regulated, determined by unique combinations of adhesion molecules and chemokines.[17] For example, certain lymphocytes may preferentially migrate across HEVs into intestinal lymphoid tissues (either Peyer patches or mesenteric lymph nodes) or into respiratory tract tissues or may specifically home to the peripheral lymph nodes or the spleen.

Separate combinations of cell-surface adhesion molecules and chemokines allow activated lymphocytes and other leukocytes to migrate into nonlymphoid tissues, especially during inflammation and in response to the release of inflammatory cytokines.[17] The difference in trafficking patterns for nonactivated (resting) versus activated lymphocytes is striking and emphasizes the importance of particular adhesion molecules in the control of lymphocyte migration.

IMMUNE RECOGNITION

B CELLS AND ANTIBODIES

Structure of Immunoglobulin and the B Cell Receptor for Antigen

Ig molecules, or antibodies, are glycoproteins that act as BCRs. These molecules can also be secreted in large quantities by activated B cells and plasma cells. Figure 16.1 shows the basic structure of an Ig molecule. Each Ig molecule is bifunctional, consisting of an antigen binding region (Fab) and a constant region (Fc) that mediates various effector functions, such as binding to host tissues and activating the first component of the complement system.

The basic structure of Ig molecules involves two identical light polypeptide chains and two identical heavy polypeptide chains linked together by disulfide bonds (see Fig. 16.1A). The isotype (class or subclass) of an Ig molecule is determined by its heavy chain type. There are five Ig classes—IgG, IgM, IgA, IgD, and IgE—corresponding to the γ, μ, α, δ, and ε heavy chain types. In humans, there are four IgG subclasses, IgG1 to IgG4. There are major differences in the structure and main functions of these different Ig classes and subtypes.

In Figure 16.1B, the IgG molecule is shown as an example of basic antibody structure. Each chain is composed of a series of globular regions or domains, and each domain encompasses about 60 to 70 amino acids connected via an internal disulfide bond. The site of antigen binding is the amino (NH_2)-terminal domain for both the *heavy* (H) and *light* (L) chains. This domain is characterized by remarkable sequence variability and is referred to as the variable region of the heavy and light chains (V_H and V_L region, respectively). The combination of V_H and V_L forms the antigen-binding site, and there are two such sites per IgG molecule (see Fig. 16.1B). The remainder of each polypeptide has a relatively constant structure. The constant domain of the light chain is termed the C_L region, whereas the heavy chain has three constant domains: C_H1, C_H2, and C_H3. The hinge region, located between the C_H1 and C_H2 domains, provides flexibility and independence to the two antigen-binding sites. In both μ and ε heavy chains, there is an additional constant domain between C_H1 and C_H2, resulting in a total of four constant domains.

The greatest variability in antibody molecules takes place in the V_H and V_L domains, and these domains are responsible for the specificity in antigen binding.[18] Within the variable domains (see Fig. 16.1C), certain short segments show exceptional variability and are called *hypervariable* regions. These regions are also referred to as *complementarity-determining regions* (CDRs) because they are directly involved in the binding to antigen. In both the V_H and V_L regions, there are three CDRs (CDR1 to CDR3) with intervening segments referred to as framework regions (see Fig. 16.1C). CDR3 (a component of the polypeptide V region) is formed by parts of the V (*variable*), D (*diversity*), and J (*joining*) gene segments. Variation within the V_H and V_L regions distinguishes one antibody molecule from another and is referred to as idiotype or idiotypic variation. Additional information on heavy chain rearrangement is shown in eFig. 16.1.

Formation of the B Cell Receptor Repertoire

The BCR repertoire and the Ig molecules are characterized by enormous diversity. The principal genetic mechanisms that are used to generate this diversity include (1) genetic

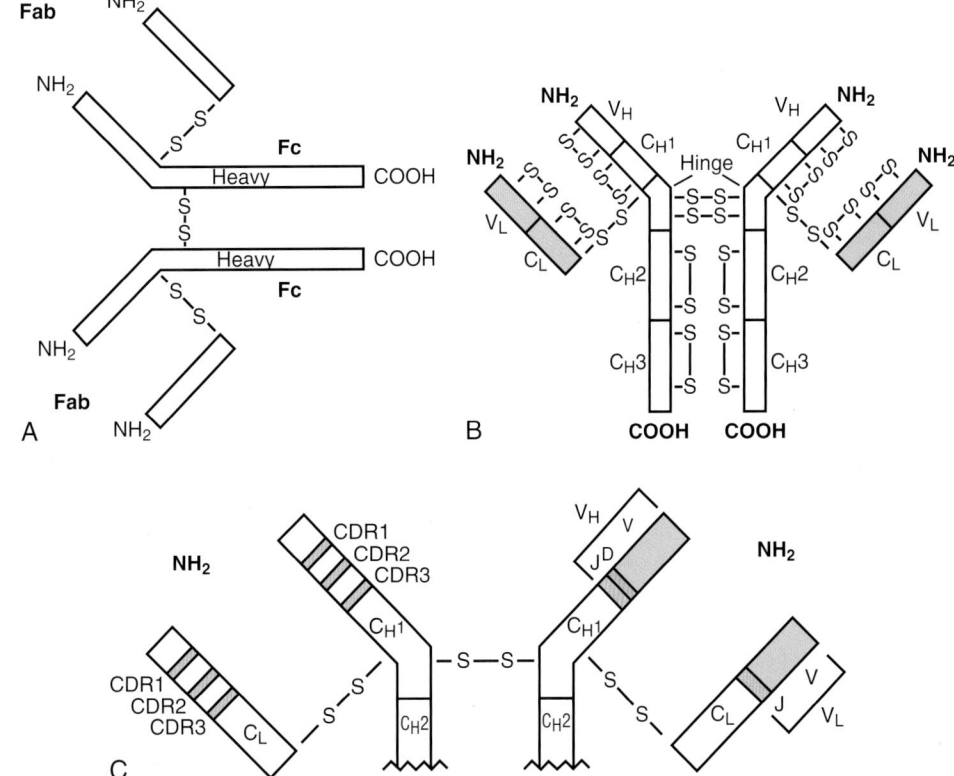

Figure 16.1 The structure of *immunoglobulin* (Ig) molecules. (A) Basic Ig structure with two heavy chains and two light chains linked together by disulfide bonds. The Fab region is involved in antigen binding, whereas the Fc region mediates various effector functions. (B) Increasing detail of IgG molecule showing domains of both heavy and light chains. Each domain has an internal disulfide bond. The sites of antigen binding involve the NH_2-terminal domains of both the heavy and the light chains and are referred to as the variable regions (V_H and V_L, respectively). The rest of each chain has a relatively constant structure (C_H and C_L domains). (C) Close-up of the antigen-binding variable regions. On the left, the complementarity-determining regions (CDRs) are shaded because they are the most variable components (i.e., hypervariable regions) and are involved in actual antigen binding. The CDRs are separated by intervening segments referred to as framework regions. On the right, the Ig polypeptide regions are correlated with the Ig gene segment (exons) that encode the variable region. Note that CDR3 corresponds to parts of the V/D/J junctional region of the rearranged heavy chain gene and the V/J junctional region of the rearranged light chain gene. D, diversity region; J, joining region; V, variable region.

recombination of gene segments to form a functional Ig gene, (2) combinatorial diversity of heavy and light chain matching, and (3) somatic hypermutation of rearranged genes.[19] Another major force in shaping the antibody repertoire has been termed *receptor editing*, which allows receptors with self-reactive potential to be modified by additional recombination events during B cell differentiation.[20,21]

Figure 16.2A illustrates the principle of genetic recombination for an Ig gene.[18] In this case, one of several V region gene segments (normally separated upstream from the *constant* [C] region gene segments on the same chromosome) can be linked to a single C region gene segment by genetic recombination. The combining of gene segments, rather than the existence of a single gene coding for every individual antibody molecule, considerably reduces the amount of genetic information required to encode many different antibody molecules. In Figure 16.2B the different gene segments that encode a κ light polypeptide chain are shown. Note that, in this case, a V region rearranges proximal to a J segment, which is linked to the C region segment. Rearrangement of κ or γ light chain genes involves V, J, and C region gene segments (see Fig. 16.2A; see also Fig. 16.1C). In the formation of a functional heavy chain gene, a successful rearrangement of gene segments includes one

V, one D, and one J region segment linked to a C region segment (compare Figs. 16.1C and 16.2B).

During genetic recombination, additional variability is generated by a process known as junctional diversification. When two gene segments are brought together during rearrangement, linking is not precise. Instead, some nucleotides are randomly inserted or deleted at the junctional site. This introduces new codons, and therefore new amino acids, into the junctional sequence. If an incorrect number of junctional nucleotides are added or deleted, functional molecules will not be encoded because the rest of the gene will be "out of frame" or a "stop" sequence will be introduced. Junctional diversification takes place in the hypervariable CDR3 region of the molecule (see Fig. 16.1C).

In general, a single B cell usually expresses an Ig molecule of only one antigen specificity, composed of one heavy chain molecule and one light chain molecule. Even though there are two chromosomal copies of the heavy chain genes in each cell, only one is usually functionally expressed. This phenomenon of using genes on only one parental chromosome is known as allelic exclusion. Once there has been a functional rearrangement of heavy chain genes on one parental chromosome, rearrangement of heavy chain genes on the other chromosome is mostly prevented. If the first rearrangement is not successful, the second one can take place. All of the genetic events described earlier happen before the B cell encounters antigen. The B cell (or antibody) response further diversifies after interaction with antigen by a process known as *somatic hypermutation*, primarily involving point mutations in the hypervariable regions of the V genes.[22] Somatic hypermutation can be viewed as fine tuning of the antibody response, taking place after the primary response to a stimulus and during the development of memory B cells. It is, therefore, mostly observed during a secondary immune response. Somatic hypermutation allows for the production of antibodies with higher affinity for antigen, that is, the ability to bind more strongly to an antigen. Although the mutations are random, B cells with high affinity are selectively expanded (referred to as affinity maturation) because the stronger binding allows preferential stimulation by the target antigen. Somatic hypermutation is closely tied to isotype switching, and T cell help is required. Somatic hypermutation usually takes place at the site of T cell–B cell interaction in the germinal centers of lymph node or spleen.

Isotype Switching and Function of the Different Immunoglobulin Classes

One B cell usually makes antibody of a single specificity that is fixed by the nature of $V_L J_L$ and $V_H D_H J_H$ rearrangements. During the lifetime of this cell, however, it can switch from making an IgM molecule to producing a different class of antibody, such as IgG or IgA, while retaining the same antigenic specificity. This phenomenon is known as class switching or *isotype switching*.[19]

Figure 16.3 shows the predominant mechanism by which a B cell switches from production of surface IgM to secretion of an IgG, IgA, or IgE molecule. The mechanism involves further DNA rearrangement (a process unique to Ig heavy chain genes), linking rearranged VDJ gene segments with a different heavy chain C region gene segment downstream. The *switch* (S) region is a stretch of repeating sequences 5′ to

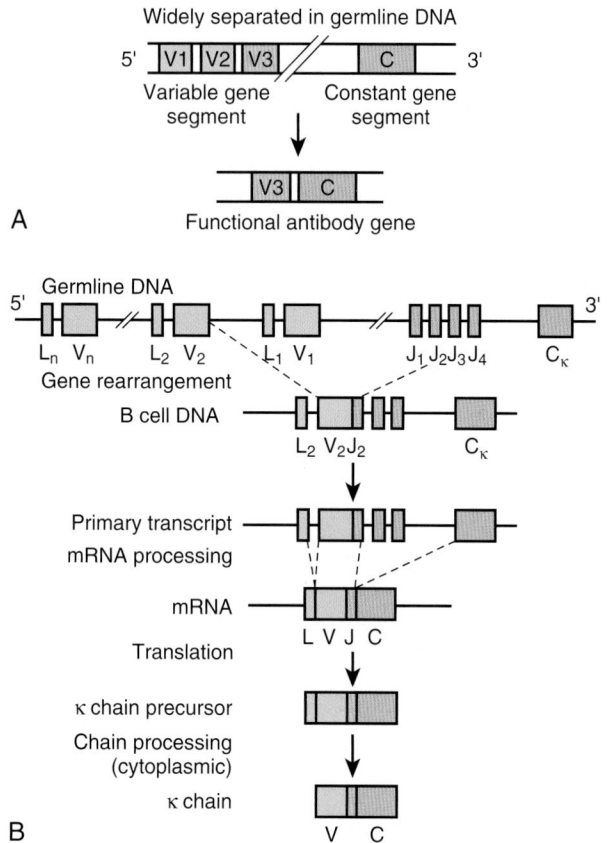

Figure 16.2 Principles of genetic recombination. (A) In the germline DNA, the V region segments are located upstream from the D, J, and C segments on the same chromosome. Recombination, which takes place only in lymphocytes, brings the V gene segments in proximity to the downstream segments. (B) In the B cell, rearrangement of gene segments separated in the germline DNA allows for the formation of a functional immunoglobulin light chain gene (compare with Fig. 16.1C) in this case, a κ light chain. mRNA, messenger RNA.

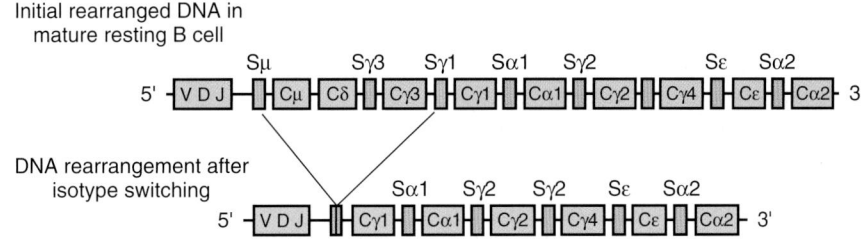

Figure 16.3 Genetic mechanisms involved in *immunoglobulin* (Ig) isotype switching. *Top,* The initial rearrangement of Ig heavy chain gene segments has already taken place in the B cell to put the V region proximal to the D, J, and Cμ segments. This latter genetic region contains other constant region gene segments farther downstream, including Cδ, various Cγ and Cα gene segments, and Cε. In the process of T cell–dependent B cell activation in the germinal centers, the B cell is signaled to undergo isotype switching to allow high-rate secretion of an IgG1 antibody. *Bottom,* This is accomplished by additional DNA rearrangements that put the VDJ unit adjacent to the Cγ1 segment downstream. The intervening DNA is deleted. S, switch region.

Table 16.4 Properties and Functional Characteristics of Immunoglobulin Classes and Subclasses*

Effector Function	IgM	IgD	IgG1	IgG2	IgG3	IgG4	IgA	IgE
Mean serum levels (mg/mL)	1.5	0.04	9	3	1	0.5	2.1	0.00003
Opsonization	—	—	+++	—	++	+	+	—
Complement fixation	+++	—	++	+	+++	—	—	—
Binding of Fc receptor on phagocytic cells	—	—	++		++	+	—	—
Induction of mast cell degranulation	—	—	—	—	—	—	—	+++

*Activity levels of immunoglobulin classes and subclasses: +++ high; ++ moderate; + low; =/— minimal; — none.
Ig, immunoglobulin.

the C region that allows a VDJ unit (previously linked to the Cμ region gene segment) to rearrange to another C region downstream. In the process the intervening DNA is deleted. The B cell, therefore, cannot return to IgM production. Class switching generally follows stimulation of the B cell by antigen and frequently is dependent on factors released by T helper cells and pathogen-associated molecular patterns present in surrounding microenvironment.

Each class of secreted Ig has a different set of functions (Table 16.4).[23] IgG is the major antibody of secondary immune responses and is most important for obtaining effective immunization to various toxins, toxoids, and certain extracellular pathogens. IgG accounts for 70–75% of the total Ig pool and is the major Ig class in the blood. It also crosses the placenta and confers immunity to newborns and neonates for the first few months of life. The interaction of IgG antibodies with antigen can have diverse consequences, including precipitation, agglutination, neutralization, complement activation, and various cellular effector functions via IgG receptors.[23–26] There are four IgG subclasses, with IgG1 and IgG3 being most effective at fixing complement and activating complement-mediated effector functions.

IgM is the predominant early-secreted antibody, frequently seen in primary immune responses. IgM is important for effective responses to antigenically complex infectious organisms, especially those with polysaccharide-containing cell walls. IgM antibodies may also be extremely effective at precipitation, agglutination, and complement activation after binding to antigen. Secreted IgM is usually found as a pentamer of the basic (four-domain) Ig unit. Polymerization is facilitated by the binding of the heavy chain tailpieces to a J peptide.

IgA plays a major role in mucosal immunity and is the predominant Ig in saliva and tracheobronchial secretions. Secretory IgA exists mainly in dimeric form and contains a secretory component, which is synthesized by epithelial cells and facilitates transport into secretions as well as protection from proteolysis. Secretory IgA is involved in the prevention of microbial adherence to mucosal cells and in the agglutination of microorganisms. IgA provides the first line of defense against a variety of pathogens.

IgE is scarce in serum. Its major importance relates to its ability to bind to FcεR1 receptors on mast cells and basophils, and cross-linking of IgE bound to these cells results in cellular activation, degranulation, and release of mediators involved in allergic responses, such as histamine and various leukotrienes.[27] IgE plays a role in immunity to parasites but, in developed countries, it is more commonly associated with allergic responses and allergic diseases, such as hay fever and asthma (see Chapters 60, 61, and 62).[28] IgE interaction with FcεR1 also promotes anti-tumor immunity by enhancing antigen cross presentation by DCs.[29]

B Cell Development

B cells are produced in the specialized microenvironments of the fetal liver and the adult bone marrow.[30] After migration from the bone marrow, the life span of mature naive B cells is limited unless there is contact with antigen. B cells interact with foreign antigen in the peripheral lymphoid tissues, particularly in germinal centers of lymph nodes and spleen.[31] The interaction with antigen, in the setting of T cell help, results in the generation of memory B cells and cells that secrete large amounts of Ig. This frequently involves class switching and somatic hypermutation, which allows a secondary antibody response to generate antibodies of a different isotype with higher affinity for the stimulating antigen. An additional view of B cell development is shown in eFig. 16.2.

The formation of the B cell repertoire in the bone marrow is mostly random, and B cells with self-reactivity are generated. Negative selection of cells capable of strongly binding to self-antigens is an important part of B cell development. This process of B cell self-tolerance involves both deletion (elimination) and functional inactivation (anergy) of self-reactive cells.[32] In addition, as mentioned, B cells with specificity for self-antigens can modify their receptors through receptor editing.[20,21] These self-reactive B cells undergo a reversible arrest of development and reinitiate light chain gene rearrangements to alter their BCR. If a B cell fails to edit its BCR, it is destined for cell death (apoptosis). Immature B cells in the bone marrow are capable of receptor editing, whereas mature B cells in the peripheral lymphoid tissues normally lose this ability to initiate a new round of Ig gene rearrangements.

Immunoglobulin Interactions with Antigen

An antigen is a molecule or molecular complex recognized by B cells or T cells. The term *immunogen* usually refers to a substance capable of eliciting an immune response, and therefore it must also be capable of being recognized as an antigen. An antigen (e.g., a protein molecule) is usually much larger than the small region fitting into the binding site of an Ig molecule or the processed peptide recognized by a TCR. This smaller region is frequently referred to as an antigenic determinant or *epitope*. In a protein, a B cell epitope can theoretically be constructed in two ways—as a continuous or a discontinuous epitope. In a continuous epitope, the amino acid residues are part of a single uninterrupted sequence, whereas, in a discontinuous epitope, residues are not contiguous in the primary structure but are brought together by the folding of the polypeptide chain. Because this kind of epitope requires a special conformation of the antigen, it is frequently referred to as a conformational epitope.

B cells and T cells usually recognize different parts of an antigen. B cells and their secreted Ig molecules most commonly recognize unprocessed or "native" antigens. These antigens have maintained their native configuration, and most of the epitopes are usually of the discontinuous or conformational type. In general, only a minor component of a B cell response is directed to small linear peptide regions of the antigen. Studies indicate that epitopes recognized by B cells are not randomly distributed throughout the antigen but rather reside in regions with particular structural features. One important feature is accessibility because epitopes normally must be on the outer surface of a protein and may protrude from an antigen's globular surface to be able to interact with the BCR.

T CELLS AND ANTIGEN-PRESENTING CELLS

In contrast to B cells, T cells recognize processed pieces of a protein antigen, which are presented to the TCR by MHC molecules on the surface of antigen-presenting cells.[3–5,33]

T Cell Receptors

The TCR shows important structural similarities with Ig molecules (Fig. 16.4).[3–5] The αβ TCR is expressed by at least 90% of peripheral blood T cells. Essentially, all CD4+ T cells and most CD8+ T cells express this form of TCR. A small percentage of αβ-expressing T cells have a double-negative (CD4− and CD8−) phenotype. As shown in Figure 16.4, each chain consists of two extracellular Ig-like domains

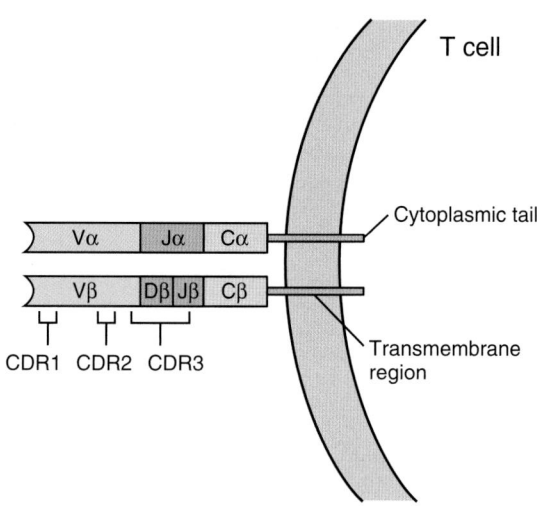

Figure 16.4 **The *T cell receptor* (TCR) α and β chains indicate the regions encoded by different TCR gene segments.** The positions of the *complementarity-determining regions* (CDRs) of both the β and the α chains are also shown. These are the most variable parts of the TCR and the most important for TCR binding to the peptide/major histocompatibility complex. CDR1 and CDR2 of both the α and the β chains are encoded within the variable region genes. CDR3 is formed by the rearrangement of V, D, and J gene segments of the β chain and V and J segments of the α chain and is encoded by the distal part of the V region segment through part of the J segment. The different parts of the TCR are not drawn to scale.

anchored into the plasma membrane by a transmembrane region and a short cytoplasmic tail. Similar to Ig molecules, the outer NH_2-terminal domain of each chain constitutes the variable region. Outside of the transmembrane region, the two chains are covalently linked together by disulfide bonds. Due to the short cytoplasmic tail, the αβ heterodimer is not capable of transmitting an intracellular signal after TCR engagement. This function is accomplished by the CD3 complex of polypeptides and other signaling proteins that are associated with the TCR.

The γδ TCR is an alternative form of TCR that is similar in overall structure to the αβ receptor.[34] Although some γδ cells express CD8, most are CD4− and CD8− (double negative). CD8 expression is largely confined to those γδ cells residing in the small intestine. The γδ TCR is also expressed in association with the CD3 complex. Although γδ T cells form a minor proportion of the T cells in the thymus and secondary lymphoid organs, they are abundant in various intraepithelial locations, such as in the skin, intestines, and lung.[35]

T Cell Receptor Structure and T Cell Receptor Repertoire Formation

Genes encoding the TCR are organized similarly to Ig genes[5,36] (eFig. 16.3). In a manner similar to that described previously for B cells, rearrangement of gene segments, junctional diversity, and combinatorial joining of the two chains are responsible for the diversity of the TCR repertoire. However, in contrast to B cells, TCR genes do not undergo somatic hypermutation. Thus, nearly the entire TCR αβ repertoire is formed during T cell development in the thymus and before any interaction with antigen. It is believed that extrathymic somatic hypermutation might result in the generation of deleterious self-reactive T cells.

The components of the αβ TCR heterodimer are shown in Figure 16.4, and the ribbon backbone structure of the Vα and Vβ portions of a human TCR are shown in Figure 16.5.[3–5,37,38] The upward-pointing loop structures are the CDRs. These regions are the most variable part of the TCR α and β chains and are most important for binding of the TCR to the MHC/peptide complex. The CDR1 and CDR2 regions of the α chain and β chain are encoded within the germline *TCRAV* and *TCRBV* gene segments, and variability in their sequences distinguishes the different V region subfamilies. The most diverse part of the α and β chains is the CDR3, which directly interacts with peptide in the binding groove of the MHC molecule.

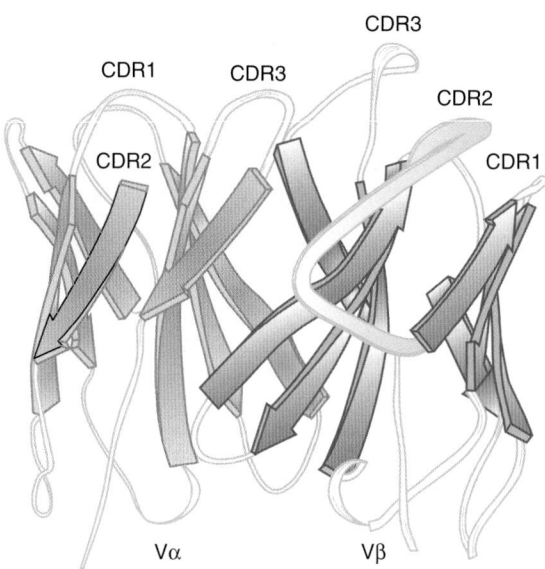

Figure 16.5 A ribbon backbone structure of the Vα and Vβ portions of a human *T cell receptor* (TCR). The upward-pointing loop structures are the *complementarity-determining regions* (CDRs). These regions are the most variable part of the TCR α and β chains and are most important for TRC binding to peptide/major histocompatibility complex. The CDR1 and CDR2 regions of the α chain and β chain are encoded within the germline *TCRAV* and *TCRBV* gene segments, respectively. The highly variable CDR3 region is formed by the rearrangement of V, D, and J gene segments. Junctional nucleotide substitutions and deletions at the margins of rearrangement add to the potential diversity of the CDR3 region. (Modified from Kotzin BL, Kappler J. Targeting the TCR in rheumatoid arthritis. *Arthritis Rheum.* 1998;41:1907.)

Antigen-Presenting Cells and the Major Histocompatibility Complex

There are two major varieties of MHC molecules (and genes) involved in the presentation of antigens to T cells. MHC class I molecules include *human leukocyte antigen* (HLA)-A, HLA-B, and HLA-C molecules. MHC class II molecules include the HLA-DR, HLA-DQ, and HLA-DP molecules. MHC class I molecules are expressed on nearly all nucleated cells. In contrast, MHC class II molecules have a limited distribution and are normally present only on cells involved in antigen presentation to T cells, including dendritic cells, macrophages, B cells, and thymic epithelial cells. The limited expression of MHC class II molecules in different tissues may be extremely important in preventing various types of autoimmune reactions. After activation or exposure to certain cytokines, such as *interferon-γ* (IFN-γ), other human cell types, such as activated T cells and epithelial cells, can express MHC class II molecules.

The general structures of the two classes of MHC molecules are shown in Figure 16.6. For MHC class I antigens, the α chain (encoded within the MHC) is complexed to beta₂-microglobulin (encoded outside the MHC). The α chain is highly polymorphic (variable between individuals), whereas beta₂-microglobulin is invariant. The extracellular portion of the α chain is divided into three domains: α1, α2, and α3. The outer α1 and α2 domains represent the polymorphic components of the molecule, and the α3 domain is relatively constant. MHC class II molecules are composed of an α and a β chain, both of which are encoded within the MHC. The NH₂-terminal domains of each chain (α1 and β1 domains) represent the polymorphic regions of the molecule and are important in antigen presentation, whereas the α2 and β2 domains are relatively constant.

The structures of MHC class I and class II molecules have provided remarkable insight into how antigenic peptides are bound and presented to T cells.[4,39–42] In Figure 16.7A, the peptide-binding groove of a class I molecule is viewed from the top, showing the surface that is contacted by a TCR. MHC class I pockets can usually bind only peptides of 8 to 10 amino acids, which are bound in a typical extended conformation with both the NH₂ terminus and the carboxy terminus anchored in the peptide-binding groove. In the case of MHC class II, the peptide-binding groove is formed by the interaction of the NH₂-terminal domains of the α and β chains (see Fig. 16.7B). The structure of MHC class

Figure 16.6 Comparison of the composition of *major histocompatibility complex* (MHC) class I and II molecules. The MHC class I α chain is variable (polymorphic) among different individuals. It is expressed with beta₂-microglobulin, which is encoded outside the MHC region and does not differ among different individuals. The MHC class II molecules are composed of α and β chains. For *human leukocyte antigen* (HLA)-DR molecules, only the β chain is variable, whereas for the HLA-DQ and HLA-DP molecules, both the α and the β chains are encoded by polymorphic alleles. In MHC class I molecules, the peptide-binding region is formed between the α1 and the α2 domains, which are polymorphic. The peptide-binding region of MHC class II is formed between the α1 and β1 domains of the α and β chains, respectively.

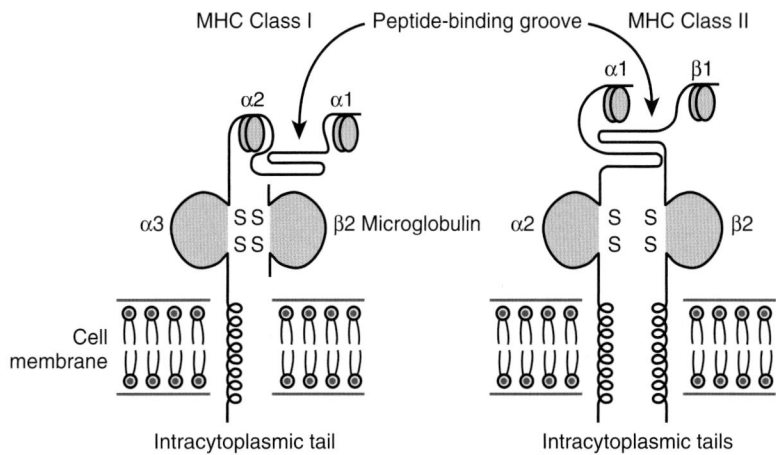

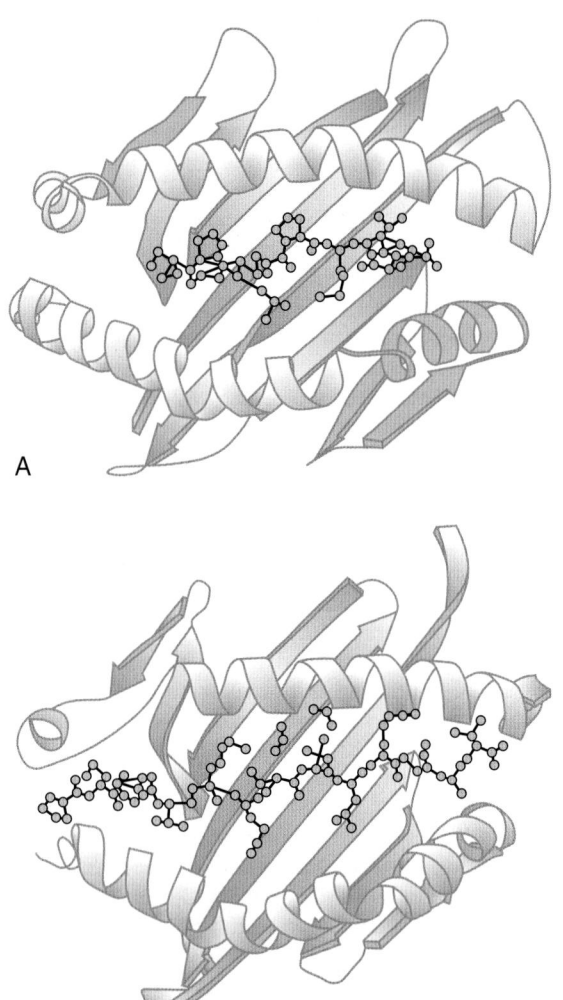

A

B

Figure 16.7 Structure of the _major histocompatibility complex_ (MHC)/ peptide complexes. (A) A schematic view of an MHC class I binding groove with peptide. The peptide is shown in ball-and-stick representation. In class I molecules, the peptide is usually of fixed length (8–10 amino acids) and bound so that both the NH_2 and carboxy termini are anchored in the peptide-binding groove. (B) A schematic view of an MHC class II (human leukocyte antigen–DR1) molecule with bound peptide in the groove. The peptide is shown in ball-and-stick representation. The peptide has the typical polyproline extended helical conformation seen in all class II bound peptides. The structure of class II allows peptides of varying lengths to bind because both ends of the peptide are free and can extend out of the groove on both sides. (From Jones EY. MHC class I and class II structures. _Curr Opin Immunol._ 1997;9:76-77.)

II allows peptides of varying lengths to bind because both ends of the peptide are free, and the peptide shown in Figure 16.7B has the typical polyproline-like extended helical conformation seen in all MHC class II-bound peptides.

Presentation and T Cell Recognition of Antigens

In contrast to B cells, T cells recognize processed peptides of a foreign antigen that are complexed to MHC molecules on antigen-presenting cells. Because of the process of thymic selection for self-MHC recognition, there is little capability for T cells to recognize intact or native protein antigens. CD4$^+$ T cells generally recognize peptides complexed to MHC class II molecules, whereas CD8$^+$ T cells interact with peptide/MHC class I molecules.[3–5,43] The purpose of this relatively complex antigen-presentation process may

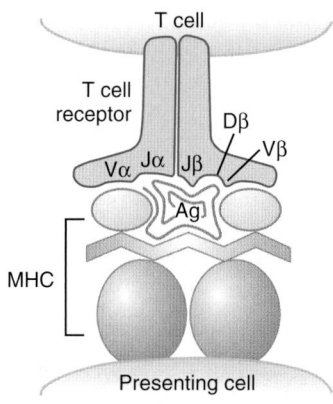

Figure 16.8 T cell recognition of a conventional peptide antigen. The _major histocompatibility complex_ (MHC) molecule on the antigen-presenting cell (_brown_) shows the peptide-binding groove with a peptide in it. The interacting _T cell receptor_ (TCR) is shown as a _blue_ structure. Note that the junctional regions of the TCR α chain (Vα/Jα) and β chain (Vβ/Dβ/ Jβ) are depicted so that they appear to have the most important interaction with the peptide. These junctional regions form the _complementarity-determining region_ (CDR) 3 of the α and β chains, which is the most variable component of the TCR. The CDR1 and CDR2 loops are encoded within the Vα and Vβ regions and may have more interaction with the MHC parts of the complex compared with CDR3. A ribbon diagram of the TCR CDR loops is depicted in Figure 16.5. (Modified from Drake CG, Kotzin BL. Superantigens: biology, immunology, and potential role in disease. _J Clin Immunol._ 1992;12:140.)

be to focus the T cell response onto cells. For example, it is much easier for a T cell to kill a virus-infected cell before the pathogen has the opportunity to multiply than it is to kill individual virus particles. The MHC class I molecules therefore focus the cytotoxic T cell response on cells infected with intracellular organisms, whereas free infectious particles are the targets of antibodies. MHC class II molecules similarly focus the delivery of T cell help on the relevant antigen-specific B lymphocytes that eventually produce antibodies. Recognition of antigen only on the surface of MHC class II–expressing cells also allows for a system by which the activation of CD4$^+$ T cells can be closely regulated.

Peptide-containing MHC class I and class II molecules on the surface of antigen-presenting cells serve as ligands for TCRs of CD8$^+$ and CD4$^+$ T cells, respectively. To present antigenic peptides effectively, antigen-presenting cells must be capable of performing at least two functions: (1) processing and displaying parts of antigens in the peptide-binding groove of MHC molecules on their cell surface and (2) providing the other accessory signals necessary for T cell activation. _Antigen processing_ refers to the series of steps that generate these peptide fragments, load them onto MHC molecules, and allow expression of the peptide/MHC complex on the cell surface.[44–48] Major differences exist in the manner in which endogenous and exogenous foreign antigens are processed and presented to T cells, which are beyond the scope of this chapter.

Figure 16.8 shows a schematic view of antigen recognition by a CD4$^+$ T cell. A foreign peptide is contained within the antigen-binding groove of an MHC class II molecule, and the TCR simultaneously recognizes the complex of peptide and MHC class II molecule. Thus, residues of the variable region of the TCR interact with the peptide and MHC residues extending out from the peptide-binding groove. The highly variable CDR 3 region of the αβ TCR is frequently most important in the binding of peptide, whereas other parts of the variable regions are more involved in interactions with MHC residues.[33,49]

Development and Selection of the TCR Repertoire

Stem cells precommitted to the T cell lineage arise in the bone marrow and migrate to the thymus. See eFig. 16.4 for additional information on T cell development and maturation. These cells do not express TCR molecules and do not express CD4 or CD8 molecules. These cells develop by rearranging TCR α and β chain genes and generating a functional αβ TCR. In the thymus, two major processes modify this repertoire.[50,51] One process positively selects cells that have some TCR affinity for self-MHC molecules. Evidence suggests that an interaction with thymic cortical epithelial cells is involved in this positive selection step. This process allows mature cells to recognize foreign antigens in the context of self-MHC antigens (a phenomenon termed self-MHC restriction). Cells that are not positively selected undergo programmed cell death (apoptosis) within the thymus. The other process deletes cells that have a high level of self-reactivity (termed negative selection or self-tolerance). This deletion process primarily involves an interaction with bone marrow–derived cells (macrophages, dendritic cells, B cells) that have migrated to the thymus and specialized cells within the thymic medulla (medullary epithelial cells) that express a variety of organ-specific antigens.[52] The transcriptional regulator, Aire, plays an important role in T cell tolerance induction in the thymus, mainly by promoting ectopic expression of a large repertoire of transcripts encoding proteins normally restricted to differentiated organs in the periphery.[52] Only a small percentage ($\approx$1–3%) of thymocytes actually survive positive and negative selection and become mature thymocytes that have a relatively high level of TCR expression and express either CD4+ or CD8+ markers. In general, cells that are positively selected by an interaction with MHC class II molecules mature into the CD4 population, whereas cells that are positively selected on MHC class I molecules become the CD8 population.[53] Mature thymocytes subsequently migrate to peripheral lymphoid tissues, where they maintain these surface characteristics.

T Cell Tolerance: Prevention of Self-Reactivity

Tolerance at the T cell level is critically important for the prevention of autoimmunity. Clonal deletion of self-reactive T cells in the thymus is a major process for eliminating T cells that are reactive to non–organ-specific cellular proteins and to circulating proteins because these self-antigens are likely to be in the thymus during T cell development. Some organ-sequestered antigens (e.g., certain uveal tract, brain, and endocrine organ antigens) are also expressed in the thymus.[52,54] However, studies have clearly shown that T cells to various self-antigens, including many organ-sequestered and posttranslationally modified antigens, are not completely deleted in the thymus. Therefore, self-tolerance must also involve the prevention of activation of these autoreactive T cells after they migrate from the thymus to the peripheral lymphoid tissues.[55,56]

Studies have shown that T cells with self-reactive TCRs are present in the peripheral lymphoid organs and the circulation of healthy individuals, but they are not sufficient

for the development of autoimmune disease. Different peripheral mechanisms appear to help prevent the generation of autoimmune responses. One process appears to prevent the self-antigen from being effectively presented to a self-reactive T cell, which maintains that T cell in an ignorant state. For example, resting T cells with self-reactive potential may not be able to traffic to the tissue that expresses the antigen, or the antigen may not be presented by antigen-presenting cells. Some studies have suggested that inappropriate expression of MHC class II antigens in a tissue can lead to autoimmunity, perhaps by circumventing this protective mechanism. T cell activation triggered by a separate process (e.g., an infectious agent) may also bypass this protective mechanism by allowing cells with self-reactive potential to traffic to tissues inappropriately. T cells that do recognize antigen without effective antigen-presenting cells and co-stimulation may also be functionally deactivated (or anergized)[57] and prevented from any subsequent stimulation by that self-antigen. These cells continue to be present in the peripheral T cell repertoire, but their prior contact with self-antigen prevents any subsequent response. Current evidence indicates that anergic T cells activate some but not other signaling pathways after TCR engagement.[57] There is also evidence that the encounter of self-reactive T cells with antigen, but without effective presentation, sometimes leads to death of the autoreactive T cell rather than just anergy.

A final mechanism to prevent activation of self-reactive T cells involves regulatory (suppressor) T cells. In experimental animal models, there is evidence that CD4+, CD8+, and γδ T cells may be involved in the down-regulation of certain immune responses, and their absence may be associated with pathologic autoimmune responses. At least two subsets of regulatory CD4+ T cells have been described that can inhibit cell-mediated immune responses and autoimmune pathologic responses: naturally occurring cells with suppressive activity and those induced by stimulation.[58,59] The naturally occurring regulatory CD4+ T cells are characterized by constitutive CD25 expression and constitute 5–10% of the circulating CD4+ population.[58–61] In murine models, depletion of these CD4+CD25+ T cells results in the spontaneous onset of multiorgan autoimmunity. These cells mediate their suppressive effects in a contact-dependent, antigen-independent manner in the absence of *interleukin-10* (IL-10) or *transforming growth factor-β* (TGF-β). A novel member of the forkhead box/winged-helix family of transcription regulators, designated FOXP3, has been identified as a specific molecular marker for this type of regulatory T cell, and its expression is essential for programming both thymic development and function of these T cells.[59,62] In sarcoidosis, FOXP3-expressing regulatory T cells accumulate at the periphery of the granuloma in subjects with active disease.[63] However, despite suppressing mitogen-induced T cell proliferation, the regulatory T cells in lung could not completely suppress *tumor necrosis factor-α* (TNF-α) and IFN-γ secretion, suggesting that the activity of this regulatory T cell subset was incapable of controlling granulomatous inflammation. The other type of regulatory CD4+ T cell is activation induced, and these cells lack CD25 and FOXP3 expression.[59] Much of the suppression from this group of regulatory cells can at least in part be attributable to cytokines such as TGF-β, because TGF-β is capable of suppressing both *type 1* (Th1) and *type 2* (Th2) *T helper* cell responses (see Th1 and Th2 responses, later). It is relevant to note that mice deficient in TGF-β show evidence of progressive inflammation and autoimmunity involving multiple organs.[64] In some cases, regulatory CD4+ T cells appear to release cytokines, such as IL-10 or even IL-4, that modulate the development and activation of Th1-type cells involved in a cell-mediated response.[58,65,66]

GENERATION OF AN IMMUNE RESPONSE

T CELL ACTIVATION AND CO-STIMULATION

Most immune responses depend on the activation of T cells and, normally, immune responses to foreign antigens are carefully orchestrated by a reciprocal communication between antigen-specific T cells and antigen-presenting cells. To be activated, naive T cells must receive several signals. One signal is antigen specific and is provided by engagement of the TCR. Additional signals are provided by co-stimulatory molecules and their interactions (Fig. 16.9). Resting antigen-presenting cells, such as resting B cells, frequently do not express significant levels of co-stimulatory molecules, and their interaction with T cells does not lead to T cell activation. Two of the most important co-stimulatory systems involve the interaction of CD28 with B7-1 (CD80) and B7-2 (CD86) and the interaction of CD40 ligand with CD40.[67] These two systems of interacting molecules also affect each other.

CD28 is constitutively expressed on CD4+ T cells. Early in the immune response, B7-1 and B7-2 are up-regulated on the antigen-presenting cells. Binding of CD28 to B7 co-stimulates T cell activation, leading to increased T cell production of IL-2 and other cytokines, increased cytokine receptor expression, increased cell survival, and increased T cell proliferation.[68-70] Occupation of the CD28

receptor alone, without TCR engagement, has little effect on T cells; therefore, signaling through CD28 is clearly a co-stimulatory event. The intracellular signaling that follows CD28 co-stimulation may overcome certain negative signals generated when the TCR is activated alone.[67,71,72]

Presentation in an inflammatory setting also leads to up-regulation of CD40 ligand (CD154) on the CD4+ T cell.[73] CD40 ligand interacts with its counter-receptor, CD40, on B cells and other antigen-presenting cells, also inducing up-regulation of B7-1 and B7-2 as well as certain adhesion molecules and cytokine production by the presenting cell.[74] The interaction of CD40 ligand with CD40 is clearly bidirectional in that it provides signals important for T cell and B cell activation. CD40 ligand is a member of the TNF receptor family, and a variety of other TNF receptor family members, such as CD134 (OX40), CD137 (4-1BB), and CD27, have also been shown to possess co-stimulatory function following T cell activation.[67,75] In chronic beryllium disease, CD137 has been shown to be a critical co-stimulatory molecule for the induction of T cell proliferation and for the prevention of activation-induced cell death in effector CD4+ T cells in lung.[76]

Following activation, T cells express *cytotoxic T lymphocyte antigen-4* (CTLA4) on their surface, which also binds B7-1 and B7-2 on the antigen-presenting cell and with stronger affinity than CD28.[77] This interaction sends a negative signal to down-regulate the T cell response after its initial activation. CTLA4 appears to be involved in the development of anergy and the generation of peripheral tolerance. CTLA4-deficient mice develop a lymphoproliferative disorder and die early, and alterations in the gene encoding CTLA4 have been associated with autoimmune endocrine diseases, further emphasizing the role of CTLA4 in the control of lymphocyte homeostasis.[78,79] *Programmed cell death 1* (PD-1) is another activation-induced inhibitory receptor that is expressed by T cells and binds the B7 family members PD-L1 and PD-L2.[80] Similar to CTLA4, PD-1 engagement by its ligands results in down-regulation of the

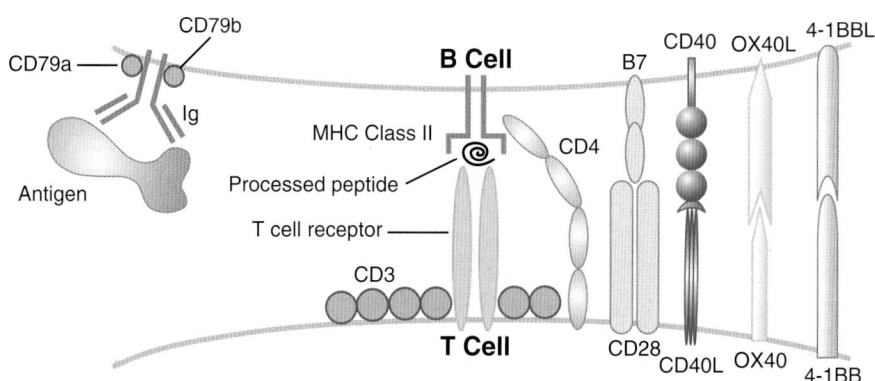

Figure 16.9 T helper cell–B cell interactions important for T cell–dependent antibody production. Antigen cross-links membrane *immunoglobulin* (Ig) on the *B cell receptor* (BCR), which provides the first signal for the B cell. CD79a (Ig-α) and CD79b (Ig-β) are Ig-accessory molecules necessary for transmitting the signal intracellularly. The antigen is internalized into an intracellular compartment in the B cell, processed to peptides, and combined with *major histocompatibility complex* (MHC) class II molecules for expression and presentation to the T helper cell. *T cell receptor* (TCR) binding to the peptide/MHC provides the first signal for the T cell. The CD3 complex allows for the TCR signal to be transmitted intracellularly. Activation of the T cell results in expression of CD40 ligand (CD40L), OX40, and 4-1BB. Interaction with CD40 provides the most important second signal to the B cell and is involved in T cell activation. In addition, B7-1 (CD80) and B7-2 (CD86) are up-regulated on the B cell. Interaction with CD28 provides an important co-stimulatory signal to the T cell. This figure does not show the release of cytokines from the T helper cell that are necessary for full activation and differentiation of the B cell. In addition, this figure does not show other cellular interactions mediated by adhesion molecules. For example, the lymphocyte function-associated antigen (LFA)-1 integrin (CD11a, CD18) on the T cell interacts with intercellular adhesion molecule-1 (CD54) on the B cell. This interaction appears to be enhanced once the TCR and BCR have been engaged. CD2 on the T cell also interacts with LFA-3 on the B cell, which provides additional cell-cell adhesion.

immune response. Deficiencies of this gene have been associated with autoimmune diseases in animals and may be a possible gene contribution to human lupus.[81,82] In contrast, blockade of CTLA4 or PD-1 signaling can activate cytolytic T cells in tumors and provides highly effective immunotherapy for a subset of patients with certain tumors, including non–small cell lung cancer.[83] In addition to these negative signals, down-regulation of the T cell response may be further ensured by decreases in surface expression of CD40 ligand, OX40, and 4-1BB after T cell activation.[70,75]

As discussed earlier in the context of self-tolerance, engagement of the TCR on a naive T cell in the absence of co-stimulation can result in different outcomes.[67] In some situations, the outcome is a failure to stimulate, and the T cell is oblivious to this encounter. At other times, recognition can induce death (apoptosis) of the responding T cells or anergy, in which case the T cells are unable to respond to a subsequent encounter with the same antigen (tolerance). Memory T cells appear to be less dependent on co-stimulatory molecules. However, antagonists that interrupt co-stimulatory interactions have been shown to have profound effects even later in the course of an established immune response. Blockers of the CD28-B7 interaction (with CTLA4-Ig, anti-B7, or anti-CD28 monoclonal antibodies) or of the CD40 ligand-CD40 interaction (with anti-CD40 ligand monoclonal antibodies), separately and together, are being investigated as therapies to treat autoimmune diseases and alloreactive responses after transplantation.[84-87] However, the development of

cytokine storm in healthy volunteers receiving an anti-CD28 monoclonal antibody demonstrates the potential risk of immunotherapy.[88]

SUBSETS OF T HELPER CELLS

Although more sharply defined in mice than in humans, it is clear that T cells after activation may evolve into at least four major subsets of T helper cells, distinguished by their secreted cytokines (Fig. 16.10).[65,66] Th1 cells are defined as a unique T helper lineage by their expression of the transcription factor T-bet and mainly synthesize IL-2, IFN-γ, and TNF-α as well as other inflammatory cytokines, such as lymphotoxin. *T follicular helper* (Tfh) cells are characterized by the ability to secrete CXCL13, IL-21, and IL-4. Th2 cells are defined by expression of the Th2 lineage-determining factor GATA-3 and are primarily distinguished by secretion of IL-4, IL-5, and IL-13. Th17 cells represent a distinct lineage of T cells from either Th1 or Th2 cells and express IL-17A, IL-17F, and IL-22 as well as the transcription factor RORγt.[89-92] These major types of T helper cells serve very different functions. Th1 cells primarily enhance cell-mediated immune responses, such as delayed-type hypersensitivity reactions, which involve activation of macrophages and effector T cells. Th2 cells appear to be important for immune responses, especially against helminths.[20] Th2 cells also drive allergic responses, such as IgE production and eosinophil activation in asthma (see Chapter 60).[20] The ability to mediate an effective immune response against certain intracellular pathogens and the pathogenesis of certain diseases

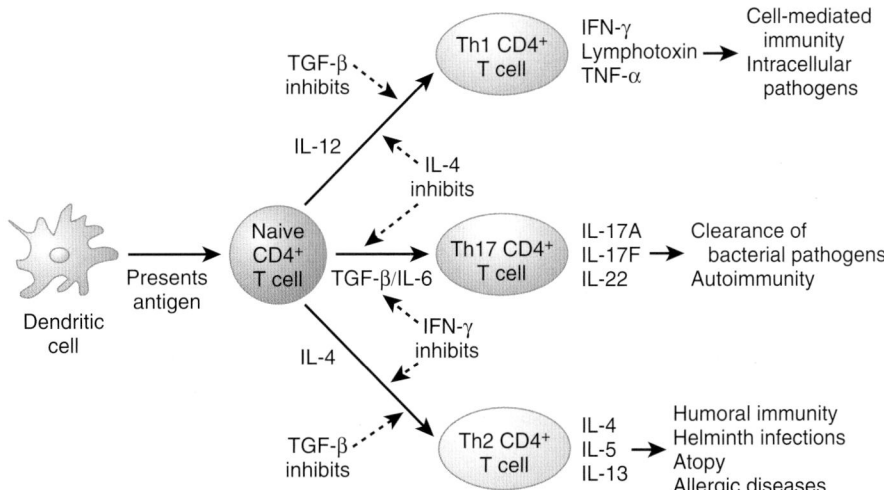

Figure 16.10 Regulation of T helper cell activation and responses. Naive CD4+ T cells can develop into *type 1 T helper* (Th1) cells if they are activated in the presence of *interleukin* (IL)-12, produced mostly by macrophages and other non–T cells. *Interferon*-γ (IFN-γ), increased by IFN-γ–inducing factor (IL-18), also enhances the development toward a Th1 response. IFN-γ appears to increase the production of IL-12 and also the expression of receptors for IL-12. The generation of a Th1 response leads to the production of IL-2, IFN-γ, lymphotoxin *tumor necrosis factor*-β (TNF-β), and TNF-α. These inflammatory cytokines are important for a successful immune response to intracellular pathogens. Inappropriate Th1 responses have also been implicated in organ-specific autoimmunity, such as in type 1 diabetes, multiple sclerosis, and rheumatoid arthritis. The early presence of IL-4 in the activation of a helper cell prevents Th1 responses and enhances the development of a type 2 T helper cell (Th2) response. The source of the early IL-4 is not clear, but it may come from Th2 cells already present, natural killer 1+ T cells, or non–T cells, such as mast cells and eosinophils. The Th2 response results in production of IL-4, IL-5, IL-10, and IL-13 and enhances humoral immunity. Although the Th2 cells are critical for the immune response to helminths, in the developed world, Th2 cells are probably most singled out for their important role in allergic disease and asthma. IL-4 and IFN-γ inhibit the development of a Th17 response that promotes bacterial clearance and may play a role in the development of autoimmunity. IL-6 and *transforming growth factor*-β (TGF-β) promote the development of Th17 cells, whereas IL-23 expressed by macrophages augments expression of Th17 cytokines by memory but not naive CD4+ T cells. Various regulatory CD4+ T cells have also been described. Regulatory CD4+ T cells secreting IL-10 have been shown to suppress Th1 responses. Regulatory T cells secreting TGF-β have the capability to suppress both Th1 and Th2 responses. Evidence suggests that, in addition to the cytokines present at the time naive CD4+ T cells are stimulated, the type of dendritic cell may regulate the differentiation of CD4+ T cells into Th1, Th2, or Th17 subsets.

are strongly influenced by the type of T helper cells involved. For example, in leishmaniasis and leprosy, the development of a response polarized toward the Th1 pathway is important for successful immune defense. The development of an early Th2 response may result in the inability to clear the pathogen. Inappropriately developed and activated Th1 cells have been implicated in the pathogenesis of certain autoimmune diseases, such as type 1 diabetes, multiple sclerosis, and rheumatoid arthritis. Th17 cells function at the interface between the innate and adaptive immune response, secreting cytokines that are important in bacterial clearance and in the pathogenesis of autoimmunity. Evidence suggests that in collagen-induced arthritis, T cell–mediated colitis, and experimental autoimmune encephalitis, Th17, as opposed to Th1, cytokines are critically important for the induction and maintenance of inflammation.[93–95] Although Th2 cells were initially described to provide help to B cells by promoting class switching and enhancing the production of certain IgG isotypes and production of IgE, it is now clear that this role is largely performed by a different subset of IL-4-expressing Tfh cells that reside in the B cell follicles.[96-98] Tfh cells are classified by expression of the follicular homing chemokine receptor CXCR5, and by PD-1 and IL-21 expression.[99–101] Tfh cells lack high expression of the T helper lineage-determining factors T-bet, GATA-3, and RORγt. Instead, this population of CD4$^+$ T cells expresses the Tfh lineage-determining factor BCL6.[102–104] Like classical Th1, Th2, and Th17 subsets, Tfh cells in humans and mice can express IFN-γ, IL-4, and IL-17, respectively, but secretion of these cytokines by Tfh is largely confined to B cell follicles and germinal centers and can be repressed by BCL6.[96,104–106] The directed secretion of these cytokines induces class switching toward distinct isotypes as discussed.

Th1, Th2, and Th17 subsets develop from the same T cell precursor, which is a naive CD4$^+$ T lymphocyte producing mainly IL-2 after stimulation with antigen. Considerable evidence indicates that the cytokine microenvironment is the primary determining factor for Th1, Th2, or Th17 differentiation (see Fig. 16.10).[65,66,90,91] IL-12 and IFN-γ are most important in directing the development of Th1 cells that then produce IFN-γ and TNF-α. IL-12 is produced by antigen-presenting cells (e.g., macrophages and dendritic cells) in response to Toll-like receptor stimulation by pathogens. IL-12 drives Th1 differentiation through signal transducer and activator of transcription 4 and the activation of a unique Th1 transcription factor known as T-box expressed in T cells (T-bet).[107,108] Certain microbial products induce macrophages and natural killer cells to release IFN-γ, which is involved in driving development of Th1 cells from their naive precursors. IFN-γ up-regulates a component of the IL-12 receptor on naive and differentiating T cells.[109] However, some pathogens, such as the measles virus, have the ability to down-regulate IL-12 production by macrophages and therefore possibly evade destruction by cell-mediated immune responses. Early production of IFN-γ by Th1 cells and natural killer cells has been related to the production of IFN-γ-inducing factor (IL-18), and this cytokine may synergize with IL-12 for maximal early production of IFN-γ and Th1 development.

In a similar but opposite manner, the presence of IL-4 early in the immune response promotes Th2 cell development from naive precursors through signal transducer and activator of transcription 6, which leads to activation of the transcription factor GATA3 and up-regulation of IL-4, IL-5, and IL-13.[88,90] The effects of IL-4 in promoting Th2 development are dominant over Th1- and Th17-polarizing cytokines.[56,57,91] Thus, if IL-4 levels exceed a threshold, Th2 commitment ensues, which leads to additional IL-4 production. Th2 cells do not respond to IL-12, which may be related to the ability of IL-4 to down-regulate expression of a component of the IL-12 receptor.

TGF-β and IL-6 are necessary for the differentiation of naive CD4$^+$ T cells into Th17 cells.[110–113] The orphan nuclear receptor, RORγt, is the master transcription factor in the differentiation of Th17 cells.[114] Expression of RORγt is TGF-β and IL-6 dependent and is both necessary and sufficient to induce Th17 development in most CD4$^+$ T cells.[91] The ligand of RORγt remains unknown. Using an IL-6–independent pathway, IL-21 and TGF-β can induce Th17 cells. IL-21 is also highly expressed by Th17 cells, and IL-21 production creates a positive feedback loop to amplify Th17 responses in vivo.[110] Despite the finding that IL-23 signaling is not required for Th17 commitment and early IL-17 secretion, IL-23 is important in amplifying and/or stabilizing the Th17 phenotype.[91]

The cytokines produced by Th1, Th2, and Th17 subsets cross-regulate one another's development and function. For example, IFN-γ produced by Th1 cells inhibits the development of Th2 and Th17 cells and certain humoral responses.[65,66,107] In a similar manner, IL-4 produced by Th2 cells inhibits Th1 and Th17 development and activation as well as macrophage activation by Th1 cytokines. IL-4 and IL-10 inhibit IL-12 production by dendritic cells and macrophages. In addition, the transcription factors GATA3 and T-bet expressed in T cells may antagonize the development of the opposite T cell subset by directly opposing each other's expression.[107,115] TGF-β also inhibits the development of Th1 and Th2 phenotypes.[107] However, separation of T cell differentiation into Th1, Th2, and Th17 phenotypes is not absolute. For example, in BAL fluid and mediastinal lymph nodes from patients with active sarcoidosis, increased proportions of T cells expressing markers consistent with Th17 and Th1 phenotypes (designated Th17.1 cells) have been defined as compared to patients undergoing disease resolution within 2 years.[116]

Following antigen exposure, naive T cells become activated, proliferate, and migrate to sites of inflammation. Although the majority of antigen-primed cells die, a population of memory T cells develops, which allows for a more rapid and effective secondary immune response upon reexposure to antigen.[117–121] There are at least three subsets of memory T cells, possessing different functional and migratory capabilities compared with naive lymphocytes. The effector memory T cell represents a terminally differentiated cell that immediately produces cytokine following antigen exposure and lacks the lymph node homing receptors L-selectin and CCR7. Conversely, central memory T cells express L-selectin and CCR7 and can differentiate into effector memory cells after subsequent antigen exposure. A third subset of tissue-resident memory T cells persists at the nonlymphoid site of infection.[122–125] These memory T cells are long-lived and do not transit back into the circulation or migrate into lymphoid tissues. Tissue-resident memory cells can be distinguished from effector memory T cells found in nonlymphoid tissues by their high expression of CD103 and CD69.[126–128] Functionally, these tissue-resident memory cells act as key early sentinels against reinfection.

CD4+ T CELL–B CELL COLLABORATION AND REGULATION OF ANTIBODY PRODUCTION

A central event in the immune response is the antigen-specific interaction between a T helper lymphocyte and a B lymphocyte, which leads to their mutual activation. Although some antigens (usually nonproteins derived from bacteria) can activate B cells in a T cell–independent fashion, the antibody response to most protein antigens requires the relevant B cell to recognize antigen with its surface Ig receptor and receive activation signals from a specialized subset of CD4+ T helper cells that reside largely in Tfh cells. These signals include both secreted T cell–derived lymphokines and those resulting from cell-cell contact. T cell recognition of antigenic peptides bound to MHC class II molecules on the B cell surface, with co-stimulatory signals, leads to T cell activation and secretion of T helper lymphokines. Secretion is directed toward the site of contact with the B cell. Thus far, no combination of known T cell–derived factors can fully replace contact with the T helper cell, indicating that the interaction of surface molecules provides additional signals to the B cell that promote its activation. Numerous interacting molecules have been identified that could transmit signals in the T cell–B cell interaction (see Fig. 16.9).

Similar to the process of effective T cell stimulation, which requires interaction of TCR with MHC/peptide and co-stimulatory signals, B cells also need more than one signal for activation to take place. The first signal is provided by antigen binding to surface Ig (BCR), and cross-linking of multiple receptors is usually required. The B cell then processes and presents the antigen via its MHC class II molecule to a cognate T helper cell that is specific for that MHC/peptide complex. A major second signal to the B cells is provided via CD40 on its surface through interaction with up-regulated CD40 ligand on the T helper cell. After receiving additional co-stimulatory signals from up-regulated B7-1 and B7-2 on the B cells, the activated T helper cell delivers cytokines in a focused manner to the antigen-specific B cell it is helping. Although many reciprocal receptor-ligand pairs are expressed on T cells and B cells, the signaling between CD40 ligand and CD40 is an obligatory and non-redundant interaction for functional T cell–dependent B cell activation.[87] The signals transduced by CD40 are essential for the prevention of apoptosis of antigen-specific B cells in the germinal center and required for B cell proliferation and differentiation, isotype switching, and formation of memory B cells. Mutations in the CD40 ligand gene cause X-linked hyper-IgM syndrome, characterized by absent or low levels of IgG, IgA, and IgE (Ig isotypes that require T cell help) but normal or elevated levels of IgM. Because T cell activation also requires co-stimulatory signals through CD40 ligand, these individuals demonstrate defects in T cell-mediated immunity and defective T cell activation.[129]

T cell help is required for effective antibody responses, especially those involving specific high-affinity antibodies of the IgG, IgA, and IgE isotypes. However, as emphasized earlier, T cell–B cell signaling is clearly bidirectional. After resting T cells are activated, which frequently requires specialized antigen-presenting cells such as dendritic cells, they migrate to the follicular border where they recognize cognate antigen presented by antigen-specific B cells. B cells may be the most efficient presenters of determinants of a specific antigen.[130] The helper CD4+ T cell recognizes a processed antigen presented on the B cell in the context of MHC class II. The B cell focuses antigen for antigen-specific help by binding antigen through its Ig receptor, internalizing and processing the antigen, and presenting the derived peptides with MHC class II molecules (see Fig. 16.9). It is important to emphasize that the epitope on the native antigen recognized by the B cell is almost always different from the peptide epitope recognized by the Tfh cell. After interacting with B cells at the follicular border, Tfh cells undergo follicular migration where they are required for productive germinal center development and high-affinity B cell selection and antibody production.[131,132]

Subsequent to recognition, the T cell is activated to provide help for B cell proliferation and differentiation. T cell help is critically dependent on the T cell release of various cytokines, as described earlier. These cytokines have marked effects on B cell maturation, especially in determining which Ig isotypes will be produced by the B cell. The reciprocal surface molecular interactions, the directed nature of T cell cytokine release, and the controlled local action of these molecules result in "focused T cell help" without generalized bystander activation of surrounding B cells.

GENERATION AND REGULATION OF CELL-MEDIATED IMMUNE RESPONSES

Cell-mediated cytotoxicity is an essential defense against intracellular pathogens, including viruses and certain bacteria and parasites. Cytotoxic T cells are stimulated by presented antigens, predominantly derived from intracellular pathogens and bound to MHC class I molecules. In contrast to most helper cells that express CD4, cytotoxic T cells are usually CD4−CD8+. The recognition of the antigen presented by MHC class I molecules triggers the T cell to express receptors for IL-2. Although some cytotoxic lymphocytes are able to produce their own IL-2, most depend on IL-2 produced by helper CD4+ T cells of the Th1 type. The binding of IL-2 and possibly other cytokines leads to some proliferation and to the development of cytotoxic function. CD4+ T helper cells (Th1 type) provide additional signals and cytokines for the generation of a maximal cytotoxic response.

Activated effector cells are capable of delivering a lethal message to a target cell, separating from their dying target, and moving on to strike a new target. This creates a very efficient system of killing unwanted cells. Several mechanisms are involved in the actual killing process.[133–136] For example, cytotoxic T cells can directly signal their targets to undergo apoptosis through the interaction of FAS ligand, expressed on the surface of activated T cells, with FAS on the target cell. The cytotoxic T cell also produces substances such as lymphotoxin (also known as TNF-β), trimers of which bind to receptors on the cellular targets and signal for apoptosis. During binding to the target cell, the cytotoxic CD8+ T cells also release the contents of their granules, which include perforins and granule-associated serine esterases (granzymes), toward the adjacent membrane of the target cell. Released perforins assemble on the surface of the target cell and perforate the target cell plasma membrane, resulting in lysis and the entry of enzymes. The transmembrane channel created by the perforins resembles the membrane attack complex of the complement cascade. After entry into the target cell, activated granzymes released from the cytotoxic T cell activate proteins that mediate apoptosis and cause other types of cell damage.

INNATE LYMPHOID CELL SUBSETS AND FUNCTION

ILCs seed peripheral tissues during fetal development and early in neonatal life.[137,138] ILCs in the fetal liver and later the bone marrow develop from a common lymphoid progenitor.[139,140] At this stage, they lose natural killer cell potential and progress through an early helper ILC precursor and finally to a common ILC progenitor that expresses the transcription factor PLZF.[139-142] However, some ILC progenitors maintain natural killer cell progenitor potential.[143] ILC progenitors give rise to ILC1/3 and ILC2 progenitors that fully mature into ILC1, ILC2, and ILC3 subsets.[144-146] Once in the peripheral tissues, ILCs acquire tissue-specific identities that modulate tissue homeostasis and act as sentinels for barrier integrity.[147,148]

The ILC1 subset secretes IFN-γ and encompasses classical natural killer cells.[7,149,150] A large proportion of natural killer cells contains numerous electron-dense granules and is recognized morphologically as large granular lymphocytes. Markers on these cells are frequently shared with T cells (e.g., CD2 and CD8) or cells of the myelomonocytic series, for example, the integrin molecule CD11b or the low-affinity receptor for IgG (FCGR3 or CD16). Natural killer cells appear to play an important role in the initial (innate) host defense against infection and tumor cells. Similar to certain phagocytes, they have the capability to destroy target cells or pathogens that have been coated with specific antibody via a process known as antibody-dependent cellular cytotoxicity. While ILC1 share expression of T-bet and IFN-γ with natural killer cells, these two cell types are distinct in a number of ways. ILC1 arise during fetal development and require GATA-3 and IL-7 receptor while natural killer cells do not depend on these factors and arise after birth.[151] Another difference relates to the dependence of ILC1 and natural killer cells on the transcription factors T-bet and Eomes.[152] While natural killer cells depend on Eomes expression, they can develop in the absence of T-bet. Conversely, ILC1 depend on T-bet but not Eomes. Lastly, natural killer cells and ILC1cells differ in their cytotoxicity and expression of perforin. Natural killer cells mediate effector function through the release of IFN-γ to promote macrophage activation and phagocytosis. Natural killer cells are directly cytotoxic via their release of perforin. In contrast, ILC1-mediated killing is largely confined to promoting macrophage engulfment of infected cells. ILC1 cells exhibit little direct cytotoxicity because they express low amounts of perforin. Despite these differences, both natural killer cells and ILC1 cells are important in type-1 immunity against intracellular pathogens such as viruses and bacteria and antitumor immunity.

The ILC2 subset modulates barrier integrity and tissue repair at mucosal sites.[153-155] ILC2 cells, similar to T

helper 2 cells, depend on the transcription factor GATA-3 during development and for ultimate commitment to the ILC2 fate.[145,156,157] These cells can be distinguished from other ILC subsets through their high expression of the surface receptor KLRG1 and cytokine receptors for IL-33, IL-25, and thymic stromal lymphopoietin.[153-155,158] Human ILC2 can be additionally identified by the expression of the chemokine receptor CRTH2 and the c-type lectin receptor CD161.[159,160] Their effector function depends on the production of IL4, IL-5, and IL-13. ILC2-derived cytokines are critical for mucosal barrier homeostasis. This is most evident in the small intestine where resident ILC2 cells sense IL-25 produced by intestinal tuft cells and in turn produce IL-13 to regulate intestinal goblet and tuft cell differentiation.[161-163] In addition, ILC2 cells are important in orchestrating early type 2 immune responses to large extracellular pathogens such as parasitic helminths. In the intestine, the presence of helminths increases IL-25 production by tuft cells, initiating a feed-forward circuit promoting ILC2-derived IL-4 and IL-13, which leads to goblet and tuft cell hyperplasia. As a result, the generation of IL-13 by ILC2 cells leads to enhanced mucus production, smooth muscle contractility, and ultimately worm clearance. In addition to their role in antiworm immunity, ILC2 cells express both arginase-1 and amphiregulin, which are important effector molecules involved in innate defense and tissue repair.[160,164-166] In combination, ILC2-derived IL-4, IL-5, IL-13, arginase-1, and amphiregulin promote the differentiation of reparative or alternatively activated macrophages, eosinophil mobilization, and tissue repair. Lastly, neuropeptide receptors are also expressed by subsets of ILC2 cells, allowing these cells to sense signals from the neuroendocrine systems of both the lung and intestine.[167-170] These neuropeptides work with alarmins to enhance ILC2 cytokine production in these mucosal tissues. This suggests that, like alarmins released by damaged epithelial cells, neuropeptides and neurotransmitters released by the neuroendocrine system may represent signals of barrier damage. When sensed by ILC2 cells, this initiates the recruitment of other immune cells for enhanced mucosal immunity and tissue repair.

ILC3 cells, like ILC2 cells, are found primarily in mucosal tissues and modulate barrier tissue homeostasis.[171-174] The ILC3 subset, like ILC1 cells, is heterogeneous. Two distinct subsets can be distinguished based on their surface expression of natural cytotoxicity receptors NKp46 (mouse) or NKp44 (human).[172,174,175] ILC3 cells produce IL-17 and/or IL-22, and *granulocyte-macrophage colony-stimulating factor* (GMCSF). All ILC3 cells in mice depend on the expression of the transcription factor RORγt similar to committed T helper 17 cells.[173,175,176] This is more variable in humans where IL-17-producing ILC3s require RORγt but IL-22-producing cells can exist in its absence.[144] Like other ILC subsets, ILC3 cells respond to various signals in the tissue microenvironment. These consist of both host-derived signals like retinoic acid, IL-1β, and IL-23, as well as exogenous, environmental signals such as microbial and dietary metabolites.[177-182] As these various tissue-specific cues suggest, ILC3 cells serve various functions in both tissue homeostasis and immunity. First, ILC3-derived IL-22 modulates intestinal stem cell differentiation and epithelial cell survival.[183-185] Second, ILC3 and IL-22 aid in modulating commensal bacteria and homeostasis at barrier tissues.[16,186-189] Third, ILC3 subsets promote mucosal immunity by promoting phagocytosis of infected cells, regulating CD4 T cell responses, and inducing epithelial cells to produce antimicrobial peptides to protect against pathogens that may breech the epithelial barrier.[12,190,191] Lastly, like ILC2 cells, ILC3 cells also recognize signals derived from the nervous system, suggesting an important role for this innate lymphocyte in neuroimmune cell communication.[192,193]

SPECIFIC IMMUNE RESPONSES IN THE LUNG

LYMPHOCYTE POPULATIONS AND TRAFFICKING IN THE LUNG

The lung in healthy individuals usually harbors only a small number of lymphocytes.[194,195] The location of CD4[+] and CD8[+] αβ T cells can be arbitrarily separated into four compartments: bronchoalveolar space, *bronchus-associated lymphoid tissue* (BALT), lung interstitial tissues, and intravascular space. Although lymphocytes from these different positions may be involved in lung immune responses, there is no clear indication that these cells represent a resident lymphocyte population in the lung in humans. In contrast, γδ T cells have been localized to intraepithelial positions in the lung, and these cells may selectively reside in the lung.[35]

In a normal nonsmoking individual, lymphocytes account for approximately 10–15% of the bronchoalveolar cells obtained during bronchoalveolar lavage.[195] The number of bronchoalveolar lymphocytes can increase markedly in inflammatory diseases involving the alveoli and the interstitium, such as in hypersensitivity pneumonitis and sarcoidosis (see Chapters 91 and 93). Most bronchoalveolar lymphocytes are T cells, and essentially all of these cells express memory cell markers (e.g., CD45RO and low CD62L), indicating previous activation.[196] In disease, a significantly increased percentage of these T cells compared with those in peripheral blood also express markers of recent activation, such as HLA-DR, IL-2 receptor (CD25), and CD69.

BALT is a localized collection of lymphocytes in the subepithelial area of bronchi, analogous to gut-associated lymphoid tissue (e.g., Peyer patches).[197] These lymphoid aggregates are separated from the airway lumen by a lymphoepithelium composed of flattened epithelial cells, which lack cilia. BALT also contains HEVs facilitating the recirculation of lymphocytes between blood and lymph. However, unlike gut-associated lymphoid tissues in the form of Peyer patches, which are present in all mammals, BALT is found only in some mammalian species. Indeed, it is usually absent in humans as long as there is no respiratory tract infection. Evidence suggests that BALT may appear in patients after chronic airway inflammation and COPD.[198,199]

The interstitium of the normal lung contains few lymphoid cells, and most of these are not T cells. The majority of interstitial lymphocytes are natural killer cells, which belong to the ILC1 subset and constitute 10–15% of circulating lymphocytes. These cells do not express TCR or Ig but express markers characteristic of both T cell and myelomonocytic lineages.[200] Natural killer cells recognize

and kill tumor cells and virus-infected cells in a nonspecific manner.[200] These cells also kill targets coated with antibodies via surface receptors for IgG (FCGR3 or CD16) in a process known as antibody-dependent cellular cytotoxicity. Furthermore, natural killer cells can also be an important source of cytokines (e.g., INF-γ, TNF-α, and GM-CSF) early in the immune response.

γδ T cells constitute only 0.5–10% of the peripheral blood lymphocyte population in humans.[35] However, they represent an enriched T cell population in the pulmonary epithelium, intestinal epithelium, and skin. Unlike αβ T cells, epithelial γδ T cells do not recirculate and appear to represent resident pulmonary lymphocytes. The population of γδ T cells in the lung of normal adult C57BL/6 mice is approximately 2 to 5 × 10⁴ cells, with the majority being either Vγ4[+] or Vγ1[+].[201] Importantly, the different γδ T cell subsets are thought to have different functional capabilities. For example, in a murine model of asthma, Vγ1[+] γδ T cells enhance airway hyperresponsiveness, whereas Vγ4[+] γδ T cells suppress this response.[202] The pulmonary γδ T cells preferentially interact with F4/80[+] macrophages and MHC class II–expressing dendritic cells, suggesting that γδ T cells represent a primitive line of defense evolved to protect epithelial integrity and provide a possible bridge between innate immunity and acquired immune responses. γδ T cells have also been implicated in the regulation of various immune responses in the lung through IL-22 expression.[203]

The distribution and trafficking of lymphocytes is governed by interactions between molecules on the lymphocyte surface and ligands present on vascular endothelial cells. The migration of lymphocytes from the bloodstream is not a random event, and this migration appears to be restricted to lymphoid tissue and areas of inflammation.[17] Naive T cells lack the ability to initiate an antigenic response until they are activated within a secondary lymphoid organ. Evidence indicates that their initial interaction with an antigen entering through the lung takes place in the surrounding lymphoid tissues and not in the lung directly. Naive and resting lymphocytes represent the major population that recirculates from blood to lymph via HEVs,[204] with the initial attachment mediated by the homing receptor L-selectin (CD62L) to peripheral lymph node addressin and glycosylation-dependent cell adhesion molecule-1 on the surface of endothelial cells.[17] This interaction results in lymphocyte tethering and rolling along the endothelial surface. Subsequent binding of chemokines (e.g., stromal cell–derived factor-1α, 6-C-kine, and macrophage inflammatory protein-3b) to G protein–coupled receptors on the lymphocyte surface leads to activation of integrin molecules (*lymphocyte function–associated antigen-1* [LFA-1]).[17] After activation, LFA-1 binds to intercellular adhesion molecule-1 on the vascular endothelium, resulting in firm adhesion.[17] This is followed by transendothelial migration of the lymphocyte into the lymphoid tissue. A second family of G protein–coupled receptors, known as sphingosine-1-phosphate receptor-1, is required for lymphocyte egress from the lymph node.[205] As stated earlier, BALT consists of diffuse lymphoid aggregates found in the bronchial mucosa of most mammals.[197] In contrast to HEVs in other secondary lymphoid organs, BALT HEVs express high levels of vascular cell adhesion molecule-1, which binds α₄β₁ integrin on T cells. Thus, an adhesion cascade exists involving

L-selectin/peripheral lymph node addressin, $\alpha_4\beta_1$ integrin/ vascular cell adhesion molecule-1, and LFA-1/intercellular adhesion molecule-1, which targets specific lymphocyte populations to BALT and other bronchopulmonary tissues.[17,197]

Effector and memory T lymphocytes have distinct pathways of lymphocyte recirculation compared with naive lymphocytes.[17] Effector T cells, especially after activation in the lymphoid tissues, travel to regions of inflammation where chemokines and other chemotactic molecules are generated by the underlying inflammatory process.[17] Expression of adhesion molecules on the lymphocyte and binding to their appropriate molecular targets expressed on inflamed vascular endothelium allow cells to enter sites of inflammation.[17] The expression of intercellular adhesion molecule-1, P-selectin, and vascular cell adhesion molecule-1 on the surface of inflamed vascular endothelium is involved in lymphocyte entry into areas of inflammation.[17] Tissue tropism is established by the expression of different combinations of adhesion molecules that allow a different subset of effector cells to home to different sites. For example, circulating memory lymphocytes specific for skin-associated antigens express the cutaneous lymphocyte antigen.[17] Conversely, memory for intestinal antigens has been localized to circulating lymphocytes expressing high levels of $\alpha_4\beta_7$ integrin.[17] Thus, memory T cells display selective homing to the tissue type where antigen was first encountered.

ILC2 and ILC3 cells represent important populations of lymphocytes in the lung. These are rare cells that acquire a lung-specific identity based on tissue-specific and environmental cues. The majority of turnover among ILC2 and ILC3 populations in the lung is a result of local homeostatic proliferation.[11,137,206] However, these cells can quickly proliferate in response to inflammation and tissue damage. In addition to local proliferation of the tissue-resident ILC2 population, a transient population of ILC2 cells migrates to the lung early after mucosal barrier disruption.[158] Unlike the tissue-resident population that is responsive primarily to IL-33, this circulating ILC2 population responds preferentially to IL-25. The small intestine has been described as one source for this migratory ILC2 population, and it has been suggested that this population can convert to a tissue-resident phenotype upon entry into the lung tissue.[207] It should be noted that IL-33 has also been shown to induce the migration of ILC2 cells to the lung from the bone marrow, indicating that migratory IL-33-responsive ILC2 cells may also play a role in immunity in the lung.[208]

ANTIBODY-MEDIATED IMMUNE RESPONSES IN THE LUNG

Immune Response to Extracellular Pathogens

The humoral immune response is adapted for elimination of extracellular pathogens. An example of an antibody-mediated immune response is that which takes place after exposure to *Streptococcus pneumoniae*. This bacterium frequently colonizes the nasopharynx and is the most common bacterial cause of community-acquired pneumonia.[209] Pneumococci gain access to the lower respiratory tract via aspiration. The upper airway is equipped with clearance mechanisms (e.g., mucociliary clearance and cough) that

effectively eliminate most inhaled or aspirated bacteria from the airways (see Chapter 4). If aspirated pneumococci evade the upper airway defenses, the pathogen first encounters the mucosal humoral immune system. IgA provides the first line of defense against infectious agents, with IgG and IgM being less important in the bronchial secretions. The major functions of secretory IgA include the prevention of microbial adherence to the epithelial surface and the promotion of the agglutination of microorganisms. The combination of inhibition of adhesion and microbial agglutination favors the clearance of pneumococci via mechanical forces. Unlike IgG, IgA is unable to activate complement and is not an effective opsonin.

The first exposure of the host to the pneumococcus generates a primary humoral response. Bacteria in the lung are bound by antigen-presenting phagocytes, which migrate to secondary lymphoid organs, where antigens are processed and presented with MHC class II molecules to CD4$^+$ T cells (Fig. 16.11). After TCR binding and effective co-stimulation enhanced by an inflammatory environment, antigen-specific T cells are activated and multiple T helper cytokines are elaborated. During this process, naive B cells in the lymph node bind unprocessed antigen via surface IgM and present peptide fragments to specific T helper cells via MHC class II molecules. T cell–B cell interactions in the germinal centers lead to additional T cell and full B cell activation, characterized by clonal proliferation, isotype switching, and differentiation of B cells into antibody-secreting plasma cells and memory cells. Subsequently, specific antibody, activated T cells, and perhaps some activated B cells circulate back to the lung to combat the pneumococcal infection.

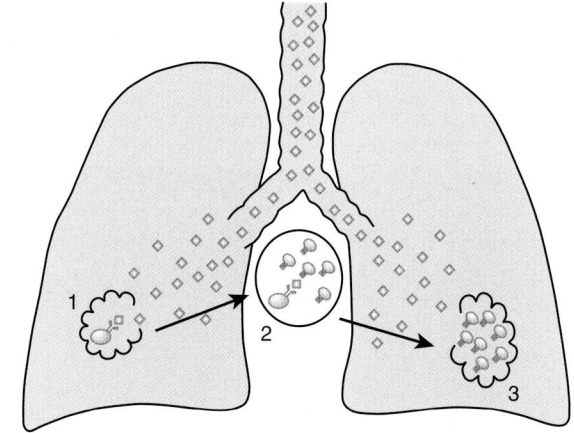

Figure 16.11 Immune responses in the lung. Antigen (e.g., bacterial pathogen) enters the lung. Microbial products create an inflammatory environment. *1,* Antigen is taken up by nonspecific phagocytic cells and transported to regional lymph nodes. *2,* In the lymph nodes, a primary immune response is generated. Antigen-specific T cells are stimulated, and initial T helper cell–B cell interactions and antibody production take place in the germinal centers. *3,* Antibodies, T helper cells, and effector cells circulate back to the lung for the immune response to target the pathogen. Trafficking of inflammatory cells is enhanced by the production of chemokines and other chemotactic factors and involves interactions of leukocytes with endothelial cells in the area of inflammation. In the process of the initial immune response, memory T cells and B cells are generated. This allows for the generation of a more effective secondary immune response if the same pathogen is encountered at a later time.

In the area of infection, IgG1, IgG3, and IgM specific for intact pneumococcal antigens activate the complement system, resulting in some bacterial cell lysis. More important, antibody and complement act as opsonins, enhancing phagocytosis of encapsulated microorganisms. The release of mediators from activated T cells also enhances the antibacterial capacity of recruited nonspecific inflammatory cells in the lung. These events take place over a 4- to 7-day period and characterize the initial phase of a primary response. The time needed for peak response is approximately 7 to 10 days. The presence of memory B and T cells ensures that repeat exposure to *S. pneumoniae* results in a secondary immune response, which is characterized by a shorter lag phase, resulting in a more rapid response of greater magnitude and longer duration. Clinically, pneumococcal vaccination, which induces a primary humoral response, has decreased the rates of invasive pneumococcal disease in both children and adults.[210]

Immune Response to Autoantigens

Autoimmune disorders result when the normal mechanisms of immune self-tolerance fail. Essentially all autoimmune diseases, including antibody-mediated autoimmune diseases, appear to be dependent on the inappropriate activation of autoreactive CD4+ T cells as well as on the autoreactive B cells responsible for the pathogenic autoantibodies. One example of an autoimmune disease involving the lung is anti-*glomerular basement membrane* (GBM) disease (also known as Goodpasture syndrome) (see also Chapter 94). This syndrome is characterized by pulmonary hemorrhage and glomerulonephritis, which are associated with elevated levels of IgG antibodies directed against basement membrane antigens. In various studies, pathologic damage has been shown to be dependent on the binding of these autoantibodies, which are primarily directed against the noncollagenous domain (α3 chain) of type IV collagen in basement membrane.[211–213] Immunofluorescent staining with anti–human IgG antibodies usually reveals a linear deposition of IgG in the glomerular and alveolar basement membranes. Despite the widespread distribution of type IV collagen in the body, disease expression is mostly limited to the lungs and kidneys. This limited disease expression suggests the possibility that other factors allow exposure of this autoantigen selectively in alveolar or glomerular basement membranes. In this regard, influenza A infection, hydrocarbon inhalation, and cigarette smoking have been associated with the initial episode of diffuse alveolar hemorrhage and exacerbation of disease in the setting of elevated levels of anti–basement membrane antibodies. Much is known regarding how autoantibodies cause damage in an autoimmune disease such as anti-GBM disease. More recently, HLA associations and the B- and T cell epitope have been identified.[214] *HLA-DRB1*15:01* is strongly associated with the development of anti-GBM disease, whereas *HLA-DRB1*07:01* and *DRB1*01:01* confer protection against development of this disease. In addition, the T cell epitope has been mapped to the amino-terminal region of the α3 chain of type IV collagen.[215] As noted earlier, activation of both autoreactive CD4+ T cells and autoreactive B cells appears to be necessary for a pathologic autoimmune response. These autoreactive CD4+ T cells require CD28 co-stimulation, because blockade of this co-stimulatory molecule reduces anti–basement membrane antibody production and prevents the development of experimental autoimmune glomerulonephritis.[216]

Studies have identified an autoimmune cause underlying the development of acquired pulmonary alveolar proteinosis.[217] This disorder is characterized by the accumulation of a periodic acid–Schiff staining, granular, eosinophilic material within the alveolar space (see Chapter 98). Based on the development of pulmonary alveolar proteinosis in mice rendered deficient in GM-CSF, a fundamental role of this factor in surfactant homeostasis has been discovered.[218] In addition, the presence of neutralizing IgG autoantibodies directed against GM-CSF has been identified in the bronchoalveolar lavage fluid and serum of all patients with acquired pulmonary alveolar proteinosis, but not in individuals with the congenital or secondary form of the disorder or in normal control subjects.[219] The detection of this IgG autoantibody is highly sensitive and specific and thus useful in the diagnosis of the acquired form of this disease. More recently, mutations in the ligand-binding α chain of the GM-CSF receptor have been identified in pediatric patients with pulmonary alveolar proteinosis.[220]

Immune Response in Allergic Disease

Atopic asthma results when an immune response and IgE antibodies are directed against normally harmless proteins present in the environment (see Chapter 60). Numerous cell types, including mast cells, eosinophils, macrophages, and CD4+ T lymphocytes, as well as IgE-secreting B cells, are important in the development of allergy and asthma. The CD4+ T cells, which accumulate in the lungs of asthmatics, display a Th2 phenotype,[221] and studies using murine asthma models have shown that allergic airway inflammation is dependent on Th2-type CD4+ T cells. As discussed earlier, the development of a Th2 response is prompted by exposure of naive CD4+ T cells to IL-4 at the beginning of an immune response.[65,66,107,109] In the presence of high expression of IL-4 and low IFN-γ, these IL-4–producing CD4+ T cells induce isotype switching in antigen-specific B cells to IgE.[222] The elevated levels of IgE in asthma are essential for the immediate hypersensitivity response. The presence of IL-4 and IL-5 and the production of various chemokines during T cell activation also enhance accumulation of eosinophils and basophils in the airways. Studies in murine models of allergic asthma have suggested an important role for another Th2 cytokine, IL-13, which is capable of inducing the pathologic features of asthma independent of IgE and eosinophils.[223] Related to the Th2 dependence of asthma in humans, susceptibility to disease has been linked to loci on chromosome 5q, which contains the genes for IL-4 and IL-13.[224] Studies also suggest that genetically determined abnormalities in antigen-presenting cells may also play a role in the development of allergic reactions. In atopic individuals, antigen-presenting cells were shown to underproduce IL-12 or overproduce prostaglandin E$_2$, which favors a Th2 response.[225]

CELL-MEDIATED IMMUNE RESPONSES IN THE LUNG
Granulomatous Lung Disease

Granulomas are characteristic of persistent infections caused by organisms that reside intracellularly, such as *Mycobacterium tuberculosis* and *Mycobacterium leprae*. There is considerable evidence to suggest that CD4[+] T cells and the elaboration of Th1 cytokines are required for maximal granulomatous inflammation in the response to these infections. The triggering event in the development of noninfectious granulomatous lung disease is the deposition of antigen in the lung parenchyma. In the case of chronic beryllium disease[226,227] and hypersensitivity pneumonitis (see Chapter 91), the antigenic stimulus is known. In sarcoidosis, the inciting agent is unknown, although the immunopathogenic events are believed to be similar (see Chapter 93).[228] Thus, the unknown antigen is likely to be engulfed by antigen-presenting cells (i.e., dendritic cells and macrophages) in the lung parenchyma and presented to naive CD4[+] T cells in peripheral lymphoid organs. In the absence of IL-4, exposure of these activated naive CD4[+] T cells to IL-12 released by macrophages directs the T cell toward a Th1 response.[65,66,107,109] The development of a Th1 response is also influenced by early release of IFN-γ through the up-regulation of IL-12 production by macrophages and through the up-regulation of receptors for this cytokine on Th1 cells.

Production of chemokines and other chemotactic factors at the site of inflammation in the lung directs migration of activated effector CD4[+] T cells to the lung. The Th1 cytokines and other mediators produced by these T cells are responsible for the recruitment and activation of macrophages and other inflammatory cells. The accumulation of inflammatory cells within the alveolus (alveolitis) appears to be the initial lesion characterizing sarcoidosis and other granulomatous lung diseases. In sarcoidosis, the accumulated CD4[+] T cells (obtained at bronchoalveolar lavage) include expanded subsets, identified by expression of particular TCR Vβ and Vα regions. Within these subsets are expansions of T cell clones, each with a unique $\alpha\beta$ TCR. The presence of these oligoclonal expansions indicates a T cell response to conventional peptide antigens, and the presence of different T cell clones with related TCRs indicates a response to the same antigen. Both the HLA allotype (the presenting MHC class II molecule) in an individual and the stimulating antigen(s) will determine the TCRs used in these T cell responses. In chronic beryllium disease, particular HLA-DP alleles (e.g., *HLA-DPB1* alleles expressing a glutamic acid residue at the 69th position of the β-chain) are the most important in the presentation of antigen to beryllium-specific T cells,[229] and this explains the increased disease susceptibility in individuals with the same HLA-DP alleles.[230] CD4[+] T cell clones expressing similar TCRs (with the same V regions and highly similar CDR3 regions) have been noted to be expanded in the lungs of different individuals with chronic beryllium disease, reflecting similarities in presenting MHC class II molecules and the same stimulating antigen (beryllium).[231] In sarcoidosis, an association between the TCR usage of Vα2.3 and HLA-DR17 (DR3) expression has been reported.[232] It is important to emphasize that the pathologic T cell responses in these diseases are compartmentalized to the lung because the same T cell clones are either absent or rare in the peripheral blood.[196] Recent evidence suggests that increased expression of inhibitory receptors (e.g., PD-1) on CD4[+] T cells in sarcoidosis results in an exhausted phenotype and that this exhaustion reverses with clinical resolution of pulmonary sarcoidosis.[233,234]

The major effector cells of inflammation in chronic beryllium disease, sarcoidosis, and other granulomatous diseases appear to be macrophages primarily derived from circulating monocytes during the process of inflammation. Activated alveolar macrophages express MHC class II molecules and may contribute to antigen presentation. Noncaseating granulomas form by coalescence of activated macrophages, which can also fuse to form multinucleated giant cells. CD4[+] T cells predominate in the center of the noncaseating granuloma, with CD8[+] T cells located at the periphery of the granulomatous response.

Cytotoxic T Cell Reactions in the Lung

Cytotoxic T lymphocytes (CTLs) are critical in the recognition and elimination of virus-infected cells and tumor cells as well as in allograft rejection. These cells predominantly express CD8, although CD4[+] CTLs and natural killer cells may also be involved in cytotoxic responses. CD4[+] T helper cells are almost always required for full expression of a cytotoxic T cell reaction. CTL responses have been detected in humans after infection with numerous viruses, including respiratory syncytial virus, parainfluenza, and influenza A and B. Once a CD8[+] CTL recognizes a respiratory syncytial virus–infected cell, there are at least three distinct mechanisms by which the CTL can induce cell death.[133-136] As discussed earlier, CTLs can secrete cytotoxic cytokines such as TNF-α and IFN-γ in the vicinity of the target cell. In addition, CTLs can release granule enzymes, including perforin and granzymes, which cause pore formation in the membrane of the target cell and enzyme-mediated apoptosis. Finally, CTLs can induce cell death via the interaction of FAS ligand on its surface with FAS on the target cell. CD4[+] CTLs do not have cytotoxic granules and primarily use FAS-mediated apoptosis as their mechanism of cytotoxicity.

Natural killer cells have a role complementary to that of CTLs in combating virus-infected cells or tumor cells.[200] Natural killer cells appear to form the first line of defense against viral infection, providing cytotoxic activity to kill virus-infected cells. These cells differ from CTLs in their lack of TCRs, and they recognize their targets in a non–MHC-restricted fashion. However, the mechanism of natural killer cell killing appears to be similar to that employed by CD8[+] CTLs. In addition, natural killer cells have receptors for IgG (FCGR3; CD16) and can bind to the Fc region of antibody attached to the surface of a target cell and mediate antibody-dependent cellular cytotoxicity.

Innate Lymphoid Cell Responses in the Lung

ILC2 cells in the lung play a role in the protective immunity against parasitic helminth infection.[154,155] After parasitic larvae enter the lung via capillaries, they migrate into the air spaces before eventual entry into the intestine. It is here that the larvae mature into adult worms and produce eggs. The migration of the larvae through the lung causes extensive damage and release of tissue alarmins such as IL-25, IL-33, and thymic stromal lymphopoietin. ILC2 cells recognize these alarmins and rapidly produce type 2 cytokines to initiate innate cell recruitment, mobilization of eosinophils from the bone marrow, and promote the mucosal response in the small intestine to eliminate worms. In addition, ILC2 cells express MHC class II molecules and promote dendritic cell generation of T helper 2 responses, which are required for protective type 2 immunity.[13,14] Lastly, ILC2 cells express factors such as amphiregulin and arginase-1, which, in addition to type 2 cytokines, promote the differentiation of reparative macrophages and tissue repair.[160,164,166,235]

In addition to their protective capacity in the context of parasitic helminth infection, ILC2 cells have been described to have a pathogenic role in other settings of type 2 inflammation. In particular, ILC2 cells have been described to play a pathogenic role in various lung diseases. These cells have been best studied in the context of allergic asthma.[14,236–239] Furthermore, ILC2 cells have been implicated in the exacerbation of asthma as it relates to respiratory viral infections. These include asthma exacerbations driven by respiratory syncytial virus, rhinovirus, and influenza.[240–245] Lastly, although less well characterized, ILCs have been implicated in driving inflammation associated with many other chronic respiratory diseases, including COPD, pulmonary fibrosis, and cystic fibrosis.[246]

Key Points

- Although a functional immune system is essential to protect against microbial invasion, dysregulated immune responses contribute to pathogenesis of diverse lung diseases.
- Protective immunity against microbial pathogens is provided by humoral immune responses and a variety of cell-mediated responses that result in activation and accumulation of leukocytes.
- T helper cells are central to all of these immune responses for their full expression and maximal effect.
- The capacity for defense against widely diverse pathogens is achieved through unique molecular mechanisms of the B cell receptor and the T cell receptor repertoire formation, which are fundamental to the adaptive immune response.
- The end results of specific immune responses depend on cytokine expression and interactions of regulatory T cells with effector T cell subsets.

- In some individuals, the defense system may break down and, in others, aberrant immune responses contribute to pathologic conditions involving the lungs.
- Granulomatous lung diseases (e.g., sarcoidosis and chronic beryllium disease) are characterized by exuberant type 1 T helper CD4+ T cell responses, whereas allergic diseases (e.g., asthma) are characterized by excessive type 2 T helper responses.
- Type 17 T helper polarized immune responses contribute to defense in bacterial pneumonia and to pathology in subjects with severe, corticosteroid-unresponsive asthma.
- Innate lymphoid cells are tissue-resident immune cells that regulate mucosal barrier homeostasis and serve as early sentinels against infection and tissue damage.

Key Readings

Barry M, Bleackley RC. Cytotoxic T lymphocytes: all roads lead to death. *Nat Rev Immunol.* 2002;2:401–409.

Chen K, Kolls JK. T cell-mediated host defenses in the lung. *Annu Rev Immunol.* 2013;31:605–633.

Chen L, Flies DB. Molecular mechanisms of T cell co-stimulation and co-inhibition. *Nat Rev Immunol.* 2013;13:227–242.

Davis MM, Boniface JJ, Reich Z, et al. Ligand recognition by alpha beta T cell receptors. *Annu Rev Immunol.* 1998;16:523–544.

Garcia KC, Teyton L, Wilson IA. Structural basis of T cell recognition. *Annu Rev Immunol.* 1999;17:369–397.

Gauld SB, Dal Porto JM, Cambier JC. B cell antigen receptor signaling: roles in cell development and disease. *Science.* 2002;296:1641–1642.

Greaves SA, Atif SM, Fontenot AP. Adaptive immunity in pulmonary sarcoidosis and chronic beryllium disease. *Front Immunol.* 2020;11:474.

Josefowicz SZ, Lu LF, Rudensky AY. Regulatory T cells: mechanisms of differentiation and function. *Annu Rev Immunol.* 2012;30:531–564.

Klose CS, Artis D. Innate lymphoid cells as regulators of immunity, inflammation and tissue homeostasis. *Nat Immunol.* 2016;17:765–774.

Lambrecht BN, Hammad H, Fahy JV. The cytokines of asthma. *Immunity.* 2019;50:975–991.

Masopust D, Schenkel JM. The integration of T cell migration, differentiation and function. *Nat Rev Immunol.* 2013;13:309–320.

Stritesky GL, Jameson SC, Hogquist KA. Selection of self-reactive T cells in the thymus. *Annu Rev Immunol.* 2012;30:95–114.

Weaver CT, Hatton RD, Mangan PR, et al. IL-17 family cytokines and the expanding diversity of effector T cell lineages. *Annu Rev Immunol.* 2007;25:821–852.

Complete reference list available at ExpertConsult.com.

17 *MICROBIOME*

GEORGIOS KITSIOS, MD, PHD • BRYAN J. MCVERRY, MD •
ALISON MORRIS, MD, MS

INTRODUCTION

The recent discovery of diverse microbial communities present in the human respiratory tract, collectively termed the *lung microbiome*, is reshaping our understanding of respiratory physiology and disease pathogenesis. Propelled by technological innovations of *next-generation sequencing* (NGS), culture-independent studies have reproducibly demonstrated the existence of a lung microbiome, which is detectable in health and altered in disease. Such findings overturned a long-standing dogma of presumed lung sterility that the normal lungs were free from bacteria and introduced new conceptual models in pulmonology. The human lung can no longer be viewed as a sterile organ, and theories of disease need to address not only host cell biology but also complex host-microbe interactions.

The lung microbiome field is nascent and rapidly evolving in scope and volume. Early observations of disease-associated microbiota and proposed mechanisms of actions will have to stand the tests of time and replication. Lung microbiome research is only a few years old, and many of the methodologies continue to develop, suggesting that our understanding of the lung microbiome and its role in health and disease will evolve in upcoming years. For these reasons, this chapter does not provide an exhaustive catalog of reported microbiota associations with lung disease. Instead, we review basic principles and important lessons learned in the first wave of lung microbiome research; provide an accessible overview of commonly used terminology, experimental and analytic approaches, and prevailing ecologic theories; and review key findings in the healthy lung microbiome and major lung diseases.

Table 17.1 provides definitions of commonly used terms necessary for understanding the lung microbiome literature.[1–5]

THE GENESIS OF THE LUNG MICROBIOME FIELD

Since the introduction of the germ theory and Koch's postulates,[6] our view of human-associated microbes has been formed primarily through the lens of a microscope focused over ex vivo cultured bacteria. After completion of the Human Genome Project, technological innovations in massive parallel sequencing of nucleic acids (via NGS) allowed a culture-independent revolution in microbiology.[7,8] With NGS studies of 18 body site specimens, the first phase of the Human Microbiome Project revealed microbial communities with enormous diversity, functional capacity, and interpersonal variability in all examined loci.[9,10] Mainly composed of bacteria, but also including fungi, viruses, and archaea, the microbiota of the entire human body are estimated to amass a total of 3.8×10^{13} cells with more than 2 million genes.[11] The human microbiome is emerging as a major contributor to human health, conceptualized as an internalized organ that helps modulate immune responses, host metabolism, mucosal barrier homeostasis, and colonization resistance against pathogens.[1] Microbiome disruptions can lead to disease via loss of commensal physiology, pathogen invasion, production of bacterial metabolites, and dysregulation of the host inflammatory response.[2,12]

The lungs were not included among the 18 body sites examined in the Human Microbiome Project published in 2012,[9,10] perhaps as a reflection of a belief of lung sterility, in addition to practical difficulties in sampling the lower airways of healthy individuals. This omission contributed to a considerable delay in systematic investigations. Early reports of culture-independent bacterial identification in bronchoscopic samples from healthy lungs were met with skepticism.[4] The detected bacterial DNA was attributed to procedural contamination of the bronchoscope during passage through the high biomass oropharynx. However,

Table 17.1 Commonly Used Terms in the Microbiome Literature

GENERAL TERMS

Human microbiome	The collection of all genomes of microbes (including bacteria, viruses, fungi, archaea, and protozoa) in the human body
Microbiota	The assemblage of microbes in a defined ecosystem
"Meta-omics": Metagenome Metatranscriptome Metaproteome Metabolome	The total content of a microbial community in terms of: Genomic DNA Transcribed RNA Entire protein complement Metabolite pool
Commensal bacteria	Bacteria that provide benefits to the human host without being affected by it
Symbiotic bacteria	Bacteria in a mutually beneficial relationship with the human host
Dysbiosis	Disruption of the normal structure and function of the microbiome that is detrimental for the host

TERMS FOR SEQUENCING TECHNOLOGIES

Culture-independent technique	Molecular technique that analyzes biologic material directly from a sample and not from cultured microbes
Marker	A DNA sequence that identifies the genome that contains it
Amplicon sequencing	Amplification (with polymerase chain reaction) and sequencing of specific markers
16S ribosomal RNA gene	16S ribosomal subunit gene, unique to prokaryotic cells, with highly preserved sequence and specific hypervariable regions used as markers for bacterial identification
Metagenomic shotgun sequencing	Sequencing of short, random DNA/RNA fragments in an undirected whole-genome fashion

BIOINFORMATICS/ECOLOGY TERMS

Operational taxonomic units	Classification for amplicon sequences clustered based on a similarity threshold (e.g., >97%) as a proxy for species-level taxonomic assignment.
Abundance	Prevalence of a particular taxonomic group in a microbial community
Richness	Number of taxonomic groups in a microbial community
Evenness	Relative abundance of different taxonomic groups
Alpha diversity	Within-sample taxonomic diversity (including richness and evenness) as a summary statistic of a single population
Beta diversity	Between-sample taxonomic diversity describing absolute or relative taxonomic overlap between samples

carefully designed, multicenter studies from the Lung HIV Microbiome Project identified bacterial DNA sequences from the *lower respiratory tract* (LRT) across different cohorts, with a minimal effect of pharyngeal carryover contamination.[13–15] After these seminal observations the field has been growing rapidly.[16] In retrospect the notion of lung sterility appears a rather implausible one. Given that bacterial communities can be found even in the most extreme environmental niches on earth,[17] it is now counterintuitive to theorize that no bacteria should be expected to be found in the warm and moist mucosal surfaces of the lower airways, centimeters away from the bacteria-rich oropharynx and subject to an influx of bacteria with breathing and with subclinical microaspiration.[18] With the concept of the lung microbiome now widely accepted, the roles of lung microbes are being examined in a wide spectrum of diseases.

TECHNOLOGIES FOR MICROBIOME STUDIES

High-throughput, culture-independent technologies have allowed comprehensive microbiota analyses that were not possible using culture-based methods. Cultures are inherently selective, identifying only the living microbes at the time of sampling that are able to grow in the specific media and incubation conditions used. Although recent methodologic developments with combinations of multiple growth conditions and prolonged incubation have increased the scope of culture-based approaches (culturomics),[19–21] such methods are laborious and not possible in large-scale lung microbiome studies. By using assays for specific molecules of interest (e.g., nucleic acids, proteins, or metabolites), culture-independent methods allow for organisms in a sample to be detected regardless of viability or specific growth conditions.[7,8,22] Such methods are advantageous in terms of comprehensiveness (capturing organisms without the need for ex vivo growth) and efficiency (ability to analyze millions of multiplexed sequences in a single experiment). An overview of the available -omics approaches for microbiome studies, moving from DNA to RNA to protein-based approaches, is provided in Fig. 17.1. DNA approaches offer information on the composition of the microbial community, whereas RNA, protein, and metabolite approaches provide functional insights about the community of interest (e.g., revealing which pathways are expressed or what metabolic products are being produced). Because most of the available literature has used the efficient and highly reproducible DNA-based methods,[16] we provide a brief overview of the two main DNA-based approaches and refer to additional resources for further details on other techniques.[7,23–26]

Amplicon sequencing methods rely on marker DNA sequences in the genome that can be used as molecular fingerprints for the organisms of interest. The most commonly used method for bacteria involves 16S *ribosomal RNA* (rRNA) gene sequencing (16S).[27] *Polymerase chain reaction* (PCR) primers amplify conserved regions of the 16S gene common to all bacteria that flank interspersed hypervariable regions (regions 1–9). These hypervariable regions are the molecular fingerprints that can allow categorization of bacteria (Fig. 17.2). With PCR amplification of the hypervariable regions, millions of short genome sequences (typically <250 base pairs) can be generated and then aligned, sorted, and classified according to publicly available databases. Sequences that are similar above a certain threshold (often >97%) are grouped together into *operational taxonomic units* (OTUs or taxa) as a proxy for bacterial species, although often these OTUs can only be identified to

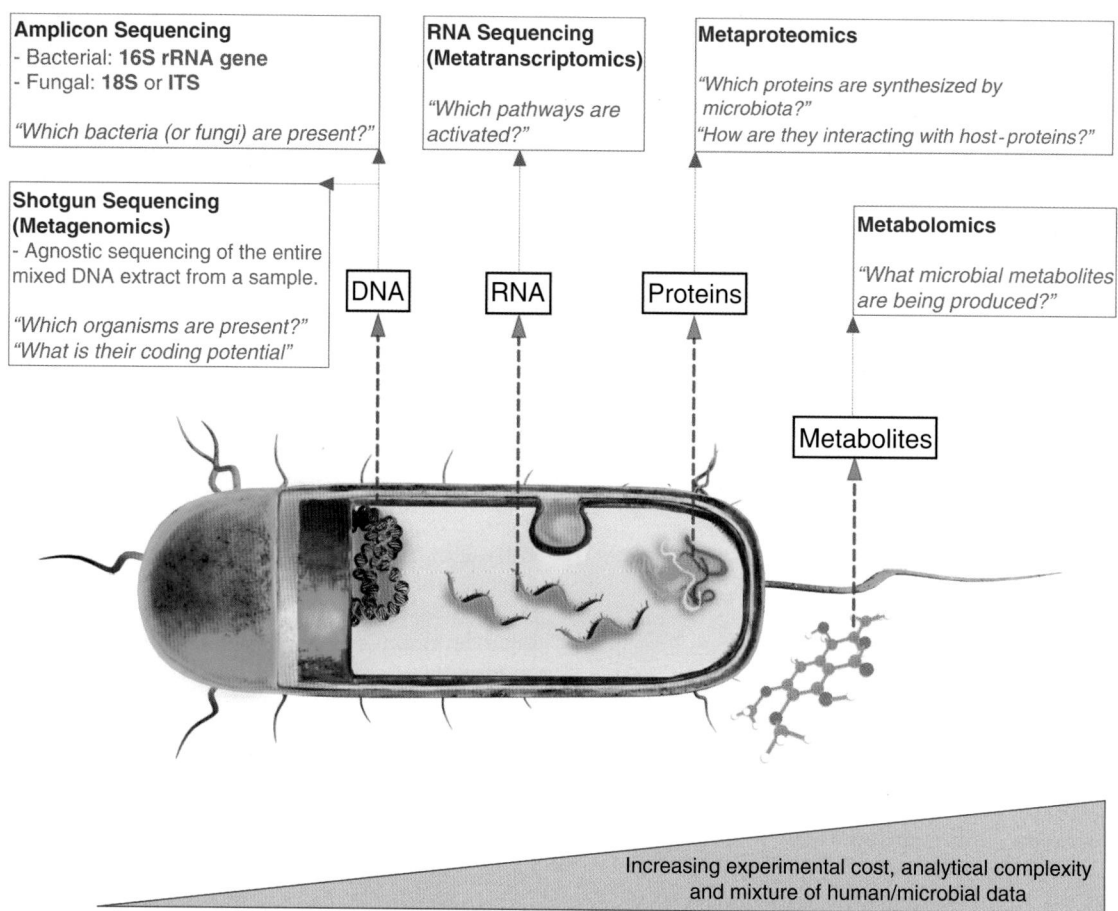

Figure 17.1 Overview of available -omics approaches for culture-independent studies of microbiota. Available technologies are structured according to the central dogma of biology, that is, from DNA- to RNA- to protein/metabolite-based approaches. DNA-based approaches are the most widely used due to the stability of DNA molecules and standardization of experimental and analytic pipelines. DNA methods include both amplicon sequencing (e.g., 16S ribosomal RNA gene sequencing for bacteria) and metagenomic shotgun sequencing for community-wide agnostic microbial detection. Metatranscriptomics, metaproteomics, and metabolomics approaches can offer more functional insights about the community of interest but are associated with higher experimental costs, analytic complexity, and difficulties in disentangling human from microbial data. ITS, internal transcribed spacer.

a genus level.[28] The end result of this approach is a population census for each sample, that is, how many times each taxonomic group was encountered, that can then be used for further analytic processing. *Quantitative PCR* (qPCR) of the 16S rRNA gene can approximate the absolute bacterial load present in each sample but, because there may be more than one 16S gene copy per bacterium, precise bacterial counts are not possible.[29] The 16S approach is reproducible and cost-effective and has become the workhorse method for large-scale microbiome studies. Drawbacks of 16S include the narrow scope (capturing only bacteria and not viruses or fungi), limited resolution (only genus-level taxonomy can be predicted accurately), lack of information on the full bacterial genome, and sensitivity to potential biases in the experimental pipeline (primer selection, amplification biases, etc.).[16] Similar amplicon sequencing approaches are available for fungi, by sequencing the 18S rRNA subunit or an internal transcriber spacer region, but not for viruses.[30]

Metagenomic shotgun sequencing techniques sequence the entire mixture of DNA present in a sample (see Fig. 17.2). The derived sequences are compared against reference genomes or gene catalogs for assignment to specific organisms and pathways. This approach allows improved

taxonomic resolution (e.g., ability to distinguish a sequence belonging to *Staphylococcus aureus* vs. *Staphylococcus epidermidis* when 16S can only identify the genus *Staphylococcus*) and can offer insights into the functional capability of a community (e.g., abundance of specific genes and pathways).[8] Metagenomics can capture DNA from all successfully extracted organisms and thus reveal comprehensive microbial profiles. However, the high abundance of human DNA present in low microbial biomass samples, such as those from the lung, makes metagenomic experiments impractical and expensive because the vast majority of sequences detected are of human origin.[31] Several methods have been developed to deplete human genomic DNA from clinical samples,[32–34] but given current technical challenges and associated costs, the lung microbiome literature contains few metagenomic studies.[16]

Regardless of the sequencing approach used, culture-independent methods are vulnerable to contamination risks in every step of the experimental pipeline.[35] Reagent contamination is a threat for generating false-positive results (type I errors) when working with low microbial biomass samples, and thus close attention is needed to minimize, identify, and account for effects of contaminating DNA in sequencing experiments.[26,35,36]

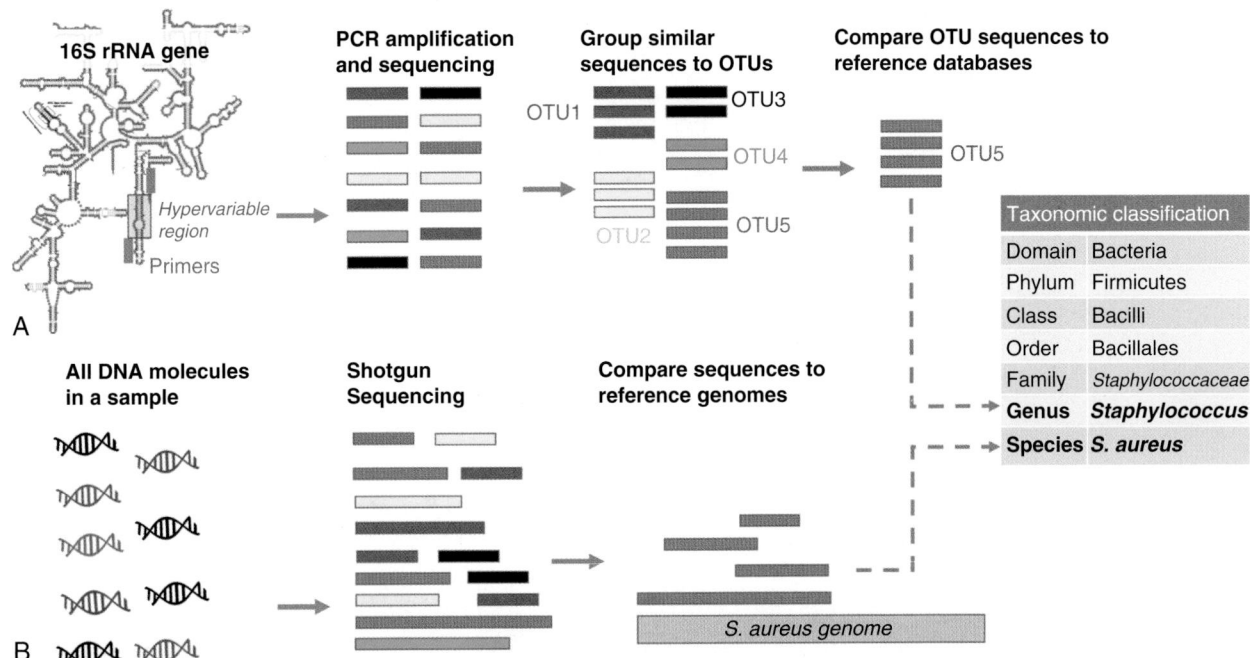

Figure 17.2 **Amplicon sequencing vs. metagenomic shotgun sequencing.** (A) Amplicon sequencing of the 16S *ribosomal RNA* (rRNA) gene for bacteria. Highly conserved regions in the 16S gene allow the design of *polymerase chain reaction* (PCR) primers *(blue vertical bars)* for amplification of interspersed hypervariable regions with informative genomic variation *(red vertical shaded bar).* The PCR amplicons are sequenced in parallel with barcoding methods to allow multiplexing of many samples, and then they are grouped together based on similarity thresholds to *operational taxonomic units* (OTUs) as proxies for bacterial taxa. An alternative method to OTU similarity thresholds applies individual comparisons between sequences for distinguishing sequence variants and inferring bacterial origin (amplicon sequencing variants). Regardless of approach used, the taxa (OTUs) are compared against reference databases to obtain taxonomic information for this group of sequences, which can typically be reliably predicted at the genus level of taxonomic classification. (B) Metagenomic shotgun sequencing involves agnostic sequencing of all DNA molecules in a sample. The derived sequences are then compared against reference genomes (or gene catalogs) to obtain more detailed, species- or strain-level identification of the organism of interest (bacterial, fungal, or viral) and protein coding potential.

SEQUENCING DATA ANALYSIS

After the completion of a sequencing experiment and appropriate bioinformatic data processing[37,38] (see Fig. 17.2), the final output consists of a taxonomic table, that is, a population census expressed as either absolute number or relative abundance of taxa for each sample. Although analyses of such multidimensional data can be undertaken at many different levels of complexity and sophistication, widely used approaches are based on main principles of microbial and environmental ecology theory.[27,39,40] Microbiome sequencing data lend themselves to analyses of diversity measures within (alpha) and between (beta) samples, as well as comparisons of taxonomic abundance, as illustrated in the example analysis in Fig. 17.3.

STUDY DESIGN APPROACHES FOR MICROBIOME STUDIES OF THE RESPIRATORY TRACT

HUMAN STUDIES

Multiple different sampling approaches have been used for direct study of *upper respiratory tract* (URT) and LRT microbiota in humans, including nasopharyngeal or oropharyngeal swabbing, induced or expectorated sputum, endotracheal aspirate, *bronchoalveolar lavage* (BAL),

bronchoscopic protected specimen brushing, and surgical lung biopsy (eFig. 17.1). Although no gold-standard approach exists, and different samples can offer complementary information, attention to procedural sterility and collection of procedural experimental controls (e.g., sterile saline, bronchoscope rinse before insertion) is essential to minimize, detect, and control procedural contamination, especially for LRT samples.[26]

ANIMAL MODEL STUDIES

Animal modeling is a powerful tool for mechanistic interrogations of lung microbiota in respiratory diseases.[41–44] This approach allows controlling microbial exposure in ways that are impossible for human studies, such as with germ-free animals, microbiota depletion with intensive antibiotic treatments, introduction of specific bacteria (e.g., gnotobiotic animals),[45] or microbial replacement (e.g., with fecal transplant or oral gavage).[16] Of note, with mice, LRT sampling is most reproducibly achieved by using whole-lung homogenate instead of BAL.[46,47] Nonetheless, animal studies are not free from confounding, because studies have shown the influences of cage and cohousing on lung microbiota of coprophagic mice, and such factors need to be taken into account in study designs.[46,48] Mice are the most commonly used animal models in this literature, but given the anatomic and ecologic differences of the mouse and human respiratory tracts, mice also present challenges in providing information relevant to human biology. In this regard,

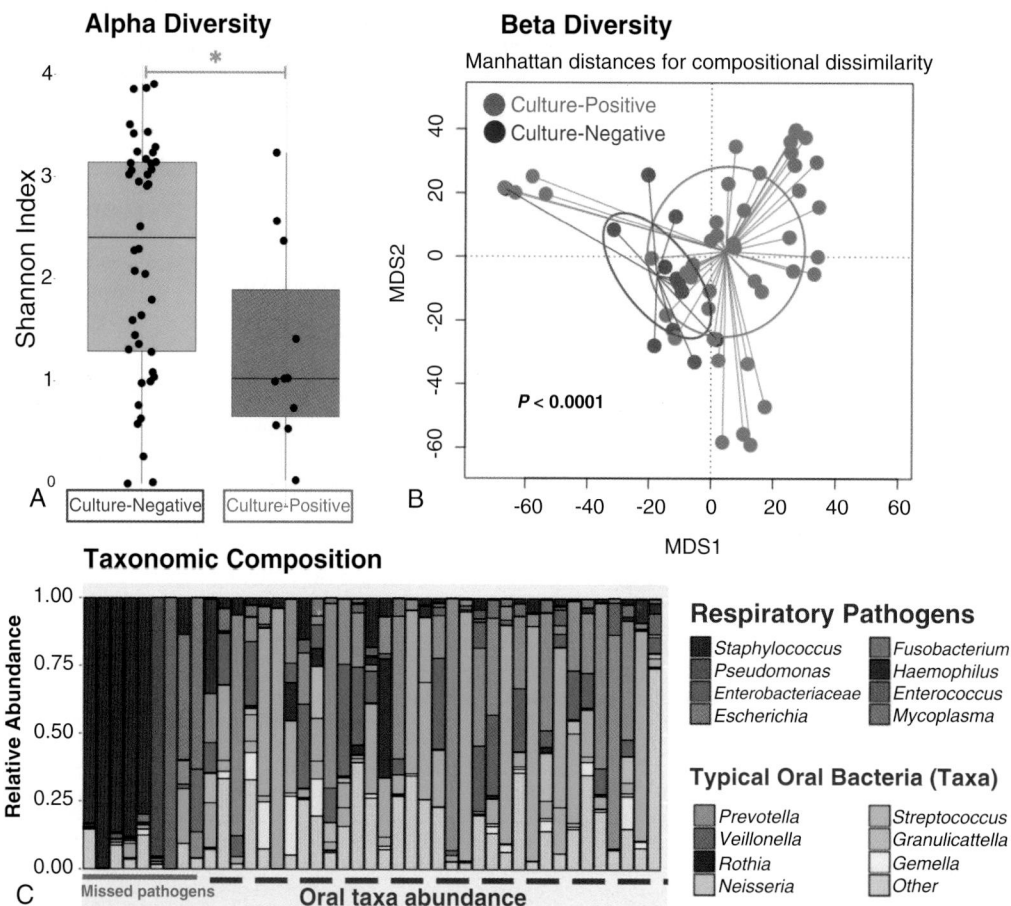

Figure 17.3 Common analytic approaches for microbiome data. Analyses applied in a study example of microbial communities analyzed with 16S sequencing from culture-positive and -negative endotracheal aspirate samples obtained from critically ill mechanically ventilated patients. (A) *Alpha diversity* examines the organismal richness of an individual sample (i.e., *How many different OTUs [i.e., taxa] are present?*) and the evenness of the organisms' abundance distribution in the sample (i.e., *How are the microbes balanced to each other, are they similar in abundance, or do some species dominate others?*). Commonly used metrics include Chao1, Shannon, Simpson, or Faith's index.[27,40] In general, for respiratory microbial communities, high alpha diversity is considered a marker of community fitness and often, but not always, associated with health. In the example of a study of mechanically ventilated patients with culture-positive and -negative endotracheal aspirates,[113] culture-positive samples had much lower alpha diversity (Shannon index) compared to culture-negative samples, indicating that culture-positive communities were dominated by fewer (pathogenic) bacterial taxa. (B) *Beta diversity* compares taxonomic dissimilarity between each pair of samples, generating a matrix of beta diversity distances between all pairs of samples in a study. Many different beta diversity metrics are available, assessing either relative abundance (e.g., Bray-Curtis, weighted UniFrac, or Manhattan) or presence/absence of taxa (e.g., Jaccard or unweighted UniFrac). With available software, beta diversity metrics can be statistically compared for differential clustering between groups of interest (e.g., *Do communities in patients with asthma differ from healthy controls?*) and can also be used for visualizing compositional differences with ordination techniques that reduce the dimensionality of data into interpretable plots, such as the *principal coordinates analysis method* (PCoA). In panel B, the PCoA plot illustrates different clustering of culture-positive versus culture-negative samples, suggesting differences in underlying taxonomic composition. Each circle represents a microbial community, and distance between individual communities on this two-dimensional plot depicts compositional dissimilarities. Formal statistical comparison with *permutation analysis of variance* (PERMANOVA) showed statistically significant differences in beta diversity by culture positivity ($P < 0.0001$). (C) *Taxonomic composition* and *differential abundance* describe individual samples in terms of their component taxa (genera or species) expressed in relative or absolute abundance. Comparisons for differentially abundant taxa or functional elements (e.g., genes or pathways) between groups of interest can reveal important organisms or other features that explain differences in communities. Nonetheless, microbiome data are compositional and interdependent in nature, requiring dedicated analytic methods for robust assessment of differential abundances.[40] In panel C the relative abundance at the genus level for culture-negative samples is shown. Each bar represents a separate sample, and the relative height of each component color represents the relative abundance for each taxon. Twenty percent of culture-negative samples were dominated by common respiratory pathogen taxa (e.g., *Staphylococcus* or *Pseudomonas*) (see "Missed pathogens" on *x*-axis), whereas the remaining 80% had high abundance of typical members of the oral microbiome (e.g., *Prevotella*, *Veillonella* and *Streptococcus*) (see "Oral taxa abundance" on *x*-axis). Overall, the analytic considerations described above apply not only to DNA sequencing data but also to functional -omics approaches, although analytic pipelines and software platforms are less standardized.

nonhuman primates can offer important experimental insights (see also Chapter 1 for comparison of human and mouse lungs).

THE HEALTHY LUNG MICROBIOME

A key question before studying the role of the microbiome in disease is its composition in health. Multicenter NGS studies

of BAL from healthy individuals reveal significant interpersonal variability in lung microbial communities,[13,14] but with some common, recognizable features.

1. *Low biomass:* BAL fluid from healthy subjects analyzed by 16S rRNA gene qPCR has a much lower bacterial load (estimated bacterial density approximately 10^{2-3} bacteria/mL of BAL fluid[3,49–52]) compared to oral wash fluid (density estimates in range of 10^{5-6} bacteria/mL of oral wash).[49,50,52] The differences are considered to be

much greater than would be accounted for by differences in dilution.

2. *High alpha diversity:* Although specific estimates of alpha diversity vary among studies based on experimental and analytic differences, BAL communities from healthy subjects are generally characterized by higher alpha diversity indices[13] compared to diseased subjects[53,54] (see Fig. 17.3).

3. *Oral similarity:* The higher compositional similarity of lung communities with corresponding oral and not nasal communities is a reproducible finding in many studies,[13,50,52,55,56] which has reinforced the notion of the mouth (and not the nose) as the source of bacteria in healthy lungs.

4. *Limited regional heterogeneity:* In healthy subjects who underwent bronchoscopic sampling of multiple sites, microbial communities differed more between than within subjects, that is, a given individual's right middle lobe community more closely resembles the same individual's left upper lobe than another individual's right middle lobe.[57]

Firmicutes and Bacteroidetes are the two dominant phyla in healthy individuals, with lower abundance of Proteobacteria phylum organisms, Actinobacteria, and Fusobacteria.[13,52,55,58,59] The number of reported unique taxa (community richness) present in BAL samples is in the range of approximately 50 taxa per sample.[13,50,56,60] Bacteria recovered by culture comprise 61% of the taxa detected by 16S sequencing, indicating that NGS-profiles in BAL specimens provide representations of viable bacterial communities.[60]

Although typical oral-origin bacteria are predominantly found in the lung microbiome, their presence is not always detected in healthy individuals. Based on unsupervised clustering techniques, there appear to be two main profiles, referred to as *pneumotypes,* with similar frequency: a supraglottic pneumotype with higher bacterial load that contains typical members of the oral microbiome, such as *Prevotella, Veillonella,* and *Rothia,* and a background pneumotype that is enriched for taxa found in background controls (i.e., experimental noise), such as *Acidocella, Pseudomonas,* and *Sphingomonas.*[52,55] A notable exception to the predominance of supraglottic bacteria is the case of *Tropheryma whipplei,* a bacterium that is detected in up to a quarter of BAL samples from healthy subjects.[13,61–63] *T. whipplei* is associated with the gut microbiome (and the pathogenesis of Whipple disease) and is generally not detected in the mouth; its presence in the lungs may indicate site-specific reproduction and selective growth.

The lung *mycobiome* has been the subject of only a few studies in healthy individuals. Nonetheless, fungal DNA has been reproducibly detected and sequenced with amplicon approaches, with distinct and variable communities between individuals.[30,64–66] Predominant fungal taxa include members of the family Davidiellaceae, and the genera *Cladosporium, Eurotium, Penicillium,* and *Aspergillus,* whereas *Pneumocystis* colonization is also found in a small proportion of healthy individuals.[49,64]

The lung virome has not yet been characterized in detail because of methodologic challenges. Amplicon sequencing has been constrained because there is no conserved genomic region in DNA or RNA viruses to enable the design of primers. With metagenomic shotgun sequencing, high prevalence of members of the *Anelloviridae* family and bacteriophages have been detected.[67,68]

DERIVATION OF THE LUNG MICROBIOME

Multiple theories have been proposed to explain the formation of the lung microbiome in health and its disruption with disease.[26] Whether the relatively low microbial population density in the LRT is resident and reproducing in the lungs or whether it represents the net result of continuous population renewal from influx and efflux of microbes from the high biomass URT is not completely established. According to the widely cited *adapted model of island biogeography,*[12,26,57,69] the URT is the primary source of microbes in the lungs (Fig. 17.4). The lungs are conceptualized as microbial islands whose members are influenced by the rates of microbial immigration from the URT "mainland" (through inhalation, microaspiration, or mucosal dispersion) and elimination from the lung "island" (through mucociliary clearance, cough, and host mucosal defense mechanisms).[12,26,57,69,70] The net balance of these opposing forces determines the formation of a highly diverse, but low biomass, lung microbiome in health. Subclinical microaspiration even in healthy asymptomatic individuals is a well-established phenomenon that likely accounts for a continuous low-grade influx of bacteria in the lungs (see Chapter 43).[56] Changes in the rates of immigration and elimination (e.g., oropharyngeal dysphagia, diminished cough reflex) could reset this equilibrium and alter the lung microbial community. The lung microbiome may also be impacted by regional reproductive rates of microbes in the lungs as determined by nutrient availability, immune defenses, and environmental conditions (see Fig. 17.4). Whereas environmental conditions may not be conducive to bacterial proliferation in health, the altered ecosystem of diseased lungs with anatomic distortion and aberrant physiology (e.g., with stagnant nutrient-rich mucus in inflamed cystic fibrosis airways) can lead to bacterial overgrowth, further mucosal injury, inflammation, and a vicious cycle for establishment of *dysbiosis*—the disruption of the normal microbiome leading to harm to the host.[69] Finally, the concept of a gut-lung axis for microbiota has been proposed, with lung communities being influenced by gut microbiota by direct translocation of intestinal organisms to the lungs in states of abnormal gut permeability,[44] by shaping of the systemic immune response from the gut microbiome, by remote effects of gut microbe-derived components and metabolites on airway physiology and microbiota, or a combination of these mechanisms.[71,72]

THE EARLY LIFE ORIGINS OF THE HUMAN LUNG MICROBIOME

From birth and delivery to the outer microbial world and throughout early childhood development, there is evidence of dynamic adaptation of respiratory communities.[73]

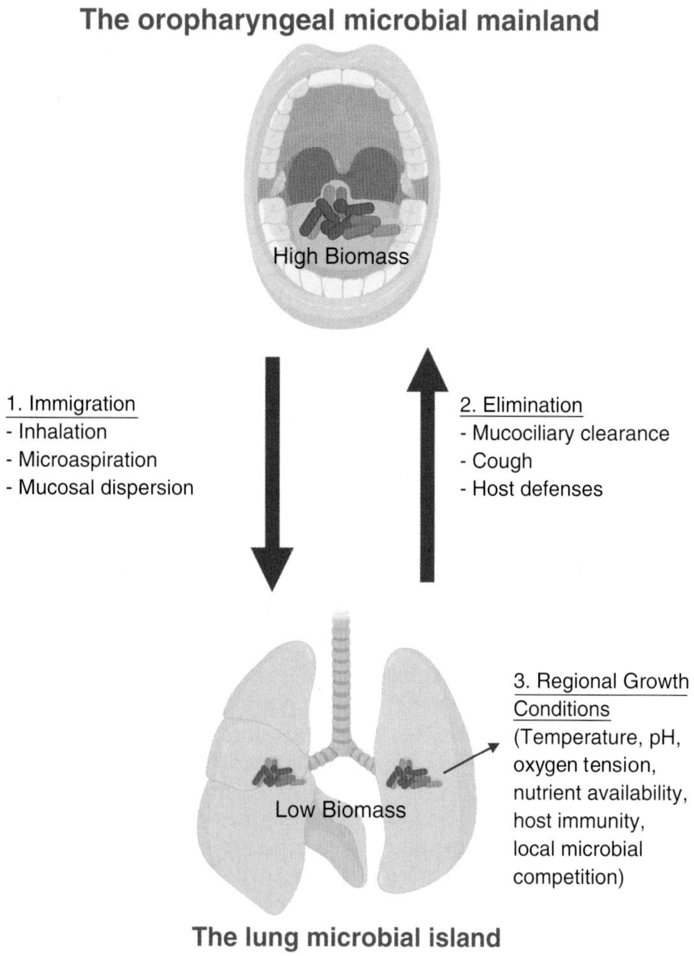

The oropharyngeal microbial mainland

High Biomass

1. Immigration
- Inhalation
- Microaspiration
- Mucosal dispersion

2. Elimination
- Mucociliary clearance
- Cough
- Host defenses

3. Regional Growth
Conditions
(Temperature, pH,
oxygen tension,
nutrient availability,
host immunity,
local microbial
competition)

Low Biomass

The lung microbial island

Figure 17.4 The adapted model of island biogeography for the formation of the lung microbiome in health and its disruption in disease. This model explains key features of the oral-lung axis: the large differences in microbial density, the taxonomic similarity of communities, and their gravitational relationship in humans, the only primates walking upright. According to the model, there is continuous influx and efflux of microbes in the lungs, with immigration from the high biomass oropharyngeal mainland (microbial source) to the low biomass lung islands (via microaspiration, inhalation, or direct mucosal dispersion) and elimination via cough, mucociliary escalator clearance, or phagocytosis. In health, the net balance between immigration and elimination determines the composition and load of microbes in the lungs. In disease, altered environmental growth conditions are expected to have a larger impact on shaping the lung microbial communities by creation of specific niches and enabling selective growth.

Vaginally born children are seeded with maternal gut/urogenital microbiota, whereas caesarean-born children carry typical skin bacteria.[74,75] Although the effects of such initial colonization appear to be transient, children who are born vaginally and/or are breastfed demonstrate more swift and predictable transition to stable microbial profiles associated with lower risk of respiratory illnesses (e.g., higher abundance of URT *Moraxella, Corynebacterium,* and *Dolosigranulum* taxa and lower abundance of *S. aureus*).[75,76] The "maturation" process of the respiratory microbiome in childhood is subject to multiple environmental influences, including infections and antibiotics, vaccination, dietary changes, daycare or school exposures, and pets in the household.[3] Although the gut microbiota matures into an adult-like profile by the first 3 years of life,[77] the time required to establish an adult-like pneumotype is unknown. Changes in the lung microbiome beyond childhood have not been defined.

THE LUNG MICROBIOME IN DISEASE

An expanding body of literature has reported associations between alterations in microbial profiles and disease. Compared with the healthy LRT, lung diseases can

be associated with a high bacterial load by 16S qPCR, lower alpha diversity of LRT communities, and higher abundance of Proteobacteria phylum organisms (instead of the normal Firmicutes and Bacteroidetes composition). However, it remains to be determined whether such microbiome perturbations are disease specific, causally related, and clinically relevant. Most evidence consists of single-center, cross-sectional, observational surveys of LRT samples with 16S sequencing.[16] Cross-sectional study designs do not allow examination of longitudinal dynamics or determining temporality and directionality of effects, that is, "Does the microbiome change before disease onset and lead to disease or vice versa?" With few exceptions,[13,14,61] the small datasets collected in different centers have not yet been synthesized in multicenter analyses to examine the robustness and generalizability of findings across populations. In addition, the descriptive nature of 16S-based studies may miss informative species-level information or functional disruptions, detection of which would require more sophisticated meta-omics approaches. Thus interpretation for much of the available evidence needs to be cautious and viewed as hypothesis-generating for subsequent studies.

In the next sections we review key findings of selected human and animal model lung microbiome studies of obstructive airway diseases, interstitial lung diseases, infectious diseases, lung cancer, lung transplantation, *acute respiratory distress syndrome* (ARDS) and other conditions.

OBSTRUCTIVE DISEASES

Asthma

Research efforts in asthma have broadly focused on two different phases of disease pathogenesis: first, on early-life interactions between microbiota (gut and URT) with risk of asthma development, and second, on associations between LRT microbiota with disease severity and response to treatment in adults.[78,79] Studies of the nasopharyngeal microbiome in children have shown associations between altered microbial communities, recurrent viral illnesses, and subsequent risk of asthma development. Alpha diversity of URT communities has been inversely associated with sensitization to house dust mites.[80] Similarly, a seminal study comparing Amish children (raised on traditional farms with low prevalence of asthma) with Hutterite children (raised on highly industrialized farms with high prevalence of asthma) found that differences in dust microbial composition and endotoxin load from the two housing environments were associated with very different innate immunity responses and with protection from asthma in Amish children.[81] Patterns of gut microbiome composition in young children have also been associated with increased risk for asthma.[82] In adults with established asthma, features of dysbiosis, including reduced alpha diversity and higher proteobacteria abundance (mainly due to enrichment for *Moraxella* and *Haemophilus*), have been associated with neutrophilic inflammation, degree of airflow obstruction, and resistance to corticosteroids.[83–86] Different microbial profiles found in different asthma subphenotypes (e.g., low bacterial load in patients with high type 2 inflammation)[87] suggest potential microbial contributors (and thus treatment targets) for observed clinical heterogeneity in asthma.

Chronic Obstructive Pulmonary Disease

Unlike asthma, where dysbiosis has been associated with future risk of disease development and severity across the entire spectrum, few differences in microbiomes have been observed among smokers, nonsmokers, and those with mild-to-moderate COPD.[79] Instead, dysbiosis in COPD has been more consistently detected in patients in severe disease by *Global Initiative for Chronic Obstructive Lung Disease* (GOLD) criteria,[4,79] with an increase of the Proteobacteria (mainly *Haemophilus* enrichment) and a decrease of the Bacteroidetes phylum.[59,88,89] Patients with acute exacerbations have shifts in the sputum microbiome, including low alpha diversity and increased abundance of *Staphylococcus*,[90,91] which may predict long-term adverse outcomes after hospital discharge.[92]

Cystic Fibrosis

Cystic fibrosis (CF) is the lung disease with the largest number of published microbiome studies in adult and pediatric populations.[16] Culture-independent methods have revealed a far greater microbial complexity than detected by cultures, and microbiome profiles are associated with host inflammation. Through early adulthood, diversity decreases and dominance develops of typical CF pathogens of the Proteobacteria phylum (*Pseudomonas*, *Burkholderia*, and *Achromobacter*) or *Staphylococcus* taxa.[53,54,93–95] With longitudinal analyses, a complex, multidirectional relationship between disease progression and airway microbiota has emerged: Airways progressively obstructed with mucus create niches for characteristic microbiota, which relate to host inflammation and infectious exacerbations, triggering repeated antibiotic exposures that further select for resistant bacteria, thereby establishing a vicious cycle of dysbiosis and inflammation.[79,96]

Non–Cystic Fibrosis Bronchiectasis

The microbiome of non-CF bronchiectatic diseases is not as well studied. Among patients with established bronchiectasis, the lung microbiome remains relatively stable over time, with separate clusters of *Pseudomonas* or *Haemophilus* dominance.[97] Of importance, patients with low-diversity communities may experience worsening airway obstruction.[97]

INTERSTITIAL LUNG DISEASES

Idiopathic Pulmonary Fibrosis

The lung microbiome has been implicated in *idiopathic pulmonary fibrosis* (IPF) pathogenesis based on the results of two cohort studies from patients with early stage IPF, in which high bacterial burden by 16S qPCR was independently associated with shorter patient survival.[43,98] Additional features of BAL microbial communities correlated with systemic and local innate immune responses and inflammation.[43,99,100] In murine models of bleomycin-induced fibrosis, lung dysbiosis preceded peak lung injury, whereas germ-free mice had longer survival.[43] These provocative findings have provided a rationale for studies of chronic antibiotic treatments in early IPF.[101,102] Nonetheless, the exact location of lung microbiota in IPF remains to be defined, with tissue-based examination suggesting that areas of end-stage honeycombing are devoid of bacterial loads above the detection threshold.[103,104]

Sarcoidosis

Despite long-standing hypotheses about potential microbial triggers and perpetuators of sarcoid-related granulomatous inflammation,[105] no reproducible microbial profile has emerged in available studies to date,[105–109] with sensitive metagenomic analyses revealing no clearly associated microbial lineages.[108]

INFECTIOUS DISEASES

Pneumonia

In multiple observational studies, NGS techniques have been leveraged for better understanding of the molecular microbiology of infectious pneumonia,[110] as well as for development of diagnostics to overcome the limitations of cultures.[31,111,112] Individual microbial profiles vary depending on the causative pathogen(s) in cases of community- or hospital/ventilator-acquired pneumonia.[32,113–125] In cases caused by a single pathogen, diversity collapses, and the community is dominated by the pathogen. However, NGS studies have also revealed more complex profiles, that is, by identifying abundant organisms not frequently considered typical respiratory pathogens, organisms that are difficult to culture, and oral bacteria, routinely dismissed as non-pathogenic contaminants of LRT samples in clinical microbiology.[113,120,123,126,127] With integration of host responses and microbial profiles,[113,125] NGS studies in pneumonia can help redefine concepts of "pathogenicity" and "colonization versus infection" for respiratory microbiota.

Nontuberculous Mycobacteria Infection

The microbial profiles of samples from patients with *nontuberculous mycobacteria* (NTM) have disclosed an ecologic profile distinct from other bacterial infections: The causative NTM DNA has low abundance, near or below the limit of detection of dedicated molecular methods,[128] suggesting that NGS approaches may have inadequate sensitivity compared to cultures for NTM.[129]

Tuberculosis

Despite the global burden of tuberculosis, very limited knowledge of LRT microbiota is available for patients with or at risk for *tuberculosis* (TB).[130–132] High abundance of oral anaerobes (*Prevotella*) and elevated serum short-chain fatty acids have been associated with diminished production of protective antituberculous cytokines (e.g., interferon-γ and interleukin-17) and increased risk for TB infection.[131] In a macaque model, TB infection led to modest shifts of lung microbiota composition with enrichment for typical oral taxa, and not with the Actinomycetales order to which the *Mycobacterium* genus belongs. Important interactions with the gut microbiome have been reported,[133–135] with risk of *Mycobacterium tuberculosis* infection and progression modified by intestinal *Helicobacter* coinfection.[136]

Human Immunodeficiency Virus Lung Disease

Systematic examination of LRT microbiota with NGS was first performed in *persons with human immunodeficiency virus* (PWH). In initial studies, no major differences in microbial communities were found between generally healthy PWH and uninfected individuals, although *T. whipplei* was more common in PWH.[13,137,138] In PWH studied before and after initiation of antiretroviral therapy, their oral taxa abundance in BAL progressively increased.[139] Systems biology approaches have identified significant correlations between BAL metabolites, microbiota, and peripheral CD4 counts in PWH, suggesting a functional impact of the lung microbiome.[140]

LUNG CANCER

Compared to animals with a normal microbiome, germ-free animals demonstrate a lower risk of spontaneous or induced carcinogenesis, suggesting a potential role for the microbiome in cancer.[141] However, analyses of microbial communities in tumors or adjacent tissue in lung cancer patients have not disclosed a clear signal.[142–146] *Streptococcus* and *Veillonella* taxa have been associated with up-regulation of carcinogenic signaling pathways (*extracellular signal-regulated kinase* [ERK] and *phosphatidylinositol-3-kinase* [PI3K]) both in vivo and in vitro, suggesting a potential mechanistic link.[145] The microbiome may also play a role in response to therapy. For example, gut microbiota appear to modulate the response to immune checkpoint inhibitor therapy for non–small cell lung cancers, suggesting potential to improve clinical response rates by targeting the gut microbiome.[147]

LUNG TRANSPLANT

Given the intensive immunosuppressive therapy and associations of prior allograft infections with rejection, the role of lung microbiota in transplant recipients is actively investigated in both short-term (primary graft dysfunction) and long-term (*chronic lung allograft dysfunction* [CLAD]) outcomes.[148,149] Lung transplant recipients with clinical suspicion of pneumonia have low lung microbial community diversity and elevated alveolar cytokine and catecholamine levels, indicative of host inflammation and injury.[150,151] Both culture-based and culture-independent studies have shown that bacterial (mainly *S. aureus* and *P. aeruginosa*), viral (cytomegalovirus), and fungal (*Aspergillus*) detection in lung allografts are associated with risk for CLAD.[148,149,152,153] BAL microbiota are also associated with proinflammatory myeloid-derived suppressor cells and catabolic lung remodeling gene expression, potentially contributing to CLAD pathogenesis.[154,155]

ACUTE RESPIRATORY DISTRESS SYNDROME

The markedly altered ecosystem of the flooded alveolar space in ARDS, with nutrient-rich edema and intense host inflammation, may support increased microbial growth and further propagation of alveolar injury.[2,156] This hypothesis is reinforced by animal models of lipopolysaccharide-induced lung injury, where bacterial load increased fivefold in BAL samples due to a bloom of proteobacteria capable of metabolizing the alveolar nutrients.[42] In the few studies available in humans, enrichment of the lung microbiome with gut-associated bacteria (e.g., *Bacteroides*[44] or Enterobacteriaceae[157]) was associated with ARDS development and increased host inflammation. Antibiotic-mediated depletion of microbiota in mice leads to more severe ventilator-induced lung injury, suggesting that a healthy microbiome may also protect the host.[158]

OTHER LUNG DISEASES

The potential role of respiratory microbiota has also been investigated in other disease entities, including obstructive sleep apnea,[159] allergic bronchopulmonary aspergillosis,[160] pulmonary complications posthematopoietic cell transplant,[161] pulmonary hypertension,[162] and bronchopulmonary dysplasia,[163] among others. The reader is referred to the primary literature referenced for discussion of these emerging associations.

FUTURE DIRECTIONS FOR LUNG MICROBIOME RESEARCH

The transition of the lung microbiome field from its current, largely descriptive, hypothesis-generating studies into more mechanistic and targeted interventional studies will be necessary for clinical translation of related discoveries.[2,16]

Multi-omics data integration approaches, including deep phenotyping of host responses with detailed profiling of microbiota, supplemented by rigorous animal modeling experiments, can uncover new mechanisms of respiratory disease pathogenesis. With the evolution of rapid NGS platforms, real-time lung microbiome profiles may offer important diagnostic or prognostic information in clinical practice, such as improved accuracy for etiologic pathogen diagnosis in pneumonia [32,112,113,125,127] or risk stratification for patients with acute exacerbations with COPD.[92] Finally, there is potential for new therapeutic interventions targeting lung microbiota, either with direct manipulations (e.g., aerosolized drug delivery or URT community decontamination/reconstitution) or with indirect mediation via the gut-lung axis (e.g., use of probiotics or dietary interventions).[164] Although formidable challenges exist for advancing the lung microbiome research agenda, methodologic rigor and transparency in this nascent research field is expected to catalyze its maturation into a transformative new frontier of pulmonary medicine.

Key Points

- The study of the lung microbiome was made feasible by the introduction of culture-independent next-generation sequencing techniques of microbial DNA.
- The lung has a detectable microbiome even in healthy individuals, which is highly diverse, has a low bacterial biomass, and resembles the oral cavity microbiome in composition.
- Continuous microaspiration and elimination of microbes via the oropharynx are considered to be the main forces shaping the lung microbiome in health.
- Fungi and viruses are also detectable in the lung, but their communities and importance are less well understood.
- Studies of the lung microbiome are susceptible to contamination because of the low biomass in the lower respiratory tract.
- The lung microbiome may impact disease via infection, metabolite production, or modulation of host inflammatory pathways.
- Common alterations of the normal communities seen in various lung diseases include increase in bacterial biomass, loss of biodiversity, and shifts in community composition favoring pathogenic proteobacteria.
- The potentially causative role of microbiome changes in disease remains to be elucidated.

Key Readings

Biesbroek G, Tsivtsivadze E, Sanders EAM, et al. Early respiratory microbiota composition determines bacterial succession patterns and respiratory health in children. *Am J Respir Crit Care Med.* 2014;190(11):1283–1292.

Carney S, Clemente J, Cox MJ, et al. Methods in lung microbiome research. An American Thoracic Society Working Group report. *Am J Respir Cell Mol Biol.* 2019.

Charalampous T, Kay GL, Richardson H, et al. Nanopore metagenomics enables rapid clinical diagnosis of bacterial lower respiratory infection. *Nat Biotechnol.* 2019;37(7):783–792.

Cookson WOCM, Cox MJ, Moffatt MF. New opportunities for managing acute and chronic lung infections. *Nat Rev Microbiol.* 2018;16(2):111–120.

Cox MJ, Ege MJ, von Mutius E, eds. *The Lung Microbiome.* Sheffield, United Kingdom: European Respiratory Society; 2019.

Dickson RP, Erb-Downward JR, Falkowski NR, Hunter EM, Ashley SL, Huffnagle GB. The lung microbiota of healthy mice are highly variable, cluster by environment, and reflect variation in baseline lung innate immunity. *Am J Respir Crit Care Med.* 2018;198(4):497–508.

Dickson RP, Erb-Downward JR, Freeman CM, et al. Bacterial topography of the healthy human lower respiratory tract. *MBio.* 2017;8(1).

Huang YJ, Charlson ES, Collman RG, Colombini-Hatch S, Martinez FD, Senior RM. The role of the lung microbiome in health and disease. A National Heart, Lung, and Blood Institute workshop report. *Am J Respir Crit.* 2013;187(12):1382–1387.

Human Microbiome Project Consortium. Structure, function and diversity of the healthy human microbiome. *Nature.* 2012;486(7402):207–214.

Kitsios GD, Fitch A, Manatakis DV, et al. Respiratory microbiome profiling for etiologic diagnosis of pneumonia in mechanically ventilated patients. *Front Microbiol.* 2018;9:1413.

Langelier C, Kalantar KL, Moazed F, et al. Integrating host response and unbiased microbe detection for lower respiratory tract infection diagnosis in critically ill adults. *Proc Natl Acad Sci USA.* 2018;115(52):E12353–E12362.

Man WH, de Steenhuijsen Piters WAA, Bogaert D. The microbiota of the respiratory tract: gatekeeper to respiratory health. *Nat Rev Microbiol.* 2017;15(5):259–270.

Morris A, Beck JM, Schloss PD, et al. Comparison of the respiratory microbiome in healthy nonsmokers and smokers. *Am J Respir Crit Care Med.* 2013;187(10):1067–1075.

Poroyko V, Meng F, Meliton A, et al. Alterations of lung microbiota in a mouse model of LPS-induced lung injury. *Am J Physiol Lung Cell Mol Physiol.* 2015;309(1):L76–83.

Salter SJ, Cox MJ, Turek EM, et al. Reagent and laboratory contamination can critically impact sequence-based microbiome analyses. *BMC Biol.* 2014;12:87.

Segal LN, Clemente JC, Tsay J-CJ, et al. Enrichment of the lung microbiome with oral taxa is associated with lung inflammation of a Th17 phenotype. *Nat Microbiol.* 2016;1:16031.

Shenoy MK, Iwai S, Lin DL, et al. Immune response and mortality risk relate to distinct lung microbiomes in patients with HIV and pneumonia. *Am J Respir Crit Care Med.* 2017;195(1):104–114.

Stein MM, Hrusch CL, Gozdz J, et al. Innate immunity and asthma risk in Amish and Hutterite farm children. *N Engl J Med.* 2016;375(5):411–421.

Venkataraman A, Bassis CM, Beck JM, et al. Application of a neutral community model to assess structuring of the human lung microbiome. *MBio.* 2015;6(1).

Yadava K, Pattaroni C, Sichelstiel AK, et al. Microbiota promotes chronic pulmonary inflammation by enhancing IL-17A and autoantibodies. *Am J Respir Crit Care Med.* 2016;193(9):975–987.

Complete reference list available at ExpertConsult.com.

PART 2

DIAGNOSIS AND EVALUATION OF RESPIRATORY DISEASE

DIAGNOSIS

18 *HISTORY AND PHYSICAL EXAMINATION*

ELAINE FAJARDO, MD • J. LUCIAN DAVIS, MD

INTRODUCTION

Today, medical technology is thoroughly integrated into medical practice, including all aspects of evaluation. The electronic medical record prepopulates much of the history with clinical problems, the past medical history, and medications. The electronic medical record often serves as the primary source of information about a patient's medical, social, and family history, thereby replacing one of the most personal aspects of the medical interview and taking away an early opportunity to establish a relationship with the patient. In many settings, laboratory and imaging tests are preemptively ordered before the medical interview and examination. Today a conscientious clinician can generate lists of differential diagnoses before the patient interview with help from various computer resources. Artificial intelligence is already entering the process of medical evaluation.[1-3] Yet, despite our adoption of technology in every aspect of everyday practice, the ancient and fundamental skill of constructing a history and performing a thorough physical examination remains the defining art of the clinician.

Inevitably, both the practice of medical interviewing and physical diagnosis, as well as the underlying goals and philosophy, have evolved significantly. One principal influence is the biopsychosocial model, which postulates that to provide comprehensive care, clinicians must consider not only the diagnosis and prognosis of the underlying condition but also how the patient experiences it. Although initially proposed in the 1970s, it is only in recent years that the tenets of the biopsychosocial model have begun to shape the way the medical interview is conceived and taught.

For example, while building a history, the physician faces the challenge of separating out the "illness"—how a patient experiences his or her condition—from the "disease"—the pattern of symptoms and signs that are observed and expected to manifest themselves in the patient's body. There are many benefits to considering the illness and disease first individually and then together. Consider a patient with locally advanced lung cancer intially experiencing the illness simply as mild dyspnea. Without significant functional limitations, the patient may feel reluctant to accept that the prognosis is life-threatening. Risky or uncomfortable treatments, including chemotherapy and surgery, could appear unnecessary in this context. Conversely, consider a patient with undifferentiated cough in whom the clinician has already excluded the most common concerns such as laryngopharyngeal reflux and sinusitis, as well as more serious ones such as asthma, interstitial lung disease, and cancer. In this scenario, the provider may feel reassured that there is no important disease present, yet the patient is left without relief for the unexplained and perhaps debilitating cough. The conventional maxim may then be reversed so that only when the illness is understood can the disease be diagnosed and treated.[4]

Providers who adopt this more holistic approach may experience higher patient satisfaction and adherence, fewer lawsuits, less doctor-shopping, and improved health outcomes.[5] The premise of this chapter is that high-quality care requires the full integration of the patient and provider perspectives into the history-building and physical examination.

COMMUNICATION SKILLS

Physicians are often better at obtaining medical information than at understanding how that information affects the patients.[6] The legendary internist Sir William Osler used to tell students "Listen to the patient, he [or she] will tell you the diagnosis." The ability to listen attentively and to communicate with the patient clearly and empathetically is the foundation for the physician-patient relationship. This can be challenging, particularly in today's environment, where long-term physician-patient relationships are less common and time pressures are ubiquitous.

Patients may communicate through both verbal and nonverbal means.[7] For example, when embarrassing or personal symptoms are discussed, patients may change topics, exhibit avoidance, or engage in spontaneous associations.[8] There may be shifts in posture, a loss of eye contact, fidgeting with the hands, or tapping of the feet, each hinting at emotional concerns and personal reactions. Taking these forms of communication into account is one way that clinicians can begin to place the medical context of the disease within the human context of the illness that the patient is experiencing.

The physician's communication should be objective, nonjudgmental, and empathetic. The clinician should also be mindful that her/his posture, gestures, and words should convey transparency and help make the patient feel secure. More directly, the clinician can acknowledge the patient's emotions and inquire about beliefs.[9] Clinicians should be aware that patients may guard or conceal certain symptoms or concerns when the physician, ignorant of these fears, takes the lead. Time constraints may pressure physicians to control or accelerate the pace of the conversation. These pressures may contribute to misjudgments and cognitive traps that are more likely to lead to medical errors. The average physician interrupts the patient's initial history in as little as 16 seconds and frequently thereafter.[10] Explicitly setting expectations at the opening of the meeting may help patients and physicians alike change this dynamic. Specifically, physicians should note the time available for the session, encourage the patient and any other attendees to begin by sharing a list of concerns, and then jointly set priorities and plans for follow-up on other matters. Facilitation techniques such as sharing silence, summarizing the concerns stated by the patient, echoing, making open-ended requests, nodding, and making neutral utterances are other ways to keep the session productive without interrupting.

CLINICAL REASONING

There is both an art and a science to clinical reasoning, and today's paradigm draws from both medieval philosophy and modern decision science.[11,12] The maxim "uncommon presentations of common diseases are

Table 18.1   Selected Biases in Judgment or Reasoning

Bias	Definition
Anchoring	Tendency to lock onto salient features in the patient's initial presentation too early in the diagnostic process, with failure to adjust initial impression in light of later information.
Confirmation bias	Tendency to look for confirming evidence to support a diagnosis rather than for evidence to refute it, despite the latter often being more persuasive and definitive.
Framing effect	Tendency to be influenced by how the available clinical information is framed or presented using a recognizable rubric (e.g., presenting a patient with fever and tachycardia as having sepsis rather than a viral syndrome may lead to initiation of potentially harmful resuscitative care).
Premature closure	Tendency to accept a diagnosis before it has been fully verified. The consequences of the bias are reflected in the maxim "When the diagnosis is made, the thinking stops."
Search satisfying	Tendency to call off a search once something is found. This may lead the clinician to overlook critical comorbidities, second foreign bodies, other fractures, and coingestants in poisoning. Also, if the search yields nothing, diagnosticians should be sure that they have been looking in the right place.
Unpacking principle	Failure to elicit all relevant information (unpacking), which may result in missing important diagnostic possibilities.

Modified from Croskerry P. The importance of cognitive errors in diagnosis and strategies to minimize them. *Acad Med.* 2003;78:775–780.

more frequent than common presentations of uncommon diseases" is likely true. More than one disease may be present, and rare diseases are diagnosed only if they are considered. Thus it is important to continue to gather information and to be open to revising diagnostic hypotheses as more information becomes available. Premature judgment or failing to consider reasonable alternatives after making an initial diagnosis is the single most common diagnostic error.[13–15] In the field of "human factors engineering," these failures are postulated to arise from "cognitive dispositions to respond" and include several of the biases in judgment or reasoning defined in Table 18.1.[16] Making clinicians more aware of these common errors of reasoning and encouraging the use of checkpoints to facilitate "cognitive debiasing" could reduce their frequency.[17] Another complementary approach is to use decision-support software to expand the differential diagnosis and consider unusual or severe conditions.[18] Finally, patient-centered conversations have the potential to empower the patient to hold the clinician accountable when the proposed diagnosis does not fully explain all symptoms or concerns.

Bayes' theorem implies that diagnostic tests can be more efficiently used if the probability of the diagnosis before testing (also called pretest probability) is considered. Specific details from the history may then raise or lower the probability of different diagnoses and help direct selective testing toward the most important diagnostic possibilities. The added value of further investigations depends on the history.

Table 18.2 Comparison of Physician-Directed and Patient-Centered Approaches to the Medical Interview

	Physician-Directed Approach	Patient-Centered Approach
Philosophy and objectives	Identify the biomedical cause of disease	Elicit the psychosocial causes and consequences of the illness
History and physical (H&P)	Take a history 1. Ask questions to characterize symptoms: location and radiation; quality; intensity; onset, frequency, and duration; aggravating or alleviating factors and associated symptoms 2. Complete all components of the H&P in the first sitting	Build a history 1. Prompt the patient to tell you how the symptoms and signs impact the patient's experiences (e.g., misses work, cannot sleep) 2. Establish rapport and return as needed for additional data collection
Tests and imaging	Order in advance to save time for physicians	Order only after discussion with patient about the goals of the testing in order to engage the patient in the diagnostic process
Assessment strategies	Redirect the patient to the clinician's agenda Provide a diagnosis and prognosis	Allow the patient to set the agenda Summarize the patient's concerns
Plan	Write prescriptions to treat the disease and to treat the symptoms	Educate and empower the patient to manage the illness

CLINICAL HISTORY

"Medical interviewing is the process of gathering and sharing information in the context of a trustworthy relationship that takes into account both disease, if present, and illness."[9] Although traditionally conceived as an interview of the patient by the clinician, we will argue here that constructing the clinical history should be framed as a patient-centered collaboration between the clinician and the patient. Its main purposes are to (1) gather useful information, (2) develop rapport between the patient and the clinician, (3) respond to patient concerns, and (4) educate the patient. Some of the differences between the physician-directed and patient-centered approaches to the clinical history are outlined in Table 18.2.

The process of building a clinical history with the patient establishes rapport and understanding. It is "a purposeful conversation...[that] reflects the respective needs of both participants—patient and physician."[8] To start, the patient is encouraged to take the lead in expressing his or her symptoms and experiences related to these symptoms.[19] There are clear benefits for both parties: Patients find satisfaction in having their problems heard and understood, whereas physicians learn which symptoms are of greatest concern.[20] In addition, the patient's adherence to diagnostic and treatment plans depends on the physician's ability to win the patient's trust.[8] In the subsequent phase of the interview, most patients want to be informed about their condition and to be involved in the deliberations and decision making.[21] The physician assists this process when he or she explains symptoms, provides a plan for physical and mental recovery, and comforts.[8] Collaborating on the care plan is another way of emphasizing the importance of the patient perspective in building the clinical history.

The physician sets the stage for the discussion by welcoming the patient, introducing herself or himself to the people in the room, and clarifying the relationship of each person present to the patient.[9] This technique helps ensure that the environment is comfortable for the patient and family and free of barriers to communication, a goal that can be emphasized by providing adequate seating and removing obstructing objects from the room. Expectations are established by setting a time limit for the visit and an agenda for the meeting. The patient's concerns should have a central place on this agenda, although it may be necessary to ask the patient to prioritize the two or three most important items, while committing to addressing other questions at a later time. The physician should then encourage the patient to talk about himself or herself, using nonfocusing communications skills, such as open-ended questions and supportive gestures. Subsequently, focusing skills can guide the patient to elaborate further. Physicians can echo the patient (e.g., "You can't breathe?") or make requests ("Can you tell me more about how your walking has changed?") to fill in missing details about the present illness, past medical history, social history, family history, and review of systems. At this point in the meeting, the physician has likely assimilated enough data to establish and explore one or more working diagnoses. It is important that the physician remain attentive to the personal and emotional context of the patient's responses, even while directing the conversation. The medical session closes with the physician summarizing the patient's concerns and explaining how they might be further explored or addressed.

CHIEF COMPLAINT AND PRESENT ILLNESS

The medical history includes the chief complaint; the present, past, social, and family histories; and the review of systems. Ideally, the chief complaint should be written in the patient's own words, lest the physician's assessment be prematurely substituted for the patient's actual concerns. After being asked about the chief complaint, the patient should be allowed a few moments to mention any other ailments. Multiple concerns are common,[22] and inviting patients to enumerate them up front does not extend the length of the session[23] but does reduce the frequency of last-minute requests.[24] As each chief complaint is explored in detail, the resulting aggregate of information constitutes the history of the present illness. The clinician should organize the information into a cogent, chronological story that incorporates all the facts that support the preliminary diagnosis and differential diagnoses. At the end of the clinical history, the review of systems is a series of questions designed to cover previously unexamined territory, especially by probing topics that may help narrow or expand the differential diagnosis.[25,26] It is also sometimes useful to ask what the patient thinks may be causing the condition under evaluation, to expose previously unexplored avenues for inquiry.

MAJOR PULMONARY SYMPTOMS

Dyspnea, cough, and chest pain are among the most common reasons for patients to visit physicians, and may portend serious underlying intrathoracic disease. Careful questioning is warranted to establish their etiology and significance. The anatomic and pathophysiologic basis of these cardinal symptoms is provided in Part 3 of the textbook. In general, an adequate assessment of any symptom takes into consideration seven basic characteristics: (1) location, (2) quality, (3) intensity, (4) temporality, (5) aggravating factors, (6) alleviating factors, and (7) related symptoms. To aid the interviewer in obtaining a medical history, a brief overview of these three common presenting symptoms is provided as follows.

Dyspnea

When a healthy person increases his or her level of physical activity sufficiently, an awareness of breathing emerges; if the intensity of activity increases further, the sensation becomes progressively more unpleasant, until it ultimately compels the individual to slow down or stop.[27] Although dyspnea, shortness of breath, and breathlessness are often used interchangeably, some purists use the term *dyspnea* only when the symptom is abnormal. Many patients describe their breathing discomfort as "tightness," "choking," "feeling unable to take a deep breath," "suffocating," "feeling unable get enough air," or occasionally even "feeling tired."

The mechanisms underlying the sensation of dyspnea remain poorly understood and are reviewed in Chapter 36. Unlike pain and cough, for which specific receptors and neural pathways have been identified, such information is lacking for dyspnea, although evidence is mounting that links the symptom with pain.[27,28] Studies of the neurophysiology of dyspnea are further complicated by the lack of objective tools to quantify a subjective sensation with interindividual variation. Rating instruments, such as the Borg scale,[29] and questionnaires, such as the British Medical Research Council questionnaire[30] and the Pulmonary Functional Status and Dyspnea Questionnaire,[31] have been validated as useful in measuring dyspnea.

Clinical Features. Patients with respiratory, cardiac, hematologic, metabolic, and neuromuscular disorders may all complain of dyspnea, which may worsen with disease progression. Others say their dyspnea has not worsened, but probing reveals that this is because they now walk more slowly or no longer climb stairs. Sometimes this slowing down is so gradual that patients are unaware of it or attribute it to aging. Thus accurately assessing the activity required to bring about dyspnea is important. How many stairs can be climbed before stopping? How far can someone walk on level ground at her or his own pace without stopping? Does talking on the phone, getting dressed, or eating cause dyspnea? Is the patient short of breath at rest?

The course of dyspnea over time should be noted. Dyspnea may be triggered by cigarette smoke, dusts, molds, and perfumes, or alleviated by staying indoors or albuterol use. Associated features, such as wheezing, productive cough, fever, or lower extremity edema, may help differentiate among the causes of dyspnea, such as airways disease, pulmonary infections, and pulmonary vascular congestion.

Special types of dyspnea are distinctive and warrant separate designations. Episodes of breathlessness that wake persons from sleep, *paroxysmal nocturnal dyspnea,* usually denote left ventricular failure. This symptom may also be described by patients with chronic lung disease because of pooling of secretions in the airways, in patients with gravity-induced decreases in lung volumes, in patients with sleep-induced increases in airflow resistance, or in those with nocturnal aspiration. *Orthopnea,* the onset or worsening of dyspnea on assuming the supine position, such as paroxysmal nocturnal dyspnea, is found both in patients with heart disease and in those with chronic lung disease.[32] The inability to assume the supine position *(instant orthopnea)* is characteristic of paralysis of both diaphragms. Dyspnea soon after assuming the supine position may also be associated with other conditions, such as arteriovenous malformation, bronchiectasis, and lung abscess. *Platypnea,* which denotes dyspnea in the upright position, and *trepopnea,* an even rarer form of dyspnea that develops in either the right or the left lateral decubitus position, suggest pulmonary vascular shunting. Both the terms *hyperpnea,* an increase in minute ventilation, and *hyperventilation,* an increase in alveolar ventilation in excess of carbon dioxide production, indicate that ventilation is abnormally increased, without any implication about the presence or absence of dyspnea.

Cough

As described in Chapter 37, coughing is an essential mechanism that protects the airways from inhaled noxious substances and from excess secretions.[33] The daily quantity of bronchial secretions produced by a nonsmoking healthy adult is not precisely known, but it is sufficiently small to be removed by mucociliary action alone: Healthy persons seldom cough.[34] Coughing can be occasional, transient, and unimportant. By contrast, it may indicate the presence of severe intrathoracic disease.

Clinical Features. Most episodes of coughing are short lived, and patients, recognizing this, seldom visit their physicians for this type of cough. Nevertheless, cough is the most common complaint for which patients seek medical attention and the second most common reason for having a general medical examination.[35] Physicians should realize that when patients seek their help for cough, it is often out of concern for something new, different, and alarming about the symptom. The evaluation of cough begins with categorizing the duration of cough as acute, less than 3 weeks; subacute, 3 to 8 weeks; and chronic, greater than 8 weeks of cough symptoms. Next, the physician must exclude any red flags that may signify severe illness: hemoptysis; a new cough in an active smoker older than 45 years; a change in the characteristics of an existing cough or a change in voice; any cough in a 55- to 80-year-old with a history of smoking of 30 pack-years or greater; and any cough in association with any of the following symptoms—prominent dyspnea at rest or at night, hoarseness, fever, weight loss, dysphagia, or vomiting—with a history of recurrent pneumonia, or with any abnormality on physical examination or imaging.

Any of these findings should prompt further investigation beyond the common causes of cough into potential underlying conditions, such as interstitial lung disease or malignancy. In endemic areas, tuberculosis should be considered during every cough evaluation. Also, environmental and occupational exposures should also be reviewed as potential culprits.[36]

Acute coughing is frequently associated with respiratory tract infections, often viral, and exacerbations of underlying illnesses, such as asthma or COPD and pneumonia.[36] Less commonly, cough may be the chief manifestation of pulmonary embolus, heart failure, or inhalation of allergenic or irritating substances. Subacute coughing can be due to postinfectious cough, exacerbations of underlying illnesses, and upper airway cough syndrome due to rhinosinus disease. Chronic coughing is often due to upper airway cough syndrome, asthma, nonasthmatic eosinophilic bronchitis,[37] and gastroesophageal reflux disease.[35,36] Other important, though less common, etiologies include the use of angiotensin-converting enzyme inhibitors[38] and sitagliptin, a dipeptidyl peptidase-4 inhibitor used to treat diabetes.[39] Of interest, dipeptidyl peptidase-4 inhibition in the mucosa promotes inflammation, and manifests as rhinorrhea, postnasal cough, and fatigue. An unsuspecting patient or physician may erroneously assume these symptoms are due to a cold or seasonal allergies. Less well known is that cough may be the sole presenting manifestation of asthma[40] or gastroesophageal reflux disease.[41] It is noteworthy that, of the various components of the workup used by the authors of a systematic anatomic investigation to determine the causes of chronic cough, the medical history alone led to the correct diagnosis in 70% of patients.[35] A careful history of patients with cough lasting at least 3 months revealed that nearly all patients misdiagnosed as "psychogenic" had one of the conditions listed previously for chronic cough.[42] Even cough made worse with psychological stress is often caused by underlying lung disease. Patients with exaggerated cough responses or habitual cough may have a "psychogenic" component; therefore, even when chronic cough has a pulmonary cause, behavioral modification may be effective.[43]

Among the many complications of persistent or recurrent cough that may present concurrently are tussive syncope; retinal vessel rupture; persistent headache; chest wall and abdominal muscle strains, including the development of abdominal wall hernia[44]; subcutaneous emphysema; pneumothorax; and even rib fractures. Severe chronic cough may create devastating personal distress, causing patients to restrict their social and professional activities.

Chest Pain

Various types of chest pain are extremely common; their mechanisms and clinical patterns are described in Chapter 38. Because there is no clear relationship between the intensity of the discomfort and the importance of its underlying cause, all complaints of chest pain must be carefully considered.[45]

Clinical Features. Pleurisy, or acute inflammation of the pleural surfaces, has several distinctive features. Pleuritic pain is usually localized and unilateral, and it tends to be distributed along the intercostal nerve zones. Pain from diaphragmatic pleurisy is often referred to the ipsilateral shoulder and side of the neck. The pain may be variously described as "sharp," "burning," or simply as "a catch." The most striking and defining characteristic of pleuritic pain is its clear relationship to respiratory movements. It typically worsens by taking a deep breath, and coughing or sneezing causes intense distress. Patients with pleurisy frequently experience dyspnea because the aggravation of their pain during inspiration makes them conscious of every breath.

Acute pleuritic pain can be found in patients with spontaneous pneumothorax, pulmonary embolism, and pneumonia, especially bacterial pneumonia, whereas a gradual onset over several days is observed in patients with tuberculosis; an even slower development is characteristic of primary or secondary malignancies. Chronic pleuritic pain is characteristic of mesothelioma. It may be difficult to distinguish pleuritic pain from the pain of a rib fracture, although point localization favors the latter. Pericardial pain is typically sharp, retrosternal in location, and relieved by sitting up and leaning forward.

The distribution and superficial knifelike quality of the pain of intercostal neuritis or radiculitis may resemble pleural pain because it is worsened by vigorous respiratory movements but, unlike pleurisy, not by ordinary breathing. A neuritic origin may be suggested by the presence of lancinating or electric shock–like sensations unrelated to movements, and hyperalgesia or anesthesia over the distribution of the affected intercostal nerve provides confirmatory evidence. In many instances of new-onset neuritic chest wall pain, the diagnosis becomes clear a day or two later when the typical vesicular rash of herpes zoster appears.[46] Among the most important types of chest pain is myocardial ischemia. Typical anginal pain is induced by exercise, heavy meals, and emotional upsets; the pain is usually described as a substernal "pressure," "constriction," or "squeezing" that, when intense, may radiate to the neck or down the ulnar aspect of one or both arms.[47] Pain from variant or Prinzmetal angina is similar in location and quality to typical anginal pain but is experienced intermittently at rest rather than during exertion.[48] Acute myocardial infarction should be considered when the pain is greater than that of angina in intensity and duration, when the pain arises without exertion or is not alleviated by rest or nitroglycerin, or when the pain is accompanied by profuse sweating, nausea, hypotension, and arrhythmias. Pain similar to that of myocardial ischemia can also be experienced by patients with aortic valve disease, especially aortic stenosis, and other noncoronary heart disease.

Inflammation of or trauma to the joints, muscles, cartilages, bones, and fasciae of the thoracic cage is a common cause of chest pain.[49] Redness, swelling, and soreness of the costochondral junctions is called Tietze syndrome. All of these disorders are characterized by point tenderness over the affected area.

Most pulmonary thromboemboli are not associated with chest pain; the hallmark of pulmonary infarction, however, is typical pleuritic pain, presumably because the infarction irritates the visceral and then the parietal pleural membranes. (The visceral pleura is now known to contain pain fibers, but most pain is still thought to arise from the parietal pleura.) Both acute and chronic causes of pulmonary hypertension may be associated with episodes of chest pain that resemble myocardial ischemia in its substernal location and pattern of radiation and in its being described as "crushing" or "constricting."[49] This type of chest pain is believed to result from right ventricular ischemia owing to impaired coronary blood flow secondary to increased right ventricular mass and elevated systolic and diastolic pressures or to compression of the left main coronary artery by the dilated pulmonary artery trunk.

FAMILY HISTORY AND SOCIAL HISTORY

The family history provides important clues to the presence of heritable pulmonary diseases, such as cystic fibrosis, alpha$_1$-antitrypsin deficiency, hereditary hemorrhagic telangiectasia, immotile cilia syndrome, and immunodeficiency syndromes, among others. Careful history taking also can uncover even more common familial disease associations, which are polygenic or in which the exact mode of genetic transmission has not yet been established. As genomic surveillance uncovers more genetic linkages, the family history assumes greater importance. The family history should encompass at least three generations to account for sex-linked traits. Family history also can identify relevant prior exposures, such as to tuberculosis or other contagious diseases.

Of course, no evaluation of pulmonary symptoms is complete without a detailed history of smoking habits. The physician should ask, "Have you ever smoked?" If a negative answer returns, this should prompt a confirmatory question such as, "So you are a lifelong nonsmoker?" If the patient has smoked, the next questions should be, "When did you start?" "When did you quit?" and "How much did you smoke when you were smoking?" Ask also about different forms of tobacco and exposure at home or workplace to other people's tobacco smoke. A history of exposure to environmental smoke is also important.[50] A separate inquiry into electronic cigarette use or vaping should be made. In many developing countries, smoke from indoor cooking and heating fires is a major cause of lung disease, especially in women. Risk factors for *human immunodeficiency virus* (HIV) infection, such as unprotected sexual activity and injection drug abuse, should be specifically queried. Finally, the amount and frequency of any alcohol or illicit drug use should be recorded.

Medications and Allergies

A complete list of medications is essential to a thorough history. Ideally, the patient should bring in all his or her medications, and the physician should carefully go through each one, checking that the prescription has been properly written and filled and that the patient understands the benefits and possible side effects of each medicine. A complete listing of supplements and herbal medications should also be recorded and reviewed for potential interactions with conventional medications. It is essential to note whether the patient has ever had an allergic or toxic reaction and what these reactions were.

Occupational History

The occupational history, which is often included as part of the social history, is an integral part of a thorough medical interview. Identifying a relevant occupational exposure may provide the only opportunity to remove the patient from the exposure and prevent progressive and irreversible lung damage. Moreover, identifying injurious occupational exposures can facilitate justifiable compensation for the patient and removal of the hazardous materials from the workplace by the industry.

The evaluation of possible occupational lung disease is discussed in Chapters 100 to 103. Although only a few questions are asked in most initial medical interviews, if occupational illness is seriously being considered, a detailed inquiry about each industry, profession, and job the patient has held needs to be performed.[51,52] Environmental exposures and associated illnesses are constantly changing; it can be valuable to consult online resources from federal agencies such as the Centers for Disease Control and Prevention's National Center for Environmental Health (https://www.cdc.gov/nceh/) or National Institute for Occupational Safety and Health (https://www.cdc.gov/niosh/index.htm), and to involve occupational health specialists to identify and learn more about possible environmental toxins.[53,54] Individual state health department occupational safety and health contacts can also be found online (https://www.cdc.gov/niosh/statosh.html).

Travel History

A review of prior places of residence can expose the possibility of endemic fungal diseases, especially histoplasmosis and coccidioidomycosis. A history of recent travel may help establish the possibility of exposure to infectious diseases restricted to specific geographic regions.[55] The physician should inquire about duration of travel. Long trips by air or car increase the risk for deep venous thrombosis and venous thromboembolism, which are reported in up to 10% of passengers on long-haul flights.[56] Of importance, these may present at variable times after the inciting event. Finally, the epidemic of severe acute respiratory syndrome in Southeast China in 2002 and the pandemic of COVID-19 in 2019 and their rapid spread throughout the world by airline passengers emphasizes the importance of obtaining a careful travel history.

PAST MEDICAL HISTORY

Previous illnesses may recur (e.g., tuberculosis), and new diseases may complicate old ones (e.g., bronchiectasis as a sequela of necrotizing pneumonia). Information about previous illnesses, operations, intubations, and trauma involving the respiratory system may be essential to understanding the current problem. Although such data may be gathered as part of the past medical history, it may also emerge while obtaining the history of present illness in chronological sequence. Prior chest radiographs are an important aid in the evaluation of any abnormal chest radiograph because of the insights they provide into the duration and trajectory of illness. Patients should be asked to bring in previous films but, if they are unavailable, physicians should make every effort to obtain them because old radiographs may save needless, costly, and sometimes risky interventions.

QUESTIONNAIRES, COMPUTER-ASSISTED AND NURSING HISTORY

Printed or computer-based questionnaires and histories taken by nurses or allied health professionals are often used to expedite history taking. Occupational questionnaires have been shown to enhance recognition of occupational illness and correlate well with the findings of an industrial hygienist.[57] Computer-based interviews can gather more

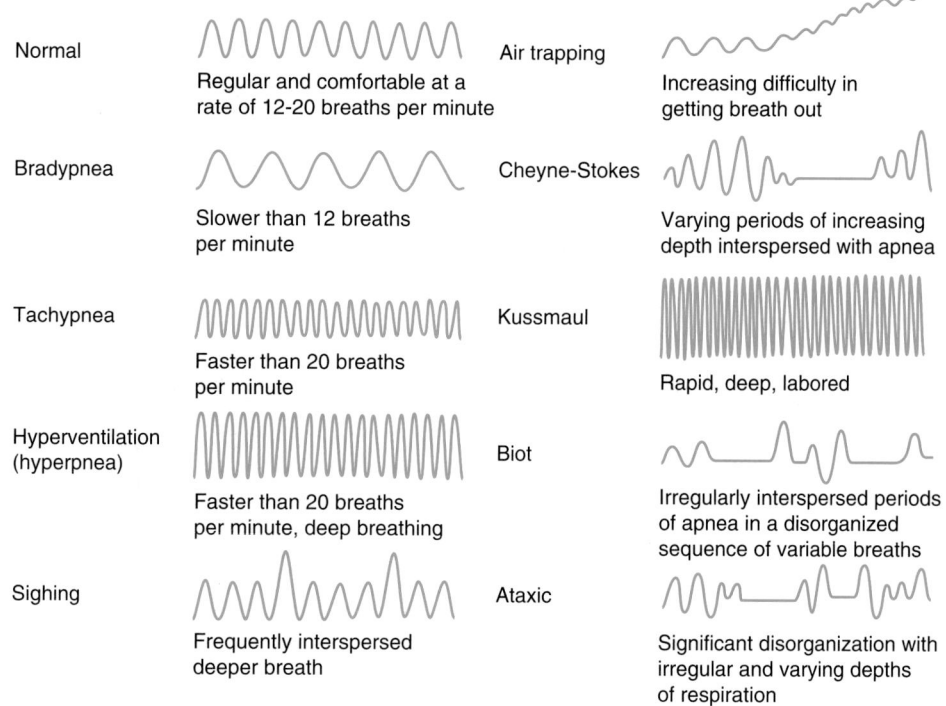

Normal — Regular and comfortable at a rate of 12-20 breaths per minute

Bradypnea — Slower than 12 breaths per minute

Tachypnea — Faster than 20 breaths per minute

Hyperventilation (hyperpnea) — Faster than 20 breaths per minute, deep breathing

Sighing — Frequently interspersed deeper breath

Air trapping — Increasing difficulty in getting breath out

Cheyne-Stokes — Varying periods of increasing depth interspersed with apnea

Kussmaul — Rapid, deep, labored

Biot — Irregularly interspersed periods of apnea in a disorganized sequence of variable breaths

Ataxic — Significant disorganization with irregular and varying depths of respiration

Figure 18.1 Waveforms in different patterns of breathing. (Modified from Wilkins RL, Hodgkin J, Lopez B. *Lung and Heart Sounds Online.* St. Louis: Mosby; 2011.)

information, allow more time to complete the interview, uncover sensitive information, and may be adaptable to the hearing impaired and to persons speaking a language different from that of the physician.[58] These forms of information gathering should be considered as adjuncts to and not as substitutes for the thorough history taken by the physician.

For monitoring the course of certain disorders such as asthma, daily recording of symptoms such as wheezing and breathlessness and objective assessments of disease severity using peak expiratory flow are preferable to a single questionnaire because recall of symptoms may be faulty, and one-time measurements may not be representative. Electronic monitors embedded within home noninvasive ventilation devices give the date and time of the respiratory events and use time of these devices. Increasingly, patients agree to real-time transmission of such measures to physicians' offices to improve routine management and early recognition of danger signs.

PHYSICAL EXAMINATION

Sadly, the declining emphasis on proficiency in physical examination during medical school and residency training and the ever-increasing reliance on technology-based diagnosis have led to a decreased interest in, some say even in the "demise" of, the physical examination.[59] However, the old observation that 88% of all diagnoses in primary care were established by taking a thorough medical history and performing a complete physical examination[60] probably still holds true today. At the very least, a carefully executed history and physical examination leads to more intelligent and cost-effective use of diagnostic testing. Moreover, a physical examination can be performed virtually anywhere, lends itself to serial observations, and increases the confidence patients have in their physicians.

EXAMINATION OF THE CHEST

Physical examination of the chest uses the four classic techniques of inspection, palpation, percussion, and auscultation. Each is described subsequently, as are the patterns of abnormalities. Apart from inspection, which may be both a visual and an olfactory tool, the other three modalities depend on the generation and the perception of sound or tactile sensations and vibrations. The optimal conditions to perform the physical examination therefore allow privacy, warmth, good light, and a quiet atmosphere.

Inspection

The physical examination begins the moment the clinician first sees the patient. Keen observations and the ability to pursue and interpret these observations are the keys to skilled clinical diagnosis. Inspection of the chest is carried out after sufficient clothing has been removed and the patient has been suitably draped to permit observation of the entire thorax. Ordinarily, inspection is performed with the patient sitting. Observing the shape and symmetry of the chest allows such abnormalities as kyphoscoliosis, pectus excavatum, pectus carinatum, ankylosing spondylitis, gynecomastia, and surgical scars or defects to become obvious. The pattern of breathing can provide immediate clues to the nature of the illness; several classic patterns of ventilation are described in Fig. 18.1.[61] Inspection, including the sense of smell, may be a clue to habits or addictions. Tobacco leaf stains may be visible on teeth, lips, fingers, or clothing, and tobacco or cannabis smoke may leave a characteristic odor on hair and clothing. The odor of ethanol or other toxic alcohols may be detected on the breath, as is the odor of ketones during diabetic crisis. Characteristic odors may also arise from certain infections, such as the foul smell of an anaerobic lung abscess, or the sweet smell of a skin and soft tissue infection caused by *Pseudomonas aeruginosa*.

Palpation

Palpation of the thorax can detect bony abnormalities, such as a cervical rib, and subcutaneous calcinosis seen with systemic sclerosis. It is essential in evaluating pain to test for point tenderness and thoracic spinal tenderness. It can detect fluctuant areas associated with *empyema necessitans* and crepitant areas associated with subcutaneous emphysema. Palpation of the trachea deviant from the suprasternal notch suggests shifts of the mediastinum. A spastic, extra-firm-feeling back muscle recognized by palpation may identify the cause of thoracic pain. A lag in movement of the chest wall can be confirmed by placing the two hands over opposite portions of each hemithorax and both feeling and observing whether or not the thorax moves symmetrically[61]; assessing symmetry is as important in palpation as it is in inspection.

A palpable vibration felt on the body, usually over the chest, is called *fremitus.* Vocal fremitus is elicited by having the patient speak "one, two, three," while the examiner's palms or sides of the hands are moved from top to bottom of the two hemithoraces. Vocal fremitus is increased over regions of lungs where there is increased transmission of sound, for example, consolidation from pneumonia. Conversely, fremitus is decreased in conditions in which sound transmission is impaired, for example, pleural effusion.

In examining the heart, the examining physician should always search for an apical impulse, heaves and lifts, thrills, and palpable valve closure. In patients with severe COPD, the abnormal cardiac movements are often better felt in the subxiphoid region than over the precordium.

Percussion

Skillful percussion depends on a uniform free and easy stroke of the striking finger (plexor) on the finger being struck (pleximeter), the ability to sense minor changes in pitch, and a keen sense of vibration; although the percussion note is heard, it is predominantly felt. Percussion of the thorax over normal air-containing lung produces a resonant note.

Pathologic processes may impair or enhance the resonating quality of the thorax. For example, the percussion note over a large pneumothorax is hyperresonant and becomes tympanitic when tension is present; in contrast, percussion over a pleural effusion or pneumonia produces dullness, which has been defined as a low-intensity sound of short duration, feeble carrying power, and rather high pitch.[62] Flatness is the nonresonant sound obtained by percussing over the liver. Three different tonal zones can thus be detected when percussing large pleural effusions: normal resonance above the fluid, dullness in the middle, and flatness when completely below the fluid.

Auscultation

A stethoscope draped around the neck has long been the badge of the medical professional, and it is worn with pride by physicians, nurses, and respiratory therapists, despite predictions such as "it, too, will someday be relegated to a museum shelf."[63] This will not happen for a long time, however, according to Murphy,[64] who mounts a spirited defense of stethoscopes backed up by analyses of breath sounds obtained by respiratory acoustic recording. The fundamentals of lung auscultation in physical examination are also covered in this review.[65]

Stethoscopes are also helpful in identifying pathology when chest radiograph findings are normal, such as detecting wheezes in asthmatic patients or crackles in patients with interstitial lung disease. Moreover, patients with cardiorespiratory complaints expect their physicians to listen to their heart and lungs.

Like any piece of medical equipment, there are a number of available choices, and the design and care of the stethoscope may have a substantial impact on performance. Electronic models promise ambient noise reduction and audio amplification, features shown in randomized trials to provide statistically significant improvements in acoustics, especially in noisy environments.[66,67] However, the magnitude of improvement is small relative to the best acoustic stethoscopes, and electronic stethoscopes have not been shown to improve trainee performance.[68] Sound quality with any stethoscope can be substantially degraded by failure to maintain the integrity of the rubber fittings, and prolonged contact of the tubing with the skin when worn around the neck can lead to hardening of the tubing and decreased performance. In any case, the stethoscope must be kept clean because it is increasingly recognized as a vector of nosocomial infection.[69] Glycerin-free isopropyl alcohol wipes are gentler on rubber and preferred to chlorine bleach except when *Clostridium difficile* colitis is possible; soap and water is an alternative, provided all internal pieces are allowed to dry.

The terminology of breath sounds has been standardized and simplified to enhance understanding and communication (Table 18.3). Although standardized nomenclature has been proposed by the American Thoracic Society[70] and the Tenth International Conference on Lung Sounds,[71] communication at the bedside often strays from recommended terminology. Although a number of other nonstandard terms (e.g., vesicular breath sounds, coarse breath sounds, rales, crepitations, sibilant and sonorous rhonchi, and high- and low-pitched wheezes) may be encountered based on historical usage, on homologies with terms used in languages other than English, or on common usage, we encourage adherence to this standard classification.[72]

The basic technique of auscultation with an ordinary stethoscope is well known to most physicians: The diaphragm detects higher-pitched sounds, and the bell detects lower-pitched sounds, although if the bell is tightly pressed against the body, the taut underlying skin itself may serve as a "diaphragm" and improve perception of higher pitches. Conversely, the bell should be applied very lightly to hear low-pitched sounds, for example, the low-pitched rumble of mitral stenosis. Full contact with the skin is necessary for best listening, which may pose a problem in a patient whose intercostal spaces are sunken from weight loss. In addition, the skin or hairs may brush against the diaphragm and produce a sound that resembles a pleural friction rub. As with examiners' hands, a warm stethoscope head is appreciated by patients. The importance of a quiet room and of applying the stethoscope directly to the skin rather than through clothing has recently been reemphasized.[73]

Table 18.3 Classification of Major Lung Sounds

Lung Sounds	Acoustic Characteristics	American Thoracic Society Nomenclature	Significance (Examples)
Normal	200–600 Hz; decreasing power with increasing Hz; soft, nonmusical sound heard on inspiration	Normal breath sounds*	
	75–1600 Hz Flat until sharp decrease in power (900 Hz); hollow, nonmusical sound heard in both inspiration and expiration just below the sternal notch	Tracheal breath Sounds	
Adventitious (abnormal)	Same as tracheal breath sounds but heard in periphery of lung; louder than normal breath sounds; equal on inspiration and expiration	Bronchial breath sounds†	Indicate airless air spaces around patent airway (e.g., atelectasis, consolidation)
	Discontinuous, interrupted explosive sounds (softer, higher in pitch, and shorter in duration than coarse crackles or crackles), middle to late inspiratory	Fine crackles	Indicate opening of collapsed distal airways (e.g., atelectasis, fibrosis)
	Discontinuous, interrupted explosive sounds (loud, low in pitch), early inspiratory or expiratory	Coarse crackles	Indicate opening of distal airways, may change after cough (e.g., distal secretions)
	Continuous sounds (>250 msec, high-pitched; dominant frequency ≥ 400 Hz, hissing in quality)	Wheezes	Indicate airway narrowing (e.g., asthma/COPD if diffuse, airway lesion if focal)
	Continuous sounds (>250 msec, low-pitched; dominant frequency < 200 Hz, a snoring sound)	Rhonchi	Indicate secretions in large airways (e.g., may clear with cough or suctioning)
Extrapulmonary	Continuous high-pitched sound mainly inspiratory, high-pitched, best heard over neck	Stridor	Indicates extrathoracic variable or fixed obstruction; needs urgent attention (e.g., anaphylaxis, epiglottitis)

*The label "vesicular" has now been shown to be inaccurate because normal breath sounds do not arise from the opening of vesicles (i.e., alveoli) but from turbulent airflow within distal airways.
†Associated with voice-generated sounds, such as egophony (Audio 18.8), bronchophony (Audio 18.9), and whispered pectoriloquy (Audio 18.10).

Careful auscultation of both front and back of the patient's chest is required for a comprehensive examination. The sections that follow include links to audio clips of many of the most important lung sounds; **these are best appreciated by listening through a stethoscope, while holding the diaphragm near your audio speaker.**

Normal Lung Sounds

Normal lung sounds, as shown in Table 18.3, are categorized as normal breath sounds (Audio 18.1) and tracheal breath sounds. Normal breath sounds were previously termed vesicular breath sounds because they were incorrectly assumed to represent air entering the alveoli or vesicles; we now know that air enters the alveoli via diffusion, a silent process. Instead, the inspiratory component arises from sounds generated by turbulent airflow within the lobar and segmental bronchi, whereas the expiratory component arises within the larger airways.[70] During normal breathing, inspiratory sounds are louder, and expiratory sounds are softer or even inaudible. Compared to inspiratory sounds, expiratory sounds are softer because the sounds are generated in the larger, more central airways, where they are dampened by the large volume of the lungs' air spaces. The intensity of normal breath sounds varies with regional ventilation and, like percussion notes, diminishes with increasing thickness of the chest wall. There is considerable variation among persons in the quality of breath sounds, which makes it essential to compare breath sounds from one hemithorax with those heard over the same location on the opposite hemithorax. Tracheal breath sounds (Audio 18.2) are tubular, nonmusical sounds heard in both phases of the respiratory cycle; their frequency pattern resembles "white noise." It is best heard below the suprasternal notch.

Auscultation of tracheal breath sounds implies open central and upper airways.

In pathologic conditions, the transmission of normal breath sounds to the chest wall may be either attenuated or exaggerated. When the lung parenchyma is consolidated, breath sounds are well transmitted to the chest wall and *bronchial breath sounds* (Audio 18.3) become audible in the peripheral areas. Bronchial breath sounds are loud, medium-pitched, tubular sounds that are as loud as or louder during expiration as during inspiration. Bronchial breath sounds are similar to *tracheal breath sounds*, but their presence in the periphery is the classic auscultatory sign of consolidation, which could be from pneumonia, pulmonary edema, or hemorrhage. The presence of this sign assumes that the sounds originate centrally at the trachea and reach the chest wall only through amplification within airways surrounded by consolidated lung.[74] Furthermore, detecting bronchial breath sounds indicates that the airway to this region is patent.

Interposition of a sound barrier between the central airways, where sounds originate, and the chest wall, where they are heard, also attenuates or interrupts transmission of normal lung sounds. In accordance, normal breath sounds are diminished or absent over a pleural effusion, pneumothorax, or peripheral bulla, or distal to an obstructing mass lesion. Conversely, they may be increased if chest wall deformity or bronchial or tracheal derangement allows movement of air to be closer than usual to the stethoscope.

Adventitious (Abnormal) Lung Sounds

The major types of adventitious, or abnormal, lung sounds are classified in Table 18.3. Two generic categories of adventitious sounds have been documented by high-speed recording techniques, and each of these has two subdivisions: discontinuous sounds, including fine crackles and coarse crackles, and continuous sounds, including wheezes and rhonchi.[75] This categorization emphasizes the relevance of noting the timing of breath sounds. Abnormal breath sounds generally have a strong expiratory component; loud expiratory sounds should raise special concern, and their type and origin should be clarified.

Fine and Coarse Crackles (Discontinuous Sounds)

Crackles, still often referred to as "rales" in the United States and "crepitations" in Great Britain, consist of a series of short, explosive, nonmusical sounds that punctuate the underlying breath sound; fine crackles (Audio 18.4) are softer, shorter in duration, and higher in pitch than coarse crackles (Audio 18.5). There is general agreement that the brief recurrent pops that characterize fine crackles are caused by the explosive openings of small airways that had closed owing to the surface forces within them.[70,76] This is also compatible with the presence of crackles in healthy elderly or obese persons in whom dependent airways close at resting lung volumes. Crackles therefore are best heard during the first deep breaths at the lung bases posteriorly. After several such breaths or intentional coughing, these fine crackles will disappear if the small airways remain open throughout the time the patient is being examined.[76] Coarse crackles are lower-frequency sounds transmitted to the mouth that indicate intermittent airway opening, such as found with secretions.[77] Coughing or deep inspiration may also change the quality of coarse crackles, but the crackles rarely disappear entirely.

The timing of crackles is also important. Fine crackles are much more common during inspiration than during expiration, which is why they are best heard over dependent lung regions—where airways are more likely to close—than over the uppermost regions. Nath and Capel[78] have shown that fine crackles heard late in inspiration are more often found in restrictive lung disease rather than in alveolar filling processes. This suggests that more tension is required to open individual airways in fibrosis than in lungs with secretions or edema. As inspiration progresses, radial traction on airway walls increase until suddenly they pop open.[78] Thus crackles heard later in inspiratory time imply that the tension required to open individual airways is greater. Expiratory crackles are much less frequent than inspiratory crackles and are often seen in obstructive lung disease.[75]

Wheezes and Rhonchi (Continuous Sounds)

The American Thoracic Society Committee on Pulmonary Nomenclature has defined wheezing as high-pitched (dominant frequency > 400 Hz) continuous adventitial lung sounds.[74] Continuous sounds are longer than 250 msec in duration. Wheezes are usually louder than the underlying breath sounds and frequently noted by patients. A leading theory is that wheezes are produced by fluttering of the airway walls and air together, induced at or above a critical flow velocity.[79] The pitch of the wheeze is dependent on the mass and elasticity of the airway walls and the flow velocity. The degree of bronchial obstruction is proportional to the amount of the respiratory cycle it occupies. There is no relationship to the intensity or pitch of the wheeze and pulmonary function. Wheezes are well heard over the trachea, and listening over the trachea may be superior to listening over the lung in most asthmatic patients[79] (Audio 18.6). Wheezing with forced expiration can sometimes be provoked in healthy subjects[70] and does not establish a diagnosis of asthma. A more specific technique for detecting pathologic wheezes is to elicit wheezing and/or coughing *without* forced expiration by having the patient breathe slowly to end-expiration. Because several disease states are associated with wheezing, additional information should be obtained to make the correct diagnosis.

Rhonchi are low-pitched continuous sounds with a dominant frequency of approximately 200 Hz or less (Audio 18.7). These sounds are likely to originate from rupture of fluid films and airway wall vibrations.[70] Rhonchi may clear with cough or with suctioning in intubated patients. Some have questioned whether the term rhonchi is needed at all, finding the substitute "low-pitched wheezes" more parsimonious.[80] However, the term retains its place in classification systems and in clinical usage.[70,71,77]

Voice-Generated Sounds

Another way of generating sounds for auscultation is to have a patient speak certain sounds (e.g., "one, two, one, two," "ninety-nine, ninety-nine," or "eee-eee.") in a quiet voice while the examiner listens to his or her chest. If enhanced responses are heard, the patient repeats the words while whispering. Because sounds of central origin are attenuated as they are transmitted peripherally through normal air-filled lung, voice-generated sounds have a muffled quality and the words are indistinct. In the presence of consolidation, the characteristics of the sounds are remarkably different. The term *egophony* (Audio 18.8) indicates sounds with a high-pitched, bleating quality; a change in sound-filtering properties of consolidated lungs accounts for the change in transmitted frequency. The classic way to identify egophony is with the "E" to "A" test. When a patient says "E" and the sound is transmitted along a patent airway through an area of consolidation, its frequency drops so that the "E" sounds more like an "A." *Bronchophony* (Audio 18.9) and *pectoriloquy* (Audio 18.10) both mean that spoken sounds are transmitted with increased intensity and pitch; when each syllable of every word, especially when whispered, is distinct and easily recognized, pectoriloquy is the preferred description. Each of these auscultatory findings is a manifestation of the same acoustic property of consolidated lungs, such as would be present in pneumonia or atelectatic lung with a patent airway.

Pleural Friction Rub

The small amount of liquid normally present in the pleural space separates the visceral and the parietal pleural layers and allows the lungs to expand and contract freely during breathing. In contrast, when the pleural surfaces are thickened and roughened by an inflammatory or neoplastic process, sliding is impaired and a pleural friction rub (Audio 18.11) may be produced. These sounds vary in intensity but often have a leathery or creaking quality that may be exaggerated by pressure with the stethoscope. Typically rubs are heard during both inspiration and expiration, but they are evanescent and variable and may be heard in only one part of the respiratory cycle. The terminology "rub" implies that friction between pleural surfaces generates the sounds. In actuality, rubs may be generated simply by the change in shape of the thickened pleura itself, because a small amount of fluid is likely always present between the pleural surfaces, preventing their direct contact. This would also explain why rubs are occasionally audible even in the presence of large pleural effusions.

Extrapulmonary Sounds

Stridor is a high-pitched continuous sound produced by turbulent flow in the extrathoracic airway, which is louder and longer during inspiration than expiration (Audio 18.12). Stridor has many causes,[81] some of which are life-threatening and demand immediate attention (see also Chapter 39). At the patient's peril, stridor is occasionally mistaken for wheezing. Wheezing is an exclusively expiratory sound that is loudest over the chest. Auscultation over the upper trachea with attention to the timing in the respiratory cycle will help identify stridor and differentiate it from wheezing. Stridor may be heard only during inspiration if the causative lesion is functional or dynamic, or in both inspiration and expiration if the lesion is fixed.

The presence of air or other gas in the mediastinum may be associated with crunching, crackling sounds that are synchronous with cardiac contraction and are audible when breathing is momentarily stopped. This association with cardiac rather than respiratory motion differentiates a crunch from a rub, and pitch is lower for crunch than a rub. The finding of a mediastinal crunch by auscultation usually signifies mediastinal emphysema, even when the chest radiograph shows no abnormalities.

Various sounds may originate from the chest wall itself. Some of these have pathologic significance; others do not. Rubbing hairs between the skin and the stethoscope produce intermittent crackling sounds that may be confused with crackles (Audio 18.13). Variable crackles are also produced when the stethoscope is placed over an area of subcutaneous emphysema and is rocked back and forth (Audio 18.14). Contracting chest wall muscles may generate sounds that have a muffled, distant, low-pitched, and rumbling quality. On occasion, it is possible to hear a snapping sound during breathing from motion of a newly fractured rib, a sound called bone crepitus (Audio 18.15).

Interpretation

When abnormalities are discovered on physical examination of the chest, it is useful to identify them by their anatomic location in the involved lung. This requires knowledge of the surface projections of the underlying bronchopulmonary lobes, which are shown in Fig. 18.2. In the presence of either distortions of pulmonary anatomy or the shape of the rib cage, the surface projections of the underlying lung also change.

The classic findings on physical examination of the chest in some common pulmonary disorders are shown in Table 18.4. Ordinarily, consolidation must be within 1 or 2 cm of the costal surface to be reliably detected. Even then, physical examination alone cannot be relied upon to diagnose or exclude pneumonia.[82] Some pneumonias, such as *Mycoplasma* pneumonia, typically cause surprisingly few physical abnormalities despite extensive radiographic involvement (see eFig. 33.9) but, even in patients with classic lobar pneumonia, the findings may

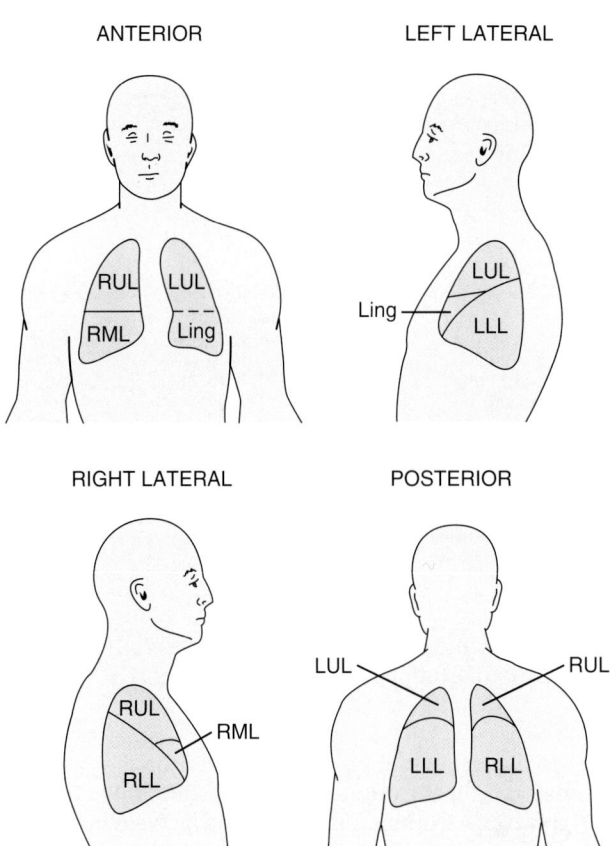

Figure 18.2 **Surface projections of underlying lobar anatomy of a healthy man.** The upper and lower lobes of both lungs are separated by the two oblique fissures, which course from the spinous process of the third thoracic vertebra posteriorly to the level of the 6th rib in the midclavicular line anteriorly. On the right side anteriorly, the upper and middle lobes are separated by the horizontal fissure, which lies at about the level of the 4th costal cartilage. Ling, lingular division of left upper lobe; LLL, left lower lobe; LUL, left upper lobe; RLL, right lower lobe; RML, right middle lobe; RUL, right upper lobe.

be nonspecific. Although unable to distinguish reliably between new-onset pneumonia and other pulmonary diseases, the findings from physical examination, including vital signs and mental confusion, are extremely important in assessing severity and in deciding whether or not to hospitalize patients with pneumonia.[83] The distinction between pleural effusion and atelectasis can be made on physical examination by determining whether the heart and mediastinal contents shift toward or away from the abnormal side, a finding that can usually be made only if the effusion is large or the atelectasis involves at least one lobe. However, the absence of these findings does not exclude an abnormality, and a chest radiograph or ultrasound image should be obtained to complete the pulmonary workup.

EXTRAPULMONARY MANIFESTATIONS

The examination of the lungs and pleura unlock only some of the clues to the presence of lung disease. Looking for extrapulmonary signs can often point toward a specific pulmonary disease or toward systemic diseases, such as lupus erythematosus, or toward diseases arising elsewhere in the

Table 18.4   Classic Physical Findings in Selected Common Pulmonary Disorders

Disorder	Inspection	Palpation	Percussion	Auscultation
Bronchial asthma (acute exacerbation)	Hyperinflation; use of accessory muscles of respiration	Impaired excursion; decreased fremitus	Hyperresonance; low diaphragm	Prolonged expiration: inspiratory and expiratory wheezes
Pneumothorax (complete)	Lag on affected side, increased size of hemithorax	Absent fremitus on affected side	Hyperresonant or tympanitic	Absent breath sounds
Pleural effusion (large)	Lag on affected side, increased size of hemithorax	Decreased fremitus, trachea and heart shifted away from affected side	Dullness or flatness	Absent breath sounds
Atelectasis (lobar obstruction)	Lag on affected side	Decreased fremitus; trachea and heart shifted toward affected side	Dullness or flatness	Absent breath sounds
Consolidation (pneumonia)	Possible lag or splinting	Increased fremitus on affected side	Dullness	Bronchial breath sounds; bronchophony, pectoriloquy, crackles

Modified from Hinshaw HC, Murray JF, eds: *Diseases of the Chest*. ed 4. Philadelphia: WB Saunders; 1980:23.

body that secondarily involve the lung. Certain extrapulmonary manifestations are particularly useful.

Clubbing

The association of clubbing of the fingers or toes with disease has caught the attention of physicians since the time of Hippocrates. Clubbing is easy to recognize when severe (Fig. 18.3), but subtle changes are more common and less reliable. The hallmarks of clubbing are (1) an increase of the normal 165-degree angle that the nail makes with its cuticle, in effect flattening it; (2) a softening and periungual erythema of the nail beds, where the nails to seem to float; (3) an enlargement or bulging of the distal phalanx, which may be warm and erythematous; and (4) a curvature of the nails themselves. Of these features, the straightening of the nail cuticle angle appears to be the most sensitive measurement.[84] The main pathologic finding in clubbing is increased capillary density stimulated by hypoxia, which intensely produces vascular growth factors.[85] With histochemical staining, Atkinson and Fox[86] showed increases in vascular endothelial growth factor, platelet-derived growth factor, hypoxia-inducible factor-1α, and hypoxia-inducible factor-2α, along with increased microvessel density in the stroma of clubbed digits. The second common characteristic of patients with digital clubbing is shunting of blood past the capillary bed of either the lung or the liver, which suggests that lack of metabolism of angiogenic factors that bypass a critical organ may be involved. Several of the conditions associated with clubbing have inflammation and shunting, such as bronchiectasis and liver cirrhosis.

Clubbing may develop rapidly, about 2 weeks in patients with new-onset empyema, and similarly reverse, also about 2 weeks in patients after corrective cardiac surgery. Clubbing was found in 1% of all admissions to an internal medicine department and was associated with "serious disease" in 40% of afflicted patients[87]; therefore new-onset clubbing always warrants a chest radiograph and, if unrevealing, a CT scan to look for a pulmonary neoplasm or other lesion, which may still be localized and curable. Clubbing has been found in many diverse conditions, such as in children with HIV[88] and in patients with hepatopulmonary syndrome[89] or with benign asbestos pleural disease[90] (eTable 18.1).

Patients with clubbing may also have *hypertrophic osteoarthropathy*: subperiosteal formation of new cancellous bone at the distal ends of long bones, especially the radius and ulna and the tibia and fibula. Hypertrophic osteoarthropathy (eFig. 18.1) is almost always associated with clubbing, particularly in patients with bronchogenic carcinoma, other intrathoracic malignancies, and cystic fibrosis. It occasionally develops in patients with bronchiectasis, empyema, and lung abscess but is rare in patients with most of the other conditions in which clubbing has been observed. Both clubbing and hypertrophic osteoarthropathy can be idiopathic, familial, or drug induced (e.g., voriconazole); the familial form is often transmitted as a dominant trait.

Other Extrapulmonary Associations

Besides clubbing, thoracic neoplasms may cause extrathoracic abnormalities that may become evident on physical examination, including anemia, Cushing syndrome, gynecomastia, and other paraneoplastic syndromes (eTable 18.2). Wasting, hoarseness, adenopathy (especially supraclavicular), and hepatomegaly are additional common extrathoracic manifestations. When evaluating patients with dyspnea, a thorough examination of the neck for increased jugular venous pressure should be performed to exclude right heart failure.[91] The extremities should also be examined for peripheral edema, venous thrombosis, chronic venous stasis, and scars that suggest injection drug abuse.

Lung disease is associated with abnormalities in other organ systems. Important lesions associated with various primary lung disorders are listed in tables available in the electronic version of the text. Included are lists of the lung diseases associated with skin and subcutaneous abnormalities (eTable 18.3); eye involvement (eTable 18.4); renal involvement (eTable 18.5); bone, joint, nerve, or muscle involvement (eTable 18.6); and gastrointestinal or hepatic involvement (eTable 18.7).

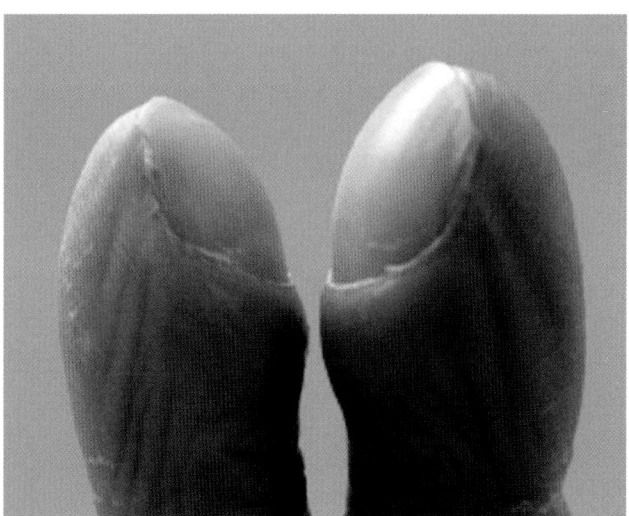

Figure 18.3 Clubbing of the digits as seen in severe diffuse interstitial pulmonary fibrosis. (From Cashman MW, Sloan SB. *Nutrition and nail disease. Clin Dermatol.* 2010;28:420–4225.)

Acknowledgment

We acknowledge Professor John F. Murray for his major contributions to earlier versions of this chapter, many of which have been retained in the current edition.

Key Points

- An integrated approach to the history and physical examination balances the concerns of patients and clinicians so that the experience of the patient's illness receives as much attention as the quest for a diagnosis for any underlying disease.
- Physical examination can be performed virtually anywhere, provides important information, lends itself to serial observations, and increases patients' confidence in their physicians.
- After the clinician arrives at a tentative diagnosis, selected radiographic, laboratory, and other tests are ordered for further and confirmatory evaluation.
- Careful questioning and further workup of patients with dyspnea, cough, and chest pain is mandatory because these symptoms are among the most common reasons for patients to visit physicians and can indicate serious underlying chest disease.
- Stridor, a high-pitched continuous sound louder and longer during inspiration than expiration, can indicate a life-threatening upper airway obstruction and requires immediate attention.
- New-onset clubbing of the digits warrants further investigation owing to its frequent association with serious underlying disease.
- After collecting high-quality data during the history and the physical examination, it is essential to remain vigilant against common errors in clinical reasoning, which are among the most common causes of diagnostic error.

Key Readings

Baraniuk JN, Jamieson MJ. Rhinorrhea, cough and fatigue in patients taking sitagliptin. *Allergy Asthma Clin Immunol.* 2010;6(1):8.

Bond WF, Schwartz LM, Weaver KR, Levick D, Giuliano M, Graber ML. Differential diagnosis generators: an evaluation of currently available computer programs. *J Gen Intern Med.* 2012;27(2):213–219.

Charon R. Narrative and medicine. *N Engl J Med.* 2004;350:862–864.

Croskerry P. The importance of cognitive errors in diagnosis and strategies to minimize them. *Acad Med.* 2003;78:775–780.

Croskerry P. From mindless to mindful practice—cognitive bias and clinical decision making. *N Engl J Med.* 2013;368:2445–2448.

Engel GL. The need for a new medical model: a challenge for biomedicine. *Science.* 1977;196(4286):129–136.

Engel GL. The clinical application of the biopsychosocial model. *Am J Psychiatry.* 1980;137(5):535–544.

Engel GL. How much longer must medicine's science be bound by a seventeenth century world view? *Psychother Psychosom.* 1992;57(1-2):3–16.

Fortin AH. *Smith's Patient Centered Interviewing: An Evidence-Based Method.* 4th ed. New York: McGraw-Hill Education; 2019.

Graber ML, Mathew A. Performance of a web-based clinical diagnosis support system for internists. *J Gen Intern Med.* 2008;23(suppl 1):37–40.

Groopman J. *How Doctors Think.* New York: Houghton Mifflin; 2007.

Haidet P, Paterniti DA. Building" a history rather than "taking" one: a perspective on information sharing during the medical interview. *Arch Intern Med.* 2003;163(10):1134–1140.

Heritage J, Robinson JD, Elliott MN, Beckett M, Wilkes M. Reducing patients' unmet concerns in primary care: the difference one word can make. *J Gen Intern Med.* 2007;22(10):1429–1433.

Hurwitz B. Narrative and the practice of medicine. *Lancet.* 2000;356:2086–2089.

Irwin RS, French CL, Chang AB, Altman KW, Panel CEC. Classification of cough as a symptom in adults and management algorithms: CHEST Guideline and Expert Panel Report. *Chest.* 2018;153(1):196–209.

Lichstein PR. The medical interview. In: Walker HK, Hall WD, Hurst JW, eds. *Clinical Methods: The History, Physical, and Laboratory Examinations.* 3rd ed. Boston: Butterworths; 1990.

Marvel MK, Epstein RM, Flowers K, Beckman HB. Soliciting the patient's agenda: have we improved? *JAMA.* 1999;281(3):283–287.

Nakamura J, Halliday NA, Fukuba E, et al. The microanatomic basis of finger clubbing—a high-resolution magnetic resonance imaging study. *J Rheumatol.* 2014;41(3):523–527.

National Academies of Sciences. *Engineering, and Medicine. Improving Diagnosis in Health Care.* Washington, DC: National Academies Press; 2015.

Pauker SG, Kassirer JP. The threshold approach to clinical decision making. *N Engl J Med.* 1980;302(20):1109–1117.

Riches N, Panagioti M, Alam R, et al. The effectiveness of electronic differential diagnoses (DDX) generators: a systematic review and meta-analysis. *PLoS One.* 2016;11(3):e0148991.

Stewart M, Brown J, Levenstein J, McCracken E, McWhinney IR. The patient-centered clinical method. 3. Changes in residents' performance over two months of training. *Fam Pract.* 1986;3(3):164–167.

William, Boehner P. *Summa Logicae.* St. Bonaventure, NY: Franciscan Institute; 1951.

Complete reference list available at ExpertConsult.com.

19 MICROBIOLOGIC DIAGNOSIS OF LUNG INFECTION

NIAZ BANAEI, MD • STANLEY C. DERESINSKI, MD •
BENJAMIN A. PINSKY, MD, PHD

INTRODUCTION

The clinical microbiology laboratory plays a critical role in diagnosis and management of patients with *lower respiratory tract* (LRT) infections. By providing pathogen detection and identification and susceptibility testing, the laboratory provides the basis of optimal empirical antimicrobial therapy and individually tailored regimens.[1] The microbiology laboratory also provides data that assist the hospital epidemiologist in the prevention, detection, investigation, and termination of nosocomial outbreaks.[2] When correctly and promptly used, the information provided by the clinical microbiology laboratory improves clinical outcomes, reduces unnecessary use of antibiotics, and prevents nosocomial transmissions.[3,4]

The primary aim of this chapter is to assist clinicians in efficient and effective use of the clinical microbiology laboratory in diagnosis and management of infections of the LRT. This chapter assumes that clinical laboratories are using validated methods and reporting quality-assured results and does not delve into technical or operational aspects of the clinical microbiology laboratory. For additional information on laboratory operation, the reader is referred to the latest edition of the *Manual of Clinical Microbiology* (American Society for Microbiology).[5]

PREANALYTIC PRINCIPLES

PRINCIPLES OF TESTING

The decision to order a diagnostic test should hinge on whether the result is likely to affect the clinician's treatment decisions. If the clinician is convinced that the patient has a particular disease based on clinical presentation and prevalence (high pretest probability), then the decision to treat will likely not be altered by the test result and testing may not be indicated. Similarly, testing should not be ordered if the clinician has a high degree of a priori certainty that the patient does not have a disease because the decision not to

treat will likely not be altered by the test result. Testing is most useful when the clinician is uncertain about the probability of disease and the result can sway the physician's decision about treatment. In addition to the pretest probability, several factors affect this decision. For example, if therapy comes at a low harm (in terms of toxicity, financial cost, and selection of resistance), then treating all patients without testing may be appropriate. If the diagnostic test has a low sensitivity (i.e., it is positive in a low percentage of patients with disease), then testing may lead to an inappropriate decision not to treat. Similarly, if a diagnostic test has a low specificity (i.e., it is positive in a high percentage of patients without disease), then testing may lead to unnecessary treatment. The determination that clinical suspicion is uncertain enough to benefit from a particular diagnostic test involves the interplay of the cost and accuracy of the test, pretest probability of the disease, and benefit and harm of treatment.

INFECTION PREVENTION

The clinician plays a critical role in notifying the microbiology laboratory (and the hospital infection control epidemiologist) when virulent and transmissible agents are suspected as the cause of disease. Alerting laboratory staff reduces the risk of exposure of laboratory staff handling specimens and cultures harboring highly virulent pathogens (listed in Table 19.1). Not all specimens from patients with infectious diseases should be handled by the on-site laboratory. According to guidelines developed by local and national public health officials, specimens potentially containing high-risk agents, such as *Bacillus anthracis* spores, *Francisella tularensis*, *Yersinia pestis*, variola major, hemorrhagic fever viruses, or *Clostridium botulinum* toxin, are directly sent to the public health laboratories, where appropriate containment facilities and diagnostic tools are applied to make a diagnosis.[6] Other pathogens that are handled by the on-site laboratory, but still require laboratory notification, include *Coccidioides* and *Brucella* species because cultures of these are associated with a high risk for

Table 19.1 Pathogens That Require Laboratory
Notification When Suspected Clinically

Bacillus anthracis
Brucella sp
Burkholderia pseudomallei
Clostridium botulinum
Coccidioides sp
Francisella tularensis
Hemorrhagic fever viruses
Yersinia pestis
Variola major

laboratory-associated infection. Although the technologists are expected to handle all specimens and microbiologic cultures using universal precautions, accidental exposures can happen, especially if the findings are unexpected. Therefore laboratory notification alerts the staff to protect themselves from exposure to highly transmissible agents.

SYNDROMIC ORDER SETS

The diversity of etiologic agents of LRT infection poses a number of diagnostic challenges for the clinician. First, the provider must formulate a comprehensive yet pragmatic differential diagnosis that takes into account the clinical presentation, immune status, and the exposure history of the patient. Then the clinician must order the correct set of laboratory tests and ensure collection of the appropriate specimens and their placement in correct transport containers for transport to the laboratory under preestablished conditions for testing. Because improper test selection and specimen collection could reduce the analytic sensitivity and specificity of assays performed in the laboratory, syndromic order sets have been designed that consider the most common pathogens for the specific syndrome. Syndromic order sets incorporate general guidelines for the types of specimen required, collection and transport, and available assays for pathogens expected in a given clinical setting or syndrome. By prioritizing diagnostics that maximize yield and avoiding the need to repeat invasive procedures, these order sets also serve to minimize risk to the patient and to lower health care costs. However, it is the responsibility of the clinician to ensure that specimen requirements are met and the most critical tests are prioritized, especially when the amount of specimen material obtained is limited and multiple tests are ordered. Tables 19.2 to 19.4 show syndromic order sets for *community-acquired pneumonia* (CAP), hospital-acquired and ventilator-associated pneumonia, and immunocompromised host pneumonia, respectively. Order sets developed to address local epidemiologic characteristics and preanalytic practices may be tailored to serve each institution. Finally, clinicians should also familiarize themselves with local sample storage practices in case additional tests need to be performed.

SPECIMEN SELECTION, COLLECTION, AND TRANSPORT

In general, sterile specimens such as tissue samples and aspirates are the most valuable diagnostically because the absence of contamination with commensal organisms ensures that any organism detected likely represents a true pathogen. Histopathologic examination of tissue also provides information on the immunopathologic characteristics of the infectious process. However, a major diagnostic challenge of LRT infection is that LRT secretions are usually obtained through the oropharynx, which normally contains 10^{10} to 10^{12} *colony-forming units* (CFU) of aerobic and anaerobic bacteria per milliliter. Therefore LRT secretions collected for microbiologic examination are commonly contaminated with diverse bacteria (Table 19.5),[7] some of which, such as *Streptococcus pneumoniae, Haemophilus influenzae, Moraxella catarrhalis*, and *Neisseria meningitidis*, can also be pathogens of the LRT.[8–10] The oropharynx can also contain *Mycoplasma pneumoniae*[11] and aerobic actinomycetes, including *Nocardia* and nontuberculous mycobacteria, in the absence of disease.[12] Aspiration of even minute amounts (0.1–1 μL) of oropharyngeal secretions can deliver 10^9 CFU to the tracheobronchial tree. The distinction in such cases between colonization of the *upper respiratory tract* (URT) and pneumonia cannot be easily made by sputum examination and culture. Another challenge is that oropharyngeal secretions, which normally contain only a few gram-negative bacilli, such as Enterobacteriaceae, *Pseudomonas*, and *Acinetobacter*, may become colonized with as many as 10^7 CFU of gram-negative bacilli per milliliter in seriously ill patients requiring intensive care,[13] patients treated with antibiotics after hospitalization for acute pulmonary inflammatory disease,[14] chronic alcoholic and diabetic patients,[15] institutionalized older adults and chronically ill patients,[16] and hospitalized patients with acute leukemia.[17] Last, *Aspergillus* spores present in the environment are commonly deposited in the LRT and may be recovered from sputum in the absence of disease, although in immunocompromised patients it is best to consider this finding seriously.[18] In summary, because LRT secretions collected through the oropharynx are nearly always contaminated with resident microflora of the oral cavity, and definitive diagnosis would require sterile lung tissue with demonstration of parenchymal invasion, appropriate steps must be taken to obtain specimens of highest quality for microbiologic testing.

Expectorated sputum is the specimen most frequently obtained for the laboratory diagnosis of LRT infection.[5] The importance of proper sputum collection was documented by Laird[19] 100 years ago in studies on the yield of *Mycobacterium tuberculosis* according to the appearance and cellular composition of the sputum examined. The first requirement for collection of a good-quality sputum specimen is an alert and cooperative patient who can be instructed to rinse out his or her mouth with water or even brush his or her teeth before producing an LRT specimen. The patient then must be encouraged to cough deeply to expectorate a sample of LRT secretions. With some infections such as *tuberculosis* (TB), a larger sputum volume (i.e., minimum of 5 mL) can improve the sensitivity of culture.[20] Specimens are to be collected in sterile, leakproof, screw-capped containers. Containers should be transported in a watertight plastic biohazard bag.

Although a single sputum specimen may be sufficient for establishing the diagnosis of an acute bacterial process, collection of a series of three sputum specimens obtained in 1 or 2 days is recommended by the *Centers for Disease Control and Prevention* (CDC) in the United States for patients

Table 19.2 Community-Acquired Pneumonia Order Set

Syndrome/Organisms	Testing Uses/Indications	Appropriate Specimens	Available Testing
TYPICAL BACTERIA			
Haemophilus influenzae *Moraxella catarrhalis* *Staphylococcus aureus* *Streptococcus pneumoniae* *Streptococcus pyogenes* Aerobic gram-negative bacilli	Outpatients: microbiologic studies optional Inpatients: ■ Sputum studies for those with defined risks, complications, and/or severity ■ Blood culture for defined risk factors, including ICU admission	Sputum Bronchoscopic specimen Tissue Blood	Gram stain Aerobic culture Aerobic culture
LESS COMMON BACTERIA			
Chlamydophila pneumoniae *Chlamydia psittaci* *Coxiella burnetii* *Legionella pneumophila* serogroup 1 *Legionella* sp—other *Mycobacterium tuberculosis* *Mycoplasma pneumoniae*	*Mycoplasma* and *C. pneumoniae*: outbreaks and familial transmission *C. psittaci*: exposure to psitaccines	Nasopharyngeal swab, throat swab or washings Sputum Bronchoscopic specimen Bronchoalveolar lavage Tissue (including FFPE) Serum	NAT (species specific): *M. pneumoniae*; *C. pneumoniae*; *C. psittaci* NAT: 16S rRNA sequencing (tissue only) DFA: *C. pneumoniae* IgM, IgG: *M. pneumoniae*; *C. pneumoniae*; *C. psittaci* IgM, IgA, IgG: *C. burnetii*
	Legionella: outbreaks, travel-associated, lack of response to cell wall–active antibiotics, severe illness	Sputum Bronchoscopic specimen Tissue (including FFPE) Urine	BCYE culture NAT: *Legionella* sp NAT: 16S rRNA sequencing (tissue only) DFA: *L. pneumophila* *L. pneumophila* serogroup 1 antigen
	M. tuberculosis complex: appropriate epidemiology	Sputum Bronchoscopic specimen Tissue Pleural fluid	Acid-fast stain Mycobacterial culture NAT
VIRUSES			
Influenza A/B Adenovirus Parainfluenza 1/2/3 Respiratory syncytial virus Human metapneumovirus Varicella-zoster virus Hantaviruses Novel coronaviruses Novel influenza viruses SARS-CoV-2	Viral testing may provide justification for discontinuing antibiotics Seasonal epidemiology Known outbreak, epidemic, or pandemic	Nasopharyngeal swab Nasal aspirates or washes Bronchoscopic specimen Tissue	NAT
ASPIRATION PNEUMONIA			
Mixed anaerobic infections	Anaerobes typically already covered by broad-spectrum antibiotics; anaerobic culture rarely changes management	Pleural fluid Bronchoscopic specimen using protected specimen brush Tissue Pleural fluid Tissue	Gram stain Aerobic culture Anaerobic culture NAT
INVASIVE FUNGI			
Dimorphic Molds			
Blastomyces dermatitidis *Coccidioides immitis* *Coccidioides posadasii* *Histoplasma capsulatum* *Paracoccidioides brasiliensis*	From area of high endemicity	Sputum Bronchoscopic specimen Tissue Tissue Tissue (including FFPE) Pleural fluid Serum Urine	Fungal stain Fungal culture Histology NAT: species specific NAT: rRNA locus sequencing Antigen: *H. capsulatum*; *B. dermatitidis*; *C. immitis/posadasii* IgG (complement fixation, EIA): *H. capsulatum*; *C. immitis/posadasii*; *B. dermatitidis* IgM (immunodiffusion, latex agglutination, EIA): *C. immitis/posadasii* Antigen: *H. capsulatum*

Table 19.2 Community-Acquired Pneumonia Order Set—cont'd

Syndrome/Organisms	Testing Uses/Indications	Appropriate Specimens	Available Testing
Cryptococcus *C. neoformans* *C. gattii*		Serum Tissue Tissue (including FFPE) Pleural fluid	Cryptococcal antigen test Fungal stain Culture NAT: species specific NAT: rRNA locus sequencing
PARASITES			
Strongyloides stercoralis *Paragonimus* sp	From area of high endemicity	Sputum Bronchoscopic specimen Tissue	Microscopic examination Histology NAT: species specific

BCYE, buffered charcoal yeast extract; DFA, direct fluorescent antibody; EIA, enzyme immunoassay; FFPE, formalin-fixed paraffin-embedded; ICU, intensive care unit; Ig, immunoglobulin; NAT, nucleic acid test; rRNA, ribosomal ribonucleic acid; SARS-CoV-2, severe acute respiratory syndrome coronavirus 2.

Table 19.3 Hospital-Acquired and Ventilator-Associated Pneumonia Order Set

Syndrome/Organisms	Testing Uses/Indications	Appropriate Specimens	Available Testing
TYPICAL BACTERIA **Aerobic Gram-Positive Cocci** *Staphylococcus aureus* *Streptococcus pneumoniae* **Aerobic Gram-Negative Bacilli** *Acinetobacter* sp *Enterobacter* sp *Escherichia coli* *Klebsiella pneumoniae* *Pseudomonas aeruginosa* *Stenotrophomonas maltophilia* **Anaerobes** Mixed anaerobic species	Refractoriness to antibiotics Clinically ill patients with suspicious respiratory or chest radiograph findings Anaerobes typically already covered by broad-spectrum antibiotics; anaerobic culture rarely changes management	Sputum Endotracheal aspirate Bronchoalveolar lavage Bronchoscopic specimen using protected specimen brush Tissue Tissue (including FFPE) Blood	Gram stain Aerobic culture Anaerobic culture NAT: 16S rRNA sequencing Aerobic culture
ATYPICAL BACTERIA *Legionella pneumophila* serogroup 1 *Legionella* sp—other	*Legionella* outbreaks Refractory to β-lactams or AGs Immunocompromised Pneumonia plus GI symptoms	Induced sputum Bronchoscopic specimen Urine Tissue (including FFPE)	BCYE culture *Legionella* sp NAT: *Legionella* PCR DFA *L. pneumophila* serogroup 1 urine antigen NAT: 16S rRNA sequencing
VIRUSES Influenza A, B Adenovirus Parainfluenza 1, 2, 3 Respiratory syncytial virus	Circulating in community/seasonality Unvaccinated host Outbreak/cluster Pneumonia despite broad-spectrum antibiotics	Nasopharyngeal swab Nasal aspirates or washes Endotracheal aspirate Bronchoscopic specimen Bronchoscopic specimen using protected specimen brush	NAT
INVASIVE FUNGI *Aspergillus* sp *Mucorales* Mold species—other	Pulmonary cavity disease Environmental exposure/outbreak Immunocompromised	Endotracheal aspirate Bronchoalveolar lavage Bronchoscopic specimen using protected specimen brush Tissue Plasma Tissue (including FFPE) Bronchoalveolar lavage Serum	Fungal stain Fungal culture NAT: species specific NAT: rRNA locus sequencing (tissue only) NAT: metagenomics sequencing (plasma) Histology NAT: 18S rRNA sequencing Galactomannan (1→3) β-D-glucan

AGs, aminoglycosides; BCYE, buffered charcoal yeast extract; DFA, direct fluorescent antibody; FFPE, formalin-fixed paraffin-embedded; GI, gastrointestinal; NAT, nucleic acid test; rRNA, ribosomal ribonucleic acid; sp, species.

Table 19.4   Immunocompromised Host Pneumonia Order Set

Syndrome/Organisms	Testing Uses/Indications	Appropriate Specimens	Available Testing
BACTERIA			
CAP and HAP/VAP bacteria	See Tables 19.2 and 19.3	See Tables 19.2 and 19.3	See Tables 19.2 and 19.3
Burkholderia cepacia complex	Cystic fibrosis, CGD	Sputum Bronchoscopic specimen	Aerobic culture
Aerobic Actinomycetes			
Nocardia sp *Rhodococcus* sp Actinomycetes—other	Soil/environmental exposure	Sputum Bronchoscopic specimen Tissue (including FFPE)	Gram stain Modified acid-fast stain Aerobic culture including BCYE plate NAT: 16S rRNA sequencing (tissue only)
MYCOBACTERIA			
M. tuberculosis complex *M. avium-intracellulare* complex *M. kansasii* *M. xenopi* *M. haemophilum*	From area of high endemicity Known exposure/outbreak Bronchiectasis Appropriate epidemiology	Expectorated sputum Bronchoscopic specimen Tissue (including FFPE)	Cytology Acid-fast stain Mycobacterial culture NAT: *M. tuberculosis*–specific NAT: nontuberculous mycobacteria–specific NAT: 16S rRNA sequencing (tissue only)
M. abscessus *M. chelonae*—other		Tissue	Histology
VIRUSES			
CAP and HAP/VAP viruses Cytomegalovirus Herpes simplex virus Varicella-zoster virus	See Tables 19.2 and 19.3 CMV 1–4 months after transplant Serodiscordant donor/recipient Skin lesions	See Tables 19.2 and 19.3 Bronchoscopic specimen Tissue Tissue (fresh and FFPE) Plasma	See Tables 19.2 and 19.3 Cytology NAT Shell vial culture: CMV; HSV Histology Immunohistochemistry: CMV; HSV NAT NAT
FUNGI			
Pneumocystis jirovecii		Sputum Bronchoalveolar lavage Bronchoscopic specimen	DFA Fungal stain NAT
Cryptococcus neoformans *C. gattii*		Serum Tissue	Cryptococcal antigen test Fungal stain Culture
Monomorphic molds *Aspergillus fumigatus* Other *Aspergillus* sp		Sputum Bronchoscopic specimen Tissue Tissue (fresh and FFPE) Pleural fluid Plasma Serum	Fungal stain Fungal culture Histology NAT: species specific NAT: rRNA locus sequencing; metagenomics sequencing (plasma) Antigen: galactomannan Antigen: (1→3) β-D-glucan
Dimorphic molds	See Table 19.2	See Table 19.2	See Table 19.2
PARASITES			
Toxoplasma gondii	Cat exposure Raw meat consumption From area of high endemicity Lymphadenopathy	Induced sputum Bronchoscopic specimen Tissue Serum	Giemsa stain NAT IgM
Strongyloides stercoralis	From area of high endemicity	Induced sputum Bronchoscopic specimen Stool Tissue	Microscopy for larvae Strongyloides culture Histology

BCYE, buffered charcoal yeast extract; CAP, community-acquired pneumonia; CGD, chronic granulomatous disease; CMV, cytomegalovirus; DFA, direct fluorescent antibody; FFPE, formalin-fixed paraffin-embedded; HAP, hospital-acquired pneumonia; HSV, herpes simplex virus; IgM, immunoglobulin M; NAT, nucleic acid test; rRNA, ribosomal ribonucleic acid; VAP, ventilator-acquired pneumonia.

Table 19.5 Oropharyngeal Bacteria That Can Be Present Without Causing Disease

Commonly Present	Less Commonly Present, Transiently Present, or Present Only in Specific Contexts
Actinomyces, Corynebacterium, Eikenella corrodens, Enterococcus, Haemophilus, Moraxella catarrhalis, Neisseria, Staphylococcus, Streptococcus, Candida	Enterobacteriaceae, Pseudomonas aeruginosa, Acinetobacter baumannii, nontuberculous mycobacteria

suspected of having TB and nontuberculous mycobacterial infections.[21,22] In patients with nonproductive cough or suspected mycobacterial, fungal, or *Pneumocystis jirovecii* infections,[23] it may be helpful to induce sputum production with an inhaled aerosol of hypertonic salt solution (3–10%).

Once collected, the specimens should be delivered rapidly to the laboratory for processing to avoid overgrowth by contaminating flora, which can compromise microscopic detection and isolation of pathogenic bacteria.[24,25] Penn and Silberman[25] found that organisms observed microscopically on Gram-stained smears of sputum specimens and their relative numbers in cultures changed dramatically between processing within an hour of collection and processing after overnight refrigeration. Although there were no significant differences in the culture results between the immediate and delayed cultures in this study, the loss of reliable microscopic features had a significant impact on the interpretation of culture results. Processing delay is particularly important for culture recovery of slow-growing mycobacteria.[26] Specimens not sent to the laboratory for processing within 2 hours should be refrigerated for no more than 5 days.[27] If refrigeration is not possible, samples should be treated first with equal volume of 0.6% cetylpyridinium bromide or 1% cetylpyridinium chloride in 2% sodium chloride, which reduces the survival of contaminating microorganisms while preserving the viability of *M. tuberculosis* for up to 8 days.[26,28–30] Although the recovery of fungi is optimal from cultures of fresh specimens, most clinically significant fungi survive storage of 16 days or longer.[31] Specimens for viral cultures should be shipped refrigerated but not frozen, whereas specimens for chlamydial culture should be placed into sucrose phosphate medium and shipped frozen.

Although there is no universal agreement on the value of anaerobic culture,[32] protected catheter brushes may be used to obtain samples for culture and identification of organisms causing anaerobic pleuropulmonary disease.[33] It is essential to transport samples in an anaerobic vial to preserve the viability of anaerobic organisms.

For detection of respiratory viruses, nasopharyngeal specimens are preferred, although LRT specimens may be necessary to detect viral infection of the LRT.[34] There are a number of methods for the collection of nasopharyngeal specimens, which includes the use of flocked and traditional swabs, as well as aspirates and washes. Flocked swabs contain perpendicular arrangements of fibers with an open structure, to create a highly absorbent thin layer capable of efficient uptake of respiratory samples and elution into viral transport media. Nasopharyngeal flocked swabs have been

shown to be more sensitive for the detection of respiratory viruses than traditional swabs.[35,36] In turn, nasopharyngeal aspirates or washes have been shown to be more sensitive than nasopharyngeal flocked swabs.[37–39] However, the modest gains in sensitivity for detection of most respiratory viruses using aspirates or washes may be offset by the ease of nasopharyngeal specimen collection using flocked swabs. Oropharyngeal specimens are less sensitive for the diagnosis than nasopharyngeal specimens, although the combination may increase respiratory virus detection.[40–43] Oropharyngeal swabs may also be used for detecting *Chlamydophila pneumoniae*,[44–47] *M. pneumoniae*,[44,48,49] and *Legionella* sp.[44]

In patients who are critically ill or immunocompromised, or who cannot expectorate, one or more invasive approaches may be necessary to obtain diagnostic samples. Specimens may include endotracheal aspirates, pleural fluids, *bronchoalveolar lavage* (BAL), percutaneous lung aspirate, or lung biopsies.[5,50] The use of BAL has also been expanded to include diagnosis of bacterial pneumonia, especially for nosocomial cases.[51–53] In patients with CAP requiring admission to the hospital, use of protected catheter brush and BAL has been shown to provide microbiologic diagnoses not obtainable by noninvasive means,[54] although there is little support for using these procedures to diagnose CAP.[55] Although the results of cultures from protected catheter brushes and BAL specimens are quantitatively similar, Meduri and Baselski[54] concluded that BAL specimens provided a larger and more representative sample of LRT secretions than the protected catheter brushes, allowing microscopic analysis of the cytocentrifuged BAL fluid to identify the type of bacteria present and to demonstrate the presence of neutrophils with intracellular organisms. These procedures may also yield additional pathogens not obtainable by noninvasive approaches. Much work has also been done with the use of BAL for the diagnosis of ventilator-associated pneumonia[53–56] (see Chapter 49).

In children younger than 7 years with suspected TB, gastric aspirate is used as a surrogate for respiratory samples. Historically, it has been recommended that the pH of gastric aspirate be neutralized with sodium bicarbonate before transport to the laboratory; however, a more recent study suggests that neutralization of gastric aspirate may reduce the recovery of *M. tuberculosis*.[57] Nasopharyngeal aspirates have also been used for diagnosis of TB, although the sensitivity for culture-confirmed TB is lower than with induced sputum.[58] Stool samples in children with pulmonary TB may become the specimen of choice if processing methods can be optimized to concentrate the tubercle bacilli.[59,60]

Other specimen types that may aid in diagnosis of LRT infection include whole blood for blood culture, serum for antibody and antigen testing, urine for antigen testing, and plasma for detection of pathogen *cell-free DNA* (cfDNA). Blood culture is recommended in cases of severe pneumonia[61] but is positive only up to 37% in CAP and in less than 25% in nosocomial pneumonia.[61–65] It is important to note that a large blood volume (60 mL or three sets of blood culture bottles in adults) is necessary to maximize sensitivity of blood culture.[66,67] Although routine blood culture systems have been shown to be highly sensitive for detection of candidemia and cryptococcemia, automated blood culture systems are insensitive for cultivation of monomorphic and dimorphic molds. Isolation of molds (and fastidious bacteria) from blood requires the lysis-centrifugation method (Isolator)[68–70] or the use of enriched fungal medium bottles.[71,72]

S. pneumoniae can be recovered from urine cultures in as many as 38% of patients with pneumococcal pneumonia.[73] Urine may be tested for the presence of pneumococcal[74] and *Legionella pneumophila* serogroup 1[75] antigens. Fungal antigen tests of urine are also available for diagnosis of histoplasmosis, blastomycosis, and coccidioidomycosis.[76–78] Antigen assays are discussed later in this chapter.

Detection of cfDNA in the acellular fraction of blood (i.e., plasma) and urine has recently emerged as a promising new modality for noninvasive testing for infectious diseases.[79–81] Several different blood collection tubes and urine preservatives are commercially available. Studies are starting to define best practices for sample collection and processing to maximize accuracy.[82]

SPECIMEN ADEQUACY

Clinical laboratories are mandated by accrediting agencies to monitor specimen quality and quantity and to enforce rejection criteria when sample requirements are not met. Common causes for rejection include insufficient sample quantity, poor sample quality, and mislabeling of samples. For bacterial cultures, microscopic examination of sputum and endotracheal aspirate with Gram stain is used to screen samples for adequate quality.[19,83] The presence of excessive squamous epithelial cells (>10–25 per low-power field) is indicative of oropharyngeal contamination and therefore grounds for rejection for bacterial culture (Fig. 19.1). Although earlier criteria for the adequacy of sputum specimens for bacterial cultures also required the presence of polymorphonuclear leukocytes (neutrophils), the number of neutrophils in a sample is no longer used to evaluate specimen adequacy.[84] Endotracheal aspirates are rejected if the screening Gram-stained smears show no organisms.[83,85] Inclusion of microscopic sputum quality characteristics, such as a high number of white blood cells and or a low number of squamous epithelial cells, was not shown to be associated with diagnostic yield (i.e., smear microscopy) of *M. tuberculosis*.[86] For mycobacterial, fungal, and viral

cultures, cytologic screening to determine specimen acceptability is not enforced because contamination with commensals does not interfere with interpretation of the culture results. However, the presence of respiratory columnar epithelial cells has been shown to improve respiratory virus detection by *direct fluorescent antibody* (DFA) testing.[87]

MICROBIOLOGIC ASSAYS

The clinical microbiology laboratory offers a broad range of assays for diagnosis of LRT infection. For any particular pathogen, multiple assays may be available, and therefore it is the responsibility of the clinician to choose the assay with the best performance characteristic for a particular specimen type. eTable 19.1 summarizes the accuracy of assays used in the diagnosis of LRT infections caused by bacteria, fungi, and parasites. In addition, the clinician must be familiar with the turnaround time for each assay to optimize use of the results in managing the patient.

MICROSCOPY

Microscopic examination of LRT specimens offers a rapid approach to detection and identification of many pathogens. However, microscopic examination cannot distinguish between infection, colonization, and contamination when the specimen is collected through the oropharynx.[88–90] In addition, microscopy lacks sensitivity in specimens with less than 10^4 CFU per milliliter. Microscopy does routinely provide valuable information on the quality of specimen and the type of inflammatory response present. Specimens demonstrating a preponderance of polymorphonuclear leukocytes, ciliated columnar epithelial cells, or alveolar macrophages with few, if any, squamous epithelial cells (<10 per low-power field) represent LRT secretions. The presence of alveolar macrophages is a more specific marker of LRT secretions than neutrophils and is more likely to be associated with a significantly lower incidence of oropharyngeal contamination.[91] The finding of neutrophils with intracellular organisms is considered indicative of an active infectious process.[92–94]

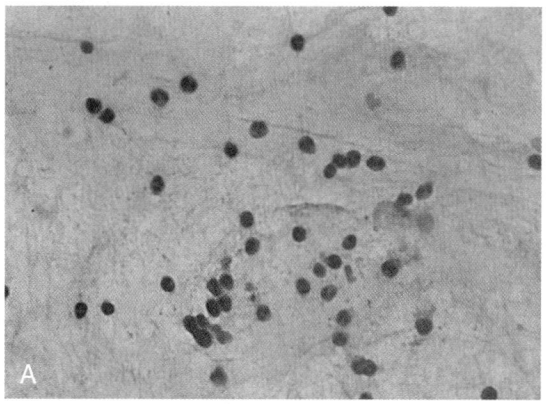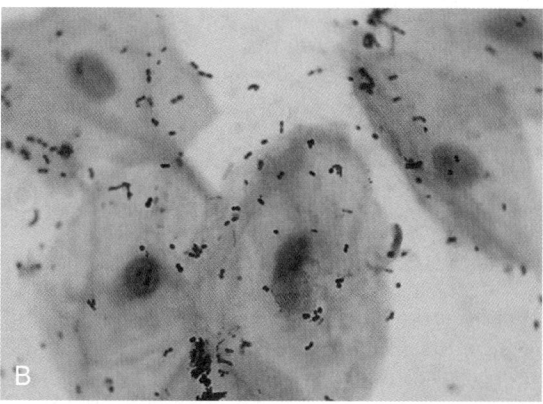

Figure 19.1 Gram stain of sputum specimens. (A) This specimen contains numerous polymorphonuclear leukocytes and no visible squamous epithelial cells, indicating that the specimen is acceptable for routine bacteriologic culture. (B) This specimen contains numerous squamous epithelial cells and rare polymorphonuclear leukocytes, indicating an inadequate specimen for routine sputum culture. (From Tille P. *Bailey & Scott's Diagnostic Microbiology,* ed 13. Philadelphia: Elsevier; 2014.)

Table 19.6 Laboratory Criteria for Reporting Gram Stain Results to the Ordering Physician

Number of Bacteria Found per Field Under Oil Immersion 100× Objective	Bacterial Quantity Reported to Clinician
0	Negative
<1	1+ (rare)
1–5	2+ (few)
6–30	3+ (moderate)
>30	4+ (heavy)

Table 19.7 Pathognomonic Gram Stain Patterns

Pattern Reported	Pathogen or Entity Suggested
Intracellular organisms	Active infection
Gram-positive cocci in pairs (lancet-shaped diplococci) and short chains	*Streptococcus pneumoniae*
Pleomorphic gram-negative coccobacilli	*Haemophilus influenzae*
Gram-negative diplococci	*Moraxella catarrhalis**
Gram-positive cocci in clusters	*Staphylococcus aureus*
Mixed morphotypes of gram-positive and gram-negative rods, cocci, and coccobacilli	Aspiration pneumonia
Beaded gram-positive or gram-variable rods	Actinomycetales order, which includes genera *Mycobacterium, Actinomyces, Corynebacterium*
Filamentous branching gram-positive or gram-variable rods	*Nocardia, Actinomyces*

*Cannot be distinguished from *Neisseria meningitidis*.

The Gram-stained smear is an essential and necessary part of the evaluation of sputum and tracheal aspirates for determining the quality and acceptability of specimens for bacterial culture[83,85] and for providing a rapid assessment of the most likely etiologic agent of the pneumonia. Although Gram stains might also suggest the presence of mycobacteria, fungi, and parasites, special stains should be ordered when those pathogens are suspected. Table 19.6 shows criteria used by the laboratory to interpret findings on Gram stain and report them to the physician. Although it is impossible to correlate every staining pattern to a particular pathogen, several Gram stain patterns are pathognomonic for a particular pathogen or clinical entity (Table 19.7).

The accuracy of Gram stain for detection of infection depends on the stringency of criteria. In assessing patients with acute CAP, Rein and colleagues[95] found that three or more gram-positive lancet-shaped diplococci (Fig. 19.2A) correctly predicted the presence of pneumococci in corresponding cultures in 90% of cases, with a sensitivity and specificity of 62% and 85%, respectively. As expected, improving the sensitivity of the Gram stain examination by lowering the criteria for positivity resulted in reduced specificity in the diagnosis of pneumococcal infection. Similar levels of sensitivity of Gram-stained smears have been reported by others in identifying pneumococci as well

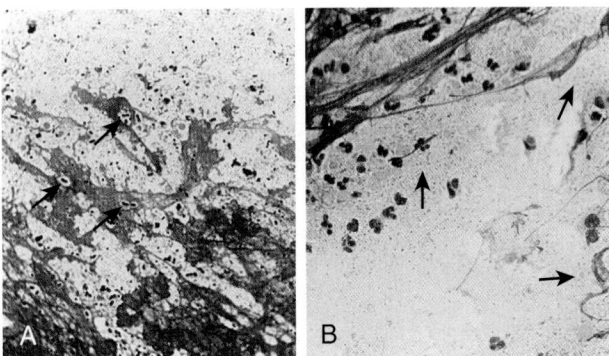

Figure 19.2 Gram stains of bacteria in sputum. (A) Lancet-shaped diplococci in Gram-stained sputum from a case of *Streptococcus pneumoniae* pneumonia. The clear "halo" surrounding some of the diplococci *(arrows)* is the consequence of the thick polysaccharide capsule. (B) Gram stain of *Haemophilus influenzae* in sputum. The small gram-negative bacilli *(arrows)* can be difficult to distinguish from debris. (From Tille P. *Bailey & Scott's Diagnostic Microbiology*, ed 13. Philadelphia: Elsevier; 2014.)

as *H. influenzae* (see Fig. 19.2B) in sputum specimens from patients with acute CAP.[96,97] For the diagnosis of pneumococcal pneumonia, a combination of Gram-stained smear and culture of sputum can yield the correct diagnosis in greater than 80% of patients who received less than 24 hours of effective antibiotic therapy.[98]

Direct examination of sputum for the identification of other organisms that can either be commensals or causes of acute bacterial pneumonia in adults, such as *H. influenzae*, *M. catarrhalis*, and *N. meningitidis*, may also be challenging.[8,88,90,99] Their role as etiologic agents of pneumonia is strongly suggested by the finding of large numbers of gram-negative coccobacilli *(H. influenzae)* and diplococci (*M. catarrhalis* and *N. meningitidis*) located within and outside of neutrophils in sputum specimens.[92–94] Because sputum microscopy (and subsequent culture) can give misleading results, the diagnosis of *Haemophilus, Moraxella*, or meningococcal pneumonia can be confirmed only by invasive techniques. Because invasive techniques are infrequently performed to identify the etiologic agents of acute CAP, the sensitivity and specificity of sputum Gram-stained smears cannot be determined reliably in such cases. A similar challenge is faced when trying to distinguish between colonization and infection by gram-negative bacilli. For example, up to 10^8 CFU of gram-negative bacilli per milliliter may be found in respiratory secretions of patients on mechanical ventilation in intensive care units without evidence of pneumonia.[13]

Acid-fast staining is the method of choice for visualization of mycobacteria in respiratory specimens. Laboratories may use either carbolfuchsin or fluorochrome to stain mycobacteria. Table 19.8 shows criteria used by the laboratory to report findings on the acid-fast stain. In most studies the carbolfuchsin-based stain has a sensitivity of 60% or lower compared with culture.[100] The fluorochrome stain, which uses a fluorescent dye such as auramine or auramine-rhodamine to highlight mycobacteria, is on average 10% more sensitive than carbolfuchsin[100] and is therefore the method recommended by the *World Health Organization* (WHO) for screening sputum smears for mycobacteria. The sensitivity of acid-fast microscopy depends on the bacillary burden, sample volume, host immune status,

Table 19.8   Laboratory Criteria for Reporting of Acid-Fast Stain Results

No. of AFB Found Under Oil Immersion 100× Objective (Carbolfuchsin Stain)	No. of AFB Found Under 10× Objective (Fluorochrome Stain)	Bacterial Quantity Reported to Clinician
0 per 300 fields	0 per 30 fields	Negative
1–2 per 300 fields	1–2 per 30 fields	± (suspicious)
1–9 per 100 fields	1–9 per 10 fields	1+
1–9 per 10 fields	1–9 per field	2+
1–9 per field	10–90 per field	3+
>9 per field	>90 per field	4+

AFB, acid-fast bacilli.
Modified from David HL. *Bacteriology of the mycobacterioses.* Publication No. CDC 76-8316. Atlanta: Department of Health, Education, & Welfare. 1976:153.

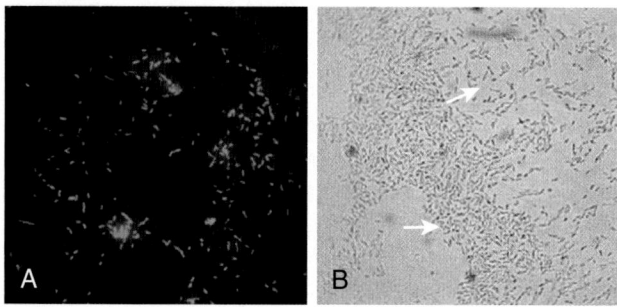

Figure 19.3 *Legionella* pneumophila detection by microscropy. (A) Direct fluorescent antibody stain. (B) Gram stain of a colony grown on agar. The organisms are thin gram-negative bacilli *(arrows).* (From Tille P. *Bailey & Scott's Diagnostic Microbiology,* ed 13. Philadelphia: Elsevier; 2014.)

staining method, and other variables.[101] The major limiting factor is that approximately 10^4 acid-fast bacilli per milliliter of sputum must be present to be visualized under light microscopy using an acid-fast stain.[101] The insensitivity of smear microscopy for TB therefore necessitates the use of more sensitive methods, such as culture and *nucleic acid tests* (NATs).[102,103] In addition, although acid-fast stains have high specificity, they cannot distinguish between *M. tuberculosis* complex and nontuberculous mycobacteria, and carbolfuchsin stains also stain *Legionella micdadei* (also known as *Tatlockia micdadei*).[104] Modified acid-fast stain, a modified carbolfuchsin stain, is used for direct staining of partially acid-fast–positive organisms, such as *Nocardia, Tsukamurella, Rhodococcus,* and *Gordonia.*[5]

Immunofluorescence examination by DFA staining is an alternative method for direct visualization of organisms. The diagnosis of legionellosis is usually made by a combination of direct immunofluorescence examination and culture of respiratory specimens, and antigen and antibody testing. DFA staining can be performed on sputum, endotracheal aspirate, bronchial washing, and lung tissue specimens, with sensitivities ranging from 25–66% and specificities of greater than 94% for the diagnosis of *L. pneumophila* pneumonia[105] (Fig. 19.3). Both clinical and technical variables account for the broad range of sensitivity of this test, and the accuracy of this method for detection of pneumonia due to other *Legionella* sp is less precisely known. In the absence of other supporting evidence, a positive DFA result is generally not accepted as sufficient for the diagnosis of *Legionella* infection, and other confirmatory measures should be undertaken.

DFA testing is sensitive and specific in detecting *Chlamydia trachomatis* in nasopharyngeal specimens from infants with pneumonia and has also been applied to sputum and BAL for detection of *P. jirovecii,* the agent of *Pneumocystis* pneumonia.[106,107] Silver stain, direct immunofluorescence, indirect immunofluorescence, and Diff-Quik (a modified Giemsa stain) have all been found to have greater than 90% sensitivity for detecting *P. jirovecii* in induced sputum and BAL samples from *human immunodeficiency virus* (HIV)-infected patients[108] (Fig. 19.4A). All of these staining techniques have lower sensitivity in patients who are not infected with HIV, but DFA is consistently more sensitive than the other staining techniques.[109,110]

DFA has also been applied to respiratory secretions for the diagnosis of respiratory virus infections. DFA testing can be performed in 1 to 4 hours and is typically more sensitive than rapid antigen tests.[87,111] However, DFA testing for respiratory viruses requires a high level of technical and interpretive expertise, is difficult to adapt to the high throughput required for pandemic or high-volume testing, and remains less sensitive than real-time *polymerase chain reaction* (PCR).[87,112] DFA for viral detection has been phased out in many clinical laboratories as rapid, sensitive, multiplexed molecular diagnostic respiratory virus tests have become available.

The visualization of fungal elements in respiratory secretions requires the use of special stains. Historically, potassium hydroxide was used to degrade host tissue and visualize fungal elements, such as *Blastomyces* (see Fig. 19.4B–C). Calcofluor white stain, a fluorochrome that binds to chitin and cellulose present in the fungal cell wall, is now commonly added to potassium hydroxide or used alone to provide better delineation of fungal elements, including *Histoplasma capsulatum* (see Fig. 19.4D).[113,114] Table 19.9 lists staining patterns suggestive of certain fungal pathogens. It is important to note that identification of fungi based on microscopic appearance of fungal elements in lung tissue or secretions is subject to error, and definitive identification must be deferred to culture or NATs.[115]

The identification of pulmonary parasites, such as *Strongyloides stercoralis* and *Paragonimus* sp, is typically made by microscopic examination of respiratory secretions. *S. stercoralis* larvae and rarely eggs can be seen on most stains but are sufficiently large that they are more likely to be found using a low-power objective (Fig. 19.5).[116] The diagnosis of microfilariae causing tropical pulmonary eosinophilia requires peripheral blood parasite examination of nightly blood samples because these parasites typically

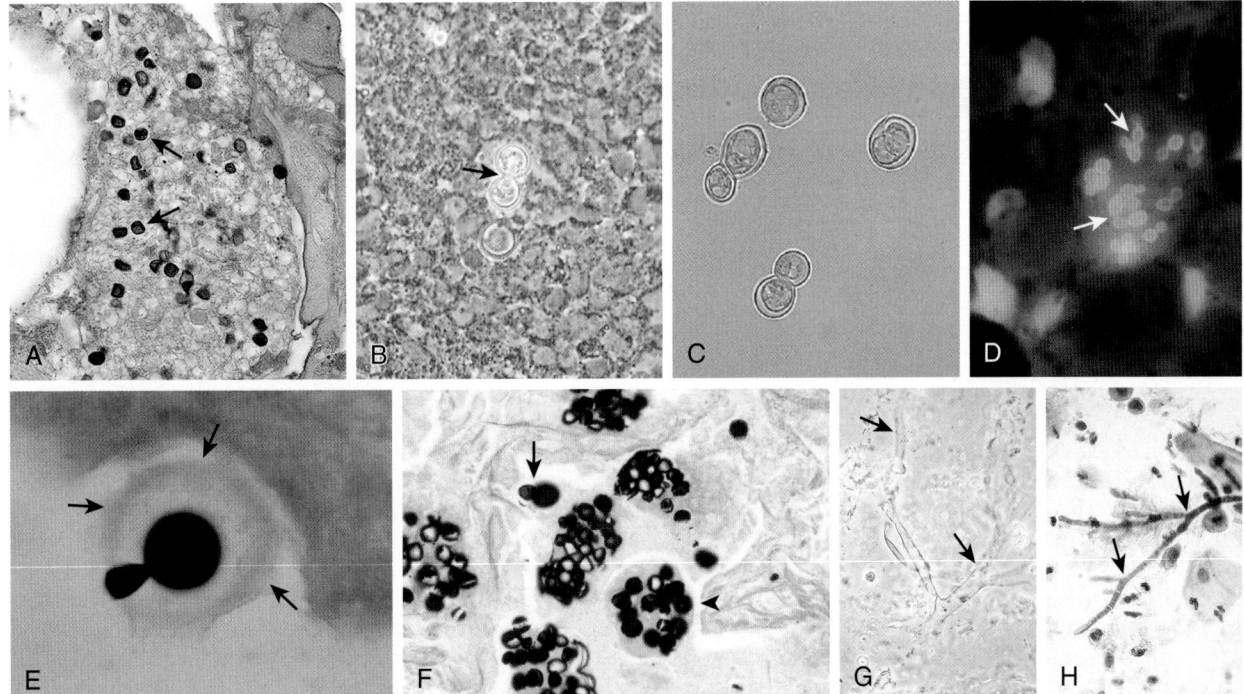

Figure 19.4 Microscopic identification of fungal pathogens. (A) Cyst forms of *Pneumocystis jirovecii (arrows)* stained with methenamine silver and hematoxylin and eosin stain (×500 original magnification). (B) *Blastomyces dermatidis*. Potassium hydroxide preparation of exudate shows a large budding yeast cell with a distinct broad base *(arrow)* between inflammatory cells (phase-contrast microscopy). (C) Thick-walled, oval to round, single-budding, yeast-like *Blastomyces dermatidis* cells from culture. (D) *Histoplasma capsulatum (arrows)* seen with calcofluor white stain of sputum showing 2- to 5-μm-diameter intracellular organisms. (E) *Cryptococcus neoformans* with narrow-based bud; silver stain. The faintly staining capsule is also visible *(arrows)*. (F) *Coccidioides immitis* spherules in a tissue biopsy. Spherules can also be found in fresh sputum samples. The internal endospores stain with silver *(arrowhead)*, whereas the external wall of the spherule does not. The endospores that have been released from a spherule resemble budding yeast *(arrow)* (GMS stain; ×400 original magnification). (G) *Rhizopus* sp in a potassium hydroxide preparation of sputum showing broad, predominantly nonseptate hyphae *(arrows)*. Phase-contrast microscopy. (H) Branching septate hyphae *(arrows)* of *Aspergillus fumigatus*. Papanicolaou staining of sputum. GMS, Gomori methenamine silver. (A–D and F–H, From Tille P. *Bailey & Scott's Diagnostic Microbiology*, ed 13. Philadelphia: Elsevier; 2014; E, From Mandell GL, Bennett JE, Dolin R. *Principles and Practice of Infectious Diseases,* ed 7. Philadelphia: Elsevier; 2010.)

Table 19.9 Microscopic Descriptions Suggestive of Certain Fungal Pathogens

Key Patterns Reported From Respiratory Specimens	Pathogens the Findings Suggest
Broad-based budding yeast (see Fig. 19.4B–C)	*Blastomyces dermatitidis*
Narrow-based budding yeast (Fig. 19.4D–E)	*Candida, Cryptococcus, Histoplasma capsulatum, Sporothrix schenckii*
Spherule (Fig. 19.4F)	*Coccidioides immitis, Coccidioides posadasii*
Nonseptate hyphal element (Fig. 19.4G)	Zygomycetes (cannot be predicted from formalin-fixed paraffin-embedded tissue)
Septate hyphal element (Fig. 19.4H)	Monomorphic hyaline and dematiaceous molds, including *Aspergillus*

circulate in the blood only at night, which coincides with activity of its insect vector.[117] *Echinococcus* cysts may be detected in pulmonary cyst fluid, and *Entamoeba histolytica* may be seen in association with pleural disease, if an amebic liver abscess erodes through the diaphragm.

CULTURE

Microbiologic culture of respiratory specimens allows definitive identification of the suspected pathogens and permits

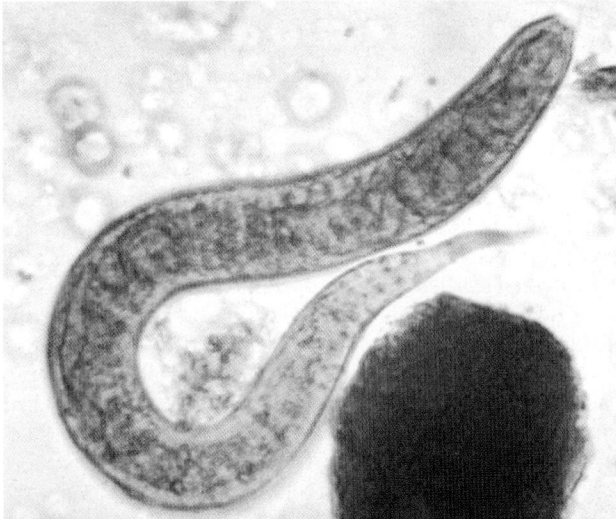

Figure 19.5 *Strongyloides stercoralis* rhabditiform larva; iodine stain. When examined under low power, staining of sputum may be unnecessary. Unfixed preparations can also show larval mobility. (From Tille P. *Bailey & Scott's Diagnostic Microbiology,* ed 13. Philadelphia: Elsevier; 2014.)

determination of susceptibility to antimicrobial agents for bacteria, mycobacteria, and yeast. For cultivation of particular groups or species of microorganisms, laboratories must inoculate processed samples on one or more culture media supplemented with nutrients suitable for cultivation of the desired

Table 19.10 Semiquantitative Scheme for Grading Bacterial Growth on Streaked Agar Plates

Grade	NO. OF COLONIES PRESENT IN CONSECUTIVE STREAKED QUADRANTS		
	First	Second	Third
1+	<10	0	0
2+	>10	<5	0
3+	>10	>5	<5
4+	>10	>5	>5

Data from Waites KB, Saubolle MA, Talkington DF, et al. *Cumitech 10A: Laboratory Diagnosis of Upper Respiratory Tract Infections.*Washington, DC: American Society for Microbiology Press; 2006.

microorganisms and inhibitors for selective inhibition of undesirable organisms. The clinician must therefore be aware that, although many organisms do grow on routine aerobic and anaerobic cultures, a number of respiratory pathogens, such as *Mycoplasma, Legionella, Mycobacterium, Nocardia, Rhodococcus,* and *H. capsulatum,* require pathogen-specific growth conditions (growth supplements, temperature and carbon dioxide requirements, and incubation times), which have to be specified when fastidious pathogens are part of the differential diagnosis.[5] For example, *Legionella* sp require culture media supplemented with L-cysteine and α-ketoglutarate (buffered charcoal yeast extract),[105] slow-growing mycobacteria require media enriched with a lipid extract and antimicrobials to limit the growth of oral commensals,[101] and *H. capsulatum* requires extended incubation time up to 4 weeks.[118] Although most *Nocardia* sp grow well on mycobacterial culture media and on ordinary bacterial and fungal culture media, optimal recovery from clinical specimens is obtained by using the same buffered charcoal yeast extract culture medium as that for the isolation of *Legionella.*[119]

Laboratories commonly use a semiquantitative culturing method and report the number of colonies present in consecutive streaked quadrants using a 1+ to 4+ grading system. Table 19.10 lists criteria for reporting of semiquantitative cultures. It is important to note that with the semiquantitative culture method, the volume of specimen cultured is not standardized. Quantitative cultures are also performed on certain respiratory specimens, such as protected catheter brush specimens and BAL fluid.[120] Nonetheless, a randomized trial found that in mechanically ventilated patients with pneumonia, the use of quantitative BAL and nonquantitative endotracheal aspirate cultures resulted in similar clinical outcomes, although patients known to be colonized or infected with *Pseudomonas aeruginosa* or methicillin-resistant *Staphylococcus aureus* were excluded, and antibiotics were withheld until the results of culture were available.[56] Bacteria present in quantities greater than 10^3 CFU/mL in cultures of protected catheter brushes[52] and in quantities greater than 10^4 CFU/mL in cultures of BAL fluids[54] are defined by the laboratory as positive and identified and tested for their susceptibility to appropriate antimicrobial agents.[121] The diagnostic value of break points of bacterial growth (i.e., 10^3–10^5 CFU/mL) depends not only on the type of microbiologic processing used but also on the relationship of two variables: The concentration of pathogens present in the BAL fluid and degree of contamination of the bronchoscopic channel through which lavage fluid was injected and aspirated. Other variables affecting the sensitivity of BAL specimens include antibiotic administration and the volume of lavage fluid injected and volume of fluid retrieved.[122] Diagnostic specificity depends greatly on techniques used to minimize contamination of the specimen by upper respiratory flora, such as discarding the first aliquot of aspirated fluid.[123]

Because many pathogens of the LRT are also members of the oropharyngeal flora, culture results must be correlated with the Gram stain findings, including the presence or absence of polymorphonuclear leukocytes. Respiratory pathogens seen to be predominant on Gram stain with typical morphologic characteristics within and outside polymorphonuclear leukocytes are reported and identified to the species level. Upper respiratory colonization with potentially pathogenic microorganisms, such as gram-negative bacilli, may not be related to the actual etiologic agents of LRT infection. Sputum specimens contaminated with Enterobacteriaceae or *S. aureus* from oropharyngeal secretions may obscure the diagnosis of pneumococcal pneumonia, anaerobic pleuropulmonary infection, or even TB.[124–127] With the exception of *Cryptococcus,* yeasts are considered to be of upper respiratory origin and are not routinely identified.[127]

The sensitivity and specificity of cultures depend on the pathogen burden, specimen type, collection method, the cytologic screening criteria applied to ensure sampling of LRT secretions, and the threshold of colony count to distinguish infection from contamination. In 1971, Barrett-Connor[124] showed that only 45% of patients with bacteremic pneumococcal pneumonia had pneumococci isolated from their sputum cultures, whereas 27% of patients had moderate to heavy growth of another potential pathogen in these cultures. In contrast, fungal cultures of respiratory specimens were positive in approximately 85% of cases with disseminated or chronic pulmonary histoplasmosis.[128,129] Careful specimen collection, cytologic screening of specimens to discard those contaminated with oropharyngeal secretions, and use of the results of the Gram-stained smear to guide identification of isolates in culture all contribute to the diagnostic value of sputum culture in acute pneumococcal pneumonia.

It is also important for the clinician to have knowledge of the turnaround time of all tests, including cultures. The time to detection of positive culture results is dependent on the number of organisms in the inoculum and the replication rate of the pathogen.[118] Table 19.11 shows typical turnaround times for LRT pathogens.

Bacterial cultures can also assist with diagnosis of certain parasitic infections. Fecal *Strongyloides* culture may be useful in cases of suspected pulmonary involvement with *S. stercoralis* when sputum cytologic examination fails to identify larvae. The agar plate method, which looks for tracking of bacteria by the motile larvae, is a useful adjunct to standard microscopic fecal examination and may be up to six times more sensitive.[130–133]

Viral culture techniques previously played an important role in the diagnosis of respiratory virus infections.[134] However, traditional viral culture is laborious, requires significant technical and interpretive expertise, allows the isolation of only a limited range of disease-causing viruses, and has a long turnaround time that limits clinical utility.[135] Shell vial culture is an improved method in which a sample is centrifuged onto a layer of cells, with subsequent detection of viral

Table 19.11 Time to Detection of Respiratory Pathogens in Culture

Key Respiratory Pathogens	Time to Detection in Culture
Acinetobacter baumannii, Aspergillus, Coccidioides immitis, Coccidioides posadasii, Cryptococcus, Escherichia coli, Haemophilus influenzae, Klebsiella pneumoniae, Moraxella catarrhalis, Mycobacterium abscessus group, *Mycobacterium chelonae, Neisseria meningitidis, Nocardia,* Pseudomonas aeruginosa, Staphylococcus aureus, Streptococcus pneumoniae, Zygomycetes*	1–3 days
Actinomyces, Legionella* Sporothrix schenckii	3–5 days
Blastomyces dermatitidis, Histoplasma capsulatum, Mycobacterium avium-intracellulare complex, *Mycobacterium tuberculosis* complex, *Mycoplasma pneumoniae*	1–4 weeks

*May take longer.
Modified from Hove MG, Woods GL. Duration of fungal culture incubation in an area endemic for *Histoplasma capsulatum. Diagn Microbiol Infect Dis.* 1997;28:41.

antigen. Shell vial cultures, particularly those using a mixture of mink lung and A549 cells, provide equivalent to improved sensitivity compared to traditional culture, with more rapid turnaround time.[136–138] Similar to respiratory virus DFA, routine respiratory viral cultures are being phased out in many clinical laboratories with the widespread availability of respiratory virus molecular diagnostic tests. However, in BAL samples from transplant recipients and other immunocompromised patients, shell vial cultures using human fibroblast cell lines may be clinically useful for detection of *cytomegalovirus* (CMV),[139,140] and traditional viral cultures may be useful for recovery of herpes simplex virus.[141–143]

ANTIMICROBIAL SUSCEPTIBILITY TESTING

Antimicrobial susceptibility testing is performed to assist clinicians with the selection of appropriately targeted antibiotic therapy to optimize clinical outcomes. There are several aspects of this in vitro testing that are important to understand. First, testing methods and interpretation of results must be done according to accepted standards, such as the *Clinical and Laboratory Standards Institute* (CLSI), the *US Food and Drug Administration* (FDA), or the *European Committee on Antimicrobial Susceptibility Testing* (EUCAST) for the various categories of organism. Second, the selection of antibiotics to test and report is determined in collaboration with CLSI/EUCAST guidelines, the hospital formulary, infectious disease specialists, the pharmacy, and the infection prevention committee. Third, antimicrobial susceptibility testing should not be performed when the pathogen has a predictable susceptibility profile (e.g., all *Streptococcus pyogenes* are currently susceptible to penicillin), nor is susceptibility testing needed for a specific antibiotic when an organism has intrinsic resistance to that antibiotic (e.g., *Enterobacter* sp, *Klebsiella* sp, *Citrobacter* sp, and *Serratia* sp are all intrinsically resistant to ampicillin). The bacterial pathogens from the LRT for which the susceptibility profile is not predictable, and thus antimicrobial susceptibility

testing is commonly performed, are *S. pneumoniae, S. aureus, H. influenzae, M. catarrhalis*, the Enterobacteriaceae, *P. aeruginosa*, and other nonfermenting gram-negative rods. Fourth, because antimicrobial susceptibility testing measures in vitro activity, other factors must be considered when determining in vivo activity, including antimicrobial pharmacokinetics and pharmacodynamics and patient-specific factors such as immune status.

Phenotypic susceptibility testing methods used by the clinical laboratory consist of the disk diffusion method, which generates a qualitative result based on the zone size of bacterial growth inhibition, and the dilution method, which generates a quantitative result: the *minimum inhibitory concentration* (MIC). Results generated by each method are reported as "susceptible," "susceptible–dose-dependent," "intermediate," or "resistant." Susceptible implies the organism will likely respond to treatment with the antibiotic at a standard dosage. Susceptible–dose-dependent implies likely response to treatment with a higher and more frequent dose than the standard dosage. Intermediate may be effective if higher dosing can be used (e.g., β-lactams) or if the antibiotic has high concentrations at the site of infection (e.g., fluoroquinolones for urinary tract infections). Resistant implies the organism is not likely to respond to therapy with that antibiotic. The interpretation criteria (susceptible, intermediate, resistant) are specific to each organism-drug combination and to the pharmacokinetics (e.g., peak serum levels, protein binding, and clearance rate of the drug) and the pharmacodynamics (e.g., whether the rate of bacterial killing is concentration dependent) of each drug. Therefore, because the measurement of the MIC alone does not capture these multiple considerations, simply choosing a drug on the basis of the lowest MIC in a susceptibility report is not recommended.

Genotypic susceptibility testing is also possible for certain pathogen-drug combinations when a monogenic mutation accurately predicts a resistant phenotype. Examples include the *mecA* gene for methicillin resistance in *Staphylococcus*,[144] *vanA* and *vanB* for vancomycin resistance in *Enterococcus*,[145] and specific *rpoB* mutations in rifampin resistance in *M. tuberculosis*.[146]

Not all pathogens isolated in the laboratory can be reliably tested for antimicrobial susceptibility. For organisms such as *Chlamydophila, Mycoplasma, Legionella*, nontuberculous mycobacteria, and molds, there are currently no standard test methods or interpretive criteria. For these pathogens, clinical experience, use of consensus guidelines, and careful assessment of patient response to antimicrobial therapy is most valuable for optimal patient management.

NUCLEIC ACID TESTS

In recent years, technological advances in NATs and instrument automation have revolutionized the simplicity, speed, and accuracy of detecting fastidious pathogens directly from respiratory specimens.[146–148] In many laboratories, these tests have replaced conventional, less sensitive, more laborious methods for routine use. With the unique capabilities of molecular diagnostic tests and the need for rapid, sensitive detection of respiratory pathogens, molecular assays will continue to gain an increasing role in the diagnosis and management of patients with opportunistic pneumonia and CAP. Most NATs are based on amplification and detection of nucleic acid targets specific to the pathogens of interest. NATs offer several advantages over conventional direct examination, microbiologic cultures, and serologic assays. First, NATs have the ability to detect and identify pathogens rapidly (in hours). Second, NATs provide the only means of direct detection for some microorganisms that are difficult or impossible to grow in culture. Certain viruses, for example, are very difficult to cultivate by conventional culture-based methods, and NATs enable detection of these organisms in clinical specimens.[149] Third, NATs make possible detection of pathogens, such as *M. tuberculosis*, in resource-limited settings where laboratory infrastructure for culture is lacking.[150,151] Finally, for some pathogens, NATs allow determination of antimicrobial susceptibility directly from respiratory tract specimens.

A number of commercial and in-house NATs are available for direct detection of *M. tuberculosis* in sputum, BAL, pleural fluid, lung tissue, and lymph node. These assays can yield results in 2 to 8 hours. For example, in comparison to conventional cultures for *M. tuberculosis*, NATs have high sensitivities (86–97%) and specificities (98%) in smear-positive respiratory samples.[101] In smear-negative, culture-positive specimens, NATs can confirm the presence of *M. tuberculosis* in 33–96% of samples, weeks earlier than culture.[101] The Xpert MTB/RIF (Cepheid) assay is a *sample-to-answer* assay, meaning it is a self-contained system that can process the sample and provide the answer without intervening steps from the laboratory personnel. The Xpert MTB/RIF has a pooled sensitivity of 98% and 67% in smear-positive and smear-negative TB, respectively.[152] The pooled specificity is 99%. Compared to Xpert MTB/RIF, the Xpert Ultra assay, designed to have higher sensitivity, has higher pooled sensitivity (88% vs. 83%) but slightly lower specificity (96% vs. 98%).[153] For smear-negative sputa, the sensitivity of NATs further improves if the assay is performed on one to two additional samples.[146] Detection of *M. tuberculosis* susceptibility to first- and second-line drugs can also be accomplished directly from sputum.[154,155] Commercial NATs detect rifampin and isoniazid resistance with sensitivity of 94–99% and 88–95%, respectively.[101,155–157] Xpert MTB/RIF has a pooled sensitivity of 95% and specificity of 98% for rifampin resistance detection.[153] Based on the improved performance of NATs over smear microscopy and the rapid turnaround time compared to culture, the CDC has recommended that NAT "testing should be performed on at least one respiratory specimen from each patient with signs and symptoms of pulmonary TB for whom a diagnosis of TB is being considered but has not yet been established, and for whom the test result would alter case management or TB control activities."[103] Further, based on a multicenter study in US patients, FDA approved the use of either one or two negative Xpert MTB/RIF result(s) as an alternative to three negative smears to remove patients from respiratory isolation.[158] In addition, WHO has recommended the use of Xpert assay as the initial diagnostic test in all individuals with presumed pulmonary TB.[159,160]

Diagnostic methods have also been described for detecting the nucleic acids of *C. pneumoniae*,[8,45,46] *M. pneumoniae*,[44,48,49] *L. pneumophila*,[44] dimorphic fungi,[161] monomorphic fungi,[162–165] *P. jirovecii*,[166] *Toxoplasma gondii*,[167,168] respiratory viruses,[149] herpes simplex virus,[142]

and CMV[169–172] directly in respiratory specimens of normal and immunocompromised hosts. Accuracy studies have indicated that most of these assays are at least comparable to, if not better than, conventional culture, direct antigen, and/or serologic detection methods, especially when examining respiratory specimens that contain low numbers of pathogens. For example, a rapid PCR assay has been applied for the diagnosis of an outbreak of *Chlamydia psittaci* that resulted from transmission to humans from birds purchased in stores; in this outbreak, PCR detected 50% more cases than did culture.[173] Compared to culture and serologic tests, PCR was also shown to be the most sensitive method for detection of *C. pneumoniae* during an outbreak of CAP.[174] For *P. jirovecii*, pooled sensitivity and specificity of PCR in BAL fluid was 98.3% and 91.0%, respectively.[166] However, NAT results should be interpreted with caution because NATs currently cannot differentiate between organisms that inhabit the upper airway without causing disease and those that are responsible for the patient's illness. For example, as mentioned, *S. pneumoniae*, *C. pneumoniae*, and *M. pneumoniae* may inhabit the upper airway without causing disease.[7,11] Similarly, the lowered diagnostic specificity of *P. jirovecii* NATs is likely due to the detection of *P. jirovecii* nucleic acid from cysts that are present in low numbers and in a latent state in pulmonary tissues of asymptomatic patients.[175–177]

In patients with infection with negative culture results or when cultures were not performed on a tissue biopsy sample before fixation, a broad-range PCR assay coupled with amplicon sequencing can be used for detection and identification of bacterial and fungal DNA from fresh or *formalin-fixed paraffin-embedded* (FFPE) specimens.[178–182] The bacterial 16S ribosomal RNA gene and the fungal ribosomal RNA operon (encoding 5.8S, 18S, 28S ribosomal subunit genes with the internal transcribed spacer regions [ITS1 and ITS2]) are the most reliable and frequently used targets for identifying bacterial and fungal sequences, respectively.[183] As with all NATs, sensitivity is higher from fresh tissue than from FFPE specimens. For example, fungal sequencing was successfully completed on 97% of specimens when performed on fresh specimens compared to 63–70% when performed on FFPE specimens.[180,182] Despite the many advantages of direct bacterial and fungal identification by sequencing, clinicians must be aware that the success of this method is dependent on the amount of specimen submitted (e.g., open biopsy vs. needle biopsy), the pathogen burden, and whether fresh versus FFPE tissue is tested.[182] It is imperative that testing is strictly limited to samples obtained from sterile sources because contamination of the sample with commensal organisms or environmental spores could yield false-positive results and lead to mismanagement of the patient.[180,181] Sequence results must always be correlated with clinical, histopathologic, and ancillary test results (antibody or antigen detection) to ensure the clinical accuracy of sequence results.

The diagnosis of respiratory virus infections (Table 19.12) has been revolutionized by NATs.[149] These tests are now considered more sensitive than all other current methods of respiratory virus detection, including viral culture and DFA testing, discussed earlier, and rapid antigen tests, discussed later. Two major groups of respiratory virus NATs are currently in widespread clinical use, with different technical

Table 19.12 Respiratory Viruses

STANDARD RESPIRATORY VIRUS TEST PANEL

Influenza A, B

Respiratory syncytial virus

EXPANDED RESPIRATORY VIRUS TEST PANEL

Parainfluenza 1, 2, 3, 4

Human metapneumovirus

Adenovirus

Human coronavirus (229E, HKU1, OC43, NL63)

Rhinovirus

Enterovirus*

ADDITIONAL VIRUSES TO CONSIDER IN THE IMMUNE COMPROMISED

Cytomegalovirus

Herpes simplex virus

Varicella-zoster virus

Human herpesvirus 6

OTHER VIRUSES THAT CAUSE LOWER RESPIRATORY TRACT INFECTION

Hantavirus

Measles virus

SEVERE ACUTE RESPIRATORY SYNDROME VIRUSES

Avian influenza (H5N1, H7N9)

SARS coronavirus

SARS-coronavirus-2 (COVID-19)

MERS coronavirus

*Commercial multiplex nucleic acid amplification tests may not distinguish between Rhinovirus and Enterovirus.

MERS, Middle Eastern respiratory syndrome; SARS, severe acute respiratory syndrome.

and personnel requirements. These requirements are defined by the test complexity, which is divided into nonwaived and waived testing according to the *Clinical Laboratory Improvement Amendments* (CLIA). Nonwaived tests include moderate- and high-complexity testing and must be performed in accredited clinical laboratories, whereas waived tests are under less stringent regulation and can be performed outside of the clinical laboratory setting, including at the point-of-care. Previous commonly used laboratory-developed and commercial FDA-cleared high-complexity, *real-time reverse-transcriptase PCR* (rRT-PCR) assays, which require separate extraction and amplification steps before nucleic acid detection,[184–187] are being phased out as laboratories implement various automated systems to detect respiratory viruses.

The first group of respiratory virus NATs include the non-waived panels performed on FDA-cleared sample-to-answer platforms (eTable 19.2). Standard panels typically target influenza A, influenza B, and *respiratory syncytial virus* (RSV), whereas extended panels add influenza A subtyping (including H1, 2009 H1, and H3); parainfluenza virus 1, 2, 3, and 4; human metapneumovirus; adenovirus; coronaviruses; and rhinovirus/enterovirus. These expanded panels may also include bacterial targets, such as *M. pneumoniae, Chlamydophila pneumoniae, Bordetella pertussis, and Bordatella parapertussis.*

A majority of the available respiratory virus tests are only approved for URT specimens, such as nasopharyngeal swabs and aspirate/washes, so it is important to verify that the local laboratory has validated the use of LRT specimens in their test system before sending such samples for testing. Currently, one nonwaived system is approved for lower tract specimens, the Biofire FilmArray Pneumonia Panel (Biofire Diagnostics). This test is approved for expectorated/induced sputum, tracheal aspirates, and BAL fluid. This panel includes qualitative detection of viruses (influenza A, influenza B, RSV, human metapneumovirus, parainfluenza virus, adenovirus, coronaviruses, rhinovirus/enterovirus), atypical bacteria, and antimicrobial resistance genes (methicillin resistance, carbapenamases, and extended-spectrum β-lactamases), as well as semiquantitative detection of 15 bacterial causes of pneumonia. The prospective study carried out by the manufacturer to obtain FDA approval demonstrated positive percent agreements ranging from 75–100%, and negative percent agreements ranging from 89–100%, depending on the target.[187a–d]

The second group of respiratory virus NATs include the CLIA-waived panels, also performed on various FDA-cleared sample-to-answer platforms (eTable 19.3). These tests include the Alere i (Abbott),[187–197] cobas Liat (Roche),[188,196,198–205] and Xpert Xpress (Cepheid)[197,201–210] rapid influenza A/B NAT assays, among several others. Rapid detection of influenza may be essential to allow prompt treatment with antiviral agents, to reduce the risk for further transmission through implementation of infection control practices, and to reduce inappropriate use of antibiotics.[211,212] Meta-analysis revealed that these rapid NATs have pooled sensitivities of 92% for influenza A and 95% for influenza B, with pooled specificities of greater than 99%.[213] Given these test characteristics, facilities using respiratory virus tests at the point-of-care no longer need to compromise performance for simplicity, ease of use, and rapid test turnaround.[214,215] Currently, one extended panel, the BioFire Respiratory Virus Panel EZ has received a CLIA waiver. This test detects influenza A (including H1, 2009 H1, and H3 subtyping), influenza B, RSV, human metapneumovirus, parainfluenza virus, adenovirus, coronaviruses, rhinovirus/enterovirus, *B. pertussis, C. pneumoniae, and M. pneumoniae.* The waived version of this test uses identical test pouches to the nonwaived version; only the software and interpretation differs.

Given the variety of NATs currently available for the diagnosis of respiratory virus infection and the ongoing development of new NATs, it is important to communicate with the laboratory to confirm the viruses included in the local panel, the expected turnaround time, and local test performance characteristics.

ANTIGEN TESTING

The diagnosis of LRT infections can be aided by detection of pathogen-specific antigens in serum or other body fluids. Antigen detection offers an alternative to direct examination of infected tissue and may play a role in the detection of pathogens that grow poorly, or not at all, in culture.

Urinary antigen assays may have value for adults with *S. pneumoniae* and *L. pneumophila* infections. In a meta-analysis of 27 studies using a composite of culture tests as the reference standard, the pooled sensitivity for direct antigen detection of *S. pneumoniae* in the urine of adults with

CAP was 74%, and specificity was 97%.[216] In children, pneumococcal antigen in urine is less specific for invasive infection because it was detected in 43% of children with only nasopharyngeal colonization.[217] Similarly, in children with pneumonia, detection of *H. influenzae* type B antigens in urine is of potential diagnostic value, but transient anti-genuria may follow immunization with *H. influenzae* type B conjugate vaccine.[218] In the evaluation of adults for Legionnaires' disease, urine *L. pneumophila* serogroup 1 antigen has a high negative predictive value with pooled sensitivity of 74% and specificity of 99%.[219] Urine antigen for *L. pneumophila* is detectable in 80–89% of patients with Legionnaires' disease, beginning with the first 3 days of symptoms and continuing for at least 14 days; the duration of antigenuria was reduced by antibiotic therapy but was detectable for up to 42 days, especially in immunocompromised patients.[220] The urinary antigen assays are limited to detection of infections due to *L. pneumophila* serogroup 1 and not other *Legionella* serogroups or species.[104]

Detection of urinary *lipoarabinomannan* (LAM), a major lipoglycan in the *M. tuberculosis* cell wall, with *lateral flow urine LAM assay* (LF-LAM) is recommended by WHO for diagnosis and screening of TB in HIV-positive individuals with a CD4 count less than or equal to 100 cells/μL.[221] In a meta-analysis of five studies, pooled sensitivity and specificity of LF-LAM were 56% and 90%, respectively, in patients with a CD4 count less than or equal to 100 cells per μL versus 26% and 92%, respectively, and in those with a CD4 count greater than or equal to 100 cells per μL.[222]

Detection of fungal antigen in serum, urine, and other body fluids is used as an aid in the diagnosis of infections due to *Cryptococcus neoformans*, *Aspergillus*, *H. capsulatum*, *Coccidioides immitis*, and *P. jirovecii*. Assays to detect capsular polysaccharides of *C. neoformans* in serum, urine, or cerebrospinal fluid are essential for rapid diagnosis of cryptococcosis. Commercially available latex agglutination assays show sensitivity ranging from 83–97% and specificity from 93–100%.[223] More recently, a simpler lateral flow immunoassay (Immuno-Mycologics) has been introduced, which shows pooled sensitivity and specificity of 98% and 98%, respectively, on serum and sensitivity of 85% on urine.[224] Cryptococcal antigen may also be detectable in pleural fluid and BAL fluid of patients with cryptococcal pneumonia.[225,226] Serial measurement of serum antigen titers over time is not useful for management of patients with pulmonary cryptococcosis.[227] Cryptococcal antigen may be falsely positive in patients infected with *Trichosporon* sp[228] or due to the presence of rheumatoid factor or heterophile antibodies (i.e., antibodies produced to poorly defined antigens with weak affinity and multispecific activities) and falsely negative due to the prozone effect (antigen excess), localized infection, infection with a poorly encapsulated strain, or low organism burden.[229]

Two commercial *H. capsulatum* antigen assays include MiraVista Diagnostics *Histoplasma* Quantitative EIA and IMMY ALPHA *Histoplasma* Antigen EIA. These tests have variable accuracies for diagnosis of histoplasmosis.[230,231] The polysaccharide antigen of *H. capsulatum* can be detected in urine in approximately 90% of patients with disseminated disease and in 75% with diffuse acute pulmonary histoplasmosis.[128,129] A meta-analysis on the performance of *Histoplasma* antigen showed pooled sensitivity and

specificity of 79% and 99%, respectively, in urine and 82% and 97%, respectively, in serum.[232] Urinary *Histoplasma* antigen levels persist during ongoing active infection, become undetectable with successful therapy, and rise with relapse of infection. The specificity of the *Histoplasma* antigen assay was 99% in patients with nonfungal infections and in healthy controls[230]; however, the assay is known to yield positive results in patients with disseminated infections caused by *Blastomyces dermatitidis*, *C. immitis*, *Paracoccidioides brasiliensis*, *Aspergillus*, and *Penicillium marneffei*.[233,234] Cross reactivity of the assay has not been observed in patients with invasive candidiasis, cryptococcosis, or other opportunistic systemic mycoses.[233]

At least one commercial laboratory offers antigen tests for the diagnosis of coccidioidomycosis and blastomycosis, but both tests exhibit significant cross reaction with *H. capsulatum*.[235] The *Coccidioides* antigen test was 93% sensitive and 100% specific on cerebrospinal fluid in patients with coccidiodal meningitis. The performance is not characterized for pulmonary infection.

Aspergillus galactomannan is a major cell wall component of the fungus, and detection of this antigen has been studied in many different clinical situations. Galactomannan detected in serum by enzyme immunoassay can aid in the early diagnosis of invasive pulmonary aspergillosis, with pooled diagnostic sensitivity of 71% and specificity of 89% and positive predictive value of 25–62% for proven invasive aspergillosis.[236] The reported sensitivity and specificity ranges are 40–100% and 56–100%, respectively, in various patient groups.[18,162,237–239] The Platelia *Aspergillus* test (Bio-Rad Laboratories), a commercially available assay that detects galactomannan from *A. fumigatus*, *A. flavus*, *A. niger*, *A. versicolor*, and *A. terres*, has been shown to yield positive results at an early stage of infection, with positive and negative predictive values of greater than 90% in high-risk patients who were tested biweekly.[237] A modeling study showed an increase in mortality of 25% per galactomannan unit increase and 22% decrease per unit decline per week.[240] However, this assay may cross-react with *Histoplasma*, *P. brasiliensis*, *Penicillium*, *Paecilomyces*, *Alternaria*, and *Cryptococcus*,[239,241,242] and false-positive galactomannan antigen assay results were observed in earlier formulations in patients receiving certain foods or intravenous piperacillin-tazobactam, amoxicillin, or ticarcillin.[242–245] Cross reactivity with *Listeria monocytogenes* has also been reported.[246] Meta-analysis of BAL fluid specimens in patients with proven or probable invasive aspergillosis showed an overall sensitivity of 87% and specificity of 89%.[247] Of note, the Plasma-Lyte (Baxter International) solution commonly used to perform BAL has been found to yield false-positive results with the Platelia *Aspergillus* test.[248] Assays for galactomannan show promise, but their utility is currently greater in hematopoietic stem cell transplant patients than in other groups (see Chapter 57).

Another fungal antigen used for the diagnosis of invasive fungal infection is (1→3)-β-D-glucan, which is a component of the outer cell wall of saprophytic and pathogenic fungi except Zygomycetes (*Mucor* and *Rhizopus* sp) and *Cryptococcus* sp.[237,249] This antigen has been detected in serum or other body fluids of patients with invasive aspergillosis, invasive candidiasis, and infections caused by *Fusarium*, *Acremonium*, *Trichosporum*, *Scedosporium*,

Saccharomyces, and *P. jirovecii*.[164,250,251] A meta-analysis for diagnosis of invasive fungal infection showed a pooled sensitivity of 77% and specificity of 85%.[252] Similar performance was reported in a more recent meta-analysis.[253] Use of different assay cutoff values may result in differences in sensitivity and specificity among the various commercially available assays for detecting this antigen.[249,253,254] For the diagnosis of *Pneumocystis* pneumonia, a meta-analysis showed pooled sensitivity and specificity of 95% and 86.3%, respectively. In HIV-positive patients the sensitivity of the (1→3)-β-D-glucan assay was 92% and specificity was 65%.[255] In *Pneumocystis* pneumonia, β-D-glucan levels do not correlate with organism burden, severity of illness, or response to therapy.[255] Cross reactivity of β-D-glucan assays has been reported with the use of cotton gauzes, swabs, packs, pads, or sponges for wound care or surgery; cellulose filters in hemodialysis patients; and various antimicrobial agents, including piperacillin-tazobactam.[249,256]

Antigen tests are commonly used for the rapid diagnosis of influenza A and B, although CLIA-waived rapid NAT tests (discussed earlier) have begun to replace antigen testing in outpatient and emergency room settings. Rapid antigen tests for influenza demonstrate poor to moderate sensitivity, depending on the particular assay and the circulating strain. Meta-analysis of conventional influenza rapid antigen tests, typically lateral flow immunoassays with visual detection of a colloidal gold reporter, revealed pooled sensitivities of 65% for influenza A and 52% for influenza B, with a combined pooled specificity of 98%. In a subsequent meta-analysis more recently developed digital antigen immunoassays, such as the Quidel Sofia and BD Veritor (Becton Dickinson) systems that use lateral flow immunoassay readers, were shown to have pooled sensitivities of 80% for influenza A and 77% for influenza B, with combined pooled specificity greater than 98%.[213] In the same meta-analysis, conventional rapid antigen immunoassays showed pooled sensitivities of 54% for influenza A and 53% for influenza B, with similarly high pooled specificity. Higher pooled sensitivity of digital antigen immunoassays compared with conventional rapid influenza antigen tests has also been observed in an additional meta-analysis.[257] Due to the overall limited sensitivity of antigen testing, the CDC recommends that patients presenting with a syndrome consistent with influenza and who have a negative rapid antigen test should receive a confirmatory NAT or be treated as if they have influenza. Influenza rapid antigen tests have been reclassified by the FDA to meet minimum performance standards.[258] Rapid antigen tests for RSV are also available and may similarly aid in patient triage, infection control, antibiotic management, and the administration of RSV passive immunization (palivizumab), particularly in high-risk pediatric patients. Meta-analysis of RSV rapid antigen tests that included digital immunoassays with automated readers revealed a pooled sensitivity of 80% and pooled specificity of 97%.

SEROLOGIC TESTING AND INTERFERON-γ RELEASE ASSAYS

Apart from assays that detect pathogens or their products, the cause of LRT infections can be suggested by detection and quantitation of humoral (e.g., antibody) responses to pathogens. In addition, *latent TB infection* (LTBI) can be diagnosed by detection of cellular immune responses to *M. tuberculosis* antigens, such as the *interferon-γ release assays* (IGRAs). Serologic testing is used commonly to identify infections due to pathogens that are difficult to detect directly by other conventional methods, to evaluate the course of an infection, and to determine the nature of the infection (primary infection vs. reinfection, acute vs. chronic infection). Serologic testing and IGRAs are less sensitive in patients with compromised immune systems and therefore cannot be used to rule out infection.[259–261] When possible, microbiologic culture and NATs on respiratory secretions or lung tissue should be performed to detect and confirm the presence of pathogens in immunosuppressed patients who may not be able to mount antibody or cell-mediated immune responses (see Chapter 42).

The serologic methods commonly used in diagnostic laboratories include enzyme immunoassay, immunoprecipitation, *immunodiffusion* (ID), *complement fixation* (CF), immunoblotting (including Western blot), agglutination, hemagglutination inhibition, and indirect immunofluorescence assay. Serologic results are often expressed as a titer, which is the inverse of the greatest dilution, or lowest concentration of a patient's serum that retains measurable specific antibody-antigen reactivity (e.g., dilution of 1:16 = titer of 16). A fourfold or greater rise in antibody titer between acute and convalescent sera is usually required for diagnosis. An elevated pathogen-specific *immunoglobulin* (Ig)M antibody titer in a single serum sample suggests recent infection, and a falling titer provides further support for the etiologic significance of this organism. However, false-positive IgM antibody tests are not rare. Thus serologic testing of pathogen-specific IgG antibody in acute and convalescent sera remains the accepted approach to establish a specific microbial cause of the infection.[262]

Various commercial assays are available for detection of specific IgM and/or IgG antibodies to respiratory tract pathogens.[263] These assays are useful for supporting or confirming the diagnosis of bacterial infections caused by *C. pneumoniae*, *Legionella* sp, *F. tularensis*, *Y. pestis*, *C. trachomatis*, *C. pneumoniae*, *C. psittaci*, and *Coxiella burnetii*. Although antibody testing is commonly used for the detection of infection with *M. pneumoniae*, it is not possible to distinguish between infection and asymptomatic colonization with this organism.[11] The diagnosis of *C. pneumoniae* infection can also be a problem. In some additional instances, such as infection with *M. tuberculosis*, commercial serologic tests have been shown to be inconsistent and imprecise, which is the basis of WHO policy statement advising against use of existing serologic tests in TB.[264]

M. pneumoniae infection is often diagnosed by the presence of specific antibodies in serum.[265] Cold agglutinins, detected by agglutination of type O Rh-negative red blood cells at 4°C, are present in the sera of approximately 50% of patients with *M. pneumoniae* infection, and levels decline to baseline within 6 weeks after acute infection.[266] However, cold agglutinins are nonspecific. Antibodies to a chloroform-methanol glycolipid extract of *M. pneumoniae* are detected by a CF test in greater than 85% of culture-positive patients; a single elevated titer of greater than 80 or a greater than fourfold rise in titer between acute and convalescent sera is required to establish a diagnosis. Enzyme immunoassays to detect IgM and IgA antibodies that specifically recognize *M. pneumoniae* membrane proteins have been developed with improved sensitivity and specificity over the CF assay.[265] Specific IgM antibodies appear during the first week of illness and reach peak titers during the third week. However, the IgM antibodies to *M. pneumoniae* are not consistently produced in adults because of prior sensitization so that a negative IgM result does not rule out acute *M. pneumoniae* infection, particularly in older adults. False-positive IgM in pediatric patients also has to be considered.[267] Detection of specific IgA antibodies in the serum has been shown by one group to be a reliable approach for diagnosis because these antibodies are also produced early in the course of disease and more reliably present in the infected individuals regardless of age.[265] Others, however, found them of little value.[11]

Serologic testing plays an important role in the diagnosis of fungal respiratory tract infections due to *C. immitis* and *H. capsulatum*.[266] For *C. immitis* a diagnosis of infection can be based on detection of antibodies to antigens derived from the coccidioidal mycelia or spherules, although there may be cross reactivity with other yeasts and dimorphic fungi. Antibodies to *C. immitis* were conventionally detected by ID and CF. Enzyme immunoassays have been shown to be as sensitive and specific as ID and CF for detection of IgG antibodies.[268] A new immunoassay was shown to be 88% sensitive and 90% specific for active disease and was also more sensitive than ID and CF.[269] Complement-fixing IgG antibodies appear later and persist in relation to the severity of disease but decline with disease remission. Titers of 32 or higher suggest the possibility of disseminated infection.[270,271] The sensitivity of serologic testing drops 8–20% in immunocompromised hosts compared to immunocompetent patients.[272]

For *H. capsulatum*, serum antibodies are detected by CF using yeast and mycelial antigens and by an ID assay, which show increased titers in greater than 90% of patients with pulmonary histoplasmosis and approximately 80% with disseminated disease.[129] The CF test is more sensitive but less specific than the ID test for the diagnosis of subclinical and acute pulmonary histoplasmosis.[273] Antibodies become detectable first by CF at 2 to 6 weeks after *Histoplasma* infection and then by ID 2 to 4 weeks later. However, the ID test remains positive longer than the CF test after resolution of infection, becoming negative 2 to 5 years later. Antibody levels remain high in those with chronic pulmonary infection, progressive disseminated disease, or fibrosing mediastinitis. Commercially available serologic tests for blastomycosis exist but have limited accuracy and are of minimal value in patient care.[274]

Serologic testing is also useful for diagnosis of parasitic infections, especially *Paragonimus*, *T. gondii*, and *S. stercoralis*,[275,276] and for diagnosis of extraintestinal *E. histolytica* disease. Serologic testing plays an especially important role for screening prospective organ transplant recipients and other patients considered for immunosuppressive therapies.

Serologic testing plays a limited role as an aid to the diagnosis of respiratory viral infections. Although detection of recent respiratory virus infection, for example with influenza A, may be determined via seroconversion or a fourfold or greater rise in antibody titer in a convalescent relative to an acute serum sample, the requirement for two temporally distinct specimens makes serologic results unlikely to factor into clinical decision making.[277] In contrast, routine CMV serologic testing in transplant donors and recipients provides valuable information about the risk for subsequent CMV-related sequelae, including the development of respiratory disease.[278]

IGRAs are in vitro assays used to measure T cell responses to *M. tuberculosis*–specific antigens, such as *early secretory antigenic target-6* (ESAT-6) and *culture filtrate protein-10* (CFP-10).[279] Two FDA-approved commercial IGRAs are currently available: the *QuantiFERON-TB Gold Plus* assay (QFT-Plus; Qiagen) and the *T-SPOT.TB* assay (Oxford Immunotec). IGRAs were developed as an alternative to the *tuberculin skin test* (TST) for diagnosis of LTBI.[279] Compared to the TST, IGRAs have improved specificity for distinguishing between the responses due to *bacillus Calmette-Guérin* (BCG) vaccination and LTBI because the antigens used in IGRAs, ESAT-6 and CFP-10, are absent from all strains of BCG. Otherwise, the specificity of IGRA in BCG-unvaccinated individuals is 98–99% for QFT and 86–92% for T-SPOT.TB.[280,281] Also, compared to the TST, IGRAs offer logistical advantages because they do not depend on accurate intradermal injection, and patients do not have to return to a health facility for the result to be read.[279] However, like TSTs, IGRAs cannot distinguish between LTBI and active disease and are not able to predict which patients with positive results develop active TB.[282–284] The sensitivity of IGRAs in culture-positive active TB cases has ranged from 65–100%,[285,286] and the sensitivity in patients with LTBI who progressed to active TB ranged from 40–100%.[287] Both IGRAs and the TST have been shown to have similar sensitivity in adults in low- and middle-income countries.[288] The accuracy of IGRA testing appears to falter at the borderline levels of positivity due to random sources of variability.[289] Studies conducted in health care workers in low-incidence settings have shown highly variable IGRA results with serial testing. The rate of conversions (negative to positive result using the manufacturer- and CDC-recommended cutoff) ranged from 2–14%, and the rate of reversions (positive to negative result) ranged from 22–77%.[290,291] Those with borderline results around the assay cutoff are more likely to revert or convert. Standardizing QFT preanalytic and analytic steps, and including an indeterminate zone bordering the cutoff, has improved the prognosis of individuals with definite conversion.[292] IGRA results have not proven useful for monitoring response to TB treatment. In summary, IGRAs are most useful as an alternative to the TST, especially in subject populations with a high incidence of BCG vaccination (see also Chapter 42).

Acknowledgment

We thank former Stanford Pathology residents Natalia Isaza, Albert Tsai, and Lee Frederick Schroeder for contributing to this chapter.

Key Points

- Diagnostic testing should be ordered only if the result will alter treatment decisions.
- The clinician plays a critical role in preventing accidental laboratory exposure by notifying the microbiology laboratory when highly virulent and transmissible agents are suspected as the cause of disease.
- Syndromic order sets can improve the accuracy and efficiency of test selection and thus facilitate accurate diagnosis of infectious diseases.
- Lower respiratory tract secretions collected through the oropharynx are nearly always contaminated with resident microflora of the oral cavity, and therefore microscopy, culture, and nucleic acid test results must be interpreted in the context of other clinical evidence and diagnostic findings.
- Nucleic acid tests can facilitate rapid and accurate diagnosis of lower respiratory tract infections, especially those caused by viruses and pathogens that are difficult to culture.

Key Readings

Banaei N, Gaur RL, Pai M. interferon gamma release assays for latent tuberculosis: what are the sources of variability? *J Clin Microbiol.* 2016;54:845–850.

Carroll KC, Pfaller MA, et al. *Manual of Clinical Microbiology.* 12th ed. Washington, DC: American Society for Microbiology Press; 2011.

Mackowiak PA, Martin RM, Jones SR, et al. Pharyngeal colonization by gram-negative bacilli in aspiration-prone persons. *Arch Intern Med.* 1978;138:1224–1227.

Mills CC. Occurrence of *Mycobacterium* other than *Mycobacterium tuberculosis* in the oral cavity and in sputum. *Appl Microbiol.* 1972;24:307–310.

Pai M, Denkinger CM, Kik SV, et al. Gamma interferon release assays for detection of *Mycobacterium tuberculosis* infection. *Clin Microbiol Rev.* 2014;27:3–20.

Pauker SG, Kassirer JP. Therapeutic decision making: a cost-benefit analysis. *N Engl J Med.* 1975;293:229–234.

Spuesens EB, Fraaij PL, Visser EG, et al. Carriage of *Mycoplasma pneumoniae* in the upper respiratory tract of symptomatic and asymptomatic children: an observational study. *PLoS Med.* 2013;10:e1001444.

Tillotson JR, Finland M. Bacterial colonization and clinical superinfection of the respiratory tract complicating antibiotic treatment of pneumonia. *J Infect Dis.* 1969;119:597–624.

Valenti WM, Trudell RG, Bentley DW. Factors predisposing to oropharyngeal colonization with gram-negative bacilli in the aged. *N Engl J Med.* 1978;298:1108–1111.

Complete reference list available at ExpertConsult.com.

20 *THORACIC RADIOLOGY: NONINVASIVE DIAGNOSTIC IMAGING*

CLINTON E. JOKERST, MD • MICHAEL B. GOTWAY, MD

INTRODUCTION
CHEST RADIOGRAPHY: TECHNIQUES
Radiographic Views and Techniques
Medical Imaging and Radiation
APPLICATIONS OF CONVENTIONAL
    CHEST RADIOGRAPHY
Screening and "Routine" Chest Radiographs
Detection of Lung Cancer and Assessment
    of Solitary Pulmonary Nodules

Evaluation of Intensive Care Unit Patients
Indications in Acute Lung Disease
APPLICATIONS OF CROSS-SECTIONAL
    IMAGING TECHNIQUES
Solitary Pulmonary Nodules
Multiple Pulmonary Nodules
Lung Cancer Staging
Lung Cancer Screening

Hilar and Mediastinal Masses
Diffuse Lung Disease
Intrathoracic Airway Disease
Cardiovascular Disease
Pleural Disease
KEY POINTS

 An expanded version of this chapter (see italicized headings in the above outline) is available at ExpertConsult.com.

INTRODUCTION

Imaging plays a major role in the detection, diagnosis, and serial evaluation of thoracic disease. The appropriate use of imaging requires a basic understanding of the technical aspects of different imaging modalities, including the diagnostic accuracy and limitations of each technique. It is not the intent of this chapter to provide a complete description of the techniques involved or an encyclopedic catalogue of radiographic abnormalities of thoracic diseases; these issues are detailed in subsequent chapters dedicated to specific disorders. Rather, this chapter is intended to provide a general survey of the imaging methods available, their most common indications, and certain principles concerning their use.

Since the late 1990s, there have been remarkable advancements in the effectiveness of cross-sectional imaging techniques for the diagnosis of thoracic diseases, particularly with the development of multislice *computed tomography* (CT), as well as improvements in *magnetic resonance imaging* (MRI) and ultrasonography (see Chapters 23 and 24). In many instances, cross-sectional methods have supplanted radiography for the diagnosis of chest diseases. As with any imaging method, the decision to use cross-sectional imaging should be based on consideration of the patient's clinical problem and the results of other imaging and laboratory testing.

Chest radiography still plays a fundamental role in the diagnosis of thoracic disease. Chest radiography is usually the initial imaging procedure performed when chest disease is suspected. Despite the proliferation of other imaging methods, chest radiography remains one of the most frequently performed imaging examinations in the United States.

The thorax is difficult to image because of large regional differences in tissue density and thickness. For example, with standard radiography, the number of x-rays passing through the lungs is more than 100 times greater than the number of x-rays penetrating the mediastinum.[1] The dynamic contrast range of conventional film-screen radiography is insufficient to demonstrate this range of x-ray transmission properly; with standard radiographic techniques, the use of exposure high enough to display the mediastinum and the subdiaphragmatic regions usually results in overexposure of the lungs (Fig. 20.1A). Conversely, an exposure designed to provide the best visualization of the pulmonary parenchyma (see Fig. 20.1B) is normally too underexposed to visualize mediastinal anatomy. One of the advantages of digital imaging is that displayed contrast and brightness are largely independent of the *peak kilovoltage* (kVp) and milliamperage values used to obtain the examination; both contrast and brightness can be manually adjusted by the user after the image has been obtained.[2] Furthermore, the dynamic contrast range (i.e., latitude) of digital radiographic techniques exceeds that of film-screen methods by a factor of 10 or more.[2]

Meticulous attention to technique is essential. Regardless of the method of recording the image, whether through standard film-screen radiography, image intensification, or digital recording, poor quality control leads to degradation of diagnostic information. Unfortunately, many technically inadequate radiographs are produced, leading either to

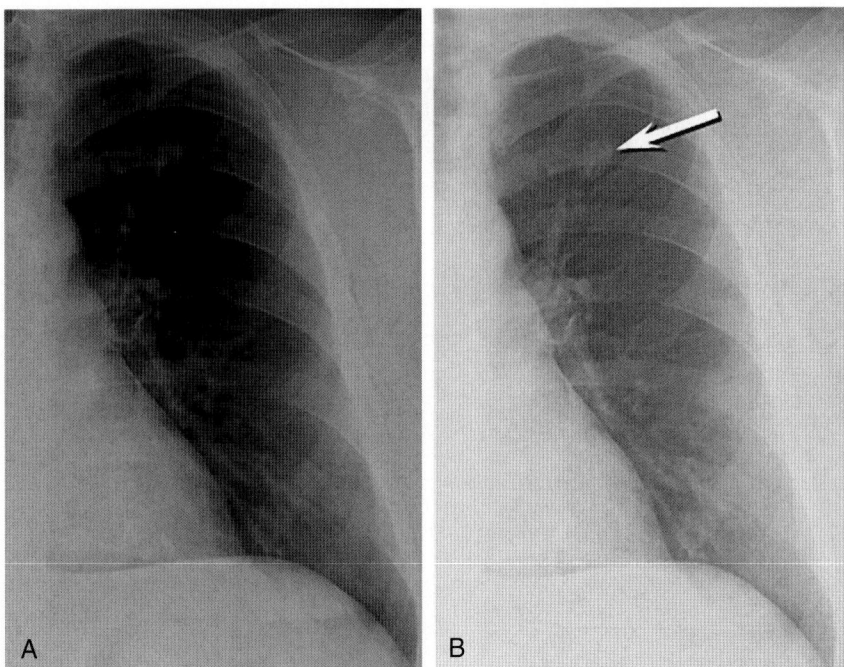

Figure 20.1 Overexposed versus properly exposed chest radiograph. (A) Frontal chest radiograph performed with overexposed technique shows relatively good visualization of the mediastinum, but the lungs are abnormally "black," which obscures fine detail. (B) Repeat frontal chest radiograph performed with proper exposure shows slightly reduced ability to "see through" the mediastinum compared with the overexposed chest radiograph, but lung parenchymal detail is clearly superior in the properly exposed image. The proper exposure allows visualization of a left upper lobe nodule *(arrow)*. (Courtesy Michael B. Gotway, MD.)

repeat studies with additional patient radiation exposure or to interpretation of the poor images, increasing the chance of diagnostic errors.

Indications for the use of chest radiography are protean and include the assessment of both acute (e.g., pneumonia) and chronic (e.g., COPD) lung diseases; assessment of dyspnea or other respiratory symptoms; evaluation of treatment success for patients with acute lung disease; follow-up of patients with a known chronic lung disease; monitoring of patients in *intensive care units* (ICUs); confirmation of life-support device placement, such as central *intravenous* (IV) lines and endotracheal tubes; diagnosis of pleural effusion; screening for asymptomatic diseases in patients at risk; monitoring patients with industrial exposure; preoperative evaluation of surgical patients; and as the initial imaging study in patients with known or suspected lung cancer or other tumors, vascular abnormalities, or hemoptysis. However, abnormal radiographic findings can be quite subtle and, in many circumstances, the sensitivity and specificity of chest radiography are limited. In such situations, other imaging modalities, especially chest CT, are performed to investigate abnormalities visible on radiographs or to evaluate patients considered high risk for a particular condition but with equivocal chest radiographic results.

The utility of chest radiography has been studied in a number of clinical settings, and the appropriate criteria for its use have been determined by the *American College of Radiology* (ACR; https://www.acr.org/Clinical-Resources/ACR-Appropriateness-Criteria). A detailed analysis of the diagnostic accuracy of chest radiography in all situations is beyond the scope of this chapter; however, for

illustrative purposes, their utility and limitations in several specific clinical settings are reviewed.

A discussion of the major technical aspects that may affect image quality is available at ExpertConsult.com.

CHEST RADIOGRAPHY: TECHNIQUES

RADIOGRAPHIC VIEWS AND TECHNIQUES

Routine Examination

A routine chest radiographic examination in an ambulatory patient usually consists of *posteroanterior* (PA) and left lateral projections. However, the utility of routine lateral radiographs has been questioned. After analyzing more than 10,000 radiographic chest examinations obtained routinely in a hospital-based population, Sagel and associates[20] concluded that the lateral radiograph could be safely eliminated in the routine examination of patients 20 to 39 years of age. Conversely, they and others[21] have concluded that the lateral radiograph should be obtained in patients with suspected chest disease and in screening examinations of patients 40 years of age or older (Fig. 20.2).

Expiratory Views

Conventional radiographs are made at total lung capacity (i.e., full inspiration), thereby permitting the greatest volume of lung to be evaluated for possible pathology and providing the most contrast between intrapulmonary

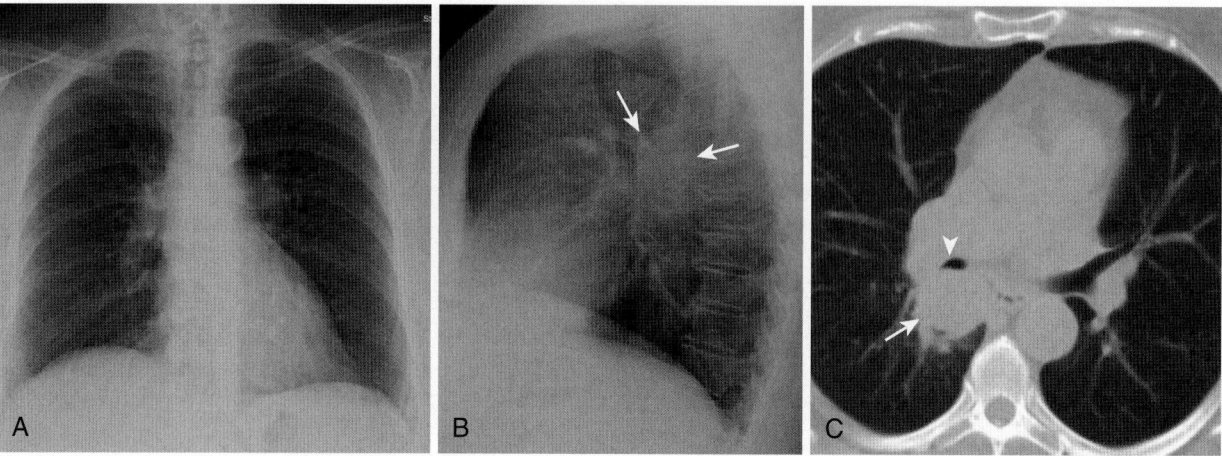

Figure 20.2 The utility of the lateral radiograph. (A) The posteroanterior radiograph shows no specific abnormalities. (B) The lateral radiograph identifies a mass (*arrows*) projected over the hilum. (C) Axial chest computed tomography confirms the presence of a mass (*arrow*) in the right lower lobe posterior to the bronchus intermedius (*arrowhead*). The lesion was found to represent bronchogenic carcinoma. (Courtesy Michael B. Gotway, MD.)

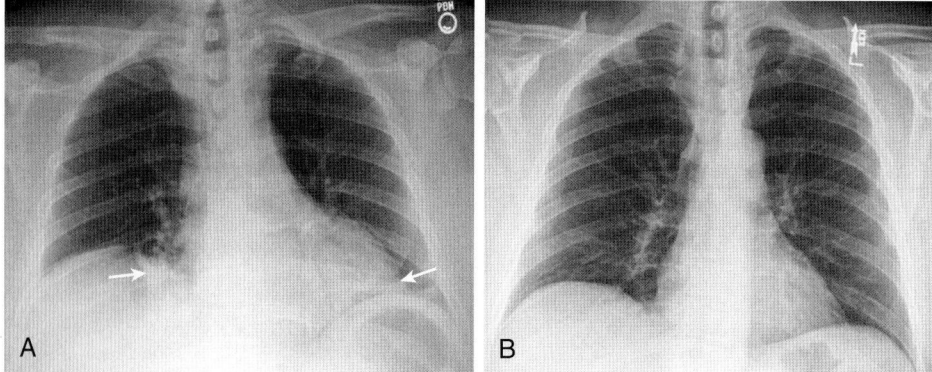

Figure 20.3 Comparison of radiographic appearances of thorax between expiratory and inspiratory radiographic techniques. (A) Frontal chest radiograph performed with expiratory technique shows basal opacities (*arrows*) bilaterally. The mediastinum is wide, and the heart size is difficult to assess. (B) Repeat frontal chest radiograph performed at full inspiratory volume made shortly after (A) now shows clearing of the basal opacities; the heart size is clearly normal, and the mediastinum now shows normal width. (Courtesy Michael B. Gotway, MD.)

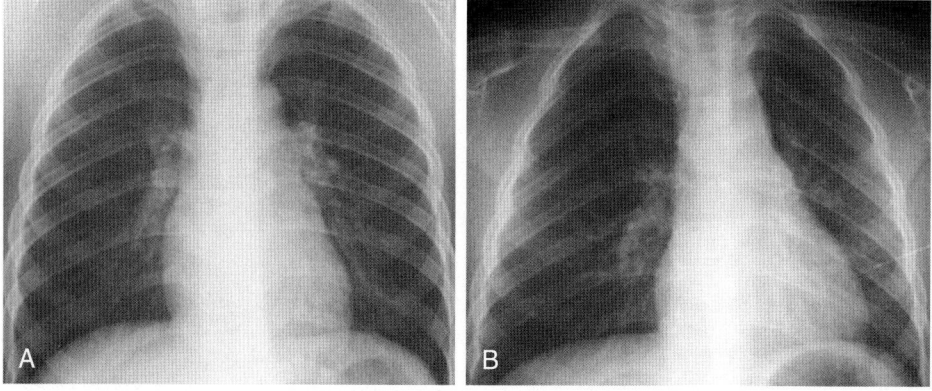

Figure 20.4 Unilateral hyperlucent lung in an 8-year-old boy with a foreign body in the right main-stem bronchus. (A) The inspiration radiograph shows mild hyperlucency of the right lung. (B) The expiration film shows that the right hemidiaphragm remains fixed in a low position, the right lung remains lucent, and the mediastinum is shifted to the left (air trapping). A foreign body was removed. (Courtesy Michael B. Gotway, MD.)

air and normal and abnormal intrathoracic structures (Fig. 20.3). However, localized or generalized air trapping in the lung or pleural space is more readily, and occasionally exclusively, detected on a radiograph made during expiration. The normal lung diminishes in volume and increases in density with expiration. Areas of air trapping retain their lucency and volume regardless of the phase of respiration. With unilateral or localized air trapping, mediastinal shift (Fig. 20.4) and failure of normal elevation of the hemidiaphragm on the affected side are frequently apparent only on expiration. Small pneumothoraces, difficult to visualize and frequently

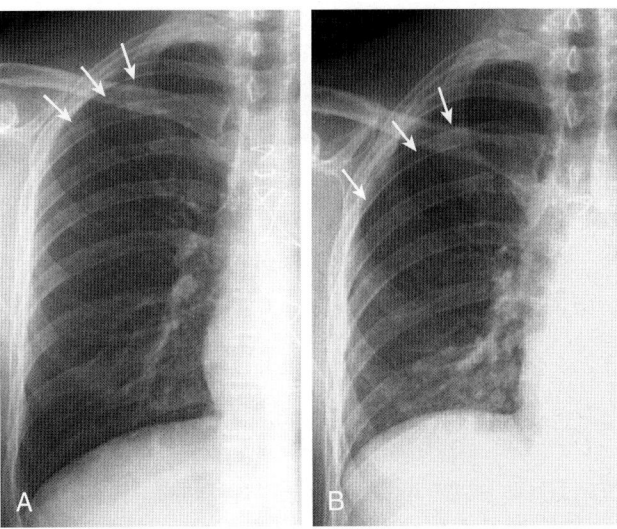

Figure 20.5 Inspiration and expiration chest radiography of pneumothorax. (A) On the inspiratory image, the right pneumothorax is difficult to visualize but is faintly seen in the right upper thorax (*arrows*). (B) On the expiratory image, the right pneumothorax (*arrows*) is outlined against denser lung and appears larger than on the inspiration study. (Courtesy Michael B. Gotway, MD.)

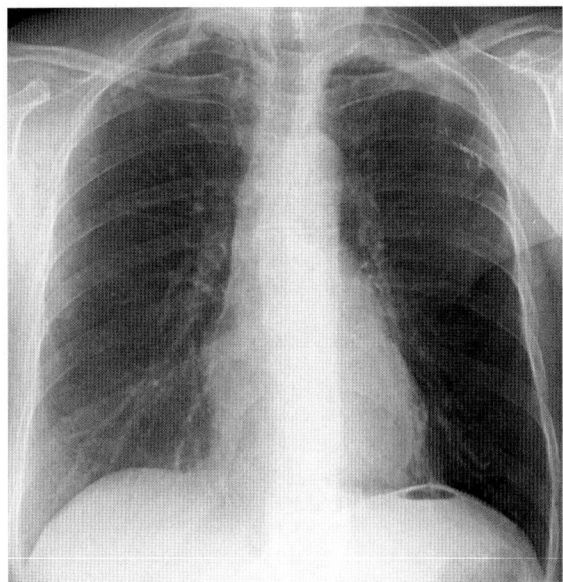

Figure 20.6 Unilateral hyperlucent lung simulating air trapping. Frontal chest radiograph shows lucency throughout the left thorax compared with the right, simulating air trapping (compare with Fig. 20.4B). Note, however, that the left thorax shows neither abnormally increased (unlike Fig. 20.4B) nor decreased lung volume. The left axillary surgical clips are a clue to the cause of left lung hyperlucency: left mastectomy for previous breast malignancy. The removal of left chest soft tissue creates less tissue density along the path of travel of the x-ray photons through the patient's left side relative to the right, resulting in relative lucency of the left thorax compared with the right. (Courtesy Michael B. Gotway, MD.)

overlooked on inspiratory radiographs, appear larger and more apparent on the expiratory study. As the thorax and underlying lung diminish in volume, the lung becomes denser, whereas the pneumothorax remains essentially unchanged in size and attenuation, thus occupying a greater proportion of the deflated hemithorax and outlined more clearly by the adjacent higher-attenuation pulmonary parenchyma (Fig. 20.5).

Localized or unilateral lucency on the radiograph may be seen without air trapping on the expiratory study. Among these are technical causes, such as patient rotation (eFig. 20.11), miscentered x-ray beam or grid, or the "anode heel" effect (i.e., an artifact of asymmetrical transmission of x-rays by the anode of the x-ray tube). Other causes of lucency without air trapping are chest wall abnormalities, either congenital or postsurgical (Fig. 20.6); areas of atelectasis with compensatory overexpansion of other portions of the lung; and primary vascular disease, such as pulmonary embolus (see eFig. 81.9). None of these causes of pulmonary lucency will show trapped air on the expiratory radiograph.

Expanded discussions of decubitus, lordotic and oblique views, fluoroscopy, bronchography, pulmonary angiography, aortography, ultrasonography, computed tomography (principles, techniques, protocols and indications) and magnetic resonance imaging (principles, techniques) are available at ExpertConsult.com.

MEDICAL IMAGING AND RADIATION

The major drawback of the increasing use of CT is radiation exposure. In 1980–82, radiation from medical imaging accounted for approximately 18% of the per capita effective radiation dose in the United States, but this value increased to 54% by 2006, largely due to increased radiation doses resulting from CT scanning and, to a much lesser extent, nuclear medicine procedures. It was recently reported that CT represents about 17% of all radiologic procedures in the world but accounts for greater than 40% of the collective

dose.[27] Given the continued increased use of CT since 2006, it is likely that these numbers are now even greater.[28]

Effective doses (scanner outputs) for CT are given in Table 20.1 and compared with nonmedical radiation exposures.

Additional material regarding radiation exposure from medical sources and on radiogenic cancer risk is available online at ExpertConsult.com.

Although conflicting interpretations are difficult to reconcile and data on both sides of the argument can be compelling, in practice, medical radiation should be used in amounts as low as reasonably achievable to answer relevant clinical questions and only in cases where other radiation-free imaging options will not suffice. Such decisions should provide an optimal approach to balancing the immediate need for diagnostic information with patient safety.

APPLICATIONS OF CONVENTIONAL CHEST RADIOGRAPHY

SCREENING AND "ROUTINE" CHEST RADIOGRAPHS

It is now generally agreed that screening chest radiographs are not indicated except in specific high-risk populations.[52] Estimates of iatrogenic disease caused by ionizing radiation from screening examinations, forecasts of possible genetic consequences, and financial concerns outweigh the medical value of such examinations. In 1973, the Department of Health, Education, and Welfare, in conjunction with the ACR and the American College of Chest Physicians, recommended the discontinuation of screening examinations. In 1985, recommendations of the ACR were more explicit:

Table 20.1 Typical Radiation Doses Associated With Background Sources and Common Thoracic Imaging Applications and Environmental Exposures

Radiation Exposure	Effective Dose (mSv)
U.S. annual per capita effective radiation dose, 2006 (background/medical/total)	2.4/3.0/5.6[27]
Posteroanterior chest radiograph*	0.02[328]
Ventilation/perfusion scan*	1.4–2[328,329]
Standard chest CT	5–8[328,329] (exposures now commonly less than this value)
"Low-dose" chest CT	2
High-resolution chest CT (1-cm noncontiguous intervals)*	1
Catheter pulmonary angiography*	2.3–4.1
Whole-body PET*	14[329]
Coast-to-coast U.S. flight (≈3000 miles)†	0.03
Living near coal-fired power plant†	0.0003
Proximity to x-ray (e.g., luggage inspectors)	0.00002
Living within 50 miles of a nuclear power plant†	0.00009
Living in Denver for 1 year	1.8
Airport backscatter device (body scanner)	0.000015–0.00088[330]
Smoking, 1 year‡	2.8

Additional comparisons are available in McCollough CH, Guimaraes L, Fletcher JG. In defense of body CT. *Am J Roentgenol* 2009;193(1):28–39.
*Values may vary according to individual equipment manufacturers, patient size, duration of study, use of dose-reduction techniques, and individual institutional protocols. Exposure for axial acquisition now similar to "standard CT," given volumetric acquisition; additional dose also from prone and postexpiratory imaging.
†Data from http://www.ans.org/pi/resources/dosechart/.
‡Data from http://web.princeton.edu/sites/ehs/osradtraining/backgroundradiation/background.htm.
CT, computed tomography; mSv, millisievert; PET, positron emission tomography.

chest radiographs obtained for routine examination, preemployment screening, prenatal or obstetric screening, and hospital admission, as well as repeated examinations of patients with positive tuberculin tests and a negative initial chest radiograph, should be eliminated. From their analysis of more than 10,000 chest radiographic examinations obtained in a hospital-based population, Sagel and associates[20] concluded that routine screening examinations done solely because of hospital admission or scheduled surgery are not warranted in patients younger than 20 years. Even in selected high-risk populations, radiographic screening for carcinoma of the lung has failed to increase longevity.

The value of the routine hospital admission chest radiograph is still controversial. Although the yield is low in asymptomatic patients, the examination can be extremely valuable as a baseline study for comparison with radiographs taken during or after the course of hospitalization in patients who develop pulmonary symptoms. In general, hospital admission chest radiographs are not recommended unless there is evidence of acute or unstable chronic cardiopulmonary disease or for elderly patients unable to provide an accurate history or undergo a reliable physical assessment.[52]

DETECTION OF LUNG CANCER AND ASSESSMENT OF SOLITARY PULMONARY NODULES

Although chest radiographs are clearly useful in the initial evaluation of patients suspected of having lung cancer, they are of limited accuracy in showing small or early cancers. At the time of their initial diagnosis, it is not uncommon for lung cancers to be visible retrospectively on prior radiographs.[53] Additional radiographic studies, such as oblique views, are cost-effective for the initial evaluation of "nodular opacities" (see eFig. 20.16) that do not clearly represent a lung nodule and are often of value in determining that a "nodular opacity" is not a true nodule. That being said, CT is superior for the detailed evaluation of a known lung nodule.[54]

EVALUATION OF INTENSIVE CARE UNIT PATIENTS

Chest radiography is generally the most common imaging study performed in the ICU. ICU radiographs are taken with portable, and therefore suboptimal, technique. Regardless, the information they provide is useful and may alter patient management.[9]

A further discussion of the indications for chest radiography in the ICU is available at ExpertConsult.com.

INDICATIONS IN ACUTE LUNG DISEASE

Dyspnea

Two studies suggest that chest radiography should be used routinely in patients with acute or chronic dyspnea.[64,65] In one study, new, clinically important radiographic abnormalities requiring acute intervention or follow-up evaluation were identified in 35% of 221 symptomatic patients.[64] Another study found that acute dyspnea was a strong predictor of a radiographic abnormality, but mainly in patients older than 40 years.[66] In this group, 86% of dyspneic patients had abnormal chest radiographs, whereas radiographs were abnormal in only 31% of patients younger than 40 years. Only 2% of patients younger than 40 years with a normal physical examination had abnormal radiographs indicative of an acute abnormality. The ACR[66a] has previously recommended chest radiography when dyspnea is chronic or severe or when additional risk factors are present, such as age older than 40 years and when there is known cardiovascular, pulmonary, or neoplastic disease, or abnormal physical findings. The ACR further suggests that chest radiography is usually an appropriate first investigation for patients with dyspnea suspected to be due to obstructive or *interstitial lung disease* (ILD), central airway disease, or diseases of the pleura, chest wall, or diaphragm.[67]

Acute Respiratory Symptoms

Opinions are also divided about the utility of chest radiographs in patients with suspected acute lung disease and symptoms other than dyspnea. In a study of 1102 outpatients with acute respiratory disease, Benacerraf and coworkers[66] found patient age, results of physical examination, and presence or absence of hemoptysis to be important factors in predicting the value of radiographs. Only 4% of patients younger than 40 years, without hemoptysis and without detectable abnormalities on physical examination, had acute radiographic abnormalities, whereas a much higher incidence of radiographic abnormalities was present if the patient was older than 40 years, had hemoptysis, or had abnormal physical findings. Heckerling,[68] in a study of 464 patients with acute respiratory symptoms, found a low incidence of pneumonia (3%) in patients with a negative physical examination, except in those with dementia. Whenever pneumonia is suspected in adults, the *American Thoracic Society* (ATS) recommends PA (and lateral when possible) chest radiography, although the impact of chest radiography on clinical outcomes in patients with lower respiratory tract infections remains unclear.[69] In this setting, chest radiography may be useful to determine which patients should be hospitalized and which patients should be classified as having "severe" pneumonia.[70] The ACR considers chest radiography appropriate in immunocompetent patients with acute respiratory illnesses when physical examination findings or vital signs are abnormal, or other risk factors or comorbidities are present, or in patients 60 years or older.[71] It has previously been thought that patients younger than 40 years with normal vital signs and physical examination findings presenting with an acute respiratory illness may not require chest radiography, but a review by the ACR[71] suggests that nearly 5% of such patients will have pneumonia, and chest radiography should therefore be deferred in this context only when reliable follow-up is ensured and there is a low likelihood of morbidity if the diagnosis of pneumonia is delayed.

Acute Asthma

In asthma, chest radiographs are often normal, and visible abnormalities in this disease are usually nonspecific.[72] Although Petheram and associates[73] reported that 9% of 117 patients with severe acute asthma had unsuspected radiographic abnormalities affecting management, and the usefulness of radiography in both adult and pediatric[74] patients with an established diagnosis of asthma who experience an acute attack is limited. Correlation between the severity of radiographic findings and the severity or reversibility of an asthma attack is generally poor,[72,73,75] and radiographs provide significant information that alters treatment in 5% or fewer patients with acute asthma.[68,76,77] Although it is difficult to generalize regarding the role of radiographs in both adults and children with acute asthma, chest imaging should be used to exclude the presence of associated pneumonia or other complications when significant symptoms and/or appropriate clinical or laboratory findings are suggestive.[72,75,77] The ACR considers chest radiography warranted in adult patients with asthma when a clinical suspicion for pneumonia or pneumothorax is present,[71] but the utility of chest radiography in otherwise uncomplicated adult acute asthma exacerbations remains controversial.[71]

Exacerbation of COPD or Cystic Fibrosis

Chest radiographs are often used in the initial assessment of patients with suspected COPD; however, they are of limited value in patients with known COPD who present with worsening of their disease.[77,78] In a study of 107 patients with COPD presenting with an exacerbation of symptoms, only 17 (16%) had an abnormal chest radiograph, and in only half of these did the radiographic findings result in a significant alteration in management.[77] In another study, including patients with both COPD and asthma, the management of 21% of patients was altered by radiographic findings.[78] The ACR indicates that chest radiography is generally appropriate for immunocompetent patients with suspected COPD exacerbations, particularly when chest pain, fever, leukocytosis, a history of coronary artery disease, or heart failure is present.[71] When such criteria are used as a guide, nearly all patients with significant findings will have radiographs performed; moreover, it should be noted that more than two-thirds of patients in one study met inclusion criteria for performing radiography.[78]

In most patients with an established diagnosis of cystic fibrosis, clinical findings and chest radiographs are often sufficient for clinical management. Conversely, it should be recognized that patients with cystic fibrosis can have a significant exacerbation of their symptoms with little visible radiographic change.

APPLICATIONS OF CROSS-SECTIONAL IMAGING TECHNIQUES

SOLITARY PULMONARY NODULES (see Chapter 41)

Assessment of a *solitary pulmonary nodule* (SPN) seen on chest radiography is a common indication for CT.[54,79] CT is used to confirm that the SPN is real, confirm that the SPN is solitary, attempt further noninvasive characterization of the lesion, guide percutaneous biopsy of the lesion, and provide staging information if the SPN is found to represent cancer.

In general, CT of a patient with an SPN should be performed with thin-section volumetric imaging to provide detailed analysis of nodule morphology and to allow identification of the presence of fat or calcium (Video 20.6, see Fig. 20.7) within the nodule, and, when the latter is present, the pattern of calcification; this is now fairly routine in the era of *multislice CT* (MSCT) technology.

In up to 20% of instances, a "lung nodule" visible on a chest radiograph actually represents an artifact, chest wall lesion (eFig. 20.28), or pleural abnormality; in some cases, CT is essential to determine the true nature of the opacity. CT can be useful to define the morphology of the SPN and suggest whether it is benign, likely malignant, or indeterminate (i.e., having neither benign nor malignant characteristics). In some patients a specific diagnosis of lesions, such as rounded atelectasis (Fig. 20.8, Video 20.7), a mucous plug, or arteriovenous malformation (Video 20.8) can be made on the basis of CT findings, indicating the benign nature of the lesion.[54,79] Other CT appearances suggest the presence of malignancy (eFig. 20.29).[54] Malignant features include spiculated (see eFig. 20.29D) or irregular margins; air bronchograms within the nodule (see eFig. 20.29A); bubbly air collections (pseudocavitation, eFig. 20.29E); cavitation; and larger size, such as diameter larger than 2 cm (Fig. 20.9, see eFig. 20.29A).[54,79] Benign features include several patterns of calcification (eFig. 20.30), such as diffuse, central, laminated, and chondroid, or "popcorn," calcification patterns (Fig. 20.10, see eFig. 20.30).[54,79] In about 30% of benign nodules, the calcium is not readily visible on chest radiographs but can be seen on thin-section CT (eFigs. 20.31 and 20.32).

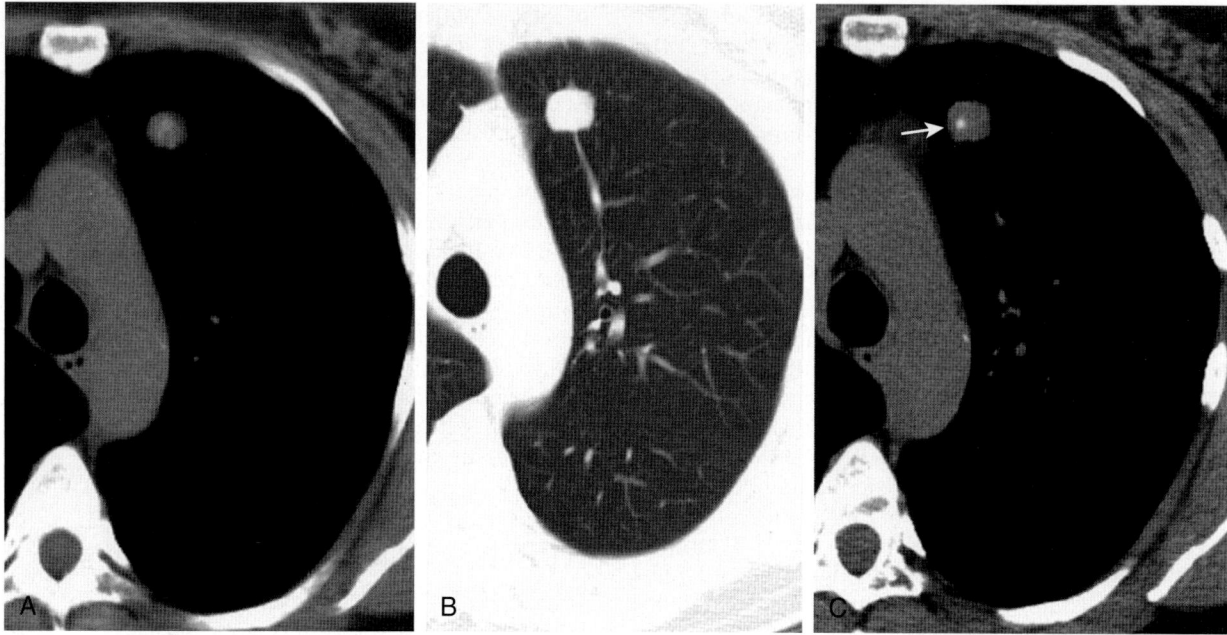

Figure 20.7 Volumetric multislice *computed tomography* (CT) imaging of a pulmonary nodule detected at chest radiography. (A) "Routine" axial 5-mm CT image shows a soft tissue nodule in the left upper lobe. Vaguely increased attenuation is seen within the nodule, suggesting calcification, but the finding is not well seen. (B) Lung window images show that the nodule is circumscribed. (C) Retrospectively reconstructed thin-section (1-mm) soft tissue image more clearly shows a small focus of calcification *(arrow)* within the lesion, suggesting a benign etiology. Coccidioidomycosis titers were elevated, and the patient is being followed. (Courtesy Michael B. Gotway, MD.)

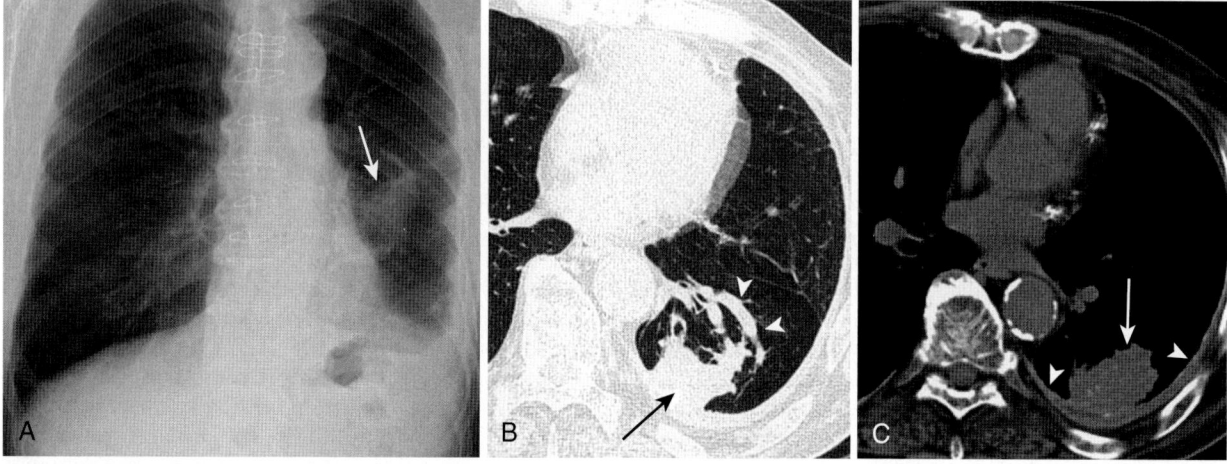

Figure 20.8 Chest *computed tomography* (CT) image shows typical findings of rounded atelectasis. (A) Frontal chest radiograph shows volume loss in the left lower lobe associated with an oblong mass *(arrow)* and left-sided pleural abnormality. (B) Axial chest CT in lung windows shows a subpleural left lower lobe mass *(arrow)* associated with left lower lobe volume loss (posterior displacement of left major fissure, small volume in the left lower lobe). Note "spiraling" appearance of left lower lobe bronchovascular bundles as they extend into the mass *(arrowheads);* this is the so-called comet-tail sign. (C) Axial chest CT displayed in soft tissue windows shows other features consistent with rounded atelectasis including abnormally thickened pleura *(arrowheads)* and contact of the mass *(arrow)* with the abnormal pleura. (Courtesy Michael B. Gotway, MD.)

Carcinomas may occasionally show calcification (eFig. 20.33), although often in an eccentric or stippled pattern. The presence of fat within an SPN, indicated by a low CT attenuation coefficient (Fig. 20.11), strongly suggests the presence of hamartoma[54,79] or lipoid pneumonia (eFig. 20.34); such nodules can be safely followed with serial radiographs.

Malignant tumors tend to show greater enhancement than benign nodules after the rapid injection of iodinated contrast material.[80–83] Because the degree of enhancement depends on the amount and rapidity of contrast infusion, it is important to use a consistent technique. Using a specific contrast enhancement CT protocol, a threshold for enhancement of 15 *Hounsfield units* (HU) or more is typically seen with malignancy, hamartoma, and some inflammatory lesions. Enhancement of less than 15 HU almost always indicates a benign lesion, usually a granuloma. Therefore, whereas positive results (enhancement of >15 HU at any time point during the study) are nonspecific, negative results are quite useful (eFig. 20.35). This technique has been shown to have a sensitivity of 98% and a specificity of 58% in diagnosing carcinoma. More important, the negative predictive value of this technique is approximately 96%.[82] CT nodule enhancement studies are most appropriately used for patients with *indeterminate* nodules (i.e., those without typical benign or malignant appearances). A

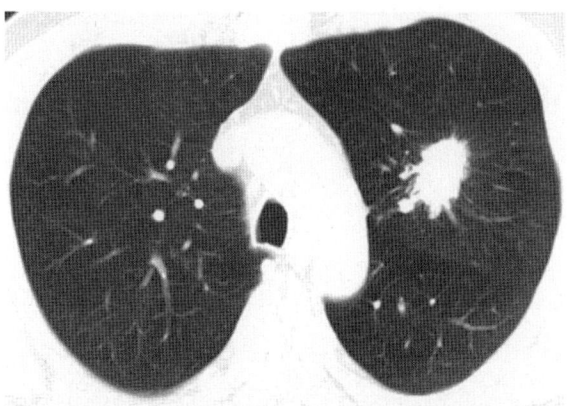

Figure 20.9 Chest computed tomography of bronchogenic carcinoma. Axial computed tomography displayed in lung windows shows a spiculated lesion within the left upper lobe. (Courtesy Michael B. Gotway, MD.)

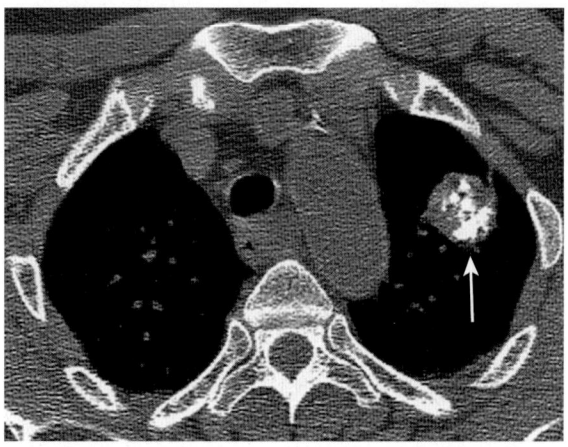

Figure 20.10 Chest computed tomography of hamartoma. Chest computed tomography showing "popcorn" (chondroid) calcification within a left upper lobe nodule (*arrow*), consistent with hamartoma. (Courtesy Michael B. Gotway, MD.)

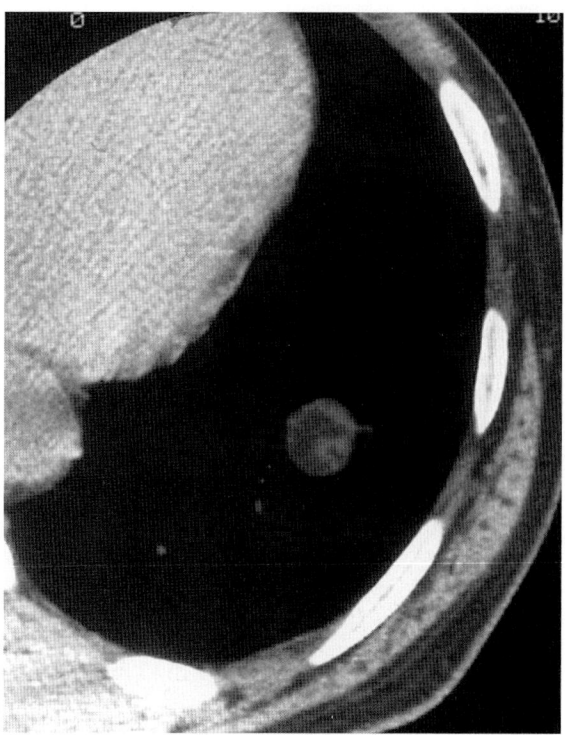

Figure 20.11 Chest *computed tomography* (CT) of a hamartoma. CT shows a low attenuation within the solitary pulmonary nodule (typical CT numbers within the lesion ranged from −90 to −100 Hounsfield units), consistent with fat. (Courtesy Michael B. Gotway, MD.)

CT, prior radiographic examinations, and the clinical presentation will improve the determination of the likelihood of malignancy.

MULTIPLE PULMONARY NODULES

CT is the favored procedure for identifying multiple pulmonary nodules or masses. It detects more and smaller metastases (Fig. 20.12, Video 20.9) than any other imaging technique, and 2- to 3-mm nodules are routinely visible.[88–90] This is most relevant for patients with extrathoracic malignancies, in whom the detection of metastatic disease has a major impact on initial staging and assessment of response to therapy. The major sources of controversy regarding the use of CT for evaluation of possible metastases have been its limited specificity and cost/benefit ratio,[89] although CT is nevertheless widely accepted for this application.

CT is clearly more sensitive than chest radiographs in diagnosing multiple pulmonary nodules in patients with suspected metastasis.[88–90] Although exquisitely sensitive for small nodule detection, CT is not infallible, and nodules, particularly small nodules, can be overlooked. Although it is likely that older reports suffer from biases, such as the possibility that surgical palpation will detect benign nodules, and may overlook some malignant nodules that subsequently manifest as growing nodules at chest CT, as well as the inherent difficulties correlating the location of nodules detected at chest CT with pathologic specimens, there are limitations of chest CT for small nodule detection and characterization.[90]

In accordance, CT results must be interpreted in light of the clinical characteristics of the patient. Primary tumors that commonly spread to the lungs, more advanced

similar use for dynamic, contrast-enhanced MRI has been reported, although data are limited.[84] Fluorodeoxyglucose *positron emission tomography* (PET) imaging (see Chapter 25) has also been shown to be useful for distinguishing benign from malignant nodules (see Fig. 25.1)[85] and is generally favored over contrast-enhanced CT for additional imaging characterization of indeterminate lung nodules. In a meta-analysis,[84] PET was shown to be 94% sensitive and 83% specific for the differentiation of benign from malignant solid nodules 1 to 3 cm in size, although specificity decreases in regions with a high prevalence of granulomatous infections. The addition of PET-CT tends to increase sensitivity with no change in specificity compared with PET alone.[86] False-positive PET results may be seen with inflammatory processes, particularly granulomatous diseases[84] such as tuberculosis, histoplasmosis, and sarcoidosis. Tumors that may be PET negative include minimally invasive adenocarcinoma (see Fig. 25.2), carcinoid tumors,[84] and some metastases (e.g., renal cell carcinoma).[87] In addition, small nodules may not be large enough to produce a positive result on PET scanning. The sensitivity of PET imaging significantly decreases with nodules measuring less than 8 to 10 mm in diameter. As with any imaging modality, the correlation of the PET results with morphologic features on

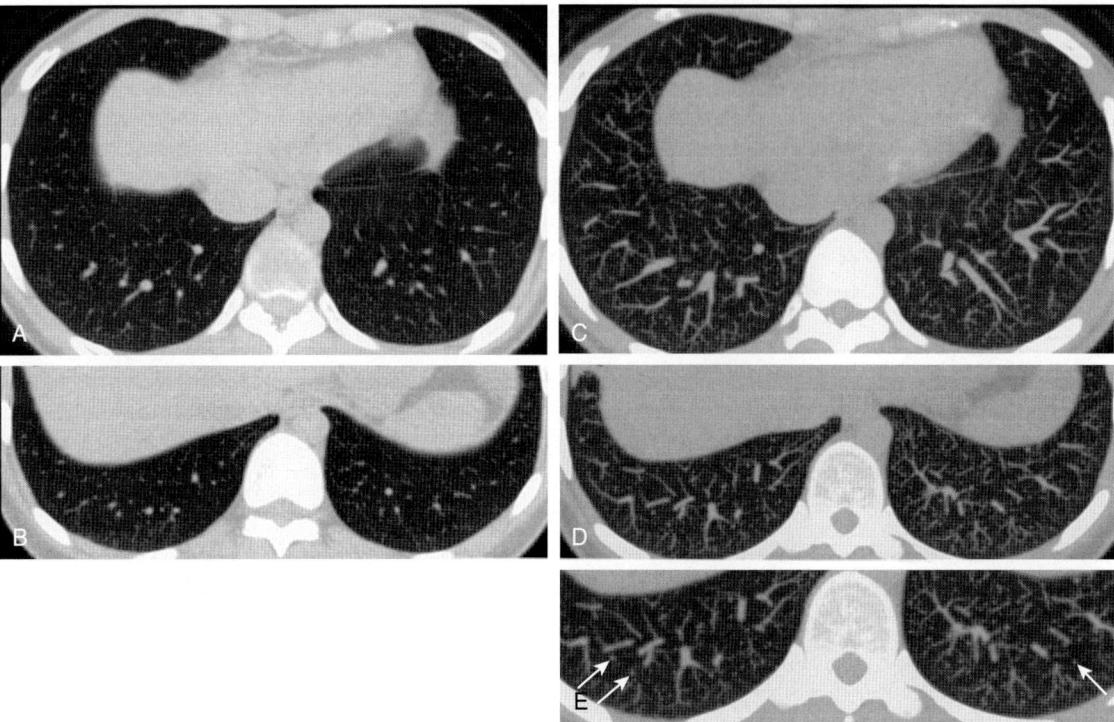

Figure 20.12 Multiple nodules representing pulmonary metastases from papillary thyroid carcinoma in a 28-year-old woman. (A–B) Axial "standard" chest *computed tomography* (CT) images (3-mm reconstruction increment) show little abnormality; some very faint nodularity may be evident in the posterior lung bases. (C–D) Maximum-intensity projected CT images (E magnified image of D) enhance the visualization of very tiny basal pulmonary nodules (*arrows*) representing metastatic disease. These nodules are difficult to visualize at "standard" chest CT (A–B) and were not visible on chest radiography. CT is more sensitive than radiography for detection of small nodules of any cause. (Courtesy Michael B. Gotway, MD.)

malignancies, and the absence of any simulators of metastases (silicosis, sarcoidosis, and prior granulomatous infection) would favor malignancy in pulmonary nodules detected by CT. Furthermore, smaller and less numerous nodules are more likely to be benign. The findings on CT are in themselves not specific, however, and follow-up may be necessary to demonstrate the growth or stability of small nodules.

LUNG CANCER STAGING

In patients with lung cancer, accurate anatomic staging is essential for planning the therapeutic approach.[91,92] CT is used in both assessment of primary tumor extent and detection of lymph node metastases. However, its accuracy in both situations is limited.[91,92] Lung cancer staging is reviewed in detail in Chapter 76.

Computed Tomography

The primary goal of CT is to help distinguish patients who likely have resectable (i.e., potentially surgically curable) tumors from those who do not.[93] Pulmonary malignancy is considered to be likely unresectable (T4) if the primary tumor (1) involves the trachea (eFig. 20.36) or carina; (2) invades the mediastinum (eFig. 20.37) with involvement of mediastinal structures (see eFig. 20.37); (3) invades the heart or great vessels (eFig. 20.38), brachial plexus (C8 or above), recurrent laryngeal nerve, esophagus, diaphragm, or vertebral column (eFig. 20.39); (4) measures more than 7 cm; or (5) is accompanied by separate tumor nodule(s) in a *different* lobe from the primary tumor but still within the *ipsilateral* lung. The tumor is also generally considered unresectable (N3 or

M1) when there is (6) contralateral hilar, peribronchial, or mediastinal lymph node involvement; (7) ipsilateral or contralateral scalene or supraclavicular lymph node involvement; (8) tumor nodules present in the lung *contralateral* to the primary tumor, (9) malignant pleural (eFig. 20.40) or pericardial effusion; (10) involvement in nonregional lymph nodes (i.e., those lymph node stations not considered among the N descriptors); and (11) metastatic disease outside the thorax or involving the osseous thorax.[93–97] Note, however, that acceptable morbidity and mortality have been reported after en bloc vertebral body resection with reconstruction for neoplasms invading the spine, particularly after induction chemotherapy, but such extensive surgeries are usually restricted to larger academic or high-volume centers. The presence of satellite nodules in the same lobe as the primary tumor is designated as T3 in the *Eighth Edition of the TNM Classification of Malignant Tumors* (TNM-8) and does not preclude surgical resection.[93–97]

Tracheal (see eFig. 20.36) or carinal invasion (eFig. 20.41) can be suggested with CT but often requires biopsy confirmation. The CT diagnosis of chest wall or mediastinal (see eFig. 20.37) invasion can sometimes be a problem, and many CT scans suggesting chest wall invasion are relatively nonspecific and can be seen with a number of inflammatory disorders. The sensitivity and specificity of CT for diagnosing T4 mediastinal or chest wall invasion are about 60% and 90%,[98,99] respectively, although some findings (e.g., vertebral body destruction, encasement of mediastinal structures, mediastinal fat infiltration) are virtually diagnostic.[98–103] Chest wall invasion is surgically resectable, and even limited mediastinal invasion is considered

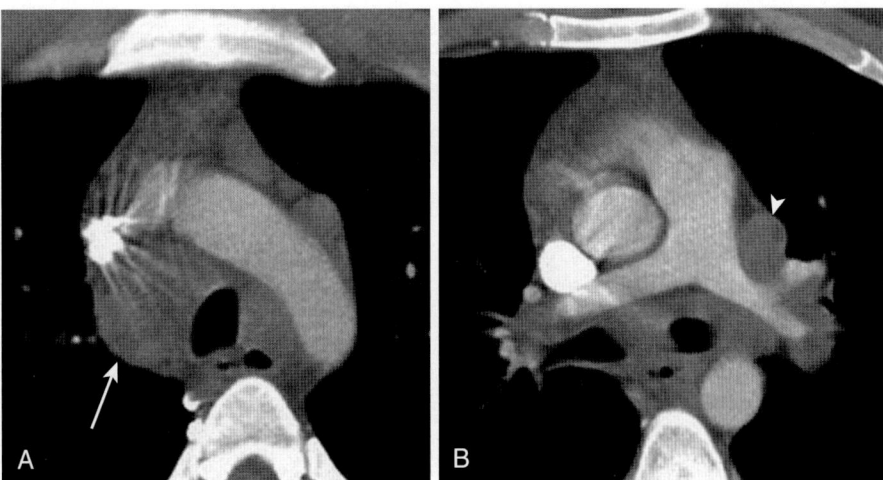

Figure 20.13 Chest computed tomography performed for staging in a patient with non–small cell lung cancer. (A) The primary tumor was present at another level in the right lung. Right paratracheal lymphadenopathy is present (*arrow*); left mediastinal nodes also appear enlarged. (B) Axial chest computed tomography at a slightly lower level shows left hilar and subaortic lymph nodes (*arrowhead*), which measure greater than 1 cm in short-axis diameter, the most widely accepted size threshold for abnormality, and would be considered suspicious for metastasis. Sampling of the left node confirmed metastatic nodal disease. (Courtesy Michael B. Gotway, MD.)

potentially resectable by many surgeons, but knowledge of tumor extent is nonetheless an important factor when planning therapy. Thoracic MRI, either without or with IV contrast, is often considered superior to chest CT for the assessment of local tumor extent when chest wall, spinal, or mediastinal invasion is suspected, particularly in the context of superior sulcus (Pancoast) tumors.[93,96]

CT findings suggesting mediastinal invasion[99,101] include (1) replacement of mediastinal fat by soft tissue attenuation; (2) compression or displacement of mediastinal vessels by tumor; (3) tumor contacting more than 90 degrees of the circumference of a structure, such as the aorta or pulmonary artery (the greater the extent of circumferential contact, the greater the likelihood of invasion); (4) more than 3 cm of contact between tumor and the mediastinum; and (5) obliteration of the mediastinal fat plane normally seen adjacent to most mediastinal structures (eFig. 20.42, see eFig. 20.37). However, individually these findings are unreliable for differentiating mediastinal invasion from anatomic contiguity.[101] Note that invasion of the mediastinal pleura, previously classified as a T3 descriptor in TNM-7, was deleted as a "T" descriptor in TNM-8 because this finding was rarely used as a descriptor in clinical staging. The presence of mediastinal pleural invasion is difficult to determine in practice, and commonly when mediastinal pleural invasion is found at pathologic staging, the primary tumor has already extended beyond the mediastinal pleura and invaded the mediastinum proper (a T4 descriptor in TNM-8).[97]

CT is often of limited value in the diagnosis of malignant pleural effusion because this diagnosis requires cytologic confirmation.[104] However, in some patients CT may show diffuse or nodular pleural thickening with or without (see eFig. 20.40) pleural liquid.[104,105] PET may show tracer uptake in patients with malignant pleural effusion, even when CT does not show evidence of nodular pleural thickening and when cytologic analysis is negative.[106]

The diagnosis of mediastinal lymph node metastasis by CT is determined largely by node size, although the preservation of fat within lymph nodes often reflects the absence of pathologic infiltration, whereas necrosis may imply pathologic

infiltration even within normal-sized lymph nodes.[92,96] By convention, a nodal short-axis diameter of greater than 1 cm is considered to be abnormal in all node stations (Fig. 20.13),[92,96] except perhaps in the subcarinal space.[107,108] In general, a tumor cannot be reliably detected in normal-sized lymph nodes by CT, nor do mildly enlarged lymph nodes always harbor tumor[96]; essentially, there are no characteristic appearances that confidently allow benign and malignant causes of nodal enlargement to be distinguished.[108–110] Pooled information from 35 studies published between 1991 and June 2006 evaluating the performance of CT scanning for noninvasive staging of the mediastinum has shown that this size threshold has a sensitivity of only about 51% and a specificity of 86% for diagnosing mediastinal lymph node metastases in patients with lung cancer.[97,111,112] Furthermore, the accuracy of CT for detecting involvement of individual node groups is low (hilar, paratracheal, subcarinal, etc.), perhaps as low as 40%.[111] In a more recent review[92] of the accuracy of mediastinal lymph node staging using CT, a combination of studies evaluating 7368 patients found the median sensitivity and specificity for mediastinal lymph node metastases detection at chest CT of 55% and 81%, respectively.

Despite its limited accuracy, CT, particularly in conjunction with PET, is useful in determining the need for preoperative invasive mediastinal lymph node staging. Furthermore, findings at CT may also be useful in deciding on the choice for a particular preoperative mediastinal staging procedure, such as endobronchial ultrasound, endoscopic ultrasound, mediastinoscopy, anterior mediastinotomy (e.g., the Chamberlain procedure), video-assisted thoracoscopy, or transthoracic needle biopsy.

Perhaps the most important contribution of CT to intrathoracic staging is precise mapping of nodes likely to be involved by tumor and directing additional diagnostic procedures required for accurate lung cancer staging.

Positron Emission Tomography and Positron Emission Tomography–Computed Tomography

The role of PET imaging in the staging of bronchogenic malignancy is explored in detail in Chapters 25 and 76.

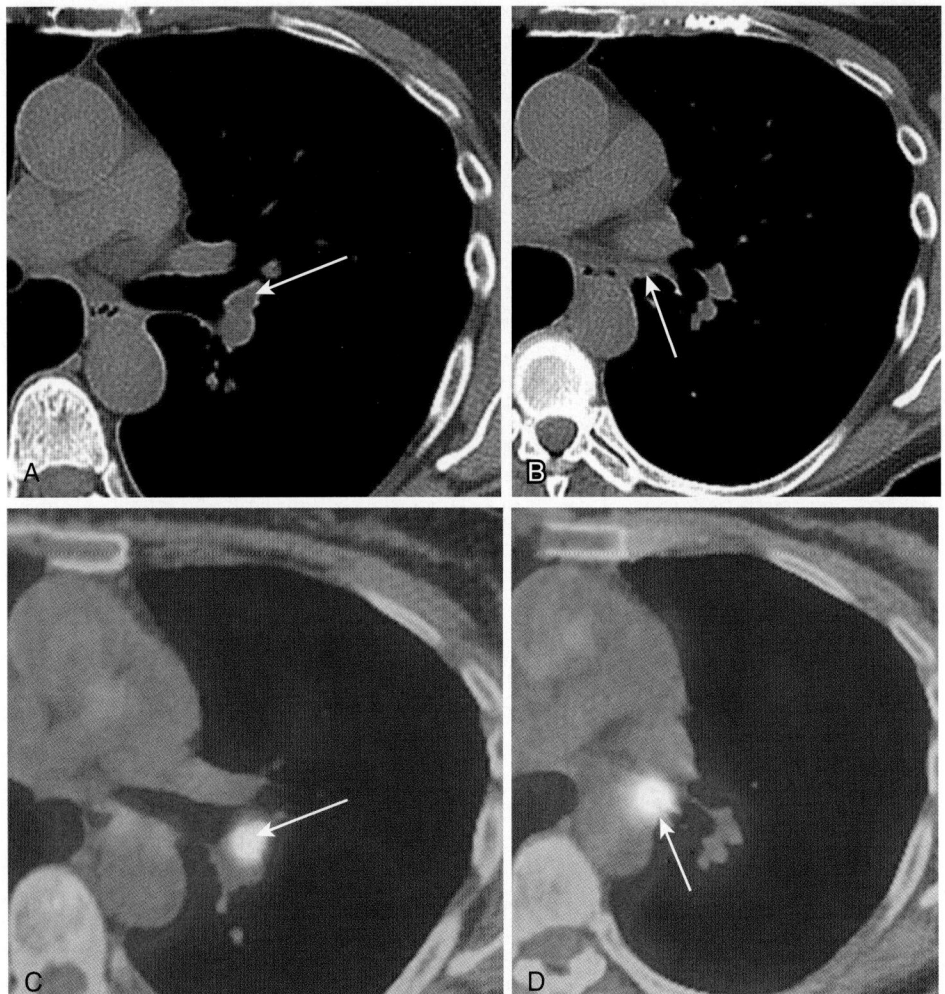

Figure 20.14 Utility of *positron emission tomography–computed tomography* (PET-CT) in the staging of pulmonary malignancy. This patient was diagnosed with left lung non–small cell lung cancer, and CT and PET-CT were performed for staging. (A–B) Axial unenhanced chest CT shows subcentimeter left peribronchial lymph nodes *(arrows)*. (C–D) Axial ¹⁸fluorodeoxyglucose-PET scan images at the same level as the CT images shows hypermetabolism within the subcentimeter left peribronchial lymph nodes, suggesting tumor involvement. Neoplastic infiltration within left peribronchial lymph nodes was confirmed at surgery. (Courtesy Michael B. Gotway, MD.)

The primary value of PET is to increase the sensitivity for the detection of local and distant malignancy to spare patients with unresectable disease from undergoing unnecessary surgery, thereby reducing the rate of futile thoracotomies.[93,96] PET and PET-CT are most useful for evaluating the N (Fig. 20.14) and M (eFig. 20.43) components of staging,[95] although PET activity in the primary tumor (T component) may provide insight into biologic aggressiveness and the chance of future spread of early localized tumors.[113]

Magnetic Resonance Imaging

There are few situations in which MRI is the preferred imaging modality for patients with primary lung cancer. The extent of chest wall, mediastinal, and great vessel invasion adjacent to a lung tumor sometimes may best be shown by MRI, and there may be some advantage to MRI over CT for assessment of mediastinal invasion, vertebral body invasion, and involvement of the chest wall.[92,93,96] Sagittal or coronal MR images can be advantageous in delineating the extent of tumors at the lung apex.[92,114] As a consequence, MRI may be more accurate than CT for determining chest wall involvement in superior sulcus tumors, and certainly

tumor involvement of the neurovascular bundle[114] is better shown with coronal and sagittal MRI than with axial or even reformatted CT images.

In most patients with primary lung cancer, MRI has little additional information to offer, and CT is the preferred imaging procedure.[92] MRI is generally similar to CT in its ability to identify mediastinal lymph nodes[92] and diagnose mediastinal metastases. Although it has been reported that MRI is more accurate than CT in detecting mediastinal[97,115] cardiac or vascular invasion by lung cancer, the reported differences in accuracy are small. In general, the MR properties of benign and tumor-bearing mediastinal lymph nodes do not differ significantly in most patients and, as with CT, node size is usually the main diagnostically useful discriminator. However, recent data with newer MR sequences—particularly diffusion-weighted imaging,[96,116] short-tau inversion recovery imaging,[117,118] and recent observations regarding findings at T2-weighted chest MRI[119]—may allow discrimination between benign and malignant lymph node involvement, even for lymph nodes with short-axis dimensions less than 1 cm. A recent meta-analysis of the performance of MR imaging for peribronchial and mediastinal lymph node status in patients with non–small cell lung carcinoma

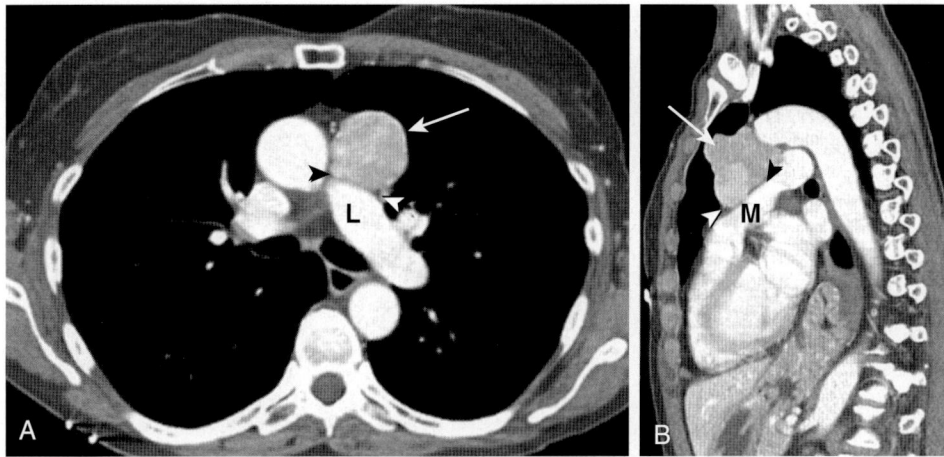

Figure 20.15 *Computed tomography* **(CT) for mediastinal mass detection and characterization.** Axial (A) and coronal (B) enhanced chest CT shows a mildly heterogeneous anterior mediastinal mass (*arrows*) subsequently shown to represent a thymoma. The CT image clearly shows a preserved fat plane (*arrowheads*) between the mass and the main (M) and left (L) pulmonary arteries. (Courtesy Michael B. Gotway, MD.)

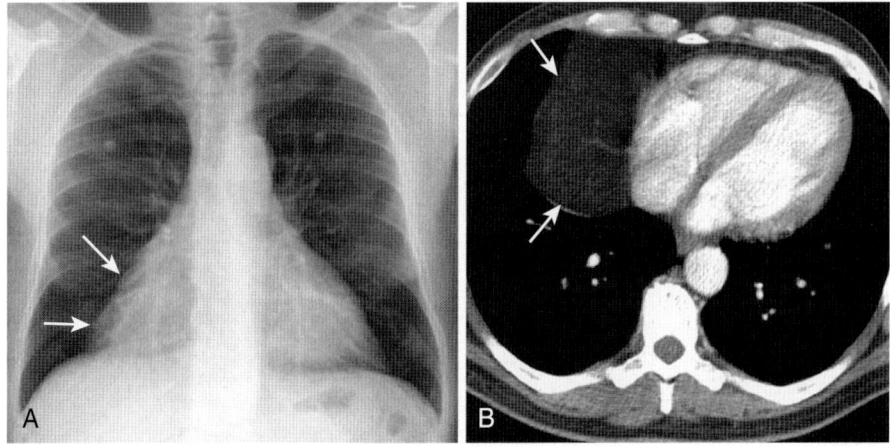

Figure 20.16 **Chest** *computed tomography* **(CT) characterization of fatty mediastinal masses.** (A) Frontal chest radiograph shows a contour abnormality (*arrows*) along the right inferior mediastinum. (B) Axial chest CT image shows a fatty right paracardiac mass (*arrows*), consistent with thymolipoma. The diagnosis was confirmed by biopsy. (Courtesy Michael B. Gotway, MD.)

indicates that the per-patient (86.5%) and per-node (87.9%) sensitivity for metastatic involvement is at least comparable to PET-CT at equivalent specificity values.[120] Furthermore, the recent development of hybrid PET-MR scanners could combine the anatomic and physiologic information available from both modalities, further improving noninvasive lung carcinoma staging (eFig. 20.44).

LUNG CANCER SCREENING

 Lung cancer screening is discussed in detail with attention to technical aspects of low-dose CT at ExpertConsult.com.

HILAR AND MEDIASTINAL MASSES

CT is indicated as the primary imaging modality in most patients with suspected hilar or mediastinal masses. The cross-sectional display and tissue discrimination of CT have revolutionized diagnostic imaging of the hilum and mediastinum.

Lesions can be detected with high sensitivity and located precisely to a particular region of the mediastinum (see Fig. 20.15, see Chapter 115). By localizing a mass to a particular

region of the mediastinum,[147,148] the differential diagnosis can be more specific and biopsy procedures can be planned with greater accuracy and safety. In addition to the information gained from the location of the mass, the density discrimination of CT enables soft tissue abnormalities, fluid collections, and fatty tissue to be distinguished accurately (Fig. 20.16).[149–151] With use of IV contrast material, masses and vascular anomalies (see eFigs. 115.47B, 115.48B–D, and 115.49B) can be accurately discriminated. CT is useful in further evaluating a mass initially detected on chest radiography, for demonstrating pathology suspected on the basis of the clinical setting (but not visible on conventional imaging studies), and for precisely delineating the location of lesions for planning therapy.

MRI may be indicated as the primary imaging modality in patients with a suspected mediastinal mass in many situations: for differentiating thymic neoplasia from thymic hyperplasia, for displaying lesions at the thoracic inlet in the coronal plane, for distinguishing cystic from solid masses (see eFigs. 115.27B–C and 115.42C–D),[152] for detecting hemorrhagic components within a mediastinal lesion (see eFig. 115.35D–E), for distinguishing between surgical (see eFigs. 115.16D–G and 115.23C–D) and nonsurgical (see eFig.

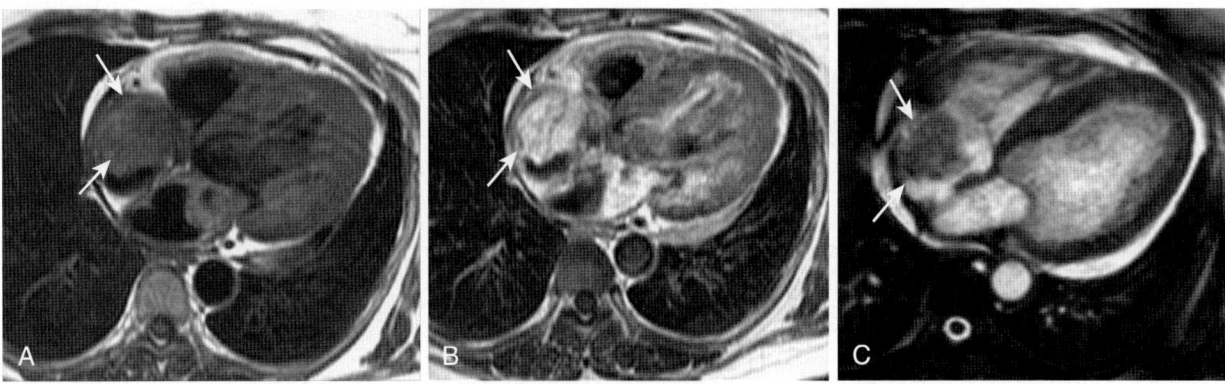

Figure 20.17 *Magnetic resolution imaging* **(MRI) characterization of cardiac masses.** (A) Axial T1-weighted image shows a soft tissue–intensity mass (*arrows*) within the right atrium. (B) Contrast-enhanced axial T1-weighted MRI shows intense enhancement of the mass (*arrows*), excluding thrombus as the diagnosis and suggesting neoplasm. (C) Balanced fast-field echo image (obtained for function) shows the mass as a low-signal lesion (*arrows*) within the right atrium. Resection confirmed right atrial myxoma. Most intracardiac right atrial tumors turn out to be thrombus (often catheter/lead related), in which case anticoagulation would be the therapy of choice, and an invasive resection would add unnecessary risk for the patient. Thus, in this case, preprocedural MRI confirmation that the right atrial lesion is indeed neoplastic is critical for guiding patient management. (Courtesy Michael B. Gotway, MD.)

115.15B–D) mediastinal masses,[153] and for evaluation of posterior mediastinal masses (see eFigs. 115.14 and 115.40D–E) and neurogenic tumors (see eFig. 115.14), which may have intraspinal components.[152,154,155] Early experience with mediastinal MRI suggested that this modality may be capable of distinguishing between a tumor mass and a benign fibrous mass[156–158] after radiation therapy, a distinction that can be difficult with CT. However, in practice the differentiation of tumor from associated inflammation or posttreatment changes is difficult with any imaging technique,[156,157] and PET is generally preferred for this distinction.

MRI is rarely indicated for imaging hilar masses; contrast-enhanced CT is usually preferred for this application. Traditionally, contrast-enhanced MR would be considered as an alternative to contrast-enhanced chest CT for the assessment of hilar or mediastinal lesions in patients with impaired renal function, however, in patients with impaired renal function, gadolinium may predispose to fibrosing dermopathy (referred to as nephrogenic systemic fibrosis).[159] Nevertheless, unenhanced MR, due to its inherent high-contrast resolution (see eFig. 115.15), may still provide valuable information regarding hilar and mediastinal masses.

Primary and metastatic cardiac tumors are often detected initially by echocardiography, but MRI is also an accurate method of delineating such lesions.[160–162] It is thus appropriate as a problem-solving technique for patients with inconclusive echocardiographic examinations, but it is also emerging as a first-line examination for a number of cardiovascular applications. Both MRI and CT can specifically demonstrate fat within cardiac lesions and fluid within pericardial cysts (see eFig. 115.42B–D). Intracardiac tumor (Fig. 20.17) and thrombus can be differentiated by MRI, particularly after contrast administration.

DIFFUSE LUNG DISEASE

The clinical assessment of a patient with suspected *diffuse ILD* (DILD) can be a difficult and perplexing problem. Imaging studies are often important in reaching a final diagnosis, suggesting appropriate diagnostic procedures, and assessing the patient's course and prognosis.

In clinical practice, the imaging studies most frequently used to evaluate patients with suspected DILD are chest radiographs and *high-resolution CT* (HRCT). HRCT is a technique that combines narrow collimation/thin-slice thickness (≈1 mm) and image reconstruction with a high-spatial-frequency algorithm to maximize sharpness in the final image—often accompanied by prone and postexpiratory imaging—and is typically used when the diagnosis is uncertain at chest radiography and clinical evaluation and further assessment is considered warranted, as well as to assess treatment response in patients with established diagnoses.

HRCT findings have been described in a wide variety of parenchymal diseases, including the idiopathic interstitial pneumonias,[163] sarcoidosis,[164–167] diffuse neoplasms, pneumoconioses,[168–172] infections, and numerous other disorders.[173–185] These studies have shown that HRCT delineates both normal anatomic structures (Fig. 20.18) and pathologic alterations in lung morphology more clearly than chest radiographs or routine CT.[167,181,186,187] Much of the basis of HRCT interpretation rests on recognition of the anatomy of the secondary pulmonary lobule (see Fig. 20.18) as reflected on HRCT images; in particular, the histopathologic patterns of disease involvement of the secondary pulmonary lobule are often reflected in HRCT images, and recognition of the HRCT correlates of these disease facilitates noninvasive diagnosis. This approach is particularly useful for the anatomic localization of small nodules at HRCT, described later.

In general, HRCT findings of lung disease can be divided into *increased* lung opacity, including reticular, linear, and nodular opacities, consolidation, and *ground-glass opacity* (GGO), and *decreased* lung opacity, including cysts, cavities, emphysema, and mosaic perfusion.[188]

Increased Lung Opacity

Linear and Reticular Opacities. Thickening of the interstitial fiber network of lung by fluid, fibrous tissue, or interstitial infiltration by cells results in an increase in both linear and reticular opacities as seen on HRCT.[188] Interlobular septal thickening is seen in patients with a variety of ILDs, but most typically with increased pressure pulmonary edema, lymphangitic spread of tumor (Fig. 20.19A),[188] and sarcoidosis,[166] in addition to a small number of rarer causes.[171,189,190] Septal thickening is not common in patients with interstitial fibrosis, except for those with sarcoidosis and

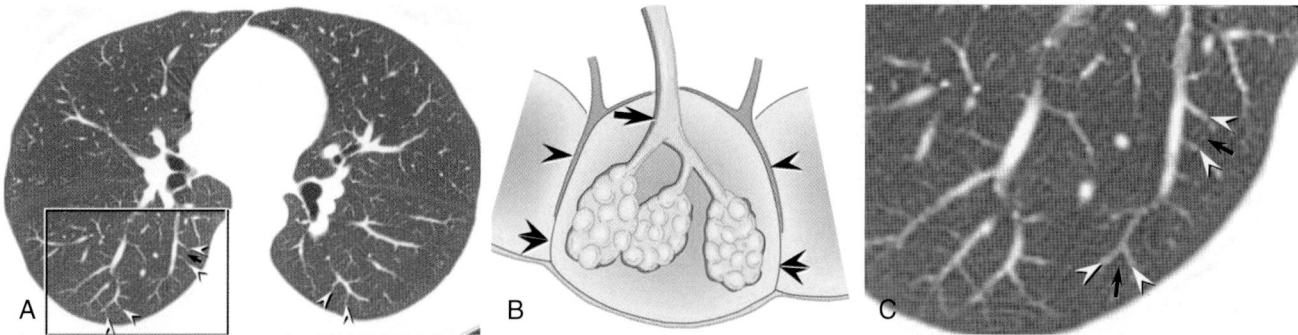

Figure 20.18 Normal high-resolution chest computed tomography (HRCT): secondary lobular anatomy. (A) Axial HRCT image through the level of the right lower lobe bronchus shows normal major (oblique) fissures, central airways, and pulmonary vessels. (Inset C is a detailed image of the area of interest in the right lower lobe.) Small peripheral pulmonary veins (*white arrowheads*) are visible. Pulmonary veins travel within interlobular septa and therefore may outline secondary pulmonary lobules (lung parenchyma between *white arrowheads*). On occasion, the centrilobular artery (*black arrows*), the artery entering the center of the pulmonary lobule, may normally be visible. An understanding of secondary pulmonary lobular anatomy underlies the anatomic approach for localization of small nodules detected at HRCT, which provides the basis for differential diagnosis of such nodules. (B) Illustration of the normal secondary pulmonary lobule. Pulmonary veins (*single arrowheads*), travel within interlobular septa (*double arrowheads*). The centrilobular artery and bronchus (*arrow*) enter the secondary lobule and branch sequentially, eventually extending to the level of gas-exchange units—respiratory bronchioles, alveolar ducts, alveolar sacs, and alveoli and the capillary network associated with these structures. (A and C, Courtesy Michael B. Gotway, MD.)

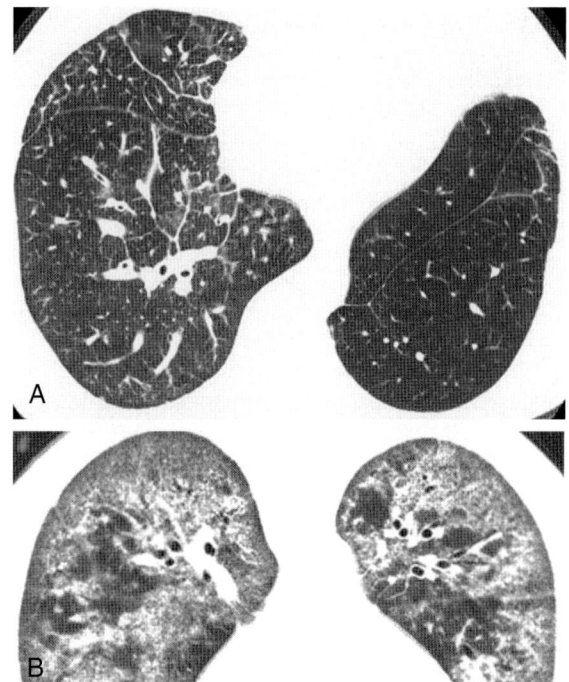

Figure 20.19 Both *interlobular* septal thickening and *intralobular* interstitial thickening. (A) Axial high-resolution computed tomography image shows smoothly thickened interlobular septa (*arrowheads*) in a patient with metastatic breast carcinoma; note asymmetry of the process. (B) Prone high-resolution computed tomography image in a patient with scleroderma shows reticular opacity resulting from numerous intralobular lines, manifesting as small, fine lines separated by a few millimeters, creating a fine, lace- or netlike pattern. Mild peripheral bronchiolectasis (*arrow*) is present. (Courtesy Michael B. Gotway, MD.)

asbestosis.[191] The term *intralobular lines* refers to a pattern of small lines within the secondary lobule separated by a few millimeters creating a reticular or netlike pattern. This finding is commonly seen in the context of fibrotic lung diseases (see Fig. 20.19B) but may also be encountered with interstitial inflammation in the absence of fibrosis. Pathologically, intralobular lines, or intralobular interstitial thickening, reflect infiltration of the distal peribronchovascular interstitium and the interstitium within the secondary lobule.

Nodules. Nodules can be classified as *perilymphatic*, *random*, or *centrilobular*, according to their distribution within the secondary pulmonary lobule (see Fig. 20.18).[188,192] Recognition of one of these distributions is fundamental to the generation of differential diagnoses.[192,193]

- *Perilymphatic* nodules affect the peribronchovascular, interlobular septal, subpleural, and, to a lesser extent, centrilobular interstitial compartments and are typical of sarcoidosis, which tends to have a peribronchovascular and subpleural predominance (Fig. 20.20, Video 20.10)[166,192–194]; silicosis and coal workers' pneumoconiosis, which predominate in the subpleural and centrilobular regions[171,176,189]; and lymphangitic spread of tumor, which is usually peribronchovascular and septal.[188]
- *Random* nodules are found both in perilymphatic and in centrilobular locations, and are defined by a broad diffuse and fairly even pattern in the lung. They are most typical of miliary infections (Fig. 20.21)[195] and hematogenous metastases.[188]
- *Centrilobular* nodules are predominantly located in the bronchovascular location in the center of the secondary lobule. They can be either well-defined or poorly defined. *Well-defined centrilobular* nodules can be seen in silicosis and coal workers' pneumoconiosis,[169] asbestosis,[168] and *pulmonary Langerhans cell histiocytosis* (PLCH).[196] *Poorly defined centrilobular* nodules often reflect bronchiolar or peribronchiolar abnormalities[193] and can be seen in silicosis and coal workers' pneumoconiosis,[169] endobronchial spread of infection,[195] pulmonary hemorrhage (Fig. 20.22), hypersensitivity pneumonitis,[197,198] and pulmonary edema.[199]

A comparison of the three nodular distributions using HRCT is shown in Fig. 20.23.

Consolidation and Ground-Glass Opacity. Air space consolidation, by definition, is seen when alveolar air is replaced by fluid, cells, or other material.[200] On HRCT, consolidation results in an increase in lung opacity associated with obscuration of underlying vessels. Among patients with chronic DILD, common causes of this pattern include chronic eosinophilic pneumonia and cryptogenic organizing

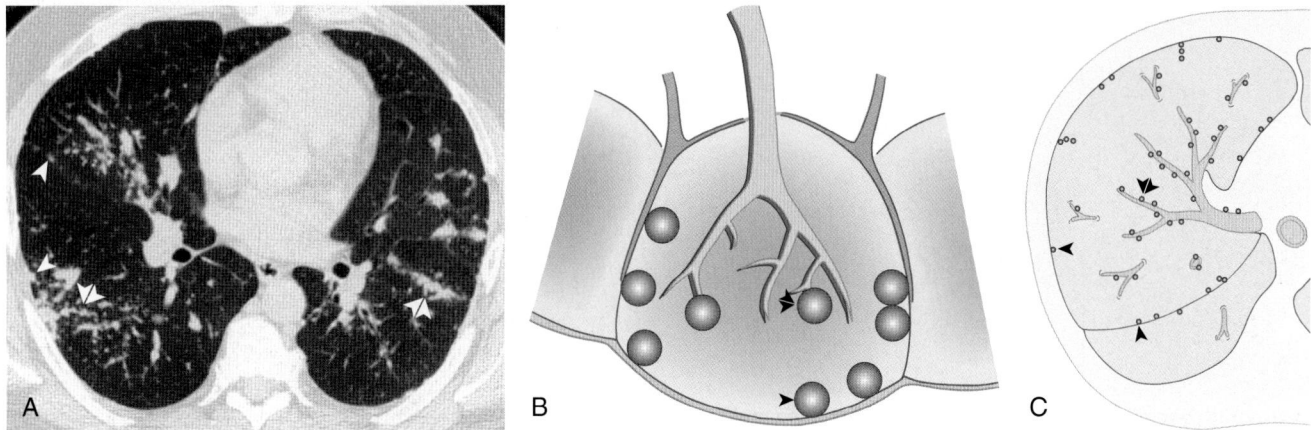

Figure 20.20 *High-resolution computed tomography* (HRCT) illustration of perilymphatic nodules: sarcoidosis. (A) Axial HRCT image of a patient with sarcoidosis shows numerous subpleural nodules in relation to costal and fissural visceral pleural surfaces (*single arrowheads*), and nodules are also clearly visible along bronchovascular bundles (*double arrowheads*). These findings, along with the patchy distribution of the nodules, are diagnostic of sarcoidosis in the appropriate clinical setting. (B) Perilymphatic nodule distribution in the secondary pulmonary lobule and (C) anatomic localization. Small nodules are primarily distributed along the visceral pleural surfaces (*single arrowhead*) and interlobular septa; to a lesser extent, they may also appear in the centrilobular area, at the bronchovascular bundles (*double arrowheads*). (A, Courtesy Michael B. Gotway, MD.)

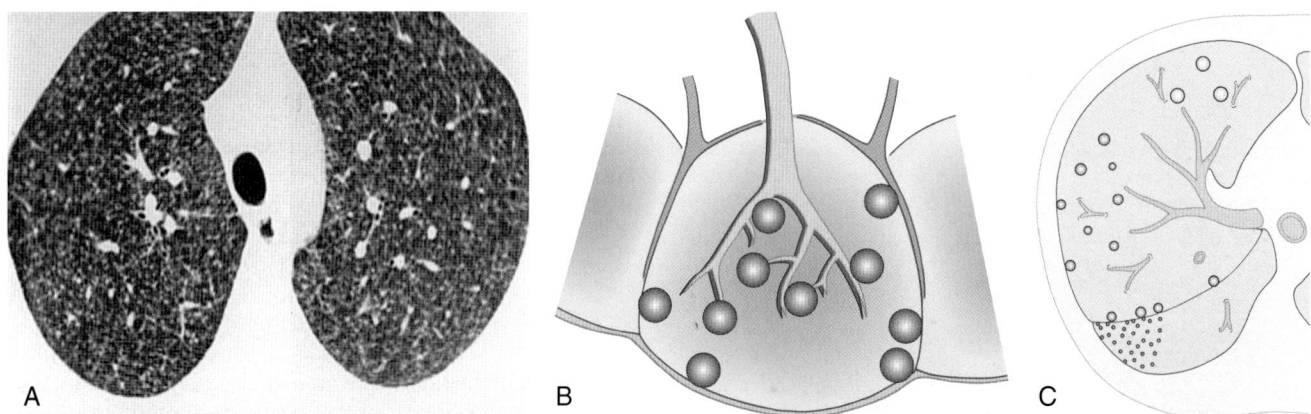

Figure 20.21 *High-resolution computed tomography* (HRCT) illustration of random nodules: miliary tuberculosis. (A) Axial HRCT image shows numerous small circumscribed nodules equally distributed throughout the lungs bilaterally, with nodules seen in contact with fissural pleural surfaces, as well as sparing the fissural surfaces. (B) Random nodule distribution in the secondary pulmonary lobule. Small nodules are seen along the visceral pleural surfaces, interlobular septa, and bronchovascular bundles. (C) Anatomic localization of small nodules at HRCT. Random nodules are distributed in a fairly even, diffuse distribution bilaterally. (A, Courtesy Michael B. Gotway, MD.)

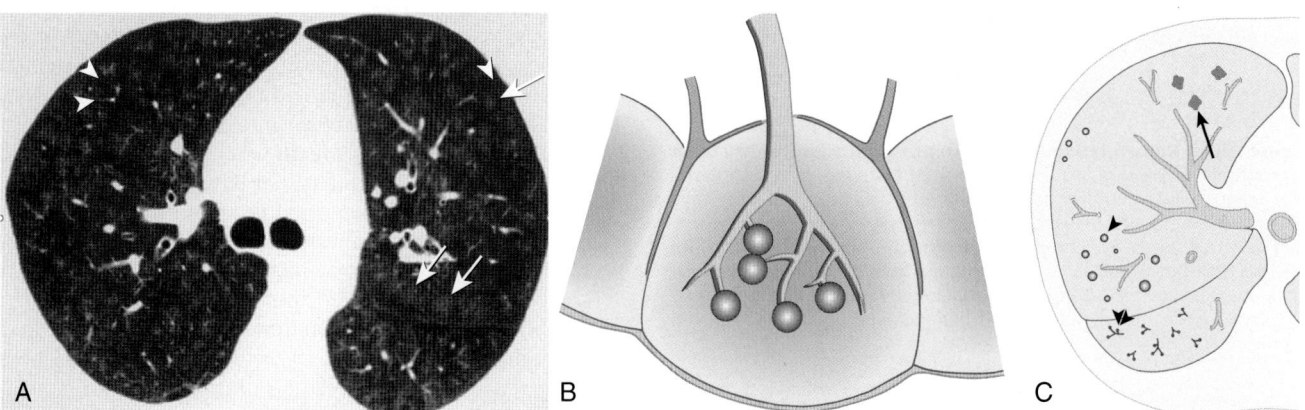

Figure 20.22 *High-resolution computed tomography* (HRCT) illustration of centrilobular nodules: diffuse pulmonary hemorrhage. (A) Axial HRCT image shows numerous bilateral poorly defined, ground-glass opacity nodules (*arrows*). Note that the nodules approach, but generally do not touch, costal and fissural visceral pleural surfaces; this relationship is particularly evident along the left major fissure. Also note that occasionally the relationship of the nodules to adjacent pulmonary veins (*arrowheads,* right upper lobe) and interlobular septa (*arrowhead,* left upper lobe) is apparent; the nodules have a small amount of "spared" lung separating them from the interlobular septa and small pulmonary veins, a key indicator of the centrilobular distribution. (B) Centrilobular nodule distribution in the secondary pulmonary lobule. Small nodules are seen primarily in the center of the lobule, along the bronchovascular bundles, largely sparing the interlobular septa, pulmonary veins, and visceral pleural surfaces. (C) Anatomic localization of small nodules at HRCT. Centrilobular nodules typically approach, but do not contact, the costal and fissural visceral pleural surfaces and interlobular septa. Centrilobular nodules may be well defined and round (*single arrowhead*) or poorly defined and irregular in shape (*arrow*), or they may show ground-glass attenuation. When centrilobular nodules show branching configurations (*double arrowhead*), the nodule morphology is often described as tree-in-bud opacity. (A, Courtesy Michael B. Gotway, MD.)

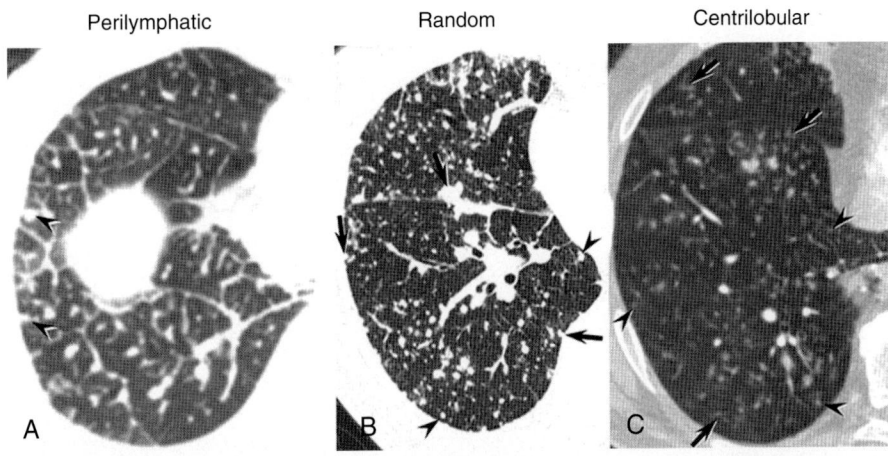

Perilymphatic   Random   Centrilobular

Figure 20.23 Comparison of nodule distribution patterns on *high-resolution computed tomography* (HRCT). (A) Axial HRCT image in a patient with lymphangitic carcinomatosis illustrates the perilymphatic small nodule distribution. Note how many of the small, circumscribed nodules are in contact with visceral pleural surfaces (*arrowheads*). Also note the presence of prominent interlobular septal thickening. (B) Axial HRCT image in a patient with metastatic malignancy illustrates the random small nodule distribution. Many nodules approach, but do not contact, the visceral pleural surfaces (*arrowheads*), consistent with a centrilobular localization, whereas other nodules (*arrows*) clearly contact the visceral pleural surfaces. Critically, the small nodules characteristic of the random distribution pattern are *diffusely distributed*—present throughout the lung parenchyma in a roughly equal manner—as opposed to the *patchy distribution* characteristic of perilymphatic processes. (C) Axial HRCT image in a patient with bronchopneumonia and centrilobular small nodule distribution shows numerous, bilateral, poorly defined nodules, most of which approach, but generally do not touch, costal and fissural visceral pleural surfaces (*arrowheads*). Several nodules also show a branching configuration—so-called tree-in-bud morphology (*arrows*)—typical of inspissated mucous and pus within small airways.

pneumonia.[201,202] GGO refers to a hazy increase in lung opacity that is not associated with obscuration of underlying vessels.[200] This finding can reflect the presence of a number of diseases and can be seen in patients with either minimal interstitial thickening or minimal air space filling.[180,182,203–206] It often reflects the presence of an active process, such as pulmonary edema (see eFig. 98.7G); alveolitis associated with some idiopathic interstitial pneumonias (see Chapters 89 and 90); pulmonary hemorrhage (see Fig. 20.22 and Chapter 94); infectious pneumonias, particularly *Pneumocystis jirovecii* pneumonia (see eFigs. 123.12B, 123.14C, 123.15B, 123.18); lipoid pneumonia (see eFigs. 43.2B and 98.7B); alveolar proteinosis (see Fig. 98.3 and eFigs. 98.5, 98.6, 98.9A–D, 98.10, and 98.11); hypersensitivity pneumonitis (see Fig. 91.4), often with a centrilobular nodular appearance (see Fig. 20.23 and eFig. 91.3C–D); and sarcoidosis.[207] However, GGO may reflect the presence of fibrosis below the resolution of HRCT, particularly when the GGO is associated with other findings of fibrotic lung disease, such as coarse reticulation, architectural distortion, traction bronchiectasis, and honeycombing.[204] Because of its potential reflection of active lung disease, the presence of GGO may lead to surgical lung biopsy depending on the clinical status of the patient.

Decreased Lung Opacity

Emphysema. Emphysema is accurately diagnosed with HRCT, and HRCT is more sensitive for the detection of emphysema than is routine CT or chest radiography.[143,183] Emphysema results in focal areas of low attenuation easily contrasted with surrounding, higher-attenuation, normal lung parenchyma (Fig. 20.24). In patients with centrilobular emphysema (see Fig. 20.24A), areas of lucency can be seen surrounding the centrilobular artery and have a patchy, upper lobe distribution. In panlobular emphysema, focal areas of lucency are usually not present, but a diffuse simplification of lung architecture and a decrease in lung attenuation are present (see Fig. 20.24B). Paraseptal emphysema is readily diagnosed at HRCT (see Fig. 20.24C),

appearing as thin-walled cystic spaces of variable size forming a single layer, usually predominating in the upper lobes. In clinical practice, HRCT is not commonly used to diagnose emphysema; usually, the combination of a smoking history, a low diffusing capacity, airway obstruction on pulmonary function tests, and an abnormal chest radiograph showing large lung volumes is sufficient to make the diagnosis. HRCT is useful for evaluating patients with COPD being considered as candidates for lung volume–reduction procedures, bullectomy, or lung transplantation. In addition, some patients with early emphysema can present with clinical findings more typical of infiltrative lung disease or pulmonary vascular disease, namely shortness of breath and low diffusing capacity, without evidence of airway obstruction on pulmonary function tests.[208] In such patients, HRCT can be valuable for detecting the presence of emphysema and excluding an interstitial abnormality. If significant emphysema is found on HRCT, no further evaluation is necessary.[209] A growing area of interest for the application of HRCT in COPD is the quantification of imaging features of obstructive pulmonary disease. Quantitative assessment of emphysema and CT measures of bronchial wall thickness in patients with COPD independently predict airflow obstruction severity at pulmonary function testing and the risk of COPD exacerbations.[210] Furthermore, the quantitative assessment of emphysema in patients with COPD is also associated with increased all-cause mortality.[210]

Further discussion of functional imaging and quantification in COPD and fibrotic lung disease is available at ExpertConsult.com.

Cystic Pulmonary Diseases. Lymphangioleiomyomatosis (see images associated with Chapter 97, eFig. 97.2, and Fig. 20.25A–B) and PLCH (see Chapter 95) often result in multiple lung cysts (see Figs. 95.1B and 20.25C), which have a distinct appearance on HRCT.[196,211–217] The cysts have a thin but easily discernible wall, ranging up to a few millimeters in thickness. Associated findings of fibrosis are usually absent or much less conspicuous than they are in patients

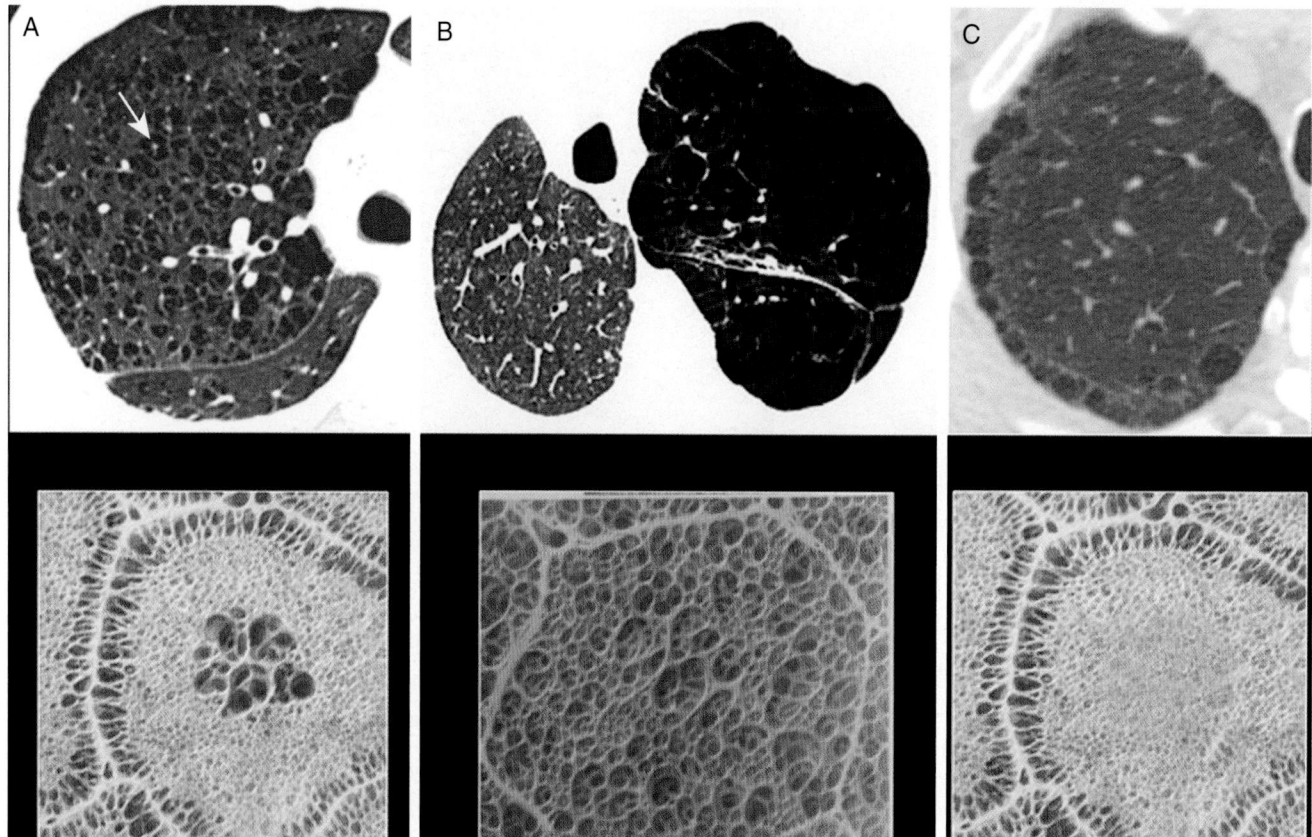

Figure 20.24 *High-resolution computed tomography* (HRCT) **appearance of emphysema and accompanying illustrations of the secondary lobule.** (A) Axial HRCT image in a patient with centrilobular emphysema shows upper lobe, well-defined, "punched-out" cystic spaces without definable walls. Note the centrilobular "dot" (*arrow*) in the center of many of the cystic spaces, representing the centrilobular artery. (B) Axial HRCT image in a patient with panlobular emphysema who underwent right lung transplantation shows the emphysematous left lung contrasted with the normal-appearing right lung. The left lung is less dense, is larger in volume, and contains fewer and smaller vessels, with "simplified" pulmonary architecture. (C) Axial HRCT image in a patient with paraseptal emphysema shows upper lobe, well-defined, thin-walled cysts lining the subpleural regions in the upper lobes, forming a single layer. Lower panels illustrate the changes at the lobular level. (Courtesy Michael B. Gotway, MD.)

with honeycombing. In these diseases, the cysts are usually interspersed within areas of normal-appearing lung. In patients with PLCH (see Fig. 95.1B–D), the cysts can have bizarre shapes and an upper lobe predominance. Numerous causes of cystic and cavitary pulmonary lesions are recognized (eFig. 20.51, see Fig. 20.25).[218,219]

Mosaic Perfusion. Decreased lung attenuation not reflecting the presence of cystic lesions or emphysema can sometimes be recognized on HRCT in patients who have diseases that produce air trapping, poor ventilation, or poor perfusion (Fig. 20.26A).* The areas of decreased lung attenuation seen on HRCT can be focal, lobular (see Fig. 20.26C),[222] lobar, or multifocal. The term *mosaic perfusion* has been used to refer to patchy decreased lung attenuation resulting from perfusion abnormalities (see Figs. 20.25K and 20.26A).[200] In patients with air trapping, this appearance can be enhanced with expiratory HRCT (see Fig. 20.26C).[183,221,223,224]

Honeycombing

The Fleischner Society defines honeycombing (Fig. 20.27A–C and G) as "the appearance of clustered cystic air spaces, typically of comparable diameters on the order of 3 to 10

mm but occasionally as large as 2.5 cm. Honeycombing is usually subpleural and is characterized by well-defined walls. It is a CT feature of established pulmonary fibrosis and is an important criterion in the diagnosis of usual interstitial pneumonia."[200] Although seemingly a straightforward imaging finding, the CT diagnosis of honeycombing is surprisingly subject to significant interobserver variability, even among experts.[225] Honeycombing is an important imaging feature for the diagnosis of the usual interstitial pneumonia pattern at CT, and hence it must be distinguished from other findings that may mimic the appearance of honeycombing (see Fig. 20.27D–F and H), particularly paraseptal emphysema (see Fig. 20.27D and H), cystic lung diseases, and traction bronchiectasis.

Important imaging features that suggest the diagnosis of honeycombing include cystic spaces with relatively thick, shared walls arranged in concentric layers, often in the subpleural regions of lung; perhaps most important, these findings should be seen in the context of other features of fibrotic lung disease, such as traction bronchiectasis, intralobular lines, and architectural distortion.

Diagnostic Utility

CT, in particular HRCT, has essentially replaced chest radiography for the detection and assessment of the treatment response for numerous causes of DILD, owing to the

---

*References 183, 201, 203, 205–209, 213–215, 220, 221.

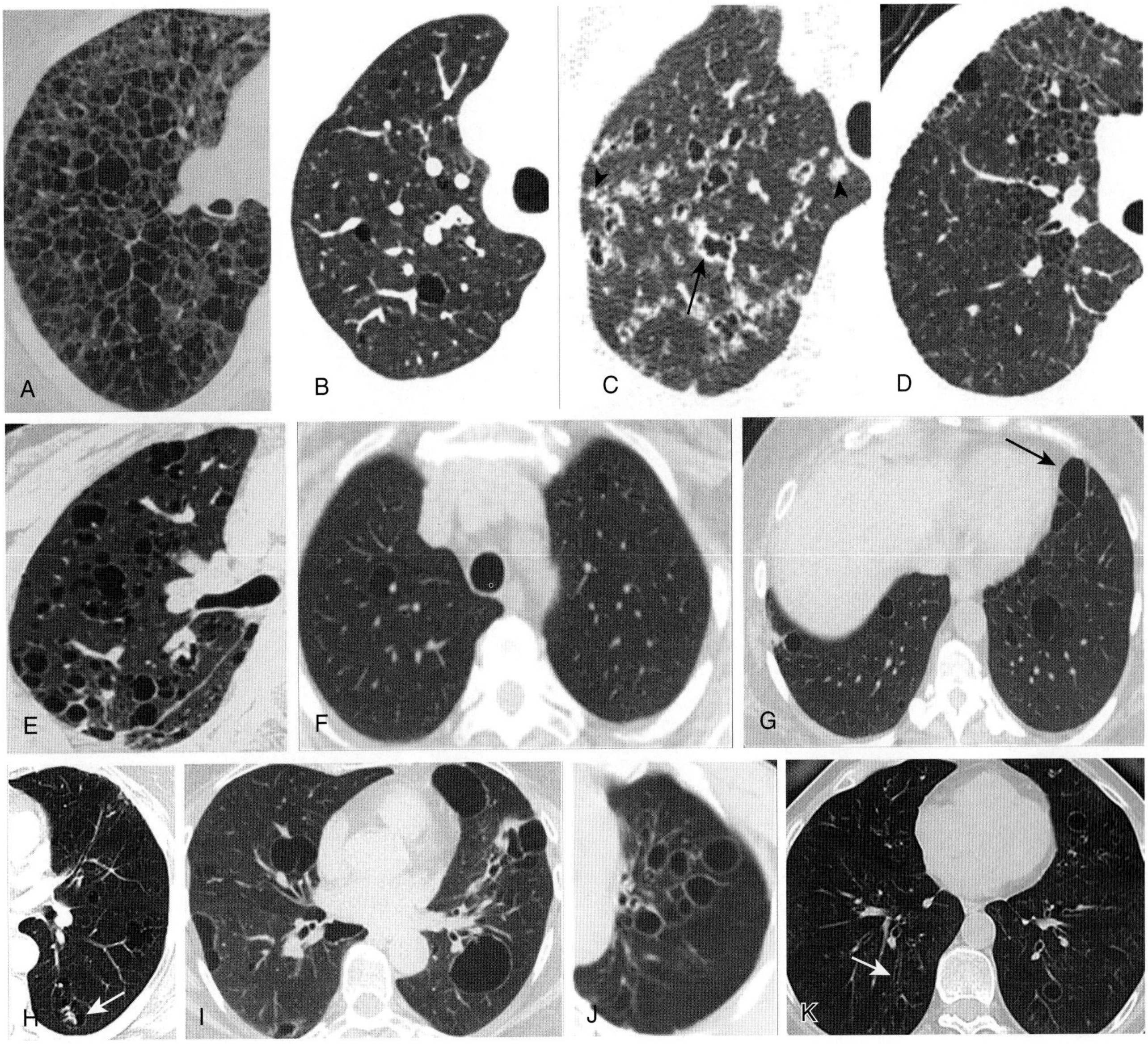

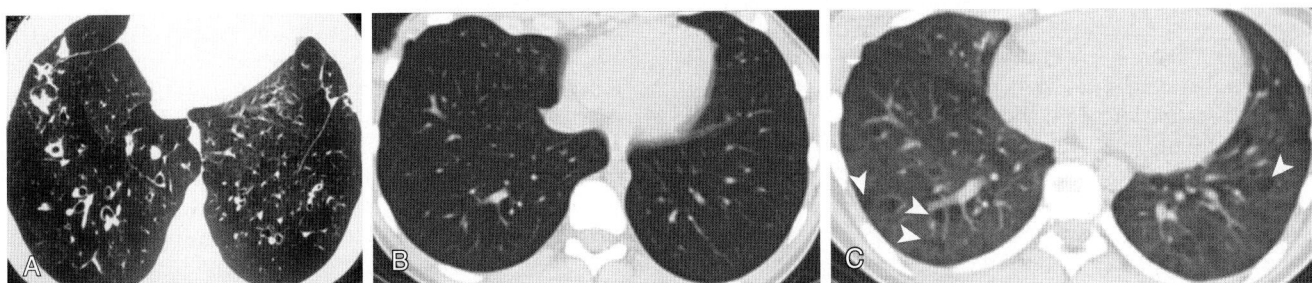

Figure 20.25 *High-resolution computed tomography* **(HRCT) appearances of diffuse cystic pulmonary diseases.** (A–B) Axial HRCT images in two patients with lymphangioleiomyomatosis, one with extensive disease (A) and the other with a paucity of cysts (B), show multiple cystic areas having clearly definable walls, in contrast to the appearance of emphysema. (C) Axial HRCT image in a 19-year-old patient with pulmonary Langerhans cell histiocytosis shows upper lobe irregular (bizarre-shaped), somewhat thick-walled cysts (*arrow*) and small nodules (*arrowheads*). (D) Axial HRCT image in a nonsmoking patient with juvenile rheumatoid arthritis and biopsy-proven follicular bronchiolitis shows uniform, thin-walled cysts in the subpleural regions of lung and more centrally located cysts. (E) Axial HRCT image in a patient with Sjögren syndrome and lymphocytic interstitial pneumonia shows uniform, thin-walled cysts in the midlung. (F–G) Axial HRCT image in a patient with Birt-Hogg-Dubé syndrome shows lower lobe predominant cysts, some with an oblong, septated appearance in a subpleural, paramediastinal location (*arrow*). (H–I) Axial HRCT images in two patients, one with amyloidosis (H) and the other with biopsy-proven pulmonary light chain deposition disease (I), show multiple pulmonary cysts. One cyst in the patient with amyloidosis shows a calcified nodule within the cyst (*arrow*). (J–K) Axial HRCT image in two patients with constrictive bronchiolitis shows multiple thin-walled cysts in addition to large airway thickening (*arrow*) and inhomogeneous lung opacity representing mosaic perfusion due to severe airflow obstruction. (Courtesy Michael B. Gotway, MD.)

Figure 20.26 Mosaic perfusion and lobular gas trapping at *computed tomography* **(CT) imaging.** (A) Axial high-resolution CT image in a patient with cystic fibrosis and mosaic perfusion shows inhomogeneous opacity in the lung bases bilaterally. The areas of decreased attenuation represent mosaic perfusion, in this patient resulting from a combination of regional air trapping due to large airway disease and hypoperfusion in the affected areas of lung. Axial inspiratory (B) and postexpiratory (C) CT images through the lower lungs in a 19-year-old patient with asthma shows relatively normal findings at inspiratory imaging (B) but, at postexpiratory imaging (C), numerous small lobular areas of low attenuation (*arrowheads*) develop, consistent with small airway obstruction. (Courtesy Michael B. Gotway, MD.)

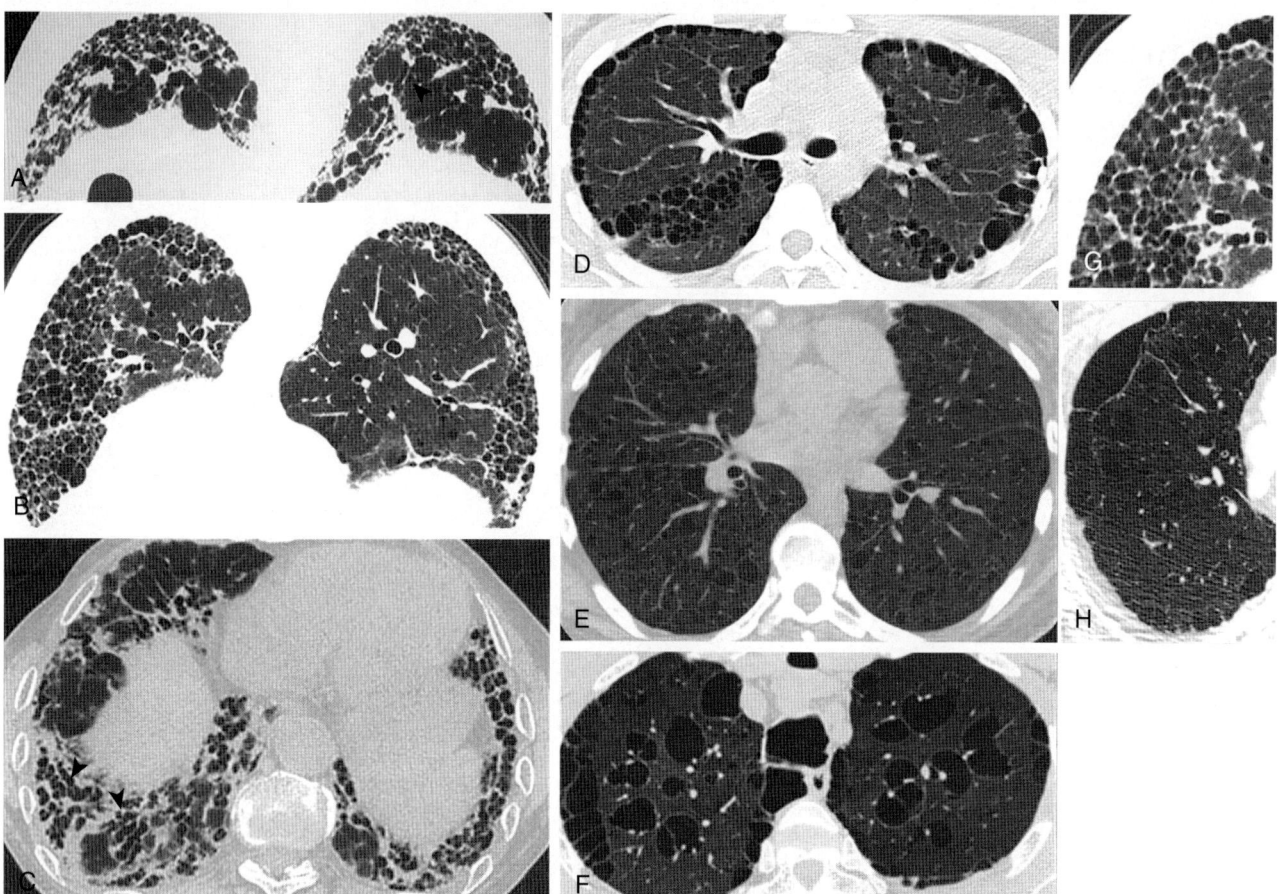

Figure 20.27 *Computed tomography* **(CT) appearance of honeycombing compared with several mimics.** Axial prone (A–B) and supine (C) CT images of honeycombing show subpleural cysts on the order of 1 to 3 mm with relatively thick walls located in the subpleural regions of lung. Note how the cysts appear to share walls and form concentric layers. Of importance, other features of fibrotic lung disease are present, such as traction bronchiectasis (*arrowheads*) and architectural distortion. (D–F), Several mimics of honeycombing. (D) Idiopathic paraseptal emphysema in a nonsmoking 17-year-old woman. Although the cysts are peripheral and even appear to stack upon themselves along the major fissures, they are all uniformly thin-walled and unassociated with other features of fibrotic lung disease. (E) Cystic lung disease due to lymphangioleiomyomatosis. Note lack of fibrotic features and normal-appearing lung intervening between the cysts. The cysts are randomly scattered throughout the lungs and do not predominate in the subpleural regions. (F) Tracheo-bronchomegaly (Mounier-Kuhn disease). Note how some cysts are thin walled, located centrally, along vessels, typical of cystic bronchiectasis. Paraseptal emphysema, forming a single layer of thin-walled cysts unassociated with features suggesting fibrosis, is also present. Detailed images of honeycombing (G) and paraseptal emphysema (H) illustrate the imaging differences between the two findings. Honeycomb cysts (G, prone image near the lung base) tend to be relatively thick-walled and may form stacked layers, whereas paraseptal emphysema cysts (H) are comparatively thin walled and form a single layer in the subpleural regions of lung. Of importance, honeycomb cysts will invariably be accompanied by other features of fibrotic lung disease, such as traction bronchiectasis, intralobular lines, and architectural distortion, whereas isolated paraseptal emphysema is typically unassociated with such findings. (Courtesy Michael B. Gotway, MD.)

ability of CT to detect the presence of lung disease (sensitivity and specificity), characterize its nature, assess disease activity, and guide lung biopsy. It is now widely recognized that CT is integral for the characterization of DILD, assessing disease activity and therapy response, and directing tissue sampling procedures. The evolution of the role CT has assumed in the evaluation of one of the most important DILDs—*usual interstitial pneumonia/idiopathic pulmonary fibrosis* (UIP/IPF)—is reviewed below as an example of how CT imaging has revolutionized DILD assessment.

CT has been widely used for the assessment of fibrotic lung disease, and it had been recognized for a number of years that the CT pattern of lower lobe–predominant honeycombing, in combination with upper lobe linear opacities,[226] is a strong predictor of the pathologic diagnosis of UIP in the proper clinical context. The 2011 ATS, *European Respiratory Society* (ERS), *Japanese Respiratory Society* (JRS), and *Latin American Thoracic Association* (LATA) statement[227] recognized that CT alone can be used to diagnose UIP without the need for tissue sampling by classifying the imaging certainty into one of three levels: definite UIP, possible UIP, and inconsistent with UIP.[227,228] A tissue sampling procedure was recommended only for the latter two patient groups. Compared to the previous clinical practice, the central role CT assumed in the diagnosis of UIP was a new approach[227] and reflected the collective accumulation of knowledge regarding the ability of the CT pattern of basal subpleural–predominant honeycombing, architectural distortion, traction bronchiectasis, and upper lobe reticulation to predict the pathologic presence of UIP.[228] Despite these advancements, a significant number of patients with UIP, particularly patients with CT findings interpreted as possible UIP, were subjected to tissue sampling procedures with the morbidity, mortality, and expense attendant to such procedures. Further

Typical UIP Pattern	Probable UIP Pattern	CT Pattern Indeterminate For UIP	CT Features Most Consistent with Non-IPF Diagnosis

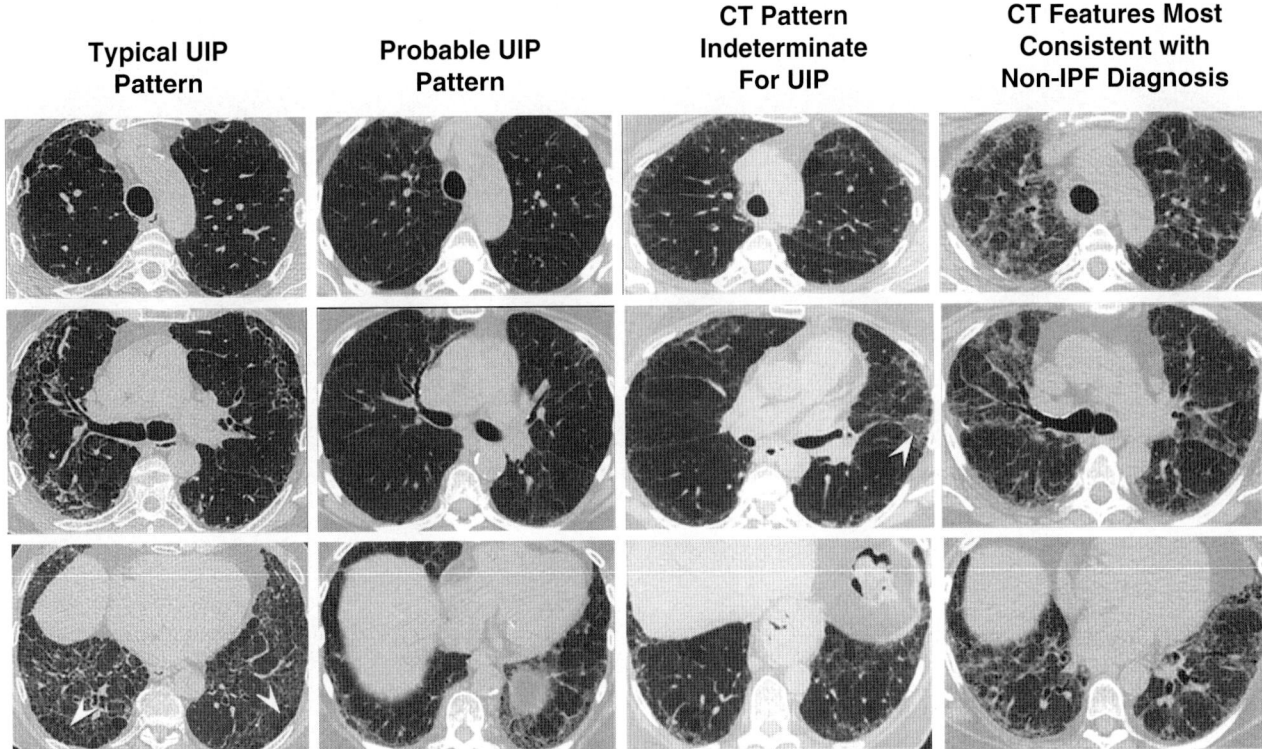

Figure 20.28 Fleischner Society diagnostic categories of usual interstitial pneumonia based on *computed tomography* (CT) patterns. *Typical usual interstitial pneumonia* (UIP) pattern: basal predominant (occasionally diffuse), subpleural and heterogeneous distribution. A reticular pattern with peripheral traction bronchiectasis or bronchiolectasis is present and honeycombing (*arrowheads*) is seen. No features to suggest an alternative diagnosis are present. *Probable UIP pattern:* basal predominant (occasionally diffuse), subpleural and heterogeneous distribution. A reticular pattern with peripheral traction bronchiectasis or bronchiolectasis is present, but honeycombing is absent. No features to suggest an alternative diagnosis are present. *CT pattern indeterminate for UIP:* diffuse or variable distribution. Evidence of fibrosis with some inconspicuous features suggestive of non-UIP pattern. In this example, some peribronchovascular ground-glass opacity extending centrally (*arrowhead*) is present, and there is slight relative basal sparing of the fibrotic findings. Surgical lung biopsy showed pathologic features characteristic of usual interstitial pneumonia. *CT features most consistent with a non–idiopathic pulmonary fibrosis (IPF) diagnosis:* Distributions atypical for usual interstitial pneumonia, such as upper lung or midlung predominant fibrosis or a peribronchovascular predominance with subpleural sparing. Any of the following findings (when they are conspicuous or predominate): consolidation, extensive pure ground-glass opacity (without acute exacerbation), extensive mosaic attenuation with extensive sharply defined lobular air trapping on expiratory CT, diffuse nodules or cysts. In this example, central peribronchovascular ground-glass opacity is present in the upper lobes, and there is basal sparing of the infiltrative lung findings, possibly with some lobular low attenuation suggesting air trapping. Surgical lung biopsy showed features consistent with hypersensitivity pneumonitis.

investigation into patients undergoing evaluation for suspected UIP lead to even greater refinements in CT interpretation; in particular, it has become widely recognized that the reliance on honeycombing to establish the presence of a UIP pattern at CT is both fraught with interobserver variability (see previous discussion regarding honeycombing and Fig. 20.27) and ultimately unnecessary, because honeycombing is a late-stage fibrosis finding, and other features of fibrosis at CT can provide equal predictive value for the pathologic diagnosis of UIP.[228] This realization lead to additional refinements in the interpretation of CT for suspected UIP/IPF, now classifying the imaging certainty into one of four levels[229,230] (Fig. 20.28): (1) typical UIP pattern, (2) probable UIP pattern, (3) CT pattern indeterminate for UIP, and (4) CT features most consistent with a non-IPF diagnosis.

These refinements have allowed tissue sampling procedures to be avoided for the first two categories—the typical UIP pattern and the probable UIP pattern—because it has been recognized that both of these CT patterns predict the pathologic diagnosis of UIP.[228,229] Although tissue sampling is still considered by some for patients with the probable UIP pattern in the proper clinical context,[230] tissue sampling is not mandatory for every patient that fits this category.[231] Furthermore, the fourth CT category of features most consistent with a non-IPF diagnosis may indicate an alternative non-IPF diagnosis and thereby direct management in an entirely different direction. This latest refinement in the CT approach to the diagnosis of UIP has significantly narrowed the number of patients with imaging that falls into the "uncertain" category (pattern indeterminate for UIP).

In addition to refining the clinical approach to the diagnosis of patients with suspected IPF, certain CT imaging findings have been shown to be important prognostic biomarkers for patients with fibrotic lung disease. In particular, the presence and severity of traction bronchiectasis[228,229] and honeycombing[228,229] have been shown to correlate with a poor prognosis in patients with IPF, and honeycombing has been further shown to be associated with a high mortality across a diverse set of non-IPF ILDs.[232] This observation suggests that the CT finding of honeycombing represents a progressive fibrotic ILD phenotype regardless of the underlying diagnosis.[232]

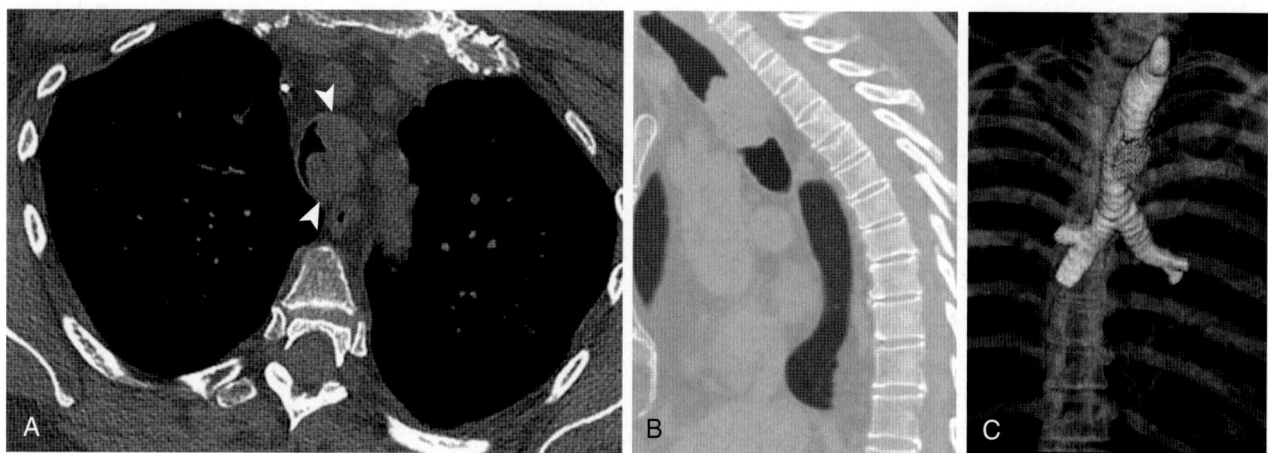

Figure 20.29 Utility of *computed tomography* (CT) for central airway lesions. (A) Axial unenhanced CT image shows a lobulated, noncalcified mass (*arrowheads*) arising from the left aspect of the trachea compromising a substantial portion of the tracheal lumen. (B) Sagittal reformatted image shows the lobulated morphology and full cephalocaudad extent of the lesion. (C) Coronal oblique volume-rendered image highlights the relationship of the lesion to the entire extent of the trachea in a single image. The diagnosis was tracheal MALT lymphoma. (Courtesy Michael B. Gotway, MD.)

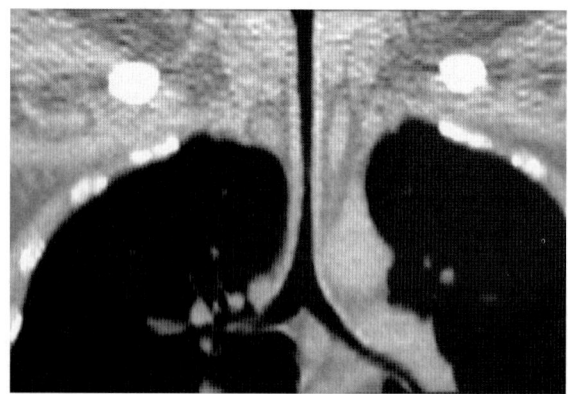

Figure 20.30 Multislice *computed tomography* (CT) for central airway evaluation. With rapid volumetric high-resolution imaging, multislice CT allows detailed three-dimensional analysis of the airways. In a patient with relapsing polychondritis, coronally reconstructed image shows diffuse thickening and narrowing of the trachea. (Courtesy Michael B. Gotway, MD.)

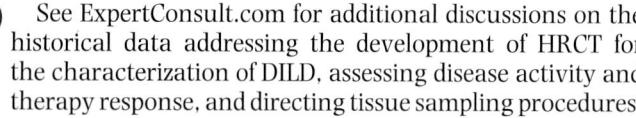 See ExpertConsult.com for additional discussions on the historical data addressing the development of HRCT for the characterization of DILD, assessing disease activity and therapy response, and directing tissue sampling procedures.

INTRATHORACIC AIRWAY DISEASE

With the development of MSCT, volumetric HRCT is now routinely performed for dedicated CT assessment of the large airways, which allows simultaneously optimized evaluation of the central airways combined with HRCT technique for evaluation of the peripheral airways in a single examination.

Central Airways

CT can effectively evaluate lesions of the trachea (Fig. 20.29) and central airways,[261] including strictures and stenoses, inflammatory diseases such as polychondritis (Fig. 20.30), some cases of extrinsic versus intrinsic obstruction,[262] aspirated foreign objects, tracheobronchomalacia (see Chapter 71), and neoplasms (Video 20.11).[261] MSCT, with its ability to acquire images rapidly with equal resolution in all planes,

is particularly useful in this assessment and can provide detailed three-dimensional analysis of the central airways (see Video 20.11B). The ability to produce excellent quality three-dimensional images aids in the evaluation of subtle airway stenoses and complex airway lesions, particularly when they are oblique with respect to the imaging plane. In the assessment of tracheal and central bronchial neoplasms, CT does not substitute for bronchoscopy and biopsy, but it can be useful to determine the extent of invasion and to direct the bronchoscopist to a particular segment or to a precise location of peribronchial disease. The major value of CT imaging is its ability to visualize the luminal contents, the airway wall, and the surrounding soft tissue. Thus, CT has the most value in circumstances that require all three of these capabilities.

Bronchiectasis

CT should be the initial investigation in all patients with suspected bronchiectasis, as discussed further in Chapter 69.[263–266] The sensitivity and specificity of HRCT for diagnosing bronchiectasis to the segmental level are 95–98% (Fig. 20.31), which is superior to thicker-section CT scans. In current medical practice, CT has replaced bronchography, and a review of the CT criteria for diagnosing bronchiectasis and the technical pitfalls that may be encountered has been published.[267] Volumetric CT scanning with narrow collimation (on the order of 1 mm) provides a larger volume of coverage and the creation of exquisite reformatted images, including volume rendering, and is now the reference standard for the diagnosis of bronchiectasis. Although there are numerous causes of bronchiectasis, certain imaging features of bronchiectasis at CT, particularly the distribution of the airway abnormalities, may suggest a specific etiology for bronchiectasis in a number of patients (eFig. 20.52, also see Fig. 69.5).[268]

Small Airway Disease

HRCT has the ability to demonstrate abnormalities of small airways having a diameter of a few millimeters or less.*

---

*References 163, 193, 199, 201, 221, 223, 224, 246, 269.

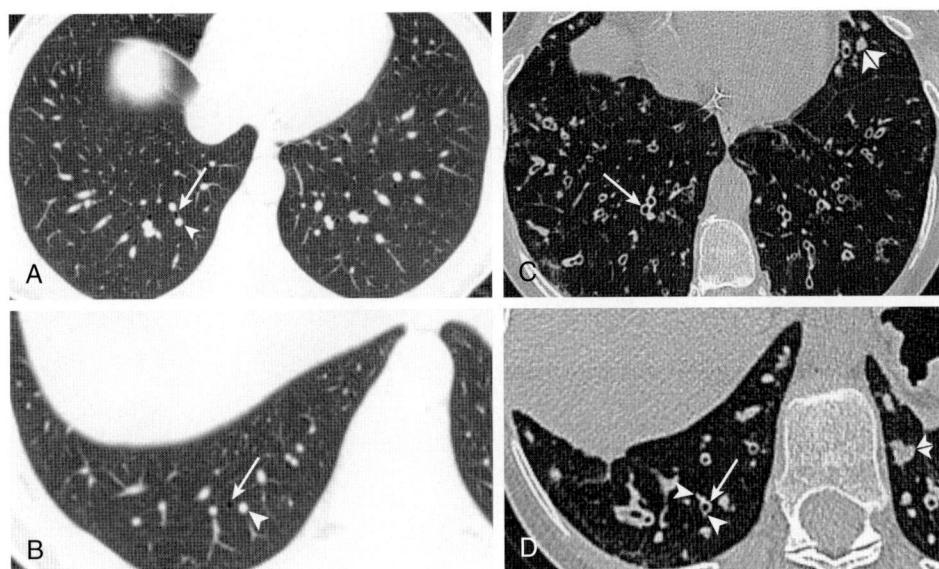

Figure 20.31 Normal appearance of bronchi at chest *computed tomography* (CT) compared with bronchiectasis. (A–B) Axial chest CT images show the appearance of normal peripheral bronchi; the internal diameter of the bronchus (*arrows*) is similar to the adjacent pulmonary artery (*arrowheads*), and the bronchi are patent and uniformly thin walled. (C–D) Detailed images through the lung bases showing CT features of bronchiectasis and large airway disease. The bronchi are abnormally dilated—the internal diameter of the bronchi (*arrows*) clearly exceeds the size of the adjacent pulmonary arteries (*single arrowheads*). The bronchi are also clearly visualized more peripherally than is normal (compare with images A and B, where peripheral bronchi are largely not visible). Finally, the bronchi (*arrows*) are visibly thick walled, and several airways show intraluminal secretions and impaction (*double arrowheads*). (Courtesy Michael B. Gotway, MD.)

Abnormalities that can be diagnosed include (1) inflammatory forms of bronchiolitis, such as cellular bronchiolitis (usually due to infection [Fig. 20.32A], aspiration, or hypersensitivity pneumonitis [see Figs. 20.23 and 20.32B]), respiratory bronchiolitis (see Fig. 20.32C), follicular bronchiolitis, and panbronchiolitis (see Fig. 20.32D), and (2) small airway diseases associated with airflow obstruction (e.g., constrictive bronchiolitis; see Fig. 20.32E–F).[269] (Cryptogenic organizing pneumonia has been previously classified as a disease of the small airways but is now considered an idiopathic interstitial pneumonia.[163,246,269]) The use of postexpiratory HRCT is particularly important in the diagnosis of small airway diseases because air trapping may be visible in the absence of other abnormalities (see Fig. 20.26B–C and eFig. 140.3).[223,224] Postexpiratory HRCT may be performed by imaging after a forced vital capacity maneuver (Video 20.12, see Videos 140.1 and 140.3)[270] or with lateral decubitus CT.[271] Compared to CT performed at a single time point, a cine CT performed during a forced vital capacity maneuver, called dynamic expiratory CT, is a more effective technique for the demonstration of subtle or transient air trapping.[270,272,273]

CARDIOVASCULAR DISEASE

Pulmonary Thromboembolism

Chest MSCT, performed with IV contrast injection using a specific *CT pulmonary angiography* (CTPA) technique, has emerged as the test of choice for the imaging evaluation of suspected *pulmonary embolism* (PE) (Fig. 20.33A, Video 20.13). Ventilation-perfusion scanning has long been used as the initial test for such patients. Its strengths and its limitations are well known and reviewed in Chapters 81 and 82. The test is extremely safe, widely available, and exceedingly sensitive; a normal perfusion scan effectively excludes PE. A high-probability scan is quite specific (97% in the *Prospective Investigation of Pulmonary Embolism Diagnosis* [PIOPED] I study).[274] However, a substantial fraction of perfusion scans yield results that are abnormal but nonspecific, which has contributed to the widespread adoption of CTPA as the first-line test for suspected thromboembolic disease.

The evolution of the adoption of CTPA for the assessment of suspected thromboembolic disease is complex and punctuated by major developments in CT technology. The brief discussion that follows focuses on several specific issues related to the use of CTPA for thromboembolic disease assessment: the negative predictive value of CTPA and the risk of "overdiagnosis" of PE at CTPA.

See ExpertConsult.com for additional discussions on the historical evolution of CTPA from single-slice CTPA to the MSCT era.

Ultimately, the main question when patients suspected of thromboembolic disease undergo CTPA is, "Can anticoagulation be safely withheld in patients with a negative result?" In other words, what is the negative predictive value of CTPA for thromboembolic disease? Several studies have addressed this question, and the negative predictive value of CTPA ranges from 95–99%.[275,276] Of importance, it has been suggested that further diagnostic testing should be pursued when CTPA results (with or without indirect CT venography, see later) are discordant with the clinical probability for PE, particularly when CTPA results are negative and the clinical probability of PE is considered high.[275]

The development of MSCT technology allowed the routine use of narrow detector configurations, resulting in improved visualization of small pulmonary arteries that were largely unapparent with single-slice CT. Although this improved resolution was initially heralded as an advance,

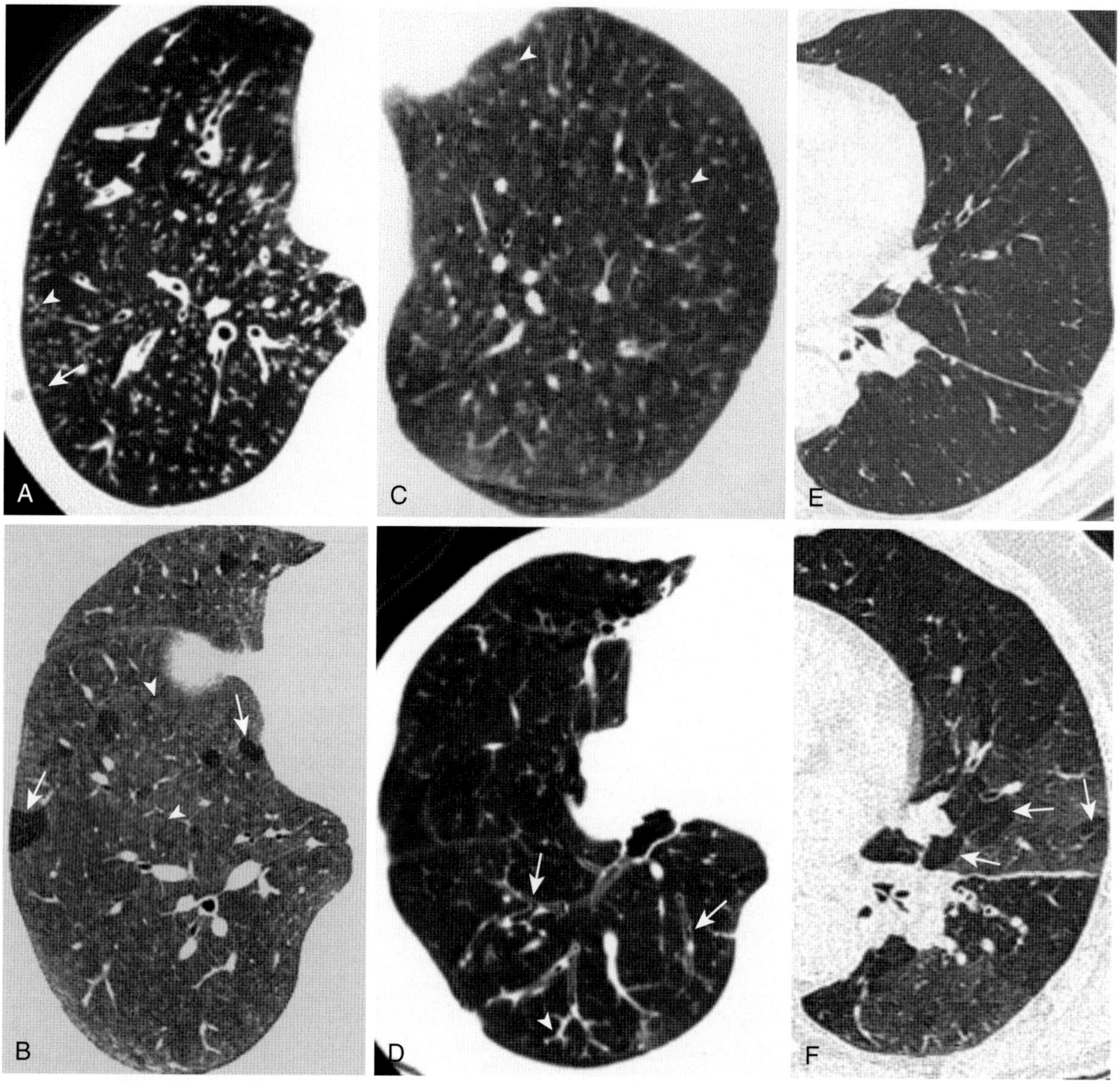

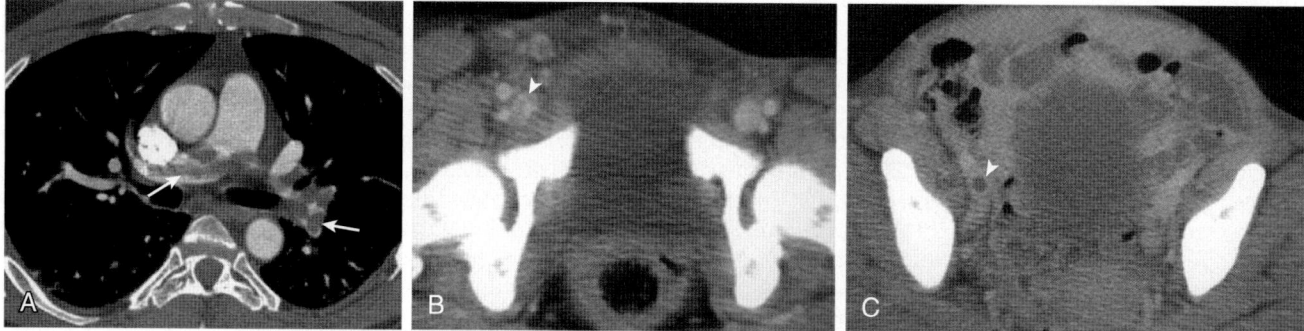

Figure 20.32 *High-resolution computed tomography* **(HRCT) manifestations of small airway disease.**   (A) Bronchopneumonia and bronchiolitis. Axial chest CT image through the right lower lobe shows numerous small, solid centrilobular nodules (*arrow*), some with branching configurations (*arrowhead*), the latter consistent with tree-in-bud opacity, representing bronchiolar impaction. (B) Cellular bronchiolitis in hypersensitivity pneumonitis. Axial chest CT image through the right lower lobe shows poorly defined ground-glass opacity centrilobular nodules (*arrowhead*). Areas of lobular low attenuation (*arrows*), representing air trapping resulting from inflammatory bronchiolitis, are present. (C) Respiratory bronchiolitis. Axial chest CT image through the left upper lobe shows faintly detectable ground-glass attenuation nodules (*arrowheads*). (D) Panbronchiolitis. Axial chest CT image through the right lower lobe shows large airway thickening and dilation (*arrows*), associated with intraluminal material and small airway impaction (*arrowhead*). (E–F) Constrictive bronchiolitis (bronchiolitis obliterans). Axial chest CT image through the left lung shows normal inspiratory scan findings (E). Postexpiratory imaging (F) shows the development of numerous areas of low attenuation consistent with air trapping, in some areas with a lobular configuration (*arrows*) due to small airway obstruction. (Courtesy Michael B. Gotway, MD.)

Figure 20.33 *Computed tomography pulmonary angiography* **(CTPA) and indirect CT venography images demonstrate pulmonary emboli and deep vein thrombosis.**   (A) CTPA image shows bilateral large filling defects (*arrows*) consistent with pulmonary emboli. (B–C) Axial indirect CT venography image (i.e., without additional contrast material injection) shows filling defects in the right common femoral and iliac veins (*arrowheads*) consistent with venous thrombi. (Courtesy Michael B. Gotway, MD.)

thereby mitigating concerns regarding insufficient sensitivity of CTPA for the diagnosis of thromboembolic disease, concerns regarding the "overdiagnosis" of pulmonary emboli soon followed. The term overdiagnosis can be interpreted to encompass two entities. On the one hand, CTPA examinations can be incorrectly interpreted as positive for pulmonary emboli, largely because of various artifacts at CT, including motion artifacts, noise, and volume averaging causing suboptimal pulmonary arterial enhancement simulating intraluminal filling defects, among others.[277] On the other hand, and possibly more important, CTPA may lead to increased detection of small, isolated subsegmental PE of uncertain clinical significance.[278] Indeed, a meta-analysis showed that that the rate of isolated subsegmental PE was twice as high for MSCT-CTPA (9.4%) compared to single-slice CT (4.7%), and there was no clear difference in the 3-month incidence of venous thromboembolism between untreated patients with negative results by single-slice CT versus MSCT.[279] Data indicating that PE-related mortality changed only minimally after the widespread adoption of CTPA for PE diagnosis (1998–2006); yet the incidence of PE increased dramatically (81%) during this time period compared with the pre–MSCT-CTPA era (2003–08),[280] which furthered this concern. Complications related to anticoagulation treatment for PE also increased in the later time period, as may be expected given the rise in number of PE diagnoses, suggesting that the possibility of overdiagnosis is not an innocuous one.[280] The conundrum of PE overdiagnosis may be multifactorial, including possible relative inexperience with the intricacies of thoracic anatomy and PE diagnosis on the part of some radiologists compared with dedicated thoracic imaging experts, overinterpretation of technically inadequate studies, and incompletely evaluated patients or frankly inappropriately ordered CTPA examinations, potentially stemming from lack of guideline adherence and from inappropriate pretest risk stratification.

However, perhaps most important among these potential causes for PE overdiagnosis is the problem of the isolated subsegmental PE.[277] Note that the term *isolated subsegmental PE* often refers to the potential identification of a single pulmonary embolus on a study that results in a positive interpretation, a situation perhaps better referred to as solitary PE,[277] but others have used this term to denote PE in the absence of deep venous thrombosis.[281] A solitary pulmonary embolus, particularly when small (distal segmental or subsegmental), is recognized as having significant potential for contributing to PE overdiagnosis because this finding is subject to significant interobserver variability (eFig. 20.53), even among experienced thoracic radiologists.[277,281] Therefore, to mitigate the potential for PE overdiagnosis, a number of measures may be undertaken[277,282]:

1. Appropriate pretest risk stratification should be used before CTPA examinations are ordered.
2. CTPA examinations should be conducted using optimized technique, and radiology reports should provide some indication of study quality. When a remark regarding study quality is lacking, it is advisable for referring clinicians to speak with the interpreting radiologist regarding their confidence in the examination interpretation, particularly when the study is rendered positive due to a solitary PE or the pretest probability is discordant with the CT interpretation.
3. When the patient's pretest probability for PE is discordant with the CTPA results, or the CTPA study is rendered positive due to a solitary PE, obtaining a second interpretation by either a dedicated thoracic radiologist, or at least a different experienced observer, is appropriate.
4. Lower extremity ultrasound examination for a potential deep venous source for thromboembolism, or an alternative study for PE, such as ventilation-perfusion scintigraphy (eFig. 20.54), may be pursued in difficult, indeterminate cases.

Various investigations also suggest that CTPA may also be able to detect deep venous thrombosis in the proximal leg and pelvic veins without injection of additional contrast material (see Fig. 20.33), a technique known as indirect CT venography.[283–285] The addition of CT venography to CTPA studies obtained for the evaluation of suspected PE allows for the simultaneous evaluation of deep venous thrombosis and PE with a single test. Combining CTPA with CT venography increased the sensitivity for the diagnosis of PE to 90%, and the negative predictive value of the combination of the examinations was 97% in the PIOPED II trial.[275] Despite these encouraging data and the appeal of a single test capable of addressing both PE and deep venous thrombosis simultaneously, indirect CT venography is not widely used, and lower extremity venous thrombosis is typically assessed with lower extremity venous ultrasound in most centers.

As for CTPA, MRI can demonstrate PE directly as intravascular filling defects on cross-sectional images (Fig. 20.34, Video 20.14).[286–298] Experience with MRI in patients suspected of having PE is more limited than that with CTPA. The two techniques are probably overall roughly similar in accuracy for the detection of PE, although MRI may show more pronounced interobserver variability than CTPA and may show slightly decreased sensitivity compared with CTPA at the segmental and subsegmental vascular levels.[296,299] The diagnostic accuracy of MRI for PE assessment is enhanced through the use of multiparametric protocols that include a combination of real-time steady-state free precession imaging (noncontrast white-blood imaging), perfusion imaging, low flip angle, three-dimensional gradient-echo imaging (a contrast-enhanced technique that allows better visualization of the vessel wall compared with MRA), and contrast-enhanced MRA (see Video 20.14)[286,287,290,293,294,300]; not all studies reporting the diagnostic accuracy of MRI for acute PE diagnosis have used a multiparametric approach.[296] In addition, MRI has been shown to be highly accurate for detecting deep venous thrombosis.[301,302]

The potential advantages of MRI are the lack of need for iodinated contrast material or ionizing radiation, ability to image the pulmonary arteries and deep venous system in a single examination, ability to assess right ventricular function simultaneously, and ability to perform perfusion imaging. The latter point is of particular significance in light of the

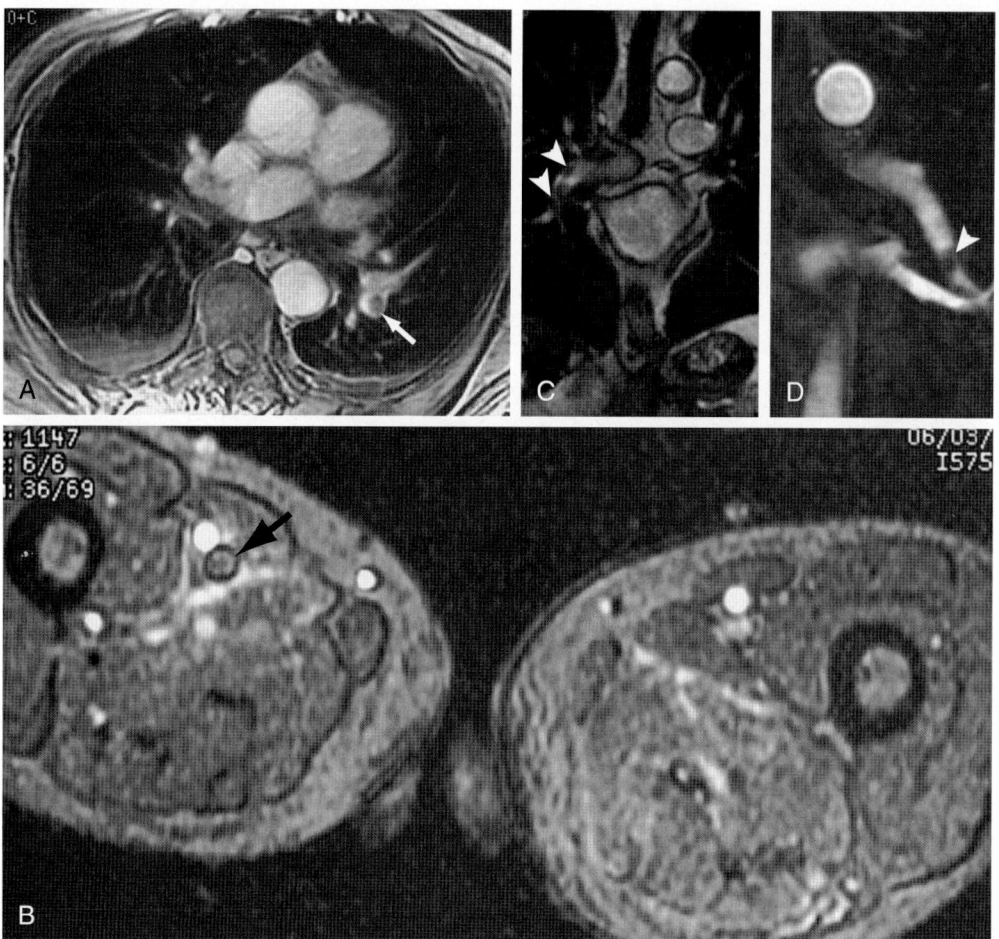

Figure 20.34 Multiparametric *magnetic resonance imaging* (MRI) demonstrating pulmonary embolism and deep vein thrombosis. (A) Contrast-enhanced fast gradient recalled-echo MRI shows a filling defect consistent with pulmonary embolus in the left lower lobe artery (*arrow*). (B) This MRI made without intravenous contrast material shows a filling defect in the right superficial femoral vein consistent with venous thrombus (*arrow*), whereas the contralateral vein is patent and without filling defects. (C) Coronal steady-state free precession image in a different patient, performed without the use of intravenous contrast, shows an intraluminal filling defect within the right interlobar and lower lobe arteries (*arrowheads*), consistent with pulmonary embolism. (D) Coronal MR angiography examination of a third patient shows a low-signal filling defect in the left lower lobe pulmonary artery (*arrowhead*) consistent with pulmonary embolism (Courtesy Michael B. Gotway, MD.)

imperfect sensitivity of CTPA. The advantages of CTPA are higher spatial resolution, wider availability, fewer artifacts, faster examination time, and simpler, more robust technology, as well as, of importance, the generation of alternative diagnoses for patients with negative results. Currently, CTPA is a realistic option in the clinical management of patients with suspected PE. The clinical use of MRI has been traditionally limited to medical centers with personnel who are highly skilled with advanced MRI technology, in part a result of the PIOPED III[296] experience; however, the data from PIOPED III[296] were limited to gadolinium-enhanced MRA only and did not use a multiparametric approach. Furthermore, MR technology has advanced significantly since the publication of PIOPED III,[300] and MRI has been successfully used for the assessment of suspected thromboembolic disease in some academic centers.[300]

See ExpertConsult.com for additional discussions on imaging acquired cardiovascular diseases and congenital anomalies of the thoracic great vessels.

PLEURAL DISEASE

Many pleural processes, as discussed further in Chapters 108 to 114, can be imaged accurately and cost-effectively with conventional radiography or ultrasonography. However, CT can be useful in evaluating several clinical problems relating to the pleura.[104,315,316] These include differentiation of pleural and parenchymal disease, including the distinction between lung abscess and empyema; detection of subtle pleural abnormalities, such as early pleural plaques or small pneumothoraces; location of pleural fluid collections and pleural tumors, including localization for interventional purposes (e.g., tube drainage, biopsy); determination of the extent of pleural tumors, in particular, metastases and mesothelioma; and on occasion, characterization of pleural lesions (Figs. 20.35 and 20.36, see Fig. 20.8) or paradiaphragmatic lesions. MRI currently has a limited role in the evaluation of pleural abnormalities, in general, but has been shown to be useful for assessment of malignant pleural mesothelioma.

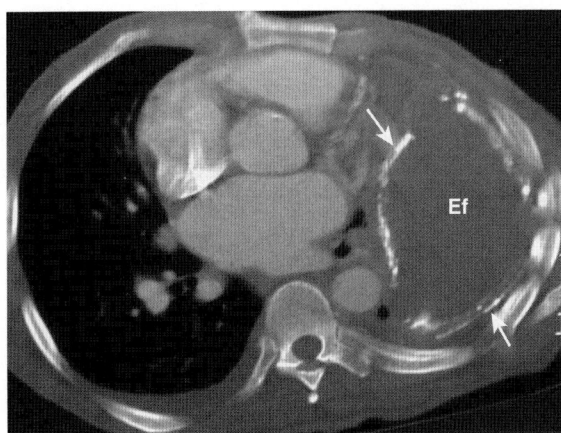

Figure 20.35 Chest *computed tomography* (CT) for pleural disease. Chest CT performed in a patient with a history of tuberculosis shows pleural thickening and calcification (*arrows*) and a residual pleural effusion (Ef) indicative of empyema. (Courtesy Michael B. Gotway, MD.)

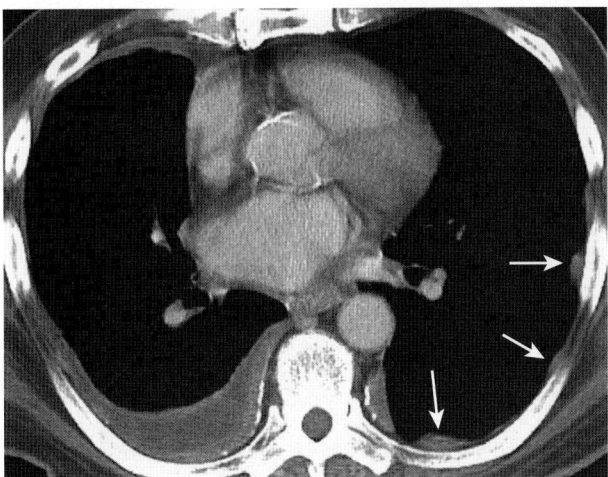

Figure 20.36 Chest computed tomography for pleural disease. A patient with prior asbestos exposure has focal areas of pleural thickening or pleural plaques within the left hemithorax (*arrows*). Pleural thickening on the right is associated with pleural effusion. This reflected the presence of early malignant mesothelioma. (Courtesy Michael B. Gotway, MD.)

Type of Fluid

Most effusions have an attenuation near to that of water; in accordance, CT numbers cannot be used to predict the specific gravity of the fluid or its cause. Exceptions include (1) acute or subacute hemothorax, which can sometimes appear inhomogeneous in attenuation, with some areas having an attenuation value higher than that of water, and (2) chylothorax, which can sometimes appear decreased in attenuation relative to water due to high fat/triglyceride content.

The presence of pleural thickening is often of value in predicting the nature of the effusion. In patients with effusion (see Chapter 108), the presence of pleural thickening on CT strongly suggests that the effusion is an exudate.[104] By definition, the pleura is considered thickened if it is visible on a contrast-enhanced or unenhanced CT. Transudative causes of pleural effusion typically do not produce pleural thickening. Conversely, the absence of pleural thickening on contrast-enhanced CT is less helpful. In this situation, the effusion can be an exudate or transudate. Only about 60% of exudates are associated with visible pleural thickening. However, the absence of pleural thickening on a contrast-enhanced scan rules out empyema; empyema is always associated with parietal pleural thickening on contrast-enhanced CT.

Pleural Versus Parenchymal Disease

Opacities detected at chest radiography can frequently be localized as either parenchymal or extraparenchymal (pleural or chest wall) in location. Chest radiographic features that favor a parenchymal location for a pulmonary opacity include a relative rounded contour, relatively acute angles between the opacity and the chest wall (Fig. 20.37, see (Figs. 50.1 to 50.6), and air-fluid levels (when present) relatively similar in length in both frontal and lateral projections (Fig. 20.38). In contrast, opacities that are extraparenchymal in location often show an elliptical or lenticular contour; the opacity forms obtuse angles at the point of contact with the chest wall (see Figs. 20.37A and 38), and air-fluid levels commonly show significantly different lengths in the frontal and lateral projections (see Fig. 20.38). However, on occasion, chest radiography may not be able to distinguish between parenchymal disease, pleural disease, and pathology affecting both compartments. CT can be useful in this setting. Pleural lesions typically have obtuse tapering margins and sharp interfaces with adjacent lung parenchyma (see Fig. 20.37 and eFig. 50.7B–E), whereas parenchymal lesions tend to blend with lung parenchyma and have acute, irregular margins (see Figs. 20.37 and 20.38, see eFigs. 50.4B–E, 50.13A, and 50.26A). One of the more common and therapeutically important problems in this category is differentiating lung abscess from empyema. Empyemas typically have smooth outer and inner margins, a lenticular shape (see Figs. 20.37 and 20.38), and a sharp interface with underlying lung; they tend to displace pulmonary vessels around them (see eFig. 50.7B–E) and often display prominent rim enhancement (the "split pleura sign") after IV administration of iodinated contrast material. Lung abscesses are characterized by spherical or polygonal shape, a thick wall with a shaggy or irregular inner margin, and destruction, not displacement, of adjacent structures (see Figs. 20.37 and 20.38). None of these features is unique but, when considered together, they permit categorization of the abnormality in most cases.

Early Detection

The contrast resolution and cross-sectional format of CT make it highly sensitive and accurate in detecting pleural thickening and early pleural plaques in patients with asbestos-related pleural disease (see Fig. 20.36).[168,316] Circumscribed plaques often are overlooked on chest radiographs unless they are calcified or attain a thickness of about 5 mm or more. Furthermore, normal extrapleural soft tissues and fat can be misinterpreted as plaques when they are prominent on chest radiography.

CT has also been shown to be accurate and more sensitive than conventional radiographs in detecting pneumothoraces. This can be of particular importance in trauma patients, who may require intubation and positive-pressure ventilation.

See ExpertConsult.com for a discussion of recent advancements and future directions.

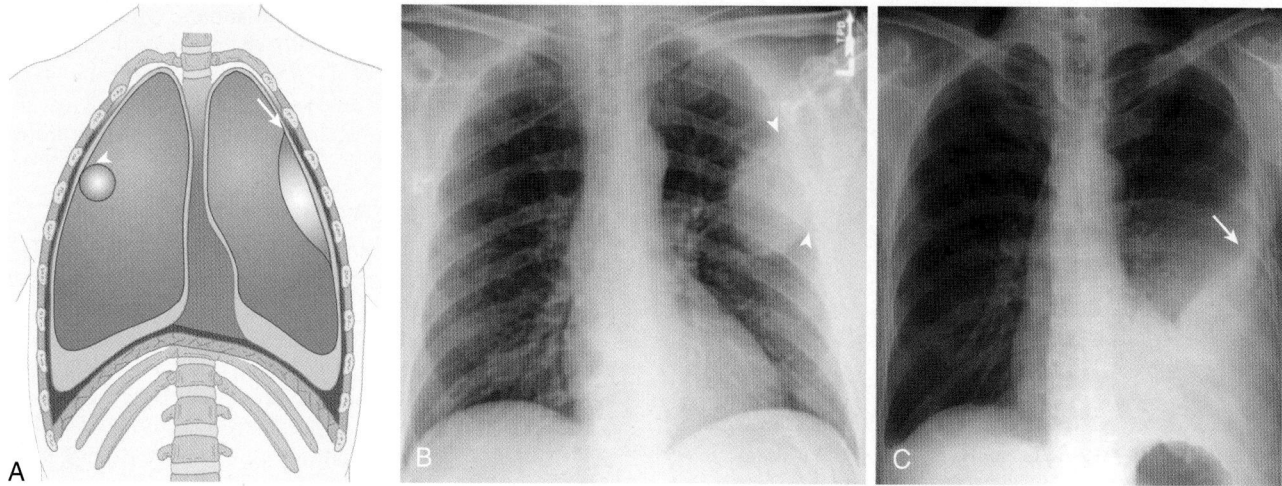

Figure 20.37 Chest radiographic localization of an opacity as parenchymal or extraparenchymal: angle of the opacity with the chest wall. (A) Illustration showing the typically *acute* angles (*arrowhead*) formed by a parenchymal process, such as a lung abscess, with the chest wall, compared with the *obtuse* angles (*arrow*) usually formed with the adjacent chest wall by an *extraparenchymal* process, such as empyema. (B) Frontal chest radiograph in a patient with a lung abscess shows the typically *acute* angles (*arrowheads*) formed with the chest wall by a *parenchymal* process. (C) Frontal chest radiograph in a patient with empyema shows the usual *obtuse* angles (*arrow*) formed with the chest wall by an *extraparenchymal* process. (B–C, Courtesy Michael B. Gotway, MD.)

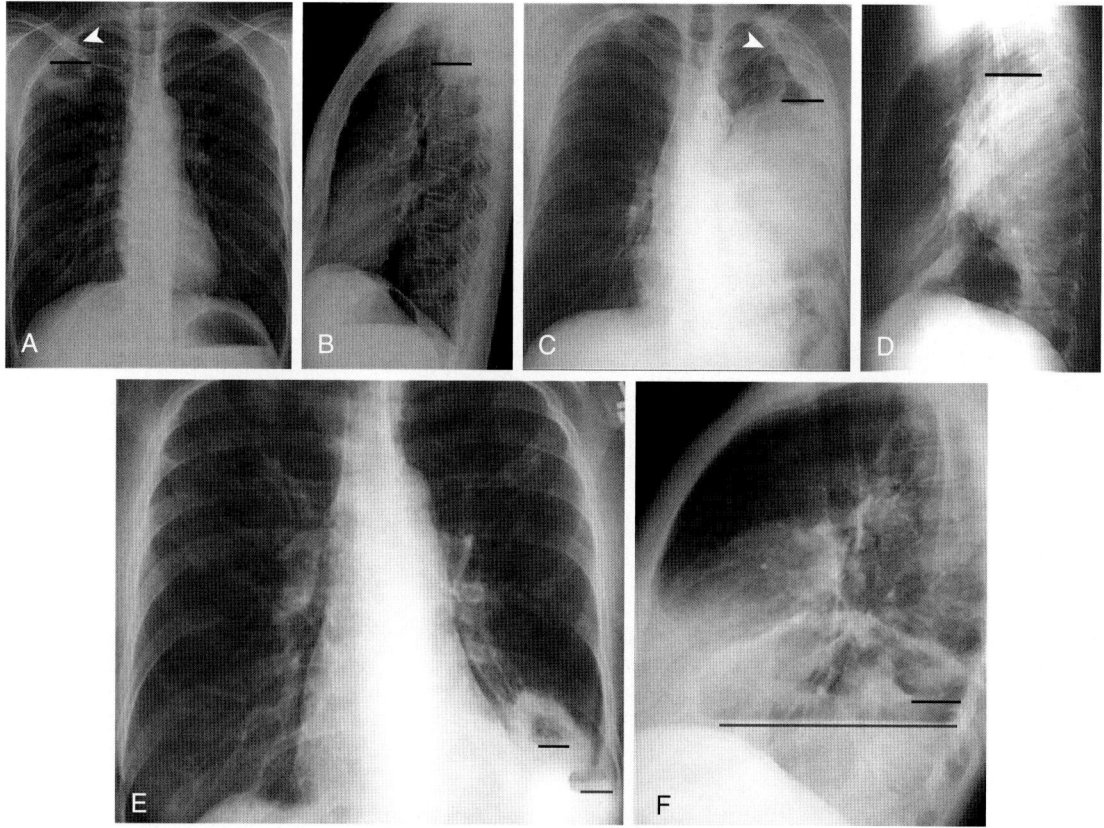

Figure 20.38 Chest radiographic localization of an opacity as parenchymal or extraparenchymal: differential air-fluid length. (A) Frontal and (B) lateral chest radiograph in a patient with lung abscess (same patient as Fig. 50.1) shows an opacity with an air-fluid level (*line*) that is roughly the same length in both projections. The typical acute angle formed by the parenchymal process with the chest wall (*arrowhead*) is evident. (C) Frontal and (D) lateral chest radiograph in a patient with empyema shows an opacity creating the obtuse angles with the chest wall characteristic of an extraparenchymal process (*arrowhead*). An air-fluid level is present (*line*) and shows a different length in both projections, which suggests extraparenchymal localization of the process. (E) Frontal and (F) lateral chest radiograph in a patient with lung abscess creating a bronchopleural fistula shows an opacity with an air-fluid level (*black line*) of roughly the same length in both projections, representing a lung abscess. Another process with air-fluid levels that differ in length markedly between the frontal (E) and lateral (F) projections (*red line*) represents empyema. (Courtesy Michael B. Gotway, MD.)

Key Points

- After the medical history and physical examination, radiography is the most commonly used technique in the evaluation of patients with known or suspected thoracic disease.
- High-quality frontal and lateral chest radiographs can address many clinical questions. Currently available techniques of digital recording of images offer many interpretive and logistical advantages.
- Helical (or spiral) *computed tomography* (CT) technology allows the entire chest to be scanned during a single breath-hold, thereby permitting volumetric imaging, which generates a continuous block of data (rather than slices) that can be reconstructed to produce images in different slice thicknesses or orientations. Multislice CT uses multiple channels during the helical acquisition, thereby dramatically increasing the amount of data acquired and the speed of acquisition.
- Multislice CT, with its rapid acquisition time and greatly improved resolution, has become the imaging method of choice for further evaluation of pulmonary nodule(s), lung cancer, mediastinal abnormalities, diffuse lung diseases, airway diseases, and suspected pulmonary embolism.
- *High-resolution CT* (HRCT) is a technique combining narrow collimation/thin-slice thickness (1 mm) and image reconstruction using a high-spatial-frequency algorithm to maximize sharpness in the final image. HRCT is best suited for analysis of the lung parenchyma in patients with diffuse lung diseases, where its findings are based on the anatomy of the secondary pulmonary lobule. HRCT findings relevant to lung disease can be broadly divided into *increased opacity*, including nodule, linear, and reticular opacities; ground-glass opacity and consolidation; and *decreased lung opacity*, including cysts, cavities, emphysema, and mosaic perfusion.
- Small nodules can be classified as perilymphatic, random, or centrilobular at HRCT, according to their distribution in the secondary pulmonary lobule. Recognition of the distribution is fundamental for generating differential diagnoses of lung disease.
- Radiation is a relatively weak carcinogen, and the risk for radiation-induced carcinogenesis from a CT scan is generally more than offset by the benefits of the information gained from an appropriately indicated study.
- Magnetic resonance imaging is useful in evaluating superior sulcus lesions, brachial plexopathy, and certain cardiac and mediastinal abnormalities. It is also useful, although less often used than multislice CT, for evaluating suspected aortic dissection and pulmonary embolism.

Key Readings

Colby TV, Swensen SJ. Anatomic distribution and histopathologic patterns in diffuse lung disease: correlation with HRCT. *J Thorac Imaging.* 1996;11(1):1–26.

Cronin P, Dwamena BA, Kelly AM, et al. Solitary pulmonary nodules and masses: a meta-analysis of the diagnostic utility of alternative imaging tests. *Eur Radiol.* 2008;18(9):1840–1856.

Gotway MB, Reddy GP, Webb WR, et al. High-resolution CT of the lung: patterns of disease and differential diagnoses. *Radiol Clin North Am.* 2005;43(3):513–542.

Hansell DM. Classification of diffuse lung diseases: why and how. *Radiology.* 2013;268(3):628–640.

Hansell DM. Thin-section CT of the lungs: the hinterland of normal. *Radiology.* 2010;256(3):695–711.

Hodnett PA, Naidich DP. Fibrosing interstitial lung disease. a practical high-resolution computed tomography-based approach to diagnosis and management and a review of the literature. *Am J Respir Crit Care Med.* 2013;188(2):141–149.

Mahesh M, Cody DD. Physics of cardiac imaging with multiple-row detector CT. *Radiographics.* 2007;27(5):1495–1509.

Mahesh M. Search for isotropic resolution in CT from conventional through multiple-row detector. *Radiographics.* 2002;22(4):949–962.

Moore EM. Percutaneous lung biopsy: an ordering clinician's guide to current practice. *Semin Respir Crit Care Med.* 2008;29(4):323–334.

Patel VK, Naik SK, Naidich DP, et al. A practical algorithmic approach to the diagnosis and management of solitary pulmonary nodules: part 1: radiologic characteristics and imaging modalities. *Chest.* 2013;143(3):825–839.

Patel VK, Naik SK, Naidich DP, et al. A practical algorithmic approach to the diagnosis and management of solitary pulmonary nodules: part 2: pretest probability and algorithm. *Chest.* 2013;143(3):840–846.

Thomson CC, Duggal A, Bice T, et al. 2018 practice guideline summary for clinicians: diagnosis of idiopathic pulmonary fibrosis. *Ann Am Thorac Soc.* 2019;16(3):285–290.

Complete reference list available at ExpertConsult.com.

21 | *THORACIC RADIOLOGY: INVASIVE DIAGNOSTIC IMAGING AND IMAGE-GUIDED INTERVENTIONS*

RYAN WALSH, MD • JEFFREY S. KLEIN, MD

INTRODUCTION

Interventional thoracic radiology can assist in the diagnosis and increasingly in the treatment of common thoracic problems. This chapter describes the indications and practical aspects of the most clinically useful procedures.

Image-guided *transthoracic needle biopsy* (TNB), which is typically performed with guidance by *computed tomography* (CT), is a minimally invasive procedure that can provide a definitive cytologic, histologic, or microbiologic diagnosis in more than 90% of patients with localized thoracic lesions.[1]

Interventional radiologists also help manage intrathoracic air and fluid collections using cross-sectional imaging to guide catheter placement and monitor response to drainage and treat massive hemoptysis by embolization of bronchial or systemic arteries. More recently, CT-guided thermal ablation of early-stage lung cancer and limited pulmonary metastatic disease has shown efficacy as a minimally invasive alternative to surgical management and external-beam radiation therapy in selected patients.

TRANSTHORACIC NEEDLE BIOPSY

INDICATIONS AND CONTRAINDICATIONS

The decision to perform TNB in lieu of alternative invasive diagnostic procedures or imaging follow-up, particularly for indeterminate lung lesions, is usually made after a multidisciplinary review of relevant clinical, laboratory, imaging, and pathologic material and requires consideration of local expertise, the availability of alternative invasive diagnostic procedures, including bronchoscopy and *video-assisted thoracic surgery* (VATS), and the needs of the referring physician and patient.

TNB is most commonly used for the diagnosis of a solitary pulmonary nodule (Fig. 21.1). Additional indications include diagnosis of a mediastinal mass,[2] enlarged hilar or mediastinal lymph nodes, chest wall mass, or a pleural mass or thickening.[3] Most often the primary diagnostic concern is malignancy, but the diagnosis of opportunistic lung infection producing focal lung lesions in immunocompromised patients is an additional indication for image-guided TNB. In these latter patients, the primary purpose for TNB is to obtain material for microbiologic stains and cultures.[4] In selected patients with suspected extensive stage *non–small cell lung cancer* (NSCLC), core tissue TNB can be performed for immunohistochemical analysis to determine if the lesion is a primary lung (squamous cell carcinoma vs. adenocarcinoma) or metastatic disease. Immmunohistochemistry can also be used to perform prognostic markers (e.g., breast cancer metastases assessed for the presence of estrogen and progesterone receptors and HER2/Neu)[5] or molecular testing for genetic alterations (e.g., epidermal growth factor receptor mutations or amplifications, echinoderm microtubule-associated protein-like 4–anaplastic lymphoma kinase fusions)[6] to help guide therapy. On occasion, a lesion thought likely to be benign, based on clinical and imaging analysis, is sampled using TNB to confirm a benign diagnosis.

The only absolute contraindication to TNB is the inability of a patient to cooperate for safe and successful sampling of the thoracic lesion in question. Most adults, even those with compromised pulmonary function, can undergo successful image-guided TNB using local anesthesia and either

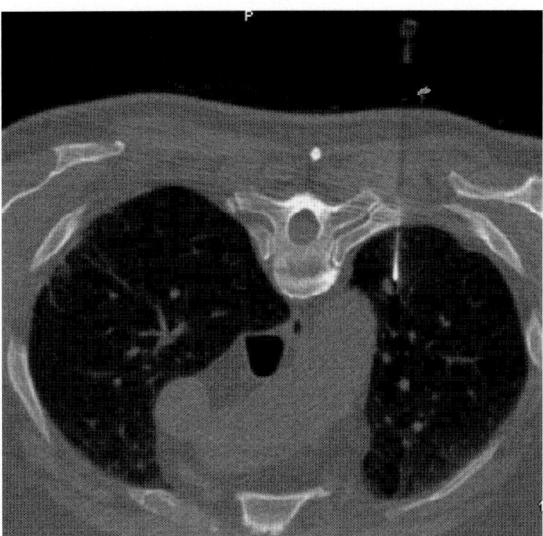

Figure 21.1 Transthoracic needle biopsy of a solitary pulmonary nodule. Computed tomography with patient prone during transthoracic needle biopsy showing the vertical course of the coaxial needle with its tip at the edge of a 1-cm left upper lobe nodule.

conscious sedation or monitored anesthesia care. For sampling of small lesions (<15 mm in diameter), the patient must be able to hold his or her breath when instructed to allow the operator to position the needle accurately within the lesion for successful retrieval of cytologic material. Precise breath-holding is less important for sampling larger lesions, particularly those at the lung periphery, or for upper lobe lesions, which move less than lower lobe lesions with normal breathing.

A bleeding diathesis is the only relative contraindication to TNB and, if identified, can usually be corrected before the procedure. Although no objective data exist showing an increased risk for bleeding from TNB in patients with abnormal clotting parameters, such as elevated international normalized ratio higher than 1.5 or a platelet count less than 50,000 cells/μL, most operators and published guidelines recommend preprocedure correction of abnormal bleeding parameters.[7] Patients receiving antiplatelet agents, including aspirin and/or P2Y12 inhibitors (e.g., clopidogrel), for prophylaxis after myocardial infarction, stroke, or recent coronary artery stent placement and who require TNB should have an assessment of the relative risks and benefits of discontinuing these agents compared with the potential bleeding complications induced by TNB. Published guidelines recommend discontinuing antiplatelet agents at least 5 days before TNB.[7] Patients considered to be at risk for thrombosis if anticoagulation or antiplatelet agents are withdrawn before biopsy can be bridged to receive intravenous heparin, which can be discontinued several hours before TNB, thereby providing a brief periprocedural window off anticoagulation. For large mediastinal masses or large peripheral lung or pleural/chest wall lesions, biopsy can be safely performed while the patient remains on anticoagulation or antiplatelet agents. Patients who have had a prior pneumonectomy are at greater risk for respiratory compromise if they develop bleeding or pneumothorax from lung biopsy. However, because these complications can usually be anticipated and managed successfully, prior pneumonectomy does not preclude TNB for evaluation of a suspicious lesion in the residual lung.

PATIENT-LESION SELECTION AND PREPROCEDURE CLINICAL AND IMAGING EVALUATION

The decision to perform a TNB follows a thorough imaging evaluation and clinical assessment of the patient (see Chapter 76). For patients younger than 35 years without significant risk factors for malignancy who have focal lung lesions, imaging follow-up is typically used because the likelihood of malignancy in such patients is very low. Conversely, for patients with localized lesions who have a high prebiopsy likelihood of NSCLC, direct referral for surgical evaluation for possible resection is reasonable and more cost-effective because the result of TNB is unlikely to obviate resection of the lesion. In patients with stage I NSCLC who are older than 75 years, sublobar resection using segmentectomy or extended wedge resection may be an effective and potentially beneficial alternative to lobectomy, particularly for patients with smaller (<2 cm in diameter) peripheral lesions (particularly if subsolid on CT) and significant medical comorbidities, such as severe COPD.[8] Nevertheless, biopsy of likely malignant nodules can be useful in several situations: for patients who are poor surgical candidates, for those whose lesion is not amenable to VATS resection, and for those with a history of prior malignancy in whom metastatic disease is a consideration but who would not be a candidate for surgical metastatectomy. For anterior mediastinal masses, core biopsy is almost always necessary for the initial diagnosis of lymphoma, particularly if diagnosis would preclude unnecessary sternotomy and resection, because these lesions are treated with radiation therapy and/or systemic chemotherapy.

All patients referred for image-guided TNB should have a recent (optimally within 4 weeks of the procedure) thin-section (<2-mm slice thickness) CT examination of the lesion to be sampled. For TNB of mediastinal masses, enlarged mediastinal nodes, or pleural and chest wall masses, a recent contrast-enhanced CT or magnetic resonance imaging study helps determine the vascularity of the lesion and its proximity to critical vascular structures.

Informed consent for TNB should include a detailed explanation of the procedure itself, the expected length of time in the department (typically 1 hour for the procedure and 3 hours of postprocedure observation), the risk of adverse events (see "Complications" section), and the benefits of the image-guided transthoracic approach compared with alternative noninvasive diagnostic options, including the option of not undergoing any further diagnostic procedures.

CHOICE OF IMAGING GUIDANCE

Although TNB can be performed under fluoroscopic, CT, or ultrasonographic guidance, most operators use standard CT-fluoroscopic or C-arm cone-beam CT guidance[9] to perform the vast majority of biopsies. CT provides rapid and precise information regarding lesion and needle location. It is the only imaging modality that allows TNB access to small central lesions and enlarged mediastinal nodes (Fig. 21.2). The ability to visualize intervening structures allows the operator to avoid bullae or large vessels in the projected needle path. Precise needle tip localization allows a more confident assessment of adequacy of needle placement, particularly for placement

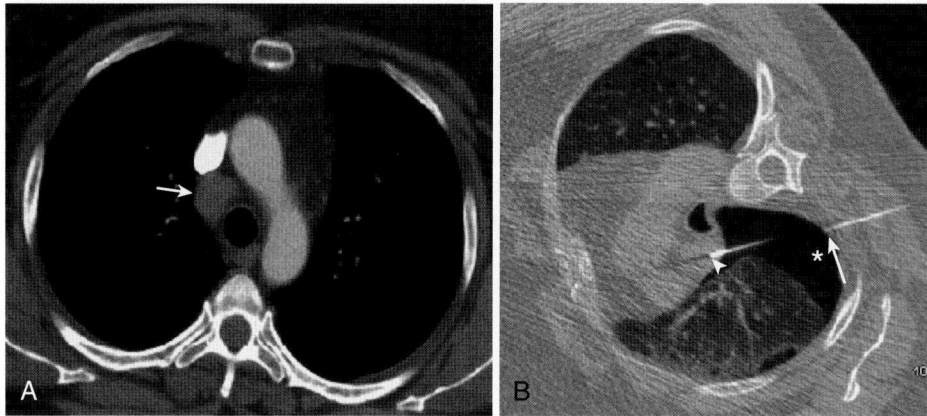

Figure 21.2 Transthoracic needle biopsy of mediastinal lymphadenopathy. (A) Contrast-enhanced computed tomography just below the level of the aortic arch shows an enlarged right lower paratracheal (4R) node *(arrow)*. The patient had a left upper lobe mass (not shown). (B) Computed tomography with the patient in the right lateral decubitus position showing the coaxial needle tip *(arrowhead)* within the enlarged right lower paratracheal node. The pneumothorax was created by a second, blunt-tipped needle *(arrow)* placed into the pleural space to inject air, allowing the coaxial needle to access the lesion without traversing the lung. Aspiration and core biopsy of the nodes confirmed the presence of contralateral (N3) nodal metastases from primary adenocarcinoma of the left upper lobe.

within small lesions or within the wall of those with central necrosis or cavitation. Complications such as bleeding or pneumothorax are readily identified and can be expeditiously managed.

Ultrasonography can be used to guide TNB in selected cases.[10] Compared to CT, its primary advantage is that it allows the operator to visualize needle placement and lesion sampling in real time. Intervening vascular structures are easily identified using Doppler ultrasonography so that they may be avoided. Although the technique is operator dependent, most radiologists have experience with diagnostic ultrasound probes and biopsy techniques that are easily applied to TNB. The use of ultrasonography to guide TNB is limited to lesions with an adequate acoustic window, such as anterior mediastinal masses and peripheral lung lesions with pleural contact (eFig. 21.1).

PROCEDURE

For CT-guided TNB, the patient is placed recumbent and positioned to provide the shortest distance from the anticipated skin puncture site to the lesion, typically with the skin puncture site nondependent, allowing a vertical needle trajectory (see Fig. 21.1). For patients unable to lie prone for the procedure because of breathing difficulties, the patient can be placed in the lateral decubitus position and a puncture performed with the needle oriented horizontally. Most patients receive local lidocaine only or conscious sedation using short-acting and readily reversible analgesic and amnestic agents, such as fentanyl and midazolam; a minority of patients require monitored anesthesia care or general anesthesia. The use of local lidocaine helps patients cooperate more consistently with breathing commands and allows the operator to position the biopsy needle accurately into smaller lesions. For TNB performed using conscious sedation, the patient should ideally be able to cooperate with consistent breath-holding, which is necessary to position the biopsy needle accurately into small lesions for successful sampling; this is particularly important for lesions near the diaphragm, which move craniocaudally even with tidal breathing.

Once the patient has been properly positioned, a scout view (a planar image of the thorax analogous to a frontal radiograph used to plan for the axial scans) is obtained at functional residual capacity (at normal end-expiration). All scans obtained through the region of interest are likewise obtained at normal end-expiration, which is a comfortable and reproducible lung volume for the patient to achieve, even when sedated. For TNB of small lung nodules, a reconstructed scan thickness of no greater than half of the diameter of the lesion should be obtained for identifying and marking the needle puncture site. This provides a detailed view of the ribs and intercostal space, helps visualize the anticipated needle path and any intervening large vessels or bullae to be avoided, and minimizes partial volume averaging when assessing the position of the needle tip relative to the lesion being sampled. Thin sections are particularly important when sampling lesions with subsolid attenuation because it is important to identify and target any solid components within the lesion to provide a more confident cytologic diagnosis of malignancy. Once the thin sections encompassing the lesion have been obtained, an electronic grid is superimposed on the image at the desired level for needle entry at the technologist's console. Measurements are then made on the console from the axis closest to the desired entry point; this point is marked on the patient's skin using a ruler and an indelible marker.

The area is then prepared and draped with a sterilizing solution, and local 2% lidocaine is administered subcutaneously to the entry site and also to the parietal pleural surface, which is heavily innervated and therefore best anesthetized before pleural transgression of the biopsy needle. In muscular or obese patients in whom the lidocaine needle may not be long enough to reach the parietal pleura, lidocaine can be administered to the pleural surface through the coaxial needle inserted to the edge of the lung. The coaxial approach involves use of an outer thin-walled guide needle, 18- or 19-gauge in diameter, placed through the chest wall and adjacent pleura and positioned with its tip at the edge of the lesion. Once positioned at the edge of the lesion, samples are obtained by placing thin 20- to 22-gauge aspiration or core biopsy needles through the outer

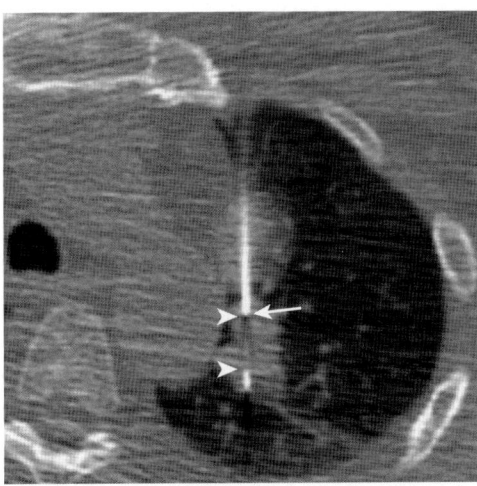

Figure 21.3 Core biopsy for molecular analysis. Computed tomography performed at the level of the aortic arch shows the coaxial guide needle *(arrow)* with its tip at the anterior edge of a lobulated left upper lobe nodule, with the receptacle stylet of the inner cutting needle (between *arrowheads*) within the nodule. Core specimens were obtained for subsequent molecular analysis of this known pulmonary adenocarcinoma.

Table 21.1   Indications for Core Needle Biopsy in the Thorax

- To obtain tissue as needed for a diagnosis of:
  - Anterior or posterior mediastinal mass
  - Probable benign lesion (hamartoma, granuloma)
  - Mesothelioma
  - Subsolid lung lesions
- To obtain sufficient tissue for molecular markers in non–small cell lung cancer
- To maximize yield for diagnosis when rapid cytolopathologic review is unavailable

---

coaxial guide needle and into the lesion. Patient breath-holding during needle placement and repositioning at the same end-expiratory volume as directed for the preliminary scans is crucial for accurate needle placement. Rapid assessment of needle position after advancement and repositioning can be obtained by repeated axial images through the region or by using CT fluoroscopy or cone-beam CT, which allows the operator to obtain several quick, contiguous, low-dose, thin-section images through the lesion and needle without having to leave the room.

Aspiration biopsy is performed by using a rapid, rotatory, and to-and-fro motion with the inner needle attached to a syringe to which suction is applied. The needle-syringe combination is removed and handed to a cytotechnologist who expresses the contents onto glass slides that are then fixed in alcohol. The slides are then stained using a rapid stain, examined with a microscope, and assessed for adequacy by a pathologist.[11] Additional aspiration samples are typically obtained for immunocytochemical analysis, cell block, molecular studies, or stains and cultures when necessary. Core tissue biopsy specimens are performed through the same coaxial needle used for the aspirates with 20-gauge or larger automated 1- to 2-cm cutting needles and are reserved for situations when histologic analysis is deemed necessary or when molecular genetic analysis is desired (Fig. 21.3; Table 21.1). A common error in sampling is to neglect to send material for culture in cases where

malignancy is not found on the initial on-site interpretation by the pathologist. Aspirates should be obtained and processed for microbiologic stains and cultures, even when infection is only remotely suspected.

The initial approach to the pathologic evaluation of a TNB specimen obtained from a lung nodule or mass is to determine whether the lesion represents a small cell lung cancer or a NSCLC. This distinction is typically made using light microscopic examination of the stained specimen.[12] In the majority of biopsy specimens showing an epithelial malignancy, additional immunocytochemical tests performed on aspirated specimens are needed for definitive determination of type and the primary site of disease (see Chapters 76 and 22 and eFigs. 21.2 and 21.3).

Neuroendocrine markers, including chromogranin and synaptophysin, are used to help confirm the diagnosis of small cell carcinoma, typical and atypical carcinoid tumors, and large cell neuroendocrine carcinoma. The markers most often used to determine the primary site of adenocarcinoma include thyroid transcription factor 1 (positive in lung and thyroid carcinoma; see eFig. 21.2), cytokeratin 7 and 20 (positive in lung and colorectal carcinoma, respectively), CDX2 (positive in colorectal carcinoma; see eFig. 21.3), and GATA3 and estrogen receptors (positive in some breast carcinomas).[13] Increasingly, core specimens for epidermal growth factor receptor, anaplastic lymphoma kinase, and programmed death ligand-1, as well as other potential molecular mutational analysis in patients with NSCLC, are obtained in patients who might benefit from targeted or immunologic therapies.

POSTPROCEDURE PATIENT MANAGEMENT

After a lung biopsy has been completed, most operators inject a pleural sealant through the coaxial needle. The most commonly used pleural sealants are an autologous blood clot obtained immediately before the biopsy, which is then injected through the coaxial needle as it is withdrawn from the chest, or a hydrogel plug that is pushed through the coaxial needle and placed at the pleural surface and hydrated before the coaxial needle is removed. These pleural sealants have been shown to reduce the rate of biopsy-induced pneumothorax and need for chest tube placement.[14] The patient is then moved by radiology personnel from the biopsy table to a stretcher, with the biopsy side placed dependently. The patient receives supplemental oxygen as a precaution while recovering from conscious sedation and also to help promote resorption of any pneumothorax (see Chapter 110).

An upright chest radiograph is obtained 2 to 3 hours after the completion of the biopsy to assess intraparenchymal or pleural hemorrhage and to exclude a pneumothorax. If no pneumothorax is detected, the patient can be safely discharged home.[15] If a small (<2 cm from chest apex to pleural line of upper lobe) pneumothorax is present and is not growing, and the patient is asymptomatic, the patient can be discharged safely. Otherwise, the patient is observed for an additional 1 to 2 hours to confirm that the pneumothorax is stable in size. Any symptomatic, moderate-sized (2–4 cm), large (>4 cm), or enlarging pneumothorax should be evacuated with placement of a pleural drainage catheter. The drainage catheter is attached to a pleural evacuation system placed on suction until the air leak ceases and resolution of the pneumothorax is confirmed on upright radiography or CT. In selected patients who have drainage of a biopsy-induced pneumothorax, the catheter can be attached to a Heimlich valve and safely managed on an outpatient basis; these patients should have no air leak, minimal to no dyspnea or pain, oxygen saturations greater than 92% or at preprocedure baseline, and have support at home with close proximity to a health care facility should symptoms worsen. The remainder of patients with pneumothorax drains are admitted for inpatient management.

DIAGNOSTIC YIELD

TNB has proven highly sensitive for the cytologic diagnosis of malignancy, with sensitivities exceeding 90% in multiple published series.[1,2] The distinction between NSCLC and small cell lung cancer is made with high accuracy (>85%).[12] A number of factors have been shown to affect sensitivity, including the patient's ability to lie still and cooperate sufficiently, the presence of underlying emphysema, operator experience, lesion size and location, lesion density, and availability of expert cytopathologic analysis. Even for lesions smaller than 10 mm, the sensitivity rate of TNB is high.[16] Certain lesions, particularly large mediastinal lymphomas, such as nodular sclerosing Hodgkin lymphoma, and certain forms of non-Hodgkin lymphoma that contain significant fibrosis, localized fibrous tumors of pleura, and neurogenic lesions can be more difficult to diagnose cytologically; core needle biopsies are typically obtained for definitive diagnosis of these lesions. For sampling of subsolid lung nodules, the yield of TNB approaches that for solid nodules.[17]

Precise cytologic diagnosis of benign pulmonary lesions, particularly granulomas, is more difficult than that of malignant lesions because their relatively small size and typically hypocellular, fibrotic matrix makes retrieval of diagnostic material from TNB difficult. Core needle biopsy as an adjunct to cytologic analysis alone can increase the diagnostic yield from TNB of benign lesions to approximately 80%.[18] Pulmonary hamartomas, particularly those with a significant cartilaginous component, can be difficult to aspirate, and core needle biopsy may be necessary for these lesions. Nevertheless, a skilled cytopathologist can make the diagnosis of a pulmonary hamartoma if provided adequate cytologic material (eFig. 21.4).

The diagnostic yield of TNB for infection is somewhat lower than for malignancy. However, TNB can identify the causative microorganisms, diagnosing focal lesions in 80% of immunocompromised patients with suspected lung infection.[19]

COMPLICATIONS

The most common complications of TNB include pneumothorax and bleeding. Pneumothorax develops in approximately 18–29% of patients undergoing TNB, of whom 4–6% require catheter or tube drainage.[20] Factors that may be associated with an increased rate of TNB-induced pneumothorax include operator inexperience, advanced patient age, smaller lesion size, greater lesion depth from the pleural surface, the presence of underlying emphysema or obstructive lung disease, larger outer coaxial needle diameter, prolonged needle dwell time, and greater obliquity of the angle between the biopsy needle and the transgressed visceral pleural surface.[21]

Hemorrhage (eFig. 21.5) with or without hemoptysis develops in approximately 6–18% of patients undergoing TNB[20,21] but is rarely the cause of prolonged observation, hospitalization, or need for transfusion. Biopsy-induced hemorrhage can preclude successful completion of TNB if it leads to intractable coughing or if blood in the lung obscures the lesion being sampled, thereby rendering further attempts at accurate sampling impossible.

Rare complications of TNB include hemothorax (0.1%) from intercostal artery damage (see eFig. 21.5), air embolism (0.06%) (eFig. 21.6), malignant seeding of the biopsy path (0.01–0.06%), and, rarely, death.[22]

CATHETER DRAINAGE OF INTRATHORACIC COLLECTIONS

Image-guided catheter or tube drainage of intrathoracic collections is an effective, minimally invasive method for treating a spectrum of intrapleural and intrapulmonary collections. This section reviews the common indications, imaging considerations, catheter placement, and postprocedure management of intrathoracic collections.

PARAPNEUMONIC EFFUSIONS: EMPYEMA

Selected patients with complicated parapneumonic effusions, defined as those unlikely to resolve spontaneously with treatment of the underlying pulmonary infection, or frank empyema can benefit from image-guided drainage, thereby avoiding prolonged hospitalization, VATS, or open surgical drainage and/or decortication procedures. Although deciding between image-guided drainage versus surgical intervention will vary by institution, there has been an overall increase in an initial trial of percutaneous drainage in recent years to treat unilocular and more complex parapneumonic effusions, typically accompanied by subsequent intrapleural fibrinolytics and DNAse[23] (see Chapter 109).

According to the American College of Chest Physicians consensus statement on the medical and surgical management of parapneumonic effusions, the anatomy of infected pleural fluid collections, the presence or absence of bacteria within the parapneumonic effusion, and pleural fluid chemistry have prognostic utility and can help determine the need for drainage.[24] Assessment of pleural fluid with ultrasonography has become the initial imaging modality of choice given its bedside utility for detection, characterization, and sampling of pleural collections.[25] Ultrasonographic findings that predict the likelihood of successful catheter or tube drainage include small to moderate size and presence of free-flowing, nonloculated fluid lacking internal echoes or septations. Alternatively,

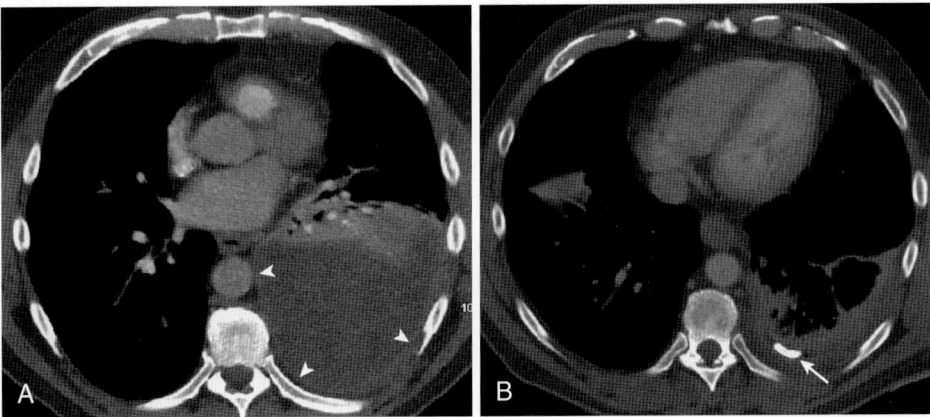

Figure 21.4 *Computed tomography* **(CT)-guided catheter drainage of loculated empyema treated with intrapleural fibrinolytics.** (A) Contrast-enhanced CT through the level of the left atrium showing a unilocular collection in the lower posterior left pleural space found to represent empyema. Note subtle enhancement of the parietal pleural surface *(arrowheads)*, suggesting presence of an exudative effusion. (B) Repeat contrast-enhanced CT scan performed through the lower lobes after placement of a 14-French pigtail drainage catheter and intrapleural instillation of recombinant tissue plasminogen activator for 5 days shows the catheter *(arrow)* in the posterior pleural space with evacuation of the pleural fluid.

ultrasonographically detected septations and multiple loculations make it more likely that a longer duration of chest tube drainage, surgical intervention, and longer hospital stay will be necessary. Similar findings can be seen with contrast-enhanced CT, which is superior to sonography for assessing the extent of pleural and parenchymal disease for planning drainage. CT findings suggesting a higher likelihood of successful percutaneous drainage include dependent meniscoid or unilocular collections; success rates were as high as 93% using small-bore (<14 French) image-guided catheter placement in one case series.[26] The presence of enhancing visceral and parietal pleural layers encompassing a loculated pleural fluid collection is relatively specific for the presence of an empyema, although the identification of this "split pleura" sign does not preclude successful catheter drainage. Selected patients with unilocular empyema or multiloculated collections can be successfully managed with one or more image-guided catheters, either as definitive therapy or as a bridge to definitive surgical treatment. Early pleural drainage is indicated for pleural fluid analysis demonstrating pus, positive Gram stain or culture or, if the effusion is associated with a pneumonia, a pH less than 7.2 or glucose less than 40 mg/dL.[24] Additional pleural fluid analysis, such as lactate dehydrogenase greater than 1000 IU/L, can also be used to guide management decisions (see Chapter 109).

After ultrasonographic or CT localization, either a Seldinger technique using a 19-gauge thin-wall coaxial needle, guidewire, and dilators or trocar catheter placement using a 14- or 16-French drainage catheter can be performed for drainage of free-flowing or unilocular, nonseptated parapneumonic collections. If a trocar placement technique is chosen, it is important to ensure that the collection has an adequate area of contact with the costal pleural surface and sufficient width of the collection to allow safe placement of the sharp-tipped trocar/catheter combination into the dependent part of the collection (Fig. 21.4). For treatment of frank empyema or large collections with septations on imaging, we prefer a 16-French pigtail drain placed with a Seldinger technique and subsequent intrapleural therapy (discussed

later). If the viscosity of the pleural fluid does not allow aspiration through the 19-gauge coaxial access needle, a larger 28-French tube is placed using a Seldinger technique. If necessary, multiple catheters or tubes can be used to drain different locules within the chest as depicted on CT, particularly for patients believed to be poor candidates for primary surgical drainage. Large-volume aspiration or an attempt at evacuation of the pleural fluid using a 60-mL syringe and a three-way stopcock or a Y-connector with a nonreturn valve at the time of catheter placement can be helpful to assess the likelihood of drainage response and need for an additional catheter placement into separate locules.

Once catheters and tubes have been placed under imaging guidance, the patient's clinical status, tube output, and radiologic studies are reviewed daily to determine the effectiveness of treatment. The tube or catheter should be flushed with saline (10 mL) three times a day to maintain patency of the lumen and prevent occlusion of the drainage holes located in the distal aspect of the device by fibrin and debris. An inadequate response to treatment is defined as a lack of improvement in fever, peripheral white blood cell count, and oxygenation, with persistent dyspnea or pain. In addition, a persistent or enlarging collection on radiography or CT warrants a reevaluation of the patient, with consideration of additional maneuvers to improve drainage or a determination to proceed to surgical management. Assuming radiologic evaluation and management demonstrates adequate positioning and functioning of the drainage catheter or tube within the collection(s), inadequate drainage in the setting of a poor clinical response may require increasing the size of the tube and/or the use of intrapleural fibrinolytic agents to promote drainage. Contrast-enhanced chest CT evaluation is helpful to detect undrained locules, to guide tube exchange when necessary, or to detect progressive pulmonary infection. Once there has been clinical and radiographic resolution of the collection and drainage has diminished to less than 100 mL/day, the catheter is removed.

Lastly, it should be reinforced that early consultation with a surgeon and consideration of surgical management (VATS or open thoracotomy) of parapneumonic effusions and empyemas are recommended in the setting of highly complex and loculated pleural collections. Early surgical management can also be considered for patients who have had documented pleural fluid or pulmonary symptoms for more than 3 weeks, have extensive pleural thickening on CT, and/or do not respond to initial percutaneous drainage (see Chapter 109 for considerations in the treatment of patients with nonresolving pleural infection).

MALIGNANT PLEURAL EFFUSIONS

A malignant pleural effusion is defined by the presence of positive cytologic results on pleural fluid analysis or positive pleural biopsy in a patient with malignancy. Malignant pleural effusion is most commonly due to lung or breast cancer, although in 10–15% of patients with malignant effusions, no primary tumor can be identified.[27] Before indwelling catheter drainage or pleurodesis is considered, the patient should be shown to be symptomatic due to the effusion by showing that symptoms of dyspnea or cough improve after a large-volume thoracentesis. Postdrainage chest radiographs and pleural manometry can be used during the evacuation of the fluid to assess for unexpandable ("trapped") lung. Catheter drainage of a malignant effusion, followed by either chemical pleurodesis or the use of an indwelling tunneled catheter, can be used to provide prolonged drainage of symptomatic malignant effusions in patients with a limited life expectancy and is a reasonable alternative to thoracoscopic or open surgical drainage and sclerosis (eFig. 21.7).[28] Patients with symptomatic malignant effusion with expandable lung may undergo talc pleurodesis or placement of an indwelling pleural catheter, whereas those with nonexpendable lungs, failed pleurodesis, or pleural loculations should be offered indwelling pleural catheters only.[29]

A drainage catheter is inserted via a lower intercostal approach to place the tip in a dependent location to facilitate drainage of dependent fluid no matter what position (i.e., supine or upright) the patient maintains. Optimally, the catheter is placed through the junction of the serratus anterior and latissimus dorsi muscles along the lower posterolateral chest wall, where it traverses the least amount of muscle and will not be compressed or kinked when the patient lies on his or her back, typically along the sixth or seventh intercostal space. For serous or thin serosanguineous effusions, a 10- or 12-French catheter allows adequate drainage, whereas a larger diameter (12- or 14-French) is used if talc slurry is to be administered for subsequent pleurodesis after adequate drainage of the pleural space and reexpansion of the underlying lung. Loculated collections can benefit from intrapleural fibrinolytics to lyse adhesions before attempts at chemical sclerosis.[30]

An indwelling pleural catheter is designed for longer-term outpatient drainage. If symptoms improve with thoracentesis, even if the lung fails to reexpand, an indwelling catheter can be useful. Of note, if the lung does reexpand, additional instillation of talc after placement of an indwelling pleural catheter has shown greater rates of pleurodesis than drainage alone.[31]

To place an indwelling pleural catheter, the patient is positioned in an oblique or decubitus position with the effusion side up. Using ultrasound, an appropriate entry site to access the pleural space and place the drain posteriorly is marked on the skin. Two skin incisions are then made—one at the aforementioned pleural insertion site and one at 5- to 8-cm lateral and caudal to the first incision for the catheter exit. The fenestrated end of a 15.5-gauge pleural catheter is then tunneled subcutaneously from the caudal lateral (catheter exit) to the cranial medial (pleural entry) incision. Using ultrasound guidance, an 18-gauge coaxial needle is used to access the pleural space through the superior skin incision, and a J-tip wire is placed under fluoroscopic guidance. The needle is removed, and a peel-away introducer is passed over the guidewire, and the guidewire is removed. The subcutaneously placed fenestrated end of the catheter is then inserted into the peel-away introducer and pleural space while the peel-away introducer is removed. The tube is connected to a drainage bag. Once patency is confirmed, both incisions are sutured, the catheter sutured to the skin, and sterile dressing placed.

If talc slurry is used for chemical pleurodesis, 4 g of talc mixed with 50 mL of normal saline is injected into the evacuated pleural space and left to dwell for 1 hour. Suction is then reinstituted, with the catheter removed once drainage has diminished to less than 150 mL/day and the patient has shown symptomatic and radiographic improvement. Complete response rates of 70% and higher have been reported for use of small-bore catheters and talc pleurodesis in selected patients.[32]

PNEUMOTHORAX (See Chapter 110)

Fluoroscopy- or CT-guided small-bore (<12-French) catheter drainage of pneumothorax can be used for management of moderate to large or enlarging pneumothoraces, or any pneumothorax that is symptomatic. Today, most often image-guided catheter drainage of pneumothorax is performed for pneumothorax that develops as a complication of TNB or thermal ablation of localized thoracic malignancy, although catheter drainage has been traditionally used to treat spontaneous pneumothorax and pneumothorax related to traumatic causes (eFig. 21.8).[33]

For pneumothorax resulting from a CT-guided procedure, catheter placement is typically performed using CT. Otherwise, fluoroscopy provides real-time visualization of catheter placement and is the preferred guidance modality. An approach via the anterior second intercostal space in the midclavicular line is typically used, although in women a lateral approach via the fifth to sixth intercostal space in the midaxillary line can be used to avoid traversing breast tissue. Conscious sedation and local anesthesia are used, with adequate numbing of the heavily innervated parietal pleura with lidocaine being the key to patient comfort during catheter placement. Similar to pleural fluid drainage, either a trocar or Seldinger techniques may be used, each with its own advantages and disadvantages. For the trocar technique, after successful pleural anesthesia, a drainage catheter with a self-retaining pigtail tip configuration loaded onto a stiffening cannula and inner sharp-tipped trocar is placed into the pleural space and positioned into the pleural apex under direct visualization. Once the catheter tip is confirmed to lie within the apex of the pleural space, the pigtail tip is "locked" into position by use of a string that opposes the catheter tip to a more proximal portion of the catheter. Lidocaine is injected, although the catheter lumen to provide local anesthesia to the apical pleura, which if contacted by the catheter, can produce significant ipsilateral shoulder pain. Alternatively, the catheter can be introduced into the pleural space in a stepwise fashion, whereby a hollow needle is initially used to access the pleural space, followed by placement of a guidewire and then progressive dilation of the track to the diameter of the catheter to be placed for drainage.

Once the catheter has been successfully placed, it is affixed to the skin using an adhesive ostomy-type dressing with ties surrounding the catheter and is attached to a chest drainage system.

Success rates for small-bore catheter drainage of iatrogenic pneumothorax exceed 85% in multiple series,[34,35] but drainage is also successful in the majority of patients when used in emergency settings for noniatrogenic traumatic and spontaneous pneumothoraces.[36]

LUNG ABSCESS (See Chapter 50)

Although postural drainage and antibiotics are the standard methods for medical management of lung abscess, collections that do not readily communicate with an airway or for which medical management is unsuccessful can be treated with catheter drainage under CT guidance. Patients who do not improve clinically or radiologically with antibiotic therapy are candidates for percutaneous drainage; those presenting with an abscess greater than 4 cm should also be considered for drainage because they have a higher rate of failure with conservative management.[36] Because most of these collections are pleural based, with intrapleural adhesions typical at the site of pleural contact, the risk for development of a pneumothorax is low. As with drainage of complex pleural collections, image-guided catheter drainage can be definitive or can be used as a bridge to surgical management.

Drainage of lung abscess or an infected bulla is best performed under CT guidance to visualize the catheter course and minimize traversal of normal intervening lung. The principles of catheter placement are similar to those for drainage of abscesses elsewhere in the body. The patient is positioned to allow access to that part of the abscess closest to a pleural surface. If possible, it is best to avoid placing the patient in the decubitus position with the unaffected side dependent because pus or blood can spill from the abscess cavity into the dependent lung during catheter placement, producing respiratory compromise. We typically use a Seldinger technique for catheter placement into the abscess, using a 19-gauge thin-wall coaxial needle, guidewire, sequential dilators, and a pigtail drainage catheter (typically 12 or 14 French). Trocar placement technique is also a reasonable option in experienced hands. The pigtail-shaped tip should be placed into the dependent part of the collection to facilitate dependent drainage of the infected fluid. Once properly positioned, we recommend attempting to aspirate as much fluid as possible with a 60-mL syringe to assess viscosity of the fluid and document residual fluid remaining in the cavity while the patient is on the

table. Due to the risk of a bronchopleural fistula, we try to aspirate and remove the tube while the patient is on the table or leave the catheter in for less than 24 hours. If the drainage catheter is to remain, it is affixed to the skin and attached to suction until fluid drainage ceases and there is evidence of clinical and radiologic improvement (eFig. 21.9).

There are only limited case series describing the success rate and complications from percutaneous catheter drainage of lung abscess. A summary of results from 21 studies showed a success rate of 84%, with a complication rate of 16%.[35] Clogging of smaller drainage tubes, pneumothorax, hemothorax, hemoptysis, and bronchopleural fistula formation are the most frequent complications after catheter abscess drainage.

BRONCHIAL ARTERIOGRAPHY

INDICATIONS AND CONTRAINDICATIONS

The most common indication for urgent or emergent bronchial arteriography is massive hemoptysis. The most commonly used criterion for massive hemoptysis is 500 mL of expectorated blood in a 24-hour period, although it has been defined variably from as low as expectoration of 100 mL to greater than 1000 mL of blood in a 24-hour period.[37] The need for emergent intervention is most commonly determined by a sudden onset of hypoxemia; hemoptysis rarely causes life-threatening exsanguination.

Massive hemoptysis most commonly results from chronic inflammatory lung diseases due to bronchiectasis, cystic fibrosis (eFig. 21.10), or complicating fungal infection.[37] Neoplasm, such as bronchogenic carcinoma or vascular metastatic disease, can also cause hemoptysis. Less common causes of hemoptysis include lung abscess, pneumonia, chronic bronchitis, ruptured bronchial artery aneurysm, pulmonary arteriovenous malformations, and traumatic or inflammatory pulmonary artery aneurysms. In resource-poor countries, pulmonary tuberculosis is by far the most common cause of massive hemoptysis.

Indications for nonemergent bronchial arteriography and intervention include patients with non–life-threatening chronic hemoptysis unresponsive to medical therapy.[38] Less frequent indications for bronchial arteriography include bronchial artery aneurysms or pseudoaneurysms and arteriovenous fistulas. Bronchial arteriography and intervention have been used for patients with lung cancer and other intrathoracic malignancies that can produce significant bleeding, such as hypervascular metastases to the chest. Relative contraindications to bronchial arteriography include severe iodinated contrast allergy and acute or chronic renal disease. Severe aortoiliac or upper extremity occlusive disease may also pose a challenge in accessing the origins of the bronchial arteries.

Conservative management of massive hemoptysis is associated with a mortality rate of 50–100%.[39] Moreover, reported mortality rates for surgery performed for massive hemoptysis are as high as 35%. Bronchial artery embolization is a safe and effective alternative to medical or surgical management of hemoptysis, with successful control of acute life-threatening hemoptysis in 73–98% of patients, although hemoptysis may recur.[38–40] Recurrence rates are 2–27% at 1 month and 10–52% at 46 months, emphasizing the point that bronchial embolization is a temporizing or palliative measure to control the bleeding but does not treat the underlying causative pathology. A preprocedure CT angiogram and/or bronchoscopy is recommended to determine laterality of the bleed, assess for hypertrophied bronchial arteries (eFig. 21.11), or exclude the rare pulmonary arterial source of the bleed.

The procedure involves obtaining aortic access and performing a descending thoracic angiogram to identify origin, number, and course of the bronchial arteries. Selective catheterization of a bronchial artery with a 5-French catheter and arteriogram is performed. A microcatheter is then advanced further to the region of presumed bleed to reduce the chance of nontarget embolization. Embolization to near stasis is performed with particulates greater than 350 μm. During bronchial artery embolization, the culprit bleeding bronchial artery or branch is typically not identified on angiography, and empirical embolization is performed to the suspected site of bleeding. Therefore, having a reasonable estimation of the source or region of bleeding via a bronchoscopy showing asymmetrical airway blood or a CT showing localized alveolar hemorrhage or other abnormalities is often needed to direct appropriate therapy.

The bronchial arteries have variable anatomy with multiple different combinations of origins, branching patterns, and vessel course (eFig. 21.12). There may also be anomalous and collateral bronchial arteries; the latter typically supply the lung after directly crossing diseased pleura (eFig. 21.13) or via the pulmonary ligament. Unlike the bronchial artery collaterals, these systemic collaterals do not follow the course of bronchi from the hila. An alternative systemic source should be considered in two main settings: when the bronchial artery supply to a known and often peripheral parenchymal abnormality is not demonstrated during angiography or when massive hemoptysis persists despite recent bronchial artery embolization. In these instances, investigating for the presence of anomalous or collateral blood supply may be necessary; unfortunately, this search for an alternative systemic source of hemoptysis can be difficult and time consuming.

PULMONARY ARTERIOGRAPHY

INDICATIONS AND CONTRAINDICATIONS

Multidetector CT pulmonary angiography has largely replaced conventional pulmonary angiography in the localization and diagnosis of pulmonary arterial pathologic conditions, particularly for pulmonary embolism (see Chapter 81). Therefore diagnostic pulmonary angiography is rarely performed in modern practice for purely diagnostic purposes.

Nevertheless, the most common indications for conventional pulmonary angiography are acute pulmonary embolism and diagnosis of pulmonary arteriovenous malformations[41] (eFig. 21.14) as discussed further in Chapter 88. Although there are no randomized trials demonstrating improved clinical outcomes, there is increasing use of catheter-directed thrombolysis and mechanical

thrombectomy for patients presenting with massive pulmonary embolism. Fibrinolytic therapy administered directly into the clot has been shown to increase the rate of lysis alone or in combination with simple mechanical techniques, such as fragmentation of the thrombus with catheter rotation or angioplasty balloons. Newer devices using different mechanisms of thrombectomy and thrombolysis include rheolytic, rotational, and ultrasonic fragmentation and aspiration may have a larger and emerging role in treating massive acute pulmonary emboli in the future.[42]

Less common indications for pulmonary arteriography include the diagnosis of chronic pulmonary embolism, pulmonary sequestration, pulmonary artery stenosis, pulmonary aneurysm or pseudoaneurysm, and pulmonary artery neoplasms.[41–43] Relative contraindications for pulmonary arteriography include severe contrast allergy, severe pulmonary hypertension, and left bundle-branch block.

THERMAL ABLATION OF LOCALIZED LUNG CANCER AND PULMONARY METASTATIC DISEASE

INDICATIONS AND CONTRAINDICATIONS

Thermal ablation of lung nodules using *radiofrequency* (RF) waves, microwaves, or a cryoprobe has been used to obtain local control of malignancy in the chest for more than 15 years.[44–46] All three minimally invasive techniques involve image-guided targeting of lung nodules or masses with needles that induce tumor necrosis via either coagulation necrosis (*radiofrequency ablation* [RFA], microwave) or freezing and thawing of tissues (cryoablation). The most extensive experience with thermal lung ablation has been with RFA. When used in the chest, the needle probes are usually placed via CT guidance, with the patient under conscious sedation or, less often, general anesthesia.

Two primary groups of patients are considered for thermal ablation of the lung: (1) those with small, stage Ia (T1 lesions ≤3 cm) NSCLC in whom surgery is contraindicated or has been declined and (2) patients with malignancy and limited (three or fewer) pulmonary metastases who are not candidates for surgical metastasectomy and have documented control of the primary tumor. For those with limited pulmonary metastases, a potential survival benefit from successful treatment of their metastases should exist to consider thermal ablation. Because many of these same patients are also candidates for external-beam radiation using stereotactic techniques, the decision for nonsurgical candidates to use one or both techniques, if available, is made by a multidisciplinary group in consultation with the patient.

There are several relative or absolute contraindications to performing image-guided thermal ablation of the lung. A patient's inability to cooperate for a prolonged (1.5 hours) procedure on the CT table despite the use of conscious sedation can be managed by the use of general anesthesia with airway maintenance. Coagulopathy is a particular concern with cryoablation, which tends to

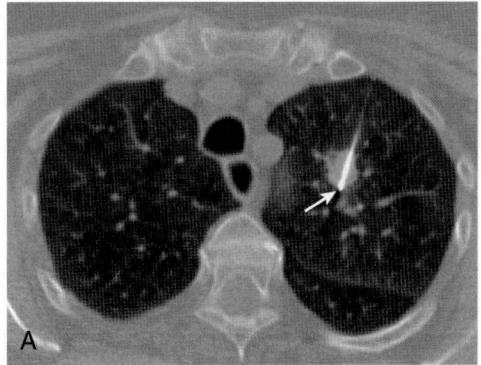
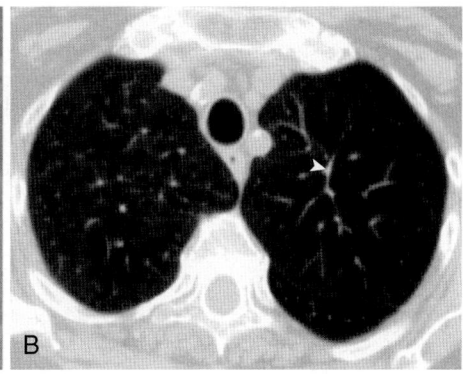

Figure 21.5 Long-term success of radiofrequency ablation for T1a non–small cell carcinoma of lung. (A) Unenhanced computed tomography performed through the upper lobes during radiofrequency ablation shows the electrode *(arrow)* placed through the left upper lobe nodule known to reflect a non–small cell lung carcinoma. (B) Computed tomography scan 5 years after ablation shows a linear scar *(arrowhead)* at the site of the previous nodule.

induce local bleeding as a result of the freezing and thawing of tissue inherent to this technique. For these reasons, any bleeding diathesis should be corrected before thermal ablation. Lesions immediately adjacent to the heart, aorta, superior vena cava, trachea, or esophagus are not amenable to thermal ablation due to concern for damage to these structures. In addition, lesions adjacent to large intrathoracic vessels may not be adequately heated (RFA, microwave) or frozen (cryoablation) because flowing blood in these vessels produces a "heat sink" effect. As a result, temperatures in the part of the lesion nearest the flowing blood may not reach the required cytotoxic temperature, and thus this component of the tumor may remain viable after ablation.

The procedure of performing RFA is similar to the other two approved thermal treatment methods. The patient is positioned as if undergoing CT-guided TNB, with the anticipated puncture site placed nondependently. Because RFA involves electrical current extending from the probe into the surrounding tissues and through the body, grounding pads are placed on the patients' thighs before the procedure to prevent the potential for skin burns by allowing safe egress of electrical current from the body.

For most lung lesions, a single needle probe is used and placed through to the center of the lesion along its long axis. For lesions smaller than 2.5 cm, a standard 14-gauge probe ablates approximately a 3- to 4-cm zone of tissue, which provides effective treatment of the lesion, and a 1-cm zone of normal lung surrounding the lesion, which should treat any microscopic disease at the margin of the tumor. For lesions larger than 2.5 cm, microwave ablation may be preferable because the ablation zone created with microwave probes tends to be larger and more spherical than with RF probes.

Successful RFA or microwave ablation produces a zone of ground-glass opacity surrounding the lesion and needle electrode on CT scans obtained immediately after ablation (eFig. 21.15). With cryoablation, CT obtained after ablation shows a decrease in attenuation of solid nodules because ice generated from pressurized, infused argon gas encompasses the lesion.

Multiple series detailing CT-guided RFA of unresectable early-stage lung cancer and limited pulmonary metastatic disease have shown the procedure to be safe with an acceptable complication rate.[44–46] The most common

complications include pneumothorax in approximately 30–40% of patients, with 10–20% of all patients requiring catheter drainage.[47,48] For lesions situated along the outer edge of the lung, pain typically develops either during the ablation procedure or within 5 days of treatment because RFA induces significant tissue infarction and secondary parietal pleural irritation. Twenty percent of patients, usually those with peripheral lesions, will develop a pleural effusion, with most remaining small and asymptomatic.

Although there are no randomized controlled trials comparing thermal ablation with standard therapies, such as surgery and radiation, multiple studies have shown 2-year survival rates of approximately 70% for the treatment of stage I NSCLC (Fig. 21.5) and for RF-treated colorectal metastases when lesions are 3 cm or smaller in diameter.[49–52] In comparing RFA to microwave ablation for lung cancer and pulmonary metastases, a recent meta-analysis showed that RFA was associated with superior 1-, 2-, 3-, 4- and 5-year survival rates compared to microwave ablation.[53] The majority of lung cancer recurrences are local and are more likely with a larger tumor, with lesions greater than 3 cm in diameter showing significantly higher recurrence rates and lower overall and disease-specific patient survival than those 3 cm or smaller.[54]

PREOPERATIVE COMPUTED TOMOGRAPHY–GUIDED LOCALIZATION FOR VIDEO-ASSISTED THORACIC SURGERY NODULE RESECTION

INDICATIONS AND CONTRAINDICATIONS

With the increased detection of small pulmonary nodules on multidetector chest CT examinations, there is a concomitant increase in the need for pathologic diagnosis of those lesions too small to characterize as definitively benign or to sample accurately with TNB. The most common clinical scenario is the patient with a small lung nodule or nodules and a known primary thoracic or extrathoracic malignancy in whom the diagnosis of metastatic disease must be excluded. A patient with a solitary small lung nodule in whom wedge resection would provide both diagnostic

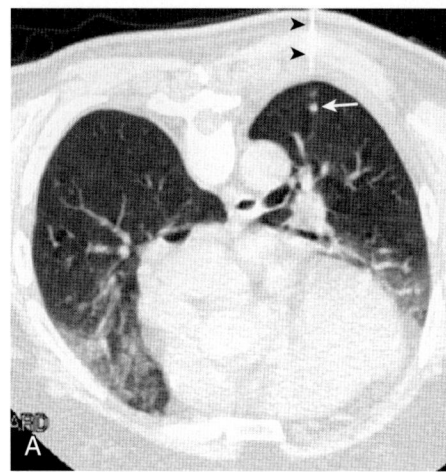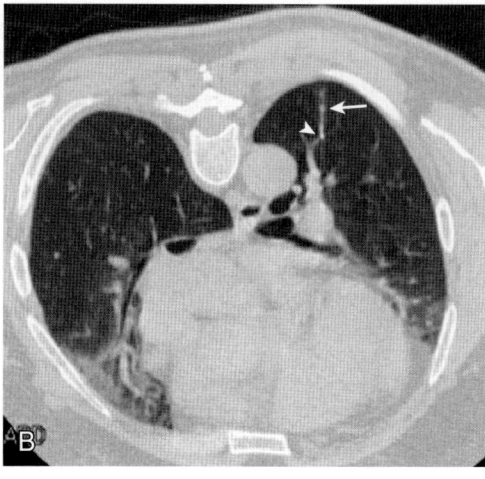

Figure 21.6 Computed tomography–guided needle localization of small peripheral nodule for video-assisted thoracic surgery resection. (A) Computed tomography performed through the mid-chest with the patient in prone position shows a 3-mm left lower lobe nodule *(arrow)* with the guide needle in the posterior chest wall *(black arrowheads)*. (B) Repeat scan after deployment of hook wire shows the wire with its tip *(arrowhead)* deep to the nodule *(arrow)*. The lesion was successfully identified and resected intraoperatively.

information and potential therapeutic benefit may also be considered for VATS resection.

Most solid nodules 1.5 cm or smaller in the lung periphery (i.e., within 1.5 cm of the costal or diaphragmatic pleural surface) can be successfully identified and resected at VATS. In certain patients with lesions smaller than 10 mm or with subsolid nodules, preoperative needle localization may aid the surgeon in identifying nodules intraoperatively. This facilitates successful intraoperative resection of these lesions, particularly if the nodule is greater than 1 cm from the visceral pleural surface and will be difficult to identify intraoperatively.

The preoperative patient preparation and basic technique of marking subpleural nodules for VATS resection is similar to that for TNB. The procedure is typically performed under CT guidance and is coordinated with the operating room so that the patient proceeds directly from radiology to the preoperative holding area and operating room immediately after image-guided localization.

The patient is positioned as if for a CT-guided TNB, with the planned needle approach being the shortest distance between the nodule and the costal pleural surface. This aids the surgeon in using the localizing needle or wire to palpate the subpleural nodule intraoperatively and resect the least amount of normal lung along with the lesion to be removed. Rarely, a biopsy of a small nodule is attempted before the localizing procedure so that a VATS planned for diagnosis can be canceled if the TNB recovers a specimen with positive cytologic results or can proceed if the TNB is nondiagnostic. For patients in whom the VATS resection will be performed regardless of the preoperative diagnosis, only a localization procedure is performed. Ordinarily, conscious sedation is used as for TNB.

Although several differential techniques have been detailed for marking small peripheral nodules to aid VATS resection, most describe placing a needle through the nodule with a hook wire deployed through the needle and positioned with the hook deep to the nodule and left in position to aid resection in the operating room (Fig. 21.6).[55] A dressing is then applied to the skin and the patient transferred to the operating room for VATS.

Additional methods include methylene blue dye injection into the nodule through the coaxial needle with or without autologous blood to reduce rapid dye diffusion. Microcoil and fiducial markers can be placed using a similar technique to the hookwire deployment, with the release of a platinum microcoil or gold fiducial marker. These markers can then be visualized with fluoroscopic guidance during the VATS procedure without the need for external wires. Instead of metallic objects, water-insoluble contrast medium, such as barium or lipiodol, have be used, also visualized by the surgeon with fluoroscopy. Radiotracer-guided localization is performed with injection of technetium-99m tagged to macroaggregated albumin into the nodule, with postprocedure scintigraphy to confirm appropriate placement and intraoperative localization with a gamma probe. Last, if the patient can tolerate complete lung deflation, an intraoperative ultrasonography for localization of lung nodule can be performed for small solid nodules; this approach is not useful for ground-glass lesions.[56]

Published success rates from multiple series detailing preoperative localization before successful VATS resection of peripheral nodules are generally around 90%.[57] Even when a wire or marker becomes displaced after deployment, the puncture site at the visceral pleura is usually visible intraoperatively and helps guide the surgeon to successful resection. Pneumothorax develops in approximately 10% of patients but rarely leads to wire displacement and is easily managed because the patients invariably proceed to thoracoscopy where a pneumothorax is induced as part of the operative procedure.

Key Points

- The most common indications for performing transthoracic needle biopsy include the definitive pathogenic diagnosis of a solitary pulmonary nodule, mediastinal mass, enlarged lymph node, chest wall mass, or pleural mass or thickening.
- Early-stage parapneumonic effusions, particularly when free flowing or unilocular, are amenable to successful image-guided catheter drainage using computed tomographic or ultrasonographic guidance; intrapleural fibrinolytic agents are considered if the patient fails to improve with drainage and antibiotics.
- Indwelling pleural catheter drainage, with or without pleurodesis, provides effective treatment of symptomatic, recurrent malignant pleural effusions, whether or not the lung reexpands.
- Small-bore catheter drainage is a particularly effective treatment for iatrogenic pneumothorax, with success rates exceeding 85%.
- When indicated, catheter drainage for lung abscesses should be performed under computed tomographic guidance, placing the catheter in that part of the abscess closest to the pleural surface, ideally avoiding traversal of normal lung.
- Image-guided thermal ablation of lung tumors is most effective for lesions less than 3 cm in diameter, with higher recurrence rates and lower overall survival for patients with lesions exceeding 3 cm.
- Needle-wire localization of lung nodules before video-assisted thoracoscopic surgical resection is most useful for lesions 1 cm or smaller and more than 1 cm from the pleural surface.

Key Readings

Bargellini I, Bozzi E, Cioni R, et al. Radiofrequency ablation of lung tumours. *Insights Imaging.* 2011;2(5):567–576.

Birchard KR. Transthoracic needle biopsy. *Semin Intervent Radiol.* 2011;28(1):87–97.

Dupuy DE, Fernando HC, Hillman S, et al. Radiofrequency ablation of stage IA non-small cell lung cancer in medically inoperable patients: results from the American College of Surgeons Oncology Group Z4033 (Alliance) trial. *Cancer.* 2015;121:3491.

Gould MK, Donington J, Lynch WR, et al. Evaluation of individuals with pulmonary nodules: when is it lung cancer? Diagnosis and management of lung cancer, 3rd ed: American College of Chest Physicians evidence-based clinical practice guidelines. *Chest.* 2013;143(suppl 5):e93S–e120S.

Kuo WT, Sista AK, Faintuch S, et al. Society of Interventional Radiology position statement on catheter-directed therapy for acute pulmonary embolism. *J Vasc Interv Radiol.* 2018;29:293–297.

Lopez JK, Lee HY. Bronchial artery embolization for treatment of life-threatening hemoptysis. *Semin Intervent Radiol.* 2006;23:223–229.

Shen KR, Bribriesco A, Crabtree T, et al. The American Association for Thoracic Surgery consensus guidelines for the management of empyema. *J Thorac Cardiovasc Surg.* 2017;153:e129–e146.

Complete reference list available at ExpertConsult.com.

22 PATHOLOGY: NEOPLASTIC AND NON-NEOPLASTIC LUNG DISEASE

ANATOLY URISMAN, MD, PHD • KIRK D. JONES, MD •
STEPHEN L. NISHIMURA, MD

INTRODUCTION

The diagnosis of both neoplastic and non-neoplastic lung disease relies heavily on pathologic evaluation of lung tissue. This chapter first reviews the types of biopsy specimens most commonly encountered by pulmonary pathologists, how these different specimens are used in specific clinical scenarios, and how the biopsy tissues are processed for histologic evaluation. The remainder of the chapter is devoted to a summary of the most common neoplastic and non-neoplastic lung lesions encountered in lung biopsies. The discussion is meant as an introduction to lung pathology, with a focus on the general approach to histologic diagnosis and emphasis on the most important clinical and radiologic correlates.

TYPES OF LUNG TISSUE SPECIMENS

Pathologic evaluation of lung tissue plays a critical role in the diagnosis of lung disease. The types of lung specimens evaluated by pathologists vary depending on the diagnostic question, type of lesion, and its accessibility for various biopsy techniques (Table 22.1).

Localized lung lesions such as consolidations or nodules (>5 to 10 mm) can be sampled using percutaneous transthoracic image-guided (most often *computed tomography* [CT]-guided) techniques. Both *fine-needle aspiration* (FNA) and/or needle core biopsy are performed via the percutaneous approach and produce samples only a few millimeters in size but sufficient for histologic classification and additional ancillary studies in many cases. Alternatively, bronchoscopic biopsy techniques can be used to target

mass lesions, particularly those located in the peritracheal or hilar regions. For example, endobronchial ultrasound–guided transbronchial FNA is often used to sample perihilar tumors as well as hilar lymph nodes for possible metastases. Lesions involving the bronchial mucosa that extend into the lumen are readily sampled by endobronchial forceps biopsy.

Diffuse parenchymal lung lesions can be targeted by transbronchial biopsy, including traditional forceps biopsy or more recently developed cryobiopsy techniques. Although transbronchial biopsy can be helpful in classifying some forms of *interstitial lung disease* (ILD), particularly acute lung injury patterns and sarcoidosis, definitive classification of interstitial fibrosis usually requires a more invasive surgical lung biopsy due to the patchy nature of the disease. At present, most surgical lung biopsies are performed via video-assisted thoracoscopic surgery and remain the gold standard for diagnosis of ILD. Although the risk of the procedure is significantly less than that of open lung biopsy, the potential risk of serious complications remains a significant barrier, particularly in patients with advanced disease.[1] More extensive procedures performed for mass lesions, most often tumors, can range in size from subsegmental wedge resections to pneumonectomies. Entire lungs are also evaluated by pathologists following lung transplantation and during autopsy.

Rapid histologic evaluation (frozen section) of tissue samples obtained during surgery is sometimes performed to guide surgical decisions. For example, an intraoperative biopsy of a solid nodule without a prior histologic diagnosis may be performed to determine whether the process is neoplastic or infectious. With this information, the surgeon is made aware of the need for further resection or staging and whether additional material is needed for flow cytometry

Table 22.1   Types of Lung Tissue Specimens Used for Pathologic Evaluation

Specimen Type	Size	Typical Use	Advantages	Limitations
Percutaneous needle ■ FNA ■ Core	1–15 mm	Localized mass lesions targetable by imaging	Safe, no need for general anesthesia	Challenging for small or central lesions
Bronchoscopic ■ Transbronchial ■ Endobronchial ■ EBUS-FNA	1–5 mm	Localized and some diffuse lung lesions, endobronchial and hilar lesions	Less invasive than surgical techniques	Low sensitivity for most diffuse interstitial processes
Surgical biopsy ■ Open lung ■ Thoracoscopy	1–5 cm per site	Diffuse ILD classification	Gold standard in diagnosis of ILD	Higher complication risk than nonsurgical techniques
Surgical resection ■ Wedge ■ Segmentectomy ■ Lobectomy ■ Pneumonectomy	From >5 cm to entire lung	Localized lesion, with or without a prior histologic diagnosis	Allows complete resection; more tissue for diagnosis and additional studies	Increased risk of complications
Autopsy	Entire lung	Evaluation of cause of death	Entire organ available for diagnosis	Postmortem preservation artifacts

EBUS, endobronchial ultrasound; FNA, fine-needle aspiration; ILD, interstitial lung disease.

for diagnosis and classification of hematolymphoid malignancies or for microbial cultures. Tissue samples requiring rapid intraoperative evaluation are snap-frozen and sections are cut in a cryostat while frozen, then briefly fixed in alcohol and stained with *hematoxylin and eosin* (H&E). The entire process is typically performed in less than 15 minutes. Other applications of intraoperative frozen sections include assessment of surgical margins to ensure complete tumor resection and confirmation that sufficient or intended target tissue is obtained. If the sampled tissue is not sufficient for diagnosis, additional diagnostic tissue can be obtained. Evaluation of frozen sections can be challenging due to freezing and sampling artifacts inherent in the method, which results in higher diagnostic uncertainty and higher frequency of misinterpretation when compared to routine histologic evaluation.[2,3] Therefore, unused frozen tissue "remnants" are formalin-fixed and processed using routine histologic techniques. These "permanent sections" have fewer histologic artifacts and allow additional special stains to be performed to help establish the final diagnosis.

TISSUE PROCESSING AND HISTOLOGIC EVALUATION

Lung tissue samples obtained via bronchoscopic biopsy and tissue cores collected by percutaneous biopsy are immediately placed in formalin to ensure optimal preservation of the tissue. Additional tissue is sometimes collected for microbial cultures or other testing such as flow cytometry or electron microscopy; these tissue samples should not be put in formalin and require special transport media for processing. Because bronchoscopic and core samples are small (<15 mm), they are generally properly fixed by formalin within hours and can be histologically examined the day after the procedure. Lung tissue samples obtained during surgical resections are generally larger (>1 cm) and are usually delivered to the pathology department for formalin fixation. Large specimens require longer fixation times for optimal penetration of formalin, which may delay histologic

examination compared to small biopsies. Large specimens, once fixed, are dissected and evaluated grossly to identify the most representative or diagnostic areas, from which sections are taken for histologic evaluation. In tumor resection specimens, in addition to sampling the tumor, sections are also taken to evaluate the margins and to assess tumor stage (e.g., invasion into adjacent structures or lymph node involvement).

The tissue sections are placed in cassettes for processing, which is usually automated and includes dehydration (with alcohol), clearing (with xylene), and paraffin wax infiltration steps. The processed *formalin fixed paraffin embedded* (FFPE) tissue blocks are then cut into 3- to 5-μm thick tissue sections, which can be stained by various histochemical techniques (Table 22.2). H&E is the mainstay of microscopic evaluation used by pathologists and is the only stain required for diagnosis in many cases. However, additional special histochemical stains may be needed to highlight specific histologic structures or cellular or extracellular components (e.g., mucin, basement membranes, collagen, elastic fibers, amyloid), elements or minerals (e.g., calcium or iron), or microbial cell wall components (e.g., mycobacteria or fungi).

Over the last several decades, *immunohistochemical* (IHC) stains targeting specific cellular proteins have been developed to aid in the diagnosis of diverse neoplastic and nonneoplastic lesions.[4] These stains employ antibodies directed against defined cellular components such as various cytokeratins, transcription factors, or surface glycoproteins. A histologic section is first incubated with a primary antigen-specific antibody, and bound antibodies are then detected by a secondary antibody conjugated to an enzyme that catalyzes a chromogenic (color-producing) chemical reaction. The resulting stable brown (or sometimes red) staining pattern can be visualized under a regular light microscope. Hundreds of IHC markers are currently used by pathology practices and are a critical component of the diagnostic workup to determine the neoplastic or infectious nature of a pathologic process. Common IHC markers used in diagnosis of lung cancer are listed in Table 22.3.

Table 22.2 Common Histochemical Stains

Stain	Purpose	Appearance
Hematoxylin and eosin	Primary histologic evaluation	Nuclei/chromatin: blue Cytoplasm, collagen, fibrin: pink
Verhoeff-Van Gieson	Highlight elastic fibers	Elastic fibers: brown-black (silver stain)
Trichrome	Highlight areas of fibrosis	Collagen fibers: blue
Periodic acid–Schiff	Highlight basement membranes, glycoproteins, mucin	Basement membranes, mucin: pink-purple
Congo red	Identify tissue amyloid deposits	Amyloid: orange-red under routine light microscopy, changes to apple-green (birefringence) under polarized light
Perls Prussian blue	Highlight ferric iron in ferritin and hemosiderin, and ferruginous bodies	Iron deposits: dark blue
Mucicarmine	Highlight mucin; identify polysaccharide capsule of *Cryptococcus* species	Mucin: pink-purple
Grocott-Gomori methenamine silver	Identify fungi (stains fungal cell walls)	Fungi: brown-black (silver stain)
Acid-fast bacilli (e.g., Kinyoun or Fite)	Identify mycobacteria (stains mycobacterial cell walls)	Pink-red
Gram (e.g., Brown-Brenn)	Identify bacteria (stains bacterial cell walls)	Gram-positive: purple-blue Gram-negative: pink

Table 22.3 Common Immunohistochemical Stains Used in Diagnosis of Lung Cancer

Target Protein	Pulmonary Cell Type	Cellular Localization	Common Diagnostic Use
Cytokeratins (multiple)	All epithelial cells	Cytoplasmic	Carcinoma (positive) vs. sarcoma (negative) Pulmonary adenocarcinoma (CK7)
TTF-1	Bronchiolar epithelial cells, alveolar epithelial type 2 cells	Nuclear	Pulmonary adenocarcinoma
Napsin A	Alveolar epithelial type 2 cells, alveolar macrophages	Cytoplasmic	Pulmonary adenocarcinoma
p63 or p40	Bronchial epithelial basal cells, squamous cells	Nuclear	Squamous cell carcinoma, other
Synaptophysin	Neuroendocrine cells	Cytoplasmic	Neuroendocrine tumors
Chromogranin A	Neuroendocrine cells	Cytoplasmic	Neuroendocrine tumors
Ki-67	All dividing cells	Nuclear	Proliferation index (% dividing cells)

Additional ancillary studies performed on tissue sections include RNA-directed in situ hybridization (e.g., to detect RNA transcripts of Epstein-Barr virus or human papillomavirus), fluorescence in situ hybridization (e.g., to detect common gene fusions or translocations in numerous malignancies), and increasingly other molecular techniques.[5] For example, tissue sections are used as starting material for isolation of nucleic acids for downstream sequencing applications, including detection of genetic alterations, evaluation of mRNA expression or DNA methylation profiles of specific genes, and detection of various pathogens. Mass spectrometry–based proteomic techniques that utilize FFPE tissue are also being developed (e.g., amyloid subtyping).[6] Many of these techniques can be applied retrospectively on archival FFPE blocks in both research and clinical applications. Further development and widespread adoption of molecular techniques are anticipated to transform the practice of pathology over the next decades and will have a major impact on how we diagnose, subclassify, and treat both neoplastic and nonneoplastic lung disease.

CYTOLOGY SPECIMENS

Cytology is a subfield of pathology that uses cells obtained from fluids or removed from tissues to determine a diagnosis. Common thoracic cytology specimens include sputum samples, pleural fluid aspirates, bronchoalveolar lavage fluid, and FNA samples collected using bronchoscopic or transcutaneous techniques. Clinicians collecting these samples must consider the differential diagnosis and plan accordingly if a sample needs to be apportioned for multiple tests in addition to the routine microscopic cytologic evaluation (e.g., microbial cultures, flow cytometry, or molecular assays).

The cytologic evaluation of fluid samples, such as pleural or bronchoalveolar aspirates, begins with sample centrifugation to concentrate the cells, after which a variety of techniques can be used to prepare slides for microscopic evaluation. Traditionally, a direct smear from the cell pellet is made, followed by air drying or alcohol fixation and staining. However, over the past 2 decades, several commercial systems for liquid-based cytology have been developed to automate the entire process of cell centrifugation, slide preparation, and staining.[7] In addition to the cytologic slide preparations, large volumes of fluid can be centrifuged into cell pellets to make FFPE histologic blocks. These so-called cell blocks have the advantage of the traditional FFPE tissue blocks because they allow the full range of conventional sectioning and staining techniques (including histochemical and immunohistochemical stains), molecular nucleic acid–based tests, and long-term archival storage.[8] However, in general, histologic sections prepared from cell blocks do not provide information about the tissue architecture.

FNA biopsies are typically more cellular than body fluid samples, and smears can be prepared directly from the aspirated material without centrifugation. A small portion of the aspirate is spread on a glass slide, which is then air dried or alcohol fixed and stained for cytologic evaluation. The remaining aspirate is typically used to prepare an FFPE cell block and used for other testing modalities (e.g., microbial cultures or flow cytometry) if needed.

Cytopathologists and trained cytology technicians often perform rapid on-site evaluation of FNA samples at the time they are being acquired by radiologists or interventional pulmonologists.[9] Rapid on-site evaluation ensures that a target lesion is adequately sampled and allows real-time decision making about sample handling. For example, if an inflammatory lesion is encountered, a portion of the sample is sent for microbial cultures. Rapid on-site evaluation has been shown to decrease the number of nondiagnostic FNAs and to reduce the need for repeat procedures.[10]

EVALUATION OF NEOPLASTIC LUNG LESIONS

Pathologic evaluation continues to be a critical component in the diagnosis, staging, prognostication, and treatment of lung cancer. This discussion focuses on the most common subtypes of primary lung cancer. Other less common lung neoplasms are discussed in Chapters 78 through 80.

A histologic (and increasingly a molecular) classification of a suspected lung neoplasm is the main objective of the initial diagnostic evaluation. Small samples, such as image-guided core biopsies or bronchoscopic FNAs, are most frequently used for this purpose.[11] In contrast, most surgical resections (both primary and post–neoadjuvant therapy) may be curative but also serve to confirm and refine the initial histologic diagnosis, determine the pathologic tumor stage, assess resection margins, and evaluate response to pre-resection therapy (when applicable).

The three most common histologic subtypes of lung cancer are adenocarcinoma and squamous cell carcinoma (comprising non–small cell lung carcinomas [NSCLCs]), and small cell lung carcinoma (SCLC), which together account for approximately 85% of all lung cancer cases.[12] Other histologic subtypes encompass a diverse list of tumors (Table 22.4), some relatively common (e.g., carcinoid tumors) and

Table 22.4 World Health Organization Classification of Tumors of the Lung (2015)[20]

Adenocarcinoma
- Lepidic adenocarcinoma
- Acinar adenocarcinoma
- Papillary adenocarcinoma
- Micropapillary adenocarcinoma
- Solid adenocarcinoma
- Invasive mucinous adenocarcinoma
- Colloid adenocarcinoma
- Fetal adenocarcinoma
- Enteric adenocarcinoma
- Adenocarcinoma in situ
- Minimally invasive adenocarcinoma

Squamous cell carcinoma
- Keratinizing squamous cell carcinoma
- Nonkeratinizing squamous cell carcinoma
- Basaloid squamous cell carcinoma
- Squamous cell carcinoma in situ

Neuroendocrine tumors
- Small cell carcinoma
- Large cell neuroendocrine carcinoma
- Carcinoid tumor
- Diffuse idiopathic pulmonary neuroendocrine cell hyperplasia

Large cell carcinoma

Adenosquamous carcinoma

Sarcomatoid carcinoma

Salivary gland–type tumors

Papillomas

Adenomas

Mesenchymal tumors

Lymphohistiocytic tumors

Tumors of ectopic origin

Metastases to the lung

some exceedingly rare. The classification of lung neoplasms continues to evolve, with molecular diagnostic techniques playing an increasingly important role in defining subcategories relevant to prognosis, treatment selection, and response to therapy (see also Chapter 73).

Historically, the most important distinction in the diagnosis of lung cancer was between SCLC and NSCLC, because SCLC often presents at advanced stage, is resistant to treatment, generally does not benefit from surgical resection, and has markedly worse prognosis compared to NSCLC.[13] However, over the past 2 decades, in addition to this distinction, more precise histologic subclassification of NSCLC has become critically important in the evaluation of lung cancer, prompted by the advances in systemic therapy for specific histologic subtypes and the introduction of targeted therapies.[14]

ADENOCARCINOMA

Adenocarcinomas account for approximately 40% of all lung cancer cases in the United States.[12] A large portion of pulmonary adenocarcinomas are thought to arise from components of the terminal respiratory unit (i.e., acinus).[15,16] These tumors arise in the peripheral lung parenchyma, and the tumor cells transcriptionally resemble

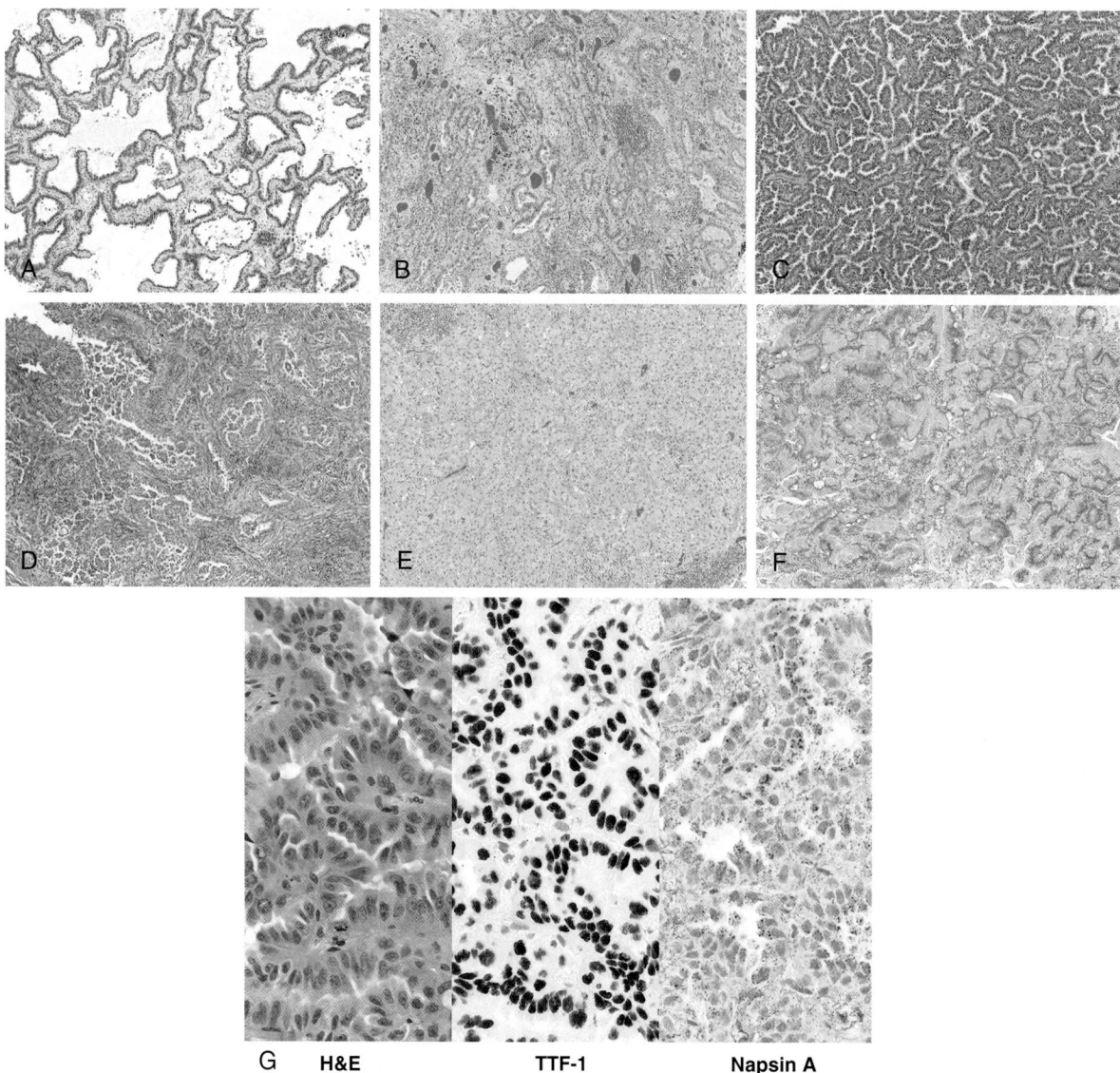

Figure 22.1 Pulmonary adenocarcinoma. Architectural patterns of growth are the basis of histologic grading of adenocarcinoma and include the following types. (A) Lepidic: neoplastic cells grow along preexisting alveolar septa without stromal invasion. (B) Acinar: neoplastic cells form irregular glands with stromal invasion. (C) Papillary: neoplastic cells line branchlike structures called papillae that grow from preexisting alveolar septa and contain fibrovascular bundles at their cores. (D) Micropapillary: neoplastic cells form small papillary-like tufts that lack a central fibrovascular core and shed extensively into alveolar spaces. (E) Solid: neoplastic cells grow as sheets or solid nests that are often invasive into the stroma. (F) Mucinous: alveoli, papillae, or acini are lined by characteristic columnar pseudostratified cells with abundant mucinous cytoplasm and basal ovoid nuclei (hematoxylin and eosin [H&E]; ×100 original magnification). (G) Immunohistochemical stains useful in diagnosis of pulmonary adenocarcinoma (×200 original magnification). TTF-1, thyroid transcription factor 1.

alveolar epithelial type 2 cells (i.e., express *thyroid transcription factor 1* [TTF1] and napsin A). In addition, adenocarcinomas can arise throughout the bronchoalveolar tree, including in association with larger caliber airways (i.e., non–terminal respiratory unit tumors). These tumors often lack expression of TTF1 and napsin A and histologically resemble bronchial columnar epithelial or mucinous cells.[17]

Conventional non-mucinous pulmonary adenocarcinoma (also called adenocarcinoma not otherwise specified) may exhibit several architectural patterns of growth such as lepidic (along the alveolar septa), acinar, papillary, micropapillary, or solid (Fig. 22.1). The predominant architectural pattern is an important predictor of survival in adenocarcinoma. Therefore, the 2011 International Association for the Study of Lung Cancer/American Thoracic Society/European Respiratory Society lung adenocarcinoma classification recommends that the diagnosis of adenocarcinoma should include the predominant histologic pattern, and enumeration of all patterns within a tumor (as percent of total in 5% increments) is encouraged in all resection specimens.[18] Tumor grading schemes use histologic features such as degree of cell differentiation (or similarity to benign counterparts) as predictors of tumor behavior. Although no universally accepted tumor grading system for adenocarcinoma has been developed, a simple system largely based on the predominant architectural pattern is in wide use today (Table 22.5). Some authors also advocate the use of mitotic count in grading pulmonary adenocarcinoma.[19]

In addition to pulmonary adenocarcinoma not otherwise specified, several distinct histologic adenocarcinoma variants are recognized by the 2015 *World Health Organization* (WHO) classification,[20] including invasive mucinous (formally mucinous bronchioloalveolar carcinoma), colloid, enteric, and fetal adenocarcinoma. These rare variants have characteristic architectural and cytologic appearance and appear to represent biologically distinct categories. For example, invasive mucinous adenocarcinomas often exhibit oncogenic *KRAS* mutations, frequently present with multifocal lung involvement which can mimic pneumonia on CT scan, and may show aggressive clinical behavior.[21]

Staging of adenocarcinoma follows the general tumor-node-metastasis guidelines for lung tumors (see later and Chapter 76). However, two categories deserve a special mention. Adenocarcinoma *in situ* (is) is defined as a tumor 3 cm or less in size and composed of lepidic growth pattern only. Minimally invasive adenocarcinoma is defined as a lepidic-predominant tumor of up to 3 cm in size, wherein the invasive component cannot exceed 5 mm. Both adenocarcinoma in situ and *minimally invasive* (mi) adenocarcinoma have excellent prognosis, with near 100% 5-year survival, and are given the pathologic stage of pT0is and pT1mi, respectively. Both adenocarcinoma in situ and minimally invasive adenocarcinoma are thought to be precursor lesions for higher-grade adenocarcinomas.[18]

Molecular profiling studies of lung adenocarcinoma have identified recurrent activating genetic alterations in several driver oncogenes, including mutations in *KRAS* (30% of cases), *EGFR* (15–30%) and *BRAF* (5–10%); and rearrangements of *ALK* (5%) and *ROS1* (<2%), among others.[22]

Table 22.5 Adenocarcinoma Grading System Based on the 2011 IASLC/ATS/ERS International Multidisciplinary Classification of Lung Adenocarcinoma[18]

Predominant Architectural Pattern	Tumor Grade
Lepidic	Low grade (G1, well-differentiated)
Acinar, papillary	Intermediate grade (G2, moderately differentiated)
Solid, micropapillary	High grade (G3, poorly differentiated)

IASLC/ATS/ESR, International Association for the Study of Lung Cancer/American Thoracic Society/European Respiratory Society.

Specific inhibitors targeting many of these oncogenes are now available and have transformed the treatment options of patients with lung adenocarcinoma. As a result, routine testing for the most common actionable mutations in adenocarcinoma is now standard practice, particularly in advanced-stage cases requiring systemic therapy.[23,24] Although single-gene testing for common genetic alterations is still in use, targeted multiplex gene sequencing panels using next-generation sequencing are now preferred. The next-generation sequencing multiplex panels provide more comprehensive coverage of known genetic alterations, do not require division of the sample for multiple tests, and offer turnaround times approaching those of single-gene assays. Both biopsy tissue blocks and cytology preparations (cell blocks or smears) are compatible with next-generation sequencing panels as long as there is sufficient tumor cellularity (at least 20%).[23]

SQUAMOUS CELL CARCINOMA

Squamous cell carcinoma (SCC) accounts for approximately 25% of all lung cancer cases in the United States.[12] Chronic smoking continues to be the most important risk factor for SCC. Smoking is thought to promote transformation of bronchial epithelial lesions from squamous metaplasia to dysplasia, to carcinoma in situ, and finally to invasive carcinoma.[25,26] Historically, up to two-thirds of SCC presented as central lung tumors in association with hilar airways.[27] However, over the past 2 decades, there has been an increase in the proportion of peripheral SCC, which also coincided with a declining proportion of SCC relative to adenocarcinoma in smokers.[28,29] Although the reasons for these trends are not well understood, the shift from unfiltered to filtered cigarettes in the 1960s and 1970s has been proposed as a possible contributor.[30]

The morphologic features of squamous cell differentiation include intercellular bridges, keratinization of individual cells, and formation of keratin pearls (Fig. 22.2). These features are readily apparent in well-differentiated tumors, can be subtle or focal in moderately differentiated tumors, and may be entirely absent in poorly differentiated tumors. The diagnosis of SCC is supported by nuclear expression of p63 (or its splice variant p40) and the lack of expression of pulmonary adenocarcinoma markers (TTF1 and napsin A) by IHC.[31] Next-generation sequencing of SCC has identified recurrent alterations in *TP53* (65%), *PIK3CA* (30%), *CDKN2A* (25%), *SOX2* (15%), and *CCND1*

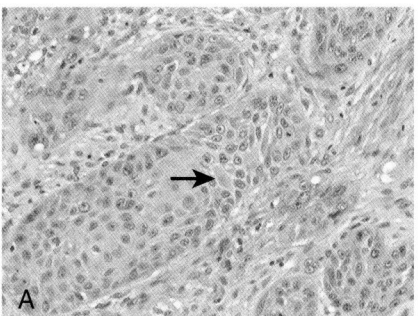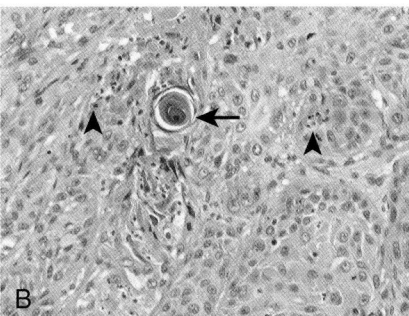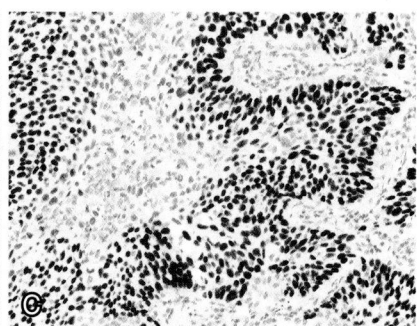

Figure 22.2 Squamous cell carcinoma. Histologic features include (A) intercellular bridges (*arrow*), (B) intracellular keratinization (*arrowheads*), and keratin pearls (*arrow*) (hematoxylin and eosin; ×100 original magnification). (C) Brown staining demonstrates expression of p40, helpful in confirming squamous differentiation, particularly in poorly differentiated tumors (×200 original magnification).

(15%), none of which are currently actionable for targeted therapy.[32,33] Although *FGFR1* amplification is observed in up to 20% of SCC, FGFR inhibitors alone have been largely ineffective.[34]

The 2015 WHO classification recognizes three histologic subtypes of SCC (keratinizing, nonkeratinizing, and basaloid), but there appears to be little prognostic significance to the three subtypes.[20] Similarly, although several grading systems (which categorize SCC as well differentiated, moderately differentiated, or poorly differentiated) have been proposed, none is uniformly accepted.

SMALL CELL CARCINOMA

SCLC accounts for 10–15% of lung cancer cases in the United States.[12] Most cases present with a perihilar mass, and over 80% of cases are at an advanced stage (III or IV) at presentation.[35] Importantly, current studies on the utility of low-dose CT screening in heavy smokers suggest that, unlike NSCLC, screening may not significantly improve the rate of detection of early-stage tumors or reduce mortality in SCLC.[36] The diagnosis is most often made using transbronchial biopsy or FNA. Surgical resections are rare and most often performed for small solitary lesions, where surgery in the context of multimodality therapy may have a role in improving survival.[37]

Histologically, SCLCs are solid neoplasms with very cellular sheetlike or nested growth architecture.[38] The tumor cells characteristically have scant pale cytoplasm, which gives an impression of "small" cell size. However, the overall cell size is still two to three times that of a lymphocyte. The nuclei usually show high pleomorphism, fragile nuclear envelopes (manifest as nuclear "smudging" and "molding"), finely granular nuclear chromatin, and absent or inconspicuous nucleoli (Fig. 22.3). Mitotic activity is characteristically high, and necrosis is usually extensive. Although not required, immunohistochemical staining is helpful in confirming the diagnosis. SCLC cells are often positive for neuroendocrine markers (e.g., synaptophysin and chromogranin A) and show a high (usually >80%) Ki-67 *proliferation index*, that is, the percentage of the malignant cells that are undergoing division, as measured by IHC staining for Ki-67, a nuclear protein expressed during cell division. Next-generation sequencing of SCLC has revealed a highly characteristic bi-allelic inactivation of *TP53* and *RB1* in approximately 90% of the tumors.[39,40]

Rarely, SCLC can present in combination with other types of NSCLC such as large cell carcinoma, adenocarcinoma, squamous cell carcinoma, or other less common histologic types. To date, no significant difference in clinical features, prognosis, or response to therapy has been demonstrated in these combined tumors compared with pure SCLC.[41,42]

LARGE CELL NEUROENDOCRINE CARCINOMA

Large cell neuroendocrine carcinoma (LCNEC) accounts for approximately 3% of resected lung cancer cases.[43] LCNEC is a high-grade neuroendocrine carcinoma that shares some morphologic and molecular similarities with SCLC.[44] However, like other types of NSCLC, LCNEC has a better prognosis than SCLC.[45] The common histologic features include nested or trabecular (cord-like) pattern of growth, frequently with peripheral palisading, and abundant central necrosis

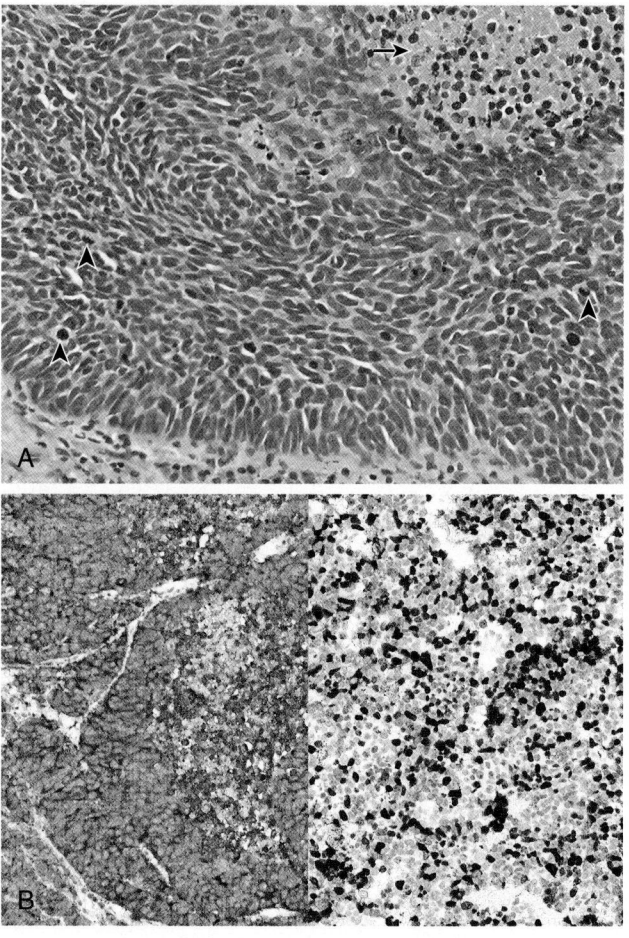

Synaptophysin   **Ki-67**

Figure 22.3 Small cell lung carcinoma. (A) Cells appear "small" due to high nucleus to cytoplasm ratio. Nuclei contain finely granular chromatin and lack prominent nucleoli. Note scattered mitotic figures (*arrowheads*) and focal necrosis (*arrow*) (hematoxylin and eosin, ×400 original magnification). (B) Expression of synaptophysin by immunohistochemical staining is helpful in confirming neuroendocrine differentiation (×200 original magnification). Ki-67 stain shows a high (>80%) proliferation rate (×200 original magnification).

within the tumor nests (Fig. 22.4). The tumor cells are large and polygonal, with abundant cytoplasm, and nuclei with frequent prominent nucleoli and neuroendocrine-like coarse or vesicular chromatin. The mitotic rate is high (11 or more per 2 mm² with a mean of 60 per 2 mm²). The diagnosis is confirmed by the presence of at least one immunohistochemical marker of neuroendocrine differentiation, such as synaptophysin, chromogranin A, or neural cell adhesion molecule (CD56). Molecular profiling of LCNEC has identified two major molecular subtypes: SCLC-like group with high frequency of *TP53* and *RB1* co-mutation or loss, and NSCLC-like group with genetic alterations characteristic of NSCLC (including *STK11, KRAS,* and *KEAP1*). However, no significant differences in clinical characteristics, including survival, have been identified between the two groups.[46]

CARCINOID TUMORS

Carcinoid tumors account for less than 5% of all invasive lung neoplasms.[12] Although SCLC, LCNEC, and carcinoid tumors are grouped together under the general category of neuroendocrine neoplasms in the 2015 WHO classification of lung tumors, it is clear that carcinoid tumors (also known as well-differentiated neuroendocrine tumors) have major biologic differences compared with the high-grade LCNEC and SCLC (Table 22.6).[47,48] Carcinoid tumors in younger patients do not have a strong association with smoking and have a significantly better prognosis than either LCNEC or SCLC.[49]

Carcinoid tumors may arise centrally, often in association with a large airway where they may have a significant luminal component, or less commonly in the distal subpleural parenchyma.[47,50] The tumors have smooth lobulated borders on imaging and may bleed during biopsy owing to their extensive vascular supply. A classic pattern shows organoid (nested) growth of cytologically uniform cells with neuroendocrine appearance (Fig. 22.5). The cells have round or ovoid nuclei with smooth nuclear envelopes, finely granular ("salt and pepper") chromatin, and moderate-to-abundant eosinophilic or granular cytoplasm. However, a variety of other growth patterns (trabecular, papillary, or rosette-like, among others) and cell features (e.g., spindle cell, acinic cell-like, signet-ring, mucin-producing, or melanocytic) have been described. These patterns do not have prognostic significance but are important for pathologists to recognize to avoid misclassification.

Lung carcinoid tumors are traditionally classified as either typical carcinoid ($\approx$90%) or the more aggressive atypical carcinoid ($\approx$10%). According to the 2015 WHO diagnostic criteria, typical carcinoids have low mitotic rates (<2 per 2 mm^2) and lack tumor cell necrosis, whereas atypical carcinoids have higher mitotic counts (2 to 10 per 2 mm^2) and/or demonstrate tumor cell necrosis, which may be focal or punctate.[20] Typical carcinoids tend to be smaller at presentation, less frequently metastasize, and have a better prognosis than the atypical carcinoids (5-year survival is approximately 90% for typical compared to 60% for atypical carcinoids). Importantly, regional lymph node involvement should not be used to distinguish between the two types of carcinoid tumors because it is present in approximately 10% of typical carcinoid as well as 50% of atypical carcinoid cases.[47,50]

Carcinoid tumors stain strongly for neuroendocrine markers such as synaptophysin, chromogranin, and CD56. The Ki-67 proliferation index in typical carcinoid is low (<5%) compared with atypical (5–20%). Ki-67 staining is particularly helpful in small biopsies for separating either of the carcinoid tumors from high-grade neuroendocrine carcinomas (LCNEC and SCLC), which have much higher proliferation rates (typically >40% and >60%, respectively).[47,51]

OTHER LESS COMMON TUMOR TYPES

Adenosquamous carcinoma accounts for 1% of lung cancer cases in the United States. It is defined by the presence of both adenocarcinoma and squamous cell carcinoma when each component comprises at least 10% of the entire tumor. This diagnosis is difficult to make definitively in small biopsies and is usually reserved for resected specimens. Molecular testing of these tumors often reveals genetic alterations commonly found in adenocarcinoma, including mutations in *EGFR* and *KRAS*.[52,53]

Large cell (undifferentiated) carcinoma is a subtype of NSCLC. It is a diagnosis of exclusion reserved for undifferentiated

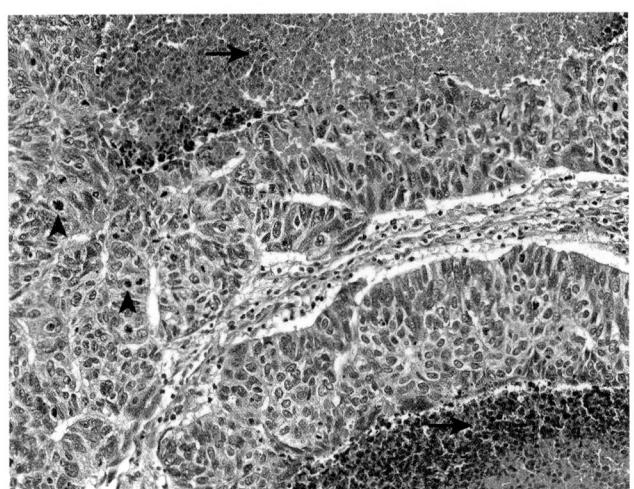

Figure 22.4 Large cell neuroendocrine carcinoma. Large cell neuroendocrine carcinoma cells have more ample cytoplasm and more frequent nucleoli than in small cell lung carcinoma. Note the ribbon-like architecture, areas of necrosis (*arrows*), and frequent mitotic figures (*arrowheads*) (hematoxylin and eosin; ×200 original magnification).

Table 22.6 Lung Neuroendocrine Tumors

	Typical Carcinoid	Atypical Carcinoid	Large Cell Neuroendocrine Carcinoma	Small Cell Lung Carcinoma
WHO grade	Low (grade 1)	Intermediate (grade 2)	High (grade 4)	High (grade 4)
Morphology/cytology	Well-differentiated/ neuroendocrine cells	Well-differentiated/ neuroendocrine cells	Poorly differentiated/non-small cells	Poorly differentiated/small cell
Mitoses (per 2 mm^2)	<2	2–10	>10	>10
Necrosis	No	May be present (focal, punctate)	Yes (extensive)	Yes (extensive)
Ki-67 index (%)	<5	5–20	40–90	60–96
Neuroendocrine markers by immunohistochemistry	Yes	Yes	Yes (required)	Absent in 10–15% of cases (not required)

WHO, World Health Organization.

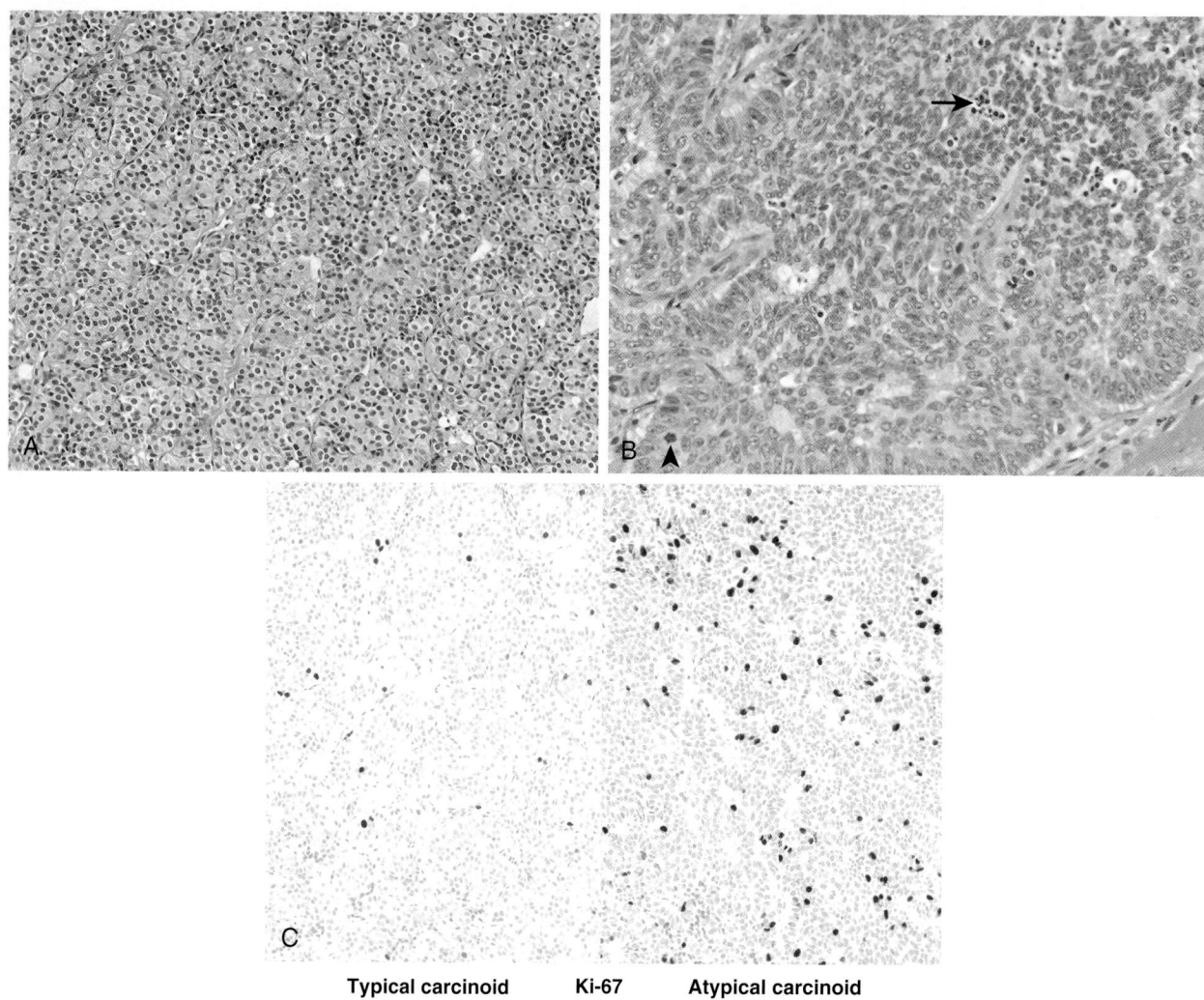

Figure 22.5 Carcinoid tumors. (A) Typical carcinoid with classic organoid architecture and cytologically uniform cells; no mitosis or necrosis is seen (hematoxylin and eosin [H&E]; ×200 original magnification). (B) Atypical carcinoid with increased nuclear pleomorphism, occasional mitoses (*arrowhead*), and small foci of necrosis (*arrow*) (H&E; ×400 original magnification). (C) Immunohistochemical staining for Ki-67 shows a lower proliferation index in typical carcinoid than in atypical carcinoid (×200 original magnification).

tumors that lack features of adenocarcinoma, squamous cell carcinoma, or neuroendocrine carcinoma. In the past 2 decades, the widespread use of IHC markers to help distinguish poorly differentiated cases of adenocarcinoma and squamous cell carcinoma has significantly reduced the number of cases diagnosed as large cell carcinoma, from about 9% of all lung cancer cases in the 1980s to less than 2% at present.[12,54] Recent molecular evidence also parallels this trend. Up to one-third of large cell carcinoma tumors that cannot be further classified histologically harbor molecular alterations characteristic of adenocarcinoma, and up to one-fourth harbor those typical of SCC. Importantly, at least 20% of the tumors do not reveal any recognizable lineage-specific genetic profiles, suggesting that large cell carcinoma will likely remain a rare histologic subtype in need of further characterization.[55]

Sarcomatoid carcinomas are the rarest histologic subgroup of the major types of lung cancer and account for 0.5% of all invasive lung malignancies in the United States. These poorly differentiated tumors histologically resemble sarcomas and may have pleomorphic, sarcomatoid, or sarcomatous elements. They are often bulky and have aggressive

invasive clinical behavior. Immunohistochemical expression of epithelial markers, particularly keratins, is helpful in confirming epithelial rather than mesenchymal origin, thus confirming the diagnosis of carcinoma rather than sarcoma. Peripheral tumors can be challenging to distinguish from sarcomatoid mesothelioma. In these cases, IHC stains for tissue-specific antigens such as TTF1 and mesothelial markers may be helpful.[56,57]

PATHOLOGIC STAGING

Staging of lung tumors is performed using guidelines provided by the American Joint Commission on Cancer in the United States and by the Union for International Cancer Control internationally.[58,59] Pathologic staging considerations are relevant to both resection specimens and some small biopsies. In resection specimens, tumor size is measured either grossly or microscopically, and the largest dimension is reported with millimeter precision. Surgical resection margins (i.e., edges of the specimen that have tissue transected by the operation, which most often include lung parenchyma, bronchi, and pulmonary vessels) are evaluated for the presence of tumor. The distance from tumor to the closest margin is measured, both grossly and microscopically, and recorded in the report. Tumor invasion into mediastinal structures, pleura, or chest wall is assessed grossly and in histologic sections. All surgically sampled lymph nodes, as well as lymph nodes identified within the resection specimen, are evaluated for the presence of metastases. Microscopic evaluation may also reveal lymphovascular or perineural invasion, both of which are markers of more aggressive tumor behavior.

Small biopsies of presumed metastatic sites (e.g., hilar lymph nodes or extrathoracic sites) may be used to stage and identify the histologic subtype of lung cancer and to provide tissue for molecular marker analysis. Similarly, sampling of two (or more) simultaneously identified lung masses may be used to distinguish between metastatic disease and synchronous primaries.

Most pathology practices follow standardized cancer reporting protocols, also known as *tumor synoptics*, such as those available from the College of American Pathologists.[60] These protocols are regularly updated and are available for the entire range of cancer types, including lung cancer. Standardized reporting facilitates data collection by local and national cancer tracking databases and enables longitudinal studies of cancer trends. Lung cancer staging is further discussed in Chapter 76.

EVALUATION OF NON-NEOPLASTIC LUNG DISEASE

Transbronchial biopsies are most useful in diagnosis of acute lung injury patterns, pulmonary sarcoidosis, some localized processes (particularly when aided by endobronchial ultrasound or electromagnetic navigation), and in evaluation of lung allograft rejection. Nodules and sometimes more diffuse consolidative processes can also be sampled by percutaneous CT-guided biopsy. However, small transbronchial biopsies are not sufficient for definitive diagnosis of most diffuse chronic patterns of ILD, particularly those with interstitial fibrosis, due to their non-uniform distribution in the lung and the difficulty in sampling subpleural parenchyma.[61,62] Recent experience from several centers shows that transbronchial cryobiopsy has improved sensitivity for ILD classification compared to conventional transbronchial biopsy and has the potential to be used as an alternative to surgical lung biopsy.[63] However, surgical lung biopsy continues to be the gold standard in ILD diagnosis. Therefore, the discussion later is focused largely on histopathologic evaluation of surgical lung biopsies.

In patients with ILD, histologic evaluation of surgical biopsies may show distinct histologic patterns useful in generating a differential diagnosis of possible etiologies or associated conditions. Liebow and Carrington published their classification of interstitial pneumonias in 1969.[64] While their classification continues to be refined by new knowledge about the underlying mechanisms and by newly recognized clinicopathologic entities,[62,65,66] the major histologic patterns of ILD (Table 22.7) have remained unchanged over several decades and continue to serve as the foundation of histologic evaluation. There are several methods of

Table 22.7 Histologic Patterns of Interstitial Lung Disease

Acute lung injury
- Diffuse alveolar damage
- Organizing pneumonia
- Acute fibrinous and organizing pneumonia

Consolidation of alveolar spaces
- Eosinophilic pneumonia
- Desquamative interstitial pneumonia
- Pulmonary alveolar proteinosis

Interstitial fibrosis
- Usual interstitial pneumonia
- Nonspecific interstitial pneumonia (fibrosing NSIP)

Interstitial inflammation
- Nonspecific interstitial pneumonia (cellular NSIP)
- Lymphocytic interstitial pneumonia
- Hypersensitivity pneumonitis

evaluating lung biopsies according to pattern of injury and distribution of disease.[67–69] The following set of questions is provided as a conceptual framework for understanding how findings in a lung biopsy can help define the disease process.

IS THERE ACUTE LUNG INJURY?

The acute lung injury patterns traditionally included *diffuse alveolar damage* (DAD) and *organizing pneumonia* (OP). *Acute fibrinous and organizing pneumonia* (AFOP) is a more recently described pattern.[70] Recognition of these patterns of lung injury is important because they are most often associated with severe acute or subacute respiratory illness. A unifying feature of acute lung injury patterns is the presence of cellular or proteinaceous exudates in the alveolar spaces, which are likely recognized on high-resolution CT as areas of consolidation.

Diffuse Alveolar Damage

The *acute phase* of DAD (Fig. 22.6A) is histologically characterized by diffuse injury of the alveolar septa.[71,72] Both alveolar epithelial and endothelial cells show changes ranging from swelling to necrosis. The alveolar septa show interstitial edema and scattered inflammatory cells in the alveolar septal capillaries. The alveolar spaces accumulate proteinaceous exudate containing serum, fibrin, scattered macrophages, and occasional neutrophils. Within several days, the fibrin-rich exudate and necrotic cellular debris form compacted linear aggregates lining the alveolar walls called hyaline membranes, a diagnostic feature of DAD.[73,74]

Over days to weeks following the injury, tissue repair mechanisms are activated. In this *organizing phase* of DAD (see Fig. 22.6B), the alveolar septa become thickened by fibroblast-rich granulation tissue and sparse chronic inflammation. Proliferation of alveolar epithelial cells (alveolar epithelial type 2 cell hyperplasia) results in re-epithelialization of the injured alveolar septa. The alveolar exudates first become more cellular, with an influx of macrophages and fibroblasts, and are then consolidated into rounded plugs of granulation tissue that resemble organizing pneumonia. Over weeks to months, there may be

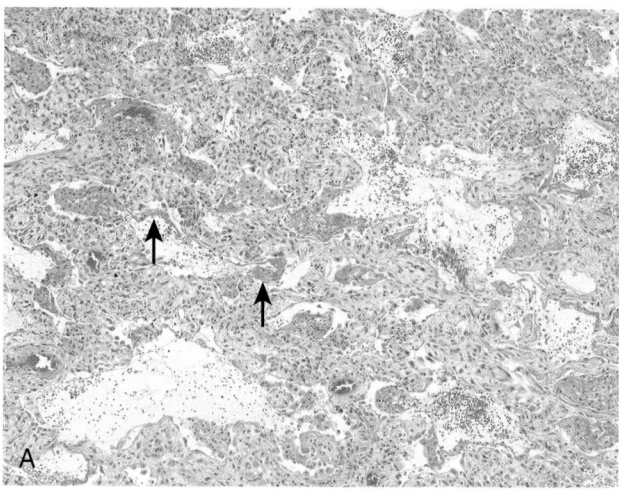

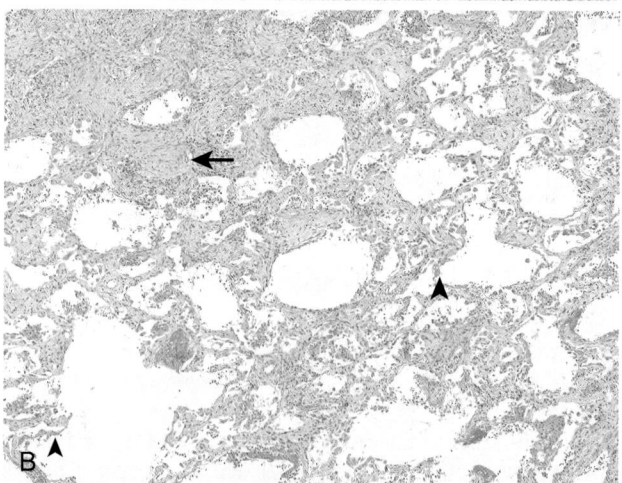

Figure 22.6 Diffuse alveolar damage. (A) Acute phase of *diffuse alveolar damage* (DAD) with prominent alveolar septal thickening by edema and early granulation tissue, alveolar epithelial type 2 cell hyperplasia, air space filling by fibrinous exudate, and occasional hyaline membranes (*arrows*). (B) Organizing phase of DAD with alveolar septal consolidation by granulation tissue and replacement of air space exudates by fibroblast-rich plugs of granulation tissue resembling organizing pneumonia (*arrow*); residual hyaline membranes are still present (*arrowheads*) (hematoxylin and eosin; ×100 original magnification).

complete or near-complete resolution or variable degrees of persistent fibrosis and alveolar septal loss.

While most cases of DAD show nonspecific histologic findings that cannot differentiate between multiple possible etiologies, biopsies may occasionally reveal histologic clues suggestive or even diagnostic of the underlying process. Examples of such findings include viral cytopathic changes in viral pneumonia, aspirated food particles in aspiration pneumonia, or characteristic lipid-filled or foamy macrophages in some drug toxicities.

Organizing Pneumonia

OP is characterized histologically by polypoid plugs of granulation tissue filling the alveolar spaces (Fig. 22.7). The plugs are bound by the surrounding alveolar septa, which gives them the characteristic rounded and branching shapes. The plugs are rich in fibroblasts, loose myxoid matrix, and often contain admixed inflammatory cells. Alveolar epithelial type 2 cell hyperplasia can be prominent in many cases.[75,76]

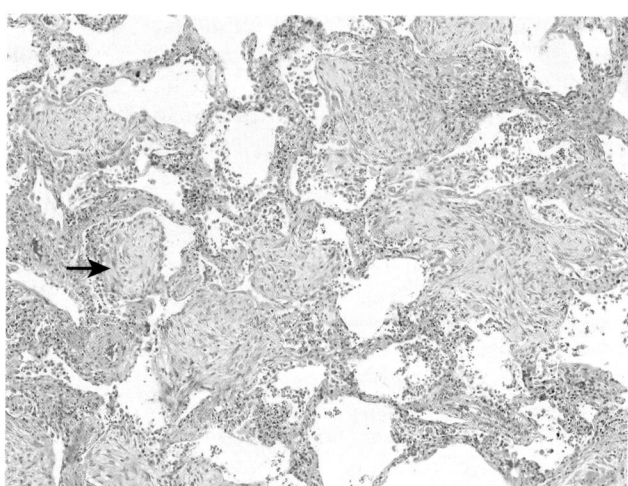

Figure 22.7 Organizing pneumonia. The air spaces contain rounded plugs of fibroblast-rich granulation tissue (*arrow*) (hematoxylin and eosin; ×100 original magnification).

As with DAD, most cases of OP lack histologic features to suggest a specific etiology. However, if present, histologic clues such as viral cytopathic changes or aspirated food material are very helpful in establishing or confirming the cause. If clinical evaluation does not reveal a specific etiology, cryptogenic organizing pneumonia is used as the diagnosis of exclusion.[77]

Acute Fibrinous and Organizing Pneumonia

AFOP is an acute lung injury pattern with histologic features resembling both DAD and OP (Fig. 22.8). Well-developed hyaline membranes are not present in AFOP, but rather the air spaces contain prominent plug-like aggregates of fibrin. Both the clinical presentation and differential diagnosis are essentially the same as those of DAD, although some of the patients appear to have a less severe clinical course compared to DAD. Therefore, AFOP is considered a variant of DAD by some authors.[78]

IS THERE CONSOLIDATION OF ALVEOLAR SPACES?

Acute lung injury is just one of the many causes of filling of air spaces. Consolidation of the air spaces may be secondary to accumulation of edema, blood, proteinaceous fluid, or various cells (e.g., neutrophils, eosinophils, or macrophages). Several of these diverse air space–filling clinicopathologic entities are briefly described later.

Eosinophilic Pneumonia

Eosinophilic pneumonia is characterized by numerous eosinophils within the air spaces (Fig. 22.9) and is divided clinically into acute and chronic forms. Like other acute lung injury patterns, acute eosinophilic pneumonia shows features of alveolar injury, including alveolar epithelial type 2 hyperplasia, interstitial edema, and alveolar accumulation of fibrin and macrophages. Chronic cases typically show findings of air space consolidation by eosinophils and plugs of granulation tissue similar to those of OP and may show variable associated fibrosis. Known etiologies include initiation of or a change in smoking habits, exposure to

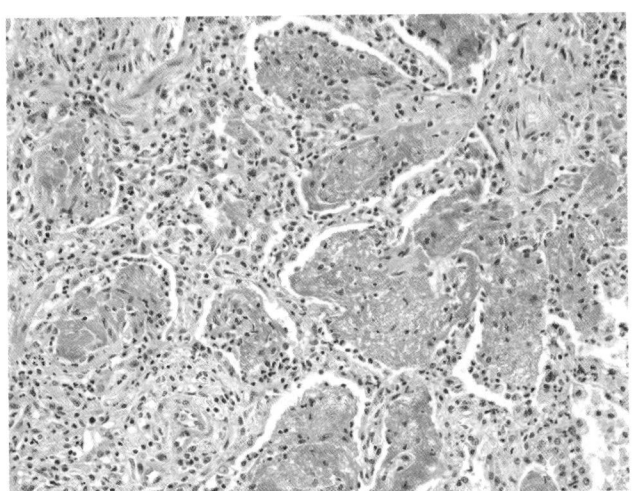

Figure 22.8 Acute fibrinous and organizing pneumonia. The alveolar septa show diffuse edema and sparse lymphocytic and neutrophilic inflammation. The air spaces are filled by fibrin with occasional inflammatory cells (hematoxylin and eosin; ×200 original magnification).

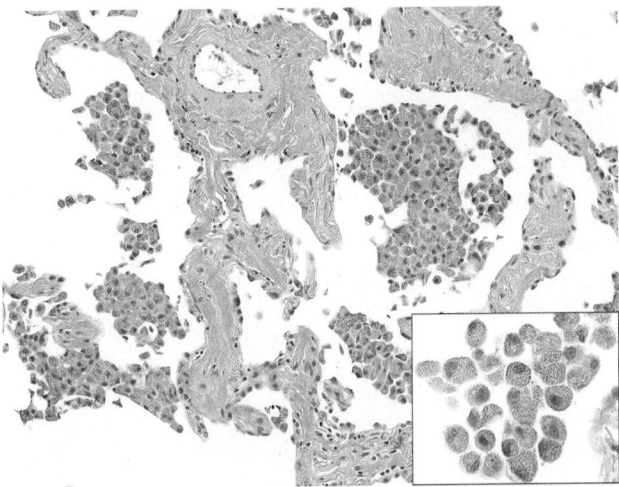

Figure 22.10 Desquamative interstitial pneumonia. The alveolar spaces are filled by large clusters of variably pigmented "smoker's" macrophages. The alveolar septa are thickened by acellular fibrosis, without significant inflammation (hematoxylin and eosin; ×200 original magnification). *Inset,* Smoker's macrophages at high magnification (×400 original magnification).

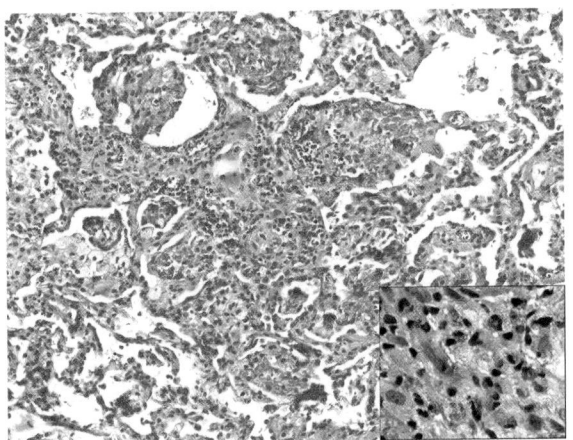

Figure 22.9 Eosinophilic pneumonia. Numerous eosinophils are seen in the fibrin-rich air space exudates and focally within the alveolar septa (hematoxylin and eosin; ×200 original magnification). *Inset,* Eosinophils at high magnification (×400 original magnification).

other inhaled substances, drug- or toxin-induced reactions, systemic hypereosinophilic syndromes, and rare infections (e.g., parasitic).[79,80]

Desquamative Interstitial Pneumonia

Desquamative interstitial pneumonia is characterized by dense alveolar filling with alveolar macrophages (Fig. 22.10). Although the term desquamative interstitial pneumonia is a misnomer because the primary process is neither desquamative nor interstitial, it nevertheless has stuck since first being coined by Liebow in the 1960s. The most common cause is smoking, and therefore desquamative interstitial pneumonia is often discussed in the context of smoking-related lung diseases. Other findings of smoking are often present, including respiratory bronchiolitis (peribronchiolar accumulation of smoker's macrophages), emphysema, and variable alveolar septal fibrosis. Smoker's macrophages characteristically have fine gray-brown and sometimes coarse black pigment in the cytoplasm. Less common causes of desquamative interstitial pneumonia include other inhaled substances,

drug reactions, and rarely autoimmune connective tissue diseases.[81,82]

Pulmonary Alveolar Proteinosis

Pulmonary alveolar proteinosis is characterized by alveolar filling and expansion by granular eosinophilic proteinaceous material. There are frequent acicular (needle-like) cholesterol clefts, rare macrophages, and scattered hypereosinophilic protein globules (Fig. 22.11).[83] The proteinaceous fluid is classically described as periodic acid–Schiff positive, but this staining may be weak to absent in some cases. Electron microscopy is used in some cases but is usually not necessary for diagnosis; it may show extracellular and macrophage accumulation of surfactant with characteristic lamellar bodies.[84,85] The most common cause of pulmonary alveolar proteinosis is acquired antibodies to granulocyte macrophage colony stimulating factor in adults. Rarer causes include genetic deficiencies of granulocyte macrophage colony stimulating factor or surfactant in neonates[86,87] (see also Chapter 98).

IS THERE INTERSTITIAL FIBROSIS?

ILD encompasses many different entities that are characterized predominantly by increased fibrosis (fibrosing interstitial pneumonias), inflammation (cellular interstitial pneumonias), or both. Fibrosing ILD patterns are characterized by accumulation of collagen in the lung interstitium. When classifying these patterns histologically, it is helpful to note the distribution of fibrosis within the pulmonary lobule (Fig. 22.12).

Usual Interstitial Pneumonia

Usual interstitial pneumonia (UIP) is the most common pattern of fibrosing ILD.[88,89] Although its most frequent clinical correlate is idiopathic pulmonary fibrosis, this pattern is also observed in some cases of familial ILD, autoimmune connective tissue disease, chronic *hypersensitivity*

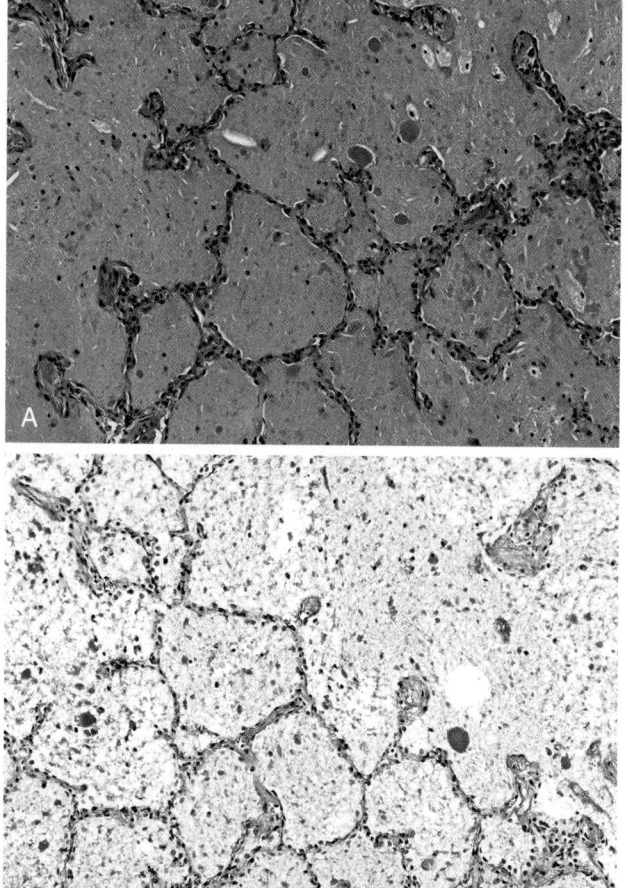

Figure 22.11 Pulmonary alveolar proteinosis. (A) The alveolar spaces are filled by brightly eosinophilic proteinaceous fluid; the alveolar septa appear normal (hematoxylin and eosin; ×200 original magnification). (B) Occasional periodic acid–Schiff (PAS)-positive precipitates (*dark pink*) are seen in the alveolar spaces (PAS; ×200 original magnification).

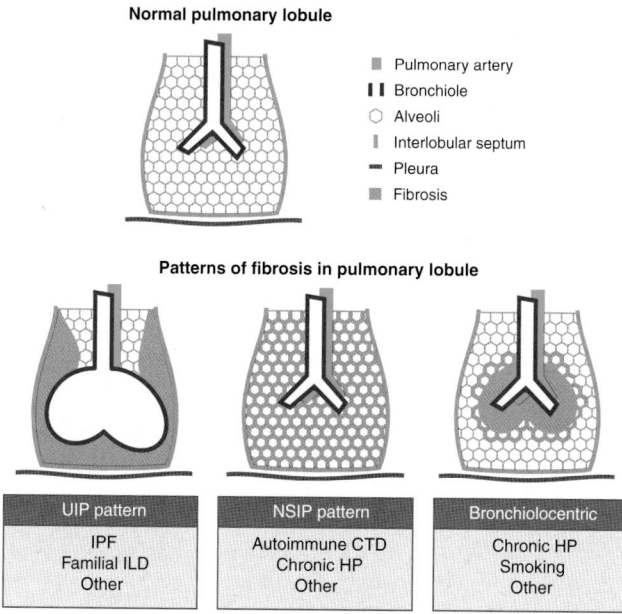

Figure 22.12 Patterns of pulmonary lobule involvement by fibrosis. The distribution of fibrosis in affected pulmonary lobules helps classify fibrosis into three histologic patterns: usual interstitial pneumonia (UIP) pattern (subpleural and interlobular septal fibrosis with microscopic honeycombing), nonspecific interstitial pneumonia (NSIP) pattern (diffuse alveolar septal fibrosis), and bronchiolocentric fibrosis (peribronchiolar fibrosis). Recognition of these patterns aids in formulating a differential diagnosis for the underlying etiology or associated condition. CTD, connective tissue disease; HP, hypersensitivity pneumonitis; ILD, interstitial lung disease; IPF, idiopathic pulmonary fibrosis.

pneumonitis (HP), some pneumoconioses (e.g., asbestosis), and rare drug toxicities (e.g., nitrofurantoin).[90] It is important to distinguish UIP from other patterns because it has the worst prognosis among all fibrosing ILD, independent of the underlying cause.[91,92] Classical high-resolution CT findings of UIP include basilar and subpleural-predominant fibrosis, honeycombing, and traction bronchiectasis. When present, these findings have approximately 90% specificity for UIP, and biopsy is usually deferred. However, in patients with less certain findings on high-resolution CT, surgical biopsy is usually sought for definitive diagnosis and to rule out other causes of ILD.[93]

Histologically, UIP is characterized by fibrosis most notable along the pleura and interlobular septa (periphery of the pulmonary lobules). Affected lobules are replaced by fibrosis from outside in, which eventually leads to cystic dilation of the distal airways surrounded by dense fibrosis. This so-called microscopic honeycombing is most notable in the distal subpleural parenchyma (Fig. 22.13).[94,95] Areas of fibrosis are juxtaposed with areas of normal lung in the more central parenchyma, producing the distinctive feature of spatial heterogeneity. Another feature of UIP is temporal heterogeneity, which refers to the coexistence of

old collagenous fibrosis as well as new fibrosis in the form of fibroblast foci. These fibroblast-rich areas are found at the interface of fibrosis with normal lung and are thought to be the sites of active collagen deposition. Fibroblast foci should not be confused with the plugs of granulation tissue in OP. Although both feature numerous fibroblast or myofibroblast-like cells within a loose myxoid matrix, fibroblast foci are located in the interstitium, while plugs of OP develop in the air spaces.

Nonspecific Interstitial Pneumonia

The term *nonspecific interstitial pneumonia* (NSIP) was initially coined to describe a histologic pattern of ILD distinct from UIP, which later was shown to have different epidemiologic and clinical features.[96] Patients with NSIP tend to be younger, are more often female, and overall have a better prognosis compared to those with UIP.[82,97]

The histologic pattern of NSIP is defined by diffuse alveolar septal involvement that lacks the temporal heterogeneity of UIP and instead appears to be more uniform (Fig. 22.14). The alveolar walls are thickened by variable proportions of chronic interstitial inflammation and fibrosis. Although areas of relative accentuation and sparing may be present, the transitions between them are more gradual, and completely normal parenchyma is most often absent. NSIP cases are a spectrum ranging from those dominated by interstitial inflammation and lacking significant fibrosis to those marked by prominent fibrosis. NSIP can be classified into three groups: cellular NSIP (with predominance of interstitial inflammation), cellular and fibrotic NSIP (with a mixture of inflammation and fibrosis), and fibrotic NSIP

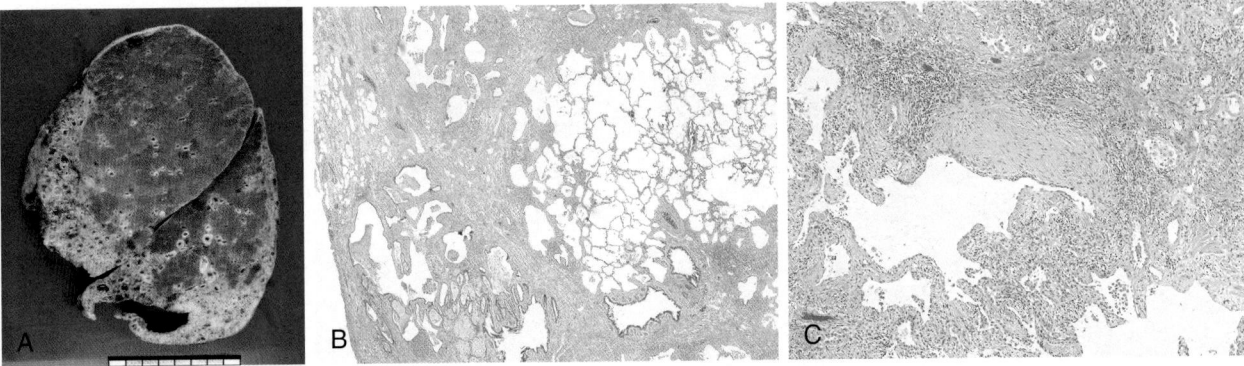

Figure 22.13 Usual interstitial pneumonia. (A) Pneumonectomy specimen from a patient who underwent lung transplantation demonstrates subpleural and lower lobe predominant fibrosis (1 cm scale at bottom). (B) A histologic section from the same specimen shows fibrosis with subpleural and interlobular septal distribution, areas of microscopic honeycombing, and abrupt transition to more central nonfibrotic parenchyma (hematoxylin and eosin [H&E]; ×20 original magnification). (C) A fibroblast focus in an area of fibrosis is seen at a higher magnification (H&E; ×100 original magnification).

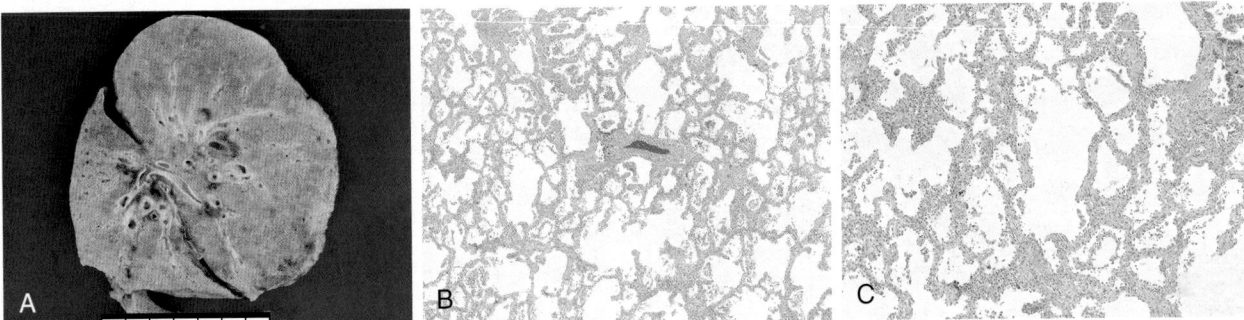

Figure 22.14 Fibrosing nonspecific interstitial pneumonia. (A) Transplant pneumonectomy specimen from a patient with autoimmune connective tissue–associated interstitial lung disease shows diffuse involvement by fibrosis (1 cm scale at bottom). (B) A histologic section from the same specimen shows diffuse widening of the alveolar septa (hematoxylin and eosin [H&E]; ×20 original magnification). (C) At higher magnification, the alveolar septa appear diffusely thickened by fibrosis (fibrosing nonspecific interstitial pneumonia) and contain occasional lymphocytes (H&E; ×100 original magnification).

(with predominance of interstitial fibrosis).[96] As one would predict, NSIP cases with a predominance of fibrosis have more advanced disease, are less responsive to treatment, and have less favorable prognoses compared to those dominated by inflammation.

A significant proportion of the patients with NSIP have identifiable associated conditions (Table 22.8), most importantly autoimmune connective tissue disease, chronic HP, viral or atypical bacterial infections, some immunodeficiency conditions, and rare drug toxicities.[98–101] Several useful histologic clues can aid in the identification of an associated condition.[102] For example, cases of autoimmune connective tissue disease more often show frequent large lymphoid follicles (sometimes with germinal centers) and involvement of other compartments such as pleura and blood vessels. Conversely, cases of chronic HP with NSIP pattern tend to have more prominent bronchiolocentric accentuation of both inflammation and fibrosis; the presence of peribronchiolar interstitial poorly formed granulomas is highly suggestive of this etiology. However, many biopsies with NSIP pattern lack distinct histologic features to implicate a specific cause. In these instances, careful correlation with the clinical features, laboratory findings, and exposure history is recommended and is best accomplished in a multidisciplinary discussion setting.[62,103] Cases without identifiable cause or associated condition are classified clinically as idiopathic NSIP.[104]

Table 22.8 Conditions Associated with Nonspecific Interstitial Pneumonitis Pattern

Autoimmune connective tissue diseases

Chronic hypersensitivity pneumonitis

Infection (e.g., viral or atypical bacterial)

Inherited or acquired immunodeficiency

Drug toxicity

Idiopathic

IS THERE INTERSTITIAL INFLAMMATION?

The distribution of interstitial inflammation can vary from diffuse involvement of the alveolar septa (as in cellular NSIP) to more variable distribution with accentuation around bronchioles, to strictly bronchiolar involvement. If inflammation is associated with interstitial fibrosis, then fibrosing ILD patterns should be the primary focus in the evaluation. On the other hand, if the inflammation is largely restricted to bronchioles, primary patterns of bronchiolitis should be considered.

Cellular Nonspecific Interstitial Pneumonia Versus Lymphocytic Interstitial Pneumonia

As discussed earlier, cellular NSIP refers to a subset of cases with an NSIP pattern in which interstitial inflammation is

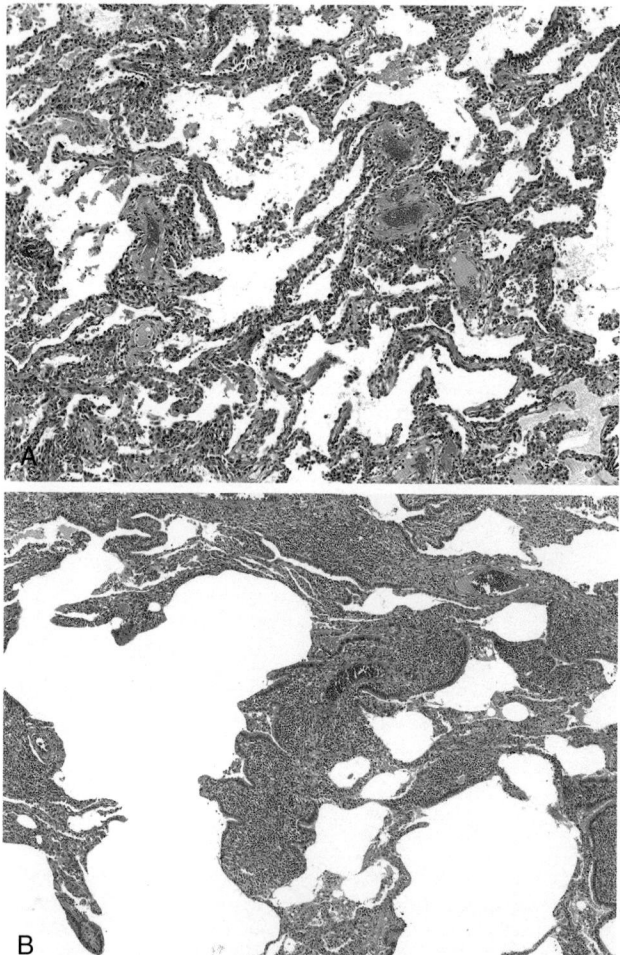

Figure 22.15 Cellular nonspecific interstitial pneumonia and lymphocytic interstitial pneumonia. (A) Cellular nonspecific interstitial pneumonia pattern is characterized by diffuse alveolar septal inflammation, most often composed of lymphocytes and occasional plasma cells, without significant fibrosis (hematoxylin and eosin [H&E]; ×100 original magnification). (B) In lymphocytic interstitial pneumonia pattern, the inflammatory infiltrate is much more prominent, resulting in marked thickening of the alveolar septa and formation of frequent lymphoid follicles (H&E; ×80 original magnification).

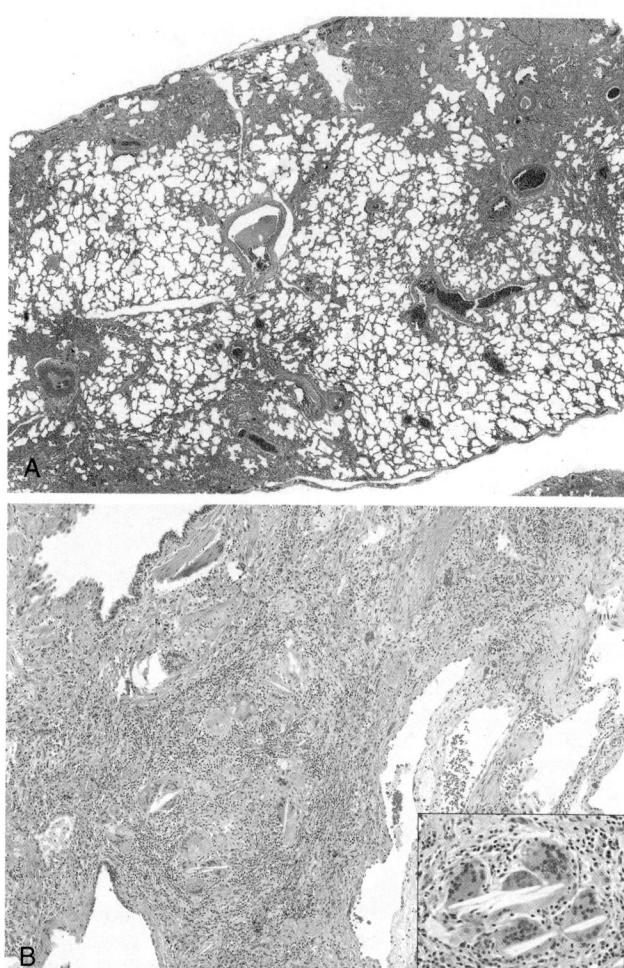

Figure 22.16 Hypersensitivity pneumonitis. (A) A low-magnification view shows a patchy parenchymal involvement with peribronchiolar accentuation (hematoxylin and eosin [H&E]; ×10 original magnification). (B) At higher magnification, peribronchiolar interstitium is expanded by fibrosis, chronic inflammation, and contains several poorly formed granulomas with giant cells and cholesterol clefts (H&E; ×100 original magnification). *Inset,* Poorly formed granuloma at high magnification (×400 original magnification).

present without significant interstitial fibrosis (Fig. 22.15A). These cases tend to represent early or less advanced disease, are more responsive to treatment, and have better long-term prognoses than fibrotic NSIP. However, the clinical differential diagnosis is essentially the same for both NSIP subtypes.[82,96,104]

Lymphocytic interstitial pneumonia is a term reserved for cases that have particularly prominent interstitial inflammation that leads to dramatic widening of the alveolar septa by a lymphocyte-predominant infiltrate (Fig. 22.15B). Some of the alveolar septa become obliterated by the inflammation, which may result in formation of parenchymal cysts (a helpful radiologic correlate of lymphocytic interstitial pneumonia). Frequent lymphoid aggregates, usually with germinal centers, are another feature of lymphocytic interstitial pneumonia. The main differential diagnosis of lymphocytic interstitial pneumonia is autoimmune connective tissue disease or immunodeficiency syndromes (e.g., congenital HIV or common variable immunodeficiency), but rare cases

of lymphoma can also present with similar histologic findings.[105–107]

Hypersensitivity Pneumonitis

The inflammatory infiltrates in HP tend to be bronchiolocentric with sparing of more distal lobular parenchyma, particularly early in the disease. However, in more advanced cases, the distribution of inflammation and fibrosis can be difficult to distinguish from fibrotic NSIP. Bronchiolocentric accentuation of inflammation remains a helpful feature, and the presence of poorly formed granulomas is highly suggestive of HP. The HP-type granulomas (Fig. 22.16) are most commonly found in the interstitium surrounding the bronchioles and are composed of epithelioid macrophages and multinucleated giant cells. The giant cells often contain needle-shaped *cholesterol clefts* likely derived from the breakdown of cellular membranes and sometimes dystrophic calcifications called Schaumann bodies.[108–110]

ARE THERE NODULES OR MASSES?

Pathologic processes that manifest as lung nodules or larger masses are sometimes considered together due to

Table 22.9 Histopathologic Entities Characterized by Lung Nodules

Malignancy
- Solid primary lung or metastatic
- Hematolymphoid

Infection
- Granulomas
- Abscess or necrobiotic nodule
- Miliary (hematogenous)

Infarct

Pulmonary Langerhans cell histiocytosis

Sarcoidosis

Beryllium lung disease

Vasculitis

Amyloidosis

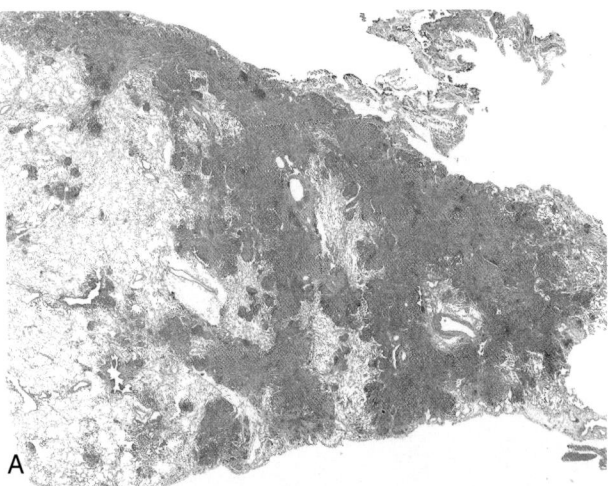
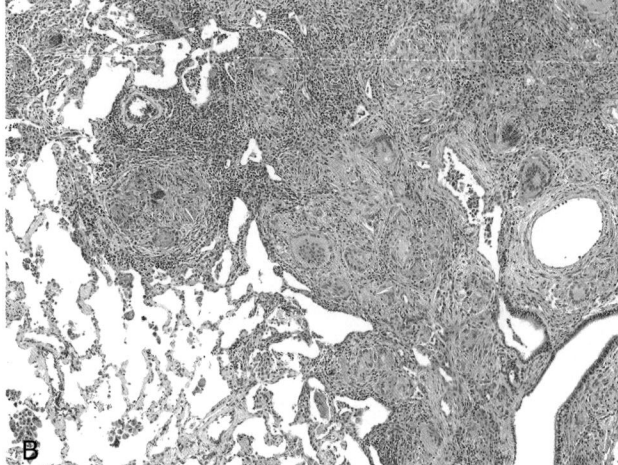

Figure 22.17 Pulmonary sarcoidosis. (A) At low magnification, the perilymphatic distribution of parenchymal nodules is apparent (hematoxylin and eosin [H&E]; ×6 original magnification). (B) The nodules are composed of well-formed granulomas, which are numerous and coalescing; they lack necrosis and are surrounded by fibrosis and chronic inflammation (H&E; ×100 original magnification).

their characteristic appearance on imaging studies and an overlapping clinical differential diagnosis. However, this group is a collection of very diverse histopathologic entities (Table 22.9). Aside from neoplasms that include both primary lung and metastatic tumors, nodules can arise in multiple infectious processes, pulmonary sarcoidosis, *pulmonary Langerhans cell histiocytosis* (PLCH), and other less common conditions.

Pulmonary Sarcoidosis

The histologic hallmark of sarcoidosis in any organ is the presence of non-necrotizing granulomas.[111,112] In the lung parenchyma, sarcoidal granulomas form nodules that have a characteristic distribution along the lymphatic routes (Fig. 22.17A). This "lymphangitic" distribution of the nodules is apparent both histologically and on high-resolution CT and includes involvement of the bronchovascular bundles, interlobular septa, and the pleura.[113,114] Mediastinal lymph node involvement is also present in most cases. The granulomatous inflammation is associated with variable amounts of fibrosis, which can be very prominent, in some cases leading to the clinical manifestations of an ILD.[115] Unlike most types of ILD that require surgical lung biopsy for diagnosis, transbronchial biopsies are often sufficient for evaluation of sarcoidosis.[116–118]

Sarcoidal granulomas are composed of well-formed rounded aggregates of epithelioid macrophages, occasional multinucleated giant cells, and few scattered lymphocytes (Fig. 22.17B). The granulomas are often numerous and coalesce to form larger aggregates. Early granulomas may show more prominent lymphocytic inflammation without much fibrosis, while more established ones are embedded in collagenous or sclerotic stoma. Importantly, sarcoidal granulomas should lack significant necrosis. If necrosis is detected, an infectious process is much more likely.[111,112]

Pulmonary sarcoidosis continues to be a diagnosis of exclusion requiring careful consideration of other possible etiologies and mimics. No immunohistochemical or molecular testing is currently available to confirm the diagnosis, and therefore the efforts are largely directed towards excluding other causes. Acid-fast and Gomori methenamine silver stains are routinely obtained to exclude mycobacterial and fungal infections, respectively. Careful correlation with the exposure and medication history is helpful in ruling out other mimics such as beryllium lung disease and drug-induced sarcoidal reaction.[112,119]

Infectious Granulomas

Numerous infectious pathogens can produce single or multiple granulomas in the lung parenchyma. The most important examples include mycobacterial species such as *Mycobacterium tuberculosis* and *Mycobacterium avium* complex, and fungal species such as *Coccidioides*, *Aspergillus*, *Histoplasma*, *Cryptococcus*, and many others. The histologic appearance of the granulomas and changes in the surrounding lung tissue may vary, but most infectious granulomas show prominent central necrosis (Fig. 22.18). When encountered grossly, the granulomas are often described as caseating, referring to their cheese-like appearance when transected. However, when evaluated histologically, the term necrotizing granuloma is preferred to describe the presence of central necrosis more specifically. Acid-fast and Gomori methenamine silver stains are very helpful in highlighting the microorganisms but, in cases where a pathogen is not readily identified, additional immunohistochemical

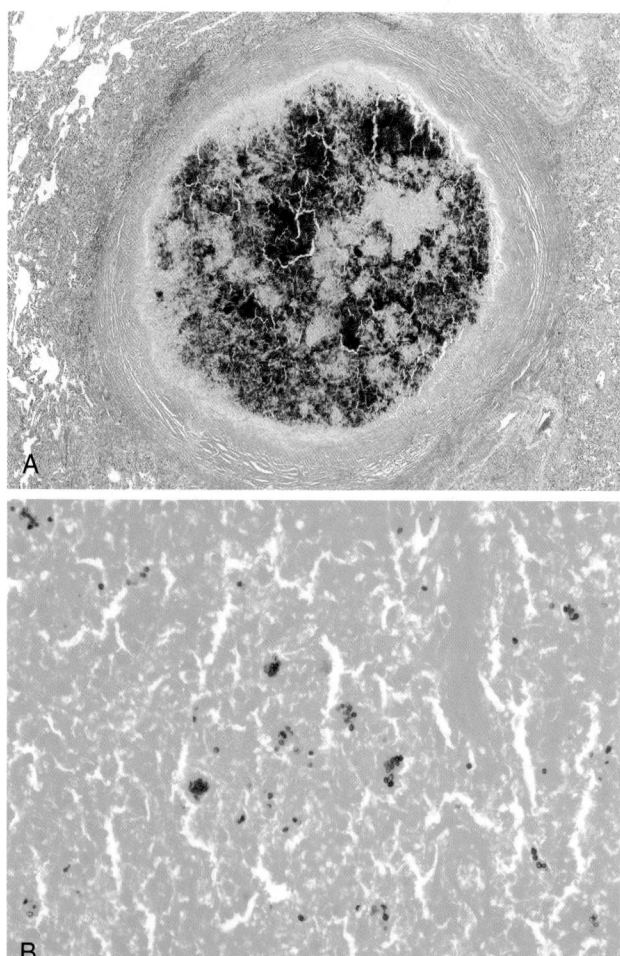

Figure 22.18 Infectious necrotizing granuloma of pulmonary histoplasmosis. (A) This granuloma forms a round solid nodule with a fibrotic rim and a partially calcified necrotic core (hematoxylin and eosin; ×50 original magnification). (B) Gomori methenamine silver stain highlights clusters of *Histoplasma capsulatum* yeast forms in the cytoplasm of macrophages within the necrotic core of the granuloma (×600 original magnification).

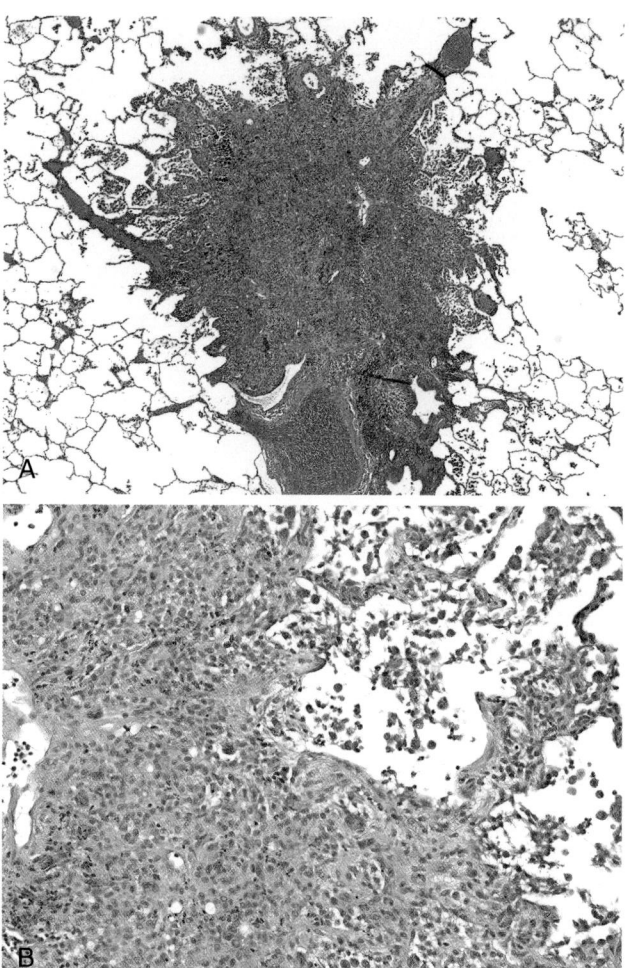

Figure 22.19 Pulmonary Langerhans cell histiocytosis. (A) At low magnification, a peribronchiolar irregularly shaped fibroinflammatory nodule is easily recognized (hematoxylin and eosin [H&E]; ×40 original magnification). (B) The nodule is composed of a cellular proliferation of Langerhans cells, pigmented smoker's macrophages, scattered eosinophils, and associated fibrosis (H&E; ×200 original magnification).

and molecular techniques (e.g., universal bacterial 16S RNA or targeted polymerase chain reaction) can be performed on the FFPE blocks.[120–122]

Pulmonary Langerhans Cell Histiocytosis

PLCH is another process that may show a nodular appearance on imaging. Histologically, it is defined by interstitial aggregates of Langerhans cells (Fig. 22.19), often with associated eosinophils.[123] Most cases are associated with cigarette smoking and resolve with smoking cessation. The lesions can be replaced by fibrosis (forming characteristic stellate scars), particularly with persistent smoking.[124] Destruction of the alveolar walls by the lesions often leads to formation of parenchymal cysts that can be an important radiologic clue to the diagnosis of PLCH.[125] Significant associated fibrosis and pulmonary hypertension can develop in rare cases. Similar lesions have been described in multiple organs, including the skin, bones, lymph nodes, brain, liver, spleen, and other sites. Most of these lesions are now known to be neoplasms of Langerhans cells or their progenitors with frequent genetic alterations involving genes of the MAPK signaling

pathway.[126,127] These extrapulmonary cases should be distinguished from those of PLCH. While cases of single-organ bone and skin disease tend to have a benign clinical course, disseminated multiorgan disease carries a poor prognosis[128,129] (see also Chapter 95).

WHAT IF THE LUNG PARENCHYMA LOOKS NORMAL?

While assessment of small airways and blood vessels is part of any surgical biopsy evaluation, it is particularly important not to overlook these compartments when the lung parenchyma appears to be normal. Some of the important entities to consider in this setting are obliterative (constrictive) bronchiolitis and vascular diseases such as pulmonary arterial hypertension and pulmonary veno-occlusive disease. The diagnosis of both small airway and vascular diseases can be challenging due to their patchy distribution in the lung. Special stains, such as Verhoeff-Van Gieson, are often helpful in identifying subtle lesions by highlighting the elastic fibers within the walls of small airways and vessels.[102,130,131]

FUTURE OUTLOOK

Pathology as a field, including thoracic neoplastic and non-neoplastic pathology, is in the process of transformation from strictly morphologically defined entities to those increasingly augmented or even redefined by molecular phenotypes. With the continued evolution of gene sequencing and protein-based detection technologies, we expect to see a shift from larger to smaller, less invasive biopsies and, in some cases, from tissue samples to liquid biopsies, such as from bronchoalveolar lavage fluid or peripheral blood. Continued developments in digital pathology and automated image analysis will reshape ways in which pathologists examine and report their findings and will revolutionize the ways in which practitioners, patients, researchers, and educators access and share pathologic imaging.

Key Points

- Histopathologic evaluation of lung tissue specimens is an integral component in the diagnosis of both neoplastic and non-neoplastic lung diseases.
- Neoplastic lung disease is evaluated either by small biopsies, to provide a histologic and/or molecular diagnosis, or by resections, which may be curative but also confirm and refine the initial histologic diagnosis, determine the pathologic tumor stage, assess resection margins, and evaluate response to preresection therapy (if any).
- Small biopsies are increasingly used for the diagnosis, staging, and molecular typing of lung neoplasms.
- Molecular characterization is used for diagnosis and therapeutic planning for both malignant (e.g., *EGFR*, *BRAF*, and rearrangements of *ALK* and *ROS1*) and nonmalignant diseases (e.g., MAPK signaling pathway in pulmonary Langerhans cell histiocytosis).
- Non-neoplastic lung disease is evaluated by considering whether there is presence of the following pathologic patterns: acute lung injury, consolidation of alveolar spaces, interstitial fibrosis, interstitial inflammation, nodules/masses, or normal lung.
- The histologic diagnosis of most diffuse patterns of interstitial lung disease, particularly usual interstitial pneumonitis, continues to be challenging in small transbronchial biopsies and often requires surgical lung biopsy.
- Correlation of a histologic pattern of interstitial lung disease encountered in a lung biopsy with clinical and radiologic findings is key to identifying the most likely etiology or underlying condition and is best accomplished in a multidisciplinary discussion setting.

Key Readings

Beasley MB. The pathologist's approach to acute lung injury. *Arch Pathol Lab Med.* 2010;134(5):719–727.

Cavazza A, Harari S, Caminati A, et al. The histology of pulmonary sarcoidosis: a review with particular emphasis on unusual and underrecognized features. *Int J Surg Pathol.* 2009;17(3):219–230.

El-Zammar OA, Katzenstein AL. Pathological diagnosis of granulomatous lung disease: a review. *Histopathology.* 2007;50(3):289–310.

Friedlaender A, Banna G, Malapelle U, Pisapia P, Addeo A. Next generation sequencing and genetic alterations in squamous cell lung carcinoma: where are we today? *Front Oncol.* 2019;9:166.

George J, Lim JS, Jang SJ, et al. Comprehensive genomic profiles of small cell lung cancer. *Nature.* 2015;524(7563):47–53.

Jones KD, Urisman A. Histopathologic approach to the surgical lung biopsy in interstitial lung disease. *Clin Chest Med.* 2012;33(1):27–40.

Lindeman NI, Cagle PT, Aisner DL, et al. Updated molecular testing guideline for the selection of lung cancer patients for treatment with targeted tyrosine kinase inhibitors: guideline from the College of American Pathologists, the International Association for the Study of Lung Cancer, and the Association for Molecular Pathology. *Arch Pathol Lab Med.* 2018;142(3):321–346.

Miller R, Allen TC, Barrios RJ, et al. Hypersensitivity pneumonitis: a perspective from members of the Pulmonary Pathology Society. *Arch Pathol Lab Med.* 2018;142(1):120–126.

Pelosi G, Rodriguez J, Viale G, Rosai J. Typical and atypical pulmonary carcinoid tumor overdiagnosed as small-cell carcinoma on biopsy specimens: a major pitfall in the management of lung cancer patients. *Am J Surg Pathol.* 2005;29(2):179–187.

Perez-Moreno P, Brambilla E, Thomas R, Soria JC. Squamous cell carcinoma of the lung: molecular subtypes and therapeutic opportunities. *Clin Cancer Res.* 2012;18(9):2443–2451.

Raghu G, Collard HR, Egan JJ, et al. An official ATS/ERS/JRS/ALAT statement: idiopathic pulmonary fibrosis: evidence-based guidelines for diagnosis and management. *Am J Respir Crit Care Med.* 2011;183(6):788–824.

Rekhtman N, Pietanza MC, Hellmann MD, et al. Next-generation sequencing of pulmonary large cell neuroendocrine carcinoma reveals small cell carcinoma-like and non-small cell carcinoma-like subsets. *Clin Cancer Res.* 2016;22(14):3618–3629.

Rekhtman N, Travis WD. Large no more: the journey of pulmonary large cell carcinoma from common to rare entity. *J Thorac Oncol.* 2019;14(7):1125–1127.

Rekhtman N. Neuroendocrine tumors of the lung: an update. *Arch Pathol Lab Med.* 2010;134(11):1628–1638.

Ryu JH, Colby TV, Hartman TE, Vassallo R. Smoking-related interstitial lung diseases: a concise review. *Eur Respir J.* 2001;17(1):122–132.

Smith M, Dalurzo M, Panse P, Parish J, Leslie K. Usual interstitial pneumonia-pattern fibrosis in surgical lung biopsies. Clinical, radiological and histopathological clues to aetiology. *J Clin Pathol.* 2013;66(10):896–903.

Travis WD, Brambilla E, Nicholson AG, et al. The 2015 World Health Organization classification of lung tumors: impact of genetic, clinical and radiologic advances since the 2004 classification. *J Thorac Oncol.* 2015;10(9):1243–1260.

Travis WD, Brambilla E, Noguchi M, et al. Diagnosis of lung cancer in small biopsies and cytology: implications of the 2011 International Association for the Study of Lung Cancer/American Thoracic Society/European Respiratory Society classification. *Arch Pathol Lab Med.* 2013;137(5):668–684.

Travis WD, Brambilla E, Noguchi M, et al. International Association for the Study of Lung Cancer/American Thoracic Society/European Respiratory Society: international multidisciplinary classification of lung adenocarcinoma: executive summary. *Proc Am Thorac Soc.* 2011;8(5):381–385.

Travis WD, Costabel U, Hansell DM, et al. An official American Thoracic Society/European Respiratory Society statement: update of the international multidisciplinary classification of the idiopathic interstitial pneumonias. *Am J Respir Crit Care Med.* 2013;188(6):733–748.

Travis WD, Hunninghake G, King Jr TE, et al. Idiopathic nonspecific interstitial pneumonia: report of an American Thoracic Society project. *Am J Respir Crit Care Med.* 2008;177(12):1338–1347.

Travis WD. Update on small cell carcinoma and its differentiation from squamous cell carcinoma and other non-small cell carcinomas. *Mod Pathol.* 2012;25(suppl 1):S18–S30.

Complete reference list available at ExpertConsult.com.

23 ULTRASONOGRAPHY: PRINCIPLES AND BASIC THORACIC AND VASCULAR IMAGING

AMY E. MORRIS, MD • ROSEMARY ADAMSON, MB, BS • JAMES FRANK, MD, MA

INTRODUCTION

Point-of-care ultrasound (POCUS) is routinely used for pulmonary and critical care procedures and diagnostic applications in pulmonary and critical care medicine. POCUS differs from comprehensive ultrasound examinations performed by technicians and interpreted by radiologists or cardiologists in at least two important ways. First, POCUS is often used to answer urgent clinical questions when comprehensive imaging may not be available, practical, or necessary. Second, POCUS is best targeted to specific questions for which a dedicated examination of a single or limited number of structures might be obtained to provide a dichotomous "yes or no" answer. An adept clinician will use POCUS in these settings, understanding that appropriate follow-up may require a traditional comprehensive diagnostic ultrasound study to address nuanced or complex questions.

This chapter covers the principles underlying thoracic ultrasound and basic thoracic and vascular applications. The following chapter, Chapter 24, covers advanced ultrasound, including cardiac evaluation.

PHYSICS OF ULTRASOUND

Humans hear sounds in the frequency range of 20 to 20,000 Hz. Ultrasound imaging uses sound pressure waves generated in a handheld transducer with frequencies of 2 to 15 MHz. In conventional ultrasound transducers, sound waves are generated by the application of an electrical current across a crystal lattice, which induces vibration and sound wave formation, a phenomenon known as the reverse piezoelectric effect.

The transducer is placed on a patient's skin with a layer of conductive gel to facilitate transmission of the sound waves into the body. Waves then travel through the tissues and are reflected back to the transducer by the underlying structures. Returning sound waves are translated by the transducer crystals into electrical signals (i.e., the piezoelectric effect), which then generate images on the ultrasound screen. The depth of structures in the body is computed using the time required for waves ("echoes") to return to the skin surface from these structures.

Acoustic impedance is the resistance to propagation of sound waves. Tissues have variable degrees of resistance to propagation and, as sound waves travel through the body, they encounter differences in acoustic impedance between adjacent tissues. These interfaces cause scatter, refraction, or reflection of sound waves. The cumulative pattern of reflected waves returning to the transducer translates into detailed images of tissue structure. For example, a wave may pass through a layer of subcutaneous fat before reaching the surface of an organ. The difference in acoustic impedance between these tissues results in increased reflection of sound waves at that depth, which appears on the ultrasound screen as the edge of that structure.

Attenuation is the loss of wave energy via absorption by the tissue as the ultrasound waves pass through the body. This results in a decrease in amplitude and the generation of a small amount of heat. Higher frequency (shorter wavelength) waves experience more attenuation and therefore exhibit less tissue penetration.

The focal zone of an ultrasound transducer is the regional distance from the transducer that allows the greatest image resolution for a given frequency and crystal/transducer diameter. On the ultrasound screen, areas proximal or distal to the focal zone are known, respectively, as the near and far fields. In general, the distance from the skin surface to the focal zone is shorter with higher frequency and narrower transducers. Resolution in the focal zone is generally sharper than in near and far fields.

Axial resolution is the ability to distinguish two structures in a line parallel to the course of the ultrasound beam (e.g., a superficial structure overlying a deeper one). Axial resolution is generally greater at higher sound frequencies. *Lateral resolution* is the ability to distinguish two structures aligned perpendicular to the ultrasound beam (side by side) (Fig. 23.1). Lateral resolution is generally better with wider ultrasound transducers. For any frequency or transducer size, lateral resolution is greatest within the focal zone.

In combination, these principles result in a tradeoff for imaging characteristics inherent to ultrasound at higher versus lower frequencies. As a rule, higher frequency, shorter wavelength transducers provide superior imaging of superficial structures, whereas lower frequency, longer wavelength transducers provide better imaging of deeper structures (see Table 23.1 for terminology used in ultrasound and the clinical applications).

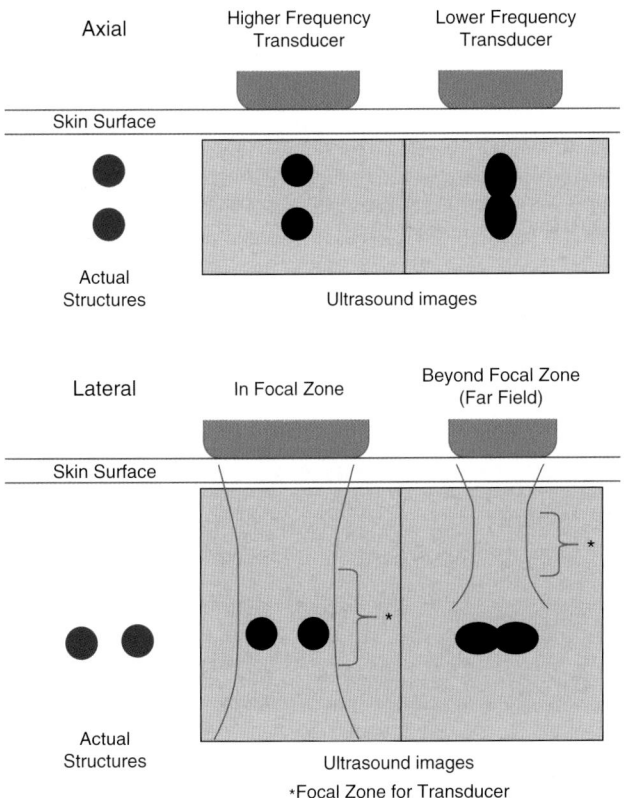

Figure 23.1 **Axial and lateral resolution in ultrasound.** Axial resolution is the ability to distinguish structures in a line parallel to the ultrasound beam and is greatest with higher frequency transducers. Lateral resolution is a property of the transducer to distinguish structures perpendicular to the axis of the beam and is dependent on frequency and crystal size. Lateral resolution is greatest within the focal zone of the transducer, often the mid-screen zone of the default settings. Distal to the focal zone, it may be more difficult to distinguish neighboring structures.

TRANSDUCER SELECTION

Transducers differ primarily in frequency and mode of crystal excitation. The optimal frequency choice for a given examination is the highest available that also provides the appropriate tissue penetration for the structure of interest. Beyond frequency, the mode of crystal excitation is relevant primarily for cardiac imaging. *Linear* transducers operate by activating crystals in a sequential fashion along the width of the transducer from one side toward to the other. *Phased array* transducers use simultaneous excitation of an array of crystals that span the transducer width to generate multidirectional, overlapping ultrasound beams. This produces *two-dimensional* (2D) imaging that is superior for the evaluation of motion and flow (see "Doppler Imaging" later). A typical configuration for a POCUS machine includes a high-frequency (5–13 MHz) linear transducer for superficial structures and at least one lower frequency (1–8 MHz) transducer for deeper structures. Ideally, for the lower frequency transducers, users will have both a phased array transducer with a small square footprint for cardiac imaging and a linear array with a curved shape to facilitate a wide field of view (*convex* or *curvilinear* transducer) (Fig. 23.2). Transducer selection for specific examinations is discussed later.

Vascular Imaging

Vascular POCUS is most often procedural in nature, to guide peripheral or central vascular access (see "Vascular Imaging" later). A high-frequency (5–13 MHz) linear array transducer provides high-resolution images of superficial structures. This transducer also is used for diagnostic imaging of the deep veins of the lower extremities to evaluate for thrombosis. In contrast, to reach an adequate depth for imaging of the *inferior vena cava* (IVC), a lower frequency (1–5 MHz) phased array or curvilinear transducer is used.

Thoracic Imaging

A phased array (1–5 MHz) transducer is used to examine the heart and great vessels (see Chapter 24). In pulmonary imaging, sliding of the parietal and visceral pleura can be evaluated with either a phased array or high-frequency linear transducer, but for deeper evaluation of pleural effusion or lung parenchyma, a low-frequency transducer, either curvilinear or phased array, is preferred.

Abdominal Imaging

Examining deeper structures, such as the liver, spleen, kidneys, or bladder, is typically performed with a low-frequency (2–5 MHz) curvilinear transducer, with a linear crystal array and a convex shape for a wide field of view. In addition to better penetration, this transducer type has a wider beam that affords greater lateral resolution than narrower phased array transducers.[1]

ULTRASOUND MODES

Two-Dimensional Mode, or B-Mode

The mode most commonly used in POCUS is 2D mode, also called B- (for "brightness") mode, in which pixel brightness is proportional to the intensity of the reflected sound waves, and a 2D image is displayed on the screen. Tissues

Table 23.1 Point-of-Care Ultrasound Terminology

Term	Definition	Clinical Application
PHYSICS OF ULTRASOUND		
Echogenicity	Interpretation of returning sound wave energy by the ultrasound machine that results from differences in tissue impedance, attenuation, reflection, and scatter of sound waves	Tissues are described as isoechoic when similar in intensity or brightness, hyperechoic when brighter than reference, hypoechoic when dimmer, and anechoic when black
Frequency	The physical property of sound waves indicating the time elapsed between wave peaks passing a specific point	Higher frequency, shorter wavelength waves attenuate more quickly in body tissues, so are best for imaging structures close to the skin surface
Focal zone	A property of the beam emitted from the transducer where it is most narrow	Lateral resolution, or the ability to distinguish objects side by side, is best for any transducer within its focal zone
Acoustic impedance	Property of a tissue that influences sound wave propagation, including transmission, reflection of waves, and energy loss over distance	Physical basis for visualizing distinct tissues with ultrasound
Acoustic enhancement	Region of increased echogenicity immediately distal to a tissue with low acoustic impedance relative to surrounding tissues, such as a cyst or blood vessel	May facilitate identification of vessels and cysts compared to soft-tissue masses or nodules, such as lymph nodes
Acoustic shadowing	Region of hypoechoic or anechoic signal immediately distal to a tissue with very high impedance relative to surrounding tissues, such as a bone	Allows identification of bones, calcifications, and certain stones
TRANSDUCER NOMENCLATURE		
Linear transducer	Transducer in which crystals are activated in a sequential, linear fashion along the length of the array. Narrow rectangular footprint	Best for examining static structures throughout the field, or motion within a single vertical line from the transducer
Phased-array transducer	Transducer in which crystals are activated in a simultaneous, sweeping fashion through the field of view	Ideal for detecting motion across an entire field of view, such as in echocardiography
Convex/curvilinear transducer	Transducer in which crystals are activated in a linear fashion but with a curved footprint; usually lower frequency for imaging deeper structures	Creates a wider field of view than linear transducer, used for imaging the abdomen or, less common, the thorax
Transducer indicator	Marker on the ultrasound screen and on the transducer that allows for orientation of image direction	Standard orientation in lung ultrasound is cephalad left on the ultrasound screen
MODES		
B-mode or two-dimensional	"Brightness" mode, or two-dimensional imaging, wherein pixel intensity corresponds to the strength of the returning sound wave energy	The most commonly used modality in point-of-care ultrasound
M-mode	"Motion" mode of imaging, wherein a signal intensity along a single line within the transducer beam is evaluated over time	Often used to detect and measure movement of structures, such as the pleura, diaphragm, vessel walls, or heart structures
KNOBOLOGY		
Depth	Distance from the transducer; shallow structures appear at the top of the ultrasound screen; deeper structures appear lower	Depth is often adjusted so that the region of interest is in the middle of the screen; in procedural ultrasound, depth may be set to maximize the operative field of view for needle passage
Far field/near field	Region distal (far) or proximal (near) to the focal zone within the ultrasound beam, a property of the transducer	Lateral resolution, or the ability to distinguish objects side by side, is poorer for any transducer outside its focal zone
Gain	Factor by which all signals received from the transducer are multiplied as to make an image appear brighter or darker	Makes the image brighter or darker
Time gain compensation	Application of increasing gain inversely proportional to the timing of signal return to the transducer so as to compensate for sound wave attenuation due to distance traveled through the tissues	Used to make a tissue appear homogeneous through the depth of the image, whereas would otherwise appear darker at increasing depth due to ultrasound attenuation

that transmit sound waves well, and therefore generate less reflected sound, appear dark. For example, simple fluid reflects very little sound and therefore appears black (anechoic) on the monitor. This includes vessels, simple pleural effusions, or urine in the bladder. Solid structures that strongly reflect and attenuate sound waves appear as bright, hyperechoic edges with deeper structures obscured by dark anechoic shadows (see "Ultrasound Artifacts"

later). All other tissues appear hypoechoic, or as shades of gray, on the ultrasound screen.

M-Mode

M- (for "motion") mode surveys a single point in the ultrasound beam over time. This mode is useful for evaluating changes in size or shape over time, such as change in diameter of the IVC with respiration (Fig. 23.3).

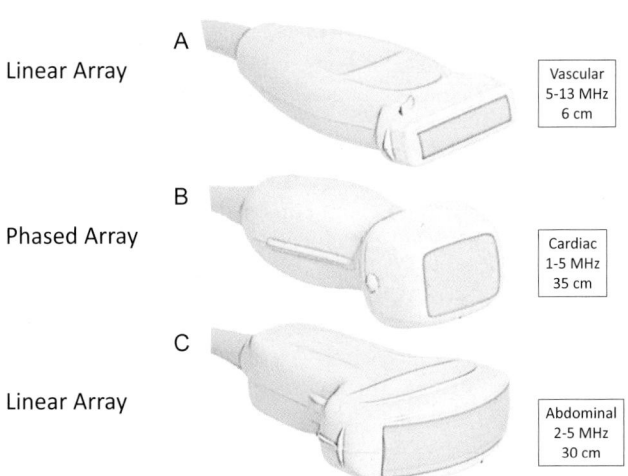

Figure 23.2 **Transducers frequently used in point-of-focus ultrasound.** A typical configuration for a point-of-focus ultrasound machine includes (A) a high-frequency (5–13 MHz) linear transducer for superficial structures, (B) a phased array transducer with a small square footprint for cardiac imaging, and (C) at least one lower frequency (2–5 MHz) transducer with a curved shape for deeper structures to facilitate a wide field of view (convex or curvilinear transducer).

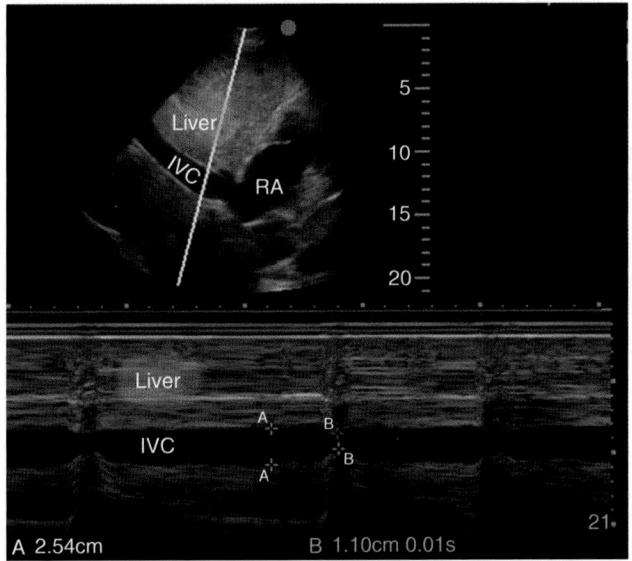

Figure 23.3 **Two-dimensional image and associated M-mode.** In the two-dimensional image at the top of the screen, a subcostal view of the inferior vena cava (IVC) is seen coursing through the liver to empty into the right atrium (RA). The white M-mode line indicates the location to be followed over time on the bottom half of the screen. The diameter of the IVC changes over time due to respiratory variation, fluctuating between 2.54 cm (measurement A) and 1.10 cm (measurement B).

Doppler Imaging

In POCUS, color flow Doppler is most often used to evaluate blood flow in vessels. Flow toward or away from the transducer is color coded on the ultrasound machine in response to the Doppler shift during 2D imaging (Video 23.1). Spectral Doppler, particularly pulse wave Doppler, is used in POCUS to detect flow velocity over time within a specific region. In this mode a sampling gate is placed over the area of interest and the angle of the gate

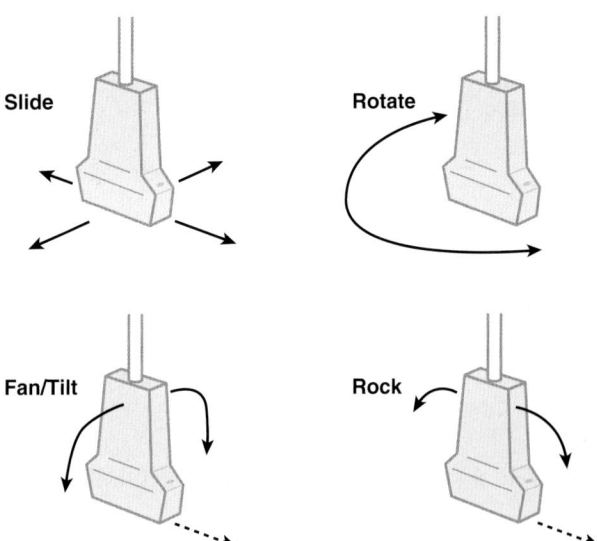

Figure 23.4 **Conventional terms for movement within planes of examination in point-of-focus ultrasound.** Sliding indicates movements across the body surface. Rotation is movement around a single point on an axis perpendicular to the skin surface. Fanning or tilting is the side-to-side movement of the distal end of the transducer in a vector perpendicular to that of the orientation marker of the transducer (*dashed line*), while maintaining the same position at the skin surface. Rocking is the side-to-side movement of the distal end of the transducer in a vector parallel to that of the orientation indicator (*dashed line*), while maintaining the same position at the skin surface.

adjusted to be parallel with flow. Pulse wave Doppler can be used to examine blood flow velocity over time within a vessel or at the left ventricular outflow tract to estimate cardiac output (see Chapter 24).

KNOBOLOGY

Knobology refers to machine settings that are adjusted by the user to optimize image quality for every ultrasound examination.

Depth, gain (essentially "brightness" control), and orientation are essential knobology functions that are discussed in detail at ExpertConsult.com.

IMAGING PLANES AND TRANSDUCER MOVEMENT

POCUS terminology includes the conventional terms for sagittal, coronal, and transverse body planes, as well as terms for planes specific to the structure being imaged. The *longitudinal* axis refers to imaging with the ultrasound beam parallel to the long axis of the structure. *Cross-sectional* or *short axis* images refer to imaging with the beam perpendicular to the long axis of the structure. Transducer movements are described in Figure 23.4.

When acquiring ultrasound images, it can be helpful to isolate transducer movements to one plane or direction at a time. Transducer movements in the *x*, *y*, and *z* axes are rocking, fanning, and rotation, respectively. *Sliding* refers to translocation of the transducer to a new acoustic window. *Rotation* around the *z*-axis is pivoting the transducer on the current point, such as when maneuvering between the long and short axis of a structure. *Fanning* is moving the plane of view (ultrasound beam) in either direction perpendicular to the rocking motion. *Rocking* is a tilting motion of the transducer along the plane of view to extend the image in either direction within the same plane.

ULTRASOUND ARTIFACTS

The term *artifact* typically connotes an undesirable effect within a measurement system; however, in POCUS, certain artifacts associated with image generation can provide useful clinical information. Commonly encountered artifacts include acoustic attenuation and enhancement, reverberation, and mirroring.

ACOUSTIC ATTENUATION AND ENHANCEMENT

Acoustic *attenuation,* or shadowing, is a reduction of signal deep to structures that strongly reflect or absorb sound waves. In thoracic ultrasound, ribs have a bright hyperechoic curved surface, casting a shadow that may impede desired imaging of other structures, such as the heart or diaphragm (Fig. 23.5, Video 23.2).

Acoustic *enhancement* is the apparent increase in signal when sound energy is minimally attenuated as it passes through a structure with less impedance than the surrounding tissues. Tissue deep to this area appears hyperechoic, as if

a bright "tail" emanates from the low-impedance structure. Acoustic enhancement can be useful to differentiate fluid-filled structures, such as cysts, which can show enhancement, from solid masses, which will not (see Fig. 23.5).

REVERBERATION

Reverberation artifacts are caused by the reflection of sound waves between two locations of tissue interface at which there is a large difference in acoustic impedance. In simple terms, the ultrasound beam "bounces" between two strong reflection points. *A-lines* represent a clinically useful example of this phenomenon. Ultrasound beams leave the transducer and travel through the skin and soft tissues to reach the pleural surface. There is large acoustic impedance difference between soft tissue and aerated lung just deep to this location, so the sound wave is strongly reflected back to the transducer, where it again encounters a strong reflector at the skin-transducer interface. Ultrasound signal reflects repeatedly between these two locations, and each time it returns to the transducer it is interpreted as another tissue plane. Because the time from beam emission to return is interpreted as distance, the ultrasound machine displays an image of equally spaced horizontal lines, representing the distance between skin and pleura (Fig. 23.6, Video 23.3).

A-lines represent either aerated lung deep to the pleura (a normal finding) or air alone (i.e., a pneumothorax). Either will

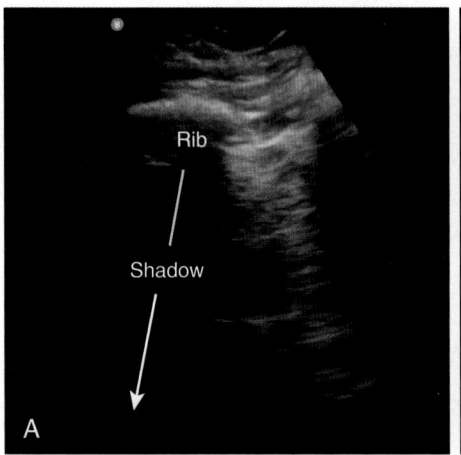
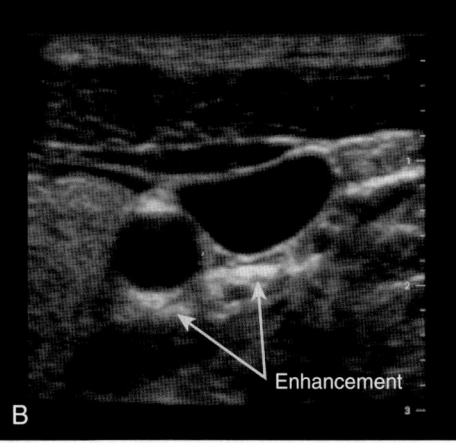

A

B

Figure 23.5 Acoustic attenuation and enhancement. (A) Acoustic attenuation, or shadowing, is seen in this thoracic image. The prominent rib casts an acoustic shadow deep to the bony cortex. Also present is a mixed pattern of horizontal A-lines and vertical ray-like B-lines in the intercostal space. (B) Acoustic enhancement is the result of sound energy passing through low-attenuation fluid, such as the blood, in this carotid artery and internal jugular vein, before encountering adjacent tissue with greater impedance. Here the tissues deep to these vessels appear as a hyperechoic "tail."

Reverberation Artifact

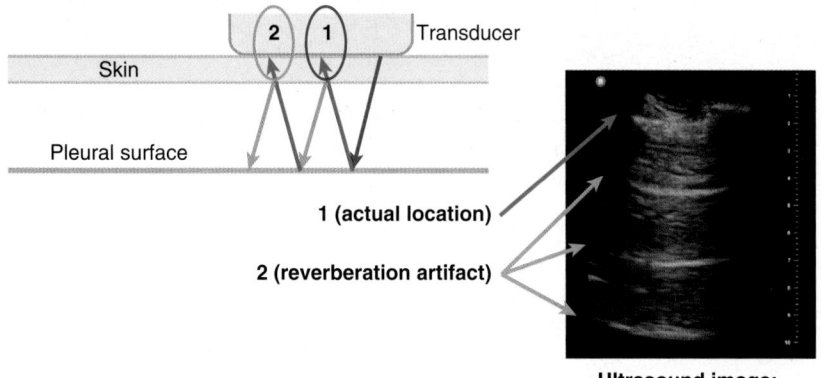

Ultrasound image: A-lines

Figure 23.6 Reverberation artifact: A-lines. An ultrasound beam (*red arrow*) leaves the transducer and reaches the pleural surface. The beam is reflected back to the transducer (*blue arrows*) and is interpreted as a bright line corresponding to the depth of the pleura relative to the skin surface (*point 1; blue arrow* on ultrasound image). Some of this reflected energy is, in turn, reflected off the inner surface of the skin (*orange arrows*) and back toward the pleural line. It takes twice as long as the first signal to return to the transducer, so it is interpreted as a second hyperechoic structure exactly twice the depth of the pleural line (*point 2*). This is the first A-line. This pattern repeats with each signal reflecting, generating multiple A-lines at equidistant depths on the ultrasound screen (*orange arrows* on ultrasound image).

produce the same pattern of reflection between skin and pleural surface (see Fig. 23.6). The presence of other normal findings, such as pleural sliding, can exclude pneumothorax and reassure the examiner that the lung parenchyma at the scanned location is normal (see "Pneumothorax" and "Use of Ultrasound in the Clinical Evaluation of Respiratory Failure" later).

B-lines are generated via complex mechanisms but are most easily understood as another type of reverberation artifact. However, B-lines represent abnormal lung. Unlike normal air-filled lung, thickened intralobular septa near the visceral pleura allow ultrasound waves to penetrate into lung tissue. Ultrasound signal will continually reverberate between the abnormal intralobular septa and collapsed or fluid-filled alveoli over small distances within the lobule below the spatial resolution of the ultrasound machine. This leads to a near-continuous stream of signal returning to the transducer that is portrayed on screen as a B-line, an uninterrupted ray of hyperechoic signal emanating from the pleural line[2] (Fig. 23.7, Videos 23.2 and 23.4). B-lines move with pleural sliding, extend to the bottom of the screen, and obliterate any A-lines they cross.

Dependent lung regions in normal patients may have small amounts of intralobular fluid or microatelectasis causing occasional thin B-lines; one or two narrow, discrete B-lines in an intercostal space can be a normal finding if it is not a widespread pattern.[2] With alveolar interstitial processes, such as pulmonary edema, interstitial fibrosis, or early pneumonia, the number of B-lines (both in a given intercostal space and distribution across lung fields) and their width increase (Video 23.5). Differentiating a predominantly A-line or B-line pattern and assessing the focality of any B-lines can be helpful in determining the cause of respiratory impairment in the acute setting (see "Use of Ultrasound in the Clinical Evaluation of Respiratory Failure" later).

MIRRORING

Mirroring artifacts may be seen in thoracic ultrasound, typically when a field of view captures structures immediately above and below the diaphragm. It is important to recognize this artifact so that "mirrored" images of abdominal structures that appear to lie superior to the diaphragm are not confused for abnormal lung tissue (Fig. 23.8).

ARTIFACTS AND IMAGE PROCESSING FEATURES

Many bedside ultrasound machines use imaging processing software that can influence the appearance of images and artifacts.[3] Tissue harmonic imaging is essentially a filter that limits certain reverberation artifacts, improves lateral resolution, and decreases beam thickness. Decreased beam slice thickness reduces speckle artifact (bright dots throughout the image) and increases acoustic enhancement, enhancing the appearance of some artifacts that are useful in thoracic ultrasound, such as B-lines.[4] Other features, such as image compounding via spatial compound imaging, reduce B-lines.[1] A detailed discussion is beyond the scope of this chapter, but POCUS providers should be familiar with these features on the machines used in practice and their impact on the obtained images.

THORACIC ULTRASOUND

NORMAL PLEURA AND LUNG

By using 2D imaging with the ultrasound transducer oriented cephalad-caudad, the pleura is visualized as a hyperechoic line in the intercostal space just deep to the ribs. When the two pleural layers are normally apposed, the movement of visceral pleura against the relatively stationary parietal pleura creates a shimmering effect on the ultrasound screen. This is the pleural "sliding" or "gliding"

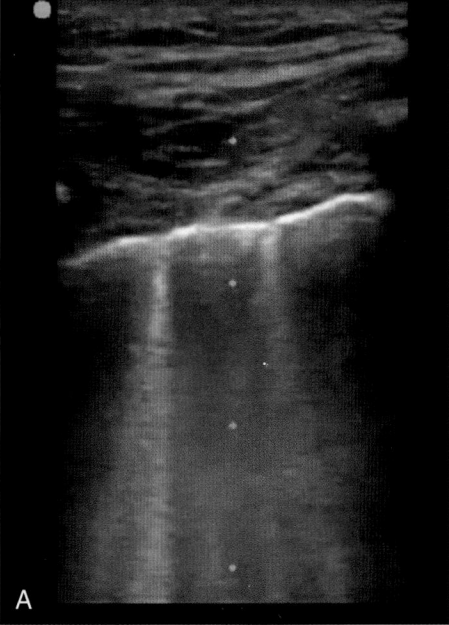
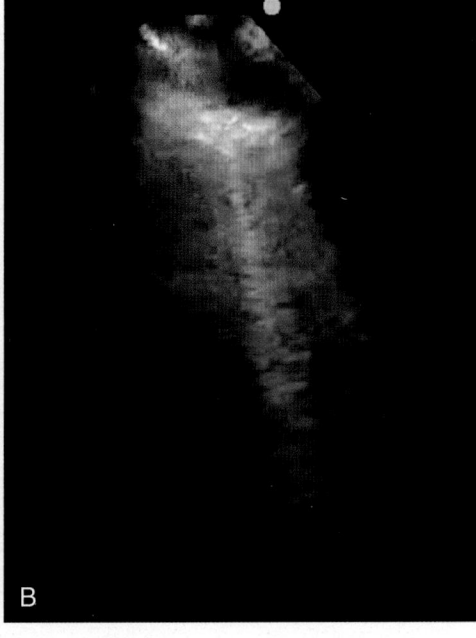

Figure 23.7 B-lines. B-lines are a type of reverberation artifact, as seen with a linear transducer (A) and phased array transducer (B). Pleura and B-lines often appear less distinct with the lower frequency, phased array transducer (B), but their recognition is the same: B-lines are hyperechoic vertical rays that extend from the pleural line all the way to the bottom of the ultrasound screen, obliterating any A-lines along the path.

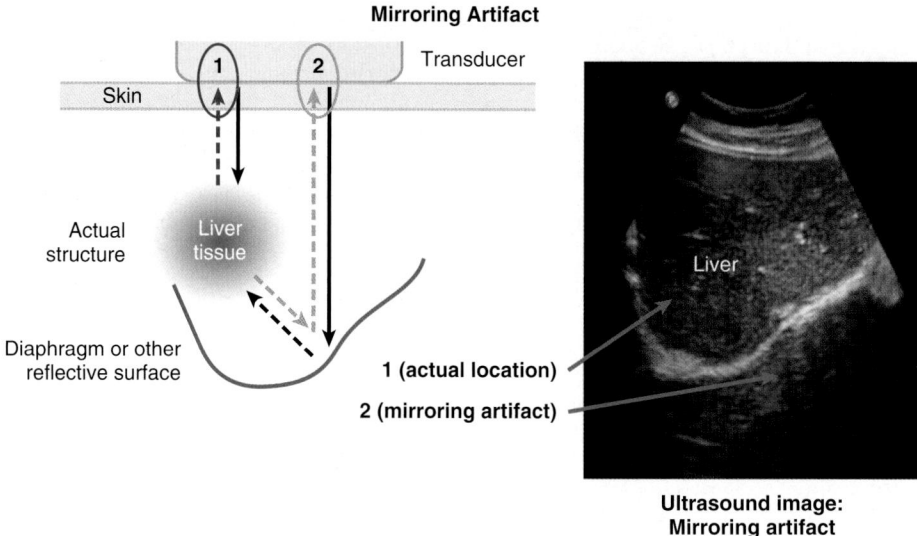

Figure 23.8 Mirroring. Mirroring is an ultrasound artifact in which duplicate structures are seen on either side of a curved, highly reflective surface. Some ultrasound waves travel to and from a structure along a direct path, reflecting off the structure (*dashed red line*) to produce an image corresponding to the depth of the structure (*point 1*). At the same time, sound wave energy from a different part of the transducer will reflect off the reflective surface at an angle, where the waves are directed to the structure (*dashed black line*) and back again (*dashed orange line*) to the reflector and then the transducer (*point 2*). The machine assumes returning echoes have traveled a direct path, and therefore, because these waves took longer to return than the direct echoes, they are interpreted as representing structures deep to the reflector. A common example in thoracic imaging is the appearance of hepatic structures both above and below the diaphragm when imaging from the abdomen. Mirroring can be mitigated by decreasing gain.

sign (also called lung sliding) (Video 23.6). Below the pleural line, normal lung is not visible, because it is fully aerated. Instead, an A-line reverberation pattern is seen on the ultrasound screen, as described earlier. In M-mode imaging of normal lung, the linear pattern seen with stationary subcutaneous tissues is interrupted at the pleural level due to pleural sliding, creating an appearance likened to lines of waves at the top of the screen meeting a sandy beach below the pleural line (the "seashore" sign; see below). Normal and abnormal ultrasound findings are listed in Table 23.2.

PNEUMOTHORAX

Because the appearance of pleural sliding represents the apposition of both pleural layers, this sign effectively excludes the presence of a pneumothorax at the imaged location.[5,6] The absence of sliding suggests either that the pleural layers are no longer in apposition at the imaged location, as seen in pneumothorax or pleural effusion, or that the pleural layers are not moving relative to each other, as seen in apnea or pleural adhesions (Video 23.7).

M-mode images may supplement B-mode evaluation of pleural sliding. In M-mode, stationary tissue has a uniform linear appearance over time. This means that the soft tissues of the chest wall create an image with a uniform linear pattern. Normally, this linear pattern is interrupted at the pleural level due to pleural sliding, creating the seashore sign as just described[7] (Fig. 23.9A). When pleural movement is absent, as in pneumothorax, apnea, or pleural adhesions, this linear pattern extends from the top to the bottom of the screen as a result of A-line reverberation artifact beyond the parietal pleura (i.e., a series of horizontal lines • throughout the depth of the ultrasound screen),

an appearance known as the "bar code" or "stratosphere" sign (see Fig. 23.9B).

Although the presence of pleural sliding excludes pneumothorax at the imaged location, a lack of sliding does not by itself confirm a diagnosis of pneumothorax because there may be alternative explanations for its absence.[8] When sliding is absent, POCUS providers can exclude pneumothorax by identifying other findings suggesting the pleural layers are in apposition. For example, the presence of B-lines indicates there is abnormal lung tissue immediately below the pleural line (see "B-Lines" earlier).[3,5,8,9] Similarly, a *lung pulse* represents the transmission of cardiac pulsations through the lung parenchyma and also indicates that lung is immediately underneath the pleura[10,11] (Video 23.8).

Although the absence of pleural sliding is not specific for pneumothorax, a "lung point" is highly suggestive of this diagnosis.[12] This finding has the appearance of sliding on one side of the ultrasound image and an absence of sliding on the other side, where the lung has fallen away from the parietal pleura. A lung point therefore represents the edge of the pneumothorax[13] (Video 23.9). The transition point from presence to absence of sliding moves with breathing. Identification of a lung point at multiple locations can allow for estimation of pneumothorax size.[14]

In practical terms, ultrasound is most easily used to exclude pneumothorax at a given location by confirming the presence of pleural sliding. Using ultrasound to diagnose pneumothorax is a more complex multistep process (Fig. 23.10). The clinical context is important in deciding how to act upon the finding of absent pleural sliding, especially if the lung point cannot be identified. For example, the pretest probability that this represents a pneumothorax is much higher in a trauma patient compared to one without

Table 23.2 Common Ultrasound Findings in Thoracic Imaging

Term	Definition	Clinical Interpretation
PLEURA		
Pleural sliding (i.e., lung sliding)	Appearance of movement in the horizontal direction along the pleural line in thoracic ultrasound.	Results from the movement of visceral pleura against the relatively stationary parietal pleura. Indicates that the two pleural layers are apposed (i.e., pneumothorax is not present).
Seashore sign	M-mode finding of normal lung and pleura in thoracic ultrasound.	M-mode correlate of pleural sliding. Indicates normal apposed pleura.
Stratosphere sign	M-mode finding in pneumothorax with exclusively horizontal lines through the field of view.	M-mode correlate of absent pleural sliding and A-line reverberation pattern. Consistent with, although not diagnostic of, pneumothorax.
Lung point	A transition involving the appearance of sliding in part of the field of view and absence of sliding in an adjacent area.	Represents the point at which inflated lung contacts the visceral pleura at the edge of a pneumothorax. Has high specificity for pneumothorax.
LINE ARTIFACTS		
A-lines	Reverberation artifact in which ultrasound beams "bounce" between two strong reflectors. Repeated signal return is interpreted by the machine as multiple equidistant structures deep to the reflector.	Seen at the interface of tissues with markedly different impedance, in thoracic ultrasound this refers to signal reverberation between the skin surface and pleura, resulting in a pattern of repeating horizontal A-lines deep to the pleural line. Present in normal lung and with pneumothorax.
B-lines	Continuous, long vertical lines that appear to move with the pleura that result primarily from reverberation artifacts near the lung surface.	Indicates lung tissue is present beyond the pleura, and is not fully aerated. B-lines increase in number and width with increased septal thickness or alveolar filling as in interstitial lung diseases, early pneumonia, pulmonary edema, and other conditions.
OTHER ARTIFACTS		
Mirroring	Interpretation by the ultrasound machine of returning sound wave signals as two images instead of one due to alternate paths of sound wave reflections returning to the transducer.	Commonly seen with the liver and spleen adjacent to the diaphragm, wherein these organs may appear both above and below the diaphragm due to its reflective properties and the limited returning signal from the lung.
Shred or fractal sign	An irregular linear interface between collapsed or consolidated lung and aerated lung within a lobe.	Diagnostic of partially collapsed or consolidated lung.

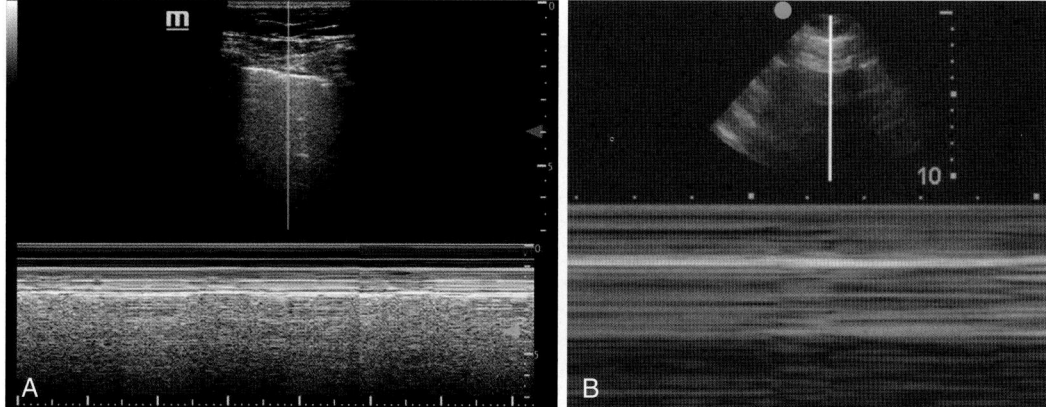

Figure 23.9 M-mode appearances of pleural sliding: normal and absent. (A) Normal pleural sliding in M-mode: "seashore" sign. Immobile soft-tissue structures of the chest wall appear as horizontal lines at the top of the image, whereas sliding at the pleural surface creates a white noise pattern lower down, in the far field. (B) Absent pleural sliding: "stratosphere sign." In comparison, when the visceral parietal pleura layers are not in apposition (as in a pneumothorax) or are affixed together (as after a pleurodesis), the M-mode panel will demonstrate a lack of movement at all depths, appearing as fixed lines in a "bar code" or "stratosphere" sign.

that history. Overall, ultrasound has been shown to have a sensitivity of 79–91% for the diagnosis of pneumothorax in meta-analyses, performing considerably better than portable chest radiographs, which have a sensitivity of 28–75%.[15–19] These studies noted that the test performance characteristics of ultrasound in the diagnosis of pneumothorax are operator dependent.

PLEURAL EFFUSION AND THORACENTESIS

Simple pleural fluid appears as an anechoic (black) space between the parietal and visceral pleura. On 2D imaging, atelectatic lung may be visible as hypoechoic tissue, often triangular in shape, moving within the pleural fluid (Videos 23.10 and 23.11). In M-mode, the respiratory motion of

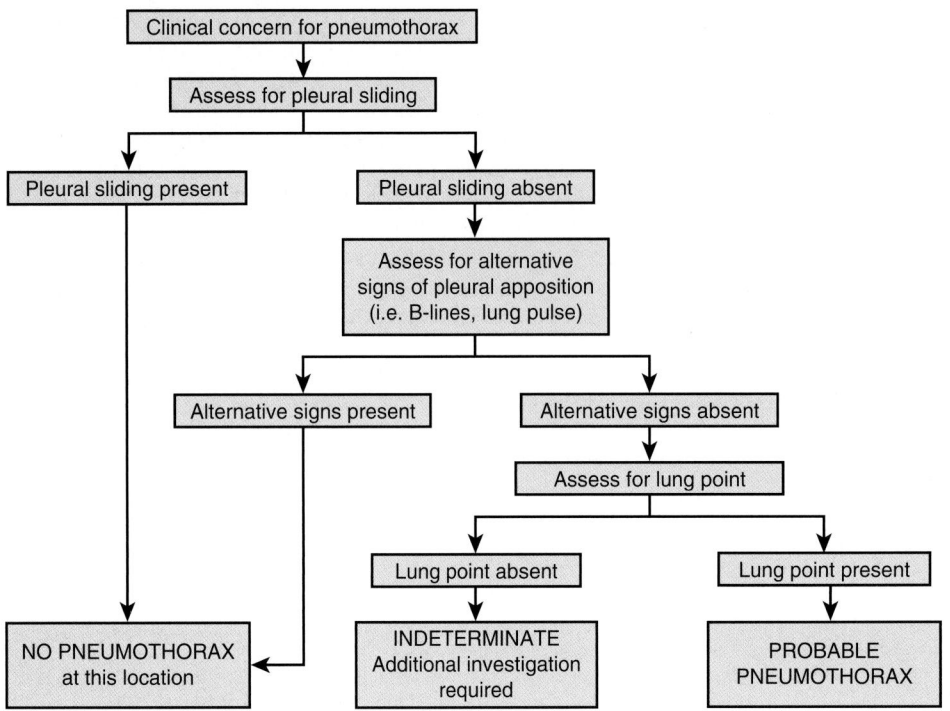

Figure 23.10 **Sample algorithm for evaluation of suspected pneumothorax using ultrasound.** The presence of pleural sliding rules out this diagnosis at the scanned location, but its absence is not confirmatory of that diagnosis. When pleural sliding is absent, one can look for alternative findings to suggest pleural apposition, such as B-lines or a lung pulse. Absent these, finding a lung point is highly suggestive of a pneumothorax; otherwise the examination is indeterminate at that location. As shown in this algorithm, it is easier to use ultrasound to exclude a pneumothorax than to make the diagnosis.

visceral pleura relative to parietal pleura creates an undulating pattern referred to as the "sinusoid" sign.[20] Pleural fluid should be distinguished from ascites by confirming that the anechoic space lies superior to the diaphragm.[21] In the absence of pleural effusion, aerated lung lies directly cephalad to the diaphragm and liver or spleen and will descend with respiration to obscure the view of these structures; a normal finding known as the "curtain" sign (Video 23.12).

Ultrasonography is more sensitive than chest radiograph but less sensitive than *computed tomography* (CT) for detecting pleural effusion.[22,23] Pleural effusion volume may be estimated using several formulas, the simplest of which involves multiplying the distance between the pleural surfaces by a constant.[24,25] Estimates are likely more accurate when the patient is upright.

The sonographic appearance of pleural fluid can help characterize the nature of an effusion; ultrasound is superior to CT for characterizing the internal structure of pleural effusions and may be more useful for following evolution over time.[26,27] Echogenic material within an effusion may indicate septations in a complex exudative process[28,29] (Videos 23.13 and 23.14). The presence of septations suggests that the fluid may be loculated and may require a different management approach than would simple pleural effusions[30,31] (Video 23.15). Pleural thickening of more than 3 mm also suggests an exudative effusion.[28,29]

Ultrasound guidance improves the success rate and safety of thoracentesis.[32,33] *Static guidance* refers to preprocedure imaging to mark the insertion site, ideally immediately before and with the patient in the same position as during the procedure. *Dynamic guidance* is used to direct needle movement in real time. In either technique, the needle insertion site should be selected to maximize the depth of pleural fluid, avoid lung and other structures, and allow the needle to pass over the top of a rib to avoid the intercostal

neurovascular bundle. The sonographer should note the limits of downward excursion of the lung and upward excursion of the diaphragm during respiration to avoid injury to this structure. If using static guidance, the operator should hold the transducer at the anticipated angle of needle insertion and note the distance from skin to pleural fluid and the depth of pleural fluid. The depth of fluid indicating a safe volume for thoracentesis depends on the skill level of the operator and the patient's clinical circumstances. British Thoracic Society guidelines suggest a minimum of 10 mm of pleural fluid depth, although other authors suggest 20 mm.[34,35] Dynamic guidance may be required for very small or loculated pleural effusions and should be performed by operators with appropriate experience.

The addition of color Doppler imaging to determine the location and course of the intercostal artery may reduce the risk of bleeding complications with thoracentesis.[36,37] A high-frequency linear array transducer is used to scan the anticipated needle course to identify any aberrant vessels within the intercostal space. As compared with CT imaging, POCUS can rule out such a vessel with a sensitivity of 0.86.[36]

PLEURA AND PLEURAL BIOPSY

Normal pleura is a thin hyperechoic line on ultrasound. Pleural irregularities may be seen in areas of inflammation, such as acute respiratory disease syndrome or pneumonia.[38,39] Pleural thickening, however, has a different significance. Pleural thickening has been defined as a focal lesion greater than 3 mm in width arising from either pleural surface.[40] Thickened pleura is typically hypoechoic and may be difficult to distinguish from pleural fluid. Because respiratory or cardiac motion will be transmitted to pleural fluid, but not to pleural thickening, the presence of a Doppler color signal may help to differentiate the two.[41] In the presence of a pleural effusion, the findings of pleural thickening greater than 1 cm, pleural nodularity, or diaphragmatic thickening greater than 7 mm all suggest the presence of malignancy[42] (Video 23.16).

Thoracoscopy is increasingly considered the gold standard for pleural biopsies but is not universally available. Closed pleural biopsy is the traditional alternative, and the widespread availability of ultrasound has improved the diagnostic yield and safety of this approach. Because it is a blind procedure, closed pleural biopsy is typically only performed in the presence of at least a moderate effusion or pneumothorax to minimize the risk of lung injury, with a diagnostic yield of less than 60% for pleural malignancy and 80–90% for tuberculous pleural effusion.[43,44] The use of ultrasound to guide the location of closed pleural biopsies to thickened areas can increase the yield for pleural malignancy and may allow performance even in the absence of a large pleural effusion.[45–47]

LUNG PARENCHYMA

Ultrasound evaluation of the lung can be a useful addition to the physical examination in the urgent evaluation of dyspnea and respiratory failure to aid in diagnostic and therapeutic decision making.[48,49] Imaging findings from multiple locations in both lungs should be interpreted together rather than relying on a single lung image. Key parenchymal findings include artifact patterns, such as B-lines, and abnormalities within the lung parenchyma, including consolidation and air bronchograms.

B-Lines

The appearance and generation of B-line artifact were described earlier. One or two individual B-lines may be seen in an intercostal space of a normal lung, particularly in more dependent regions. However, if multiple scanned locations demonstrate this pattern, it may represent pathology. As parenchyma becomes increasingly abnormal with interstitial thickening or alveolar filling, B-lines become more numerous, widen, and may coalesce into broad beams extending from the pleural line (see Video 23.5). B-lines correlate with extravascular lung water and can be quantified to follow dynamic changes, such as increases in pulmonary edema.[50,51] Of importance, B-lines are not specific to a single diagnosis; early pneumonia, pulmonary edema, interstitial fibrosis, or acute respiratory disease syndrome will all cause B-line artifacts. The term *alveolar interstitial syndrome* originally described a nonspecific chest radiograph finding of alveolar filling and interstitial thickening that correlated well with the presence of B-lines, and this term is similarly used by point-of-care sonographers.[2] Clinicians must interpret B-line patterns in light of the full clinical context, including history, physical examination, and additional studies, such as echocardiography, to make a clinical diagnosis.

Consolidation

When B-lines are seen, there is at least some air in the lung. However, when air spaces become completely fluid filled (consolidated) or degassed (atelectasis), the lung is easily penetrable to ultrasound and appears as a solid organ

with a similar echogenic texture as the liver. It is therefore described as "hepatized" on ultrasound. Air bronchograms may be visible as branching shapes of hyperechoic signal that move with respiration (Video 23.17). In the absence of any aerated lung, B-lines are not seen.

At the interface between normally aerated lung and an area of dense consolidation or atelectasis, there may be a transition zone of partially air-filled lung. This area is sometimes visualized as a "fractal" or "shred" sign: an irregular hyperechoic border with B-lines emanating from it. This finding may be seen in pneumonia or atelectasis (Video 23.18).

DIAPHRAGM

The diaphragm is best imaged with a high-frequency linear transducer at the point of diaphragm apposition with the chest wall. This is typically at approximately the tenth rib interspace along the midaxillary line. The diaphragm appears as two hyperechoic parallel lines deep to the ribs and intercostal muscles. The diaphragm thickens during inspiration from 1.6 to 2.9 mm at functional residual capacity to approximately 4.5 mm at total lung capacity[52,53] (Video 23.19). Paralyzed hemidiaphragms are thinner at rest, demonstrate little change during inspiration, and may move paradoxically cephalad with inhalation.[54] The contralateral working hemidiaphragm typically thickens even more than in normal subjects.

Increased diaphragm thickness during inspiration correlates with the pressure generated during a maximal inspiratory pressure maneuver in normal subjects and with respiratory effort in ventilated patients.[52,55] Diaphragm thickening and excursion, particularly in combination with other measures of readiness, has been shown to improve prediction of successful extubation in some studies[56–58] but not in others.[59]

In patients with neuromuscular disease, diaphragm thickness on inspiration correlates closely with other measures of respiratory muscle strength. In patients with amyotrophic lateral sclerosis, diaphragm thickening correlated with forced vital capacity, maximal inspiratory pressure, and sniff nasal inspiratory pressure.[60] Decreased diaphragm thickening, measured as a fraction of the resting thickness, may predict the need for noninvasive ventilation in patients with amyotrophic lateral sclerosis, performing similarly to measurements of forced vital capacity.[61]

USE OF ULTRASOUND IN THE CLINICAL EVALUATION OF ACUTE RESPIRATORY FAILURE

Diagnostic POCUS may be used to answer isolated questions or can be applied using a systematic approach to aid in the assessment of seriously ill patients with a broad differential diagnosis. POCUS does not replace a careful physical examination but can greatly augment the traditional bedside evaluation to narrow the differential diagnosis or confirm a specific diagnosis and direct further evaluation and urgent clinical intervention.

Several algorithmic approaches have been developed to evaluate patients with acute respiratory failure alone or as part of multisystem critical illness. The *Bedside Lung Ultrasound in Emergency* (BLUE) protocol is one of the best-known examples.[48,62] This and other published protocols use the recognition of thoracic ultrasound patterns at a standard set of examination points on the thorax to determine likely clinical diagnoses (Fig. 23.11). A thorough thoracic ultrasound protocol can be performed with a lower frequency (1–8 MHz) phased array or linear transducer that allows imaging depths up to 17 cm, but some providers also choose to use a higher frequency linear transducer for better resolution of the pleura. Published protocols and consensus guidelines call for a minimum of three or four scanned intercostal spaces per hemithorax.[63] The BLUE protocol includes one upper anterior location just caudal to the clavicle in the mid-clavicular line, one anterolateral location at the fifth intercostal space between the mid-clavicular and anterior axillary lines, and a third dependent location as far posterior as possible.

At each examination point, the operator first identifies the pleural line and examines for sliding. If absent, additional evidence will be sought to evaluate for pneumothorax (see "Pneumothorax" earlier and Fig. 23.10). The clinician then determines whether the lung parenchyma in each examination location has only A-lines throughout (A-pattern), B-lines in all locations (B-pattern), a combination of only A-lines in some fields and B-lines in others (A-B pattern), or consolidated lung in any location. When a B-line pattern is present in a single field, the full assessment should include the patterns identified in the other fields also examined (e.g., B-lines localized to some, but not all fields, or widespread) and severity (e.g., few or many B-lines, narrow/discrete or coalescent).

In some cases, these elements alone may be enough to solidify a clinical diagnosis (see Fig. 23.11). For example, a dyspneic patient who has a history of both heart failure and obstructive lung disease, with intact pleural sliding and a widely distributed B-line pattern, likely has pulmonary edema and not an isolated COPD exacerbation. Among patients with acute hypoxemic respiratory failure, the finding of B-lines in all six locations has been reported to have a positive predictive value of 87% for acute cardiogenic pulmonary edema.[48] In contrast, the same patient with intact pleural sliding and a normal aerated A-line pattern in all locations more likely has an exacerbation of underlying obstructive lung disease.

In other situations, the clinical context may necessitate further investigation. For a dyspneic patient with diffuse B-lines but no history of heart failure, echocardiography should be considered. Similarly, hypoxemia in a postoperative patient with intact pleural sliding and a diffusely normal A-line pattern should prompt further evaluation for pulmonary embolism. The presence of a widespread A-line pattern and a deep venous thrombosis has a positive predictive value of 94% for pulmonary embolism.[48] The combination of A-lines only in some areas and B-lines in others (mixed A-B pattern) requires further investigation and can

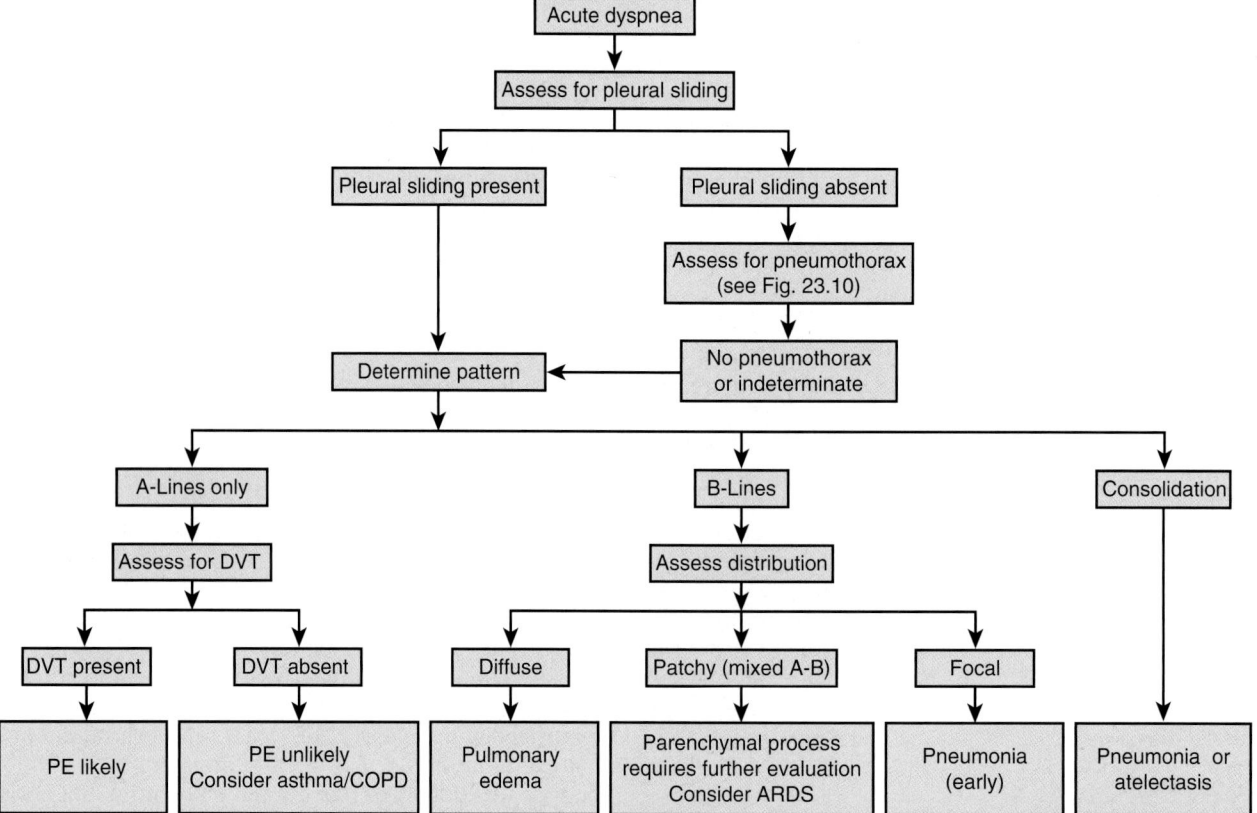

Figure 23.11 Sample algorithm for the use of ultrasound to evaluate a patient with acute dyspnea. After evaluating for pleural sliding (see Fig. 23.10), ultrasound can be used to differentiate between A-lines, B-lines, or mixed A-B line patterns and to identify areas of consolidation. The overall pattern identified in multiple scanned areas can guide the operator toward additional investigations, if needed, and direct early treatment. ARDS, acute respiratory distress syndrome; DVT, deep venous thrombosis; PE, pulmonary embolism.

be seen in pneumonia, acute respiratory distress syndrome, or limited cardiogenic pulmonary edema, for example.

In all of these cases, a thorough history and detailed physical examination provide context for the findings of a protocolized ultrasound examination to narrow the differential diagnosis for the presenting complaint and to guide clinical decision making.

VASCULAR IMAGING

CENTRAL VENOUS CATHETER PLACEMENT

The use of ultrasound to guide central venous catheterization is a recommended standard practice endorsed by many professional society guidelines.[64–70] It has been demonstrated to improve the success rate and decrease the complications of this procedure, particularly for less-experienced practitioners, in both adult and pediatric patients.[71–75]

Because the *internal jugular vein* (IJV) overlies the carotid artery in greater than 50% of patients, the increased safety provided by the use of ultrasound is at least partly related to visualization of the adjacent artery.[76–79] The position of the subclavian vein posterior to the clavicle is less easily amenable to ultrasound guidance, but this technique can be used by experienced providers in a supraclavicular or infraclavicular approach.[75]

Technique

Before the procedure, a preliminary scan of the relevant vascular structures should be performed to assess vessel patency. For IJV and subclavian vein catheters, it may be helpful to document the presence of sliding lung in the anterior thoracic field in the event of patient deterioration raising the question of pneumothorax (see "Pneumothorax" earlier). The operator should choose the insertion site based on external patient anatomy and imaging because the IJV often appears largest inferiorly on the neck, where it is also closest to the lung apex. Dynamic ultrasound guidance is recommended over a static approach.[65,66,71,75] The vessel and needle may be visualized using a short-axis (transverse, or out of plane) or long-axis (longitudinal, or in plane) approach; neither is conclusively superior.[80–82] The short-axis view allows visualization of the vein and accompanying artery but requires the operator to translocate, or fan, the transducer (see Fig. 23.4) in small movements, alternating with advancement of the needle, to visualize the needle tip throughout the procedure. The longitudinal approach does not require alternating movements of the ultrasound and needle, but the needle must remain precisely in plane with the ultrasound beam, which may be more challenging for novices. A short neck length or inguinal crease, in the case of femoral vein catheterization, may not allow a longitudinal approach.

Despite ultrasound guidance, arterial puncture and occasionally cannulation happen rarely.[74,75] To avoid malposition, the operator should visualize the guidewire in the short and long axis to confirm venous placement before dilation and catheter insertion (Fig. 23.12). After the procedure is completed, chest radiography is traditionally used to confirm catheter position, but ultrasound can also be used with a combination of vascular and cardiac views.[83,84]

PERIPHERAL VASCULAR ACCESS

Ultrasound may be used to facilitate catheterization of the peripheral venous and arterial system. The relative ease of compressibility of the venous lumen with gentle pressure aids in the differentiation of peripheral veins and arteries. In patients with difficult venous access, ultrasound guidance reduces the number of attempts and the time to successful placement of peripheral intravenous catheters compared to traditional blind technique. Improved success with ultrasound-guided peripheral intravenous catheter placement may reduce the need for central venous catheters.[85–89] In addition to traditional antecubital fossa and forearm locations, the use of ultrasound allows providers to access brachial or proximal basilic vessels. However, these locations require careful consideration because standard 3 to 5 cm length catheters have a high rate of dislodgement and early failure.[90] As in central venous catheter guidance, providers may use a short- or long-axis approach to peripheral vessels.

DEEP VENOUS THROMBOSIS ASSESSMENT

Limited sonography of the lower extremity deep veins is a useful adjunct in the assessment of dyspnea when pulmonary embolism is suspected. Clinicians can diagnose deep venous thrombosis by performing a two-point compression examination at the femoral and popliteal locations with a sensitivity and specificity of 96% and 97%, respectively, compared to gold-standard formal duplex examinations or

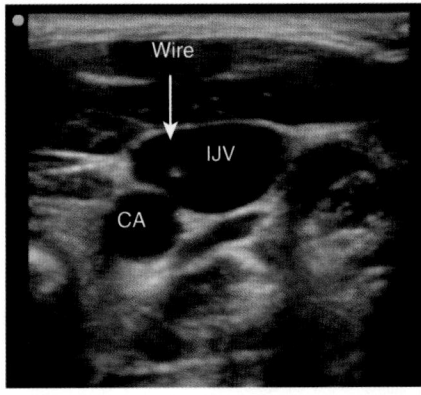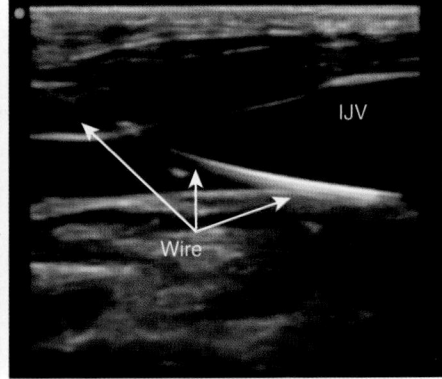

Figure 23.12 Central venous catheter placement. To ensure proper placement before dilating and catheter insertion, visual confirmation of the wire within the target vessel should be confirmed as shown in both the short (A) and long (B) axes. CA, carotid artery; IJV, internal jugular vein.

venography.[91,92] To perform the examination, the supine patient's leg is externally rotated slightly at the hip and flexed at the knee. The common femoral vein is identified above the inguinal ligament using a high-frequency linear transducer in the transverse plane. The operator follows its course to the bifurcation into the superficial and deep femoral veins, compressing every 2 cm along the course of the veins. This is repeated for the popliteal vein from just above the popliteal fossa to its distal trifurcation.

Normal veins are easily completely collapsed with light pressure (Video 23.20). If adequate pressure is applied to deform the accompanying artery slightly and the vein is *not* completely collapsed, even if no material is visible in the lumen, it suggests the presence of a fresh acute thrombus that is not yet organized and therefore less echogenic (Video 23.21). Absence of Doppler signal at this location, with or without augmentation by calf compression, may help confirm presence of thrombosis. Larger and older, organized thrombus may be visible within a vein as a hypoechoic structure (Video 23.22).

Key Points

- Point-of-care ultrasound is increasingly used for diagnostic purposes in pulmonary and critical care medicine and is the standard of care for several common procedures.
- Ultrasound signal travels through the body, reflects off internal structures, and returns to the transducer, where it is interpreted as images. The time required to complete this journey is interpreted as depth.
- Tissues have variable acoustic impedance, which determines how ultrasound signal travels through the body and the echogenicity, or brightness, with which they appear on screen.
- Lung ultrasound images are often generated by artifacts, but these patterns can provide useful information even if they are not a true picture of the underlying tissues.
- The presence of pleural sliding rules out pneumothorax at the imaged location with high accuracy.
- B-lines, which indicate the underlying lung parenchyma is not normally aerated, can be seen in pulmonary edema or interstitial fibrosis but are not specific for any one diagnosis.
- Ultrasound guidance for thoracentesis, pleural biopsy, and central venous catheter placement increases the success and safety of these procedures and is the standard of practice.

Key Readings

American Society of Anesthesiologists Task Force on Central Venous Access, Rupp SM, Apfelbaum JL, Blitt C, et al. Practice guidelines for central venous access: a report by the American Society of Anesthesiologists Task Force on Central Venous Access. *Anesthesiology.* 2012;116(3):539–573.

Baad M, Lu ZF, Reiser I, Paushter D. Clinical significance of US artifacts. *Radiographics.* 2017;37:1408–1423.

Frankel HL, Kirkpatrick AW, Elbarbary M, et al. Guidelines for the appropriate use of bedside general and cardiac ultrasonography in the evaluation of critically ill patients—part I: general ultrasonography. *Crit Care Med.* 2015;43(11):2479–2502.

Havelock T, Teoh R, Laws D, Gleeson F, BTS Pleural Disease Guideline Group. Pleural procedures and thoracic ultrasound: British Thoracic Society pleural disease guideline 2010. *Thorax.* 2010;65(suppl 2):ii61–ii76.

Lamperti M, Bodenham AR, Pittiruti M, et al. International evidence-based recommendations on ultrasound-guided vascular access. *Intensive Care Med.* 2012;38(7):1105–1117.

Lichtenstein DA, Mezière GA. Relevance of lung ultrasound in the diagnosis of acute respiratory failure. The BLUE protocol. *Chest.* 2008;134:117–125.

Lichtenstein DA. Ultrasound in the management of thoracic disease. *Crit Care Med.* 2007;35(suppl 5):S250–S261.

Soni N, Arntfield R, Kory P. *Point of Care Ultrasound.* 2nd ed. St. Louis: Elsevier; 2019.

Volpicelli G, Elbarbary M, Blaivas M, et al. International Liaison Committee on Lung Ultrasound (ILC-LUS) for International Consensus Conference on Lung Ultrasound (ICC-LUS). International evidence-based recommendations for point-of-care lung ultrasound. *Intensive Care Med.* 2012;38(4):577–591.

Complete reference list available at ExpertConsult.com.

24 ULTRASONOGRAPHY: ADVANCED APPLICATIONS AND PROCEDURES

CHRISTOPHER F. BARNETT, MD, MPH • DANIEL A. SWEENEY, MD • LINDSEY L. HUDDLESTON, MD

INTRODUCTION

The use of ultrasound machines in *intensive care units* (ICUs) is common. Noncardiologists can learn to acquire images and interpret them rapidly and correctly to answer common clinically relevant questions, such as determining a patient's left ventricular systolic function. The answers to these questions can alter treatment and optimize patient care. This chapter reviews the data to support training in critical care echocardiography for noncardiologists. It then reviews how to acquire basic views and how to interpret these images to be used in clinical decision making. The chapter concludes with a suggested approach to combining all of the ultrasound assessments described in Chapter 23 and this chapter for use in the evaluation and management of a patient with shock.

Critical care ultrasound (CCU), defined as point-of-care ultrasound performed by intensivists, has become a widely embraced technology in the ICU to aid with procedures, diagnosis, and treatment. *Critical care echocardiography* (CCE), a subdivision of CCU, can be further divided into basic and advanced skill sets. Basic CCE is largely limited to B- and M-mode imaging, addresses specific clinical questions (e.g., whether pericardial effusion is present), and generates qualitative findings (e.g., the systolic function is hyperdynamic, nearly normal, reduced, or severely reduced). Basic CCE has lent itself to the development of a number of systematic approaches (with acronyms such as FEEL, FATE,

and RUSH) for addressing specific critically ill groups of patients, including, most notably, patients with shock.[1-3] Advanced CCE, conversely, is quantitative and goes beyond basic CCE to include Doppler ultrasound for the purpose of evaluating valvular function, cardiac output, and left heart diastolic function. Advanced CCE is beyond the scope of this chapter. In contrast, basic CCE has been promoted by the Accreditation Council for Graduate Medical Education and is quickly becoming an expected skill set for all intensivists.[4]

CRITICAL CARE ECHOCARDIOGRAPHY AS A DIAGNOSTIC TOOL FOR INTENSIVISTS

Noncardiologist physicians from different specialties (emergency medicine, internal medicine, and surgery) at different levels of training (resident or attending) can perform and accurately interpret focused cardiac ultrasound examinations.[5-9] Shared characteristics across studies support the diagnostic use of basic CCE. In most studies, training was limited to 1 day and included both didactic and hands-on sessions. Most of these studies, using complete or formal echocardiographic examinations as the comparator, demonstrated that noncardiologists are able to use a portable or handheld ultrasound device to make a qualitative assessment of left ventricular function, identify the presence or absence of a pericardial effusion, and evaluate the size of the *inferior vena cava* (IVC) with good interrater agreement. Basic CCE estimations of left ventricular function can be performed in less than 15 minutes.[7,9] Moreover, the basic CCE examination is almost always performed in conjunction with a pulmonary ultrasound examination. When the findings of these two examinations are integrated, a more complete clinical picture can be achieved, especially in cases of undifferentiated shock or when there is concern for heart failure with pulmonary edema.[10]

Judging whether a hypotensive patient would be responsive to fluids is an ongoing challenge for critical care practitioners. The use of central venous pressure, a static measure, to predict fluid responsiveness is inferior to dynamic measurements, such as assessing the changes of IVC diameter with breathing.[11] Nonetheless, even when performed in sedated, mechanically ventilated patients, measurements of IVC diameter variation are imperfect in predicting fluid responsiveness.[11] Advanced CCE skills such as measuring stroke volume variation have been shown to be superior to assessing IVC variation in some studies, although this examination requires more time at the bedside and can be technically challenging.[12] In addition, the practitioner of advanced CCE should be cautious when assessing valvular disease because this can be demanding even for experienced echocardiographers.[13]

IMPACT OF CRITICAL CARE ECHOCARDIOGRAPHY ON THE MANAGEMENT OF CRITICALLY ILL PATIENTS

The impact of CCE on the management of critically ill patients has been studied, with mixed results. In one study, CCE evaluation changed the working diagnoses and the corresponding management plans in 37% (33 of 90) of critically ill patients.[7] Typical management changes after the CCE examination included starting or stopping diuretic agents, fluid resuscitation, or inotropic therapies. In a study of trauma patients (n = 240), CCE assessment led to a decrease in intravenous fluid administration, a quicker time to the operating room, and a trend toward a lower mortality rate (11% vs. 19.5%; $P = 0.09$).[14] In a retrospective study of patients with subacute septic shock (N = 220), CCE led to less fluid administration, increased use of inotropic therapies, and improved 28-day survival (66% vs. 56%; $P = 0.04$) compared with historic control subjects.[15] Unfortunately, not all studies of point-of-care ultrasound in critically ill patients have shown benefit, including one retrospective report (n = 5441) that found care delays and a higher in-hospital mortality rate (29% vs. 22%; $P < 0.001$) if bedside ultrasound examination was performed before initiating a fluid bolus or a vasoactive medication.[16]

CRITICAL CARE ECHOCARDIOGRAPHY TRAINING, COMPETENCY, AND CERTIFICATION

Various education and clinical care regulatory bodies, along with surveyed critical care fellowship directors, have acknowledged the importance of point-of-care ultrasound in the care of critically ill patients. However, there is no consensus on how best to train intensivists, determine competency, and ultimately award certification for CCU.[3,4,17] In general, most CCU training includes a short focused course (1 to 2 days), with the majority of the time dedicated to CCE. Typically, didactic lectures constitute 50% of the training time, with the other 50% of the course dedicated to hands-on training using task trainer simulation, ultrasound simulation, and live ultrasound scanning of volunteer individuals. Hands-on training is generally performed in small groups usually consisting of one model, one instructor, and five or fewer learners.[18] For critical care fellows in training, a comprehensive CCU program also entails regular image review sessions and documentation by the trainee of successfully performed point-of-care ultrasound examinations and ultrasound-guided procedures.

Despite recognition of the importance of all of these elements, it is rare that a fellowship program can achieve such a comprehensive CCU educational experience. In a 2014 survey of critical care program directors, 42% (25 of 60) lacked a formal curriculum.[19] Limited numbers of faculty proficient in point-of-care ultrasound and limited time to teach CCE are among the barriers to developing a CCU program.[17] Despite these shortcomings in training, multiple societies have produced position papers establishing standards for CCU, including CCE training and competency.[20–22] Beginning in 2019, The National Board of Echocardiography began offering an Examination of Special Competence in Critical Care Echocardiography. The examination was developed with input from the National Board of Medical Examiners and representation from eight medical societies, with the aim of establishing an objective means of identifying individuals with expertise in CCE.[23]

IMAGE ACQUISITION AND INTERPRETATION OF THE CRITICAL CARE ECHOCARDIOGRAM

The following sections describe the four standard cardiac views that we suggest should be obtained during a cardiac critical care echocardiogram. We then share the approach that we recommend for use in interpreting the images obtained. We favor a simple subjective evaluation of the images that can be easily performed without additional image processing. Acquiring CCU skills requires adequate training. Professional society guidelines vary; however, we recommend a structured program of didactic and hands-on instruction followed by a longitudinal curriculum that incorporates proctored ultrasound examinations and image interpretation.[24]

DATA QUALITY, CONFIDENCE OF INTERPRETATION, AND RESPONSIBILITY FOR UNEXPECTED FINDINGS

Similar to the physical examination, cardiac ultrasound image acquisition and interpretation are subjective, and the value of the interpretation is markedly affected by the quality of the data acquired. Operators should incorporate an assessment of the quality of the data and confidence in their interpretation into the report of their findings. For example, during assessment of left ventricular function, if only two of four recommended assessments can be performed, it should be clearly noted that the data were inadequate to perform a complete evaluation and the interpretation may be adversely affected. These limitations should then be considered when making patient care decisions. At times, it is appropriate to conclude that the data from the ultrasound examination are of poor quality, cannot be interpreted, and should not be used for clinical decisions. Assessment of the data quality is an important skill that must be learned and practiced and will improve as operators accumulate experience.

Another important aspect of data collection and interpretation is recognizing when an acquired image shows an unexpected finding that may have clinical significance but that the operator does not know how to interpret.[25] We recommend that, in this setting, the operator immediately contact an imaging expert to review the stored images or to perform a complete examination.

PREPARATION FOR THE CRITICAL CARE ECHOCARDIOGRAM

Similar to other ICU procedures, spending adequate time to gather all needed equipment and prepare for the ultrasound examination will increase the possibility of successful image acquisition and greater likelihood that the examination will be useful in patient care. Needed equipment includes ultrasound gel, towels for removing ultrasound gel at the completion of the examination, the ultrasound machine with ultrasound probes needed for the planned examination, a wedge or pillows to position the patient and, ideally, an assistant who can manage the controls on the ultrasound machine during the examination so the operator can focus on image acquisition and interpretation.

Less experienced operators will benefit if the ultrasound machine is positioned so that the patient and ultrasound probe are in the same line of sight as the ultrasound machine. Typically, this means that the machine will be positioned on the side of the patient opposite to the position of the operator. The patient's bed should be raised or lowered so that the operator can acquire images without bending or reaching. Sometimes this is best accomplished with the operator sitting on a chair or standing on a step. The bed height should be adjusted during the examination as needed to optimize patient positioning with respect to the operator.

For acquiring parasternal long, short, and apical views, patients should be in the left lateral decubitus position (eFig. 24.1). Although it may be possible to acquire these images in the supine patient, it is often much more difficult and may significantly degrade data quality, particularly when acquiring an apical view in which foreshortening (see later for a description of foreshortening) can go unnoticed. Echocardiography laboratories often use beds with a breakaway panel to facilitate imaging of the patient in a decubitus position. Although this is not possible in an ICU bed, wedges, pillows, or towels can all be used to provide space for the probe. In contrast, the subcostal view requires the patient to be supine. When possible, having patients bend their knees can result in relaxation of abdominal muscles and improved imaging.

PROBE MANIPULATION

Familiarity with how to manipulate the ultrasound probe and the terminology that describes these maneuvers can markedly improve the ability of the operator to acquire high-quality ultrasound images. It is important that the operator analyze the image on the screen, determine how image quality can be optimized, and then carefully and deliberately manipulate the probe to achieve the desired image.

Four basic probe movements can be described using agreed-upon terminology (eFig. 24.2). When the foot (the part of the probe in contact with the patient's skin) of the ultrasound probe is moved to a new location on the chest (e.g., when moving from a parasternal to an apical view, or moving along a rib space in the parasternal view), this is referred to as "sliding." All other movements should be performed while keeping the foot of the probe anchored in place on the patient's chest. "Rocking" is changing the angle of the probe along the long axis of the probe foot while maintaining contact with the patient in a fixed position. "Fanning" is changing the angle of the probe interface along the short axis of the probe foot while maintaining contact with the patient in a fixed position. "Rotating" is turning the probe clockwise or counterclockwise while keeping the foot of the probe in contact with the skin. In general, these maneuvers should be performed sequentially rather than simultaneously (i.e., fan only; do not also rock or tilt in the same maneuver) to obtain and optimize an image in a stepwise fashion.

BASIC CRITICAL CARE ECHOCARDIOGRAM VIEWS

Basic CCE uses four ultrasound views to answer clinically relevant questions (Fig. 24.1). These four views exclude significant portions of the heart, such as segments of the anterior and inferior wall, that would be seen in a complete echocardiogram.

Obtaining images of the heart in all four views is important for several reasons. First, not all cardiac structures are present in all views, so all of the views described here are needed to view all relevant cardiac structures. Second, it is often difficult to see all of the cardiac structures expected in a view because of the limitations of ultrasound physics (see Chapter 23 for a discussion of basic ultrasound physics) or because of a patient's anatomy. For example, the endocardial borders (where the cardiac wall ends and the left ventricular cavity starts) are better visualized when the ultrasound beam is perpendicular to the cardiac walls versus when the ultrasound beam is parallel to cardiac walls. Third, it is necessary to confirm findings in multiple views because images may be affected by artifact or other imaging errors that are recognized only when the same structure is seen in a different view.

Obtaining high-quality images and recognizing normal cardiac structures and function require proctored ultrasound scanning and repetitive scanning of many patients with normal hearts. Comparison with gold standard images, hands-on instruction, and review of saved images with an expert are all approaches that we recommend so

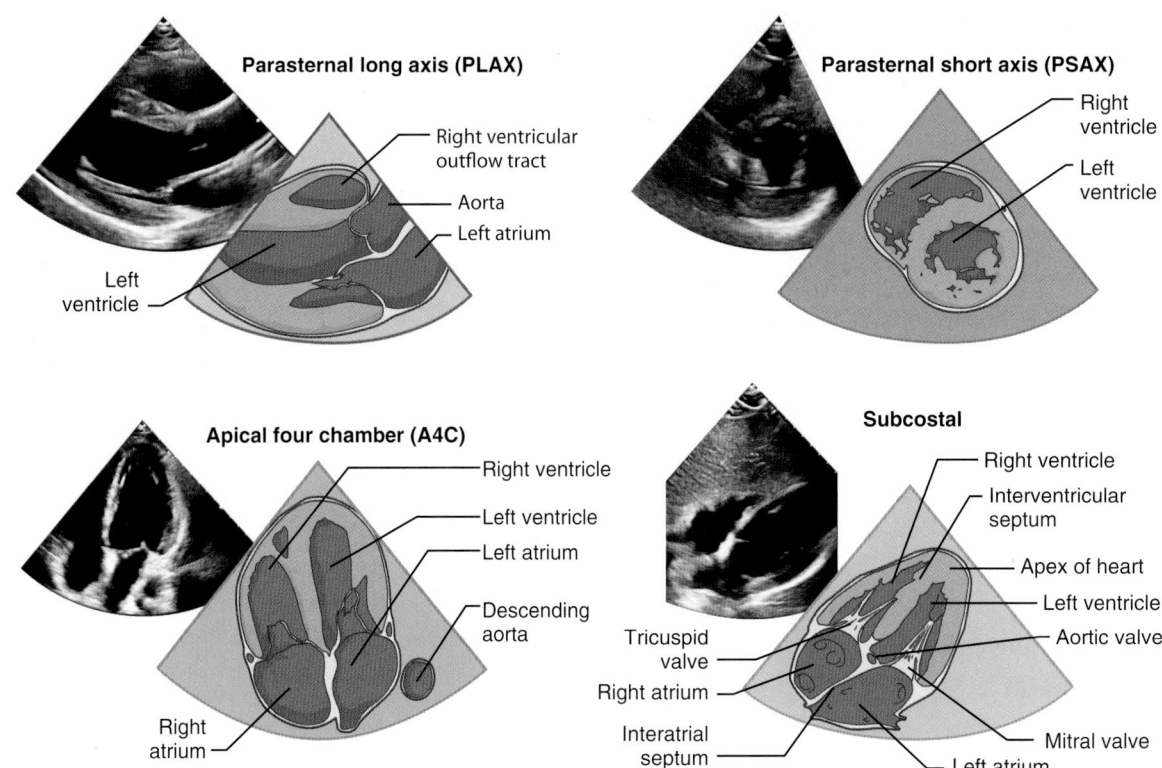

Figure 24.1 The four basic critical care echocardiography views. Careful attention should be paid to the ultrasound images to ensure that only good-quality data are incorporated into clinical decision making. If image quality is not adequate, the image should be discarded and other ultrasound views should be obtained. Multiple views should be interrogated in all patients to ensure that findings are consistent across views and do not represent artifact or result from poor data quality.

learners will come to recognize what a healthy heart looks like and therefore will recognize abnormalities. To achieve proficiency in identifying healthy and abnormal hearts, we recommend 50 or more proctored cardiac examinations; however, skills will continue to improve with additional practice.

Although a few high-quality images obtained from these four basic views are typically adequate to answer the clinically relevant questions posed by an intensivist, for complete assessment of cardiac structure and function, a complete echocardiogram requires between 70 and 125 images.

PARASTERNAL LONG-AXIS VIEW

The *parasternal long-axis* (PLAX) view is obtained by placing the foot of the ultrasound probe in the third or fourth intercostal space adjacent to the sternum with the long axis of the probe in line with the patient's right shoulder (Video 24.1). Sliding the probe laterally along the rib space may improve image quality. The probe is sequentially rotated and fanned until all of the desired structures are optimally viewed. A good-quality image of the heart in the PLAX view has the following characteristics: (1) the heart will appear horizontal on the screen; (2) the walls of the myocardium will be parallel; (3) the two leaflets of the mitral valve along with the posterior papillary muscle and two of three leaflets of the aortic valve will be seen; and (4) the complete left atrium will be seen. Frequently, the heart will appear to point up to the top of the screen. This is an indication that the probe is too low on the chest, thus placing the apex

too close to the transducer. To remedy this issue, the probe should be moved up an intercostal space.

In this view, segments of the anteroseptal and posterior walls are seen perpendicular to the ultrasound beam, so this view is useful to assess for wall thickening. This view is frequently the optimal view for assessment of mitral valve opening and mitral annular excursion, which are important for determining left ventricular systolic function.

PARASTERNAL SHORT-AXIS VIEW

The *parasternal short-axis* (PSAX) view is a view through the midwalls of the myocardium at the level of the papillary muscles (Video 24.2). An optimal PSAX view is obtained by starting with an optimal PLAX view and then rocking the probe so a line dropped from the apex of the image intersects perpendicularly with both walls of the myocardium and passes through the papillary muscle. Many ultrasound machines can display a line on the screen that can be turned on to facilitate this maneuver. The probe is then rotated clockwise 90 degrees with care not to rock or fan. The resulting image of the left ventricle is a circle with the papillary muscles in the short axis evident at approximately the 3 and 7 o'clock positions. Because there are few asymmetric structures in the PSAX view useful to guide probe movement for image optimization, we recommend returning to a PLAX view as needed to optimize the image, then using the same rock-then-rotate maneuver, returning to the PSAX view.

The PSAX view shows the midsegments of all of the myocardial walls. Because the mitral valve is not visualized, the view is of limited utility in assessing left ventricular dysfunction. The PSAX view provides important clues to the presence of right ventricular dysfunction because it is the best view to identify flattening of the septal wall of the left ventricle caused by right ventricular abnormalities.

APICAL FOUR-CHAMBER VIEW

The *apical four-chamber* (A4C) view is obtained by positioning the ultrasound probe as close as possible to the apex of the heart, which can be located by palpation of the point of maximum impulse (Video 24.3). The probe is then rotated and fanned until both ventricles, both atria, and the mitral and tricuspid valve leaflets can be seen fully opening and closing.

It is important to recognize and avoid foreshortening of the left ventricular image in the A4C view (Fig. 24.2). Foreshortening results when the ultrasound beam does not pass through the left ventricular apex but instead passes through a wall of the left ventricle. The apex of the left ventricle is normally thin, and it thickens only minimally during ventricular systole. If the apex appears thick in an A4C view, then the image is likely foreshortened. If an image is foreshortened, abnormalities of the left ventricular apex will not be seen. Foreshortening can also make left ventricular systolic function appear better than it actually is, thereby leading to misinterpretation of data. Additionally, a foreshortened A4C results in artifactual enlargement of the right ventricle, so a normal, healthy right ventricle may appear dilated with reduced function. To obtain a proper image of the right ventricle in the A4C view, a non-foreshortened image of the left ventricle must first be obtained, and then the probe should be rotated until the right ventricle is as large as possible.

This view shows the basal, middle, and apical segments of the septal and lateral walls, as well as the right ventricular chamber, which is not seen in the parasternal views. This view also provides another view of the mitral valve annulus, which is important in the evaluation of left ventricular dysfunction.

SUBCOSTAL VIEW

The subcostal view (or the subxiphoid view) is obtained by placing the probe inferior to the xyphoid process and slightly lateral (right) to the midline with the probe foot in a horizontal position (Video 24.4). The ultrasound probe is oriented so the beam passes through the liver, and the probe is then rotated, fanned, and rocked until the heart can be identified.

As in the A4C view, both ventricles, both atria, and the tricuspid and mitral valves should be seen on the subcostal view. The IVC can be imaged by manipulating the probe so the right atrium is in the center of the screen. The probe is then rotated counterclockwise and manipulated to be perpendicular to the abdominal wall.

The structures seen in the subcostal view are the same as the structures seen in the A4C view. At times, these structures are better visualized from the subcostal view. The subcostal view is often the best view for assessing right

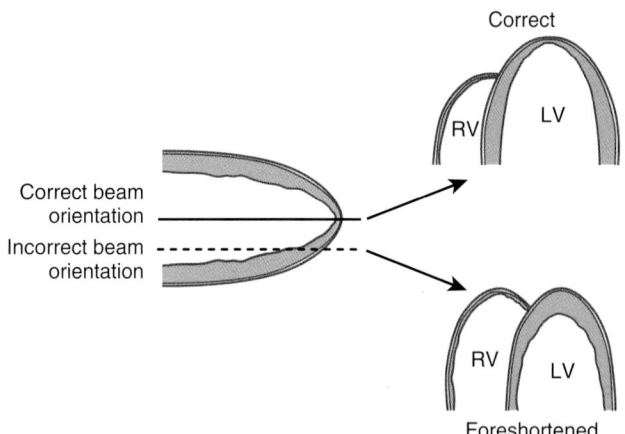

Figure 24.2 Foreshortening. Foreshortening results when the ultrasound beam does not pass through the left ventricular apex but instead passes through a wall of the left ventricle (LV). With foreshortening, the true apex of the left ventricle is not imaged, and the right ventricle (RV) falsely appears enlarged; this may lead to incorrect image interpretation and inappropriate patient care decisions.

ventricular function because the ultrasound beam is perpendicular to the right ventricular free wall.

INTERPRETATION OF ULTRASOUND IMAGES

LEFT VENTRICULAR FUNCTION

For evaluation of the left ventricular systolic function, we recommend combining four subjective assessments into an overall impression and suggest that each of the four assessments should be performed as completely as possible in each of the four basic ultrasound views. Furthermore, we recommend grading systolic function into one of three broad categories: (1) normal or hyperdynamic, (2) reduced systolic function, or (3) severely reduced systolic function (Videos 24.5 through 24.8).

1. The first assessment is an evaluation of the change in the size of the cavity of the ventricle. This is a subjective assessment of the ejection fraction that is made by simply examining the left ventricular cavity during systole and diastole and noting whether the cavity decreases in size and by how much (Table 24.1).
2. The second assessment is an evaluation of wall thickening. Even though the term *wall motion* is in common use, it is important to understand that myocardial segments are functioning normally when the myocardium thickens. (Dysfunctional myocardial segments may "move" because they are adjacent to other normally functioning myocardial segments.) The visible walls should be examined to determine whether the wall is thickening.
3. The third assessment is an evaluation of the motion of the anterior leaflet of the mitral valve in the PLAX view. This is a subjective assessment of the E-point septal separation, a measure commonly used to assess systolic function before the availability of two-dimensional echocardiographic imaging.[26] In a heart with normal systolic function, the mitral valve should open wide

Table 24.1 Assessments of Left and Right Ventricular Function*

LEFT VENTRICULAR FUNCTION

1. Change in the size of the left ventricular cavity
2. Thickening of the walls of the myocardium
3. Opening of the mitral valve
4. Movement of the mitral valve annulus toward the apex

RIGHT VENTRICULAR FUNCTION

1. Movement of the tricuspid annulus toward the apex
2. Motion of the right ventricular free wall
3. Change in the size of the right ventricular cavity
4. Flattening of the interventricular septum

*Recommended assessments to use for evaluating ventricular systolic function. Each of these assessments should be performed in as many of the four views as possible and integrated for a final conclusion about ventricular function.

during diastole so the anterior mitral leaflet is close to the interventricular septum.

4. The final assessment is evaluation of the motion of the mitral valve annulus; this is best assessed in either the PLAX view or the A4C view. The movement of the myocardium at the point that it joins the posterior mitral valve leaflet is assessed. In a heart with normal systolic function, the mitral valve annulus moves vigorously from the base of the heart toward the apex. In a complete echocardiographic evaluation of this function, the equivalent objective measurement is referred to as the *mitral annular plane systolic excursion.*

Because no single view and no single assessment are reliable, all four of these assessments should be performed in all four basic views (with the exception of the PSAX view, in which only two of the assessments are possible). For example, in a patient with mitral valve disease, the mitral valve may not appear to open fully, but the provider can conclude that systolic function is normal on the basis of the other three assessments.

There are several technical pitfalls in assessing left ventricular systolic function. As previously discussed, a foreshortened view may cause systolic function to appear better than it actually is because the cavity size appears smaller during systole. A similar problem arises if the heart moves out of the ultrasound imaging plane during image acquisition.

There are also pitfalls in interpretation of left ventricular systolic function when other pathologic conditions are present. For example, hypovolemia may falsely create the appearance of normal systolic function because there is little intracavitary volume. Another potential pitfall is the presence of severe mitral valve regurgitation. Assessment of mitral valve disease is beyond the scope of this chapter; however, when there is severe mitral regurgitation, left ventricular systolic function may appear normal because much of the blood ejected during systole is ejected into the low-pressure left atrium. Nonetheless, there may still be significant myocardial dysfunction. In fact, a patient may present in cardiogenic

shock resulting from severe mitral regurgitation, but myocardial function on the standard views as described earlier will appear normal.

RIGHT VENTRICULAR FUNCTION

Right ventricular systolic function is evaluated using a set of assessments similar to those used for left ventricular systolic function. Because right ventricular function is more difficult to evaluate, we recommend grading the right ventricle as "normal" or "not normal." In the PSAX and PLAX views, the right ventricle is typically not well visualized, and only a portion of the right ventricular outflow tract can be seen. The A4C and subcostal views are therefore needed for a meaningful evaluation of right ventricular function (Video 24.9).

1. The first assessment is evaluation of the motion of the tricuspid valve annulus in the A4C or subcostal views. The movement of the myocardium at the point that the right ventricular free wall joins the tricuspid valve leaflet is assessed. In a heart with normal systolic function, the tricuspid valve annulus moves vigorously from the base of the heart toward the apex. In a complete echocardiographic evaluation of this function, the equivalent objective measurement is referred to as the *tricuspid annular plane systolic excursion*[27] (see Table 24.1).

2. The second assessment is an evaluation of the motion of the right ventricular free wall. However, the right ventricular free wall is often not well visualized, especially in a healthy right ventricle, so this assessment cannot always be incorporated into the final conclusions about right ventricular function.

3. The third assessment is an evaluation of the change in the size of the cavity of the ventricle. This assessment is made by examining the right ventricular cavity during systole and diastole and noting whether the cavity decreases in size and by how much. Given the shape of the right ventricle, it is not possible to calculate an ejection fraction without three-dimensional imaging. The analogous objective assessment performed in the echocardiography laboratory is the *fractional area change.*

4. The fourth assessment is an evaluation of the shape of the interventricular septum. In the PSAX view, the left ventricle should appear round. Flattening of the septum (so the left ventricle appears D-shaped) suggests that there may be an abnormality of the right ventricle. Evaluation of the right ventricle in other views is needed to confirm and characterize the abnormality more clearly.

RIGHT ATRIAL PRESSURE

Determining the IVC diameter and the change in diameter with breathing is a useful technique for estimating right atrial pressure.[28] There are several approaches to obtaining this view. We recommend starting with a good-quality subcostal view of the heart. The probe is then rotated counterclockwise and manipulated so the probe is perpendicular to the abdominal wall. During this motion, the right atrium is kept in the center of the screen. As

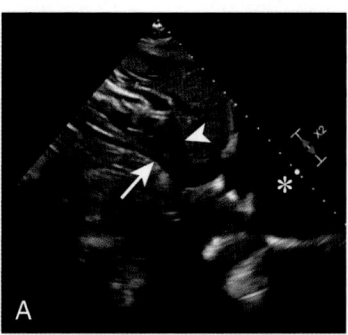 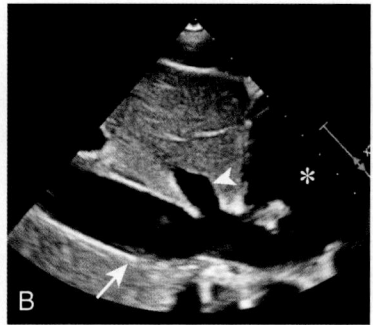 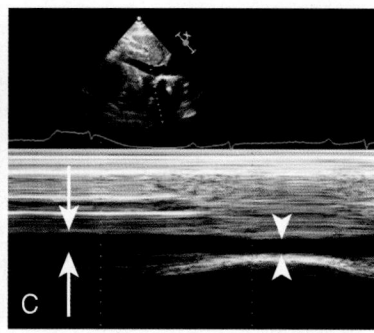

Figure 24.3 Images of the inferior vena cava. These images show (A) a small, nearly completely collapsed inferior vena cava compared with (B) a large, dilated inferior vena cava. (C) Application of M-mode imaging just distal to the hepatic vein to visualize inferior vena cava diameter over time and identify maximum (*arrows*) and minimum (*arrowheads*) inferior vena cava diameter. The appearance of the inferior vena cava reflects right atrial pressure. An inferior vena cava that is less than 2 cm in diameter and collapses by 50% (to a diameter of 1 cm) corresponds to a right atrial pressure of approximately 5 mm Hg, which is normal. The relationship between right atrial pressure and inferior vena cava diameter is lost in patients treated with positive-pressure ventilation. The assessment of inferior vena cava diameter may be used to make predictions about hemodynamic response to fluid administration for patients in shock and is addressed in the text. *Arrow*, inferior vena cava; *arrowhead*, hepatic vein; *asterisk*, right atrium.

the probe is rotated, the image of the IVC in long axis will come into view. The aorta lies just medial to and can easily be confused with the IVC. Definitive identification of the IVC requires seeing it enter the right atrium and seeing it connect with the hepatic vein. The diameter of the IVC and the change in diameter with breathing are used to assess right atrial pressure (Fig. 24.3). The significance of right atrial pressure depends on the clinical scenario, which must be carefully considered when using IVC imaging to make patient care decisions (see the later discussion of assessment of volume status).

PERICARDIAL EFFUSION AND CARDIAC TAMPONADE

Pericardial tamponade is a life-threatening emergency typically identified by findings on echocardiography interpreted in combination with the clinical status. A complete echocardiographic hemodynamic assessment for pericardial tamponade is beyond the scope of this chapter; however, it is reasonable for intensivists to identify a pericardial effusion, as well as features suggestive of pericardial tamponade. Pericardial fluid usually appears as an echo-free (hypoechoic) space around the heart. Identifying fluid anterior to the aorta in the PLAX view is useful as a way to differentiate pericardial from pleural and peritoneal fluid; fluid seen anterior to the aorta in the PLAX view is pericardial, and fluid seen posterior is pleural or peritoneal. Fat in the pericardial space is common, but it is typically seen primarily anterior to the heart and is bright in appearance (hyperechoic). It is important to remember that the size of a pericardial effusion is not necessarily related to the risk of pericardial tamponade. Small amounts of fluid accumulating quickly may cause tamponade, whereas large pericardial effusions accumulating slowly typically do not (Video 24.10).

Several findings suggest a diagnosis of pericardial tamponade. In tamponade physiology, the pressure inside the pericardial space exceeds the diastolic pressure inside the cardiac chambers. This results in compression of the right ventricle and right atrium during diastole. Because the heart rate is typically high during pericardial tamponade, the compression may be difficult to appreciate and may not

be visible in all cardiac cycles and in all portions of the respiratory cycle. We recommend recording long clips with multiple cardiac cycles and then reviewing these clips slowly to look for evidence of right heart chamber diastolic collapse (Video 24.11). Although not always present, the associated finding of a plethoric IVC that does not collapse with breathing would further support the diagnosis of cardiac tamponade. In this context, the high right atrial pressure indicated by assessment of the IVC is caused by the elevated pericardial pressure.

THE USES OF CRITICAL CARE ULTRASOUND

Perhaps the most studied and validated role for CCE is its use in detecting the cause of undifferentiated shock. It is often difficult to determine the reason for undifferentiated shock with traditional invasive monitoring and physical examination alone. Furthermore, transporting unstable patients to remote locations for imaging studies is not always feasible or safe. Ultrasound has the advantage of being portable, noninvasive, and repeatable, and it allows critical care physicians to make rapid assessments of pulmonary and cardiac physiology. Focused CCE has been shown to be reliable in providing rapid assessments of volume status, left ventricular function, the presence or absence of pericardial effusion, and right ventricular size and function and thereby aids in the diagnosis of undifferentiated shock.[25,29,30]

ASSESSMENT OF VOLUME STATUS

Determining volume status in critically ill, hemodynamically unstable patients is complex, and volume responsiveness (defined as a 10–15% increase in stroke volume or cardiac output with a crystalloid or colloid bolus of 250 to 500 mL[31]) is often difficult to predict. Although optimization of volume status improves outcomes, excessive fluid administration can lead to increased morbidity and mortality.[32–34] In addition, studies have shown that only one-half of hemodynamically unstable patients will respond to a fluid challenge.[11,35] Historically, intensivists have used a variety of invasive monitors, laboratory studies, diagnostic studies, and physical examination maneuvers to predict volume responsiveness. In more recent times, IVC measurements, both static and dynamic, have emerged. Measured at one time point, IVC diameter, a surrogate for central venous pressure, is a static measure. Measuring the respiratory variation in the IVC diameter over time is a dynamic measure that has been found to have some success as a means of estimating fluid responsiveness in critically ill patients.[11,36,37]

Inferior Vena Cava Diameter and Collapsibility and/or Distensibility

When imaging the IVC for the purpose of estimating fluid responsiveness, both the absolute greatest diameter and the change in diameter with breathing should be assessed. IVC diameter and collapsibility (decrease in diameter of the IVC) in spontaneously breathing patients can be used to estimate right atrial pressure and, by extrapolation, central venous pressure. If the IVC is small (<2.0 cm) and collapses more than 50% with inspiration, the central venous pressure is low or normal. If the IVC is large (>2.0 cm) and does not collapse, the central venous pressure is elevated. Three indices have been studied with regard to respiratory variation of the IVC and prediction of fluid responsiveness: the IVC collapsibility index, the IVC distensibility index, and IVC diameter variation (Table 24.2). All three of these dynamic IVC measurements have been studied in mechanical ventilation; only the IVC collapsibility index has been studied in spontaneously breathing patients.[35,38–41]

Inferior Vena Cava and Volume Status

There is extensive literature on the accuracy of the IVC examination (in both spontaneously breathing and mechanically ventilated patients) in predicting volume responsiveness. Early studies on mechanically ventilated patients showed that an IVC distensibility index greater than 15% was suggestive of fluid responsiveness.[38,41] However, patients in these studies were receiving large tidal volumes (10 mL/kg) and were heavily sedated and/ or paralyzed, which is uncommon in current critical care management. In some small studies of spontaneously breathing patients, higher values of the IVC collapsibility index (>40%) have been predictive of fluid responsiveness.[39,40] The change in IVC diameter with assisted ventilation (continuous positive airway pressure, bilevel positive airway pressure, supportive mechanical ventilation modes, high-flow nasal cannula) is much more difficult to predict and standardize given multiple confounding factors, including patient effort, chest wall compliance, and degree of positive end-expiratory pressure. In addition, there are many pitfalls associated with measuring the IVC and interpreting the examination. For example, movement of the IVC during inspiration can lead to misalignment of the scanning plane and over-estimation of collapsibility. Imaging the aorta instead of the IVC can lead to the mistaken conclusion that there is an absence of respiratory variability. Finally, in several clinical conditions, IVC size and respiratory variability may not accurately predict preload or volume responsiveness.[42,43]

Because of inconclusive existing evidence on the accuracy of predicting volume responsiveness and the

Table 24.2 Three Different Dynamic Inferior Vena Cava Measurements*

Measure	Formula	Study Patients
IVC collapsibility index (cIVC)	$\dfrac{(IVC_{max} - IVC_{min})}{IVC_{max}} \times 100$	Spontaneously breathing, mechanically ventilated
IVC distensibility index (dIVC)	$\dfrac{(IVC_{max} - IVC_{min})}{IVC_{min}} \times 100$	Mechanically ventilated
IVC diameter variation (ΔD_{IVC})	$\dfrac{(IVC_{max} - IVC_{min})}{(IVC_{max} + IVC_{min})/2} \times 100$	Mechanically ventilated

*Multiple different cutoff values have been reported for each of the measurements above in defining which patients in shock are more likely to respond favorably to administration of fluids. However, all of these measures have limited predictive utility.

IVC, inferior vena cava; max, maximum; min, minimum.

potential for misinterpretation, it is paramount to recognize the limitations of the IVC examination and to interpret images accordingly.[44] IVC examination is more useful with serial examinations and at the extremes (i.e., very collapsible or very dilated). In this context, we recommend the following approach for specific clinical scenarios:

- *Large IVC that does not collapse with respiration (patient not undergoing mechanical ventilation):* The patient is unlikely to benefit from additional fluid (except in the case of cardiac tamponade). Obtain cardiac views to evaluate for tamponade or obstructive shock. Perform a pulmonary ultrasound examination to evaluate for prominent B-lines suggestive of pulmonary edema. Consider diuresis if concern exists for decompensated heart failure or pulmonary edema causing respiratory failure.
- *Small IVC that collapses with respiration (patient not undergoing mechanical ventilation):* The patient may benefit from a fluid bolus. Evaluate the patient for deep breathing, which may exaggerate IVC collapsibility. If the patient is in shock, consider fluid administration.
- *Large IVC that does not collapse with respiration (patient undergoing mechanical ventilation):* In this scenario it is unclear whether the patient will benefit from additional fluid or whether additional fluid will be harmful. Do not use an IVC examination alone to determine whether the patient will be volume responsive. We recommend performing a full CCU examination and using other clinical data to help determine volume status.
- *Small IVC that collapses with respiration (patient undergoing mechanical ventilation):* The patient is likely to be volume responsive. We recommend administering a fluid bolus if the patient is in shock if the respiratory status allows.

OTHER CRITICAL CARE ULTRASOUND EXAMINATIONS TO EVALUATE SHOCK AND ASSESS VOLUME STATUS

Basic Critical Care Echocardiography

Assessment of left ventricular function, presence or absence of pericardial effusion, and assessment of right ventricular size and function are all useful measurements

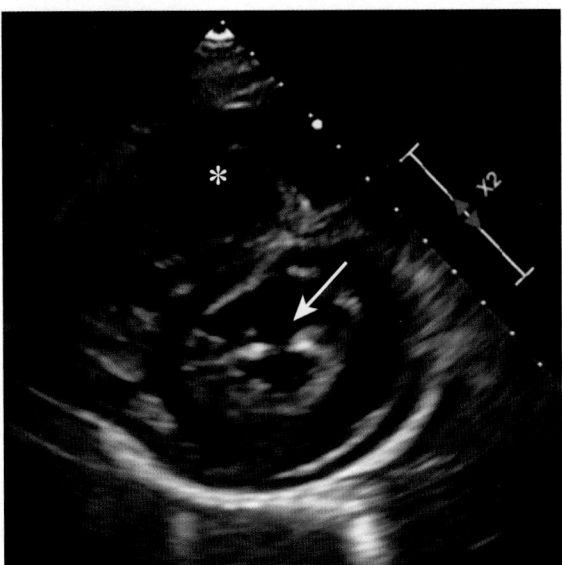

Figure 24.4 Underfilled left ventricle. The heart seen in a parasternal short axis view shows "kissing" papillary muscles (*arrow*) suggestive of an underfilled left ventricle. *Asterisk,* right ventricle.

to help determine the etiology of undifferentiated shock. A hyperdynamic left ventricle with complete obliteration of the left ventricular cavity in systole ("kissing" papillary muscles on the PSAX view) may be suggestive of an underfilled left ventricle and predict that a patient would benefit from fluid administration (Fig. 24.4). In the setting of hemodynamic instability, hemorrhagic shock from blood loss and distributive shock from sepsis should be considered as potential causes. Alternatively, decreased left ventricular function and/or the presence of obvious wall motion abnormalities may suggest that cardiac dysfunction is contributing to shock. This can be seen in the setting of myocardial infarction, myocarditis, chronic heart failure, and various other clinical settings such as sepsis-induced cardiomyopathy. Detecting the presence of left ventricular dysfunction can help guide decisions about using inotropic agents and vasopressors, withholding fluids to avoid volume overload, or obtaining more definitive diagnostic studies (e.g., complete echocardiography, cardiac catheterization). If a pericardial effusion is present in a patient with hemodynamic instability, the diagnosis of tamponade should be considered (Fig. 24.5). Depending on the clinical scenario, further imaging with complete echocardiography and consultation with cardiology or emergency pericardiocentesis may be indicated. An enlarged right ventricle seen in the A4C and/or subcostal view or flattening of the intraventricular septum in the PSAX view may indicate right ventricular dysfunction. When coupled with a positive deep venous thrombosis ultrasound examination in a patient with shock, these findings are highly suggestive of an acute pulmonary embolism (Fig. 24.6 and eFig. 24.3; see also Fig. 81.2).

Advanced Critical Care Echocardiography

Basic CCE can answer many questions about a patient in shock, but some cardiac causes of shock and/or respiratory failure may not be identified by this limited approach. For example, as mentioned, a patient with cardiogenic shock resulting from severe acute valvular regurgitation

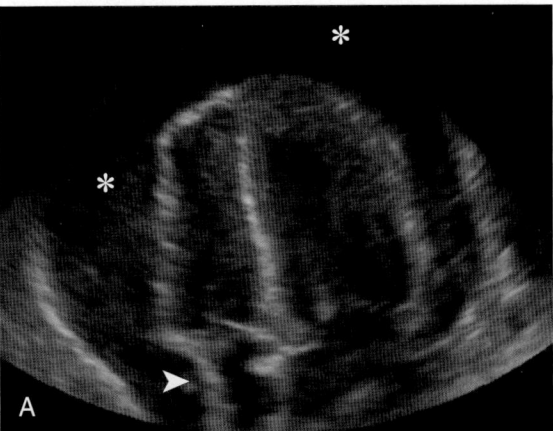
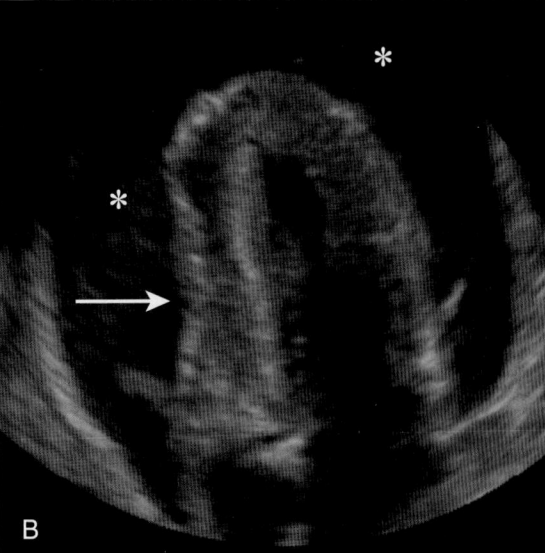

Figure 24.5 Cardiac tamponade. The heart is seen in an apical four-chamber view. The images show a large pericardial effusion with diastolic collapse of the (A) right atrium (*arrowhead*) and (B) right ventricle (*arrow*) suggestive of tamponade. *Asterisk,* pericardial fluid.

may show normal left ventricular function on a basic CCE examination. Advanced CCE can address some of these shortcomings. For example, using advanced CCE, one can perform cardiac ultrasound examinations to obtain quantitative measures such as cardiac output that can be repeated over time to assess the efficacy of therapeutic interventions.[45,46] Additional applications of advanced CCE include evaluation for severe valvular disease, noninvasive cardiac output measurement, identification of regional wall motion abnormalities, and measurement of pulmonary artery systolic pressure. A detailed description of these applications is beyond the scope of this chapter. It is important to recognize that competence in advanced CCE requires significantly more training and experience than required for basic CCE.[22]

Pulmonary Ultrasound

The pulmonary ultrasound examination is an important, simple, and sometimes underused tool for evaluating the patient in shock and/or respiratory failure. Pneumothorax is common in the ICU and can be related to trauma, underlying lung disease, mechanical ventilation, or procedural complications. The pneumothorax examination is fast and easy to

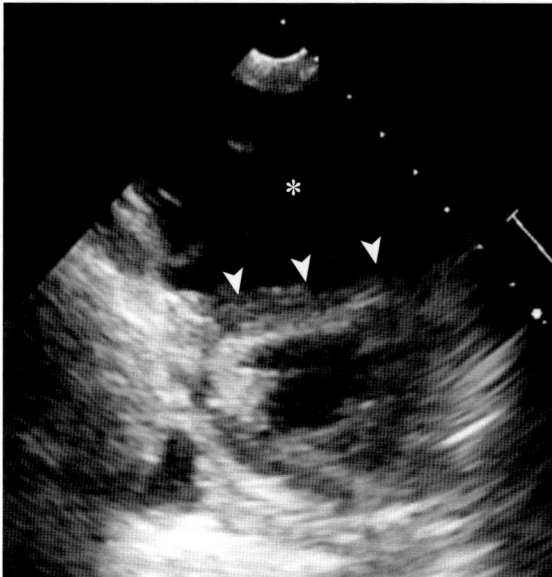

Figure 24.6 Flattening of the interventricular septum. The heart in the parasternal short-axis view shows a flattened or D-shaped septum (*arrow-heads*) suggestive of right ventricular pressure or volume overload. *Asterisk,* right ventricle.

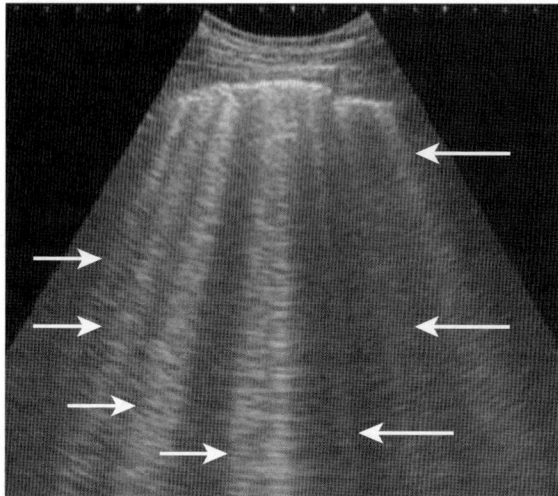

Figure 24.7 Lung ultrasound showing multiple B-lines (*arrows*) suggestive of interstitial edema. (From Blum M, Ferrada P. Ultrasound and other innovations for fluid management in the ICU. *Surg Clin North Am.* 2017;97:1323–1337.)

perform, and it can lead to an immediate intervention with chest tube placement, with resolution of shock. As detailed in Chapter 23, pneumothorax would be suspected if there is an absence of lung sliding and/or an absence of B-lines on pulmonary ultrasound examination. If a lung point is seen during the examination, then pneumothorax can be definitively diagnosed. Diffuse B-lines emanating from the lung parenchyma can aid in the diagnosis of respiratory failure and guide diuresis in patients with significant pulmonary edema (Fig. 24.7). The use of ultrasound to assess for pleural fluid in the setting of respiratory failure can lead to potential therapeutic interventions such as thoracentesis to improve clinical status. In the setting of shock, diagnostic sampling of

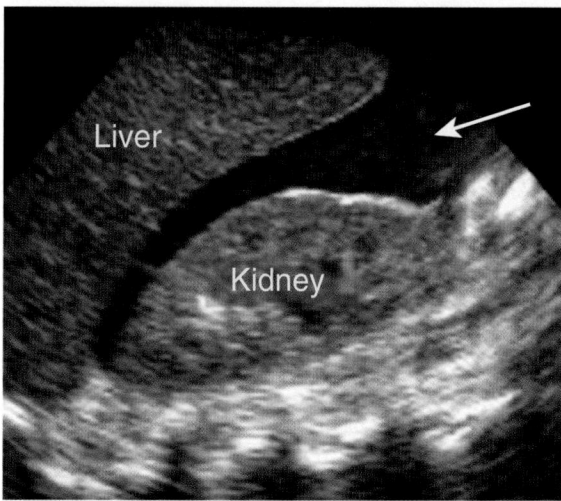

Figure 24.8 Examination of the right upper quadrant demonstrating free fluid between the liver and kidney. The potential space between the liver and the kidney, known as Morison's pouch, is the most common place for fluid to accumulate in the right upper quadrant view. If there is no fluid, there will be no space between the liver and the kidney. Free fluid appears either anechoic (*arrow*, as demonstrated in this figure) or hypoechoic (clotted blood, ascites). In an unstable trauma patient, a positive result of a *focused assessment with sonography in trauma* (FAST) examination is extremely sensitive and specific for intra-abdominal bleeding. In the intensive care unit setting, a positive result of a FAST examination is less specific and sensitive for acute hemorrhage (ascites and normal post-surgical changes may appear similar).

pleural fluid may yield the source of infection in sepsis and lead to source control with drainage of infected fluid. Finally, consolidations viewed on lung ultrasound examination suggest respiratory failure from pneumonia and, in the patient with shock, potential sepsis from a pulmonary source.

Abdominal Ultrasound

Abdominal ultrasound can detect the presence of intra-abdominal hemorrhage, aortic abnormalities, and potential sources of septic shock. The *focused assessment with sonography in trauma* (FAST) examination has been used and validated extensively in trauma to detect the presence of free fluid suggestive of active bleeding in hemodynamically unstable patients with blunt injury.[47] Although a "positive" FAST examination result in the ICU is much less specific, some findings can be helpful. Serial abdominal ultrasound examinations showing increasing size of fluid pockets in an unstable patient suggests intra-abdominal hemorrhage as a cause of shock (Fig. 24.8). Abdominal ultrasound with examination of the aorta may reveal an enlarged abdominal aorta or aortic dissection. Finally, in patients with suspected septic shock, abdominal ultrasound may reveal hydronephrosis or other fluid collections concerning for abscesses when looking for sources of infection (Fig. 24.9).

PUTTING IT ALL TOGETHER: A SYSTEMATIC APPROACH

Given the limitations and pitfalls of using any one measurement to elucidate the etiology of shock in critically ill patients, we recommend completing a comprehensive

CCU examination on patients in shock. This includes not only cardiac ultrasound, but pulmonary ultrasound, abdominal ultrasound, and the deep venous thrombosis examination when indicated. Each of these examinations has unique findings depending on the etiology of shock and, when combined, will provide a clearer clinical picture and help yield a diagnosis (Table 24.3). For example, a patient with cardiogenic shock may have decreased left ventricular function and a dilated, noncollapsing IVC on cardiac ultrasound and prominent B-lines on pulmonary ultrasound. A patient with hemorrhagic shock may have hyperdynamic left ventricular function, a small and collapsible IVC, and free fluid on abdominal ultrasound.

Numerous protocols for ultrasound in shock and critical illness have been developed as CCU has become more ubiquitous in critical care. Each protocol uses some combination of the core ultrasound examinations described previously (e.g., cardiac, pulmonary, abdominal) to create a fast and systematic way to use ultrasound to aid in diagnosis and guide resuscitation in shock.[48] In addition, each protocol prescribes the order in which the different ultrasound examinations should be performed. Because of the complex nature of critically ill patients across different ICUs (e.g., cardiac, medicine, surgical), we do not recommend a single protocol for CCU.[48] Instead, we suggest tailoring each CCU examination to the patient's real-time clinical scenario and adding additional ultrasound examinations as needed to enhance clinical understanding. For example, in a patient with acute respiratory distress, hypotension, and high peak pressures immediately after a central line was placed in the internal jugular vein, the highest priority and most appropriate ultrasound examination to perform would be the lung ultrasound to evaluate for pneumothorax. In a more complex patient with hypoxemia, hypotension, elevated lactate, and fever who has just had major abdominal surgery, a more comprehensive examination, including cardiac, IVC, FAST, and potentially deep venous thrombosis examinations, would be appropriate.

When performing CCU, it is important to know the limitations of each component of the ultrasound examination. Findings should always be interpreted in the context of the patient's entire clinical picture. Examinations should be repeated as indicated to evaluate for both the efficacy of therapeutics and the need for further interventions. Any unclear or clinically relevant findings should prompt more complete diagnostic studies. Guidelines for the use of ultrasound in the critical care setting have been developed by professional societies with expert consensus.[49–51] It is essential that training programs adhere to these guidelines and establish robust, longitudinal ultrasound curricula that ensure competency of trainees. CCU is a valuable tool to improve patient care when used in the appropriate scope of practice by competent providers. As this section has described, CCU is vital in the setting of undifferentiated shock and/or respiratory failure, and it should be incorporated into daily practice in the critical care setting.

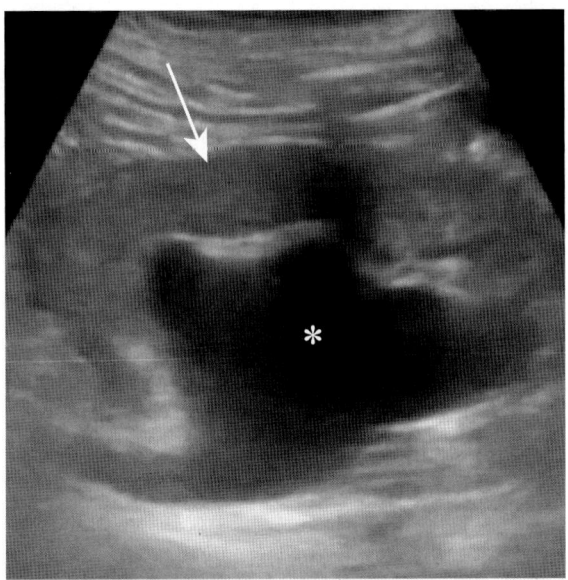

Figure 24.9 Hydronephrosis. Left kidney ultrasound examination shows severe hydronephrosis with a severely dilated renal pelvis. In a patient with sepsis, this finding could suggest a urinary source of infection. *Arrow,* renal parenchyma; *asterisk,* renal pelvis.

Table 24.3 Patterns of Findings on Critical Care Ultrasound in Shock

Parameter	Cardiogenic	Hypovolemic or distributive	Obstructive*
Cardiac function	Abnormal	Normal or hyperdynamic	Hyperdynamic LV RV dysfunction
Cardiac filling	Full	Underfilled RV and LV	Underfilled LV
Other cardiac findings	Wall motion abnormalities Valvular disease	—	Pericardial effusion
Inferior vena cava	Enlarged, noncollapsible	Collapsible	Enlarged, noncollapsible
Pulmonary	Pulmonary edema	Consolidation or pleural effusion (source of sepsis)	Pneumothorax
Vascular	—	—	Deep venous thrombosis
Abdominal or FAST	—	Free fluid Hydronephrosis	—

*Ostructive shock is considered to be mostly extracardiac, usuallly due to pulmonary vascular obstruction but also tamponade or pneumothorax.
FAST, focused assessment with sonography in trauma; LV, left ventricle; RV, right ventricular.

Key Points

- Noncardiologists can learn to acquire and interpret cardiac ultrasound images and use their findings to make patient management decisions.
- Critical care echocardiographic images should be carefully evaluated and, if image quality is not adequate for interpretation, the data should be discarded and not incorporated into patient care decisions.
- The four assessments used to determine the left ventricular systolic function are (1) change in the left ventricular cavity size, (2) thickening of the left ventricular myocardium, (3) opening of the mitral valve, and (4) motion of the mitral annulus.
- Foreshortening of the left ventricle in the apical four-chamber view is important to recognize and avoid because it can lead to overestimation of left ventricular systolic function and to underestimation of right ventricular systolic function.
- The clinical meaning of right atrial pressure determined by imaging of the inferior vena cava varies depending on the clinical context. For example, elevated right atrial pressure is a feature of both decompensated heart failure and cardiac tamponade.
- Ultrasound examination of the inferior vena cava has limitations for use in predicting which patients will improve hemodynamically following fluid administration. Our approach is to emphasize the value of either a very collapsed or a dilated inferior vena cava, serial inferior vena cava examinations, and incorporation of other clinical data into clinical decision making about fluid administration.
- When assessing a patient in shock, examinations of multiple body areas (critical care echocardiography, pulmonary ultrasound, abdominal ultrasound) should be combined to make the correct diagnosis and treatment decisions.
- It is important to know the limitations of critical care ultrasonography. Complete imaging or consultation with specialty services should be considered to evaluate further or to clarify clinically significant or unexpected findings or when critical care ultrasonographic images are not adequate for diagnosis.

Key Readings

Accreditation Council for Graduate Medical Education. ACGME program requirements for graduate medical education in pulmonary disease and critical care medicine; 2020. https://www.acgme.org/Specialties/Program-Requirements-and-FAQs-and-Applications/pfcatid/16Julie/Specialties.

Bentzer P, Griesdale DE, Boyd J, MacLean K, Sirounis D, Ayas NT. Will this hemodynamically unstable patient respond to a bolus of intravenous fluids? *JAMA.* 2016;316:1298–1309.

Dinh VA, Giri PC, Rathinavel I, et al. Impact of a 2-day critical care ultrasound course during fellowship training: a pilot study. *Crit Care Res Pract.* 2015;2015:675041.

Kanji HD, McCallum J, Sirounis D, MacRedmond R, Moss R, Boyd JH. Limited echocardiography-guided therapy in subacute shock is associated with change in management and improved outcomes. *J Crit Care.* 2014;29:700–705.

Kirkpatrick JN, Grimm R, Johri AM, et al. Recommendations for echocardiography laboratories participating in cardiac point of care cardiac ultrasound (POCUS) and critical care echocardiography training: report from the American Society of Echocardiography. *J Am Soc Echocardiogr.* 2020;33(4):409–422, e404.

Levitov A, Frankel HL, Blaivas M, et al. Guidelines for the appropriate use of bedside general and cardiac ultrasonography in the evaluation of critically ill patients-part ii: cardiac ultrasonography. *Crit Care Med.* 2016;44(6):1206–1227.

Melamed R, Sprenkle MD, Ulstad VK, Herzog CA, Leatherman JW. Assessment of left ventricular function by intensivists using hand-held echocardiography. *Chest.* 2009;135:1416–1420.

Millington SJ. Ultrasound assessment of the inferior vena cava for fluid responsiveness: easy, fun, but unlikely to be helpful. *Can J Anaesth.* 2019;66(6):633–638.

Spencer KT, Kimura BJ, Korcarz CE, Pellikka PA, Rahko PS, Siegel RJ. Focused cardiac ultrasound: recommendations from the American Society of Echocardiography. *J Am Soc Echocardiogr.* 2013;26(6):567–581.

Complete reference list available at ExpertConsult.com.

25 POSITRON EMISSION TOMOGRAPHY

CHRISTOPHE M. DEROOSE, MD, PHD • CHRISTOPHE DOOMS, MD, PHD

INTRODUCTION

Positron emission tomography (PET) is a noninvasive imaging technique allowing depiction of molecular targets or metabolic processes. Its main clinical applications are in the field of respiratory medicine, where PET has evolved from a tool for in vivo research to a routine imaging test for patients with lung tumors at many different stages of disease. The main use currently is for staging of lung cancer, where it is a crucial tool for determining the *tumor, nodal, and metastatic* components of cancer stages. However, it has important applications for other cancers, such as small cell lung cancer, mesothelioma, and neuroendocrine tumors. It is increasingly used to follow response to therapy and monitor patients in follow-up after therapy with curative intent. New tracers are also being developed. Because ^{18}F-*fluorodeoxyglucose* (^{18}F-FDG) is by far the most commonly used tracer for this purpose, the term PET refers to ^{18}F-FDG-PET unless stated otherwise.

PRINCIPLES

POSITRON EMISSION TOMOGRAPHY CAMERA

A PET camera produces tomographic images that represent the three-dimensional distribution of radioactivity within the body of a patient. Any molecule labeled with a positron-emitting radionuclide can be used to generate PET images. The PET camera consists of a number of rings containing several thousands of scintillation detectors that detect high-energy photons resulting from the annihilation of the emitted positrons when the radionuclide decays. To identify the direction of the incoming rays, a conventional gamma camera uses lead collimators that block photons from directions. A PET camera does not need physical collimators to generate an image and uses a complex algorithm to trace the high-energy photons back to their source in the body, an "electronic" collimation. As a result, instead of losing more than 99% of the emitted photons to absorption from the collimators, PET has higher sensitivity (counts per unit of radioactivity) and higher spatial resolution. The spatial resolution of contemporary PET cameras is about 3 to 4 mm, allowing characterization of lesions larger than 6 to 8 mm. Smaller lesions cannot be accurately depicted except for strongly FDG–avid lesions. Images can be acquired with or without respiratory gating.[1]

Modern PET cameras are hybrid systems in which a PET camera is combined with a morphologic imaging modality, either *computed tomography* (CT)[2] or a *magnetic resonance* (MR) camera. The morphologic imaging modality adds the following to the PET image: (1) increased accuracy of the exact position of the lesion and morphologic characterization of the underlying correlate, reducing equivocal findings; (2) increased confidence of the reporting physician; (3) in the case of PET/CT, CT-based attenuation correction, which corrects for absorption of signal by the body of the patient. To match the respiratory phase of PET, which is expiration dominated, the CT is often performed in expiration, which can lead to limited depiction of small lesions and increase in density of ground-glass lesions compared to inspiratory CT.

PET/MR imaging and PET/CT show an equivalently high diagnostic and *tumor-node-metastasis* (TNM) staging performance in *non–small cell lung cancer* (NSCLC).[3] The main disadvantages of PET/MR are its higher cost, lesser availability, smaller bore size, more difficult imaging of lung parenchyma, and typically longer scan times. On the other hand, it offers better assessment of thoracic wall and diaphragmatic invasion than PET/CT, and MR of the brain, the test of choice for detecting brain metastasis, can be performed simultaneously. Due to current limited availability of PET/MR (one system for each 20 to 50 PET/CT scans performed[4]), PET/CT is the current modality used to evaluate lung cancer patients.

In a recent trend, the PET camera rings are increased, leading to a larger *field of view* (FOV) and allowing shorter scan times, less injected activity, or both. Typical scan times are 10 to 15 minutes for PET/CT cameras with an FOV of approximately 20 cm and skull-to-thigh imaging. Total-body PET scanners, using cameras with a very large FOV, up to greater than 190 cm,[5] allow acquisition of a whole-body image (skull-to-toe) and completion of imaging within 1 minute. PET is preferably combined with a high-dose, contrast-enhanced diagnostic CT for more precise TNM staging, because localization and interpretation of the CT is superior compared to that of low-dose CT.[6]

METABOLIC TRACER: 18F-FLUORODEOXYGLUCOSE

For clinical cancer imaging, the glucose analog FDG is by far the most common tracer. Its use is based on the observation that cancer cells have an increased cellular uptake of glucose, due to an increased expression of facilitative *glucose transporters* (GLUTs), and a much higher rate of glycolysis.[7] FDG is a glucose analog in which the oxygen molecule in position 2 is replaced by a positron-emitting fluorine-18 atom, undergoes the same uptake as glucose, but it is metabolically trapped and accumulated in the neoplastic cell after phosphorylation by hexokinase.[8] The radiation dose for a typical examination is in the order of 5 to 8 mSv.[9]

The image units with FDG-PET can be quantitative in nature (expressed in mmol glucose used per minute per gram of tissue), but this requires time-consuming dynamic scanning (continuous imaging of a lesion for about 60 minutes). In clinical practice, FDG uptake is expressed as the *standardized uptake value* (SUV), a semiquantitative measure of tracer uptake that normalizes the uptake within a lesion by the injected activity per unit of body weight. The SUV is thus the ratio between the observed radioactivity concentration in a specific tissue (e.g., primary tumor) and the virtual concentration that would be observed if the full amount of the injected tracer spread evenly in the entire body. SUV can be determined in the voxel (i.e., a volume unit of information, a volumetric pixel) with the *highest value of a volume of interest in the image* (SUV_{max}) or on the whole lesion (SUV_{mean}).

INTERPRETATION OF PET IMAGES

For tumor detection, visual analysis focuses on the detection of lesions with activity higher than background not caused by physiologic processes, both for the discrimination of nodules and for the evaluation of mediastinal involvement. Non–attenuation correction images should be examined to detect small lung lesions because they have a higher contrast than corrected images. High physiologic FDG uptake is present in the brain (cortex > white matter), kidney, and urinary tract (due to urinary excretion) and can be present in the heart.[10] There is a low degree of physiologic uptake of FDG in the other thoracic structures. The high uptake in the brain interferes with lesion detection in the brain, which is one of the weaknesses of PET.

False-positive findings can be anticipated because FDG uptake is not tumor specific. Uptake of FDG can be found in all active tissues with high glucose metabolism, particularly in those with inflammation. Therefore, clinically relevant FDG–positive findings, especially if isolated and decisive for patient management, require confirmation. The differentiation between metastasis, a benign[11] or inflammatory lesion, or even an unrelated second malignancy should be made by other tests or tissue diagnosis. The major causes of false-positive results in chest pathology are infectious, inflammatory, and granulomatous disorders (Table 25.1) and recent iatrogenic procedures.[12] An emerging class of nonmalignant uptake is seen in patients treated with immuno-oncologic drugs, where immune-related side effects can cause inflammation in a range of organs and be detected by FDG-PET imaging.[13]

Table 25.1   Reasons for False-Positive and False-Negative PET Findings.

FALSE-POSITIVE FINDINGS

Infectious/Inflammatory Lesions

(Postobstructive) pneumonia/abscess
Mycobacterial or fungal infection
Granulomatous disorders (sarcoidosis, granulomatosis with polyangiitis)
Chronic nonspecific lymphadenitis
Rheumatoid arthritis
Occupational exposure (anthracosilicosis)
Bronchiectasis
Organizing pneumonia
Reflux esophagitis

Iatrogenic Causes

18F-FDG embolus
Invasive procedure (puncture, biopsy)
Talc pleurodesis
Radiation esophagitis and pneumonitis
Bone marrow expansion postchemotherapy
Colony-stimulating factors
Thymic hyperplasia postchemotherapy

Benign Mass Lesions

Salivary gland adenoma (Whartin)
Thyroid adenoma
Adrenal adenoma
Colorectal dysplastic polyps
Focal physiologic 18F-FDG-uptake
  ■ Gastrointestinal tract
  ■ Muscle activity
  ■ Brown fat
  ■ Unilateral vocal cord activity
  ■ Atherosclerotic plaques

FALSE-NEGATIVE FINDINGS

Lesion Dependent

Small tumors (<8–10 mm)
Ground-glass opacity neoplasms
Carcinoid tumors
Lower lobe lesions (with greater respiratory motion)

Technique Dependent

Hyperglycemia
Paravenous 18F-FDG injection
Excessive time between injection and scanning

FDG, fluorodeoxyglucose; PET, positron emission tomography.

False-negative findings are less common and may be due to lesion-dependent or technical factors (Table 25.1). Early lesions in the development of lung adenocarcinoma can rely on intracellular glucose transport mediated by the *sodium-glucose cotransporter* (SGLT), not GLUT, resulting in low FDG avidity.[14] Certain tumors are also known to have decreased FDG uptake, such as small-sized very well-differentiated adenocarcinoma, adenocarcinoma with lepidic growth, or carcinoid tumors (see eFig. 78.6). Small lesions, less than 5 mm, may be falsely negative due to the limitations in spatial resolution. Lesions in the lower lung fields, where respiratory motion exceeds that in the apices, may be more difficult to detect due to motion, and the detection limit may even be 10 mm.[15] High blood glucose levels can reduce ^{18}F-FDG uptake through competitive inhibition of GLUT and hexokinase, and blood glucose should be measured and confirmed to be within an acceptable range (typically 60–180 mg/dL) before tracer injection.

DIAGNOSIS

Noncalcified *solitary pulmonary nodules* (SPNs) are a common finding on radiograph or CT in clinical practice and have become even more common with the increasing use of low-dose spiral CT for early lung cancer detection.[16] FDG-PET/CT is a routine technique in the determination of a malignant etiology of these nodules[17] (see also Chapters 41 and 75).

Initial PET studies in the diagnosis of SPNs used a threshold value of greater than 2.5 for the SUV_{max} for the diagnosis of malignancy. With this criterion, overall sensitivity, specificity, and positive and negative predictive values of 96%, 78%, 91%, and 92%, respectively, were reported in a meta-analysis based on series with nodules larger than 1 cm[18] (Fig. 25.1).

The use of SUV_{max} of less than 2.5 to exclude malignancy has been challenged. Solid malignant lesions of at least 1 cm will usually have an SUV_{max} greater than 2.5, but smaller cancers, lesions with ground-glass appearance on CT (e.g., the lepidic type of adenocarcinoma[19,20]; Fig. 25.2), or tumors with low metabolic activity (e.g., typical carcinoid tumors[21,22]) may be missed. Early lesions in pulmonary adenocarcinoma development, such as adenocarcinoma in situ, minimally invasive adenocarcinoma, mucinous adenocarcinoma, and lepidic adenocarcinoma, can have SUV_{max} values less than 2.5, with a stepwise increase in SUV from adenocarcinoma in situ to micropapillary invasive adenocarcinoma.[23,24] A large prospective study with PET/CT scanning in indeterminate SPNs

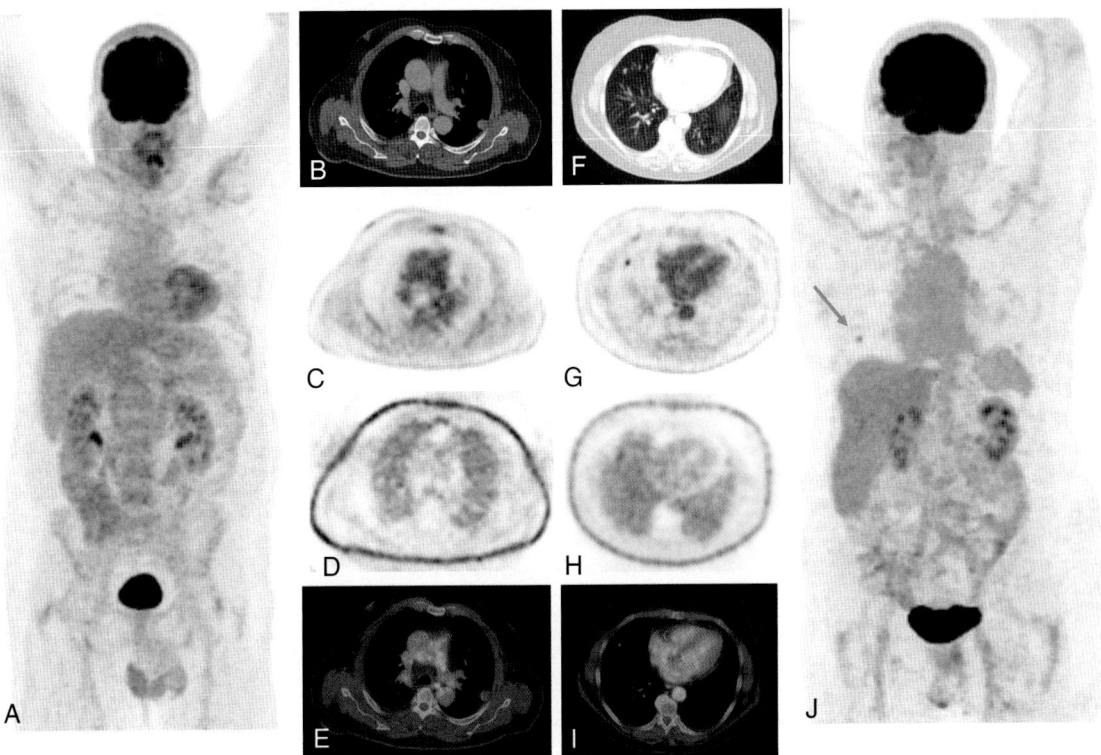

Figure 25.1 Solitary pulmonary nodules in two patients: value of *positron emission tomography* (PET) in diagnosis. Two patients with a solitary pulmonary nodule lesion differentiated by [18]F-*fluorodeoxyglucose* (FDG) PET/*computed tomography* (CT). (A–E) The first patient, a 60-year-old man, presented with a smooth juxtapleural nodule in the left upper lobe on CT (B), with limited growth over a 4-month period up to 19 mm. Both the attenuation-corrected and non–attenuation-corrected transverse FDG-PET images (C and D, respectively) show absence of increased FDG uptake, with a maximum standardized uptake value of 2.1. The fusion image shows uptake within the lesion lower than in the mediastinal vessels (E). Histology after wedge resection demonstrated a pulmonary fibrous hamartoma. (F–J) The second patient, a 69-year-old woman, had a history of chemoradiation treatment for a bronchial squamous cell carcinoma 6 years before presentation with a slowly growing 7 mm large, irregularly delineated lesion on CT (F). FDG-PET/CT showed focal increased uptake, on both the attenuation-corrected (G) and non–attenuation-corrected (H) images, corresponding to the nodule on the fusion images (I). The maximum standardized uptake value was 3.9, and the lesion was clearly visible on the maximum intensity projection images (J, *arrow*). Pathology after right middle lobe lobectomy showed bronchial adenocarcinoma.

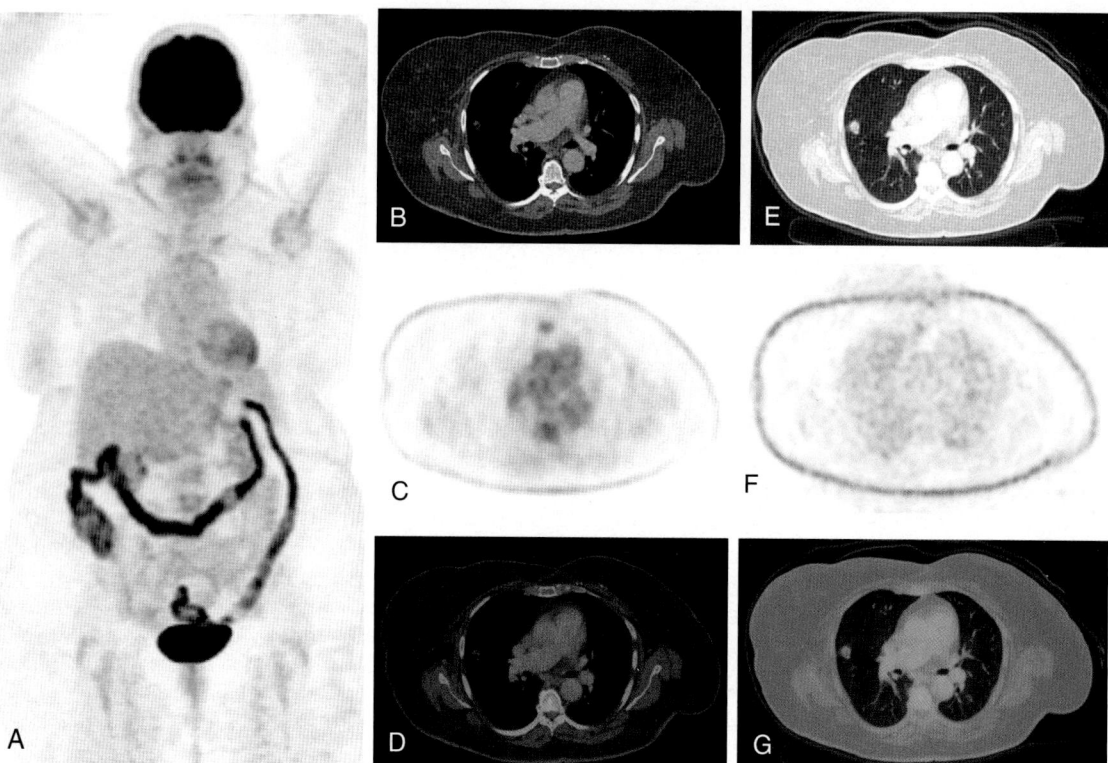

Figure 25.2 False-negative ^{18}**F-*fluorodeoxyglucose* (FDG) positron emission tomography finding.** (B and E) A 65-year-old woman with a 17-mm part-solid nodule with central lucency in the right upper lobe. There is absence of FDG uptake in the lesion on the maximum intensity projection image (A), attenuation-corrected (C) and non–attenuation-correction image (F), confirmed by the fusion images (D and G). The maximum standardized uptake value was 0.84. Pathology after lobectomy showed a bronchial mucinous adenocarcinoma with lepidic growth pattern.

less than 2.5 cm reported a 24% chance of a malignant nodule when SUV_{max} was between 0 and 2.5, 80% if between 2.6 and 4.0, and 96% if 4.1 or more.[25]

Rather than using the SUV_{max} criterion as a threshold, the visual information from PET images (lesions with any increased FDG-uptake being potentially malignant) should be added to the comprehensive nodule assessment based on clinical characteristics (smoking and age being core factors), imaging characteristics (aspect and margins on CT), and growth pattern if available. With this approach, PET improves standard prediction models to estimate the chance of malignancy in an SPN. The added benefit of PET in this setting was examined in a series of 106 radiologically indeterminate SPNs (61 malignant).[26] PET improved the accuracy over a clinical and radiographic prediction model[27] by 13.6% when measured as improvement in area under the receiver operating characteristic curve. This so-called Herder model, which uses FDG-PET information in addition to clinical and radiologic data, is recommended by several guidelines, including those from the British Thoracic Society.[28]

Recent meta-analyses have shown that the positive predictive value of FDG-PET evaluation of SPNs is dependent on the incidence of known causes of false positives, in particular endemic infectious lung disease. In a large meta-analysis including 70 studies (of which 10 were in areas of endemic fungi) evaluating 8511 nodules (60% cancer incidence), there was a 16% lower average- adjusted specificity for malignancy in regions with endemic infectious lung disease (61%) compared with nonendemic regions (77%).[29] As expected, sensitivity was not influenced

by endemic infections (88% in nonendemic vs. 94% in endemic regions).

STAGING

According to the extent of the primary *tumor* (T), the spread to locoregional *lymph nodes* (N) and the presence of distant *metastasis* (M), lung cancer patients of different TNM subsets with similar prognosis are grouped into stages. Stage is the most important factor in prognosis and choice of treatment[30,31] (see also Chapter 76). Therefore, reliable noninvasive methods for accurate staging are very important. CT scan, endoscopic techniques, and surgical staging procedures are key players, but addition of PET to these conventional methods has been shown to improve the staging process substantially by distinguishing patients who are candidates for curative approaches, such as surgical resection or intense multimodality treatment, from those who are not.[32]

For the T factor, detailed images of modern multislice CT allow the reviewer to evaluate the relationship of the tumor to fissures, mediastinal structures, and the pleura and chest wall, determining the type of resection most appropriate, if any. Integrated PET/CT images may allow more precise evaluation of chest wall and mediastinal infiltration or correct differentiation between tumor and peritumoral inflammation or atelectasis[33–35] (Fig. 25.3).

For the N factor, initial studies[36,37] indicate the addition of PET to CT results in more accurate lymph node staging than CT alone, with an overall sensitivity of 80–90% and specificity of 85–95%.[38–40] The absence of mediastinal lymph node

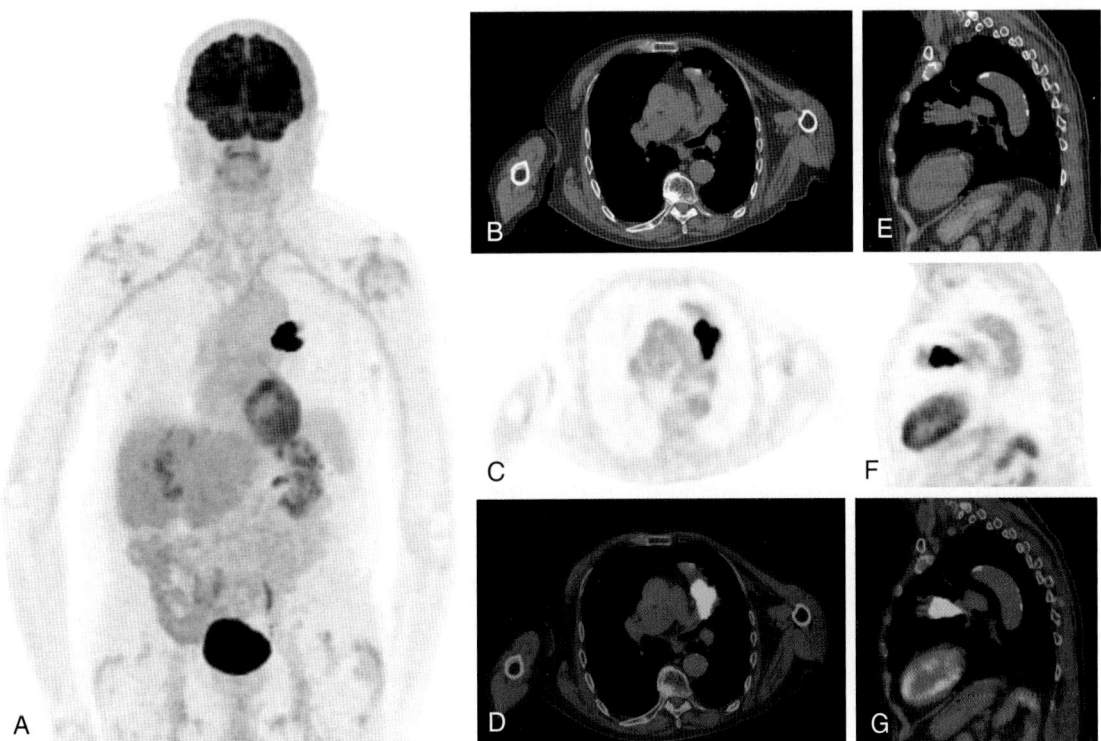

Figure 25.3 Usefulness of [18]**F-*fluorodeoxyglucose* (FDG)** *positron emission tomography* **(PET)/*computed tomography* (CT) in determination of T stage.** An 84-year-old man presented with an increasing consolidation (81 mm longest diameter) in the left upper lobe visualized on unenhanced CT (B and E). On FDG-PET/CT, the mass showed very intense FDG avidity (maximum standardized uptake value of 59.4) in the central part, with only very limited uptake in the more distal part, in line with the mediastinal blood pool (A, C, D, F, G). The distal part was caused by postobstructive mucus plugging. The longest diameter of the FDG-avid part was 48 mm, leading to a T2B stage instead of a T4. Biopsy showed bronchial squamous cell carcinoma.

disease on PET/CT has a high negative predictive value; invasive lymph node staging tests may thus be omitted in these patients, who can proceed straight to surgical resection. Exceptions to this include a primary tumor greater than 3 cm, insufficient FDG-uptake in the primary tumor, hilar nodal disease (N1), or a centrally located tumor that may obscure coexisting N1 or N2 disease on PET. When PET/CT is suggestive of lymphatic spread, images may direct tissue sampling procedures, such as *endobronchial ultrasound* (EBUS)-guided or *esophageal ultrasound* (EUS)-guided transbronchial needle aspiration or cervical mediastinoscopy. Because there may be false-positive images in lymph nodes (based on the conditions listed in Table 25.1), pathologic proof of lymph node involvement should be sought in most patients with positive mediastinal nodes on PET, except those with obvious bulky nodes on imaging.

For the M factor, PET added to CT is almost uniformly superior to CT alone, except for brain imaging, where sensitivity is unacceptably low due to the high glucose uptake of normal cortical brain tissue. For detecting extrathoracic metastases, the pooled sensitivity and specificity for PET/CT were 77% (95% confidence interval [CI], 47 to 93) and 95% (95% CI, 92 to 97), respectively, in a recent meta-analysis.[41] MRI remains the method of choice for brain imaging.

For bone metastases, which are actually bone *marrow* metastases not necessarily affecting the mineral content of bone tissue, PET is more accurate than *technetium-99m–methyl diphosphonate* (^{99m}Tc-MDP) bone scintigraphy; sensitivity is at least as good (90–95%), and specificity is far superior (95% vs. 60%).[42,43] Limitations are the limited FOV when PET images

only from the head to just below the pelvis, and possible false-negative findings in osteoblastic lesions, which are nonetheless rare in untreated lung cancer. A series of PET/CT-guided bone biopsies has shown very high diagnostic yields (>95%) and confirmed bone metastases in 48 out of 51 patients, with other non-NSCLC malignant lesions confirmed in the remaining three patients.[44]

For adrenal gland metastases, PET has a high sensitivity of detection so that an equivocal lesion on CT without corresponding FDG uptake on PET has a low probability of being metastatic. PET may also be of help in evaluating hepatic lesions that remain indeterminate by conventional studies. PET may reveal metastases in sites that escape attention or are outside the FOV in conventional staging (Fig. 25.4), including soft tissue lesions, retroperitoneal lymph nodes, hardly palpable supraclavicular nodes, and painless bone lesions. Exclusion of malignancy requires caution in case of smaller lesions (<1 cm) (see Table 25.1). A particular example is the finding of small contralateral lung nodule(s), common in the era of spiral multislice CT, where PET/CT often does not give certainty so that invasive sampling by, for instance, thoracoscopy or rigorous follow-up, is still needed.

For pleural metastases, the use of PET/CT has shown promising results[45–47] because small pleural deposits, especially without an associated pleural effusion, can be missed on CT imaging alone due to low tumor load and/or partial volume effects. Inflammatory pleural lesions can cause false-positive findings, such as pleurodesis-induced inflammation. A recent meta-analysis of 323 lung cancer patients has shown an acceptable diagnostic accuracy, with a sensitivity of 86% and specificity of 80%.[48] If pleural abnormalities determine the choice for curative treatment, pathologic verification with cytology or thoracoscopy is needed.

INFLUENCE ON TREATMENT CHOICES AND PLANNING WITH CURATIVE INTENT

PET has a significantly complementary role to CT for two reasons. First, unexpected lymph node or distant organ metastatic spread (see Fig. 25.4) may be detected. After a negative conventional staging, unknown metastases are found on PET/CT in 5–20% of the patients, in increasing numbers from clinical stage I to III tumors.[49–57] Second, PET is able to determine the nature of some equivocal lesions on conventional imaging.[49,50,52,53] Interpretation is indisputable when whole-body PET shows multisite metastases, but an isolated suspect lesion that would exclude candidacy for curative treatment should always be verified by other tests or tissue sampling because of the risk of a false-positive finding (see Table 25.1) or a second primary tumor. In one large retrospective series of NSCLC patients, solitary extrathoracic lesions were documented in about 20% of the patients.[53] About half of these were metastatic, whereas the other half were not related to lung cancer; they were either inflammatory, other benign lesions, or second primary tumors. In nonrandomized studies, PET induced a change of stage in 27–62% of NSCLC patients, in general more often upstaging than downstaging, mainly due to the detection of unexpected distant lesions.

The effect of adding PET or PET/CT to a standard lung cancer staging algorithm has been investigated in several randomized controlled trials.[58,59] In an early Dutch trial,[58] patients with stages IIIA and IIIB were included (29% of total) and the end point of "futile thoracotomy" (a surgical procedure deemed not to result in benefit to the patient) was clearly defined (i.e., benign disease, explorative thoracotomy, pathologic stage IIIA–N2/IIIB, or postoperative relapse or death within 12 months). In the PET arm of this trial, a reduction in futile thoracotomies of 20% in all patients was observed. Selection of surgical candidates using PET reduced the frequency of futile thoracotomies by 50% in those who underwent surgery.

Three later trials used PET/CT imaging in addition to standard workup, two of which were in the surgical setting. The study by Fischer and colleagues[60] largely reproduced the Dutch experience, with a significant reduction of futile thoracotomies (42% of all patients in the control group underwent a futile thoracotomy vs. 21% in the PET/CT group; 52% of performed thoracotomies in the control group were futile vs. 35% in the PET group). The study by Maziak and colleagues[61] mainly looked at improved correct upstaging in resectable stage I to III NSCLC and met this primary end point. Overall, there was a 4–11% increased detection rate of stage IV disease.[60,61] The use of PET/CT led to a positive change in patient management, both in intent (curative vs. palliative) and modality (chemotherapy vs. other modalities). In a study in unresectable stage III NSCLC, upstaging was correct in 21 of 140 (15%) patients with PET/CT versus 4 of 149 (2.7%) with CT only (P = 0.0002). Thus, the evidence shows significantly more accurate TNM staging with PET/CT compared to conventional imaging alone, influencing treatment decisions (e.g., the avoidance of futile surgery) and goals of therapy (curative or palliative intent). Although more accurate staging and resulting treatment recommendations are recognized benefits of PET/CT,[62] improved overall outcomes[63,64] have

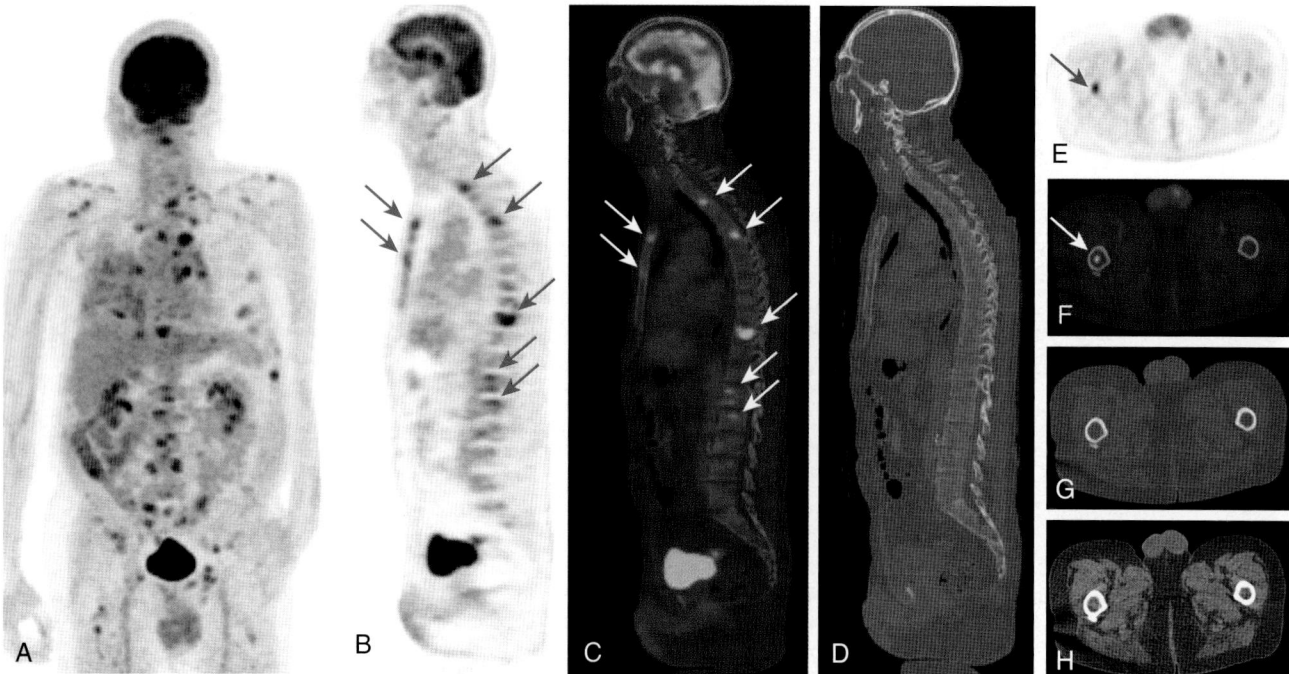

Figure 25.4 Detection of radio-occult bone marrow metastases. A 72-year-old man underwent a [18]F-*fluorodeoxyglucose* (FDG) *positron emission tomography* (PET)/*computed tomography* (CT) scan for an adenocarcinoma of the right lung. (A) In addition to strong uptake in the central primary tumor, the maximum intensity projection image showed multiple skeletal foci with pronounced FDG avidity. Sagittal PET image (B, *red arrows*) shows multiple lesions in the thoracic and lumbar vertebrae and in the sternum, confirmed by the fusion image (C, *white arrows*). (D) The corresponding CT image does not show alterations of the bone mineral content (no osteolysis, no sclerosis). (E–H) Similar findings are seen in the proximal left femur, where PET imaging showed a focus of increased FDG uptake (E and F, *arrows*) without abnormalities on CT (G and H).

yet to be observed because randomized controlled trials were underpowered to assess this end point.

It has been shown in many radiotherapy planning studies that PET/CT influences the accurate delineation of target volumes for radiotherapy.[65–67] The PET-based volume delineations were in general smaller than those with CT alone, mainly due to the possibility of more selective nodal irradiation.[65] The more selective radiation field allowed for an escalation of the radiation dose to the tumor in a substantial number of patients. Prospective clinical trials using PET/CT-based selective nodal irradiation reported isolated nodal failures in less than 5% of patients treated with (chemo)radiotherapy.[66,67] PET/CT-based delineation may also be crucial to avoid geographical misses (i.e., misses of the target) leading to treatment failures. Because of the possibility of false-positive lymph nodes on PET, invasive nodal staging using EBUS or mediastinoscopy may be warranted if malignant involvement of the nodes concerned would have a major impact on the radiation treatment field. We recently proposed an algorithm on how to incorporate EBUS findings in patients staged with PET/CT (Fig. 25.5).[69]

For the primary tumor, the gain of PET-based delineation compared to CT-based delineation is in general smaller, except in situations with postobstructive atelectasis. The optimal method of delineation still remains to be defined. In recent studies, automated PET/CT delineation reduced the interobserver variability in treatment planning compared to CT alone.[70] PET may also identify radio-resistant areas within the primary tumor (e.g., areas with higher FDG uptake requiring higher radiation doses) before and during treatment with high accuracy.[71,72] Guidance on using this information to plan higher radiation doses to these areas to improve outcomes is under investigation. Radiation dose escalation using an integrated boost to the high FDG-uptake region inside the primary tumor proved to be safe and feasible in a small cohort of a randomized phase II study.[73] A recent update on the toxicity of this integrated boost strategy in 107 patients showed increased toxicity compared to standard treatment but lower than the study predefined stopping rules.[74]

PROGNOSIS AND SURVIVAL

Several studies clearly demonstrated stage migration (i.e., reclassification into different prognostic groups based on recognition of disease or disease manifestation) when PET

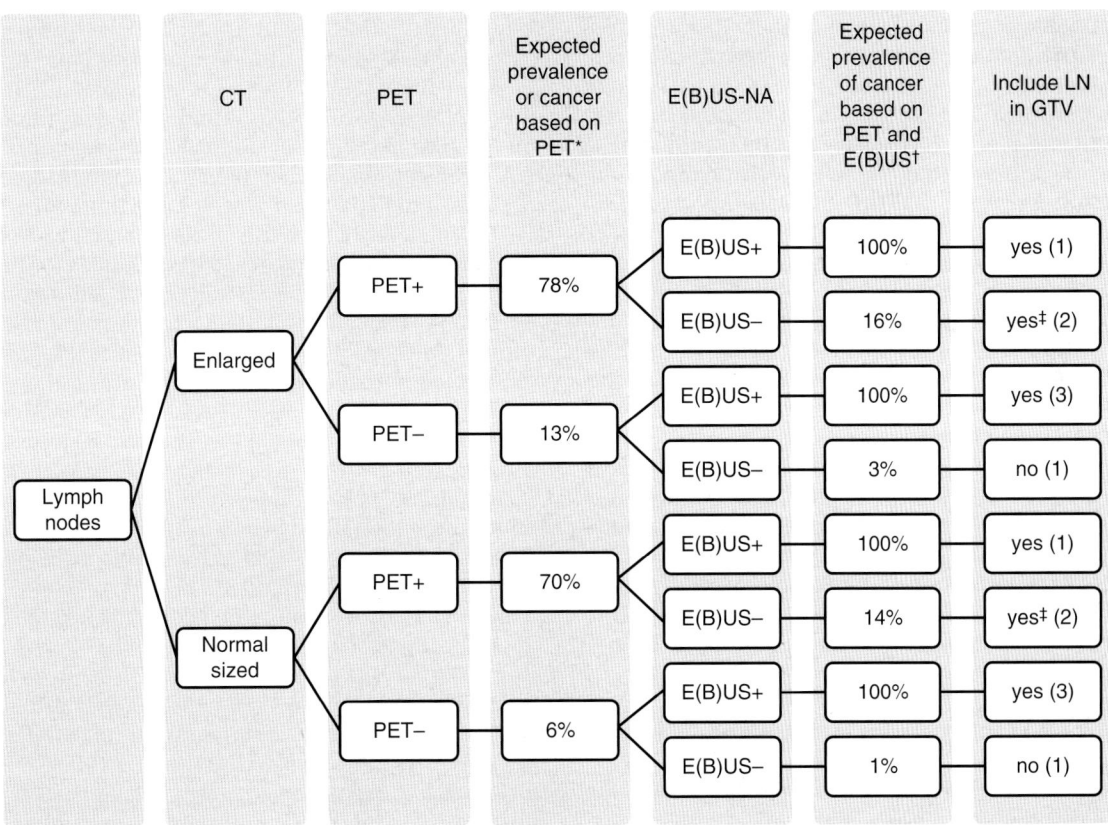

Figure 25.5 Inclusion of lymph nodes in radiotherapy target volume based on [18]F-*fluorodeoxyglucose* (FDG) *positron emission tomography* **(PET)/***computed tomography* **(CT) and** *endobronchial/esophageal ultrasound* **(E[B]US) findings.** Expected prevalence of cancer for different findings on CT, FDG-PET, and E(B)US needle aspiration (NA). The last column indicates whether the lymph node (LN) should be included in the gross tumor volume (GTV) for radiation planning: (1) E(B)US does not change GTV compared to PET-CT only; (2) E(B)US sometimes changes GTV; and (3) E(B)US increases GTV. *Based on Hellwig and colleagues.[169]
[†]Prevalence of cancer, taking into account a false-negative rate of E(B)US of 20%.
[‡]With the exception of symmetrical FDG-PET–positive LN with a nonmalignant diagnosis (anthracosis, silicosis, granulomatous disease, etc.) after adequate E(B)US mapping.
(From Peeters ST, Dooms C, Van Baardwijket A, et al. Selective mediastinal node irradiation in non–small cell lung cancer in the IMRT/VMAT era: how to use E(B)US-NA information in addition to PET-CT for delineation. *Radiother Oncol.* 2016;120[2]:273–278.)

was used.[62] The effect of stage migration in part accounts for improvements in survival of treated patients both in early and in advanced disease stage cohorts, widely referred to as the "Will Rogers phenomenon" of the PET scan era.[75] Will Rogers, the American humorist, was believed to have said, "When the Okies left Oklahoma and moved to California, they raised the average intelligence level in both states." This phenomenon suggests that, if patients are moved from one group, where their survival is below the average, to another, where their survival is above the average, they can increase the average survival of each group. Examples can be found in the prospective multicenter trials on the use of PET in patients with stage III NSCLC, where 25–30% of patients had upstaging confirmed and where there was a significantly longer overall survival ($P = 0.006$) in patients staged by PET than in those without PET. However, the randomized controlled trials in NSCLC were underpowered to evaluate the potential individual patient survival benefit attributable to PET. Smaller studies in *small cell lung cancer* (SCLC) have shown similar stage migration effects to those observed in NSCLC.[76]

PET has also been shown to predict the prognosis of patients with NSCLC.[77] SUV of the primary tumor at diagnosis may predict outcome in NSCLC, especially in earlier stages.[78] Recent meta-analyses on individual patient data have confirmed that SUV_{max} has prognostic value in stage I to III NSCLC.[79] These studies consistently found a better overall survival among patients with a metabolic activity lower than the threshold SUV value, which itself is determined by post hoc analysis and thus varies from study to study. Although SUV may be a way to assess prognosis, there is no true cutoff point suitable for broad clinical use. Instead of a true cutoff point, there is a continuous SUV spectrum of a gradually worsening prognosis. Baseline SUV, incorporated as a continuous variable in a Cox proportional hazards model, showed a 7% increase in hazard of death after a one-unit increase in SUV in resected stage I to III NSCLC[80] and a 6% increase in hazard of death after a one-unit increase in SUV in inoperable NSCLC patients treated with radiotherapy.[81] In patients treated with surgery, SUV_{max} is similarly prognostic, but a recent meta-analysis points to potential superior (and potentially complementary) prognostic value of the determination of the volume with increased FDG uptake (*metabolic tumor volume* [MTV]) and the total glucose consumption of tumoral tissue (*total lesion glycolysis* [TLG]).[82] Recent studies have confirmed the utility of TLG assessment, with a markedly different prognosis in stage III patients based on wholebody TLG.[83] Similar effects have been observed in other tumor types, and this is a very active area of research.[84]

INDICATIONS BEYOND INITIAL EVALUATION OF NON–SMALL CELL LUNG CANCER

SMALL CELL LUNG CANCER

SCLC typically shows very high FDG accumulation. The data on the use of PET in the management of SCLC are less robust than in NSCLC because the emphasis on systemic and radiation therapy provides less histologic data to serve as the gold standard. Furthermore, most studies are

rather small (mean, $n = 40$) and retrospective in nature. A review of 14 studies comparing FDG-PET with conventional staging procedures found an overall cumulative staging concordance between PET and conventional imaging in 84%.[85] Based on PET, limited-stage SCLC was upstaged to extensive-stage SCLC in 18%, and extensive-stage SCLC was downstaged to limited stage in 11%. The information on PET could result in considerable changes in patient management, ranging from 27%[86] to 47%[87] across studies. A recent meta-analysis in SCLC[88] concluded that PET/CT is more sensitive for detecting bone metastases than bone scintigraphy or CT alone and is more sensitive for detecting any distant metastases. Another meta-analysis, focusing on detection of extensive disease, showed a sensitivity of 97.5% and specificity of 98.2% for extensive disease, based on a pooled analysis of 369 patients.[89]

The use of PET/CT resulted in changes to the threedimensional conformal radiation therapy plan in 58% of patients with SCLC in a small pilot study, mainly by decreasing the target volume (in case of atelectasis) or detecting unsuspected nodal or pulmonary foci.[90] Complete metabolic response on posttreatment PET/CT was associated with better outcome in retrospective analyses.[91]

MESOTHELIOMA

Integrated PET/CT imaging has an increasing role in the assessment of suspected or known *malignant pleural mesothelioma* (MPM; Fig. 25.6) (see also Chapter 114). PET/CT is an effective tool in differentiating malignant (mainly MPM) and benign pleural diseases in asbestos-related CT findings with an overall accuracy of greater than 90% and a high negative predictive value of greater than 90%.[92,93] PET/CT is significantly more accurate in baseline TNM staging of patients who are appropriate candidates for multimodal therapy based on CT scan alone.[94–96] Although PET/CT does not provide additional information about the primary tumor compared to CT alone, it identifies a higher number of metastatic mediastinal lymph nodes and/or unknown distant metastatic disease in up to two-thirds of patients, resulting in a significant clinical impact on treatment planning. Because of the greater accuracy of MRI than CT for T staging, MPM is a disease entity where PET/MRI could outperform PET/CT, as shown by small pilot studies.[97,98] One particular pitfall in MPM is chronic iatrogenic inflammation after talc pleurodesis on FDG-PET[99] (see Fig. 114.2).

Early evidence also suggests that PET/CT may have a role in evaluating response to therapy in MPM,[100] with changes in MTV and TLG correlated with overall survival. This is interesting because the assessment of response in patients with MPM according to standard response criteria on CT is far from simple, with potential for PET/CT to outperform *response evaluation criteria in solid tumors* (RECIST)[101] imaging criteria[102] commonly used to evaluate treatment responses in oncology clinical trials and clinical practice. More work to define response criteria for MPM on PET is needed. Furthermore, a prospective study in patients with nonsarcomatoid malignant pleural mesothelioma observed that baseline MTV on PET was more predictive of survival than CT-assessed TNM stage in a multivariate analysis.[103] These observations of prognostic potential show considerable promise but still require prospective validation.

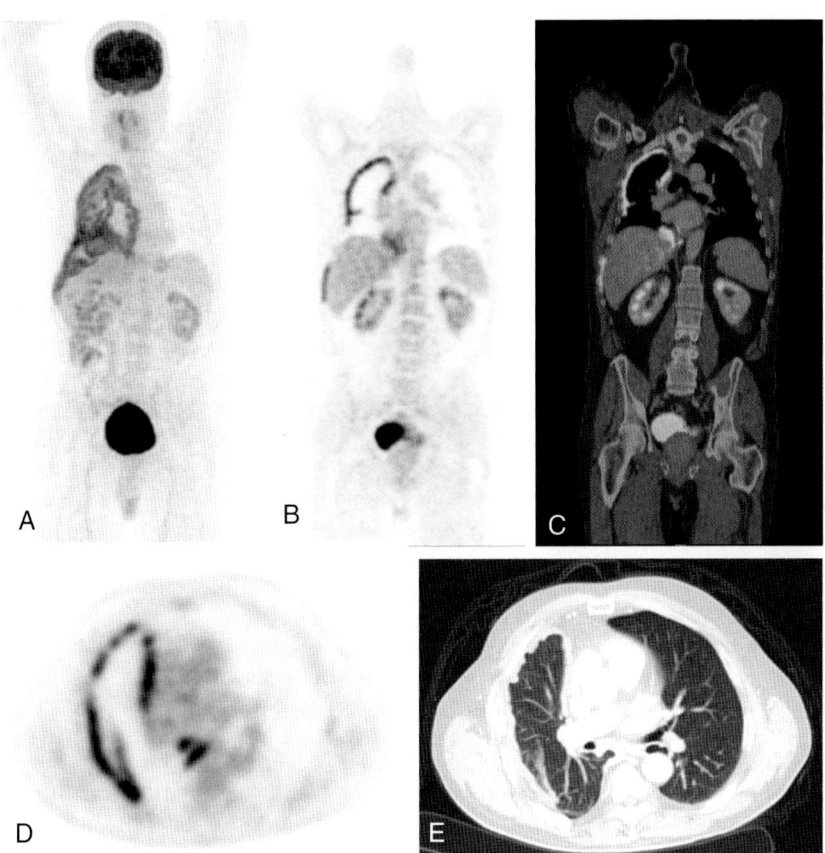

Figure 25.6 **¹⁸F-*fluorodeoxyglucose* (FDG) *positron emission tomography* (PET)/*computed tomography* (CT) in mesothelioma.** A 67-year-old patient underwent FDG-PET/CT for staging of a primary epithelioid pleural mesothelioma. (A) The maximum intensity projection images show diffuse strong uptake in the right chest cavity. (B–C) Coronal sections show linear strong uptake on a large portion of the lateral and medial pleura, with a small area on the lateral side without increased uptake. (D) Transverse section shows increased uptake of most of the pleura, corresponding to tumoral irregular thickening of the pleura (E).

NEUROENDOCRINE TUMORS

Neuroendocrine tumors (NETs) arise in cells of the diffuse neuroendocrine system, also known as the amine precursor uptake and decarboxylation system. NETs of the lung are divided into four categories: *typical carcinoid* (TC), *atypical carcinoid* (AC), *large cell neuroendocrine carcinoma* (LCNEC), and small cell neuroendocrine carcinoma (i.e., SCLC).[104] FDG uptake is often low in TC and is known as a cause of false negatives on FDG-PET. In contrast, in higher-grade NETs (AC, LCNEC), the FDG-uptake can be similar to NSCLC and SCLC.[105] (See Chapter 78.)

Alternative tracers have been studied for the detection and staging of the NETs with low FDG avidity. Neuroendocrine cells synthesize and secrete a range of peptide hormones. The molecular substrate of this hormone production has been harnessed to provide imaging targets. The most studied target is the *somatostatin receptor* (SSTR), a seven-transmembrane G-coupled peptide receptor that plays a role in the control of hormone secretion and cell growth[106] and is internalized upon ligand binding.[107] Synthetic peptides derived from the somatostatin hormone have been derived with chelators and radiolabeled with a range of different radionuclides, of which the most interesting for PET are the so-called *gallium-68–dodecanetetraacetic acid* (⁶⁸Ga-DOTA) peptides labeled with the generator-derived gallium-68.[108] They consist of a positron-emitting radionuclide (⁶⁸Ga), a chelator (DOTA), and a *somatostatin analog* (SSA) vector molecule binding the SSTR (e.g., *d-Phe¹-Tyr³-octreotide* [TOC], *Tyr³-octreotate* [TATE], *¹-Nal³-octreotide* [NOC]). Three of these are currently in clinical use: ⁶⁸Ga-DOTA-TOC,

⁶⁸Ga-DOTA-TATE, and ⁶⁸Ga-DOTA-NOC. These tracers all have a high affinity for subtype 2 of the SSTR, the SSTR2A (in the low nanomolar range), varying affinity for subtypes 3 and 5, and low affinity for subtypes 1 and 4.[109]

Many studies have documented the increased diagnostic performance of these ligands for detection of NETs in general.[110,111] A recent study documented expression of SSTR2A, the prime target for these radioligands, in more than 80% of patients with bronchial carcinoid, with similar mean immunohistochemistry scores for SSTR2A in TC and AC.[112] There are very high uptake rates in TC and AC, with median SUV$_{max}$ of about 15, 20, and 25, respectively, for ⁶⁸Ga-DOTA-TATE,[105] ⁶⁸Ga-DOTA-TOC,[113] and ⁶⁸Ga-DOTA-NOC[114] (Fig. 25.7). Somatostatin-based tracers may have advantages compared to FDG tracers in imaging of NETs. In a large series of 207 patients, FDG-PET showed a sensitivity for mediastinal lymph nodes of 33%.[115] SSTR-PET, on the other hand, has been shown to provide additional information for staging compared to CT in 37% of patients, with impact on patient management, including 21% of patients in which occult metastatic disease was detected.[116] Also, in 16% of early postsurgical patients, metastatic disease was detected. Comparing FDG and ⁶⁸Ga-DOTA-TATE uptake, an interesting observation has been made regarding central bronchial carcinoids,[117] which often present with postobstructive atelectasis. ⁶⁸Ga-DOTA-TATE consistently showed low uptake in the area of atelectasis, whereas FDG could yield moderate to even very high uptake due to postobstructive inflammation or infection, and low uptake in the primary tumor.[105] Based on these data, international guidelines recommend the use of ⁶⁸Ga-DOTA-SSA PET if available.[118] A recent review of seven studies concluded that somatostatin analogs and FDG gave complementary information in patients with NETs.[118a] Further strategies for increasing availability include commercial kit development and use of longer–half-life radionuclides, such as fluorine-18 and copper-64.[119] This tracer is also used to select patients for radionuclide therapy with SSA that include beta- or alpha-emitters, a concept called peptide receptor radionuclide therapy; selecting patients for therapy using imaging with very similar radiopharmaceuticals is referred to as *theranostic* use.

RESPONSE TO THERAPY

FDG uptake in tumors is related to (1) the number of viable cancer cells, (2) their metabolic activity and proliferation capacity, and (3) the presence of inflammatory cells.[120] In many clinical settings, the metabolic changes caused by cancer therapy precede morphologic changes. The discrimination of viable tumor from nonviable tumor is the basis for the use of PET for the determination of response to therapy. Whenever PET scans will be compared at different time points, it is crucial to perform the entire PET procedure using the same methodology (interval from last therapy, patient preparation, camera setting, reconstruction parameters, image analysis).[121,122]

For early-stage NSCLC, the assessment of response and prediction of outcome after *stereotactic ablative radiotherapy* (SABR) have become very important. Retrospective data regarding the value of pretreatment FDG uptake on PET in the prediction of response to SABR are too conflicting to be used in clinical practice.[123–125] On the other hand, the potential of semiquantitative FDG uptake on posttreatment PET at 3, 6, and 9 months after SABR for stage I NSCLC has been evaluated in both retrospective and prospective studies. For posttreatment follow-up, CT is the standard

and, if suspicious findings are observed, PET/CT should be performed.[126] A systematic literature review suggests that recurrent disease is highly likely if these high-risk CT changes correlate on PET with an SUV_{max} of 5 or greater or an SUV_{max} higher than the pre-SABR value in tumors with low FDG avidity. If the SUV values are below these values, there is a low suspicion of recurrence, and close follow-up or biopsy should be used.[126] PET/CT has a high specificity of 94% and complements CT.[127] Further studies are, however, needed to validate these findings.

For potentially resectable stage III NSCLC, the evaluation after induction chemo(radio)therapy is crucial in deciding whether to resect. Several studies addressed restaging after induction therapy. In the restaging of mediastinal lymph nodes, integrated PET/CT has a sensitivity of up to 70%, with a specificity of up to 90%. Mediastinal restaging with PET/CT thus reaches an accuracy level of some clinical value, but tissue confirmation is still mandatory to certify the real nodal status. New positive lesions, especially lymph nodes, need to be interpreted carefully because new findings in this setting have a high false-positive rate.[128] The findings of the value of PET/CT on prediction of outcome after induction therapy are even more interesting. The classical prognostic parameters for surgery in these patients are obtained from the resection specimens: (1) downstaging of mediastinal nodes and (2) the pathologic response in the primary tumor. These histologic features are poorly predicted by clinical symptoms or evolution of CT findings during induction therapy. In these prospective studies, both the residual FDG uptake in the primary tumor after induction, as well as the change in FDG uptake when comparing preinduction and postinduction values, had strong power to predict outcome after combined modality treatment (Fig. 25.8). With the advent of minimally invasive EBUS/EUS baseline mediastinal staging to confirm N2/N3 disease, the postinduction assessment can be based on

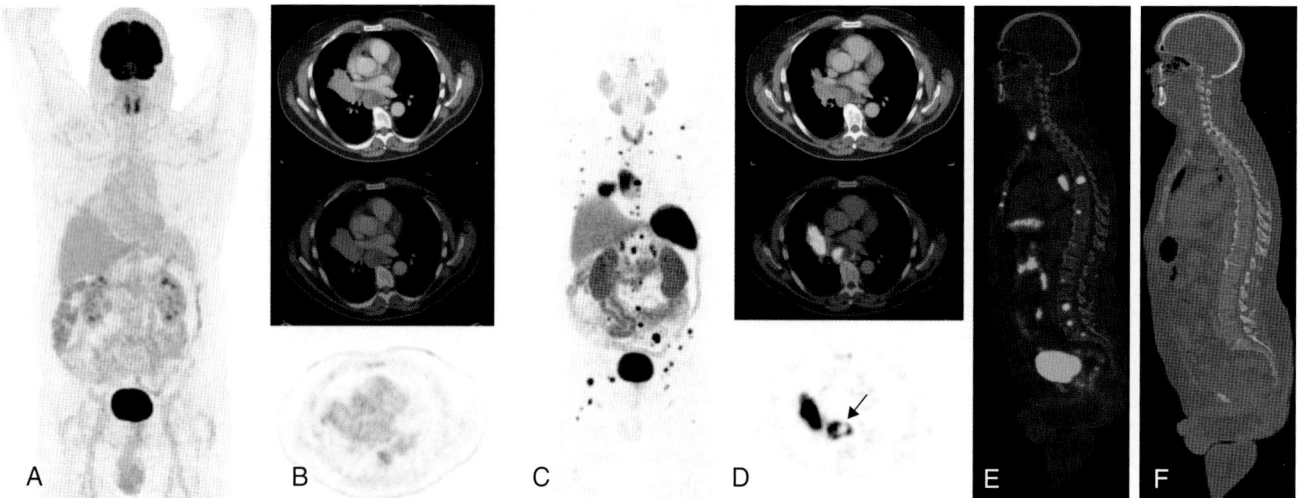

Figure 25.7 **Additional value of ^{68}Ga-DOTA-TATE *positron emission tomography* (PET)/*computed tomography* (CT) in bronchial neuroendocrine tumor.** A 62-year-old man, a former smoker with 20 pack-years, was treated for a right-sided pulmonary infection. Chest radiography and CT showed a mass in the right lung hilum associated with hilar and subcarinal lymphadenopathy. (A–B) [18]*F-fluorodeoxyglucose* (FDG)-PET/CT showed consolidation adjacent to the right hilum and lymphadenopathy with only faint FDG uptake, similar to the mediastinal blood pool (B). Transbronchial biopsies showed a bronchial neuroendocrine tumor, positive for synaptophysin and chromogranin A, with a Ki-67 index less than 2% and without necrosis or mitosis figures, compatible with a typical carcinoid. Based on these findings, ^{68}Ga-DOTA-TATE PET/CT was performed. (C) The maximum intensity projection image shows intense uptake in the tumor in the right middle lobe and the subcarinal lymph nodes, with necrosis-induced central photopenia in the latter (D, *arrow*), as well as multiple foci with strong to intense uptake in the skeleton (E), with no changes on the corresponding CT to indicate osseous metastases (F). Based on these findings, no surgery was performed, contrary to the initial CT and FDG-PET/CT–based treatment plan.

primary tumor response information on serial comparison of PET or lymph node assessment by EBUS/EUS or mediastinoscopy. In one model, the combination of lymph node involvement and primary tumor response on PET could discriminate "good prognosis" patients (5-year survival, 62%) from "poor prognosis" patients (only 6%; hazard ratio, 0.18).[129] Other studies have shown a similar separation in prognosis based on similar cutoff values in a setting of induction chemoradiotherapy, with 5-year survival of approximately 70% in the group with good PET response and approximately 22% survival in the group with poor PET response.[130] Thus, PET/CT can be regarded as a key tool for the planning of preoperative induction therapy, for following response to treatment, and for determining overall prognosis.

For nonresectable stage I to III NSCLC treated with curative radiotherapy, the data are in line with the findings described earlier for operable disease.[131] Indeed, patients undergoing radiotherapy alone or sequential/concurrent chemoradiotherapy had a markedly different prognosis based on their metabolic response status 2 weeks into radiotherapy[132] (e.g., 2-year survival 92% for responders vs. 33% for

nonresponders in one study).[133] PET obtained after completion of (chemo)radiotherapy also allows for strong discrimination of prognosis, with complete metabolic responders having a median survival of 31 months versus 11 months for incomplete metabolic responders.[134] When compared to CT alone, PET enables more accurate determinations of response to treatment and is a better predictor of survival than baseline stage response on CT or performance status.[135] In locally advanced patients treated with concurrent chemoradiotherapy, PET after completion of treatment has an accuracy of approximately 90% for predicting subsequent tumor response after treatment.[136] PET has also been used to predict recurrent tumor growth and spread after radiotherapy or chemotherapy, enabling a more personalized approach by guiding the need for and timing of supplemental therapy on an individual basis.[137] One study suggests improved outcomes when the decision to perform salvage lung resection after curative-intent radiation in patients with locally advanced NSCLC is guided by abnormal FDG-PET findings rather than the more traditionally used obvious relapse by CT (overall median survival, 43 vs. 12 months).[138]

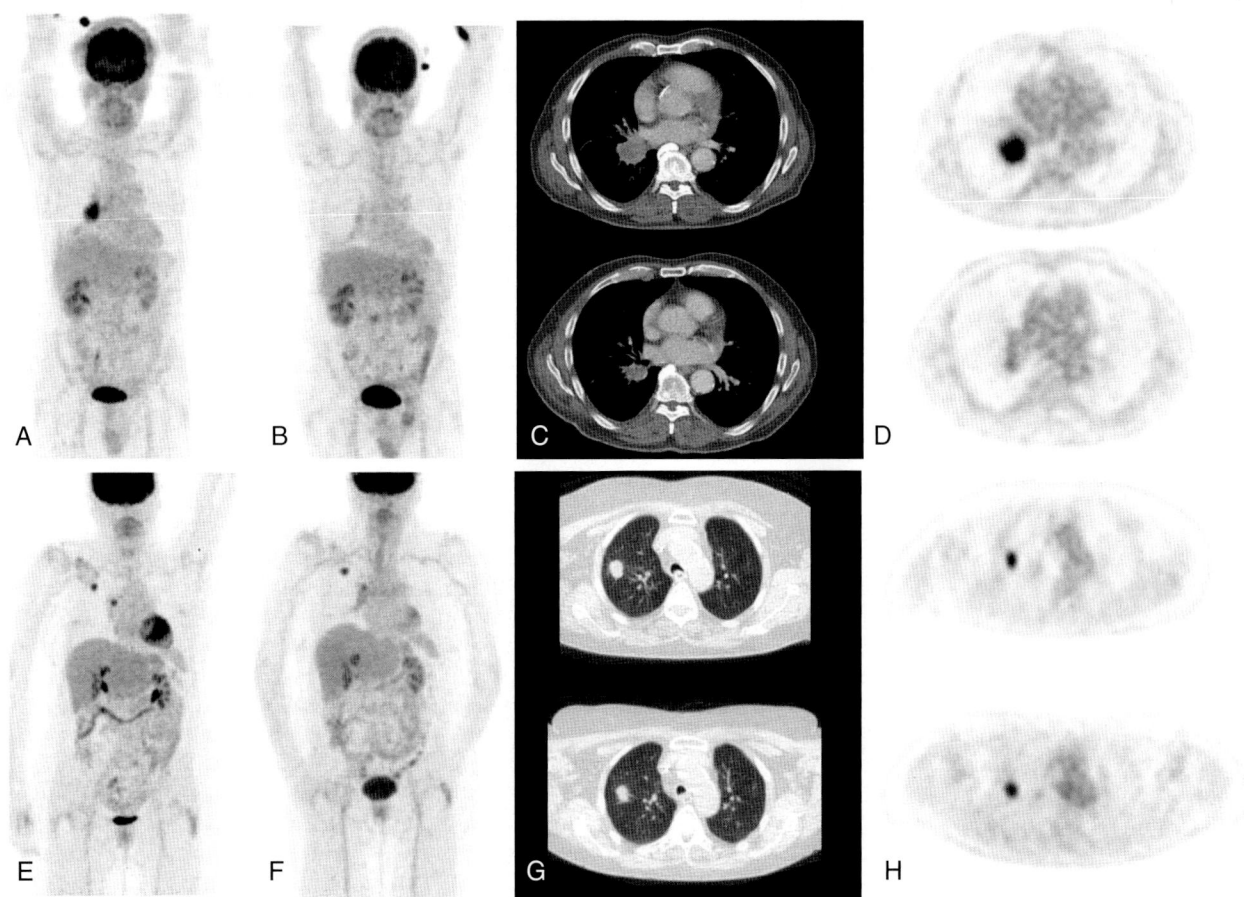

Figure 25.8 **¹⁸F-*fluorodeoxyglucose* (FDG) *positron emission tomography* (PET)/*computed tomography* (CT) after induction chemotherapy.** Two patients with histologically proven N2 disease treated with induction chemotherapy and surgery are shown. (A–D) The first patient was a 67-year-old man with a cT2N2M0 adenocarcinoma. Baseline images (A; C–D *upper row*) showed intense uptake in the tumor in the right lower lobe (SUV$_{max}$, 13.5). Images after three cycles of cisplatinum-gemcitabine doublet (B; C–D *lower row*) showed a near normalization of FDG uptake in the primary tumor (*maximum standardized uptake value* [SUV$_{max}$], 3.45; ΔSUV$_{max}$, −74.5%), compatible with a metabolic response. Surgery showed ypTisN1M0 disease. He was alive 7 years later with no evidence of recurrence. (E–H) The second patient is a 73-year-old woman with a cT1aN2M0 tumor in the right upper lobe. Baseline images (E; G–H, *upper row*) showed intense uptake in the tumor in the right upper lobe (SUV$_{max}$, 9.80) and in hilar lymph nodes. Images after three cycles of cisplatinum-pemetrexed doublet (F; G–H, *lower row*) showed a persistent elevated uptake in the primary tumor (SUV$_{max}$, 8.12; ΔSUV$_{max}$, −17%), compatible with metabolic nonresponse. Mediastinoscopy demonstrated persistent multilevel N2 disease after which she was treated with radiotherapy. She died from progressive disease 7 months after the initial PET/CT scan.

In patients with stage IV NSCLC, effective systemic chemotherapy causes a rapid decrease in FDG uptake during the first cycle and therefore could potentially identify chemotherapy responders and nonresponders at an early treatment stage.[139] Targeted therapies are a cornerstone of modern respiratory oncology and conceptually PET might be of great interest in the assessment of these agents. Two independent studies have shown that early PET can predict progression-free and overall survival in patients treated with erlotinib, even in the absence of a response based on imaging criteria (RECIST).[140,141] A systematic review of *epidermal growth factor receptor* (EGFR) inhibitors showed that patients who were responsive to this therapy presented with a metabolic response within the first 2 weeks and had a durable response to treatment. Patients without early response had a low probability of benefit.[142] In a small study evaluating the role of PET/CT versus CT in determining tumor response to anaplastic lymphoma kinase inhibitors, PET/CT detected progression earlier than CT in almost half of progressive events and simultaneously with CT for the other events.[143] PET/CT could be of benefit in the detection of oligoprogressive disease, where disease is stable at some sites but progresses in others, in oncogene-addicted NSCLC. A recent study showed that patients with oligoprogressive disease detected by PET/CT could be treated with ablative therapies in a higher fraction, leading to greater progression-free survival and overall survival.[144] PET/CT can be of particular value in the follow-up of patients with disease burden difficult to assess with CT alone (e.g., patients with predominant bone [marrow] involvement) with few target lesions for imaging-based (RECIST) follow-up.

The rapid advent of immuno-oncologic treatment in both nonmetastatic and advanced-stage lung cancer provides promising opportunities for FDG-PET/CT, such as assessment of response to neoadjuvant treatment, discrimination of pseudoprogression, or the detection and characterization of immune-related adverse events.[13,145–147]

FOLLOW-UP AFTER CURATIVE-INTENT TREATMENT

After curative therapy of NSCLC, early detection of recurrence is important because salvage therapies can be rewarding, especially in asymptomatic locoregional recurrences.

Selective use of PET can be recommended for the evaluation of a suspect local recurrence on conventional radiologic imaging in lung cancer patients previously treated for early stage NSCLC with curative intent. Two prospective studies compared the differential diagnostic performance of PET and CT in the early detection of local recurrence.[148,149] In both, the accuracy of PET was better than that of CT (93% vs. 82%; 96% vs. 84%). Several prospective series in patients with a residual thoracic abnormality after treatment addressed the value of PET to differentiate between local recurrence versus residual nonspecific posttreatment changes.[148–153] A cutoff for SUV of 2.5, differentiating benign from malignant lesions, just as suggested for newly diagnosed lung lesions, had a sensitivity ranging from 97–100% and a specificity ranging from 62–100%.

Surveillance by PET/CT every 6 to 12 months after a treatment with curative intent (surgery or SABR) for early-stage NSCLC cannot be recommended. Despite several reports of a better sensitivity to detect disease recurrence on PET/CT in asymptomatic patients compared to chest CT scan alone, no survival benefit has been demonstrated in the postoperative follow-up setting.[154,155] However, PET/CT can be used in patients showing suspicious findings on follow-up CT in patients treated with SABR.[126]

HEALTH ECONOMICS

As respiratory oncologists, we aim for the best-quality health care for our patients, while acknowledging the need for financial prudence. The major cost of modern oncology practice, however, does not lie in the baseline diagnostic process but in the delivery of expensive treatments and in caring for morbidity related to side effects. Therefore, application of economic modeling to the use of PET has to be based on both diagnostic and therapeutic aspects of health care expenditure within a routine clinical setting.

In a recent overview of all economic evaluations on PET in oncology performed between 2005 and 2010, it was concluded that the strongest evidence for cost-effective use of PET was the staging of NSCLC, where there may be a benefit for patients in terms of a slight increase in life expectancy and for the health care system in terms of avoiding invasive procedures.[156] Taking into account the superior accuracy of PET/CT compared to PET alone in lung cancer staging, the cost-effectiveness can probably be extended to PET/CT. Since the introduction of PET/CT technology in 2001, additional studies in respiratory oncology have confirmed the cost-effectiveness of this integrated scanning method.[157,158] Furthermore, PET was shown to be cost-effective for characterizing SPNs and the most cost-effective diagnostic strategy for nodules of low to moderate pretest probability of malignancy on CT.[159]

NEW TRACERS

The vast majority of PET imaging in pulmonary medicine is performed with FDG. However, many new tracers are being developed to expand the uses of PET (eTable 25.1). One recently developed category of tracers could potentially outperform FDG as a general cancer detection tracer: radiolabeled *fibroblast-activation protein inhibitors* (FAPIs). These tracers, for instance, ^{68}Ga-FAPI-04, target fibroblasts in the tumoral stroma. They have very low background uptake in lung, mediastinum, liver and, in contrast with FDG, normal brain, which can improve staging in NSCLC patients.[160] Initial studies in 25 lung cancer patients have shown high tumoral SUV values,[161] and comparison with FDG has shown significantly higher SUV values in 14 lung cancer patients compared to FDG-PET (12.0 vs. 4.5, respectively).[162] The increased lesion to background of ^{68}Ga-FAPI-04 compared to FDG might be one advantage of this tracer but, similar to FDG, this tracer also shows uptake in inflammatory processes, so little improvement in specificity is expected. The low background in virtually all normal organs will allow for development of therapeutic radiopharmaceuticals and theranostics imaging.

PET tracers have been developed for a whole range of biologic and pathophysiologic processes.[163]

These tracers are described at ExpertConsult.com and in eTable 25.1.

Key Points

- ^{18}F-*fluorodeoxyglucose* (FDG) is the most common tracer used for clinical cancer *positron emission tomography* (PET) imaging and reflects cellular uptake of glucose.
- FDG-PET/*computed tomography* (CT) results in better *tumor-node-metastasis* (TNM) staging in *non–small cell lung cancer* (NSCLC) than conventional imaging alone and may alter treatment choice or intent in a substantial proportion of patients.
- Limitations to FDG-PET should be well understood. False-negative PET findings can result from slow-growing tumors, small tumors (<8–10 mm), or hyperglycemia. False-positive PET findings can result from increased metabolic activity from inflammation, infection, autoimmune processes, sarcoidosis, talc pleurodesis, or some benign tumors.
- Higher uptake of FDG by NSCLC is often associated with greater aggressiveness and poorer prognosis.
- FDG-PET is useful in assessments of response to therapies, particularly in patients with locally advanced NSCLC, with combined modality treatment. PET/CT should not be used for surveillance after curative intent in early-stage NSCLC but can be useful to characterize abnormal findings detected on conventional imaging during follow-up.
- PET/*magnetic resonance imaging* (MRI) and PET/CT have equivalent staging performance for NSCLC. PET/MRI offers superior assessment of disease involving the chest wall or diaphragm but is suboptimal for imaging of the lung parenchyma and is less widely available.
- PET imaging may be similarly useful in the assessment of small cell lung cancer and mesothelioma (using FDG) and bronchial carcinoid tumors (using radiolabeled somatostatin analogs).
- Other tracers beyond FDG are emerging to detect tumor metabolic activity based on sodium-dependent glucose transporters, mitochondrial membrane potential, tumor hypoxia, epidermal growth factor receptor mutation status, and immune system imaging, which may potentially guide immuno-oncologic therapy.
- The most cost-effective role of PET is in staging NSCLC, where PET reduces the number of invasive procedures and improves staging accuracy of disease. Use of FDG-PET in NSCLC patients with a potential for cure is evidence based and cost effective.

Key Readings

Aide N, et al. FDG PET/CT for assessing tumour response to immunotherapy: report on the EANM symposium on immune modulation and recent review of the literature. *Eur J Nucl Med Mol Imaging.* 2019;46(1):238–250.

Bensch F, et al. ^{89}Zr-atezolizumab imaging as a non-invasive approach to assess clinical response to PD-L1 blockade in cancer. *Nat Med.* 2018;24(12):1852–1858.

Callister ME, et al. British Thoracic Society guidelines for the investigation and management of pulmonary nodules. *Thorax.* 2015;70(suppl 2):ii1–ii54.

Caplin ME, et al. Pulmonary neuroendocrine (carcinoid) tumors: European Neuroendocrine Tumor Society expert consensus and recommendations for best practice for typical and atypical pulmonary carcinoids. *Ann Oncol.* 2015;26(8):1604–1620.

Deppen SA, et al. Accuracy of FDG-PET to diagnose lung cancer in areas with infectious lung disease: a meta-analysis. *JAMA.* 2014;312(12):1227–1236.

Dooms C, Verbeken E, Stroobants S, et al. Prognostic stratification of stage IIIA-N2 non-small cell lung cancer after induction chemotherapy: a model based on the combination of morphometric-pathologic response in mediastinal nodes and primary tumor response on serial 18-fluoro-2-deoxy-glucose positron emission tomography. *J Clin Oncol.* 2008;26:1128–1134.

Fischer B, Lassen U, Mortensen J, et al. Preoperative staging of lung cancer with combined PET-CT. *N Engl J Med.* 2009;361:32–39.

Gorospe L, Raman S, Echeveste J, et al. Whole-body PET/CT: spectrum of physiological variants, artifacts and interpretative pitfalls in cancer patients. *Nucl Med Commun.* 2005;26:671–687.

Gregory DL, et al. Effect of PET/CT on management of patients with non-small cell lung cancer: results of a prospective study with 5-year survival data. *J Nucl Med.* 2012;53(7):1007–1015.

Herder GJ, et al. Clinical prediction model to characterize pulmonary nodules: validation and added value of 18F-fluorodeoxyglucose positron emission tomography. *Chest.* 2005;128(4):2490–2496.

Hoekstra CJ, Stroobants SG, Smit EF, et al. Prognostic relevance of response evaluation using [18F]-2-fluoro-2-deoxy-d-glucose positron emission tomography in patients with locally advanced non-small cell lung cancer. *J Clin Oncol.* 2005;23:8362–8370.

Huang K, Dahele M, Senan S, et al. Radiographic changes after lung stereotactic ablative radiotherapy (SABR)—can we distinguish recurrence from fibrosis? A systematic review of the literature. *Radiother Oncol.* 2012;102:335–342.

Kirchner J, et al. Prospective comparison of (18)F-FDG PET/MRI and (18)F-FDG PET/CT for thoracic staging of non-small cell lung cancer. *Eur J Nucl Med Mol Imaging.* 2019;46(2):437–445.

Lardinois D, Weder W, Hany TF, et al. Staging of non-small cell lung cancer with integrated positron-emission tomography and computed tomography. *N Engl J Med.* 2003;348:2500–2507.

Nakamura H, et al. Close association of IASLC/ATS/ERS lung adenocarcinoma subtypes with glucose-uptake in positron emission tomography. *Lung Cancer.* 2015;87(1):28–33.

Ng TL, et al. Detection of oligoprogressive disease in oncogene-addicted non-small cell lung cancer using PET/CT versus CT in patients receiving a tyrosine kinase inhibitor. *Lung Cancer.* 2018;126:112–118.

Turgeon GA, et al. What (18)F-FDG PET response-assessment method best predicts survival after curative-intent chemoradiation in non-small cell lung cancer: EORTC, PERCIST, Peter Mac Criteria, or Deauville Criteria? *J Nucl Med.* 2019;60(3):328–334.

Van Tinteren H, Hoekstra OS, Smit EF, et al. Effectiveness of positron emission tomography in the preoperative assessment of patients with suspected non-small cell lung cancer: the PLUS multicentre randomised trial. *Lancet.* 2002;359:1388–1393.

Vansteenkiste JF, Stroobants SG, De Leyn PR, et al. Lymph node staging in non-small cell lung cancer with FDG-PET scan: a prospective study on 690 lymph node stations from 68 patients. *J Clin Oncol.* 1998;16:2142–2149.

Vansteenkiste JF, Stroobants SG, De Leyn PR, et al. Prognostic importance of the standardized uptake value on FDG-PET-scan in non-small cell lung cancer: an analysis of 125 cases. *J Clin Oncol.* 1999;17:3201–3206.

Wauters I, Stroobants S, De Leyn P, et al. Impact of FDG-PET induced treatment choices on long-term outcome in NSCLC. *Respiration.* 2010;79:97–104.

Complete reference list available at ExpertConsult.com.

DIAGNOSTIC BRONCHOSCOPY: BASIC TECHNIQUES

ELIF KÜPELI, MD, FCCP • ATUL C. MEHTA, MBBS, FACP, FCCP

INTRODUCTION AND HISTORICAL BACKGROUND	Monitoring	Endobronchial Biopsy
INDICATIONS	**BASIC TECHNIQUES**	Transbronchial Biopsy
PROCEDURE	Bronchoalveolar Lavage	Conventional Transbronchial Needle Aspiration
Sedation and Anesthesia	Bronchial Washings	**KEY POINTS**
	Bronchial Brushings	

INTRODUCTION AND HISTORICAL BACKGROUND

Flexible bronchoscopy (FB) is one of the most frequently performed invasive procedures in pulmonary medicine. It is increasingly being performed for its diagnostic and therapeutic potentials. Recently, the introduction of novel technologies, such as electromagnetic navigation and robotic bronchoscopy, has further increased the reach of the instrument and increased the diagnostic yield. This chapter deals with the basics of the FB procedure; the advanced diagnostic techniques and therapeutic applications are presented in the successive chapters of this textbook.

Gustav Killian performed the first bronchoscopy in 1897 to extract a piece of a pork bone from the right main bronchus.[1] From that meager beginning, the technology in bronchoscopy has advanced exponentially. In 1966 the flexible bronchoscope was introduced into clinical practice by Shigeto Ikeda.[2] Currently, this instrument is one of the most important tools for diagnosis and treatment of pulmonary diseases.

FB can be performed in an outpatient setting, under moderate sedation and local anesthesia. Compared with FB, rigid bronchoscopy is now primarily used for selective indications, such as massive hemoptysis and therapeutics.[3–6]

INDICATIONS

The indications for diagnostic FB are broad and growing (Table 26.1). Nonetheless, certain conditions are not considered indications for FB. For example, FB is not indicated to evaluate patients with cough unless the cough fails to respond to conventional treatment or if there is a change in its character. Similarly, bronchoscopy is not indicated to evaluate patients with isolated pleural effusion or atelectasis,[7–9] and its use to remove secretions during acute exacerbations of chronic obstructive lung disease is also considered inappropriate.[10] FB also has little role in finding synchronous lesions in patients undergoing lung resection of a solitary pulmonary nodule suspected to be primary bronchogenic carcinoma.[11] Absolute and relative contraindications to performing FB are presented in Table 26.2.

PROCEDURE

The nasal and oral routes provide excellent access to the lower airways. By either route, attention should be given to the upper airway. In particular, bronchoscopy performed for the evaluation of hemoptysis or wheezing should also include a careful evaluation of the upper airway, including the nasopharynx, oropharynx, and vocal cords. FB is often performed via the nasal route.[12] The nasal route is avoided in patients suspected to have foreign body aspiration, to have sufficient room to remove the object, and among those with coagulopathies, because of the risk of epistaxis.

SEDATION AND ANESTHESIA

The need for sedation during FB remains a matter of some debate in the literature.[13–15] The purpose of sedation is to improve patient comfort and add to the ease of the procedure for the bronchoscopist.[16,17] Although bronchoscopy can be carried out without sedation,[18,19] most are performed under moderate sedation.[20–23] Of interest, according to some surveys, 16% to 21% of physicians use deep sedation or general anesthesia for FB.[20,22]

Intravenous (IV) preparations of various sedatives, such as diazepam, midazolam, lorazepam, morphine sulfate, fentanyl, and hydrocodone, have been used either alone or in combination based on the bronchoscopist's preference and the availability of the drug.[24–29] Fentanyl has a greater analgesic potency than morphine.[25] Hydrocodone has a greater antitussive property than codeine but less than that of morphine.[30] Due to its rapid onset and anxiolytic and amnestic properties, midazolam is one of the most commonly used sedatives; sedation with midazolam in FB improves the patient's comfort and decreases recall without causing significant hemodynamic compromise. It should be offered to the patient on a routine basis.[31,32]

TABLE 26.1 Indications for Diagnostic Flexible Bronchoscopy (Adult)

Hemoptysis

Wheeze and stridor: suspected stricture, upper airway obstruction

Lung opacities of unknown cause
- Suspected pulmonary infections not responding to conventional treatment
    Localized
    Diffuse
- Lung opacities in an immunocompromised host
- Recurrent or unresolved pneumonia
- Cavitary lesion
- Interstitial opacities
- New pulmonary nodule

Unexplained lung collapse without air bronchograms

Suspected or known bronchogenic carcinoma
- Positive or suspicious sputum cytologic findings
- Staging of known bronchogenic carcinoma
- Follow-up after endobronchial treatments

Mediastinal and hilar lymphadenopathy and masses

Lung transplantation
- Inspect airway anastomosis
- Rejection surveillance

Esophageal cancer evaluation

Endotracheal intubation
- Confirm tube position
- Evaluate for tube-related injury

Evaluation for foreign body aspiration

Chest trauma
- Rule out rupture of central airways
- Examine for aspirated contents

Evaluation following burns or chemical injury to the airways

Unexplained superior vena cava syndrome

Unexplained vocal cord paralysis or hoarseness

Suspected fistulas
- Bronchopleural
- Tracheoesophageal and bronchoesophageal
- Tracheoaortic or bronchoaortic
- Iatrogenic (postsurgical)

Table 26.2 Contraindications for Flexible Bronchoscopy

ABSOLUTE

Uncorrectable hypoxemia
Lack of patient cooperation
Lack of skilled personnel
Lack of appropriate equipment and facilities
Unstable angina
Uncontrolled arrhythmias

RELATIVE

Unexplained or severe hypercarbia
Uncontrolled asthma
Uncorrectable coagulopathy
Unstable cervical spine
Need for a large tissue specimen for diagnosis
Debility, advanced age, malnutrition

The combination of a benzodiazepine and an opioid has been shown to be safe and synergistic for the purposes of sedation during FB.[28,33] Because the combination of benzodiazepines and opiates may cause hypoventilation, particularly in patients with preexisting respiratory failure, patients should be appropriately monitored.[34] The combination of hydrocodone and midazolam reduces cough during FB without causing significant desaturation and improves the patient's tolerance for the procedure.[28,33] Dexmedetomidine (Precedex, Dexdomiror) also has favorable properties of sedation, sympatholysis, analgesia, and a low risk for apnea. These properties suggest that dexmedetomidine may be useful in procedural sedation. However, it has been shown that dexmedetomidine as a sole agent is unable to provide adequate sedation for awake diagnostic FB without the need for rescue sedation in a large proportion of patients.[35] Dextromethorphan can also be given orally 90 minutes before the procedure to improve cough suppression during the procedure.[36]

Propofol has come into use, both alone and in combination. For conscious sedation, propofol alone has been shown to be as effective and safe as combined sedation in patients undergoing FB, thus representing an appealing option if timely discharge is a priority.[37] Deep sedation with propofol for bronchoscopy has gained popularity in recent years, although concern has been raised regarding its potential to induce severe respiratory depression. In one prospective study, the use of small boluses of propofol at short intervals, with monitoring of transcutaneous carbon dioxide level, was found to be safe; the authors concluded that propofol used in this manner does not cause excessive respiratory depression and represents an excellent alternative to traditional sedation agents.[38] In another prospective study, the combination of propofol and hydrocodone was safe and better for cough suppression than propofol alone during FB.[39] Fospropofol disodium is a water-soluble prodrug of propofol. In a subset analysis among elderly patients (≥65 years) undergoing FB, fospropofol provided safe and effective sedation, rapid time to fully alert status, and high satisfaction, outcomes which were comparable to those in younger patients.[40]

Higher-than-usual doses of sedatives are usually required for patients with human immunodeficiency virus infection, recipients of stem cell transplantation, lung transplant recipients for cystic fibrosis, and drug users.[31-43] In addition, because protease inhibitors used in patients with human immunodeficiency virus infection have been shown to extend the half-life of benzodiazepines significantly, many institutions in the United States instead encourage the use of deep sedation in these patients.

Local Anesthesia

Although nerve blocks can be used to provide excellent analgesia to the airway, physicians generally rely on topical administration of local anesthetic agents. Lidocaine is the most commonly used drug for providing topical anesthesia.[44] It offers a relatively wide margin of safety, with a rapid onset and sufficient duration of action to allow completion of most bronchoscopic procedures. The gel preparation of lidocaine is preferred over the spray for nasal anesthesia.[45-47] Given that sensory anesthesia is not dependent on the concentration of lidocaine, 1% is preferred because larger volumes can be instilled to cover a greater surface area of the mucosa before toxic dosages are reached.[48,49] The oropharynx can be anesthetized with 2-4% lidocaine applied as a spray, nebulized solution, or gargles.

The vocal cords and the endobronchial tree are anesthetized by direct instillation of lidocaine via the working channel of the bronchoscope. The total dose of lidocaine should be limited to 8.2 mg/kg in adults, with extra caution in the elderly or those with liver, renal, or cardiac impairments.[24]

Anticholinergic agents, such as atropine and glycopyrrolate, have been commonly used as premedication for FB,[50,51] with the aim to reduce the bronchial secretions and suppress vagal overactivity. Several studies have shown that anticholinergics offer little advantage as premedications, and their use should be abandoned.[52–54]

MONITORING

To ensure adequate oxygenation (oxygen saturation of >92%) and hemodynamic stability, pulse oximetry, heart rate, and blood pressure are monitored throughout the procedure. There should be IV access and equipment for resuscitation readily available. Supplemental oxygen should be administered to all patients undergoing bronchoscopy. In October 2010, the American Society for Anesthesiology updated their statement on basic anesthesia monitoring to include capnography in addition to clinical assessment to monitor ventilation during moderate sedation. It has been realized that sedation to anesthesia is a continuum, and patients can slip into a deeper-than-intended plane of sedation without any prior warning. In fact, it has been shown that the majority of patients undergoing moderate sedation may enter a state of deep sedation, at least for a short duration, and the use of capnography can improve safety[55] (see also Chapter 44). All FB procedures are performed observing universal precautions. After each procedure, the instrument is thoroughly disinfected or sterilized according to published consensus statements.[56–59]

Approach

The standard procedure for FB involves a thorough examination of the entire tracheobronchial tree in a systematic fashion, from the upper airway and vocal cords to the trachea and carina, major bronchi, and the segmental bronchi in each of the five lung lobes. A thorough understanding of normal features can allow detection of abnormalities in anatomy (e.g., missing or duplication of bronchi), shape (e.g., narrowing or distortion), changes in the anatomy with breathing (e.g., collapse), or endobronchial mucosa (e.g., induration, friability, erythema, lesions). A bronchoscopy of a patient with a relatively normal tracheobronchial tree is shown in Video 26.1. The bronchoscopist aims to maintain the bronchoscope in the center of the airway to avoid cough and endobronchial trauma, which can also obscure airway lesions, and away from major and minor carinae where the cough fibers are concentrated.

Inspection

Examination of the upper airway can be instructive. The vocal cords may be involved with infections (Fig. 26.1) or malignancy; the cords may be paralyzed as a result of interruption of the recurrent laryngeal nerve or be erythematous or edematous due to gastroesophageal reflux. The trachea may be abnormal owing to either congenital or acquired conditions (Fig. 26.2A–B). The endobronchial

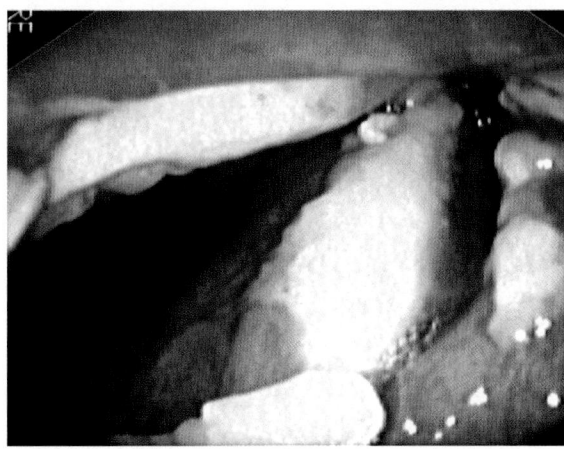

Figure 26.1 Vocal cord abnormality on inspection. Vocal cord candidiasis in an immunocompromised host.

mucosa exhibits characteristic changes due to infiltrative or systemic conditions (Fig. 26.2C–D). Endobronchial lesions may be caused by a multitude of conditions, including inflammatory, malignant, or infectious disease, or by foreign bodies (Fig. 26.3). Attention should also be paid to the normal expiratory collapse of the central airway as well as to the presence of excessive dynamic airway collapse/tracheobronchomalacia.[60–65]

During the inspection of the airways, the bronchoscopist should remain vigilant for any endobronchial anomalies, such as tracheal bronchus (Fig. 26.4). The bronchial wall mucosa should be thoroughly inspected for neovascularization, submucosal infiltration, or depigmentation. Yellowish pigmentation of the mucosa may suggest endobronchial amyloidosis, whereas black pigmentation may suggest tuberculosis (Fig. 26.5). Cobblestoning involving the bronchial mucosa, resembling a "pebbly mural," is nearly pathognomonic for endobronchial sarcoidosis[66–69] (Fig. 26.2C).

Narrow-band imaging, a feature often supplementing videobronchoscopy, lacks both specificity and sensitivity in detecting carcinoma in situ and hence is not a part of routine airway examination.

BASIC TECHNIQUES

BRONCHOALVEOLAR LAVAGE

Bronchoalveolar lavage (BAL) is an important clinical and investigational tool.[70,71] It is a standard diagnostic procedure in all patients with diffuse lung abnormalities of unknown cause, whether an infectious, noninfectious, immunologic, or malignant cause is suspected.[72,73] BAL allows the recovery of both cellular and noncellular components of the epithelial (alveolar) lining fluid and epithelial surface of the lower respiratory tract. Components of the BAL fluid represent the inflammatory and immune status of the lower respiratory tract and the alveoli[70,74] (Fig. 26.6). BAL, which samples the distal air spaces, differs significantly from a bronchial washing, which samples the large airways via aspiration of small amounts of instilled saline.[73,75,76] BAL should be considered a standard procedure in the evaluation of diffuse lung diseases, suspected infection, or malignancy, especially when the bleeding risk

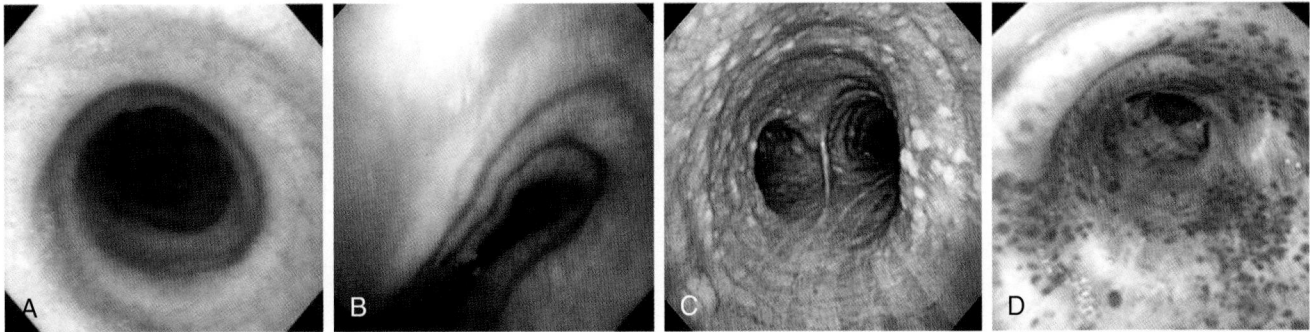

Figure 26.2 Tracheal abnormalities on inspection. (A) Complete tracheal ring, also called a "stovepipe trachea." Note the absence of the posterior membrane. (B) A "saber-sheath" trachea in a patient with emphysema. (C) Diffuse "pebbly mural" appearance of endobronchial sarcoidosis. (D) Endobronchial petechiae in a patient receiving clopidogrel. (A, Courtesy Dr. James Stoller.)

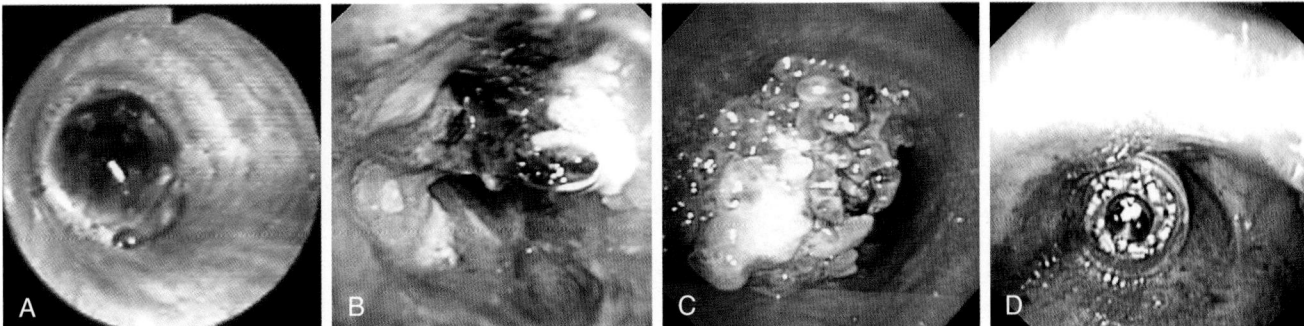

Figure 26.3 Endobronchial lesions. (A) Metastatic melanoma involving the left main bronchus. Note the black pigmentation of the tumor. (B) *Aspergillus niger* infection in a lung transplant recipient. The black pigment indicates the fungus, and the white pigment indicates calcium oxalate crystals produced by the fungus. (C) Recurrent respiratory papillomatosis involving the trachea. Note the typical mulberry appearance. (D) A foreign body in the left main bronchus. The object is a camera used for capsule endoscopy that was aspirated into the lungs. (D, Courtesy Dr. Thomas Gildea.)

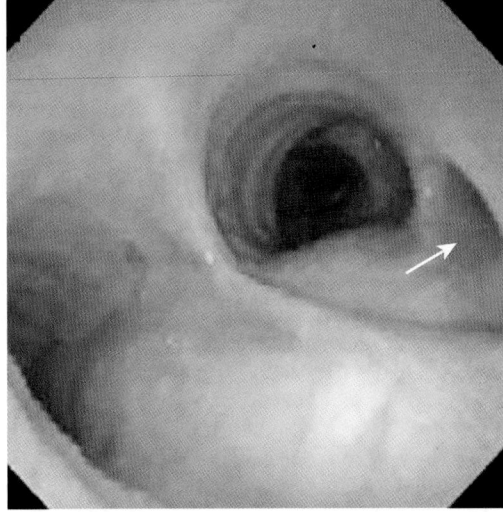

Figure 26.4 Tracheal bronchus. The view from a bronchoscope at a level above the major carina *(center)*. Note right upper lobe bronchus arising from the right lateral tracheal wall *(arrow)*. (From Mehta AC, Thaniyavarn T, Ghobrial M, Khemasuwan D. Common congenital anomalies of the central airway in adults. *Chest.* 2015;148:274–287.)

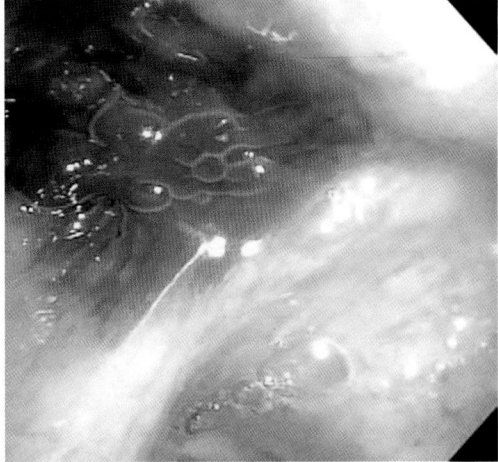

Figure 26.5 Appearance of endobronchial tuberculosis. Black, velvety, irregular mucosa involving the superior segment of the left lower lobe from *Mycobacterium tuberculosis.*

prohibits either bronchial brushing, *transbronchial biopsy* (TBB), or *transbronchial needle aspiration* (TBNA).

For diffuse opacities, any area can be chosen for BAL; however, in such cases, either the right middle lobe or the lingula is preferred because, in a supine patient, gravity assists the recovery of a maximal amount of BAL fluid

return.[70,72,77] In the case of localized disease, lavage should be performed in the area of focal radiographic abnormality[73,75,77] and, for maximal recovery, the patient can be positioned appropriately to improve recovery from the desired segment. For example, the patient's head can be elevated to improve recovery from the upper lobes, or the patient can be turned sideways to improve recovery from the lateral segments. "Good wedge" position usually means that the bronchoscope is advanced as far as possible without losing

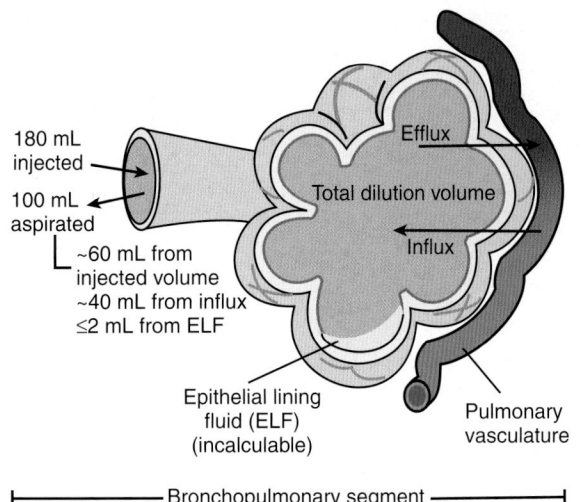

Figure 26.6 Schematic presentation of the constituents of the bronchoalveolar lavage fluid. The fluid samples the cellular and noncellular components of the lower respiratory tract. (From Kuvuru MS, Dweik RA, Thomassen MJ. Role of bronchoscopy in asthma research. *Clin Chest Med.* 1999;20:153–189.)

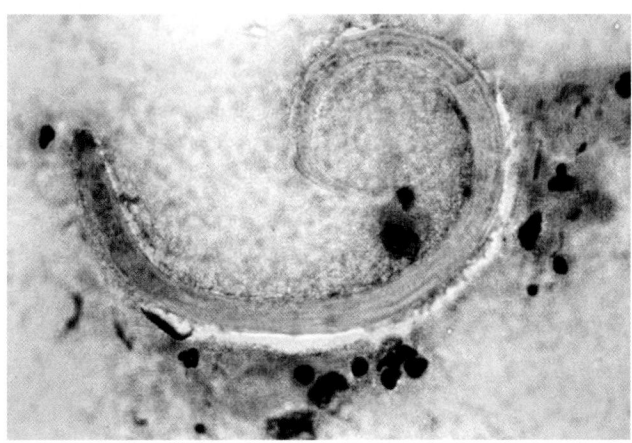

Figure 26.7 Bronchoalveolar lavage can be diagnostic for infection. Bronchoalveolar lavage specimen reveals a larva of *Strongyloides stercoralis*. (Courtesy Dr. Suhail Raoof.)

TABLE 26.3 Diseases in Which Bronchoalveolar Lavage Can Be Diagnostic

Opportunistic infections (*Pneumocystis jirovecii,* fungi)
Invasive aspergillosis (via galactomannan levels)
Pulmonary alveolar proteinosis
Diffuse alveolar hemorrhage
Malignant opacities (solid tumors, lymphoma, leukemia)
Eosinophilic lung disease
Chronic beryllium disease
Pulmonary Langerhans cell histiocytosis

the view of the distal lumen. In this optimal position, a slow, manual gentle aspiration, without allowing the airway walls to collapse, tends to maximize the lavage return.[78]

BAL has significantly improved the diagnostic workup of lung diseases, whether diffuse or localized. In pulmonary alveolar proteinosis, it has both diagnostic and therapeutic values.[72,79–82] In an international statement on the major interstitial lung diseases, BAL is considered to be helpful in strengthening the diagnosis of sarcoidosis in the absence of a tissue diagnosis, by finding a lymphocytosis (>25%) and a CD4/CD8 ratio greater than 4.[83,84] BAL may be a useful tool in the diagnosis of peripherally located primary lung cancer, with an overall diagnostic yield range of 33–69%, being exclusively diagnostic in 9–11% of cases.[85–92] Numerous case reports confirm the ability of BAL to diagnose leukemia and lymphomatous pulmonary involvement, as well as plasma cell dyscrasia.[93–95] Finding asbestos bodies in BAL fluid may correlate with occupational exposure, yet in itself, it is not proof of an asbestos-related lung disease.[96,97] The presence of greater than 25% eosinophils in the BAL fluid confirms the diagnosis of eosinophilic lung diseases, and the presence of greater than 4% CD1+ Langerhans cells confirms a diagnosis of pulmonary Langerhans cell histiocytosis, albeit with low sensitivity.[98] In chronic beryllium disease, lymphocytes from the BAL proliferate when stimulated in vitro with soluble beryllium salts, with a sensitivity and specificity approaching 100%; this lymphocyte stimulation test has become a valuable diagnostic tool for this condition and has replaced open-lung biopsy.[99,100]

In patients with ventilator-associated pneumonia, a positive quantitative culture (>10^4 *colony-forming units* (CFU)/mL) on BAL fluid may be clinically useful, with a sensitivity of 22–93% and a specificity of 45–100%, depending upon the clinical status of the patient.[101–108] BAL is also a useful tool in the diagnosis of pulmonary infections in immunocompromised patients, with the reported yield as high as 93%[109–116] (Fig. 26.7). Thus, in certain conditions, BAL findings can be diagnostic and thus avoid the need for either TBB or open-lung biopsy (Table 26.3). In other settings, although not diagnostic, BAL can be used as an adjunct to

the diagnosis when interpreted in the context of the entire clinical picture and can be used to exclude infection before starting immunosuppressive therapy.

While performing BAL in an immunocompromised host and if invasive *Aspergillus* infection is suspected, the fluid should be submitted for galactomannan cell wall antigen detection using an enzyme immunoassay. The sensitivity and specificity of elevated galactomannan levels in BAL fluid are of value in immunocompromised patients; according to two meta-analyses in immunosuppressed populations, the sensitivity ranged from 71–92%, and the specificity was 89–98%.[117,118] It needs to be pointed out that concomitant use of certain antibiotics, such as piperacillin-tazobactam, amoxicillin, or amoxicillin-clavulanate, may produce false-positive results. Besides, the test may also have cross reactivity with *Histoplasma capsulatum* and *Penicillium* species cell wall antigens. Hence the results should be interpreted in the context of the total clinical picture and rechecked if clinically indicated.[119]

The most common complications associated with BAL are fever, which can be seen in up to 30% of patients, and transient hypoxemia, which is readily handled with supplemental oxygen. Rare cases of pneumothorax after BAL have also been reported.[120]

BRONCHIAL WASHINGS

Bronchial washings are obtained by advancing the bronchoscope into an airway, instilling 10 to 20 mL of sterile saline, and then quickly aspirating the instilled saline into a specimen trap. The utility of bronchial washings is largely for the diagnosis of airway diseases, including primary or metastatic lung carcinoma and fungal or mycobacterial infection. Of the various bronchoscopic procedures, bronchial washing is the easiest to perform but has the lowest yield (sensitivity, 27–90%),[121–126] with a higher yield for central lesions.[124,127–129] Bronchial washings are an inexpensive adjunct and should be collected during a diagnostic bronchoscopy when appropriate because, even though by a small percentage, they can increase the overall diagnostic yield of the procedure.[124,130,131]

BRONCHIAL BRUSHINGS

Bronchial brushings were analyzed for the first time in 1973 and showed highly suspicious cytologic findings in most cases with lung cancer.[132] In general, bronchial brushings provide diagnostic material in 72% (44–94%) of patients with central lung cancers and 45% of patients with peripheral lesions, when obtained under fluoroscopic guidance.[133] When bronchial brushing is combined with *endobronchial biopsy* (EBB) of central lesions, the diagnostic yield of FB increases to between 79% and 96%.[134] We usually perform brushing after obtaining all the other bronchoscopy specimens because the bleeding caused by the brushing can interfere with obtaining or interpreting subsequent samples. The diameter or the length of the brush has not been shown to affect the diagnostic yield from the bronchial brushing.

Protected Specimen Brush

Protected specimen brush was first described in 1979 by Wimberley and coworkers[135] as a technique to establish an accurate diagnosis in patients with suspected pneumonia. Brushing specimens are collected using a brush that is enclosed within a double catheter sheath, capped at its distal end by a wax plug that can be easily dislodged before obtaining the specimen. The purpose of the catheter sheath and wax plug is to prevent contamination of the brush with oropharyngeal flora inside the working channel of the bronchoscope.

In patients with ventilator-associated pneumonia, the sensitivity of protected specimen brush sampling ranges from 58–86% and the specificity from 71–100%.[136,137] For now, the procedure appears to have lost popularity against empiricism for the diagnosis of ventilator-associated pneumonia; however, when it is used, protected brush samples should be analyzed using quantitative cultures with a cutoff value of greater than 10^3 CFU/mL.

ENDOBRONCHIAL BIOPSY

EBB is an essential and technically simple technique in the diagnosis of endobronchial neoplasms and for inflammatory conditions involving the airways, such as sarcoidosis and amyloidosis. For tissue sampling using EBB, the cusps of the forceps are opened, advanced onto the target and closed, thereby gripping the target. The forceps are then briskly pulled back, taking a sample of the endobronchial lesion 2 to 4 mm in diameter. The forceps and biopsy specimen are then pulled out through the working channel, and the tissue sample is collected in saline or fixative. EBB is used for

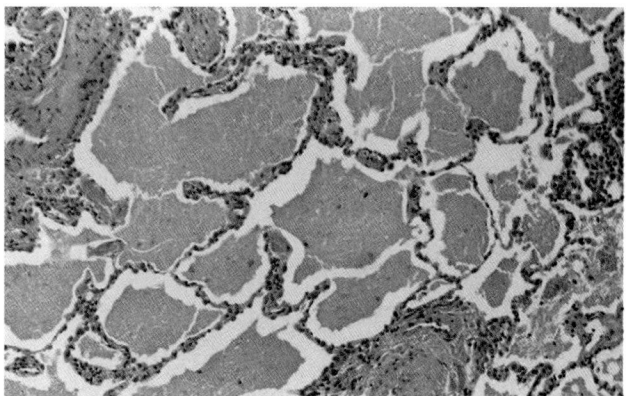

Figure 26.8 Transbronchial biopsy specimen confirms the diagnosis of pulmonary alveolar proteinosis. Note periodic acid–Schiff stain–positive material filling up the alveolar spaces.

lesions directly visualized during bronchoscopy. It provides histologic specimens, whereas bronchial washing provides only cytologic samples. The reported diagnostic yield of EBB is 80%, with a range of 51–97%, depending upon the patient population.[121,122,133,138–140] The number of biopsy specimens required for optimal diagnostic yield varies according to the suspected diagnosis. Three biopsy specimens of an endobronchial lesion suspected to be bronchogenic carcinoma can provide a diagnostic yield of greater than 97%.[141] Care should be taken to prevent excessive bleeding after an endobronchial biopsy of a lesion that appears very vascular, such as carcinoid. One can instill a small amount of ice cold saline before obtaining the biopsy or may consider performing TBNA instead. A deep biopsy of a necrotic-looking tumor is essential to obtain a viable and diagnostic tissue. On the contrary, biopsy of a lesion exhibiting vascular hue and pulsation should be avoided (i.e., Dieulafoy lesion of the bronchus). Endobronchial ultrasound can be helpful in identifying an increased risk of bleeding after EBB.

TRANSBRONCHIAL BIOPSY

TBB is the technique by which a piece of lung parenchyma is obtained using flexible forceps positioned distally via FB. TBB specimens can be obtained blindly or with guidance by fluoroscopy, computed tomography, or radial-probe endobronchial ultrasonography. In many instances TBB can obviate the need for an open-lung biopsy; however, certain conditions, such as interstitial lung diseases, generally require larger tissue samples than those that can be obtained bronchoscopically. TBB is diagnostically useful in 38–79% of patients (average sensitivity, 52%), depending upon the underlying disease.[142–146] For example, in sarcoidosis, TBB has a diagnostic yield of 40–90%,[147,148] although later studies have indicated that endobronchial ultrasound–guided TBNA of mediastinal/hilar nodes may have a greater diagnostic yield.[149] TBB has also been shown to be diagnostic in up to 10–40% of cases of pulmonary Langerhans cell histiocytosis,[150] 88–97% in *Pneumocystis jirovecii* pneumonia,[111,151] and 57–79% in lung infections caused by *Mycobacterium tuberculosis*.[152] In patients suspected of having pulmonary alveolar proteinosis, its diagnostic yield has been reported to be as high as 100% (Fig. 26.8).

The diagnostic yield of TBB increases with the number of biopsy specimens obtained.[153] Usually, 6 to 10 biopsy specimens are obtained under fluoroscopic guidance. However, the use of fluoroscopy is not mandatory in patients with diffuse parenchymal disease, and biopsy specimens can be obtained by assessing the proximity to the pleura as guided by the patient's perception of chest pain. It is highly recommended that a large (7.3-mm cusp size), fenestrated, crocodile-type biopsy forceps should be used to obtain tissue of an adequate size without crush artifact. Compared to cutting forceps, crocodile forceps are considered to provide larger pieces of tissue by tearing rather than cutting. The yield of TBB for malignant peripheral lesions more than 2 cm in diameter was also reported to be 70% in one study, even without fluoroscopic guidance.[154] When performed in association with bronchial brushings and TBNA, TBB adds to the diagnostic yield of FB for peripheral lung cancers.[128,133,155–160]

The success of lung transplantation cannot be imagined without the contributions from FB and especially TBB. In lung transplant recipients, TBB helps in diagnosing or ruling out acute cellular rejection. It also helps establish the diagnosis of antibody-mediated rejection and chronic rejection, albeit with lower yield. To date, however, there are no gold standard findings for diagnosing rejection in the lung transplant population.

Pneumothorax and hemorrhage are the most feared complications after TBB, with an incidence of up to 5% of cases. Renal insufficiency (blood urea nitrogen level >30 mg/dL [10.7 mmol/L] and creatinine level >3 mg/dL [0.27 mmol/L]) and other coagulopathies are considered risk factors for bleeding after TBB.[161,162] Although there are no scientific data, there is a prevailing notion among bronchoscopists that IV vasopressin (desmopressin, DDAVP [1-deamino-8-D-arginine vasopressin]) 3 to 4 hours before TBB in patients with uremia or those who are on dialysis may reduce the risk of bleeding. Bleeding after the TBB is from the bronchial circulation, and moderate pulmonary hypertension is not a contraindication for the procedure.[163]

TBB can be safely performed while patients are receiving aspirin or nonsteroidal anti-inflammatory drugs; however, clopidogrel bisulfate should be withheld for at least 5 to 7 days before the procedure.[164–166] Wedging the tip of the bronchoscope in the segment of interest before obtaining a TBB is highly recommended to prevent spilling of the blood in other areas and resultant hypoxemia. A 4-minute wait before dislodging the bronchoscope allows enough time for clot formation and adds to the safety of the procedure. Other management of hemoptysis is discussed in Chapter 40.

Use of fluoroscopy during TBB may reduce the rate of pneumothorax. After the procedure, a repeat fluoroscopy is sufficient to rule out pneumothorax. A chest radiograph is not essential unless the complication is suspected. A thoracic ultrasound can be used for the confirmation, yet could be redundant.

CONVENTIONAL TRANSBRONCHIAL NEEDLE ASPIRATION

Conventional TBNA (C-TBNA) is a sensitive, accurate, safe, and cost-effective technique in the diagnosis and staging of

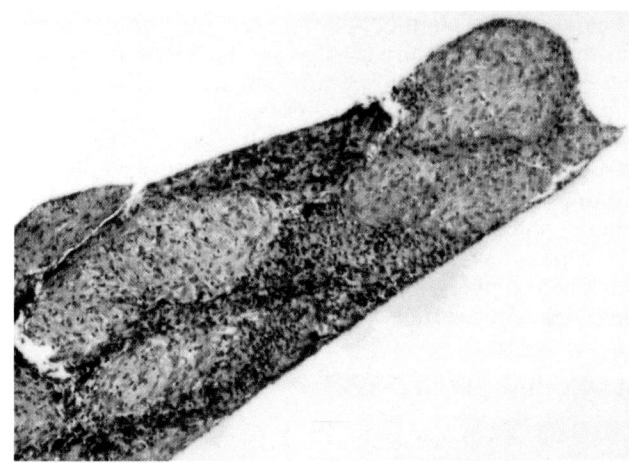

Figure 26.9 Transbronchial needle aspiration specimen in sarcoidosis. A tissue sample obtained using a 19-gauge histology needle reveals noncaseating granulomas under high-power magnification (×200 original magnification) after hematoxylin and eosin stain.

lung cancer.[160,167–172] It can also be applied for the diagnosis of nonmalignant diseases, such as sarcoidosis[173–178] (Video 26.2). Despite proven advantages, C-TBNA remains underutilized.[179–181] Needless to say, the advantages of the C-TBNA have been heavily overshadowed by the introduction of endobronchial ultrasound–guided TBNA. There are no absolute, specific contraindications for C-TBNA.

Diagnosis and staging of bronchogenic carcinoma, lymphoma, and sarcoidosis can be established using 21- or 22-gauge cytology needles.[149,180,182,183] For the diagnosis of lung cancer, the reported sensitivity, specificity, and accuracy of C-TBNA are 60–90%, 98–100%, and 60–90%, respectively.[182–187,193] For mediastinal staging of lung cancer, the overall sensitivity, specificity, and accuracy of C-TBNA are 50%, 96%, and 78%, respectively.[133] Judicious use of C-TBNA can thus reduce the need for surgical staging. In the diagnosis of involvement of mediastinal or hilar lymph nodes by sarcoidosis or tuberculosis, C-TBNA can be useful as well[173–177] (Fig. 26.9). In cases with pulmonary nodules, C-TBNA increases the diagnostic yield of FB by 25%.[149] C-TBNA can also be safely performed in mechanically ventilated patients.[187]

The procedure of C-TBNA is safe, with an overall major complication rate of approximately 0.26%. Complications include fever, bacteremia, bleeding from the puncture site (Fig. 26.10), and damage to the working channel of the bronchoscope.[155,160,180] Use of computed tomography, fluoroscopy, and ultrasonographic guidance has been shown to improve the yield of C-TBNA.[190–195]

Low-grade postbronchoscopy fever has been reported in up to 50% of patients within first 24 hours. It is more frequent when a BAL specimen is obtained. It is postulated that the release of cytokines, such as tumor necrosis factor and interleukins (IL-1, -6, and -8), into the bloodstream from the alveolar cells is responsible for the phenomenon. There are no data to suggest that the postbronchoscopy fever is related to transient bacteremia, and hence there is no indication for prophylactic antibiotics.[196]

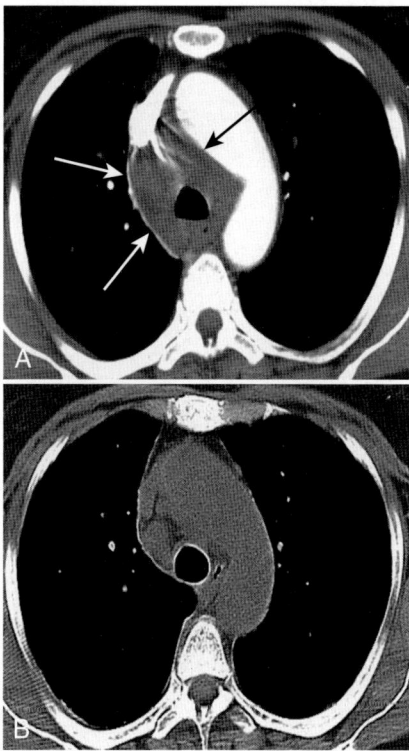

Figure 26.10 Complication of transbronchial needle aspiration. (A) On day 1 mediastinal hemorrhage is noted *(arrows)*. (B) By day 6 the abnormality has resolved. (Courtesy Dr. Stefano Gasparini.)

Key Points

- Since its introduction in 1966, flexible bronchoscopy has replaced rigid bronchoscopy for most diagnostic and therapeutic indications; rigid bronchoscopy has a continued role for unique indications, such as massive hemoptysis and removal of large foreign bodies.
- Bronchoalveolar lavage, which samples the distal air spaces, can be used to diagnose several diseases that involve the air spaces, including opportunistic infections, eosinophilic pneumonia, and pulmonary alveolar proteinosis.
- Bronchial brushing can add to the diagnostic yield of bronchoscopy, particularly for the diagnosis of endobronchial neoplasms.
- Endobronchial biopsy is a high-yield procedure for all types of airway neoplasms and for infiltrative processes.
- Transbronchial biopsy has value in the diagnosis of diffuse pulmonary diseases. With the advent of novel guidance techniques, such as electromagnetic navigation, transbronchial biopsy may also become accurate at sampling distal focal lesions.

Key Readings

Ali SR, Mehta AC. Alive in the airways, live endobronchial foreign bodies. *Chest.* 2017;151(2):481–491.

Antoniades N, Worsnop C. Topical lidocaine through the bronchoscope reduces cough rate during bronchoscopy. *Respirology.* 2009;14:873–876.

Carmi U, Kramer MR, Zemtzov D, et al. Propofol safety in bronchoscopy: prospective randomized trial using transcutaneous carbon dioxide tension monitoring. *Respiration.* 2011;82:515–521.

Cases Viedma E, Pérez Pallarés J, Martínez García MA, et al. A randomized study of midazolam for sedation in flexible bronchoscopy. *Arch Bronconeumol.* 2010;46:302–309.

Choudhury M, Singh S, Agarwal S. Efficacy of bronchial brush cytology and bronchial washings in diagnosis of non-neoplastic and neoplastic bronchopulmonary lesions. *Turk Patoloji Derg.* 2012;28:142–146.

Deshwal H, Avasarla S, Ghosh S, Mehta AC. Forbearance with bronchoscopy: a review of gratuitous indications. *Chest.* 2019;155(4):834–847.

Dooms C, Seijo L, Gasparini S, et al. Diagnostic bronchoscopy: state of the art. *Eur Respir Rev.* 2010;19:229–236.

Fujitani S, Yu VL. Diagnosis of ventilator-associated pneumonia: focus on non-bronchoscopic techniques (nonbronchoscopic bronchoalveolar lavage, including mini-BAL, blinded protected specimen brush, and blinded bronchial sampling) and endotracheal aspirates. *J Intensive Care Med.* 2006;21:17–21.

Khemasuwan D, Farver C, Mehta AC. Parasites of the air passages. *Chest.* 2014;145(4):883–895.

Kumar A, Raju S, Das A, Mehta AC. Vessels of the central airways: a bronchoscopic perspective. *Chest.* 2016;191(3):869–881.

Küpeli E, Khemasuan D, Lee P, Mehta AC. "Pills" and the air passages. *Chest.* 2013;144(2):651–660.

Küpeli E, Khemasuan D, Tunsupon P, Mehta AC. "Pills" and the air passages: a continuum. *Chest.* 2015;147(1):242–250.

Lee GD, Kim HC, Kim YE, et al. Value of cytologic analysis of bronchial washings in lung cancer on the basis of bronchoscopic appearance. *Clin Respir J.* 2013;7:128–134.

Lee K, Orme R, Williams D, et al. Prospective pilot trial of dexmedetomidine sedation for awake diagnostic flexible bronchoscopy. *J Bronchology Interv Pulmonol.* 2010;17:323–328.

Mehta AC, Taniavarn T, Ghobrial M, Khemasuan D. Common congenital anomalies of the central airway in adults. *Chest.* 2015;148(1):274–287.

Meyer KC, Raghu G, Baughman RP, et al. An official American Thoracic Society Clinical practice guideline: the clinical utility of bronchoalveolar lavage cellular analysis in interstitial lung disease. *Am J Respir Crit Care Med.* 2010;185:1004–1014.

National Lung Screening Trial Research Team, Aberle DR, Adams AM, et al. Reduced lung-cancer mortality with low-dose computed tomographic screening, The National Lung Screening Trial Research Team. *N Engl J Med.* 2011;365:395–409.

Panchabhai T, Mehta AC. Historical perspective of bronchoscopy: connecting the dots. *Ann Am Thorac Soc.* 2015;12(5):631–641.

Panchabhai T, Mukhopadhyay S, Sehgal S, Bandyopadhyay D, Erzurum S, Mehta AC. Plugs of the air passages: a clinicopathologic review. *Chest.* 2016;150(5):1141–1157.

Rolo R, Mota PC, Coelho F, et al. Sedation with midazolam in flexible bronchoscopy—prospective study. *Rev Port Pneumol.* 2012;18:226–232.

Schlatter L, Pflimlin E, Fehrke B, et al. Propofol versus propofol plus hydrocodone for flexible bronchoscopy: a randomised study. *Eur Respir J.* 2011;38:529–537.

Shabini K, Ghosh S, Arrossi VA, Mehta AC. Broncholithiasis: a review. *Chest.* 2019;156(3):445–455.

Stolz D, Kurer G, Meyer A, et al. Propofol versus combined sedation in flexible bronchoscopy: a randomised non-inferiority trial. *Eur Respir J.* 2009;34:1024–1030.

Tunsupon P, Panchabhai T, Khemasuwan D, Mehta AC. Black bronchoscopy. *Chest.* 2013;144(5):1696–1707.

Wahidi MM, Jain P, Jantz M, et al. American college of chest physicians consensus statement on the use of topical anesthesia, analgesia, and sedation during flexible bronchoscopy in adult patients. *Chest.* 2011;140:1342–1350.

Wheat LJ, Walsh TJ. Diagnosis of invasive aspergillosis by galactomannan antigenemia detection using an enzyme immunoassay. *Eur J Clin Microbiol Infect Dis.* 2008;27:245–251. 2008.

Complete reference list available at ExpertConsult.com.

27 DIAGNOSTIC BRONCHOSCOPY: ADVANCED TECHNIQUES (EBUS AND NAVIGATIONAL)

A. CHRISTINE ARGENTO, MD, FCCP • AJAY WAGH, MD, MS, FCCP • DAVID FELLER-KOPMAN, MD, FCCP

INTRODUCTION

Gustav Killian performed the first bronchoscopy in 1897 to extract a piece of a pork bone from the right main bronchus. From that meager beginning, the technology in bronchoscopy has advanced exponentially. In 1966, the flexible bronchoscope was introduced into clinical practice by Shigeto Ikeda. Currently, this instrument is one of the most important tools for diagnosis and treatment of pulmonary diseases.

Following publication of the National Lung Screening Trial[1] and the increasingly common use of *computed tomography* (CT) scans in general, more pulmonary nodules are found and the requirement for biopsy, especially for peripheral nodules, has increased.[2] Likewise, bronchoscopy is often performed to investigate lung opacities in immunocompromised patients, search for sources of hemoptysis, and evaluate interstitial lung disease and mediastinal/hilar adenopathy.

Previously, the diagnostic yield for peripheral nodules with bronchoscopy ranged from 20–80%. Historically, these biopsies used a bronchoscope with an outer diameter of 5 to 6 mm, often under fluoroscopic guidance. Limitations included the restricted depth of bronchoscope insertion due to a relatively large diameter, difficulty in guiding the bronchoscope and biopsy instruments to smaller peripheral lesions, and lack of real-time confirmation of target localization.[3,4] This chapter reviews the many advances in diagnostic bronchoscopy. More "basic" bronchoscopic procedures and therapeutic bronchoscopy are discussed in other chapters.

ENDOBRONCHIAL ULTRASOUND

Endobronchial ultrasound (EBUS) is a bronchoscopic approach that offers sonographic assessment of parenchymal lesions and tumors compressing/invading the central airways as well as real-time localization and sampling of mediastinal, hilar, or parenchymal lesions. There are two forms: convex EBUS evaluates the mediastinum, hilum, and central pulmonary lesions, and radial EBUS evaluates lesions that involve the airway itself or peripheral pulmonary lesions.

CONVEX

The convex EBUS bronchoscope, introduced in 2004, has a convex ultrasound probe at the tip of the bronchoscope and provides sonographic, real-time visualization during *transbronchial needle aspiration* (TBNA) of lymph nodes and peribronchial lesions.[5] Convex EBUS has revolutionized the diagnosis and staging of lung cancer and extrathoracic malignancies. EBUS has become standard of care with such widespread acceptance that it has largely replaced conventional TBNA and even mediastinoscopy as the gold standard for lung cancer staging.[6,7]

Other entities commonly diagnosed with convex EBUS include lymphoma and nonmalignant diseases such as sarcoidosis. The *American College of Chest Physicians* (ACCP) has published guidelines and evidence-based recommendations regarding the technical use of EBUS.[8] A needle-based approach (EBUS-TBNA) is recommended in the 2013 ACCP Guidelines for Lung Cancer as a first-line intervention for

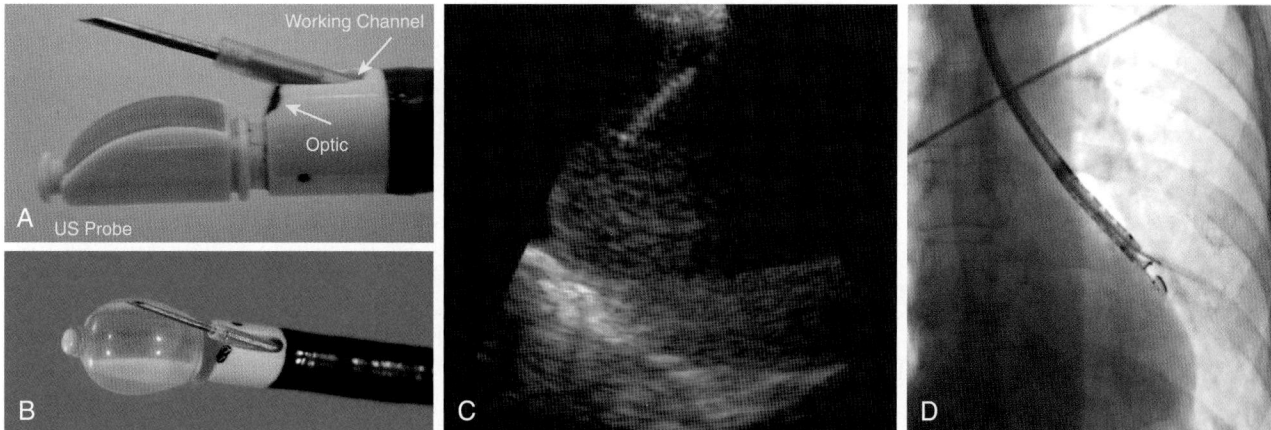

Figure 27.1 **Convex *endobronchial ultrasound* (EBUS).** (A) EBUS scope is shown with the probe, working channel and optic portions labeled. (B) EBUS scope shown with balloon filled with saline, used to improve probe contact with airway wall for better image quality. (C) EBUS *transbronchial needle aspiration* (TBNA) of a mediastinal lymph node showing needle within node. (D) Fluoroscopic view of EBUS-TBNA of a central pulmonary lesion. (A–B, Courtesy Olympus Medical.)

invasive mediastinal staging of *non–small cell lung cancer* (NSCLC).[9,10]

Convex EBUS incorporates a 7.5 MHz ultrasound transducer on the tip of a bronchoscope used to guide TBNA (Fig. 27.1). The EBUS sonographic footprint lies parallel to the long axis of the bronchoscope and provides a 50-degree field of view. Depending on the location of the lymph node or lesion, the ultrasound may not have adequate contact with the airway wall, a technical problem that can substantially affect the ultrasound image quality. In that case, a latex balloon at the tip of the ultrasound probe can be inflated with saline to assist in probe contact and improve image acquisition. However, it is unclear if the balloon tip improves diagnostic yield. Its use should be avoided in patients with a latex allergy.[8]

Diagnostic Yield for Lung Cancer

Many studies, systematic reviews, and meta-analyses have demonstrated a pooled sensitivity of EBUS for mediastinal staging of lung cancer of approximately 90%,[6,7,11,12] which is comparable to that from video mediastinoscopy.[9] However, it should be noted that after neoadjuvant chemotherapy and radiation, the sensitivity of EBUS-TBNA is only approximately 67%, and thus a nondiagnostic EBUS in that setting may need to be followed by surgical restaging.[13] Additionally, EBUS-TBNA has also been found to have a high yield for intrathoracic lymph node metastases from extrathoracic malignancies with a pooled sensitivity of 85%, though with a sensitivity of only 55% for occult metastatic disease (pathologic disease without suggestive radiographic findings such as a lung mass or lymphadenopathy that is pathologic by radiographic criteria).[14] Therefore, minimally invasive mediastinal and hilar lymph node investigations should be considered for both intrathoracic and extrathoracic disease.

Many techniques and factors can affect results and improve diagnostic yield with EBUS:

- *Number of passes:* The diagnostic yield for detection of malignant cells does not increase above three passes.[15] If *rapid on-site evaluation* (ROSE) by cytology is available, a reasonable approach is to perform aspirations until adequate cell material (i.e., sufficient for a specific diagnosis or a good recovery of lymphocytes) is obtained or a minimum of four to five passes are completed to ensure a diagnosis and adequate material for specific molecular testing.[6,16,17]

- *Size of needles:* EBUS needles of several sizes are currently commercially available. Guidelines recommend the use of either a 21- or 22-gauge needle as acceptable, though newer studies would suggest that 19- and 25-gauge options are equally effective. In selected cases, additional tissue obtained with a 19-gauge needle may increase the diagnostic yield.[18–24]

- *Suction:* One prospective, single-blinded, randomized control trial looked at 115 patients who underwent EBUS-TBNA with passes taken with or without suction. Results showed no difference in diagnostic yield regardless of the size of lymph node (greater or less than 1 cm).[25]

- *Use of stylet:* The EBUS needle stylet helps reduce needle contamination with airway epithelial debris and mucosa. It can also be used to assist in providing suction via capillary action when it is withdrawn from the needle during sampling. Another study evaluated TBNA samples with and without the stylet using an EBUS-TBNA needle for a prospective, single-blind, randomized control trial with 121 patients and 194 lymph nodes sampled. Results reported no difference in sample adequacy or diagnostic yield.[26]

- *Sedation:* Several studies have looked at different sedation strategies for EBUS (moderate sedation vs. general anesthesia using either a laryngeal mask airway or endotracheal tube), and the data are conflicting without a significant benefit to any one strategy. The EBUS guidelines therefore recommend that either sedation strategy can be used, based on operator comfort level and institutional preferences.[27–30]

Central lesions (within the inner one-third of the lung) in a peribronchial location can often be sampled using EBUS-TBNA. Two studies retrospectively evaluated the yield of EBUS for centrally located pulmonary lesions and found the diagnostic yield to be greater than 84%, even when there was no visible airway leading into the lesion (i.e., a bronchus sign).[31,32]

Additionally, performing concurrent *endoscopic ultrasound* with fine-needle aspiration via the esophagus using an EBUS scope or a gastrointestinal endoscope has demonstrated improved diagnostic yield.[9,33]

Ultrasound Features That Predict Malignancy

EBUS ultrasound characteristics of lymph nodes have been shown in several studies to be predictive of malignancy.[34,35] Fujiwara et al.[34] reported that several signs were independent risk factors for malignancy: round shape, distinct margin, heterogeneous echogenicity, and the coagulation necrosis sign. When all four signs were absent, there was a 96% negative predictive value for metastases. Another cohort by Memoli et al.[35] showed that increased size and a round or oval shape are risk factors for malignancy. Also, increased vascularity in specific patterns may be useful in identifying malignant lymph nodes.[36,37] Finally, the absence of a central nodal vessel on ultrasound may also be predictive of malignant involvement.[38] However, despite such ultrasound imaging characteristics, tissue diagnosis is still necessary.[8]

Molecular Markers

Molecular marker testing is considered standard of care and necessary for the consideration of tailored therapy in every locally advanced or metastatic NSCLC (see also Chapter 73). Since EBUS is increasingly used for the diagnosis and staging of lung cancer, many studies have now emerged demonstrating the ability of EBUS-TBNA to acquire samples with enough cellularity to perform all of the necessary immunohistochemistry, molecular, and next-generation sequencing required, including PD-L1 testing. In several studies, PD-L1 expression in NSCLC was compared from different biopsy samples (cytology, small biopsy, and surgical biopsy) and found to be adequate with comparable results among all specimen types.[39–51]

Diagnostic Yield for Diagnoses Other Than Lung Cancer

Lymphoma. For diagnosing and subtyping lymphoma, the yield for EBUS has been around 70%, though with considerable variation reported.[52–54] Despite the lower diagnostic yield, EBUS-TBNA is still recommended as an initial minimally invasive evaluation.[8] EBUS has been reported to have a lower sensitivity for Hodgkin lymphoma compared with non-Hodgkin based on sample size along with cytopathology expertise and comfort level.[54,55] Reed-Sternberg cells within the needle aspirates are usually scarce, and the evaluation of lymphoid background architecture is often difficult. It is noted that recurrence of lymphoma is more easily diagnosed by EBUS than a de novo diagnosis (91% vs. 79%).[54]

Sarcoidosis. The sensitivity of EBUS-TBNA for pulmonary sarcoidosis is 85–90% as opposed to transbronchial biopsy and endobronchial biopsy, which have a combined diagnostic yield of only 35%. Combining all three modalities of biopsy can increase the yield to 93–95%.[8,56–59]

Infection. Although EBUS-TBNA is suggested for evaluation of patients with mediastinal or hilar adenopathy concerning for tuberculosis or possible histoplasmosis, the value in respiratory infection is unproven but understudied. In one retrospective study, routine microbiologic results of EBUS-TBNA samples from 82 patients showed very little evidence of infection. The authors concluded that EBUS did not have sufficient sensitivity to rule out infectious causes of adenopathy.[60] Another study demonstrated that polymerase chain reaction for *M. tuberculosis* using EBUS-TBNA samples is a useful laboratory test for evaluating intrathoracic granulomatous lymphadenopathy. Moreover, this technique can prevent further invasive evaluation in patients whose histologic and microbiologic tests are nondiagnostic.[61] Dhooria et al. reported that a cartridge-based nucleic acid amplification test has good specificity and positive predictive value in the diagnosis of tuberculosis and is a useful investigation in separating tuberculosis from sarcoidosis.[62]

More sensitive methods of detection will be needed to improve the usefulness of EBUS in this population of patients.

Rapid On-Site Evaluation

Multiple conflicting studies have been published on the utility and importance of ROSE, whereby a pathologist/cytopathologist or cytotechnologist prepares slides for immediate visualization and interpretation during the procedure. In the setting of traditional TBNA, ROSE has been performed routinely to ensure adequate sampling by confirming location within a lymph node.[8] With EBUS-TBNA, because the needle is visualized within the target lesion in real time, this benefit of ROSE is not as clear cut. Though ROSE may not improve the diagnostic yield of EBUS-TBNA, it does reduce the number of aspirations or passes required, can reduce overall procedure time, and may reduce the need for other procedures such as transbronchial biopsy of a parenchymal lesion, thus decreasing complications such as bleeding and pneumothorax. Notably, if ROSE is available, it can help determine the sample adequacy for immunohistochemistry, molecular, and next-generation sequencing testing. Thus, the value of ROSE with EBUS-TBNA lies in a timely and accurate diagnosis with streamlined care and a decrease in unnecessary procedures, thereby minimizing complications and cost.[63–67]

Complication Rate and Safety

A large systematic review of more than 1500 patients identified no serious adverse events with EBUS-TBNA and only agitation, cough, and blood at the puncture site as minor complications.[68] Prospective database analyses report complication rates of EBUS to be approximately 1%, though there are individual reports of more serious complications such as mediastinitis, pericarditis, and death.[69,70]

With respect to EBUS and anticoagulation, only two studies have evaluated the safety of performing EBUS in patients taking clopidogrel. The first was a retrospective review of 12 patients on clopidogrel who underwent EBUS-TBNA, 67% of whom were also taking aspirin; there were no bleeding complications. The more recent study accrued 42 patients for a prospective, multicenter cohort, all of whom were unable to stop therapy with clopidogrel and aspirin for

5 days. Only 1 of the 42 patients had significant bleeding; this was controlled with instillation of 30 mL of cold saline at the needle insertion site. No long-term or serious complications were reported.[71,72] Convex EBUS can be considered in a patient taking clopidrogel and aspirin if the patient is at high risk for discontinuation.

Cost

There are cost data to support the use of EBUS for mediastinal sampling. A large retrospective database review compared EBUS-TBNA with mediastinoscopy using claims data. Of 30,570 patients, 49% underwent EBUS. Severe adverse events were similarly low between the groups. Compared with mediastinoscopy, EBUS was associated with less vocal cord paralysis (odds ratio, 0.57) and less expense.[73] Another study looked at the cost of performing EBUS-TBNA under monitored anesthesia care versus moderate sedation. They found no difference in diagnostic yield, significant complications, or procedure duration, but the cost was $245 more for the monitored anesthesia care cases.[74] Finally, Steinfort et al. proposed a minimally invasive staging strategy in which patients are first biopsied using EBUS and, if they have a negative result, proceed to mediastinal staging with mediastinoscopy. This EBUS/mediastinoscopy strategy was compared to performing EBUS without surgical confirmation of negative results, conventional TBNA alone, and mediastinoscopy alone. The costs were AU$2691, AU$3344, AU$3754, and AU$8859, respectively, demonstrating cost-effectiveness of a thoughtful, minimally invasive approach to staging of patients with NSCLC.[75]

Education and Competency

Because the safety and value of EBUS are now well known, more Pulmonary and Critical Care fellowship programs are aiming to have their trainees certified in EBUS prior to graduation. The number of procedures required to perform EBUS competently is unknown, though 50 supervised procedures has been cited by the ACCP.[76] Previous data have shown that the number of procedures needed to reach this level of proficiency is variable from person to person and can take up to 120 procedures or more depending on the operator and his or her experience and training.[77–81] A key factor, however, is not merely acquiring "minimal competency," but rather mastery; in addition, as with any other procedure, key knowledge as well as procedural competence determine procedure success. A recent study, for example, found that interventional pulmonologists have a much higher rate of "appropriate mediastinal staging" than general pulmonologists,[82] presumably because of their greater procedural experience and competence.

There has been increased interest in simulation-based learning and the development of combined cognitive and skills assessments validated for EBUS.[83,84] These tools may assist in the development and assessment of the detailed anatomic knowledge and procedural skills required to evaluate and sample using EBUS-TBNA to ensure standardization and ability. Such skills are particularly important when staging for cancer because this requires diligence and precision and should not be performed without the necessary expertise.

In sum, convex EBUS is a minimally invasive, safe tool that has revolutionized the evaluation of mediastinal, hilar, and central pulmonary disease for a variety of both benign and malignant conditions. Successful use is dependent on operator training and skill.

RADIAL

Introduction

Radial EBUS was first described in 1992 and was initially used to locate mediastinal lymph nodes and guide conventional TBNA as well as to distinguish tumor invasion from compression in the central airways.[5] Radial EBUS provides a circumferential or 360-degree ultrasound image around a small probe inserted through the working channel of a bronchoscope and allows the bronchoscopist to characterize the tissue densities surrounding the probe in real time (Fig. 27.2). A standard frequency of 20 MHz is used, providing a spatial resolution of less than 1 mm and penetration depth up to 5 cm. Unfortunately, it is currently not possible to biopsy with direct visualization using the radial EBUS image because the probe must be removed from the working channel to allow the biopsy instrument to be introduced.

Imaging Techniques

When radial EBUS is used to evaluate the multiple layers of the bronchial wall, the probe has an integrated water-filled balloon sheath to ensure "acoustic coupling." This approach allows evaluation of the depth of central lesions in the tracheobronchial wall.[85] Distinguishing central tumor invasion from compression was the initial use of radial EBUS and, for this use, radial EBUS was found to be more accurate than chest CT imaging.[86]

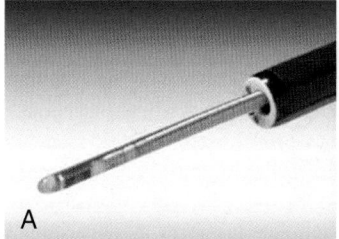 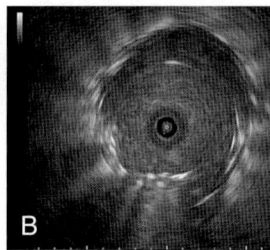 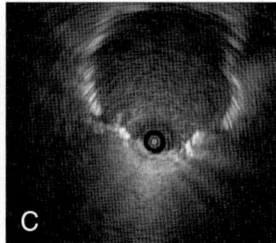 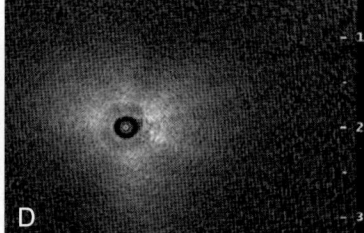

Figure 27.2 **Radial *endobronchial ultrasound* (EBUS).** (A) Radial EBUS probe extended through a bronchoscope channel showing circumferential imaging surface at tip. (B) Radial EBUS concentric view of peripheral lesion. (C) Radial EBUS eccentric view of a peripheral lesion. (D) Radial EBUS "blizzard" appearance of an area of a ground-glass opacity. (A, Courtesy Olympus Medical.)

More recently, radial EBUS is used for localization and to guide sampling of peripheral pulmonary lesions. Radial EBUS is typically directed to the lesion in conjunction with navigation modalities including virtual bronchoscopic navigation, *electromagnetic navigation bronchoscopy* (ENB), or robotic bronchoscopy, which are all discussed in further detail later in this chapter. Normal lung parenchyma has a "snowstorm" appearance due to air-filled alveolar tissue, whereas nodules and masses appear as hypoechoic lesions with a bright and well-defined border. Even ground-glass opacities can be visualized using radial EBUS because they are now recognized to create a "blizzard sign," which is an enlarged hyperintense acoustic shadow.[4,87]

There are two methods of utilizing the radial EBUS ultrasound. Either the probe can be advanced through the working channel of a bronchoscope directly or through a separate sheath, also known as a guide sheath. The value of the guide sheath is that, once the radial probe is removed, the sheath secures the location for subsequent biopsies of the lesion.

Utilizing ultrathin bronchoscopes may obviate the need for a guide sheath because such bronchoscopes can be advanced much deeper into the periphery of the lung (discussed in more detail later in this chapter). Although radial EBUS can provide real-time imaging, it cannot provide actual real-time biopsy visualization because the probe is withdrawn from the bronchoscope or guide sheath before sampling.[4]

Diagnostic Yield

A randomized trial comparing radial EBUS-guided transbronchial biopsy for malignancy by Paone and colleagues demonstrated a sensitivity of 79% compared with 55% using conventional transbronchial biopsies.[88] Another prospective study utilizing radial EBUS for small peripheral pulmonary lesions, which were invisible on fluoroscopy, demonstrated an 89% localization and 70% diagnosis for lesions averaging 2.2 cm in size.[89] The overall sensitivity of radial EBUS for the diagnosis of peripheral lung lesions is around 70%.[90]

Localization and diagnostic yield of radial EBUS is dependent on several factors, including lesion location, size, the presence of a "CT bronchus sign" (i.e., an airway that goes directly to the target lesion), and location of the probe relative to the lesion. Based on a multivariate analysis in a retrospective study, Tay and colleagues concluded that lesions less than 2 cm and more than 5 cm from the hilum were significantly less likely to be localized by radial EBUS.[91] Kurimoto and colleagues demonstrated that diagnostic yield was significantly higher when the radial probe was within a lesion (87%, concentric view) compared with when the probe was adjacent to it (42%, eccentric view).[92] Of note, a concentric view may not guarantee a high diagnostic yield in a malignant nodule because the malignant cells may not be homogeneously present in the lesion. Other studies have demonstrated that the diagnostic yield with radial EBUS increases with nodule size and the presence of a CT bronchus sign.[93–95]

The diagnostic yield is lower for ground-glass opacities compared with solid lesions despite using radial EBUS for localization. One retrospective study evaluated 67 patients with ground-glass opacities with a mean diameter of 21 mm who underwent radial EBUS with a guide sheath and fluoroscopy. This study found a 57% diagnostic yield using this radial EBUS method.[96] Another retrospective study of 40 patients with ground-glass opacities with a mean diameter of 22 mm (90% were partly solid) undergoing radial EBUS bronchoscopy and tomosynthesis guidance found a diagnostic yield of 65%.[97] Tomosynthesis refers to the technique by which a limited-angle image reconstruction is performed from images acquired from a two-dimensional method such as fluoroscopy or cone beam, thereby improving the appreciation of three-dimensional anatomy.[98]

Complications

The complication rate of radial EBUS is low, with one meta-analysis reporting a pneumothorax rate of 1% and only 0.4% requiring a chest tube.[90] Additionally, the guide sheath may be used to tamponade biopsy-related bleeding.[4]

Conclusion

In summary, radial EBUS has helped improve peripheral bronchoscopic evaluation and diagnostic yield of biopsies of peripheral pulmonary lesions. Notably, a certain amount of skill and learning are required to utilize and interpret the information gathered from this tool.

CONFOCAL BRONCHOSCOPY

Fibered confocal fluorescence microscopy is a technique that produces microscopic imaging of living tissue via a small probe introduced through the working channel of a conventional bronchoscope. Fibered confocal fluorescence microscopy can analyze human airway wall architecture and endobronchial abnormalities with near-histologic detail in vivo.[99] Thiberville and colleagues used fibered confocal fluorescence microscopy to examine two bronchial specimens ex vivo and in vivo for 29 individuals at high risk for lung cancer.[100] Alterations of the microstructure were observed in 19 of 22 metaplastic or dysplastic samples, 5 of 5 carcinomas in situ, and 2 of 2 invasive lesions. The authors suggest this could potentially be a minimally invasive method to study specific basement membrane alterations associated with premalignant bronchial lesions in vivo.

Another prospective, observational study evaluated ex vivo transbronchial biopsy samples of 36 patients using a 1.4-mm diameter confocal mini-probe.[101] Once the biopsy samples were obtained, they were placed in formalin for fixation, then removed and placed on gauze for assessment with the confocal probe. The stroma and parenchyma were examined and the carcinoma samples were found to have a highly fluorescent field penetrated by dark hollows. The sensitivity for malignancy was 91%, and the specificity was 77%. Both interobserver and intraobserver agreement was moderate. The authors concluded that this method could be used as a form of ROSE because it could be used to provide immediate feedback on specimen adequacy and preliminary diagnosis.

This technology continues to be evaluated as a form of "optical biopsy" that can help direct appropriate sampling in the future.

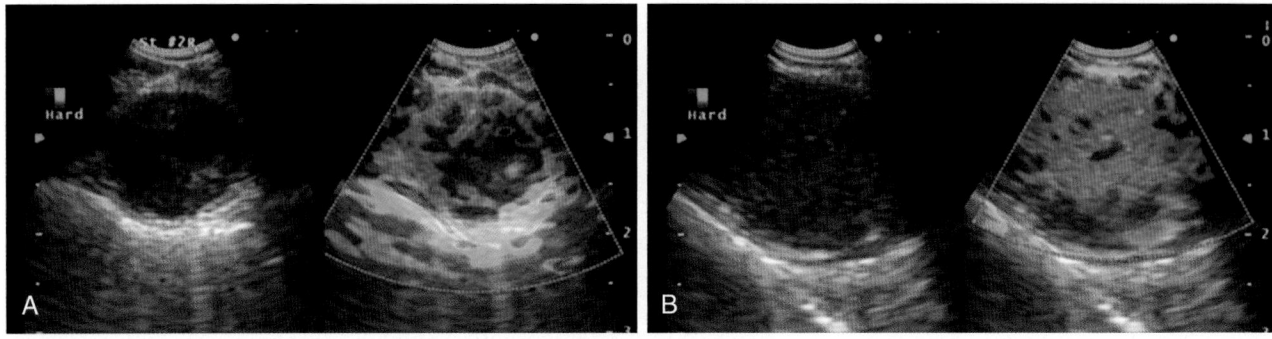

Figure 27.3 Elastography added to standard endobronchial ultrasound. (A) A lymph node demonstrating a malignant elastography pattern showing areas of stiffness (blue predominant). (B) A lymph node demonstrating a benign elastography pattern (green and red predominant). (From Fujiwara T, Nakajima T, Inage T, et al. The combination of endobronchial elastography and sonographic findings during endobronchial ultrasound-guided transbronchial needle aspiration for predicting nodal metastasis. *Thorac Cancer.* 2019;10[10]:2000–2005.)

ELASTOGRAPHY

Elastography is an ultrasonic technique that measures tissue compressibility and is an add-on feature to standard EBUS bronchoscopy. Because pathophysiologic processes such as malignancy generally make tissues more stiff, detecting stiffness can assist tumor location. With elastography, the stiffness of tissue is translated into a color signal overlaid onto the B-mode image. The colors associated with stiff, intermediate, and soft tissue are blue, green, and yellow/red, respectively. Normal and inflammatory lymph nodes have been shown to have a deformable medulla and hilum, with stiffness localized to the cortex. In early metastatic infiltration of a lymph node, stiffness can be detected in localized areas of the node; such imaging characteristics may help direct biopsies to the more abnormal areas. In advanced-stage cancer, stiffness will be increased throughout the lymph node (Fig. 27.3).[102]

Early endoscopic ultrasound elastography studies used a combination of color and color pattern homogeneity to differentiate benign from malignant lesions; however, better results have been obtained when the strain ratio is calculated (see below). Combining elastography with EBUS-TBNA may allow for the lymph node(s) most affected and even small areas within individual nodes to be targeted for optimal results.[103]

Various studies have evaluated the usefulness of elastography. In a study of 94 patients, 206 lymph nodes were evaluated by EBUS-TBNA and elastography. B-mode and elastography patterns were used to distinguish between benign and malignant nodes; sensitivity for malignancy was found to be 91%.[102]

Another study published in 2015 by He et al. performed EBUS-guided elastography of lymph nodes prior to EBUS-TBNA.[104] Elastography data were given a grading score of 1 to 4, with higher values being more likely to represent malignancy. Strain ratio was then calculated by quantifying the strain value of the target lymph node and comparing it to a similar area of normal tissue. Pathologic determination of malignant or benign lymph nodes was used as the gold standard. Results of this study showed that elastography images and strain ratio are well correlated and, when verified against pathologic data, the sensitivity,

specificity, positive predictive value, negative predictive value, and accuracy were 88% (37/42), 81% (21/26), 88% (37/42), and 85% (58/68), respectively. The authors thus determined that elastography and strain ratios can be used effectively to predict mediastinal and hilar lymph node metastases.

Finally, Fujiwara et al. published their experience with lung cancer or suspected lung cancer patients undergoing EBUS-TBNA.[105] Sonographic, B-mode, and elastography findings were independently evaluated for each lymph node. Benign features on EBUS included oval shape, indistinct margins, and homogeneous echogenicity. Lack of coagulation necrosis on B-mode and less than 31% of the lymph node appearing malignant on elastography were also considered benign features. The results of these imaging interpretations were compared with a final pathologic diagnosis. B-mode predicted benign lymph nodes 96% of the time, and elastography predicted malignant lymph nodes 72% of the time. The combination of sonographic evaluation, B-mode, and elastography predicted malignant nodes 83% of the time and benign lymph nodes 96% of the time, showing benefit of a combined approach.[105]

Pitfalls when using elastography are anatomic location and pathologic changes that create significant artifact of the ultrasound image and compromise compressibility.[106]

THIN AND ULTRATHIN BRONCHOSCOPY

The thin bronchoscope has an outer diameter of 4 mm and a working channel of 2 mm. The most recent ultrathin bronchoscope on the market has a distal tip outer diameter of 3 mm and a working channel diameter of 1.7 mm (Fig. 27.4). This device has been developed to overcome the low diagnostic yield of bronchoscopy for peripheral lesions less than 20 mm in diameter.[107–110] Complexities of the distal airway anatomy often requires fluoroscopic, electromagnetic/virtual bronchoscopic navigational, or CT guidance to direct the bronchoscope to peripheral lesions.[111] Given the 1.7-mm working channel on the new ultrathin bronchoscope, radial EBUS can also be inserted and used for real-time confirmation of location within the lesion.

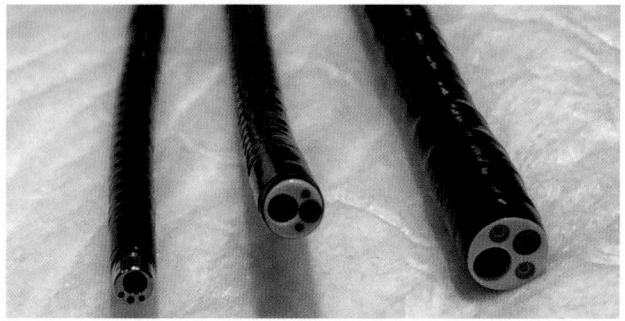

Figure 27.4 Ultrathin and thin bronchoscopes. *Left to right,* ultrathin, thin, and regular bronchoscopes. The outer diameters are 3 mm, 4.2 mm, and 6.2 mm, respectively.

Ultrathin bronchoscopes allow greater penetration into the lung. Whereas a conventional bronchoscope can navigate to the fourth-generation airways, the ultrathin bronchoscopes can navigate to a median of the fifth and up to the ninth-generation airways.[112] Oki and colleagues reported a diagnostic yield for peripheral nodules of 59% with a thin (4 mm) bronchoscope versus 70% using the ultrathin (3 mm) bronchoscope in combination with virtual bronchoscopy and fluoroscopic guidance.[113]

Aside from the ability to navigate more distally in the airways, the thin and ultrathin bronchoscopes can be used to evaluate the nature and extent of central airway obstruction where there is a risk for completely obstructing the airways with standard-sized bronchoscopes.[107] An ultrathin bronchoscope can define the distal extent of endobronchial tumor because it is more easily able to traverse the lesion, even when the lesion causes significant airway obstruction.[111] These smaller bronchoscopes can also be used for mechanically ventilated patients despite small endotracheal tubes.

Although most reports show these bronchoscopes to be safe, there have been case reports of visceral pleural perforation caused by the ultrathin bronchoscope. Care should be taken to monitor the location of the scope at all times when in the distal bronchi.[114]

VIRTUAL BRONCHOSCOPY

Virtual bronchoscopy uses a thin-slice CT scan to create a three-dimensional map of the airways using proprietary software that enables the user to create a virtual pathway through the tracheobronchial tree. The software is mainly limited by the quality of the CT scan used to create the three-dimensional airway model as well as the ability to differentiate distal airway and emphysematous lung. Ideally, CT slices should be less than 1 mm in thickness with some overlap (slice spacing <0.625 mm). The virtual images of the proposed pathway can be displayed during bronchoscopy and synchronized with the endoscopic images in real time (Fig. 27.5).

Asano et al. published their series on 38 peripheral pulmonary lesions measuring less than 30 mm using a combination of virtual bronchoscopy, ultrathin bronchoscopy, and fluoroscopic guidance. Virtual bronchoscopic images

were generated to a median of sixth-generation bronchi. The ultrathin bronchoscope could be inserted into 95% of the planned airways, and diagnostic yield was 82%.[115] The diagnostic yield in a meta-analysis was found to be 74% for lesions less than 3 cm and 67% for lesions less than 2 cm.[116]

Finally, another study compared the use of radial EBUS with and without virtual bronchoscopy. Virtual bronchoscopy increased the diagnostic yield from 78% to 94% in patients who had lesions smaller than 2 cm located in the outer third of the lung where an airway could be seen leading to the nodule (CT bronchus sign) but invisible on fluoroscopy.[117]

ELECTROMAGNETIC NAVIGATION

Like virtual bronchoscopy, *electromagnetic navigation* (EMN) utilizes CT data to reconstruct the tracheobronchial tree and identify a lung nodule. However, with EMN, the patient lies in an electromagnetic field and a sensor can be tracked during the bronchoscopic procedure in space and time, with the goal of improving navigation to the target lesion. In principle, the device is similar to the global positioning system used in automobiles.

Two systems are currently available in the United States: SuperDimension (Medtronic) and SPiNDrive (Veran Medical Technologies).[118] To date, there have been no comparative efficacy trials between these systems.

Preprocedure planning differs slightly between the two systems. The SuperDimension system uses a chest CT scan obtained while the patient is in an inspiratory hold for preprocedure planning, and the movement of target related to breathing is estimated by a preprogrammed algorithm. The magnetic field is generated by a board placed underneath the patient. The SPiNDrive System uses both inspiratory and expiratory chest CT images. Respiratory motion is accounted for by using fiducial pads on the chest during the procedure. The magnetic field is generated by a pad over the patient.

The instruments used by the two systems are also different. SuperDimension uses a sensor placed within a locatable guide loaded into an extended working channel passed through the working channel of a therapeutic bronchoscope. The locatable guide and extended working channel are then steered to the target and the locatable guide is removed, leaving the extended working channel in place through which standard bronchoscopic sampling tools (i.e., needle, brush, forceps) are passed. In contrast, the SPiNDrive sensor is located on the tip of its instruments and allows for "always on" tracking during navigation as well as during the sampling process[5] (Fig. 27.6).

ENB may have a better yield for the diagnosis of peripheral lung lesions, especially when combined with radial EBUS. Eberhardt et al. compared the use of radial EBUS alone, ENB alone, and the combination of radial EBUS with ENB in 118 patients followed by surgical resection.[119] The diagnostic yield of the combination of radial EBUS/ENB was 88% as opposed to radial EBUS alone (69%) or ENB only (59%) ($P = 0.02$).

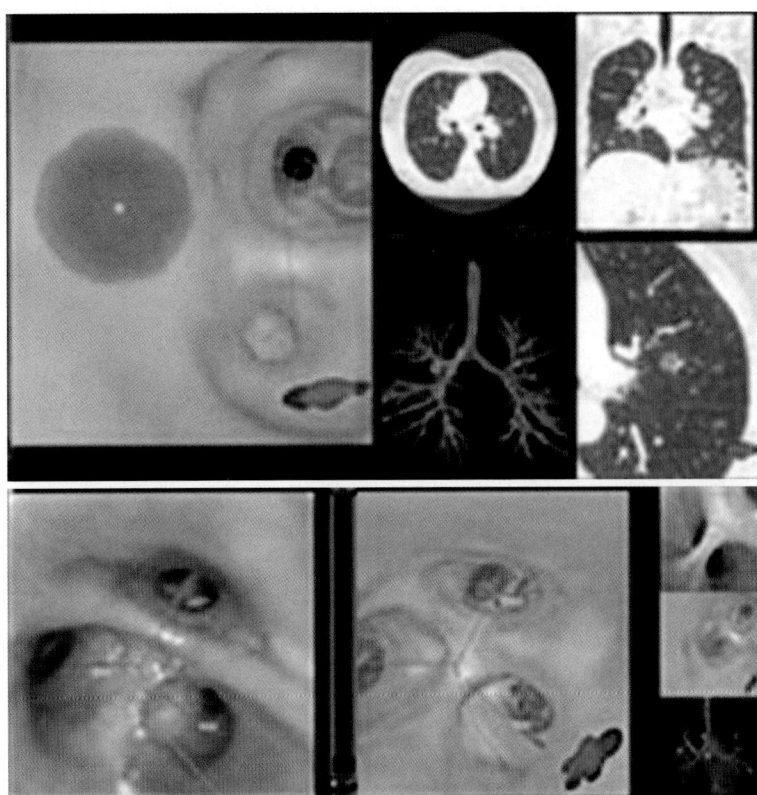

Figure 27.5 Virtual bronchoscopy platform. The broncho-scopic navigation pathway was created to access the lesion (*shown in pink*). This platform shows a virtual endoscopic view and three views of the patient's uploaded computed tomography scan (axial, coronal, and sagittal), followed by a pathway (*blue line*) superimposed upon the virtual endoscopic image.

In 2012, a large meta-analysis of more than 3000 cases found that the diagnostic yield of all advanced bronchoscopic techniques, including radial EBUS and ENB for peripheral lung nodules (malignant or nonmalignant), was roughly 70%.[121] A more recent meta-analysis with inclusion of 15 trials reported an overall diagnostic yield of ENB to be 65%.[120] Analysis of a prospectively gathered, multicenter registry indicates a considerably lower diagnostic yield of only 39% for EMN.[122] Another prospective, multicenter (academic and community centers) registry of 1092 patients reported an overall diagnostic yield of 73% for EMN cases at 12 months.[123] Such widely divergent diagnostic yield is unexplained but may relate to various factors.

Predictors of improved diagnostic yield include operator experience (independent of lesion size and location),[124] presence of a CT bronchus sign (i.e., a visible airway leading into the lesion), the addition of TBNA, and larger size of nodule.[125,126]

Many hypotheses for the relatively poor diagnostic yield have been suggested. There could be a bias for using ENB only for the smaller or more difficult to localize lesions or lesions without a CT bronchus sign. In addition, several studies have demonstrated the variability in nodule location during breathing.[127,128] Protocols for mechanical ventilation during bronchoscopy have been published to minimize nodule motion and atelectasis, both of which can significantly alter the location of the nodule to be sampled.[129] Navigation without real-time guidance certainly limits the chances of adjustment for changes in nodule location. Finally, on occasion, nodules have been shown to regress or resolve between the time of CT scan and bronchoscopy.[130]

Overall, ENB is a safe procedure. A meta-analysis reported complications of ENB including pneumothorax in 3.1% (1.6% requiring chest tube insertion) as well as bleeding in 0.9% that was either minor or moderate.[121] In the NAVIGATE study, the pneumothorax rate requiring either admission or chest tube placement was found to be 2.9%. Grade 2 or higher bleeding was 1.5% and grade 4 or higher respiratory failure was 0.7%.[123]

ENB is also used to place fiducial markers to guide stereotactic body radiation therapy, to mark with dye to guide video-assisted or robotic-assisted thoracoscopic resection of lesions not palpable by the surgeon, such as ground-glass nodules/carcinoma in situ,[131,132] and to retrieve foreign bodies.[133]

ELECTROMAGNETIC NAVIGATIONAL TRANSTHORACIC NEEDLE ASPIRATION

In combination with ENB, *electromagnetic navigational transthoracic needle aspiration* (ETTNA) has been introduced as an application of the EMN (SPiNDrive) system. This procedure uses a sensor-tipped ("always-on") transthoracic needle guided within the same electromagnetic field generated for ENB to provide guidance for transthoracic biopsy. A single-center, prospective pilot study examined safety, feasibility, and diagnostic yield of combined EMN and ETTNA. A total of 24 patients underwent EBUS for staging

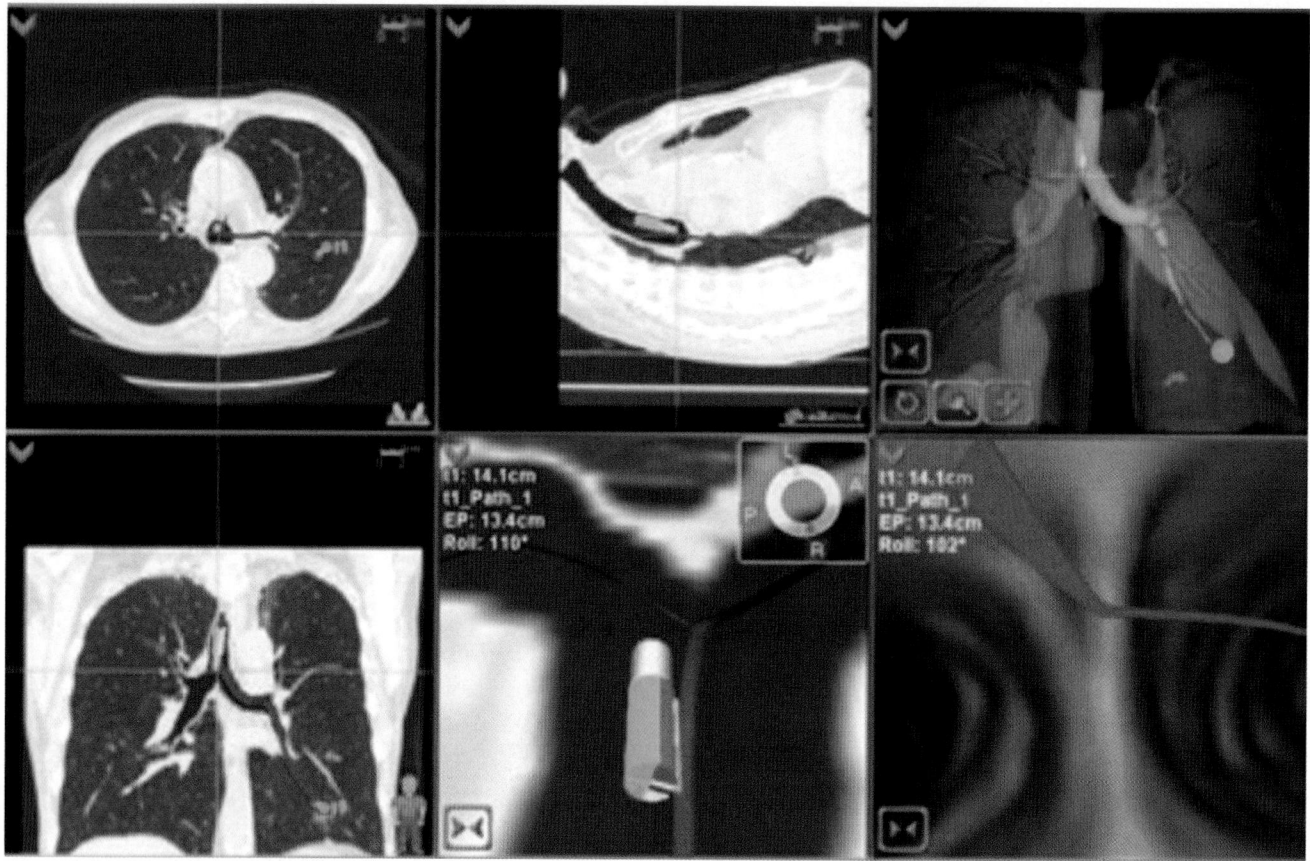

Figure 27.6 Electromagnetic navigation bronchoscopy. This system demonstrates preprocedural planning with computed tomography in three views (axial, coronal, and sagittal) with a three-dimensional airway reconstruction overlay and a pathway to the lesion (*pink line*). (From Arias S, Yarmus L, Argento AC. Navigational transbronchial needle aspiration, percutaneous needle aspiration and its future. *J Thorac Dis.* 2015;7[S4]:S317–S328.)

followed by EMN with ETTNA for sampling of a peripheral lesion. The diagnostic yield for ETTNA alone was 83% and increased to 87% when combined with EMN. With all three modalities combined, the diagnostic yield increased to 92%[134] (Fig. 27.7). A multicenter randomized study is currently underway to validate these results (All in One Study: A Prospective Trial of Electromagnetic Navigation for Biopsy of Pulmonary Nodules; NCT03338049).[5,135]

BRONCHOSCOPIC TRANSPARENCHYMAL NODULE ACCESS

Bronchoscopic transparenchymal nodule access (BTPNA) uses virtual bronchoscopy to identify and create a pathway from the central airways to a peripheral pulmonary lesion based on a preprocedure CT scan. The previously discussed navigational platforms help guide biopsy of lesions that have a CT bronchus sign but, for those without a bronchus leading directly into the lesion, the Archimedes system (Broncus Medical, Inc.) allows biopsy via a BTPNA. The system will identify the target nodule as well as the pulmonary vasculature to plan a safe biopsy pathway.[4] Once the target has been selected, the proprietary software calculates two suitable points of entry with straight-line access to the targeted lesion. The path is then fused to a fluoroscopic image. Users are able to "visualize" the blood vessels, points of entry, and target lesion on the virtual pathway. A needle is then used to create a hole in the airway, and a balloon catheter is inserted to dilate the hole. A sheath with a blunt-tipped stylet is advanced under fused fluoroscopic guidance through the lung parenchyma to the lesion. Once in the lesion, as seen on fused fluoroscopy in multiple views, needle aspirates, brushings, and biopsies are taken (Fig. 27.8). The feasibility study for BTPNA showed that tunneled pathway creation was successful in 10 of 12 (83%) patients with peripheral pulmonary lesions. The inaccessible lesions were in the left apex, and the process was limited by bronchoscope angulation. No complications were noted in these procedures. These patients then underwent surgical resection of their lesions, and there was no evidence of hemorrhage or parenchymal laceration.[136] A subsequent report of BTPNA showed that after successful biopsy in 5 of 6 (83%) patients, 2 patients developed iatrogenic pneumothoraces (only 1 required chest tube insertion).[137]

Although this approach is helpful for lesions without a CT bronchus sign, there are still lesions out of reach, particularly in the lung apices or superior segments, due to limitations in bronchoscope angulation.[135]

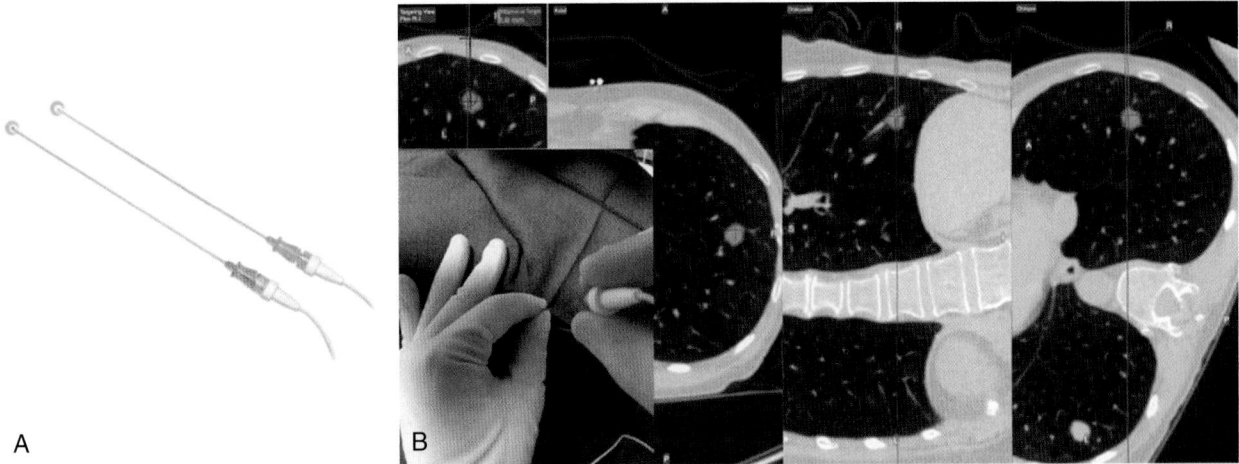

Figure 27.7 *Electromagnetic navigational transthoracic needle aspiration* (**ETTNA**). (A) ETTNA needle with the sensor-tipped needles. (B) ETTNA procedure showing the needles directed using an electromagnetic navigation system. (A, Courtesy Veran Medical Technologies. B, From Arias S, Yarmus L, Argento AC. Navigational transbronchial needle aspiration, percutaneous needle aspiration and its future. *J Thorac Dis.* 2015;7[S4]:S317–S328.)

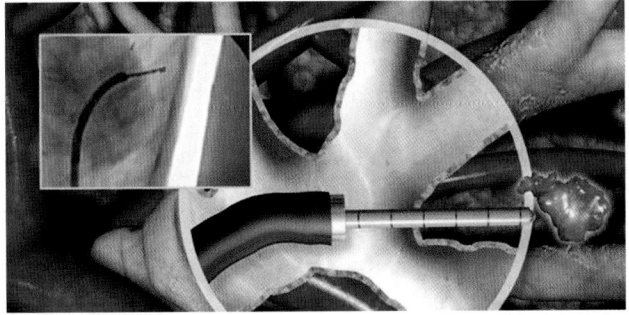

Figure 27.8 Bronchoscopic transparenchymal nodule access. Based on a preprocedure computed tomography scan, virtual bronchoscopy is used to create a pathway from the central airways to a peripheral lesion. The path through the airway wall is opened and dilated to allow access for the biopsy. *Inset,* Fluoroscopic view. (From Herth FJF, Eberhardt R, Sterman D, et al. Bronchoscopic transparenchymal nodule access [BTPNA]: first in human trial of a novel procedure for sampling solitary pulmonary nodules. *Thorax.* 2015;70[4]:326–332.)

AUGMENTED FLUOROSCOPY NAVIGATION

Augmented fluoroscopic navigation enhances nodule as well as airway visualization in an attempt to improve sensitivity of navigation-guided bronchoscopy. As discussed above, the diagnostic yield of guided bronchoscopy (via radial EBUS, virtual bronchoscopy, or ENB) is approximately 50–70%. This is significantly worse than CT-guided biopsy (sensitivity of ≈90%), though the latter is associated with a higher pneumothorax rate (approximately 15%).[2,138] The reduced diagnostic yield of guided bronchoscopy is likely secondary to the reliance on preoperative CT planning and virtual navigation as opposed to real-time image guidance. As a result, there can be significant divergence between the CT and the body. Suggested possibilities contributing to divergence include the difference in lung volume at the time of CT scan compared with the time of the procedure, influence of general anesthesia, and the development of atelectasis.[127] Augmented fluoroscopic

navigation is designed to minimize these problems. There are three available augmented fluoroscopic platforms currently available.

The first and most established is Fluoroscopic Navigation (SuperDimension-Medtronic), which utilizes digital tomosynthesis by conventional fluoroscopy to visualize and reregister the target nodule location. As described, tomosynthesis refers to a sweep arc of a fluoroscopic C-arm around the chest wall with continuous image acquisition, obtaining multiple image projections. The goal is to improve positional accuracy of the navigation catheter due to real-time changes and assist with path correction if the nodule has changed locations during the procedure. One retrospective study utilizing this technology demonstrated a 25% absolute increase in diagnostic yield (79%) compared with using standard navigation bronchoscopy (54%). In this study, the majority of nodules (64%) were less than 20 mm in diameter and only 22% had a CT bronchus sign.[139]

Another augmented fluoroscopy platform, LungVision (BodyVision), enables enhanced fluoroscopic visualization of airways with predetermined pathways as well as target lesions. These enhanced views are obtained by utilizing preoperative CT planning software along with fluoroscopic registration; the platform has demonstrated improved diagnostic yield in small case series.[140]

Finally, a third system by SONIALVISON (Shimadzu) was studied in 40 patients with radial EBUS with sheath guide combined with preprocedural chest tomosynthesis to serve as a map. The nodules were ground-glass opacities with a mean average diameter of 22 (±10) mm. Overall diagnostic yield was 65%, which improved to 79% if a radial EBUS view of the lesion was obtained. The ability to detect the nodule on tomosynthesis was not predictive of improved diagnostic yield.[141]

CONE BEAM CT FOR BRONCHOSCOPY

Cone beam CT (CBCT) is another imaging modality that may improve the diagnostic yield for bronchoscopic lung biopsy. It is a compact CT system with a moving C-arm that can be used during bronchoscopy to provide real-time confirmation of biopsy device location. This modality has previously been widely adopted in many fields of interventional radiology, including intravascular and hepatobiliary interventions. Similar to the aforementioned fluoroscopic tomosynthesis approach, the C-arm of the CBCT performs a single rotation around a stationary patient to obtain volumetric data. After image acquisition, the biopsy device location can be reviewed and adjusted to a new target location as needed with repeat scans.[142]

A prospective study of bronchoscopy with a thin bronchoscope, radial EBUS, and CBCT in 20 patients demonstrated that by redirecting sampling tools to the lesion based on CBCT images, the diagnostic yield increased from 50% to 70%.[143] In a prospective study of 20 patients, Casal and colleagues concluded that CBCT-guided bronchoscopy demonstrated a 25% absolute increase in navigation yield and 20% absolute increase in diagnostic yield of peripheral lung nodules. Additionally, they noted that the use of CBCT was associated with acceptable radiation doses (11 to 29 mSv).[144] Hohenforst-Schmidt and colleagues conducted a prospective feasibility study combining CBCT with conventional bronchoscopy without radial EBUS. In the 33 patients with peripheral pulmonary lesions, the overall diagnostic yield was 70%.[145]

Adoption of CBCT may be difficult given its cost, lack of availability in most endoscopy suites, and increased radiation exposure when compared to other enhanced navigation technologies.

ROBOTIC BRONCHOSCOPY

Robotic bronchoscopy has better maneuverability, enabling navigation further into the periphery of the lung, and can remain static once a desired position is reached. There are currently two companies in the market: the Monarch (Auris), which was approved by the U.S. Food and Drug Administration in 2018, and the Ion (Intuitive), which was approved in 2019. Research is underway to demonstrate diagnostic yield and peripheral reach of these systems. Large prospective data, however, are lacking.[146,147]

The Monarch system robotic arms are operated with a small handheld controller similar to that for a videogame. The controller guides an outer sheath that is wedged in a proximal position and then steers an inner scope to the biopsy site. Chen et al. evaluated this robotic platform using human cadavers to compare how far the scope could reach compared to a thin scope driven by expert bronchoscopists.[148] The robotic bronchoscope was able to be advanced farther into the lung periphery compared to a thin bronchoscope despite the scopes having the same outer diameter. The outer sheath design provides support for the inner scope and allows for improved maneuverability. A subsequent cadaver study reported that lesional tissue was able to be acquired in 65 of 67 (97%) human cadavers when using the robotic platform with EMN guidance and radial EBUS confirmation.[149]

The Ion platform uses an ultrathin robotic catheter with a 3.5-mm outer diameter. EMN is not required because the catheter is fitted with shape-sensing technology to provide accurate positional information. The catheter is advanced with a trackball and wheel controller. In order to have such a small outer diameter, the optic is removed once the target is reached, and the catheter (with shape-sensing technology) is used as a guide sheath through which various sampling instruments are introduced.

The early data using these systems are encouraging. A pilot study of 15 patients with the Monarch system reported safety and feasibility with no major bleeding events or pneumothorax despite biopsies having been performed in 93% of patients.[147] The first human study for Ion robotic bronchoscopy by Fielding and colleagues[150] was performed in 30 patients with small peripheral nodules (12.5 mm mean diameter). Radial EBUS was used to confirm the location of the target lesion, and flexible TBNA needles, forceps, and brushes were used for sampling. The overall diagnostic yield was 83%, and there were no device-related adverse events.

CRYOBIOPSY

Cryobiopsy has emerged as a technique for sampling tissue in diffuse parenchymal lung disease. Cryobiopsy has been shown to obtain larger pieces of tissue than standard transbronchial biopsies and minimize crush artifact, thereby leaving intact parenchymal architecture and a potentially higher overall diagnostic yield than standard bronchoscopic techniques. Unfortunately, complications such as pneumothorax and massive hemorrhage have been reported in up to 20% of cases. For years, the technique of cryobiopsy varied widely among practitioners, including whether they used fluoroscopy or bronchial blockers, the duration of freeze time, and other factors. A recent consensus statement has been published with the goals of standardizing the procedure and minimizing complications.[151]

The technique requires a cryotherapy probe, for which there are currently two sizes: 1.9 mm and 2.4 mm. The probes are introduced through the working channel of a bronchoscope and extended into the periphery of the lung, ideally 1 to 2 cm from the pleural surface, as seen on fluoroscopy. The cryoprobe is then cooled for 3 to 6 seconds, causing lung tissue to adhere to the tip. Finally, the probe is removed en bloc along with the adherent tissue and the bronchoscope to obtain a large piece of lung tissue (Fig. 27.9). Ideally, the

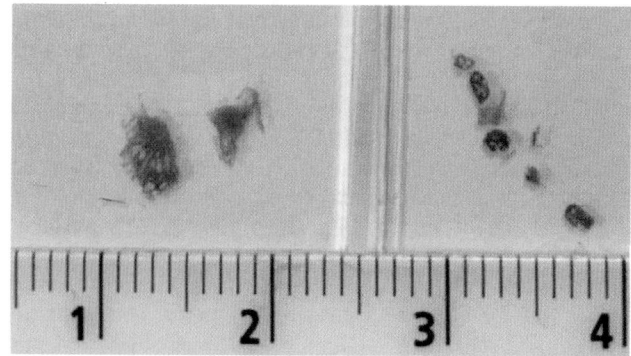

Figure 27.9 Cryobiopsy. Cryobiopsies *(left)* are larger than transbronchial biopsies *(right)*. Measurements are in centimeters. (From Lentz RJ, Argento AC, Colby TV, Rickman OB, Maldonado F. Transbronchial cryobiopsy for diffuse parenchymal lung disease: a state-of-the-art review of procedural techniques, current evidence, and future challenges. *J Thorac Dis.* 2017;9[7]:2186–2203.)

patient is intubated and under general anesthesia for the procedure. A bronchial blocker should also be positioned into the target airway ahead of time and, once the biopsy, probe, and bronchoscope are removed, the blocker is inflated in case bleeding results. When the sample is collected and the bronchoscope is back in the airway, the blocker can be deflated and bleeding can be assessed. Pneumothorax and significant bleeding are reported to range from 9–10% and from 14–20%, respectively. For these reasons, cryobiopsy should only be performed in experienced centers with the ability to manage these complications.[152–154]

In 2018, an international conference on transbronchial cryobiopsy published an expert statement on safety, utility, and the need for standardization of this procedure.[151] They report that despite a substantial and expanding body of literature, the technique has not yet been standardized and its place in the diagnostic algorithm of diffuse parenchymal lung disease remains to be defined. A meta-analysis of 27 studies demonstrated a yield of 73% for cryobiopsy in the diagnosis of diffuse parenchymal lung disease, together with a lower complication rate than for surgical lung biopsy.[155] They concluded that cryobiopsies have a good diagnostic yield but a significant risk for complications and that outcomes vary markedly across institutions, indicating that standardization of the procedure is required. Romagnoli et al. published a prospective two-center study comparing specimens obtained in a single setting: cryobiopsy and surgical biopsy obtained by video-assisted thoracic surgery for patients with interstitial lung disease. Their pathologic results were compared to consensus from a multidisciplinary discussion that demonstrated poor concordance between cryobiopsies and surgical biopsies, with surgical biopsy results more frequently consistent with the multidisciplinary conference diagnosis. The group concluded that surgical biopsies should remain the gold standard for interstitial lung disease.[156] Thus, cryobiopsy in its current form is not ready for routine use outside of the research setting. In addition to interstitial lung disease, information about the utility of cryobiopsy in cancer, post–lung transplant, and immunocompromised hosts is emerging.[157–160]

Finally, in a recent study using an animal model, a mini-cryoprobe that can acquire samples through the working channel of a bronchoscope showed preservation of histologic quality with the promise of improved safety. Clinical trials are underway.

Key Points

- Endobronchial ultrasound, both convex probe and radial probe, has revolutionized the diagnosis and staging of lung cancer and replaced surgical mediastinoscopy as first-line approach for this indication.
- Certain techniques, such as confocal bronchoscopy and elastography, may help direct biopsy to areas of the tumor or lymph node based on imaging characteristics.
- Thin and ultrathin bronchoscopes offer advantages for deeper penetration into the lung, for evaluating obstructing lesions, and for use in mechanically ventilated patients with small endotracheal tubes.
- Recent advances in technology, including radial probe endobronchial ultrasound and virtual and electromagnetic navigation, have increased the diagnostic yield for peripheral pulmonary nodules to approximately 70%.
- Robotic bronchoscopy shows promise because it allows for improved localization and stability of the bronchoscope for biopsy of peripheral lung nodules.
- Cryobiopsy needs to be standardized to benefit from improved diagnostic yield for diffuse parenchymal lung disease while avoiding a greater risk of complications.

Key Readings

Chen AC, Pastis NJ, Machuzak MS, et al. Accuracy of a robotic endoscopic system in cadaver models with simulated tumor targets: ACCESS study. *Respiration*. 2020;99(1):56–61.

Detterbeck FC, Lewis SZ, Diekemper R, Addrizzo-Harris D, Alberts WM. Executive summary: diagnosis and management of lung cancer, 3rd ed: American College of Chest Physicians evidence-based clinical practice guidelines. *Chest*. 2013;143(suppl 5):7S–37S.

Fujiwara T, Nakajima T, Inage T, et al. The combination of endobronchial elastography and sonographic findings during endobronchial ultrasound-guided transbronchial needle aspiration for predicting nodal metastasis. *Thorac Cancer*. 2019;10(10):2000–2005.

Hetzel J, Maldonado F, Ravaglia C, et al. Transbronchial cryobiopsies for the diagnosis of diffuse parenchymal lung diseases: expert statement from the Cryobiopsy Working Group on Safety and Utility and a call for standardization of the procedure. *Respiration*. 2018;95(3):188–200.

Izumo T, Sasada S, Chavez C, Matsuoto Y, Tsuchida T. Radial endobronchial ultrasound images for ground-glass opacity pulmonary lesions. *Eur Respir J*. 2015;45(6):1661–1668.

Matsuno Y, Asano F, Shindoh J, et al. CT-guided ultrathin bronchoscopy: bioptic approach and factors in predicting diagnosis. *Intern Med*. 2011;50(19):2143–2148.

Silvestri GA, Gonzalez AV, Jantz MA, et al. Methods for staging non-small cell lung cancer: diagnosis and management of lung cancer, 3rd ed: American College of Chest Physicians evidence-based clinical practice guidelines. *Chest*. 2013;143(suppl 5):e211S–e250S.

Wahidi MM, Herth F, Yasufuku K, et al. Technical aspects of endobronchial ultrasound-guided transbronchial needle aspiration: CHEST guideline and expert panel report. *Chest*. 2016;149(3):816–835.

Complete reference list available at ExpertConsult.com.

28

THERAPEUTIC BRONCHOSCOPY: INTERVENTIONAL TECHNIQUES

DAVID FELLER-KOPMAN, MD, FCCP • SAMIRA SHOJAEE, MD, MPH

INTRODUCTION AND HISTORICAL BACKGROUND

Gustav Killian performed the first rigid bronchoscopy in 1897 to extract a piece of a pork bone from the right main bronchus.[1] Because this was in the preantibiotic era, this innovation resulted in a dramatic decrease in the mortality from aspiration pneumonia. In 1966 the flexible bronchoscope was introduced into clinical practice by Shigeto Ikeda.[2] Currently, the majority of pulmonologists are trained in *flexible bronchoscopy* (FB), whereas only a minority have been trained in rigid bronchoscopy.[3,4] With the advent of formalized fellowship training programs in interventional pulmonology, training in rigid bronchoscopy has made a comeback. The rigid bronchoscope is an extremely valuable instrument in the management of central airway obstruction[5] (Video 28.1). Whereas FB remains invaluable for the diagnosis of lung masses, parenchymal disease, and mediastinal/hilar adenopathy, the rigid bronchoscope offers the ability to provide an airway allowing oxygenation and ventilation, as well as the passage of large-bore suction catheters and a variety of tools, including the flexible bronchoscope, that can aid in the destruction and excision of tumor. In addition, because silicone stents can be placed only via the rigid bronchoscope, rigid bronchoscopy allows the physician more options and therefore the ability to place the "best" stent in a selected patient as opposed to being limited to stents that can be placed solely via FB.

Central airway obstruction, from both malignant and nonmalignant causes (Table 28.1), is associated with significant morbidity and mortality and often presents a great challenge to physicians. It is estimated that 20–30% of patients with lung cancer will develop complications associated with airway obstruction, and the incidence of nonmalignant causes, such as postintubation/posttracheostomy

stenosis, is likely to increase due to the increasing use of artificial airways in an ever-aging population.[6]

It should be noted that designing large randomized trials to investigate comparative treatment efficacy is extremely difficult and potentially unethical in patients with central airway obstruction. Limitations include selecting patients with comparable disease and comorbidities, as well as the fact that many of these patients present in respiratory distress. Double blinding is also clearly impossible. Therefore the literature supporting therapeutic bronchoscopy is primarily based on large case series/registries and retrospective analyses. That being said, the impact of therapeutic bronchoscopy on quality and length of life is impressive.[7–12] In addition, improvements in dyspnea and health-related quality of life are maintained long term.[11] Therapeutic bronchoscopy has also been associated with immediate reductions in the level of care required for patients with acute respiratory failure from central airway obstruction.[13]

Training in advanced diagnostic and therapeutic bronchoscopy tends to be limited to the centers that have dedicated interventional pulmonology training programs.[14] Over the last decade, however, dedicated training in interventional pulmonology has become more popular, with 37 dedicated programs currently available in the United States, adding more than 40 interventional pulmonologists into the workforce annually[15,16] (aabronchology.org). With this expansion, standardized interventional pulmonology fellowship training requirements, curricula, and in-service examinations have been developed.[5,17,18]

Even with the recent increase in training in rigid bronchoscopy, the flexible bronchoscope remains an essential tool in therapeutic bronchoscopy. It is used in almost every rigid bronchoscopic procedure and, when rigid bronchoscopy is not available, can also be used as the only bronchoscope for foreign body removal, tumor excision/tumor destruction, bronchial thermoplasty, bronchoscopic lung volume reduction, and balloon dilation. There are several therapeutic techniques, each with its own associated risks and benefits, advantages, and disadvantages (Table 28.2). Because comparative data are lacking, the technique of choice often depends on equipment availability and the bronchoscopist's expertise. Two of the most important considerations in the care of patients with central airway obstruction are assessing the stability of the patient for the planned procedure and having a realistic understanding of the local resources and skill set. Clearly, all efforts should be made to ensure that a patient with a relatively stable airway does not develop an unstable airway during the procedure because such patients can deteriorate quickly. These patients are often best cared for in a multidisciplinary approach in centers of excellence that routinely evaluate and manage such complex patients.[6]

REMOVING FOREIGN BODIES

INDICATIONS

Foreign body aspiration is one of the most common indications for therapeutic bronchoscopy. There is a bimodal incidence of airway aspiration, peaking in children 1 to 2 years of age and in adults older than 70 years. Risk factors for aspiration in adults include alcohol intoxication, sedative and hypnotic drug use, poor dentition, senility, seizure, trauma, swallowing impairment, parkinsonism, and general anesthesia. In adults foreign bodies are most commonly found in the right-sided airways but in children are found equally in the left and right owing to the equal size and angulation of the main bronchi. Because a history

Table 28.1 Causes of Central Airway Obstruction

Nonmalignant	Malignant
Vascular	Primary airway tumors
Sling	Bronchogenic
Cartilage	Mucoepidermoid
Relapsing polychondritis	Adenoid cystic
Lymphadenopathy	Carcinoid
Infectious (e.g., histoplasmosis, tuberculosis)	Tumors metastatic to the airway
Sarcoidosis	Bronchogenic
Granulation tissue associated with:	Renal cell
	Breast
Artificial airways	Melanoma
Airway stents	Thyroid
Aspirated foreign bodies	Colon
Surgical anastomosis	Esophageal
Inflammatory lesions	Lymphadenopathy from any malignancy
Granulomatosis with polyangiitis	Mediastinal tumors
Amyloidosis	Thyroid
Papillomatosis	Thymus
Tracheobronchomalacia	Germ cell
Other:	Lymphoma
Goiter	
Secretions/blood clot	

Table 28.2 Advantages and Disadvantages of Therapeutic Modalities

Modality	Time to Achieve Results	Advantages	Disadvantages	Comments
Electrocautery	Immediate	Inexpensive Multiple accessories	Often need to couple with mechanical débridement	Need to deactivate pacemaker/AICD Keep F_{IO_2} <0.4
Argon plasma coagulation	Immediate	Inexpensive Can treat at an angle to electrode	Risk for gas embolization with higher flow rates Often need to couple with mechanical débridement	Need to deactivate pacemaker/AICD Depth of penetration 2–3 mm Keep F_{IO_2} <0.4
Laser photoresection	Immediate	Extensive data supporting its use	Need laser safety precautions	Depth of penetration up to 10 mm Keep F_{IO_2} <0.4
Stent	Immediate	Only bronchoscopic modality for extrinsic compression	All stents have associated complications of granulation tissue formation, infection, and migration	Metallic stents should be used with caution in patients with nonmalignant disease
Microdébrider	Immediate	Can use in high-F_{IO_2} environments Can provide tissue for pathology	May need additional tools to provide hemostasis	Cannot reach distal airways
Cryotherapy	48–72 hr	Normal airway is cryoresistant Can use in high-F_{IO_2} environments	Delayed maximal effect Requires "cleanout" bronchoscopy	Cryoadhesion can remove organic foreign bodies
Photodynamic therapy	48–72 hr	Can destroy submucosal tumor Can use in high-F_{IO_2} environments	Delayed maximal effect Requires "cleanout" bronchoscopy Systemic photosensitivity Need laser safety precautions	Swelling of tumor can cause obstruction
Brachytherapy	Delayed: days to weeks	Can destroy submucosal tumor	Coordination with radiation oncology	Radiation bronchitis Risk for erosion into vessels Swelling of tumor can cause obstruction

AICD, automatic internal cardiac defibrillator; F_{IO_2}, fractional concentration of oxygen in inspired gas.

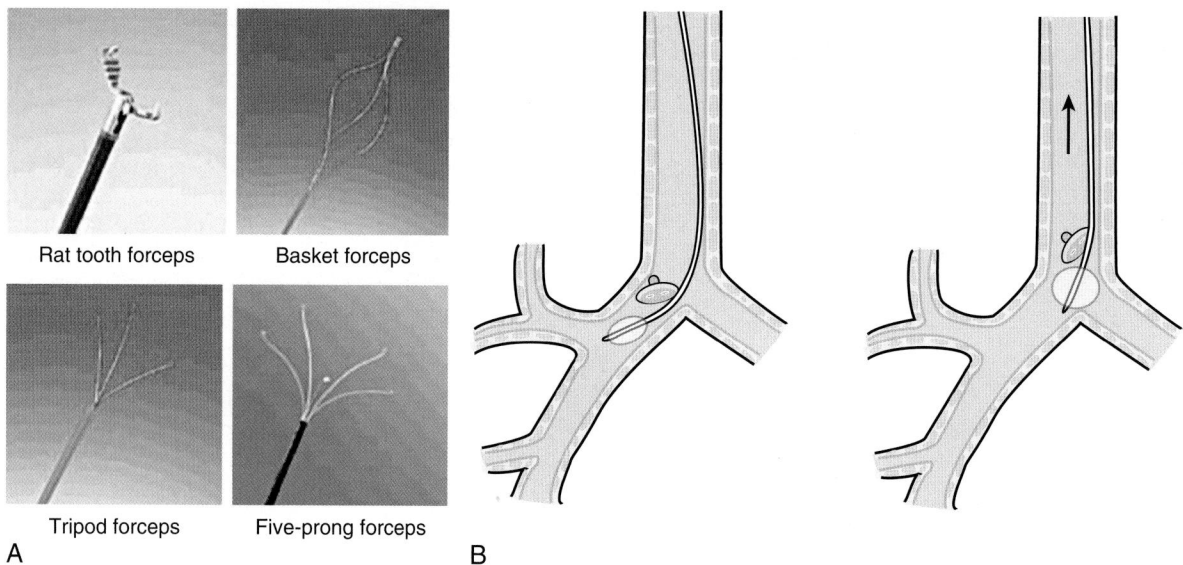

Figure 28.1 Tools and schematic diagram of the method used for foreign body removal. (A) Examples of foreign body retrieval tools: rat tooth forceps, basket forceps, tripod forceps, five-prong forceps. (B) The use of a balloon catheter for dislodging a foreign body by a retrograde pull *(arrow).* (B, Courtesy Dr. Eric Folch.)

of aspiration is obtained in less than 50% of patients, and visible foreign bodies can be identified on chest radiography in less than 10% of cases, a high index of suspicion is required.[19–22]

CONTRAINDICATIONS, PROCEDURE, RESULTS, AND COMPLICATIONS

All contraindications that apply to routine FB also apply to the removal of a foreign body. Lack of experience and lack of availability of all necessary endobronchial accessories are the more important considerations. Removal of a foreign body using FB should be attempted only by or under the supervision of an expert bronchoscopist. The removal of foreign bodies can be performed successfully with either the flexible or rigid bronchoscope. Flexible bronchoscopy is successful in 86–91% of cases, whereas rigid bronchoscopy is successful in 99.9%.[20,21,23–29] If available, rigid bronchoscopy should be used in all cases of acute respiratory distress caused by foreign body aspiration, given the near 100% success rate. The benefits of FB include its widespread availability and its lack of a requirement for general anesthesia. Despite these benefits, however, in the setting of acute respiratory distress or large foreign body aspiration, the extraction of the foreign body is much more efficient with rigid bronchoscopy because it can be accomplished often on a first attempt, using rigid graspers and removal through the large lumen of the rigid scope.

Foreign body removal using FB is carried out in stages: first, dislodging the foreign body; then, grasping or securing the object; and finally, removing it along with the flexible bronchoscope as a single unit. A variety of ancillary accessories (forceps, grasping claws, snares, baskets, and magnets) are available for foreign body extraction (Fig. 28.1). A cryoprobe passed through the flexible bronchoscope can be especially useful for the removal of blood clots, mucous plugs, and organic material because the extreme cold can cause immediate and strong adherence ("cryoadherence")

to the biologic materials.[30] Once the object is grasped and secured, care must be taken to avoid losing it at the level of the vocal cords. If necessary, the patient can also be asked to cough to expel the foreign body once it has been brought into the mid-upper trachea.

Serious complications can accompany removal of a foreign body, including central airway obstruction, hypoxemia, bronchospasm, and bleeding. Objects can also migrate, and their fragments can impact in distal airways resulting in postobstructive pneumonia.

MANAGING CENTRAL AIRWAY DISORDERS

A variety of techniques have been developed for managing central airway obstructions usually due to malignant or benign tumors. Each technique has its own advantages and disadvantages, and special considerations for its use (see Table 28.2). Of course, only some of these techniques may be used at any one institution. The indications for the use of therapeutic bronchoscopy for central airway disorders include malignant airway obstruction, postintubation tracheal stenosis and other nonmalignant etiologies of central airway strictures and stenosis, massive hemoptysis with or without central airway tumors, and foreign body extraction as discussed earlier. The specific indications and complications of these procedures are discussed in turn.

ELECTROCAUTERY

Endobronchial electrocautery is the application of heat produced by high-frequency electrical current to cut or destroy tissue. It involves the use of special accessories, such as blunt probes, forceps, knives, and snares introduced through the bronchoscope. These function as an active electrode that focuses energy at the point of contact, leading to tissue cutting, coagulation, or

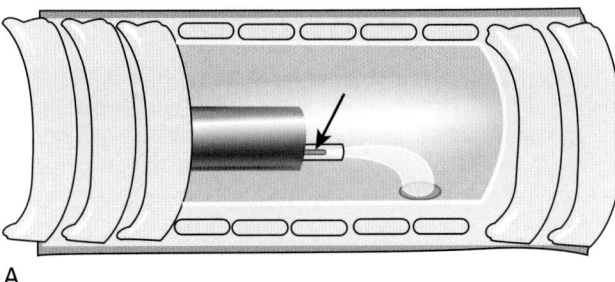

A

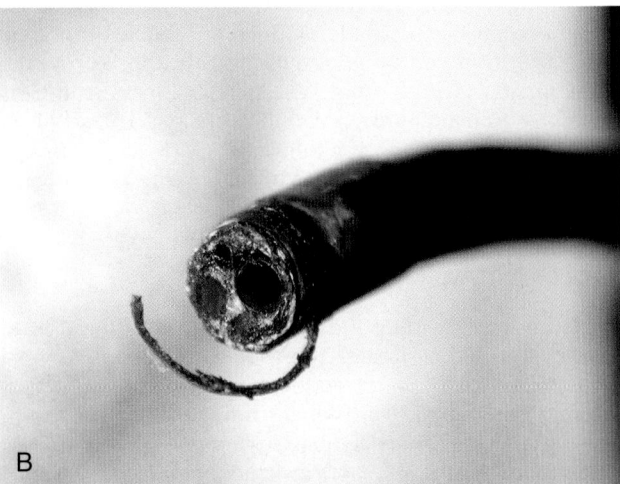

B

Figure 28.2 Argon plasma coagulation and a complication. (A) Argon plasma coagulation can be used to treat lesions tangential to the bronchoscope. *Arrow* shows the tungsten carbide electrode. Positively charged argon gas automatically flows radially to the negatively charged bleeding tissue. (B) Damage to the tip of the bronchoscope caused during argon plasma coagulation by having the catheter too close to the tip of the bronchoscope during activation. Note the charred tip along with the frayed rubber sheath. (A, Courtesy Dr. Eric Folch.)

vaporization. The degree of tissue destruction depends on the power used, duration of contact, surface area of contact, and water content of the tissue. Use of the snare device is especially suited for the removal of a pedunculated airway lesion because cauterization of the stalk can allow removal of the majority of the tumor for pathologic review (Video 28.2).

To avoid endobronchial ignition, the *fractional concentration of oxygen in inspired gas* (FIO_2) should be kept less than 0.4, requiring active communication with the anesthesiologists. Insulated bronchoscopes, compatible with electrocautery, are used to prevent leakage of electrical current, avoiding burns or electrical shock to the patient and the bronchoscopist.

Indications and Contraindications

Electrocautery is used for either coagulation or vaporization of malignant or nonmalignant disease within the airways and may be curative in patients with carcinoma in situ. Coagulation is achieved by gently touching the tumor tissue and applying 1- to 2-second bursts of 20- to 40-W energy until blanching or destruction of the mucosa becomes apparent. Additional contact time can result in vaporization of the tissue as desired. The tumor area should be kept free of blood or mucus by continuous suctioning to prevent dissipation of the electric current. The coagulated

tissue can then be removed using biopsy forceps or suction. The use of electrocautery is considered a relative contraindication in patients with pacemakers and/or defibrillators because of the potential for electrical interference with these devices.[31]

Results and Complications

Electrocautery has been used effectively and safely as an ablative modality in both malignant and nonmalignant airway obstruction. In several studies electrocautery has been shown to achieve luminal patency and symptomatic improvement at rates similar to *laser* (light amplification by stimulated emission of radiation) and other ablative airway modalities.[32–36] Moreover, electrocautery is a cost-effective bronchoscopic intervention due to the low cost of the unit and the reusable nature of its accessories.[32] In a selected group of patients with small, polypoid endobronchial lesions, Coulter and Mehta[37] showed that electrocautery had a high success rate (89%) under local anesthesia, thereby eliminating the need for the more costly laser therapy. Complications are rare in experienced hands: The most common ones are bleeding (2–5%), endobronchial fire in a high-FIO_2 environment, and electrical shock to the operator should the cautery probe touch an ungrounded bronchoscope. It should be noted, however, that in a multicenter study, Ost and colleagues[38] showed that, after multivariate analysis of many factors, electrocautery use was associated with increased likelihood of requiring escalation in the level of care.

ARGON PLASMA COAGULATION

Argon plasma coagulation (APC) is a noncontact form of electrocautery that uses ionized argon gas (plasma) to conduct electrical current from the probe to the tissue. Because positively charged argon gas flows toward the negatively charged tissue, treatment can be directed in an axial or tangential fashion (Fig. 28.2A). As the tissue becomes desiccated, it offers more resistance to the electrical current, limiting its penetration to approximately 2 to 3 mm.[31,32] APC probes can be passed via a rigid or flexible bronchoscope.

Indications and Contraindications

APC is frequently used for palliation of malignant airway obstruction as part of multimodality therapy, including mechanical débridement. APC is also extremely useful for the control of bleeding in the central airways and has been used for the treatment of excess granulation tissue (including stent-related granuloma), postinfectious airway stenosis, and endobronchial papillomatosis (Video 28.3).[31,32] The most important advantages of this technique are the ability to treat lesions tangential to the tip of the probe, to treat lesions in close proximity to airway stents, and to achieve hemostasis. The major limitation of APC is the depth of penetration of less than 3 mm; however, this also may reduce the risk for airway perforation. Its only absolute contraindication is the presence of a pacemaker or implantable defibrillator susceptible to electrical interference. As with electrocautery and laser use in the airway, APC requires that the FIO_2 be less than 0.4.

Results and Complications

In properly selected cases, APC in conjunction with other modalities, such as mechanical tumor debulking, provides symptomatic relief in almost 90% of patients with central airway obstruction.[31,32] It is also portable, less expensive than laser, and typically available in most operating rooms, although the bronchoscopic probes that carry the current through the bronchoscope to the endobronchial tumor at the desired location may need to be purchased. Potential complications include gas embolization,[39] airway fire, postprocedure stenosis, and injury to deeper structures or to the flexible bronchoscope (see Fig. 28.2B). The observed mortality and overall complication rates are 0.4% and 3.7% of cases, respectively.[40,41]

LASER PHOTORESECTION

Laser light has three unique characteristics—monochromaticity, coherence, and collimation—that permit controlled delivery of a well-defined energy. Laser light causes thermal, photodynamic, and electromagnetic changes in living tissue. Laser energy can cut, coagulate, or vaporize endobronchial lesions in a predictable manner, depending on the wavelength used. Although many types of laser systems exist, the *neodymium:yttrium-aluminum-garnet* (Nd:YAG) and *neodymium:yttrium-aluminum-perovskite* (Nd:YAP) lasers are most commonly used in the airways because of their ability to coagulate and vaporize tissue, with a depth of penetration of 5 to 10 mm.[32] Another laser, the carbon dioxide laser, provides minimal hemostasis but is extremely precise (depth of penetration of <1 mm). Such precision can permit fine procedures, such as those needed to incise weblike stenoses or to remove granulation tissue surrounding airway stents.

Indications

The main indications for *laser photoresection* (LPR) are relief of central airway obstruction from exophytic obstructive neoplasms and from tracheal stenosis (Video 28.4). An ideal lesion for LPR is an endobronchial tumor that arises from a single wall of a central airway and has a visible distal lumen, with a duration of distal lung collapse of less than 4 to 6 weeks. LPR can be performed using either a rigid or flexible bronchoscope. The end results and the complication rates are similar with both types of instruments. The selection of the scope mainly depends upon personal preference, availability of the instruments, and training. Bronchoscopists proficient in rigid bronchoscopy typically prefer to use the rigid scope because of the ease of mechanical debulking and superior suction capabilities.

Contraindications

Lesions not amenable to LPR are extrinsic or submucosal, primarily involving lobar or segmental bronchi, and those for which the operator is unable to identify a patent airway distal to the obstruction. As with other forms of heat therapy, laser is contraindicated in patients with a high oxygen requirement.[32]

Results and Complications

LPR can restore airway patency with immediate symptomatic improvement in 93% of cases (Fig. 28.3).[32,42] It can be combined with other techniques, such as mechanical debulking, using the rigid bronchoscope, microdébrider, APC, or stent placement to achieve full patency of major airways. This technique palliates symptoms of cough, dyspnea, and hemoptysis along with documented benefits in radiographic, spirometric, and quality-of-life parameters.[11] LPR is generally a very safe procedure; however, bleeding, endobronchial ignition, pneumothorax or barotrauma, bronchopleural or bronchoesophageal fistula, and hypoxemia have been reported.[43] Extensive knowledge of the anatomy of the tracheobronchial tree is mandatory before performing the procedure. Accumulation of blood and secretions can lead to rapid desaturation. Tracheobronchial tree perforation can be fatal owing to the close proximity of the airways to the great vessels. While performing the procedure, one must take precautions to avoid airway fires, activating the laser only when the F_{IO_2} is less than 0.4. Laser safety precautions for the bronchoscopist and operating room personnel are also required.[43]

STENT PLACEMENT

Stents are devices used for the internal splinting of luminal structures. The first stents that were used in the trachea were silicone T-tubes developed by Montgomery.[44] Although they require a tracheostomy for their placement, these stents are still widely used, primarily in patients with high tracheal stenosis and/or tracheomalacia. Westaby and colleagues[44a] modified this stent and designed a T-Y prosthesis, which enabled splinting of the distal trachea and carina. Dumon[45] later developed the first stents that could be inserted through a bronchoscope without a tracheostomy. Over the years, several other stents have been developed, including "dynamic" stents made to mimic the airway with a "posterior longitudinal membrane," stents made of steel or nitinol (a nickel-titanium alloy), and newly developed (although not commercially available) bioabsorbable and drug-eluting varieties (Fig. 28.4).[46] Unfortunately, there is no perfect stent. The ideal stent would be easy to insert and remove, strong enough to support the airway yet flexible enough to mimic normal airway physiology and promote secretion clearance, biologically inert to minimize the formation of granulation tissue, and available in a variety of sizes and shapes. Self-expanding metallic stents can be placed with flexible bronchoscopy. However, silicone stents require rigid bronchoscopy because the silicone stent is thick walled and requires manual folding and loading into a stent loader, which can only fit within the lumen of a rigid bronchoscope. Many bronchoscopists feel that metallic stents are also best placed via rigid bronchoscopy because the larger rigid forceps allow easier stent manipulation, and the patients are under general anesthesia. All currently available stents have their own advantages and disadvantages, and thus it is most important to select the best stent for the individual patient. This requires the bronchoscopist to be familiar with and be able to place a variety of stents.

Indications and Contraindications

Airway stents may be indicated for (1) counteracting extrinsic compression from tumors or lymph nodes (Video 28.5), (2) preventing regrowth of intraluminal tumor that will compromise an airway, (3) maintaining airway patency in patients with significant and symptomatic malacia, or (4) sealing

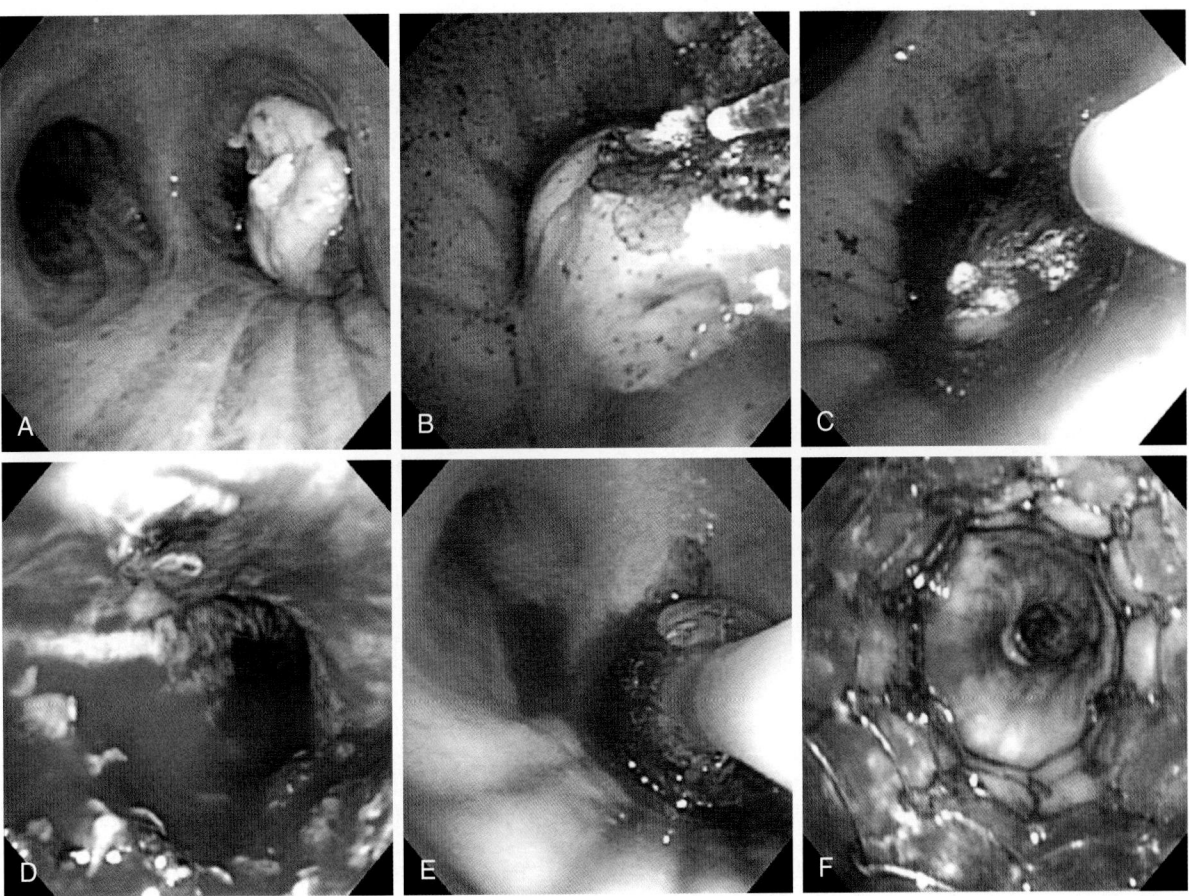

Figure 28.3 Bronchoscopic images of multimodality palliative therapy for a patient with a malignant lesion obstructing the right mainstem bronchus. (A) Pretreatment. (B) Laser photoresection (note the laser fiber). (C) Argon plasma coagulation (note the blue argon plasma coagulation catheter). (D) After mechanical débridement. (E) Balloon dilation. A silicone balloon is fully inflated in the right mainstem bronchus location. (F) Stent placement. Note the self-expanding metallic stent in place. (Courtesy Dr. Eric Folch.)

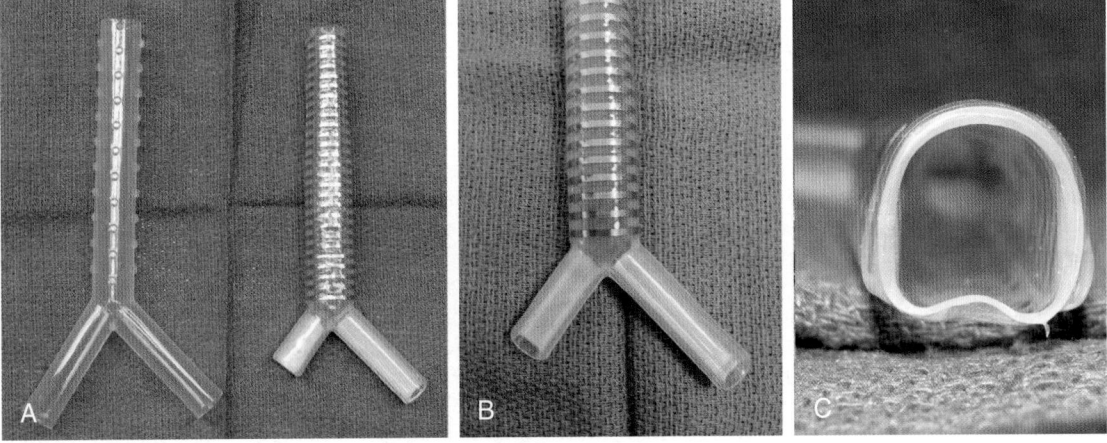

Figure 28.4 Various airway stents. (A) Silicone Y stent and Rusch Y stent. (B) Rusch Y stent (with metal anterior rings to mimic the normal trachea). (C) Rusch Y stent on end. Note the dynamic nature of the stent with a "posterior membrane."

malignant fistulas.[32] Because one of the major complications of metallic stents is epithelialization, which makes removal extremely difficult, the *U.S Food and Drug Administration* (FDA) has issued a warning against the use of metallic stents in patients with benign conditions until all therapeutic options, including use of silicone stent and surgery, have been explored. Although many of the other modalities described in this chapter can be used to treat patients with intraluminal or transmural disease, airway stents are the only bronchoscopic modality that can treat extrinsic airway compression.

Results and Complications

Airway stenting has been associated with improved quality and length of life in patients with malignant airway obstruction[11,32,47,48]; improved quality of life in patients with tracheobronchomalacia[49]; an increased ability to be liberated from the ventilator, even in patients with nonmalignant disease[50]; and improved lung function and pulmonary infection rates in patients with airway stenosis after lung transplantation.[51]

Retained secretions, bacterial colonization, migration, stent fractures, and development of granulation tissue are frequent complications, and all can be seen with any type of stent. Silicone stents tend to have a higher incidence of migration, whereas covered metallic stents are more prone to infection.[52–54] Silicone stents and the presence of lower respiratory tract infections were also found to increase the risk for granulation tissue formation. Although typically requiring rigid bronchoscopy, removal of silicone stents is a relatively easy procedure. Removal of metallic stents on the other hand, especially the uncovered/partially covered varieties, can be extremely difficult and associated with significant complications and cost.[55,56] Surveillance bronchoscopy within 4 to 6 weeks of stent placement may be useful for early detection of complications and their subsequent management because the complications, if present, are often easier to manage earlier rather than later after the patient develops symptoms.[57]

MICRODÉBRIDER

The microdébrider is a form of "powered instrumentation" that uses a spinning blade contained within a rigid suction catheter to cut tissue while providing suction to remove blood and tumor/granulation tissue[58,59] (Video 28.6). We generally use a 45-cm-long, 4-mm-wide angle-tip blade, allowing it to reach lesions in the trachea, mainstem bronchi, and bronchus intermedius. Advantages of the microdébrider are that it can be used in high-FIO_2 environments, and because it does not vaporize tissue, a specimen trap can be connected in line so that tissue can undergo pathologic analysis. The continuous suction also provides a clean operating environment. Because the microdébrider does not use any thermal energy, it is often necessary to use additional modalities, such as APC, to achieve complete hemostasis. When used by skilled operators, adverse events are rare but can include airway perforation and bleeding.

CRYOTHERAPY

Cryotherapy relies on repeated freeze-thaw cycles to cause tissue damage. Maximal cellular damage results from rapid and deep cooling and a relatively slow thaw. The Joule-Thompson effect describes the drop in temperature that develops as a gas expands from a high-pressure to a low-pressure environment. The most commonly used cooling agents (cryogens) available are nitrous oxide and carbon dioxide. The cryoprobe can be used through rigid or flexible bronchoscopes. When nitrous oxide is used, the temperature at the tip of the probe falls to −89°C within several seconds. The temperature increases approximately 10°C per mm from the tip ("warming effect"), so the effective killing zone is approximately 5 to 8 mm. Because freezing and recrystallization depend on cellular water content, cartilage and fibrous tissue are relatively cryoresistant, making it more difficult to damage the normal airway with this therapy than with other forms of thermal energy. Repeated cycles of freezing and thawing are applied to the endobronchial tissue in a contiguous fashion to cover the entire surface of the lesion. Tissue necrosis and sloughing take place within 24 to 48 hours, and a "cleanup" bronchoscopy is

usually required to remove necrotic tissue. This delayed tissue effect is one of the shortcomings of cryotherapy.[60]

Indications and Contraindications

Cryotherapy has been used for the destruction of endobronchial lesions when immediate results are not mandatory and "hot" therapies are contraindicated (Video 28.7). For example, cryotherapy is ideal for treating stent-related granulomas when the stent is made of a flammable material.[32,60] Cryotherapy can be used with excellent results in removing organic foreign objects, blood clots, and mucous plugs by cryoadhesion, as described earlier. Advantages of cryotherapy include its ability to be used in a high-oxygen environment and its limited bronchial wall damage.[60] Cryoextraction describes the related technique in which tumor in the central airways is frozen to the cryoprobe and removed en bloc with the bronchoscope.[61,62]

Results and Complications

In most cases cryotherapy offers a safe and inexpensive alternative for ablation of endobronchial tumor, with success rates up to 80%.[63,64] Kuo and colleagues[62] noted that reobstruction after cryotherapy was significantly associated with nonsquamous cell carcinoma (65.7 vs. 16.7%, $P = 0.001$). As mentioned, tumor sloughing requiring a repeat bronchoscopy and delayed maximal effect are the two major downsides of using cryotherapy for tumor excision. As a result, in the setting of acute central airway obstruction, cryotherapy should be used in conjunction with other modalities. Moderate bleeding, mediastinitis, and fistula formation after cryotherapy have also been encountered in few cases, although the risk for bleeding is likely less than with other therapies due to the vasoconstrictive and platelet-aggregating properties of cryotherapy.[11,60,62] Likewise, the risk for airway fire is nonexistent. It should be noted that the risk for bleeding may be higher when the tumor is removed by cryoextraction than when the tumor is destroyed by cryotherapy.

PHOTODYNAMIC THERAPY

Photodynamic therapy (PDT) refers to a process by which a photosensitizing drug is activated by a nonthermal laser light to induce a phototoxic reaction leading to cell death. PDT is a three-step process. On day 1 a photosensitizing agent (typically porfimer sodium) is administered intravenously. Forty-eight hours after injection, when the drug has been preferentially retained by tumor cells and cleared from most healthy tissues, the tumor is exposed to a nonthermal laser light introduced via a flexible bronchoscope. Exposure of the drug to light of wavelength 630 nm results in a photochemical reaction, including generation of oxygen radical species, direct damage to cells and organelles, indirect ischemic effects, apoptosis, and inflammatory effects. One to 2 days later, a cleanup bronchoscopy is necessary to remove the devitalized tissue, which can be difficult to expectorate and cause complications, such as postobstructive pneumonia, respiratory distress, or respiratory failure.[32]

Indications and Contraindications

PDT is indicated for the palliation of advanced non–small cell lung cancer obstructing the tracheobronchial tree and appears to be effective for superficial and submucosal disease. Curative treatment for early lung cancer/carcinoma in situ is another indication for PDT. On occasion, it is also used preoperatively to reduce the extent of surgical resection by rendering the line of resection free of disease.

Owing to its delayed effect and to possible edema after the therapy, PDT is relatively contraindicated for treatment of tracheal and carinal lesions or lesions in postpneumonectomy patients (i.e., lesions for which any swelling might precipitate total lung obstruction).[65] PDT is also contraindicated if the tumor invades vascular structures or if there is a history of porphyria and/or porphyrin hypersensitivity.

Results and Complications

PDT has been used to treat advanced lung cancer,[66] to treat multiple malignancies alone or in combination with surgery,[67] and to pretreat to reduce the extent of the surgical resection.[68] In superficial tumors a complete remission rate between 64% and 98% with PDT has been described, and balloon-sheath endobronchial ultrasonography can be invaluable in determining lack of transmural spread.[66,67,69]

Compared to other therapies, PDT is not immediately effective and therefore should not be used for acute central airway obstruction. In addition, cleanup bronchoscopy is required, and the induced systemic photosensitivity mandates that the patient avoid sunlight for 4 to 6 weeks, a potentially major drawback for those with limited life expectancy.[65,70] The most common complications include photosensitivity, local airway edema, strictures, hemorrhage, and fistula formation.[32]

BRACHYTHERAPY

Brachytherapy refers to a technique in which the radiation source is placed within or in close proximity to the target to deliver the maximum dose of radiation to the tumor while sparing the normal surrounding tissues. The radiation dose to the surrounding tissue is dictated by the inverse square law, according to which the radiation dose decreases as a function of the inverse square of the distance from the center of the source. Thus this mode of radiation therapy allows the tumor to receive significantly higher radiation doses than the surrounding healthy tissues, such as lung parenchyma and mediastinal vasculature.

For central airway lesions, a polyethylene catheter is placed adjacent to the lesion via FB and its position verified by fluoroscopy. The catheter is then loaded with the radioactive source while it is secured in position adjacent to the tumor. Low-dose-rate, intermediate-dose-rate, and high-dose-rate treatments imply a dose of less than 2 Gy/hr, 2 to 12 Gy/hr, and greater than 12 Gy/hr, respectively, to a target at a distance of 10 mm. High-dose-rate brachytherapy, which uses iridium-191 as the radiation source, is the most common form of brachytherapy and is typically applied in three treatment sessions over a week in the outpatient setting.[71] Brachytherapy requires close collaboration between the bronchoscopist and the radiation oncologist. The role of the bronchoscopist is to identify appropriate patients and place a catheter into the tracheobronchial tree, whereas the radiation oncologist calculates the radiation dose and guides the actual delivery of radiation to the tumor. The catheter may be removed after each treatment session, as in high-dose-rate brachytherapy, or left in place for the few days of treatment, as in low-dose-rate brachytherapy, an approach that often requires inpatient care.

Indications

Brachytherapy is most useful for endobronchial tumors with a component of submucosal/peribronchial disease. Brachytherapy is also useful for recurrent tumors after maximally tolerated external beam radiation. The primary goal of brachytherapy is palliation of tumor symptoms, such as cough, dyspnea, and hemoptysis. Because it requires up to 3 weeks for the tumor to regress, brachytherapy is not suitable for immediate relief of obstructive symptoms.[71] Brachytherapy is a therapeutic option for occult early-stage central lung cancers when surgery cannot be performed. Brachytherapy has also been used in management of excessive granulation tissue at the site of anastomosis in lung transplant recipients.[71]

Contraindications

Few absolute contraindications for endobronchial brachytherapy exist; one of these is the presence of fistulas involving the airways. To avoid life-threatening complications, one should exclude tumors directly involving the major vessels. Patients with endotracheal carcinoma causing high-grade obstruction should not be treated with brachytherapy because of the delayed effects and potential postradiation edema that could lead to total airway obstruction.

Results and Complications

When compared to external beam radiation, brachytherapy produced similar symptom relief but no survival benefit; thus the role of brachytherapy is mainly for palliation.[72] Brachytherapy is reported to improve cough in 20–70%, dyspnea in 25–80%, and hemoptysis in 70–90% of patients.[73] For patients who have not yet received radiation, external beam radiation therapy offers improved duration of response and survival compared with brachytherapy alone; thus external beam radiation therapy should be selected as first-line therapy instead of brachytherapy for lung cancer patients with central lesions.[72] In patients with inoperable early-stage cancer of the central airways, brachytherapy has been reported to produce a complete endoscopic response in up to 60–90% with 5-year survival rates of 30–80%.[71,74,75]

Complications include respiratory compromise, massive hemoptysis, fistula formation, radiation bronchitis, and airway stenosis. Fatal hemoptysis has been reported in up to 5–10% of patients.[74,75] The risk for late exsanguination has been found to be highest in patients receiving brachytherapy to the right upper lobe, owing to its close proximity to the pulmonary artery.[71,74]

MANAGING OTHER INDICATIONS

Bronchoscopy has emerged as a therapeutic option for some of the most common respiratory diseases, such as COPD and asthma. The emergence of new technology and its utility in small obstructive airway disease management is supported by ongoing research focused on appropriate patient selection, and short- and long-term outcomes.

BRONCHOSCOPIC LUNG VOLUME REDUCTION

Until recently the only options for patients with advanced emphysema in the United States were the use of supplemental oxygen, lung volume-reduction surgery, and lung transplantation.[76] The National Emphysema Treatment Trial demonstrated that, in patients with heterogeneous emphysema with upper lobe predominance and low exercise capacity, lung volume-reduction surgery significantly improves lung function, exercise tolerance, quality of life, and survival.[77] Unfortunately the associated morbidity and mortality of the procedure have limited its widespread application. Bronchoscopic treatments of emphysema were introduced to achieve the beneficial physiologic changes seen with surgical lung volume reduction. In June 2018 the FDA approved endobronchial Zephyr valves manufactured by Pulmonx, as the first bronchoscopic treatment in the United States for patients with heterogeneous emphysema and minimal collateral ventilation.

Indications and Contraindications

Endobronchial treatment of severe emphysema has been studied for over a decade and has been approved in several countries around the world. Due to the lack of data on long-term and clinically meaningful benefits of bronchoscopic lung volume reduction, endobronchial treatment was not approved for use by the FDA until recently.[76] Various devices and chemical agents have been used via the endobronchial route to reduce lung volumes in a relatively noninvasive fashion.[78-83] The majority of studies have focused on patients with heterogeneous (i.e., upper lobe predominant) emphysema, although some have also investigated patients with homogeneous disease. Due to scarcity of long-term outcome data for most of these techniques and devices, the ideal patient population for each specific approach will need to be defined. The following section provides a brief review of current knowledge related to concepts of bronchoscopic lung volume reduction.

Endobronchial Valves

Endobronchial valves are one-way valves designed to allow air to exit the targeted lung segment without allowing reentry of the inspired air, thus leading to deflation of the emphysematous portion of the lung and volume reduction (Fig. 28.5). Two different types of valves, the Zephyr valve and *intrabronchial valve* (IBV; Olympus), have been recently approved by the FDA. For either of these valves, the ability to deflate the lung, and thus the benefit of their use, may depend on the lack of collateral ventilation to the abnormal segment (Videos 28.8 and 28.9).

The *Pulmonx Endobronchial Valves Used in Treatment of Emphysema Study* (LIBERATE) randomized, multicenter, international study was conducted in patients with severe heterogeneous emphysema. Before randomization, all patients were shown to have little or no collateral ventilation by use of a bronchoscopic system (Chartis; Pulmonx) that has an effectiveness of approximately 75% in predicting clinical improvement after lobar occlusion.[83] LIBERATE examined the safety, efficacy, and durability of benefits of Zephyr endobronchial valves for 12 months in comparison to optimal medical care without valves.[84] Compared to those without valves, patients with endobronchial valves

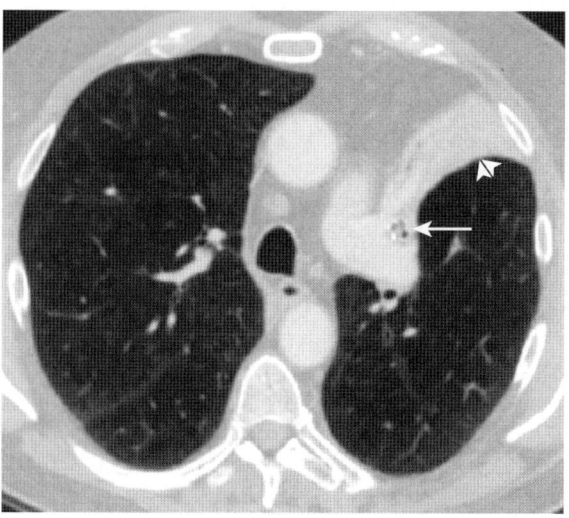

Figure 28.5 Complete left upper lobe collapse after endobronchial valve placement. The valve was placed in a patient with COPD for lung volume reduction. Axial chest computed tomography displayed in lung windows shows complete collapse of the left upper lobe (*arrowheads*) after placement of left upper lobe endobronchial valves (*arrow*). (Courtesy Steve Tseng, DO, Pulmonary and Critical Care Medicine, University of Arizona College of Medicine—Phoenix.)

were more likely to have at least a 15% improvement in postbronchodilator *forced expiratory volume in 1 second* (FEV$_1$) (47.7% endobronchial valve and 16.8% control, P < 0.001). The endobronchial valve group also showed significant improvements in secondary outcomes, including absolute changes in postbronchodilator FEV$_1$, 6-minute walk distance, and St. George's Respiratory Questionnaire scores. Pneumothorax, the most common serious adverse event, was seen only in the endobronchial valve group (26.5%, all during the first 45 days).

The IBV Valve for Emphysema to Improve Lung Function Study (EMPROVE) was another randomized multicenter study in emphysema patients with heterogeneous emphysema and no evidence of collateral ventilation via a chest computed tomography assessment of fissure integrity. The results of EMPROVE achieved the primary end point, and the valve was also approved by the FDA in December 2018.[85]

Bronchial Lung Volume-Reduction Coils

The bronchial lung volume-reduction coil (PneumRx) is made of nitinol wires that, when deployed by advancing into the bronchus via the bronchoscope, retract and fold the parenchyma, thus reducing lung volume in abnormal areas. The benefit of this approach is that the presence of collateral ventilation does not affect its efficacy. A single-center open-label pilot study in Germany using lung volume-reduction coils showed improved quality of life, pulmonary function, and 6-minute walk distance.[86] The *Lung Volume-Reduction Coil for Treatment in Patients with Emphysema Study* (RENEW), a multicenter, randomized phase III trial, was conducted in patients with severe emphysema and evidence of severe air trapping.[87] The primary outcome was the difference in absolute change in 6-minute walk distance between baseline and 12 months. The study showed that among patients with emphysema and severe hyperinflation treated for 12 months, the use of endobronchial coils compared with usual care resulted in an improvement in median exercise tolerance that was modest and of uncertain clinical importance, with a higher likelihood of major complications, such as pneumonia, requiring hospitalization and other potentially life-threatening or fatal events. As such, this device was not approved by the FDA for use in the United States; however, it is available in Europe.

Biologic Sealant

Bronchoscopic lung volume reduction using direct application of a biologic sealant to collapse areas of emphysematous lung has been reported. Initial tests of a synthetic polymeric foam sealant (emphysematous lung sealant, AeriSeal; Aeris Therapeutics) have shown improvements in pulmonary function, exercise capacity, and quality of life.[81] It should be noted that fissure integrity may not be as important with this method of achieving bronchoscopic lung volume reduction because the sealant may block sites of collateral ventilation.[88] A pivotal trial, study of the *AeriSeal System for Hyperinflation Reduction in Emphysema* (ASPIRE), was terminated for financial reasons.[76]

Bronchoscopic Thermal Vapor Ablation

Bronchoscopic thermal vapor ablation involves delivery of a precise dose of steam water vapor at a precise temperature directly into the targeted lung segments via a specialized catheter. The thermal reaction produces a localized inflammatory response leading to fibrosis and atelectasis. This results in complete and permanent lung volume reduction. Improvements in pulmonary function and quality of life have been reported with this technique in preliminary studies.[89] As with the coils and biologic sealants, a potential advantage of bronchoscopic thermal vapor ablation is that success is independent of the presence or absence of collateral ventilation.[90]

Complications

Because these procedures are performed in patients with severe underlying emphysema, complications can be expected. The more common complications include transient reductions in lung function, flares of bronchitis or pneumonia, and pneumothorax. Whereas placement of valves is reversible, the placement of coils, instillation of sealant, and ablation via bronchoscopic thermal vapor are irreversible.

BRONCHIAL THERMOPLASTY FOR SEVERE ASTHMA

Bronchial thermoplasty (BT) is a novel bronchoscopic treatment for patients with severe asthma aiming to reduce the airway smooth muscle mass, therefore diminishing bronchial constriction and improving asthma symptoms.[91] This is accomplished by delivering controlled heat to the airway walls via a radiofrequency electrical generator and a disposable catheter with an expandable four-electrode basket at its distal tip (Fig. 28.6). BT is performed in three bronchoscopy sessions, 2 to 3 weeks apart. The first two sessions treat each lower lobe separately, and the third session treats both upper lobes; the right middle lobe is not treated because it was not included in the original study protocols, although inclusion of the right middle lobe has been shown to be feasible.[92] Radiofrequency energy is delivered in a systematic fashion at 5-mm intervals, starting from just beyond the endoscopic visual limit sequentially to the proximal lobar bronchi.

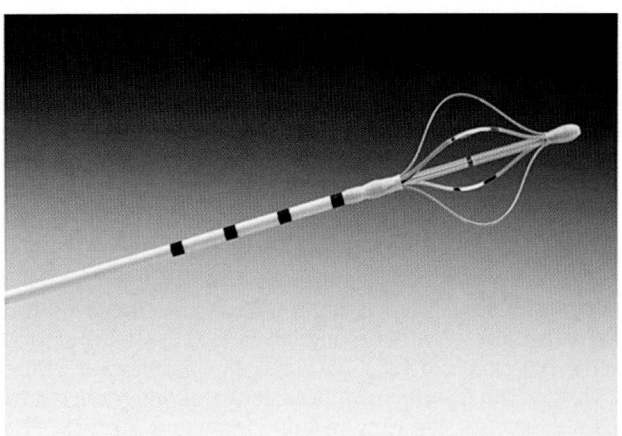

Figure 28.6 Catheter used for bronchial thermoplasty. The disposable catheter contains a four-electrode basket that delivers controlled heat to the airways.

Indications and Contraindications

BT is indicated in adult patients with severe persistent asthma who remain symptomatic despite maximal medical treatment. Concomitant medical conditions that can contribute to asthma symptoms should be sought and treated before resorting to this treatment. In addition, BT should not be used as a substitute for medication compliance. Contraindications for BT include the presence of an implantable electronic device and severe comorbid conditions that increase the risk of the procedure. In children (age < 18 years), the procedure has not been studied and is not approved.

Results and Complications

In multiple studies performed in patients with asthma of various severity, BT has been shown to reduce asthma exacerbations and improve quality of life.[93–97] Adverse events were limited to an increase in asthma exacerbations in the perioperative period.[93–97]

The definitive study of BT, which led to FDA approval, used a randomized double-blind, sham-controlled design of 288 subjects with severe persistent asthma.[97] Patients receiving BT had improvement in quality of life based on a questionnaire but, most important, had a 30% reduction in severe exacerbations, an 80% reduction in emergency department visits, and a decrease in days missed from work or school. The short-term adverse events included airway inflammation and upper respiratory infections that resolved with conventional treatment. There was a higher rate of hospitalization in the BT group in the postprocedure period. In a 5-year follow-up of 162 patients enrolled in the study, the procedure was shown to be safe and its benefits durable.[98] In a similar multicenter study of 279 patients, the findings were reproduced; at the 3-year follow-up, there was a 45% reduction in severe exacerbation, 55% decrease in emergency department visits and 40% decrease in hospitalization rate compared to the control group.[99]

No comparative data between BT and biologic therapy, such as targeted monoclonal antibodies, are currently available.[100]

ENDOBRONCHIAL VALVE PLACEMENT FOR PERSISTENT AIR LEAKS

Persistent air leaks after thoracic surgery are a common complication, reported in up to 18% of patients undergoing lobectomy or lesser resections, and are associated with prolonged hospitalizations, morbidity, and considerable health care costs.[101–103] The usual management of these patients includes prolonged tube thoracostomy drainage, pleurodesis, or attempts at surgical repair. The IBV endobronchial valve, initially developed as an approach to achieve bronchoscopic lung volume reduction in patients with emphysema, has received FDA approval as a humanitarian use device for the treatment of persistent leak after lobectomy, segmentectomy, or lung volume-reduction surgery. The procedure is performed under deep sedation/general anesthesia and begins with selective balloon occlusion of the suspected airways; when the culprit airway is occluded, a significant reduction or cessation of the leak can be visualized in the water-seal chamber of the chest drainage system. A calibrated balloon is used to select the proper-sized valve, which is then placed under bronchoscopic control. It is common that multiple valves are used in each case because many patients have a degree of collateral ventilation. After 6 weeks the valves are removed. IBV use in this patient population has been associated with cessation of the air leak as soon as 1 day after placement and hospital discharge within 3 days in the majority of patients. Although complications can theoretically include postobstructive pneumonia, hypoxemia, and valve migration, these seem to be quite rare. In a recent systematic review of available literature in the form of case reports and case series comprising 208 patients, the most common underlying etiologies were emphysema and cancer, and valves were used most often in postlobectomy and other causes of persistent air leak.[104] In their analysis, upper lobes were found to be the most frequent location of air leaks. Complete resolution was gained within less than 24 hours in the majority of patients, and no deaths were reported due to valve implantation. The most common complications were migration or expectoration of valves, moderate oxygen desaturation, and infection of the treated lung. More data are required before the use of endobronchial valves can be recommended for other causes of persistent air leaks, such as in the setting of secondary spontaneous pneumothorax.

Key Points

- Rigid and flexible bronchoscopy are essential tools for the interventional pulmonologist.
- Therapeutic bronchoscopy can improve quality and length of life in patients with central airway obstruction.
- Each therapeutic bronchoscopic modality has its own advantages and disadvantages; it is hoped that, with ongoing research, the best use of these techniques will be determined.
- Patients with central airway obstruction are best served by a multidisciplinary team of an interventional pulmonologist, thoracic surgeon, head and neck surgeon, anesthesiologist, and medical and radiation oncologist.
- Central airway obstruction with tumor can be approached by immediate (e.g., laser, stent) or delayed approaches (e.g., cryotherapy, photodynamic therapy). Techniques with immediate action should be selected when urgent therapy is needed or when any swelling would compromise ventilation.
- The hot techniques (electrocautery, argon plasma coagulation, laser photoresection) have immediate effects but cannot be used in a high-FIO_2 environment because of the risk for fire. For immediate therapy in a high-FIO_2 setting, a stent or microdébrider can be considered.
- Stent placement is the only technique that can treat extrinsic airway compression.
- Lung volume reduction can now be achieved via bronchoscopic techniques, including one-way endobronchial valves. One-way valves are reversible and affected by collateral flow; lung volume-reduction coils, biologic sealants, and thermal vapor ablation are irreversible and may be useful even in the presence of collateral air ventilation.
- Bronchial thermoplasty is indicated only in adult patients with severe persistent asthma who remain symptomatic despite maximal medical treatment and consideration of other causes of asthma exacerbation, such as acid reflux or chronic respiratory infections.

Key Readings

Amjadi K, Voduc N, Cruysberghs Y, et al. Impact of interventional bronchoscopy on quality of life in malignant airway obstruction. *Respiration.* 2008;76:421–428.

Becker HD. Gustav Killian: a biographical sketch. *J Bronchol.* 1995;2:77–83.

Bolliger CT, Sutedja TG, Strausz J, et al. Therapeutic bronchoscopy with immediate effect: laser, electrocautery, argon plasma coagulation and stents. *Eur Respir J.* 2006;27:1258–1271.

Castro M, Rubin AS, Laviolette M, et al. Effectiveness and safety of bronchial thermoplasty in the treatment of severe asthma: a multicenter, randomized, double-blind, sham-controlled clinical trial. *Am J Respir Crit Care Med.* 2010;181:116–124.

Chhajed PN, Baty F, Somandin S, et al. Outcome of treated advanced non-small cell lung cancer with and without central airway obstruction. *Chest.* 2006;130:1803–1807.

Colt HG, Harrell JH. Therapeutic rigid bronchoscopy allows level of care changes in patients with acute respiratory failure from central airway obstruction. *Chest.* 1997;112:202–206.

Cox G, Thomson NC, Rubin AS, et al. Asthma control during the year after bronchial thermoplasty. *N Engl J Med.* 2007;356:1327–1337.

Criner GJ, Sue R, Wright S, et al. A multicenter randomized controlled trial of Zephyr Endobronchial Valve Treatment in Heterogeneous Emphysema (LIBERATE). *Am J Respir Crit Care Med.* 2018;198(9):1151–1164.

Ernst A, Feller-Kopman D, Becker H, et al. State of the art: central airway obstruction. *Am J Respir Crit Care Med.* 2004;169:1278–1297.

Grosu HB, Debiane L, et al. Long-term quality-adjusted survival following therapeutic bronchoscopy for malignant central airway obstruction. *Thorax.* 2019;74(2):141–156.

Lamb C, Feller-Kopman D, Ernst A, et al. An approach to interventional pulmonary fellowship training. *Chest.* 2010;137:195–199.

Ost D, Ernst A, Grosu HB, et al. Complications following therapeutic bronchoscopy for malignant central airway obstruction: results of the AQuIRE Registry. *Chest.* 2015;148(2):450–471.

Ost DE, Shah AM, Lei X, et al. Respiratory infections increase the risk of granulation tissue formation following airway stenting in patients with malignant airway obstruction. *Chest.* 2012;141:1473–1481.

Pastis NJ, Nietert PJ, Silvestri GA. Variation in training for interventional pulmonary procedures among US pulmonary/critical care fellowships: a survey of fellowship directors. *Chest.* 2005;127:1614–1621.

Sciurba FC, Criner GJ, Strange C, et al. Effect of endobronchial coils vs usual care on exercise tolerance in patients with severe emphysema: the RENEW randomized clinical trial. *JAMA.* 2016;315(20):2178–2189.

Seijo LM, Sterman DH. Interventional pulmonology. *N Engl J Med.* 2001;344:740–749.

Complete reference list available at ExpertConsult.com.

29 *THORACOSCOPY*

NAJIB M. RAHMAN, BM, BCH, MA(OXON), MSC, FRCP, DPHIL • MOHAMMED MUNAVVAR, MD, DNB, FRCP(LON), FRCP(EDIN)

INTRODUCTION

Biopsy procedures play an essential role in the diagnostic evaluation of patients with respiratory diseases. Most of the techniques used today were developed and refined during the 20th century. Recently, significant advances in endoscopic technology have provided sophisticated endoscopic instruments and endoscopic telescopes with extremely high optical resolution and small diameters. In addition, developments in anesthesiology offer a wide range of alternatives, from procedures performed under local anesthesia to selective double-lumen intubation under general anesthesia.

As with all medical procedures, the risk/benefit ratio of invasive methods must be considered for each individual patient by weighing the risk for morbidity and mortality against the benefit of obtaining the diagnosis either to guide correct therapy or to provide clarity on prognosis and clinical trajectory. More invasive procedures are used if less invasive methods have failed and if therapeutic options can be combined with a diagnostic modality.

This chapter reviews the more invasive procedures associated with pleural disease, performed thoracoscopically and by pulmonologists. Other invasive pulmonary methods, including bronchoscopic biopsies, thoracentesis, needle biopsy of lung lesions, and nonthoracoscopic biopsy of the pleura, are described in other chapters.

THORACOSCOPY (PLEUROSCOPY/ MEDICAL THORACOSCOPY)

 A brief history of the use of thoracoscopy is available at ExpertConsult.com.

The terms *thoracoscopy*, *medical thoracoscopy*, and *pleuroscopy* are used interchangeably in the literature. To avoid confusion, this chapter uses the term *thoracoscopy* for the procedure performed by the pulmonologist, and consequently the terms *thoracoscopist* and *thoracoscope*, whether rigid or semirigid. For the thoracoscopic procedure performed by a surgeon, the term *video-assisted thoracic surgery* (VATS) is used. This procedure is technically very similar to thoracoscopy, with some important differences. First, the surgeon can perform procedures on the lung, whereas the pulmonologist usually, but not always, confines the biopsies and interventions to the pleura. Second, VATS is usually performed with the patient under general anesthesia and intubated and ventilated using a double-lumen endotracheal tube that allows selective blockage of a main bronchus and thus collapse of the lung. Although VATS has significant advantages, producing a pneumothorax cavity in which to operate regardless of the state of the lung, it is associated with the normal risks of general anesthesia and may not be suitable in all patients.

In both Europe and the United States, thoracoscopy is part of the training program of interventional pulmonary medicine.[15] According to a national survey in 1994, thoracoscopy was used frequently by 5% of all pulmonary physicians.[16] The interest in the technique seems to be increasing.[17] However, training is lagging: In an American College of Chest Physicians survey of U.S. pulmonary/critical care fellowship programs in 2002–03, only 12% of the directors stated that thoracoscopy was offered in their programs.[18] In the United Kingdom, where thoracoscopy has been increasing compared with the rest of Europe, there is also growing interest, with a doubling in the number of centers offering thoracoscopy over a 5-year period.[19–21] In 2010, the *British Thoracic Society* (BTS) published a guideline on thoracoscopy using local anesthetic, which has driven further interest and quality standards.[22] In this guideline, three levels of competence in thoracoscopy are defined, of which level 1 includes basic diagnostic and therapeutic techniques and level 2 including the more advanced techniques, whereas level 3 covers all VATS techniques (e.g., lung resection) and is considered the province of the thoracic surgeon.[22]

Meanwhile, the technique has been introduced successfully in many Asian countries and in other parts of the world, particularly with the introduction of the semirigid (semiflexible) thoracoscope.[11,23–25]

TECHNIQUES

Thoracoscopy is an invasive technique that should be used to obtain a diagnosis when other simpler methods are nondiagnostic, in case of pleural exudates, or to achieve pleurodesis, in case of recurrent pleural effusion or pneumothorax.[26] As with all technical procedures, there is a learning curve before full competence is achieved,[27–29] and appropriate training is mandatory.[10,29,30] The technique involves insertion between the ribs into the pleural space of a rigid or semirigid trocar, through which fluid is aspirated and air is allowed to enter. The thoracoscope is then inserted to visualize the pleural cavity and conduct biopsies or other interventions. Insertion of the trocar is conducted with a thorough local anesthetic technique and then blunt dissection, using an incision in the skin of no more than 1 cm; as such, this part of the technique is very similar to insertion of a "surgical" or large-bore chest tube. Once the scope is in the pleural space, the thoracoscopist can visualize and obtain biopsies as appropriate from all areas of the pleural cavity, including the chest wall, diaphragm, mediastinum, and lung, under direct visual control. When indicated, talc poudrage can be performed.

There are two different techniques of diagnostic and therapeutic thoracoscopy, as performed by the pulmonary physician.[10,27,31–33] In the first technique, a single entry site is usually produced with a trocar for a thoracoscope with a working channel for accessory instruments and optical biopsy forceps.[5] This approach can be modified for use of a semirigid thoracoscope, also called the pleuroscope.[11,23] In the other technique, two entry sites are used: one with a trocar for the examination telescope and the other with a smaller trocar for accessory instruments, including the biopsy forceps. For both techniques, adequate local anesthesia and conscious sedation are used, with some operators preferring deep sedation or general anesthesia.[12,27] In some countries the use of heavily sedating medications, such as propofol, even in the absence of intubation, requires the presence of an anesthesiologist.

With increasing data on the use of thoracic ultrasound, it is generally agreed that ultrasound should be performed "live" just before the procedure to identify the best entry site and the presence of septations and adhesions.[22,31,34,35]

EQUIPMENT

Rigid

Rigid instruments are still used for thoracoscopy,[32] although more recently the semirigid thoracoscope has become an attractive option. The requirement for full sterilization of the equipment had been a limitation in the use of semirigid tools until the development of a modified semirigid thoracoscope with a flexible tip that could tolerate sterilization.[23,24]

The single entry site technique is usually performed via a 7 or 9 mm diameter trocar and a cannula. Trocars are available with diameters of 5 and 3.75 mm for performing thoracoscopy in children. Optical devices exist with various fields of view (0, 30, and 90 degrees) (Fig. 29.1).

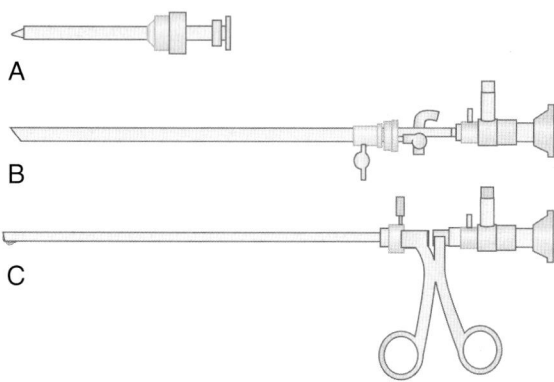

Figure 29.1 Instruments for thoracoscopy. (A) Trocar and cannula with valve. (B) Single-incision thoracoscope (9 mm diameter). (C) Biopsy forceps with straight optics. (Modified from Loddenkemper R. Thoracoscopy—state of the art. *Eur Respir J.* 1998;11:213–221.)

Alternatively, a mini-thoracoscope is available, requiring two ports for biopsy, with the use of a rigid optical telescope of 3 mm and a trocar with a diameter of 4 mm, providing somewhat limited views but a similar size to a needle aspiration catheter.[33] This instrument is particularly helpful in the initial evaluation of small pleural effusions or in the presence of a narrow intercostal space. A second port of entry is necessary in these cases to obtain biopsy specimens. For talc pleurodesis, a talc atomizer is used.[27]

The two-entry-site technique uses a 7-mm trocar for the first site of entry for appropriate telescopes and forceps and similar accessory instruments. For the second site of entry, a 5-mm trocar is used for insertion of instruments designed for its smaller bore, including a loop for dividing adhesions and a double-lumen insufflator.[27]

Semirigid

The semirigid (semiflexible) thoracoscope offers several useful features.[11,23,24] The design, including the handle, is similar to that of a standard flexible bronchoscope; however, the proximal 22 cm is stiff, and the distal 5 cm is bendable with an angulation of 160 and 130 degrees (Fig. 29.2). The outer diameter of the shaft is 7 mm, and a working channel of a diameter of 2.8 mm allows the use of standard instruments available for flexible bronchoscopy. The scope is inserted using a dedicated, soft trocar/cannula of approximately the same size as that used for a rigid procedure. The skills involved in operating the instrument are already familiar to the practicing bronchoscopist. Because the shaft is rigid, it can be moved like the rigid thoracoscope without losing the orientation, and it is compatible with the video processors and light sources of the same manufacturer. The flexible tip permits easier visualization of the entire pleural cavity and permits a homogeneous distribution of talc on all surfaces.[11] The potential easier navigation technique around the pleural space, using the flexible tip, may put less pressure on the surrounding ribs and thus result in a more comfortable procedure. In addition, more advanced imaging techniques, such as narrow band imaging, are feasible through the semirigid thoracoscope, which may have the potential to increase diagnostic yield by better identification of early malignant change,[36,37] although prospective data are currently lacking.

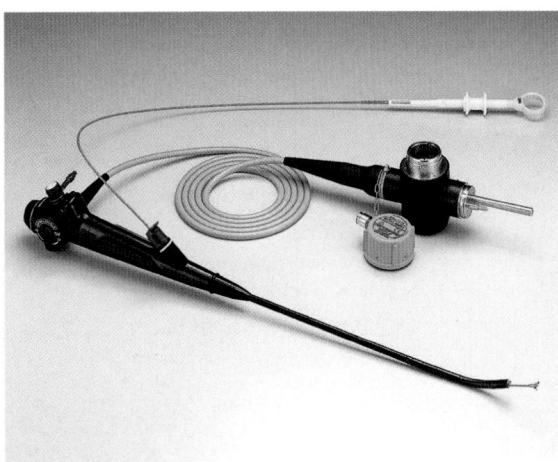

Figure 29.2 The semirigid (semiflexible) thoracoscope (Olympus Corporation). The control section allows handling as with the flexible bronchoscope. (Copyright Olympus SE & Co. KG.)

There are some disadvantages of the semirigid instrument compared to more traditional rigid scopes. The flexible scope is more costly and there may be smaller biopsy specimens, although the diagnostic yield in pleural disease has been shown to be comparable with that of the conventional rigid thoracoscope.[11,38] It should be noted that the only direct randomized trial of the two techniques showed a higher diagnostic yield using the rigid scope in the intention-to-treat population,[39] although there were methodologic issues with this study. In some cases, the flexible forceps used with the thoracoscope may not have the mechanical strength to obtain pleural biopsy specimens of sufficient depth, which may reduce the diagnostic yield in mesothelioma. This technical problem can be overcome by the use of a various techniques (diathermic knife, cryobiopsy),[40–42] which may also have a role in lysing pleuropulmonary adhesions.

Environment

The procedure suite should be equipped with monopolar or bipolar electrocoagulation (in units where adhesion division is practiced, with bipolar electrocautery having the advantage of not requiring grounding unlike monopolar), as well as equipment for resuscitation and assisted ventilation; electrocardiography; blood pressure monitoring; and a defibrillator, an oxygen source, and vacuum generators.[22,27] Thoracoscopy can be performed in the operating room or in an environment dedicated to invasive procedures.[10,24] Besides the physician, there should be an endoscopy nurse (or an endoscopy assistant) to assist with the instrumentation and an additional assistant outside the sterile field to bring necessary equipment.[22,29] Ideally, an additional person sits at the patient's head end and monitors his or her overall condition. In an emergency, thoracoscopy can be performed with only a physician and a nurse, but this is less efficient and prolongs the procedure. There is now increasing evidence that medical thoracoscopy can be performed safely in an entirely outpatient setting.[43,44]

INDICATIONS

Thoracoscopy today is primarily a diagnostic procedure but can also be applied for therapeutic purposes (Table 29.1).[10,12,45] Thoracoscopy is mainly used for diagnosis of exudates of unknown cause, for staging of diffuse malignant mesothelioma or lung cancer, and for treatment by talc pleurodesis of malignant or other recurrent effusions.[46] Thoracoscopy is also a possible technique for diagnostic biopsies from the diaphragm, lung, mediastinum, and pericardium, and for more elaborate procedures; although, because of the increased risk of complications, these applications should be restricted to highly expert individuals.[13,14] As mentioned earlier, there is an overlap of indications between thoracoscopy and VATS (see later discussion and Table 29.1). In addition, thoracoscopy offers a remarkable tool for research in the study of pleural effusions.

Diagnostic thoracoscopy has its main and oldest use for the diagnosis of pleural effusions, as described by Jacobaeus himself in his earliest articles.[2] The diagnostic value of thoracoscopy grew to include evaluation and diagnosis of spontaneous pneumothorax, focal pulmonary disease, diseases of the chest wall, mediastinal tumors, diseases of the heart and great vessels, and thoracic trauma. Later, these indications were expanded to include performing biopsies for localized and diffuse lung diseases.[10] Today the use of thoracoscopy for diagnosis of lung diseases has decreased owing to the improvements in less invasive pulmonary biopsy techniques, such as flexible bronchoscopic biopsy and *computed tomography* (CT)-guided biopsy, as well as higher confidence in diagnosis of interstitial lung disease from CT imaging and clinical features alone.

In the past, *therapeutic* thoracoscopy was used extensively for collapse treatment of *tuberculosis* (TB) to sever adhesions that prevented a complete artificial pneumothorax.[3,47] This indication disappeared after the successful introduction of chemotherapy for TB. Today the main indication for therapeutic thoracoscopy is talc poudrage in malignant or other chronic and recurrent pleural effusions.[48] The first report on *talcage* was published in 1935[46] and, in 1963, it was first used for treating recurrent effusions.[47] Since then, talc poudrage performed during thoracoscopy for pleurodesis in malignant pleural effusions has been widely applied, especially in Europe. Talc pleurodesis via thoracoscopy has been thought to have advantages over pleurodesis with talc slurry via a thoracostomy tube: simultaneous drainage of pleural fluid, visualization of the visceral pleura to ensure that the lung is not encased by pleural thickening or tumor that could prevent reexpansion (Video 29.1), and guidance of chest tube placement.[49]

However, increasing data, including high-quality randomized studies, demonstrate that the overall pleurodesis success rate in malignant pleural effusion is not higher via poudrage than slurry and, in our view, should not be preferred over talc slurry as a stand-alone therapeutic procedure (see later for a review of the data). The main advantage of talc poudrage via thoracoscopy is the single-procedure approach, whereby, if there is clear macroscopic evidence of tumor, the malignant effusion can be fully drained, high-yield biopsies obtained, and talc poudrage performed at one time. In addition, talc pleurodesis can be used to prevent recurrent pneumothorax, although it should be noted

Table 29.1 Indications for Thoracoscopy (Medical Thoracoscopy) vs. VATS (Surgical Thoracoscopy)

Thoracoscopy	Thoracoscopy or VATS (Gray Area)	VATS
PLEURAL EFFUSIONS	**SPONTANEOUS PNEUMOTHORAX**	**LUNG PROCEDURES**
■ Pleural effusions of unknown cause ■ Staging of lung cancer ■ Staging of tumor in diffuse malignant mesothelioma ■ Pleurodesis by talc poudrage	■ Inspection/evaluation ■ Pleurodesis by talc poudrage	■ Lung biopsy ■ Lobectomy ■ Lung volume-reduction surgery
	EMPYEMA (STAGE I/II)	**PLEURAL PROCEDURES**
	■ Drainage	■ Pleurectomy (pneumothorax) ■ Drainage/decortication (empyema stage III)
	DIFFUSE PULMONARY DISEASES	
	■ Biopsy	**ESOPHAGEAL PROCEDURES**
	LOCALIZED LESIONS	■ Excision of cyst, benign tumors ■ Esophagectomy ■ Antireflux procedures
	■ Chest wall, diaphragm ■ Sympathectomy ■ Splanchnicectomy	**MEDIASTINAL PROCEDURES**
		■ Resection of mediastinal mass ■ Thoracic lymphadenectomy ■ Thoracic duct ligation ■ Pericardial window ■ Sympathectomy

VATS, video-assisted thoracic surgery.

that the presence of normal parietal pleura in these cases means that the procedure is potentially very painful, and deep sedation or general anesthesia should be considered for these cases.[50]

Other indications for therapeutic thoracoscopy are the drainage of early empyema[12] or dorsal sympathectomy in patients with hyperhidrosis.[14] Anecdotal reports describe its use for removal of foreign bodies,[51] for removal of benign tumors, and for the production of pericardial fenestrations, although we believe that these techniques are best conducted in the highly controlled environment of VATS.

CONTRAINDICATIONS

Contraindications to thoracoscopy are few and rarely absolute.[22] The main limitation is the size of the free pleural space. If extensive adhesions prevent the lung from collapsing away from the chest wall, thoracoscopy can still be performed, using *extended thoracoscopy*, where manual dissection is used to create a pleural space to conduct biopsies, but this requires special skill and should not be undertaken without appropriate training.[52]

Although the majority of thoracoscopy cases are performed in patients with pleural effusion, the technique is possible in cases with small or no pleural effusion, for example, where there are pleural nodules or thickening in the absence of pleural fluid. This technique requires induction of a pneumothorax, which is performed using a pneumothorax induction needle, known as the Boutin needle, in which there is a front- and side-facing opening to allow entrainment of air. Increasing evidence demonstrates that the use of preprocedure ultrasound can predict the presence of a freely moving lung and therefore a nonadhered pleural space.[35]

Several factors are relative contraindications to thoracoscopy; these include a persistent cough, hypoxemia, hypocoagulability (prolonged international normalized ratio or platelet count <40,000–60,000/μL), and cardiac abnormalities. Hypercarbia indicative of respiratory failure may

prove to be an absolute contraindication, except in patients with a tension pneumothorax or massive pleural effusion, in whom it can be anticipated that thoracoscopy would provide therapeutic benefit in addition to a possible diagnosis. Under these conditions, premedication should be administered judiciously to minimize respiratory center depression. In cases of respiratory compromise, consideration should be given to conducting VATS in preference, with the advantage of full anesthetic control, but with the understanding that this will require complete single-lung ventilation and general anesthesia.

Concerning lung biopsy via thoracoscopy, contraindications include suspicion of arteriovenous pulmonary aneurysm, vascular tumors, hydatid cysts, or a stiff fibrotic lung because of a higher risk for persistent bronchopleural fistulae. After lung biopsy in patients with interstitial lung disease, Vansteenkiste and coworkers[53] found that the pleural drainage time was on average 5.3 ± 4.7 days and was related to the total lung capacity, which mirrors the severity and stiffness of interstitial lung disease. Relative contraindications for lung biopsy include previous systemic steroid or immunosuppressive therapy because, under these circumstances, bronchopleural fistulas resulting from lung biopsy may heal poorly. However, due to increased risk of fistula and the increased need to handle complications such as bleeding, we do not recommend lung biopsy via thoracoscopy be performed by physicians except in specific circumstances and by specific operators.

COMPLICATIONS

Thoracoscopy is a safe and effective modality in the diagnosis and treatment of several pleuropulmonary diseases if certain standard criteria are fulfilled.[22,55] In the most thorough review, there was only one death among 8000 cases, for a mortality rate of 0.01%.[54] In another series reviewing 4300 cases, the mortality rate was 0.09%.[27] The reported mortality rate of thoracoscopy is thus roughly equivalent to or less than that of transbronchial biopsies. The major complication rate in a series of 102 patients was 1.9% and included ventricular tachycardia responding to resuscitation, subcutaneous emphysema, and persistent air leak.[56] The minor complication rate was 7.5%, including transient air leak, fever, and minor bleeding at biopsy sites. Another large series including 360 patients reported morbidities of fever in 9.8%, empyema in 2.5%, pulmonary infection in 0.8%, and malignant invasion of the scar in 0.3%.[57] Major uncontrollable bleeding requiring thoracotomy was not reported in any of these large series and appears to be extremely rare. In case of persistent bleeding, electrocoagulation may become necessary,[27] and operators should have a plan of escalation in case of uncontrolled bleeding, such as involvement of interventional radiology or surgery.

Reexpansion pulmonary edema from the removal of large pleural effusions is infrequent; this is likely to be because immediate equilibration of the pleural pressure is provided by direct entrance of air through the cannula into the pleural space, with the lung allowed to expand only at procedure end. Bronchopleural fistulas may follow lung biopsies; if the lungs are stiff, a fistula may require longer to heal than the usual 3- to 5-day period of chest tube drainage.[27] Local site infection is uncommon, and empyema has been reported rarely.[54] In cases of mesothelioma, the late complication of tumor growth at the site of entry has been observed after thoracoscopy and also after thoracentesis or closed-needle biopsy. Radiation therapy 10 to 12 days after thoracoscopy has been used to prevent this late complication,[58] although adequately powered randomized trials indicate that the routine use of prophylactic radiation therapy in these cases is not required.[59] After talc poudrage, any postprocedure fever, such as a nonspecific inflammatory reaction, and pain can be treated symptomatically.

In the studies reviewed in the evidence-based BTS medical thoracoscopy guideline review of 2010,[22] the mortality from thoracoscopy was low and, for diagnostic procedures only (i.e., not using poudrage), was close to 0%. The reported mortality rate in this review was largely driven by the large randomized trial of thoracoscopy poudrage[60] in which small-particle talc was used; small-particle talc has been shown to be associated with lung inflammation and acute respiratory distress syndrome, most likely because of dissemination of the smaller talc via the lymphatics to the circulation.[61] Studies have demonstrated that use of large-particle (graded) talc is not associated with lung inflammation[62]; thus, if poudrage is conducted, graded talc should be used. With the use of graded, larger-particle talc, the mortality rate from thoracoscopy should be quite low, nearly 0%.

In conclusion, the overall mortality rate with thoracoscopy is extremely low. Morbidity, which is mainly due to benign postprocedural fever, is minimal.

PATIENT PREPARATION

Before planning thoracoscopy, the patient should provide informed consent and receive information on major and minor complication rates; diagnostic sensitivity and the rationale for treatment should also be discussed. Radiologic tests should have confirmed the presence of pleural effusion or thickening and, in the presence of fluid, a previous pleural aspiration without a definitive diagnosis is often required. Because thoracoscopy in this situation is

an elective procedure, the clinician should consider stopping anticoagulation and antiplatelet agents as long as this does not risk other complications, including considering low-molecular-weight heparin bridging if required. It is our practice to stop clopidogrel for 7 days before such procedures and aspirin for 5 days, but this is not based on evidence.

Evaluation of the patient's respiratory status requires basic observation and consideration of arterial blood gas analysis in cases where hypercarbia is considered possible. An electrocardiogram should be obtained to exclude recent myocardial infarction or significant arrhythmia. The clinical laboratory will provide the coagulation parameters, serum electrolyte levels, and blood glucose level, as well as blood group typing, platelet count, results of liver function studies, and serum creatinine level. We would recommend a platelet transfusion if the platelet count is less than 50×10^9 cells per milliliter and that the international normalized ratio be corrected to below 1.5. Patients with renal dysfunction can safely undergo thoracoscopy, but caution must be used with sedative drugs, and it should be noted that there is a higher risk of bleeding; the risk benefit of biopsy should be openly discussed with the patient.

Immediately before the procedure, ultrasonography for localization of the pleural fluid and for diagnosis of potential fibrinous membranes or adhesions in the pleural space is now considered mandatory (see Chapter 23). In an observational study, thoracic ultrasonography localized a safe site for thoracoscopy, when not clinically apparent, in 11 of 80 cases (14%) and detected unexpected septations in 7 (9%).[63] According to the guidelines of the BTS on pleural procedures and ultrasonography, thoracic ultrasonography is strongly recommended before all pleural procedures to localize the site of pleural fluid.[64] A CT scan is not mandatory before thoracoscopy but is usually performed. CT scans can be helpful to localize abnormalities, such as loculated empyema or localized lesions (tumors) of the chest wall or diaphragm.

ANESTHESIA

Thoracoscopy by the single-entry-site technique is usually done under local anesthesia with premedication, together with an antianxiolytic, a narcotic, or both (e.g., midazolam and hydrocodone).[32] If necessary, additional pain medication should be given during the procedure, as required. With the use of conscious sedation, an anesthesiologist is usually not needed. However, there are circumstances where the presence of an anesthesiologist is very helpful as, for example, with rare idiosyncratic or allergic sensitivities to typical anesthetics, very anxious patients or patients unable to cooperate, including children, and patients with severe hypercarbia. An alternative is sedation by propofol with or without premedication[65]; however, the use of propofol for moderate sedation is not approved in some countries, including the United States, without the supervision of an anesthesiologist.[66] General anesthesia with intratracheal intubation and ventilation is used in some centers, as it is for VATS, but is not generally necessary for thoracoscopy.

Monitoring devices such as a cardiac monitor, oxygen saturation monitor, and automatic blood pressure monitor are applied. Some advocate the simultaneous measurement of cutaneous or exhaled carbon dioxide tension because sedation may lead to significant hypoventilation.[67] An intravenous line is maintained, both for intravenous sedation and for possible resuscitation medications.

ACCESS TO THE PLEURAL SPACE

Because it is impossible to perform the procedure if the pleural cavity is completely obliterated, a sufficiently large pleural space is an essential prerequisite, allowing the introduction of the trocar and thoracoscope without injuring the lung or other organs.

The simplest access is available in the setting of a preexisting complete pneumothorax or large pleural effusion, in which the trocar can be introduced directly into the pleural space without risk of injuring the lung. In the setting of a small or moderate-size pleural effusion, a needle puncture should be performed at the level of greatest opacification/dullness or, ideally, under ultrasonographic guidance. After pleural fluid is aspirated, the syringe is removed from the needle, and air enters the pleural space either spontaneously or after the patient takes a few deep breaths. The entry of air causes the lung to collapse away from the chest wall and creates a larger pleural space for safe trocar insertion. Alternatively, if the needle is well positioned in the pleural fluid (e.g., not in the lung), air can be injected into the pleural space by syringe. Most often, a few milliliters of air are sufficient to create a good separation of the lung from the chest wall. Greater safety is provided under ultrasonographic guidance, which allows the operator to localize the pleural effusion and to exclude thick septations/adhesions, which may prevent a sufficient collapse of the lung and thus may cause possible complications, such as bleeding and injury to the lung, diaphragm, and other thoracic structures, when introducing the trocar at the site of the septations/adhesions.[68] Another option is fluoroscopy of the patient "on the table," which can show the air-fluid level caused after injection of air and the presence of any adhesions.

If neither effusion nor pneumothorax is present, an artificial pneumothorax must be created either by the blunt dissection technique using the finger[52] or by the technique of pneumothorax induction. The blunt dissection technique (i.e., extended thoracoscopy) involves gentle dissection of the pleural adhesions with a finger to advance the thoracoscope into the pleural space.[52] Some operators introduce carbon dioxide, which is absorbed more rapidly than air, and would maximize absorption rates in the unlikely event of air embolism. If so, the pneumothorax should be induced immediately before undertaking thoracoscopy, because the pneumothorax will be absorbed rapidly. Some thoracoscopists induce a pneumothorax the day before the procedure, allowing more time to obtain pressure measurements and to determine if the pleural space is patent, as indicated by a fluctuation of pressure with breathing between −15 and −5 cm H_2O (1 cm H_2O ≅ 1 mbar). A direct ultrasound-guided technique to induce pneumothorax can also assist in prediction of where the lung will fail to collapse.[35] In cases where the ultrasound predicts that thoracoscopy will not be possible, a real-time image-guided cutting-needle biopsy is an alternate approach, and can provide high diagnostic yields. This allows the pulmonologist to obtain tissue without the patient needing to reattend for a further procedure.[69]

POSITION AND ENTRY SITE

Thoracoscopy is usually performed with the patient in the lateral decubitus position with the intended procedural site facing upward.[5,27,45] The site of introduction of the thoracoscope should be chosen to access the location of presumed abnormalities and to avoid potentially hazardous areas, such as the midanterior line, where the internal mammary artery lies; the axillary region with the lateral thoracic artery; and the infraclavicular region with the subclavian artery. The region of the diaphragm is unsuitable, not only because adhesions are frequent there but also because the liver or spleen may be injured.[5,27] For general applications, the trocar is introduced in the lateral thoracic region between the midaxillary and the anterior axillary line in the fourth to seventh intercostal space (i.e., the triangle of safety); for pleural effusions, in the sixth or seventh intercostal space; and for pneumothorax, in the fourth intercostal space. After preparation with a surgical disinfectant and local anesthesia, using 1% or 2% lidocaine, a small skin incision is made, and blunt dissection using scissors or a blunt pair of forceps is used to create a tract. The trocar is advanced with a corkscrew motion until the detectable resistance of the internal thoracic fascia has been overcome. The cannula of the trocar should lie at least 0.5 cm within the pleural space. Pleural effusions should be removed by using a suction tube that does not occlude the cannula so that air may rapidly enter the pleural space and avoid generating large negative pleural pressures. After complete removal of the effusion or, in cases without effusion, the optical device is then introduced through the cannula, and the pleural space is inspected (eFig. 29.1). A second trocar can be safely placed using direct vision via the thoracoscope once a suitable position has been found (Video 29.2).

THORACOSCOPIC TECHNIQUE

The pleural space can be inspected directly through the thoracoscope or indirectly by viewing the image on a screen via videothoracoscopy. The advantages of videothoracoscopy over direct thoracoscopy are multiple: the view is better when projected on a screen and the other participants of the procedure (fellow, nurse, anesthesiologist) can watch the thoracoscopy, which is also important for teaching purposes.

Anatomic relationships and intrathoracic structures are usually well recognized (Video 29.3). Biopsies of the pleura and, if needed, the lungs, can be performed easily and safely by means of the biopsy forceps (Video 29.4). In the presence of undiagnosed pleural effusions, biopsy specimens should be taken from macroscopic lesions at the anterior chest wall, the diaphragm, and the posterior chest wall for histologic evaluation and, usually, for mycobacterial culture. If no macroscopic abnormalities are visible, several biopsy specimens should be taken from different sites of the parietal pleura. Pleural biopsies should be taken down to the fat, because this is helpful for the pathologist to comment on invasion.

Biopsy specimens are not routinely taken from the lung because of the risk of creating a fistula but may be necessary when abnormalities are seen only on the lung surface. The likelihood of creating a bronchopleural fistula can be reduced by the use of an electrocautery biopsy forceps. In cases of inflammatory pleural exudates or when several therapeutic thoracenteses have already been performed, fibrinous membranes or adhesions may be present that hinder examination. If so, these can be severed by using blunt forceps or by cutting with electrocautery.

Although a single site of entry is generally sufficient, a second site may be useful for biopsies or to coagulate.[27] A second port of entry is mandatory to introduce a biopsy forceps in case of mini-thoracoscopy, in which the scope is too small to accommodate a forceps.[33] The position of the second site of entry can be determined by viewing through the 50-degree scope while depressing the possible entry site with the index finger. It may be helpful to insert a needle through the same site while viewing its precise location through the thoracoscope. After administration of a local anesthetic, a 5-mm incision is made, and the 5-mm trocar is inserted directly. Its cannula will accommodate many instruments designed for its smaller bore.

The semirigid technique is very similar to the earlier description and usually does not require a second port. Using a combination of the flexible tip and angular movements of the entire scope, the entire pleural cavity can be visualized. A flexible large-jaw biopsy forceps (2.2–2.6 mm diameter) is introduced via the working channel of the scope to perform biopsies of visualized abnormalities or of thickened parietal pleura.

TALC POUDRAGE PLEURODESIS

Talc poudrage is the most widely reported method of talc instillation into the pleural space.[46] It is mainly used for pleurodesis in malignant or recurrent pleural effusions[46,48] but also in persistent or recurrent spontaneous pneumothorax.[50] Thoracoscopic talc pleurodesis can be performed under local anesthesia but generally requires additional pain medication.[32]

Talc poudrage is conducted during thoracoscopy under a number of circumstances. Most commonly, poudrage is conducted when there is evidence during thoracoscopy of macroscopically obvious malignancy, usually manifested as multiple and different-sized pleural nodules. In cases where there is no evidence of macroscopic malignancy, but the pleura is not normal (e.g., diffuse pleural thickening, which can be caused by either benign or malignant conditions), the decision is more challenging. In our practice, we tend to use poudrage in cases where any further pleural intervention is not an option (e.g., the elderly, in whom thoracic surgery is not possible), but this does risk introducing talc in those who are subsequently shown to have a benign cause of their effusion. This decision is now somewhat more complex, because there is also the possibility of insertion of an indwelling pleural catheter (as a definitive pleural intervention) during thoracoscopy.

Before poudrage, it is important to confirm that the lung can completely expand because contact of the lung with the chest wall is necessary for a successful pleurodesis.[46,48,49] Failure to expand fully may indicate a trapped lung caused

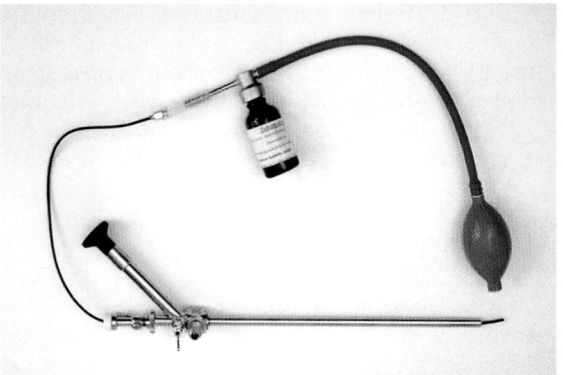

Figure 29.3 Apparatus for talc poudrage. The flexible catheter, connected to a small bottle containing talc and to a pneumatic atomizer (manual insufflator), is introduced through the working channel of the rigid thoracoscope. This allows talc to be sprayed on the pleural surface under direct vision during thoracoscopy.

by thickening of the visceral pleura, which can be suspected at thoracoscopy, although blinded video studies have shown that this is not detected reliably by expert operators.[70] Most reliably, lung expansion is confirmed with a large-volume pleural aspiration before the thoracoscopy, conducted to obtain samples for cytology.

The optimal dose of talc for poudrage is not known, but usually a dose of 4 g is recommended for malignant or recurrent effusions,[48,49] whereas, for pneumothorax patients, 2 g is usually sufficient.[50] The pleural cavity should be inspected during insufflation of the talc to ensure that the talc is uniformly distributed (Video 29.5). For this purpose, one can use a thoracoscope with an angled optical device and a flexible suction catheter connected to a small bottle containing talc and to a pneumatic atomizer introduced through the working channel of either the thoracoscope[27] (Fig. 29.3) or the semirigid thoracoscope.[11,17]

After talc poudrage, a 10- to 24-French chest tube should always be inserted. We recommend a tube of at least 20-French size to ensure that air leak does not result in the creation of subcutaneous emphysema leaking around the chest tube and the port site. The use of suction postprocedure is controversial, and no clear data exist to demonstrate its utility. If suction is applied, the use of high-volume, low-pressure systems is recommended, with a gradual increment in pressure to about −20 cm H_2O.[48] The introduction of digital suction, which is more accurate and highly portable, may be an important direction in the future, but more data demonstrating utility are required.

After the procedure, chest tube removal has been recommended when the daily amount of fluid production is less than 150 mL, but there is little evidence to support this practice.[48] One report suggests that the chest tube can be removed within 24 hours after talc slurry pleurodesis without regard to daily fluid production; however, this was an underpowered study.[71]

Talc is inexpensive and highly effective.[72] Its most common short-term adverse effects include fever and pain. Cardiovascular complications, such as arrhythmias, cardiac arrest, ischemic chest pain, myocardial infarction, and hypertension, have been noted. Acute respiratory distress syndrome, acute pneumonitis, and respiratory failure have also been reported after talc poudrage and slurry, especially in the United States, where only talc including small-particle sizes was available. The use of graded, larger-size talc appears to be absolutely safe, both in the treatment of recurrent pleural effusions and spontaneous pneumothorax.[62,73] More recently, large-particle size-calibrated talc has been approved for use in the United States.

RESULTS

Pleural Effusions

Even after extensive diagnostic workup of the pleural fluid, the cause of a number of pleural effusions may remain undetermined. Blind needle biopsies may establish the diagnosis in some additional cases, particularly in tuberculous pleurisy. In a 1981 series by Boutin and colleagues[74] of 1000 consecutive patients with pleural effusion, 215 cases remained undiagnosed after repeated pleural fluid analysis and performance of pleural biopsies. This has been supported by the results of several other authors who, without the use of thoracoscopy, report that at least 20–25% of pleural effusions remain undiagnosed, although this certainly depends strongly on the particular patient populations.[10] Because of the higher diagnostic yield and ability to induce pleurodesis in a single setting, it has been estimated in a theoretical cost analysis in the United Kingdom that medical thoracoscopy may save considerable costs in the evaluation of unexplained pleural effusions compared with other tests, including transthoracic image-guided pleural biopsy.[75]

Several studies have tried to determine the diagnostic accuracy of thoracoscopy in the setting of undiagnosed pleural effusion, but the results vary, with a range of 60–90%, as is well summarized in the evidence-based BTS guidelines of 2010.[22] One well-designed study of thoracoscopy in 102 patients reported by Menzies and Charbonneau,[56] with follow-up periods between 1 and 2 years, found a sensitivity of 91%, a specificity of 100%, accuracy of 96%, and a negative predictive value of 93%. Boutin and colleagues[74] reported a false-negative rate of 15% within 1 year of follow-up. In a retrospective study of 709 patients who underwent thoracoscopy for diagnosis of unexplained exudative effusions, Janssen and Ramlal[76] also found a 15% false-negative rate in a long-term follow-up (minimum, 24 months) of 208 patients with initial negative results; the overall sensitivity of thoracoscopy was 91%, the specificity was 100%, the positive predictive value was 100%, and the negative predictive value was 92%. This finding has been replicated in several other well-designed studies since.[77–80]

Of note, even surgical thoracotomy can "miss" the diagnosis. In a study of the results of thoracotomy in patients with pleural effusion of undetermined cause, even after a pathologic diagnosis of a benign pleural process, 25% of patients were diagnosed with a malignancy over a period of follow-up. The diagnoses most often missed were malignant pleural mesothelioma and lymphoma.[76,81] We believe that a certain small proportion of such patients are, in fact, not diagnosable using any form of biopsy or histologic analysis, requiring further follow-up and later biopsy; whether these cases are truly false-negative rather than "undiagnosable" at the time is not clear.

Because of its high diagnostic accuracy, diagnostic thoracoscopy is an excellent option in cases of exudates in which the cause remains undetermined after pleural fluid analysis

and radiology (usually CT).[22,48] The procedure allows fast and more definite biopsy diagnosis, including a high yield for TB cultures, and determination of hormone receptors and molecular targets in malignancies. Furthermore, staging in lung cancer and diffuse mesothelioma is possible. The exclusion of an underlying malignancy or of TB is provided with high probability. Surgery, including surgical thoracoscopy, not only is more invasive and expensive but also does not produce better results than thoracoscopy.

Malignant Pleural Effusions

Diagnosis. Malignant pleural effusions are the leading diagnostic and therapeutic indication for thoracoscopy[82] (Fig. 29.4A and eFig. 29.2). In a prospective comparison of diagnostic tests, each performed in every patient, the diagnostic yield of nonsurgical biopsy methods in malignant pleural effusions was studied simultaneously in 208 patients, including 116 metastatic pleural effusions (from 28 breast cancers, 30 cancers of various other organs, and 58 cancers of undetermined origin), 29 cancers of the lung,

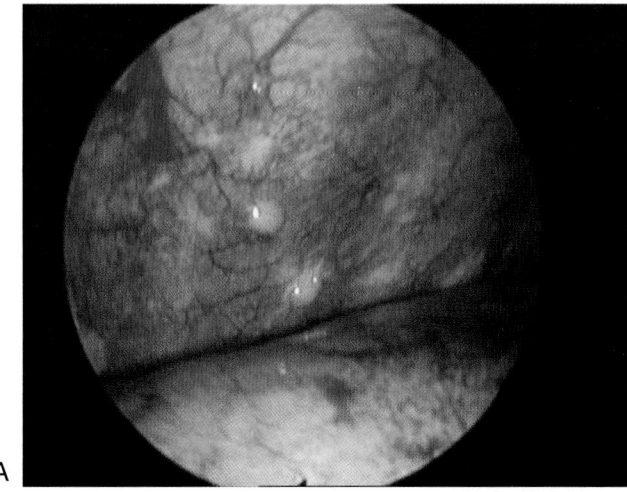

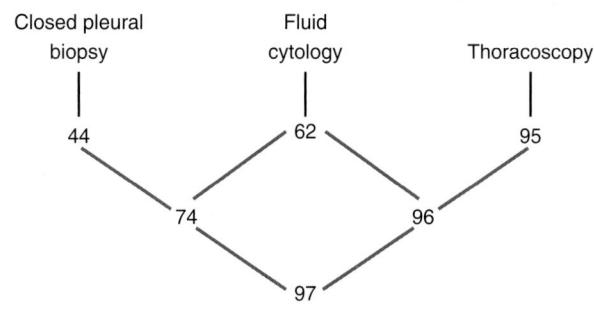

Figure 29.4 Thoracoscopy for diagnosis of malignancy. (A) View through the thoracoscope in a patient with a malignant pleural effusion due to breast cancer. Small whitish tumor nodules are present on the parietal (chest wall) pleura (*top of photograph*). The lung surface (*bottom of photograph*) demonstrates some anthracosis. (B) Sensitivity of different biopsy methods (cytologic and histologic results combined) for the diagnosis of malignant pleural effusions. Numbers represent sensitivity (%) of tests, either alone or combined, in a prospective intrapatient comparison of 208 patients. Thoracoscopy alone has 95% sensitivity for the diagnosis of malignancy; cytology and closed pleural biopsy contribute little to the total sensitivity of 97% for all three tests. (A, From Loddenkemper R, Mathur PN, Noppen M, Lee P. *Medical Thoracoscopy/Pleuroscopy: Manual and Atlas.* New York: Thieme; 2011. B, Modified from Loddenkemper R, Boutin C. Thoracoscopy: present diagnostic and therapeutic indications. *Eur Respir J.* 1993;6:1544–1555.)

58 diffuse malignant mesotheliomas, and 5 malignant lymphomas.[54] The diagnostic yield of pleural fluid cytologic examination was 62%, of closed pleural biopsy was 44%, and of thoracoscopy was 95%. The sensitivity of thoracoscopy was higher than that of cytologic examination and closed pleural biopsy combined (95% vs. 74%; $P < 0.001$). The combined methods were diagnostic in 97% of malignant pleural effusions (see Fig. 29.4B). In 6 of the 208 cases (2.9%), an underlying neoplasm was suspected at thoracoscopy but confirmed only by thoracotomy or autopsy. Similar results have been reported by other investigators.[77–79]

The diagnostic sensitivity of thoracoscopy is similar for all types of malignant effusion. In one study, the overall yield in 287 cases was 62% for cytologic examination and 95% for thoracoscopy; the relative yields for cytologic examination and thoracoscopy did not vary greatly for lung carcinomas ($n = 67$), at 67% and 96%, respectively; for extrathoracic primaries ($n = 154$), at 62% and 95.5%, respectively; or for diffuse malignant mesotheliomas ($n = 66$), at 58% and 92%, respectively.[54]

Staging. Thoracoscopy may be useful in staging lung cancer, diffuse malignant mesothelioma, and metastatic cancer. In lung cancer patients, thoracoscopy can help to determine whether the effusion is malignant or paramalignant.[54] As a result, it may be possible to avoid exploratory thoracotomy for tumor staging. Canto and associates[83] found no thoracoscopic evidence of pleural involvement in 8 of 44 patients with lung cancer and pleural effusion; 6 proceeded to resection, where the lack of pleural involvement was confirmed.

In diffuse malignant mesothelioma (Videos 29.6 and 29.7), thoracoscopy can provide an earlier diagnosis and better histologic classification than closed pleural biopsy because of larger and more representative biopsy specimens and more accurate determination of the extent of tumor.[84,85] Earlier diagnosis and staging may have important therapeutic implications either for surgery or for local immunotherapy or local chemotherapy because better clinical outcomes have been observed for patients detected in earlier stages; thoracoscopy provides information on T stage, although this technique cannot be used to assess lymph node involvement.[85]

Thoracoscopy is also helpful in the diagnosis of benign asbestos-related pleural effusion by excluding mesothelioma or malignancies. Fibrohyaline, or calcified, thick, and pearly white pleural plaques, may be found (Video 29.8), indicating possible asbestos exposure.

A further advantage of thoracoscopy in metastatic pleural disease is that biopsies of the visceral and diaphragmatic pleura are possible under direct observation. In addition, the larger size of thoracoscopic biopsy specimens may provide easier identification of primary tumor, including hormone receptor determination in breast cancer,[86] and improved morphologic classification in lymphomas.[87]

The assessment of specific mutations in lung cancer cells can increasingly direct targeted therapy. In pleural biopsy specimens, Guo and colleagues[88] found a rate of 70% of epidermal growth factor receptor mutations and concluded that pleural biopsy specimens, in this case obtained by VATS, provided better material than other techniques. Adequate tissue may be important for these assays;

however, the reliability of cytologic examination for demonstration of epidermal growth factor receptor mutations does have a growing evidence base and is recommended in guidelines.[89,90]

Therapy. The relative utility of thoracoscopic talc poudrage pleurodesis has been mentioned above. In summary, despite high success rates reported in case series using poudrage, which will suffer from selection bias, randomized trials have failed to demonstrate a consistent benefit of talc poudrage over talc slurry, with overall success rates of 70–80%.[60] Thus, we suggest that talc poudrage is an effective method of pleurodesis in malignant effusion but should not be promoted in isolation (i.e., where a biopsy is not required) as a therapeutic procedure over talc slurry, which is less invasive.

In chylothorax due to lymphoma, Mares and Mathur[91] showed excellent results of talc poudrage, all in cases refractory to chemotherapy or radiation therapy. All 19 patients with 24 hemithoraces involved had no recurrence after 30, 60, and 90 days (8 patients died during the 90 days of follow-up).

The development of "tunneled" or *indwelling pleural catheters* (IPC) has challenged the position of talc pleurodesis as the first option of treatment for malignant pleural effusion.[92–94] The primary goal of an IPC is symptom relief by repeated drainage of pleural fluid in the home setting. In addition, the IPC can induce a spontaneous pleurodesis at mean rate of 46%,[95] although this rate is less in randomized studies.[96–98] Spontaneous pleurodesis is increased by active management of the indwelling catheter, including daily drainage,[96,98] and the administration of talc through the indwelling catheter.[97] However, the drainage bottles are expensive, and reimbursement by health insurance companies is not provided in many countries. Reported complications include malfunctioning of the catheter (9.1%), pneumothorax requiring chest tube (5.9%), pain (5.6%), and blocked catheter (3.7%). Less common complications are catheter fracture, empyema, cellulitis, and tumor metastasis along the catheter tract.[95]

No randomized studies are yet available comparing thoracoscopic talc poudrage and IPC placement. In a randomized controlled trial, talc slurry pleurodesis and an IPC were compared with a primary end point of patient-reported relief of dyspnea; in this study, no significant difference between the two methods was found in dyspnea or in quality of life. Twelve patients (22%) in the talc slurry group required further pleural procedures, compared to three patients (6%) in the IPC group. On the other hand, fewer patients in the talc group had adverse events (13%) than in the IPC group (40%).[93] In a cost-analysis study, talc slurry pleurodesis was found to be more cost-effective than the IPC if the patient survived for more than 6 weeks,[99] and a number of other analyses have supported the relative cost-effectiveness of indwelling catheters in the absence of long survival.[100,101]

In a noncomparative study, thoracoscopic talc poudrage and IPC placement were combined in 30 patients.[102] Successful pleurodesis was obtained in 92%; the IPC could be removed at a median of 7.5 days. The authors stated that both length of hospital stay and duration of IPC use could be reduced significantly compared to either procedure alone.

This finding has since been replicated in a similar observational study.[103]

An IPC placement is a better treatment option in patients with a trapped lung.[104] For all other patients, the advantage of placement of an IPC as opposed to thoracoscopic talc pleurodesis, or the combination of both, remains to be established. A major advantage of thoracoscopic talc pleurodesis is the possibility of obtaining a histologic diagnosis of the pleura in the same session. In future studies comparing IPC and thoracoscopic talc pleurodesis, assessment of this advantage should be included in the design of the study.

In real-life practice, if a patient requires fluid control in a case of established malignant effusion, patient choice is crucial when deciding between talc- and IPC-based treatment. We tend to discuss patient preference in terms of "outpatient" or "inpatient" treatment and proceed accordingly. It is also, of course, perfectly feasible to place an IPC at the completion of a thoracoscopic biopsy procedure; we tend to follow this procedure in patients who do not wish to stay in the hospital and in those with a known or recognized trapped lung.[70]

Tuberculous Pleural Effusions. Although the diagnostic yield of pleural fluid culture combined with closed-needle biopsy for the diagnosis of TB is quite high, there may be indications for thoracoscopy in otherwise uncertain pleural effusions (Fig. 29.5). The diagnostic accuracy of thoracoscopy is almost 100% because the pathologist is provided with multiple selected biopsy specimens, and there is a higher likelihood of obtaining the tubercle bacilli on culture. In a prospective comparison in which diagnostic procedures were compared in each patient, an immediate diagnosis of *Mycobacterium tuberculosis* infection in 100 cases was established histologically in 94% with thoracoscopy but in only 38% with needle biopsy.[54] This may be of clinical importance because a proper histopathologic diagnosis allows antituberculous chemotherapy to be started without delay. The combined yield of histologic diagnosis and bacteriologic culture was 99% for thoracoscopy and 51% for needle biopsy, increasing to 61% when culture results from effusions were added (see Fig. 29.5B). The percentage of positive *M. tuberculosis* cultures from thoracoscopic biopsies (78%) was twice as high as that from pleural fluid and needle biopsies combined (39%), allowing bacteriologic confirmation of the diagnosis and, importantly, drug susceptibility testing. In 5 of the 78 positive cases (6.4%), resistance to one or multiple antituberculous drugs was found and influenced therapy and prognosis.

Closed-needle biopsy can have high yield in areas with a high prevalence of TB but, even then, thoracoscopy can have benefits. In a prospective study of 40 cases from South Africa, thoracoscopy had a diagnostic yield of 98% compared with an 80% diagnostic yield from pleural biopsies performed with an Abrams needle.[105] In addition, thoracoscopy can allow complete drainage of the effusion; initial complete drainage of the effusion, performed during and after thoracoscopy, has been associated with greater symptomatic improvement than subsequent pleural therapy.[106] The positive role of early removal of the pleural fluid has also been shown in a double-blind, randomized, placebo-controlled trial from Taiwan.[107] No studies are known that compare the potential benefits of

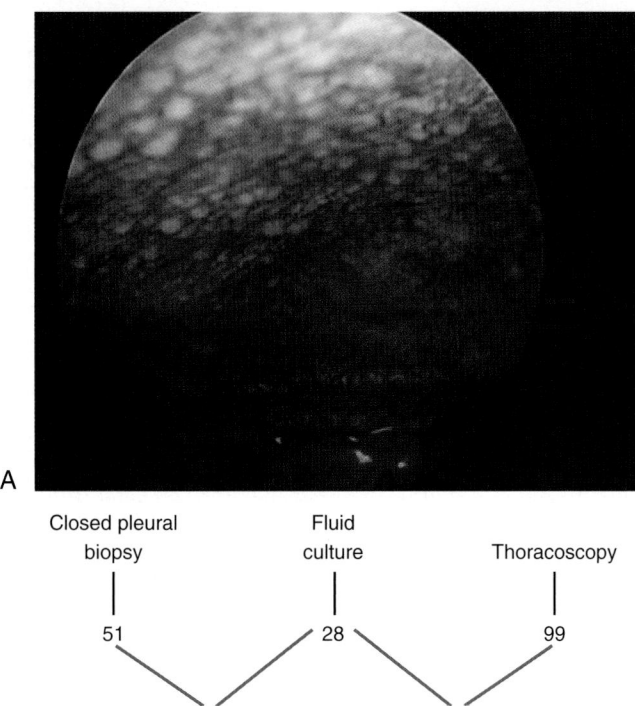

Figure 29.5 Thoracoscopy for diagnosis of tuberculosis. (A) View through the thoracoscope in a patient with a tuberculous pleural effusion. Note the numerous small whitish nodules on the parietal (chest wall) pleura. The histologic examination revealed florid exudative tuberculous pleurisy with epithelioid cell granulomas, numerous multinucleated giant cells, and necrosis. *Mycobacterium tuberculosis* cultures from the biopsy specimens were positive, whereas those from the effusion were negative. (B) Sensitivity of different biopsy methods (histologic and bacteriologic results combined) for the diagnosis of *M. tuberculosis* infection. Numbers represent sensitivity (%) of tests, either alone or combined, in a prospective intrapatient comparison of 100 patients. Thoracoscopy alone has 99% sensitivity for the diagnosis of tuberculosis. (A, From Loddenkemper R, Mathur PN, Noppen M, Lee P. *Medical Thoracoscopy/Pleuroscopy: Manual and Atlas.* New York: Thieme; 2011. B, Modified from Loddenkemper R, Boutin C. Thoracoscopy: present diagnostic and therapeutic indications. *Eur Respir J.* 1993;6:1544–1555.)

thoracoscopy, allowing early diagnosis, complete drainage, and early drug treatment with those of empirical drug treatment alone.

It is debatable whether to treat patients with antituberculous medication merely on the suspicion of tuberculous pleurisy if they present with a high lymphocyte count in the pleural fluid and a positive skin test. In countries with a low prevalence of TB, supportive tests such as for adenosine deaminase have low specificity and should not be used for the diagnosis of TB pleuritis. In these circumstances, pleural biopsy (thoracoscopic or blind) is indicated. The high yield for *M. tuberculosis* cultures from thoracoscopic biopsy specimens increases the possibility of obtaining susceptibility tests, which, in cases of drug resistance, may influence therapy and prognosis.[105]

Other Pleural Effusions. For diagnosis in cases with effusions that are neither malignant nor tuberculous, thoracoscopy may give visual clues to the cause, such as revealing thick white fibrin deposits seen in rheumatoid effusions, calcifications in effusions after pancreatitis, dilated veins in liver cirrhosis, or signs of trauma.[54] Although for these entities the history, pleural fluid analysis, and physical and other examinations are usually helpful, thoracoscopy may be indicated to confirm the clinical suspicion. Thoracoscopy is well suited for determining that a patient with a history of asbestos exposure likely has benign asbestos-related pleural effusion, which, by definition, is a diagnosis of exclusion of other causes, in particular malignancies.[84]

For diagnosis in the setting of other undiagnosed pleural effusions, the main diagnostic value of thoracoscopy lies in its ability to exclude malignant and tuberculous disease.[108] By means of thoracoscopy, the proportion of so-called idiopathic pleural effusions usually falls below 10%, whereas, in studies that have not used thoracoscopy, failure to obtain a diagnosis can exceed 20% of cases. However, this certainly also depends on the selection of patients and on the definition of "idiopathic." Even after surgical exploration—the gold standard—there are still undiagnosed effusions.[79]

For treatment, talc pleurodesis can be considered in some cases of nonmalignant pleural effusions that are recurrent and symptomatic and do not respond to medical therapy. Such effusions may include those due to hepatic and renal hydrothorax, chylothorax, yellow nail syndrome, and systemic lupus erythematosus.[109–111] In such patients with recurrent benign undiagnosed effusions, Vargas and colleagues[112] achieved successful pleurodesis in 20 of 22 patients by using talc poudrage.

Empyema

Thoracoscopy can also be used in the management of early empyema, mainly to achieve early and complete drainage[12,27] (Video 29.9). As a procedure intermediate between tube thoracostomy and VATS, thoracoscopy has the potential to be effective and, compared with surgical drainage, is less costly and avoids general anesthesia; however, choice of patients at an early stage of pleural infection is likely a key factor for success. In cases with multiple loculations, it is possible to open these spaces to remove the fibrinopurulent membranes by forceps and to create a single cavity that can be successfully drained and irrigated.[113] If performed for this indication, thoracoscopy should be carried out early in the course of empyema, before the adhesions become too fibrous and adherent to perform thoracoscopy. As mentioned, adhesions can be evaluated before the procedure by ultrasonography; thick dense adhesions may preclude thoracoscopy or talc pleurodesis.[31] In fact, ultrasonographic imaging before thoracoscopy significantly reduces the number of pleural access failures; it helps locate the optimal site for thoracoscopy and, in case of complete adhesion of the pleura, indicates the need for another procedure, such as VATS or a CT-guided biopsy.[31]

If the indication for placement of a chest tube is present and if the facilities are available, thoracoscopy can be performed at the time of chest tube insertion. In effect, thoracoscopy is a procedure similar to chest tube placement but one that enables the creation of a single pleural cavity, allowing potentially more effective drainage.[34,113] In a retrospective study of 41 patients, thoracoscopy was successful without further intervention in 35 (85%)[114]; this was mainly successful in free-flowing fluid (100%) and multiloculated empyema (92%), but in only 4 of 8 patients with an empyema in the organizational stage. However,

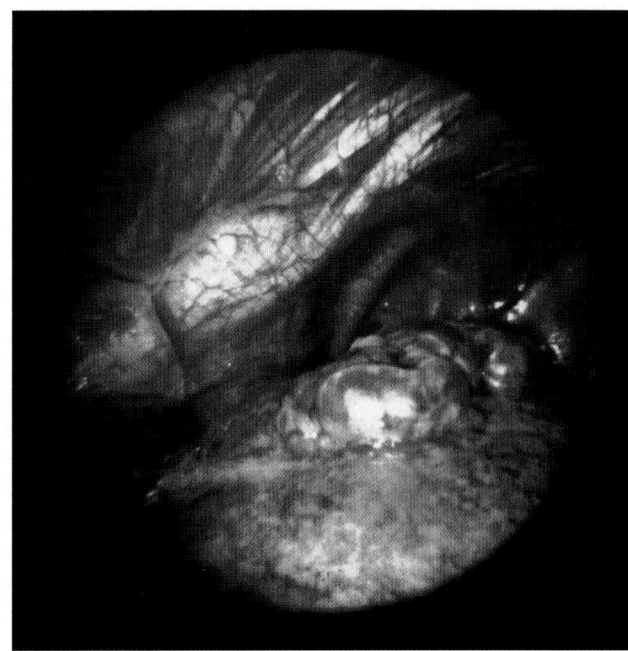

Figure 29.6 View through the thoracoscope in a patient with a spontaneous pneumothorax. On the surface of the lung (*lower part of image*), large apical blebs are visible.

prospective comparative studies on the role of thoracoscopy in the treatment of early empyema in adults are currently lacking, and the evidence from retrospective case-selected noncomparative studies should be interpreted cautiously. We suggest that only early-stage pleural infection should be considered for thoracoscopic intervention because later-stage disease may require decortication of the lung surface, which can only be performed surgically. In addition, there are now other nonthoracoscopic options in pleural infection treatment, such as combined tissue plasminogen activator/DNAse and saline irrigation,[115,116] which are proven in randomized trials to improve outcomes and, in our view, should be used preferentially.

Spontaneous Pneumothorax

In spontaneous pneumothorax, thoracoscopy has both diagnostic and therapeutic purposes[5,27,54,117–119] (Fig. 29.6). Whenever a chest tube is introduced by the trocar technique, it is easy to use an optical device for visual inspection of the lung and pleural cavity before insertion of the chest tube. Special techniques, including fluorescence thoracoscopy, have been used to identify blebs and other porosities (Video 29.10).[120] By inspection during thoracoscopy, the underlying lesions can be directly assessed for the presence of bullae and blebs.[117] In 1047 cases of pneumothorax in which thoracoscopy was used by three different teams, pathologic lesions were detected in approximately 70%.[10]

Treatment by thoracoscopy may include electrocautery of blebs and bullae and pleurodesis using talc poudrage (Video 29.11).[10] Talc poudrage achieves excellent results, with recurrence rates reported as less than 10%.[50] A prospective study showed that, for complicated pneumothorax, defined as recurring or persistent pneumothorax, simple talc poudrage under local anesthesia prevented recurrence in a large proportion of patients.[121] In a prospective, randomized, multicenter comparison, talc poudrage for primary spontaneous pneumothorax proved more efficient (only 1 of 61 patients with talc poudrage had a recurrence, compared with 10 of 47 with simple pleural drainage) and more cost-effective than drainage alone.[122] The recurrence rate after thoracoscopic talc poudrage is 5%, which is similar to the recurrence rate after VATS.[123] An important disadvantage of VATS is long-term postoperative pain, which may develop in more than 30% of patients and may last for 3 to 18 months.[124] Currently there is no study directly comparing efficacy and complication rates of VATS and thoracoscopy for pneumothorax management.[123]

Other types of pneumothorax treated successfully by thoracoscopy have included those due to *Pneumocystis jirovecii* pneumonia, metastatic osteosarcoma, pleural endometriosis, lymphangioleiomyomatosis, and cystic fibrosis.[125]

In talc poudrage for pneumothorax, 2 to 4 g of talc can be sufficient for effective pleurodesis.[50] The short-term safety of insufflation of large particle size talc in patients with spontaneous pneumothorax has been shown in a prospective multicenter study.[62] In a study of patients 22 to 35 years after talc poudrage, there were no long-term sequelae; total lung capacity averaged 89% of the predicted value in 46 patients, whereas it was 97% of the predicted value in 29 patients treated with tube thoracostomy alone.[126] In this long-term follow-up, none of the poudrage group developed mesothelioma. Although talc poudrage may result in minimally reduced total lung capacity, as well as pleural thickening on chest radiography, these changes appear to be clinically unimportant.[127,128] Talc poudrage may be relatively contraindicated for patients who may become candidates for lung transplantation, although it is not considered an absolute contraindication to lung transplantation.[129]

In some centers, apical bullectomy followed by mechanical abrasion or resection of the pleura is considered the procedure of choice for treatment of recurrent spontaneous pneumothorax, if apical blebs or bullae are present. It is important to add pleurodesis, chemical or mechanical, to a VATS procedure because the recurrence rate after bullectomy alone is unacceptably high—27.5% after 10 years of follow-up in one study.[130] Mechanical pleurodesis can include abrasion or a partial parietal pleurectomy. There are a few studies comparing these approaches. When talc pleurodesis was added to the VATS procedure, Bridevaux and colleagues[73] found a significantly lower recurrence rate of 1.8% compared to 9.2% after partial parietal pleurectomy. In a review by Sepehripour and associates,[131] recurrence rate after VATS pleurectomy was demonstrated to be lower than after pleural abrasion; however, there were slightly better results with talc pleurodesis than with either of the mechanical techniques.

Therefore, if the facilities are available, thoracoscopy may be performed in patients with spontaneous pneumothorax, but, as mentioned earlier, thought should be given to adequate heavy sedation during the poudrage procedure.

Diffuse Pulmonary Diseases

Previously, diagnosis of diffuse lung diseases has been considered an indication for diagnostic thoracoscopy[5,27,54,53,132,133] (Fig. 29.7). An overview of the entire lung surface, assisted by the magnification of the

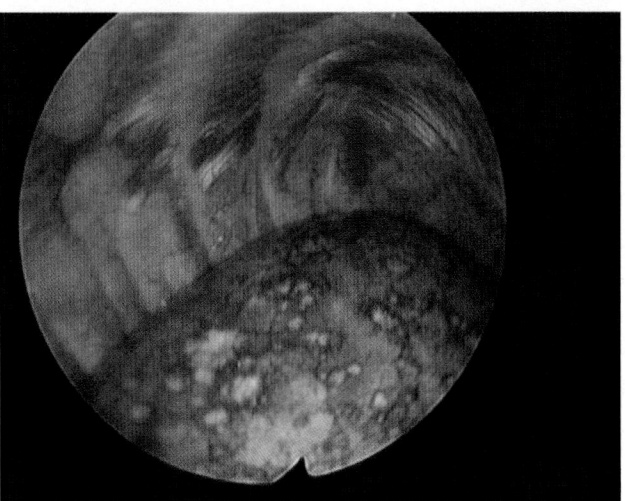

Figure 29.7 A view through the thoracoscope in a patient with diffuse lung infiltration. The abnormalities were found to represent multiple pulmonary metastases due to ovarian cancer (*lower part of image*).

thoracoscope, allows harvesting of representative samples of abnormal areas of parenchyma. In a review of the literature, the sensitivity of thoracoscopic lung biopsy specimens was 93% in 1031 cases with varying causes.[27] In a large series of 419 patients with diffuse lung diseases, the overall sensitivity was 85%, with different yields depending upon the underlying disease: 98% in sarcoidosis stage II and III, 88% in malignant diseases, 85% in diffuse pulmonary fibrosis/interstitial pneumonia, and 42% in pulmonary Langerhans cell histiocytosis.[54] Thoracoscopy has also been used with a high diagnostic yield in immunocompromised patients.[133]

In comparison with bronchoscopy, thoracoscopy is more invasive (see "Contraindications" section) but presents several advantages. It provides significantly larger samples and allows the physician to choose the biopsy site. Unlike transbronchial biopsy, thoracoscopy enables electrocautery so that bleeding after a thoracoscopic parenchymal biopsy can be managed without difficulty.

With regard to diagnostic sensitivity and invasiveness, thoracoscopy ranks between transbronchial biopsy and open-lung biopsy.[54] In an experimental animal study, subpleural and deep-lung biopsy specimens were taken during thoracoscopy in six sheep.[134] No significant differences were found between subpleural and deep biopsies regarding the mean quality scores of the tissue obtained. According to this study, subpleural biopsy specimens obtained during thoracoscopy might be sufficient for establishing an accurate diagnosis in diffuse parenchymal lung disease, where the subpleural layers are involved.

With better radiologic techniques and reclassification of interstitial lung disease, the reliance on lung biopsy in general has waned in the last few years, meaning that this biopsy technique is required less often. The innovation of transbronchial cryobiopsy to obtain lung parenchymal tissue for diagnosis of interstitial lung disease[135] may well decrease the need for thoracoscopic lung biopsy even further.

Localized Diseases

Localized abnormalities of the chest wall, diaphragm, and thoracic spine may be diagnosed using thoracoscopy if the pleural space is not obliterated.[5,54] Hyaline pleural plaques, localized pleural mesothelioma, lipoma, neurinoma, rib metastasis, rib erosions, and the like can be examined and, if necessary, biopsied. Very discrete metastases are sometimes found in the region of the diaphragm and the posterior chest wall, with or without associated pleural effusion. Chest wall lesions may be easier to diagnose than lung lesions. In a retrospective study in which 109 cases with chest wall lesions of different causes were analyzed, the diagnostic sensitivity was 83%,[54] whereas, in solitary lung lesions, the overall diagnostic sensitivity was only 46%.

Currently, the application of thoracoscopy has decreased substantially for localized disease because of better imaging techniques, such as CT, magnetic resonance imaging, and ultrasonography, which allow image-guided biopsies. Alternatively, VATS will now be used for these indications because the technique not only is diagnostic but also allows the complete resection of benign or malignant lesions.

DIFFERENCES BETWEEN THORACOSCOPY AND VIDEO-ASSISTED THORACIC SURGERY

As described in the preceding sections, thoracoscopy is used mainly for diagnosis of pleural diseases. The most common indications for thoracoscopy are diagnosis of pleural effusion with inspection of the pleural cavity, combined with biopsy specimens from the parietal pleura, as well as treatment of malignant or other therapy-refractory effusions by talc poudrage. It is a relatively simple and inexpensive technique because it can be performed in an endoscopy room, under local anesthesia or conscious sedation, and through a single-entry site with nondisposable instruments.

VATS, conversely, has now been technically developed to the point that it can replace thoracotomy for most indications, if certain limitations, such as dense pleural symphysis, are not present. VATS requires an operating room, general anesthesia with single-lung ventilation, more than two (usually three) entry sites, and complex instruments. Overall, it is a more invasive and expensive technique with a higher risk than thoracoscopy; however, in experienced hands and in the proper setting, VATS is less invasive, is less expensive, and has a lower risk than thoracotomy.

The different clear-cut indications for either thoracoscopy or VATS are listed in Table 29.1. However, there remains a gray area of indications for which method can be used (see Table 29.1). Gray areas include treatment of pneumothorax, drainage of early empyema, biopsies in diffuse parenchymal lung diseases, and sympathetic nerve interventions. For these indications, the choice of the medical or the surgical approach depends on local expertise, availability of the technique, and performance status and prognosis of the patient.

Key Points

- Thoracoscopy (medical thoracoscopy/pleuroscopy) is less invasive than video-assisted thoracic surgery (surgical thoracoscopy) because it is performed under local anesthesia and conscious sedation, most commonly through a single entry port; it is less expensive because it can be performed in an endoscopy suite and usually does not require an anesthesiologist.
- Thoracoscopy is used mainly for diagnostic purposes, in particular in pleural effusions of otherwise indeterminate origin, with very high sensitivity and specificity for the diagnosis of malignancy and tuberculosis.
- Thoracoscopy is the investigation of choice in patients with cytology-negative undiagnosed effusion, either by obtaining a diagnosis or by providing reassurance with negative biopsies in benign disease.
- Thoracoscopy allows definitive pleural intervention to prevent fluid recurrence by the use of talc poudrage, used in malignant and recurrent pleural effusions, or by the placement of an indwelling catheter.

Key Readings

Ali MS, Light RW, Maldonado F. Pleuroscopy or video-assisted thoracoscopic surgery for exudative pleural effusion: a comparative overview. *J Thorac Dis.* 2019;11(7):3207–3216.

Bridevaux PO, Tschopp JM, Cardillo G, et al. Short term safety of thoracoscopic talc pleurodesis for recurrent primary spontaneous pneumothorax. *Eur Respir J.* 2011;38:770–773.

DePew ZS, Wigle D, Mullon JJ, Nichols FC, Deschamps C, Maldonado F. Feasibility and safety of outpatient medical thoracoscopy at a large tertiary medical center: a collaborative medical-surgical initiative. *Chest.* 2014;146(2):398–405.

Havelock T, Teoh R, Laws D, et al. Pleural procedures and thoracic ultrasound: British Thoracic Society pleural disease guideline 2010. *Thorax.* 2010;65(suppl 2):ii61–ii76.

Hooper CE, Lee TCG, Maskell NA, et al. Setting up a specialist pleural disease service. *Respirology.* 2010;15:1028–1036.

Janssen J, Collier G, Astoul P, et al. Safety of pleurodesis with talc poudrage in malignant pleural effusion: a prospective cohort study. *Lancet.* 2007;369:1535–1539.

Kyskan R, Li P, Mulpuru S, Souza C, Amjadi K. Safety and performance characteristics of outpatient medical thoracoscopy and indwelling pleural catheter insertion for evaluation and diagnosis of pleural disease at a tertiary center in Canada. *Can Respir J.* 2017;2017:9345324.

Lee P, Folch E. Thoracoscopy: advances and increasing role for interventional pulmonologists. *Semin Respir Crit Care Med.* 2018;39(6):693–703.

Loddenkemper R, Mathur PN, Noppen M, et al. *Medical Thoracoscopy/Pleuroscopy: Manual and Atlas.* New York: Thieme; 2011.

Psallidas I, Corcoran JP, Fallon J, et al. Provision of day-case local anesthetic thoracoscopy: a multicenter review of practice. *Chest.* 2017;151(2):511–512.

Rahman NM, Ali NJ, Brown G, et al. Local anaesthetic thoracoscopy: British Thoracic Society pleural disease guideline 2010. *Thorax.* 2010;65(suppl 2):ii54–ii60.

Skalski JH, Astoul PJ, Maldonado F. Medical thoracoscopy. *Semin Respir Crit Care Med.* 2014;35(6):732–743.

Tschopp JM, Purek L, Frey JG, et al. Titrated sedation with propofol for medical thoracoscopy: a feasibility and safety study. *Respiration.* 2011;82:451–457.

Complete reference list available at ExpertConsult.com.

30 *THORACIC SURGERY*

SHAMUS R. CARR, MD • JOSEPH FRIEDBERG, MD

PREOPERATIVE EVALUATION

Before thoracic surgery where pulmonary resection will be performed, all patients should be seen by a thoracic surgeon. In addition to recent axial imaging (i.e., *computed tomography* [CT] scan), all patients should have a cardiopulmonary workup and examination. This will almost always include *pulmonary function testing* (PFT). In patients with cardiac issues, obtaining consultation with a cardiologist can be of benefit in determining the cardiac risk to the patient. Additional testing, such as *positron emission tomography* (PET) scans, magnetic resonance imaging, *ventilation-perfusion* (V/Q) scans, and other tests (e.g., echocardiogram), are ordered on a case-by-case basis.

LUNG RESECTION: PULMONARY FUNCTION TESTING

Because the majority of pulmonary surgeries involve anatomic lung resections, such as a lobectomy for lung cancer, the pulmonary workup is essential before surgery. The initial, and often sole, component of this evaluation is PFT that includes both spirometry and diffusion. On the spirometry side, the *forced expiratory volume in 1 second* (FEV$_1$) has the most predictive value for the ability to tolerate a resection. In general, a patient with an FEV$_1$ greater than 2 L should be able to tolerate any resection. A patient with an FEV$_1$ greater than 1.5 L should be able to tolerate a lobectomy.[1,2] In addition to predicting if a patient will tolerate a resection, these tests are predictive for postoperative complications. Studies have shown pulmonary complications are more frequent when the preoperative FEV$_1$ is less than or equal to 60% and *diffusing capacity for carbon monoxide* (DL$_{CO}$) is 50% or less, and when the estimated postoperative FEV$_1$ or DL$_{CO}$ is 50% or less.[3]

To calculate a postoperative predictive FEV$_1$ from PFT is relatively straightforward. As discussed elsewhere in this textbook, the lung is made up of lobes that are further subdivided into segments. In general, there are 9 to 10 segments in each lung, for a total of 19. The clinician needs to determine how many segments will be resected (e.g., three from the right upper lobe) and use this as a fraction to calculate the predictive postoperative value.

The following equation is most commonly used to calculate estimated postoperative FEV$_1$:

$$epoFEV_1 = preFEV_1 \times \frac{19 - \text{segments to be removed}}{19}$$

where *epoFEV$_1$* is estimated postoperative FEV$_1$ and *preFEV$_1$* is preoperative FEV$_1$. Segments include right (upper 3; middle 2; lower 5) and left (upper 3; lingula 2; lower 4).

Using this equation, the following example is given. A patient with an FEV$_1$ of 1.3 L is planning to undergo a right upper lobectomy. Resection of the right upper lobe will result in removal of three segments. Therefore, at the conclusion of the resection, the patient will retain 84% of the original lung parenchyma ([19 − 3]/19 = 84%). Thus, the expected postoperative FEV$_1$ should be about 1.1 L, and thus the patient should be able tolerate the resection.

When PFTs are marginal, judgment is required when determining a patient's candidacy. A commonly encountered scenario is one in which a patient with marginal PFTs would require an upper lobectomy. Such a patient is likely to have emphysematous changes in the lungs, which, if homogeneous, would mean the patient would likely have inadequate lung function after surgery. If, however, the patient has heterogeneous distribution of emphysema, with compressed parenchyma in the bases and overt bullous disease in the upper lobe, the patient might tolerate an upper lobe resection that would be contraindicated by the calculations just listed. Embarking on these high-risk cases that rely on a "lung volume reduction effect" requires mature judgment.

Previously, it was accepted that an epoFEV$_1$ less than 800 mL was a contraindication to surgery.[4] This value has been called into question because extrapolating from studies on lung volume reduction surgery, such as the National Emphysema Treatment Trial,[5] and calculating *maximal oxygen consumption* ($\dot{V}O_{2max}$) and quantifying split lung function (while taking into account the area of the lung to be resected) has allowed surgery to be performed on patients who previously would have been considered inoperable. Nonetheless, although there is no set "lower limit," care must be exercised when operating on patients for whom the epoFEV$_1$ is likely to be less than 800 mL.

In these cases of marginal PFTs, the quantitative V/Q scan may also contribute useful information. Quantitative V/Q scans can allow the clinician to calculate postoperative values more accurately. Using the perfusion portion of the scan, preferably done with both anterior-posterior and posterior-oblique views, an estimate can be made of the exact amount of perfusion to each lobe of the lung. This test can complement the PFTs to help render a more accurate prediction of postoperative predicted lung function. An example would be a patient with moderate COPD with significant disease only in the upper lobes. It is not uncommon to see perfusion to the upper lobes less than 5% of the overall perfusion. Thus, if the patient has a tumor that requires resection of the upper lobe, it can be expected that the overall PFTs will decrease by only 5% after a right upper lobectomy. In addition, it is known that after some resections, such as a pneumonectomy, the final decrease in pulmonary function testing is less then would be predicted, likely due to increased inflation of the remaining lung parenchyma.[6,7]

Quantitative V/Q scan is most commonly used when the estimated postoperative predictive value for either FEV$_1$ or DL$_{CO}$ is less than 40%. This does not mean that surgery cannot be performed but that the plan must be highly individualized. When the estimated values are less than 40%, studies show minimally invasive surgery can be used to perform lung resections with complication risks that are the same as patients with values closer to 60% done by open thoracotomy.[8] In patients with a value less than 40% or when there are other concerns about suitability for surgery, additional testing should be performed.[9] Cardiopulmonary testing with measurement of the $\dot{V}O_{2max}$ has been shown to be helpful; in a prospective study, patients with a $\dot{V}O_{2max}$ less than 16 mL/min/kg were significantly more likely to suffer complications and death.[10]

In patients where there is concern about postoperative lung function, another option is for surgeons to limit the amount of lung resected. Whereas lobectomy currently remains the gold standard for lung cancer resections, there are two potentially appropriate parenchymal-sparing approaches: anatomic segmentectomies and nonanatomic wedge resections.

Anatomic segmentectomy allows preservation of lung parenchyma and, in the appropriate setting, has been shown to be equivalent to a lobectomy in oncologic outcomes.[11,12] Although lobectomy is currently the standard of care for an early stage *non–small cell lung cancer* (NSCLC), anatomic segmentectomy may prove an appropriate option for a patient with compromised pulmonary function, by providing equivalent oncologic outcomes. A clinical trial evaluating this issue has recently closed to accrual. It will

TABLE 30.1 Common Complications for Different Lung Resections

	Wedge Resection*	Lobectomy/ Segmentectomy	Pneumonectomy
Atrial fibrillation	1.2%	7.3–12.3%	19.9–34%
Air leak > 5 days	1.9%	7.6–8.7%	1–4%
Bleeding	0.5–1.9%	1.1–4.7%	2%
Any pulmonary complication	5.6%	6.8–12.6%	23%
Any complication	12–19%	26.2–36.6%	48.2%
Mortality (30 day)	0.5–1.5%	0.9–1.8%	2.4–11.1%

*Wedge resection includes lung biopsy for interstitial lung disease.
Data from references 3, 6, 30, 31, 39, and 40.

be a few more years before these prospective results are available. The results will hopefully show what role exists for anatomic segmentectomy and whether perhaps it will be considered the standard of care for some lung cancers.

A retrospective review of patients who had PFT, before and between 6 and 36 months after surgery, demonstrated that parenchymal-sparing resection results in better preservation of pulmonary function at a median of 1 year. However, the benefit appeared to be greatest when only one to two segments were resected.[13]

LUNG RESECTION: ADDITIONAL WORKUP AND EVALUATION

In addition to the standard PFTs that should be done for all patients undergoing lung resection, any additional testing should be tailored to each individual patient's physiologic and oncologic circumstances. This can vary considerably for benign and malignant conditions. If there are any concerns about a patient's cardiac status, in addition to an electrocardiogram, an echocardiogram and/or stress test can be obtained along with cardiac risk stratification by a cardiologist. Some refer to this as "cardiac clearance." This term should, arguably, be abandoned because the cardiologist provides insightful risk stratification, but the onus for "clearance" ultimately lies with the surgeon taking the patient to the operating room. In general, common rates of complications are known for most pulmonary operations (Table 30.1).

For cases of malignancy, a PET scan is a standard preoperative test to screen for metastatic disease throughout the body, except the brain. Although some surgeons obtain magnetic resonance imaging of the brain with contrast for all patients with lung cancer, others only get it for tumors greater than 3 cm or in cases with concern for neurologic symptoms.[14] For lung tumors greater than 3 cm, there is an increased incidence of spread beyond the lung to both mediastinal lymph nodes and distant sites, such as the liver, adrenal glands, bone, and brain.[15] Staging of the mediastinum before surgery is mandatory when a PET scan shows increased uptake in mediastinal lymph nodes. Studies demonstrate that mediastinoscopy and *endobronchial ultrasound*

(EBUS) with transbronchial fine-needle aspiration, in the hands of a skilled bronchoscopist, are essentially equivalent.[16] Some surgeons, particularly since the emergence of EBUS, tend to obtain invasive staging by EBUS on most patients, to avoid the very small, but real, risk of false-negative radiographic staging. A current trend, where navigational bronchoscopy is used to diagnose lung nodules, is to perform mediastinal staging with EBUS at the same setting if intraoperative cytology reveals the lung nodule to be malignant. Staging the mediastinum is essential whenever there is concern for stage 3A(N2) disease because this may serve as an indication for nonoperative therapy in a marginal surgical candidate or as an indication for neoadjuvant chemotherapy or chemoradiotherapy in a good surgical candidate who understands the potential risks and benefits of the proposed operation.[17]

The need for biopsy of the primary lung tumor is to be considered on a case-by-case basis. The role for CT-guided biopsy has decreased with the advent of navigational bronchoscopy, where it is available. Compared to CT-guided biopsy, navigational bronchoscopy does have a slightly lower overall diagnostic yield (88% vs. 69%). However, the risk of complications is lower with navigational bronchoscopy.[18] Instead of thinking of the two modalities as competitive, it is better to think of them as complementary. In central lesions or when a fissure is likely to be crossed using CT-guided biopsy, navigational bronchoscopy may be a better choice. However, when nodules that are within 2 cm of the visceral pleura, the reverse may be true, and CT-guided biopsy is likely preferable. The current success of navigational bronchoscopy, to a great extent, hinges on having the target nodule in proximity to a navigable airway. Even peripheral nodules, if favorably located, can sometimes be accessed with navigational bronchoscopy. As previously noted, another potential advantage of navigational bronchoscopy is that that it can be combined with EBUS, at the same setting, both to establish a diagnosis and stage the mediastinum (see Chapters 21 and 27).

Establishing a tissue diagnosis before consideration for surgery is not mandatory. Clinical suspicion of a nodule growing on serial imaging with increased uptake on PET scan should be considered highly suspicious for malignancy in most patients. When nodules are near the visceral surface, a frozen section via a wedge resection at the time of surgery carries very low morbidity and mortality with far greater accuracy of establishing a diagnosis compared to preoperative biopsy techniques, such as CT-guided biopsy or navigational bronchoscopy. Concerns have also been raised about whether CT-guided biopsy leads to pleural dissemination.[19] A meta-analysis[20] concludes that CT-guided biopsy does not increase overall risk of total recurrence compared to other strategies; however, in the subgroup of patients with subpleural lesions compared to those without subpleural lesions, there was an increase in pleural recurrence. The researchers concluded that CT-guided biopsy should not be performed for subpleural lesions and only on non-subpleural lesions where a pathologic diagnosis is necessary. Further studies are needed on this issue. The final point in considering foregoing a CT-guided diagnostic test depends on the pretest probability of cancer. The context of the evolution and appearance of the mass needs to be considered but, in some cases, it is completely appropriate to proceed to surgery without a diagnosis if the lesion is highly suspicious for a cancer and, especially, if a negative biopsy result would be considered likely to be a false negative. In either case, the patient would still require surgery: for an excisional biopsy if malignancy is not proven preoperatively or for resection if the diagnosis is established. In either case, surgery would be an appropriate step without subjecting the patient to the risk and discomfort of a preoperative invasive diagnostic procedure.

The argument that a diagnosis must be established to "rule out small cell cancer" is passé. In a patient with a solitary pulmonary nodule that is PET avid and without radiographic findings concerning for either distant or lymphatic spread, surgery for small cell lung cancer treated with lobectomy has been retrospectively shown in large databases to have superior overall survival compared to chemoradiotherapy alone.[21,22] Therefore, in patients who are clinically stage 1 with pulmonary nodules that can be localized, surgical resection carries certain advantages, such as decrease in the time from clinically finding the tumor to treatment.

SURGICAL PROCEDURES ON THE LUNG

Multiple different surgical procedures can be performed on the lung for a variety of reasons, both oncologic and noncologic. The appropriate procedure to perform is based upon the underlying disease process and the patient's physiologic status. Some of these factors include, but are not limited to, the indications (e.g., oncologic vs. benign), the intent (e.g., diagnostic and/or therapeutic), the pulmonary status (e.g., PFTs or on a ventilator), and the location of a nodule. Clearly communicating the decision making and the details of the operation is important for the surgeon in working together with the pulmonologists and other specialists, and in educating the patient and the family.

When pulmonary surgery is performed for cancer, it is important to understand if it is for primary disease (e.g., lung cancer) or secondary disease (e.g., pulmonary metastasis). For both, the first principle is to achieve negative margins. In addition, resection of primary lung cancer requires an anatomic resection and resection of the lymph nodes that drain the lung and evaluation of mediastinal lymph nodes. Anatomic resections (e.g., segmentectomy, lobectomy, and pneumonectomy) all remove associated lymph nodes both individually and en bloc with the resected lung parenchyma. As for mediastinal lymph nodes, a prospective trial of sampling versus complete resection only demonstrated equivalence.[23] For primary lung cancer, it is generally accepted that at least five separate stations need to be evaluated and greater than 14 total lymph nodes need to be examined by pathology for it to be considered an adequate resection.[24] In contrast, resection of pulmonary metastases generally does not require a lobectomy, pneumonectomy, or removal of lymph nodes.

WEDGE

Wedge resection is a nonanatomic resection of lung (Fig. 30.1A). It is considered therapeutic when it includes a

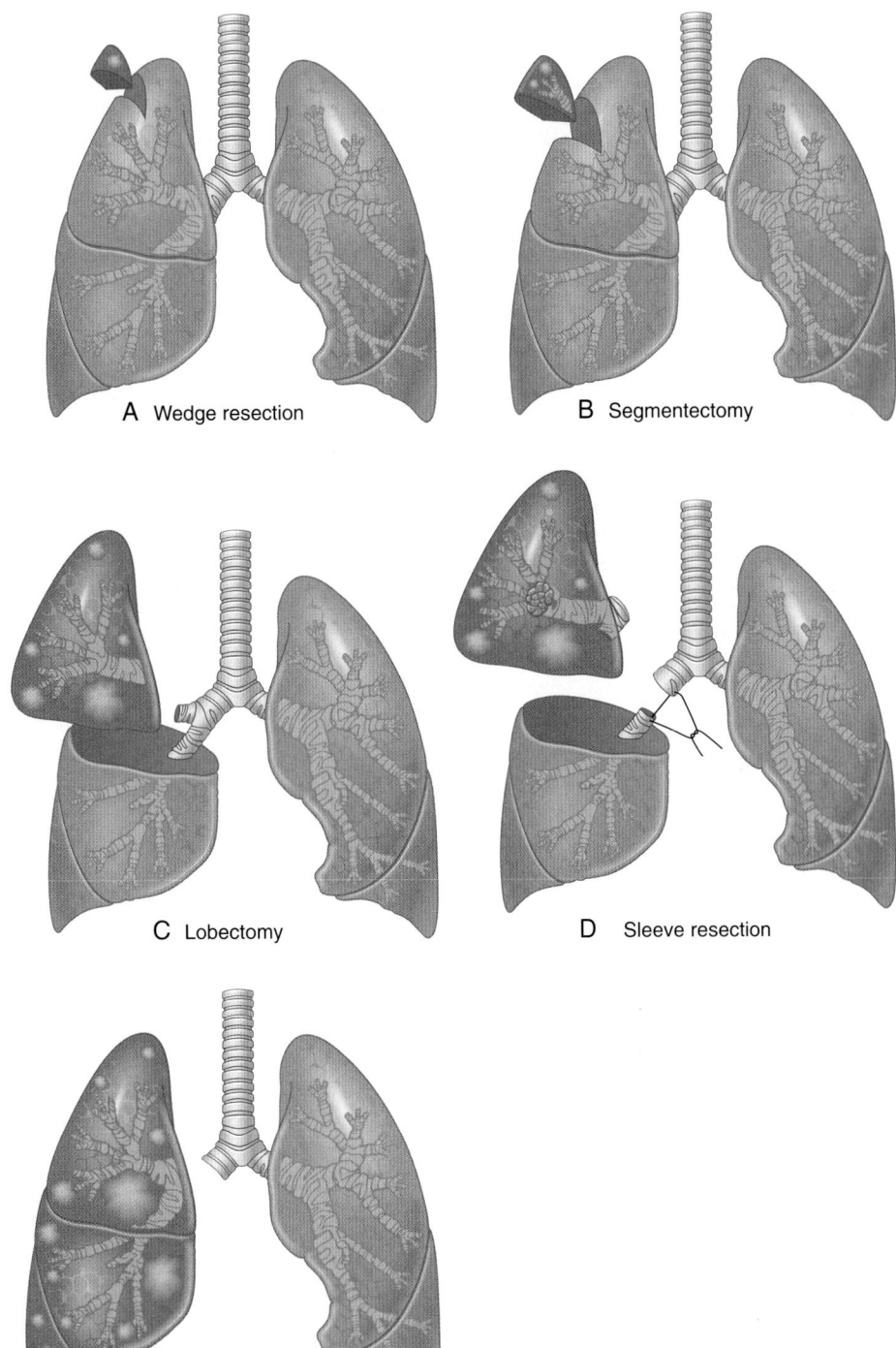

A Wedge resection

B Segmentectomy

C Lobectomy

D Sleeve resection

E Pneumonectomy

Figure 30.1 Standard lung resections. (A) Wedge resection. A nonanatomic resection, usually used for diagnosis of diffuse lung disease. (B) Segmentectomy. An anatomic resection of one of the 19 pulmonary segments, increasingly used for lung-sparing resections of lung cancer. (C) Lobectomy. An anatomic resection of one of the five pulmonary lobes. It remains the standard for curative lung cancer surgery. (D) Sleeve resection. A reconstruction of the bronchus to spare a lobe not involved in tumor, thereby avoiding a pneumonectomy. (E) Pneumonectomy. Resection of an entire lung. (Modified from Chabner DE. *The Language of Medicine*, 11th ed. St. Louis: Elsevier; 2017.)

nodule that is sent for diagnosis. It is considered diagnostic when performed for a diffuse or localized process, such as for interstitial lung disease. This is generally done near the periphery of the lung and has a very low complication rate, and air leaks are generally not expected. This is almost always performed with a specialized stapler that staples and cuts simultaneously. There is another technique known as a Perelman resection.[25] This technique uses electrocautery dissection to perform a nonanatomic resection in certain circumstances in which the location of the lesion makes a stapled wedge resection difficult or impossible. In the Perelman technique, the raw surface of

the lung is left charred and allows minimum to no air leak after the procedure.

SEGMENTECTOMY

Each of the five lobes of the lungs is made up of a number of individual segments. Each lobe has a unique number of segments, discussed earlier. A segmentectomy is an anatomic resection where both the bronchus and pulmonary artery are individually divided, similar to a lobectomy (see Fig. 30.1B). The pulmonary vein is occasionally divided independently but can also be resected as part of the intersegmental fissure. Segmentectomy, like wedge resection, is a parenchymal-sparing operation. As opposed to wedge resection, segmentectomy is anatomically based with resection of the pulmonary vessels and airway at their respective origins and, depending upon the scenario, has been shown to be both equivalent to a lobectomy for both cancer-specific and overall survival. As opposed to wedge resection, which may still be appropriate in highly selected situations, a proper segmentectomy adheres to the same oncologic principles of lobectomy or pneumonectomy.[11]

LOBECTOMY

This is the most common oncologic resection performed by thoracic surgeons. It has been the backbone of lung cancer surgery since publication of the Lung Cancer Study Group results in 1995.[26] This operation consists of complete and independent division of all bronchovascular structures leading to one of the five anatomic lobes of the lung, and separation of the operative lobe from those around it by dissection of any incomplete intralobar fissures (see Fig. 30.1C).

BILOBECTOMY

Bilobectomy is a right-sided operation that consists of removal of either the upper or lower lobe, along with the middle lobe. Preservation of only the middle lobe is typically considered ill advised because the middle lobe is small and would be unable to fill the hemithoracic space; as such, it would be prone to significant complications, such as torsion.

SLEEVE RESECTION

A sleeve resection may be indicated to spare lobes not involved in tumor to avoid pneumonectomy (see Fig. 30.1D). This can become useful when the tumor involves the main bronchus or is too close to the lobar bronchial orifice to close and maintain a negative airway margin. In such situations, the option is typically to go more proximally on the airway and perform a pneumonectomy, or to perform a sleeve resection by removing that part of the airway (which looks like a short tube or "sleeve" of bronchus) and to reattach the distal airway from the remaining lobe(s) to the divided end of the proximal airway. The most common is a right upper lobe sleeve resection. In this operation, the distal divided bronchus intermedius is anastomosed to the proximal right mainstem bronchus. Any lobe can be "sleeved." In addition, there are more complex operations involving sleeve resections involving the carina. In addition to a sleeve resection of the airway, sometimes it is necessary to perform sleeve resections of the pulmonary artery or to remove a portion of the pulmonary artery and reconstruct it to maintain a normal caliber. These can be complex operations, sometimes requiring advanced reconstructive techniques on both the artery and airway to preserve a lobe. In general, the pulmonary veins will not tolerate reconstruction, and whatever portion of the lung is supplied by invaded veins will need to be removed.

PNEUMONECTOMY

Pneumonectomy, that is, complete removal of a lung, was the first successful operation for NSCLC and was performed by Dr. Evarts Graham in 1933 on a physician from Pittsburgh. This operation involves individual ligation and division of all bronchial and vascular structures to the resected lung (see Fig. 30.1E). One of the key technical points of this procedure is to ensure that the bronchial stump is as flush as possible to the carina, to prevent pooling of secretions that can lead to infection and possible stump breakdown leading to bronchopleural fistula. Bronchopleural fistula and the resultant empyema, after pneumonectomy, is a devastating complication and accompanied by a significant mortality rate. Pneumonectomy is also the main thoracic operation in which the remaining lung is most vulnerable to hydrostatic edema from volume overload, for which fluid restriction during and immediately postsurgery is thought to be protective. This complication is rare but is likely the genesis of the misperception that all "thoracic surgical patients" be run very dry. Diuresis and volume depletion is rarely indicated for patients other than pneumonectomy patients and can, in some thoracic surgical patients, such as those having nonpulmonary surgery, actually be harmful.

INTUBATION AT THE TIME OF SURGERY

The overwhelming majority of pulmonary operations require lung isolation, that is, the ability to ventilate one lung while allowing the other to collapse. There are two standard ways to isolate the two lungs during general anesthesia.

DOUBLE-LUMEN ENDOTRACHEAL TUBE

This approach is the same as a standard endotracheal intubation, except that the endotracheal tube is divided into two separate channels. One of the channels, the bronchial side, is longer and seats in either the right or left mainstem airway (Fig. 30.2). The shorter channel terminates in the distal trachea. The most commonly used *double-lumen tube* (DLT) is a left-sided DLT, owing to the greater length of the left mainstem airway, which makes it easier to maintain the tube in position while the lung is manipulated during surgery. A right-sided double-lumen tube can be much harder to position and maintain and is typically only used for left pneumonectomy or left-sided sleeve resections. There are two separate cuffs on the DLT, with the more proximal cuff referred to as the tracheal balloon. There is a separate cuff to inflate on the bronchial lumen that allows isolation of the left lung from the right. By opening either the tracheal or bronchial lumen to the atmosphere, while ventilating the other lumen, one lung can be allowed to collapse while the other is maintained on positive-pressure ventilation. Because most thoracic surgery cases are performed with the patient in the lateral decubitus position, the isolated lung will be the "up" lung, the

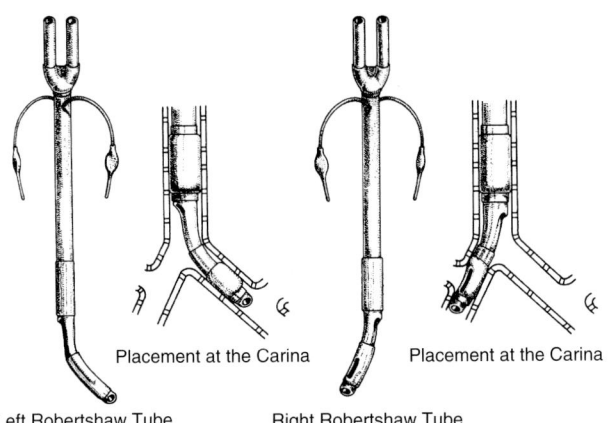

Figure 30.2 Left- and right-sided double-lumen endotracheal tubes. The left-sided double-lumen tube is easier to insert because it can be seated in the longer left main bronchus. The right-sided double-lumen tube is more difficult to position because it sits in the shorter right main bronchus and must be aligned so its side hole faces the orifice of the right upper lobe. (Modified from Benumof JL. *Anesthesia for Thoracic Surgery*. Philadelphia: WB Saunders; 1987.)

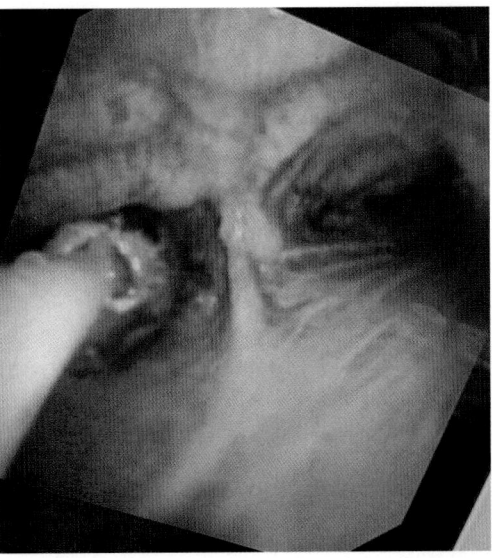

Figure 30.3 Single-balloon blocker in place in the left mainstem bronchus.

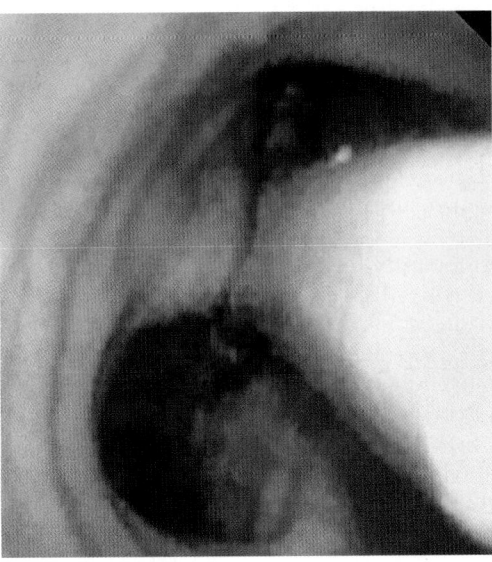

Figure 30.4 Dual-balloon blocker in place in the airway. Once placed in the airway, with one balloon in each major bronchus, the blocker can be used to isolate each lung separately.

lung facing the ceiling, and the ventilated lung will be the "down" lung, the lung facing the floor. A DLT must always be placed under bronchoscopic visualization to confirm that the tube is in the correct position. This is accomplished after the patient is intubated and still in the supine position. The bronchoscope is passed down the tracheal lumen; the carina should be clearly seen and the bronchial lumen should be seen in the left mainstem bronchus. Then the right upper lobe orifice, with its classic appearance, should be identified. The tube placement position should be rechecked after the patient is placed in lateral decubitus position because the tube can migrate.

The right-sided DLT is placed in exactly the same way as just described, except that the bronchial lumen is placed in the right mainstem bronchus, with a side hole cut into the lumen to allow the right upper lobe to be ventilated. This tube requires a more fastidious placement to avoid obstructing the right upper lobe orifice. It is important to recall that some patients may have a *bronchus suis*, an accessory bronchus sometimes supplying the entire right upper lobe, which originates from the trachea. A patient with *bronchus suis* can present a challenge for DLT placement.

BRONCHIAL BLOCKERS

The other option for isolation of the lungs is with a bronchial blocker. There are two types: the conventional single-balloon bronchial blocker (Cook) (Fig. 30.3) and dual-balloon blocker (EZ-Blocker, Teleflex Medical) (Fig. 30.4).

The blocker is placed via a *single-lumen endotracheal tube* (SLT), which must be at least an 8.0 endotracheal tube. The conventional blocker is placed under direct visualization into the mainstem to be isolated (see Fig. 30.3). The dual blocker is designed with two separate lumens, with one branch going down each mainstem bronchus (see Fig. 30.4). Once in place, a cuff is inflated and the selected lung is isolated. The lung isolation can be confirmed with either bronchoscopy or auscultation.

SEGMENTECTOMY VERSUS LOBECTOMY

Any lung resection results in a decrease in lung capacity due to resection of lung parenchyma, with the exception of those done for volume reduction. Although it seems obvious, the larger the resected section of lung, the greater the decrease in lung function for a patient. However, there are certain situations when this is not the case, such as when the resection is for a patient with apical-predominant heterogeneous emphysematous lungs who would be eligible for lung volume reduction surgery. But in general, for those with marginal lung function, sublobar resections are considered, to avoid damaging the quality of life or causing a major pulmonary disability. In addition, sublobar resections are considered in patients with excellent lung function if they have disease that appears likely to recur and may require more surgery in the future. Sublobar is generally defined as less than lobar but can either be wedge resection, which is nonanatomic, or segmentectomy, which is anatomic (see earlier).

As of this writing, the current standards of care for surgical treatment of NSCLC are still dictated by the results of the Lung Cancer Study Group[26] published in 1995. This is the trial that established lobectomy as the appropriate oncologic operation for lung cancer. Although there are many limitations of this prospective, randomized controlled trial, the conclusion was that local recurrence rates were significantly higher after sublobar resection than anatomic lobectomy. Unfortunately, in this trial both nonanatomic wedge resections and anatomic segmentectomies were combined as sublobar resections, which together were found to be inferior to lobectomy. In the more than 25 years since this publication, many investigators have sought to understand the role of anatomic segmentectomy.[11,27–29]

In one of the largest series, a single-institution retrospective review demonstrated equivalent recurrence and survival for segmentectomy compared to lobectomy for patients with NSCLC less than 3 cm in size, when all lymph nodes were negative.[11] In a separate study, a previously unrecognized variable that independently influences recurrence rate was the ratio of the margin (i.e., the distance from the tumor to the stapled bronchovascular margin) to the tumor diameter (M:T). In segmentectomy patients, when M:T was greater than 1, patients had significantly lower local recurrence rates compared to those with M:T less than 1.[12] Although all currently published studies are observational, a prospective randomized controlled trial, CALGB 140503, has completed enrollment of 701 patients who were randomized to either lobectomy or sublobar resection, which could have been either a wedge or a segmentectomy. The primary end point is to determine whether disease-free survival after sublobar resection is noninferior to that after lobectomy in patients with small peripheral NSCLC less than or equal to 2 cm in size. The results of this trial are not yet available but are eagerly anticipated.

MINIMALLY INVASIVE SURGERY VERSUS OPEN THORACOTOMY

Essentially any thoracic surgery procedure can be performed either by open or minimally invasive approaches. The benefits of minimally invasive surgery are essentially the same, no matter the operation, and may include shorter length of stay, less postoperative pain, quicker recovery, and, possibly, decreased cost.

In thoracic surgery, minimally invasive surgery can be done in one of two different ways: *video-assisted thoracoscopic surgery* (VATS) or *robotic-assisted thoracoscopic surgery* (RATS). At the present time, there are no prospective trials comparing the two; however, there is currently an international trial looking into that question (*Robotic Approach for Lobectomy or Anatomical Segmentectomy* [ROMANS] Trial; estimated completion date in 2023).

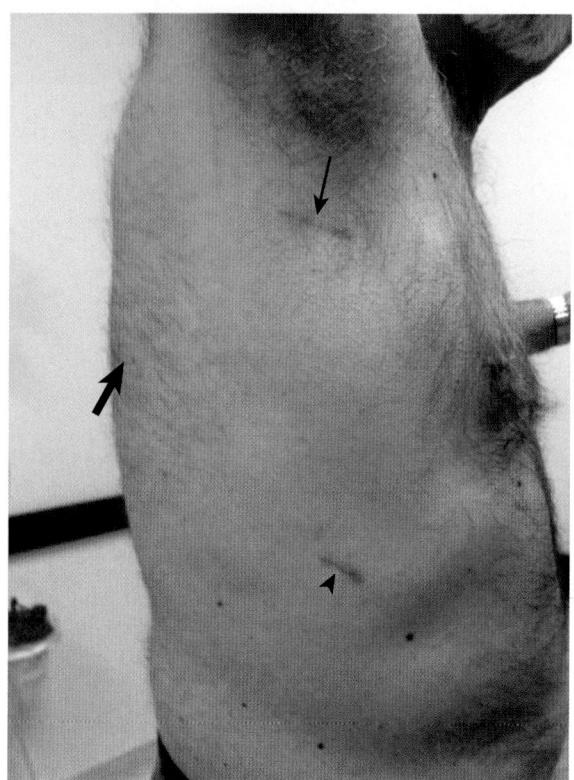

Figure 30.5 Traditional video-assisted surgery port sites on right chest. Access port is near axilla *(arrow)*, camera port is at the level of the eighth intercostal space *(arrowhead)*, the third port is to allow the assistant to aid with retraction *(thick arrow)*. This third port is posterior and at about the same level at the anterior camera port and is usually in line with the tip of the scapula.

This trial is randomizing patients to either of the two minimally invasive techniques and assessing both short- and long-term outcomes, except disease-free survival, for which the studies are not adequately powered.

However, there are several studies that support the purported benefits of either minimally invasive platform compared to open procedures.[30–33] Currently the recommendation from the Society of Thoracic Surgeons is that all early stage lung cancers should be performed in a minimally invasive fashion. The decision of VATS versus RATS is deferred to the surgeon in discussion with the patient.

In general, a patient who undergoes VATS surgery will have three incisions. (Fig. 30.5) There will be an access incision near the axilla that is set at the level of the hilum. This incision is normally between 2 to 5 cm in length. The other two incisions are smaller, both less than 10 mm, because they are used for the camera and assistant ports. They are at about the same level in approximately the eighth intercostal space, with one anterior and the other posterior, usually in the line of the tip of the scapula. A newer technique for VATS, preferred by some surgeons, involves using just one incision, "uniportal" VATS.[34] This technique is only practiced in very few centers and seems to have a steep learning curve. With the wider adoption of robotic approaches, which are easier to learn, the future of uniportal VATS is unclear.

RATS normally requires five incisions. There are four incisions to accommodate the individual arms of the robotic platform. There is also an assistant port to aid with retraction, passing of surgical sponges, and suction. All the robotic ports are placed in the same intercostal space to minimize pain. One of these ports is enlarged, if needed, at the end of the procedure to retrieve the specimen.

In comparing VATS to open lobectomy, a propensity-matched analysis of the Society of Thoracic Surgeons General Thoracic Surgery Database[31] demonstrated a reduction in length of stay by 2 days and in duration of chest tube by 1 day. Later studies continue to demonstrate the same results. Regardless of the particular minimally invasive approach, it is the prevailing opinion of thoracic surgeons and a consensus opinion by the Japanese Association of Chest Surgery[35] that all early stage lung cancers be resected in this manner. Although multiple studies and case reports have been published on successful completion of essentially every thoracic surgical operation in a minimally invasive fashion, experience and clinical judgment should help guide which cases should go "straight to open." Some very experienced thoracic surgeons are able to do sleeve resections either by VATS or on the robotic platform. However, one should accrue significant experience with less complex operations before attempting highly technically advanced cases.

INTRAOPERATIVE LOCALIZATION OF NODULES

Palpation of the lung during surgery can generally identify most nodules in the lung. One of the drawbacks of robotic surgery is the lack of haptic feedback, which makes the ability to find subpleural nodules harder. In addition, due to nodule size, sometimes even manual palpation of the lung is not successful in finding the nodule. In cases where these concerns exist, there are a few options for helping to identify the pulmonary nodule so that a therapeutic wedge resection can be performed to secure a diagnosis on frozen section.[36–38]

Needle localization with a wire placed by radiology under CT imaging, similar to wire localization for breast cancer, has been performed for many years. Although this technique is not new, it does still have a few limitations. The biggest limitation is that it can be dislodged, especially when the chest is opened with the patient on single-lung ventilation. At this point the lung collapses, and the wire can be pulled from the lung parenchyma. Although it may provide an idea of the area to evaluate the lung for the nodule, the wire then does not actually locate the lesion.

Navigational bronchoscopy is being used more often now either to place a fiducial radiographic marker or inject dye for visualization. When a fiducial marker is used, it can be placed at the time of the initial navigational biopsy, and surgery can be on a different day. The use of a marking dye can be either methylene blue or indocyanine green. Either dye must be placed at the beginning of the surgical case. Then, once the chest is entered, the area with the nodule can be visualized. Indocyanine green is a fluorescent dye that requires use of a near-infrared light with a wavelength of around 800 nm to visualize (Fig. 30.6). Of note, if the injection breaches the visceral pleura, it can dye the entire pleural space and interfere with localization.

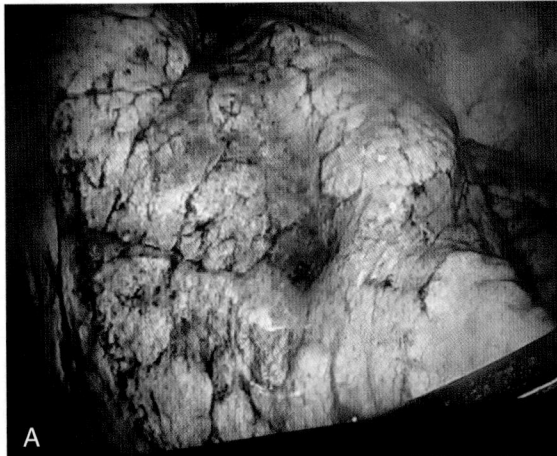
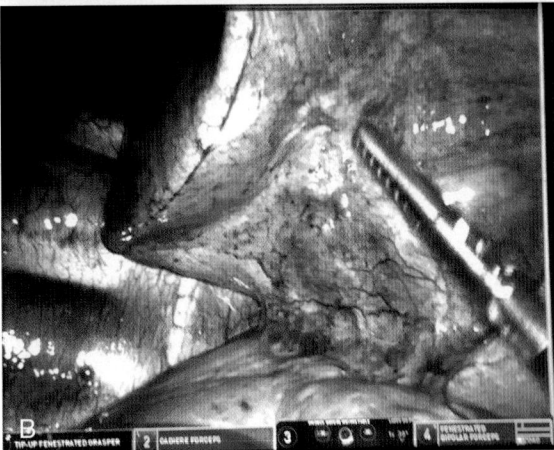

Figure 30.6 Methylene blue and indocyanine green dye marking for a pulmonary nodule. These dyes were placed at the site of a pulmonary nodule via navigational bronchoscopy. (A) Methylene blue can be detected with white light. (B) Indocyanine green requires near-infrared light to visualize.

WEDGE RESECTION FOR INTERSTITIAL LUNG DISEASE

There are times when a patient has a diffuse lung process that cannot be diagnosed by any means other than a surgical biopsy. This operation is historically, and still commonly, referred to as an open lung biopsy. However, an open procedure should be extremely rare. Indeed, there are dire circumstances where a patient is unstable and cannot be moved from the intensive care unit or will not tolerate any element of decreased ventilation from intrathoracic gas insufflation during VATS and, in these situations, an open biopsy through an inframammary incision with the patient supine may be all that can be offered. However, the vast majority of these operations should be performed using a VATS approach.

In attempting to predict if an intubated patient will tolerate single-lung ventilation, it is our practice to place an intubated patient on 100% FIO_2 and, after about 15 minutes, obtain an arterial blood gas. If the arterial PO_2 is greater than 120 mm Hg, patients will usually tolerate single-lung ventilation long enough to allow a biopsy.

The procedure is relatively straightforward. After a patient is intubated, the two lungs are isolated. As long as the disease process is equally distributed to both lungs and the patient will tolerate having the right lung collapsed, then the right side is generally preferred because there is more space to operate in the right chest. A 5-mm incision is made, and a port is introduced through the seventh intercostal space at the anterior axillary line. Carbon dioxide is insufflated to 8 mm Hg pressure. This initial port site can be used for a chest tube at the conclusion of the case. The second port site is posterior near the level of the diaphragm in line with the tip of the scapula. The stapler can be introduced through this port. On occasion, an additional 5-mm port needs to be inserted anteriorly to allow insertion of an instrument to manipulate the lung. Ports are placed for two reasons. First, they allow instruments to be inserted and removed quickly and easily, thus speeding up the operation. The second reason is that with instrument ports in place and the hemithorax insufflated with carbon dioxide, the patient can by placed back on two-lung ventilation if needed, without complete visual loss of the operative field. The positive pressure of the insufflated gas allows the lung to be inflated and ventilated partially, thereby allowing the procedure to be completed in a minimally invasive fashion.

Separate biopsies of each lobe are performed that are each about 1 × 3 cm in size. This allows plenty of tissue for both pathology and microbiologic studies while allowing ease of extraction from the chest. Review of the imaging with radiology and pulmonary medicine before surgery allows directed biopsies of the lung that correspond to areas of concern for active disease. At the conclusion of the case, a 24-Fr chest tube can be placed and attached to a chest drainage unit, commonly known as a Pleur-evac (Teleflex Medical). As long as the lung remains expanded, the chest tube can be left on water seal.

Lung biopsy entails some risks of complications. In a review of the Society of Thoracic Surgeons General Thoracic Database, the overall complication rate was less than 10%. The composite rate of postoperative respiratory failure, defined as pneumonia, initial ventilator support of more than 48 hours, acute respiratory distress syndrome, reintubation, or tracheostomy, was 2.9%. The rate of any pleural complication was 5.6%. In this database, the operative mortality was 1.5% at 30 days after an operation.[39,40] Risk factors for morbidity and mortality were pulmonary hypertension, preoperative corticosteroid use, and low diffusion capacity. Although all patients are different, careful consideration and multidisciplinary discussion can result in a safe procedure that provides answers to allow optimal treatment of the patient. The utility of lung biopsies is a question that generates debate. Discussion with pulmonary medicine and radiology of the radiographic findings with the clinical picture generally narrows the differential diagnosis. When the results of the biopsy can change treatment and help to provide a guide to prognosis, lung biopsy can be extremely helpful.

POSTOPERATIVE MANAGEMENT

The management of patients after surgery is as critically important as good surgical technique and preoperative decision making. This can even begin before surgery with the application of *enhanced recovery after surgery* (ERAS) protocols. After pulmonary resections, there are particular issues to manage. For one, all patients will have a chest tube. For another, pain control allows patients to take deep breaths, ambulate, and clear secretions with coughing. How these two issues are managed can have a profound impact on patient outcomes. In some situations, a patient may remain intubated after surgery. In these instances, ventilator management strategies focusing on airway pressures need to be considered.

CHEST TUBE MANAGEMENT

Overall, the management of chest tubes after surgery does have some individual variations, but there is literature to support an overall approach. Some practice variation concerns different views about the use of a clamp trial to ensure that there is no air leak and different end points for the appropriate output before removing the tube.

First, after surgery, placing a chest tube to water seal initially is ideal, regardless of whether or not there is an air leak.[41,42] This begs the question: when should the chest tube be on suction?

For all patients after thoracic surgery, a chest radiograph should be obtained in the recovery area. If the lung is not full expanded, and it is the expectation of the surgeon that the residual lung should fill the entire pleural space, then suction should be applied. A repeat radiograph can then confirm that the lung is expanded. At that point, suction should be applied until at least the next day and then placed back to water seal. A follow-up radiograph can confirm that the lung remains expanded. The underlying principle behind the preference for water seal is that it minimizes the pressure gradient across fresh staple lines and bronchial stumps. Thus, in deciding to apply suction for a pneumothorax, one cannot refer to an algorithm. The decision is based on the degree of postoperative air leak, the lobe removed and the expected lung volume loss (e.g., lower lobectomy patients can often have some residual space), and the patient's pulmonary status. Most current pleural evacuation systems have a regulator to titrate the suction from none (water seal) to −10, −20, −30, or −40 cm of water suction. If the goal is to reexpand the lung in the immediate postoperative setting, then one should use the least amount of suction necessary to accomplish this.

The other immediate postoperative indication for placing the chest tube to suction is to deal with increasing amounts of subcutaneous air. Although this is very rarely dangerous to the patient, it does cause discomfort and, when extreme, is reversibly disfiguring and often quite disconcerting to the patient, the patient's family, or even medical staff unfamiliar with this condition. Patients can, literally, inflate from head to toe. One of the only scenarios where this can be life threatening is if the air actually dissects into the oropharynx, compressing the tissue and limiting air flow through the trachea. The subcutaneous air can cause a condition known as Hamman syndrome and creates the characteristic crackling feeling, or subcutaneous crepitation, under the skin of the patient to the examiner's touch. Changes in voice normally manifest as an increase in pitch. Without placing the chest tube to suction, the air can continue to accumulate until the eyes swell shut. Even this degree of subcutaneous air is almost never dangerous. Development of subcutaneous emphysema in the setting of an indwelling chest tube is the result either of the chest tube not able to access the air (by perhaps being clogged, kinked, or walled off by expanded lung), the chest tube unable to handle a massive air leak, or often the chest tube with one of the ports outside the pleural space and providing access of the pleural air to the subcutaneous tissue. The initial steps are to ensure the tube is patent and functioning and has all ports within the pleural space. Then suction is gradually increased until the process appears to arrest. If maximal suction is reached and the situation is progressive, then another tube will be required. It is much more common in the perioperative period for there to be an issue with the tube than for it to be functioning perfectly and overwhelmed by the size of the leak. If an additional tube is required, a CT scan might be helpful in determining the optimal location. Once the air leak stops, in general it takes about 7 to 10 days for the subcutaneous air to resolve.

Starting on postoperative day 1, the indications for chest tube removal are the same: no air leak and appropriate chest tube output.

To check for an air leak, drain all the fluid from the tubing into the collection chamber and then have the patient perform a vigorous cough. There should be no bubbles coming through the water-seal chamber. The tube can then be safely removed. If there is an air leak, the tube should not be removed. On occasion a patient may generate a cough that moves a bubble or two across the water seal. This generally happens only on the first cough and a series of coughs can help to determine if there is or is not an air leak.

If there is any concern, a clamp trial may be of benefit. This is done by clamping the chest tube and getting serial radiographs. Individuals may want a different protocol, but in general a tube is clamped for 4 to 6 hours and, if there is no change in radiographs compared to the one before clamping, the chest tube can be removed. If the radiographs appear equivocal, then leaving the tube clamped longer, typically 24 hours, may be advised. It is important to emphasize that, when a chest tube is clamped, the patient should remain closely monitored. If there are any concerns, such as increasing subcutaneous air, hypotension, acute tachycardia, or hypoxia, the tube should be unclamped immediately.

The recent advancement of digital pleural drainage systems may change the need for clamp trials.[43,44] They provide real-time objective measurements and digitally track both fluid output rates and air leaks. The precise time when the air leak resolves can be identified with the digital readout, thus decreasing unexpected pneumothorax after removal of the chest tube caused by a failure to appreciate a small air leak.

The appropriate chest tube output acceptable for removal is not certain.[45–47] Most thoracic surgeons use an amount between 250 and 400 mL per day. Studies looking at correlating chest tube output with weight and body mass index have not shown that using the amount of output as a ratio to another variable adds anything to the actual output.

Pneumonectomy Patients

There are some unique postoperative concerns for patients who undergo pneumonectomy. First, chest tube management differs. Although chest tubes are not usually removed until the output decreases to an appropriate level, after a pneumonectomy, the chest tube is removed relatively early to allow the pleural space to fill completely with fluid. The chest eventually needs to fill with fluid that will then form a fibrothorax and allow the mediastinum and heart to remain in their appropriate anatomic position. Issues can come up when the chest fills too fast, too slow, stops filling up, or fully empties.

When the chest fills too fast, this can cause a tension hydropneumothorax because the fluid has nowhere to go, and the air is not able to be reabsorbed fast enough by the body. Just like a tension pneumothorax, it presents clinically with tachycardia, hypotension, and shift of the mediastinum away from the side of the pneumonectomy. This complication can be treated by placing a central venous catheter directly into the pleural space to "balance the mediastinum." This is done normally through the second or third intercostal space anteriorly at the midclavicular line. Then the air and some fluid are withdrawn until the symptoms are relieved. The benefit is nearly instantaneous. The catheter is left in place for a few days to provide access for repeated treatment, if necessary. Repeat radiographs will demonstrate return of the heart to the center of the chest.

When the chest takes an excessive length of time to fill up completely (>2 weeks), one must consider a possible mechanism limiting fluid accumulation. The diagnosis of greatest concern to thoracic surgeons is the development of a bronchopleural fistula at the bronchial stump staple line. If not diagnosed and treated immediately, it can result in a postpneumonectomy empyema. This should be considered when the fluid forms a horizontal line on radiograph at the level of the carina. Confirmation is made with bronchoscopy and evaluation and interrogation of the staple line stump. If this diagnosis is suspected or confirmed, thoracic surgery should be consulted immediately.

Rarely after a pneumonectomy, when the pleural space does not fill up with fluid or the fluid is slowly reabsorbed over years, a patient can develop a postpneumonectomy syndrome. With this syndrome, the mediastinum shifts to that side, leading to partial or complete obstruction of the contralateral airway and/or pulmonary venous system. This can acutely or progressively cause significant cardiopulmonary impairment (Fig 30.7). If this should happen, management involves surgery to recenter the mediastinum. We prefer to use adjustable saline breast implants in the pleural space to maintain the position of the heart and allow relief of the obstruction of the bronchus and/or pulmonary veins[48,49] (Fig. 30.8).

PAIN

Postoperative pain can lead to various serious complications, including atelectasis, mucous plugging, pneumonia, blood clots, and pulmonary embolism. Pain also interferes with deep breathing, coughing, and mobility. Atelectasis is a particular issue for thoracic surgery patients, all of whom experience single-lung isolation during surgery and thus decruitment of alveoli. Mucous plugging can lead to hypoxia and increased risk of cardiac arrhythmias. If a patient is unable to cough and clear the plug, bronchoscopy is then routinely performed. Certain operations, such as sleeve resection, typically have higher rates of patients requiring postoperative bronchoscopy, both because of plugging and ciliary dysfunction after the resection. Thus postoperative pain control is paramount in a thoracic surgery patient.

Various steps to prevent or treat postoperative pain are used, and more are under investigation. If an open thoracotomy is being planned, before induction of anesthesia, the placement of a thoracic epidural is highly encouraged. This

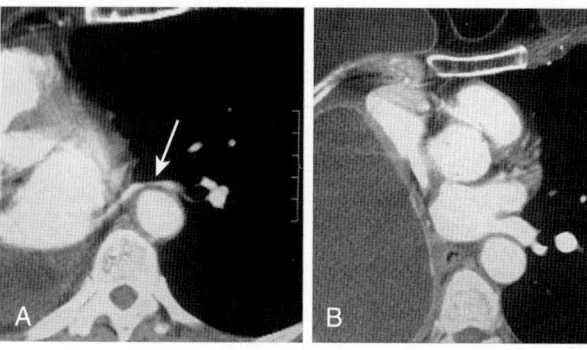

Figure 30.7 *Computed tomography* **(CT) scans demonstrating change in the caliber of the inferior pulmonary vein before (A) and after (B) placement of adjustable implants.** (A) Two years after a right pneumonectomy, the patient had progressive dyspnea, dysphagia, and reflux. CT scans showed a gradual shift of the mediastinum to the right with increasing compression of the left inferior pulmonary vein *(arrow)* and left lower lobe bronchus. During thoracotomy, two saline implants were placed, and their volume was adjusted to move the mediastinum medially. Upon recovery, the patient's symptoms were completely resolved. (B) Six months later, repeat CT scan shows significant increase in size of the inferior pulmonary vein. (From Encarnacion CO, Deshpande SP, Mondal S, Carr SR. Surgical correction of postpneumonectomy syndrome with adjustable saline implants and transoesophageal echocardiography. *Eur J Cardiothorac Surg.* 2020;57:1224–1226.)

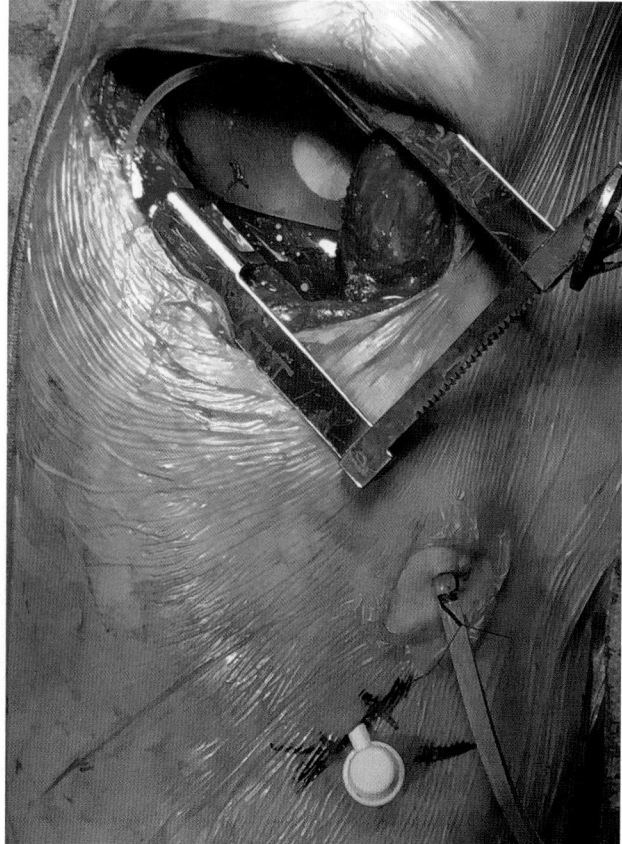

Figure 30.8 Intraoperative picture of the implants and adjustable access reservoir. An adjustable saline breast implant is seen through the incision in the right hemithorax. The access port for postoperative adjustments is the white-colored structure next to the pleural drain. (From Encarnacion CO, Deshpande SP, Mondal S, Carr SR. Surgical correction of postpneumonectomy syndrome with adjustable saline implants and transoesophageal echocardiography. *Eur J Cardiothorac Surg.* 2020;57:1224–1226.)

allows excellent pain control for patients without oversedating them, which aids in their ability to ambulate and participate in maneuvers for improving their pulmonary toilet. However, these can cause issues with hypotension, epidural headaches, and urinary retention. When a patient experiences hypotension, decreasing the epidural analgesic flow rate can allow improvement in blood pressure but may come at the cost of pain control. In a prospective study in thoracic surgery patients from the Mayo Clinic, leaving Foley catheters in place until the epidural was removed resulted in few complications, which generally runs counter to most hospital policies of removing Foley catheters within 24 hours of surgery to decrease the risk of catheter-associated urinary tract infections. In this study, the opposite was seen, mainly thought to be because, in the setting of urinary retention, maintaining the Foley catheter in place avoided multiple instrumentations of the bladder.

Paravertebral blocks are becoming more popular. Although more challenging to place than an epidural, they can provide equivalent pain relief without the side effects of hypotension and spinal headache commonly seen with epidurals. Hypotension, the most common side effect with an epidural, is due to a bilateral effect on the sympathetic nerves. This is uncommon with paravertebral blocks because they only affect the sympathetic nerves on the side of the block. Spinal headache from an epidural is due to its intrathecal location; this is also less common with the paravertebral block because the catheter is extrathecal.

Recently, the use of cryoablation has been proposed. In this procedure a cryoprobe is used to freeze the intercostal nerves at their emergence from the spine. Early nonrandomized preliminary data suggest that this may be effective, but this has not been demonstrated in a conclusive way.[50] Studies are ongoing. Of note, the effect does not start until 24 to 48 hours after cryoablation, so early pain control measures are needed, but the hope is that this approach could allow decreased use of postoperative narcotics and early recovery.

There has been a recent push to adopt ERAS protocols.[51,52] In addition to early mobilization, the protocols support the use of adjuvants for pain control to include nonsteroidal anti-inflammatory drugs, acetaminophen, and gabapentin. Studies of ERAS protocols have shown decreased use of opiates after surgery. There are a few studies on this topic in thoracic surgery patients, but all are favorable. In addition to ERAS protocols, a current study is underway at the University of Maryland School of Medicine, the WINNERS Trial, that, in addition to using ERAS protocols, helps to educate patients on what to expect and set goals and expectations for after discharge. The aim is to determine if preoperative education can also help to decrease hospital readmission rates.

Patients who are mobilized early and often decrease their risks for blood clots and pulmonary embolism. Pulmonary embolism is generally poorly tolerated in this population and, particularly after pneumonectomy, is accompanied by a significant mortality rate. Mobilization allows increased ventilation and recruitment of lung.

VENTILATOR MANAGEMENT

In general, every attempt is made to extubate thoracic surgery patients at the conclusion of the operation. Patients who undergo decortication are sometimes the exception, where the patient is left on positive-pressure ventilation to help reexpand a lung that has been entrapped for a significant period of time. Even when a significant air leak is present while a patient is on positive-pressure ventilation, extubation greatly reduces the air leak. It is rare for a patient to require reintubation for an air leak. The main reason to strive for extubation is to decrease the pressure on the bronchial stump, staple lines, and/or airway anastomosis.

When a patient must remain intubated, it is imperative to minimize airway pressure. Pressure-control modes of ventilation are generally preferred to volume-controlled modes. Although there are no data providing exact target values, we generally aim for peak airway pressures of less than 24 cm H_2O and plateau pressures in the teens. We have unpublished data demonstrating that the peak inspiratory pressures are most damaging to a fresh staple line and therefore recommend ventilator management geared toward limiting peak inspiratory pressures. Permissive hypercapnia is tolerated and worth trying to keep airway pressures low, as long as the arterial blood gas pH remains greater than 7.30. Allowing for spontaneous ventilation with minimal pressure support to provide adequate ventilation should be the goal. On occasion, a patient may develop acute respiratory distress syndrome after pulmonary surgery. In this type of scenario, extracorporeal membrane oxygenation may provide the only option to support gas exchange while minimizing ventilation and airway pressures.

Patients who undergo decortication are occasionally left intubated for 24 to 48 hours after surgery to help with alveolar recruitment from a lung that has been very atelectatic for a long period of time. Providing a patient with a low level of pressure support and setting the positive end-expiratory pressure at 8 to 10 cm H_2O helps with lung expansion in the immediate postoperative period.

Key Readings

British Thoracic Society, Society of Cardiothoracic Surgeons of Great Britain and Ireland Working Party. BTS guidelines: guidelines on the selection of patients with lung cancer for surgery. *Thorax.* 2001;56(2):89–108.

Brunelli A, Xiumé F, Refai M, et al. Evaluation of expiratory volume, diffusion capacity, and exercise tolerance following major lung resection: a prospective follow-up analysis. *Chest.* 2007;131(1):141–147.

Cao C, Louie BE, Melfi F, et al. Impact of pulmonary function on pulmonary complications after robotic-assisted thoracoscopic lobectomy. *Eur J Cardiothorac Surg.* 2020;57(2):338–342.

Carr SR, Schuchert MJ, Pennathur A, et al. Impact of tumor size on outcomes after anatomic lung resection for stage 1A non–small cell lung cancer based on the current staging system. *J Thorac Cardiovasc Surg.* 2012;143(2):390–397.

Durheim MT, Kim S, Gulack BC, et al. Mortality and respiratory failure after thoracoscopic lung biopsy for interstitial lung disease. *Ann Thorac Surg.* 2017;104(2):465–470.

Ginsberg RJ, Rubinstein LV. Randomized trial of lobectomy versus limited resection for T1 N0 non–small cell lung cancer. lung cancer study group. *Ann Thorac Surg.* 1995;60(3):615–622; discussion 622–623.

Loewen GM, Watson D, Kohman L, et al. Preoperative exercise Vo_2 measurement for lung resection candidates: results of Cancer and Leukemia Group B Protocol 9238. *J Thorac Oncol.* 2007;2(7):619–625.

Marshall MB, Deeb ME, Bleier JIS, et al. Suction vs water seal after pulmonary resection: a randomized prospective study. *Chest.* 2002; 121(3):831–835.

Paul S, Altorki NK, Sheng S, et al. Thoracoscopic lobectomy is associated with lower morbidity than open lobectomy: a propensity-matched analysis from the STS database. *J Thorac Cardiovasc Surg.* 2010;139(2):366–378.

Wang T, Luo L, Zhou Q. Risk of pleural recurrence in early stage lung cancer patients after percutaneous transthoracic needle biopsy: a meta-analysis. *Sci Rep.* 2017;7(1):42762.

Yasufuku K, Pierre A, Darling G, et al. A prospective controlled trial of endobronchial ultrasound-guided transbronchial needle aspiration compared with mediastinoscopy for mediastinal lymph node staging of lung cancer. *J Thorac Cardiovasc Surg.* 2011;142(6). 1393–400.e1.

Complete reference list available at ExpertConsult.com.

Key Points

- Minimally invasive surgery should be the initial approach for nearly all thoracic surgery pulmonary resections because the risk of complication and recovery time are usually less compared to open surgery.
- Whereas lobectomy is the gold standard for oncologic resections, anatomic sublobar resection (e.g., segmentectomy) appears to have a role in early stage lung cancer by preserving pulmonary parenchyma.
- Thoracoscopic wedge resections for interstitial lung disease are safe and provide high diagnostic yield compared to other approaches.
- Postoperative pain management is paramount to helping decrease complications after surgery.
- Chest tubes in patients after thoracic surgery should ideally be on water seal, with the exception of patients where achieving pleural to pleural apposition is essential (e.g., decortications and pleurodesis).
- In patients requiring ventilation after pulmonary resection, pressure-control modes of ventilation are preferred to decrease overall airway pressure on surgical staple lines.

EVALUATION

31 *PULMONARY FUNCTION TESTING: PHYSIOLOGIC AND TECHNICAL PRINCIPLES*

NIRAV R. BHAKTA, MD, PHD • DAVID A. KAMINSKY, MD

INTRODUCTION

Pulmonary function tests (PFTs) permit accurate, reproducible assessment of the functional state of the respiratory system. PFTs do not diagnose specific diseases. Different diseases cause different patterns of abnormalities in a battery of PFTs. These patterns allow us to quantify the severity of respiratory disease, which enables us to detect disease early and characterize the natural history and response to treatment. The accuracy of interpretation depends on a complete knowledge of the physiologic basis of the functions tested, properly validated equipment, and appropriate protocols. The purpose of this chapter is to describe these PFTs, reviewing briefly their physiologic basis, their equipment and protocol requirements, and their clinical implications. The next chapter, Chapter 32, covers the clinical interpretation and application of PFTs in more detail.

This chapter has an extended online version. A wealth of details of procedures, normal and predicted values, equations, and descriptions of techniques can be found at ExpertConsult.com.

MECHANICAL PROPERTIES OF THE RESPIRATORY SYSTEM

The physiologic determinants of airflow during quiet breathing, maximal airflow, lung volumes, and elastic recoil are introduced in Chapter 11. Figure 31.1 reviews the equal pressure point theory for limitation of maximal airflow in more detail.

FORCED SPIROMETRY

Spirometry is the measurement of the volume of air inhaled or exhaled. Spirometry is commonly performed with a pneumotachometer that measures flow rates and integrates flow to obtain the volume of air inhaled and exhaled during a series of ventilatory maneuvers. Lung volumes and capacities are defined in Figure 31.2. Recommended criteria for acceptable performance standards for equipment have been published, as well as criteria for an acceptable maneuver.[1] Although the maneuver appears quite simple, the initial 25–30% of the maximal expiratory maneuver is effort dependent, and these measurements depend heavily on patient understanding and

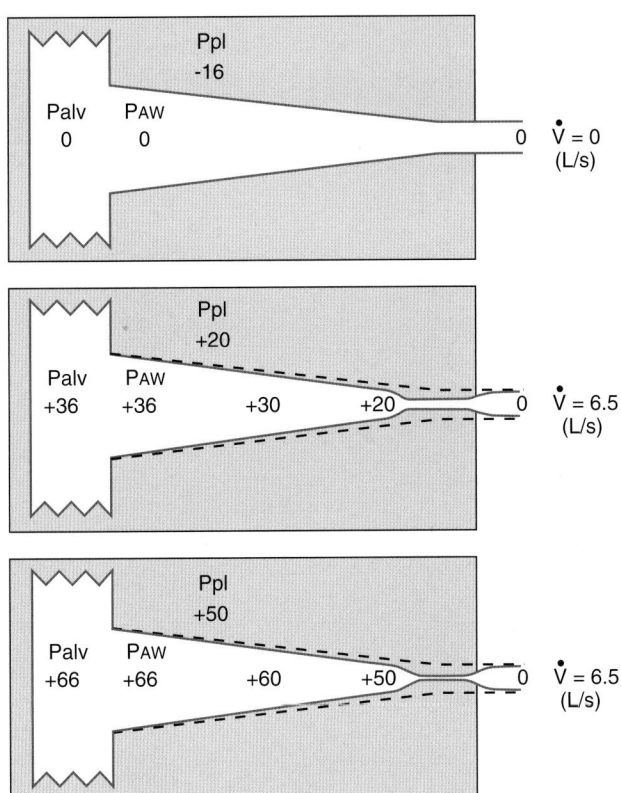

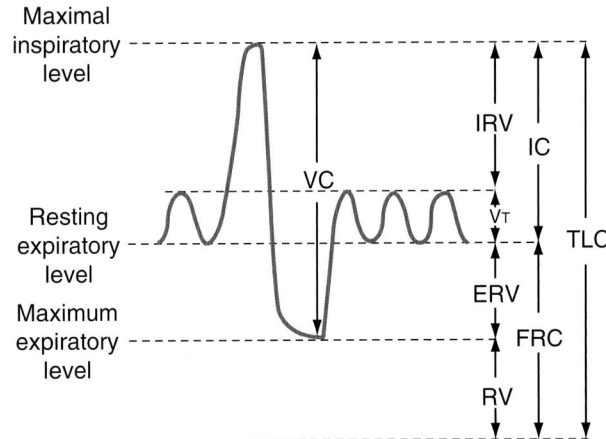

Figure 31.2 Lung volume and capacity. *Volumes:* There are four volumes, which do not overlap: (1) tidal volume (VT) is the volume of gas inhaled or exhaled during each respiratory cycle; (2) inspiratory reserve volume (IRV) is the maximal volume of gas inspired from end inspiration; (3) expiratory reserve volume (ERV) is the maximal volume of gas exhaled from end expiration; and (4) residual volume (RV) is the volume of gas remaining in the lungs after a maximal exhalation. *Capacities:* There are four capacities, each of which contains two or more primary volumes: (1) total lung capacity (TLC) is the amount of gas contained in the lung at maximal inspiration; (2) vital capacity (VC) is the maximal volume of gas that can be expelled from the lungs after maximal inspiration, without regard for the time involved; (3) inspiratory capacity (IC) is the maximal volume of gas that can be inspired from the resting expiratory level; and (4) functional residual capacity (FRC) is the volume of gas in the lungs at resting end expiration.

Figure 31.1 Model of expiratory flow limitation. *Top:* The static relationships of pleural pressure (Ppl), alveolar pressure (Palv), intraluminal airway pressure (PAW), and airway dimensions at a fixed lung volume. *Middle and bottom:* Conditions at the onset of maximal flow and with increased expiratory effort, respectively. *Dotted lines* show static airway dimensions for comparison with the dynamic state. All three panels show pressures (cm H_2O) at the same lung volume: 60% of total lung capacity where lung elastic recoil pressure is +16 cm H_2O and equals the transpulmonary pressure (PL): (PL = Palv – Ppl). *Top:* When conditions are static, Palv is zero (i.e., atmospheric) and flow (V̇) at the mouth is zero. *Middle:* The subject makes a forced expiratory effort at the same lung volume. Now V̇ is 6.5 L/sec driven by Palv of +36 cm H_2O. Because of the resistances down the airways from alveolus to mouth, PAW decreases to the point where PAW = Ppl (+20 cm H_2O, which is called the equal pressure point [EPP] because Ppl = PAW). Between the alveolus and the EPP, the airways are not compressed, but distal to the EPP there is compression and airway narrowing because Ppl exceeds the pressure within the airways. For this lung volume, 6.5 L/sec is the maximal flow possible. *Bottom:* The subject makes a forced expiratory effort starting at the same volume as in the top and middle panels (PL = Palv – Ppl = +16). In this instance, the expiratory effort is markedly increased, reflected by the increased Ppl (+50 cm H_2O) and Palv (+66 cm H_2O). However, the flow generated is still only 6.5 L/sec because the increased effort succeeds only in compressing the airways more, dissipating the increased driving pressure across the increased resistance offered by the more narrowed airways; thus, flow is maximum for this particular lung volume. (Modified from Rodarte JR: Respiratory mechanics. In: Rodarte JR, Hyatt RE. *Basics of Respiratory Disease.* New York: American Thoracic Society; 1976.)

cooperation and must be conducted by a well-trained technician able to communicate instructions clearly.

Comparison of the resulting tracings of volume versus time and flow versus volume, as well as the numbers derived from these tracings, to expected values from healthy reference populations, determines whether the subject has a normal ventilatory reserve or an abnormal pattern characteristic of obstructive, restrictive, or mixed ventilatory abnormalities. None of these patterns is specific, although most diseases cause a predictable type of ventilatory defect. Spirometry alone cannot establish a diagnosis of a specific disease, but it is sufficiently reproducible to be useful in following the course of many different diseases. In addition, the results of

spirometry make it possible to estimate the degree of exercise limitation due to a ventilatory defect (e.g., *maximal voluntary ventilation* [MVV] can be predicted from the *forced expiratory volume in 1 second* [FEV$_1$])[2] and to identify the type of patient likely to develop ventilatory failure after pneumonectomy.[3,4]

Indications for spirometry are reviewed at ExpertConsult.com and in society guidelines.[1] Definitions are reviewed at ExpertConsult.com.

Maximal-Effort Expiratory Vital Capacity

To obtain a maximal-effort expiratory *vital capacity* (VC), the subject inhales maximally to *total lung capacity* (TLC) and then exhales as rapidly and forcefully as possible. When volume is recorded on the *y*-axis and time on the *x*-axis, the resulting curve is called the *forced vital capacity* (FVC) curve (Fig. 31.3). Analysis of this curve permits computation of the volume exhaled during the time after the start of the maneuver (*forced expiratory volume over time* [FEV$_t$]), the ratio of FEV$_t$ to total FVC, and average flow rates during different portions of the curve. The terms used in clinical spirometry, including these different components, are summarized in Table 31.1.[7]

Forced Expiratory Volume Over Time

The FEV$_1$ is the measurement of dynamic volume most often used in conjunction with the FVC in analysis of spirometry (see Fig. 31.3). The measurement incorporates the early, effort-dependent portion of the curve and enough of the midportion to make it reproducible and sensitive for clinical purposes. The *forced expiratory volume exhaled in 6 seconds* (FEV$_6$) approximates FVC, and FEV$_1$/FEV$_6$ ratio has been shown to be a valid alternative to the conventional FEV$_1$/FVC ratio and is easier for patients with severe airflow obstruction to attain.[8] In addition, the end of the test is more clearly defined, permitting more reliable correspondence between measured and referenced values.[9]

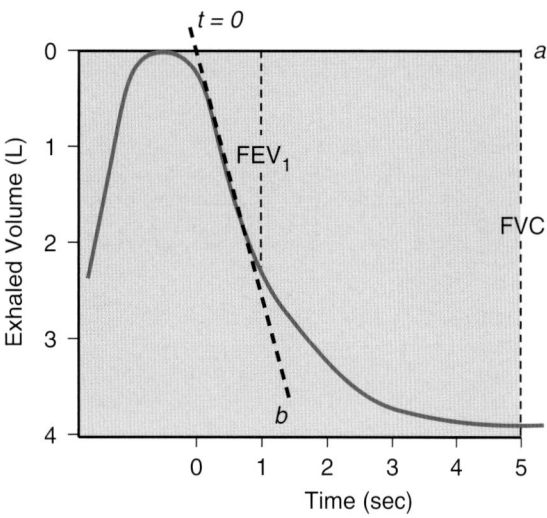

Figure 31.3 Measurement of *forced expiratory volume in 1 second* (FEV₁). This diagram illustrates measurement of FEV_1 using the back-extrapolation method to define time zero (i.e., the point during the forced vital capacity [FVC] maneuver when the subject began to blow as hard and as fast as possible). A solid horizontal line (*a*) indicates the level of maximal inhalation. A heavy dashed line (*b*) passes through the steepest portion of the volume-time tracing. The intersection point of these two lines becomes time zero, from which timing is initiated, as indicated; 1 second after time zero, the vertical dashed line is drawn, indicating FEV_1, and 5 seconds later, another vertical dashed line is drawn, indicating FVC.

Table 31.1   Terms Used for Spirometric Measurements

Term	Description
Vital capacity (VC)	Largest volume measured on complete exhalation after full inspiration
Forced VC (FVC)	VC performed with forced expiration
Forced expiratory volume with subscript indicating interval in seconds (FEV_t) (e.g., FEV_1)	Volume of gas exhaled in a given time during performance of FVC
Percentage expired in time (seconds) ($FEV_t\%$) (e.g., $FEV_1\%$)	FEV_t expressed as percentage of FVC
Forced midexpiratory flow ($FEF_{25\%-75\%}$)	Maximal midexpiratory flow
Forced expiratory flow with subscript indicating volume segment (FEF_{V1-V2}) (e.g., $FEF_{200-1200}$)	Average rate of flow for a specified segment of FVC, most commonly 200–1200 mL in adults
Maximal voluntary ventilation (MVV)	Volume of air a subject can breathe with voluntary maximal effort for a given time

Modified from Kory RC. Clinical spirometry: recommendation of the Section on Pulmonary Function Testing, Committee on Pulmonary Physiology, American College of Chest Physicians. *Dis Chest.* 1963;43:214.

Forced Expiratory Volume Over Time as a Percentage of Forced Vital Capacity

The ratio of FEV_1 to total FVC has been defined precisely in healthy subjects.[10] It declines with age, but abnormally decreased ratios indicate airway obstruction; normal or increased ratios do not reliably exclude airway obstruction, particularly in the presence of a decreased FVC. When the FVC is decreased by an interstitial process or by chest wall restriction and the airways are normal, the FEV_1/FVC ratio is

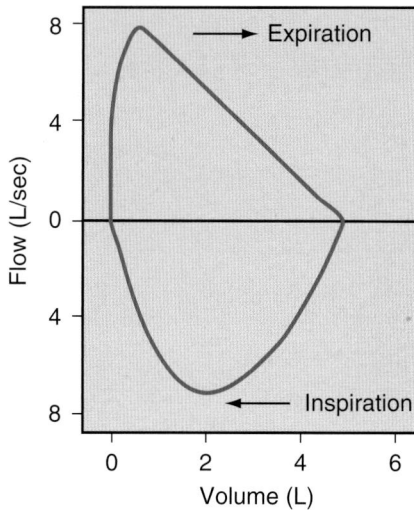

Figure 31.4 The flow-volume curve. The tracing of the flow-volume curve is recorded during maximal inspiration and expiration in a normal subject.

increased. (The FEV_1/FVC ratio may also be increased in subjects who are not able to sustain a maximal effort throughout the expiratory maneuver.) The absence of an increased ratio in patients in whom one would expect the ratio to be increased suggests the presence of concomitant airway obstruction.

Average Forced Expiratory Flow Between 25% and 75% of Forced Vital Capacity

The average *forced expiratory flow between 25% and 75%* ($FEF_{25\%-75\%}$) of FVC was introduced as the maximal midexpiratory flow rate (eFig. 31.1). This measurement was intended to reflect the most effort-independent portion of the curve and a portion more sensitive to airflow in peripheral airways, where diseases of chronic airflow obstruction are thought to originate.[11] These properties have gained support from clinical experience and theoretical analysis.[12] However, the $FEF_{25\%-75\%}$ shows marked variability in studies of large samples of healthy subjects, and the 95% confidence limits for normal values are so large that they limit its sensitivity in detecting disease in an individual subject.[4,13]

Maximal Voluntary Ventilation

The *maximal voluntary ventilation* (MVV) measurement is defined as the maximal volume of air that can be moved by voluntary effort in 1 minute. Subjects are instructed to breathe rapidly and deeply for 12 seconds, ventilatory volumes are recorded, and the maximal volume achieved over 12 consecutive seconds is expressed in liters per minute. Lung volumes are reported at the largest size possible within the chest and at body temperature (37°C) and standard pressure fully saturated with water vapor (760 mm Hg). MVV in L/min can be estimated as FEV_1 (L) × 40, and in the absence of inspiratory airflow obstruction, neuromuscular weakness or morbid obesity, is a reasonable alternative.

For additional information, see ExpertConsult.com.

FLOW-VOLUME RELATIONSHIPS

Most commonly, spirometry data are visualized by plotting flow versus volume data obtained while a subject inspires and expires fully with maximal effort (Fig. 31.4). As summarized in Figure 31.1, analysis of these curves has contributed to the basic understanding of the mechanical events that limit maximal exhalation. Maximal flow clearly depends on lung volume: for every point on the lower two-thirds of VC, a maximal flow exists that cannot be exceeded regardless of the effort exerted by the subject. Thus maximal flow must depend on mechanical characteristics of the lungs. Flow-volume curves also provide a useful way to display ventilatory data for diagnostic purposes.

On forced exhalation, the flow-volume curve has a characteristic appearance. The curve shows a rapid ascent to peak flow and subsequently a slow linear descent proportional to volume. The curve over the initial quarter to one-third of vital capacity exhaled depends on effort. As a subject exerts increasing effort during exhalation, associated with increasing intrathoracic pressure, increasing flow is generated. This portion of the curve has limited diagnostic use because its appearance depends primarily on the subject's muscular effort and cooperation rather than on the mechanical characteristics of the lung.

Shortly after development of peak flow, the curve follows a remarkably reproducible, effort-independent envelope as flow diminishes in proportion to volume until *residual volume* (RV) is reached. For each point on the volume axis, a maximal flow exists that cannot be exceeded regardless of the pressure generated by the respiratory muscles. Although this portion of the curve is very reproducible in a given patient from time to time, it is altered in a characteristic manner by the effect of diseases on the mechanical properties of the lungs. In most subjects older than 30 years and in patients with pulmonary disease, RV is determined by airway closure, so the flow-volume curve shows a gradual downward slope in flow until RV is reached. In some young individuals, however, and perhaps in some patients with chest wall disease, RV is determined by chest wall rigidity, which limits maximal exhalation. In such cases, expiratory flow abruptly decreases to zero at low lung volumes.

On forced inhalation, the flow-volume curves are normally entirely effort dependent. The shape of the inspiratory portion is symmetric with flow, increasing to a maximum midway through inspiration and then decreasing as inhalation proceeds to TLC. It is less influenced by diffuse airway or parenchymal disease. When central airway obstruction is suspected, however, the inspiratory limb of the flow-volume curve has great diagnostic usefulness, whereas ordinary spirometry reveals a nonspecific pattern. See the section on "Large Airway Obstruction: Stenosis and Malacia" in Chapter 32.

See ExpertConsult.com for discussion on other measurements derived from the flow-volume curve.

LUNG VOLUMES

Vital Capacity and Other Static Lung Volumes

The measurement of VC requires the subject to inhale as deeply as possible and then to exhale fully, taking as much time as required. Figure 31.2 illustrates the subdivisions of lung volume.[20] The measurement can also be obtained by adding two of its components: the *expiratory reserve volume* (ERV), obtained by having the subject exhale maximally from the resting end-tidal level; and the *inspiratory capacity* (IC), obtained by having the subject inspire fully from the resting end-tidal level. The sum of these two measurements

yields the "combined VC"; as long as the resting end-tidal lung volume is the same for the two component maneuvers, the combined VC and the VC are equal. In patients with severe airflow obstruction, the combined VC appears to be larger than the VC, suggesting the presence of poorly ventilated regions of lungs, or so-called trapped gas. This result probably reflects increased transmural pressure, which tends to cause airway closure during a large portion of the single maneuver—but only in the portion near RV during the combined VC maneuver.

A similar inference can be made by comparing the "slow VC" (performed without regard to time) and FVC, or by comparing inspired VC (maximal volume inhaled from RV to TLC) with the expired VC maneuver just described. Except for those subdivisions involving RV, each of the defined volumes can be recorded and measured by simple spirometry. The RV can be measured only by indirect methods (e.g., nitrogen [N_2] washout, helium (He) dilution, or body plethysmography). Figure 31.2 illustrates the fact that VC can be decreased in two different ways: by a decrease in TLC or by an increase in RV. Only by measuring RV and TLC can these two causes be differentiated.

Gas Dilution Methods

The two most commonly used gas dilution methods for measuring lung volume are the open-circuit N_2 method and the closed-circuit He method. Both methods rely on the use of a physiologically inert gas that is poorly soluble in alveolar blood and lung tissues. These methods most often make a primary measurement of *functional residual capacity* (FRC), the volume of gas remaining in the lung at the end of a normal expiration. Other lung volumes are subsequently derived by asking the subject to breath out to RV and in to TLC in linked maneuvers through a spirometer.

In the original open-circuit method, all exhaled gas is collected while the subject inhales pure oxygen. By assuming values for the initial concentration of N_2 in the lungs (alveolar N_2 fraction varies slightly with the respiratory quotient but is assumed to be approximately 0.81) and, for the rate of N_2 elimination from blood and tissues (about 30 mL/min, or estimated from a formula based on body surface area), measurement of the total amount of N_2 washed out from the lungs permits the calculation of the volume of N_2-containing gas present at the beginning of the maneuver, usually FRC (Fig. 31.5). In the modern era of rapid N_2 analyzers, the total amount of N_2 washed out is calculated as the sum of the within-breath product of tidal volume and the fraction of exhaled gas that is N_2, across all breaths until the fraction of N_2 is below some threshold (e.g., <1.5%) for at least three breaths.[21] With rapid analyzers, rather than assuming a value, the initial concentration of N_2 in the lungs is measured.

In the closed-circuit He dilution method (Fig. 31.6), the theory is similar. The subject rebreathes a gas mixture containing He, a physiologically inert tracer gas, in a closed system until equilibration is achieved. If the volume and concentration of He in the gas mixture rebreathed are known, measurement of the final equilibrium concentration of He permits calculation of the volume of gas in the lungs at the start of the maneuver, usually FRC.

See ExpertConsult.com for further details on gas dilution methods.

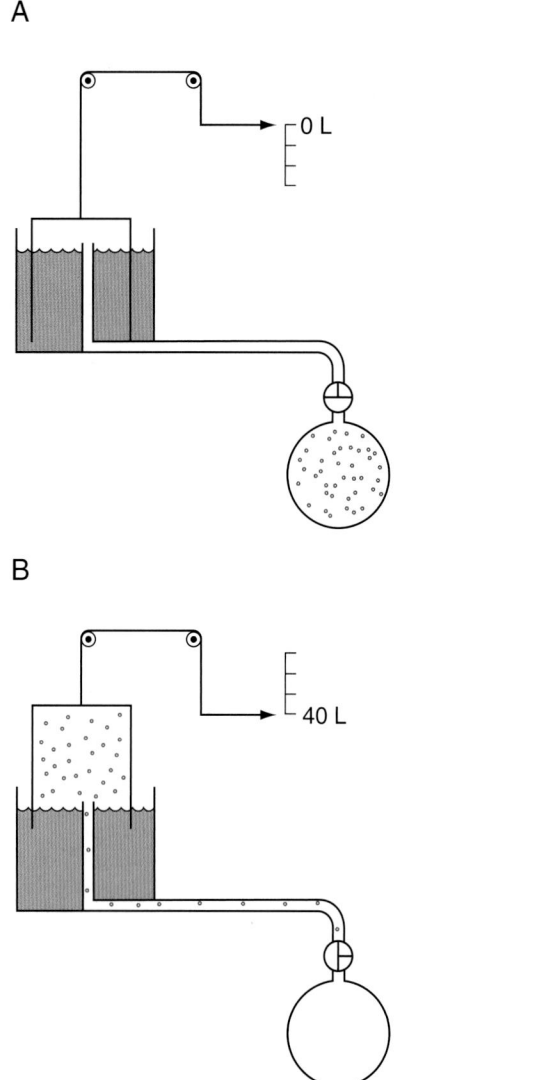

Figure 31.5 Open-circuit nitrogen method to measure functional residual capacity. Dots represent nitrogen (N_2) molecules. (A) Initially, all the N_2 molecules are in the lungs (as 80% N_2). (B) When N_2-free oxygen ("pure O_2") is breathed, the N_2 molecules are washed out of the lungs and collected with the O_2 as expired gas in the spirometer. The spirometer contains 40,000 mL of mixed expired gas with a N_2 concentration of 5%. Thus, the spirometer contains $0.05 \times 40,000 = 2000$ mL of N_2; the remaining 38,000 mL of gas is mainly O_2 used to wash the nitrogen out of the lungs, plus some carbon dioxide. The 2000 mL of N_2 was distributed within the lungs at a concentration of 80% N_2 when the washout began; therefore, the alveolar volume in which the N_2 was distributed was 2000 mL/0.8 = 2500 mL. (Corrections must be made for the small amount of N_2 washed out of the blood and tissue when O_2 is breathed and for the small amounts of N_2 in "pure O_2.")

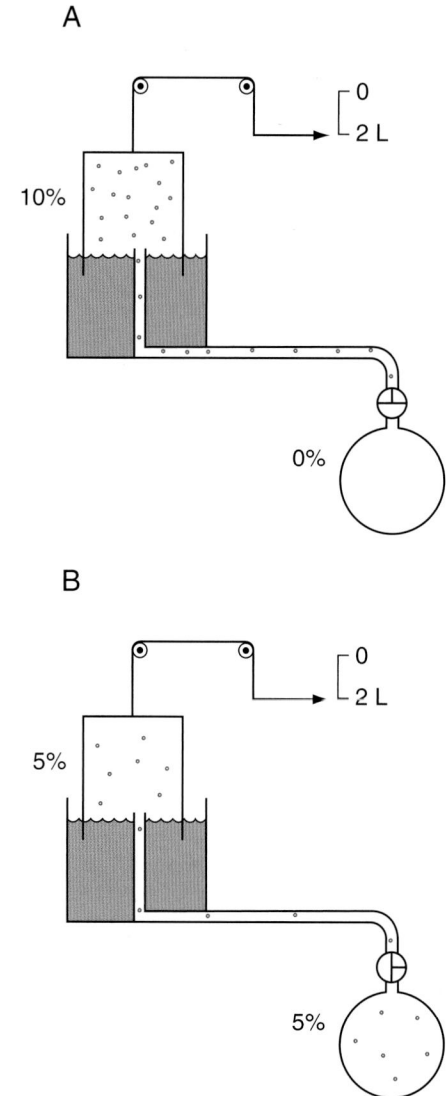

Figure 31.6 Closed-circuit helium method to measure functional residual capacity. Dots represent molecules of helium (He). (A) Initially, all He molecules are in the spirometer and tubing (as 10% He), and no molecules are in the lungs. If the spirometer and tubing contain 2000 mL of gas, of which 10% is He, then 2000 mL × 0.1, or 200 mL, of He is present in the spirometer and tubing before rebreathing. (B) Rebreathing results in redistribution of the He molecules until equilibrium develops, at which time lung volume can be calculated. At the end of the test, the same amount of He (200 mL) must be redistributed in the lungs, tubing, and spirometer, assuming that He is inert and not soluble in blood or tissues. At equilibrium, the concentration of He is 5%. The spirometer and tubing then account for 0.05 × 2000 mL = 100 mL He; the lung accounts for the remainder of the He: 200 − 100 mL = 100 mL. Therefore, the lung volume is 100 mL/0.05 = 2000 mL.

Body Plethysmography

There are three types of plethysmographs: pressure (most commonly used in clinical practice), volume, and pressure-volume.

Pressure (Closed-Type) Plethysmograph. This type of plethysmograph has a closed chamber with a fixed volume in which the subject breathes the gas in the plethysmograph (or body box) (Fig. 31.7). Volume changes associated with compression or expansion of gas within the thorax are measured as pressure changes in gas surrounding the subject within the box. Volume exchange between lung and box does not directly cause pressure changes, although thermal, humidity, and carbon dioxide–oxygen exchange differences between inspired and expired gas do cause pressure changes. Thoracic gas volume and airway resistance are measured during rapid maneuvers, so small leaks are tolerated; in fact, small leaks may be introduced to allow the pressure to equalize to the outside as air warms in the body box. This device is best suited for measuring small volume changes because of its high sensitivity and excellent frequency response. It need not be leak-free, absolutely rigid, or refrigerated because the measurements are usually brief and are used to study rapid events.

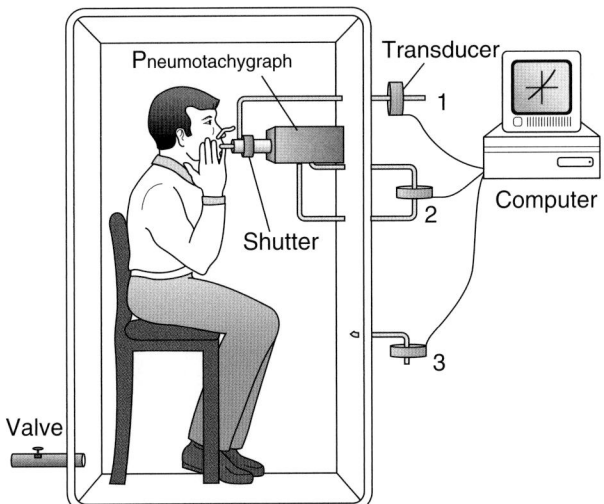

Figure 31.7 Pressure (closed-type) plethysmograph. The subject breathes through a shutter/pneumotachygraph. The shutter is open during tidal breathing and for measurements of airway resistance and closed for measurements of thoracic gas volume. When the shutter is closed, mouth pressure (equal to alveolar pressure at no flow) is measured by a pressure transducer (*1*). The pneumotachygraph measures airflow with another transducer (*2*), and the flow signal is integrated to volume electronically. The plethysmograph pressure is measured by a third transducer (*3*). The signals from the three transducers are processed by a computer. Excess box pressure caused by temperature changes when the subject sits in the closed box is vented through a valve.

Volume (Open-Type) Plethysmograph. This type of plethysmograph (eFig. 31.2) has constant pressure and variable volume. When thoracic volume changes, gas is displaced through a hole in the box wall and is measured either with a spirometer or by integrating the flow through a pneumotachygraph (or flowmeter). This device is suitable for measuring small or large volume changes. For a good frequency response, the impedance to gas displacement must be very small. This requires a low-resistance pneumotachygraph, a sensitive transducer, and a fast, drift-free integrator, or meticulous use of special spirometers; in consequence, this form of plethysmography is challenging and is used in the research setting only.

Pressure-Volume Plethysmograph. This device (eFig. 31.3) combines features of both the closed and open types. As the subject breathes from the room, changes in thoracic gas volume compress or expand the air around the subject in the box and also displace it through a hole in the box wall. The compression or decompression of gas is measured as a pressure change; the displacement of gas is measured either by a spirometer connected to the box or by integrating airflow through a pneumotachygraph in the opening. At every instant, all of the change in thoracic gas volume is accounted for by adding the two components (pressure change and volume displacement) (eFig. 31.4). This combined approach has a wide range of sensitivities, permitting all types of measurements to be made with the same instrument (i.e., thoracic gas volume and airway resistance, spirometry, and flow-volume curves). The box has excellent frequency response and relatively modest requirements for the spirometer. The integrated flow version dispenses with water-filled spirometers and is tolerant of leaks.

Measurement of Thoracic Gas Volume in a Pressure (Closed-Type) Plethysmograph. The *thoracic gas volume*

(V, also often referred to as TGV) is the compressible gas in the thorax, whether or not it is in free communication with airways. In the process of determining the V, the airway is occluded, and the subject makes small inspiratory and expiratory efforts against the occluded airway. The thoracic gas volume usually measured is slightly larger than FRC unless the shutter is closed precisely after a normal tidal volume is exhaled. Connecting the mouthpiece assembly to a valve and spirometer (or pneumotachygraph and integrator), or using a pressure-volume plethysmograph, makes it possible to measure TLC and all its subdivisions in conjunction with the measurement of thoracic gas volume.

During inspiratory efforts against the closed shutter, the thorax enlarges (ΔV) and decompresses intrathoracic gas, creating a new thoracic gas volume ($V' = V + \Delta V$) and a new pressure ($P' = P + \Delta P$), where P is atmospheric pressure. A pressure transducer between the subject's mouth and the occluded airway measures the new pressure (P'). It is assumed that the *mouth pressure* (Pmouth) equals *alveolar pressure* (Palv) during compressional changes as long as there is no airflow at the mouth because pressure changes are equal throughout a static fluid system (Pascal's principle). By Boyle's law, pressure multiplied by the volume of the gas in the thorax is constant if its temperature remains constant ($PV = P'V'$). In accordance,

$$PV = P'V' = (P + \Delta P)(V + \Delta V) \qquad \text{Eq. 1}$$

$$0 = P\Delta V + \Delta P V + \Delta P \Delta V \qquad \text{Eq. 2}$$

$$\text{If } \Delta P \ll P, \text{ then } \Delta P \Delta V \approx 0 \qquad \text{Eq. 3}$$

$$V = -\frac{\Delta V}{\Delta P}P \qquad \text{Eq. 4}$$

where P equals atmospheric pressure minus water vapor pressure (in mm Hg), assuming that alveolar gas is saturated with water vapor at body temperature; ΔV equals change in thoracic gas volume; and ΔP equals change in Pmouth, which is equal to the change in alveolar pressure (ΔPalv). Note that ΔP is a negative value during inspiratory efforts. Then the thoracic gas volume is calculated as follows:

$$V = -\frac{\Delta V (mL)}{\Delta Palv (cm\,H_2O)} \times (P - 47\,mm\,Hg)(1.36\,cm\,H_2O/mm\,Hg) \qquad \text{Eq. 5}$$

If a closed plethysmograph is used, ΔV is detected by measuring plethysmographic pressure with a sensitive pressure transducer. If plethysmographic pressure is displayed on the *x*-axis and Pmouth = Palv is displayed on the *y*-axis (Fig. 31.8), the slope of the line (α) can be measured during panting efforts against the closed airway. In the following equations, the term *box calibration* refers to an empirically derived constant relating how changes in box volume reflect proportional changes in box pressure.

$$V = \frac{(P - 47\,mm\,Hg)(1.36\,cm\,H_2O/mm\,Hg) \times box\,calibration\,(mL/cm\,H_2O)}{\alpha} \qquad \text{Eq. 6}$$

$$V = \frac{970 \times box\,calibration}{\alpha} \qquad \text{Eq. 7}$$

Technical issues are discussed at ExpertConsult.com.

Lung Volume

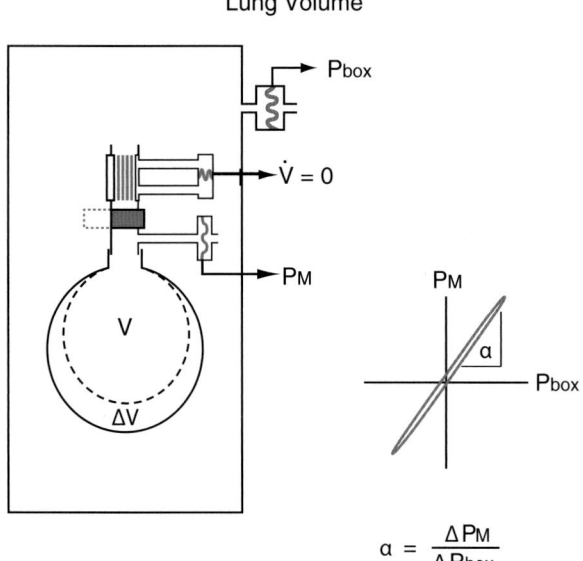

$$\alpha = \frac{\Delta P_M}{\Delta P_{box}}$$

Figure 31.8 A closed, constant-volume, variable-pressure whole-body plethysmograph. As described in eFig. 31.4, at end-expiration airflow ($\dot{V}$) is zero, thoracic gas volume (V) = functional residual capacity, and alveolar pressure (Palv) = mouth pressure (P_M) = barometric pressure (Pbar). The rectangle represents the plethysmograph. When the subject inhales against an occluded shutter in the airway, airflow remains zero, but V increases by ΔV to V′ and P_M (= Palv) changes by ΔP (P + ΔP) to equal P′. When P_M is plotted against box pressure (Pbox), the slope of the line (α) yields ΔPalv/ΔPbox, and V is derived, as indicated in the text. $\dot{V}$, airflow. (Modified from Comroe JH Jr, Forster RE 2nd, DuBois AB, et al. *The Lung: Clinical Physiology and Pulmonary Function Tests.* 2nd ed. Chicago: Year Book; 1962.)

AIRWAY RESISTANCE

General Principles

Airway resistance (Raw) is always related to the lung volume at which it is measured. It is useful to detect diseases such as asthma, which are associated with increased airway smooth muscle tone, as well as diseases such as COPD, in which there is a loss of airways or narrowing of airways due to secretions or edema. Increased tone can be shown by demonstrating that Raw is abnormally increased relative to lung volume and can be significantly reduced by administration of bronchodilator drugs. The measurement of Raw can also detect increased airway smooth muscle tone induced by provocative stimuli such as exercise, cold air, or specific agents, including allergens and chemicals (e.g., isocyanates) associated with occupational asthma (see "Bronchial Provocation" section).

Raw is measured during airflow and represents the ratio of the driving pressure (between the alveoli [Palv] and mouth [Pmouth]) and instantaneous airflow ($\dot{V}$). In a closed plethysmograph, inspiration of gas from the box into the lungs increases plethysmographic pressure, because to reduce Palv to subatmospheric pressure and drive air into the lungs, the expansion of the lungs slightly exceeds the volume of air drawn into the lungs from the box. This decompression of thoracic gas is equivalent to adding a small volume of gas to the plethysmograph around the thorax, so its pressure increases, as measured by a sensitive

Airway Resistance

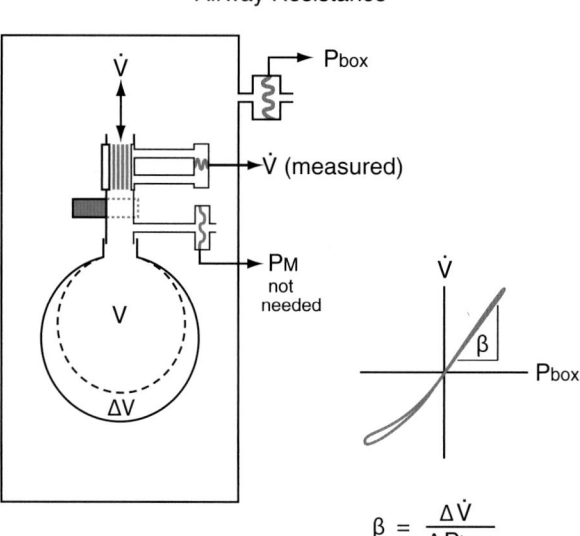

$$\beta = \frac{\Delta \dot{V}}{\Delta P_{box}}$$

Figure 31.9 Measurement of airway resistance by plethysmography. The rectangle represents a closed, constant-volume, variable-pressure, whole-body plethysmograph. The subject is represented by a single alveolus and its conducting airway. The top pressure transducer measures pressure within the plethysmograph, or box pressure (Pbox). The middle pressure transducer measures the pressure drop across the pneumotachygraph connected in series with the open shutter to the airway, which yields airflow ($\dot{V}$). During inspiration, the alveolus enlarges by ΔV from the original volume (*dashed line*) to a new volume (*solid line*); during expiration, the alveolus returns to its original volume. Throughout inspiration, alveolar gas (previously at atmospheric pressure) is subatmospheric and therefore occupies more volume. This is the same as adding this increment of gas volume resulting from decompression of the alveolar gas to the plethysmograph, so Pbox increases and is recorded by the sensitive Pbox transducer. The reverse happens during expiration when alveolar gas is compressed. Thus alveolar pressure can be monitored throughout the respiratory cycle. When $\dot{V}$ is plotted against Pbox, the slope of the line (β) yields the ratio of $\Delta\dot{V}$/ΔPbox as indicated in the text. (Modified from Comroe JH Jr, Forster RE 2nd, DuBois AB, et al. *The Lung: Clinical Physiology and Pulmonary Function Tests.* 2nd ed. Chicago: Year Book; 1962.)

pressure transducer. The reverse results during exhalation, when alveolar gas is compressed. Thus $\dot{V}$ is measured continuously with a pneumotachygraph, Pmouth is measured with a pressure transducer connected to a side tap in the mouthpiece, and Palv is estimated continuously with the body plethysmograph (Fig. 31.9).

In practice, Raw is determined by measuring the slope (β) of a curve of plethysmograph pressure (*x*-axis) displayed against airflow (*y*-axis) on a computer monitor during rapid, shallow breathing (panting) through a pneumotachygraph within the plethysmograph. Air is exchanged between the lungs and the box without communication to the air outside the box. Then a shutter is closed across the mouthpiece, and the slope (α) of plethysmographic pressure (*x*-axis) displayed against Pmouth (*y*-axis) is measured during panting under static conditions. Because Pmouth equals Palv in a static system, the closed shutter step serves two purposes. First, it relates changes in plethysmographic pressure to changes in Palv in each subject. Palv is thus effectively calculated from plethysmographic pressure changes with the shutter open, provided that the ratio of lung to plethysmographic gas volume is constant; this is true because Palv for a given plethysmographic pressure is the same whether or not flow is interrupted. Second, it relates RAW to a particular thoracic gas volume.

$$RAW = (Palv - Pmouth)/\dot{V} = (Palv - 0)/\dot{V}$$
$$= Palv/\dot{V} = \Delta Palv/\Delta \dot{V} \qquad \text{Eq. 8}$$

For Δ Palv, substitute $\Delta Palv_{open} = \dot{V}box_{open} \times$
$(\Delta Pmouth_{closed}/\Delta \dot{V}box_{closed}) = \Delta \dot{V}box_{open} \times \alpha$.

$$RAW = \Delta \dot{V} box_{open} \times \alpha/\Delta \dot{V}$$
$$= \alpha/(\Delta \dot{V}/\Delta \dot{V} box_{open})$$
$$= \alpha/\beta \qquad \text{Eq. 9}$$

The resistance of breathing through the mouthpiece and pneumotachygraph is subtracted from the result above. The units of RAW are cm H_2O per L/sec. The inverse of RAW, 1/RAW, is airway conductance, GAW. GAW increases, and RAW decreases, as lung volume increases. Therefore a value that is normalized for and independent of lung volume is made by dividing GAW by the thoracic lung volume at which it was measured and is called specific airway conductance: sGAW = GAW/TGV. The inverse of sGAW is specific airway resistance, sRAW, which can be interpreted as the work of breathing through a fixed resistance.[36,37] Although there is no universally accepted method by which to measure the slope β on the panting loops, common approaches have been described.[36,37] Inspiratory and expiratory resistance, and hence slope β, can differ in some obstructive airway diseases, further complicating the determination of a single β.

See ExpertConsult.com for physiologic factors that affect the measurement of airway resistance.

Forced Oscillation Methods

DuBois and colleagues[42] described an oscillatory method to measure the mechanical properties of the lung and thorax. In contrast to the methods already described, the *forced oscillation techniques* (FOT) use an external loudspeaker or similar device to generate and impose flow oscillations on spontaneous breathing, rather than using the respiratory muscles, and is measured during quiet tidal breathing. The FOT measures *respiratory system impedance* (Zrs),[45] which is the sum of all forces that must be overcome to cause airflow.[46] These forces include resistance and reactance, the latter of which is composed of elastance and inertance. Sound waves at various frequencies (typically 4–35 Hz) are applied to the entire respiratory system (airways, lung tissue, and chest wall). With computer methods, the slow frequency changes in pressure, flow, and volume generated by the respiratory muscles during normal breathing are subtracted from the raw data, permitting analysis of the pressure-flow-volume relationships imposed by the oscillation device (eFig: 31.6). Clinically, the FOT is mostly used for the assessment of pulmonary function in children, but it is expected to have expanded use in adults as research increasingly shows a value for the detection of abnormal function in this group. The European Respiratory Society recently released updated technical standards for oscillometry covering hardware, software, testing protocols, and quality control.[47] Technical details are reviewed at ExpertConsult.com.

LUNG ELASTIC RECOIL

Lung elastic recoil is an important physiologic characteristic of the lungs, which may change in qualitatively different ways in various diseases. In general, elastic recoil is increased in a restrictive ventilatory defect associated with decreased lung volumes. Conversely, in almost all forms of airflow obstruction, elastic recoil is decreased. Testing for elastic recoil is time consuming, difficult to perform, expensive, and invasive. Thus the test may not be practical for the routine evaluation of patients with restrictive ventilatory defects but may be of great value in the assessment of various obstructive ventilatory defects, including those with isolated bullae or advanced emphysema, to determine whether patients will benefit from resection of nonfunctioning or very poorly functioning lung tissue. In other patients, it may be useful to differentiate emphysema from asthma or bronchitis. In evaluating patients with mixed ventilatory defects (e.g., emphysema plus fibrosis), the test may confirm the presence of both disorders.

Principles, protocols, and analysis of the measurements are presented at ExpertConsult.com.

EXPIRATORY FLOW LIMITATION

Obstructive airway disease is associated with a reduced reserve between maximal flow rates and those achieved during tidal breathing. This reduced flow reserve often presents as a superimposition of tidal breathing loops on the maximal expiratory limb of the flow-volume curve. In the research setting, this overlap has been quantified as shown in Figure 31.10 and termed *expiratory flow limitation* (EFL). EFL has also been quantified by a reduced augmentation of flow during tidal breathing with applied negative pressure at the mouth (eFig. 31.9).[63]

Further details regarding comparison of tidal and maximal flow-volume curves are given at ExpertConsult.com.

The degree of expiratory flow limitation has been found to be associated with dyspnea in obstructive airway diseases independent of FEV_1. Expiratory flow limitation may develop with exercise even if not present at rest. An important physiologic consequence of expiratory flow limitation is the inability to exhale the inhaled tidal volume completely as respiratory rate and tidal volume increase during exercise, a phenomenon known as *dynamic hyperinflation*.

Dynamic hyperinflation is a progressive increase in *end expiratory lung volume* (EELV, synonymous with FRC), typically during exercise, although it may also manifest with any increase in respiratory rate or tidal volume, such as from pain, anxiety, or hypoxemia. Assuming TLC does not change, an increase in EELV is linked to a decrease in IC, which can be easily measured during exercise to infer changes in EELV. There are a number of negative consequences of dynamic hyperinflation with exercise, including increased work of breathing due to increased elastic load at higher lung volumes, increased dyspnea, early ventilatory limitation to exercise, reduced maximum oxygen consumption, *carbon dioxide* (CO_2) retention, and potential adverse cardiac consequences. Although airway resistance decreases slightly at higher operating lung volumes, this change is usually not enough to prevent expiratory flow limitation. Of importance, dynamic hyperinflation

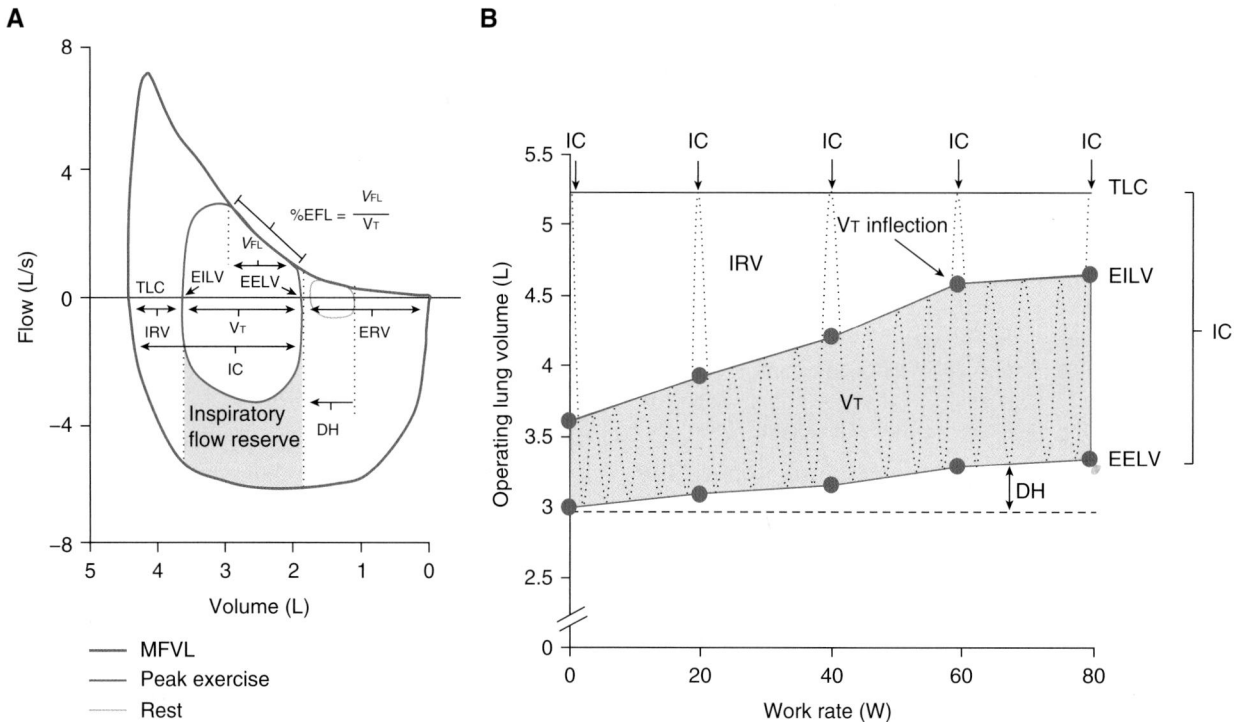

Figure 31.10 *Dynamic hyperinflation* **(DH) with exercise, showing the** *expiratory flow limitation* **(EFL) and decrease in** *inspiratory capacity* **(IC).** (A) Example of a resting (*lighter line*) and peak exercise (*darker line*) tidal breath superimposed within a maximum flow-volume loop (*thick black line*). The position of the tidal breaths along the x-axis is based on the measurement of end-expiratory lung volume as determined from inspiratory capacity maneuvers. (B) Operating lung volume plot versus cycle work rate. IC maneuvers are performed at rest (0 W) and every 20 W throughout exercise. Note how the IC decreases with DH. EELV, end-expiratory lung volume; %EFL, percentage of expiratory flow limitation; EILV, end-inspiratory lung volume; ERV, expiratory reserve volume; MFVL, maximum flow-volume loop; VFL, volume of the tidal breath that is flow limited on expiration; VT, tidal volume. (From Guenette JA, Chin RC, Cory JM, et al. Inspiratory capacity during exercise: measurement, analysis, and interpretation. *Pulm Med.* 2013;2013:956081.)

may even be present in mild COPD, causing dyspnea and reduced exercise tolerance independent of the severity of airflow obstruction as assessed by other parameters such as FEV_1. Supplemental oxygen, via a reduction in respiratory rate, and bronchodilators, via an increase in expiratory flow, have been shown to improve exercise capacity in COPD in part through reduced dynamic hyperinflation.

DISTRIBUTION OF VENTILATION

For discussion of ventilation, blood flow, and gas exchange, see Chapter 10. eFigure 31.10 illustrates the concept of uneven distribution of inspired gas.

Additional information on the single-breath N_2 washout test is available at ExpertConsult.com.

Measurements of Distribution Of Ventilation

The physiologic determinants of distribution of ventilation are reviewed in Chapter 10. eFigure 31.10 illustrates the concept of uneven distribution of inspired gas.

Tests that measure distribution of ventilation are very sensitive to abnormalities in lung structure and function but are nonspecific. Thus they are useful for detecting the presence of abnormal function early when other test results are normal or to confirm the presence of airflow obstruction when other test results are only mildly abnormal. They may be very useful in epidemiologic studies, such as evaluation of the effects of smoking or air pollution in large populations.

Multiple-Breath Nitrogen Washout

The measurement of residual N_2 after *multiple-breath, open-circuit N_2 washout* (MBNW) is used to assess the uniformity of the distribution of ventilation.[82] In the MBNW, continuous breath-by-breath measurement of N_2 concentration at the mouth during tidal breathing of pure oxygen is performed until end-tidal N_2 concentration falls to less than 1%. The fall in end-tidal N_2 concentration on a breath-by-breath basis is related to the cumulative volume of ventilation or breath number. By extending the N_2 washout time to 30 minutes or more in subjects with severe chronic airway obstruction, estimates of lung volume may be obtained that compare favorably with those calculated by plethysmographic or radiographic methods.[83]

There are three major indexes derived from the MBNW.[84] The *lung clearance index* (LCI) is the total number of FRC-sized breaths (termed lung turnovers) that are required to reduce the N_2 concentration down to $\frac{1}{40}$ of its starting value. As ventilation becomes more uneven, the measured LCI increases, because more lung turnovers are required to dilute the ambient N_2. The LCI is abnormal in obstructive airways disease, such as asthma, COPD, and *cystic fibrosis* (CF). The LCI is a global measure of ventilation heterogeneity but does not allow any specific anatomic localization of the site of heterogeneity. Two other indices, S_{cond} and S_{acin}, attempt to do this, based on modeling the lung in terms of the two types of mechanisms of gas transport. The first mechanism is gas transport due to convection, driven by pressure gradients, which takes place in the conducting airways; this is quantified by S_{cond}. The second mechanism is gas transport due to diffusion-convection flow driven by concentration gradients, which takes place in the extreme periphery of the lung, likely beginning at the entrance to the portion of lung distal to a terminal bronchiole (the last purely conducting airway), also called an acinus; this is quantified by S_{acin}. During MBNW, the slope of the phase III (alveolar gas plateau; see eFig. 31.10) of each breath is measured, normalized by the N_2 concentration in that breath, and plotted against the number of lung turnovers. The slope of the regression of the normalized phase III slopes between 1.5 and 6 lung turnovers is thought to represent convection-dependent ventilation heterogeneity in the conducting airways, and is termed S_{cond}. This value (S_{cond}) is subtracted from each measurement of normalized phase III slope to derive the contribution of the diffusion-convection–dependent heterogeneity of ventilation, termed S_{acin}. The clinical significance of S_{cond} and S_{acin} is just beginning to be appreciated, particularly as they relate to asthma severity and control.[85]

DIFFUSION

Tests for measuring diffusing capacity permit diagnosis of an impaired surface area for the transfer of gases from the alveoli to the pulmonary capillaries, sometimes even during early stages of disease. Many pulmonary diseases may manifest by a diffusion defect when there is no abnormality apparent in other routine PFTs. These include interstitial lung diseases, asbestosis, scleroderma, lupus erythematosus, emphysema, pulmonary thromboembolism, diffuse metastatic cancer of the lungs,[86] *Pneumocystis jirovecii* pneumonia, and rejection of a transplanted lung. There is now considerable evidence correlating the diffusing capacity and its subdivisions (*membrane diffusing capacity* [DM] and *pulmonary capillary blood volume* [Vc]) with the morphometric study of normal lungs.[87] Similar correlative studies of the lungs of patients with emphysema[38] document the structural basis for the abnormal alveolar-capillary interface as a result of decreased numbers of patent pulmonary capillary segments.[88] Finally, the tests are relatively simple (as far as the patient is concerned) and easy to repeat, making it practical to study the diffusing capacity frequently and to evaluate the effects of therapy or the natural history of the disease.

GENERAL PRINCIPLES

The measurement of pulmonary diffusing capacity (also known as transfer factor) requires the use of a gas that is more soluble in blood than in lung tissues. Oxygen and carbon monoxide are two such gases, and their chemical reaction with hemoglobin is responsible for this unusual pattern of "solubility." Both molecules measure the same process, and estimates of DL_{O2} can be made by multiplying the *diffusing capacity for carbon monoxide* (DL_{CO}) by 1.23. However, the more difficult and time-consuming method of measurement by oxygen has been displaced by the carbon monoxide method.

For the standard DL_{CO} method, a low concentration of carbon monoxide is added to inspired air. Molecules of

carbon monoxide diffuse across the alveolar capillary membrane, dissolve in the plasma, cross the *red blood cell* (RBC) membrane, and then combine with hemoglobin. The DL_{CO} is often thought of as a measure of gas exchange or the ability of the lungs to oxygenate blood. In Europe, the test is called the transfer factor for carbon monoxide. The term transfer factor is actually more accurate because the movement of gas from air to blood depends not only on diffusion but also on hemoglobin concentration. The measurement is typically measured at rest, thus yielding a result much less than the maximal capacity for transfer. *Carbon monoxide* (CO) was chosen as the test gas nearly 100 years ago because it has a high affinity for hemoglobin, 210 times that of oxygen; thus CO in the vicinity of a hemoglobin molecule binds avidly to it, and the partial pressure of dissolved CO remains very low. With such a high affinity, it was assumed that CO instantaneously combined with hemoglobin, maximizing the gradient for diffusion. In that case, changes in the DL_{CO} would only reflect changes in the total surface area and thickness of the alveolar-capillary membrane. Unfortunately, the noninstantaneous reaction between CO and hemoglobin makes interpretation of the test more complicated. In fact, some studies estimate that less than 50% of the measured DL_{CO} is determined by the surface area the lung provides to diffusion. The remainder is determined by the limited hemoglobin reservoir: As CO diffuses, it accumulates in the plasma during the maneuver. The more hemoglobin available to bind CO, the lower the accumulation of soluble CO concentration in the plasma during the test and the higher the concentration gradient for diffusion across the barrier. The hemoglobin reservoir is determined by pulmonary capillary blood volume and hemoglobin concentration. The extent to which the membrane affects the measured DL_{CO} is determined principally by the available capillary surface area exposed to the test gas; the membrane itself is very thin and likely affects CO diffusion minimally in health or disease. The transfer of carbon monoxide therefore can be considered a measure of the surface area and volume of blood-containing capillaries available for gas exchange.

DL_{CO} is calculated as follows:

$$DL_{CO} = \frac{\text{CO transferred from alveolar gas to blood (mL/min)}}{\text{Mean alveolar CO pressure} - \text{Mean capillary CO pressure (mm Hg)}} \qquad \text{Eq. 13}$$

To determine the amount of carbon monoxide transferred from alveolar gas to blood per minute, it is necessary to measure the mean alveolar carbon monoxide pressure and the mean pulmonary capillary carbon monoxide pressure. The technical factors that can affect the measurement of DL_{CO} are in Table 31.2. There are several tests available.

The standard single-breath DL_{CO} test is probably the most widely used and the best standardized of the various methods described. It has been used in the largest number of normal subjects and has been corrected for the effects of age, body size, sex, ethnic background, cigarette smoking, and physiologic factors.

Table 31.2   Technical Factors That Affect Measurement of $D_{L_{CO}}$

Factor	Effect on $D_{L_{CO}}$	Mechanism
Incomplete maximal inspiration	Reduced*	Reduced alveolar surface area and capillary blood volume
Incomplete exhalation before maximal inspiration	No change	
Valsalva maneuver during breath hold	Reduced	Less capillary blood volume
Mueller maneuver during breath hold	Increased	More capillary blood volume
Carboxyhemoglobin (without adjustment)	Reduced	Fewer heme sites available to bind CO
Anemia (without Hb adjustment)	Reduced	Fewer heme sites available to bind CO
Polycythemia	Increased	More heme sites available to bind CO
Altitude (low inspired partial pressure of oxygen)	Increased	More heme sites available to bind CO
Supine position, exercise, left-to-right shunt	Increased	Capillary recruitment/filling

Although changes in $D_{L_{CO}}$ during the menstrual cycle, independent of hemoglobin concentration, have been reported, the results are inconsistent. Reports of diurnal variation and the effect of β_2-agonists (in health and in patients with airflow obstruction) on $D_{L_{CO}}$ and V_A are also inconsistent. ATS/ERS guidelines conclude that the weight of evidence is against a significant effect of β_2-agonists on the $D_{L_{CO}}$. Some carbon monoxide sensors may be affected by exhaled ethanol and ketones.

*The effect of incomplete inspiration is nonlinear, with small changes in $D_{L_{CO}}$ near TLC. This nonlinear relationship between lung volume and $D_{L_{CO}}$ likely reflects the complex effects of alveolar and capillary unfolding and stretching as lung volume increases.

ATS, American Thoracic Society; CO, carbon monoxide; $D_{L_{CO}}$, diffusing capacity for carbon monoxide; ERS, European Respiratory Society; Hb, hemoglobin; TLC, total lung capacity; V_A, alveolar volume.

SINGLE-BREATH METHOD

In the single-breath method the patient inhales a gas mixture containing 0.3% carbon monoxide and a low concentration of inert gas (0.3% neon, 0.3% methane, or 10% helium), then holds his or her breath for approximately 10 seconds. During the breath-hold, carbon monoxide leaves the air spaces and enters the blood. The larger the diffusing capacity, the greater the amount of carbon monoxide that enters the blood in 10 seconds. In the single-breath test, alveolar P_{CO} is not maintained at a constant concentration, because carbon monoxide is absorbed during the period of breath-holding.

The equation used in the single-breath method is as follows:

$$D_{L_{CO}} = \frac{V_A \times 60}{(Pbar - 47) \times t} \ln \frac{F_{A_{CO_0}}}{F_{A_{CO_t}}} \qquad \text{Eq. 14}$$

where $F_{A_{CO_t}}$ is fractional alveolar carbon monoxide concentration at time (t), t is breath-hold time in seconds, $Pbar$ is barometric pressure (in mm Hg), V_A is alveolar volume (in mL, in *standard temperature, pressure, and dry* [STPD]) obtained from the ratio of inspired and expired inert gas concentrations and inspired volume, $F_{A_{CO_0}}$ is the inspired carbon monoxide concentration corrected for dilution by the RV as estimated by the ratio of inspired and expired inert gas concentrations, and 60 is the conversion factor for seconds to minutes.

Analyses are performed with an infrared analyzer or gas chromatograph, and no blood samples are needed. An inert gas such as helium, methane, or neon must be inhaled with carbon monoxide to correct for dilution of inspired carbon monoxide.

Factors such as inhalation time, breath-holding time, breath-holding lung volume, exhalation time, and the size and portion of alveolar gas sampled have all been shown to affect the single-breath $D_{L_{CO}}$. Ogilvie and colleagues[89] recognized that these discrepancies could exist either because diffusing capacity is not distributed homogeneously within the lung or because the single-breath equation ignores the fact that carbon monoxide uptake takes place during inhalation

and exhalation as well as during breath-holding. They tried to circumvent these problems by standardizing the test.

Jones and Mead[90] showed that, because the diffusion equation was valid only for breath-holding, there are errors in calculation of single-breath $D_{L_{CO}}$ owing to the nature of carbon monoxide uptake during inhalation and exhalation. Because delay in collection of the alveolar sample has been shown to cause an apparent increase in $D_{L_{CO}}$, the *American Thoracic Society* (ATS) Epidemiology Standardization Project[14] developed a variation of the Jones and Mead method that took this problem into account and placed strong emphasis on an automated system, which standardized the procedure and is available in most commercial systems.

Standardization of the Single-Breath Methods

The ATS has recommended standardization of the test using acceptability criteria, including rapid inspiration, inspired volume at least 90% of largest VC, breath-hold time between 8 and 12 seconds, sample collection completed within 4 seconds of the start of exhalation, and adequate washout and sample volumes.[91] At least two acceptable $D_{L_{CO}}$ measurements within 2 mL/min per mm Hg are required to meet criteria for repeatability (at STPD). The mean of the acceptable tests is reported. Calculations are standardized for breath-hold time and adjusted for dead space, gas collection conditions, and carbon dioxide concentration.

Refer to ExpertConsult.com for three additional methods to measure the diffusing capacity (steady-state, rebreathing, and intrabreath).

TECHNICAL AND PHYSIOLOGIC FACTORS

Hemoglobin. Adjustment for hemoglobin is not mandatory but is desirable. Unadjusted values must always be reported even if the adjusted values are also reported. The adjustment should be made on the observed, not the predicted, value. Hemoglobin is reported in grams per deciliter, and the method of Cotes and associates[123] should be used to make the adjustment, where DM is the membrane diffusing capacity and VC is the pulmonary capillary blood volume.

Carboxyhemoglobin. Heavy smokers may have as much as 10–12% carboxyhemoglobin in their blood, and therefore the back-pressure of carbon monoxide in mixed venous blood entering the pulmonary capillaries cannot be assumed to be zero in such individuals. The steady-state method is more sensitive to errors caused by this problem than the single-breath technique. Carbon monoxide back-pressure may be estimated, and $D_{L_{CO}}$ calculations may be corrected for back-pressure of carbon monoxide using the Haldane equation.[123,124] Alternatively, carboxyhemoglobin may be measured directly.[125] In either case, the measured $D_{L_{CO}}$ is adjusted, and both the unadjusted and the adjusted values are reported. $D_{L_{CO}}$ measurements should not be performed on patients who have been breathing oxygen-enriched mixtures immediately before the test; at least 20 minutes of breathing room air should be allowed before measurement of $D_{L_{CO}}$.

Graham and associates[126] demonstrated that carbon monoxide back-pressure has a more complex effect than suggested in the ATS standardization statement. To adjust properly for the effect of carbon monoxide on the diffusing capacity, not only must the direct effect of carbon monoxide back-pressure build-up be corrected, but also the indirect anemia effect of increasing carboxyhemoglobin.

Altitude. As altitude increases and *fractional concentration of inspired oxygen* (FIO_2) remains constant, *pressure of inspired oxygen* (PIO_2) decreases and $D_{L_{CO}}$ increases approximately 0.35% for every 1-mm Hg decrease in alveolar PO_2.

If alveolar PO_2 is not available, adjustments may be made for interpretative purposes, assuming a mean PIO_2 of 150 mm Hg at sea level and assuming PIO_2 = 0.21(Pbar − 47).

Lung Volume. Adjustment of the $D_{L_{CO}}$ for lung volume is a controversial issue. A primary measurement from the single-breath $D_{L_{CO}}$ is K$_{CO}$ (the CO transfer coefficient), the portion of equation (Eq. 14) that is multiplied by the computed VA, which is reported at *body temperature (37°C) and standard pressure fully saturated with water vapor (760 mm Hg)* (BTPS) but converted to STPD to calculate $D_{L_{CO}}$. K$_{CO}$ can be computed from reported data as $D_{L_{CO}}$/VA, which leads to the suggestion that $D_{L_{CO}}$ can be corrected or normalized for the lung volume accessible to test gas. However, $D_{L_{CO}}$/VA fails to correct for inadequate inspired vital capacity because $D_{L_{CO}}$ decreases far less than the amount of lung volume below TLC. This finding may be due to the complex relationship between increasing lung volume, alveolar-capillary surface area, and capillary blood volume as the membrane unfolds and stretches.[91] In disease states, the intent of the $D_{L_{CO}}$ is to quantify the capability of the lung as a whole—healthy and diseased portions together—to participate in gas exchange. One cannot assume that areas of lung inaccessible to test gas have a normal capillary bed. The variability in VA and K$_{CO}$ within diseases[127] and the low predictive value of K$_{CO}$ for hypoxemia[128] further limit the clinical utility of K$_{CO}$. Even after lung resection, changes in blood flow make an abnormal K$_{CO}$ an unreliable parameter by which to detect disease in the remaining lung tissue. Examination of K$_{CO}$ and VA separately may aid in

interpretation of the pathophysiology behind a reduced or increased $D_{L_{CO}}$, but as of yet the evidence base for its clinical utility is not robust.[129,130] A somewhat related parameter, FVC%/$D_{L_{CO}}$%, has promise as part of a multivariate screening tool for pulmonary hypertension in scleroderma[131] but may increase cost of screening compared to echocardiography alone. A method to adjust $D_{L_{CO}}$ and K$_{CO}$ to actual lung volume has been derived from healthy humans, but its role in clinical decision making remains to be established.[132]

Additional physiologic factors affecting the diffusing capacity are discussed at ExpertConsult.com.

REGULATION OF VENTILATION

Ventilatory regulation may be assessed by measuring the ventilator response to hypoxia or hypercapnia or by measuring the overall respiratory drive. The response to hypoxia and hypercapnia has been assessed using rebreathing methods, which are less time-consuming and tiring than classic steady-state methods. In one rebreathing method described by Severinghaus and associates,[144] rapid step changes in the patient's PO_2 while PCO_2 is stabilized offer the advantage of a brief stable period of hypoxia. Respiratory drive can be assessed by measuring the *inspiratory occlusion pressure* at 100 msec (0.1 second), which is thought to reflect the entire neural output of the respiratory center. It is not influenced by conscious muscle effort and is less influenced by abnormal mechanical properties of the respiratory system than is measurement of ventilation. Other methods, including electromyographic measurements of the diaphragm, the measurement of isometric inspiratory loads, and the use of drugs that stimulate the carotid body, have not been used often enough to establish their clinical utility.[145]

See ExpertConsult.com for protocols for the measuring of regulation of ventilation.

VENTILATION-PERFUSION RELATIONSHIPS

For discussion of ventilation, blood flow, and gas exchange, see Chapter 10.

MEASUREMENTS OF VENTILATION-PERFUSION RELATIONSHIPS

Inhaled air and pulmonary capillary blood flow are not distributed uniformly or in proportion to each other, even in the normal lung. Distributions of ventilation and blood flow are altered by posture, lung volume, and exercise not only in healthy subjects but even more so in patients with respiratory disease. The most common cause of arterial hypoxemia is increased mismatching of ventilation and perfusion, resulting in regional hypoventilation relative to perfusion (eTable 31.1). Whereas samples of alveolar gas and pulmonary capillary blood cannot be obtained to analyze gas exchange, inspired and expired gas (gas entering and leaving the alveoli), mixed venous (blood entering the pulmonary capillaries), and arterial blood can be obtained and analyzed.

Specific measurements of ventilation-perfusion measurements are discussed at ExpertConsult.com.

Arterial Blood Gases

The physiologic determinants of arterial oxygen levels and acid-base balance are reviewed in detail in Chapters 10 and 12, respectively.

The technical aspects of these measurements are discussed at ExpertConsult.com.

OTHER PULMONARY FUNCTION TESTS

BRONCHIAL PROVOCATION

Provocation tests may be extremely useful in the diagnosis and management of patients with asthma or occupational asthma and in the differential diagnosis of patients with chronic cough, wheezing, or intermittent dyspnea. Although most laboratories use spirometry to evaluate the airway response, the measurement of RAW in a body plethysmograph is more sensitive, more specific for abnormalities in airway tone, and usually easier for the patient to perform than spirometry, which depends on inspiration to TLC followed by a forced exhalation. In limited numbers of patients, tests with exposure to specific allergens may be helpful in the evaluation of allergic asthma. Similarly, in a small number of patients suspected of having occupational asthma, specific challenge with agents found in the workplace may be useful in the diagnosis. However, the referring physician should be aware that these challenge tests are dangerous and tedious, usually require hospitalization for observation, and may not be useful if the patient is exposed to multiple agents in the workplace.

TESTS OF NONSPECIFIC AIRWAY RESPONSIVENESS

Abnormal airway responsiveness is viewed by many as a characteristic feature of asthma. It may also be found in patients with chronic bronchitis and CF. Although a variety of stimuli have been used to induce airway response, including exercise and eucapnic ventilation (see later in discussion of indirect tests), the most common stimulus is methacholine.

Methacholine is an acetylcholine agonist that causes constriction of airway smooth muscle through direct stimulation of M3 receptors. The test begins with baseline measurement of spirometry and in some cases sRAW.[216] Next, the patient is asked to inhale a control aerosol consisting of the diluent, and responses are reported relative to the diluent value. Then the patient inhales a methacholine aerosol at increasing doses, starting from a low dose to avoid an inordinately severe reaction. Inhalation should take place through tidal breathing, avoiding deep inhalations, and over a period specified by the aerosol characteristics of the nebulizer. Approximately 1 minute of tidal breathing is recommended for each dose. Spirometry is then measured at 30 and 90 seconds after completion of the inhalation period, and FEV_1 recorded. If the requisite 20% or more fall in FEV_1 is not seen, then the next dose is prepared and administered, maintaining a consistent 5 minutes between doses. A dose-response plot is constructed depicting the dose of agonist on the logarithmic abscissa as amount of agonist (in micromoles) delivered from the nebulizer, and the response as the FEV_1 on the ordinate. The end point for the test is the dose causing a decrease in FEV_1 of 20% or causing a doubling of sRAW.

FEV_1 is the most common test used to evaluate the outcome of this procedure, although sRAW may be more sensitive. Medications, baseline airway function, respiratory infections, and exposure to specific allergens and chemical sensitizers influence responses. Bronchodilators, antihistamines, and other agents that decrease bronchial responsiveness should be withheld before the test.[217]

Compared to methacholine, which has *direct* effects on airway smooth muscle to cause airway narrowing, so-called *indirect* challenge tests, which cause airway narrowing indirectly by triggering mast cell degranulation by osmotic stimuli, or mediator release from inflammatory cells, may have an important place in the assessment of asthma.[218] Such indirect challenge tests, including exercise-induced bronchoconstriction, eucapnic voluntary hyperpnea, hypertonic and hypotonic aerosols, and mannitol, are useful for monitoring treatment with inhaled corticosteroids.[219] Indirect tests identify subjects with the potential for exercise-induced bronchoconstriction and therefore are useful for members of the armed services, firefighters, police, and elite athletes. A positive indirect test result suggests that inflammatory cells and their mediators are present in sufficient numbers and concentration to indicate that asthma is active at the time of the test. A negative test result in a known asthmatic patient means good control or mild disease. Healthy subjects do not experience significant bronchoconstriction during indirect tests.[219]

More information on the advantages of indirect tests and specific airway responsiveness is available at ExpertConsult.com.

RESPIRATORY MUSCLE FUNCTION TESTS

Respiratory muscle function may be tested clinically by measuring muscle strength or endurance. Common measurements include maximally negative inspiratory and positive expiratory airway pressure, sniff nasal inspiratory pressure, maximum transdiaphragmatic pressure, maximum voluntary ventilation, diaphragmatic electromyography, and fluoroscopy.

For more details about these measurements of muscle function, see ExpertConsult.com.

For a discussion about pulmonary function testing in children, see ExpertConsult.com.

PULMONARY FUNCTION LABORATORY MANAGEMENT

GENERAL STRUCTURE: PERSONNEL, EQUIPMENT, AND QUALITY CONTROL

The pulmonary function laboratory is an essential component of any diagnostic laboratory service. Surprisingly, at the present time, a pulmonary function laboratory is not overseen for quality by any formal accreditation body, unlike any other diagnostic laboratory. Many of the following general principles are outlined in detail in such references as the ATS Pulmonary Function Laboratory Manual (http://store.thoracic.org/product/index.php?id=a1u3300 0000ye1TAAQ).

The PF laboratory must have a medical director who oversees the proper management of the laboratory, supervises laboratory personnel, develops policies and procedures, maintains ongoing quality control, and ensures timely and accurate reporting and interpretation of results. Working closely with the medical director will be a laboratory manager, who typically has direct experience in pulmonary function testing and equipment, as well as supervising personnel and maintaining standard operating procedures. The laboratory manager and all laboratory personnel must be familiar with policies and procedures, including all facility procedures related to safety, hygiene, and infection control, and those related to scheduling and billing. The PF laboratory technologists must be certified as competent in performing PFTs, typically through accredited respiratory care training and credentialing by the National Board for Respiratory Care. All equipment must be in good working order and pass regular calibration checks and quality control for accuracy and safety.[1,238] Quality control should be performed both mechanically, to test the accuracy of equipment, and by testing of healthy, normal biologic controls to check the entire testing process. Quality control analysis should be as rigorous as that found in any laboratory, including careful logs and plotting of longitudinal data to inspect for "out-of-control" conditions.[239]

SAFETY AND CONTRAINDICATIONS TO TESTING

The physical demands and potential hemodynamic consequences of forced exhalation can be challenging for patients with selected conditions. Expert opinion lists recent myocardial infarction, pneumothorax, abdominal surgery, eye surgery, brain surgery, and sinus or middle ear surgery or infection as contraindications; suggested recovery periods before testing vary.[238,240,241] Other safety concerns include pregnancy with cervical incompetence, severe hypertension or hypotension, and history of syncope with forced exhalation or cough. A sensitivity to develop tachyarrhythmia may increase the risk of bronchodilator administration. Interrupting supplemental oxygen for the recommended greater than or equal to 10 minutes before measurements of DL_{CO} may not be tolerated by patients with certain conditions; oxygen saturation should be monitored during the wait time and during testing with a minimum value protocolized at which time testing is aborted. Of note, for the few cases where evidence has accumulated, such as with aortic aneurysms, prior concerns with testing that arose from expert opinion have been tempered.[242]

INFECTION CONTROL

When patients with communicable infectious diseases are referred for PFTs, they always present a potential risk for transmission of infectious diseases to the technical and administrative staff, as well as to other patients who may be in the laboratory for studies at the same time. Pulmonary laboratory directors are familiar with the risk for spreading tuberculosis by aerosols produced by sputum-positive patients. There has also been the more theoretical possibility of transmitting tuberculosis from one patient to another via infected secretions, which may contaminate pulmonary function equipment. The increasing number of immunosuppressed patients in cancer treatment and transplantation programs has raised the possibility of increased risk for transmission of infection to such patients. In most

circumstances, testing of patients with active communicable respiratory infection is delayed until the risk of transmission no longer poses a significant threat.

All studies are performed with the patient breathing through a filter that traps particles as small as 0.2 μm in diameter without affecting the results of the physiologic tests performed. It is assumed that infectious particles, whether bacterial, fungal, parasitic, or viral, will be carried in respiratory secretions of such a large size that all of them will be trapped by these filters. However, not all such filters are perfect, and it should not be assumed that they remove the need for regular decontamination.[238] For testing patients with CF, who are at risk of being colonized with multidrug-resistant organisms, special protocols are followed, including circulation of air through a high-efficiency particulate air filter before and after testing; use of gloves, gown, and mask by technical staff; and external cleaning of equipment.

Key Points

- Because pulmonary function testing is effort dependent, technicians must be trained and laboratories must adhere to high standards to obtain the most accurate and reproducible results possible.
- Measurements from spirometry alone, including the flow-volume curve, can be useful in patients whose main physiologic impairment is airway obstruction. The findings from spirometry can provide clues that concomitant restriction is present; however, for assessment of restriction, lung volumes must be measured.
- Gas dilution methods to measure lung volumes are accurate except in patients with airflow obstruction in whom lung volumes may be underestimated. If airflow obstruction is suspected, body plethysmography will yield more accurate measures of functional residual capacity, reserve volume, expiratory reserve volume, and total lung capacity.
- In patients with reversible mild airway disease, the results of pulmonary function tests may be normal. Assessment of spirometry and airway resistance (e.g., by body plethysmography or forced oscillation) before and after bronchodilation may be needed.
- Tests of the distribution of ventilation can provide additional evidence of abnormal structure of the airways or lung parenchyma. They may be more sensitive than spirometry or lung volumes but less specific.
- Methacholine provocation testing is used to identify abnormal airway responsiveness. Usually this indicates a diagnosis of asthma, but the clinician must understand that other conditions that involve airway inflammation may also show abnormal airway responsiveness.
- The diffusing capacity measurement is used to determine defects of the alveolar-pulmonary capillary unit. An abnormal diffusing capacity alerts the physician that the alveolar-capillary membranes and/or pulmonary capillaries may not be normal, and further evaluation of the underlying cause of this defect should be pursued.

Key Readings

Bates HT, Ramon CG, Farré R, Hantos Z. Oscillation mec-hanics of the respiratory system. *Compr Physiol.* 2011;1(3):1233–1272.

Berger AJ, Mitchell RA, Severinghaus JW. Regulation of respiration. *N Engl J Med.* 1977;297:92–97.

Buist AS, Vollmer WM, Johnson LR, McCamant LE. Does the single-breath N_2 test identify the smoker who will develop chronic airflow limitation? *Am Rev Respir Dis.* 1988;137(2):293–301.

Coates AL, Wanger J, Cockcroft DW, et al. ERS technical standard on bronchial challenge testing: general considerations and performance of methacholine challenge tests. *Eur Respir J.* 2017;49(5):1601526.

Dubois AB, Botelho SY, Bedell GN, Marshall R, Comroe Jr JH. A rapid plethysmographic method for measuring thoracic gas volume: a comparison with a nitrogen washout method for measuring functional residual capacity in normal subjects. *J Clin Invest.* 1956;35(3):322–326.

Dubois AB, Botelho SY, Comroe Jr JH. A new method for measuring airway resistance in man using a body plethysmograph: values in normal subjects and in patients with respiratory disease. *J Clin Invest.* 1956;35(3):327–335.

Giustini D, Giuntini C. Relationship between extent of pulmonary emphysema by high-resolution computed tomography and lung elastic recoil in patients with chronic obstructive pulmonary disease. *Am J Respir Crit Care Med.* 2001;164:585–589.

Graham BL, et al. 2017 ERS/ATS standards for single-breath carbon monoxide uptake in the lung. *Eur Respir J.* 2017;49(1).

Graham BL, Steenbruggen I, Miller MR, et al. Standardization of spirometry 2019 update. An official American Thoracic Society and European Respiratory Society technical statement. *Am J Respir Crit Care Med.* 2019;200(8):e70–e88.

Guenette JA, Chin RC, Cory JM, Webb KA, O'Donnells DE. Inspiratory capacity during exercise: measurement, analysis, and interpretation. *Pulm Med.* 2013;2013:956081.

Hughes JM, Bates DV. Historical review: the carbon monoxide diffusing capacity (Dl_{CO}) and its membrane (DM) and red cell (Theta.Vc) components. *Respir Physiol Neurobiol.* 2003;138(2-3):115–142.

Janssens JP, Pache JC, Nicod LP. Physiological changes in respiratory function associated with ageing. *Eur Respir J.* 1999;13:197–205.

Kaminsky DA. What does airway resistance tell us about lung function?. *Respir Care.* 2012;57(1):85–96; discussion 96-9.

Krogh M. The diffusion of gases through the lungs of man. *J Physiol.* 1915;49(4):271–300.

Laveneziana P, Albuquerque A, Aliverti A, et al. ERS statement on respiratory muscle testing at rest and during exercise. *Eur Respir J.* 2019;53(6):1801214.

Mead J, Turner JM, Macklem PT, et al. Significance of the relationship between lung recoil and maximum expiratory flow. *J Appl Physiol.* 1967;22:95–108.

Nadel JA, Gold WM, Burgess JH. Early diagnosis of chronic pulmonary vascular obstruction. *Am J Med.* 1968;44:16–25.

Oostveen E, MacLeod D, Lorino H, ERS Task Force on Respiratory Impedance Measurements, et al. The forced oscillation technique in clinical practice: methodology, recommendations and future developments. *Eur Respir J.* 2003;22(6):1026–1041.

Roughton FJ, Forster RE. Relative importance of diffusion and chemical reaction rates in determining rate of exchange of gases in the human lung, with special reference to true diffusing capacity of pulmonary membrane and volume of blood in the lung capillaries. *J Appl Physiol.* 1957;11(2):290–302.

Wanger J, Clausen JL, Coates A, Pedersen OF, Brusasco V, et al. Standardisation of the measurement of lung volumes. *Eur Respir J.* 2005;26(3):511–522.

Complete reference list available at ExpertConsult.com.

32

PULMONARY FUNCTION TESTING: INTERPRETATION AND APPLICATIONS

NIRAV R. BHAKTA, MD, PHD • SURYA P. BHATT, MD, MSPH

INTRODUCTION

Pulmonary function tests are a core tool in the diagnostic approach to common signs and symptoms that bring patients to the pulmonary consultant (Table 32.1). These reasons include cough, shortness of breath, wheezing, hypoxemia, and imaging abnormalities. The results of pulmonary function tests sometimes are a core part of disease definitions, as in the case of asthma and COPD and, in many other cases, narrow the differential diagnosis and suggest further specific testing. Pulmonary function tests also provide objective data for physicians to monitor disease activity and response to treatment. This chapter addresses the applications of pulmonary function tests; the underlying principles are covered in Chapter 31.

MAJOR PATTERNS ON PULMONARY FUNCTION TESTS

Pulmonary function test results can be classified into the following major patterns: normal, obstructive ventilatory defect, restrictive ventilatory defect, mixed pattern (when lung volumes are available) or a pattern that is not clearly obstructive or restrictive (when lung volumes are not available), and a nonspecific pattern (Fig. 32.1). Patient effort and cooperation are essential for acquiring valid spirometry; hence spirometry efforts should be assessed for quality

before interpretation. The *American Thoracic Society* (ATS) and *European Respiratory Society* (ERS) guidelines recommend that at least three acceptable spirograms should be obtained.[1,2] Testing should be repeated until the two largest *forced vital capacity* (FVC) measurements and the two largest *forced expiratory volume in 1 second* (FEV$_1$) measurements from acceptable spirograms are within 150 mL of each other, or, if this is not achieved, until a practical upper limit of eight efforts have been made.[1,2] Failure to meet acceptability criteria should be noted in the report and considered when interpreting results.

OBSTRUCTIVE VENTILATORY DEFECT

Obstruction to airflow is characterized by a decrease in FEV$_1$/FVC, reduced FEV$_1$, normal (or reduced) FVC, normal (or reduced) *vital capacity* (VC), and a decrease in measures that may reflect small airway disease (Table 32.2). It is also characterized by an upward concavity in the expiratory flow-volume curve (also described as curvilinear) (Fig. 32.2). Supplementary data supporting airflow obstruction include increased *residual volume* (RV), RV/*total lung capacity* (TLC) ratio and *airway resistance* (RAW), uneven distribution of ventilation, and significant reversibility of airflow obstruction, with or without decreased diffusing capacity. Examples of diseases that manifest with airflow obstruction are shown in eTable 32.1.

Table 32.1   Indications for Pulmonary Function Tests

SPIROMETRY

Diagnose obstruction
Quantify severity
Assess effects of occupation/environment
Assess effects of therapy
Assess preoperative eligibility
Assess disability/impairment

LUNG VOLUMES

Diagnose restriction
Assess hyperinflation and air trapping

DIFFUSING CAPACITY

Diagnose early or mild parenchymal lung disease
Assess progression of parenchymal lung disease
Assess pulmonary involvement in systemic diseases
Differentiate obstructive diseases
Assess pulmonary vascular disease
Assess cardiovascular disease
Assess drug toxicity

Although lung function varies along a continuum, categorization of lung function using thresholds aids in clinical decision making and in recognizing major disease patterns, with the caveat that caution should be exercised in the interpretation of borderline results.

The first step in the interpretation of spirometry is to evaluate the ratio of the FEV_1 to the FVC (see Fig. 32.1). FEV_1/FVC should be interpreted as an absolute ratio and not its percentage of predicted. If this ratio is less than 0.70, it indicates that less than 70% of the VC was exhaled in the first 1 second during a forced exhalation maneuver. FEV_1/FVC less than the fifth percentile is a statistical definition of abnormality recommended by the ATS/ERS document that can reduce bias (e.g., a change associated with age but not disease),[3] although recent data suggest a fixed threshold of less than 0.70 may be more suitable for diagnosing COPD and the associated clinically relevant outcomes, such as hospitalizations and mortality.[4–7] The Global Initiative for Chronic Obstructive Lung Disease document and other respiratory society statements suggest a threshold of less than 0.70 for the postbronchodilator FEV_1/FVC ratio to diagnose COPD.[8–10] A fixed approach posits a uniform threshold below which normal physiologic reserves are overcome. The diagnosis of airflow obstruction should be made using postbronchodilator values because a substantial number of individuals have reversibility of airflow obstruction, and prevalence estimates can vary by as much as 33% depending on whether prebronchodilator or postbronchodilator values are used.[11]

Because the end of a test is sometimes hard to detect or achieve, FVC can be substituted by FEV_6, the forced expiratory volume in the first 6 seconds, thus setting time as the end-of-test criterion rather than plateaued low flow. FEV_6 is generally lower than FVC, especially in those with obstructive lung diseases[12,13]; hence, a ratio of FEV_1/FEV_6 less than 0.73 is equivalent to FEV_1/FVC less than 0.70 for the diagnosis of airflow obstruction.[13,14] Reference equations are also available for FEV_1/FEV_6.[15,16]

When FEV_1/FVC is low, the next step is to evaluate FEV_1 and FVC. A reduced FEV_1 further supports the presence of airflow obstruction, especially when the FVC is normal. The degree of impairment of FEV_1 can be used to grade the severity of airflow obstruction (Table 32.3). An isolated decrease in FEV_1/FVC without abnormalities in FEV_1 or FVC suggests early or mild airflow obstruction.[17] This may also represent *dysanaptic* lung growth leading to a high FVC with a normal FEV_1.[18] Dysanapsis, a mismatch of airway tree caliber to lung size, was historically thought to be a physiologic variant but has now been shown to be associated with symptoms and outcomes.[19,20] Demonstration of bronchodilator responsiveness also supports a diagnosis of airflow obstruction (see section "Bronchodilator Responsiveness").

VC measurements can be obtained while performing a *slow* (SIVC) or a *fast* (FIVC) *inspiratory vital capacity* maneuver or a *slow* (SVC) or *fast* (FVC) *expiratory vital capacity* maneuver. Given that airflow resistance is greater during forced exhalation than during slow inhalation, FIVC > SIVC > SVC > FVC in individuals with obstructive lung disease.[21] FVC is the most commonly reported measure of VC because inspiratory maneuvers are not always performed in pulmonary function testing laboratories, and reference values are most reliably available for FVC. Although either SVC or FIVC can be substituted for FVC in the FEV_1/FVC ratio, there are no normative data available to interpret these ratios adequately.

A number of additional tests may be needed to confirm airflow obstruction in cases in which spirometry results are borderline, or when clinical features suggest an obstructive airway disease but FEV_1 and FEV_1/FVC are normal. A commonly used metric is the *forced expiratory flow at 25% to 75% of the FVC* ($FEF_{25\%-75\%}$), also called the maximum mid-expiratory flow.[22] The physiologic basis for this metric is that the lung elastic recoil is lower and airway dimensions are smaller at lower lung volumes; hence, this metric has been postulated to reflect abnormalities in small airways and to be sensitive to early changes in lung elastic recoil. $FEF_{25\%-75\%}$ has high variability, however, due to its dependence on the FVC, and normal values range from 60–140% of predicted. Although a value of less than 60% predicted has often been used to diagnose mild airflow obstruction, its utility in the presence of a normal FEV_1/FVC is questionable. The $FEF_{25\%-75\%}$ is highly correlated with FEV_1 and FEV_1/FVC, and there is minimal discordance between these metrics in population studies.[23] Prediction equations are hard to interpret for this metric because $FEF_{25\%-75\%}$ is measured at a different lung volume in patients with disease (in whom FVC is abnormal) than in healthy subjects (in whom FVC is normal). Mild airflow obstruction can also be detected by the low flow at end expiration. Lung segments with longer time constants, and therefore slower to empty, are represented in the latter part of the spirometry curves. By including a larger component of the distal segment of the expiratory curve, the FEV_3 appears to be more sensitive to mild airflow obstruction than FEV_1/FVC. Compared with FEV_1/FVC, FEV_3/FVC is more sensitive in identifying reductions in terminal expiratory flow.[24,25]

Visual inspection of the flow-volume curve can also aid detection of an obstructive pattern in a few ways. Both

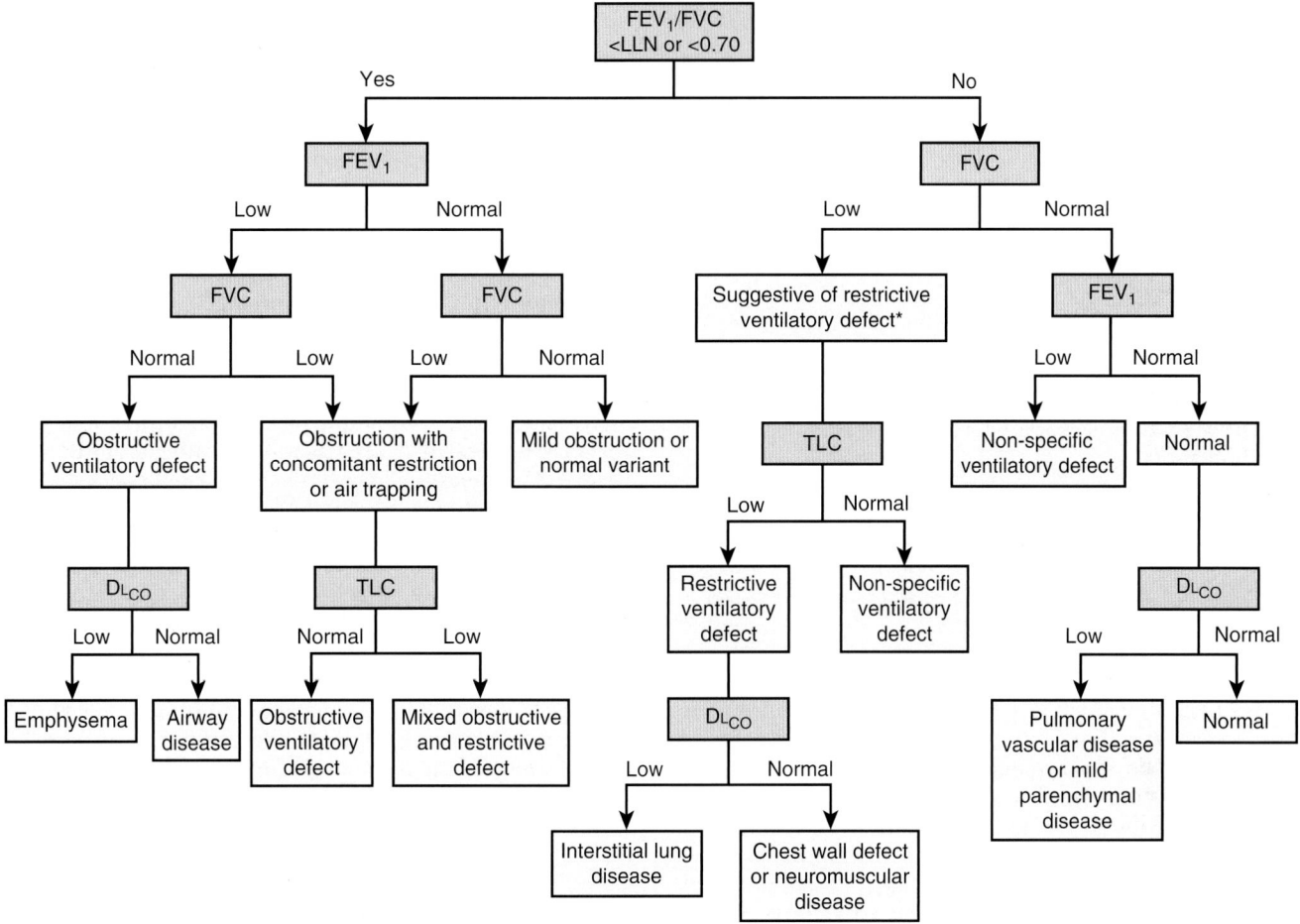

Figure 32.1 Algorithm for interpretation of pulmonary function tests. The major pulmonary function tests include spirometry, lung volumes, and diffusing capacity. The figure provides a simplified schema for interpretation of common lung function patterns. Before interpreting lung function tests, evaluate the flow-volume and volume-time curves to ensure quality of the maneuver(s) and to identify patterns suggestive of obstructive ventilatory defect, restriction, or large airway obstruction. The first step in the interpretation is consideration of the *forced expiratory volume in 1 second* (FEV$_1$) to the *forced vital capacity* (FVC) ratio. Low FEV$_1$ and low FVC will lead to a consideration of an obstructive ventilatory defect. *Total lung capacity* (TLC) is necessary for confirmation of a restrictive ventilatory defect. *Diffusing capacity of carbon monoxide* (DL$_{CO}$) helps assess presence of parenchymal disease in the setting of both obstructive and restrictive patterns; however, as noted in the text, the sensitivity and specificity of the DL$_{CO}$ for detection of emphysema, interstitial lung disease, or pulmonary vascular disease is not high near the LLN. Not infrequently, individuals have features of a mixed obstructive and restrictive pattern. A nonspecific pattern results when the FEV$_1$/FVC is normal and either the FEV$_1$ is low or the FVC is low and the TLC is normal. All patterns other than an obstructive ventilatory defect should be either confirmed or further evaluated with sequential testing as suggested in the schema. The schema gives a sequential approach that does not capture all combinations of test results. For combinations not represented (e.g., TLC < LLN and normal FVC, or DL$_{CO}$ and FEV$_1$ < LLN with normal FEV$_1$/FVC), the individual abnormalities may require further evaluation. *Low* indicates a value below the LLN; *normal* means at or above the LLN. *When FEV$_1$/FVC is above LLN and FVC is low but the FEV$_1$/FVC ratio is lower than expected—for example, considerably lower than the predicted value for the ratio—this can be interpreted as not clearly obstructive or restrictive. This pattern on spirometry alone should be investigated with further lung volume testing or imaging and followed closely.

small airway obstruction and poor elastic recoil due to emphysema can result in reduced flow at lower lung volumes with relatively preserved flows at higher lung volumes, and a resultant concave upwards pattern on the distal part of the flow-volume curve (see Fig. 32.2).[26] Also, when expiratory airflow rates during quiet breathing exceed those during maximal effort, it is attributed to abnormal compressibility or collapse of the airway walls; in this situation, tidal breathing involves less expiratory force, less collapse of highly collapsible airways, and slightly greater flow than seen with a maximal forced expiratory maneuver (see Fig. 32.2). This pattern has been termed *negative effort dependence* and may be seen in

diseases associated with airflow obstruction, including emphysema, cystic fibrosis, and bronchiolitis obliterans; small amounts of negative effort dependence may be an artifact of gas compression.[27] Finally, a number of metrics have been derived by mathematically quantifying the shape of the flow-volume and volume-time curves; these include the estimation of the angle between the first and second slopes in the descending part of the flow-volume curve or the "spirographic kink,"[28–31] quantification of the curvature of the expiratory curve,[32,33] the slope-ratio of the middle 20–80% of the expiratory curve to quantify its concavity,[34] flow ratio expressed as a percentage of the instantaneous flow at 75% of the expired vital capacity

Table 32.2 Obstructive Ventilatory Defect

CHARACTERISTICS OF OBSTRUCTIVE VENTILATORY DEFECT

Decreased FEV_1/FVC
Decreased FEV_1
Normal or decreased FVC or VC

OTHER DATA SUPPORTING OBSTRUCTION

Concave upward flow-volume curve (i.e., curvilinear)
Increased forced expiratory time
Decreased $FEF_{25\%-75\%}$
Decreased FEV_3/FVC
Increased RV
Increased TLC
Increased RV/TLC
Increased airway resistance (plethysmography, oscillometry)
Significant response to bronchodilator
Ventilation inhomogeneity on gas dilution (lung clearance index)
Decreased DL_{CO}
Decreased MVV

DL_{CO}, diffusing capacity of carbon monoxide; $FEF_{25\%-75\%}$, forced expiratory flow at 25–75% of FVC; FEV_1, forced expiratory volume in 1 second; FEV_3, forced expiratory volume in the first 3 seconds; FVC, forced vital capacity; MVV, maximal voluntary ventilation; RV, residual volume; TLC, total lung capacity; VC, vital capacity.

Modified from Welch MH. Ventilatory function of the lungs. In: Guenter CA, Welch MH, eds. *Pulmonary Medicine*. Philadelphia: JB Lippincott; 1977: 72–123.

(i.e., FR75),[35] and parameter D, a measure of the rate of rise of volume on the volume-time curve.[36] These measures are sensitive to mild disease and detect additional subjects with normal FEV_1/FVC who have an obstructive ventilatory defect; however, these metrics have not been adapted into clinical practice, in part due to a lack of reference values.

There is growing interest in using *inspiratory capacity* (IC) as an indirect measure of air trapping. With progressive airflow obstruction, FRC increases and results in a reduction in IC, whereas TLC does not change significantly until later stages of the disease.[37] In individuals with COPD, the ratio of IC/TLC (the inspiratory fraction) is associated with survival independently of the BODE (*body mass index, airflow obstruction, dyspnea, and exercise capacity*) index,[38,39] with exacerbations[40] and with exercise capacity.[41,42] An inspiratory fraction less than 0.25 is considered low.[39] Change in IC after bronchodilator therapy is also more closely associated with improvement in symptoms than is change in FEV_1.[37,43] However, when determining eligibility for interventions aimed at reducing air trapping, such as surgical and endoscopic lung volume reduction procedures, the actual measurement of RV should be performed.

R_{AW} and *airway conductance* (G_{AW}), measured using body plethysmography, are rarely used for diagnosis in clinical practice but can be used to support a diagnosis of airflow obstruction in borderline cases and in situations where individuals are unable to perform a forced expiratory maneuver.[44] Assessment of airway resistance can also be made through a forced oscillometry technique and impulse oscillometry.[45] The respiratory resistance at 5 Hz (R5) represents the total airway resistance, and the resistance at 20 Hz (R20) represents the resistance of the large airways. The difference between these two resistances (R5 − R20) is the resistance in the small airways.[45]

Lung volumes can provide supportive evidence for the presence of obstructive lung disease. Lung hyperinflation (TLC > *upper limit of normal* [ULN]) and air trapping (RV or RV/TLC ratio > ULN) may be seen in individuals with more advanced obstructive disease. In individuals at risk for COPD but with normal spirometry, an increased RV/TLC is associated with higher health care use, mortality, and risk for progression to COPD.[46] It should be noted that lung volumes estimated using gas dilution or washout techniques are usually lower than those estimated using body plethysmography, either due to noncommunicating airways, alveolar units with very slow time constants, or overestimation of volumes on plethysmography.[47] A ratio of single-breath alveolar volume measured during a diffusing capacity test (V_A, which is an estimate of TLC minus anatomic dead space) to the TLC measured by multibreath gas dilution less than 0.85 suggests heterogeneous distribution of ventilation.[48] In addition, MVV can be low in obstructive disease, but poor patient effort or a neuromuscular disorder should be considered when MVV is low in the setting of a normal FEV_1 and FVC.

The single-breath *diffusing capacity of the lung for carbon monoxide* (DL_{CO}) can be used to differentiate airflow obstruction associated with intrinsic airway disorders from airflow limitation related to emphysema. A normal single-breath DL_{CO} in the setting of an obstructive pattern argues against the presence of a large amount of emphysema but does not rule out a small amount.[49–51] Several studies have demonstrated a correlation of DL_{CO}, not only with the presence of emphysema, but also with the amount of emphysema.[50,52–54] In fact, a normal or increased single-breath DL_{CO} associated with airflow obstruction is often associated with asthma.[55] The single-breath DL_{CO} may be abnormal in patients with emphysema when there is no evidence of airflow obstruction, and it may decrease more rapidly than tests of airway function.[56–58] Individuals with normal spirometry but an isolated reduction in DL_{CO} are at higher risk of developing airflow obstruction over time than those with a normal DL_{CO}.[59]

RESTRICTIVE VENTILATORY DEFECT

A restrictive ventilatory defect is suggested by a parallel decrease in FEV_1 and FVC with a normal or increased FEV_1/FVC ratio, but this diagnosis requires confirmation with a decreased TLC using plethysmography or using the multiple-breath gas dilution method (Table 32.4). Examples of diseases that may manifest with a restrictive ventilatory defect are shown in eTable 32.1.

In many restrictive disorders, the increased elastic recoil at higher lung volumes leads to a convex upward pattern in the descending limb of the maximal expiratory flow-volume curve (also described as steep and vertically oriented) (see Fig. 32.2). Because spirometry does not estimate RV, a restrictive ventilatory defect on spirometry alone has a low sensitivity for correctly diagnosing restrictive lung disease; only up to 50% of those with this pattern have true restriction on lung volume assessment.[60–62] However, when the VC is normal, spirometry has a 96–97% negative predictive value in ruling out true restriction.[60,63] A TLC less than the *lower limit of normal* (LLN) defines a restrictive ventilatory defect. A reduced RV is also seen in the restrictive diseases

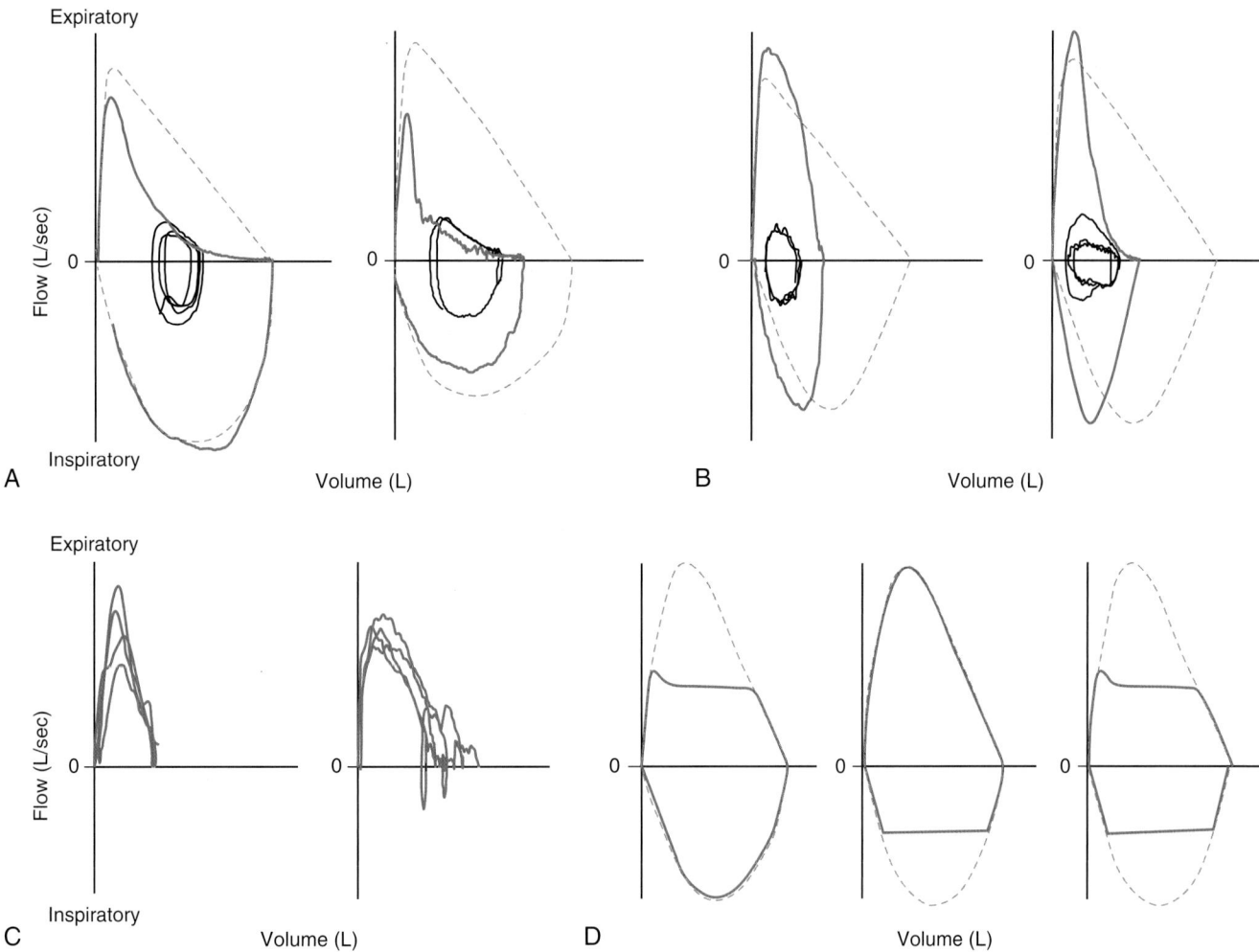

Figure 32.2 Typical flow-volume curves of major pulmonary function test patterns. *Solid lines* indicate curves obtained from patients. *Dashed lines* represent curves derived from the predicted flows and volumes for the corresponding patients. Tidal breathing appears in *gray*. The aspect ratio between the flow and volume axes is 2:1, consistent with standard practice and guidelines.[1] (A) COPD. With an obstructive ventilatory defect, maximal expiratory flow is concave upward, also called curvilinear; this shape reflects a greater reduction in flow at low compared to high lung volumes and can be understood in terms of the inverse relationship between lung elastic recoil and lung volume. Compared to predicted values, expiratory flow is usually reduced more significantly than inspiratory flow. In the example on the right, vital capacity is reduced due to air trapping; flow during tidal breathing (*gray tracing*) exceeds that observed with maximal effort—at low and midlung volumes in this example—a pattern called negative effort dependence. (B) Interstitial lung disease. In restrictive ventilatory defects associated with increased lung elastic recoil, maximal expiratory flow appears steep and vertically oriented (also described as convex upward) with increased flow at high lung volumes. Vital capacity is reduced. In the example on the right, the curve becomes concave upward at low lung volumes, a finding likely due to concomitant airway disease or loss of lung elastic recoil associated with aging. (C) Suboptimal effort manifests as uneven, slurred, or notched curves without repeatability across maneuvers. (D) Large airway obstruction: variable intrathoracic obstruction (*left*), variable extrathoracic obstruction (*middle*), and fixed obstruction (*right*).

associated with increased lung elastic recoil or in situations in which lung units are either collapsed or filled (e.g., pneumonia or hemorrhage). However, an isolated decrease in RV can be due to true restriction (i.e., TLC is read as normal due to small technical or biologic variations, or inaccuracy of predicted values) or obesity, or it could be a normal variant. Unlike in obstructive disease, lung volumes assessed using either dilution methods or plethysmography should be similar in those with a restrictive ventilatory defect.[64] A normal lung volume using either single-breath or multibreath dilution methods rules out restriction.[65] Although lung volume testing is required for the confirmation of spirometric restriction, once a diagnosis of restriction has been made, spirometry alone can be used for follow-up of lung volumes and is preferred due to better repeatability compared to TLC.

In true parenchymal restriction, the high FEV_1/FVC ratio arises from the reduction in FVC and the disproportionately lower decrease in FEV_1 due to a high lung elastic recoil. In these cases, DL_{CO} is usually decreased. In extraparenchymal restriction, however, the high FEV_1/FVC ratio results from the decreased VC. DL_{CO} may be normal in neuromuscular weakness and structural extraparenchymal restriction, such as scoliosis and kyphosis, but can be low when associated with markedly reduced lung volumes and/or basal atelectasis. A pattern of a normal or elevated RV, low TLC, and high RV/TLC ratio suggests a possible neuromuscular or chest wall etiology.[66,67] The flow-volume curve in neuromuscular weakness is not expected to have a convex upward pattern. Rather, it often maintains a nearly normal shape but with reduced flow rates and can feature a sudden drop in forced expiratory flow near RV.[68]

Table 32.3   Severity of Pulmonary Function Impairment*

Impairment	FEV$_1$[†]	TLC[‡]	VC[‡]	DL$_{CO}$
Abnormal	<LLN	<LLN	<LLN	<LLN
SEVERITY GRADING				
Mild	≥70%	≥70%	≥70%	≥60%
Moderate	60–69%	60–69%	60–69%	40–60%
Moderately severe	50–59%		50–59%	
Severe	35–49%	<60%	35–49%	<40%
Very severe	<35%		<35%	

*Grading scheme for FEV$_1$ follows the American Thoracic Society guidelines from 2005[3]; VC limits mirror those for FEV$_1$.
[†]Airflow obstruction is based on a decreased FEV$_1$/VC ratio. If the ratio is decreased below fifth percentile, the severity of airflow is graded on the percentage of predicted FEV$_1$. The FEV$_1$/VC ratio itself is not graded.
[‡]Pulmonary restriction is based on decreased TLC. If TLC is not available, a reduction in VC without a reduction in the FEV$_1$/VC ratio is considered a restriction of the volume excursion of the lung.
DL$_{CO}$, diffusion capacity of carbon monoxide; FEV$_1$, forced expiratory volume in 1 second; LLN, lower limit of the 95% confidence interval; TLC, total lung capacity; VC, vital capacity.

Table 32.4   Restrictive Ventilatory Defect

CHARACTERISTICS OF RESTRICTIVE VENTILATORY DEFECT

Normal or high FEV$_1$/FVC
Decreased VC
Decreased TLC

OTHER DATA SUPPORTING RESTRICTION

Convex upward flow-volume curve*
Decreased RV[†]
Decreased DL$_{CO}$[‡]
Increased (A–a)PO$_2$

*A convex upward flow-volume curve is not expected with a restrictive ventilatory defect due to extraparenchymal causes such as neuromuscular weakness, chest wall or spine diseases.
[†]RV may be normal or increased with extraparenchymal causes of a restrictive ventilatory defect, leading to an elevated ratio of RV to TLC.
[‡]DL$_{CO}$ can be normal or decreased in extraparenchymal diseases.
(A–a)PO$_2$, alveolar-arterial PO$_2$ difference; DL$_{CO}$, diffusing capacity of carbon monoxide; FEV$_1$, forced expiratory volume in 1 second; FVC, forced vital capacity; PO$_2$, partial pressure of oxygen; RV, residual volume; TLC, total lung capacity; VC, vital capacity.
Modified from Welch MH. Ventilatory function of the lungs. In: Guenter CA, Welch MH, eds. *Pulmonary Medicine*. Philadelphia: JB Lippincott; 1977: 72–123.

As mentioned, in approximately 50% of cases where spirometry is suggestive of a restrictive ventilatory defect, lung volumes do not show restriction.[60–62] In this situation, the forced expiratory time and the end-of-test criteria should be evaluated to ensure that the restrictive pattern is not due to inadequate exhalation. In cases of significant air trapping, the FVC may be artificially low and the FEV$_1$/FVC ratio may be artificially normal or elevated, resulting in a pseudorestrictive pattern. This pseudorestrictive pattern is often interpreted as a mixed obstructive/restrictive process. Pseudorestriction should be suspected when the clinical indication for spirometry is an obstructive airway disease or when the expiratory flow-volume curves show a concave upward obstructive pattern and can be confirmed by demonstrating a normal TLC on lung volume measurement. RV and RV/TLC ratio will also be elevated in this condition. There is, however, no linear relation between the degree of air trapping and the magnitude of decrease in FVC.

A special type of restriction termed *complex restriction* has been described, wherein the reduction in FVC is out of proportion to the reduction in TLC (a >10% difference between the percentage of predicted TLC and percentage of predicted FVC). In one study, approximately 4% of all pulmonary function tests and 33% of restrictive pulmonary function tests showed complex restriction.[69] This pattern was associated with diseases classically associated with restriction and also with a significant number of obstructive diseases, such as COPD, likely due to impaired emptying of the lung during a forced exhalation maneuver. Care should be taken to ensure the disproportionately low FVC is not due to incomplete exhalation. Recognition of this pattern should prompt evaluation for an additional process, such as chest wall limitation, neuromuscular weakness, poor performance, or occult obstruction.

A brief discussion on diffusion capacity in interstitial lung disease is available at ExpertConsult.com.

MIXED VENTILATORY DEFECTS

A mixed obstructive and restrictive ventilatory defect is present when both the FEV$_1$/FVC and TLC are less than the LLN (see eTable 32.1 for examples). In these cases, both the obstructive and restrictive processes are expected to reduce the FEV$_1$. In accordance with guidelines, it is reasonable to quantify the total ventilatory impairment by the FEV$_1$ percentage of predicted.[3] It is logical to assume that using the FEV$_1$ percentage of predicted to grade the severity of obstruction in a mixed disorder will overestimate the severity due to the concomitant loss of volume contributed by restriction. To address this issue, an FEV$_1$ percentage of predicted adjusted for the degree of restriction was defined as the FEV$_1$ percentage of predicted divided by the TLC percentage of predicted.[75] In a cohort of 199 subjects with a mixed ventilatory defect, with use of this *adjusted* FEV$_1$ percentage of predicted, 33% were classified as having severe or very severe obstruction, whereas, with the *unadjusted* FEV$_1$ percentage of predicted, 76% were classified in this category.[75] The correlation between the adjusted FEV$_1$ percentage and RV/TLC was better than with the unadjusted FEV$_1$ percentage. Because this work has not been validated, there is no consensus on its use in clinical practice; however, it is important for the clinician to be cognizant of the possibility of overestimating the severity of obstruction in a patient when restriction is also present.

In the presence of a restrictive ventilatory defect, the sensitivity of the FEV_1/FVC ratio to detect an obstructive ventilatory defect may be reduced; findings other than a reduced FEV_1/FVC ratio can suggest airflow obstruction. Caution must be exercised in diseases with opposing effects on FEV_1/FVC and TLC, such as combined pulmonary fibrosis and emphysema. In this condition both FEV_1/FVC and TLC can appear to be preserved due to the effects of airflow obstruction and air trapping counterbalanced by the increased elastic recoil of fibrosed lung regions. The only pulmonary function defect observed in this situation may be a disproportionately decreased DL_{CO}.[76]

NONSPECIFIC PATTERNS

When the FEV_1/FVC ratio is normal with a low FVC and/or low FEV_1, but with a normal TLC, this is indicative of a nonspecific pulmonary function test pattern. Although the 2005 ATS/ERS document recommends interpreting this pattern as obstructive, a substantial proportion of individuals with this pattern do not have evidence of obstruction, but rather chest wall limitation, including obesity and muscle weakness, or poor test performance.[3] In a study of 80,929 subjects, a nonspecific pattern was identified in 7702 subjects (≈10%).[77] Longitudinal study of 1284 of these subjects who had one or more pulmonary function tests performed 6 months or more after initial testing, with a median follow-up of 3 years, revealed that the nonspecific pattern was stable and persistent in 64%.[78] Roughly equal numbers of subjects (≈15%) developed a restrictive or obstructive pattern, whereas 3% normalized and 2% showed a mixed pattern. Of note, the definition of the nonspecific pattern differed slightly between the initial (low FVC and FEV_1) and follow-up (low FVC and/or FEV_1) reports.

Due to the absence of measurements of TLC in many datasets, the prevalence and associated patient characteristics of nonspecific patterns on spirometry alone have also been investigated.[79] The definitions share the requirement for a normal FEV_1/FVC ratio but differ in whether the FEV_1, FVC, or both are reduced. A number of conditions have been reported to be associated with these patterns. In particular, a low FVC and normal FEV_1/FVC ratio with or without low FEV_1, termed a restrictive spirometric pattern, has been associated with risk for cardiovascular disease[80,81] and diabetes mellitus.[82] Another nonspecific pattern, a normal FEV_1/FVC ratio with an isolated FEV_1 reduction, was found in 2.1% of 15,192 subjects.[83] Compared to normal subjects, this category included a higher proportion of smokers; individuals with radiologic abnormalities, including emphysema and tuberculosis; and those with a history of respiratory disease, including asthma, chronic bronchitis, and tuberculosis. These data highlight the importance of obtaining a measure of TLC if a restrictive ventilatory defect is suspected and of following patients with nonspecific spirometry patterns. In the setting of a normal TLC, patients with these patterns may have worse outcomes than those with normal spirometry and, in the appropriate

clinical context, an evaluation for parenchymal, pleural, chest wall, and neuromuscular disease may be indicated. Tests of airway resistance can also help distinguish obstructive from restrictive processes.

PULMONARY VASCULAR DISEASE

In patients presenting with dyspnea during exertion, a decreased DL_{CO} without evidence of obstructive or restrictive ventilatory defects should raise suspicion for disorders of pulmonary circulation. A decreased DL_{CO} is not a sensitive test to detect pulmonary vascular disease. For example, many patients with elevated pulmonary arterial pressure and pulmonary vascular resistance will have a normal DL_{CO}.[84-86] In systemic sclerosis, an autoimmune condition associated with pulmonary hypertension and *interstitial lung disease* (ILD), two screening algorithms incorporate the DL_{CO} percentage predicted and the ratio of DL_{CO} percentage predicted to FVC percentage of predicted to trigger further testing, including echocardiography or right heart catheterization.[87-89] Because most studies have not reported the reference values used, one should be cautious in applying the literature on the performance of the DL_{CO} in detecting disease. The published reference values for DL_{CO} differ significantly, limiting the applicability of studies that report on the performance of DL_{CO} as a percentage of predicted.

In general, when pretest probability is more than minimal, a normal DL_{CO} should not preclude the pursuit of more detailed pulmonary function studies of the pulmonary circulation. These studies include exercise tests, which are especially useful when signs of pulmonary hypertension are absent and radiographic methods fail to demonstrate obstruction of large pulmonary arteries.

See ExpertConsult.com for a discussion of the changes seen in DL_{CO} in the setting of pulmonary vascular obstruction.

RESPIRATORY MUSCLE WEAKNESS

Tests of respiratory muscle weakness should be considered in individuals in whom neuromuscular disease is known or suspected, such as in cases of weak cough, spirometric restriction, unexplained dyspnea or orthopnea, and hypercapnic respiratory failure. Causes of respiratory muscle weakness are listed in eTable 32.1. Routine pulmonary function tests can provide significant information about neuromuscular disease. Upright and supine VC testing can be used to obtain a global assessment of inspiratory and expiratory muscle function.[96] Unilateral diaphragm weakness is associated with a modest decrease in the VC, whereas severe bilateral diaphragmatic weakness can result in a VC of less than 50% predicted. Repeating VC testing in the supine position can unmask diaphragmatic weakness. A postural decrease in VC of 25% or more is suggestive of diaphragmatic weakness, but a normal supine VC does not rule out clinically significant diaphragmatic weakness.[97-99] The VC does not decrease until substantial inspiratory muscle weakness has set in because only very small pressures are required to inflate the lung fully. MVV is also low in neuromuscular disease, and neuromuscular disease should be suspected when the reduction in MVV is disproportionate to the reduction in FEV_1 and FVC.[66,100]

TLC decreases in parallel with VC, but RV frequently stays normal or elevated. This pattern of an isolated decrease in TLC with normal or elevated RV should raise suspicion for neuromuscular disease.

The initial assessment of muscle strength in individuals with suspected neuromuscular disease is by voluntary tests of respiratory muscle strength. These include the *maximum static inspiratory pressure* (MIP, or PI_{max}) and *maximum expiratory pressure* (MEP, or PE_{max}) at the mouth. These tests offer a simple assessment of overall respiratory muscle strength. The MIP reflects the strength of the diaphragm and other inspiratory muscles and is usually measured at RV. Care should be taken to observe the patient performing the test because involvement of the cheeks can help generate a significant negative inspiratory pressure. The MEP reflects the strength of the abdominal and other expiratory muscles and is usually measured at TLC. The ATS guidelines recommend that the highest 1-second average should be recorded for both MIP and MEP.[101] Lower limits of normal have not been clearly defined for MIP and MEP, and the large variations mean that the LLNs are usually approximately 50% predicted. A normal MIP is 80 cm H_2O or more in men and 70 cm H_2O or more in women.[101] Values greater than these will rule out clinically significant inspiratory muscle weakness. Values less than 60% predicted suggest unilateral diaphragmatic weakness, and those less than 30% predicted suggest bilateral diaphragmatic weakness.[102,103] However, reference data for MIP and MEP vary, and the choice can significantly impact the diagnosis of neuromuscular weakness.[104] These normal ranges can be significantly affected by the presence of underlying obstructive disease, such as COPD, because hyperinflation-induced diaphragmatic flattening can decrease the MIP without true weakness of the diaphragm.

The maximal sniff nasal inspiratory pressure is slightly more invasive in that it requires a transducer catheter to be placed in the nostril. The inspiratory effort usually starts at FRC. The ATS recommends that the highest pressure should be recorded.[101] Normal values for men and women are 70 cm H_2O or more and 60 cm H_2O or more, respectively.[101] Testing maximal sniff nasal inspiratory pressure may be easier to perform for many patients with neuromuscular disease because, unlike MIP, this maneuver is not affected by ineffective mouth seal or having to sustain a maximal inspiratory effort.

Peak cough flow (PCF) provides a measure of expiratory muscle strength and the effectiveness of mucus clearance in neuromuscular disorders. PCF can be measured using a spirometer or handheld peak flowmeter. Normal values in healthy subjects range from 290 to 880 L/min.[105] A PCF less than 270 L/min is associated with a higher likelihood of pulmonary complications in neuromuscular disease.[106]

When these noninvasive measures of muscle strength are equivocal, more invasive assessments, including the measurement of esophageal, gastric, and transdiaphragmatic pressures while sniffing and coughing, may be required (see Chapter 31). Advanced testing, including phrenic nerve stimulation and electromyography, may be required in some cases. These measures are discussed in more detail in Chapter 130. Measures obtained in the pulmonary function laboratory can be complemented by radiographic and imaging measures to track diaphragm movement and thickening while sniffing (see Video 20.1).

LARGE AIRWAY OBSTRUCTION: STENOSIS AND COLLAPSIBILITY (See Chapter 39)

Flow-volume curves may be especially helpful in identifying tracheal or other upper airway lesions as a cause of obstruction.[107] Large (also called central) airway obstruction (i.e., proximal to the tracheal carina) located within the thorax produces a repeatable plateau during forced exhalation instead of the usual rise to and descent from peak flow (see Fig. 32.2). Peak flow is also usually blunted. When more than 50% of the VC has been exhaled, the curve then follows the usual flow-volume curve to RV. In patients with stridor, particular attention should be paid to the configuration of the inspiratory portion as well as the expiratory portion of the flow-volume curve. Lesions that cause either stenosis or collapsibility located in the trachea *inside* the thorax decrease airflow, particularly during exhalation; during inhalation, the posterior tracheal membrane is pulled outward by negative intrathoracic pressure, so increased effort increases airflow rates and the inspiratory limb of the flow-volume curve can appear normal. Conversely, tracheal lesions that cause stenosis or collapsibility located *outside* of the thorax decrease airflow during inhalation; during inhalation, the tracheal membrane is sucked in and is usually associated with stridor, whereas during exhalation, the lesion may be stented open by positive airway pressure and the expiratory limb of the flow-volume curve can appear normal (see Fig. 32.2). When the inspiratory and expiratory limbs are differentially affected, the obstruction is referred to as variable. In contrast, if a lesion is fixed and not altered by surrounding pressures, whether intrathoracic or extrathoracic, airflow should be limited equally during inhalation and exhalation (see Fig. 32.2). Similarly, because a flow-limiting orifice located at the thoracic outlet is not affected by pressure above or below the lesion, airflow is limited equally during both inhalation and exhalation.[108] The diameter of a stenotic lesion can be estimated by analysis of the flow-volume curve (eFig. 32.3), but the length of the flow-limiting segment must be confirmed by computed tomography scan to plan surgical correction, if required. A plateau in maximal expiratory flow associated with central airway obstruction that reduces the size of the tracheal lumen significantly below normal is expected to reduce flow to approximately 4 L/sec or less (see eFig. 32.3). In contrast, normal variants sometimes seen in young adults lead to plateaus at high lung volumes with higher flow.[109,110]

Although the finding of a repeatable plateau on forced inspiratory or expiratory flow suggests central or upper airway obstruction, the FEV_1, FVC, and FEV_1/FVC are not sensitive.[111,112] Ratios derived from individual spirometric variables, such as FEV_1/*peak expiratory flow rate* (PEFR) greater than 10, *forced expiratory flow at 50% lung volume* (FEF_{50})/*forced inspiratory flow at 50% lung volume* (FIF_{50})

greater than 1.2, $FIF_{25\%-75\%}/FEF_{25\%-75\%}$ less than 1, and MVV/FEV_1 less than 25 perform better at identifying large airway obstruction than FEV_1, FVC, or FEV_1/FVC.[112–115] The presence of chronic airflow obstruction from diseases that affect the airways diffusely and heterogeneously (e.g., asthma, COPD) decreases the sensitivity of spirometry to detect concomitant large airway obstruction.[116]

REFERENCE VALUES

Reference values derived from a population without lung disease can yield equations for expected values for a given height, sex, and age. Reference values allow comparison of results between individuals and make it possible to follow the trend of values across time within an individual while removing the average effect of aging. Publications describing reference populations should include not only the prediction equations but also a means to define their lower limits. A lower limit can be estimated from a regression model: for spirometry, where a clinical concern arises from abnormally reduced but not elevated values, the fifth percentile is usually considered the LLN.[117] For some tests in which both high and low values are considered abnormal, the 2.5th and 97.5th percentile define the lower and upper limits of normal, respectively. There is no statistical basis for the common practice of using 80% of the predicted normal values for FEV_1 and FVC as the LLN in adults. A study of 11,413 patients found that using fixed cut points to determine whether lung function is abnormal could misdiagnose more than 20% of patients and could be avoided by using the LLN based on the fifth percentile values. The use of cutoffs based on a percentage of the predicted value has the potential for age and height bias because the spread of the distribution often varies with these parameters,[118] whereas the use of percentile cutoffs (or equivalently, z-scores, which represent the number of standard deviations above or below the mean) avoids this problem. When the standing height cannot be measured accurately, as in those with an inability to stand or with thoracic spine abnormalities, height should be estimated from arm span with the use of regression equations accounting for the effects of age, sex, and ethnicity.[119]

The clinical application of pulmonary function tests requires the recognition of the limitations of reference values (eTable 32.3). Although the fifth percentile is often chosen to define the LLN, adjustments can be made depending on the prevalence of the disease in the target population and the desired sensitivity and specificity. Furthermore, reference ranges are derived from healthy individuals, whereas in disease, lung function at 70% of predicted but above the LLN may nonetheless have an impact on symptoms, hypoxemia, and exacerbations or mortality risk.[6,120,121] Values in the normal range might reflect the variability of expression of a disease across patients. This last point is used as an argument for the use of percentage of predicted for disease severity classifications rather than z-scores, and there is limited evidence that such an approach is valid in COPD.[122] The causes of differences in lung function between ethnic groups are diverse, not completely understood, and include exposures such as pollution, stress including

discrimination, and early-life nutritional differences.[123–125] Large variability within traditionally defined ethnic groups limits the perceived advantages of using specific equations within groups. Chest size is only partially associated with differences within or between groups and confounded with exposures and early life events.[124,126–128] Clinicians and investigators are increasingly grappling with the use of population-specific reference equations—both the potential harms (e.g., underdiagnosis, underestimation of severity, denial of access to therapies, disability, and masking of modifiable risks for reduced lung function) and potential benefits (e.g., avoidance of overdiagnosis, and inclusiveness to meet requirements to work or receive therapies such as resection of lung cancer, stem-cell transplantation, and chemotherapy).

Additional information on reference values can be found at ExpertConsult.com.

GENERAL APPROACH TO INTERPRETATION

Figure 32.1 depicts an algorithm for the interpretation of pulmonary function tests. For this algorithm, we suggest that postbronchodilator spirometry values be used. Prebronchodilator spirometry is the most commonly performed pulmonary function test but, in cases where airflow obstruction is suspected, postbronchodilator spirometry should be performed and be used for interpretation.[8] Although reference equations were derived using prebronchodilator values, LLNs can be applied to postbronchodilator spirometry. In cases of borderline significance, close follow-up and repeat testing are recommended.

The first step in the interpretation of spirometry is visual inspection of the flow-volume curves, which may give clues regarding test quality and the presence of large airway obstruction.

The second step is to assess the FEV_1/FVC ratio. If the FEV_1/FVC ratio is low, the next step is to evaluate the FEV_1. If the FEV_1 is also low, this confirms obstruction. At this point, the FVC is useful: if the FVC is normal, this confirms a simple obstructive defect; if the FVC is also low, this indicates an obstructive ventilatory defect associated with either a concomitant restrictive ventilatory defect or with air trapping. If the FEV_1/FVC ratio is low and the FEV_1 is normal, this could indicate early or mild airflow obstruction or be a normal variant due to dysanaptic lung growth. Lung volumes may support the diagnosis of obstruction when TLC and RV are high or a mixed obstructive and restrictive ventilatory defect when TLC is low.

If the FEV_1/FVC ratio is normal, this could indicate normal spirometry or a restrictive ventilatory defect. The next step is to evaluate the FVC. A low FVC can be due to restriction or due to air trapping and should be investigated with lung volume testing. A low TLC confirms restriction, whereas a normal TLC can often be seen with a low FVC and should be interpreted as a nonspecific pulmonary function pattern. A normal TLC and a high RV suggests air trapping as the etiology of the low FVC (pseudorestriction). If the FEV_1/FVC ratio is normal, a normal FVC essentially rules out restriction, and lung volume testing is not recommended unless clinical suspicion is very high for a restrictive ventilatory defect.

Spirometry with an isolated reduction in FEV_1 or FVC with normal FEV_1/FVC ratio should be interpreted as not clearly obstructive or restrictive in the absence of a TLC for further clarification. This pattern can also be read as a nonspecific ventilatory defect and investigated further with lung volume and DL_{CO} testing. The FEV_1/FVC ratio is expected to be higher than normal in cases of parenchymal restriction where there is increased elastic recoil. A high FEV_1/FVC should also be followed up with lung volume testing.

A restrictive ventilatory defect should be further evaluated with DL_{CO}. A low DL_{CO} suggests an intraparenchymal process, but a normal DL_{CO} suggests an extraparenchymal process, such as a chest wall defect or neuromuscular disease. DL_{CO} may be low in neuromuscular disease as well as when there is basal atelectasis. A low DL_{CO} in the setting of normal spirometry and normal lung volumes may be indicative of pulmonary vascular disease, or mild emphysema or ILD.

Once the major pulmonary function pattern has been recognized, the severity is graded using FEV_1 percentage predicted, irrespective of pattern. Restriction can also be graded using percentage predicted TLC. Table 32.3 shows the severity grading recommended by the ATS.[3]

FACTORS AFFECTING PULMONARY FUNCTION TESTING AND INTERPRETATION: CAVEATS AND PRECAUTIONS

A number of factors can affect test results, and care should be taken in the performance and interpretation of pulmonary function tests.

TEST PERFORMANCE CHARACTERISTICS

Pulmonary function tests in general depend heavily on the cooperation of the subject. The following factors should be kept in mind when making decisions about response to therapy and for comparisons on follow-up. If a competent technician performs the procedures and if recordings of the test tracings accompany the measurements, it is usually possible to determine the validity of the data. Suboptimal effort can usually be identified on the basis of the features listed in eTable 32.4. Supplemental data confirming invalid test results include uneven, slurred, or notched curves on inspection; poor repeatability of maximal expiratory flow (see Fig. 32.2), FEV_1, and FVC within a test session; poor agreement between measures of VC across spirometry, lung volumes, and diffusing capacity maneuvers; and poor reproducibility on repeated testing. FVC can be underestimated when end-of-test criteria are not met or when inhalation is incomplete before the forced expiratory maneuver. A valid restrictive pattern differs from a test with poor effort in that it is repeatable, shows smooth expiratory curves on

direct examination, a steep slope at the start of the volume-time curve, and a normal or nearly normal MVV. FEV_1 can be frequently underestimated in the setting of significant hesitancy or an incomplete full inhalation before the forced expiratory maneuver. The back extrapolated volume on the volume-time curve should be less than 5% of the FVC or 100 mL, whichever is greater, to ensure that the start of test criteria is satisfactory. The inspiratory curve should be evaluated to confirm a full inhalation.

It should be noted that although lung volumes can be reliably measured using body plethysmography or gas dilution techniques (helium dilution or nitrogen washout), significant differences may be observed in estimates of lung volumes in individuals with obstructive lung disease. Plethysmography can overestimate thoracic gas volume at FRC, but this can be mitigated by coaching patients to pant slowly at 0.5 to 1.0 Hz.[138] Nonetheless, plethysmography is likely more accurate because, unlike the gas dilution estimates of lung volumes, it is not affected by noncommunicating airways. Milite and colleagues[139] reported that the difference in measured thoracic gas volume between the commonly used plethysmography and nitrogen washout methods is approximately 0.5 L in patients with emphysema.

The gas dilution methods are sensitive to leaks, which can result in overestimation of FRC and hence TLC and RV. A leak during plethysmography can result in either overestimation or underestimation of FRC. A leak most often happens during the closed-valve panting phase and tends to shift the baseline of the subsequent tidal breathing. Because the slow expiratory VC maneuver is performed after the panting phase, an upward shift will cause an overestimation of TLC, and a downward shift will result in an underestimation of TLC. Air trapping can be overestimated if the effort-dependent ERV measurement is suboptimal. DL_{CO} can be underestimated if the inspiratory capacity maneuver is submaximal.

SUBJECT CHARACTERISTICS

Medications

Caffeine and alcohol are bronchodilators and hence should not be consumed within 4 hours of testing; the effects are unlikely to be clinically significant with moderate consumption.[140] Alcohol also affects patient cooperation and can interfere with the methane sensor and the measurement of diffusing capacity.[141] When postbronchodilator testing is indicated, short-acting β-agonists and antimuscarinic agents should be withheld for at least 4 hours before testing. Long-acting β-agonists should be withheld for at least 12 hours, whereas long-acting anticholinergics and ultra-long-acting β-agonists should be withheld for at least 24 to 48 hours before testing.

Obesity

The prevalence of obesity is increasing, and hence it is important to consider the effects of obesity on lung function. Due to mechanical constraints, the increased mass of the chest wall decreases ERV, subsequently FRC, and then TLC.[142] Despite a decrease in TLC with obesity, TLC is still most often within the normal range.[143,144] As the ERV diminishes, tidal volume is shifted toward RV, graphically depicted when the tidal volume loop is superimposed on the flow-volume loop at low lung volumes. Morbid obesity is often associated with basal atelectasis and decreased DL_{CO}. These effects are worsened in the supine posture. Obesity affects the detection of airflow obstruction in two competing directions. On one hand, because of extrathoracic restriction, individuals with obesity breathe at lower lung volumes where airway diameters are narrower, with resulting higher airway resistance. On the other hand, the detection of this airway resistance is complicated due to the decrease in FVC, which can raise the FEV_1/FVC ratio and thus mask airflow obstruction. Reference equations do not take obesity into account. Furthermore, obesity is commonly measured using the body mass index, which does not specifically reflect the mechanical constraints on the chest.

INTERPRETATION OF CHANGES IN FUNCTION OVER TIME

VARIATION BETWEEN TESTS WITHIN A YEAR

Changes in spirometric measurements may represent a true change or merely variability. A real change is more likely when a series of tests shows a consistent trend. A change varies in significance depending on the variable measured, the time period, and whether the individual has normal or abnormal lung function. The variability is greater with increasing intervals between tests and in individuals with established lung disease. When the FEV_1 and FVC are followed in healthy, normal subjects, within-day changes of 5% or more, between-weeks changes of 11–12% or more, and yearly changes of 15% or more are probably clinically significant.[3] Data are limited for lung volume variability over time and also vary with the method of determination of lung volume. Current guidelines suggest that 5–10% and 200 to 400 mL are thresholds that can be used clinically.[145] For DL_{CO}, within-year changes of greater than 10% or 5 units (mL/min/mm Hg) are likely significant; within-day variability is 5–10% or 2 to 2.5 units.[3,146,147] Other than a change in lung function, sources of fluctuation in DL_{CO} include increased depth of inspiration during the test, changes in altitude, and changes in hemoglobin concentration (for which the DL_{CO} can be adjusted).

AGING LUNG

Aging is associated with a decrease in lung elastic recoil pressure at all lung volumes. Morphologic studies have confirmed increased alveolar dimensions. VC decreases with age, whereas RV and closing volume increase with age,[148] suggesting that lung emptying is limited with increasing age because of airway closure.[149] The consequence of increasing airway closure and loss of elastic recoil is a progressive decline in FEV_1 and FVC beginning in the mid 20s to 30s, with a subsequent linear decline in FEV_1/FVC.[117,150] The rate of decline in FEV_1 and FVC varies, ranging from 17.7 to 46.4 mL/year (median, 22.4 mL/year) for FEV_1 in healthy nonsmokers. Higher rates are observed among current

and recent smokers, people with asthma or obesity, those with occupational exposures or who live near traffic, people of certain ethnic backgrounds, and the elderly.[151–155] Differences in the relative decline in FEV_1 are not different between men and women.[155] Application of these average rates to the individual, particularly over short time frames and in those with lung disease, is challenging due to episodic loss of lung function associated with respiratory events. MVV decreases approximately 30% between 30 and 70 years of age, probably as a consequence of decreased maximal respiratory pressures, decreased distensibility of the total respiratory system, decreased lung elastic recoil, and impaired coordination of the respiratory muscles. TLC and RAW are independent of age.[137,148,156] DL_{CO} decreases with advancing age. Experiments with the series resistance model of Roughton and Forster[157] suggest possible mechanisms. The decreases in membrane diffusing capacity after 40 years of age more likely reflects loss of alveolar-capillary surface area than a change in membrane thickness; pulmonary capillary blood volume is maintained until the seventh decade and then decreases rapidly.[158]

BRONCHODILATOR RESPONSIVENESS

Another approach to the differential diagnosis of the obstructive pattern is the assessment of responsiveness of impaired expiratory airflow to acute administration of a bronchodilator. The ATS recommends that VC (slow or forced) and FEV_1 be the primary spirometric indices used to determine bronchodilator response.[3] Total expiratory time should be considered when using FVC to assess the bronchodilator response because in obstructed patients FVC increases when expiratory time increases. A 12% increase above the prebronchodilator value *and* a 200-mL increase in either FVC or FEV_1 indicate a positive bronchodilator response in adults.

BRONCHODILATOR RESPONSIVENESS IN ASTHMA

Variable airflow obstruction is a core functional criterion by which to make a clinical diagnosis of asthma. Variable airflow obstruction can be established by variation over time in peak flow, variation over time in FEV_1,[159] or bronchodilator responsiveness. Repeatable peak flow measurements are very dependent on effort and thus are inherently more variable than other measures of airflow. Often, repeated measures of FEV_1 over time are not available. Therefore, the assessment of bronchodilator responsiveness at a single testing session is a useful test by which to make a diagnosis of asthma. Of importance, one must first consider whether other conditions are present that feature a bronchodilator response before making a diagnosis of asthma. For example, bronchodilator responsiveness is common in COPD.[160]

Failure to demonstrate significant responses to acute bronchodilator therapy does not rule out bronchodilator-responsive airflow obstruction. For example, many reports confirm that asthmatic patients with completely reversible airflow obstruction may fail to respond to inhaled bronchodilators until after corticosteroid treatment.[161] Bronchodilator response is a continuous phenomenon, and therefore there is uncertainty about the significance of the finding near the threshold. Related to this, there are many reasons why a patient may not have a significant response at any one session: recent use of a short or long-acting bronchodilator, not enough abnormal smooth muscle contraction on that particular day, intraluminal mucus and/or airway edema as the predominant cause of obstruction, limitations of FEV_1 in assessing airflow obstruction, and the effect of a deep breath on airway caliber. The presence or lack of a significant bronchodilator response to short-acting albuterol during one testing session is poorly predictive of the long-term response to bronchodilator treatment in terms of change in FEV_1, symptoms, or exacerbations in asthma or COPD.

BRONCHODILATOR RESPONSIVENESS IN COPD

Between 35–60% of individuals with COPD show a bronchodilator response in FEV_1.[162–164] Hence, bronchodilator reversibility does not differentiate asthma from COPD. Patients with COPD are more likely to show a bronchodilator response in FVC than in FEV_1, likely due to a reduction in air trapping, especially in more severe disease; an FVC response is seen in up to 67% of individuals with COPD.[162] Also, compared to the FEV_1 response, an FVC response is more common in individuals with hyperinflation[43,165] and is more strongly associated with gas trapping.[166] Approximately 5% of individuals with COPD display a paradoxical bronchoconstriction in response to administration of a bronchodilator; this is associated with worse respiratory outcomes, including dyspnea, functional capacity, and exacerbations.[167,168]

Bronchodilator reversibility can change with repeated testing in parallel with the day-to-day variation in lung function and hence may not be a stable phenotype. In the *Inhaled Steroids in Obstructive Lung Disease in Europe* (ISOLDE) study, approximately 50% of subjects changed bronchodilator reversibility status between visits.[169] In the *Evaluation of COPD Longitudinally to Identify Predictive Surrogate End-Points* (ECLIPSE) study, only 16% of subjects considered to have reversibility at the first visit met reversibility criteria at all subsequent visits over the next 3 years.[170] The clinical utility of a positive bronchodilator response in COPD is thus unclear. Multiple studies have also shown that a lack of reversibility does not preclude response to long-acting bronchodilators.[160]

 Additional information on bronchodilator responsiveness can be found at ExpertConsult.com.

BRONCHIAL CHALLENGE TESTING

Increased smooth muscle responsiveness is a core pathologic and clinical feature of asthma. Therefore, when patients do not have variable airflow obstruction or bronchodilator responsiveness, a bronchial challenge test can fulfill the functional criteria for asthma. This may be important to do because 25–40% of individuals with physician-diagnosed asthma in the community do not have evidence of airway hyperreactivity.[177] They may be taking medications for asthma unnecessarily and may have another diagnosis that is not being managed.

An abnormal/positive provocation test supports an asthma-focused diagnostic and treatment program but, of note, is frequently seen in other airway diseases (e.g., COPD,[178] sarcoidosis[179]), in the setting of allergic rhinitis without lower airway symptoms, or after recent upper respiratory tract infection or smoking. Airflow limitation in response to methacholine can reflect not only increased smooth muscle responsiveness, but also airway wall edema, luminal mucus, and changes in smooth muscle content and geometry.[180]

A normal/negative test argues strongly against asthma as a cause of current symptoms, except when there is exercise-induced asthma, early occupational asthma, or recent systemic corticosteroid treatment. If there are no symptoms currently, then it may have been some time since exposure to the right trigger/allergen, and a methacholine challenge may be negative. In this case, it can be argued that the patient does not currently have asthma, which highlights alternatives to a categorical asthma versus no-asthma interpretation: features of asthma can wax and wane, and there may be uncertainty in the diagnosis of asthma at any one time point.

The most frequently used type of positive bronchial challenge result is an abnormal increase in airflow limitation after exposure to sequential doses (doubling of concentration between doses) of inhaled methacholine, a direct smooth muscle agonist. The result is often reported as the concentration in mg/mL that leads to a 20% decrease in FEV_1 relative to the value after inhaling a saline control (*provocative concentration* [PC20]; usually extrapolated between doses if FEV_1 falls by more than 20%). Recommendations for a categorical interpretation of methacholine challenge results that nonetheless reflect the continuous relationship between dose/concentration and certainty of asthma are reproduced in eTable 32.5.[181] A significant change in PC20 from one test to another is considered 1.5 dose doublings, a figure informed by short-term repeatability of the test in stable asthma. Recently updated ATS/ERS guidelines recommend reporting the cumulative *provocative dose of methacholine delivered* (PD20), rather than PC20, to ensure reproducibility and comparability across delivery devices and protocols.[181]

An alternative or additional measure of response to methacholine is serial measurement of airway resistance after each dose of methacholine. An increase in specific airway resistance (equivalently, a decrease in *specific airway conductance* [sGAW]) is more sensitive than a decrease in FEV_1 because measurement of FEV_1 necessarily involves a deep inspiration. Deep inhalations are known to reduce smooth muscle tone and have a bronchodilatory effect on airways, although this effect is reduced or absent in asthma.[182,183] Although some data suggest FEV_1 is more specific for asthma than airway resistance, another report suggests that among patients referred for testing, those without a significant change in FEV_1 but with a significant change in airway resistance ($\approx$20% of referrals in this study) have a similar symptom burden as those with a significant decrease in FEV_1.[184] A common threshold for a significant change in sGAW after inhalation of methacholine is a greater than or equal to 40% decrease.[175]

Vocal cord dysfunction is in the differential diagnosis of asthma and may coexist with asthma. Vocal cord dysfunction can be induced by methacholine challenge and can cause a decrease in sGAW and abnormal flattening of the inspiratory limb on spirometry. Of note, FEV_1 is expected to be normal.[175]

ADDITIONAL APPLICATION OF PULMONARY FUNCTION TESTS IN DECISION MAKING

In addition to enabling the differential diagnosis of lung disease by recognizing major patterns, pulmonary function testing aids clinical decision making in a number of situations.

INHALER SELECTION

In addition to using appropriate inhaler technique for the proper deposition of inhaled medication into the lung, there is growing evidence that the *peak inspiratory flow* (PIF) is an important factor in the ability to actuate inhalers. This is especially true in the case of dry powder inhalers, where a patient-generated PIF of 60 L/min or greater is considered ideal for actuation of the device and deaggregation of the medication formulation,[185] and PIF less than 30 L/min may be insufficient for optimal delivery of medication.[186] PIF measured using a device with resistance modified to match the specific inhaler resistance is likely to result in more accurate identification of inadequate inspiratory force.[187,188] The most important factors associated with low PIF are age, female gender, and lower lung function.[188]

ASTHMA CONTROL

Stabilization of asthma can be estimated by frequent measurement of the *peak expiratory flow* (PEF). PEF variation correlates strongly with symptom burden as assessed using the Asthma Control Test.[189] PEF is predominantly a reflection of large airway patency and hence can underestimate the involvement of small airways in asthma. It can be measured during spirometry or using a peak flowmeter. Spirometry values are approximately 7% lower than PEF measured using peak flowmeters; hence, peak flowmeters should be used for measuring diurnal variation.[190] Diurnal variability greater than 20% suggests suboptimal asthma control and a higher risk of exacerbations.[191] Baseline PEF is affected by demographics and also restrictive processes that affect full inspiration, such as obesity, chest wall disease, and neuromuscular disease. For these reasons, a baseline *personal best* PEF should be estimated individually in each subject after a period of optimal therapy and should be reevaluated at frequent intervals. Peak flowmeters offer advantages of convenience and portability; however, results from peak flowmeters are also less reproducible than those from standard spirometry. Thus, it is essential that physicians recognize the importance of the use of spirometers in the initial assessment of the patient suspected of having asthma and in periodic monitoring.

LUNG VOLUME REDUCTION

Both surgical and endoscopic lung volume reduction procedures are now available for a subset of patients with severe emphysema who have significant air trapping. The evaluation of patients suitable for these therapies starts with spirometry. The National Emphysema Treatment Trial enrolled patients with FEV_1 of 15–45% predicted and with an RV of 150% or greater than predicted.[192] More recent endobronchial valve trials included patients with various thresholds for air trapping, for instance, RV ranging from 150–200% or greater than predicted.[193-195] Individuals with DL_{CO} less than 20% predicted were excluded from these trials. It is recommended that body plethysmography be used for estimation of lung volumes in these individuals with severe COPD due to concerns of underestimation of lung volumes with gas dilution techniques. Although no thresholds have been defined, an elevated RV/TLC ratio correlates with an improvement in FVC and in FEV_1 post–lung volume reduction.[196-198] The improvement in FEV_1 is partially due to a reduction in airflow obstruction as indicated by the FEV_1/FVC ratio, likely resulting from improvement in elastic recoil, improved matching of the lung and rib cage size, and an improvement in the length-tension relationship of the diaphragm and other respiratory muscles.[196,199]

LUNG TRANSPLANTATION (See Chapter 140)

Spirometry after transplantation shows a characteristic increase in FVC and FEV_1 that on average approaches a plateau at 3 to 6 months after transplantation, with additional smaller increases at 6 to 12 months.[200,201] As expected, the increases in FVC and FEV_1 are greater with double-lung transplantation than with single transplantation. Post-transplantation morbidities, such as acute rejection, infection, pleural effusion, diaphragm injury, myopathy, anastomotic complications, and delayed chest wall healing can influence the trajectory of lung function changes. In relation to predicted values based on characteristics of the transplant recipient, FVC and FEV_1 do not always increase to the normal range, a condition termed *baseline lung allograft dysfunction* (BLAD). Many variables, including donor-recipient size mismatch, have been implicated but, in a multivariable model of data from recipients of bilateral lung transplantation, only heavy donor smoking and ILD as an indication for transplantation were predictors of BLAD; BLAD was also associated with impaired survival.[202] A plateau in expiratory flow at high to mid lung volumes on the flow-volume curve is not unusual after transplantation. This plateau in flow after the initial peak may be due to denervation of the lung and alterations of the large airway(s) at the site of anastomosis.[203,204] Transplantation of two lungs results in a normal TLC in patients with pre-existing chronic hyperinflation (e.g., COPD and cystic fibrosis) but with a persistent increase in FRC and RV.[205]

REJECTION OF TRANSPLANTED LUNGS

A major cause of morbidity and mortality after lung transplantation is *bronchiolitis obliterans* (BO), a progressive obstruction and destruction of bronchioles that may in part be due to an alloimmune response.[206] Histopathologic diagnosis from bronchoscopic biopsies is difficult. Therefore, the *International Society for Heart and Lung Transplantation* (ISHLT) recommends a clinical surrogate for BO termed *bronchiolitis obliterans syndrome* (BOS), which is defined as a 20% decrease in FEV_1 from the best baseline post-transplantation value.[207] The total cross-sectional area of the numerous bronchioles results in a relatively small overall contribution to resistance to airflow. Thus, early in disease, when there is patchy narrowing, standard tests of pulmonary function, such as FEV$_1$, are not expected to be abnormal.[208,209] The distribution of ventilation assessed via single- and multiple-breath nitrogen washout has been shown to change earlier than FEV$_1$ in patients who develop BOS, although this awaits larger-scale validation before becoming part of routine monitoring.[210,211]

The obstructive defect in bronchiolitis obliterans is often accompanied by a decline in FVC due to air trapping. A concurrent decline in FEV$_1$ and FVC has a poorer prognosis than a subsequent decline in FVC, which is consistent with disease progression.[212] A concurrent decline in FVC can alternatively reflect restrictive allograft syndrome, a form of rejection with parenchymal fibrosis, which may have worse prognosis than bronchiolitis obliterans.[213] Given that FEV$_1$ may fall in the setting of either BO or restrictive allograft syndrome, an umbrella term was developed to refer to any sustained decrease in FEV$_1$: *chronic lung allograft dysfunction.*[207] Trending of the ratio of FEV$_1$ to FVC aids in the distinction between obstructive and restrictive changes after transplantation.

A major limitation to the use of simple lung function monitoring in single-lung transplant patients is the bias caused by the contribution of the native lung to measured lung function. Imaging techniques can help localize function to the transplanted lung.[214]

A brief discussion of the assessment of capacity in lung resections, high altitude, and air travel can be found at ExpertConsult.com and in Chapters 105 and 106.

SHUNT

In understanding the measurement of shunt, one starts with a model of the lung with two compartments, in which one has matched ventilation and perfusion and the other has blood flow but no ventilation (i.e., shunt). In this model, the shunt fraction reflects the fraction of otherwise normal lung that would have to be operating as a pure shunt to explain a deficit in the ability of the lung to oxygenate blood. Using this model, the shunt fraction is calculated from an arterial blood gas measurement after breathing 100% oxygen (see Chapter 31 for details of the calculation[227]). Inhalation of 100% oxygen achieves an oxygen tension in areas of low *ventilation-perfusion* (V/Q) that is nearly the same as in areas with normal V/Q ratios, thereby removing the effect of low V/Q on arterial oxygenation and isolating the effect of the shunt on oxygenation. Measurement after breathing 100% oxygen also ensures that arterial hemoglobin oxygen saturation from the perfused alveoli is 100%, a required assumption in the calculation. The classic textbook normal value for the anatomic shunt fraction is 2–5%.[228,229] However, we recommend using a higher cutoff for the 100% inspired oxygen-based calculation of shunt fraction for a number of reasons. First, 100% oxygen may alter the shunt fraction by changing pulmonary microcirculation vasomotor tone or by inducing reabsorption microatelectasis.[230] Second, the calculation assumes a fixed value for the arterial-venous oxygen content difference (D(A–V)O$_2$), which may not apply to every individual, leading to overestimation of shunt if the D(A–V)O$_2$ is underestimated. Finally, technical factors that

may overestimate the shunt fraction are air leaks in the blood gas collection device and decreases in accuracy and precision of blood gas analyzers at the higher than normal arterial PO$_2$ values. A reasonable threshold to trigger further workup is a shunt fraction of 10.5%, which is the average of two studies that used the 100% oxygen-based method.[228,231]

A relatively high shunt fraction is required to affect arterial oxygen saturation while breathing ambient air. Assuming a negligible contribution of dissolved non–hemoglobin-bound oxygen to blood oxygen content, the mixed venous oxygen saturation and shunt fraction can be used to calculate estimated arterial oxygen saturation as in the nomogram in Figure 32.3. For example, at an average mixed venous oxygen saturation of 70%, a shunt fraction of 15% is expected to yield an arterial oxygen saturation of 95%; a shunt fraction of 20% would yield an arterial oxygen saturation of 94%; and a shunt fraction of 30% would yield an arterial oxygen saturation of 91%. This exercise highlights a key difference between this quantitative measurement of shunt and qualitative studies, such as the abnormal passage of saline contrast on an echocardiogram or other quantitative studies, such as abnormal passage of radiolabeled albumin macroaggregates from the right-sided to left-sided circulation. The quantitative measurement of shunt from breathing 100% oxygen provides information about

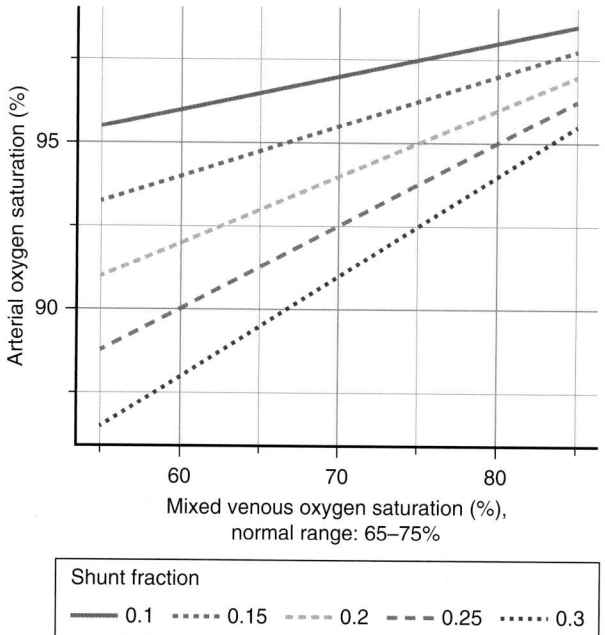

Figure 32.3 A nomogram for estimating the effect of a shunt on arterial oxygen saturation while breathing ambient air. To use the nomogram, first assume a normal mixed venous oxygen saturation of 70%. Then, of the two remaining variables—SaO$_2$ or shunt fraction—use the measured value of one to locate the curve that allows estimation of the remaining variable. To derive the relationship, an assumption was made that any defect in oxygenation is only due to a fraction of the lung operating as a shunt, and the rest of the lung is normal (see main text and Chapter 31 for the principles of shunt measurement). Dissolved oxygen contributes very little to blood oxygen content, and therefore SaO$_2$ is simply a weighted sum of blood from the shunt and normal portions of the lung: SaO$_2$ = (1 – Qs/Qt) × 100% + (Qs/Qt) × S$\bar{v}$O$_2$. A limitation of this nomogram is that with reduced SaO$_2$, mixed venous oxygen saturation may be lower than normal; nonetheless, the nomogram can give a rough estimate as to whether the measured shunt fraction accounts for the observed arterial oxygen saturation. Qs, total shunted blood flow; Qt, total blood flow; SaO$_2$, arterial oxygen saturation; S$\bar{v}$O$_2$, mixed venous saturation of oxygen.

the effect of the shunt on oxygenation, whereas the other diagnostics do not. The measurement of shunt with the body in different positions has been used to localize areas for embolization that will optimize benefit on oxygenation. In hepatopulmonary syndrome, the 100% oxygen breathing method is expected to give smaller values for the shunt fraction than radiolabeled perfusion scans because the increased alveolar PO_2 can overcome the diffusion defect related to diffuse microvascular dilation at the alveolar level (type 1, parenchymal shunts); convergence in the results between the tests is expected when the predominant lesions are discrete precapillary macrovascular (i.e., anatomic) shunts (type 2, vascular lung shunts).[232] (See Chapter 44.)

Key Points

- There are two main ventilatory patterns measured by pulmonary function tests: obstructive and restrictive. Mixed and nonspecific patterns are frequently observed as well, and these need further evaluation and follow-up. The shape of the flow-volume curve can alert the clinician to large airway obstruction.

- Because pulmonary function testing is effort dependent, the clinician must ensure the data meet quality standards for accuracy and repeatability before interpretation.

- Measurements from spirometry alone can be useful in individuals whose main physiologic impairment is airflow obstruction. The findings from spirometry can provide clues that concomitant restriction is present; however, for assessment of restriction, lung volumes must be measured.

- Lung function is different across age, sex, height, and ethnicity. Therefore, interpretation should be based on comparison of test results to reference values that adjust for these effects. The limitations of reference values underscore the importance of correlating pulmonary function test results with other clinical information, as well as testing repeatedly when signs or symptoms of disease persist. Accounting for differences across ethnic groups may have the unintended consequence of hiding causes for these differences, including those due to structural racism, and potentially leads to underdiagnosis and underestimation of severity of disease.

- In individuals with reversible mild airway disease, the results of pulmonary function tests may be normal because the disease is dynamic and individuals with mild airflow obstruction may spontaneously return to normal.

- Methacholine provocation testing is used to identify whether abnormal airway responsiveness is present. Its most important clinical utility is that a negative test makes bronchial asthma highly unlikely.

- In addition to diagnosis, pulmonary function testing is useful for monitoring disease activity and progression, as well as for following the response to or side effects of therapy.

- Pulmonary function testing is also useful for specific applications, such as inhaler selection, candidate selection for lung volume reduction and lung transplantation, and post-transplantation evaluation and monitoring.

Key Readings

Agusti AG, Barbera JA. Contribution of multiple inert gas elimination technique to pulmonary medicine. 2. Chronic pulmonary diseases: chronic obstructive pulmonary disease and idiopathic pulmonary fibrosis. *Thorax.* 1994;49(9):924–932.

Chiang ST. A nomogram for venous shunt (Qs-Qt) calculation. *Thorax.* 1968;23(5):563–565.

Coates AL, Wanger J, Cockcroft DW, et al. ERS technical standard on bronchial challenge testing: general considerations and performance of methacholine challenge tests. *Eur Respir J.* 2017;49(5).

Godfrey MS, Jankowich MD. The vital capacity is vital: epidemiology and clinical significance of the restrictive spirometry pattern. *Chest.* 2016;149(1):238–251.

Graham BL, Steenbruggen I, Miller MR, et al. Standardization of spirometry 2019 update. An official American Thoracic Society and European Respiratory Society technical statement. *Am J Respir Crit Care Med.* 2019;200(8):e70–e88.

Hanania NA, Celli BR, Donohue JF, Martin UJ. Bronchodilator reversibility in COPD. *Chest.* 2011;140(4):1055–1063.

Jones RL, Nzekwu MM. The effects of body mass index on lung volumes. *Chest.* 2006;130(3):827–833.

Laveneziana P, Albuquerque A, Aliverti A, et al. ERS statement on respiratory muscle testing at rest and during exercise. *Eur Respir J.* 2019;53(6).

Meyer KC, Raghu G, Verleden GM, et al. An international ISHLT/ATS/ERS clinical practice guideline: diagnosis and management of bronchiolitis obliterans syndrome. *Eur Respir J.* 2014;44(6):1479–1503.

Ming DK, Patel MS, Hopkinson NS, Ward S, Polkey MI. The "anatomic shunt test" in clinical practice; contemporary description of test and in-service evaluation. *Thorax.* 2014;69(8):773–775.

Nadel JA, Gold WM, Burgess JH. Early diagnosis of chronic pulmonary vascular obstruction. Value of pulmonary function tests. *Am J Med.* 1968;44(1):16–25.

Pellegrino R, Viegi G, Brusasco V, et al. Interpretative strategies for lung function tests. *Eur Respir J.* 2005;26(5):948–968.

Shrikrishna D, Coker RK, Air Travel Working Party of the British Thoracic Society Standards of Care Committee. Managing passengers with stable respiratory disease planning air travel: British Thoracic Society recommendations. *Thorax.* 2011;66(9):831–833.

Complete reference list available at ExpertConsult.com.

33 EXERCISE TESTING

ANDREW M. LUKS, MD • ROBB W. GLENNY, MD

INTRODUCTION

Sustained exercise requires tight integration of the cardiac, neuromuscular, and respiratory systems. Diseases affecting any of these systems can manifest as dyspnea or exercise limitation. In addition to other modalities commonly used to assess patients with these complaints, *cardiopulmonary exercise testing* (CPET) provides a systematic means to evaluate exercise responses, unravel the interacting components, and determine which system contributes the most to the exercise limitation. CPET has other important uses, including quantifying maximal exercise capacity, assessing functional limitation, prescribing rehabilitation and training regimens, and guiding clinical decisions, such as the timing of transplant listing or fitness for surgery.

This chapter describes the clinical application of CPET and assists the reader in understanding the role of CPET in the evaluation of dyspnea and exercise limitation. Because CPET interpretation requires an understanding of the physiologic responses to exercise, the chapter begins with a review of exercise physiology that sets the foundation for the balance of the content. The review includes exercise responses in healthy individuals and those with various forms of cardiopulmonary disease. The chapter then describes the indications and contraindications of CPET, the options for conducting exercise tests, and an approach to test interpretation. It concludes by describing alternative modalities for assessing exercise responses in clinical practice.

PHYSIOLOGIC RESPONSES TO EXERCISE

EXERCISE AS A MULTISYSTEM PROCESS

To support vigorous aerobic exercise, the respiratory system works as a ventilatory pump to move oxygen from the atmosphere into the bloodstream where it binds to hemoglobin, whereas the heart pumps the oxygenated blood to the exercising muscles, which extract oxygen to support *adenosine triphosphate* (ATP) generation and muscle contraction. Muscle activity generates *carbon dioxide* (CO_2), which must be delivered by the circulatory system to the lungs, where it diffuses across the alveolar walls and is eliminated via the ventilatory pump. The nervous system contributes at multiple stages in this process, providing signals to raise ventilation and signals to exercising muscles that drive contractions. All of these systems work in a coordinated manner to support exercise, and problems in one or more of them may manifest as dyspnea or exercise limitation.

HEALTHY INDIVIDUALS

To appreciate changes in exercise tolerance in cardiopulmonary disease, it is helpful to examine the normal physiologic responses to progressive exercise in four major areas: metabolic activity, hemodynamic responses, ventilatory responses, and gas exchange. The major parameters within each area and the expected responses are described later and in other resources.[1]

Metabolic Activity

Oxygen Consumption. *Oxygen consumption*, denoted as $\dot{V}O_2$, (a volume per time, e.g., mL/min) is the most useful parameter for assessing overall exercise capacity. In essence, $\dot{V}O_2$ is the amount of fuel consumed in conducting work; the stronger the motor, the greater the maximal fuel consumption. To understand this concept, consider the determinants of $\dot{V}O_2$ using the Fick equation:

$$\dot{Q} = \dot{V}O_2 \div (CaO_2 - C\bar{v}O_2) \qquad [1]$$

where $\dot{Q}$ is cardiac output (mL/min), CaO_2 is arterial oxygen content (mL/dL), and $C\bar{v}O_2$ is mixed venous oxygen content (mL/dL). Rearranging the relationship as follows,

$$\dot{V}O_2 = \dot{Q}(CaO_2 - C\bar{v}O_2) \qquad [2]$$

demonstrates that oxygen consumption is dependent on cardiac output, oxygen content, which is related to the concentration of hemoglobin and the PO_2, and tissue oxygen utilization. As a result, $\dot{V}O_2$ provides useful information about many of the systems required for sustained high-level exercise.

In addition to providing information on overall exercise capacity, *maximal oxygen consumption* ($\dot{V}O_{2max}$) is useful for assessing cardiac function. Given that the arteriovenous oxygen content difference at maximal exercise is largely the same in healthy individuals and in those with cardiac disease,[2] the wide variation in $\dot{V}O_{2max}$ across individuals is primarily determined by the variation in cardiac output. The greater the $\dot{V}O_{2max}$, the greater the cardiac output and vice versa.

Oxygen consumption can also be used to estimate stroke volume at maximal exercise. To understand this, Eq. 2, where *HR* is heart rate and *SV* is stroke volume, can be rewritten:

$$\dot{V}O_2 = HR \times SV \times (CaO_2 - C\bar{v}O_2) \qquad [3]$$

and then rearranged as:

$$\dot{V}O_2/HR = SV \times (CaO_2 - C\bar{v}O_2) \qquad [4]$$

Given that the arteriovenous oxygen content difference is largely the same across healthy individuals at maximal exercise, the term $\dot{V}O_2/HR$, referred to as the *oxygen pulse* or O_2 *pulse*, represents a surrogate for stroke volume. The O_2 pulse should increase throughout exercise due to both the increasing stroke volume and the arteriovenous oxygen content difference.

During progressive exercise to a symptom-limited maximum, $\dot{V}O_2$ increases linearly relative to workload from resting values near 250 mL/min for an average-sized person until a plateau is reached at maximum effort ($\dot{V}O_{2max}$). If a plateau is not identified, the term $\dot{V}O_{2peak}$ is applied instead to denote that it may not represent the individual's potential maximum. In average sedentary individuals, $\dot{V}O_{2max}$ is roughly 30 to 40 mL/kg/min at end exercise, whereas very fit athletes can attain values as high as 80 to 90 mL/kg/min. $\dot{V}O_{2max}$ is influenced by many factors, including age and sex, which are discussed further later. With intensive training, unfit subjects can increase their $\dot{V}O_{2max}$ by 15–25%[3,4] but cannot raise their $\dot{V}O_{2max}$ from an average to an elite level. What improves with training is the efficiency of work and the ability to sustain high levels of work. Genetic factors also affect an individual's $\dot{V}O_{2max}$[5] and his or her response to training regimens.[6] In clinical exercise testing, an individual's $\dot{V}O_{2max}$ is typically expressed in reference to that predicted for his or her age and sex based on data from large population studies. Reference values have been published, but methodologic issues limit the wide applicability of many of them.[7] As with all reference values, the normal range is dependent on the population studied.

Carbon Dioxide Output.
In early exercise, *CO2 output* ($\dot{V}CO_2$) increases linearly relative to workload from resting values near 200 mL/min for an average-sized person at about the same rate as oxygen consumption. Above the *ventilatory threshold*, an important time point described later, the rate of CO2 output steepens as bicarbonate buffering of increasing lactate production leads to CO2 elimination beyond that generated by aerobic metabolism.[7]

Respiratory Exchange Ratio.
Defined as CO2 elimination divided by oxygen uptake ($\dot{V}CO_2/\dot{V}O_2$), the *respiratory exchange ratio* (R) remains stable between 0.8 and 0.9 in

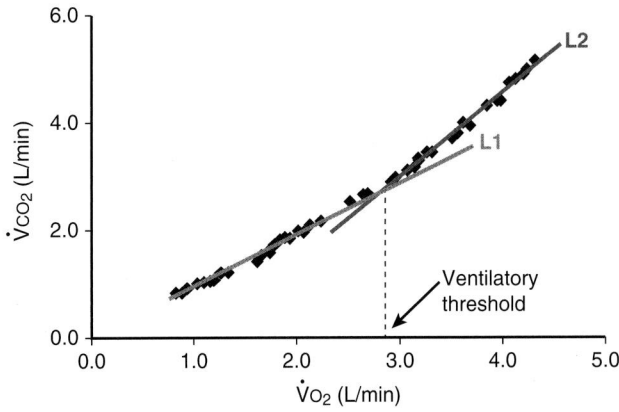

Figure 33.1 The V-slope method for identifying the first ventilatory threshold. Before the threshold, $\dot{V}O_2$ and $\dot{V}CO_2$ rise at the same rate. A best-fit line through these points is labeled L1 and is denoted in *brown*. After the threshold, $\dot{V}CO_2$ rises faster than $\dot{V}O_2$. A best-fit line through these points is labeled L2 and is denoted in *blue*. The point at which the two lines intersect denotes the $\dot{V}O_2$ at which the ventilatory threshold is reached. $\dot{V}CO_2$, carbon dioxide output; $\dot{V}O_2$, oxygen consumption.

early to mid-exercise, with slight variation between individuals depending on their balance of dietary fats and carbohydrates. It is important to note that R is measured using exhaled gases, in contrast to cellular R, otherwise known as the *respiratory quotient* (RQ), which is measured at the tissue level. Just before and in the early stages of exercise, R may transiently increase due to anticipatory hyperventilation. Above the ventilatory threshold, $\dot{V}CO_2$ increases markedly, and R increases above 1.0. With cessation of exercise, $\dot{V}O_2$ decreases abruptly, whereas $\dot{V}CO_2$ remains high as tissue CO2 stores continue to be eliminated. R can subsequently increase over 1 to 2 minutes to values as high as 1.3 to 1.5 before finally decreasing.

Ventilatory Thresholds.
Healthy individuals demonstrate a phenomenon termed the *ventilatory threshold* at about 50–60% of the $\dot{V}O_{2max}$, although there is interindividual variability in the timing of this phenomenon.[7,8] This threshold marks a critical point in progressive exercise where blood flow to the exercising muscle is no longer sufficient to meet metabolic demands and the individual transitions from light-moderate to moderate-high intensity exercise.[9] Alternatively referred to as the *lactate threshold*, *gas exchange threshold*, or *anaerobic threshold*, the phenomenon is temporally related to an increase in lactic acid production and a decrease in pH, with considerable debate regarding the mechanisms for the increased lactate production[10,11] and whether it happens suddenly or in a more continuous manner throughout exercise.[12–14] As lactic acid dissociates, hydrogen ions are buffered by intracellular bicarbonate, leading to further CO2 generation beyond that associated with aerobic metabolism.[9,15] This causes a steep rise in the $\dot{V}CO_2$ versus work relationship as well as the $\dot{V}CO_2$ versus $\dot{V}O_2$ relationship (Fig. 33.1). Identifying the change in slope of the latter relationship is referred to as the *V-slope method* and is a key step in CPET interpretation, as described later.

As work increases beyond the ventilatory threshold, many individuals demonstrate a second ventilatory threshold, sometimes referred to as the *respiratory compensation point*, at which rising lactate concentrations cannot be buffered by intracellular bicarbonate, and *minute ventilation* ($\dot{V}E$) increases beyond that expected for the increase in $\dot{V}CO_2$, thereby causing a respiratory alkalosis.[9,15] This point, which is not visible in all individuals due to interindividual variation in ventilatory responses to metabolic acidosis, can be identified by finding threshold responses in several ventilatory parameters, as described further later.

Hemodynamic Responses

Cardiac Output. Cardiac output (mL/min) increases linearly with workload before plateauing near peak exercise; it can be estimated from $\dot{V}O_2$ using the Fick principle, measured invasively with a *pulmonary artery* (PA) catheter or estimated noninvasively using inert gas rebreathing techniques.[16,17] The initial increase is due to increasing stroke volume and heart rate, whereas changes near peak exercise result from increases in heart rate.[18]

Heart Rate. Due initially to decreased vagal tone and later to increases in sympathetic activity, heart rate (beats/min) increases linearly with increasing $\dot{V}O_2$. The *heart rate reserve*, defined as the difference between the maximum predicted heart rate and the heart rate achieved at peak exercise, is typically very small in healthy individuals (<20 beats/min), but this parameter is difficult to use in exercise test interpretation due to significant variability in maximum heart rates in healthy age-matched individuals.[7,19] Another measure of heart rate response, also termed the *heart rate reserve*, is the difference between the resting and maximum heart rate. This chapter uses the former definition.

Pulmonary Arterial Pressure. PA pressure rises only modestly with progressive exercise in healthy individuals due to recruitment and distention of the pulmonary vasculature and decreased pulmonary vascular resistance. There is interindividual variability in observed responses,[20] with greater variability in older individuals.[21]

Stroke Volume. Characterized during CPET by the O_2 pulse, stroke volume increases in early exercise before leveling off in late exercise.[18] Initial increases are driven largely by mobilization of blood from lower extremity venous capacitance vessels, whereas later smaller increases result from increased inotropic activity.

Systemic Blood Pressure. Due to increases in cardiac output and vascular resistance in the skin, renal, and splanchnic circulations, systemic blood pressure increases with progressive exercise. Although exercising muscle vasodilation limits the rise in diastolic pressure, systolic pressure rises significantly, particularly after the ventilatory threshold, and may reach values greater than 200 mm Hg at peak exercise.

Ventilatory Responses

Minute Ventilation. Due to an increase in respiratory rate and tidal volume, *minute ventilation* ($\dot{V}E$, mL/min) rises throughout exercise with large increases seen after the ventilatory threshold. The tidal volume plateaus at 50–60% of vital capacity, after which the $\dot{V}E$ increases further due to increases in respiratory rate.[22,23] At peak exercise, $\dot{V}E$ is typically less than 80% of the predicted maximum, as estimated by the *maximum voluntary ventilation* (MVV) or *forced expiratory volume in 1 second* (FEV$_1$) × 40.[24]

Ventilatory Equivalents for Oxygen and Carbon Dioxide. The ventilatory response can be expressed as a function of the amount of ventilation per liter of oxygen consumed ($\dot{V}E/\dot{V}O_2$, unitless) or per liter of exhaled carbon dioxide ($\dot{V}E/\dot{V}CO_2$, unitless). Both ratios remain relatively steady (~24–30) through early exercise as ventilation rises proportionately with $\dot{V}O_2$ and $\dot{V}CO_2$ and then increases after the ventilatory threshold, peaking around 35 to 40, with slightly greater increases seen in $\dot{V}E/\dot{V}O_2$.[7] Both parameters may be elevated in early exercise in highly fit or anxious individuals but typically return to normal as exercise progresses, reaching a nadir just before the ventilatory threshold. The range of ventilatory equivalents seen across healthy individuals reflects the variability in respiratory drives in the population.

Dead-Space Fraction. Due to increased tidal volume and recruitment of the pulmonary vasculature resulting from increased pulmonary blood flow, the *dead-space fraction* (VD/VT, unitless) decreases from 0.3 to 0.4 at rest to less than 0.3 at peak exercise.[7]

Gas Exchange

Arterial and End-Tidal Partial Pressures of Carbon Dioxide. Despite the increasing $\dot{V}CO_2$, the *arterial* PCO$_2$ (mm Hg) and *end-tidal* PCO$_2$ (mm Hg) remain constant and near normal through early exercise due to the fact that alveolar ventilation rises proportionally with $\dot{V}CO_2$. These values may decrease in individuals who hyperventilate at the start of exercise but typically normalize over the first few minutes of work. After the ventilatory threshold is reached, minute and alveolar ventilation rise out of proportion to $\dot{V}CO_2$. As a result, both arterial PCO$_2$ and and end-tidal PCO$_2$ decrease so that both values are nearly always less than 40 mm Hg at $\dot{V}O_{2max}$.[25]

Arterial and End-Tidal Partial Pressures of Oxygen and the Alveolar-Arterial Oxygen Difference. Below the ventilatory threshold, the *end-tidal* PO$_2$ (mm Hg), a surrogate measure of alveolar PO$_2$, and the arterial PO$_2$ remain constant in the normal range, as do *arterial oxygen saturation* (SO$_2$, %) and the *alveolar-arterial PO$_2$ difference* ([A−a]PO$_2$, mm Hg). Beyond the ventilatory threshold, end-tidal PO$_2$ increases due to alveolar ventilation increasing out of proportion to $\dot{V}O_2$. Although alveolar PO$_2$ increases, arterial PO$_2$ remains unchanged due to a lower C$\bar{v}$O$_2$ and normal physiologic shunting. As a result, the (A−a)PO$_2$ increases slightly with heavy exercise. In a minority of highly fit individuals with high $\dot{V}O_{2max}$, arterial PO$_2$, and arterial SO$_2$ can decline in late exercise, a phenomenon referred to as *exercise-induced arterial hypoxemia*.[26-28]

In CPET, the changes in many of the parameters described above can be identified from tabular data or graphically using an approach developed by Wasserman and colleagues[29] in which nine separate graphs are displayed in a standardized format (Fig. 33.2).

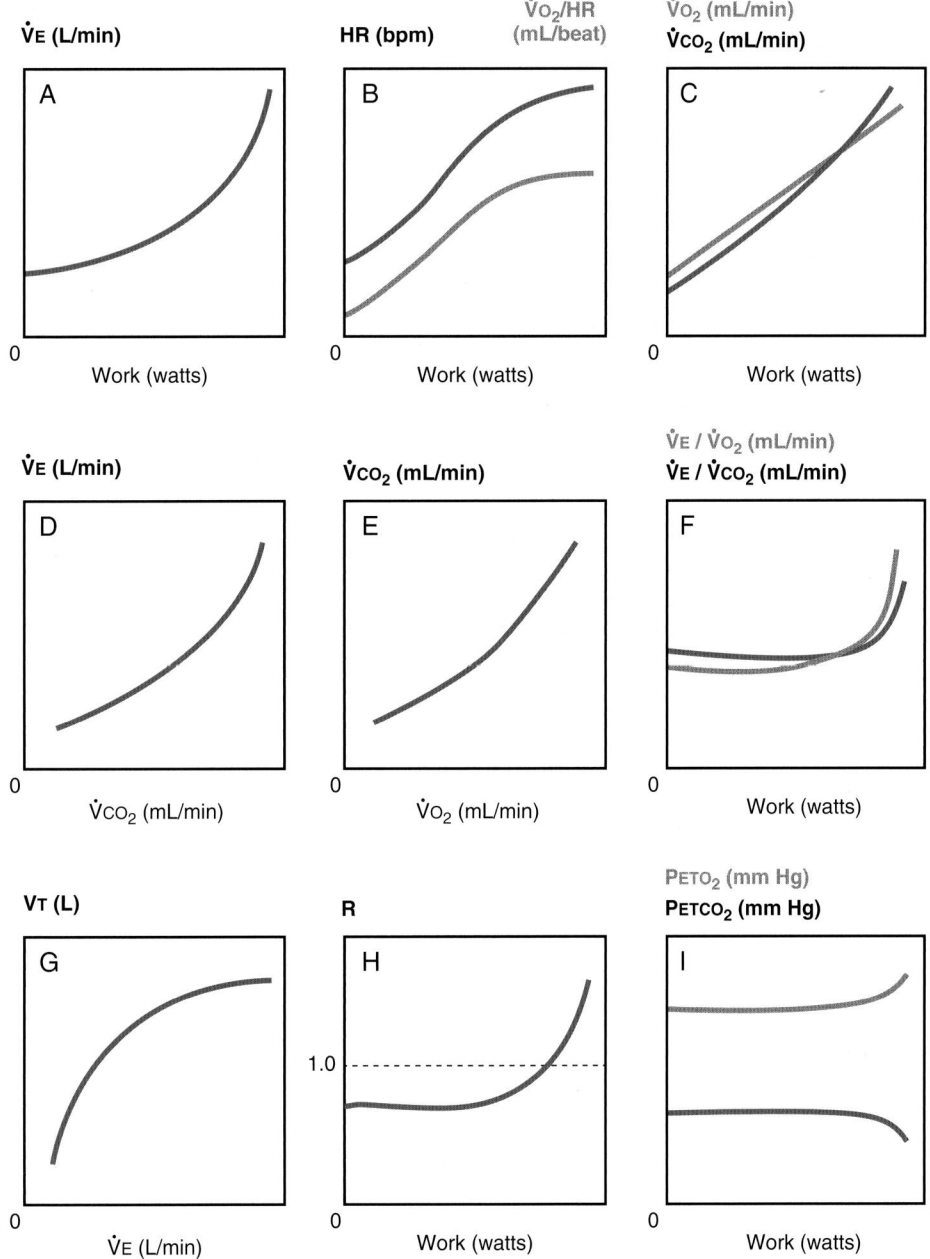

Figure 33.2 Normal pattern of responses to exercise in healthy individuals shown in a nine-box plot. (A) $\dot{V}_E$ vs. watts. (B) Heart rate (HR) and $\dot{V}_{O_2}$/HR vs. watts. (C) $\dot{V}_{O_2}$ and $\dot{V}_{CO_2}$ vs. watts. (D) $\dot{V}_E$ vs. $\dot{V}_{CO_2}$. (E) $\dot{V}_{CO_2}$ vs. $\dot{V}_{O_2}$. (F) $\dot{V}_E$/$\dot{V}_{O_2}$ and $\dot{V}_E$/$\dot{V}_{CO_2}$ vs. watts. (G) Tidal volume (VT) vs. $\dot{V}_E$. (H) Respiratory exchange ratio (R) vs. watts. (I) PETO$_2$ and PETCO$_2$ vs. watts. Labels for the y-axis variables are presented on the top of each graph. Note that for the variables on the x- and y-axes the lowest values are in the lower left corner of each plot. PETCO$_2$, end-tidal partial pressure of CO_2; PETO$_2$, end-tidal partial pressure of O_2; $\dot{V}_{CO_2}$, carbon dioxide output; $\dot{V}_E$, minute ventilation; $\dot{V}_{O_2}$, oxygen consumption.

Changes With Age

A decrease in $\dot{V}_{O_2max}$ with increasing age has been consistently reported in cross-sectional[30,31] and longitudinal studies,[32,33] with documented rates of decline in $\dot{V}_{O_2max}$ varying from as low as 0.28 mL/kg/min/yr[32] to as high as 1.04 mL/kg/min/yr.[34] Although some studies demonstrate a slower rate of decline in active individuals compared to sedentary individuals,[32] others[35] report no effect of activity level on age-related declines in $\dot{V}_{O_2max}$. Training programs in older sedentary individuals may reverse much of the age-related decline,[36] which accelerates in the later stages of life.[37]

Between 20 and 50 years of age, the decline in $\dot{V}_{O_2max}$ is attributable to impaired peripheral oxygen extraction,[33] whereas changes later in life relate to impaired peripheral extraction and decrements in maximal cardiac output due to an inability to raise stroke volume at maximal exercise.[38] Observed changes in peripheral extraction may be due to decreased lean body mass, age-related changes in skeletal muscle, or blood flow distribution at peak exercise,[33] whereas the decline in cardiac output may represent increasing incidence of comorbid conditions affecting cardiac performance.[38]

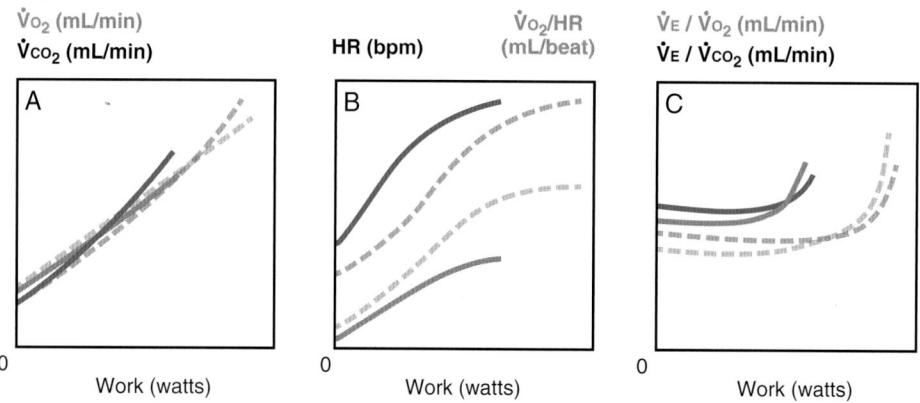

Figure 33.3 **Heart failure pattern of responses to exercise compared to normal shown on three key figures from the nine-box plot.** The responses for cardiac limitation in heart failure *(solid lines)* are compared to healthy individuals *(dotted lines)*. (A) $\dot{V}O_2$ and $\dot{V}CO_2$ vs. watts. (B) Heart rate (HR) and $\dot{V}O_2$/HR vs. watts. (C) $\dot{V}E/\dot{V}O_2$ and $\dot{V}E/\dot{V}CO_2$ vs. watts. A complete nine-box plot for this pattern of limitation is shown in eFig. 33.1. $\dot{V}CO_2$, carbon dioxide output; $\dot{V}E$, minute ventilation; $\dot{V}O_2$, oxygen consumption.

Sex Differences

Comparisons of exercise responses in men and women are difficult because most studies of physiologic responses to exercise have been performed in men. The available evidence demonstrates that women have the same qualitative responses to exercise as men but have lower $\dot{V}O_{2max}$, even after accounting for differences in lean body mass and training status.[39–41] The mechanism for these differences remains unclear but may relate to differences in blood volume, heart size, hormonal and metabolic status, or autonomic nervous system regulation of the heart and vascular system.[39] Some studies report slower age-related rates of decline in $\dot{V}O_{2max}$ in women compared to men, whereas others have not found such a differences.[37]

Ventilatory responses and gas exchange may also differ by sex, with some studies noting higher $\dot{V}E/\dot{V}O_2$ and $\dot{V}E/\dot{V}CO_2$ in women[37,40,42] and others reporting higher $(A-a)PO_2$ in fit women at very high levels of oxygen consumption.[43] At high exercise intensities, women may also rely more heavily than men on fat oxidation as a fuel source and thus have a lower respiratory exchange ratio.[44,45]

Obesity

Obese individuals with normal underlying cardiac or pulmonary function display a lower $\dot{V}O_{2max}$ than predicted for age and sex when expressed per kilogram of actual body weight but normal values when adjusted for ideal body weight. Because of the increased metabolic requirements resulting from increased weight, however, several important differences are observed relative to nonobese individuals. $\dot{V}O_2$ for any given level of work is higher than in the nonobese, although the *rate of change in oxygen consumption per given change in work rate* ($\Delta\dot{V}O_2/\Delta WR$) remains the same.[46,47] Obese individuals also have increased $\dot{V}O_2$ when pedaling without resistance (unloaded pedaling) due to the energy demands of moving heavier legs against gravity,[48] which is not reflected in the WR on the cycle ergometer.

$\dot{V}E$ is also increased for a given WR compared to the nonobese due to the added CO_2 production from the additional tissues.[46] This is typically achieved by increasing respiratory rate rather than tidal volume, which some data

suggest is decreased during exercise relative to nonobese individuals,[49,50] possibly due to the increased inspiratory load associated with extra chest wall soft tissue. Obese individuals also have difficulty decreasing end-expiratory lung volume during exercise, likely due to expiratory flow limitation.[50,51]

The presence and magnitude of differences in these parameters may be a function of the degree of obesity, with greater differences in heavier individuals, as well as the baseline level of fitness[52] and the presence of comorbid conditions, such as obstructive sleep apnea.[53]

INDIVIDUALS WITH UNDERLYING CARDIOPULMONARY DISEASE

Underlying cardiopulmonary disease alters these physiologic responses to exercise with different responses seen depending on the particular disease process.

Heart Failure

As in healthy individuals, maximal exercise in patients with heart failure is limited by the amount of blood that can be delivered to exercising muscle (i.e., a cardiac limitation to exercise). As a result, patients with heart failure demonstrate a similar pattern of physiologic responses during progressive exercise to a symptom-limited maximum, albeit with significant differences in the magnitude of many responses. Selected graphs from a nine-box plot demonstrating key differences relative to healthy individuals are shown in Figure 33.3 (the full nine-box plot can be seen in eFig. 33.1).

The most important difference relative to healthy individuals is the decrease in $\dot{V}O_{2max}$ and peak WR. The decrease in $\dot{V}O_{2max}$, which is similar between patients with systolic or diastolic dysfunction,[54,55] results from an inability to raise cardiac output due to impaired stroke volume responses with progressive exercise, denoted by decreased $\dot{V}O_2$/HR. The ventilatory threshold is still usually reached at 50–60% of $\dot{V}O_{2max}$ but at a lower absolute $\dot{V}O_2$ compared to healthy individuals.

Many patients with heart failure compensate for decreased stroke volume with an increase in heart rate for any given level of work. As a result, the heart rate reserve at peak exercise is usually small (<20 beats/min). There is considerable variability in these responses, however, with some patients manifesting an inability to raise heart rate with progressive exercise (*chronotropic incompetence*), which persists even after discontinuation of β-blockers.[56] In addition, heart rate recovery, which happens as a result of reactivation of vagal tone[57] and is defined as the difference between peak heart rate and heart rate 1 minute into recovery, is decreased compared to healthy individuals.

Patients with heart failure also have altered ventilatory responses, including increased airway resistance,[58] expiratory flow limitation at low WRs,[59] and a larger ventilatory reserve due to the fact that they cannot do as much work and therefore do not require a high $\dot{V}E$. Perhaps the most important difference, however, is increased ventilatory inefficiency in patients with moderate to severe systolic or diastolic dysfunction, as indicated by an increased $\dot{V}E/\dot{V}CO_2$ at the ventilatory threshold or an increased slope of the relationship between these parameters ($\Delta\dot{V}E/\Delta\dot{V}CO_2$).[54,55] The most likely cause of this phenomenon, which worsens with aging,[60] is an increase in physiologic dead space due to impaired lung perfusion.[61] Studies have shown, for example, that ventilatory inefficiency is related to abnormal pulmonary vascular tone[62] or right ventricular dysfunction[63] and improves after treatment with phosphodiesterase inhibitors and improvements in right ventricular function even when left ventricular function is unchanged.[64] Abnormal peripheral and central chemoreceptor sensitivity may also augment ventilation above that necessary for a given level of CO_2 production.[65]

Some patients with severe heart failure demonstrate exercise oscillatory ventilation, an abnormal ventilatory response in which exercise ventilation demonstrates periodicity similar to that seen in central sleep apnea (eFig. 33.2).[66,67] The mechanism is not clear but may relate to increases in circulatory times, peripheral chemoreceptor sensitivity, ventilatory responses related to pulmonary congestion, and signaling related to muscle metabolic abnormalities.[67] Exercise oscillatory ventilation may be a marker of reduced cardiac index both at rest and during exercise,[68] is associated with an increased risk of cardiovascular death,[69] and may improve with exercise training,[70,71] administration of acetazolamide,[72] or other therapeutic interventions directed at the underlying heart failure.[73] Despite these altered ventilatory responses, patients with heart failure may have a normal $(A-a)PO_2$ and may not develop hypoxemia during exercise even though PA occlusion pressure is elevated.[74,75]

Pulmonary Vascular Disease

Patients with pulmonary vascular diseases, such as *pulmonary arterial hypertension* (PAH) and *chronic thromboembolic pulmonary hypertension* (CTEPH), demonstrate physiologic responses to progressive exercise that are similar to those seen in patients with heart failure. Relative to healthy individuals, $\dot{V}O_{2max}$, peak WR, and $\dot{V}O_2/HR$ are decreased, and the ventilatory threshold is reached at a lower $\dot{V}O_2$. Similar to patients with heart failure, the observed decline in $\dot{V}O_{2max}$, which correlates inversely with mean PA pressure,[76] is due to an inability to raise cardiac output during exercise. The cardiac output is limited because the right ventricle cannot adequately preload the left ventricle due

to high pulmonary vascular resistance.[77] The fact that treatment with a pulmonary vasodilator, such as sildenafil, over several months improves both $\dot{V}O_{2max}$ and $\dot{V}O_2/HR$ supports this concept.[78]

These patients also demonstrate abnormal ventilatory responses, including increases in $\dot{V}E/\dot{V}O_2$ and $\dot{V}E/\dot{V}CO_2$ [79,80] of greater magnitude than those seen in patients with heart failure of similar *New York Heart Association* (NYHA) functional class.[81] This ventilatory inefficiency is due to increased VD/VT, as well as increased peripheral chemoreceptor stimulation from exercise-induced hypoxemia, and improves after treatment with sildenafil.[78] Depending on the extent of vascular occlusion and subsequent differences in VD/VT, the degree of ventilatory inefficiency, as measured by $\Delta\dot{V}E/\Delta\dot{V}CO_2$, may vary in magnitude between types of pulmonary vascular disease, with higher values seen in CTEPH than PAH.[82]

Aside from these similarities, an important difference between heart failure and pulmonary vascular disease pertains to the PA pressure responses. Unlike in healthy individuals or patients with heart failure, where PA pressure rises only modestly with increasing exercise, patients with pulmonary vascular disease experience large rises in PA pressure with increasing blood flow due to impaired pulmonary vascular recruitment and distention.[83,84]

In addition, whereas VD/VT decreases from 0.3 to 0.4 at rest to less than 0.3 at peak exercise in healthy individuals and patients with heart failure, it decreases only mildly and may even increase in pulmonary vascular disease,[82,85] with some variation in observed changes based on the cause of pulmonary hypertension.[86] This response is abnormal because perfusion of many lung units does not increase proportionately with alveolar ventilation due to impaired recruitment and distention. In addition, if patients develop right-to-left shunting by opening a patent foramen ovale during exercise, mean expired CO_2 decreases, leading to a higher calculated VD/VT (based on the Enghoff modification of the Bohr dead-space equation).[87] As a result of the abnormal VD/VT, end-tidal PCO_2 is decreased relative to normal individuals at all stages of exercise in proportion to the patient's functional limitation.[76]

A final difference is the fact that patients with pulmonary vascular disease develop hypoxemia and a widened $(A-a)PO_2$[25,85] with progressive exercise even in the absence of resting hypoxemia. In some patients hypoxemia develops due to right-to-left shunting through an existing right-to-left communication or through a foramen ovale that opens during exercise due to the rise in PA pressure, a finding predictive of death or need for transplant.[88] In other cases hypoxemia develops due to diffusion limitation; red blood cell capillary transit time decreases with increasing pulmonary blood flow and is no longer sufficient to ensure full equilibration between the capillary and alveolar PO_2 when the functional capillary bed is decreased.[89] This latter phenomenon is accentuated by the low $C\overline{v}O_2$ resulting from the low cardiac output in these patients.

Selected graphs from a nine-box plot demonstrating key differences relative to healthy individuals are shown in Figure 33.4 (the full nine-box plot can be seen in eFig. 33.3).

Interstitial Lung Diseases

Patients with *interstitial lung disease* (ILD) manifest physiologic responses during progressive exercise similar to

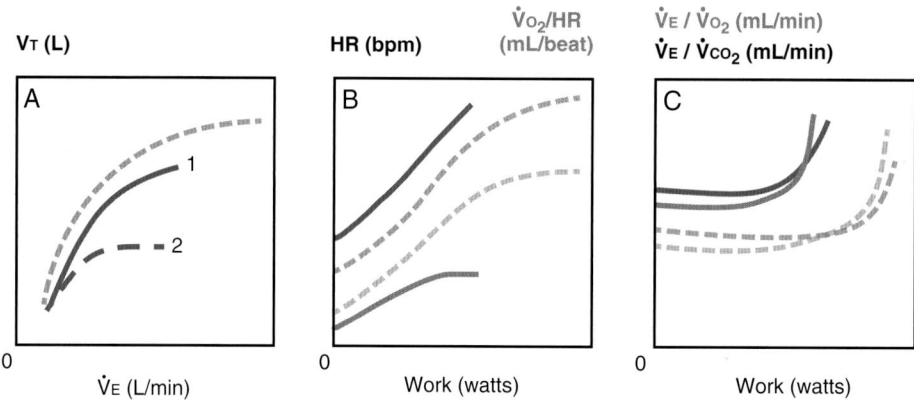

Figure 33.4 Pulmonary vascular or interstitial lung disease patterns of response to exercise compared to normal shown on three key figures from the nine-box plot. Pulmonary vascular or interstitial lung disease patterns of limitation *(solid lines)* are compared to healthy individuals who demonstrate a normal cardiac pattern of limitation *(dotted lines)*. Because the patterns of responses to exercise in each disease are similar, they are represented in parts B and C by a single line. (A) Tidal volume (VT) vs. $\dot{V}$E. The *solid blue line* (line 1) represents the expected response for a patient with pulmonary vascular disease, whereas the *dashed blue line* (line 2) represents the expected response for a patient with interstitial lung disease. (B) Heart rate (HR) and $\dot{V}O_2$/HR vs. watts. (C) $\dot{V}$E/$\dot{V}O_2$ and $\dot{V}$E/$\dot{V}CO_2$ vs. watts. A complete nine-box plot for this pattern of limitation is shown in eFig. 33.3. $\dot{V}CO_2$, carbon dioxide output; $\dot{V}$E, minute ventilation; $\dot{V}O_2$, oxygen consumption.

those seen in patients with pulmonary vascular disease. In particular, they demonstrate reduced $\dot{V}O_{2max}$ and *maximum WR*, increased $\dot{V}$E/$\dot{V}O_2$ and $\dot{V}$E/$\dot{V}CO_2$, reduced tidal volumes and increased respiratory rates, stable or increased VD/VT at end exercise as well as reduced arterial PO_2, and increased (A−a)PO_2. Although patients with ILD may not have a decreased $\dot{V}O_2$/HR, and the ventilatory threshold may not be decreased relative to their $\dot{V}O_{2max}$, these differences are usually not sufficient to distinguish between ILD and pulmonary vascular disease on the basis of CPET alone, and further studies such as pulmonary function tests (PFTs) and computed tomography imaging are necessary.

Debate exists regarding the underlying mechanism for the reduction in maximal exercise capacity. Hansen and Wasserman,[90] for example, demonstrated that abnormal cardiac function due to pulmonary vascular pathology was more important than respiratory system factors in limiting exercise, whereas Marciniuk and colleagues[91] used dead-space loading during exercise to show that abnormal respiratory mechanics were more important. Ventilatory equivalents are increased due to the increased dead space and the hypoxic ventilatory response, whereas exercise-induced hypoxemia is due to a combination of $\dot{V}A/\dot{Q}$ inequality and diffusion limitation.[92]

Because the term ILD represents a heterogeneous group of disorders, the physiologic responses to exercise vary based on the specific disease. Wells and colleagues,[93] for example, found increased dyspnea and hypoxemia in *idiopathic pulmonary fibrosis* (IPF) compared to systemic sclerosis with ILD, whereas other studies have also shown worse hypoxemia and increased PA pressure responses in patients with IPF compared to sarcoidosis and other forms of ILD.[94,95] The onset of pulmonary hypertension as a complication of ILD or an underlying systemic illness is associated with worse exercise tolerance, hypoxemia, and ventilatory inefficiency compared to otherwise similar patients with normal pulmonary artery pressures.[96,97]

Selected graphs from a nine-box plot demonstrating key differences relative to healthy individuals are shown in Figure 33.4 (full plot can be seen in eFig. 33.3).

Adult Congenital Heart Disease

Similar to patients with heart failure, adults with congenital heart disease demonstrate reductions in $\dot{V}O_{2max}$ that correlate with NYHA functional class,[98] peak WR and maximum heart rate, and increases in $\dot{V}$E/$\dot{V}CO_2$ compared to healthy individuals.[99] In contrast, however, many congenital heart disease patients develop hypoxemia at end exercise.[100] Given that many patients have coexisting pulmonary hypertension, one might also expect unchanged or increased VD/VT at end exercise in many patients, but this variable has not been reported in major series of adult patients.

Owing to the diversity in the type and severity of congenital lesions, there is variability in the magnitude of changes in $\dot{V}O_{2max}$ and $\dot{V}$E/$\dot{V}CO_2$ with the most serious abnormalities seen in those patients with Eisenmenger syndrome and complex lesions, such as double-outlet ventricle or univentricular physiology.[99,101] Patients with cyanosis and/or pulmonary hypertension also demonstrate greater reductions in these parameters when compared with patients lacking these problems.[101,102] Of importance, functional impairment is not limited to those with significant lesions, as even reportedly asymptomatic patients[103] or those with mild lesions, such as repaired coarctation of the aorta, demonstrate decreased $\dot{V}O_{2max}$ and increased $\dot{V}$E/$\dot{V}CO_2$ compared to healthy individuals.[99] Surgical repair improves exercise capacity,[104,105] with the degree of improvement related in some cases to whether the abnormality is repaired in childhood or in adulthood.[106]

Although much of the decrement in exercise capacity in these patients is attributable to cardiac and pulmonary vascular dysfunction related to the underlying defect or its repair, some patients are also limited by abnormal respiratory mechanics. Up to 50% of patients who have undergone surgical repairs have findings suggestive of restrictive physiology on spirometry,[107,108] resulting sometimes from

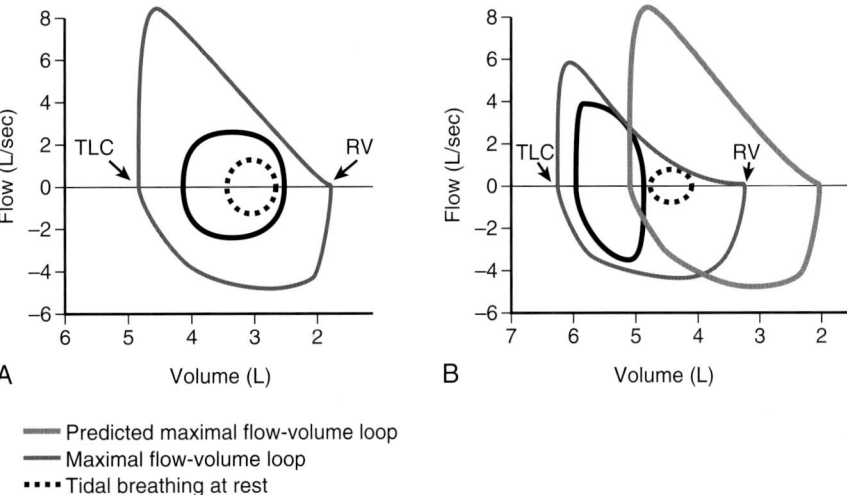

Figure 33.5 Expiratory flow limitation in COPD. (A) The typical pattern in healthy individuals. During exercise, the expiratory flow *(solid black line)* remains below the expiratory flow obtained in a forced vital capacity maneuver *(blue line)*. (B) Similar data are shown for a patient with COPD and expiratory flow limitation. The flow volume loop obtained in a forced vital capacity maneuver *(blue line)* is shifted to the left (higher volumes) relative to the healthy individual *(brown line)*. With exercise, expiratory flow during tidal breathing *(black line)* is equal to maximum expiratory flow over a portion of exhalation. TLC, total lung capacity; RV, residual volume.

━━━ Predicted maximal flow-volume loop
━━━ Maximal flow-volume loop
▪▪▪▪ Tidal breathing at rest
━━━ Tidal breathing with exercise

multiple thoracotomies and sternotomies and demonstrate worse exercise capacity and NYHA functional class compared to those with normal spirometry.[108]

Chronic Obstructive Pulmonary Disease

Patients with mild COPD may actually have normal exercise capacity, whereas patients with moderate to severe COPD demonstrate decrements in $\dot{V}O_{2max}$ and peak WR proportional to disease severity, as measured by *Global Initiative for Obstructive Lung Disease* (GOLD) stage.[109,110] Of importance, the pattern of physiologic responses to progressive exercise in COPD is very different than it is in patients with heart failure. Whereas exercise is limited in heart disease by an inability to deliver oxygenated blood to exercising muscles, patients with moderate-severe COPD are limited by altered respiratory mechanics; their ventilatory pump fails before the heart does.

The hallmark of this ventilatory limitation is the fact that both arterial PCO_2 and end-tidal PCO_2 remain stable or increase at end exercise due to an inability to raise alveolar ventilation in response to increasing $\dot{V}CO_2$ and, when present, a metabolic acidosis. This phenomenon, which is present to a greater extent at higher GOLD stages,[110] arises due to mechanical constraints from dynamic hyperinflation during exercise and altered $\dot{V}A/\dot{Q}$ relationships.[111,112]

In addition, $\dot{V}E$ at peak exercise will be at or close to the maximum predicted ventilation as measured by the MVV or $FEV_1 \times 40$, a marked contrast from healthy sedentary individuals and those with heart failure in whom $\dot{V}E/MVV$ is normally less than 75–80%. Ventilation is typically higher for any given WR and is usually marked by a high respiratory rate, low tidal volume, higher end-expiratory volume, and lower inspiratory capacity compared to healthy individuals.[113] Although patients with mild disease may still develop a metabolic acidosis[114] and even manifest a ventilatory threshold at lower levels of $\dot{V}O_2$ than normal individuals,[113] most patients with severe disease lack a ventilatory threshold.[115] Along with the fact that peak heart rate is typically well below the maximum predicted heart rate, this finding strongly indicates that the ventilatory pump is failing before the heart.

An important reason for these manifestations of ventilatory limitation is a phenomenon referred to as *dynamic hyperinflation*. Due to expiratory flow limitation that develops even at low-moderate levels of exercise, patients with COPD must increase end-expiratory lung volumes and encroach on their inspiratory reserve volume to raise $\dot{V}E$ as metabolic activity increases (Fig. 33.5). The resulting hyperinflation causes flattening and decreased contractile strength of the diaphragm, increases respiratory muscle fatigue, and increases dyspnea for any given level of ventilation.[116] One contributor to development of this problem is the increase in minute ventilation as compensation for a higher VD/VT than in healthy control subjects.[117] Of interest, patients with dynamic hyperinflation have less locomotor muscle fatigue with exercise[118] because the ventilatory pump fails before the nonrespiratory muscle groups face significant loads.

Dynamic hyperinflation also has hemodynamic effects, including alterations in cardiac preload and afterload that subsequently impair cardiac function and manifest as a decrease[119] in $\dot{V}O_2/HR$. These changes inversely correlate with the increase in end-expiratory lung volumes,[120] and improvement can be seen after interventions that decrease dynamic hyperinflation, such as *lung volume reduction surgery*.[121] Right ventricular function is also impaired by increased pulmonary vascular resistance due to hypoxic pulmonary vasoconstriction and structural changes in the pulmonary circulation.[122] In fact, in patients with COPD and mean pulmonary artery pressure greater than or equal to 40 mm Hg, impaired circulatory function is often the primary factor limiting exercise rather than the ventilatory constraints.[123]

Another important feature of progressive exercise in COPD is the onset of hypoxemia with a widened $(A-a)PO_2$. This problem correlates with reductions in diffusion capacity,[124] is more likely when patients have emphysema rather than chronic bronchitis as the etiology of their COPD, is more severe in patients with pulmonary hypertension,[125] and is more prominent with walking compared to cycling.[126] The predominant mechanism is $\dot{V}A/\dot{Q}$ inequality, the effects of which are magnified by reductions in $C\bar{v}O_2$ during exercise.[92] Depending on the distribution of blood flow and ventilation, however, $\dot{V}A/\dot{Q}$ inequality and arterial PO_2 may actually improve during exercise.[127,128]

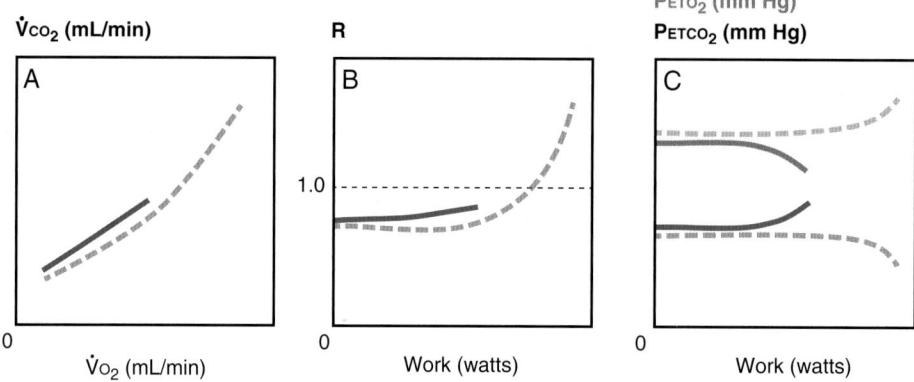

Figure 33.6 Ventilatory limitation pattern of responses to exercise compared to the normal cardiac limitation pattern shown on three key figures from the nine-box plot. The expected physiologic responses to exercise in patients with ventilatory limitation *(solid lines)* are compared to healthy individuals who demonstrate a cardiac pattern of limitation *(dotted lines)*. (A) $\dot{V}CO_2$ vs. $\dot{V}O_2$. (B) Respiratory exchange ratio (R) vs. watts. (C) P_{ETO_2} and P_{ETCO_2} vs. watts. A complete nine-box plot for this pattern of limitation is shown in eFig. 33.4). P_{ETCO_2}, end-tidal partial pressure; P_{ETO_2}, end-tidal partial pressures of O_2; $\dot{V}CO_2$, carbon dioxide output; $\dot{V}E$, minute ventilation; $\dot{V}O_2$, oxygen consumption.

Selected graphs from a nine-box plot demonstrating key differences relative to healthy individuals are shown in Figure 33.6 (the full nine-box plot can be seen in eFig. 33.4).

CARDIOPULMONARY EXERCISE TESTING

INDICATIONS AND CONTRAINDICATIONS

The indications for CPET sort into five general areas: determining the etiology of exercise limitation, assessing functional status, stratifying risk for surgery, prognosticating outcomes in specific diseases, and creating individualized exercise prescriptions for rehabilitation programs. The list of indications for CPET is largely compiled from expert opinions, and the evidence for the utility of CPET varies by indication, each of which is reviewed later.

Determining the Etiology of Dyspnea and Exercise Limitation

Evaluating Dyspnea. When the cause of dyspnea is not apparent from history, physical examination, laboratory testing (including a hemoglobin and resting arterial blood gas), chest imaging, and PFTs, CPET can be used to (1) quantify a patient's exercise limitation and (2) determine the system limiting exercise. Although CPET can narrow the differential list down to a single limiting system, such as in patients with chronotropic incompetence or myocardial ischemia, it is most useful in identifying the best avenue of investigation in making a definitive diagnosis.

The first step in using CPET to evaluate dyspnea is to determine if the patient's subjective description of his or her limitations are aligned with the ability to do work. It is therefore imperative that the patient gives a maximal effort during the CPET. An arterial blood gas at the end of exercise can be very helpful to determine whether the individual gave a good effort, was limited by ventilation, had excess dead space, or was hyperventilating. It is also important to ask the patient if the CPET reproduced their symptoms. In a group of 50 patients referred for CPET with unexplained

dyspnea,[129] for example, broad diagnoses of cardiac limitation, pulmonary limitation, obesity and/or deconditioning, and psychogenic dyspnea were identified.

Evaluating Exercise Limitation. Patients presenting with exercise limitation rather than dyspnea state that they just are not able to perform the amount of work that they could do in the past. CPET is useful in this setting to quantify the amount of work individuals can perform and compare it to what they say they can do during activities of daily living. eTable 33.1 provides a rough estimate of the maximal oxygen consumption that correlates with the level of exercise patients state they are able to perform.[130] It is important to keep in mind that there is a broad spectrum of exercise capabilities across the normal population. Although an individual may have a "normal" exercise study as judged by the maximal oxygen consumption, the observed response for any individual may represent a significant decline in exercise performance from a previous supranormal level and hence evidence of pathology.

Evaluating Combined Cardiovascular and Pulmonary Disorders. When individuals have disease in more than one system, CPET can determine which system is primarily responsible for their exercise limitation. For example, in a patient with both aortic stenosis and COPD, CPET can determine whether or not to proceed with valve repair. Were such a patient to be primarily limited by ventilatory capacity, repairing the aortic valve may not be indicated because after surgery the individual would still be significantly limited. Although it can assist in identifying the primary limiting system, CPET cannot quantitatively partition the degree of limitation due to each of the affected systems.

Diagnosing Exercise-Induced Bronchoconstriction. CPET can be used to diagnose exercise-induced bronchoconstriction, a transient bronchoconstriction that develops during or after strenuous exercise, which is present in greater than 10% of the general population and up to 90% of persons previously diagnosed with asthma.[131] Although administration of inhaled bronchoprovocatory agents, such as methacholine or mannitol, can be used to make the diagnosis, exercise challenge using free running, treadmill, or cycle ergometry has been used to elicit exercise-induced bronchoconstriction since the 1970s[132] and, along with eucapnic voluntary hyperventilation, is a more sensitive and specific testing modality.[133] Exercise testing for this purpose requires specialized equipment, personnel, and the ability to exercise at 85–95% maximum heart rate with dry medical grade air and high flow rates (>100 L/min)[134] and should be performed according to published guidelines.[135,136]

Due to the logistical issues associated with exercise challenges, the International Olympic Committee Medical Commission recommends eucapnic voluntary hyperventilation[133] as the initial testing modality, followed by CPET if eucapnic voluntary hyperventilation is nondiagnostic.[137]

Assessing Functional Status and Degree of Impairment

Quantitative measures of exercise capacity are also useful in determining eligibility for disability because static tests, such as PFTs and ejection fraction on echocardiography, do not correlate well with exercise capacity.[138–140] Despite these issues, the American Thoracic Society statement on the evaluation of impairment and disability[141] states that impairment can be determined from standard PFTs in most cases and that further testing with CPET may be helpful in selected situations. Of importance, quantifying impairment informs but does not define disability, because disability assessment requires social, economic, environmental, and other input.[142] Largely based on empirical knowledge, rough estimates of the work an individual should be able to perform were proposed (eTable 33.2).

Risk Stratification

Risk Assessment for Thoracic Surgery. Multiple studies have looked at preoperative CPET to determine if patient outcomes can be predicted based on exercise capacity.[143–146] Although the available studies have not used randomized, controlled designs and generally involve small numbers of patients from single centers, they do show an association between exercise capacity and postsurgical outcomes. Drawing on this evidence, an expert panel of the American College of Chest Physicians[147] devised an algorithm that incorporates CPET along with the *Thoracic Revised Cardiac Risk Index* (ThRCRI),[148] spirometry, diffusing capacity for carbon monoxide, and performance on stair climbing or shuttle walk testing to guide selection of the appropriate therapeutic approach in lung cancer patients (eFig. 33.5). The general approach can likely be used as a foundation for any lung resection surgery. Patients who require CPET as part of this algorithm are deemed low risk (expected risk of mortality < 1%) if the $\dot{V}O_{2max}$ is greater than 20 mL/kg/min or greater than 75% of predicted, and considered high risk (expected mortality > 10%) if their $\dot{V}O_{2max}$ is less than 10 mL/kg/min or less than 35% of predicted. The ThRCRI has been shown to be an independent prognostic factor after lung resection for early-stage lung cancer.[149]

Evaluation for Lung Volume Reduction Surgery (LVRS). The landmark National Emphysema Therapy Trial[150] demonstrated that LVRS was of benefit but only to the subset of patients defined by their exercise capacity using a modified but formalized exercise protocol. The study participants underwent a maximal CPET on a cycle ergometer while wearing a face mask delivering a fractional concentration of oxygen in inspired gas of 0.30 and pedaling for 3 minutes without resistance, followed by increasing the wattage by 5 or 10 W/min. Those patients with a low exercise capacity, defined as less than 25 W for women and less than 40 W for men, benefited the most from LVRS.

Risk Assessment for Extrathoracic Surgery. A number of studies have investigated the utility of CPET for risk stratification or identification of other comorbidities that could be addressed in the perioperative period in a variety of major surgeries, including abdominal-aortic repair,[151,152] hepatic transplantation,[153] upper gastrointestinal surgery,[154] and in elderly patients undergoing intra-abdominal surgery.[155] Seven of the nine studies included in a review of this issue[156] found higher mortality in patients with lower $\dot{V}O_{2max}$. In one of the studies[155] $\dot{V}O_2$ at the ventilatory threshold was used to determine the appropriate hospital location for postoperative care with $\dot{V}O_2$ less than 11 mL/kg/min being the cutoff for postoperative intensive care and a marker of increased mortality. Despite this evidence, there are no prospective studies documenting survival benefit or cost-effectiveness for using CPET in this manner.

Prognosticating Clinical Outcomes

In healthy individuals without specific diseases and in general among individuals with disease, improved survival is associated with a higher exercise capacity.[157,158] Interventional studies have not been conducted, however, to demonstrate whether training to improve $\dot{V}O_{2max}$ increases life expectancy. Some of the patient populations for whom $\dot{V}O_{2max}$ and other data derived from CPET provide prognostic information are described later.

Heart Failure. $\dot{V}O_{2max}$ is the most objective data available for assessing exercise capacity in individuals with heart failure. Both the American College of Cardiology and the American Heart Association recommend CPET in patients presenting with heart failure to guide management and determine whether heart failure is the cause of exercise limitation when the contribution of heart failure to exercise limitation is uncertain.[159] A number of early studies[160–162] documented a progressive decline in survival with decreasing $\dot{V}O_{2max}$ and indicated that a $\dot{V}O_{2max}$ greater than 14 mL/kg/min identified a population with a 94% 1-year survival and should be used as a criterion to defer heart transplantation. More recent studies have shown similar relationships between $\dot{V}O_{2max}$ and mortality.[163,164] Of importance, the inclusion of patients on β-blocker therapy in recent series[165–167] suggests a threshold less than 14 mL/kg/min should be considered for heart transplantation. Most studies investigating the utility of $\dot{V}O_2$ for prognostication in heart failure use the traditional weight normalized values (mL/kg/min) but due to the obesity "epidemic," the reported oxygen consumption data may be inappropriately low, and decisions for heart transplantation may be skewed toward the obese. Correcting $\dot{V}O_2$ for lean body mass may improve prognostication.[168,169]

Other CPET variables may augment the predictive value of $\dot{V}O_{2max}$. A series of studies, for example, demonstrate that $\dot{V}E/\dot{V}CO_2$ or the $\dot{V}E/\dot{V}CO_2$ slope[170–175] are accurate predictors of mortality and may improve predictive capabilities of models used in heart failure management.[176] Although most of these studies identify a single threshold above which the $\dot{V}E/\dot{V}CO_2$ indicates a higher mortality in patients with heart failure, a more recent analysis by Arena and colleagues[170] created four classes based on the $\dot{V}E/\dot{V}CO_2$ slope and demonstrated that event-free survival was significantly different across the four classes. When combined with the peak $\dot{V}O_2$, the $\dot{V}E/\dot{V}CO_2$ slope further differentiates which patients are at risk for major cardiac events (eFig. 33.6). The available literature suggests individuals with a $\dot{V}O_{2max}$ less than 10 mL/kg/min or a $\dot{V}E/\dot{V}CO_2$ slope greater than 40 have the poorest prognosis.[177]

Other parameters shown to be associated with outcomes such as mortality, need for transplantation, or need for device implantation in patients with heart failure, include heart rate recovery,[178–181] oxygen uptake efficiency,[182–184] exercise oscillatory ventilation,[66,67,185] heart rate variability,[186,187] and blood pressure response.[188,189] A number of different groups have attempted to use multiple CPET parameters[190–192] or combined CPET parameters with other medical information (e.g., renal function, echocardiography, questionnaires)[164,193] to guide prognostication as an alternative to the traditional strategy of using a single parameter.

Adult Congenital Heart Disease. CPET has become a valuable tool in the management of patients with congenital heart disease because it aids in risk stratification and determining the need for and timing of therapeutic interventions.[98,99,194] Whereas NYHA class provides a simple way to assess functional status, CPET provides more specificity regarding the source of exercise limitation in these patients. CPET[195] is thought to be of special importance in this patient population because self-reported exercise capacity is of poor predictive value,[196] and functional limitation can be identified in those who are asymptomatic.[103] Similar to patients with heart failure, $\dot{V}O_{2max}$[103] and $\dot{V}E/\dot{V}CO_2$[197] are strong predictors of mortality. Due to a variety of factors, including the significant heterogeneity of adult congenital heart disease, the decision about when to consider heart transplantation in adult congenital heart disease is particularly complex but can be informed by CPET.[101,198,199]

Pulmonary Arterial Hypertension. Assessment of exercise capacity can also be used to assess prognosis and response to treatment in patients with PAH.[200] Sun and colleagues,[80] for example, found that peak WR, $\dot{V}O_{2max}$, ventilatory threshold, O_2 pulse, and slope of $\dot{V}E/\dot{V}CO_2$ were all correlated with NYHA class, whereas Yasunobu and colleagues[76] demonstrated that end-tidal PCO_2 progressively decreased as the disease severity increased and directly correlated with changes in mean PA pressure. Other studies have demonstrated a relationship between survival and $\dot{V}O_{2max}$ and $\dot{V}E/\dot{V}CO_2$,[77,201,202] and that persistent exercise-induced right-to-left shunting and poor ventilatory efficiency during serial assessments were highly predictive of poor outcomes in patients with PAH.[88]

Although CPET is a safe[80,203] and effective means to grade the severity of exercise limitation, assess prognosis,

and measure response to therapy,[204] the use of CPET is limited in most PAH trials due to a number of practical issues. Instead, most trials rely on the simple, less expensive and reproducible *6-minute walking test* (6MWT, described in greater detail later), which, like CPET, provides prognostic information.[205–207] Improvement in the 6MWT after therapeutic intervention may also be associated with decrease in mortality,[208,209] although not all studies have validated this finding.[210]

Exercise Prescriptions for Cardiac and Pulmonary Rehabilitation Programs

Given that the aerobic exercise intensity prescription is directly linked to both the amount of improvement in exercise capacity and the risk of adverse events during exercise, a joint position statement of the European Association for Cardiovascular Prevention and Rehabilitation, the American Association of Cardiovascular and Pulmonary Rehabilitation, and the Canadian Association of Cardiac Rehabilitation stressed the importance of functional evaluation through exercise testing before starting an aerobic training program.[9] Although there are many methods for creating individualized training programs, these guidelines propose that CPET be the gold standard for comprehensive exercise intensity assessment and prescription. The committee's goal is to shift from a "range-based" to a "threshold-based" aerobic exercise intensity prescription to maximize the benefits obtainable by the use of aerobic exercise training in cardiac rehabilitation.[9]

Similarly, the American Thoracic Society and the European Respiratory Society statement on pulmonary rehabilitation[211] states that before initiating rehabilitation for COPD, CPET should be considered as part of a thorough assessment to identify factors contributing to exercise limitation, determine the exercise prescription, and evaluate safety by monitoring electrocardiography and blood pressure for potential risks.[212] Casaburi and colleagues,[213] for example, have shown that high-intensity training programs (80% of *maximum work rate* [W_{max}] in the incremental test) are more effective than less intense programs (50% of W_{max}) in patients with COPD. From a practical standpoint, a formal CPET study may not be necessary to build a tailored exercise program, and others have used variables obtained in the 6MWT, such as peak heart rate,[214] to target exercise levels.

Despite expert opinion that CPET or 6MWT should be used to create individualized training programs, and some evidence that use of CPET to individualize home exercise is safe in certain classes of patients, such as those with heart failure and implanted defibrillators,[215] there are no data demonstrating the exercise prescription derived by these means improves quality of life or survival.

SAFETY CONSIDERATIONS AND CONTRAINDICATIONS TO CARDIOPULMONARY EXERCISE TESTING

CPET is not without risk, and the decision to conduct the test must reflect consideration of those risks relative to the benefits in terms of information gained. Multiple contemporary surveys indicate that the risks of complications that require hospitalization, including serious arrhythmias, acute myocardial infarction, or sudden cardiac death during or immediately after a CPET, are less than 0.2%, 0.04%, and 0.01%, respectively.[216] These estimates capture the risk for the entire population of individuals performing CPET and likely vary in a given patient based on the underlying disease. Unfortunately, risk estimates are not available for every possible condition, and the clinician must use clinical judgment in assessing risk.

Some diseases carry significantly higher risks and represent absolute or relative contraindications to performing CPET (Table 33.1). Patients with implantable cardiac defibrillators also require special attention. Documentation of the defibrillator settings should be reviewed before exercise to ensure that the peak heart rate during the test does not encroach on the rate at which the defibrillator is set to discharge. The defibrillator should also not be disabled in case the patient has a shockable arrhythmia during the CPET.

CONDUCTING EXERCISE TESTS

Exercise Equipment

There are a number of commercially available exercise monitoring systems that allow breath-by-breath measurements of exhaled gases. The general components of these systems include an airflow transducer to measure the volumes of each inhalation and exhalation and rapid gas analyzers to measure the O_2 and CO_2 during inspiration and expiration. As technologies have improved, these components have become more reliable but still require strict and daily calibration tests to ensure accurate readings. Multiple resources are available with recommendations for calibration procedures and quality control.[7,8,177] Gas exchange measurements during exercise are very reproducible; however, a good practice is to have one or two individuals in the exercise laboratory perform monthly CPET to confirm that

their data remain stable over time. Both maximal and submaximal tests can be used for this purpose because reproducible data are generated in either case.

EXERCISE MODALITIES AND PROTOCOLS

Cycle Ergometer Versus Treadmill

Functional capacity is usually assessed in CPET by having the individual exercise on a stationary cycle ergometer or motorized treadmill. Progressive work is performed on the cycle ergometer by increasing the resistance to pedaling and quantifying work over time as a rate in *watts* (W). Work rate on the treadmill is primarily determined by the grade and speed of the treadmill. Because arm movement and the uplift of body weight while walking/running on the treadmill add to the work performed, work on a treadmill is more dependent on an individual's weight and, as a result, is harder to quantify than with cycle ergometry, where leg muscles do the vast majority of the work and the individual's weight is supported by the bicycle. Treadmill work is measured relative to each individual's resting energy expenditure and is typically expressed in terms of *metabolic equivalents* (METs). One MET represents the amount of oxygen consumed at rest and each successive stage achieved in a given treadmill protocol corresponds to a higher level of METs that can, in turn, be related to the individual's oxygen consumption (1 MET = 3.5 mL O_2/kg/min in the average adult).[217] As discussed previously, $\dot{V}O_2$ is tightly linked with WR on a cycle ergometer, with $\dot{V}O_2$ increasing 10 mL/min/W above the resting value. Hence watts and METs can be roughly compared through the shared $\dot{V}O_2$ and are dependent on the individual's weight. Table 33.2 provides examples of watts, oxygen consumption, and METs for two individuals of different weights to give the reader a general idea of how these measures of work compare.

Both exercise modalities impose progressively increasing WRs that provide a range of oxygen consumptions to identify exercise patterns described earlier in this chapter. The resistance, and therefore watts, in cycle ergometry can be increased in either a continuous or stepwise manner over time. Treadmill WRs are usually increased according to specific protocols, such as the Bruce,[218] Balke,[219] or Naughton[220] protocols, which define how to change the speed and inclination of the treadmill over time. The WR ramp or steps should be chosen so that the subject can perform 10 to 12 minutes of exercise before reaching $\dot{V}O_{2max}$ because this timeframe usually provides the temporal resolution necessary to identify patterns of exercise responses. $\dot{V}O_{2max}$ estimates tend to be 10–15% higher using a treadmill compared to a cycle ergometer due to the extra work performed by the arms when walking or running. Each modality offers advantages depending on the patient and goals of the test. Whereas cycle ergometry tends to be better for patients who are obese or have gait problems and is more suited for drawing arterial blood gases, treadmill testing may be preferred in patients whose symptoms are elicited with walking and running or in patients with exercise-activated pacemakers that sense arm movement.

Invasive Cardiopulmonary Exercise Testing

When competing comorbidities make it difficult to determine the primary cause of exercise limitation, exercise with a right

Table 33.1 Contraindications for Cardiopulmonary Exercise Testing

Absolute	Relative
Active myocardial ischemia (unstable angina, myocardial infarction within 30 days)	Severe pulmonary hypertension
Acute heart failure exacerbation	Left main coronary artery stenosis
Exercise-induced syncope	Moderate stenotic valve disease
Uncontrolled arrhythmias	Severe hypertension (SBP > 200 mm Hg, DBP > 120 mm Hg)
Severe aortic stenosis	Hypertrophic cardiomyopathy
Acute endocarditis, myocarditis, pericarditis	High-degree atrioventricular block
Acute aortic dissection or suspected dissecting aortic aneurysm	Severe electrolyte abnormalities
Acute pulmonary embolism or lower extremity deep venous thrombosis	Tachyarrhythmias or bradyarrhythmias
Active COPD exacerbation or uncontrolled asthma	Advanced or complicated pregnancy
Active pulmonary edema	Implanted cardiac defibrillator that cannot be interrogated or temporarily reset due to inaccessibility of an individual qualified to do this (e.g., device manufacturer representative)
Oxygen saturation < 85% breathing air at rest	
Acute respiratory failure	

DBP, diastolic blood pressure; SBP, systolic blood pressure.

Table 33.2 Comparison of Oxygen Consumption and Metabolic Equivalents at Different Levels of Work in Individuals of Two Different Weights

| Watts | 70-KG PERSON | | 100-KG PERSON | |
	$\dot{V}O_2$ (mL/min)	METs	$\dot{V}$ (mL/min)	METs
0 (rest)	250	1.0	350	1.0
25	500	2.0	600	1.7
50	750	3.1	850	2.4
100	1250	5.1	1350	3.9
200	2250	9.2	2350	6.7
300	3250	13.3	3350	9.6
400	4250	17.3	4350	12.4

METs, metabolic equivalents; $\dot{V}$, ventilation flow; $\dot{V}O_2$, oxygen consumption.

heart catheter can provide additional data to help separate out the cardiac and pulmonary systems, further differentiate the broad category of "cardiac limitation" as either right or left heart failure, and identify muscle deconditioning.[221] The data available from the right heart catheter include mixed venous oxygen saturation and content, PA pressure, PA occlusion pressure, and thermodilution cardiac output. With increasing exercise to exhaustion in a normal individual, cardiac output should increase fourfold to fivefold, but the mean PA pressure should remain less than 30 mm Hg.[222] In patients with left heart failure or pulmonary vascular disease, the mean PA pressure may increase above this level and, if associated with symptoms of dyspnea, may give a clue to underlying mechanisms. Pulmonary vascular resistance can be calculated to determine if elevated PA pressures are due to left-sided heart failure or pulmonary vascular disease. Because intrathoracic pressure affects right heart catheterization measurements, the PA occlusion pressure may be difficult to measure accurately. Stroke volume can be calculated from the heart rate and cardiac output rather than assessed through a surrogate measure, the O_2 pulse. Placement of an arterial line with the right heart catheter allows calculation of cardiac output using the Fick equation and determination of the arteriovenous oxygen content difference, with narrow values of the latter providing evidence of deconditioning as a cause of exercise limitation.

Noninvasive Estimates of Cardiac Output During Cardiopulmonary Exercise Tests

A number of noninvasive commercial methods are also available for estimating the cardiac output during exercise, which rely on a variety of technologies, including CO_2 rebreathing,[223] pulse contour analysis,[224] chest bioreactance,[225] echocardiography,[226] and inert gas rebreathing.[227] The technology that has been most rigorously evaluated in exercise[228] is the inert gas rebreathing method using the Innocor Rebreathing System (Innovision A/S). Whereas the available evidence demonstrates these measurements are feasible and that cardiac output and $\dot{V}O_2$ are tightly correlated in both normal subjects and individuals with heart failure,[229] their clinical utility remains unclear.[227]

Indications for Arterial Blood Gases

Arterial blood gases provide additional data that assist in differentiating the causes of exercise limitation and dyspnea.

In particular, they allow the determination of the $(A-a)P_{O_2}$ to evaluate gas exchange, the arterial P_{CO_2} as the gold standard for identifying ventilatory limitation, V_D/V_T as an indicator of pulmonary vascular disease, and base deficit as a surrogate for lactic acidosis. Arterial blood gases can be obtained throughout the CPET to identify the position of the ventilatory threshold or one time at the end of exercise. The former approach requires an arterial line, whereas a single needle puncture can be used for the latter. The operator should be aware that arterial puncture after maximal exertion can cause a vagal reaction and hypotension, especially in younger subjects.

INTERPRETING CARDIOPULMONARY EXERCISE TESTS

Figure 33.7 describes a basic approach to interpreting the results of CPET. Because CPET interpretation is highly dependent on the data quality, before assessing the physiologic responses to exercise, it is important to ensure there are no systematic data collection errors and that the patient gave a full effort. Several key aspects of the interpretation process are considered later.

Reference Values

As is the case in pulmonary function testing, many of the measured parameters and, in particular, the $\dot{V}O_{2max}$, are not assessed by looking at the absolute value of the parameter and, instead, are judged based on comparison of that value to that expected for an individual of that age, sex, body habitus (weight and/or height), and mode of exercise. In conducting and interpreting a CPET, it is essential to use reference values appropriate to the patient undergoing evaluation. A comprehensive list of reference values is available elsewhere.[7]

Identifying the Ventilatory Threshold

One of the important steps in CPET interpretation is identifying whether the patient reached a ventilatory threshold, because it is one of the primary means of distinguishing between cardiac or pulmonary vascular limitation, on the one hand, and ventilatory limitation on the other. The ventilatory threshold can be identified by invasive and noninvasive means. The former involves measurement of arterial lactate or bicarbonate concentrations. A single

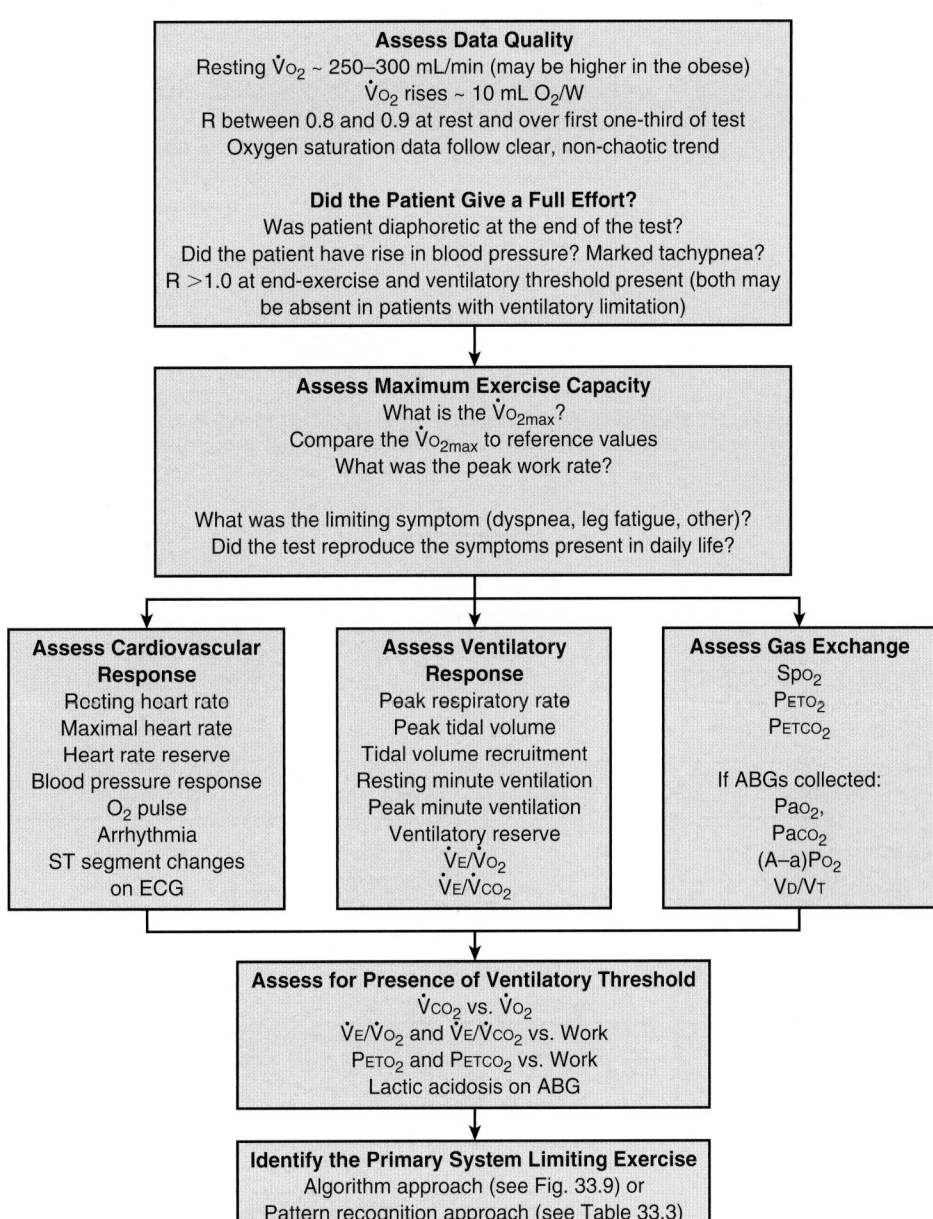

Assess Data Quality
Resting $\dot{V}O_2$ ~ 250–300 mL/min (may be higher in the obese)
$\dot{V}O_2$ rises ~ 10 mL O_2/W
R between 0.8 and 0.9 at rest and over first one-third of test
Oxygen saturation data follow clear, non-chaotic trend

Did the Patient Give a Full Effort?
Was patient diaphoretic at the end of the test?
Did the patient have rise in blood pressure? Marked tachypnea?
R >1.0 at end-exercise and ventilatory threshold present (both may
be absent in patients with ventilatory limitation)

Assess Maximum Exercise Capacity
What is the $\dot{V}O_{2max}$?
Compare the $\dot{V}O_{2max}$ to reference values
What was the peak work rate?

What was the limiting symptom (dyspnea, leg fatigue, other)?
Did the test reproduce the symptoms present in daily life?

Assess Cardiovascular Response
Resting heart rate
Maximal heart rate
Heart rate reserve
Blood pressure response
O_2 pulse
Arrhythmia
ST segment changes
on ECG

Assess Ventilatory Response
Peak respiratory rate
Peak tidal volume
Tidal volume recruitment
Resting minute ventilation
Peak minute ventilation
Ventilatory reserve
$\dot{V}E/\dot{V}O_2$
$\dot{V}E/\dot{V}CO_2$

Assess Gas Exchange
SpO_2
$PETO_2$
$PETCO_2$

If ABGs collected:
PaO_2,
$PaCO_2$
$(A–a)PO_2$
VD/VT

Assess for Presence of Ventilatory Threshold
$\dot{V}CO_2$ vs. $\dot{V}O_2$
$\dot{V}E/\dot{V}O_2$ and $\dot{V}E/\dot{V}CO_2$ vs. Work
$PETO_2$ and $PETCO_2$ vs. Work
Lactic acidosis on ABG

Identify the Primary System Limiting Exercise
Algorithm approach (see Fig. 33.9) or
Pattern recognition approach (see Table 33.3)

Figure 33.7 A general approach to cardiopulmonary exercise test interpretation. Because data interpretation is highly dependent on the quality of the data, the initial steps involve ensuring there are no systematic data errors and that the patient gave a complete effort. Once this is done, the next tasks are to assess maximal exercise capacity and the cardiovascular, ventilatory, and gas exchange responses and then identify whether a ventilatory threshold is present and determine the primary system limiting exercise.

measurement at end exercise is sufficient for a binary decision as to whether the threshold was reached, whereas serial measurements every other minute during exercise can be used as part of several different techniques to determine the $\dot{V}O_2$ at which the threshold was reached.[12,230] Several noninvasive methods can also be used, including the V-slope method described earlier (see Fig. 33.1), identification of the point at which $\dot{V}E/\dot{V}O_2$ and $\dot{V}E/\dot{V}CO_2$ reach their nadir and begin to increase or the point at which the end-tidal PO_2 starts to rise or and end-tidal PCO_2 starts to decrease (Fig. 33.8). The accuracy of the different methods varies based on operator experience, the testing protocol, and the data collection system,[7] and there is no evidence that any particular noninvasive method is superior to the others.[231,232] This is not a critically important issue in most of CPET interpretation, where the key question is whether or not the threshold was reached rather than the specific time point.

Identifying the Primary System Limiting Exercise: Algorithmic Versus Pattern Recognition Approaches

Perhaps the most important aspect of CPET interpretation is identifying the primary reason for exercise limitation. One approach, first introduced by Wasserman and colleagues,[29] uses a binary tree algorithm and flow charts that direct the interpretation though a series of decision points to specific causes of exercise limitation. A simplified flow chart is shown in Figure 33.9 to demonstrate the concept. The advantages of this approach are that the decision points and values are well defined so that there is no ambiguity in the direction to branch in the flow chart. This strategy is likely easier to follow for the novice interpreter than the pattern recognition approach outlined later. The primary disadvantage is that the interpretation is dependent on a single data point at each bifurcation. Any error in data

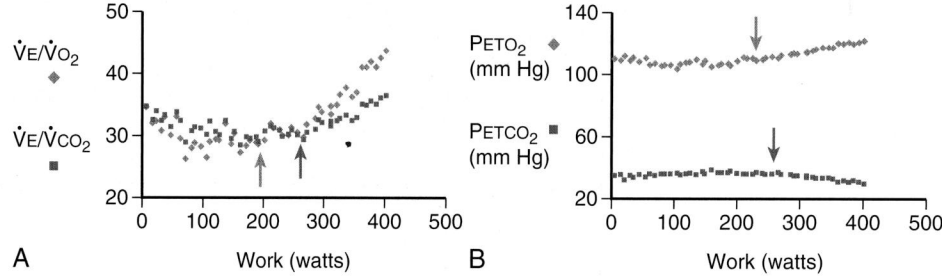

Figure 33.8 Two methods to identify ventilatory threshold during exercise test interpretation. (A) Analysis of ventilatory equivalents to identify whether a ventilatory threshold is present. After the increase in minute ventilation at the ventilatory threshold, $\dot{V}E/\dot{V}O_2$ (noted in *brown*) and $\dot{V}E/\dot{V}CO_2$ (noted in *blue*) begin a steady rise. The point at which each variable starts to rise is marked by an *arrow* in the respective colors. The start of the rise in $\dot{V}E/\dot{V}O_2$ is associated with the first ventilatory threshold, which is expected before the rise in $\dot{V}E/\dot{V}CO_2$. (B) Using changes in P_{ETO_2} and P_{ETCO_2} to identify whether a ventilatory threshold is present. At the ventilatory threshold, $\dot{V}E$ increases out of proportion to the changes in $\dot{V}O_2$ and $\dot{V}CO_2$. As a result, P_{ETO_2} (noted in *brown*) begins a steady rise *(brown arrow)*, whereas P_{ETCO_2} (noted in *blue*) begins a steady decrease *(blue arrow)*. P_{ETCO_2}, end-tidal partial pressure; P_{ETO_2}, end-tidal partial pressures of O_2; R, respiratory exchange ratio; $\dot{V}$, ventilation flow; $\dot{V}CO_2$, carbon dioxide output; $\dot{V}E$, minute ventilation; $\dot{V}O_2$, oxygen consumption; V_T, tidal volume.

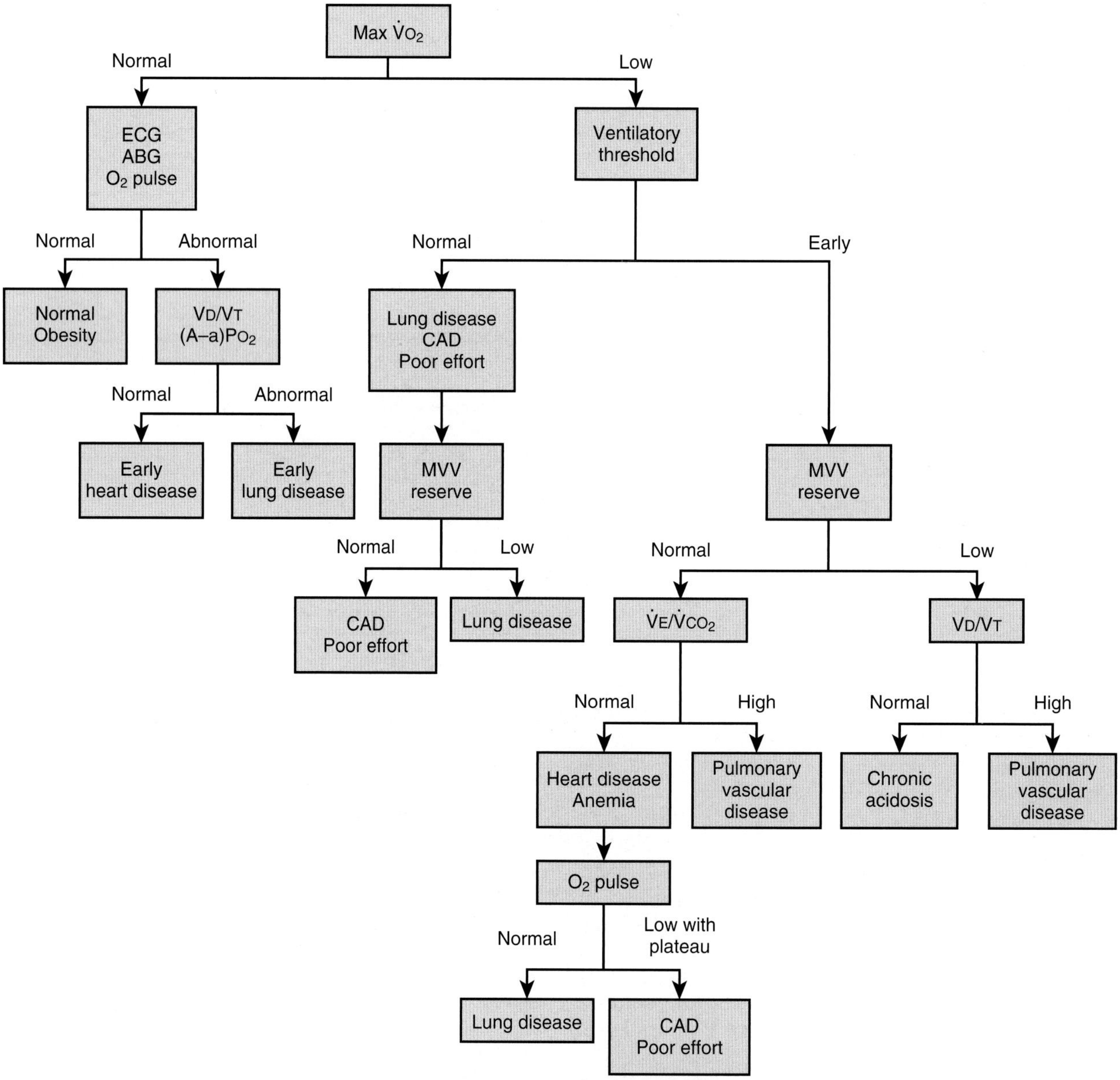

Figure 33.9 Simplified flow chart demonstrating decision making in CPET interpretation. The decision tree begins at the top with the $\dot{V}O_{2max}$ compared to predicted values. ABG, arterial blood gases; CAD, coronary artery disease; ECG, electrocardiogram; $\dot{V}O_{2max}$, maximum oxygen consumption. (Modified from Wasserman K, Hansen JE, Sue DY, et al. *Principles of Exercise Testing and Interpretation.* 5th ed. Philadelphia: Lippincott Williams & Wilkins; 2012.)

collection or misinterpretation at one bifurcation can direct the interpretation down a wrong pathway toward an incorrect diagnosis.

An alternative method is one of pattern recognition that uses the expected trends for multiple variables over the course of progressive exercise to identify the organ system limiting exercise. As discussed earlier, general disease categories, such as heart failure, pulmonary vascular disease, or ventilatory insufficiency, have expected patterns of exercise response (Table 33.3). These patterns can be weighted by their relative specificity for each organ system and then examined in sum to suggest the most likely organ system to be limiting exercise. Patients with cardiac limitation, for example, will demonstrate a ventilatory threshold, decreased end-tidal P_{CO_2} and arterial P_{CO_2}, and increasing ventilatory $\dot{V}_E/\dot{V}_{O_2}$ and $\dot{V}_E/\dot{V}_{CO_2}$ at end exercise. Patients with pulmonary hypertension demonstrate many similar findings but will manifest hypoxemia and a fixed V_D/V_T in late exercise. Other potential findings considered to be specific for an organ system failure, such as exercise oscillatory ventilation in heart failure, can be seen with exercise but not regularly enough to warrant listing in Table 33.3.

Because the various observations listed in Table 33.3 are not necessarily present in every patient, a useful approach in the pattern recognition method is to conceptualize it as a scale on which the different observations are shown as blocks that are placed on the side of the scale representing the potential limiting pattern (Fig. 33.10). Each block may be of different size, representing the relative weight placed

Table 33.3 Identifying the Pattern of Limitation on Cardiopulmonary Exercise Testing

Observation	PATTERN OF LIMITATION		
	Cardiac	Pulmonary Vascular	Ventilatory
Clear ventilatory threshold	◉	◉	
Plateau in O_2 pulse late in exercise	●	●	◉*
High $\dot{V}_E/\dot{V}_{CO_2}$	●	●	
High $\dot{V}_E/\dot{V}_{O_2}$	●	●	
$\dot{V}_{E_{max}}$ far below MVV	●		
Metabolic acidosis by arterial blood gas late in exercise	●	●	
Decreasing P_{ETCO_2} late in exercise	●	●	
R clearly rises above 1.0	●	●	
Stop exercising due to leg fatigue	●	●	
Heart rate near predicted maximum late in exercise	●		
ST changes on electrocardiography	●		
Inappropriate blood pressure response	●		
Increasing or unchanged V_D/V_T by arterial blood gas late in exercise		●	
Absent ventilatory threshold			◉
Decrease in oxygen saturation		●	●
Heart rate far below predicted maximum late in exercise			●
Increasing or unchanged P_{ETCO_2} late in exercise			◉
Pa_{CO_2} > 40 mm Hg by arterial blood gas (end-exercise)			◉
$\dot{V}_{E_{max}}$ near MVV			●
Decreasing tidal volume			◉
R does not increase above 1.0			●
Stop exercising due to dyspnea			●

The size of the marker indicates the relative importance of the observation.
*Can be seen if air-trapping affects cardiac function.
Modified from Luks A, Glenny R, Robertson H. *Introduction to Cardiopulmonary Exercise Testing*. New York: Springer; 2013.
MVV, maximum voluntary ventilation; P_{ETCO_2}, end-tidal partial pressure of carbon dioxide; Pa_{CO_2}, arterial partial pressure of carbon dioxide; R, exchange ratio; V_D/V_T, dead-space fraction; $\dot{V}_{E_{max}}$, maximum minute ventilation.

on that particular factor. With this method, the presence or absence of a ventilatory threshold would be the biggest block. The side of the scale with the greatest weight (number of blocks) is most likely to be the limiting organ system. By being less dependent on single parameters to make a decision throughout a binary tree, pattern recognition may be less prone to misclassifications of the limiting organ system.

ALTERNATIVE METHODS OF ASSESSING EXERCISE TOLERANCE

THE SIX-MINUTE WALK AND SHUTTLE WALK TESTS

The 6MWT is a widely available, inexpensive, and reproducible submaximal exercise test during which subjects walk back and forth along a flat indoor course varying in length between 30 and 100 m for a period of 6 minutes under the supervision of a trained technician using a specified testing protocol.[233] Individuals move at their own pace, can use supplemental oxygen, and, unlike in CPET, may stop to rest if needed. The primary measurements obtained during the test include the distance walked, heart rate, oxygen saturation, blood pressure, and subjective ratings of dyspnea and leg fatigue.

A primary purpose of the 6MWT is to monitor response to interventions or follow disease activity over time as demonstrated by the extensive use of the distance walked as an outcome in PAH[234] and IPF trials.[235] Studies done in patients with COPD,[236] PAH,[237] IPF,[238] and silicosis[239] have also shown associations between the distance walked or development of hypoxemia and outcomes such as mortality risk. Whether the distance walked is an adequate surrogate for $\dot{V}O_{2max}$ remains unclear, however, because studies have reported varying degrees of correlation between these two variables.[240] Of importance, the 6MWT cannot be used to determine the etiology of exercise limitation and is only useful to assess individuals who are unable to maintain a normal or brisk walking pace, rather than fit individuals.

Use of the test for the purposes noted earlier requires recognition of several important issues. First, the utility of published reference values[241,242] is limited by the fact that test results vary based on differences in testing methodology and in the population under consideration. Second, subject performance is affected by learning, verbal encouragement, and course layout, necessitating strict adherence to published testing protocols.[233] Finally, when using the 6MWT as part of patient assessment, clinicians must understand the minimal clinically important difference, the threshold at which a change in 6MWT is recognized as either important by the patient or associated with other outcomes. Minimal clinically important difference values have been published but vary across studies.[238,243,244]

The incremental shuttle walk test is a less widely used alternative to the 6MWT and requires the patient to walk at a specified pace that increases over time until the individual can no longer maintain the pace or stops due to symptoms.

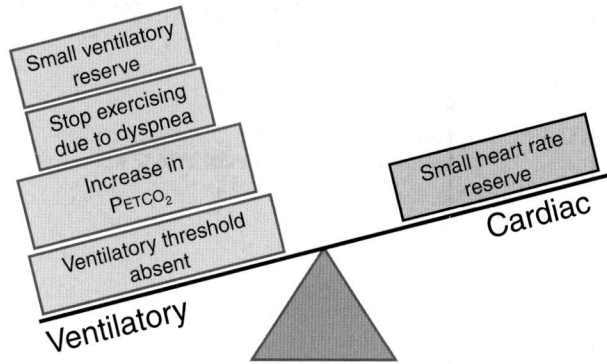

Figure 33.10 The "balance" approach to identifying the pattern of exercise limitation. In this example, the patient has many features consistent with ventilatory limitation due to COPD and only one aspect of the data consistent with a cardiac limitation. Because the preponderance of data favors the left side of the balance, this patient would be best labeled as having a ventilatory limitation pattern.

Designed as a less invasive assessment of maximal exercise capacity, the test correlates reasonably well with $\dot{V}O_{2max}$[245] and can be used to monitor responses to therapeutic interventions[246] and predict mortality in certain patient groups.[247] Only a few sets of reference values have been published,[248] and its use is largely limited to following changes over time in a given patient.

EXERCISE TREADMILL TESTING

In addition to its role in cardiopulmonary testing described earlier, *exercise treadmill testing* (ETT) is also commonly performed without exhaled gas collection. Because data collection is limited in such cases to assessment of symptoms, blood pressure, heart rate, oxygen saturation electrocardiography, and exercise duration, ETT cannot identify the system limiting exercise but can serve other important purposes.

The primary use is to identify coronary artery disease in low- to intermediate-risk individuals capable of exercise who have normal baseline electrocardiograms. The test can be performed in the outpatient setting, and it can be a part of diagnostic protocols for low-risk patients admitted to chest pain units from the emergency department.[249] Myocardial perfusion imaging is combined with ETT for patients with abnormal baseline electrocardiograms and is often necessary when evaluating female patients because the predictive capability of routine ETT is limited by the lower pretest probability of coronary artery disease in these patients.[250]

Using the concept of METs rather than direct measurement of $\dot{V}O_{2max}$, ETT can also be used to assess exercise capacity. Although this approach is less precise than measurements using exhaled gas collection, various studies demonstrate its utility in patient assessment and prognostication.[157,158,251,252] Other variables measured during ETT, such as impaired heart rate recovery,[253] and heart rate or blood pressure responses to increasing work rates,[254,255] have also been linked to various outcomes.

Key Points

- Performance of sustained exercise requires tight integration of multiple systems. Disease within any of these systems can manifest as dyspnea on exertion or exercise limitation.
- Assessment of maximal oxygen consumption provides insight into maximal exercise capacity and important aspects of cardiac function.
- Normal individuals demonstrate a characteristic pattern of responses to progressive exercise to a symptom-limited maximum. Characteristic patterns of deviation from these normal responses are seen in various diseases, including heart failure, pulmonary vascular disease, interstitial lung disease, and COPD.
- Cardiopulmonary exercise testing can be used to characterize the pattern of responses to progressive exercise and identify the primary organ system limiting exercise capacity.
- Cardiopulmonary exercise testing can be used to prognosticate and guide clinical decisions in certain patient groups, guide perioperative management in thoracic and other major surgical procedures, assess disability, and develop exercise prescriptions in rehabilitation programs.

Key Readings

American Thoracic Society, American College of Chest Physicians. ATS/ACCP statement on cardiopulmonary exercise testing. *Am J Respir Critic Care Med.* 2003;167(2):211–277.

Balady GJ, Arena R, Sietsema K, et al. Clinician's guide to cardiopulmonary exercise testing in adults: a scientific statement from the american heart association. *Circulation.* 2010;122(2):191–225.

Bruce RA, Kusumi F, Hosmer D. Maximal oxygen intake and nomographic assessment of functional aerobic impairment in cardiovascular disease. *Am Heart J.* 1973;85(4):546–562.

Dempsey JA, Reddan W, Balke B, Rankin J. Work capacity determinants and physiologic cost of weight-supported work in obesity. *J Appl Physiol.* 1966;21(6):1815–1820.

Guazzi M, Adams V, Conraads V, et al. EACPR/AHA scientific statement. clinical recommendations for cardiopulmonary exercise testing data assessment in specific patient populations. *Circulation.* 2012;126(18):2261–2274.

Jones NL. Quality control in exercise studies. In: Jones NL, ed. *Clinical Exercise Testing.* Philadelphia: Saunders; 1997:164–166.

Mezzani A, Agostoni P, Cohen-Solal A, et al. Standards for the use of cardiopulmonary exercise testing for the functional evaluation of cardiac patients: a report from the exercise physiology section of the european association for cardiovascular prevention and rehabilitation. *Eur J Cardiovasc Prev Rehabil.* 2009;16(3):249–267.

Saltin B, Blomqvist G, Mitchell JH, Johnson Jr RL, Wildenthal K, Chapman CB. Response to exercise after bed rest and after training. *Circulation.* 1968;38(suppl 5):VII1–78.

Wasserman K, Hansen JE, Sue DY, et al. *Principles of Exercise Testing and Interpretation.* 5th ed. Philadephia, PA: Lippincott Williams & Wilkins; 2012.

Complete reference list available at ExpertConsult.com.

34 PREOPERATIVE EVALUATION

KURT PFEIFER, MD, FACP, SFHM • GERALD W. SMETANA, MD, MACP

INTRODUCTION

A common activity for both general internists and pulmonologists is to provide a medical consultation before surgery. This evaluation may be challenging and seem foreign to many consultants because aspects of the care provided differ from those in the nonsurgical setting. The most important elements to include in all preoperative consultations are estimation of pulmonary risk, cardiac risk, and risk of perioperative venous thromboembolism. In each instance, the consultant estimates risk based on patient-related and procedure-related risk factors, determines the need (if any) for diagnostic testing, and proposes interventions to minimize risk and improve perioperative outcomes. In this chapter we focus on preoperative pulmonary evaluation. This chapter defines *postoperative pulmonary complications* (PPCs), estimates risk for different types of surgery, enumerates risk factors, discusses risk prediction scores, and establishes the value of pulmonary function testing to refine the risk estimate. We also discuss strategies to reduce the risk of PPCs in the preoperative, intraoperative, and postoperative settings. Finally, separate sections are devoted to the impact of sleep-disordered breathing (*obstructive sleep apnea* [OSA]) and considerations specific to airway management. The primary focus is on patients undergoing noncardiothoracic surgery, because the approach to preoperative pulmonary evaluation for patients undergoing lung resection differs (see Chapter 30).

DEFINITION AND MORBIDITY OF POSTOPERATIVE PULMONARY COMPLICATIONS

Although a definition for postoperative cardiac complications (major adverse cardiovascular events, perioperative myocardial infarction, heart failure, cardiac death, etc.) is straightforward, the definition of PPCs is less intuitive. Most authors consider only those events that are morbid, prolong hospital stay, require an intervention to treat, or increase the risk for perioperative mortality. In most research, PPCs are grouped together, and risk factor analysis does not address the risk of specific events separately. Studies of interventions more commonly address strategies that focus on one or several specific outcomes, rather than all types of PPCs. For purposes of our discussion, we consider the following to be the most important PPCs:

- Pneumonia
- Respiratory failure
- Atelectasis
- COPD exacerbation
- Bronchospasm
- Respiratory arrest due to sleep-disordered breathing
- Perioperative pulmonary mortality

Respiratory failure is commonly defined as mechanical ventilation for more than 48 hours after surgery or unplanned reintubation. Unless specifically stated otherwise, the discussion of risk factors and preoperative testing considers all PPC outcomes together, rather than a single outcome.

PPCs are morbid, increase length of stay, often require unplanned intensive care unit stays, and increase perioperative mortality. For example, a recent study evaluated the incidence and morbidity of PPCs among *American Society of Anesthesiologists* (ASA) physical status class III patients,[1] who have severe systemic disease.[2] Excluding the minor outcome of need for postoperative oxygen by nasal canula, 14% of patients had at least one PPC. The length of stay for patients with no PPCs compared to those with three PPCs increased from 3 to 8 days. The need for intensive care unit stay increased by more than three-fold. Seven-day mortality increased from 0% to 7%. In a large database study of unselected patients undergoing abdominal surgery, 6% of patients had at least one PPC.[3]

TABLE 34.1 Patient-Related Risk Factors for Postoperative Pulmonary Complications

Risk Factor*	ADJUSTED ODDS RATIOS FOR PPCS	
	Smetana et al, 2006[5]	Yang et al, 2015[3]
Age		
60–69	2.3	
70–79	3.9	
≥80	5.6	2.4
ASA class ≥3	3.1	2.8
Abnormal chest radiograph	4.8	
Heart failure	2.9	
Arrhythmia	2.9	
Total functional dependence	2.5	2.8
COPD	2.4	

*Risk factors listed are for those with odds ratios ≥2.
ASA, American Society of Anesthesiologists; PPCs, postoperative pulmonary complications.

TABLE 34.2 Procedure-Related Risk Factors for Postoperative Pulmonary Complications

Risk Factor*	ADJUSTED ODDS RATIO FOR PPCS	
	Smetana et al, 2006[5]	Yang et al, 2015[3]
Surgical site		
Aortic	6.9	
Nonresective thoracic (mainly esophageal)	4.2	5.1
Any abdominal	3.1	
Upper abdominal	3.0	2.0
Neurosurgery	2.5	
Head and neck	2.2	
Vascular	2.1	
Emergency surgery	2.5	
Prolonged surgery (>3–4 h)	2.3	2.1
General anesthesia	2.4	

*Risk factors listed are for those with odds ratio ≥2.
PPCs, postoperative pulmonary complications.

In a study of costs associated with postoperative complications, PPCs were the most costly and were more expensive than infectious, cardiovascular, and thromboembolic complications.[4] Mean costs were $54,430 (PPC), $8209 (infectious), $13,256 (cardiovascular), and $28,355 (thromboembolic).

PATIENT-RELATED RISK FACTORS

It is customary to divide risk factors for PPCs into those that are specific to the patient and those that are intrinsic to the type of surgery and anesthesia. Many patient-related risk factors are not modifiable; hence the approach to risk reduction will be a general one rather than a specific effort to eliminate or reduce a particular risk factor. This subject has been researched extensively, so confident estimates of the relative importance of individual patient-related risk factors are available.

When evaluating a patient before major noncardiac surgery, the first step is to establish the presence of patient-related risk factors for PPCs (Table 34.1). ASA classification and age dominate the patient-related risk factors. Even after adjusting for conditions more common among older patients, age remains a powerful risk factor. With each decade older than 50 years, the risk increases. Therefore even a healthy older patient who is free of other patient-related risk factors is at increased risk for PPCs. This contrasts with postoperative cardiac complications where age drops out of the analysis after multivariable adjustment for confounders.

ASA physical status classification is an important factor. This classification is broadly written to allow a general classification of risk groups based on the presence and severity of major illness.[2] For example, class 2 describes a patient with mild systemic disease, whereas class 4 is a patient with severe systemic disease that is a constant threat to life. The classification allows for clinical judgment in assigning risk class and estimating major disease severity. Several studies have shown that ASA class is an important risk factor for PPCs even after multivariable adjustment for conditions that would be more common among patients with higher ASA class scores.[3,5]

Total functional dependence is the need for assistance with activities of daily living, typically with needs for home care services, such as a visiting nurse or caregiver. This important predictor most likely results from decreased functional capacity and physiologic reserve in such patients. Surprisingly, although COPD is a patient-related risk factor, it is less important than age or ASA class. Other risk factors include an abnormal chest radiograph (discussed later), congestive heart failure, and arrhythmia.

PROCEDURE-RELATED RISK FACTORS

Procedure-related risk factors are those that are specific to the procedure, regardless of the patient's intrinsic risk (Table 34.2). In general, procedure-related risk factors are more important than patient-related factors. Among procedure-related factors, the single most important factor is surgical site. The old adage that the risk increases as the incision becomes closer to the diaphragm is generally true. Aortic and nonresective thoracic (primarily esophageal) surgeries carry the greatest risk, with *odds ratios* (ORs) for PPCs in the range of 4 to 7. Abdominal surgery is the next most important surgical site risk factor. Many studies have shown that upper abdominal surgery, such as cholecystectomy, carries more risk than lower abdominal surgery, such as gynecologic or urologic surgery. Neurosurgery, head and neck, and nonaortic vascular surgeries are additional high-risk surgical sites, although less so than aortic, thoracic, or abdominal. Orthopedic surgery, although a risk factor for perioperative thromboembolism, is not a risk factor for PPCs.

All other procedure-related risk factors are less powerful than surgical site. Emergency surgery increases PPC rates as does prolonged surgery. Prolonged surgery is generally defined as more than 3 to 4 hours.

The impact of general anesthesia on PPC rates has been the subject of substantial debate. The relevant comparison is to neuraxial anesthesia, which includes spinal and epidural anesthesia. In an early review, general anesthesia was a modest PPC risk factor, with an OR of 2.4.[5] In a recent review of patients with COPD undergoing a variety of surgical procedures, general anesthesia was likewise a modest risk factor for PPCs.[6] Rates of pneumonia (3.3% vs. 2.3%), prolonged mechanical ventilation (2.1% vs. 0.9%), and unplanned reintubation (2.6% vs. 1.8%) were all higher for patients undergoing general anesthesia. There was, however, no difference in mortality between the general anesthesia and the neuraxial anesthesia groups.

A recent systematic review of 20 studies of general anesthesia versus neuraxial anesthesia also found neuraxial blockade to be associated with reductions in several adverse outcomes. Rates of pneumonia (*relative risk* [RR], 0.56) and mortality (RR, 0.71) were lower for neuraxial anesthesia.[7] A query of the National Surgical Quality Improvement Program database revealed similar findings.[8] Although regional anesthesia had no impact on mortality, the RR for respiratory complications was 0.76. It is now possible to state confidently that epidural anesthesia confers fewer PPCs than general anesthesia.

PULMONARY RISK PREDICTION TOOLS

Multifactorial risk indices to predict postoperative cardiac complications have been used for decades.[9] More recently, several investigators have developed risk scoring systems using multivariable analysis to determine the independent contribution of patient-related, procedure-related, and diagnostic test results. In one of the first such studies, Arozullah and colleagues published multivariate risk scores separately for pneumonia[10] and respiratory failure.[11] Both tools effectively stratified patients into five risk classes that accurately discriminated high- versus low-risk scores. The pneumonia risk index was complex and not easily adapted to clinical use. The respiratory failure index was the simpler of the two and provided a useful tool for clinicians.

Building on this methodologic approach, other authors have developed multivariable risk indices for the prediction of PPC rates. Gupta and colleagues developed separate multivariable indices for postoperative pneumonia and respiratory failure. To calculate risk, a spreadsheet can be downloaded at http://www.surgicalriskcalculator.com/home. For patients and physicians who are particularly concerned about one or the other specific outcomes, these are useful tools.

We recommend the *Assess Respiratory Risk in Surgical Patients in Catalonia* (ARISCAT) tool first derived by Canet and colleagues.[12] This index was derived from a study of 2464 patients undergoing a broad variety of surgery types.

PPC outcomes included respiratory infection, respiratory failure, pleural effusion, atelectasis, pneumothorax, bronchospasm, and aspiration pneumonitis. The PPC rate was 5.0% and similar to other published estimates. Median length of stay was four times higher for those with a PPC than those without (12 vs. 3 days, respectively). Mortality at 90 days was 24.4% among patients with a PPC and 1.2% without. This study reconfirmed the morbidity associated with PPCs. After multivariable analysis, seven groupings of risk factors appear in the final risk index (Table 34.3). Risk can be stratified into three categories that effectively discriminate between risk groups. The PPC rates in the validation cohort were low risk (1.6%), intermediate risk (13.3%), and high risk (42.1%). This tool has the potential to become the gold standard multivariable risk index to predict PPCs.

ROLE OF PULMONARY DIAGNOSTIC TESTING

Although the utility of functional and anatomic pulmonary diagnostic testing before lung resection is clear, the value of such testing before nonthoracic surgery is limited. In the vast majority of nonthoracic surgery, preoperative diagnostic testing has the same indications as in the nonsurgical setting.

CHEST RADIOGRAPHY

Essentially all thoracic surgery patients undergo chest radiography due to the nature of their surgical disease. Yet, even in cardiac surgery patients, the value of chest radiographs has been debated. Although half of such studies will be abnormal, the results very rarely change management.[13] For nonthoracic surgery, this dilemma is even more pronounced, with routine preoperative chest radiographs being abnormal in 3–20% of patients and changing management in less than 3%.[14] Based on these data, the American College of Physicians, American College of Surgeons, and American College of Radiology all provided American Board of Internal Medicine Choosing Wisely recommendations to limit the use of preoperative chest radiography in noncardiothoracic surgery.[15] Specifically, the American College of Surgeons and American College of Radiology recommend chest radiography only for patients with evidence of acute cardiopulmonary disease or those older than 70 years with a history of chronic stable cardiopulmonary disease who have not had imaging within 6 months.

PULMONARY FUNCTION TESTING

Spirometry and diffusing capacity measurement are standard for preoperative evaluation of patients scheduled for lung resection. For other procedures, the benefit of these tests is questionable. Although spirometry has long been considered standard before cardiac surgery, it rarely alters management in patients without acute symptoms or changes in known pulmonary disease. Most often, the results of spirometry confirm the risk established by a careful history and physical examination. The Society of Thoracic Surgeons provided American Board of Internal

TABLE 34.3 ARISCAT Multivariable Risk Index for Prediction of Postoperative Pulmonary Complications

	Multivariate Analysis OR (95% CI) (n = 1624*)	β Coefficient	Risk Score†
Age (yr)			
≤50	1		
51–80	1.4 (0.6–3.3)	0.331	3
>80	5.1 (1.9–13.3)	1.619	16
Preoperative SpO$_2$ (%)			
≥96	1		
91–95	2.2 (1.2–4.2)	0.802	8
≤90	10.7 (4.1–28.1)	2.375	24
Respiratory infection in the last month	5.5 (2.6–11.5)	1.698	17
Preoperative anemia (≤10 g/dL)	3.0 (1.4–6.5)	1.105	11
Surgical incision			
Peripheral	1		
Upper abdominal	4.4 (2.3–8.5)	1.480	15
Intrathoracic	11.4 (4.9–26.0)	2.431	24
Duration of surgery (h)			
≤2	1		
>2–3	4.9 (2.4–10.1)	1.593	16
>3	9.7 (4.7–19.9)	2.268	23
Emergency procedure	2.2 (1.0–4.5)	0.768	8

Risk score: low risk, <26 points; intermediate risk, 26–44 points; high risk, ≥45 points.
*Because of a missing value for some variables, three patients were excluded.
†The simplified risk score was the sum of each logistic regression coefficient β multiplied by 10, after rounding off its value.
ARISCAT, Assess Respiratory Risk in Surgical Patients in Catalonia; CI, confidence interval; OR, odds ratio; SpO$_2$, oxyhemoglobin saturation by pulse oximetry breathing air in supine position.
From Canet J, Gallart L, Gomar C, et al. Prediction of postoperative pulmonary complications in a population-based surgical cohort. *Anesthesiology.* 2010;113(6):1338–1350.

Medicine Choosing Wisely recommendations to avoid obtaining routine spirometry on patients scheduled for cardiac surgery without signs or symptoms of new or worsened cardiopulmonary symptoms. In the setting of nonthoracic surgery, abnormal spirometry results have been shown to correlate with PPCs. However, when added to clinical assessment, they do not provide clear additional risk prediction benefit.[5] Thus preoperative pulmonary function testing should be reserved for patients undergoing lung resection or with evidence of acute or worsened cardiopulmonary disease.

For patients undergoing lung resection, please refer to Chapter 30 for details on preoperative diagnostic testing.

OTHER LABORATORY TESTING

Arterial blood gas analysis provides limited value for perioperative management, even before lung resections.[16] Identification of hypercapnia during preoperative evaluation does not substantially alter clinical risk stratification or perioperative management in most patients with chronic lung disease. Patients with hypercapnia at baseline would rarely escape clinical detection. As in the nonoperative setting, obtaining an arterial blood gas to evaluate new or worsened respiratory symptoms is reasonable. For patients with suspected or known untreated sleep apnea, serum bicarbonate may provide useful risk stratification

information. Elevated serum bicarbonate in these patients suggests chronic *carbon dioxide* (CO_2) retention and the presence of obesity hypoventilation syndrome or overlapping obstructive lung disease. The risk of perioperative complications is substantially higher in such patients, and the *Society of Anesthesia and Sleep Medicine* (SASM) recommends delaying nonurgent surgery for further evaluation of suspected sleep apnea with evidence of hypoxemia or CO_2 retention.[17–19]

Some studies have identified an association between PPCs and elevated blood urea nitrogen and low serum albumin.[5] However, the additive prognostic value of these tests in addition to clinical assessment is uncertain.

PREOPERATIVE RISK REDUCTION STRATEGIES

As much as the necessary surgical timeline will allow, clinicians should fully optimize pulmonary function before surgery and delay elective procedures if acute or worsening respiratory problems are present. Furthermore, all medications (except theophylline) used for chronic pulmonary disease are safe to continue through the perioperative period. Providing education to patients and their families about expectations after surgery can improve compliance with postoperative therapies, including lung expansion

TABLE 34.4 Preoperative Interventions for Reduction of Postoperative Pulmonary Complications

Optimization of chronic lung disease

Education about postoperative care

Smoking cessation

Inspiratory muscle training or cardiopulmonary rehabilitation (e.g., prehabilitation)

Oral hygiene

methods. In addition to these basic care methods, other preoperative interventions may also be beneficial in reduction of perioperative pulmonary risk (Table 34.4).

SMOKING CESSATION

Current or recent history of smoking is a risk factor for multiple postoperative complications, including wound infection and respiratory infections (see Chapter 65). Although the risks related to wound infection may be abated with as few as 3 weeks of cessation, available literature suggests that an optimal reduction of PPCs requires cessation for at least 4 to 8 weeks.[20] This is often beyond the timeframe for preoperative planning, but interventions for smoking cessation are still valuable even shortly before surgery. As previously described, these interventions can reduce other perioperative risks. Furthermore, studies have shown that perioperative smoking cessation counseling can increase the chances of long-term abstinence from cigarettes.[21,22] Contrary to older data, recent meta-analyses have found no increased pulmonary risk from quitting smoking less than 4 weeks before surgery, so smoking cessation should be pursued at any stage of the perioperative setting.[20,23]

Similar to the nonsurgical population, strategies for preoperative smoking cessation include behavioral and pharmacologic interventions (see Chapter 66). All perioperative providers should begin with obtaining a complete tobacco use history and then use the "5A's" model for smoking cessation: ask, advise, assess, assist, and arrange.[24] Intensive behavioral counseling, including motivational interviewing, is superior to more moderate methods, but even brief interventions are beneficial.[25,26] Paired with behavioral counseling, nicotine replacement therapy may provide additional benefit in reducing smoking and postoperative complications and does not increase perioperative risks.[25] Varenicline in the perioperative setting has also been associated with increased long-term abstinence and does not increase perioperative risk.[25] The role of electronic cigarettes/vaporized nicotine in perioperative risk remains unknown.

PREHABILITATION

Prehabilitation, the process of improving the patient's physical function *before* surgery, has shown great promise for reducing PPCs. Pulmonary prehabilitation incorporates methods designed to increase inspiratory muscle strength, lung capacity, and mucociliary clearance. In particular, inspiratory muscle training and cardiopulmonary

rehabilitation before major abdominal and cardiac surgery have been associated with significant reductions in PPCs.[27,28] The majority of studies have used inspiratory muscle training for at least 1 to 2 weeks before surgery with use of an inspiratory threshold device, most often with initial instruction from or under the direction of respiratory therapists. Such interventions require significant resources and time, but the potential benefit is substantial: PPCs are reduced by up to 50%, with an absolute risk reduction of 15% and the number needed to treat of 7.[29]

ORAL HYGIENE

Substantial reduction in PPCs can also be achieved by promoting good oral hygiene perioperatively. Several studies of daily oral care (toothbrushing and antigingivitis rinse use) for up to 2 weeks preoperatively found decreased rates of pneumonia in patients undergoing cardiac surgery, lung resection, esophagectomy, and other abdominal procedures.[30–32] Given the minimal cost and lack of adverse effects, good oral hygiene should be encouraged in all surgical patients.

INTRAOPERATIVE RISK REDUCTION STRATEGIES

ANESTHESIA

Although decisions regarding type of anesthesia are fully under the discretion of the anesthetist/anesthesiologist, other care providers should be aware of the impact of different anesthetic approaches on pulmonary physiology. Current literature suggests that general anesthesia contributes to the risk of PPCs.[5,8,33] Conversely, neuraxial (spinal or epidural) anesthesia reduces the risk of postoperative PPCs, even when used in combination with general anesthesia.[8,33,34] As noted above, a recent meta-analysis found an OR of 0.38 (99% confidence interval [CI], 0.36–0.40) for PPCs with neuraxial/regional anesthesia compared to general anesthesia.[33]

NEUROMUSCULAR BLOCKADE

When general anesthesia is used, neuromuscular blockade is an intraoperative management element that impacts the risk of PPCs. Use of *neuromuscular blockade* (NMB) is associated with increased risk of postoperative respiratory failure and pneumonia and should be used only when necessary.[35] When NMB is necessary, we recommend avoidance of long-acting neuromuscular blocking agents (e.g., pancuronium) due to the greater risk for residual NMB and PPCs.[36] Controversy remains over the best methods of prevention of residual NMB, including monitoring neuromuscular recovery and using routine pharmacologic reversal of NMB. Routine reversal of NMB with neostigmine and sugammadex, which act by binding blocking agents, is associated with increased risk. Neostigmine given to patients who have near-complete recovery of neuromuscular function can result in impaired upper airway muscle activity and lead to airway collapse.[37] Sugammadex requires proper dosing based on the determination of the depth of NMB; if underestimated, recurrent NMB may result in respiratory compromise.[37] These issues highlight the importance of effective NMB monitoring. Unfortunately, studies of quantitative NMB monitoring have provided mixed results, and the lack of reliable, easy-to-use technology has impeded its development. Suffice it to say, for patients at increased risk for PPCs, NMB monitoring and reversal are worthy of additional attention by anesthetists/anesthesiologists, and postoperative care providers should be aware of residual NMB as a cause of respiratory failure in the immediate postoperative setting.

MECHANICAL VENTILATION

Intraoperative mechanical ventilation management is also an opportunity for reducing perioperative risk, but much debate on best methods remains. Some studies have suggested that use of lung-protective ventilation reduces the risk of PPCs, whereas others have found no benefit or increased mortality and cardiovascular complications. Significant variability in the methods used in individual studies, including *tidal volume* (VT), *positive end-expiratory pressure* (PEEP), alveolar recruitment maneuvers, and combinations of these elements, has contributed to these conflicting results.

Available data suggest that use of supraphysiologic VT (i.e., ≥10 mL/kg) without other methods, such as "open lung" approaches, including PEEP and alveolar recruitment, to prevent atelectasis, is inferior to provision of near-physiologic VT (i.e., 6–8 mL/kg) with these open lung interventions.[38–40] The two primary concerns for the ventilated patient are barotrauma from excess airway pressure and atelectasis, and achieving the best balance of these opposing negative consequences may be guided by monitoring of airway pressures. One study identified a direct correlation between high airway driving pressure and risk for PPCs, and a large registry study that examined plateau pressures and ventilation strategies found that plateau pressures less than 16 cm H_2O were associated with the lowest risk of PPCs.[41,42] However, a recent interventional trial failed to find an improvement in PPCs with lower driving pressures and higher levels of PEEP.[43] It is reasonable to avoid extremes of VT (<6 or >10 mL/kg), PEEP, and airway pressures, and emphasize open lung techniques, such as PEEP and alveolar recruitment maneuvers, to balance the risks of alveolar collapse, barotrauma, and impaired hemodynamics.

POSTOPERATIVE RISK REDUCTION STRATEGIES

In the postoperative period, the primary focus of pulmonary risk reduction efforts is on prevention and treatment of atelectasis (Table 34.5). Unless required by surgical restrictions, early and frequent patient ambulation decreases PPCs and increases lung expansion.[44] Adequate pain control is important to allow deep breathing to avoid atelectasis. However, opioid and other sedative use should be minimized; use of epidural-based or *patient-controlled analgesia* (PCA)-administered opioids can limit systemic opioid

TABLE 34.5 Postoperative Interventions for Prevention of Postoperative Pulmonary Complications

Early and frequent ambulation/mobilization

Lung expansion maneuvers (cough/deep breathing exercises, IS, IPPB, CPAP)

Adequate pain control

Minimization of systemic opioids (including by the use of nerve blocks, epidural analgesia, and PCA)

Maximization of nonopioid analgesia (acetaminophen, nonsteroidal anti-inflammatory drugs, and application of ice)

CPAP, continuous positive airway pressure ventilation; IPPB, intermittent positive-pressure breathing; IS, incentive spirometry; PCA, patient-controlled analgesia.

exposure and reduce PPCs.[36,45] Nonopioid analgesia should also be maximized with acetaminophen, nonsteroidal anti-inflammatory drugs, and application of ice.

The evidence to support the benefit of other lung expansion methods is mixed. The simplest way to expand the lungs is by cough and deep breathing exercises, but data on effectiveness are limited. Available meta-analyses of incentive spirometry suggest it provides no benefit in preventing PPCs.[46] However, these studies have had a majority of low-risk patients and used mixed methodologies. Incentive spirometry has been incorporated into risk reduction protocols that utilize preoperative education on its use, and these protocols have demonstrated reductions in PPC rates. Intermittent positive-pressure breathing is another option for lung expansion, but it entails additional costs and side effects (abdominal distention) and has not demonstrated better efficacy than incentive spirometry. Intermittent positive-pressure breathing is likely best reserved for patients at high risk for PPCs who are unable or unwilling to comply with incentive spirometry or deep breathing exercises. Stronger efficacy data come from studies of the use of continuous positive airway pressure after abdominal procedures. Application of continuous positive airway pressure immediately after extubation and continued for as little as an hour significantly reduces the incidence of PPCs after major abdominal surgery (OR, 0.37; 95% CI, 0.24–0.56).[47,48]

PERIOPERATIVE RISK REDUCTION PROTOCOLS

Implementation of the above risk reduction measures into perioperative protocols (i.e., bundles) has become increasingly common, and studies of these combined interventions have demonstrated improvement in multiple outcomes, including decreased PPCs. Enhanced recovery programs incorporate several perioperative risk reduction interventions, including smoking cessation, use of regional anesthesia, minimally invasive surgical approaches, goal-directed fluid therapy, opioid-sparing analgesia, and early ambulation, and have demonstrated efficacy in reducing pneumonia and other respiratory complications after multiple types of surgery.[49–54] Other protocols focused on pulmonary risk, including the I COUGH (*i*ncentive spirometry, *c*ough and deep breathing exercises, *o*ral care [brushing teeth and

TABLE 34.6   I COUGH Pulmonary Risk Reduction Protocol

I	Incentive spirometry
C	Cough and deep breathing exercises
O	Oral care (brushing teeth and using mouthwash twice daily)
U	Understanding (patient and family education)
G	Getting out of bed frequently (at least three times daily)
H	Head of bed elevation

Modified from Cassidy MR, Rosenkranz P, McCabe K, Rosen JE, McAneny D. I COUGH: reducing postoperative pulmonary complications with a multidisciplinary patient care program. *JAMA Surg.* 2013;148(8):740–745.

TABLE 34.7   STOP-BANG Questionnaire for Sleep Apnea Risk Assessment

S	Snoring loudly
T	Tired, fatigued, or sleepy during the daytime
O	Observed episodes (by others) of stopped breathing during sleep
P	High blood pressure history or treatment
B	Body mass index > 35 kg/m^2
A	Age > 50 years
N	Neck circumference > 17 inches for a man or > 16 inches for a woman
G	Male gender

Low risk for sleep apnea: yes to 0–2 questions. *Intermediate* risk: yes to 3–4 questions. *High* risk: yes to 5–8 questions.
Modified from University Health Network, www.stopbang.ca.

using mouthwash twice daily], *u*nderstanding [patient and family education], *g*etting out of bed frequently [at least three times daily], *h*ead of bed elevation) perioperative pulmonary care program, have shown similar benefits (Table 34.6).[55]

SLEEP-DISORDERED BREATHING CONSIDERATIONS

Sleep-disordered breathing is an increasingly prevalent condition in the general population. The incidence of moderate or severe OSA has been found to be as high as 40% of surgical patients and is undiagnosed in the majority of patients.[56,57] Patients with OSA have increased risk of multiple complications, including infections, respiratory failure, cardiac events, and mortality.[17,57]

The ASA and SASM have both produced guidelines for the perioperative management of patients with known or suspected sleep apnea.[17,58,59] Both societies recommend using a high-sensitivity tool to screen all surgical patients for the presence of sleep apnea. Several tools are available, including the Flemons, Berlin, and STOP-BANG (*s*noring loudly; *t*ired, fatigued, or sleepy during the daytime; *o*bserved episodes [by others] of stopped breathing during sleep; high blood *p*ressure history or treatment; *b*ody mass index > 35 kg/m^2, *a*ge > 50 years; *n*eck circumference > 17 inches for a man or > 16 inches for a woman; male *g*ender) questionnaires, but the majority of recent literature has focused on STOP-BANG (Table 34.7). Patients with known OSA or an elevated STOP-BANG score are at increased risk for perioperative complications and should receive risk reduction interventions.[17,58] When one counts the number of questions that apply to the patient, the STOP-BANG cutoff score to use for determining high risk with a reasonable balance of sensitivity and specificity is 5 or greater (out of a total of 8).[60,61]

Before surgery in patients with known OSA, clinicians should obtain their previous sleep study reports and document the severity and recommended *positive airway pressure* (PAP) settings.[17] Patients using home PAP therapy should be encouraged to maintain compliance and instructed to bring their device to the hospital for perioperative use.[17] For patients without diagnosed sleep apnea who have high

STOP-BANG scores, SASM does not recommend delaying all surgical procedures for further sleep evaluation.[17] Clinicians should advise patients and the perioperative team of the elevated risks related to potential undiagnosed and untreated sleep apnea and only delay surgery for patients with elevated STOP-BANG scores plus one of the following: uncontrolled or severe systemic disease (e.g., pulmonary hypertension), hypoxemia, or evidence of CO_2 retention (elevated arterial blood CO_2 or serum bicarbonate).[17]

For all patients with known or suspected OSA, a number of intraoperative and postoperative care strategies are recommended to reduce risks related to sleep apnea. The anesthesia team should consider use of regional anesthesia methods and be prepared for a difficult airway.[59] Both intraoperatively and postoperatively, clinicians should use benzodiazepines and opioids with caution and be prepared for variable responses to each.[17,59] After surgery, nonopioid analgesia should be fully utilized, and patients should be kept in a nonsupine position (i.e., head of bed elevated) unless contraindicated by postoperative requirements.[58] Continuous pulse oximetry or capnography during hospitalization is also recommended for all patients with known or suspected sleep apnea for early detection of respiratory insufficiency.[58] Note that continuous pulse oximetry is not sensitive for hypoventilation when the patient is on supplemental oxygen (see Chapter 44).

In ambulatory surgery, special attention to perioperative planning is required for patients with known or suspected OSA. The severity of sleep-disordered breathing is increased perioperatively, and this worsening reaches a peak at 3 days after surgery and persists for up to several days.[62] Thus clinicians need to consider the severity of sleep apnea, intensity of the procedure (depth of anesthesia and duration), and postoperative opioid requirements to determine if alterations in operative and postoperative triage are required. For instance, patients with severe, untreated sleep apnea undergoing a surgery under general anesthesia that will require postoperative opioid treatment may not be good candidates for surgery at an ambulatory surgical center. Surgery at a hospital with appropriate backup mechanisms may be a better choice. Furthermore, some patients with severe sleep apnea undergoing major operations or who will not be able to use PAP after surgery (e.g., some

TABLE 34.8 Predictors of Difficult Endotracheal Intubation

Finding	Sensitivity	Specificity
Inability to bite lower teeth over upper lip (upper lip bite test)	60%	95–96%
Hyomental distance <3 to <5.5 cm	20%	97%
Retrognathia (mandible length < 9 cm)	19%	98%
Decreased neck range of motion	28%	93%
Interincisor gap <2 to 5 cm	36%	90%
Mallampati class III or IV airway	55%	87%
Thyromental distance <4 to <7 cm	45%	86%

Data from Detsky ME, Jivraj N, Adhikari NK, et al. Will this patient be difficult to intubate? The rational clinical examination systematic review. *JAMA*. 2019;321(5):493–503.

ear, nose, and throat and ophthalmologic procedures) may benefit from hospital admission rather than discharge on the same day as surgery.

AIRWAY MANAGEMENT CONSIDERATIONS

Like anesthesia selection and administration, intraoperative airway management is the primary responsibility of the anesthetist/anesthesiologist, but recognition of airway abnormalities and challenges by other perioperative care providers is still essential to provide the anesthesiology team with advance warning. For endotracheal intubation, several different tools have been studied for the prediction of difficulty (Table 34.8). No single tool is sufficiently sensitive and specific to rule in or rule out a challenging intubation; most experts recommend using a combination of these anatomic markers and tests.

For mask ventilation, several factors have been found to be predictors of difficulty, including age 45 years or older, male gender, elevated body mass index, previous difficult intubation, decreased thyromental distance, Mallampati class III or IV, full beard, snoring, sleep apnea, and neck radiation skin changes.[63] Similarly, detection of a combination of more than one of these is most suggestive of increased risk.

Key Points

- Postoperative pulmonary complications are morbid and increase length of stay, the potential for intensive care unit transfer, and mortality.
- Patient-related factors are known to increase risk of postoperative pulmonary complications. The most important patient-related risk factors are age older than 50 years, American Society of Anesthesiologists class greater than 2, and functional dependence.
- Procedure-related risk factors are more important than patient-related risk factors. Surgical site is the single most important predictor, and the highest risk surgeries include aortic, thoracic/esophageal, and upper abdominal.

- Multifactorial risk indices exist to predict postoperative pulmonary complications. Among these, we recommend the Assess Respiratory Risk in Surgical Patients in Catalonia (ARISCAT) tool.
- Preoperative pulmonary diagnostic testing, including chest radiography, spirometry, and blood gas analysis, rarely adds to risk stratification and management.
- Preoperative pulmonary risk reduction methods include optimization of chronic lung disease, patient education, smoking cessation, inspiratory muscle training, and oral hygiene promotion.
- Intraoperative risk reduction methods include use of neuraxial (spinal or epidural) anesthesia, lung-protective mechanical ventilation, and judicious use of neuromuscular blockade.
- Postoperative pulmonary risk reduction methods include early mobilization, lung expansion modalities (e.g., cough/deep breathing exercises, incentive spirometry, intermittent positive-pressure breathing, and continuous positive airway pressure), and adequate pain control with minimization of systemic opioids and sedatives and maximization of nonopioid analgesia.
- Obstructive sleep apnea is a significant risk factor for postoperative complications. Patients with high risk on screening for obstructive sleep apnea should be counseled on their risks and, if they have evidence of uncontrolled or severe systemic disease, hypoxemia, or carbon dioxide retention, delay of nonurgent surgery for further sleep medicine evaluation should be considered.

Key Readings

Brunelli A, Kim AW, Berger KI, Addrizzo-Harris DJ. Physiologic evaluation of the patient with lung cancer being considered for resectional surgery: diagnosis and management of lung cancer, 3rd ed: American College of Chest Physicians evidence-based clinical practice guidelines. *Chest*. 2013;143(suppl 5):e166S–e190S.

Canet J, Gallart L, Gomar C, et al. Prediction of postoperative pulmonary complications in a population based surgical cohort. *Anesthesiology*. 2010;113(6):1338–1350.

Chung F, Memtsoudis SG, Ramachandran SK, et al. Society of Anesthesia and Sleep Medicine guidelines on preoperative screening and assessment of adult patients with obstructive sleep apnea. *Anesth Analg*. 2016;123(2):452–473.

Detsky ME, Jivraj N, Adhikari NK, et al. Will this patient be difficult to intubate? The rational clinical examination systematic review. *JAMA*. 2019;321(5):493–503.

Fernandez-Bustamante A, Frendl G, Sprung J, et al. Postoperative pulmonary complications, early mortality, and hospital stay following noncardiothoracic surgery: a multicenter study by the Perioperative Research Network investigators. *JAMA Surg*. 2017;152(2):157–166.

Katsura M, Kuriyama A, Takeshima T, Fukuhara S, Furukawa TA. Preoperative inspiratory muscle training for postoperative pulmonary complications in adults undergoing cardiac and major abdominal surgery. *Cochrane Database Syst Rev*. 2015;(10):CD010356.

Lawrence VA, Cornell JE, Smetana GW. Strategies to reduce postoperative pulmonary complications after noncardiothoracic surgery: systematic review for the American College of Physicians strategies to reduce postoperative pulmonary complications after noncardiothoracic surgery. *Ann Intern Med*. 2006;144(8):596–608.

Smetana GW, Lawrence VA, Cornell JE. Preoperative pulmonary risk stratification for noncardiothoracic surgery: systematic review for the American College of Physicians. *Ann Intern Med*. 2006;144(8):581–595.

Wong J, Lam DP, Abrishami A, Chan MTV, Chung F. Short-term preoperative smoking cessation and postoperative complications: a systematic review and meta-analysis. *Can J Anesth*. 2012;59(3):268–279.

Complete reference list available at ExpertConsult.com.

EVALUATION OF RESPIRATORY IMPAIRMENT AND DISABILITY

ANNYCE S. MAYER, MD, MSPH • LISA A. MAIER, MD, MSPH, FCCP

INTRODUCTION

Respiratory impairment refers to an alteration in lung structure and/or lung function that results in decreased or limited functional ability and is usually manifested by dyspnea on exertion. Many respiratory diseases may cause impairment, from airway disease such as asthma and COPD to interstitial lung diseases. A pulmonary physician may be asked to evaluate impairment and/or disability, either for his or her own patients or for others in the context of an independent medical examination through a benefits or compensation program and/or to provide a statement about ability to work.

This chapter reviews the elements of an impairment evaluation. An overview of the major programs in the United States is presented. Impairment ratings are described using the framework for the assessment of respiratory impairment set forth by the *American Thoracic Society* (ATS)[1,2] along with an overview of the most commonly used impairment rating methodology contained in the *American Medical Association [AMA] Guides to the Evaluation of Permanent Impairment*, hereafter referred to as the *AMA Guides*. However, the *AMA Guides* are not used by every benefit and compensation system. The evaluating physician must understand and follow the rules and specific requirements of the program under which the patient is being evaluated. The final determination on the award is usually made by personnel in the program or a judge, but the thoroughness of the medical report and its consistency with the program requirements will increase the weight given to the physician's medical opinion. Finally, an overview of workplace protections for workers with lung disease is covered.

Program details, including how impairment and/or disability is determined under specific programs, are available at ExpertConsult.com.

Additional relevant information about specific diseases can be obtained in other chapters, including Chapters 91, 100, 101, 102, and 103.

DEFINITIONS

There is a critical distinction between the terms *impairment* and *disability*. The terms *impairment* and *disability* are often used interchangeably, perhaps made more confusing by the fact that different benefits and compensation programs may use both terms but focus on one more than the other. *Impairment* takes place at the organ or organ system level. *Whole-person impairment* refers to the loss relative to the functioning of the body as a whole. *Disability*, in contrast, refers to the person in terms of limitation in the ability to perform normal activities, including personal, social, and work activities.

Physicians should understand that such determinations are medicolegal decisions that can have additional ramifications for the patient beyond that of providing a diagnosis. The physician may be asked to address causation (i.e., opine on whether the respiratory condition was caused or at least aggravated by a certain factor, most commonly work, on a more-likely-than-not basis).

Although the terms "impairment" and "disability" are related, it is important that each term be applied in accordance with its precise definition. The definitions used in most existing benefits and compensation programs in the United States are based on the *World Health Organization's* [WHO] *International Classification of Impairment, Disability, and Handicap* (ICIDH) model from 1980.[3] This model was replaced by the *International Classification of Functioning, Disability, and Health* (ICF)[4] in 2001, which uses different definitions of these words. Because these programs have not been updated to incorporate the ICF definitions, the definitions from the ICIDH are presented here to avoid confusion. The ICF model is presented in the "Future Directions" section.

IMPAIRMENT

Impairment refers to the degree of loss of normal use or function of a body part or organ. It is defined by the WHO as "any loss or abnormality of psychological, physiologic, or anatomic structure or function."[3] It is defined by the AMA as "a loss, loss of use, or derangement of any body part, organ system or organ function."[5]

The essential elements that make up an impairment evaluation will vary to some degree according to the program or system through which the evaluation is being performed. Standard components typically include history, with occupational and environmental history and description of limitations in *activities of daily living* (ADLs), physical examination, and review of medical records and diagnostic test results that establish the respiratory condition.

Although *pulmonary function test* (PFT) results are the primary factor that determines the presence and degree of pulmonary impairment, some systems will specify that particular tests should be used for assessment of impairment or disability, whereas others allow physician discretion in choosing another test if he or she believes it to be a more accurate reflection of the patient's true respiratory impairment. Some programs only allow physicians with certain qualifications to perform impairment ratings. Before a physician can determine that a condition has resulted in permanent impairment or disability, the diagnosis should be well defined, the condition stable, and medical treatment either optimized or reasonable options exhausted. When these criteria are met, this point is termed *maximum medical improvement* (MMI).

DISABILITY

Disability refers to any resulting alteration in the individual's capacity to perform customary activities. It was defined by the WHO as "any restriction or lack of ability to perform any activity within the range considered normal for a human being."[3] The AMA defined *disability* as an "alteration of an individual's capacity to meet or perform personal, social, or occupational demands or statutory or regulatory requirements because of an impairment."[5]

Although the degree of impairment frequently correlates with the degree of disability, this is not always the case. The classic example of this is the loss of the fifth finger of the nondominant hand. Under the typical impairment rating system, the loss of this finger would be associated with a small impairment of the whole person. For the average person, this small impairment would result in a correspondingly small disability. For a concert pianist, this small impairment would be associated with significant disability, particularly in the context of work activities.

ADDITIONAL TERMS

Temporary impairment refers to impairment that exists only for a limited period of time after an injury or illness.

Temporary disability insurance covers partial compensation for loss of wages due to a *non–work-related* injury or illness. For *work-related* injuries and illness, partial compensation for lost wages, as well as medical benefits, are covered by workers' compensation.

Permanent impairment can be assessed only once the patient has reached MMI. MMI is defined in the *AMA Guides*, Sixth Edition,[6] as the "point in time in the recovery process…when further formal medical or surgical intervention cannot be expected to improve the underlying impairment" and "symptoms can be expected to remain stable with the passage of time, or can be managed with palliative measures that do not alter the underlying impairment substantially." This is termed "permanent and stationary" in some systems.

Whole-person impairment refers to the alteration in the functioning of the body as a whole and therefore can range from 0% (no impairment) to 100% (essential cessation of all body functions).

Permanent partial impairment is the numeric percentage of the loss of body functioning due to the loss or limited functioning of the affected organ system(s). For most respiratory conditions, the primary organ involved is the lung, but it can include the pulmonary arteries or nose and throat.

Permanent total disability is the medicolegal determination that a person's impairment precludes future gainful employment.

Handicap refers to the societal disadvantage caused by an impairment or disability. It was defined by the WHO in the ICIDH model as "a disadvantage for a given individual that limits or prevents fulfillment of that person's normal role depending on sex, age, social and cultural factors."[3]

CLINICAL APPROACH TO IMPAIRMENT EVALUATIONS

Although the term *impairment rating* is sometimes used interchangeably with the term *impairment evaluation*, the impairment rating itself is but a small part of what should be a comprehensive medical evaluation[7] (Table 35.1). The physician must first fully understand the purpose and requirements of the program for which the evaluation is being conducted. The initial goal of the impairment evaluation should be to confirm the medical diagnosis,[2] through a thorough, detailed patient history, physical examination, and review of diagnostic testing results that established

Table 35.1   Components of a Respiratory Impairment Evaluation

1. Clear understanding of the rules and specific requirements of the program under which the individual is being evaluated.
2. Complete medical history
   a. Complete occupational and environmental exposure history
   b. Limitations in activities of daily living
3. Physical examination
4. Diagnostic testing
   a. Tests that establish the diagnosis
   b. Tests that identify extrapulmonary conditions contributing to impairment
   c. Results used in the assessment of impairment
      i. Pulmonary function tests
         A. Spirometry
         B. Single-breath diffusing capacity (DL_{CO})
      ii. Cardiopulmonary exercise test (when indicated)
      iii. Arterial blood gas measurement (when indicated)
5. Diagnosis
   a. Assessment of causation, usually relationship to work (when indicated)
6. Impairment assessment
   a. Statement of maximum medical improvement
   b. Impairment rating
   c. Ability to work/work restrictions (when indicated)
   d. Apportionment (if requested)
   e. Future medical treatment

the diagnosis. The diagnosis or diagnoses should be clearly stated, along with extrapulmonary conditions that may be contributory to symptoms, limitations in ADLs, and/or impairment. There should also be a review of the treatment and an opinion on MMI. Factors important to the impairment rating itself include items from history, physical examination, and diagnostic testing results that reflect disease severity, including impact on normal ADLs,[5] and current treatment requirements. The physician may be asked to make a statement on causation or apportionment. An outline of reasonably anticipated future medical course and treatment requirements should be given. The following sections describe the various aspects of an impairment evaluation, including the history to be taken, the examination to be conducted, and the testing to be obtained depending on the diagnosis considered and the type of evaluation being performed.

HISTORY

The *history of present illness* (HPI) is the standard, detailed respiratory history used by most pulmonologists, including symptoms of cough, cough with phlegm, wheeze, chest tightness, and shortness of breath. If present, details should be provided that include when the symptom started, exacerbating and alleviating factors along with temporal relationship, progression over time, and current status including frequency, severity, and response to any medication. A scale for the rating of dyspnea is suggested in the *AMA Guides*, based on the Epidemiology Standardization Project,[8] which also provides standardized questions for the assessment of other symptoms. Questions about conditions such as chronic rhinitis, postnasal drip, gastroesophageal reflux disease, cardiac disease, and other lung diseases, including smoking- and vaping-related lung disease, may help the physician understand other possible contributors

to respiratory symptoms. Although dyspnea is the primary limiting symptom of respiratory impairment, dyspnea can also result from extrapulmonary causes including cardiovascular disease, obesity, and deconditioning. Frequency, severity, treatment requirements, and duration of periodic exacerbations of diseases such as asthma and bronchiectasis should be well documented. Medications used or tried in the past for the treatment of the respiratory conditions should be described, along with a description of the relief afforded.

Constitutional symptoms are relevant in the HPI in patients with certain diseases, such as fever, sweats, chills, and fatigue in patients with hypersensitivity pneumonitis; chest pain, weight loss, and malaise in patients with asbestos-related lung disease; and night sweats and fatigue in patients with chronic beryllium disease.

A standard detailed past medical and surgical history, list of medications and allergies, family history, and review of systems will provide a good understanding of the patient as a whole. It will also allow the physician to identify other possible diseases that may be contributory to the patient's current status, as well as to assess potential treatment-related side effects. The standard social history should include smoking history, including amount, duration, and current smoking status, as well as a history of vaping or drug use.

An element that may be new to most pulmonologists is the need to obtain a detailed occupational and environmental history. This is necessary to help the physician address whether there is a relationship between a respiratory condition and past or ongoing workplace exposures. The occupational history is most easily performed in chronological order starting from childhood. Details about the period of time spent at each job, the job title, description of the work performed, and details about jobs or processes that may have produced dust, fumes, gas, or smoke should be described, including estimation of intensity, frequency, and duration of exposure. Questions about ventilation and use of respiratory protection can provide helpful clues, as well as whether any immediate symptoms were noted. Chemical exposures, particularly any heavy exposures or exposures that resulted in symptoms, should be detailed. If available, the *Safety Data Sheet* (SDS), formerly called the Material Safety Data Sheet, may be reviewed because it can provide helpful information on the components of the chemicals used in the workplace and potential associated health effects. Unfortunately, SDSs are not required to provide complete information, and thus some are more reliable than others.

An environmental history including questions about heating, cooling, and humidification sources; pets, including birds; hot tubs; water-damaged areas; and exposures from hobbies should also be obtained to determine whether there is a relationship between the disease and any environmental exposures.

In addition, the history should also include a description of how the condition affects the person's ability to perform normal ADLs. Questions most relevant to patients with pulmonary disease include ability to perform basic self-care such as showering; ability to walk, including estimated distance at own pace and at a fast pace or up a hill, estimated pace compared with others one's own age, and number of flights of stairs that can be climbed; and ability to perform indoor and outdoor home maintenance chores, as well as customary hobby, exercise, and job-related activities. A number of standardized methods can assess ability to perform ADLs, some of which are disease specific. A list of ADLs suitable for all conditions is outlined in the *AMA Guides*.[5,9] Symptoms and limitations in ADLs consistent with the lung disease and objective testing data provide useful supporting information for the impairment rating. Dyspnea scales are often used and can be a helpful way to summarize the relative degree of symptomatology or activity limitation.[8] However, the degree to which dyspnea correlates with objective measures of pulmonary function and exercise performance is variable.[10–13]

PHYSICAL EXAMINATION

A complete physical examination should be performed, with focus on the respiratory and cardiovascular systems.[2,7] A detailed description of the chest should be made, including any deformities or scars, abnormal motion, respiratory rate and effort, breath sounds, and percussion, which can help support the diagnosis. Vital signs should be documented including blood pressure and heart rate, which may affect ability to perform pulmonary function and exercise tests, as well as height and weight, because obesity can cause PFT and exercise test abnormalities and contribute to pulmonary symptoms. Signs of hypoxemia, such as cyanosis and clubbing, should be documented. Signs of right heart failure, such as jugular venous distention, right ventricular heave, and liver engorgement, and peripheral edema provide evidence of severe respiratory impairment in patients with respiratory disease.[2]

DIAGNOSIS, CAUSATION, AND MAXIMUM MEDICAL IMPROVEMENT

Any available or provided medical records should be summarized, with focus on the results of the diagnostic testing that help establish the diagnosis and/or severity of the condition. Medicolegal cases may often involve the review and summarization of large volumes of records. Some independent medical examinations require that only the records provided through the program be reviewed.

The list of medical diagnoses should start with the diagnosis of the condition for which the patient is being evaluated, including disease severity. The diagnosis of asthma associated with workplace exposures may fall under one of three different diagnoses: occupational asthma (new-onset asthma caused by a workplace exposure), work-aggravated asthma (existing asthma aggravated by a workplace exposure), and *reactive airways dysfunction syndrome* (RADS), which can result from a single high-level irritant exposure (see Chapter 100). Other diagnoses that may be contributory to symptoms, limitations in ADLs, or testing abnormalities should be clearly delineated.

If relevant, the diagnosis should also include a statement on *causation*, the physician's opinion as to whether or not a given workplace exposure has caused or aggravated an illness. This is a medicolegal determination, also known as *attribution*, made on a medically probable basis (i.e., "more-likely-than-not"). That is, the physician can opine with greater than 50% certainty that the exposure(s) in the

workplace caused the respiratory condition or worsened an underlying condition on the basis of objective criteria, such as change in treatment requirements. This criterion is less rigorous than that required for scientific proof of a hypothesis (i.e., 95% certainty). This is important because, in cases of respiratory illness, there may be multifactorial causation, frequently a long latency between initial exposure and clinical onset of disease, nonspecific clinical manifestations, incomplete understanding of dose-response relationships from epidemiologic studies, and lack of individual exposure data. Although recognition of these limitations is necessary, causation can be attributed in most cases on a more-probable-than-not basis by applying reasonable judgment. This process is easier when the exposure is known, the dose-response relationship is well characterized, and competing diagnoses are unlikely. The physician should clearly describe the specific substances at the workplace; their known health effects according to the medical literature; the relative dose, based on estimated intensity, frequency, and/or duration of exposure; and finally, why it is medically probable that the exposure(s) caused or resulted in permanent aggravation of the diagnosed medical condition in this worker. When one or more of these conditions are not met, attribution should be based on the answers to the following questions.

- Is the diagnosis clearly established, and is it biologically plausible (or consistent with the available epidemiologic data) that the disease could have been caused or aggravated by the exposure in question?
- Have competing diagnoses been adequately considered?
- Is the exposure of sufficient intensity and duration to have caused or aggravated the disease?
- Has there been an adequately long latent period, or is there a temporal relationship between onset of exposure and clinical manifestation of disease?

When the examining physician believes the diagnosis is in question, or the condition is not stable, or the condition may improve with additional treatment, this should be stated, along with recommendations for what is needed to address these issues. If the conditions for MMI are met, a statement of MMI is indicated, and it is appropriate to consider whether there is permanent impairment. What happens logistically following determination of the MMI will depend on the specific program. The examining physician should be aware of the ramifications of making these medicolegal determinations. For example, in workers' compensation systems, determination of MMI allows the worker to be awarded permanent impairment but will also result in the cessation of temporary benefits such as compensation for lost wages, as the case is closed by the workers' compensation insurance company.

GUIDES TO RESPIRATORY IMPAIRMENT RATINGS

AMERICAN THORACIC SOCIETY GUIDELINES FOR EVALUATION OF IMPAIRMENT OR DISABILITY

Many systems have been used to determine respiratory impairment. Most base impairment primarily on lung function. In their "Guidelines for the Evaluation of Impairment/

Table 35.2 American Thoracic Society Impairment Categories, With Corresponding Description of Ability to Perform Job Demands

Category	Criteria	Ability to Perform Job Demands
Normal	FVC ≥ 80% of predicted *and* FEV$_1$ ≥ 80% of predicted *and* FEV$_1$/FVC×100 ≥ 75% *and* DL$_{CO}$ ≥ 80% of predicted	
Mildly impaired	FVC 60–79% of predicted *or* FEV$_1$ 60–79% of predicted *or* FEV$_1$/FVC×100 60–74% *or* DL$_{CO}$ 60–79% of predicted	Usually not correlated with diminished ability to perform most jobs
Moderately impaired	FVC 51–59% of predicted *or* FEV$_1$ 41–59% of predicted *or* FEV$_1$/FVC×100 41–59% *or* DL$_{CO}$ 41–59% of predicted	Progressively lower levels of lung function correlated with diminishing ability to meet the physical demands of many jobs
Severely impaired	FVC ≤ 50% of predicted *or* FEV$_1$ ≤ 40% of predicted *or* FEV$_1$/FVC×100 ≤ 40% *or* DL$_{CO}$ ≤ 40% of predicted	Unable to meet the physical demands of most jobs, including travel to work

DL$_{CO}$, single-breath carbon monoxide diffusing capacity; FEV$_1$, forced expiratory volume in 1 second; FVC, forced vital capacity.
From American Thoracic Society (ATS). Evaluation of impairment/disability secondary to respiratory disorders. *Am Rev Respir Dis.* 1986;133:1205-1209.

Disability Secondary to Respiratory Disorders," the ATS recommends that impairment due to most lung diseases be rated on the basis of PFT results.[2] PFT is described in detail in Chapters 31 and 32. The results of the ATS impairment system, based on PFTs, place individuals into four impairment categories. Each of these categories provides a corresponding description of the associated ability to perform job demands (Table 35.2). The ATS did not include a system by which to assign an associated numerically derived percentage of whole-person impairment, on which monetary awards are typically based. Therefore, the ATS guidelines did not lend themselves to use in most compensation systems.

AMERICAN MEDICAL ASSOCIATION GUIDES TO THE EVALUATION OF PERMANENT IMPAIRMENT

The *AMA Guides,* Fifth Edition, adapted the ATS Guidelines into a formula by adding a system through which to assign a numerically derived percentage of whole-person impairment within each of the four impairment classes.[14] Although the *AMA Guides,* Fifth Edition, is no longer the most current edition, the methodology is presented here because it is directly based on ATS Guidelines and because not all compensation systems have adopted the Sixth Edition. The *AMA Guides,* Fifth Edition, assigned the following associated ranges of whole-person respiratory impairment to each of the four ATS classes: class 1 impairment, 0%; class 2 (mild), 10–25%; class 3 (moderate), 26–50%; and class 4 (severe), 51–100% whole-person impairment. After determining the class of impairment based on *forced vital capacity* (FVC), *forced expiratory volume in 1 second* (FEV$_1$), FEV$_1$/FVC, *single-breath diffusing capacity* (DL$_{CO}$), or *maximal oxygen consumption* ($\dot{V}O_{2max}$), the physician determines the final numeric percentage of whole-person impairment on the basis of where the test results fall within that range of impairment as well as other factors, including impact of the respiratory condition on the ability to perform ADLs.

The *AMA Guides,* Sixth Edition, adopts a different methodology, defining four classes of impairment: class 0, 0%; class 1 (minimal), 2–10%; class 2 (mild), 11–23%; class 3 (moderate), 24–40%; and class 4 (severe), 45–65% whole-person impairment.[15] The key factor is the objective test data, FVC, FEV$_1$, FEV$_1$/FVC, and DL$_{CO}$, using the measurement most relevant to the disease process.[15] $\dot{V}O_{2max}$ may be considered as the key factor if one of the

other pulmonary function test results is abnormal. The specific value within the impairment class is determined by the physical examination findings, dyspnea, and treatment requirements. The maximum whole-person impairment in the *AMA Guides,* Sixth Edition, for most respiratory disorders is 65% whole-person impairment, rather than 100% whole-person impairment in previous editions, although this rating may still be combined with impairment in other organ systems.

Because a person can never have more than 100% impairment of the body, impairment in any additional organ system needs to be combined rather than added to the respiratory impairment. Each edition of the *AMA Guides* contains a special combining table for this purpose.

CLASSIFICATION OF IMPAIRMENT RESULTING FROM SPECIFIC PULMONARY DISEASES

Regardless of the rating system used, the greatest weight should be placed on objective data.

Asthma

For diagnosis and management of asthma, see Chapter 62. Rating asthma according to the standard respiratory disorder methodology can both underestimate and overestimate impairment, given the episodic and variable nature of airflow limitation and bronchial hyperresponsiveness.[16] The ATS developed "Guidelines for the Evaluation of Impairment/Disability in Patients with Asthma" in 1993 to reflect the true impairment due to this condition.[1] First, a worker with objectively confirmed asthma must be determined to be at MMI and to have achieved optimal therapeutic goals (i.e., minimum medication required and optimal time to allow medication effect).[15] To rate asthma impairment according to ATS methodology (Table 35.3), the postbronchodilator FEV$_1$, reversibility (% change with bronchodilator), or methacholine challenge results (provocative concentration of methacholine inducing a 20% drop in FEV$_1$ [PC$_{20}$ in mg/mL]), and minimum medications required to maintain this status are assigned scores using Table 35.3 parts A–C. The class of impairment is defined by the sum of the asthma scores based on Table 35.3 part D. The *AMA Guides,* Fifth Edition, adopted this ATS methodology and assigned a numeric range of whole-person impairment for each impairment class, which is equivalent to the

Table 35.3 American Thoracic Society Impairment Rating Guidelines for Asthma

A. POSTBRONCHODILATOR FEV$_1$

Score	FEV$_1$ (% Predicted)
0	> lower limit of normal
1	70–lower limit of normal
2	60–69
3	50–59
4	<50

B. REVERSIBILITY OF FEV$_1$ OR DEGREE OF AIRWAY HYPERRESPONSIVENESS*

Score	% FEV$_1$ Change	PC$_{20}$ (mg/mL or Equivalent)
0	<10	>8
1	10–19	8– >0.5
2	20–29	0.5– >0.125
3	≥30	≤0.125
4	—	—

C. MINIMUM MEDICATION NEED†

Score	Medication
0	No medication
1	Occasional bronchodilator, not daily, and/or occasional cromolyn,‡ not daily
2	Daily bronchodilator and/or daily cromolyn‡ and/or daily low-dose inhaled steroid (<800 µg beclomethasone or equivalent)
3	Bronchodilator on demand and daily high-dose inhaled steroid (>800 µg beclomethasone or equivalent) or occasional course (1–3/year) systemic steroid
4	Bronchodilator on demand and daily high-dose inhaled steroid (>1000 µg beclomethasone or equivalent) and daily systemic steroid

D. SUMMARY OF IMPAIRMENT RATING CLASSES§

Impairment Class	Total Score
0	0
I	1–3
II	4–6
III	7–9
IV	10–11
V	Asthma not controlled despite maximal treatment (i.e., FEV$_1$ remaining < 50% despite use of ≥20 mg prednisone/day)

*When FEV$_1$ is above the lower limit of normal, the PC$_{20}$ value should be determined and used for rating of impairment; when FEV$_1$ is < 70% predicted, the degree of reversibility should be used; when FEV$_1$ is between 70% predicted and the lower limit of normal, either reversibility or the PC$_{20}$ can be used. Reversibility with bronchodilator is calculated as:

$$\frac{FEV_1\ postbronchodilator - FEV_1\ prebronchodilator}{FEV_1\ prebronchodilator} \times 100\%$$

Airway responsiveness is expressed as that concentration of bronchoconstrictor agents that will provoke a fall in FEV$_1$ of 20% from the lowest postsaline value. Plot the concentration of methacholine or histamine against the fall in FEV$_1$ using a logarithm scale for the doubling concentrations. The PC$_{20}$ is obtained by interpolation between the last two points. The formula for linear interpolation of the PC$_{20}$ from the log dose response curve is as follows:

$$PC_{20} = antilog\ C1 + \frac{(\log C2 - \log C1)(20 - R1)}{(R2 - R1)}$$

where *C1* is the second last concentration (<20% FEV$_1$ fall), *C2* is the last concentration (>20% FEV$_1$ fall), *R1* is the percentage fall FEV$_1$ after C1, and *R2* is the percentage fall FEV$_1$ after C2.
†The need for minimum medication should be demonstrated by the treating physician, e.g., previous records of exacerbation when medications have been reduced.
‡Very limited current use.
§The impairment rating is calculated as the sum of the patient's scores from parts A, B, and C.
From the American Thoracic Society, Medical Section of the American Lung Association. Guidelines for the evaluation of impairment/disability in patients with asthma. *Am Rev Respir Dis.* 1993;147:1056-1061.

impairment assigned for general respiratory conditions.[14] Additionally, the ATS added a fifth class of impairment, defined as asthma not controlled despite maximal treatment (i.e., FEV_1 remaining <50% despite use of ≥20 mg of prednisone daily). The *AMA Guides*, Sixth Edition, additionally recommends that an impairment rating be performed after the patient has achieved optimal therapeutic goals, and that it is prudent to wait at least 2 years after diagnosis and removal from exposure in cases of occupational asthma.[15] If a physician determines that the MMI has been achieved for a patient before then, the report should clearly detail the rationale behind the departure from the 2-year time period. PC_{20} is used as the primary "key factor" by which the class of asthma impairment is determined. Although postbronchodilator FEV_1 may be used as an alternative, there is impairment only if the maximum postbronchodilator FEV_1 is 80% or greater than predicted, which will afford no impairment for the patient with complete reversibility. Minimum medication requirements and frequency of attacks are used to determine the specific numeric rating within the class.[15]

Bronchiectasis (See Chapter 69)

Rating conditions such as bronchiectasis by standard pulmonary function testing methods can underestimate impairment because recurrent episodes of infection and inflammation cause intermittent respiratory symptoms, respiratory dysfunction, and limitations in ADLs, often with normal lung function in between episodes. The *AMA Guides*, Fifth Edition, acknowledge that this method will be applicable only in "limited cases," but they allow the physician to assign a rating on the basis of the extent and severity of these episodes and their impact on ADLs, with objective supporting evidence documented.[14] The *AMA Guides*, Sixth Edition, does not delineate a specific methodology for this condition.[15]

Sleep Disorders (See Chapters 117–122)

Sleep disorders are recognized in the *AMA Guides*, Sixth Edition, as a condition that may cause impairment not well estimated by standard pulmonary function testing or exercise testing.[15] Both the *AMA Guides*, Fifth and Sixth Editions, describe the importance of obtaining sleep testing in an accredited laboratory, and grading severity based on the number of apnea and hypopnea episodes observed during polysomnography and the severity of hypoxemia.[14,15] However, there are no standardized, well-documented criteria for determining level of impairment. Treatment, weight loss, and repeat polysomnography is recommended prior to impairment rating, which should be performed by a sleep specialist. The *AMA Guides*, Sixth Edition, specifies that the rating should not exceed 3% whole-person impairment; however, additional impairment may be assigned for secondary conditions, such as right heart failure and polycythemia.

Lung Cancer (See Chapters 76 and 77)

The *AMA Guides*, Fifth and Sixth Editions, recommend one of two methods be used for rating permanent impairment due to lung cancer.[14,15] All individuals with lung cancer are considered severely impaired at the time of diagnosis. At 1 year after diagnosis, if there is still evidence of tumor or tumor recurrence, the person is considered to be severely

impaired. If there is no residual tumor or recurrence, the impairment rating is performed according to the standard rating methodology for respiratory diseases.

Diseases of the Pulmonary Arteries

For discussion of disorders of the pulmonary vascular bed, see Chapters 81 through 88. Diseases rated by this methodology include pulmonary artery hypertension, right heart failure, and pulmonary emboli. In the *AMA Guides*, Fifth Edition,[17] the rating is determined by the presence or absence of physical examination signs (right ventricular heave, increased pulmonic component [P_2] of the second heart sound [S_2], peripheral edema) and symptoms of right heart failure (dyspnea), as well as the observed elevated *pulmonary artery pressure* (PAP). In the *AMA Guides*, Sixth Edition,[9] the objective findings, including PAP, B-type natriuretic peptide, and $\dot{V}O_{2max}$, are the key factors that determine the class of impairment. The specific percentage assigned within the class is determined by history (dyspnea and activity limitations) and physical examination findings (signs of right heart failure).

Conditions of the Upper and Lower Airways (See Chapters 70 and 71)

The *AMA Guides*, Fifth Edition,[18] contain methodology by which to assign impairment due to physical obstruction or scarring of the upper airway, larynx, trachea, and/or bronchi, based on degree and location(s) of the obstruction, nature of the activities that trigger dyspnea, as well as need for ventilation. The *AMA Guides*, Sixth Edition, uses the nature of the activities that trigger dyspnea as the key factor in determining impairment class, and physical examination findings and objective test results, such as sinus computed tomography or findings on laryngoscopy, in determining the final numeric rating.[19] There are also methods for the rating of voice/speech impairment based on audibility, intelligibility, and functional efficiency in the *AMA Guides*, Fifth Edition. These factors are also used to define the key factor for impairment class in the *AMA Guides*, Sixth Edition, as well as consideration of strobovideolaryngoscopy, objective voice and speech measures, and Voice Handicap Index. It is important to note that there are differences in what defines impairment within a given class in the two editions. Impairment related to bronchiectasis is described above.

ROLE OF DIAGNOSTIC TEST RESULTS IN IMPAIRMENT RATINGS

RADIOGRAPHIC DATA

Documentation of chest radiograph or *computed tomography* (CT) scan abnormalities consistent with the lung disorder is frequently required to establish evidence of disease, particularly for diseases such as pneumoconiosis. The chest imaging findings may correlate poorly with the physiologic findings, especially in patients with obstructive lung disease.

Some programs require that chest radiographs be read by a *National Institute of Occupational Safety and Health*

(NIOSH)-certified B Reader and classified according to the *International Labour Organization* (ILO) classification system.[20] This radiographic interpretation system was devised in an attempt to report the presence, appearance, and extent of radiographic changes consistent with pleural and parenchymal evidence of pneumoconiosis in an objective and consistent manner. Chest radiographic findings of opacities with an ILO profusion score of at least 1/0 are "consistent with" asbestosis and are accepted for compensation purposes by programs such as the Department of Labor for that condition. If the opacities are small and irregular (classified as "s" and "t") and are found predominantly in the middle and lower lobes or are found in conjunction with pleural plaques, these findings are highly consistent with a diagnosis of asbestosis.

Whereas the ILO interpretation may help raise suspicion of pneumoconiosis or provide sufficient evidence of disease in the correct clinical situation/compensation program, the physician must determine on a clinical basis whether additional testing is necessary to establish a medical diagnosis and determine whether treatment is necessary. The physician should note that additional testing may or may not be covered by the benefits or compensation program. Because of the variability in the extent of radiographic findings and the degree of physiologic impairment, none of the major programs or rating systems uses radiographic findings in the assessment of impairment due to lung disease. The NIOSH website provides a search tool by which to find certified B Readers by state and country.[21]

A standardized CT classification system similar to the ILO system called the International Classification of High-Resolution Computed Tomography for Occupational and Environmental Disease has been proposed.[22] Although this CT classification system was found to have satisfactory inter-reader reliability by an international panel of experts,[23] the assessment mainly focused on one lung disease, asbestos-related lung disease, so the generalizability of this system is not clear. Neither this nor any other standardized system for reporting CT findings of pneumoconiosis is currently in widespread use.

PULMONARY FUNCTION TESTING (See Chapters 31 and 32)

PFTs are the most important tests, both from a diagnostic standpoint and in their use to determine impairment for most respiratory conditions. Both the ATS[2] and the *AMA Guides* specify the use of FVC, FEV_1, FEV_1/FVC, and DL_{CO}. Some programs mandate that pulmonary function testing be performed pre- and post-bronchodilator and should be done in patients with low FEV_1 or diagnoses of reversible airflow limitation. The ATS specifies that individuals should be evaluated only after they have received an accurate diagnosis and while they are receiving optimal therapy.[2] This is consistent with the *AMA Guides* requirement that the patient be at MMI, as described previously. Measurement of height without shoes is recommended, as is measurement of arm span (distance between the tips of the middle fingers with arms outstretched) in cases of spinal deformity.[2,24]

Both ATS and the *AMA Guides* emphasize the importance of only using test results that meet the quality standards

defined in the latest ATS statement "Standardization of Lung Function Testing."[25] This document governs the equipment, quality assurance, and techniques that should be used to perform lung function testing, in addition to the assessment of the quality of the test and the method of interpretation. If a physician has concern that the PFTs were not performed in a manner consistent with the ATS Guidelines, including acceptability and reproducibility, then the physician should request repeating the test. An exception happens when the patient has consistently demonstrated less than optimal technique on past tests despite language-appropriate education and encouragement. The physician may decide not to repeat testing if consistent, unacceptable test performance appears to be due to overall debilitation, pain, or language barrier or when it is unlikely that repeating the test will yield better results. Test results markedly worse than those of prior tests raise concern regarding an exacerbation of the underlying condition and that the patient is not at MMI, or it may be that the patient gave less than full effort; regardless, such results would not be considered to reflect the patient's permanent impairment status. Options include informing the subject of the discrepancy and repeating the test or using the results "as a subsidiary and not the main criterion."[26]

When evaluating PFTs for impairment, the normal values of the laboratory performing the test should not be used, but rather the normal values of the impairment rating system. For example, the ATS and *AMA Guides*, Fifth Edition, use the normal values derived from Crapo and colleagues,[27] while the *AMA Guides*, Sixth Edition, use National Health and Nutrition Examination Survey III–derived prediction equations.[28]

DL_{CO}, measured by the single-breath method of Ogilvie and colleagues[29] and interpreted according to Crapo and Morris,[30] is suggested by both ATS and the *AMA Guides*. Both recommend correction by the methodology of others for factors including hemoglobin, carboxyhemoglobin,[2,14] and altitude and alveolar volume,[2] but correction methodology and interpretive strategies are not explicitly described in the rating criteria. The most recent ATS statement on DL_{CO} describes explicit criteria for evaluating acceptability and repeatability, as well as adjustment for hemoglobin, supplemental oxygen, altitude, and carboxyhemoglobin, while noting that further study is necessary before specific recommendations for lung volume adjustment can be made.[31] In a separate statement, the ATS has noted that low DL_{CO} along with low DL_{CO} *corrected for alveolar volume* (DL_{CO}/VA) suggest parenchymal abnormalities as the cause of the impairment but recommends examining the two separately.[25] Neither the ATS nor the *AMA Guides* utilize DL_{CO}/VA in assessing impairment.

Maximal voluntary ventilation and $FEV_{25\%-75\%}$ are not recommended for use by ATS or the *AMA Guides* in impairment evaluation. ATS defines a restrictive ventilatory defect as a reduction in total lung capacity below the lower limit of normal (i.e., below the fifth percentile of the predicted value), with a normal FEV_1/FVC ratio.[25] Total lung capacity is not included in the standard rating criteria in either the ATS or the *AMA Guides*. Although the *AMA Guides*, Sixth Edition, cautions that a true restrictive defect may not be present even with a reduced FVC in the setting of a normal

Table 35.4 American Thoracic Society Interpretation of Exercise Test Results Using $\dot{V}O_{2max}$

$\dot{V}O_{2max}$	METS	Estimated Work Ability
≥25 mL/kg/min	≥7.1	Continuous heavy exertion throughout an 8-hour day in all but the most physically demanding jobs
15–25 mL/kg/min *and* Metabolic demands of the work ≤ $\dot{V}O_{2max}$		Able to perform that job comfortably, assuming there are no frequent or extended periods (5 min) requiring exertion substantially >40% $\dot{V}O_{2max}$
≤15 mL/kg/min	≤4.3	Unable to perform most jobs because they would be uncomfortable traveling back and forth

METS, the energy demand in liters of oxygen consumption per minute/basal oxygen consumption (3.5 mL/kg/min); $\dot{V}O_{2max}$, maximal oxygen consumption.
From American Thoracic Society. Evaluation of impairment/disability secondary to respiratory disorders. *Am Rev Respir Dis.* 1986;133:1205-1209.

or increased FEV_1/FVC, FVC alone continues to be the test used in the rating of impairment of restrictive lung disease.

CARDIOPULMONARY EXERCISE TESTING (See Chapter 33)

Neither the ATS nor the *AMA Guides* recommend the routine use of exercise test results in the determination of permanent impairment; however, maximal exercise test results, specifically $\dot{V}O_{2max}$, should be considered in specific circumstances. ATS recommended that exercise test results be used in cases where the resting PFTs do not reflect the true impairment present.[2] For example, studies have demonstrated that *alveolar-arterial oxygen pressure difference* [(A–a)PO_2] during exercise is a better reflection of impairment due to gas exchange abnormality than DL_{CO} in many patients with interstitial lung disease.[32] Although exercise limitation does not necessarily correlate with resting lung function testing,[33,34] exercise testing can be helpful in cases where there is a large discrepancy between symptoms and resting physiology,[32] providing a more precise measurement of work capacity.[35]

Airflow limitation and gas exchange abnormality help define the relative degree to which respiratory disease contributes to exercise limitation. When exercise limitation is present, nonrespiratory causes of exercise limitation should be considered as well, including cardiovascular disease, deconditioning, and neuromuscular disease.[36] The ATS guidelines for respiratory impairment note that exercise testing can be used as a valid measure of respiratory impairment when the following criteria are met: (1) exercise testing is not terminated for another extrapulmonary reason, (2) there is low breathing reserve at termination, and (3) there is absence of erratic overventilation at submaximal levels with failure to achieve anaerobic threshold (i.e., there is an absence of evidence of psychogenic dyspnea). However, no details are provided on how these criteria should be met, and the *AMA Guides* do not delineate a specific methodology. The reason for test termination should be noted because tests terminated early due to nonrespiratory causes such as excessive blood pressure, cardiac abnormality, or leg pain do not reflect maximum exercise tolerance.

To determine work capacity, and thus impairment, ATS requires use of $\dot{V}O_{2max}$ to place workers into one of three categories of work tolerance, assuming that workers can comfortably perform sustained work at 40% of $\dot{V}O_{2max}$ and

that O_2 requirements of the workers' jobs are known (Table 35.4). The *AMA Guides*, Fifth and Sixth Editions, both consider a $\dot{V}O_{2max}$ greater than 25 mL/kg/min to place one into the lowest (least) category of impairment (class 1 and class 0, respectively) and a $\dot{V}O_{2max}$ less than 15 mL/kg/min to place one into the highest (greatest) category of impairment (class 4). This approach has major limitations, which are detailed below.

BLOOD GAS ANALYSIS

Arterial blood gas analysis is not used for impairment rating purposes on a routine basis. Resting arterial PO_2 does not necessarily correlate with exercise capacity. Arterial hypoxemia at rest by itself is not evidence of severe impairment in exercise tolerance. ATS recommends it only be used in "selected patients" under "rigidly controlled laboratory conditions" and should be documented on at least two occasions separated by at least 4 weeks.[2] They consider hypoxemia to be evidence of severe impairment only when accompanied by evidence of right heart failure. Arterial blood gas analysis was considered to be a test infrequently indicated in the evaluation of impairment in the *AMA Guides*, Fifth Edition.[14] It is not included in the Sixth Edition.[15]

ADDRESSING DISCREPANCIES BETWEEN OBJECTIVE AND SUBJECTIVE DATA

A description of the severity of the disease or condition should be given. This can be difficult when there is a discrepancy between the severity reported by the patient and the severity of the disease based on the results of the diagnostic testing. It is important that the physician distinguish between *objective* data (findings evident to the examiner in a reproducible manner and not dependent on only the patient's perceptions), including physical signs and diagnostic testing results, and *subjective* data, which are reported by the patient, such as symptoms perceived by the patient only and not evident to the examiner. Normally, the two are similar, making the history, physical examination, and diagnostic testing findings all helpful in the assessment of true functional impairment. If the subjective complaints are not consistent with the objective findings, the physician should first be sure there is no coexisting disease process responsible for the symptoms. For example, dyspnea may also be caused by nonrespiratory disorders such as cardiac disease and anemia. *Organic impairment* refers to the presence of objective findings of respiratory dysfunction or disease. *Functional impairment* refers to dyspnea for which an objectively measured abnormality of organ function cannot be identified. Recognizing that tests for organic impairment are not perfectly sensitive, the contribution of functional impairment can range from "negligible" to "perhaps accounting for the entire extent of a patient's dyspnea." When there is a discrepancy between the subjective and the objective data, and other medical conditions have been excluded as possible contributors to the subjective complaints, several steps should be taken. The first and foremost is to review the purpose of the evaluation with the patient to ensure comprehension of questions and performance of PFTs. Second, an evaluation of test performance, including cooperation and the results of effort-independent tests such as functional residual capacity, may be of some use. Examination of test results for comparability over time may show evidence of consistency or the lack thereof. Finally, exercise testing may shed considerable light on a patient's level of effort by demonstrating the relationships of heart rate and ventilatory rate at workloads actually achieved to the predicted maximal values.

Dyspnea due to functional impairment may result from subconscious effects on the perception of symptoms or from outright malingering. Because of the inability of PFTs and other tests to be perfectly sensitive in diagnosing organic causes of impairment, the diagnosis of malingering should be made with caution. The *Diagnostic and Statistical Manual of Mental Disorders, Fifth Edition* (DSM-5), classifies malingering as a condition "that may be a focus of clinical attention."[37] Furthermore, malingering is described as "the intentional production of false or grossly exaggerated physical or psychological symptoms, motivated by external incentives." Specific listed examples of these external incentives include avoiding work and obtaining financial compensation. The DSM-5 recommends that malingering should be strongly suspected if any combination of the following is noted: (1) there is a medicolegal context of presentation, (2) a marked discrepancy between the person's claimed stress or disability and the objective findings is noted, (3) a lack of cooperation during the diagnostic evaluation and a lack of compliance with the prescribed treatment regimen are observed, and (4) there is the presence of antisocial personality disorder. Malingering is differentiated from a factitious disorder in that the motivation for the symptom production is external, rather than an intrinsic need to maintain the sick role. Malingering may also be differentiated from conversion disorder and other somatoform disorders by the intentional production of symptoms and the obvious external incentives associated with it.

Although it is important to identify frank malingering, which represents fraud, it must be emphasized that malingering is relatively rare and should remain a diagnosis made through exclusion and with extreme caution.

APPORTIONMENT AND FUTURE MEDICAL TREATMENT

APPORTIONMENT

When multiple disease processes are present that may contribute to respiratory impairment, the physician may be asked to apportion or make a statement of the relative contribution of each disease process to the total impairment. This is usually performed in the context of workers' compensation in an effort to limit the amount of the monetary award to that specifically attributed to the workplace exposure or event. It does not typically reduce medical treatment benefits or wage compensation. Unfortunately, the scientific basis for this level of precision is rarely present and thus must be acknowledged as arbitrary even if required by the entitlement system.

Cigarette smoking and its sequelae is the most common condition taken into account when considering apportionment of respiratory impairment. For example, much has been written about the difference in symptoms and physical limitations in smoking compared with nonsmoking asbestos workers,[38] and the observation that the most common cause of exercise limitation in one group studied was the cardiovascular system rather than the respiratory system.[39] Specific methods for apportionment have been proposed,[40] but none has been validated scientifically or considered generally accepted. If objective evidence of prior impairment exists, such as diagnostic testing results performed before the work-related exposure or development of disease, some states will allow apportionment to be performed by subtracting the preexisting impairment from the current total impairment.

EXPECTED FUTURE MEDICAL TREATMENT

A description of the expected natural history of the condition, that is, if the condition is expected to remain stable or potentially to deteriorate over time, should be provided. In addition, the recommended medical follow-up and anticipated treatment requirements can provide a helpful measure of reasonably anticipated future medical expenses. This is of value to the worker as well as insurance adjusters and attorneys.

MAJOR STATE AND FEDERAL BENEFIT AND COMPENSATION PROGRAMS

Most impairment and disability evaluations will be performed under the context of a particular state or federal program. A number of different programs exist for individuals and workers in specific employment settings. Some of the larger programs include the Federal Black Lung Program for coal mine workers, Social Security Disability for disabled workers, Workers' Compensation for ill and injured workers through their employers, and the Veterans Administration for veterans with service-related conditions. There are several related programs for workers at Department of Energy sites and uranium workers under the Energy Employees

Occupational Illness Compensation Program. Most of these programs refer to both impairment and disability. In some programs, the primary determination to be made by the physician is disability, usually in the context of making the dichotomous determination of "disabled" or "not disabled" and, in others, the primary determination is impairment. Each system has its own rules by which to establish patient eligibility and rules for assignment of disability and/or impairment. Most major compensation systems require physicians to undergo special training and/or approval before they are permitted to perform these evaluations for benefits programs.

Detailed descriptions of these programs are available at ExpertConsult.com.

WORKPLACE PROTECTIONS

RESPIRATORY PROTECTION

In considering whether respiratory protection may be required in the workplace, it is important to consider NIOSH's recommended hierarchical approach to reducing workplace exposures including (1) elimination, (2) substitution, (3) engineering controls, such as improving ventilation or enclosing exposures, (4) administrative controls, and, as a last resort, (5) personal protective equipment such as respirators.[49] Medical clearance for the use of respirators is mandated by the Occupational Safety and Health Administration, either through use of their standard questionnaire or through a comparable medical examination.[50] Before using a respirator, the worker should undergo tests with the specific make and model of the respirator to be used to ensure proper fit and protection. Fit testing is also regulated by the Occupational Safety and Health Administration.

WORK RESTRICTIONS

Some compensation systems, such as workers' compensation, require a statement on ability to work and whether there are any physical activities or exposures the worker should avoid. Treating physicians may recommend temporary work restrictions for their patients during exacerbations of illness; these restrictions may or may not be accommodated by the workplace because there is no requirement for them to do so. Physicians may also assign permanent work restrictions, which employers are obligated to consider for reasonable accommodation under the *Americans with Disabilities Act Amendments Act* (ADAAA).[51] Restrictions may include limitations in the ability to perform a specific physical activity, perform it safely on a sustained or repeated basis, and/or to be able to work in the presence of certain dust, fume, gas, chemical, and/or antigen exposures, as in the case of occupational allergic asthma and hypersensitivity pneumonitis.

In order for the physician to determine whether the worker can perform job tasks and if restrictions are needed, both the physical requirements of the job and the worker's capabilities need to be ascertained. Exercise testing, with its limitations noted previously, is a standard approach used in this assessment. Although submaximal testing has been used and does have some advantages in terms of administration

and merits in terms of demonstrating a worker's ability to sustain activity at a predetermined level of exertion, maximal exercise testing is normally used. Accuracy of exercise testing to predict functional performance can be increased by combining exercise testing with measures of pulmonary function[33] and with heart rate monitoring during the performance of work activities.[52] Actual simulation of work may be performed by a physical or occupational therapist, called a functional capacity evaluation. Interpretation of results and formulation of formal work restrictions should be performed in a manner consistent with the ADAAA considerations, including suggesting possible methods of reasonable accommodation in the workplace.

AMERICANS WITH DISABILITIES ACT AMENDMENTS ACT

The *Americans with Disabilities Act* (ADA) of 1990 and the ADAAA of 2008 prohibit discrimination against a qualified individual with a *disability*, defined as "a physical or mental impairment that substantially limits a major life activity."[51,53]

A brief discussion of the definitions of impairment and accommodation as it relates to this Act and the Family and Medical Leave Act is available at ExpertConsult.com.

A preemployment physical is not permitted under the ADA; an employer may not ask questions about disability or require a medical examination until after a conditional job offer has been made. A postoffer, preplacement medical evaluation is permitted, as long as the employer does this for all employees entering the same job category; if doing so is job related and consistent with business necessity on the basis of objective evidence that a worker will be unable to perform essential job functions or will pose a direct threat because of a medical condition; or when an employer receives a request for reasonable accommodation and the disability or the need for the accommodation is not obvious.

FUTURE DIRECTIONS

AN UPDATED FRAMEWORK OF DISABILITY

As noted above, the WHO replaced the ICIDH model with the ICF in 2001. The ICIDH model had been recognized as problematic in a number of respects, including an implied unidirectional relationship from impairment to handicap, limited definition of the role of the environment, and focus on the disability, rather than the factors that may enable functional ability. The ICF is an international consensus framework constructed in two parts,[4] designed to be used in conjunction with the International Classification of Diseases 10 codes as a uniform description of health and well-being. The first part of the ICF is most familiar to physicians, combining consideration of *body functions and structure, activity,* and *participation* in a cohesive manner. The term *functioning* according to the ICF combines the positive aspects of body functions, activities, and participation, whereas the term *disability* is used to describe the combination of the negative aspects of structural/functional loss (impairment), activity limitation, and participation restriction. Part 2 of the ICF encompasses an additional dimension called *contextual factors,* which are divided into *personal factors,* such as age, education, and attitudes, and *environmental factors*. *Facilitators* are contextual factors that enhance functioning and *barriers* are contextual factors that restrict or limit functioning. This model is a framework by which to describe health status, functioning, and disability in a uniform manner across a wide range of medical disorders on an international level, in the context of a given patient's health condition(s).

Implementation and, in particular, clinical use of the ICF framework has been very limited; the development of tools by which to apply it are complex and there are no tools for many medical conditions. Considerations for use include the ICF domains to be documented (activities and participation, body functions, and/or environmental factors), the perspectives to take (patient, clinician, etc.), the data collection tools to use (when they exist), and how to report the assessment.[55] Several different classification systems have been developed called *sets*, which include generic sets and core sets, which are condition- and/or population-specific lists of ICF codes that limit the categories of the ICF to those considered to be directly relevant. The development of sets is done through a multistage, multidisciplinary consensus and validation process.[56,57] The WHO Disability Schedule 2.0 is a generic set that measures six domains (cognition, mobility, self-care, getting along, life activities, and participation) to assess health status and disability generically among patients with different medical conditions.[58] The data are subjective and many of the questions relate to basic ADLs. Its use as a stand-alone tool in the description of respiratory conditions has been limited to a population of patients with pulmonary hypertension.[59] *ICF core sets* for respiratory diseases are also limited. A core set was developed for patients with cardiopulmonary conditions in rehabilitation facilities.[60] The only disease-specific core set is for obstructive pulmonary diseases. This was developed through a consensus process in 2004, including both a *comprehensive ICF core set*, which encompassed all relevant categories, and a *brief ICF core set*, which encompassed the minimum categories that need to be considered.[61] During validation in 2013 and 2014, most of the categories in the comprehensive ICF core set were confirmed from the patient's perspective, although additional categories were also identified by them.[62] Similar results were found in a validation study of the brief ICF obstructive pulmonary disease core set.[63] The core set was recently revised and applied in a pilot study of patients with respiratory diseases in the rehabilitation setting.[64] Thus, there remains no consensus set that has been validated from multiple perspectives. Core sets for other respiratory diseases need to be developed. Subsequently, consideration of how this schema would be applied within benefits and compensation systems would need to be determined. Use of the ICF has been endorsed in the occupational setting, specifically review of personal and environmental contextual factors to identify facilitators and barriers to recovery, which can help identify additional treatment that is needed or help determine when there is no additional treatment likely to improve the condition (i.e., the patient is considered to be at MMI).[65] We would recommend that the latter be applied with caution, and only under the rubric of specific consensus guidelines developed from a multidisciplinary perspective.

The Institute of Medicine had developed alternative models to update the ICIDH that included pathology, impairment, functional limitation, and disability.[66,67] While their most recent report *Future of Disability in America* (2007) ultimately endorsed the ICF as the basic framework, it called for further refinement of the model to address its shortcomings.[68] One of its authors and others in the United States continue to call for refinement and updating of the ICF model; concerns include the limited distinction between activity and participation in the model, lack of quality of life measures, need for a dynamic model to include factors that affect change of an individual into different levels of functioning and disability, and an updated model to reflect current understanding of both the determinants and consequences of health conditions, not only for patients generically, but also within the context of activity and participation important to the individual patient.[69–71]

Consideration of limitations in the current assessment of respiratory impairment include the following:

1. Use of FVC as the basis for impairment in restrictive lung disease instead of total lung capacity. Low FVC can be caused by submaximal inspiratory or expiratory effort and/or peripheral airflow obstruction.[25] One study showed the predictive value of reduced FVC to be less than 60% for the presence of a true restrictive deficit.[72] Others report concern about reduced lung function test results, including FVC, in obesity,[73,74] but there are no established criteria by which to account for obesity in testing.

2. Use of $\dot{V}O_{2max}$ in isolation without consideration of the criteria listed in the ATS guidelines for respiratory impairment based on exercise physiology, including reason for test termination. The average energy requirements of a number of jobs are listed in eTable 35.4. Major limitations to this approach include the following: (1) little published data that substantiate its use; (2) heterogeneous methods of assessing maximal oxygen uptake[75]; (3) the actual work performed by workers with the same job title can vary markedly from employer to employer or among employees with differing seniority working for the same employer; (4) the questionable relationship between exercise tolerance on the treadmill or bicycle and performance on the job[76]; and (5) the lack of consideration of modifying factors such as the need to talk or use personal protective equipment while performing the work.[77] Additionally, these existing tables are decades old and often no longer reflect the work environment. Other than specifying $\dot{V}O_{2max}$, the *AMA Guides* do not provide any details for how it should be interpreted, including the predicted normal values of the specific test performed (i.e., cycle ergometry versus treadmill, or delineation of the reason for test termination), because nonrespiratory causes such as excessive blood pressure, cardiac abnormality, leg pain, or suspicion of inadequate effort should clearly not form the basis for assignment of impaired ability due to respiratory impairment. The use of exercise testing and $\dot{V}O_{2max}$ overestimates impairment in older workers. As an alternative, it has been proposed that $\dot{V}O_{2max}$ be expressed as percentage of predicted,[78] although this is not in standard use at this time. Although advances have been

made, the recent ATS Statement on Cardiopulmonary Exercise Testing[36] noted that a comprehensive updated framework for impairment/disability is needed urgently.

3. Mandating the use of outdated reference equations that apply to fewer ethnic groups. Neither the Fifth Edition or Sixth Edition of the *AMA Guides* uses the most recent recommended reference values. The ATS/ERS now recommends the use of the *Global Lung Function Initiative* (GLI) 2012 predicted normal values for spirometry that are applicable globally to different ethnic groups. This includes reference equations for whites, Blacks, and North and Southeast Asians up to 95 years of age. A composite equation is used for those of mixed ethnic origin or not represented by one of those four groups.[79] Reference values for DL_{CO} up to age 85 years were also developed.[80]

4. Use of bronchodilator response based on change in FEV_1 from baseline. The assessment of bronchodilator response is based on percent change in FEV_1 from baseline. The ATS guidelines recommend a postbronchodilator change of 12% and 0.2 L increase in FEV_1 or FVC.[25] Change in FVC may be a better measure in some patients, such as those with more severe airflow obstruction.[81,82] Expressing bronchodilator response in terms of percent of baseline can bias impairment toward those with lower baseline values.[82,83] Expressing change in terms of difference in percent of predicted avoids this bias, as well as bias towards taller men when absolute change in volume is used; however, there is not agreement on the value that establishes a bronchodilator response.[82–84]

5. There may be better methods of relating impairment to disability. Consideration of multiple facets of this complex topic has been outlined.[85]

Key Points

- *Impairment* refers to the degree of loss of normal use or function of a body part or organ.
- *Disability* refers to any resulting alteration in the individual's capacity to perform customary activities. That definition has been expanded by the Institute of Medicine to include the "gap between a person's capacities and the demands of relevant, socially defined roles and tasks in a particular physical and social environment," emphasizing the bidirectional nature of the model and the importance of factors in the environment that facilitate or present obstacles to functioning and participation.
- *Maximum medical improvement* (MMI) is the point at which permanent impairment can be assessed. MMI is achieved when the diagnosis has been well defined, the condition is stable, and medical treatment has either been optimized or reasonable options have been exhausted.
- The Americans with Disabilities Act Amendments Act of 2008 greatly expanded the definition of disability to focus on workplace accommodation of "qualified individuals." A qualified individual is a person who has the requisite skills and experience to do the job and "can perform the essential job tasks with or

without reasonable accommodation" without risk of direct threat to self or others.

- *Reasonable accommodation* is defined as a modification or adjustment to the job, work environment, or the way things are usually done that enables a person with a disability to perform an essential job function.
- An *impairment evaluation* is a medical evaluation that typically includes history, including a detailed occupational and environmental history and description of limitations in activities of daily living; physical examination; and review of medical records and diagnostic test results that establish the respiratory condition. If the worker is at MMI, a permanent impairment rating can be performed. The physician may be asked to address causation, which is usually the relationship of the disease to workplace exposures, the need for work restrictions, future medical needs, and possibly apportionment of impairment.
- An *impairment rating* is a numeric value from 0–100% that represents the percent loss of total body function due to the respiratory system. This numeric value helps form the basis for the monetary award given to workers with permanent impairment that remains after reaching MMI.
- In addition to state and federal workers' compensation programs, other special benefit and compensation programs exist for certain groups of workers, including miners, Department of Energy workers, veterans, and radiation-exposed workers.

Key Readings

American Thoracic Society (ATS). Evaluation of impairment/disability secondary to respiratory disorders. *Am Rev Respir Dis.* 1986;133:1205–1209.

American Thoracic Society (ATS). Guidelines for the evaluation of impairment/disability in patients with asthma. *Am Rev Respir Dis.* 1993;147:1056–1061.

Becklake MR, Rodarte JR, Kalica AR. NHLBI workshop summary. Scientific issues in the assessment of respiratory impairment. *Am Rev Respir Dis.* 1988;137:1505–1510.

Chan-Yeung M. Evaluation of impairment/disability in patients with occupational asthma. *Am Rev Respir Dis.* 1987;135:950–951.

Cieza A, Ewert T, Ustün TB, Chatterji S, Kostanjsek N, Stucki G. Development of ICF Core Sets for patients with chronic conditions. *J Rehabil Med.* 2004;44:9–11.

Cocchiarella L, Andersson GBJ, eds. *Guides to the Evaluation of Permanent Impairment.* 5th ed. Chicago: AMA Press; 2001.

Cotes JE, Zejda J, King B. Lung function impairment as a guide to exercise limitation in work-related lung disorders. *Am Rev Respir Dis.* 1988;137:1089–1093.

Eisner MD, Iribarren C, Yelin EH, et al. Pulmonary function and the risk of functional limitation in chronic obstructive pulmonary disease. *Am J Epidemiol.* 2008;167:1090–1101.

Harber P, Tamimie J, Emory J, et al. Effects of exercise using industrial respirators. *Am Ind Hyg Assoc J.* 1984;45:603–609.

Harber P. Respiratory disability and impairment: what is new? *Curr Opin Pulm Med.* 2015;21:201–207.

Huang J, Reinhardt JD, Dai R, Wang P, Zhou M. Validation of the brief international classification of functioning, disability, and health core set for obstructive pulmonary disease in the Chinese context. *Chron Respir Dis.* 2019;16:1479973119843648.

Jette AM. The utility of and need for improving the ICF. *Phys Ther.* 2018;98(8):629–630.

Marques A, Jácome C, Gonçalves A, et al. Validation of the Comprehensive ICF Core Set for obstructive pulmonary diseases from the patient's perspective. *Int J Rehabil Res.* 2014;37:152–158.

McDermott S, Turk MA. Support for reevaluation of the International Classification of functioning, disability, and health (ICF): a view from the US. *Disabil Health J.* 2019;12(2):137–138.

Mitra S, Shakespeare T. Remodeling the ICF. *Disabil Health J.* 2019;12(3):337–339.

Reis A, Santos M, Furtado I, et al. Disability and its clinical correlates in pulmonary hypertension measured through the World Health Organization Disability Assessment Schedule 2.0: a prospective, observational study. *J Bras Pneumol.* 2019;45(4):e20170355.

Rondinelli RD, ed. *Guides to the Evaluation of Permanent Impairment.* 6th ed. Chicago: AMA Press; 2008.

Rondinelli RD, Eskay-Auerbach M. Healthcare provider issues and perspective: impairment ratings and disability determinations. *Phys Med Rehabil Clin N Am.* 2019;30(3):511–522.

Selb M, Escorpizo R, Kostanjsek N, Stucki G, Ustun B, Cieza A. A guide on how to develop an international classification of functioning, disability and health core set. *Eur J Phys Rehabil Med.* 2015;51(1):105–117.

Sood A. Performing a lung disability evaluation: how, when, and why? *J Occup Environ Med.* 2014;56(suppl 10):S23–9.

Spieler EA, Barth PS, Burton Jr JF, et al. Recommendations to guide revision of the guides to the evaluation of permanent impairment. *JAMA.* 2000;283:519–523.

Stucki A, Stoll T, Cieza A, et al. ICF Core Sets for obstructive pulmonary diseases. *J Rehabil Med.* 2004;(suppl 44):114–120.

Stucki G, Prodinger B, Bickenbach J. Four steps to follow when documenting functioning with the International Classification of Functioning, Disability and Health. *Eur J Phys Rehabil Med.* 2017;53(1):144–149.

Verbrugge LM, Jette AM. The disablement process. *Soc Sci Med.* 1994;38:1–14.

Vitacca M, Giardini A, Corica G, et al. Implementation of a real-world based ICF set for the rehabilitation of respiratory diseases: a pilot study. *Minerva Med.* 2019.

Wildner M, Quittan M, Portenier L, et al. ICF Core Set for patients with cardiopulmonary conditions in early post-acute rehabilitation facilities. *Disabil Rehabil.* 2005;27(7-8):397–404.

Complete reference list available at ExpertConsult.com.

PART 3

CLINICAL RESPIRATORY MEDICINE

EVALUATION OF COMMON PRESENTATIONS OF RESPIRATORY DISEASE

36 *DYSPNEA*

RICHARD M. SCHWARTZSTEIN, MD • LEWIS ADAMS, PHD

INTRODUCTION

Each minute of every day, we initiate approximately 10 to 16 breaths. Most of the time, we give little thought to this process, but when there are alterations in the respiratory system, from central control to the ventilatory pump to gas exchange, severe physical discomfort and emotional distress may result. The uncomfortable or unpleasant sensations associated with breathing are termed dyspnea, and as many as one-quarter of middle-aged and older adults may suffer from this experience.[1] The prevalence of dyspnea in noncritically ill hospitalized patients is reported in 16% of admissions in the first 24 hours, with higher numbers (23%) for patients admitted via the emergency department[2] and 49% in critically ill patients.[3]

The impact of breathing discomfort on one's functional status can be significant, and dyspnea is routinely used as a component of quality-of-life measures. In addition, there are increasing data demonstrating that dyspnea is an independent predictor of mortality in patients, with particular emphasis on those at risk for and/or suffering from cardiorespiratory diseases.[4–6] Consequently, identification of patients with breathing discomfort becomes important. Efforts to elicit this symptom, however, may be impaired by the tendency of patients to avoid activities that provoke breathing discomfort by altering their lifestyle or avoiding physical exertion.[7] These reductions in physical activity may lead to ever-worsening cardiovascular and muscular deconditioning, which intensifies dyspnea, leading to additional limitations and a vicious cycle in which

TABLE 36.1　Relationship Among Qualities of Dyspnea, Physiology, and Disease States

Quality of Dyspnea	Physiology	Disease States
Air hunger, urge to breathe, need more air	Stimulation of respiratory controller via chemoreceptors, pulmonary receptors, vascular receptors	Pneumonia, pulmonary edema, pulmonary embolism, COPD with acute gas exchange abnormalities, asthma, pleural effusion, toxic inhalations
Chest tightness	Stimulation of pulmonary receptors	Asthma, pulmonary edema with bronchospasm, toxic inhalations with bronchospasm
Cannot get a deep breath	Stimulation of respiratory controller; dynamic hyperinflation	COPD, asthma
Increased work or effort to breathe	Mechanical load on the respiratory system; neuromuscular weakness	COPD, asthma, obesity, kyphoscoliosis, Guillain-Barré, myasthenia gravis
Breathing more	Increased ventilation; stimulation of metaboreceptors in muscles	Exercise, cardiovascular deconditioning

breathlessness leads to diminished exercise, which leads to greater deconditioning and finally to more breathlessness.[8]

In the *intensive care unit* (ICU), as our understanding of ventilator-induced lung injury has led to strategies of mechanical ventilation that emphasize low tidal volume, we must be cognizant of the impact of these strategies on dyspnea. In the face of a high drive to breathe, constrained tidal volume is a powerful provocation for dyspnea[9] and may contribute to some of the patient ventilatory dyssynchrony seen in these individuals. In addition, breathing discomfort during mechanical ventilation may be a factor in the emotional and behavioral complications seen in survivors of acute respiratory failure.[10]

The physiologic stimuli that provoke dyspnea are varied but have a common effect of increasing the output from the central controller and increasing the drive to breathe. Although inputs from a range of receptors throughout the body may contribute to the perception of dyspnea and the verbal phrases or descriptors used by patients to characterize their sensations, the increased neural output from the controller is most closely associated with the sensation of "air hunger" or a need or urge to breathe. The various descriptors used by patients may provide insights into the pathophysiologic conditions contributing to breathing discomfort. Furthermore, various psychological factors may have an impact on the perception and interpretation of sensations (e.g., "Is this 'normal'?" or "Is this a 'symptom' of a disease?"), and the sensations of breathing discomfort may evoke fear and anxiety.[11–13] This interplay of sensation and emotional or affective state of the individual may explain, in part, the variability between physiologic measures of the severity of cardiorespiratory disease and the intensity of the associated breathing discomfort.

DEFINITION OF DYSPNEA

Many words have been used by patients and doctors to describe breathing discomfort, from shortness of breath to breathlessness to dyspnea. Although the medical term *dyspnea* derives from the Greek word for "difficulty breathing," the most widely used definition was promulgated in a consensus statement of the American Thoracic Society,[14] which states: "Dyspnea is a term used to characterize a subjective experience of breathing discomfort that is comprised of qualitatively distinct sensations that vary in intensity. The experience derives from interactions among multiple physiological, psychological, social, and environmental factors, and it may induce secondary physiological and behavioral responses." The emphasis on a "subjective experience" makes clear that dyspnea is a symptom that can only be described by the patient; it is distinct from physical findings or signs observed and interpreted by doctors or families as evidence of "respiratory distress." The definition further reinforces the complex interplay of physiologic changes, the psychological state of the patient, and the social and environmental conditions leading to the symptom.

LANGUAGE OF DYSPNEA

Doctors have been trained for years to inquire about the quality of pain when caring for a patient with complaints such as headache, abdominal, or chest pain; the characteristics of the pain provide clues to the etiology of the problem.[15] Less well known is a growing body of literature showing a similar range of verbal descriptors used to characterize breathing discomfort. As with pain, the descriptors may provide clues to the underlying physiologic derangements and diagnoses contributing to dyspnea, as well as the emotional and behavioral responses to the discomfort.

QUALITATIVE PHRASES—THE DESCRIPTIVE DIMENSION OF DYSPNEA

For the healthy individual, breathing is taken for granted; we are generally unaware of it. With exercise, we are cognizant of "breathing more" or that our breathing becomes "heavy." But what does it feel like to have dyspnea due to airway resistance or a stiff lung or chest wall, or due to muscle weakness? The only way to answer that question is to inquire systematically about the qualities of the sensation in individuals experiencing dyspnea.

Early investigations proceeded in two directions: (1) systematic questioning of patients with a variety of cardiorespiratory diseases who were experiencing dyspnea and (2) laboratory studies in which investigators induced dyspnea in healthy individuals using interventions to increase respiratory drive or by imposing mechanical loads on the respiratory system and inquired about the resulting sensations.[16–18] From these and subsequent studies, relationships between disease states (e.g., asthma, COPD), physiology (e.g., increased respiratory drive, dynamic hyperinflation), and descriptors began to emerge (Table 36.1). "Air hunger" or "not getting enough air" was associated with stimulation of the respiratory controller, that is, an increased drive to breathe. "Chest tightness" was quite specific for bronchoconstriction, and an "unsatisfied inspiration" or "inability to get a deep breath" was associated with dynamic hyperinflation. A sense of "increased effort or work of breathing" is characteristic of mechanical loads on the respiratory system or of inspiratory muscle weakness or fatigue. None of these is absolutely sensitive or specific for a particular condition, of course, and multiple physiologic derangements may be present in a single patient. Nevertheless, awareness of these aspects of a patient's dyspnea may be quite helpful in a physician's analysis of the patient's problem.[19]

The few cross-cultural studies performed to investigate the qualitative sensations of dyspnea have found similar associations. Many of the dyspnea questionnaires that have been developed have been translated into different languages and are being used and tested around the world.[11,13] Children also appear to be capable of making qualitative distinctions among different types of dyspnea.[20]

EMOTIONAL PHRASES—THE AFFECTIVE DIMENSION OF DYSPNEA

As noted in the discussion of the definition of dyspnea, breathing discomfort may be affected by one's psychological state, and the experience of dyspnea may provoke strong emotional responses. As we assess the quality and severity of dyspnea, we note that both of these components of breathing discomfort can have implications for the emotional response of the patient. For example, air hunger evokes a stronger affective response than does an increase in the work of breathing.[12] As the intensity of air hunger becomes very high, patients may describe a suffocating feeling; this word is rarely invoked for mild dyspnea. The Multidimensional Dyspnea Profile and the Dyspnea-12 instruments have attempted to quantify and characterize the affective dimension of dyspnea.[11,13]

Because dyspnea can invoke such strong emotional reactions, patients often avoid activities that can provoke the sensations. Individuals with COPD, for example, may limit their activity at home to avoid dyspnea ratings greater than 3 (on a 0–10 scale).[7] Pulmonary rehabilitation programs have been shown to increase exercise capability in patients with COPD without altering lung function; this benefit is likely multifactorial and may include a degree of desensitization to dyspnea by providing patients with a sense of control or mastery over their symptom,[21] that is, by reducing the affective component of the dyspnea. As we increasingly take a patient-centered approach and make greater efforts to relieve discomfort, particularly for individuals with refractory cardiopulmonary disease, we must incorporate considerations of the emotional domain of dyspnea.[22]

MECHANISMS OF DYSPNEA

Perception of breathing discomfort (dyspnea) is an interoceptive process resulting from complex neurophysiologic processing that is incompletely understood.[23] Figure 36.1 is a schema of experimentally established components of this perception; variation in both the number and relative contribution of these elements likely accounts for the differing qualities of dyspnea and the widely observed established disjunction between symptom severity and objective clinical impairment.[24]

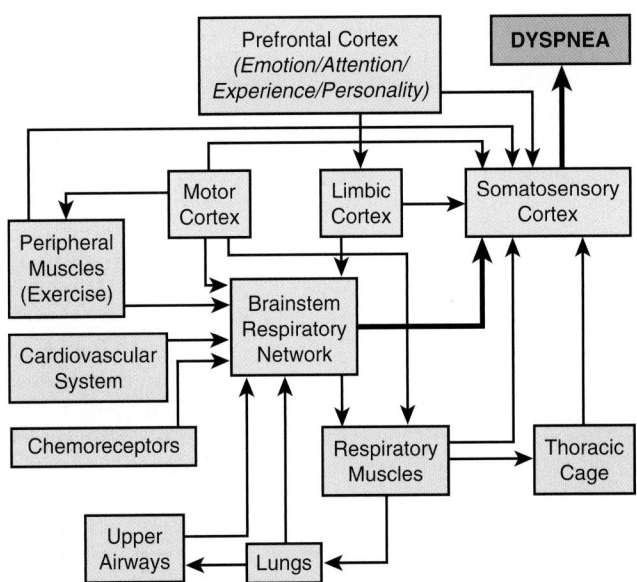

Figure 36.1 Neural basis of dyspnea perception. This schematic summarizes the key elements of the neural substrate for dyspnea perception derived from experimental and clinical studies. Dyspnea perception in the somatosensory cortex primarily reflects the degree of centrally generated drive to respiratory muscles from brainstem respiratory neurons. Respiratory drive emanating from the motor cortex and/or limbic cortex may modulate dyspnea either by direct innervation of the somatosensory cortex or via the brainstem. The primary inputs increasing reflex respiratory output are the central and peripheral chemoreceptors, pulmonary irritant and C fibers, peripheral muscle mechanoreceptors and metaboreceptors, and cardiac receptors. Slowly adapting pulmonary stretch receptors, thoracic cage mechanoreceptors, and upper airway flow receptors may ameliorate dyspnea by direct or indirect (via brainstem) innervation of the somatosensory cortex. Higher central neural activity from the prefrontal cortex can modulate dyspnea in either direction. Peripheral and central neural components of dyspnea are identified in orange and blue, respectively.

Although dyspnea can be experienced at rest, it typically presents clinically as a problem when it first appears at uncharacteristically low levels of exertion. With exertion, sensations of air hunger (also identified as "uncomfortable need to breathe" or "unsatisfied inspiration") and of the work of breathing increase together.[25] They can be separated experimentally, with the former being reported as more unpleasant than the latter in healthy subjects.[12] Similarly, patient populations identify greater morbidity associated with the air hunger component along with increasing disease severity.[25,26] Studies evaluating respiratory discomfort during exertion usually measure unimodal ratings of its intensity as exercise progresses. Such ratings, typically reported as dyspnea intensity, capture an individual's common experience of shortness of breath but not its qualitative components.

When studying dyspnea, investigators may use nonexercise stimuli to induce the sensation, notably constrained ventilation or the addition of an external respiratory load. Although the former produces marked air hunger, the latter is likely perceived as predominantly increased work of breathing at lower loads, with air hunger appearing with more severe loading. Again, these estimates of perceived respiratory discomfort are usually reported as dyspnea intensity. In reviewing the mechanism of dyspnea, this chapter will summarize findings from both healthy and dyspnea-prone populations in whom respiratory discomfort has been induced in a variety of ways.

Like all symptoms, dyspnea results from changes in neural activity within the cortical and subcortical structures of the brain involved in perception (see Fig. 36.1). Respiratory-related afferent information from the upper airway, lungs, chest wall, and chemoreceptors, as well as other signals from the cardiovascular and skeletal muscle systems, provide peripheral inputs that can contribute to the perception of dyspnea. A consistent finding is that, during ventilatory stimulation (e.g., exercise), the intensity of dyspnea correlates with the level of ventilation and that this relationship becomes steeper in the presence of respiratory mechanical impairment.[25] However, when examined relative to central respiratory drive (assessed from measures of esophageal pressure or diaphragmatic electromyography), dyspnea shows a strong correlation to central respiratory drive, independent of mechanical constraints.[27] This supports the view that the central motor command to breathe (respiratory drive) constitutes a key component of the experience of dyspnea.[28] This concept is able to explain the dyspnea noted in nonrespiratory conditions associated with increased respiratory stimulation; these include cardiac arrhythmias, deconditioning, anemia, and anxiety.

The importance of activation of respiratory-related neurons in the brainstem for the genesis of dyspnea is apparent from observations that, in healthy persons, experimental hypoxia, hypercapnia, metabolic acidosis, and exercise all result in an equivalent level of dyspnea relative to the level of ventilatory stimulation.[29] However, the relevance of increased ventilatory drive in the genesis of dyspnea is less clear. On the one hand, volitional isocapnic hyperpnea in patients with COPD causes little dyspnea compared with the same ventilation induced by hypercapnia.[30] On the other hand, in amyotrophic lateral sclerosis, dyspnea is exacerbated in the presence of cortically induced accessory muscle activation.[31] The multifactorial nature of dyspnea perception could accommodate these different observations.

The role of afferent information from respiratory-related receptors in the genesis of dyspnea is variable. As noted earlier, ventilatory activation via central and/or peripheral chemoreceptors or ill-defined ergoreceptors is associated with a level of dyspnea closely linked to the stimulus-independent degree of reflex (brainstem) respiratory drive. Moreover, in the absence of a ventilatory response to a given level of reflex stimulation, the intensity of dyspnea is potentiated.[32,33] This mismatching of ventilatory response to the ventilatory stimulus has been termed *efferent-afferent dissociation*, or neuromechanical dissociation.[25] Indeed, increasing afferent feedback can lessen the sensation of dyspnea. This concept is exemplified by volume-related feedback, with breath-holding as an extreme example. This inflation-related attenuation of dyspnea has been observed in the absence of mechanoreceptor feedback from the chest wall,[9] implicating pulmonary vagal receptors. Support for this comes from the observation that inhalation of furosemide, which potentiates slowly adapting stretch receptor activity in an animal model, has been shown to ameliorate the sensation of experimental dyspnea in healthy subjects.[34] On the other hand, volume-related relief of dyspnea has been documented in the presumed absence of pulmonary vagal afferent feedback,[35] implicating chest wall receptors. A role for afferent feedback from the respiratory system in the relief of dyspnea is consistent with clinical reports of the benefits of using a facial fan[36] (albeit via stimulation of trigeminal [not vagal] receptors) or chest wall vibration.[37] By contrast, conditions thought to activate lung irritant receptors and/or pulmonary C fibers (e.g., pulmonary edema, atelectasis, congestive heart failure) may contribute to dyspnea via vagal nerve afferents either directly or by modulating other sensory inputs that give rise to dyspnea.[38]

In light of the above, dyspnea accompanying respiratory impairment can be accounted for as the perception of the increased respiratory drive necessary to achieve adequate ventilation by a mechanically constrained respiratory apparatus. This would encompass both obstructive and restrictive disorders, including extrinsic restriction, for instance, or amyotrophic lateral sclerosis or myasthenia gravis. This concept fits with the observation that, in COPD patients, progressive hyperinflation is associated with increasing dyspnea because ventilatory demands require greater respiratory muscle activity to overcome increased elastic work at high lung volumes and to offset the foreshortening of inspiratory muscles that places them at a mechanical disadvantage.[25] Moreover, an increased end-expiratory lung volume is likely to exacerbate dyspnea via increased efferent-afferent dissociation.

The idea that dyspnea is the perception of centrally generated respiratory neural activity extends to conditions in which lung disease is not the primary problem. Thus the dyspnea of heart failure might be accounted for in terms of a heightened respiratory drive secondary to expiratory flow limitation[39] or poor peripheral muscle function.[40] Poor peripheral muscle function might also explain the dyspnea seen with anemia and deconditioning.

The sensation of dyspnea, like pain, has a psychological dimension. Dyspnea is worse when it is unexpected, when it happens in inappropriate situations, and when it is perceived by the patient to be dangerous.[41] Studies in healthy subjects and in patients with underlying disease have suggested that the perception of the intensity of breathlessness may be influenced by their prior experience of the sensation.[42] Moreover, experimentally induced changes in mood[43] have been shown to modulate exertional dyspnea independent of respiratory drive. Anxiety is an established cause of dyspnea and can affect pulmonary rehabilitation outcomes.[44] In patients with the hyperventilation syndrome, both dyspnea and ventilation can increase dramatically in the absence of any known physiologic stimulus to breathe[45] and, in patients with panic attacks, most report troublesome dyspnea.[46]

Neuroimaging technologies, principally positron emission tomography and functional magnetic resonance imaging, have been applied to study the neural basis of experimentally induced dyspnea. Despite methodologic differences in dyspnea genesis, a consistent pattern of activation of limbic and paralimbic structures, especially the anterior insular cortex, anterior cingulate gyrus, amygdala, and cerebellum, has been observed.[47] Activation of these phylogenetically ancient regions of the brain has been seen in brain imaging studies of pain, thirst, and hunger and is consistent with the idea that dyspnea is a primal experience associated with behaviors intended to counteract a threat to survival.[48] Whether these areas constitute the primary neural substrate for dyspnea or are more reflective of a generalized morbid experience is unclear. Recent commentary suggests that a more sophisticated approach to the analysis of functional brain mapping data is needed to gain improved insights into the neural basis of the complex perceptual experience of dyspnea.[49]

In summary, dyspnea may develop when there is an (1) increased central respiratory drive secondary to exercise, hypoxia, hypercapnia, or other afferent input; (2) increased requirement for the respiratory drive to overcome mechanical constraints or weakness; and (3) altered central perception in the presence of efferent-afferent dissociation.

ASSESSMENT OF DYSPNEA

PSYCHOMETRIC MEASUREMENT OF DYSPNEA INTENSITY

Like many clinical symptoms, dyspnea severity can be quickly assessed using a simple unidimensional scale. Numerical rating scales (0–10) and visual analog scales (a horizontal or vertical line usually 10 cm in length) have been widely used in clinical practice and adapted for quantifying dyspnea. The Borg Scale (modified from a preexisting scale for perceived exertion) is a variant of the numerical rating scales with verbal descriptors placed at appropriate points along the scale. All scales request a rating of dyspnea intensity between the extremes of "none" and "maximal." All scales have been validated and compared with one another and, in practice, any one of them should provide a reliable "single point in time" estimate of an individual's dyspnea intensity.[50] Variations on numerical-based assessment of dyspnea have been developed using pictorial representations for use in children[51] and scaling of observed distress in individuals unable to provide a report of their dyspnea (e.g., in the ICU).[52]

MULTIDIMENSIONAL ASSESSMENT OF DYSPNEA

There has been a growing focus on extending the assessment of dyspnea beyond the intensity domain to include the qualitative and affective components of this complex symptom. Using a multidimensional approach, modeled on those used in pain research, investigators have developed a number of validated instruments that are being used in research and clinical studies. A number of these are referenced in the earlier "Language of Dyspnea" section and have been reviewed in the overall context of dyspnea assessment.[11]

EXERCISE PERFORMANCE AS AN INDICATION OF DYSPNEA

Exercise testing is frequently used to assess the causes and functional impact of an individual's dyspnea. Cardiopulmonary exercise testing requires specialized facilities but offers the most definitive approach in evaluating the functional pathophysiologic basis of unexplained dyspnea.[53] Two widely used field tests are the 6-minute walk test and shuttle walking test,[54] which are easy to perform and require minimal equipment. When an exercise test is limited by symptoms, it is important to ask the patient the exact reason for stopping. Although the patient may appear to be in respiratory distress, often joint pain, leg fatigue or discomfort, or generalized weakness is the actual limiting factor.

REPORTED EXERCISE LIMITATION DUE TO DYSPNEA

Early attempts to evaluate the severity of dyspnea involved patient assessments of their own exercise tolerance (e.g., the five-point Medical Research Council scale[55] and its modified version, the American Thoracic Society scale); it is important to remember that such measures assess the impact of dyspnea rather than dyspnea directly. More recently, this simple assessment of *dyspnea* (D) has been supplemented with measures of *body mass index* (B), FEV_1 (O = *obstruction*), and 6-minute walk distance (E = *exercise capacity*) to yield a BODE index, a validated prognostic indicator in COPD.[56] The Baseline Dyspnea Index, a rater-administered test, was developed to rate patients with regard not only to the "magnitude of the task" that elicits dyspnea (e.g., hills compared with level ground) but also to the impact of dyspnea on activities of daily living and the effort required to produce dyspnea.[57] Measurements can be repeated over time or in response to interventions. Several easy-to-use self-administered questionnaires have been developed to assess functional limitation due to dyspnea but in general have not found widespread use.[58]

QUALITY OF LIFE AND DYSPNEA

The negative impact of dyspnea on an individual's quality of life has been increasingly recognized since the mid-1980s and now is an important outcome measure in studies of therapeutic intervention for COPD/dyspnea. Two questionnaires, the Chronic Respiratory Disease Questionnaire and the St. George's Respiratory Questionnaire, are used most often. The Chronic Respiratory Disease Questionnaire is a rater-administered questionnaire with 20 items that focus on four aspects of illness: dyspnea, fatigue, emotional function, and the patient's feeling of control over the disease.[59] Dyspnea is evaluated on a seven-point scale in relation to the five most important activities provoking dyspnea during the previous 2 weeks. In effect, the Chronic Respiratory Disease Questionnaire assesses how breathing sensations alter the quality of the patient's life. The St. George's Respiratory Questionnaire is a self-administered questionnaire with 76 items addressing symptoms, activity, and the impact of disease on daily life. Dyspnea is not evaluated specifically but is included with other respiratory symptoms, such as cough, sputum production, and wheezing.[60]

DIAGNOSTIC APPROACH TO THE PATIENT WITH DYSPNEA

PHYSIOLOGIC CATEGORIES OF DYSPNEA IN THE CONTEXT OF THE RESPIRATORY SYSTEM

Because dyspnea is an integrated sensation that reflects a range of sensory inputs (e.g., from lungs, chest wall, airways, vascular structures, chemoreceptors) and motor outputs to the ventilatory muscles, it is best to consider dyspnea

TABLE 36.2   Relationships Among Physical Examination, Physiology, and Disease States

Physical Examination	Physiology	Disease States
Tachypnea, use of accessory muscles of inhalation	Stimulation of respiratory controller via chemoreceptors, pulmonary receptors, vascular receptors	Pneumonia, pulmonary edema, pulmonary embolism, COPD with acute gas exchange abnormalities, asthma, pleural effusion, toxic inhalations
Pulsus paradoxus, tripod position, wheezes	Stimulation of pulmonary receptors and increased airway resistance	Asthma, pulmonary edema with bronchospasm, toxic inhalations with bronchospasm
Pulsus paradoxus, accessory muscles of inhalation	Increased airway resistance, decreased respiratory system compliance, neuromuscular weakness	COPD, asthma, kyphoscoliosis, Guillain-Barré, myasthenia gravis, diaphragmatic paralysis
Expiratory abdominal rounding	Creation of intrinsic positive end-expiratory pressure	Pulmonary edema
Paradoxical motion of abdomen or rib cage	Movement of abdomen and chest due to changes in intrathoracic pressure and weakness of either the diaphragm (inward movement of abdomen on inspiration) or the intercostal muscles (inward movement of rib cage on inspiration)	Diaphragm paralysis (paradoxical abdominal motion); spinal cord injury (paradoxical rib cage motion)
Kussmaul breathing	Increased alveolar ventilation (with a lower V_D/V_T ratio) to compensate for metabolic acidosis.	Diabetic ketoacidosis, severe lactic acidosis, ingestions leading to anion gap acidosis
Dullness on percussion	Absence of air in thorax	Pleural effusion; dense consolidation/pneumonia
Hyperresonance on percussion	Diminished lung parenchyma	Pneumothorax, bullous emphysema
Crackles/rales	Reduced compliance of the lung	Interstitial lung disease, pneumonia, pulmonary edema
Rhonchi	Turbulent flow secondary to airway inflammation	Pneumonia, bronchitis

V_D/V_T, ratio of dead space to tidal volume.

initially in terms of the respiratory system and of the ways in which a multitude of diseases can manifest via derangements in the components of that system. This will help us make sense of what is otherwise a long list of possible diagnostic considerations, particularly for the evaluation of the patient with chronic dyspnea.

In concert with the cardiovascular system, the ultimate goal of the respiratory system is to get oxygen from the atmosphere to alveoli to the blood to the organs and cells of the body and then to eliminate carbon dioxide, the product of metabolism. Clinically, dyspnea can be thought to arise in one of four major ways:

1. When the elements of the respiratory system (the respiratory controller, the ventilatory pump, and the gas exchanger) are altered in a way that leads to the development of hypoxemia and/or hypercapnia, with consequent stimulation of chemoreceptors and the respiratory controller;
2. When there is stimulation of discrete sensory receptors throughout the airways, lungs, chest wall, and vasculature;
3. When a mechanical load is imposed on the respiratory system (e.g., increased airway resistance, decreased lung or chest wall compliance); or
4. When neuromuscular weakness arises and inhibits the ability of the body to handle even normal mechanical loads.

Thus, rather than approach the patient by asking which organ system is causing the problem, consider these physiologic categories and the underlying pathology that might contribute to them (Table 36.2).

The first major cause of dyspnea is disease of the respiratory system, leading to abnormal blood gases. Hypoxemia and hypercapnia can be the result of derangements of the gas exchanger (the alveoli and pulmonary vasculature) or due to hypoventilation consequent to suppression of the respiratory control system and/or neuromuscular weakness. The last two can be easily distinguished by the respiratory rate (reduced rate when there is suppression of the controller; rapid rate when there is neuromuscular weakness). The *alveolar to arterial oxygen tension difference* [(A–a)PO$_2$] is also a key indicator of whether the gas exchanger itself is abnormal; when the (A–a)PO$_2$ is greater than normal (i.e., larger than 0.3 × age of the patient), a gas exchanger abnormality is contributing to the problem. One should remember, however, that hypoxemia alone is a relatively weak stimulus for the controller and leads to relatively low intensity dyspnea, and acute hypoxemia secondary to suppression of the controller will not typically lead to breathing discomfort. Acute hypercapnia (or metabolic acidemia), in contrast, can lead to more significant change in ventilation and dyspnea. As noted earlier, the dyspnea associated with stimulation of the controller is generally characterized as a sensation of air hunger, urge to breathe, or "I cannot get enough air."

The second cause of dyspnea comes from stimulation of various sensory receptors. There are multiple receptors throughout the cardiorespiratory system that can stimulate or reduce the drive to breathe from the respiratory controller and contribute to or lessen the intensity of dyspnea. Some of the best studied are unmyelinated nerve endings, stretch receptors, pressure receptors, flow receptors, and metaboreceptors. Pulmonary C fibers (also known as juxtacapillary receptors) are *unmyelinated nerve endings* that may be triggered by inflammation and inhaled chemicals or toxins, as well as by increased pulmonary capillary pressures associated with left heart failure. Airway rapidly adapting *stretch receptors* (also known as irritant receptors), in addition to responding to inhaled irritants, are triggered by deflation of the lung (e.g., atelectasis), which can cause an intense sensation of a need to take a deep breath. The dyspnea associated with large pleural effusions, for example, is likely due in part to atelectasis of underlying lung tissue, as well as displacement outward of the chest wall, which increase the mechanical load on the respiratory system. In contrast, lung inflation with large tidal volumes activates slowly adapting stretch receptors in the airways and may diminish the sensation of air hunger (see discussion of efferent-afferent dissociation in the section "Mechanisms of Dyspnea"). The sense of "tightness" associated with bronchospasm most likely originates with receptors stimulated by bronchospasm, most likely irritant receptors. *Pressure receptors* throughout the pulmonary vasculature and right heart may lead to dyspnea associated with primary pulmonary vascular disease (e.g., pulmonary emboli) and left ventricular failure. *Flow receptors* are essentially temperature receptors in the airways (higher flow on inspiration leads to cooling of the receptors); they provide information on inspiratory flow, which assists the brain in monitoring the response of the ventilatory pump to efferent messages from the controller (central drive) and the degree of efferent-afferent matching. There is one additional set of receptors, the *metaboreceptors* or ergoreceptors, located in skeletal muscle, which are apparently stimulated in the setting of low oxygen delivery and play a particular role in the dyspnea arising when we reach the limits of our cardiovascular fitness during exercise and in heart failure.[61]

The third cause, increased mechanical loading on the respiratory system, comprises some of the most common diseases we encounter clinically, that is, COPD and asthma, as well as chest wall problems, such as obesity and kyphoscoliosis. Increased airway resistance and/or decreased respiratory system compliance may lead to a need to exert greater effort to maintain normal alveolar ventilation.

Finally, the fourth cause of dyspnea arises from abnormalities of the neuromuscular system. Diseases that impair neuromuscular function, for instance, Guillain-Barré and myasthenia gravis, lead to dyspnea when the controller attempts to maintain normal alveolar ventilation.

HISTORY

As with all of medicine, a careful history, guided by one's understanding of the pathophysiology of the underlying symptom, is key to creating a differential diagnosis that leads to an efficient yet complete evaluation (see also Chapter 18). When evaluating a patient complaining of breathing discomfort, the history should be focused on five types of information: (1) the language used by the patient to describe his or her dyspnea, (2) the timing of the dyspnea, (3) the positional nature of the symptom, (4) the associated symptoms, and (5) the intensity.

Language

As described earlier, the qualitative descriptors used by patients to characterize their breathing discomfort can provide clues to the underlying problem (see Table 36.1). It is best first to ask the patient to tell you, "What does the breathing discomfort actually feel like?" Some patients are

bemused by this question, and it can be helpful to use the analogy to the different types of pain they may have experienced in the past, for instance, sharp, dull, burning, aching. Alternatively, one may ask the patient to choose the terms from a list of phrases[18,19]; if the patient chooses multiple phrases, then ask them to identify the three best descriptors of their breathing discomfort.

Timing

The timing of the dyspnea (acute, intermittent, chronic) adds important information to the story. *Acute* dyspnea is associated with diseases such as asthma; pulmonary edema; mucous plugs leading to hypoxemia in bronchitis or pneumonia, which are conditions also associated with increased airway resistance and/or reduced pulmonary compliance; and pulmonary embolism.

Intermittent dyspnea most commonly reflects dyspnea in association with exercise, that is, the patient has a chronic problem that is not of sufficient severity at rest to lead to breathing discomfort but experiences dyspnea with exercise, with its associated increased demands on the cardiorespiratory system. Patients with asthma, COPD, interstitial lung disease, chest wall abnormalities, pulmonary vascular disease, chronic heart failure, and supply-demand ischemic heart disease may all present with intermittent dyspnea. When confronted with a patient with intermittent dyspnea, one should also inquire about factors or conditions other than exercise that precipitate the symptom, for instance, environmental exposures at work or at home.

Chronic dyspnea at rest typically signifies severe, end-stage cardiopulmonary disease, such as severe COPD or heart failure. Progressive neuromuscular diseases, for instance, amyotrophic lateral sclerosis, can also present in this way.

Position

Positional dyspnea is a subset of intermittent dyspnea. Orthopnea is the consequence of increasing pulmonary vascular pressures (and stimulation of associated lung and vascular receptors) when the patient is in the recumbent position. Bendopnea, breathing discomfort when bending over, is associated most commonly with central obesity; the positional change reduces the compliance of the abdominal compartment and compromises the ability of the diaphragm to descend during inhalation. Platypnea, which is dyspnea associated with moving from the lying to sitting position, is usually associated with orthodeoxia and may be seen with arteriovenous malformations at the base of the lung, interatrial shunts, and dilated pulmonary vasculature, as seen in some patients with severe liver disease.

Associated Symptoms

Because dyspnea may arise from multiple disease states, it is important to inquire about other symptoms associated with these conditions. A patient with peripheral edema and awakening at night with shortness of breath is likely to have heart failure. Alternating chills and sweats, along with cough, may provide clues about a respiratory infection. Complaints of diffuse muscle weakness may be associated with respiratory muscle dysfunction. Symptoms of heartburn and gastroesophageal reflux could be a clue to the presence of recurrent aspiration. Skin changes may be associated with interstitial lung diseases; lower extremity lesions (erythema nodosum) or pain and blanching of the fingers in cold weather (Raynaud syndrome) can be a sign of sarcoidosis or scleroderma in a patient with exertional dyspnea.

Intensity

Finally, it is important to ask the patient to rate the intensity of dyspnea. We should not confuse the presence or absence of physical signs of "respiratory distress" (see later) with dyspnea, which can only be quantified by the patient. Studies have shown that both doctors and nurses are frequently inaccurate in estimating a patient's dyspnea, most commonly by underestimating the intensity of breathing discomfort.[62] In addition, beware of changes that patients make in their lifestyle to avoid dyspnea; these changes may mask worsening of their underlying physiologic problem. For example, if walking up a flight of stairs provokes breathing discomfort, the patient may move from a house to a one-floor apartment; if walking to the grocery store is a burden because of dyspnea, the patient may have a friend or family member do the shopping for them. Consequently, they may deny worsening dyspnea, even while they have had a marked decrease in functional status.

PHYSICAL EXAMINATION

As with the medical history, we should make attempts to link our observations with the underlying pathophysiology (Table 36.2). Vital signs can provide evidence of the state of the respiratory controller and the ventilatory pump. Tachypnea is indicative of an increased drive to breathe, although it is not necessarily evidence of alveolar hyperventilation, which is determined by rate and alveolar volume. In the absence of cardiac tamponade, pulsus paradoxus above 10 mm Hg is indicative of a derangement of the ventilatory pump; the individual must increase ventilatory muscle exertion to compensate either for increased airway resistance or decreased respiratory system compliance. Use of accessory muscles of inhalation (e.g., sternocleidomastoid, scalene) is also seen with increased respiratory drive and abnormalities of the ventilatory pump. Kussmaul breathing (very deep breathing with mild increase in rate) is typical of severe metabolic acidosis (the large tidal volume decreases the dead space to tidal volume ratio, thereby increasing the efficiency of breathing). Measurement of oxygen saturation by pulse oximetry, which is now considered a vital sign by most providers, is important to determine if oxygenation at rest and with activity is normal.

Next, look at the patient's breathing pattern from the bedside. Use of accessory muscles of ventilation in the upper chest and neck can be indicative of increased ventilation (increased drive to breathe) and/or a problem with the mechanical pump (e.g., increased airway resistance, decreased respiratory system compliance, diaphragmatic weakness). Paradoxical motion of the abdomen or rib cage during the respiratory cycle is another indicator of respiratory muscle weakness. Abdominal rounding (inward movement of the lateral abdomen with outward movement of the periumbilical region on exhalation) is characteristic of acute pulmonary edema; the maneuver is hypothesized to be an attempt by the patient to generate intrinsic positive end-expiratory pressure, thereby reducing afterload for the left ventricle.[63]

Inspection of the chest may reveal the Hoover sign (inward motion of the lower lateral rib cage on inspiration), indicative of hyperinflation and underlying emphysema with a flattened diaphragm pulling the lateral rib cage inward with each inspiration. Percussion can be used to identify pleural effusions and motion of the diaphragm. Auscultation may reveal diminished or absent breath sounds (pleural effusion, pneumothorax, bullous emphysema), wheezes (increased airway resistance), crackles (diminished lung compliance), and rhonchi (turbulence from airway secretions). Cardiovascular examination is focused on assessment of intravascular and total body volume (e.g., jugular venous pulse, S3, peripheral edema) and pulmonary artery pressure (e.g., loud P2).

The assessment of dyspnea in patients with respiratory failure treated with mechanical ventilation in the ICU is particularly challenging when they are not able to communicate with the team. In these cases, recognition of vital sign abnormalities, observation of facial expressions, and examination of ventilator tracings for evidence of patient-ventilator dyssynchrony may provide insights into the causes of patient respiratory discomfort.[63]

LABORATORY ASSESSMENT

The assessment of all the diseases that can contribute to dyspnea is beyond the scope of this chapter. Instead, this chapter concentrates on the initial tests that will help the physician focus the subsequent evaluation.

Assessment of the hematocrit and hemoglobin is important to exclude anemia; the mechanism by which anemia leads to dyspnea is not fully established; low oxygen delivery to the tissue may stimulate metaboreceptors in muscle tissue. Polycythemia can be an indicator of chronic hypoxia. Blood chemistries can detect metabolic acidosis or the elevated bicarbonate seen with compensation for a chronic respiratory acidosis, and B-naturetic peptide can be a clue to underlying heart failure. An arterial blood gas is necessary to detect hypercapnia and to calculate the $(A-a)P_{O_2}$, which assists in the evaluation of the causes of hypoxemia and the status of the patient's gas exchanger.

A chest radiograph is an important screening tool for both respiratory and cardiovascular causes of dyspnea. One may see evidence for COPD, interstitial lung disease, pleural effusions, pneumothorax, pneumonia, and heart failure. Enlarged pulmonary arteries can be a clue for thromboembolic and other pulmonary vascular diseases. Computed tomography scan of the chest with contrast, including computed tomography angiography, is more sensitive for many of these diseases and should be pursued when the evaluation has not excluded these diagnostic considerations. Echocardiography is indicated when there is concern for more subtle abnormalities of valvular and ventricular function and to estimate the pulmonary artery pressure.

PULMONARY FUNCTION TESTING

Spirometry is a useful screening test for both airway and parenchymal lung disease. Because airway obstruction in asthma may be intermittent and absent at the time the patient is in your office, monitoring the patient's peak flow

TABLE 36.3 Relationships Among Qualities of Dyspnea, Physiology, and Symptomatic Treatment

Quality of Dyspnea	Physiology	Symptomatic Treatment
Air hunger, urge to breathe, need more air	Stimulation of respiratory controller via chemoreceptors, pulmonary receptors, vascular receptors	Supplemental oxygen; nasal flow of gas; cool air on the face; chest wall vibration; inhaled furosemide; opiates
Chest tightness	Stimulation of airway receptors	Inhaled bronchodilators (beta agonists, anticholinergics, steroids)
Cannot get a deep breath	Stimulation of respiratory controller; dynamic hyperinflation	Breathing retraining (slower breathing); pursed lips breathing
Increased work or effort to breathe	Mechanical load on the respiratory system; neuromuscular weakness	Inspiratory muscle training; noninvasive ventilation/BPAP
Breathing more	Increased ventilation; stimulation of metaboreceptors in muscles	Exercise training
All qualities	Altered perception/processing of information centrally	Desensitization treatment in pulmonary rehabilitation; morphine

BPAP, bilevel positive airway pressure.

at home and at work may detect occult asthma. In those cases where there is still a high suspicion despite normal spirometry/peak flow measurements, methacholine inhalation challenge is indicated.

Lung volume measurements are critical for determination of restrictive pulmonary problems and to assess flow limitation and hyperinflation in patients with obstructive lung disease. For those patients in whom ventilatory muscle weakness is being considered, measurement of maximal inspiratory and expiratory pressures can be useful. Diffusing capacity of the lung should be assessed whenever hypoxemia is present at rest or with exercise.

SPECIAL STUDIES

For patients with new or worsening dyspnea in the setting of chronic respiratory and cardiovascular disease, determining which organ system is responsible for the onset of the symptom can be challenging. Cardiopulmonary exercise tests, during which data are collected on both pulmonary and cardiac function, can be particularly helpful in determining the specific defect at the time dyspnea begins.[64] These tests can involve progressively invasive data gathering, culminating in a level 3 test, which is performed with an arterial and pulmonary artery catheter in place. These advanced studies are particularly useful if there is a concern for diastolic heart failure and/or pulmonary vascular disease as the cause of dyspnea (see Chapter 33).

TREATMENT OF DYSPNEA

Having determined the cause of a patient's dyspnea, the first and most effective approach to treatment is to alleviate the underlying cause of the symptom. Unfortunately, many of the chronic cardiorespiratory conditions that lead to dyspnea are not curable and are often refractory to pharmacologic therapy. In the case of severe emphysema, lung volume reduction surgery has been shown to alleviate dyspnea in a subset of patients, but recurrence of symptoms within several years is common. Increasingly,

nonsurgical approaches using endobronchial valves are substituting for lung volume reduction surgery with promising results.[65]

When dyspnea persists despite optimal treatment of the underlying disease, treatment should focus on the symptom rather than the disease. In part, this leads back to the underlying physiologic mechanisms of dyspnea (Table 36.3) and our ability to manipulate them (e.g., activity of the controller, oxygenation, and respiratory muscle function).[66]

DECREASING RESPIRATORY DRIVE

An increase in the drive to breathe is a key feature of the physiology of many diseases that lead to a sense of air hunger. Reducing stimulation of the chemoreceptors with supplemental oxygen in hypoxemic patients may reduce dyspnea. A secondary effect is obtained with use of nasal cannula because activation of flow receptors in the nose may further relieve the drive to breathe. Blowing cool air on the face with a fan may have similar effects, via activation of facial sensors innervated by the trigeminal nerve.[67] Further efforts to stimulate receptors that will alleviate the drive to breathe have included chest wall vibration,[68] although the means to provide this clinically await development, and activation of slowly adapting stretch receptors in the lung with inhaled furosemide[34]; the latter has had mixed results in a number of studies and may be effective in only a subgroup of patients.[34,69,70]

REDUCING RESPIRATORY EFFORT AND IMPROVING RESPIRATORY MUSCLE FUNCTION

Patients with COPD have significant mechanical loads on the respiratory system. Abnormal airways lead to a resistive load; hyperinflation, which worsens with activity in the face of flow limitation, results in an elastic load. Both of these increased loads burden the inspiratory muscles and contribute to the increased work and effort of breathing. To address this physiology, breathing retraining, including pursed-lips breathing, can mitigate these problems by slowing and prolonging exhalation, which may reduce dynamic hyperinflation.

By providing inspiratory muscle support with noninvasive mechanical ventilation, such as bilevel positive airway pressure, one can also relieve some of the burden on the inspiratory muscles and reduce the work of breathing and muscle fatigue. This intervention has been used extensively for acute dyspnea in the emergency department and in the ICU and is being attempted increasingly in the outpatient setting. In COPD patients with muscle weakness, nutritional supplementation and inspiratory muscle training may be tried, although evidence for the efficacy of this strategy remains scarce. Although theophylline has been shown experimentally to enhance muscle function, clinical studies in COPD have not demonstrated significant benefit. Data supporting a role for systemic inflammation in COPD are growing; this may be an explanation for some of the muscle dysfunction noted in this disease. To date, however, there are no data supporting the chronic use of systemic steroids or other anti-inflammatory agents in this population.

ROLE OF EXERCISE TRAINING IN RELIEVING DYSPNEA

Exertional dyspnea is a common feature of chronic cardiorespiratory disease, and patients may consciously or unconsciously reduce their activities to avoid breathing discomfort. Not only may this contribute to depression and social isolation, patients are likely to become deconditioned, develop early onset of lactic acidosis during exercise, and demonstrate worsening symptoms when they are active. Pulmonary rehabilitation programs that include exercise, patient education, and breathing retraining have been shown to reduce dyspnea, increase exercise capacity, and improve quality of life.[71] In addition to the physiologic benefits described earlier, reassuring support during exercise training can lead to desensitization to the breathing discomfort; patients may still experience dyspnea, but they no longer have as much anxiety or fear of the sensation and can persist in their activity longer.

ALTERING CENTRAL PERCEPTION

If we can do nothing to change physiology, perhaps we change the perception of dyspnea as sensations are processed in the brain. Desensitization to dyspnea, which has been postulated as part of the effect of pulmonary rehabilitation programs as noted, is one way to alter perception. Viewing the discomfort of breathing as analogous to pain, can we provide a pharmacologic intervention to alter the perception of the dyspnea?

It is interesting that analgesics (a drug to relieve pain) have been with us for centuries, but there is no word for a medication that relieves breathing discomfort. Physicians have used opiates for relief of dyspnea for some time,[72,73] although there is concern about the side effects associated with these drugs, including respiratory depression[74] and,

more recently, the fear of developing drug dependence. Although opiates can certainly cause a decrease in ventilation, the doses needed to relieve dyspnea may be associated with relatively minor changes in breathing.[75] When opioids have been used in interstitial lung disease, there was no association with increased admission to the hospital or mortality.[76]

Opiates may have particular benefit in the management of a patient with flow limitation due to asthma or COPD in the acute setting, when one is trying to buy time for standard direct treatment of the disease to take effect. The tachypnea associated with the acute onset of airway obstruction may lead to dynamic hyperinflation, more dyspnea, increased anxiety, and worsening tachypnea; this cycle can lead to intubation and mechanical ventilation. A small dose of opiates in these circumstances may slow breathing, reverse hyperinflation, reduce dyspnea and anxiety, and allow bronchodilators to take effect without the need for intubation.[77] However, there are no large-scale studies of opiates for the management of acute or chronic symptoms in COPD patients.

Although anxiety may lead to tachypnea, increased ventilation, and dyspnea, and dyspnea may lead to anxiety, formal studies of the use of anxiolytics in the treatment of dyspnea have failed to show benefit. In patients with hyperventilation or sighing syndrome—a possible subset of hyperventilation in which patients take intermittent, very large breaths similar to "sighs" and complain of dyspnea—psychological counseling, cognitive behavioral therapy, and anxiolytics may be helpful.

RELIEF OF DYSPNEA IN END-STAGE LUNG DISEASE

Unfortunately, many patients with end-stage lung disease move from intermittent, exercise-induced dyspnea to chronic debilitating dyspnea at rest as their disease progresses. Patients develop a fear of suffocating.[78–80] National respiratory societies have called for more attention to relieving suffering for these patients[37,81,82] as goals of care shift away from extending life to maximizing comfort. Pulmonologists have begun working more closely with palliative care experts to devise the best approach for these patients, particularly with respect to use of pharmacologic and nonpharmacologic interventions (see Table 36.3).

Barriers to effective symptom relief have included lack of provider skill in having conversations about goals of care with patients and families, the fear of using opioids in patients with chronic lung disease, and the fear of taking hope away from patients and families.[83] Nevertheless, coordination of pulmonary and palliative care services has been demonstrated to enhance the patient's sense of breathlessness mastery and to prolong survival,[84] and we all must do better to alleviate suffering in our patients.

Key Points

- Dyspnea is a complex symptom arising from the central processing of information relayed from the central ventilatory control centers with modifying information from numerous afferent sources.
- Breathing discomfort can be affected by behavioral factors and can lead to strong emotional responses.
- The words and phrases used by patients to describe the quality of dyspnea can provide clues to the underlying pathophysiology.
- Most dyspnea is the consequence of problems arising in the respiratory and cardiovascular systems and frequently persists despite acceptable levels of arterial oxygen and carbon dioxide. Conditions that stimulate the drive to breathe, activate receptors in the lungs and pulmonary vasculature, or impair the mechanical response of the ventilatory pump to a given level of central drive should be considered.
- Diagnosis of the underlying cause(s) of dyspnea depends on a careful history, a physical examination that links findings to underlying physiologic derangements, and targeted laboratory studies; cardiopulmonary exercise testing may be particularly helpful in determining the reason why a patient's functional status is limited when both cardiovascular and respiratory problems are present.
- It is important to consider that a patient may gradually limit activities to avoid dyspnea, thereby becoming deconditioned, depressed, and isolated, with progressively worse symptoms when active. Physical rehabilitation can help desensitize a patient to the sensation of dyspnea.
- Treatment of dyspnea begins with interventions directed at correcting the underlying disease state. When this is inadequate, one should consider interventions that reduce the intensity and/or unpleasantness of the symptom.

Key Readings

Banzett RB, O'Donnell CR, Guilfoyle TE, et al. Multidimensional dyspnea profile: an instrument for clinical and laboratory research. *Eur Respir J.* 2015;45:1681–1691.

Bausewein C, Farquhar M, Booth S, Gysels M, Higginson IJ. Measurement of breathlessness in advanced disease: a systematic review. *Respir Med.* 2007;101:399–410.

Faull OK, Hayen A, Pattinson KTS. Breathlessness and the body: neuroimaging clues for the inferential leap. *Cortex.* 2017;95:211–221.

Gentzler ER, Derry H, Ouyang D, et al. Underdetection and undertreatment of dyspnea in critically ill patients. *Am J Respir Crit Care Med.* 2019;199:1377–1384.

Guell MR, Cejudo P, Ortega F, et al. Benefits of long-term pulmonary rehabilitation maintenance program in patients with severe chronic obstructive pulmonary disease. *Am J Respir Crit Care Med.* 2017;195:622–629.

Loring SH, Townsend SR, Gallagher DC, et al. Expiratory abdominal rounding in acute dyspnea suggests congestive heart failure. *Lung.* 2006;184:324–329.

O'Donnell DE, James MD, Milne KM, Neder JA. The pathophysiology of dyspnea and exercise intolerance in chronic obstructive pulmonary disease. *Clin Chest Med.* 2019;40:343–366.

O'Donnell DE, Milne KM, Vincent SG, Neder JA. Unraveling the causes of unexplained dyspnea: the value of exercise testing. *Clin Chest Med.* 2019;40:471–499.

O'Donnell, Elbehairy AF, Faisal A, et al. Exertional dyspnea in COPD: the clinical utility of cardiopulmonary exercise testing. *Eur Respir Rev.* 2016;141:333–347.

Parshall MB, Schwartzstein RM, Adams L, et al. An official American Thoracic Society statement: update on the mechanisms, assessment and management of dyspnea. *Am J Respir Crit Care Med.* 2012;185:435–452.

Pattinson KT, Johnson MJ. Neuroimaging of central breathlessness mechanisms. *Curr Opin Support Palliat Care.* 2014;8:225–233.

Soffler MI, Rose A, Hayes MM, et al. Treatment of acute dyspnea with morphine to avert respiratory failure. *Ann Am Thorac Soc.* 2017;14:584–588.

Yourke J, Moosavi SH, Shuldham C, Jones PW. Quantification of dyspnea using descriptors: development and initial testing of the Dyspnea-12. *Thorax.* 2010;65:21–26.

Complete reference list available at ExpertConsult.com.

37 COUGH

KIAN FAN CHUNG, MD, DSC, FRCP • STUART B. MAZZONE, PHD

INTRODUCTION

Cough is a protective mechanism, often present for transient (acute) periods of time to facilitate the removal of mucus, noxious substances, or pathogens from the airways and lungs. Impairment of coughing can be harmful or even fatal. Epidemiologic surveys have shown that 11–18% of the general population report a chronic cough,[1] which may be due to cigarette smoking, increased exposure to environmental irritants and pollution, or chronic diseases associated with cough. Chronic cough and cough hypersensitivity syndrome are therefore commonly presented to the clinician. In the United States, cough is the most common complaint for which patients seek medical attention and the second most common reason for a general medical consultation. Many people self-medicate to try to relieve their cough, and over-the-counter cough and cold medicines sold in the United States alone amounted to $2.3 billion between 2007 and 2012. Cough may also be a sign of chronic disease in which patients typically present with chronic cough, defined as a cough lasting for more than 8 weeks. Typically, chronic cough is accompanied by increased sensitivity to cough triggers, a clinical phenomenon known as cough hypersensitivity syndrome.[2–4] Patients with cough hypersensitivity syndrome often complain of a persistent tickling, irritating, or choking sensation in the throat, which often leads to paroxysms of uncontrollable coughing. Of note, chronic cough can be harmful and does not always respond to disease-modifying therapies, needing to be suppressed directly as part of disease management. New therapies to suppress cough have been recently introduced (termed *neuromodulators*), with the prospect of more effective therapies to be introduced in the coming decade.[5]

DEFINITION OF COUGH

Cough usually starts as a deep inspiration, followed by a strong expiration against a closed glottis (compression phase), which then opens with an expulsive flow of air, producing a characteristic cough sound (Fig. 37.1). (Audios 37.1 and 37.2). An initial cough may be followed by a series of expiratory efforts, with closures of the glottis but no intervening inspirations—a "cough bout" or an "epoch." There can be variations of the respiratory pattern, including an expiration-only pattern, or "huff," associated with throat clearing. Cough sounds may have clear harmonic patterns, but their significance has not been established (eFig. 37.1). Cough is usually accompanied by an awareness of airway irritation and the feeling of an "urge to cough," indicating that cough sensations are processed in the higher brain.[6,7] Cough can either be reflexively or voluntarily initiated, and habit or behavioral cough is not uncommon, especially in children.[8]

DEFINITION OF COUGH HYPERSENSITIVITY SYNDROME

The concept of cough hypersensitivity encompasses the abnormal state of chronic coughing, which is often accompanied by other sensations. Thus, many describe a persistent or intermittent tickling, irritating sensation, rawness or itch, or a choking sensation in the throat, with repeated throat clearing, chest tightness, hoarse voice and dysphonia, vocal cord dysfunction, a globus feeling in the throat, and dysphagia. In addition, innocuous triggers of cough include changes in ambient temperature, taking a deep breath, laughing, talking, cigarette smoke, aerosol sprays, and perfumes. Therefore, the cough hypersensitivity syndrome has been defined as a disorder characterized by troublesome coughing, often triggered by low levels of thermal, mechanical, or chemical exposure. There is increasing evidence that this is caused by a disordered sensory neural function, both at the peripheral and *central nervous system* (CNS), with an underlying neuropathy.

PHYSIOLOGY AND NEUROBIOLOGY

MECHANICS OF COUGHING

The inspiratory phase of cough consists of a deep inspiration through a widely opened glottis. The inhaled volume varies greatly, from a low to a nearly complete vital capacity. The inspiration may draw material into the lungs; however, the large lung volume provides a better mechanical efficiency for the expiratory muscles of cough because they are stretched, their stretch reflex is activated, and there is a stronger elastic recoil of the lung to aid expiration. Furthermore, the deep inspiration opens the airways in preparation for their clearance during the expiratory phase.[9]

In the compressive phase of cough, lasting about 200 ms, the glottis closes while the expiratory muscles contract, and the intrapleural and intra-alveolar pressures rise rapidly to a range of values that can vary from 40 to 400 cm H_2O. The expulsive phase follows when the glottis opens. The expiratory flow rate depends on the driving pressure established during the compressive phase and on resistance to airflow, largely reflective of the diameter of the central airways, which are dynamically collapsed as a result of high intrathoracic pressure. The expulsive phase of coughing may be long lasting, with a large expiratory tidal volume, or it may be interrupted by glottic closures into a series of short expiratory efforts, each having a compressive and an expulsive phase.

Maximum expiratory flow is independent of effort because it is limited by dynamic compression of the airways.[9] This compression starts immediately downstream from the equal pressure point, at which intraluminal and extraluminal pressures around the bronchial wall are equal. The effectiveness of cough depends on peak airflow and will therefore be greater with a larger elastic recoil of the lung, *which creates the driving pressure*, and a greater stiffness of the central airways, *which prevents dynamic collapse*. Dynamic compression of the airways downstream from the equal pressure point increases velocity, kinetic energy, and turbulence of the air passing through the proximal airways. Thus, the clearing capacity of the cough is improved. If cough consists of a series of expiratory efforts, with lung volume decreasing with each effort, dynamic compression is predicted to move into the more peripheral

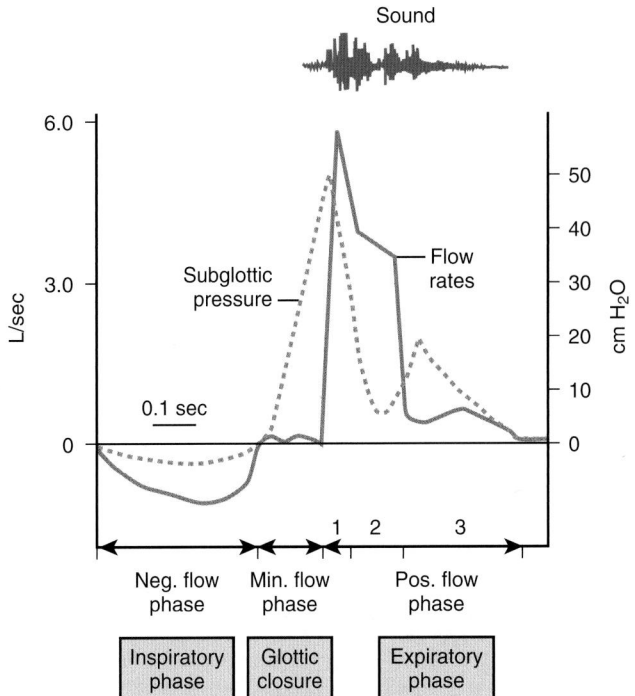

Figure 37.1 **Diagrammatic representation of the changes of the following variables during a representative cough: sound, flow rate, and subglottic pressure.** During inspiration, the flow rate is negative; at the glottic closure, the flow rate is zero; and during the expiratory phase, the flow rate is positive. The expiratory phase can be divided into three parts: during the first expulsive phase *(1)*, there is an explosive cough sound, the first cough sound; during the second phase *(2)*, as the expulsive airflow diminishes, the sound amplitude diminishes; and during the third phase *(3)*, the vibration of a partly closed glottis produces a regular periodic sound, the second sound. Refer to eFig. 37.1 for a representation of the cough waveform. Min., minimal; Neg., negative; Pos., positive. (From Bonica JJ. *Obstetric Analgesia and Anesthesia.* Amsterdam: World Federation of Societies of Anaesthesiologists; 1980.)

bronchi, which will be progressively cleared of intraluminal material.

Whereas mucociliary transport is the major method of clearing the airway lumen in healthy subjects, cough is an important reserve mechanism. However, in those with lung disease, cough plays a larger role in airway clearance. In many lung diseases, mucociliary clearance is impeded and cough is necessary to remove the increased amount of secretions and debris. Healthy subjects have twice the mucociliary clearance rate of that in patients with chronic bronchitis; with cough, whereas healthy subjects will increase their clearance by only 2.5%, patients with chronic bronchitis can increase their clearance by 22%.[10] As would be expected, all studies point to the fact that cough is effective in causing clearance if there is hypersecretion of mucus; by definition, a dry cough is an unproductive one.

COUGH MOTOR CONTROLS

The inspiratory and expiratory phases of cough rely on coordinated activity of the multiple respiratory muscle groups that ordinarily control breathing. Although glottic closure is usually regarded as definitive of cough, in both human and experimental animals the closure may be incomplete or absent, and this does not seem to impair the effectiveness of the cough in clearing the airway. Coughing is associated with respiratory actions other than those of the respiratory skeletal muscles.[11] There is usually bronchoconstriction, although this may be masked or reversed by the dramatic changes in lung volume. Bronchoconstriction increases the linear velocity of airflow and lessens the inflow of irritant material to deeper parts of the airways. Cough is also accompanied by reflex secretion of mucus from airway submucosal glands. Mucus entraps inhaled particles and irritant chemicals, and the material is thus cleared from the airways by mucociliary transport and by the cough itself. Mucus also can act as a physicochemical barrier between the luminal irritants and the airway wall.

SENSORY RECEPTORS FOR THE COUGH REFLEX

Involuntary coughing can be initiated only from those structures innervated by the vagus nerve.[12] These include the larynx and tracheobronchial tree, the lower part of the oropharynx, tympanic membrane, and the external auditory meatus. The one clear exception to vagally-mediated coughing is voluntary coughing. The most sensitive sites for initiating cough are the larynx and tracheobronchial tree, especially the carina and points of bronchial branching, areas richly innervated by cough-inducing receptors associated with vagal sensory nerve fibers.[12] It is worth noting that it is difficult or impossible to induce coughing from the smaller airways and alveoli. This is teleologically understandable because even a vigorous cough would not produce sufficient airflow to clear substances from the most distal airways. Different types of stimuli induce coughing by acting on at least two types of cough-evoking sensory nerve fiber types, broadly categorized as either vagal *nociceptors*, which detect a range of noxious chemical irritants, including inflammatory mediators, or vagal *mechanoreceptors*, which are highly sensitive to mechanical stimuli, such as particulate matter entering the airways or accumulated intraluminal mucus (Fig. 37.2 and eFig. 37.2).

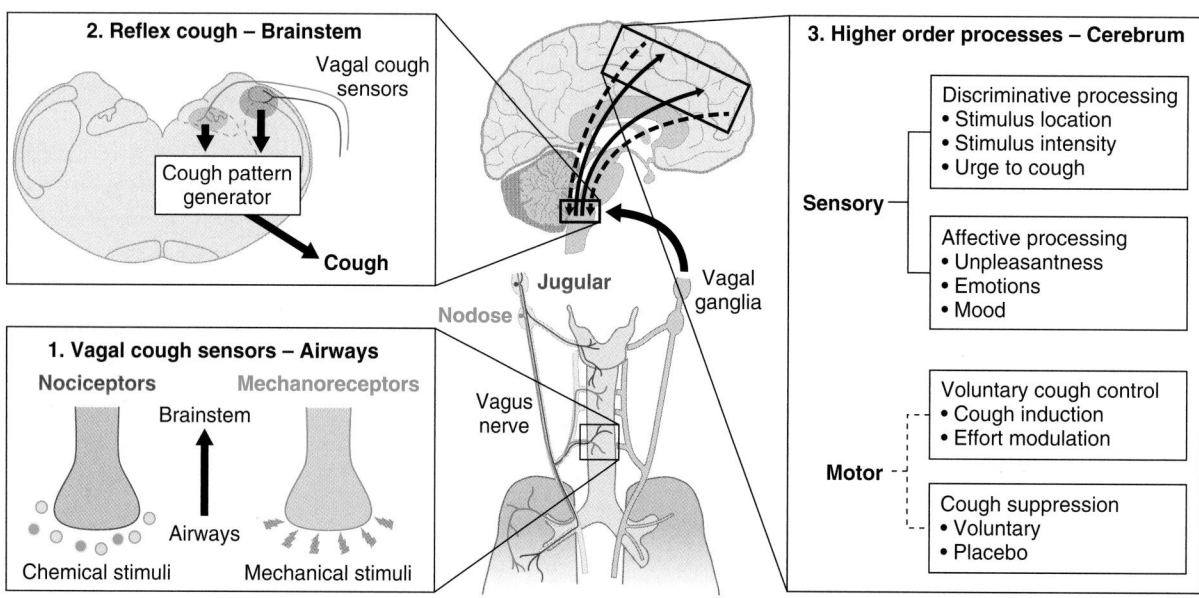

Figure 37.2 Two types of vagal sensory neurons in the airways and lungs can mediate cough. Those sensitive to chemical stimuli are termed nociceptors; those sensitive to physical stimuli are termed mechanoreceptors. Both sensory neuron types connect to the brainstem and send information that can be processed by local circuits to initiate a reflex cough. Sensory information can also ascend into the higher brain, where it encodes more complex aspects of cough, including the accompanying experience of an urge to cough. Higher brain circuits also descend upon the brainstem sites that regulate reflex coughing and can be enlisted to induce a voluntary cough, to modulate cough intensity, or to suppress a cough altogether. Inflammation can alter the sensitivity of these cough-evoking pathways because the vagal sensory neurons express a wide variety of receptors for cytokines and other chemical mediators. (Modified from Mazzone SB, Undem BJ. Vagal afferent innervation of the airways in health and disease. *Physiol Rev.* 2016;96:975–1024; and Mazzone SB, Farrell MJ. Heterogeneity of cough neurobiology: clinical implications. *Pulm Pharmacol Therap.* 2019;55:s62–s66.)

Vagal *nociceptors* are unmyelinated slow-conducting C fibers characterized by their responsiveness to the chemical capsaicin, the active ingredient in hot chili peppers. Nociceptors are also responsive to a wide range of proinflammatory molecules, which notably include bradykinin, prostaglandins, leukotrienes, proteases, and cytokines, as well as noxious irritants, such as capsaicin, acid, nicotine, and acrolein.[12] When inhaled, many such chemicals are a powerful stimulus for coughing.

Vagal *mechanosensors* are myelinated fast-conducting Aδ-fibers that are normally silent, unlike other myelinated vagal mechanosensors in the lung that monitor lung volume. Their stimuli include acid solutions, such as that aspirated from the stomach, hypotonic solutions including inhaled fog, and mechanical stimulation by catheter, mucus, or dust (but not stretch or bronchospasm). All these stimuli can provoke cough.

MEMBRANE RECEPTORS/CHANNELS FOR COUGH TRANSDUCTION

Extensive studies exist on the sensory nerve membrane channels and receptors involved in coughing.[12–14] The details are complex, so they are summarized only briefly. However, the results are of considerable importance as they indicate how chronic coughing manifests and provide a rationale for the antitussive therapeutics available or in development.

Vagal *nociceptors* express several *transient receptor potential* (TRP) channels. Capsaicin and temperature-sensitive *transient receptor potential vanilloid-1* (TRPV1) receptors are directly activated by capsaicin, used commonly as a tussive agent in clinical studies of cough; these receptors are additionally sensitized or indirectly activated by heat, protons, bradykinin, arachidonic acid derivatives, *adenosine triphosphate* (ATP), and phosphokinase C. TRPV4 is osmotically sensitive and mostly found on epithelial cells but also on a subset of vagal sensory nerve fibers, whereas TRP ankyrin 1 is often coexpressed with TRPV1 on many vagal nociceptors in the airways and is activated by allyl isothiocyanate (mustard oil), cinnamaldehyde (from cinnamon), and acrolein (from cigarette smoke). C fibers also express tetrodotoxin-insensitive voltage-gated sodium channels, many G protein–coupled receptors for inflammatory mediators, and receptors for neurotrophins, such as nerve growth factor.

Vagal *mechanosensors* are thought to express mechanically gated membrane ion channels that are unique to this class of airway sensory fibers but have yet to be identified. In addition, they have other channels that can be activated by acids and belong to the *acid-sensing ion channel* (ASIC) family. They possess different types of voltage-sensitive ion channels needed for action potential formation and conduction, including the NaV1.7 subtype of voltage-gated sodium channels, characterized by sensitivity to the neurotoxin tetrodotoxin. However, the vagal mechanosensors lack several TRP channels found in vagal nociceptors, although these TRP channels may be induced during inflammation.

Both nociceptors and mechanosensors often also express receptors for ATP and other purines. Of note, P2X2 and P2X3 purinergic receptors can be expressed alone or in combination, and it is thought that local release of ATP from the injured or inflamed airways is a major contributor to cough hypersensitivity syndrome acting via these receptors.[3]

CENTRAL NERVOUS SYSTEM CONTROL

Reflex coughing is integrated in the brainstem, where the vagal sensory fibers for coughing first terminate (see Fig. 37.2).[15–17] Recipient neurons within these sensory integration sites connect with a collection of respiratory control neurons in the brainstem, loosely defined as the cough pattern generator. Outputs from the cough pattern generator are sent to motoneurons of the respiratory muscles, larynx, and bronchial tree to actuate the cough respiratory pattern.

Vagal sensory inputs to the brainstem are also relayed to higher brain regions where inputs are integrated in pontine, subcortical, and cortical nuclei.[6,7,16] These anatomic pathways have been reasonably well defined in animals, demonstrating several different circuits important for encoding cough sensations. Studies with functional magnetic resonance imaging of the human brain during airway irritation with capsaicin and induced cough have delineated those areas involved in the different sensory discriminative and motor aspects of noxious airway stimulation (see Fig. 37.2 and eFig. 37.3). For example, the anterior insula cortex is thought to play a role in monitoring the amount of sensory input arising from the airways, whereas the primary sensory cortex is involved in assimilating sensory inputs and coding them for the urge-to-cough sensation. The posterior parietal and prefrontal cortices may provide spatial awareness (i.e., where the stimulus is coming from), and the orbitofrontal cortex in the limbic brain helps shape the affective dimensions of cough (i.e., how does it make you feel).[16]

Cough can also be behaviorally induced or modified via higher brain circuits. For example, cough can be initiated voluntarily, a process that originates in motor and premotor cortical brain regions (see Fig. 37.2).[15,18,19] These voluntary descending pathways may bypass brainstem integrative centers because some patients with brainstem damage lack a cough reflex but can voluntarily induce coughing to clear the airways.[20] The motor cortex and inferior frontal gyrus can generate voluntary cough suppression to inhibit reflex coughing temporarily.[19] The placebo effect is prominent in cough, and this involves the dorsolateral prefrontal cortex and an inhibitory pathway that reduces vagal sensory processing in the brainstem, much like the endogenous analgesia system that is proposed to mediate the placebo effect for pain.[15,18] This endogenous inhibitory system relies on endogenous opioids to induce suppression, explaining how opiates can be effective at suppressing cough. Of importance, chronic cough in disease is not simply a matter of too much sensory input from the airways and lungs but also involves a reduction in central cough suppressive mechanisms that ordinarily help to reduce unwanted coughing.[7,19]

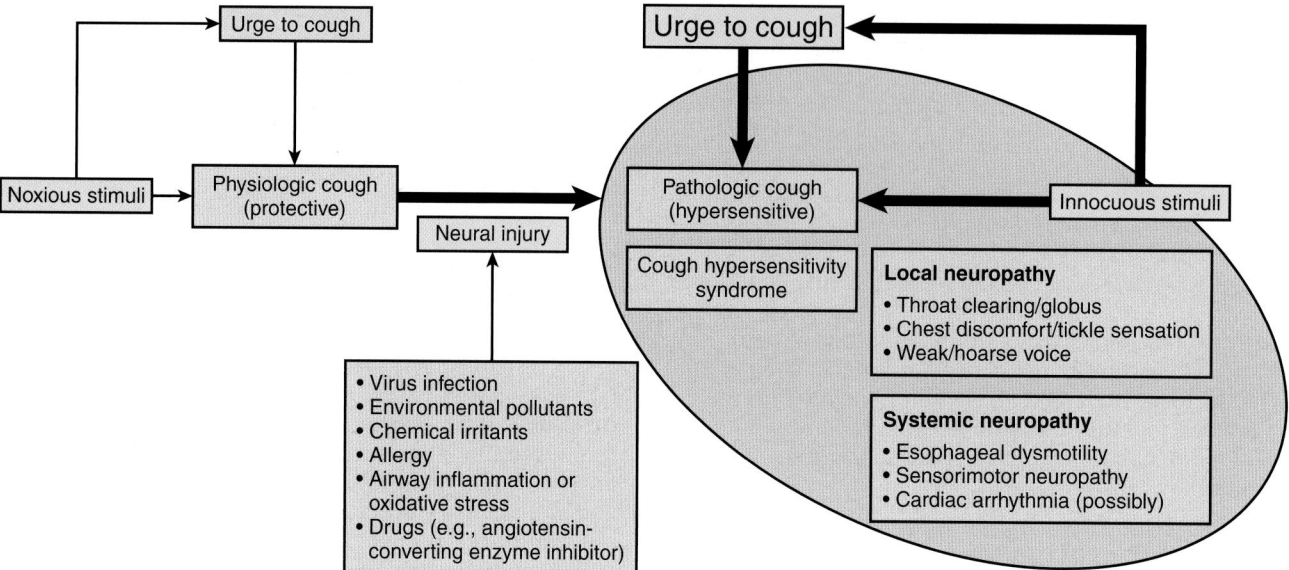

Figure 37.3 Cough hypersensitivity syndrome. On the left is a normal cough response. The proposed effect of vagal nerve injury arises from inflammation caused by airway exposure to infective, physical, chemical, and allergic insults. With neural injury (*arrow to right*), the cough progresses to a pathologic cough. The *blue oval* emphasizes the pathology (neuropathy) of the cough hypersensitivity syndrome. (From Chung KF, McGarvey L, Mazzone S. Chronic cough as a neuropathic disorder. *Lancet Respir Med.* 2013;1:414–422.)

MECHANISMS OF COUGH HYPERSENSITIVITY

In the cough hypersensitivity syndrome, the sensory receptors for cough can show an exaggerated response to stimuli that would normally be harmless or mildly irritating. This increase in sensitivity, termed *peripheral sensitization*, can be caused by allergens, viral infections, ozone, cigarette smoke, and a variety of inflammatory mediators.[12] Vagal mechanosensors can also be sensitized by mucus in the airways, smooth muscle contraction, and mucosal edema. Increases in sensitivity have been related to *neuroplasticity* in the vagal sensory fibers. Thus, terminals of vagal sensory fibers in the airways and lungs can sprout and increase their area of innervation, as well as change their expression of neurotransmitters, ion channels, and receptors, leading to alterations in their normal physiologic properties. This *peripheral sensitization* can be accompanied by *central sensitization*, a neuroinflammatory process in the CNS that amplifies incoming sensory inputs and produces hyperreflexic states.[4,16] The alterations in the structure and function of vagal sensory neurons and central processing pathways in cough hypersensitivity syndrome lead to the clinical symptoms *hypertussia* (increased cough sensitivity to known stimuli) and *allotussia* (cough in response stimuli that do not normally cause cough). This clinical presentation is analogous to a neuropathy, for example, similar to that seen in many patients with chronic pain (Fig. 37.3).[4]

APPROACH TO THE PATIENT WITH COUGH

As emphasized in national cough guidelines,[21–23] the approach to the management of a patient with cough is first to identify the cause(s) of the cough and then to treat the cause(s) (Fig. 37.4). Cough may be indicative of trivial or serious airway or lung diseases, including infections, inflammatory and neoplastic conditions, and many pulmonary and extrapulmonary conditions (Table 37.1). The foremost consideration for the clinician at the first visit is to (1) determine the severity, (2) assess the possible cause(s) of the cough, and (3) plan investigations and treatment. Various indicators in the history and examination of the patient may provide clues to the diagnosis, although these may not be entirely reliable or specific and may be absent in many cases.

The timing and selection of various investigations may vary according to presentation (Table 37.2). Initial investigations may be limited to a chest radiograph, particularly in a cigarette smoker, where abnormalities can be found in 10–30% of chest radiographs. Further investigations (e.g., *computed tomography* [CT] or fiberoptic bronchoscopy) may be pursued despite a "normal" chest radiograph. Often, the cause may not be found, the treatment of the putative cause may not suppress or improve the cough, or the cause may have no effective treatment. In those cases, therapy that suppresses cough by inhibiting the cough pathway without treating the cause is necessary.

The protocol for investigating a chronic cough takes into account several factors pertaining to the pathophysiology of cough and to the most common causes of cough. Postnasal drip ("nasal catarrh" or "upper airway cough syndrome"), asthma, and *gastroesophageal reflux disease* (GERD) are the three most common conditions associated with a chronic cough. Therefore, an initial diagnostic approach to exclude these conditions is sensible. Bearing in mind that there are also myriad other less common causes of a cough, further investigations may be indicated. Lung function tests, including lung volumes and diffusing capacity, as well as CT imaging of the lungs, should be considered to check for bronchiolar or parenchymal disease or unsuspected bronchiectasis. Fiberoptic bronchoscopy should be considered and,

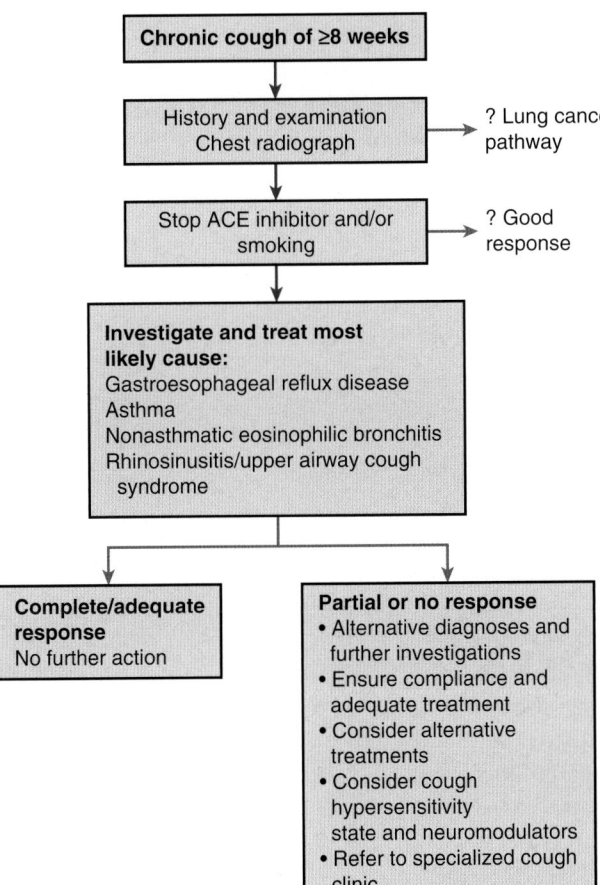

Figure 37.4 Algorithm for the management of chronic cough in adult patients. For a chronic cough lasting for >8 weeks, the evaluation and management should be methodical. After a thorough history and physical examination and chest imaging to exclude lung cancer or other intrathoracic pathology, and after stopping *angiotensin-converting enzyme* (ACE) inhibitor and/or smoking, the workup proceeds through the most common likely entities. These are listed as gastroesophageal reflux disease, asthma, non-asthmatic eosinophilic bronchitis and rhinosinusitis, or upper airway cough syndrome. Exclusion can be determined either by investigations or trial of therapy or both. Ultimately, patients with persistent chronic cough can be referred to specialized cough clinics for alternative diagnosis and treatment.

Table 37.1 Common Causes of Cough

ACUTE INFECTIONS
Tracheobronchitis
Bronchopneumonia
Viral pneumonia
Acute-on-chronic bronchitis
Pertussis

CHRONIC INFECTIONS
Bronchiectasis
Tuberculosis
Cystic fibrosis

AIRWAY DISEASES
Asthma
Eosinophilic bronchitis
Cough-variant asthma
Chronic bronchitis
COPD
Chronic postnasal drip

PARENCHYMAL DISEASES
Interstitial pulmonary fibrosis
Emphysema
Sarcoidosis

TUMORS
Lung cancer
Benign airway tumors
Mediastinal tumors

ASPIRATED FOREIGN BODIES

MIDDLE EAR PATHOLOGY

CARDIOVASCULAR DISEASES
Left ventricular failure
Pulmonary infarction
Aortic aneurysm

OTHER DISEASES
Gastroesophageal reflux disease
Laryngopharyngeal reflux
Recurrent microaspiration
Endobronchial sutures
Obstructive sleep apnea
Laryngeal dysfunction

DRUGS
Angiotensin-converting enzyme inhibitors

apart from excluding small central tumors, mucosal biopsies may be taken for histologic diagnosis (e.g., to diagnose eosinophilic infiltration or sarcoidosis). Lower airway samples can also be obtained for culture for infectious agents. As a result, a protocol based on systematic evaluation using history, physical examination, and laboratory investigations focusing on the anatomic sites of cough receptors that constitute the afferent limb of the cough reflex is the most widely advocated approach to diagnosis and treatment.[21]

Cough with usually clear sputum production often points toward conditions such as chronic bronchitis and bronchiectasis or other causes of bronchorrhea. However, the diagnostic value of knowing that the cough is productive is probably limited because similar causes are often found for both productive and dry cough.[24] For example, an enhanced cough reflex may be present in both productive and nonproductive cough. Features associated with an enhanced cough reflex include cough triggered by taking a deep breath, laughing, inhaling cold air, and prolonged talking. Although the diagnostic approach may be similar

whether or not the cough is productive, any change in the color of the sputum that indicates purulence must be considered as potential evidence of a bacterial infection, such as bronchiectasis or bronchitis.

MEASURING COUGH SEVERITY AND FREQUENCY

Cough can be measured by assessing its severity, frequency, intensity, and impact on quality of life. First, assessment of cough severity can be obtained from the history; complications such as vomiting, rib fractures, fatigue, urinary incontinence, and syncope (Table 37.3) can indicate chronicity

Table 37.2 Diagnostic Evaluation of Chronic Cough

1. History and physical examination.
2. Chest radiograph, particularly in smokers.
3. Initial evaluation may lead to diagnosis of chronic bronchitis in cigarette smokers and of angiotensin-converting enzyme inhibitor cough. Discontinue cigarette smoking and offending drug.
4. Further diagnostic evaluation on basis of initial evaluation:
   a. If suggestive of postnasal drip, order a computed tomography (CT) scan of sinuses, and allergy tests.
   b. If suggestive of asthma, request a record of peak expiratory flow measurements at home for 2 weeks and a bronchoprovocation test with histamine or methacholine, and/or a trial of antiasthma treatment.
   c. If suggestive of gastroesophageal reflux disease, request 24-hour pH monitoring and, if necessary, an endoscopic examination of the esophagus or a barium swallow series.
   d. If the chest radiograph is abnormal, consider examination of sputum and a fiberoptic bronchoscopy. A high-resolution CT scan of the thorax and further lung function evaluation may be necessary.
5. Treat specifically for associated conditions. The cause(s) of cough is (are) determined when specific therapies eliminate or improve the cough. There may be more than one associated cause for the cough.

Table 37.3 Potential Complications From Excessive Cough

RESPIRATORY
Pneumothorax
Subcutaneous emphysema
Pneumomediastinum
Pneumoperitoneum
Laryngeal damage

CARDIOVASCULAR
Cardiac dysrhythmias
Loss of consciousness

CENTRAL NERVOUS SYSTEM
Syncope
Headaches
Cerebral air embolism

MUSCULOSKELETAL
Intercostal muscle pain
Rupture of rectus abdominis muscle
Increase in serum creatine phosphokinase
Cervical disc prolapse

GASTROINTESTINAL
Esophageal perforation

OTHER
Social embarrassment
Depression
Sleep disruption
Urinary incontinence
Disruption of surgical wounds
Subconjunctival hemorrhage
Petechiae
Purpura

and intensity. Another indication of severity is the effect on lifestyle and psychological well-being, such as the development of anxiety and depression.

Cough severity can be measured by a *visual analogue scale*, on which the patient records his or her perception ranging from mild to severe or on a nominal line of 10 cm. Severity of cough can also be evaluated using quality-of-life questionnaires specific for the evaluation of the impact of chronic cough. The Leicester Cough Questionnaire uses a seven-point Likert response scale for 19 items from three domains (physical, psychological, and social) and has been shown to be repeatable and sensitive in patients with chronic cough.[25] The Cough-Specific Quality of Life Questionnaire with 28 items in six domains is validated for both acute and chronic cough.[26]

Cough frequency can be measured using a recording device of the cough sound using a microphone.[27] The coughs can either be counted by listening or by using cough detection software. There is a weak correlation between cough frequency and subjective scoring systems measured by the cough visual analogue scale or the Leicester Cough Questionnaire.[28,29]

MEASURING COUGH REFLEX

The *cough reflex* is measured by counting the number of coughs after inhalation of tussive agents, such as capsaicin, the pungent extract of peppers, or citric acid– or low-chloride-content solutions. Chronic cough may result from an increase in the sensitivity of the cough sensors. Due to a variety of causes, most patients with a chronic cough have an enhanced cough reflex when compared with healthy non-coughing subjects, but there is a significant degree of overlap between these groups.[30–33] There is also a heterogeneity of cough responses to different agents that work through different receptors. Thus, cough reflex results may reflect the underlying hypersensitive state to a particular stimulus. A combination of both subjective and objective measurements should ideally be used to assess a patient's cough. These measurements have proven to be useful in assessing the response of patients to antitussive therapies both in the clinic and in randomized controlled studies of antitussives.

ACUTE, SUBACUTE, AND CHRONIC COUGH

Cough may be divided according to its duration. An *acute* cough is defined as lasting less than 3 weeks, a *subacute* cough as lasting between 3 and 8 weeks, and a *chronic* cough as lasting more than 8 weeks.[21]

Acute cough is usually due to a viral or bacterial upper respiratory tract infection. The cough of the common cold is usually self-limiting and usually starts within the first 48 hours with accompanying symptoms of postnasal drip, throat-clearing, sore throat, nasal obstruction, and nasal discharge, which usually resolve within 2 weeks. Acute cough could also be caused by an exacerbation of underlying diseases, such as an upper airway cough syndrome secondary to rhinosinusitis, asthma, COPD, or pneumonia. Patients with the common cold usually self-medicate with over-the-counter antitussive preparations, despite a lack of good evidence for their effectiveness in acute cough.[34] Codeine is ineffective, although dextromethorphan had some variable but small effect. Honey can provide symptomatic relief.[35] The efficacy of antitussive preparations in children is lacking and, because these medications may be potentially harmful,[36] cough due to acute viral airway infections should be treated only with fluids and humidity, although honey may be tried.[34]

Subacute cough is most commonly due to a prior infection or exacerbations of underlying diseases, such as asthma, COPD, and upper airway cough syndrome. Pertussis should be considered in the differential diagnosis, particularly if the cough has a whooping quality (Audios 37.3 and 37.4) and is associated with vomiting. In adults, the presence of whooping or posttussive vomiting increases the likelihood of the diagnosis of pertussis, whereas a lack of paroxysmal cough or the presence of fever should rule it out.[37] In children, posttussive vomiting is less helpful as a diagnostic test.[37]

Chronic cough can be caused by many diseases, but it is most commonly due to postnasal drip, asthma, GERD, chronic bronchitis, and bronchiectasis.[21] Each of these will be considered along with their specific therapies (Table 37.4).

POSTNASAL DRIP (RHINOSINUSITIS, UPPER AIRWAY COUGH SYNDROME)

Postnasal drip or the upper airway cough syndrome is a common cause of chronic cough.[21,38] Postnasal drip (nasal catarrh) is characterized by a sensation of nasal secretions or of a "drip" at the back of the throat, accompanied by a frequent need to clear the throat. There may also be a nasal quality to the voice due to concomitant rhinonasal blockage and congestion, together with hoarseness. Physical examination of the pharynx is often unremarkable, although a "cobblestoning" appearance of the mucosa and draining secretions may be observed. CT of the nasal passages and sinuses may reveal rhinosinusitis with mucosal thickening or sinus opacification and air-fluid levels. Extrathoracic variable upper airway obstruction is sometimes present.[39]

The best treatment is topical administration of corticosteroid drops in the head-down position, often with the concomitant use of antihistamines.[38] Topical steroids offer a local effect with a minimum of side effects. On occasion, severe symptoms may be controlled initially by a short course of oral steroids, followed by topical therapy. A topical anticholinergic spray to the nose, such as ipratropium bromide, to dry excessive nasal secretions may provide additional benefit. A combination of topical corticosteroid, antihistamine, and anticholinergic treatments has been shown to benefit the chronic cough accompanying postnasal drip, along with an improvement in nasal discharge and endoscopic appearances.[40] Topical decongestant vasoconstrictor sprays may be useful adjunct therapy for a few days, but rebound nasal obstruction may develop after prolonged use. Antibiotic therapy is necessary in the presence of acute sinusitis involving bacterial infection with mucopurulent secretions that have persisted for at least 10 days.

ASTHMA AND ASSOCIATED EOSINOPHILIC CONDITIONS

Asthma may present with chronic cough under different clinical settings. Asthma may present predominantly with cough, often nocturnal, and the diagnosis is supported by the presence of reversible airflow limitation, bronchial hyperresponsiveness, and often elevated fractional levels of nitric oxide in the exhaled breath. This condition of "cough-variant" asthma is a common type of asthma in children.[41] Elderly asthmatics may also give a history of chronic cough before a diagnosis of asthma is made. Cough as the only presenting symptom of asthma has been reported in up to 57% of patients and is often its most prominent symptom.[42] Cough may also be present as a first sign of worsening asthma; the cough usually presents first at night, associated with other symptoms, such as wheeze and shortness of breath with reduction in early morning peak flows. Some patients with asthma may also develop a chronic dry cough despite good control of their asthma, which may be the sign of a cough hypersensitivity syndrome.

Atopic cough is recognized in Japan as an isolated chronic cough characterized by an atopic background, sputum eosinophilia, cough hypersensitivity, normal pulmonary function, and airway hyperresponsiveness.[43] A related entity, eosinophilic bronchitis, is characterized by cough without asthma symptoms or bronchial hyperresponsiveness but with eosinophilia in sputum.[44]

An enhanced cough reflex may be seen in a subgroup of asthmatics with chronic cough.[45] In these patients, cough sensors may be sensitized by inflammatory mediators, such as bradykinin, tachykinins, and prostaglandins. Cough in asthma may also be due to bronchial smooth muscle contraction, which may activate cough receptors through physical deformation. Another potential mechanism for the enhanced cough reflex observed in asthma is the presence of eosinophils. It is of interest to note that, in two conditions presenting with chronic cough, cough-variant asthma and eosinophilic bronchitis, eosinophils predominate in the airways, and inhaled corticosteroids, which inhibit the eosinophilia, are effective in controlling the cough.[46] Recent evidence indicates that eosinophils may be responsible for increasing the airway sensory nerve density that may account for an increase of cough sensitivity in airway conditions associated with cough.[47]

Cough associated with asthma should be treated with a combination of inhaled corticosteroid therapy and long-acting β_2-adrenergic agonists, treatments that should be maintained over a prolonged period (3–6 months). In some patients with cough-variant asthma, β-adrenergic bronchodilators are effective antitussives.[48] Often, a trial of oral corticosteroids (e.g., prednisolone 40 mg/day for 2 weeks) may be recommended, particularly in those asthmatic patients who have had a cough despite being on adequate inhaled antiasthma medication. Cough-variant asthma may respond to leukotriene receptor antagonists.[49] Eosinophilic bronchitis responds well to inhaled or oral corticosteroid therapy.[50]

GASTROESOPHAGEAL REFLUX DISEASE

GERD, the movement of gastric contents from the stomach into the esophagus, usually causes heartburn, chest pain, a sour taste, regurgitation, and often a chronic cough. The mechanisms that link cough with reflux remain unclear. An esophageal-tracheobronchial cough reflex mechanism triggered by acid is based on the observation that cough can be induced by perfusion of the distal esophagus with acid solutions and can be suppressed by perfusion of the distal esophagus with lidocaine and by inhalation of an anticholinergic agent, ipratropium bromide.[51] In addition, the majority of cough episodes are temporally related to reflux episodes. A heightened cough reflex to capsaicin in GERD patients provides evidence for sensitization of this pathway. Not only the acid but the non–acid reflux components, such as the liquid, gas, and pepsin, have been proposed as stimulating cough.

Patients with GERD may have laryngopharyngeal reflux with evidence of inflammation in the upper airway[52] and, in these patients, cough may result from a direct effect of refluxate reaching the cough receptors in the larynx and trachea. In symptomatic GERD, increases in tracheal acidity with a fall in pH to less than 4 are reported during episodes of reflux.[53] In the presence of reflux and microaspiration, laryngeal symptoms may be present, with dysphonia, hoarseness, frequent throat clearing, a globus sensation (e.g., a feeling of a lump in the throat), and sore throat. Often, posterior vocal cord laryngeal inflammation with edema, erythema, contact ulceration, pachydermia (a thickened mucosa), and/or granuloma is visible. Ineffective esophageal peristalsis has been reported in chronic cough, and this may increase the exposure time of the larynx and pharynx to any refluxate.

Monitoring acid reflux by 24-hour ambulatory pH, together with monitoring non–acid reflux by intraluminal impedance in the proximal and distal esophagus, with analysis of the temporal relationship between the reflux episodes and cough, may be useful. A positive association between acid reflux, non–acid reflux, and cough sounds on an ambulatory cough counter has been reported, together with a heightened cough reflex sensitivity.[54] Other tests include esophageal manometry to measure dysmotility, particularly associated with reflux episodes; upper *gastrointestinal* (GI) contrast series; or an upper GI endoscopy.

Conservative measures, such as weight reduction; a high-protein, low-fat diet; elevation of the head of the bed; and avoidance of coffee and smoking, may be useful. Reduction of acid production from the stomach can be achieved with either H_2-histamine blockers or proton pump inhibitors but, of interest, these agents have not been shown to benefit the chronic cough.[55] It is recommended that those with objective evidence of heightened esophageal acid exposure on pH monitoring or with complaints of heartburn should benefit from acid-suppressive therapy provided for 2 months. There is no good evidence for the use of prokinetics, such as domperidone or metoclopramide, which are associated with potential side effects. The effectiveness of antireflux surgery, such as laparoscopic fundoplication in patients with chronic cough associated with GERD disease whose cough has failed to respond to medical therapy, is unclear.

CHRONIC BRONCHITIS/COPD

Chronic bronchitis is diagnosed in patients who produce sputum on most days over at least 3 consecutive months, particularly during the winter months, over at least 2 consecutive years. Although up to 30% of the community smokes tobacco, chronic bronchitis is only reported in 5% of the patients seeking medical attention for cough. In a smoker, the presence of chronic bronchitis may be predictive of progressive irreversible airflow obstruction, leading to COPD. The cough of chronic bronchitis may result from excessive sputum production associated with mucus cell hyperplasia and bronchiolar inflammation. In addition, there is evidence of an increase in capsaicin cough hypersensitivity in patients with COPD.[33]

The productive cough in chronic bronchitis is exacerbated by upper respiratory infections with common viruses or respiratory bacteria or by exposure to irritating dusts or environmental pollutants. Cessation of cigarette smoking is usually accompanied by a reduction in cough, most often within 4 to 5 weeks. Treatment of chronic airflow obstruction with short-acting and/or long-acting β_2-adrenoceptor agonists and anticholinergic agents should be considered, particularly in the presence of dyspnea. Suppression of the inflammatory process in the small airways may be tried with the combination of inhaled corticosteroids and long-acting β-agonists. Mucolytic therapy may reduce the incidence of exacerbations.

In smokers, a change in the pattern or characteristics of their cough, such as an increase in intensity or an accompanying hemoptysis, should lead to an evaluation to exclude the presence of lung cancer. A chest radiograph is mandatory in this situation, with consideration of CT imaging of the chest.

BRONCHIECTASIS

The cough of bronchiectasis is associated with overproduction of airway secretions together with a reduced clearance, often within a vicious circle of recurrent bacterial infections.[56] Usually, the patient produces 30 mL or more of mucoid or mucopurulent sputum per day, sometimes accompanied by fever, hemoptysis, and weight loss. Early- onset bronchiectasis may present solely as a chronic productive cough. Bronchiectasis may be associated with postnasal drip and rhinosinusitis, asthma, GERD, and chronic bronchitis. Common pathogens cultured from sputum include *Haemophilus influenzae*, *Staphylococcus aureus*, and *Pseudomonas aeruginosa*. The chest radiograph may show increased bronchial wall thickening, particularly in the lower lobes in advanced cases, but thin-section CT of the chest can reveal early changes of airway wall thickening, dilation, and distortion, with mucus plugging, and evidence of bronchiolitis. There is an increased capsaicin cough response in bronchiectasis.[57]

Cough in bronchiectasis is the most effective mechanism for clearing airway secretions. Chest physiotherapy to improve airway clearance remains essential. Cough during infective exacerbations of bronchiectasis may become a tiring symptom. Long-term macrolide therapy may lead to an improvement in exacerbations and lung function. The cough due to bronchiectasis may be controlled by the use of inhaled β_2-agonists to improve mucociliary clearance and reverse any associated bronchoconstriction, by postural drainage of airway secretions, and by the use of intermittent antibiotic therapy. Use of antitussives is not recommended but, in the context of severe cough, some suppressive effect may be clinically beneficial.

ANGIOTENSIN-CONVERTING ENZYME INHIBITORS

Angiotensin-converting enzyme (ACE) inhibitors, often prescribed for the treatment of hypertension and heart failure, produce cough in 2–33% of patients. The cough is typically described as "dry" and associated with a tickly irritating sensation in the throat. It may appear within a few hours of taking the drug or only after taking the drug for weeks or even months. After withdrawal of the drug, the cough disappears within days or weeks. Patients with ACE inhibitor cough demonstrate an enhanced response to the capsaicin inhalation challenge. Accumulation of bradykinin and prostaglandins, which sensitize cough receptors directly, has been implicated. The best course of action for ACE inhibitor cough is to discontinue the treatment and replace it with alternative therapies, such as angiotensin II receptor antagonists. In any patient with cough who is taking an ACE inhibitor, the first step in the workup is to stop the drug and reevaluate if the cough persists.

POSTINFECTIOUS

Postinfectious cough has been reported in up to a quarter of patients with chronic cough, with up to half of patients after *Mycoplasma* or *Bordetella pertussis* infection.[58] *B. pertussis* infection is now increasingly recognized as a cause of a cough that can last for 4 to 6 weeks, particularly in older children and adults. In children, other respiratory infections associated with chronic cough include viruses (respiratory syncytial virus and parainfluenzae), *Mycoplasma*, and *Chlamydiae*. In most patients with a postinfectious cough, the initial trigger is usually an upper respiratory tract infection; the accompanying cough that would have been expected to last for only a week persists for many months. Such patients are often referred to a cough clinic and are usually investigated for the more commonly associated causes of cough. Inhaled corticosteroids are often prescribed but with variable success. Oral steroids may be successful. Macrolide antibiotics or trimethoprim-sulfamethoxazole are effective in eliminating *B. pertussis* but do not alter the subsequent clinical course.[59]

IDIOPATHIC PULMONARY FIBROSIS

Idiopathic pulmonary fibrosis (IPF) is a progressive lung disease characterized by scarring of the lungs. The main symptoms are dyspnea on exertion and a chronic dry or mildly productive cough.[60] The cough is refractory to antitussive therapy and harms the quality of life. Often cough is the first symptom and is more common during the day than at night. Compared to other conditions of chronic cough, IPF patients usually experience higher rates of cough. The cough is often associated with other comorbidities, such as postnasal drip, GERD, or cough-variant asthma. Cough reflex sensitivity to capsaicin is increased in IPF, which could result from fibrotic distortion of the lungs or by the increased levels of neurotrophins.[61] Of note, perhaps because of the added mechanical stress on the lungs, cough has been found to be an independent predictor of progression in IPF.[62]

The cough of IPF can be debilitating and difficult to treat. Comorbid conditions need to be treated. Conventional antitussive therapies, such as opiates, are often not effective. Corticosteroid therapy may sometimes work. The new antifibrotic treatment for IPF, pirfenidone, has been shown in an observational study to reduce cough frequency and subjective cough measures.[63] A trial of thalidomide has indicated some beneficial effect on the cough of IPF.

OTHER CONDITIONS

Other conditions causing cough include bronchogenic carcinoma, metastatic carcinoma, sarcoidosis, chronic aspiration, interstitial lung disease, or left ventricular failure, conditions that can usually be excluded with a normal chest radiograph. Chronic cough may also be associated with obstructive sleep apnea and chronic tonsillar enlargement. Nocturnal cough associated with obstructive sleep apnea usually presents in patients with snoring, nocturnal heart burn, and symptoms of rhinitis.[64] Continuous positive airway pressure therapy with humidification is usually effective. Psychogenic or habit cough is common, particularly in children, and is usually a diagnosis arrived at after exclusion of other causes. Habit cough is a throat-clearing noise made by a person who is nervous and self-conscious. Cough may be associated with a depressive illness, and long-standing cough may in turn cause depression. In the pediatric population other cough etiologies specific for this age group need to be considered: congenital abnormalities, including vascular rings and tracheobronchomalacia (eFig. 37.4); pulmonary sequestration or mediastinal tumors; foreign bodies in the airway (eFig. 37.5) or esophagus; aspiration due to poor coordination of swallowing or esophageal dysmotility; and heart disease.

CHRONIC COUGH OF UNKNOWN CAUSE (IDIOPATHIC COUGH)

Up to 46% of patients with chronic cough have been identified as having idiopathic cough. Patients should be diagnosed with idiopathic cough or unexplained cough only after an intensive diagnostic evaluation and empirical trial of therapies. Also within this group is the chronic refractory cough when the patient does not respond to treatments for an associated cause, such as postnasal drip or GERD. Idiopathic cough is more commonly found in women aged between 50 and 70 years with a cough onset at menopause and associated with autoimmune disorders.[65] They present with an enhanced cough reflex to capsaicin or citric acid and present with features associated with the cough hypersensitivity syndrome,[4] with a persistent tickling sensation in the throat that leads to paroxysms of coughing triggered by changes in ambient temperature, taking a deep breath, laughing, talking, and exposure to cigarette smoke or aerosol sprays or perfumes or to certain odors. Mucosal biopsies from nonasthmatic patients with idiopathic cough showed increased mast cell numbers and airway wall remodeling with sub-basement membrane thickening, increased airway smooth muscle mass, goblet cell hyperplasia, and increased number of blood vessels.[66] There is an increase in the expression of the neuropeptide, calcitonin gene-related peptide, and the calcium channel, TRPV1, in the airway epithelium that could contribute to the increased cough reflex.[67,68]

Idiopathic cough may also be caused by an increased sensitivity of the larynx to innocuous stimuli that causes the symptoms of laryngeal paraesthesia with cough associated with dyspnea, dysphonia, and laryngeal spasms.[69] Related disease associated with chronic cough may act as triggers to laryngeal hypersensitivity, such as GERD, rhinosinusitis, and asthma. Assessment of laryngeal dysfunction is becoming an important aspect of the management of chronic idiopathic cough.[70] The treatment of chronic idiopathic or refractory cough is dealt with in the next section.

COUGH SUPPRESSION THERAPIES

When the treatment of the cause of cough is not effective or not available, therapies directed at eliminating the symptom of cough irrespective of the cause of the cough should be tried[71] (Table 37.4).

NONPHARMACOLOGIC APPROACH: SPEECH PATHOLOGY MANAGEMENT

Speech pathology management or cough suppression therapy consisting of breathing exercises, cough suppression therapy, vocal and laryngeal hygiene training, and psychoeducational counseling has been shown to be effective in improving cough symptom scores and cough counts, as well as breathing, voice, and upper airway symptoms.[72] Some studies also report a reduction in capsaicin cough sensitivity and in cough severity. This treatment administered by a speech therapist or respiratory physiotherapist is now offered for patients with refractory chronic cough in specialized cough clinics. Patients with chronic cough who also present with concomitant muscle tension dysphonia and/or vocal cord dysfunction appear to be those who do particularly well with this approach.

PHARMACOLOGIC APPROACH: ANTITUSSIVE THERAPIES

Antitussives may work by inhibition of central mechanisms within the brainstem or of mechanisms involving the peripheral cough sensors in the airways. An ideal antitussive would be one that suppresses the hypertussive component of cough in disease yet allowing the protective cough to be active.

NARCOTIC AND NON-NARCOTIC ANTITUSSIVES

Opiates including morphine, diamorphine, and codeine are often used as antitussive agents.[73–75] (Diamorphine is not prescribed in the United States). At their effective doses, they cause physical dependence, sedation, respiratory depression, and GI constipation. Morphine and diamorphine are usually reserved for the palliative control of

Table 37.4 Treatments for Chronic Cough

TREATING THE SPECIFIC UNDERLYING CAUSE(S)

Asthma, cough-variant asthma	Bronchodilators and inhaled corticosteroids
Eosinophilic bronchitis	Inhaled corticosteroids; leukotriene inhibitors
Allergic rhinitis and postnasal drip	Topical nasal steroids and antihistamines Topical nasal anticholinergics (with antibiotics, if indicated)
Gastroesophageal reflux	Conservative measures Histamine H$_2$-antagonist or proton pump inhibitor
Angiotensin-converting enzyme inhibitor	Discontinue and replace with alternative drug such as angiotensin II receptor antagonist
Chronic bronchitis/COPD	Smoking cessation Treat for COPD
Bronchiectasis	Postural drainage Treat infective exacerbation and airflow obstruction
Infective tracheobronchitis	Appropriate antibiotic therapy Treat any postnasal drip

SYMPTOMATIC ANTITUSSIVE TREATMENT: NEUROMODULATORS (ONLY AFTER CONSIDERATION OF CAUSE OF COUGH)

Chronic cough (all)	Speech and language therapy
Chronic cough affecting quality of life	Amitryptiline Gabapentin
Chronic refractory cough	Slow-release morphine

cough and pain of terminal cancer patients. Slow-release morphine can be partially effective in controlling severe chronic idiopathic cough without altering the cough reflex response. These opioids also relieve anxiety and pain. Opioids can exacerbate wheezing through the release of histamine, but this is rare.

Codeine, the methylether of morphine, has long been the standard centrally acting antitussive drug against which the pharmacologic and clinical effects of newer drugs have been measured. However, it has mixed antitussive efficacy activity. Although codeine has activity against pathologic cough and cough in normal volunteers, it has little activity on cough in COPD patients or against acute cough of the common cold.[73]

Dextromethorphan is a non-narcotic antitussive, a synthetic derivative of morphine with no analgesic or sedative properties and is usually included as a constituent of many compound cough preparations sold over the counter. It is as effective as codeine in suppressing acute and chronic cough when given orally[73] and has antitussive efficacy against cough associated with upper respiratory tract infections in adults but not in children. Because of the potential adverse effects and of overdosage associated with antitussive preparations containing dextromethorphan in children, it should be avoided in that group. Side effects are few at the usual dose but, at higher doses, dizziness, nausea, vomiting, and headaches may be reported. Dextromethorphan should be used with caution in patients on monoamine oxidase inhibitors in whom central nervous depression and death has been reported. Levodropropizine, a nonopioid antitussive with peripheral inhibition of sensory cough receptors, has a favorable benefit/risk profile compared with dextromethorphan.[76]

NEUROMODULATORS

Neuromodulatory agents act on the enhanced neural sensitization that underlies idiopathic or refractory cough. Centrally acting neuromodulators, such as amitriptyline, gabapentin, and morphine, have positive effects on cough-specific quality of life. A prospective, randomized, controlled open trial comparing the effectiveness of amitriptyline versus codeine/guaifenesin for chronic cough after an upper respiratory tract infection showed that amitriptyline led to a complete response of the cough in most subjects, whereas none in the codeine/guaifenesin group had a complete response.[77] In a randomized controlled double-blind trial in patients with refractory cough, gabapentin was effective in reducing cough frequency and visual analogue scores while improving Leicester Cough quality-of-life scores, without affecting the capsaicin cough response.[78] In another randomized, controlled trial of patients with refractory cough, a combination of speech pathology therapy and pregabalin, which is related to gabapentin, reduced cough severity and cough frequency and improved quality of life when compared to speech pathology therapy alone.[79] Both amitriptyline and gabapentin have central antinociceptive actions and may modulate presynaptic N-methyl-D-aspartate receptors, leading to reduced transmitter release and postsynaptic excitability. In addition, gabapentin may have an action on gamma-aminobutyric acid neurotransmission or voltage-gated ion channels in the spinal cord and brain. The effectiveness of neuromodulators suggests that chronic cough can be a neuropathic condition in some patients.[4]

EXPECTORANTS AND MUCOLYTICS

Expectorants and mucolytics may alter the volume of secretions or their composition. Despite a lack of good evidence, mucolytic agents such as acetylcysteine, carbocysteine, bromhexine, and methylcysteine are often used to facilitate expectoration by reducing sputum viscosity in patients with chronic bronchitis. A small reduction in the number of exacerbations of bronchitis has been reported with oral acetylcysteine, accompanied by small improvement in cough, a decrease in volume of sputum, and some ease of expectoration.[80] Aromatic agents such as eucalyptus and menthol have decongestant effects in the nose and may be useful in short-term relief of cough.[73] Menthol inhibits capsaicin-induced cough in normal volunteers and acts through a cold-sensitive TRP receptor, TRPM8. Demulcents also form an important component of many proprietary cough preparations and may be useful because the thick sugary preparation may act as a protective layer at the mucosal surface.

POTENTIAL NEUROMODULATORS

New cough suppressants in development include blockers of ion channels on vagal afferent endings and centrally acting agents.[5,14,74] Preclinical studies have identified TRP channels as an exciting target for cough suppression. However, TRPV1, TRPA1, and TRPV4 antagonists all failed in clinical trials for chronic refractory cough. The most promising target currently is the ATP P2X2/3 receptor. A P2X2/3 antagonist, gefapixant, has shown efficacy in suppressing chronic cough in phase II clinical trials with a reduction in cough frequency of 75%[81] and it is currently undergoing phase III testing. The most notable side effect of gefapixant is a reduction in taste because P2X2 receptors are not only expressed by airway sensory nerves but also by gustatory nerves involved in taste processing. More selective P2X3 antagonists are in early phases of development and may reduce the off-target effects further.[5,82] Voltage-gated sodium channels, channels that initiate and conduct action potentials, are also a promising target. Lidocaine is a nonselective blocker of this family of sodium channels and displays some efficacy for cough reduction. The NaV1.7 subunit has been found to be involved in the control of cough responses to citric acid in guinea pigs,[83] but as yet there are no specific blockers of NaV1.7. Centrally acting agonists of the alpha-7 nicotinic acetylcholine receptor are also undergoing development for cough. This target arose from studies demonstrating that nicotine exposure acutely reduced cough sensitivity in humans[84] through an action believed to reside within the CNS. Alpha-7 cholinergic receptors may be expressed on central pathways that mediate cough inhibition.[85] Finally, centrally acting neurokinin 1 receptor antagonists are also currently in trial for chronic refractory cough, showing improvements in cough frequency and patient quality of life in early phase II trials.[86]

Key Points

- Cough may be a sign of disease inside or outside the airways and lungs and a useful indicator for both patient and physician for initiating a diagnostic evaluation and treatment of disease processes.
- Impairment or absence of coughing can be harmful or even fatal in disease. On the other hand, when cough is chronic and excessive, it can itself be harmful and deleterious and may need to be suppressed directly.
- The most sensitive sites for initiating cough are the larynx and tracheobronchial tree.
- In the management of a patient with cough, the first step is to identify the cause(s) of the cough and then treat the cause(s).
- Postnasal drip, asthma, and gastroesophageal reflux are the three most common conditions associated with a chronic cough, and a diagnostic approach to exclude these conditions early on is sensible.
- Many cigarette smokers have a chronic cough, but a change in the pattern or characteristics of their

cough, such as an increase in intensity or an accompanying hemoptysis, should lead a smoker to seek medical attention. A chest radiograph is mandatory in this situation.

- Patients with chronic cough while on angiotensin-converting enzyme inhibitor therapy should discontinue such therapy, with replacement by other appropriate treatments.
- The cough hypersensitive syndrome is defined as a disorder characterized by troublesome coughing triggered by low levels of thermal, mechanical, or chemical exposure, with a persistent tickling sensation in the throat that leads to paroxysms of coughing triggered by changes in ambient temperature; taking a deep breath; laughing; talking; and exposure to cigarette smoke, aerosol sprays, perfumes, or certain odors.
- When the treatment of the cause of cough is not effective, neuromodulatory therapies directed at controlling the hypersensitive cough, irrespective of the cause of the cough, should be tried.

Key Readings

Chung KF, McGarvey L, Mazzone S. Chronic cough as a neuropathic disorder. *Lancet Respir Med.* 2013;1:414–422.

Chung KF, Pavord ID. Prevalence, pathogenesis, and causes of chronic cough. *Lancet.* 2008;37:1364–1374.

Chung KF, Widdicombe JG, eds. *Pharmacology of Cough.* Berlin: Springer-Verlag; 2009:1–389.

Gibson P, Wang G, McGarvey L, Vertigan AE, Altman KW, Birring SS. Treatment of unexplained chronic cough: CHEST guideline and expert panel report. *Chest.* 2016;149(1):27–44.

Kahrilas PJ, Altman KW, Chang AB, et al. Chronic cough due to gastroesophageal reflux in adults: CHEST guideline and expert panel report. *Chest.* 2016;150(6):1341–1360.

Mazzone SB, Undem BJ. Vagal afferent innervation of the airways in health and disease. *Physiol Rev.* 2016;96(3):975–1024.

Mazzone SB, Chung KF, McGarvey L. The heterogeneity of chronic cough: a case for endotypes of cough hypersensitivity. *Lancet Respir Med.* 2018;6(8):636–646.

McGovern AE, Short KR, Kywe Moe AA, Mazzone SB. Translational review: neuroimmune mechanisms in cough and emerging therapeutic targets. *J Allergy Clin Immunol.* 2018;142(5):1392–1402.

Ryan NM, Vertigan AE, Birring SS. An update and systematic review on drug therapies for the treatment of refractory chronic cough. *Expert Opin Pharmacother.* 2018;19(7):687–711.

Complete reference list available at ExpertConsult.com.

38 CHEST PAIN

BRETT E. FENSTER, MD • TEOFILO L. LEE-CHIONG JR, MD •
G.F. GEBHART, PHD • RICHARD A. MATTHAY, MD

INTRODUCTION

Pain is a complex, subjective experience that varies from person to person in its quality, intensity, duration, location, frequency, and associated features. Its perception is influenced by a subject's culture, emotional and cognitive states, socioeconomic status, familial background, psychological factors, anticipation and previous experience, and the clinical context.

Chest pain is characterized by an unpleasant sensation either localized to the thorax or believed to originate from structures located there. It may announce the presence of severe, occasionally life-threatening disease. Diagnosis of chest pain is often complicated by the vague presentations and indistinct anatomic localization of many of its causes.

Given the wide variety of causes and seriousness of chest pain, considerable clinical judgment is required to decide which patients should be thoroughly evaluated and which tests should be used in the workup. In many instances, empirical therapy may need to be initiated even as evaluation proceeds, with subsequent readjustments in treatment protocols as more information is obtained that clarifies the clinical picture.

The most definitive treatment of chest pain, whatever its origin, is to find its cause and to cure it. The general principles of evaluation for respiratory, cardiac, musculoskeletal, esophageal, and panic disorders are available, and the clinician is encouraged to refer to them. Chronic noncardiac chest pain is more difficult to manage, especially when its trigger cannot be found. Because of the complexities and difficulties in dealing with patients who have chronic, severe, and often refractory pain, referral to special pain centers staffed by a multidisciplinary team of specialists is recommended. At times, psychiatric consultation for specific therapies may be helpful.

EPIDEMIOLOGY

Chest pain is often an important factor in studies of acute pain that warrants medical attention. In a study of randomly selected Canadian households, 16% of respondents reported experiencing pain within the 2 weeks preceding the survey.[1] Chest pain was the fifth most common type of temporary pain. Another survey involving selected enrollees of a health care plan revealed a high incidence of pain lasting a whole day or more, several times during the previous 6 months.[2]

Chest pain accounted for 12% of the reported cases but was the most common site of pain that prompted respondents (35%) to seek medical attention. Pain is also a common reason for visits to hospital emergency departments. In one study, stomach pain, other abdominal pain, and chest pain were the most often cited reasons and together accounted for 10.7% of all emergency department visits.[3]

NEUROBIOLOGY OF PAIN

Pain is not a simple sensation. The neurobiologic and functional components of the sensory channels for pain are neither fixed nor immutable. The nervous system, from the level of the nociceptor (the receptor that responds to noxious stimuli) to the supraspinal sites of integration, is characterized by a dynamic response (plasticity) to tissue insult.

Pain arising from *visceral* organs, such as the heart or *gastrointestinal* (GI) tract, differs in many ways from pain originating from *somatic* structures, such as the skin. Visceral pain is difficult to localize, is diffuse in character, and is typically *referred to* somatic structures. Pain is referred when pain is perceived to be arising from a different location from the original source of the pain (Fig. 38.1).

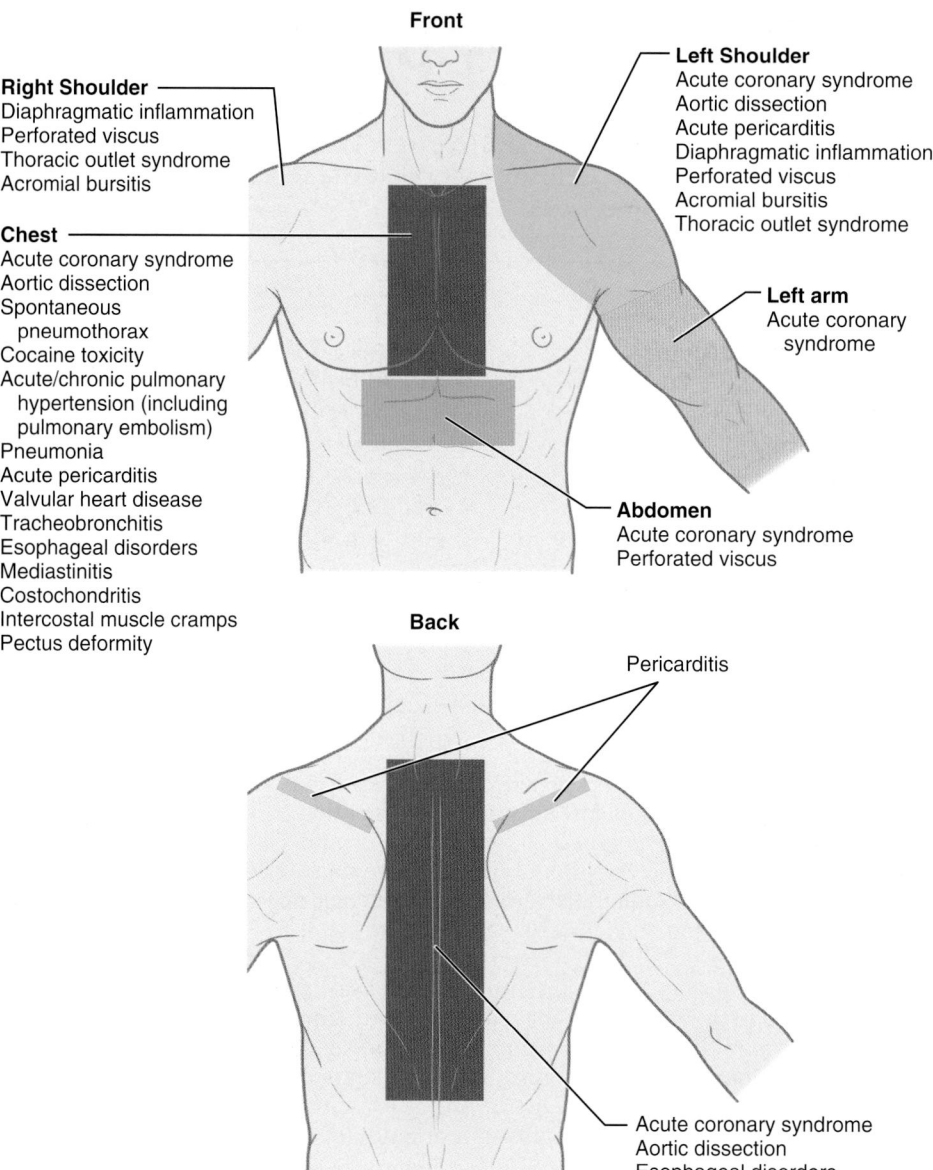

Front

Right Shoulder
Diaphragmatic inflammation
Perforated viscus
Thoracic outlet syndrome
Acromial bursitis

Chest
Acute coronary syndrome
Aortic dissection
Spontaneous
   pneumothorax
Cocaine toxicity
Acute/chronic pulmonary
   hypertension (including
   pulmonary embolism)
Pneumonia
Acute pericarditis
Valvular heart disease
Tracheobronchitis
Esophageal disorders
Mediastinitis
Costochondritis
Intercostal muscle cramps
Pectus deformity

Left Shoulder
Acute coronary syndrome
Aortic dissection
Acute pericarditis
Diaphragmatic inflammation
Perforated viscus
Acromial bursitis
Thoracic outlet syndrome

Left arm
Acute coronary
   syndrome

Abdomen
Acute coronary syndrome
Perforated viscus

Back

Pericarditis

Acute coronary syndrome
Aortic dissection
Esophageal disorders
Mediastinitis

Figure 38.1 Sites of referred pain in the chest. Some conditions are shown that should be considered as sources of referred pain in certain locations of the chest. Referred pain is generally due to viscerosomatic convergence, in which spinal cord neurons receive input from both visceral and somatic sources so that visceral pain can be interpreted as coming from a somatic source. Not shown are psychological causes of pain, which may constitute one of the most common entities, although it should remain a diagnosis only after considering and excluding these sources of pain.

In addition, visceral pain is often associated with greater autonomic and motor responses than is somatic pain. These differences between visceral and somatic pain are related to the characteristic features of sensory innervations that are unique to the viscera.

SOMATIC PAIN

Somatic structures, such as the skin, are invested with a wide variety of nociceptors, each with selective sensitivities to mechanical, thermal, or chemical stimuli, in addition to the polymodal nociceptor that responds to multiple modalities of noxious stimuli.[4,5] Cutaneous nociceptors are characterized by very infrequent or no spontaneous discharges, an ability to encode stimulus intensities in the noxious (but not innocuous) range, and most important, sensitization.

Sensitization refers to an increase in the magnitude of response after tissue insult, sometimes associated with an increase in spontaneous activity and a decrease in response threshold. This attribute of nociceptors contributes to development of hyperalgesia, or an increased response to a painful stimulus.[6] When a tissue is injured, a host of sensitizing chemicals are synthesized at the site of injury or released from circulating cells attracted to the site of injury. These include amines (e.g., histamine and serotonin), peptides (e.g., substance P and calcitonin gene-related peptide), kinins (e.g., bradykinin), neurotrophins, cytokines, prostaglandins, leukotrienes, excitatory amino acids (e.g., glutamate), and free radicals. It is unlikely that any one putative chemical mediator is responsible for nociceptor sensitization.

VISCERAL PAIN

Normal input to the *central nervous system* (CNS) from aortic baroreceptors, gastric chemoreceptors, and pulmonary stretch receptors is rarely perceived. Nevertheless, visceral afferents possess many of the characteristics of nociceptors and may be perceived when abnormal.

All viscera possess a dual innervation. Organs of the thoracic cavity are innervated by vagal afferent fibers with cell bodies in the nodose and jugular ganglia and by spinal afferent fibers with cell bodies in the thoracic dorsal root ganglia. Unlike their somatic counterpart, spinal visceral afferent fibers typically traverse either or both prevertebral and paravertebral ganglia en route to the spinal cord. Thus, in contrast to somatic input to the CNS, which has a single, usually spinal, destination, input to the CNS from organs in the thoracic cavity arrives at two locations, namely the brainstem nucleus tractus solitarii (vagal afferent input) and the thoracic spinal cord (spinal afferent fibers). In accordance, the potential exists for interaction in the CNS from inputs arising from the same thoracic organ. The esophagus and heart also possess an intrinsic nervous system with cell bodies in the organ wall or in ganglia in the epicardial fat.[7]

Somatic and visceral afferents also have a different density of innervation and spinal pattern of termination. In general, the number of visceral afferent fibers is much less than the number of somatic afferent fibers. Although this means that there are fewer central visceral terminals in the spinal cord, visceral afferent fiber terminals have many more terminal swellings (suggestive of synapses) than somatic nociceptor terminals, and they spread their afferent impulses over several spinal cord segments.[8] The obvious consequence of the low number of visceral afferents and greater intraspinal spread is loss of spatial discrimination, consistent with the diffuse, difficult to localize nature of visceral pain.

The axons of visceral sensory neurons are, with rare exception, either thin myelinated Aδ fibers or unmyelinated C fibers. In general, Aδ fibers, having some myelin, carry moderately fast impulses, usually of acute or sharp pain but also of temperature. C fibers, without myelin, carry slow impulses, usually of burning pain. In general, the proportion of Aδ fibers in visceral sensory nerves is less than the proportion of C fibers. In addition, Aδ fibers are fibers with a low threshold for response to mechanical stimulation, whereas C fibers have high thresholds; however, this is not universal.

Unlike tissue-damaging stimuli that produce pain in somatic structures, tissue injury is not required for production of pain in the viscera. For the lower airways, irritants contained in smoke, ammonia, and other inhaled substances are capable of producing discomfort and pain. For the heart and mesentery, ischemia can be an adequate stimulus.[9] For hollow organs of the GI tract, distention of the lumen of the organ, which activates stretch and tension receptors in the smooth muscles, is typically sufficient.

Hollow viscera, including the esophagus, are innervated by two populations of mechanosensitive afferent fibers, namely a larger group (70–80%) of fibers that have low thresholds for response (i.e., within the physiologic range) and a smaller group (20–30%) of fibers that have thresholds for response that fall in the noxious range.[10] All mechanosensitive visceral afferent fibers may function in some circumstances as nociceptors, and low- and high-threshold mechanosensitive fibers contribute to discomfort and pain that arise from the viscera.

Silent nociceptors, a relatively new category of receptor/afferent fibers, may also contribute to altered sensations from visceral structures.[11] Silent nociceptors, more appropriately termed *mechanically insensitive afferents,* have no spontaneous activity and do not respond to acute, high-intensity mechanical stimulation in normal circumstances. After tissue insult, mechanically insensitive afferents typically begin to discharge spontaneously and acquire sensitivity to mechanical stimulation. The contribution of such "silent" or "sleeping" afferent fibers to altered sensations that arise from the viscera continues to be studied.[12,13]

HYPERALGESIA

Some individuals are uniformly more sensitive (i.e., have lowered thresholds for stimulus-produced pain) than others. *Hyperalgesia,* the enhanced response to a stimulus that is normally noxious, consists of primary and secondary components. *Primary hyperalgesia* is the enhanced sensitivity to stimuli applied at the site of tissue injury (e.g., an incision). *Secondary hyperalgesia,* conversely, is the enhanced sensitivity to stimuli applied to uninjured tissue adjacent to, and occasionally distant from, the site of injury. Peripheral mechanisms (sensitization of nociceptors and afferent fibers innervating the insulted tissue) contribute to primary hyperalgesia and central mechanisms (changes in the excitability of spinal and supraspinal neurons) contribute to secondary hyperalgesia.[14] In the spinal cord, glutamate and substance P are co-contained in many small-diameter dorsal root ganglion cells and presumably are concurrently released in the spinal dorsal horn, where N-methyl-D-aspartate receptors on nociceptor terminals may act as autoreceptors to facilitate the further release of both glutamate and substance P.[15] In addition, substance P can act synergistically with glutamate to enhance the responses of spinal neurons.[16]

Virtually all spinal cord neurons that receive a visceral input also receive input from somatic structures, including the skin, muscle, and joints. This convergence of inputs in the spinal dorsal horn is believed to be the basis of the referred sensation that characterizes visceral pain. Such convergence suggests that injury to somatic tissue could lead to visceral hyperalgesia and, conversely, that injury to a viscus could lead to somatic hyperalgesia.

Spinal nociceptive transmission can be modulated by electrical or chemical stimulation in the midbrain or medulla.[17] Both facilitatory and inhibitory influences on spinal nociceptive transmission are present and likely play important roles in the maintenance of secondary hyperalgesia.[18] Electrical activation of vagal afferent fibers similarly engages descending facilitatory and inhibitory modulation of spinal nociceptive transmission. In studies of rats, responses of neurons in the thoracic dorsal horn to either esophageal distention[19] or lower airway irritation caused by ammonia or smoke[20] are altered when the cervical spinal cord is blocked or transected or when the vagi are cut. Responses to esophageal or respiratory stimulation would be expected to increase when the cervical spinal cord is blocked because tonic descending inhibitory influences usually present would be removed. Unexpectedly, responses were found to be more commonly reduced, suggesting the presence of a descending facilitatory influence associated with vagal input to the brainstem. Both vagal afferent input and spinal cardiac nerve afferent inputs contribute to the sensation of cardiac pain, particularly referral of such pain to the neck and jaw.[21]

MEASURING PAIN

Pain has proved to be both hard to define and difficult to measure. Because pain can be quantified only indirectly, it has been difficult to determine the optimal measuring tool for all types of pain sensations. Two widely used techniques, namely rating scales and questionnaires, are often used in clinical and epidemiologic studies of chest pain.

Rating scales constitute the simplest measurement of pain. One of the easiest to use is the quantification of pain intensity by a graded rating scale, such as the popular visual analogue scale.[22] However, the sensation of pain has many more components than just its intensity. Thus a single-dimensional rating scale leaves many aspects of the sensation undocumented.

To address the multidimensional qualities of pain, questionnaires have been developed.[23,24] Although questionnaires are a powerful way of obtaining data on both the qualitative and the quantitative aspects of pain, it is not always possible to compare the results of studies using the same questionnaire because of differences in the way they have been used.

CHEST PAIN SYNDROMES

Given the proximity of the various organs and the vagaries of perception of pain of visceral origin, pain arising from the various viscera in the thoracic cavity and from the chest wall is often qualitatively similar and exhibits overlapping patterns of referral, localization, and quality. This leads to difficulty in the differential diagnosis of chest pain (Table 38.1). Nevertheless, many chest pain syndromes are so distinctive that diagnostic efforts often rely on accurate description of the characteristic pattern of pain. The importance of the medical history in unraveling the various causes of chest pain cannot be overemphasized. The locations to which various pain syndromes are referred in the chest are illustrated in Fig. 38.1 (see also Chapter 18).

PLEUROPULMONARY DISORDERS

Although the lung parenchyma and visceral pleura are considered to be insensitive to ordinary noxious stimuli, immunohistochemical studies from vagal denervation and talc-pleurodesis animal models indicate the presence of nerve fibers in the visceral pleura that may be capable of conducting pain stimuli.[25,26] Pain does arise from stimulation of the mucosa of the trachea and main bronchi.[25] The lungs and bronchi are innervated with mechanoreceptors that respond to stretch (inflation or deflation of the lungs) and chemoreceptors called J receptors that respond to a variety of pain-inducing chemicals, including bradykinin, prostaglandins, serotonin, and capsaicin.[27,28] Inhalation of irritant substances, such as ammonia, can trigger a cough reflex and can produce a sensation of rawness, tightness in the chest, and pain. In addition, rapidly adapting mechanoreceptors that respond to lung deflation are also "irritant receptors" and signal respiratory pain. The J receptors have been proposed to contribute to discomfort and pain that accompanies breathlessness.[27–29]

Table 38.1 Common Causes of Chest Pain

PLEUROPULMONARY DISORDERS

Collagen vascular disease
Familial Mediterranean fever
Malignancy (e.g., mesothelioma)
Pleurisy
Pneumothorax
Pulmonary embolism
Pulmonary hypertension
Sickle cell disease

TRACHEOBRONCHITIS

Infection
Inhalation of irritants
Malignancy

INFLAMMATION OR TRAUMA OF THE CHEST WALL

Herpes zoster infection
Infection
Malignancy
Muscle injury (myalgia)
Neuritis-radiculitis
Rib fracture
Sickle cell disease

CARDIOVASCULAR DISORDERS

Angina pectoris
Angina (variant)
Aortic valve disease
Cocaine toxicity
Eisenmenger syndrome
Hypertrophic cardiomyopathy
Mitral valve prolapse
Myocardial infarction
Pericarditis

DISORDERS OF THE AORTA

Aortic dissection

GASTROINTESTINAL DISORDERS

Cholecystitis
Disorders of intestinal motility
Esophageal motility disorders
Pancreatitis
Peptic ulcer disease
Reflux esophagitis

MISCELLANEOUS

Iatrogenic
Mediastinitis
Thoracic outlet obstruction

These receptors are, in turn, innervated by vagal and spinal splanchnic afferent fibers. Most important are the nerve fibers that travel in the vagus nerves, including myelinated axons that carry impulses from slowly adapting stretch receptors in the conducting airways, myelinated axons that lead from rapidly adapting irritant cough receptors in the trachea and bronchi, and unmyelinated axons that subserve the extensive network of C fiber receptors (e.g., "pulmonary" J receptors and "bronchial" C fibers).[30]

The pulmonary causes of chest pain may be related to the pleural tissue, pulmonary vessels, or lung parenchyma. Causes of chest pain related to the lung parenchyma include infection, cancer, or chronic diseases, such as sarcoidosis.

Pleurisy

Pleurisy is a pain typically worse with breathing, which results from inflammation of the parietal pleura.

Inflammatory processes in the periphery of the lung that involve the overlying visceral pleura (e.g., pneumonia) frequently cause inflammation of the adjacent parietal pleura that, in turn, provokes pleuritic pain conveyed by somatic nerves. The portion of the parietal pleura that lines the interior of the rib cage and covers the outer portion of each hemidiaphragm is innervated by the neighboring intercostal nerves. When pain fibers in these regions are stimulated, pleuritic pain is localized to the cutaneous distributions of the involved neurons over the chest wall. In contrast, the parietal pleura that lines the central region of each hemidiaphragm is innervated by fibers that travel with the phrenic nerves. When this portion of the diaphragm is stimulated (e.g., by contiguous inflammation), the resulting pain is referred to the ipsilateral shoulder or neck. This pain referral likely arises because visceral afferent input carried by the phrenic nerve converges with somatic input carried by the supraclavicular nerves that innervate the skin of the shoulder onto C3–C5 spinal dorsal horn neurons (i.e., viscerosomatic convergence, a common feature of visceral pain leading to referred sensations). Thus, when this portion of the diaphragm is stimulated, the resulting pain is referred to the ipsilateral shoulder or neck.

Because of the somatic innervation of the parietal pleura and the localization of most diseases of the lungs or chest wall to one hemithorax or the other, pleuritic pain tends to be limited to the affected region rather than be diffuse, with the exception of referral to the ipsilateral neck or shoulder. Pain may be variously described as "sharp," "dull," "achy," "burning," or simply a "catch." There is a distinctive and unmistakable relationship to breathing movements, and taking a deep breath typically aggravates pleuritic pain.[31] Coughing and sneezing can cause intense distress. Movements of the trunk, such as bending, stooping, or turning in bed, worsen pleuritic pain, so much so that patients often prefer the body position that minimizes the motion of the affected region.

An immediate onset of pleuritic pain suggests traumatic injuries or spontaneous pneumothorax. A sudden onset, often associated with dyspnea and tachypnea, also characterizes the clinical presentation of *pulmonary embolism* (PE).[32] A slower, but still acute, onset over minutes to a few hours often heralds the development of community-acquired bacterial (typically pneumococcal) pneumonia, especially when accompanied by fever and chills. Recurrent acute pleuritic pain is a feature of familial Mediterranean fever.[33] Finally, a gradual onset over days or weeks, often associated with features of chronic illness, such as low-grade fever, weakness, and weight loss, suggests tuberculosis or malignancy.

Pulmonary Hypertension

Persons with pulmonary hypertension may experience crushing or constricting substernal pain that, at times, radiates to the neck or arms, resembling the pain of myocardial ischemia.[34] Pain from pulmonary hypertension has been reported in patients with conditions that are acute (e.g., multiple or massive pulmonary emboli) and chronic (e.g., Eisenmenger syndrome, pulmonary vasculitis, or mitral stenosis). In addition, approximately half of the patients with primary pulmonary hypertension may experience substernal chest pain.[35]

In acute pulmonary hypertension resulting from massive PE, the pain may be caused by sudden distention of the main pulmonary artery and stimulation of mechanoreceptors. In pulmonary arterial hypertension, chest pain may be related to either (1) right ventricular ischemia because coronary blood flow is unable to meet the metabolic needs of the overloaded right ventricular muscle mass as the latter strives to maintain sufficient systolic and diastolic pulmonary arterial pressures[36] or (2) compression of the left main coronary artery by the dilated pulmonary artery trunk.[37]

Although substernal pain related to the sudden onset of pulmonary hypertension can develop in cases of acute PE, embolism-associated pain is much more likely to be pleuritic in character, whether or not there is pulmonary infarction.[38] Pulmonary artery stenosis may also cause substernal pain, presumably by the same pressure-overload mechanism through which pulmonary hypertension with right ventricular hypertrophy provokes pain.[39]

TRACHEOBRONCHITIS

Pain of tracheal origin is generally felt in the midline, anteriorly, from the larynx to the xyphoid. Conversely, pain from either main bronchus is felt in the ipsilateral anterior chest near the sternum or in the anterior neck near the midline.[40] Whatever its origin, pain related to tracheobronchitis is typically described as "raw" or "burning" but may be "dull" or "achy" and is exaggerated by deep breathing. This type of discomfort usually denotes the presence of viral or bacterial tracheobronchitis or, less often, a malignancy but can also be experienced during exposure to noxious gases. Tracheobronchial pain is thought to be mediated by bronchial C fibers, and experimentally induced tracheal pain can be abolished by vagal blockade[41] or by vagotomy.[42]

INFLAMMATION OR TRAUMA OF THE CHEST WALL

Inflammation of, or trauma to, the joints, muscles, cartilages, bones, and fasciae that constitute the thoracic cage can cause chest pain.[43–45] Fibromyalgia, fibrositis, and other rheumatologic disorders of the thoracic cage, such as ankylosing spondylitis, are known to cause pain and discomfort in the chest.[46] Acute or chronic inflammation of the xiphoid process (xiphodynia)[47] and superficial thrombophlebitis of the chest wall (Mondor syndrome)[48] may also be uncommon sources of chest pain. On occasion, pain related to breathing may be experienced along the costal margins after vigorous exercise.[49] In addition, metastatic malignancy may present as painful lesions of the chest wall or with pain from a related rib fracture. Another source of chest pain is infectious arthritis of the sternoclavicular joint or costochondral junctions, which is a known problem among injection drug users.[50]

With *costochondritis,* chest wall pain arises from the costochondral cartilaginous junctions. It is usually described as "dull with a gnawing, aching quality." There is little, if any, relationship to breathing or other body movements. Tenderness to palpation is clearly localized to one or more of the costal cartilages.[51] There may be redness, swelling, and enlargement of the costal cartilages (Tietze syndrome). The most common sites of costosternal perichondritis are the second, third, and fourth cartilages, but any part of the sternum along the central and lower portions of the anterior thoracic cage may be involved.

The pain of *intercostal neuritis* or *radiculitis*, which often originates from disorders of the cervicodorsal spine or nerve roots, is usually perceived in the rib cage. The superficial, spontaneous lancinating or electric shock-like pain of intercostal neuritis is typically felt over the cutaneous distribution of the involved nerves and may be worsened by taking deep breaths, coughing, and sneezing. Unlike pleurisy, neuritic pain is usually not aggravated by ordinary breathing, and the diagnosis is supported by the presence of hyperalgesia or anesthesia on examination of the skin. In some patients with neuritis/radiculitis, the diagnosis becomes evident 2 or 3 days later with the development of the characteristic vesicular rash of herpes zoster over the involved dermatome. Painful radiculitis is also recognized as an important early manifestation of Lyme disease.[52]

Injuries to the ribs (fracture) and thoracic cage muscles (strain, tears, or hematoma) are common causes of localized chest pain. The relationship of the pain to trauma is obvious in most instances, but diagnosis may be elusive, particularly if the inciting event is relatively minor (e.g., unnoticed episode of coughing) or when the onset of pain is delayed.

CARDIOVASCULAR DISORDERS

Mechanosensitive and chemosensitive afferent fibers are present in the myocardium.[27,53] Chemical stimuli are believed to be the most important causes of cardiac pain, but mechanical distention or distortion may also play a role.[54] Sensory fibers travel from the heart to the spinal cord through the several cardiac nerves, the upper five thoracic sympathetic ganglia, and finally, the upper five thoracic dorsal roots. Afferent fibers also reach the brain through the vagus nerves.[55] Activity in these afferent fibers contained in the spinal afferent innervation of the heart contributes to location of perceived and referred chest pain symptoms.

Acute Coronary Syndrome

Acute coronary syndrome includes all conditions with myocardial ischemia caused by obstruction to coronary blood flow. *Angina pectoris* due to myocardial ischemia is typically described as severe "pressure," "squeezing," or "constriction" with maximal intensity retrosternally or over the left parasternal border. Radiation to the neck, jaw, shoulder, or down the inner aspect of one or both arms may be present. It is usually induced by exercise but may be provoked by heavy meals, excitement, or extreme emotion. Pain tends to recur with repeated provocation, although its severity may vary. Pain usually subsides within 2 to 10 minutes with rest, and relief is accelerated by treatment with sublingual nitroglycerin.[56,57]

Prinzmetal or variant angina is similar in quality and location to typical angina pectoris but appears at rest rather than during exercise or during times of increased myocardial oxygen needs.[58] In this syndrome, the imbalance between myocardial oxygen supply and demand is postulated to arise from epicardial coronary artery vasospasm, usually superimposed on noncritical atheromatous vessel narrowing.

Stress cardiomyopathy, also known as takotsubo cardiomyopathy, apical ballooning syndrome, or broken heart syndrome, can present with similar clinical features to an acute coronary syndrome, including anginal-like chest pain, ischemic *electrocardiogram* (ECG) changes, and elevated cardiac biomarkers. However, a hallmark of stress cardiomyopathy is the absence of a culprit obstructive coronary lesion at the time of coronary angiography. Moreover, the distal left ventricle becomes akinetic with compensatory hypercontractility of the base of the heart (also known as apical ballooning) in a manner atypical for acute myocardial ischemia. Stress cardiomyopathy is often associated with an inciting emotional or physical stress. It is treated with supportive care (including β-blockers and angiotensin-converting enzyme inhibitors) and typically resolves in the weeks to months that follow.

Pain does not always accompany myocardial ischemia, and many electrocardiographically detectable episodes of ischemia in patients with stable angina pectoris are asymptomatic ("silent" ischemia).[59] Conversely, many individuals with angina-like chest pain have normal or nearly normal coronary arteries when studied by arteriography,[60] with the development of chest pain attributed to either coronary microvascular spasm or heightened pain perception.[60,61]

The pain of *acute myocardial infarction* is similar in location to that of angina pectoris but is typically much more severe in intensity, is not relieved by rest or nitroglycerin, often requires large doses of opiates for control, and is frequently associated with profuse sweating, nausea, dyspnea, and profound weakness.[56] Acute myocardial infarction may also be silent,[62] especially in patients with diabetes mellitus.[63]

Valvular Heart Disease

Chest pain can also arise from other *non–coronary artery disorders*, including mitral valve prolapse, myocarditis,[56] pericarditis, and hypertrophic cardiomyopathy.[64] It can also be related to cocaine use.

Patients with aortic stenosis may complain of angina-like pain on exertion. The frequency of chest pain is higher with aortic stenosis than with any other valvular heart disease and is found in two-thirds of patients with severe disease.[56] Aortic stenosis should be considered whenever a patient presents with progressive angina, dyspnea, or syncope. In contrast, patients with mitral stenosis or pulmonic stenosis infrequently experience chest pain.

Pericarditis

The pain of *pericarditis* is most commonly pleuritic and arises from spread of the inflammatory process across the pericardium to the adjacent parietal pleura. Typically, pain is worse in the recumbent position and while lying on the left side, and is partially or completely relieved by sitting up, leaning forward, or lying on the right side. Radiation to the arms is uncommon. Although there are few nociceptors in the pericardium, there appear to be nociceptors in the diaphragmatic portion of its parietal layer, which is innervated by sensory axons that travel in the phrenic nerves.[65] Stimulation of these fibers causes pain that may be sharp, steady, and referred to the margins (ridge) of the trapezius muscles. Pain in this location is claimed to be specific for pericarditis because other diseases seldom cause discomfort in that area[56] (see Fig. 38.1).

Pericardial friction rubs, presumably indicating underlying pericarditis, are more common than pericardial pain during the first few days after acute myocardial infarction or with worsening uremia.[56,66] Other causes of pericarditis, usually associated with pericardial pain, are infections[67] and connective tissue diseases (e.g., lupus erythematosus). Pericarditis, usually with fever, can also develop after open-heart surgery (post-pericardiotomy syndrome) and after myocardial infarction (Dressler syndrome).[68] Often, no diagnosis can be made, and pericarditis in these cases is considered idiopathic.

Cocaine Toxicity

Chief among the presenting complaints of *cocaine toxicity* is chest pain.[69] Cocaine-associated chest pain typically begins approximately 60 minutes after injection or inhalation of the substance and lasts for about 120 minutes.[70] Pain is most frequently substernal in location and pressure-like in character. It may be accompanied by shortness of breath and diaphoresis.

Cocaine-induced chest pain is likely due to the combined effects of an increase in myocardial oxygen demand owing to an increase in heart rate and in systolic and mean arterial pressures and a decrease in myocardial oxygen supply due to vasoconstriction of the epicardial coronary arteries.

Disorders of the Aorta

Dissection of the aorta is usually associated with pain that is nearly always sudden and extremely severe at onset. Pain may be described, aptly, as "tearing" or "ripping" and often spreads widely to the neck, throat, jaw, back, or abdomen, as the dissection extends distally from its point of origin.[71] Frequent associated features are drenching sweats, nausea, vomiting, and lightheadedness. Angina-like chest pain can also arise secondary to aortic dissection or any aortic condition that reduces coronary artery blood flow, such as syphilitic aortitis or Takayasu's vasculitis.

NONCARDIAC CHEST PAIN

The term *noncardiac chest pain* is used to describe entities with pain resembling angina. There are three main categories of extracardiac disease that cause angina-like chest pain, namely (1) musculoskeletal disorders of the chest wall, which may account for 10–20% of cases; (2) a variety of esophageal disorders, particularly gastroesophageal reflux, which may cause 30–40%; and (3) psychological factors, which may explain up to 50% of the total.

MUSCULOSKELETAL DISORDERS

Of the musculoskeletal causes of chest pain, the ones most commonly confused with angina are cervical neck disease, costochondritis, subacromial bursitis, intercostal muscle cramps, or congenital malformations, such as pectus excavatum or carinatum. The best way to distinguish musculoskeletal pain from true angina is by reproduction of the pain with palpation or manipulation of the affected area. A history of recent trauma, chest infection, or coughing can also support this diagnosis.

GASTROINTESTINAL DISORDERS

Receptors are present in the esophagus and may cause pain when activated by mechanical (spasm), chemical (acid reflux), or thermal (hot liquids) stimuli. Afferent nerves travel in both vagal and spinal (T3–T12) pathways.[72] Pain originating from the esophagus is usually referred to midline structures, such as the throat, neck, and sternal regions, but may involve the arms as well. Stimulation of the distal end of the esophagus can cause pain directly over the heart.

Chest pain may arise either from esophageal reflux (the most common identifiable esophageal cause of chest pain) or from disorders of esophageal motility, such as diffuse esophageal spasm, achalasia, hyperactive lower esophageal sphincter, or nutcracker esophagus (a dysmotility disorder with high peristaltic pressures).[73-75] Esophageal pain may mimic angina pectoris by its radiation to the neck and arms and relief by nitroglycerin.[56] Chest discomfort that lasts an hour or more, that leaves a residual dull achy discomfort, or that is associated with heartburn, odynophagia, or dysphagia should suggest pain of esophageal origin.

Last, other GI disorders, such as cholecystitis, peptic ulcer disease, and acute pancreatitis, may present with pain that is perceived in the lower thorax.[65]

PSYCHOLOGICAL FACTORS

Psychological factors clearly affect each person's interpretation of bodily sensations, and a psychiatric cause should be excluded in undiagnosed cases of chest pain.

An association between noncardiac chest pain and anxiety disorders, particularly panic disorder, has been reported. This is particularly well described in patients with mitral valve prolapse.[76] Patients with demonstrable heart disease may also have panic attacks. Alternatively, persons with chest pain may have psychological distress related to the panic syndrome and not to a cardiac condition.

Mediastinitis

Mediastinitis can produce pain that mimics several other serious chest conditions, such as myocardial infarction, aortic dissection, or PE. The chest pain from mediastinitis can be severe, interscapular back or anterior pain, which is sometimes pleuritic. The association with fever or odynophagia can point to mediastinal inflammation or infection. Associated physical signs may include crepitus from subcutaneous emphysema or a crackling sound with the heartbeat on auscultation. Mediastinitis can be the clinical presentation of a silent esophageal perforation, a descending neck infection, or an iatrogenic complication of esophagoscopy or paraesophageal surgery. Other causes of acute mediastinitis include cardiac surgery and tracheal intubation (see Chapter 116).[77]

Thoracic Outlet Syndrome

Thoracic outlet syndrome is usually caused by compression of the neurovascular bundle by a cervical rib or a structural abnormality of the first rib or clavicle.[78,79] The pain can be caused by diverse entities that compress or invade structures in the thoracic outlet, structures including the brachial plexus, subclavian artery, and subclavian vein. Causes can

Table 38.2 Differential Diagnosis of Chest Pain

Diagnosis	Pain	Characteristics	ECG	CXR	Associated Features
Angina pectoris	Substernal, constricting	Transient, effort-related	Local ST depression; occasional elevation	Normal	Relief with NTG
MI	Substernal, crushing	Persistent, severe	Local ST elevation or depression	Possible vascular congestion or cardiomegaly	Relief with opiates; possible hypotension; ↑ troponin
Pulmonary embolism	Pleuritic	Sudden onset with dyspnea	Nonspecific; occasional RV strain	Normal or opacities ± small pleural effusion	Risk factor(s) for venous thrombosis
Pulmonary hypertension	Gradual onset	Associated with dyspnea, fatigue, and edema	Tall right precordial R waves, right axis deviation, RV strain	Prominent pulmonary arteries	Exclude pulmonary thromboembolism and interstitial lung disease
Bacterial pneumonia	Pleuritic	Onset in minutes to hours	Normal	Consolidation	Fever, productive cough
Pneumothorax	Sharp, unilateral	Sudden onset with dyspnea	Normal	Collapsed lung	Asthenic habitus, recurrence
Pericarditis	Pleuritic	Either side; gradual onset; pain referred to trapezius	Generalized ST elevation	Possible enlarged silhouette	Friction rub
Aortic dissection	Substernal, severe	Radiation to the back	Nonspecific; LVH or inferior MI	Widened mediastinum	Prostration, loss of pulse, aortic insufficiency
Esophageal spasm/reflux	Substernal	May mimic angina; burning	Normal or ST-T changes	Normal	Relief with NTG or antacids
Costochondritis	Dull-achy, localized	↑ by cough or deep breath	Normal	Normal	Localized tenderness
Mediastinitis	Interscapular, upper back, can be pleuritic.	Severe	Normal	Widened mediastinum, mediastinal emphysema	Associated with fever, odynophagia
Herpes zoster	Sharp, unilateral	Dysesthesia	Normal	Normal	Vesicular rash

CXR, chest radiograph; ECG, electrocardiography; LVH, left ventricular hypertrophy; MI, myocardial infarction; NTG, nitroglycerin; RV, right ventricular.

include trauma, repetitive injury, anatomic variations, and tumors, such as the Pancoast tumor or superior pulmonary sulcus tumor. Most commonly, symptoms arise from nerve compression, with pain often reproducible when performing certain activities and associated with paresthesias and weakness.

Miscellaneous Causes

Chest pain may also arise from iatrogenic causes, such as pneumothorax after bronchoscopy or central venous catheter malposition.[80]

EVALUATION OF CHEST PAIN

The evaluation of chest pain begins with a complete medical interview.[81] The history may reveal nuances in the quality, location, duration, provoking events, and relieving measures, which serve to focus the subsequent evaluation. However, with few exceptions, such as evident injury to the chest wall, a specific diagnosis cannot be made with complete confidence from the clinical history alone. Physical examination may reveal evidence of pleural, lung parenchymal, or airway disease; localized chest wall involvement; or signs of mitral valve prolapse, aortic valve stenosis, or other cardiac abnormalities.[82–87]

For adults who present to the emergency department with new-onset chest pain, the immediate concern is to identify and characterize potentially life-threatening conditions, such as myocardial infarction, acute pulmonary embolism, or tension pneumothorax, which require urgent management. Some diagnostic features are listed in Table 38.2.

A standard 12-lead ECG, appropriate chest imaging, measurement of oxygen saturation and arterial blood gas levels, and blood chemistry profiles (e.g., troponin, D-dimer) often provide important data. In the appropriate clinical setting, some patients may require echocardiography or pulmonary function testing. Many other noninvasive or invasive tests are available for the evaluation of pain believed to be of respiratory, cardiac, or GI origin. If the diagnosis remains uncertain, admission to chest pain observation units may be considered.

CARDIAC ISCHEMIA

Initial evaluation of patients with suspected acute coronary syndrome, such as unstable angina or myocardial infarction, should always include a 12-lead ECG. Serial ECGs may be considered if the initial ECG is not diagnostic or if the patient is thought to have evolving myocardial ischemia or injury. Biomarker assessment for myocardial injury should include cardiac-specific troponin; creatine kinase–MB may be measured if troponin is not available. Patients who are chest pain–free and have no ischemic ECG changes or cardiac biomarker elevation should be considered for risk stratification with a cardiac functional study, including exercise stress electrocardiography, stress echocardiography, or myocardial single-photon emission *computed tomography* (CT) imaging. The indications for stress echocardiography include the evaluation of acute chest pain and other chest pain syndromes, such as anginal equivalent, with or without heart failure, and risk assessment in symptomatic patients after revascularization procedures.

Acute ECG changes, such as ST segment deviations or deep T wave inversions, positive cardiac biomarkers or stress test results, or hemodynamic instability, should prompt admission to an intensive care unit. Hospital admission may also be considered if the diagnosis remains uncertain despite initial limited evaluations. Available risk stratification models may aid in the evaluation of patients presenting with undifferentiated chest pain. The North American Chest Pain Rule score; History, ECG, Age, Risk factors, and Troponin (HEART) score; and Thrombolysis in Myocardial Infarction score have been demonstrated to be useful in detecting low-risk patients. The HEART score may assist in differentiating persons with ischemic chest pain from those with noncardiac chest pain.[88,89]

Evaluation and management of variant or Prinzmetal angina consists of coronary angiography in patients with chest pain accompanied by transient ST segment elevation. Provocative testing may be considered in cases of diagnostic uncertainty if no contraindications exist.

For cardiac ischemic chest pain related to the use of cocaine or methamphetamine, immediate coronary angiography could be considered if electrocardiographic ST elevation (or new ST segment depression or T wave changes) persists despite pharmacologic intervention.

Intracoronary ultrasonography, coronary angiography, 24-hour ambulatory ECG, provocative testing, or coronary flow reserve measurement may be considered to aid with difficult diagnoses.

Risk stratification with exercise ECG (using the Bruce protocol or Duke treadmill score), exercise perfusion imaging, or exercise echocardiography should be considered for patients with symptomatic chronic stable angina who are able to exercise and have no contraindications to such testing. For those who are unable to exercise, pharmacologic stress testing with dipyridamole, adenosine, dobutamine or regadenoson nuclear myocardial perfusion imaging, or dobutamine echocardiography is recommended unless contraindications to such testing exist.[90]

PULMONARY EMBOLISM

PE is a life-threatening feature of venous thromboembolism and most frequently originates from deep venous thrombosis in the lower extremities.

Patients with acute PE who have elevated levels of troponin are at high risk for short-term mortality and adverse outcome events (see Chapter 81).[91,92]

PERICARDIAL DISEASE

Acute pericarditis is often associated with a pericardial effusion, diffuse concave ST segment elevation, and/or PR segment depression. It is essential to search for any underlying cause of the condition (e.g., infection or malignancy). In constrictive pericarditis, echocardiography can demonstrate the presence of pericardial thickening and calcification that limits diastolic filling of the ventricles and causes a characteristic biphasic pattern of venous return with a diastolic component equal to or greater than the systolic component.[93]

CARDIAC TAMPONADE

Cardiac (or pericardial) tamponade is the presence of fluid within the pericardial sac, leading to cardiac compression. This, in turn, impairs ventricular diastolic filling and gives rise to the sensation of chest pain and dyspnea, and signs of tachycardia, falling systemic blood pressure, elevated venous pressure (characteristic loss of the atrial y-descent with maintenance of both the systolic atrial filling wave and the x-descent), and pulsus paradoxus (an exaggerated inspiratory decrease in arterial systolic pressure >10 mm Hg).[94]

Cardiac tamponade should be suspected whenever a patient presents with unexplained hypotension and/or pulsus paradoxus after myocardial infarction, chest trauma, percutaneous coronary intervention, or cardiac surgery. Other risk factors include anticoagulation therapy, malignancy, or an underlying connective tissue disease. A pericardial rub may be appreciated during physical examination.[95] ECG changes compatible with acute pericarditis may be present along with an enlarged cardiac silhouette on chest films.

Diagnosis is generally determined by two-dimensional echocardiography that demonstrates a large pericardial effusion with an inspiratory increase of right ventricular dimensions and decrease of left ventricular dimensions, compression of the right atrium, right ventricular diastolic collapse, and a heart that swings with cardiac contractions. Left atrial collapse is less common than right atrial collapse but is very specific for cardiac tamponade. There is commonly also an abnormal inspiratory increase of blood flow velocity through the tricuspid valve accompanied by a decrease in mitral valve flow velocity and dilation of the inferior vena cava with lack of inspiratory collapse.[96]

PULMONARY HYPERTENSION

Initial evaluation of suspected pulmonary hypertension generally consists of ECG, determination of arterial blood gas levels, a chest radiograph, pulmonary function testing, exercise capacity (6-minute walk test), brain natriuretic peptide or N-terminal brain natriuretic peptide, and noninvasive Doppler echocardiography with and without saline contrast. Chronic thromboembolic disease is evaluated with ventilation-perfusion scanning and chest CT pulmonary angiography. Ultimately, right heart catheterization is required both to confirm the diagnosis and to assess the severity of the pulmonary hypertension.

Testing for connective tissue disease or human immuno-deficiency virus infection may be considered in patients with suggestive clinical histories for these disorders. Acute vasoreactivity testing using inhaled nitric oxide (or other pulmonary vasodilators, including epoprostenol, adenosine, or sodium nitroprusside) can be performed for patients with pulmonary arterial hypertension to guide therapy.[97] Polysomnography is indicated for patients with a clinical history suggestive of obstructive sleep apnea (see Chapters 83 and 120).

THORACIC AORTIC DISSECTION

Rapid diagnosis and management are critically important for patients with thoracic aortic dissection. Invasive aortography for the diagnosis of thoracic aortic dissection has been replaced by less invasive imaging techniques, including transesophageal echocardiography, contrast-enhanced chest CT scan, and *magnetic resonance imaging* (MRI). All of these modalities yield clinically reliable data for both confirming and ruling out this condition.[98] The major advantage of CT is its ready availability in most emergency departments, its speed of acquisition, and its ability to assess alternative causes of pain.[99]

PNEUMOTHORAX

Spontaneous pneumothorax can be either primary or secondary, and, if sufficiently large, can be visualized with imaging tests. A tension pneumothorax is a life-threatening condition that requires urgent management. High intrathoracic pressures develop because of ingress of air into the pleural space via a one-way valve process, which, in turn, prevents egress of air. This gives rise to vena caval compression, reduction in venous return, and diminished cardiac output. Radiographically, a tension pneumothorax presents as a complete collapse of the ipsilateral lung, depression/flattening of the ipsilateral hemidiaphragm, and shift of the mediastinum to the contralateral hemithorax (see Chapter 110).[100]

THORACIC OUTLET SYNDROME

Determining the cause of a thoracic outlet syndrome can be challenging and may involve a careful physical examination, electrophysiology, ultrasonography, and imaging via CT or MRI.[79] Superior sulcus tumors (Pancoast tumors) require a definitive tissue diagnosis before initiation of therapy. MRI, with imaging of both mediastinal and extrathoracic structures, is frequently performed to rule out involvement of adjacent neurovascular structures (brachial plexus, vertebral column, or subclavian vessels) that will influence surgical approaches.[101]

CHEST TRAUMA

Blunt and penetrating chest trauma can give rise to chest pain related to hemothorax (bleeding into the pleural space), pneumothorax, rib, sternal or clavicular fractures, or injury to the chest wall musculature.

As little as 5 mL of hemothorax can be appreciated on a decubitus chest radiograph, but a size of approximately 200 mL is required for it to be readily identified on an upright chest radiograph, where it will appear as blunting or, with a greater volume of bleeding, a concave upward sloping of the fluid in the ipsilateral costophrenic angle. In the setting of hemothorax, the presence of an air-fluid level indicates a hemopneumothorax. Chest CT is more sensitive than chest radiographs in detecting a small hemothorax and can offer clues to the origin of the bleeding (see Chapter 113).

Rib fractures may be associated with injuries to the brachial plexus and subclavian veins (upper rib fractures) or spleen and liver (lower rib fractures). A flail chest resulting from at least two fracture sites on at least three consecutive ribs can create regional chest wall instability and respiratory distress. The sternum tends to fracture most commonly at the body or manubrium, generally after direct trauma to the anterior chest or from deceleration. Significant posterior displacement of the sternum may be associated with trauma to the underlying cardiovascular structures. Chest CT is more sensitive than plain chest radiographs for detecting rib and sternal fractures (see Chapter 131).[100]

GASTROESOPHAGEAL REFLUX

Dyspepsia secondary to gastroesophageal reflux can be managed with pharmacologic agents. An empirical trial with these medications may be considered if the clinical history strongly supports the diagnosis of gastroesophageal reflux and if the patient is not at high risk for a GI malignancy. Risk factors, such as use of nonsteroidal anti-inflammatory agents, should be investigated. Endoscopy may be necessary in some patients with unexplained dyspepsia and persistent symptoms. Impedance-pH monitoring may also be indicated in persons with negative endoscopy who fail to respond to antireflux therapy.[102] High-resolution manometry is particularly useful for excluding spastic motor disorders and achalasia, whereas pH monitoring can help identify esophageal acid exposure (see Chapter 126).[103]

PANCREATITIS

Common causes of acute pancreatitis include gallstone disease ($\approx$50% of cases) and alcohol abuse (20–25%). Patients typically complain of abdominal pain and vomiting, but chest pain may develop as well. Elevation of lipase has a higher sensitivity and specificity for pancreatitis than elevation of amylase, perhaps because, compared to amylase, lipase is produced only by the pancreas. In addition, the half-life of lipase is longer than that of amylase. Other helpful laboratory tests include liver chemistry determinations, triglyceride level, and calcium level. When diagnostic doubt exists, abdominal imaging by contrast-enhanced CT may be beneficial (see Chapter 126).

Key Points

- Chest pain is characterized by an unpleasant sensation that is either localized to the thorax or believed to originate from structures located there. It may announce the presence of severe, occasionally life-threatening disease.
- Pain arising from *visceral* organs (e.g., heart or gastrointestinal tract) differs in many ways from that arising from *somatic* structures, such as the skin. Visceral pain is difficult to localize, is diffuse in character, and is typically referred to somatic structures. Visceral pain is also often associated with greater autonomic and motor responses than is somatic pain.
- Visceral and somatic innervations differ in relation to the density of innervations and spinal pattern of termination. In general, the number of visceral afferent fibers is less than the number of somatic afferent fibers, and the rostrocaudal spread of visceral afferent fiber terminals in the spinal cord is considerably greater than the spread of central terminals from somatic afferent fibers. The low number of visceral afferents and greater intraspinal spread is responsible for loss of spatial discrimination, consistent with the diffuse, difficult to localize nature of visceral pain.
- Pain is both hard to define and difficult to measure. Two widely used techniques, namely rating scales and questionnaires, are often used in clinical and epidemiologic studies of chest pain. Although rating scales constitute the simplest measurement of pain, the sensation of pain has many more components than just its intensity. Thus a single-dimensional rating scale leaves many aspects of the sensation undocumented.
- Because of the proximity of the various organs and the vagaries of perception of pain of visceral origin, pain arising from the various viscera in the thoracic cavity and from the chest wall is often qualitatively similar and exhibits overlapping patterns of referral, localization, and quality. This leads to difficulty in the differential diagnosis of chest pain.

Key Readings

Dezman ZD, Mattu A, Body R. Utility of the history and physical examination in the detection of acute coronary syndromes in emergency department patients. *West J Emerg Med.* 2017;18(4):752–760.

Fanaroff AC, Rymer JA, Goldstein SA, et al. Does this patient with chest pain have acute coronary syndrome? The rational clinical examination systematic review. *JAMA.* 2015;314(18):1955–1965.

Gómez-Escudero O, Coss-Adame E, Amieva-Balmori M, et al. The Mexican consensus on non-cardiac chest pain. *Rev Gastroenterol Mex.* 2019;84(3):372–397.

Kamali A, Söderholm M, Ekelund U. What decides the suspicion of acute coronary syndrome in acute chest pain patients? *BMC Emerg Med.* 2014;14:9.

Ruane L, H Greenslade J, Parsonage W, et al. Differences in presentation, management and outcomes in women and men presenting to an emergency department with possible cardiac chest pain. *Heart Lung Circ.* 2017;26(12):1282–1290.

van der Meer MG, Backus BE, van der Graaf Y, et al. The diagnostic value of clinical symptoms in women and men presenting with chest pain at the emergency department, a prospective cohort study. *PLoS One.* 2015;10(1):e0116431.

Wamala H, Aggarwal L, Bernard A, et al. Comparison of nine coronary risk scores in evaluating patients presenting to hospital with undifferentiated chest pain. *Int J Gen Med.* 2018;11:473–481.

Wertli MM, Ruchti KB, Steurer J, et al. Diagnostic indicators of non-cardiovascular chest pain: a systematic review and meta-analysis. *BMC Med.* 2013;11:239.

Complete reference list available at ExpertConsult.com.

WHEEZING AND STRIDOR

JESSICA B. BADLAM, MD • DAVID A. KAMINSKY, MD

LUNG SOUNDS	Approach	Approach
WHEEZING	**STRIDOR**	**THE FUTURE OF LUNG SOUND**
Definition	Definition	**ANALYSIS**
Evaluation	Evaluation	**KEY POINTS**

LUNG SOUNDS

Auscultation of the chest has long been useful in diagnosing pulmonary illness and remains an essential part of the physical examination (see also Chapter 18). The usefulness of this component of the physical examination depends on understanding the physiologic basis of respiratory function and proper correlation with the available clinical data. Lung auscultation is low cost, noninvasive, safe, and relatively easy to perform. However, lung auscultation is limited by interobserver variability, inadequate understanding of the physiologic basis of respiratory function, and imprecise nomenclature. These discrepancies in nomenclature should not overshadow the clinical importance and pathogenesis of these valuable diagnostic tools.[1]

Lung sounds heard on chest auscultation can be classified as normal or adventitious. These sounds are characterized by their frequency, intensity, and quality, which help the listener differentiate them and determine the clinical correlation.[2] Abnormal or adventitious respiratory sounds are those heard superimposed on normal breath sounds and are further classified as continuous and discontinuous. Discontinuous sounds (duration < 15 msec) are typically described as "fine or coarse crackles," whereas continuous musical sounds (duration > 80 msec) are known as "wheezes," "rhonchi," or "stridor."[3,4] This chapter focuses on these continuous adventitious sounds and addresses the evaluation and approach to a patient with this problem.

Although there is no one correct way to listen to lung sounds, certain basic principles are important. Ideally, the patient should be in a quiet environment so that the breath sounds can be heard over any ambient noise. The patient should be upright if possible, and the stethoscope should be placed directly on the skin. Overlying clothing will mask or interfere with many breath sounds, particularly crackles. One can begin on the front or back, but it is good to try to be consistent with technique so that a thorough and complete examination is performed every time. Listen to at least one complete breath, including inspiration and expiration, at each level of the lung (apex to base, or vice versa), and compare each side. Examine both the anterior and posterior chest, where the upper and lower lobes, respectively, are best heard. Also examine just under the axilla on both sides, where the lingula on the left and the right middle lobe

on the right can be appreciated. Focus on both the quality and intensity of the breath sounds—whether heard better on inspiration or expiration—and try to distinguish normal breath sounds from adventitial sounds. One should listen over the neck and trachea as well, which may help in determining the origin of the adventitial sound; this is a particularly good location to appreciate stridor, but wheezes can be heard well there also. Remember to try to categorize any adventitial sounds as to their persistence within the breath cycle (continuous or interrupted/discontinuous) and their timing (inspiratory, expiratory or both), as well as their intensity (soft or loud) and frequency (low or high pitch).

WHEEZING

DEFINITION

Wheeze is an easily recognized adventitious sound due to its musical quality and long duration (see Audio 18.6).[5] Wheezes are typically louder than underlying breath sounds, expiratory in nature, and largely signify airflow limitation. Wheezes are thought to be produced by the fluttering or resonant vibration of the airway walls at the site of airflow limitation, a result of the driving pressure exceeding the pressure required to produce maximal flow.[6] They are likely generated in the branches of the larger airways, second through seventh generation.[7] The pitch of the wheeze depends on the mass and elasticity of the airway walls and the flow velocity, not on the length or size of the airway. In addition, the volume (intensity) of the sound is not an indicator of degree of airway obstruction, because severe obstruction may limit flow to such a degree that wheezes may be absent. Very high frequency (>1000 Hz) wheezes are usually best heard over the trachea rather than the lung parenchyma and chest wall due to better transmission through the airway tree.[7] Wheezes may be monophonic or polyphonic, which are distinguished by having a single musical note or multiple musical notes, respectively.[5] Classically, monophonic wheezing, which may be inspiratory or expiratory, is associated with asthma. Polyphonic wheezes are thought to arise mainly within the larger, more central airways. A rhonchus is considered a variant of the wheeze, differentiated by a lower pitch similar to snoring (see Audio 18.7). It appears to share a similar mechanism of generation to wheezing but frequently clears with coughing, suggesting a significant role of secretions in the mechanism.[6] Wheezing, by causing mechanical perturbations of the airways, has been speculated to produce airway injury[8] based on studies of vibration of cultured human bronchial epithelial cells[9] and of the upper airway soft palate in a rat snoring model.[10] In both settings the vibration led to increases in inflammatory cytokine production.

EVALUATION

The clinical significance of wheezing depends on the mechanism of the airflow limitation. The broad differential for wheezing in adults can be seen in Table 39.1. Certain characteristics of the wheeze can give clues as to the underlying etiology. Most commonly, airflow limitation from obstructive lung disease, such as asthma or COPD, results in diffuse expiratory and also inspiratory wheezing. On the basis of auscultation alone, it is

frequently difficult to distinguish obstructive airway disease from other causes of diffuse wheezing, such as pulmonary edema or aspiration. Localized or focal wheeze may help identify the etiology and tends to indicate an abnormality, such as an aspirated foreign body, endobronchial tumor, or congenital anomaly. A short, late inspiratory wheeze may also be recognized and is called a "squawk" or "squeak"; these may be found in patients with pulmonary fibrosis, hypersensitivity pneumonitis, pneumonia, or bronchiolitis obliterans.[4]

Because wheezing may be heard during forced exhalation in healthy people,[11] wheezing during forced exhalation is neither sensitive nor specific for asthma.[12] However, more wheezes are generated during forced exhalation in patients with COPD and asthma than in healthy people,[13] and in patients with unstable asthma compared to stable asthma and healthy persons.[14] Cough is a frequent accompaniment to wheezing in asthma patients. In a study of 1701 patients with asthma, cough and wheezing in asthma were closely correlated; some patients had mostly cough, generally the older overweight women, and some had mostly wheeze, generally the older men.[14a] Monitoring lung sounds may be useful in determining the effect of therapy in asthma[15] or assessing bronchodilator response.[16] It is important to remember that wheezes may be absent in severe airway obstruction due to absolute reduction in airflow; reappearance usually indicates improvement in the underlying obstruction.

Various causes of wheezing not due to asthma or COPD include bronchial carcinoid[17,18] or compression of airways by mediastinal tumor,[19] uncommon causes such as pulmonary embolism,[20] or compression of airways by large vessel vascular malformations[21] (Fig. 39.1) or atrial myxoma.[22] Other mimics of asthma are well described and include anaphylaxis, angioedema, foreign body aspiration, and vocal

Table 39.1 Common Causes of Wheezing in Adults

Lower Airway	Intrathoracic Upper Airway
Asthma	Tracheal stenosis
COPD	Angioedema
Pulmonary edema	Foreign body aspiration
Aspiration	Benign or malignant tumors
Bronchiolitis	Tracheobronchomalacia
Cystic fibrosis	
Carcinoid	
Bronchiectasis	
Lymphangitic carcinomatosis	
Parasitic infection	
Vascular malformations	
Anaphylaxis	

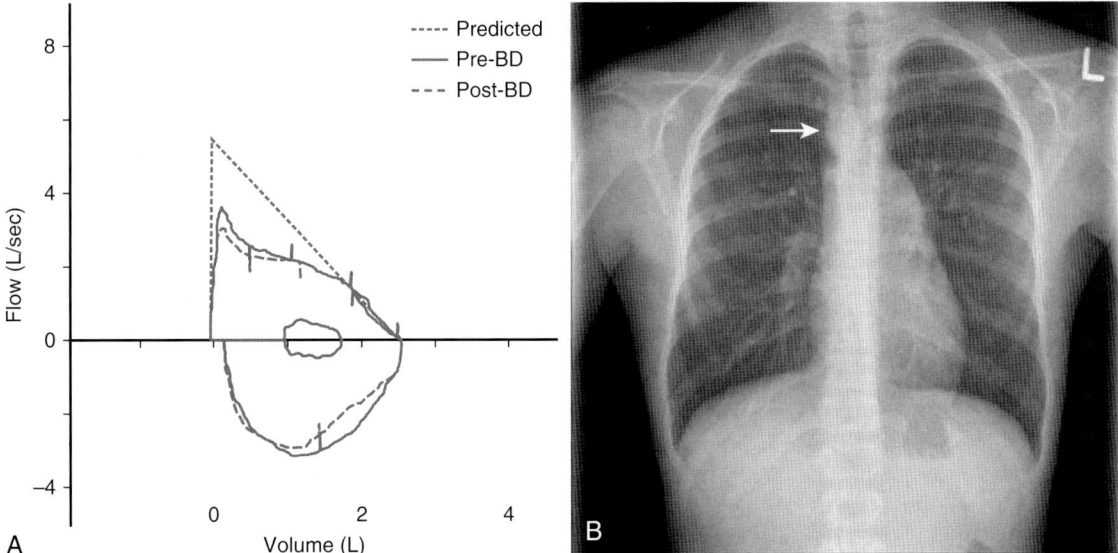

Figure 39.1 Variable intrathoracic obstruction due to right-sided aortic arch and its effect on the flow-volume loop. This patient presented with wheezing but did not respond to bronchodilators and inhaled steroids. (A) Spirometry showed limitation of expiratory flow suggestive of a variable intrathoracic obstruction, with the greatest impact at high flow rates. (B) Frontal chest radiograph showed a mass-like abnormality *(arrow)* found to be a right-sided aortic arch. BD, bronchodilator. (From Nataraj RT, Cockcroft DW, Fladeland DA. An uncommon cause of wheeze. *J Allergy Clin Immunol Pract.* 2014;2:616–617.)

cord dysfunction.[23] In addition, more than one disease may be present causing wheezing, such as tracheal stenosis in a patient with asthma.[24] As Chevalier Jackson reportedly said in 1865, "all that wheezes is not asthma."[25]

It is important to know that wheezing is very common in young children, present in up to 30% of children until age 3 years.[26] Wheezing in children may not indicate disease because the young child's respiratory system is more prone to wheezing due to more compliant and narrower airways.[27] Thus it can be difficult to recognize disease in the very young. Multiple phenotypes of childhood wheezing have been described, which differ in their clinical expression of traits such as atopy, time course, and persistence.[28] Biopsy data indicate that children with persistent, or in some cases even transient, wheezing may develop early pathologic changes of airway inflammation and remodeling, which may be associated with later development of asthma.[28] Acoustical analysis has indicated that high-pitched wheezing in asymptomatic children with asthma may indicate small airways obstruction.[29] However, such analysis was not able to distinguish wheezing from exercise-induced bronchospasm versus histamine-induced bronchospasm.[30] Wheezing in children may be used to determine response to methacholine during bronchoprovocation challenge.[31] A recent review has highlighted the features of six lung function tests that may be used in the clinical evaluation and monitoring of infants and children younger than 6 years with recurrent wheezing, in addition to bronchopulmonary dysplasia and cystic fibrosis; only some of these tests are able to distinguish children with recurrent wheeze from healthy control children.[32] Ongoing research is exploring the use of noninvasive biomarkers from blood, exhaled breath, or urine to help diagnose asthma in preschool children with recurrent wheezing.[33]

Most pathologic wheezing in children is due to acute viral illness, and among children presenting clinically with community-acquired pneumonia, wheezing independently predicted viral infection.[34] Rhinovirus-associated wheezing in the first 3 years of life has been associated with the subsequent development of asthma.[35] Other causes of childhood wheezing include asthma, allergies, gastroesophageal reflux disease, cystic fibrosis, congenital airway abnormalities, obliterative bronchiolitis, and chronic lung disease of immaturity.[36] Sudden onset of wheezing should raise concern for foreign body aspiration.[37]

Evaluating a patient, either a child or an adult, with wheezing involves multiple modalities in addition to the specific findings on lung auscultation. Indeed, one study in young children revealed poor interobserver reliability of clinical assessment of children with acute wheezing and dyspnea, emphasizing the importance of objective testing.[38] However, auscultation for wheezes in adults was rated as the most useful and frequent physical examination finding by more than 2600 internal medicine physicians.[39] Pulmonary function testing, imaging, and direct visualization with laryngoscopy or bronchoscopy are frequently used to evaluate stable patients with wheezing to make the correct diagnosis. Spirometry, including bronchodilator challenge, can be useful in the diagnosis of expiratory airflow limitation but may not be able to distinguish among the various causes. Reversible obstruction is frequently seen in asthma, whereas expiratory airflow limitation that persists despite bronchodilators is more indicative of COPD or other entities such as bronchiectasis (Fig. 39.2). Investigating the flow-volume loop in those that do not meet criteria for asthma or COPD is important in identifying other etiologies of airflow limitation. A variable intrathoracic obstruction, such as tracheobronchomalacia, can produce variable blunting, notching, or oscillations of the expiratory flow loop (Fig. 39.3). An increase in airway obstruction when supine compared to sitting may also be a clue to tracheobronchomalacia.[40] Conventional chest imaging with chest radiograph can be particularly helpful in those patients with acute respiratory distress or focal persistent wheeze. *Computed tomography* (CT) is helpful in evaluating central airway pathology, such as tracheal stenosis or entities that may be extrinsically compressing the airways and may provide valuable information about small airway or parenchymal abnormalities, such as bronchiectasis or bronchiolitis. Dynamic CT with inspiratory and expiratory imaging may be diagnostic for tracheobronchomalacia.[41] Flexible or rigid

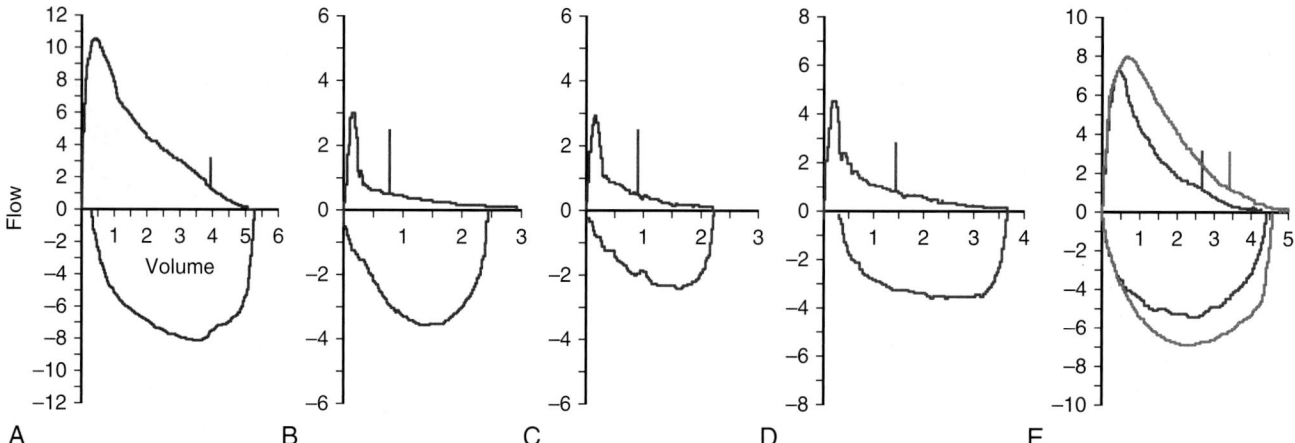

Figure 39.2 Flow-volume loops showing expiratory flow limitation from various causes. Normal (A) and flow-volume loops demonstrating classic expiratory airflow limitation in COPD/severe emphysema (B), bronchiectasis (C), and cystic fibrosis (D), as well as improvement in expiratory airflow limitation after bronchodilator *(blue)* in asthma (E). Note that short vertical lines indicate forced expiratory volume in 1 second. (Courtesy David Kaminsky, MD.)

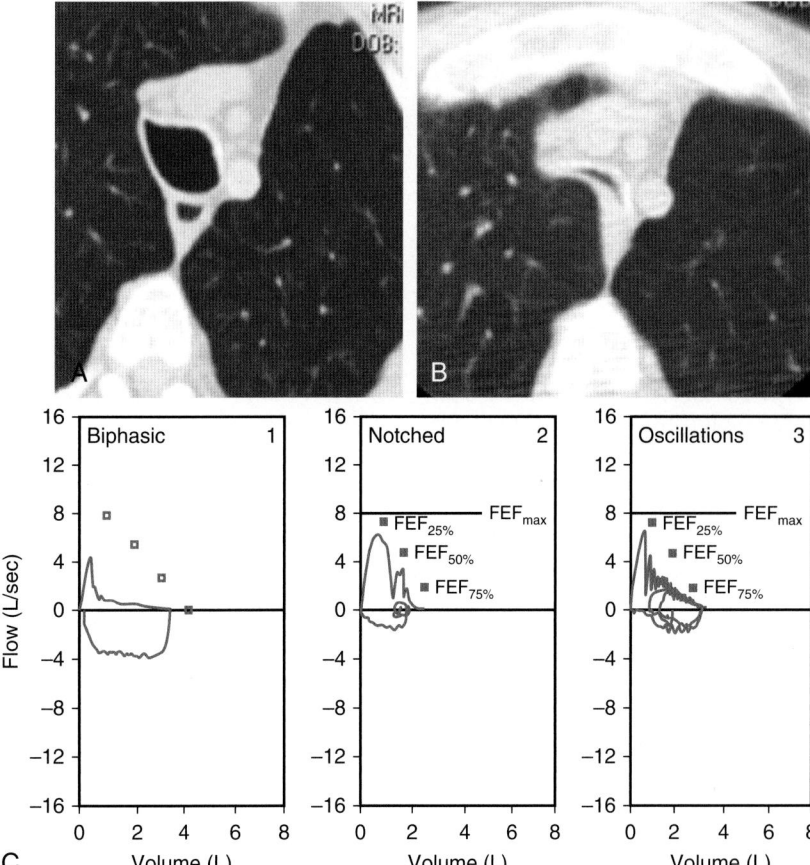

Figure 39.3 Tracheobronchomalacia shown with inspiratory (A), postexpiratory dynamic computed tomography (B), and examples of flow-volume loop patterns (C). The variable intrathoracic airway obstruction can produce findings on the flow volume loop (C) including biphasic (inspiratory and expiratory) blunting (*left*), notching of the expiratory flow (*middle*), or oscillations of the expiratory flow loop (*right*). FEF, forced expiratory flow. (From Majid A, Sosa AF, Ernst A, et al. Pulmonary function and flow-volume loop patterns in patients with tracheobronchomalacia. *Respir Care.* 2013;58:1521–1526.)

bronchoscopy may then be necessary to confirm a diagnostic suspicion of a tracheal or bronchial mass, foreign body, or tracheobronchomalacia.

APPROACH

The approach to wheezing is dictated by the patient's presentation and the breadth of possible diagnoses being considered. Although asthma and COPD remain the most common causes of wheezing, other conditions should be kept in mind, especially if the wheezing is of new onset or has not responded as expected to bronchodilator therapy. As described earlier, history, physical examination, functional studies such as spirometry, and imaging all play an initial role in determining the cause of wheezing. Because wheezing is principally caused by airway narrowing, empirical treatment of wheezing with inhaled bronchodilators to relax airway smooth muscle makes sense. However, due to airway narrowing being contributed to by airway inflammation and smooth muscle constriction, treatment of wheezing with anti-inflammatory therapy is also indicated. The mainstay of treatment of wheezing due to chronic asthma is inhaled corticosteroids with or without inhaled long-acting bronchodilators, depending on asthma severity and control (*Global Initiative for Asthma* [GINA] 2019; www.ginasthma.org). In wheezing due to COPD, the recommended treatment starts with one or two long-acting bronchodilators, before adding inhaled corticosteroids or other drugs (*Global Initiative for Chronic Obstructive Lung Disease* [GOLD] 2019; www.goldcopd.org).

In the patient with acute wheezing without previous history of obstructive lung disease, it is essential to maintain an open mind about the underlying cause. Certain causes require immediate treatment.[23] For example, wheezing may be associated with anaphylaxis, which will be recognized by multiple organ involvement in the presence of hypotension or shock. Congestive heart failure may present with wheezing (so-called "cardiac asthma"), but additional clues related to heart failure, such as orthopnea and pulmonary edema, should reveal the diagnosis. Uncommonly, pulmonary embolus may present with wheezing[20] and may require pulmonary vessel imaging to confirm a diagnosis. Focal wheezing should raise suspicion for foreign body aspiration as a cause of acute wheeze. When wheezing appears to be due to asthma or COPD, the use of *continuous positive airway pressure* (CPAP) or bilevel positive airway pressure may be beneficial to offset dynamic hyperinflation and reduce the work of breathing.[42,43] There is some evidence that CPAP may also reduce airway reactivity by causing sustained stretch of airway smooth muscle,[44] although the effect may be due, at least in part, to the application of the mask to the face and not specifically to the positive airway pressure.[45]

As with adults, the approach to diagnosis and treatment of preschool wheezing should be guided by appropriate clinical circumstances and testing, such as spirometry[46] or exhaled nitric oxide.[47] In children with recurrent wheezing and asthma and evidence of atopy, inhaled corticosteroids are indicated to reduce the risk of exacerbation.[48,49] For the treatment of acute exacerbation of wheezing and shortness of breath, the addition of high-dose inhaled budesonide has been shown to reduce hospitalization rates compared to standard therapy (short-acting β-agonist plus intravenous steroid).[50] The mechanism is postulated to be an acute anti-inflammatory and vasoconstrictive response. Another acute therapy for wheezing is the use of heliox, a helium-oxygen gas mixture. Although typically advocated for stridor, it may also be useful in pediatric patients with bronchiolitis (see later).[51]

STRIDOR

DEFINITION

Stridor is a type of adventitious sound with a very characteristic high-pitched musical sound predominantly heard during inspiration, frequently without a stethoscope (see Audio 18.12). The term *stridor* originates from the Latin verb *stridere*, meaning "to creak," and indicates a harsh or grating sound. The intensity, location over the anterior neck, and inspiratory predominance helps distinguish it from lower airway wheezing. It is produced as turbulent flow passes through a narrowed segment of the upper respiratory tract.[52] Similar to wheezing, it indicates flow limitation but with a distinct clinical presentation. It is also clinically necessary to distinguish stridor from stertor (patient awake) or snoring (patient asleep), which is a much more low-pitched noise generated from upper airway narrowing in the nasopharyngeal or oropharyngeal areas and is frequently associated with sleep-disordered breathing.[53]

The upper airway is a complex structure comprising muscles and soft tissue involved in a variety of functions, such as the passage of air, swallowing, and phonation. The lack of a rigid cartilaginous or bony structure predisposes the structure to collapse on inspiration.[54] If the obstruction is "variable" and can respond to the pressures generated during inspiration, the obstruction to airflow is also variable. During inspiration, airway pressure becomes negative relative to the surrounding atmospheric pressure, creating a gradient tending to pull the tissues inward and narrowing the lumen of the extrathoracic airways. On expiration intratracheal pressure becomes positive, lessening the obstruction and improving flow. This leads to the classic stridor typically heard only or mainly on inspiration. If the obstruction is caused by a "fixed" or rigid lesion, which does not respond to these changes in airway pressure, then the obstruction remains fixed as well. The stridor may then be heard almost equally on inspiration and expiration. Typically, lesions that reduce the upper airway diameter to about 8 mm cause symptoms with exercise.[55] Once the airway is narrowed to 5 mm, symptoms and signs of obstruction may develop at rest.[56]

EVALUATION

Stridor requires rapid evaluation and may require immediate intervention.[57] The history, including the age of the patient and acuity of onset, can help narrow the differential diagnosis. Stridor is more commonly encountered in the pediatric population due to the smaller diameter and less cartilaginous support of the upper airway. In children one must consider both congenital and acquired etiologies of stridor. Acute causes include foreign body aspiration,[58] anaphylaxis,[59]

Table 39.2   Common Causes of Stridor in Adults

Benign or malignant upper airway tumors
Vocal cord dysfunction/paralysis
Goiter
Epiglottitis
Laryngeal edema
Laryngostenosis or subglottic stenosis
Postextubation edema/granuloma
Deep neck infections (e.g., Ludwig angina)
Anaphylaxis
Obesity

bacterial tracheitis,[60] or epiglottitis.[61] If the presentation of stridor is more subacute, the most common causes are infectious, with croup (a respiratory illness of the upper airway, e.g., viral laryngotracheitis) accounting for 90% of all cases of stridor in children.[62] Croup is characterized by a gradual onset of symptoms, including fever, hoarseness, barking cough, and progression to inspiratory and sometimes expiratory stridor. Croup and epiglottitis are often confused because they both present with infectious symptoms and stridor. In a prospective study of children presenting to a pediatric hospital with stridor, croup was associated with coughing and absence of drooling and epiglottitis with an absence of coughing but with drooling.[63] Retropharyngeal and peritonsillar abscesses are also subacute infectious etiologies that tend to present with fever, "hot potato" voice, drooling, and inspiratory stridor. Chronic causes of stridor in children tend to be more congenital or structural in nature, such as laryngomalacia or tracheomalacia, subglottic stenosis, vascular ring, or bronchogenic cyst.[64]

In adults extrathoracic upper airway obstruction and stridor can result from a variety of etiologies (Table 39.2). Some of the most common acute causes in adults are infections (epiglottitis[65] and deep neck infection with Ludwig's angina[66]), laryngeal edema (especially postextubation[67] or due to anaphylaxis [68]), *vocal cord dysfunction* (VCD),[69] and subglottic tracheal stenosis after tracheostomy or prolonged intubation. More chronic causes include tumors/goiters and vocal cord paralysis. Less commonly seen chronic causes may include relapsing polychondritis, cricoarytenoid arthritis, fibromas, granulomatous inflammation, or amyloid involvement. Similar to children, the history and acuity/timing of presentation can be especially helpful in determining the etiology.

Additional diagnostic testing, including radiography, pulmonary function testing, or direct airway visualization, can be useful to identify the cause of stridor. Assessment of a stable patient with stridor involves similar diagnostic modalities as used in patients with wheezing. Pulmonary function testing, specifically the flow-volume loops, can be particularly helpful in diagnosis. Variable extrathoracic obstruction, such as VCD, can manifest as intermittent blunting of the inspiratory loop.[69] Similarly, a large thyroid goiter can flatten the inspiratory loop (Fig. 39.4). Alternatively, a fixed extrathoracic obstruction can flatten both the inspiratory and expiratory loops. Imaging with neck radiographs or CT

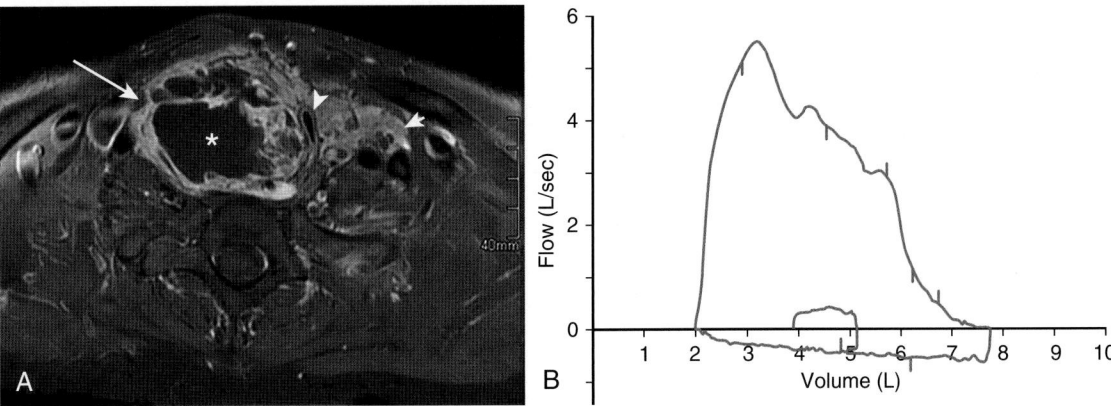

Figure 39.4 Extrathoracic obstruction causing inspiratory flow limitation due to goiter as seen on axial magnetic resonance imaging. (A) A large thyroid goiter *(asterisk)* had produced gradually increasing symptoms of dyspnea and stridor over years, associated with compression of the trachea *(arrowhead)*. (B) The thyroid gland extends from the long arrow to the short arrow. The flow-volume loop demonstrated significant reduction of inspiratory flow with fairly normal expiratory flow, characteristic of a variable extrathoracic obstruction. (Courtesy V. Courtney Broaddus, MD, Khai Vu, MD, and Michael B. Gotway, MD.)

(depending on the clinic stability of the patient) can help to characterize the obstruction further. Frequently, flexible or rigid laryngoscopy is used to visualize the upper airway to determine the specific diagnosis and provide opportunity for biopsy if necessary.

APPROACH

Patients with stridor need to be evaluated rapidly for impending airway closure, especially if the stridor has arisen acutely. Key observational findings include degree of respiratory effort and any evidence of hypoxemia or fatigue, which may suggest the need for close monitoring in the intensive care unit or immediate maintenance of the airway with endotracheal intubation or tracheostomy.

Flexible or rigid laryngoscopy and/or bronchoscopy are appropriate for the patient with an unstable airway or suspected foreign body aspiration. These procedures should ideally be performed in the intensive care unit or operating room with clinicians adept at intubation, anesthesia, and continuous monitoring. A Swiss study investigated chin lift and jaw thrust maneuvers combined with CPAP in anesthetized spontaneously breathing children to perform flexible laryngoscopy. Combining these techniques improved the view of the glottic opening and decreased stridor.[70]

Postextubation laryngeal edema (PLE) with stridor and/or respiratory difficulty is a frequent complication encountered in the critically ill adult patient.[67] This situation also requires rapid evaluation and efforts to prevent further respiratory failure because reintubation is associated with increased morbidity and mortality.[71] Many studies have identified risk factors for postextubation laryngeal edema or stridor that include female gender, longer duration of intubation, use of large tube size/high cuff pressure, and difficult intubation, but unfortunately the data are insufficient to identify high-risk patients for targeted preventative therapies.[72] The current treatment algorithm for postextubation stridor includes reintubation, if necessary, and/or using intravenous methylprednisolone, nebulized budesonide, or epinephrine to reduce inflammation and induce vasoconstriction to reduce the PLE.[72] The optimal dosages of these medications is currently unknown. The use of these strategies has also been extrapolated to other common causes of laryngeal edema, such as anaphylaxis, and may be used as temporizing measures when necessary.

For those patients with stridor without impending airway closure or in whom endotracheal intubation is not advisable or immediately available, there are two approaches to improve airflow past the obstruction: CPAP and heliox. CPAP can quickly pressurize and, in effect, splint open the upper airway to reduce stridor and dyspnea. CPAP in this setting can maintain a higher level of alveolar partial pressure of oxygen, improve ventilation by decreasing work of breathing, and increase airway compliance and positive distending pressure.[54] The resultant increase in lung volume can also reduce the collapsibility of the upper airway.[73] For these reasons, the use of CPAP in the patient presenting with stridor and without the need for an emergent airway may be beneficial as a temporizing measure to allow time to investigate the etiology further and determine an appropriate treatment strategy.

Heliox is a mixture of helium and oxygen that lowers the density of the gas and improves flow without any change in the airway diameter. Heliox, especially if the helium content is as high as 70–80%, can enable airflow to become laminar or, even if turbulence continues, can decrease the pressure required to move the gas through a small orifice. It was first described for therapeutic use in the 1930s[74] and has been used for decades in the treatment of acute upper airway obstruction,[75] but there is a paucity of randomized trials of its use in adults. The inhalation of a heliox mixture decreases airway resistance and work of breathing, but there is currently no evidence on the efficacy of administration in adults, and it has not been shown to change outcomes in children.[76] However, heliox may be of immediate benefit in the setting of upper airway obstruction by facilitating ventilation in patients until further medical or surgical intervention is available or necessary.[77]

THE FUTURE OF LUNG SOUND ANALYSIS

Although the human ear can remarkably distinguish the many types of lung sounds described in the medical literature, including wheezing and stridor, there are inherent limitations to detection sensitivity and accuracy of classification. Confusion of these two sounds can lead to serious consequences, especially if there is a failure to recognize stridor as a sign of impending airway closure. Recordings of lung sounds by electronic stethoscopes and other devices can now be made and analyzed for specific sound features, including intensity, frequency, and amplitude. Such properties may be depicted visually to allow further understanding of the difference between lung sounds. Machine learning may also be applied to lung sound data, in which different analysis methods, such as support vector machine and artificial neural network, are used to learn to distinguish lung sounds from large data sets of examples. A recent comprehensive review of this field found accuracy of wheeze detection ranging from 71–98%.[78] Such methods may prove useful not only in diagnosis but also in training and education. In particular, this technology might be useful for continuous, ambulatory monitoring for earlier detection of disease.

Key Points

- Wheezes and stridor are types of continuous adventitial lung sounds caused by fluttering of airway walls at sites of airflow limitation.
- The differential diagnosis of wheezes and stridor is broad, and making a diagnosis typically requires confirmation by other functional or imaging studies.
- Common causes of wheezing include asthma, COPD, and focal airway obstruction by mucus, tumor, or foreign body.
- Although asthma and COPD remain the most common causes of wheezing, other conditions should be considered, especially if the wheezing is of new onset, does not follow the typical pattern expected with asthma or COPD, or does not respond as expected to bronchodilator therapy.
- Common causes of stridor include vocal cord pathology, epiglottitis, goiter, laryngeal edema, and subglottic stenosis.
- Stridor may represent a medical emergency and needs to be evaluated rapidly for impending airway closure. Immediate measures to secure the airway with endotracheal intubation or tracheostomy may be necessary. Alternatives to improve airflow include continuous positive airway pressure to stabilize airway diameter during inspiration and heliox to improve airflow.

Key Readings

Baughman RPLR. Stridor: differentiation from asthma or upper airway noise. *Am Rev Respir Dis.* 1989;139:1407–1409.

Bohadana A, Izbicki G, Kraman SS. Fundamentals of lung auscultation. *N Engl J Med.* 2014;370:744–751.

Hollingsworth H. Wheezing and stridor. *Clin Chest Med.* 1987;8:231–240.

Pasterkamp H, Brand PL, Everard M, Garcia-Marcos L, Melbye H, Priftis KN. Towards the standardisation of lung sound nomenclature. *Eur Respir J.* 2016;47:724–732.

Pfleger A, Eber E. Assessment and causes of stridor. *Paediatr Respir Rev.* 2016;18:64–72.

Sarkar M, Madabhavi I, Niranjan N, Dogra M. Auscultation of the respiratory system. *Ann Thorac Med.* 2015;10:158–168.

Complete reference list available at ExpertConsult.com.

40 *HEMOPTYSIS*

YARON B. GESTHALTER, MD • FAYEZ KHEIR, MD, MSCR

INTRODUCTION

Hemoptysis is a potentially life-threatening condition that can often prove to be clinically challenging. It is defined as expectoration of blood originating from the tracheobronchial tree or pulmonary parenchyma with varied quantitative definitions of severity. However, any concern for cardiac or respiratory compromise should receive immediate attention. The diagnostic and therapeutic workup of mild hemoptysis should be geared toward identifying and correcting underlying causes, whereas massive hemoptysis should be approached in a multidisciplinary fashion involving pulmonologists, radiologists, thoracic surgeons, and intensive care providers, with the primary aim to stabilize the patient and control the airway.

DEFINITION OF SEVERITY OF BLEEDING

There is no consensus on how to stratify the severity of hemoptysis. Classically, hemoptysis has been defined according to the volume of blood expectorated over 24 hours.[1-3] However, this approach does not account for the patient's susceptibility to the harm of hemoptysis, which may stem from underlying lung and/or cardiac disease (see "Prognostic Indicators" later). In addition, the difficulty of quantifying the volume of expectorated blood further limits the utility of using volumes alone. A more practical approach to grading the degree of hemoptysis is by taking into consideration the clinical relevance of the hemoptysis, whereby severe or massive hemoptysis is any potentially life-threatening bleeding, compared to mild nonmassive hemoptysis. This accounts for additional features, such as the bleeding rate and other medical comorbidities. Any respiratory or hemodynamic instability must be used to prioritize immediate interventions (e.g., endoscopic or arterial embolization, airway, and hemodynamic stabilization).[4,5]

Mild (or nonmassive) hemoptysis is typically the manifestation of an underlying disease process and might not require admission if appropriate diagnostic and therapeutic interventions can be conducted in a reasonable time on an outpatient basis. Furthermore, in contrast to massive hemoptysis, mild hemoptysis is typically self-limited and holds a good prognosis with conservative treatment alone. Therapeutic interventions, such as bronchial artery embolization or surgery, are reserved for those who fail conservative medical management (see "Treatment" later).

EPIDEMIOLOGY AND OUTCOME

A large European epidemiologic study showed that hemoptysis accounted for 0.2% of all hospitalizations.[6] The most common etiologies for hemoptysis in high-income countries are respiratory infections (16–22%), followed by lung cancer (4–19%) and bronchiectasis (6–15%).[6-9] However, in regions with higher *tuberculosis* (TB) prevalence, TB remains a leading cause of hemoptysis (15–25%).[10-12]

In addition to the volume of expectorated blood, morbidity and mortality from hemoptysis depends on the acuity of bleeding, the ability of the patient to protect the airway by coughing blood from the airways, and the extent and severity of additional medical comorbidities. Hemoptysis, especially severe hemoptysis, carries a substantial overall mortality rate ranging from 9–38%.[1,13-16] Risk of death persists beyond the initial episode, with large epidemiologic studies reporting a 10% in-hospital mortality from non–lung cancer–related hemoptysis that increased to 16% and 20% at 1 and 3 years, respectively.[6] Idiopathic or cryptogenic hemoptysis also carries a significant risk of death (9–52%).[6-8,17] The underlying causes of hemoptysis may involve the airway (most common), the pulmonary parenchyma, or the pulmonary vessels (Table 40.1).

VASCULAR ORIGIN OF HEMOPTYSIS

The lung is supplied by both the pulmonary arterial system (a low-pressure circuit) and the bronchial artery system (a high-pressure circuit). Most hemoptysis arises from the bronchial circulation (90%),[18] whereas less common causes of hemoptysis (10%) stem from the pulmonary circulation

Table 40.1   Etiology of Hemoptysis

Airway disease	Cancer (endobronchial metastases, primary tumors)
	Inflammatory (bronchiectasis, cystic fibrosis, chronic bronchitis)
	Bronchovascular fistula
	Airway trauma
	Foreign body
Pulmonary parenchymal disease	Infections (pneumonia, tuberculosis, fungal, lung abscess, septic emboli)
	Inflammatory (vasculitis or collagen vascular disease)
	Lung contusion
	Drugs (cocaine inhalation, anticoagulation, antiplatelet, bevacizumab)
	Idiopathic pulmonary hemosiderosis
	Iatrogenic (lung biopsy)
	Clotting disorders
	Diffuse alveolar hemorrhage or damage
	Catamenial hemoptysis
Vascular disease	Pulmonary embolism/infarct
	Arteriovenous malformation
	Pulmonary artery pseudoaneurysm
	Dieulafoy lesion
	Pulmonary veno-occlusive disease
	Hereditary hemorrhagic telangiectasia
	Cardiac (mitral stenosis, heart failure)
	Iatrogenic (pulmonary artery catheter perforation)

and from nonbronchial systemic vessels, such as the aorta (aortobronchial fistula and ruptured aortic aneurysm), intercostal arteries, coronary arteries, axillary and subclavian arteries, and the upper and inferior phrenic arteries. It should be noted that bleeding from bronchial vessels is typically due to the neovascularization resulting from inflammation (e.g., bronchiectasis, abscess, and tuberculosis). Pulmonary arterial bleeding is usually due to ulceration of vessels caused by parenchymal destruction (cancers, necrotizing bacterial pneumonias, and mycetomas).

PROGNOSTIC INDICATORS

Prognostic scores have been developed to facilitate triage in the *emergency department* (ED) and to predict mortality in the *intensive care unit* (ICU).

Patients presenting to the ED with a score greater than 0 warrant additional in-hospital diagnostic tests, such as a chest CT scan, bronchoscopy, or bronchial artery angiography.[8] This score counts any of the following as warranting hospitalization:

- Systolic blood pressure less than 100 mm Hg
- History of malignancy

- Expectoration of pure blood
- Two or more episodes of hemoptysis in the prior 24 hours

For an ICU patient with hemoptysis, a mortality risk score consists of[19]:

- Need for mechanical ventilation (2 points)
- Malignancy (2 points)
- *Aspergillus* infection (2 points)
- Opacities involving greater than or equal to two quadrants on admitting radiograph (1 point)
- Involvement of pulmonary blood vessels (1 point)
- Chronic alcoholism (1 point)

The predicted probability of death upon ICU admission was as follows: score 0 = 1%; score 1 = 2%; score 2 = 6%; score 3 = 16%; score 4 = 34%; score 5 = 58%; score 6 = 79%; and score 7 = 91%.

DIAGNOSIS

INITIAL EVALUATION

Suspected hemoptysis must be confirmed and distinguished from pseudohemoptysis that may arise from epistaxis or hematemesis. Both severe epistaxis and upper gastrointestinal bleeds can have a similar presentation to hemoptysis and are potentially life threatening as well. In a large retrospective case series, pseudohemoptysis from upper airway or gastrointestinal bleeding was identified in 10% of patients presenting with presumed hemoptysis.[20] Careful history, physical examination, and laboratory tests are required to determine whether the bleeding originates from the upper airway—associated with bleeding gums, epistaxis, history of prodromal cough, sputum, sore throat, or pharyngitis—or the gastrointestinal tract—associated with coffee-ground vomitus, black tarry stools, epigastric pain, signs of chronic liver disease, abdominal pain, or nausea. Early consultation with otolaryngologists and gastroenterologists should be sought when the bleeding source is unclear.

Once pseudohemoptysis is excluded, targeted clinical history and physical examination can provide important clues concerning the etiology of hemoptysis, detail the bleeding severity, and guide diagnostic and therapeutic interventions. The general approach to mild and to massive hemoptysis is shown in Figure 40.1.

The directed history for patients presenting with hemoptysis should include questions about the duration of symptoms, frequency of hemoptysis, associated dyspnea, quantity coughed by patient during 24 hours, and any recent injury to the airway, such as diagnostic procedures, chest injury, or foreign body aspiration. A history of immobilization might be important because pulmonary embolism can present initially as hemoptysis. Also, history of tobacco, antiplatelet, or anticlotting agents, as well as recent toxic inhalants exposure, such as organic chemicals, are important to discern during initial evaluation. Furthermore, concomitant diseases, such as respiratory illness (chronic bronchitis, bronchiectasis, cystic fibrosis, pneumonia, cancer) or other diseases, such as heart disease (e.g., mitral stenosis), venous thromboembolic disease, immunosuppression, renal, hematologic, autoimmune, or systemic

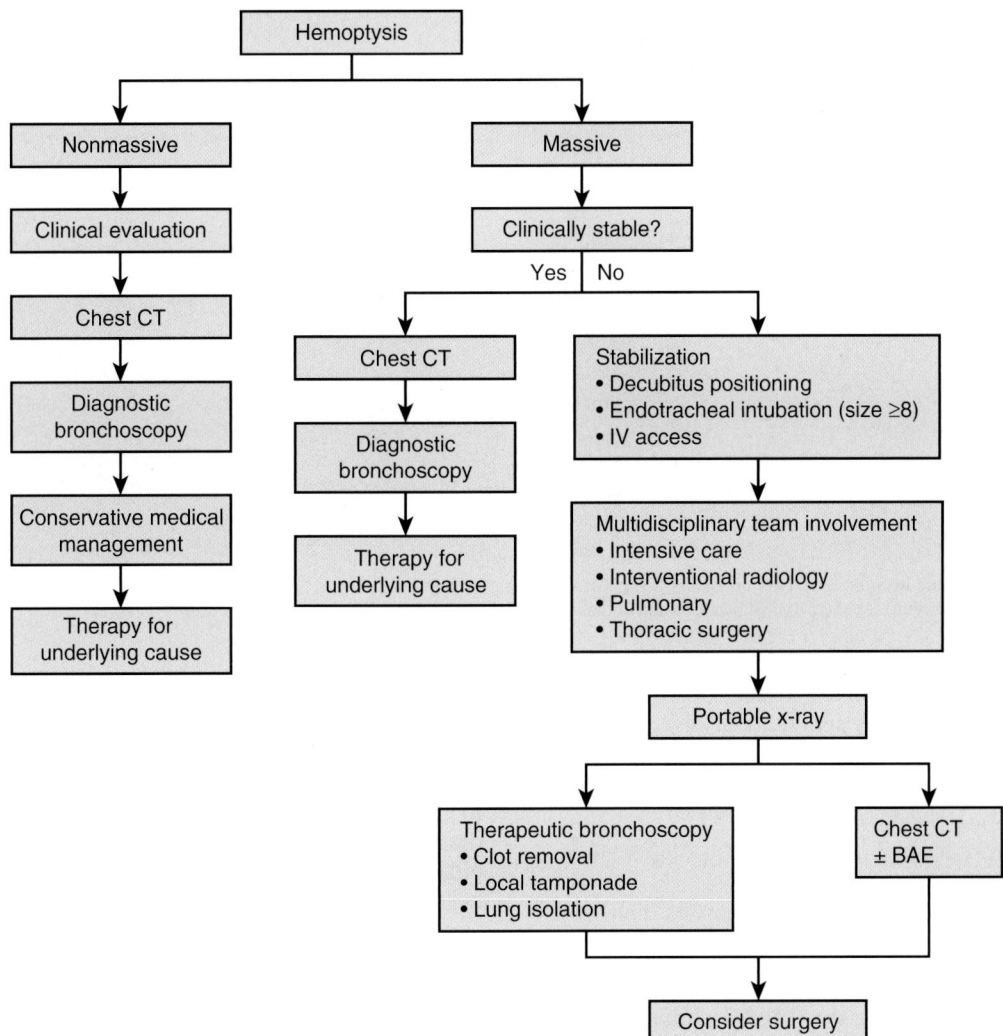

Figure 40.1 Proposed algorithm for the management of the patient with hemoptysis. BAE, bronchial arterial embolization; CT, computed tomography; IV, intravenous.

disease can help differentiate multiple causes of hemoptysis and appropriately guide laboratory work and management.

The physical examination can sometimes be useful for the assessment of the cause and the severity of bleeding but can be normal with most causes of hemoptysis. Careful inspection of the thorax can be very helpful in the setting of trauma because the signs of blunt or penetrating injury are likely to provide information regarding the site of bleeding. Stridor, crackles, wheezing, or diminished breath sounds can suggest the presence of a focal obstruction due to a foreign body, bronchiectasis, or pneumonia. Auscultation of the heart can detect the presence of murmurs for mitral stenosis or mitral regurgitation. Skin inspection for bruising can potentially suggest coagulopathy, telangiectasia of hereditary hemorrhagic telangiectasia or purpura caused by possible cutaneous vasculitis.

A comprehensive laboratory panel including chemistries, blood counts, and coagulation tests should be reviewed to identify potential reversible systemic bleeding dyscrasias. However, it is important to note that coagulation disorders alone are rarely primarily responsible for hemoptysis and, even in the setting of a coagulation disorder, an underlying disease should be thoroughly investigated. Specific studies such as N-terminal pro-B-type natriuretic peptide or D-dimer may direct attention toward specific underlying etiologies, such as congestive heart failure or pulmonary embolism, respectively, as an etiology for hemoptysis. Serologic studies, such as antinuclear antibody and anti-neutrophil cytoplasmic antibody, might uncover an underlying systemic process manifesting with hemoptysis. When a pulmonary infection is suspected, sputum cultures, including for acid-fast bacilli, are warranted. Despite diagnostic evaluations, an underlying etiology of bleeding will not be found in 5–10% of evaluations for hemoptysis.[21]

RADIOLOGY

The initial radiographic investigation of choice to diagnose and localize the source of hemoptysis should be guided by a focused medical history and physical examination. Chest radiographs perform poorly in lateralizing and identifying the cause of bleeding,[1] especially in non–life-threatening hemoptysis. *Computed tomography* (CT) of the chest plays a crucial role in localizing the site and can identify the cause of bleeding in up to 70–88% of the cases.[22,23]

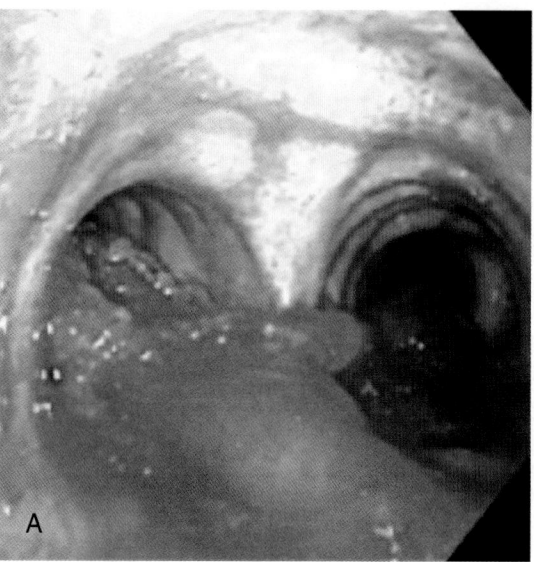 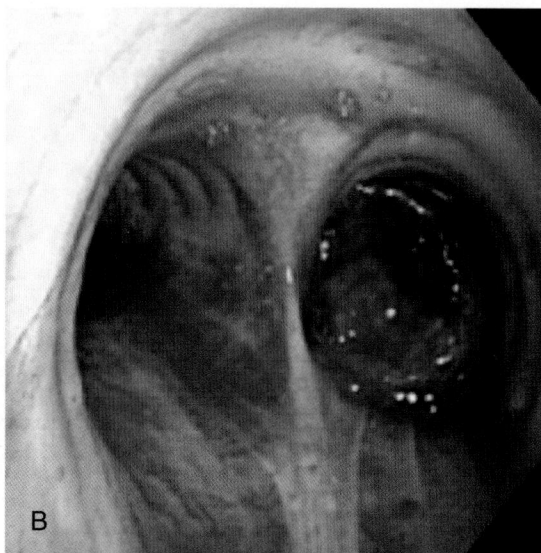

Figure 40.2 Bronchoscopic images of occlusive clots. A patient with massive hemoptysis due to severe bronchiectasis and a large obstructing clot overlying the main carina before (A) and after (B) bronchoscopic clearance of the left mainstem airway.

Chest CTs should be obtained in each of the following clinical situations in patients with hemoptysis:

- Patients suspected of having an underlying lung cancer or other thoracic malignancy, or those with pathologic findings on chest radiographs
- Patients with suspected bronchiectasis or cavitary lung disease
- Patients with life-threatening hemoptysis and active bleeding (after airway stabilization) who are candidates for embolization

CT scans acquired during the arterial phase with multiplanar reconstruction can help visualize the bronchial, nonbronchial arteries, and pulmonary circulation.[24] This detailed visualization of the thoracic vasculature can guide the optimal angiographic approach by identifying the origin and course of the bleeding arterial vessel. Intravenous contrast-enhanced CT chest angiography increases the sensitivity and specificity of hemoptysis localization relative to a non-contrast CT and should be done when feasible. Relevant findings that can be revealed by CT with contrast include bronchial arterial hypertrophy; aneurysm formation and/or tortuosity with artery diameter of 2 to 3 mm or greater; presence of pleural thickening measuring 3 mm or more adjacent to a parenchymal abnormality due to underlying chronic pulmonary inflammatory disease, for instance; and tortuosity along with enhancing vessels within extrapleural fat.[25]

Angiography of either the pulmonary or bronchial arteries has several limitations. It cannot be readily done in unstable patients or in patients with active bleeding who may require immediate endobronchial management. In patients with bilateral lung abnormalities without localizing signs, finding the site of bleeding may be time consuming and challenging.

DIAGNOSTIC BRONCHOSCOPY

The role of diagnostic bronchoscopy for hemoptysis evaluation is controversial. In patients without life-threatening hemoptysis, bronchoscopy has not been shown to increase the diagnostic yield of either benign or malignant causes of hemoptysis in comparison with CT[9,26] and has been shown to have limited ability in visualizing the bleeding source.[27] In patients with massive hemoptysis, it has been argued that early bronchoscopy, either during the active bleeding phase or within 48 hours of hemoptysis termination, can help localize the bleeding source in the airways and guide angiographic embolization.[26,28,29] However, early endoscopic examination does not seem to influence the clinical management and outcome even when it identifies the site of bleeding. Compared to bronchoscopy, CT scans have shown a higher accuracy in detecting the source of hemoptysis when bronchiectasis, pulmonary infections, or lung cancer are the underlying cause of bleeding.[9] Chest CT also has the advantage of characterizing airways that are distal to the level of bronchoscopic inspection, although CT scans are limited in their ability to differentiate between blood clots or an endobronchial tumor. Therapeutic bronchoscopy may have a role in airway management and stabilization, as well as ablative interventions as discussed later.

TREATMENT

GENERAL CONSIDERATIONS

The unpredictable clinical course for patients with hemoptysis mandates a timely evaluation with prioritization of the patient's hemodynamic and respiratory stability. A patient can asphyxiate quickly from bleeding and clotting in the airways even before there is enough blood loss to lead to hemodynamic compromise (Fig. 40.2). Thus the major goal is to protect the airway. Resuscitation should be anticipated with establishment of intravenous access and planning for close patient monitoring, usually in the ICU. Early involvement of different specialties, such as pulmonary, interventional radiology, thoracic surgery, and intensive care, for a multidisciplinary approach is important.

Beyond reversal agents for anticoagulants, no systemic therapies have been shown to be beneficial for hemoptysis

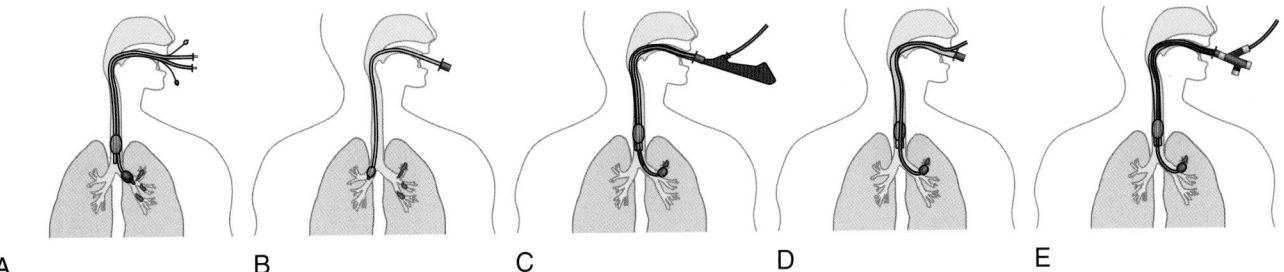

Figure 40.3 Isolation of bleeding using endotracheal tubes and airway blockers. The first two panels demonstrate the isolation of a bleeding left lung using a (A) double-lumen endotracheal tube and (B) right mainstem intubation of a single-lumen endotracheal tube to the nonbleeding lung. The last three panels demonstrate peripheral airway blockage using a balloon. A balloon catheter can be used for temporary tamponade by occluding the bleeding airway through the working channel of a bronchoscope or can be fixed in place after bronchoscopic guidance (C–D). The blocking balloon catheter can be fixed to the proximal end of the endotracheal tube (E). (Courtesy Arnon Brand, PhD.)

in general, and targeting specific underlying causes of hemoptysis should be prioritized. Therapies may include replacement of blood products (e.g., fresh frozen plasma or platelets), desmopressin to improve platelet function in the setting of renal dysfunction, or immunosuppressive therapy in the setting of vasculitis. Use of antitussive agents has been proposed as a means to minimize local irritation of friable blood vessels.[30]

Systemic therapies have been tested. Inhibiting systemic fibrinolytic activity with agents such as tranexamic acid to arrest pulmonary bleeding has been of interest based on data from other fields, such as cardiac or obstetric surgery, where antifibrinolytic use has been shown to decrease blood loss. However, a Cochrane meta-analysis demonstrated insufficient evidence for use of antifibrinolytic agents in hemoptysis, although some decrease in the duration of hemoptysis was suggested.[31] Nebulized tranexamic acid versus inhaled placebo was compared in a randomized controlled trial,[32] where nebulized tranexamic acid therapy was associated with a lower volume of blood loss, a higher rate of resolution of hemoptysis, and fewer procedures and fewer hospitalization days. Systemic use of factor VII has also been proposed, given its hemostatic properties for patients with hemophiliac disease. Experience with its use has been anecdotally reported in cases of life-threatening hemoptysis related to blunt and penetrating thoracic trauma, refractory thrombocytopenia, necrotizing infections, and cystic fibrosis.[33–37] However, concerns for adverse thromboembolic events have focused attention on local administration, although data are limited to small studies or case series.[38] Systemic use of vasopressin has also been suggested as a means to vasoconstrict hemorrhaging vessels, although concerns for the systemic side effects of vasoconstriction have been raised.[39,40]

AIRWAY MANAGEMENT

The potential compromise of the patient's respiratory status requires early consideration of airway protection. If the bleeding side is known, placing the patient in a lateral decubitus position with the affected side down can minimize spillage of blood to the unaffected lung. When the rate of bleeding overwhelms the ability of the patient to clear the airway by coughing, endotracheal intubation is indicated. Although intubation may be beneficial before blood spills to other parts of the lung, the complexity of such intubations may require some delay until the patient can be moved to a controlled environment, such as the operating room, where experienced

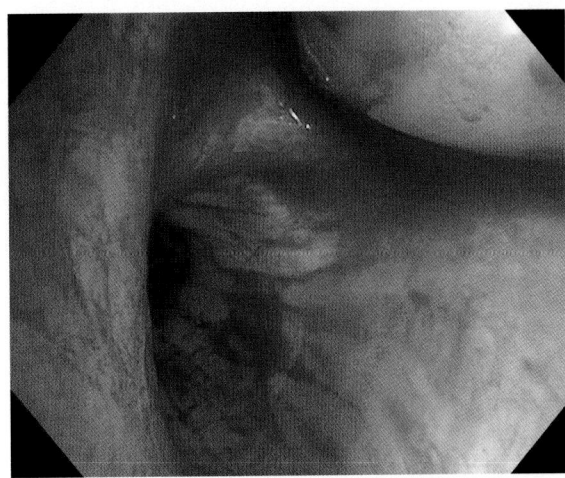

Figure 40.4 Endobronchial blocker in place. Endobronchial blocker inflated in the right upper lobe to occlude it after a lung biopsy, with protection of the bronchus intermedius from bloody spillage. (Courtesy Michael B. Gotway, MD.)

team members can manage a potentially compromised airway despite impaired visualization. Sedating a patient for intubation should be done cautiously because inhibiting the cough reflex may worsen the respiratory status by disabling the patient's own airway clearance mechanisms.

Although the airway can be secured in different ways, the unifying goal is to isolate the bleeding airway segment and ventilate as much of the uninvolved lung as possible (Figs. 40.3 and 40.4). Lung isolation can be achieved with either single- or double-lumen endotracheal tubes. *Double-lumen endotracheal tubes* (DLTs) have two parallel lumens, each cuffed with a tracheal and a bronchial side (either left or right). When the tube is correctly positioned and both balloons are inflated, the DLT effectively isolates each hemithorax (see Fig. 40.3A), allowing parallel and independent ventilation of each side and providing a conduit through which each lung can be suctioned separately. However, DLT placement requires a high level of expertise, and incorrect placement can lead to obstruction and spillage, and airway trauma.[41] In addition, their lumens are relatively narrow, thus limiting suction capacity and potential bronchoscopic interventions.

Single-lumen endotracheal tubes (SLTs) are readily available and easily placed, making them an appropriate choice for intubation for massive hemoptysis, especially if larger tube sizes (≥8) are used, which can facilitate possible bronchoscopic interventions and airway clearance. Different lung

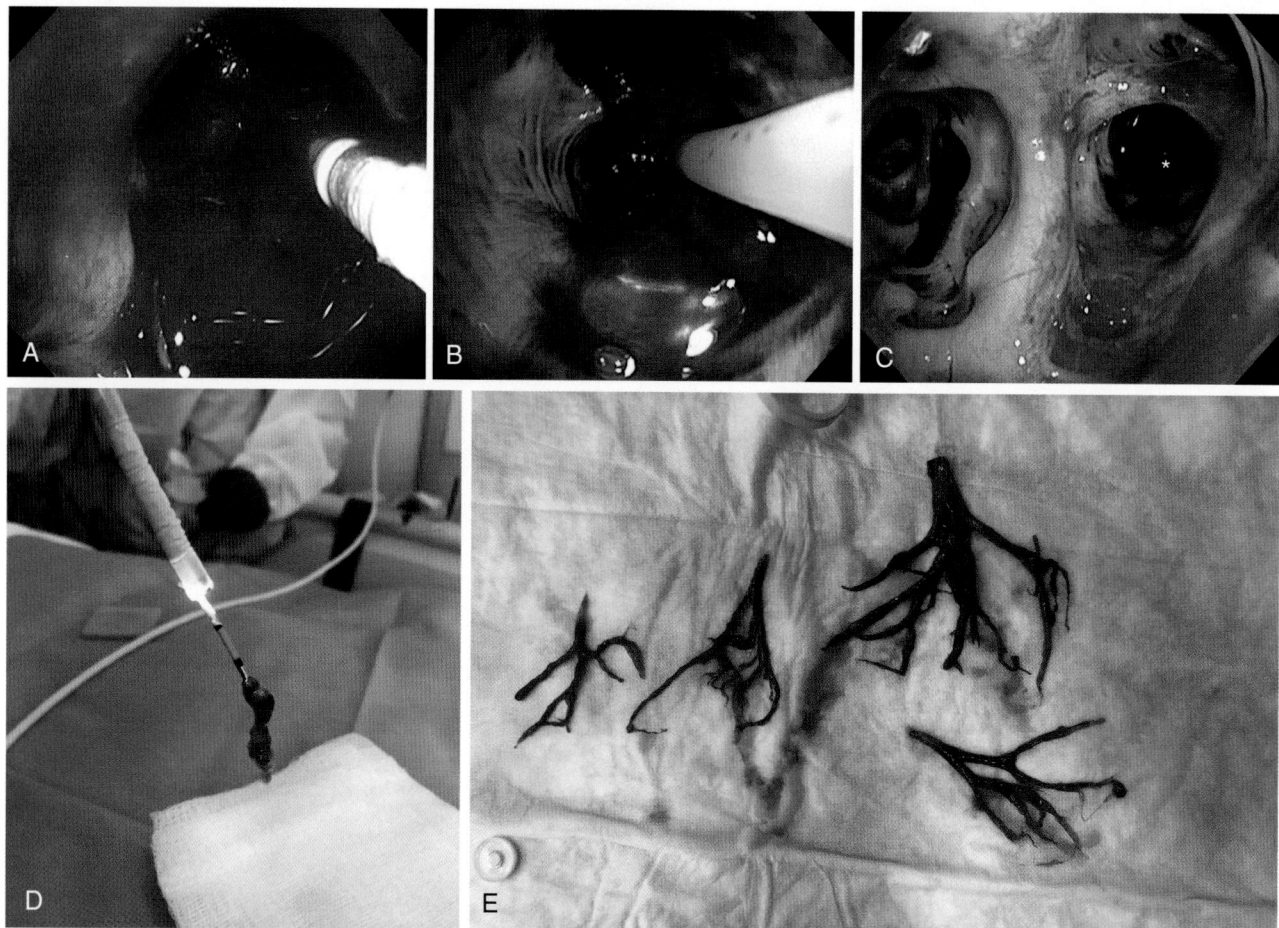

Figure 40.5 Therapeutic bronchoscopic management. Active bleeding originating from the right upper lobe (A) was controlled with a Fogarty balloon through the working channel of a bronchoscope (B). The bleeding was localized to the posterior subsegment of the right upper lobe denoted by the *asterisk* (C). Blood clots were removed from airway segments using a cryoprobe (D–E).

isolation strategies can be used via SLT to minimize lung contamination with blood. Lung isolation with SLT can be achieved through selective intubation of the uninvolved mainstem (see Fig. 40.3B), which will isolate the intubated lung from bleeding from the opposite lung. Alternatively, the SLT can be positioned as usual in the trachea, and the bronchoscope can be used to attempt selective airway tamponade with soft balloons, such as Fogarty balloons, or with blockers (see Fig. 40.3C–E; see "Endoscopic Approach" later).

ENDOVASCULAR APPROACH

Bronchial artery embolization (BAE) can both localize and embolize bleeding vessels (see also Chapter 21). The frequent involvement of the bronchial arteries in hemoptysis and the ability to perform minimally invasive bronchial arteriography in critically ill patients makes BAE an appealing approach. Radiologists can identify suspicious hypertrophic vessels and contrast extravasation, which requires a minimal rate of active bleeding to visualize. Occlusive materials, such as gelfoam, tris-acryl microspheres, coils, or alcohol particles, are then injected to block the bleeding vessel. Arteriography is considered

highly effective for a wide variety of underlying causes of bleeding, including tuberculosis, bronchiectasis, and tumors.[42] Initial success rates have been reported to be as high as 85%; however, bleeding recurs in as many as 42% of cases.[43] Radiographic features cannot predict rebleeding, although the underlying etiologies may be more predictive: BAE for hemoptysis due to active tuberculosis and amenable to therapy may be associated with higher success rates, whereas BAE for hemoptysis due to aspergillomas may have a higher chance of recurrence.[44] Recurrence of bleeding after BAE has been associated with coexistent diabetes, with the need for blood transfusion after BAE, and with angiographic evidence of a bronchial artery–pulmonary artery shunt.[44,45] Adverse effects of arterial embolization are rare but include subintimal vascular dissection and neurologic defects due to inadvertent embolism of the anterior spinal artery.[42,46]

ENDOSCOPIC APPROACH

Beyond localization, bronchoscopy can provide therapeutic benefit by controlling the source of bleeding and by preventing asphyxiation by removal of clots and minimizing spillage of blood into uninvolved portions of the lung (Fig.

40.5).[47] Flexible bronchoscopes can be limited in their field of view and have inadequate suctioning capacity, making rigid bronchoscopy advantageous when available. Rigid bronchoscopy has the added advantage of securing the airway and allowing simultaneous ventilation and oxygenation while providing a conduit for ablative tools. Blood and clots can be removed using larger-caliber suctioning catheters that can range up to 4 mm in diameter and various tools, such as cryoprobes, which can extract larger clots en bloc (see Fig. 40.5D–E). However, rigid bronchoscopy requires additional training and typically requires the setting of an operating room.

Local instillation of topical medications can provide a respite in bleeding through clot stabilization until a definitive approach can be decided upon. In their review of cases of massive hemoptysis, Conlan and colleagues[48] reported that bleeding could be stopped in 23 patients by endobronchial instillation of 50 mL aliquots of iced saline, with sustained effect in all but two patients who rebled within days of bronchoscopy. Use of topical vasoconstrictors, such as epinephrine, has been described as a means to minimize bleeding after transbronchial biopsy and is often used for hemoptysis control in other settings.[49] Agents with chronotropic effect should be used with caution because ventricular arrhythmias have been reported.[50]

Local clot stabilization has been attempted using topical application of fibrinogen and thrombin mixtures.[51,52] Clinical experience with this method is limited to small retrospective case series, which report an overall high success rate of immediate bleeding cessation. Tsukamoto and colleagues[52] reported their 5-year experience with instillation of either thrombin or a fibrinogen-thrombin combination with 5-minute bronchoscopic wedging. In a small series of 33 patients with some degree of hemoptysis, of whom 19 had massive bleeding, this approach was deemed effective in all but two patients who ultimately required surgery. Similarly, de Gracia and colleagues[51] reported that all 11 patients treated with a fibrinogen-thrombin mixture had immediate control of bleeding; three of the 11 experienced an early or late recurrence of massive hemoptysis.[51] Anecdotal experience of two patients with biopsy-related bleeding controlled with local instillation of tranexamic acid has also been reported.[53]

Tamponade of the bleeding segments has been achieved by creating an airway plug in situ. Thrombin mixed with gelatin to achieve a viscous sealant has been delivered to the bleeding airway through endobronchial blockers.[54] Airway packing with polymers such as *n*-butyl cyanoacrylate has also been described, with immediate and sustained effect in as many as 90% of patients.[55,56] Valipour and colleagues[57] reported successful tamponade using oxidized regenerated cellulose (Surgicel; Ethicon) in 56 of 57 patients who had persistent massive bleeding despite local treatment with iced saline and vasoconstrictors. However, they also noted mild to moderate recurrence of bleeding in six and obstructive pneumonias in five of those treated.

Local tamponade can also be achieved using endobronchial balloons or prosthetic devices.[58,59] Cheap and readily available balloons, such as Fogarty balloons or pulmonary angiography balloons, have been used.[60] These soft and conforming balloons can occlude distal and segmental airways to prevent bloody spillage from bleeding segments and minimize the loss of healthy lung function while awaiting definitive therapy. They can be deployed through the bronchoscope's working channel as a short-term solution or directed alongside the bronchoscope, either inside or outside of the endotracheal tube, and bronchoscopically guided to the desired airways using forceps to provide longer-term blockade (see Fig. 40.3C–D).

Dedicated commercial bronchial blockers with inflatable cuffs of varying diameter sizes are available and can be inserted into the airway and fixed in place by attaching to an endotracheal tube (Figs. 40.3E and 40.4). Although highly effective at isolating bleeding segments, these are used as temporizing measures until a definitive intervention can be undertaken. Given the potential risk of mucosal injury from prolonged balloon inflation, the airways should be inspected intermittently (every 24–36 hours) to survey the airways and confirm cessation of bleeding. Longer-term prosthetic occlusive devices can be used when other interventions, such as BAE or surgery, have either failed or are contraindicated. Airway blockade can be achieved using prosthetic occlusive devices, such as small caliber silicone spigots. Spigots are pluglike devices that can be delivered to subsegmental airways using flexible bronchoscopy, but unfortunately these are unavailable in the United States.[61] One-way endobronchial valves were originally developed for lung volume reduction and persistent air leaks; however, these have also been used to produce selective atelectasis of the bleeding segments in patients with recurrent hemoptysis.[62] With the one-way valves, there has been success in cases of hemoptysis refractory to BAE in patients who are not surgical candidates.[63,64] As a result of these promising findings, a randomized controlled trial aimed at determining the effectiveness of endobronchial valves in refractory hemoptysis patients, when surgery is not possible and embolization has either failed or is deemed not feasible, is planned.[65] "Jailing" with endobronchial stents, which refers to placing a stent across the orifice of a bleeding airway and thereby blocking it, has also been used successfully to control bleeding when bronchial artery embolization and surgery were not an option.[66,67]

Thermal ablative modalities have been reported as highly effective for the local and immediate control of bleeding (Fig. 40.6). Thermal modalities can be categorized as contact versus noncontact, referring to whether there is a need for physical interaction with tissue to exert an ablative effect. Lasers are an example of a noncontact modality for which there is now a wealth of experience in palliating hemoptysis caused by endobronchial tumors.[68] The *neodymium:yttrium-aluminum-garnet* (Nd:YAG) laser is commonly used in the airway and has been effective in the management of life-threatening hemoptysis.[69] Efficacy in controlling hemoptysis can vary, with success rates from 60–77% in patients with bleeding due to cancer.[70,71] *Argon plasma coagulation* (APC) is another noncontact thermal tool that can be deployed through a flexible scope in the peripheral airways. APC delivers

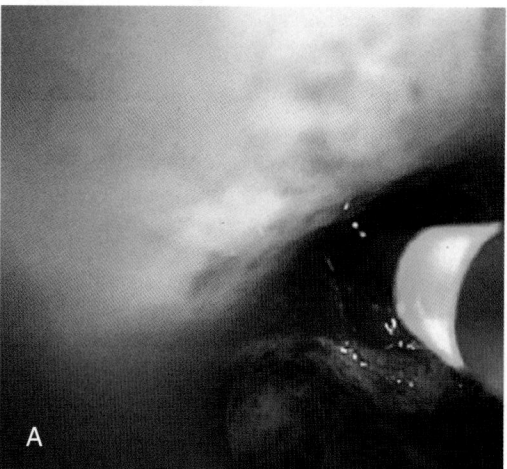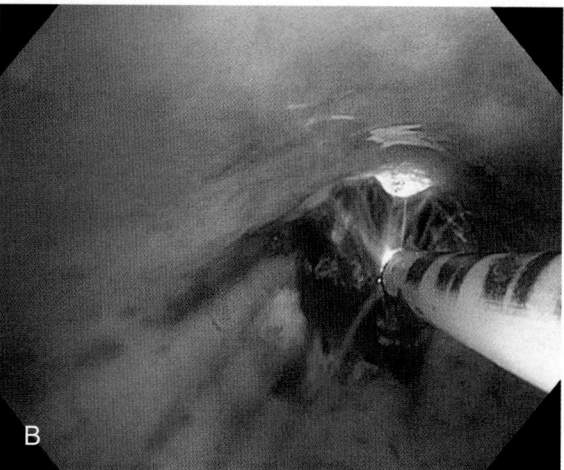

Figure 40.6 Bronchoscopic images of ablation used to stop bleeding. Ablation of a bleeding airway with a bronchoscopic-guided contact electrocautery blunt probe (A) and a noncontact argon plasma coagulation catheter (B). (A, Courtesy Yaron Gesthalter, MD. B, Courtesy Michael B. Gotway, MD.)

an electrical current along a plasma stream that conducts electricity to nearby areas of low resistance, which can superficially cauterize relatively large sections of the airway. Morice and colleagues[72] described their experience using APC in 56 hemoptysis patients in whom all had immediate and sustained effect at the site of treatment. Case reports of the effectiveness of APCs in benign vascular Dieulafoy lesions has also been described.[73,74] Contact electrocautery tools, such as blunt probes, can easily be used through a flexible bronchoscope; however, they require precise application and clear visualization of the bleeding target, given their limited surface area of application (see also Chapter 28).

Ablative modalities with delayed effect have also been used for the management of nonacute hemoptysis. Photodynamic therapy, which requires infusion with a photosensitizer 24 to 48 hours before the procedure, has been reported as having a sustained beneficial effect in patients with pulmonary hereditary hemorrhagic telangiectasia and small vessel bleeding.[75] Brachytherapy has been described in patients with hemoptysis due to endobronchial malignancy.[76,77] However, in a Cochrane review, there was no benefit to brachytherapy over external beam radiation, chemotherapy, or Nd:YAG in hemoptysis control.[78]

SURGICAL APPROACH

Surgical resection may be definitive in the prevention of bleeding recurrence; however, this is typically reserved for cases refractory to all nonsurgical approaches. Postsurgical complications can be seen in a quarter of patients, with mortality ranging from 6–15%.[16,79] Emergent surgical resection for hemoptysis is associated with poorer outcomes than nonemergent resections. Andréjak and colleagues[80] described their experience with surgical treatment of hemoptysis in which 111 of 813 patients admitted for massive hemoptysis underwent surgical lung resection. Emergent resections were associated with higher mortality rates (35%) compared to scheduled procedures (after initial bleeding control, 4%) and planned procedures (after discharge, 0%). Although these data are observational only, they highlight the benefit of preoperative stabilization and early consultation with a thoracic surgeon.

PREVENTIVE STRATEGIES FOR BLEEDING DURING LUNG BIOPSY

Bleeding during bronchoscopy is uncommon, reported in 0.26–5% of cases.[81] *Transbronchial biopsy* (TBB) increases bleeding risk through inadvertent damage to pulmonary or bronchial vessels. New techniques such as larger cryobiopsies for interstitial lung disease, may increase the need to be aware of how to prevent and manage iatrogenic bleeding.[82] Prophylactic instillation of vasoconstrictors, such as epinephrine in the airways, is not well studied and can be associated with adverse cardiac events.[49,50,83] A randomized trial assessing the utility of prophylactic topical vasoconstrictors is subject to an ongoing clinical trial.[84] In cases where TBB is being performed, most experts recommend wedging the bronchoscope into the airway of the biopsied area immediately before biopsy and leaving the bronchoscope wedged for several minutes after the biopsies until hemostasis is achieved. An additional preventive strategy includes the introduction of a deflated bronchial blocker proximal to the airway where the TBB is planned, with balloon inflation in the event of bleeding. Perhaps the most important measure for bleeding prevention is patient selection and preparation, with appropriate discontinuation of antiplatelet medicines and anticoagulants before the procedure, which should be coordinated with the patient's primary providers.[85,86] The risks and benefits of TBB in patients with pulmonary hypertension should be considered carefully and TBB avoided if possible.

Key Points

- Hemoptysis is commonly encountered and can present with a wide range of severity.
- The most common causes for hemoptysis globally include tuberculosis, bronchiectasis, and carcinoma involving the airways.
- Severity of bleeding should be assessed both by the quantity of blood expectorated and its effect on the patient's cardiopulmonary function.
- Mild hemoptysis could suggest an underlying process, such as an endobronchial tumor, and should prompt further investigation. Chest computed tomography has been shown to be more useful than bronchoscopy for identifying the underlying etiology.
- Severe or massive hemoptysis is life-threatening and warrants immediate multidisciplinary attention involving interventional radiologists, pulmonologists, thoracic surgeons, and intensive care doctors.
- Initial workup includes exclusion of pseudohemoptysis, a focused history and physical examination, and basic laboratory studies, especially for causes of coagulopathy. Although it is valuable to determine the underlying etiology, the primary focus in the setting of massive hemoptysis should be airway stabilization and cardiopulmonary support.
- Temporizing measures to spare uninvolved regions of the lung from spillage may involve decubitus positioning of the patient, with the bleeding side down, selective endotracheal intubation, or isolation of bleeding segments with balloons or other airway prosthetics.
- More definitive management can include bronchial artery embolization or endoscopic interventions.
- Surgical resection has an increased morbidity and mortality when used emergently. However, it has a role in the nonurgent setting to prevent bleeding recurrence.

Key Readings

Abdulmalak C, et al. Haemoptysis in adults: a 5-year study using the French nationwide hospital administrative database. *Eur Respir J.* 2015;46:503–511.

Cordovilla R, et al. Diagnosis and treatment of hemoptysis. *Arch Bronconeumol.* 2016;52:368–377.

Fartoukh M, et al. Early prediction of in-hospital mortality of patients with hemoptysis: an approach to defining severe hemoptysis. *Respir Int Rev Thorac Dis.* 2012;83:106–114.

Mondoni M, et al. Bronchoscopy to assess patients with hemoptysis: which is the optimal timing? *BMC Pulm Med.* 2019;19:36.

Complete reference list available at ExpertConsult.com.

41 *PULMONARY NODULE*

NICHOLE T. TANNER, MD, MSCR, FCCP • MICHAEL GOULD, MD, MS •
CHRISTOPHER G. SLATORE, MD, MS

INTRODUCTION

A pulmonary nodule is a discrete radiographic density measuring less than 3 cm, surrounded by aerated lung without associated lymphadenopathy or pleural effusion. Pulmonary nodules are often incidentally detected due to increased use of *computed tomography* (CT) scanning for a variety of clinical presentations. With the advent of *low-dose CT* (LDCT) screening for lung cancer, the incidence of pulmonary nodules will continue to rise. The majority of nodules are not malignant; however, they often pose a diagnostic dilemma for clinicians and have the potential to cause distress for patients. This chapter reviews the epidemiology, evaluation, and management of a pulmonary nodule.

EPIDEMIOLOGY

Historically, interest in the "coin lesion" first blossomed in the fifth and sixth decades of the 20th century with the publication of multiple case series that described a high prevalence of cancers among resected pulmonary nodules.[1] Most of these cases were probably identified sporadically, although at least one paper described the incidental detection of pulmonary nodules in a mass screening program for tuberculosis.[2] The subsequent accumulation of evidence linking cigarette smoking and lung cancer in the mid-1960s stimulated early studies of lung cancer screening with chest radiography. In this era, most nodules identified by radiography were relatively large (>10 mm in diameter) and presumed to be cancer until proven otherwise, often leading to unnecessary surgical resection of a benign nodule. In the 1980s, chest CT became widely used and, by virtue of its exquisite sensitivity, unintentionally launched an epidemic of incidental findings, including small, previously unrecognized pulmonary nodules.[3,4]

Chest CT is a ubiquitous presence in clinical chest medicine. In one population-based study of diagnostic imaging in six different health systems, the use of diagnostic CT increased at a rate of approximately 8% per year between 1996 and 2010, with an average rate of 23 chest CT scans per 1000 enrollees in 2008.[5] In another study from a different health system, the rate of chest CT scanning was remarkably similar (24.5 per 1000) in the 7-year period between 2006 and 2012.[6] As might be expected, greater use of imaging begets more incidental findings. In the latter study, at least one nodule measuring between 4 and 30 mm was identified in greater than 28% of diagnostic chest CT scans. Among almost 69,000 persons with an incidentally detected nodule, 3557 (5.2%) had a new diagnosis of lung cancer within 2 years of the index chest CT scan.[6] Even before the advent of lung cancer screening, the incidence of pulmonary nodules was increasing exponentially with wide availability and use of chest CT.

As demonstrated in the *National Lung Screening Trial* (NLST),[7] the introduction of lung cancer screening with LDCT has the potential to reduce lung cancer mortality, but it will simultaneously exacerbate the epidemic of nodules requiring evaluation. Randomized trials and nonrandomized cohort studies of lung cancer screening performed over the last 20 years have used slightly varying inclusion criteria to enroll high-risk current and former smokers who subsequently underwent two or more rounds of LDCT. In a systematic review from 2012,[8] the average prevalence of one or more nodules on the baseline round of screening was 20%. However, the prevalence varied from 3–30% in eight randomized controlled trials and from 5–51% in 13 cohort studies. In general, fewer nodules were identified on subsequent rounds of screening, especially in studies that only reported new (incident) nodules. In most studies, less than 5–10% of nodules were malignant; thus approximately 90–95% of all screening-detected nodules represent a false-positive finding.

Comparing and contrasting the results of studies of screening-detected nodules with more limited evidence from studies of incidentally detected nodules, it appears that nodules are found with similar frequency on both screening and diagnostic CT scans. The main source of variation in detection appears to be the individual radiologist, at least among the mostly expert radiologists who participated in the NLST, who on average identified false-positive nodules in 29% of all screening LDCT scans, with a range of 4–69%.[9] Other, less important, sources of variability in this analysis included patient characteristics, such as female sex, older age, body mass index less than 30 kg/m², current smoking, and greater than 50 pack-years smoking history, all of which were associated with a greater frequency of nodule detection. Nodule detection was similar for academic compared with nonacademic centers, and (surprisingly) for centers inside compared with outside the histoplasmosis belt.

Another potential source of variation in nodule detection arises from differing definitions of a positive screening test result. In the NLST, a positive finding was defined as any noncalcified nodule measuring at least 4 mm in any dimension. One goal of the *Lung Imaging Data and Reporting System* (Lung-RADS) classification scheme is to reduce the percentage of false positives by adjusting the nodule size threshold that defines a positive test result.[10] Thus, instead of using the NLST definition of a positive test result, a positive (category 3) Lung-RADS finding is defined as a solid nodule of undetermined age measuring 6 mm or greater or a nodule known to be new (e.g., not seen on a prior scan) measuring 4 mm or greater. In a secondary analysis of data from the NLST, using Lung-RADS criteria instead of the initial NLST criteria for nodules detected on the initial (baseline) round of screening, the specificity for identifying cancer improved from 73.4% to 87.2%, resulting in an improvement in the positive predictive value from 3.8% to 6.9%, with little change in the negative predictive value.[11] In other words, post hoc classification by Lung-RADS criteria reduced the rate of false-positive findings at baseline scan in the NLST from 27% to 13%, with a slight reduction in test sensitivity (93% to 85%).[11] Lung-RADS is the most widely adopted structured reporting system used for lung cancer screening and will require continued evaluation and updates as large registry data become available.

Most screening-detected nodules are solid in their attenuation characteristics. However, a certain number are nonsolid or part solid. Among 57,496 participants with baseline LDCT scans in the International Early Lung Cancer Action Program, nonsolid (pure ground glass) and part-solid nodules were found in 4.2% and 5.0%, respectively.[12,13] Among 64,677 annual repeat screening examinations, new nonsolid and part-solid nodules were identified in 0.7% and 0.8% of examinations, respectively. The clinical importance of distinguishing between nodules of different types of attenuation is discussed later in this chapter.

EVALUATION AND MANAGEMENT

Most nodules, whether detected incidentally or from lung cancer screening, are benign. However, the most worrisome potential cause is primary lung cancer.[7,14–16] For an individual patient with a nodule, the clinician's overarching management goal is to balance the benefits and harms of immediate versus delayed detection and treatment. Clinical decision-making needs to incorporate multiple factors, such as the likelihood of malignancy; the patient's ability and desire to undergo treatment (surgical resection or curative radiotherapy, usually *stereotactic body radiotherapy* [SBRT]); the risks of diagnostic procedures, including pneumothorax, hemorrhage, and obtaining a nondiagnostic sample; and the patient's distress induced by uncertainty and waiting for a diagnosis. Several management options usually are considered when a patient is first diagnosed with a pulmonary nodule: (1) no further workup; (2) active surveillance by waiting a period of time to obtain repeat radiographic imaging, usually a CT scan; (3) performing a *positron emission tomography* (PET) scan; (4) obtaining a biopsy specimen through a bronchoscopic or percutaneous route; or (5) proceeding directly to curative therapy, with surgical resection or SBRT. The benefits of having a quicker and more definitive diagnosis, with the earliest possible treatment, increases across this spectrum. Unfortunately, the likelihood and magnitude of harms also increase along this spectrum, most important, the unnecessary harm if the nodule is benign.

In general, clinicians and patients do not need to know if a nodule is cancer *at the moment* of detection. On the one hand, the clinician and patient want to detect a cancerous nodule before it increases in size or metastasizes to lymph nodes or other organs, and then treat it at the earliest stage possible, when patients have the highest chance for survival.[17,18] On the other hand, clinicians do not want to harm a patient from the complications of additional radiation, invasive biopsies, and surgical resection or radiation therapy for a benign nodule. Thus, the clinical question hinges on whether it safe to perform further noninvasive testing to establish the malignant potential of a cancerous nodule by showing growth on serial CT scans or by finding metabolic evidence of growth based on a PET scan. The clinician must determine whether the benefit of detecting a cancer at the earliest possible stage is worth the risks of proceeding directly to invasive biopsies or curative therapies.

Certain radiographic findings of a pulmonary nodule definitively indicate that the lesion is benign. The presence of calcification within a pulmonary nodule that takes on one of five appearances is highly suggestive that the nodule is benign. These include diffuse, central, laminar, concentric, and popcorn calcification.[19] These patterns of calcification can indicate postinfectious granuloma and hamartoma. Patterns of calcification that appear stippled or eccentric are more concerning for malignancy and should be followed. Pulmonary hamartoma is a benign lesion that can be composed of various tissues, including fat, epithelial tissue, fibrous tissue, and cartilage. Although not all densities are always present, fat and calcification seen within a nodule is diagnostic for pulmonary hamartoma (see Figs. 20.10 and 20.11).[20] In addition, nodules located within the perifissural area are commonly identified as intrapulmonary lymph nodes. Figure 41.1 demonstrates radiographic features of benign nodules.

Even for those few nodules that are cancer, most are relatively slow growing, so there is usually time to "watch and wait" with a low likelihood that a cancer starting as a nodule will increase in stage.[18] Pulmonologists now widely recognize that it is safe to follow cancerous nodules (e.g., adenocarcinoma in situ) radiographically than proceed directly to a potentially harmful diagnostic procedure.[21] In addition, there is evidence to suggest that not all "early" lung cancers are the same because patients with squamous cell and small cell lung cancers may have less benefit from early detection with formal lung cancer screening than patients with adenocarcinoma.[22,23]

Several organizations have created expert-based follow-up and surveillance guidelines for incidental and screen-detected nodules, which are based on the pretest probability that a nodule is cancerous. As will be discussed further, these guidelines attempt to balance the chance of benefit, treating lung cancer at a stage that is most curable versus the chance of harm, subjecting patients to needlessly harmful tests for benign lesions.

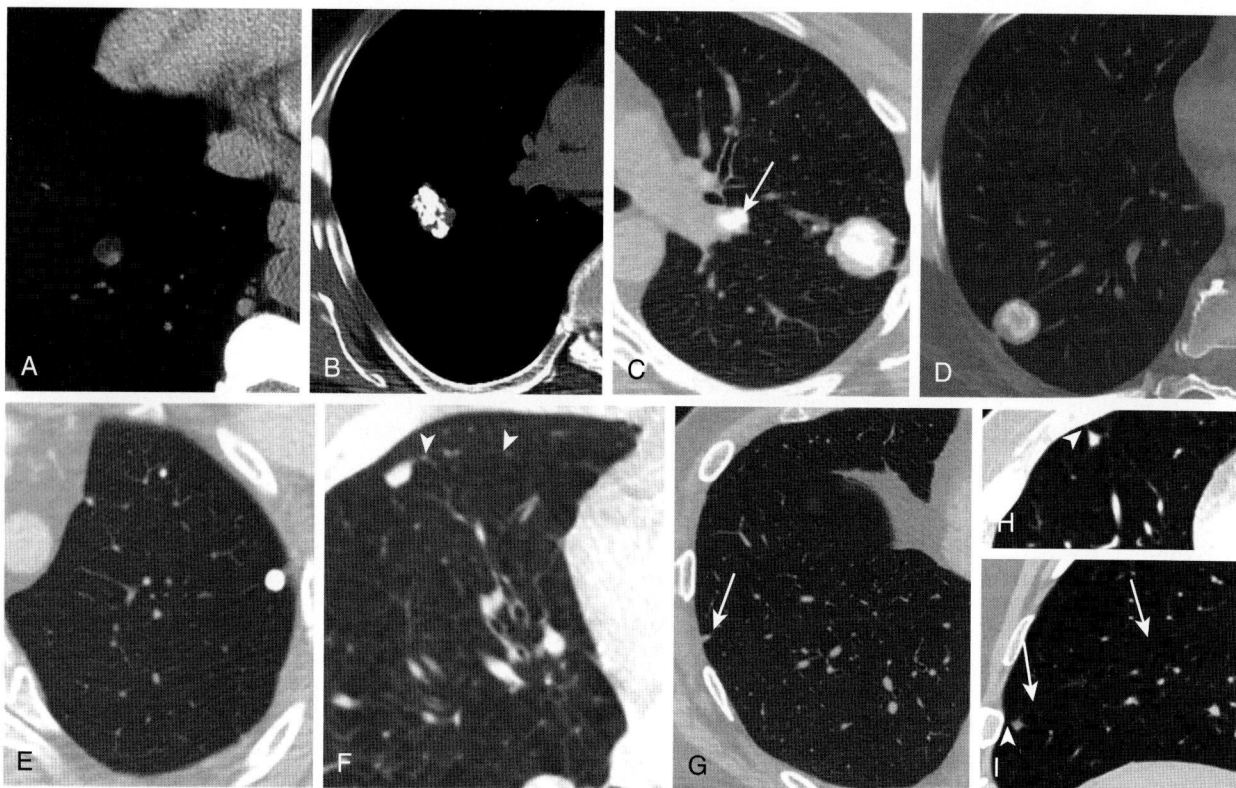

Figure 41.1 Nodules showing benign *computed tomography* (CT) features. (A) Fat within the lesion: hamartoma. (B) Chondroid ("popcorn") pattern of calcification: hamartoma. (C) Benign pattern of calcification (also see eFig. 20.30): central calcification in a postinfectious granuloma. Also note calcified left peribronchial lymph node *(arrow)*. (D) Laminar ("target") calcification: one or more concentric rings of calcium. (E) Diffuse calcification (histoplasmosis). (F–I) Perifissural nodules (also see eFig. 20.48). Note nodule in (F) abuts the right minor fissure *(arrowheads)*. Nodule in (G) *(arrow)* displays the common triangular shape, with broad-based contract with the visceral pleural surface. Axial (H) and sagittal (I) CT show a 6-mm peripheral nodular opacity with a thin septum *(arrowhead)* connecting the nodule to the visceral pleural surface. The nodule contacts, but does not distort, the adjacent minor fissure *(arrows)*. (Courtesy Michael B. Gotway, MD.)

The Fleischner guidelines offer an example of this tradeoff when they suggest that nodules with less than 1% pretest probability of being malignant do not need to be surveilled.[24]

Multiple studies have been conducted to assess the pretest probability that a patient with a pulmonary nodule will be diagnosed with cancer.[15,25–28] Many models include known risk factors for cancer, such as age, smoking history, and other exposures such as asbestos exposure and a personal history of cancer. In general, the size of the nodule at the time of detection contributes the most information to the model. No trials have been performed to evaluate the clinical usefulness of one model over the other. However, in two analyses, the Brock model, developed from data from patients undergoing screening in the Pan-Canadian Early Detection of Lung Cancer Study, was most accurate.[29,30] This model includes an online calculator that can be downloaded from https://brocku.ca/lung-cancer-screening-and-risk-prediction/risk-calculators/, which may be helpful in communicating the risk of cancer to a patient.

GUIDELINES FOR NODULE MANAGEMENT

The first set of recommendations for lung nodule evaluation was published by the Fleischner Society in 2005.[31] Before this time, there was little or no consensus about the frequency or timing of surveillance CT scans in patients with small nodules measuring less than 8 mm in diameter, which typically are not reliably characterized by PET and too small to biopsy or resect. Fortunately, these recommendations

defined a reasonable standard of care and probably reduced the frequency of unnecessary surveillance imaging among patients with small nodules. In the absence of moderate- or high-quality direct evidence from randomized trials or even large observational studies that compared different practices for follow-up, the recommendations were predicated on two reasonable assumptions; (1) nodules more suspicious for cancer should be followed earlier and more frequently; and (2) owing to imprecision in measurement, it is difficult to identify growth over short time intervals in smaller nodules. Thus, the original Fleischner Society recommendations were stratified by nodule size and the presence or absence of (unspecified) risk factors for lung cancer. In 2013, additional recommendations were made for nonsolid and part-solid nodules.[32] Because cancers presenting as nonsolid nodules tend to grow slowly, they were felt to require less intensive but perhaps longer follow-up. As for the part-solid nodules, sometimes they resolve, but the nonresolving ones are likely to be cancer; hence short-interval (3-month) follow-up was recommended.

Subsequently, the existing Fleischner Society recommendations were combined, clarified, and updated in 2017, with the goal to "reduce the number of unnecessary follow-up examinations while providing greater discretion to the radiologist, clinicians and patient to make management decisions."[24] New recommendations for patients with multiple nodules were also included, and it was clarified that the guidelines applied only to incidental nodules found in adults who were at least 35 years of age and not for patients who

Table 41.1   Fleischner Society 2017 Guidelines for Management of Incidentally Detected Pulmonary Nodules in Adults

Nodule Type	SIZE			Comments
	<6 mm (<100 mm³)	6–8 mm (100–250 mm³)	>8 mm (>250 mm³)	
SOLID NODULES				
Single				
Low risk*	No routine follow-up	CT at 6–12 mo, then consider CT at 18–24 mo	Consider CT at 3 mo, PET/CT, or tissue sampling	Nodules <6 mm do not require routine follow-up in low-risk patients (recommendation 1A).
High risk*	Optional CT at 12 mo	CT at 6–12 mo, then CT at 18–24 mo	Consider CT at 3 mo, PET/CT, or tissue sampling	Certain patients at high risk with suspicious nodule morphology, upper lobe location, or both may warrant 12-mo follow-up (recommendation 1A).
Multiple				
Low risk*	No routine follow-up	CT at 3–6 mo, then consider CT at 18–24 mo	CT at 3–6 mo, then consider CT at 18–24 mo	Use most suspicious nodule as guide to management. Follow-up intervals may vary according to size and risk (recommendation 2A).
High risk*	Optional CT at 12 mo	CT at 3–6 mo, then at 18–24 mo	CT at 3–6 mo, then at 18–24 mo	Use most suspicious nodule as guide to management. Follow-up intervals may vary according to size and risk (recommendation 2A).

Nodule Type	SIZE		Comments
	<6 mm (<100 mm³)	≥6 mm (>100 mm³)	
SUBSOLID NODULES†			
Single			
Ground-glass	No routine follow-up	CT at 6–12 mo to confirm persistence, then CT every 2 yr until 5 yr	In certain suspicious nodules <6 mm, consider follow-up at 2 and 4 yr. If solid component(s) or growth develops, consider resection (recommendations 3A and 4A).
Part-solid	No routine follow-up	CT at 3–6 mo to confirm persistence. If unchanged and solid component remains <6 mm, annual CT should be performed for 5 yr	In practice, part-solid nodules cannot be defined as such until ≥6 mm, and nodules <6 mm do not usually require follow-up. Persistent part-solid nodules with solid components ≥6 mm should be considered highly suspicious (recommendations 4A–4C).
Multiple	CT at 3–6 mo. If stable, consider CT at 2 and 4 yr	CT at 3–6 mo. Subsequent management based on the most suspicious nodule(s)	Multiple <6 mm pure ground-glass nodules are usually benign, but consider follow-up in selected patients at high risk at 2 and 4 yr (recommendation 5A).

These recommendations do not apply to lung cancer screening, patients with immunosuppression, or patients with known primary cancer. For specific recommendations (1A-5A), see table source.
*Consider all relevant risk factors, as outlined in table source.
†Dimensions are average of long and short axes, rounded to the nearest millimeter.
CT, computed tomography; PET, positron emission tomography.
From MacMahon H, Naidich DP, Goo JM, et al. Guidelines for management of incidental pulmonary nodules detected on CT images: from the Fleischner Society 2017. *Radiology.* 2017;284:228–243.

were immunocompromised or with a known extrathoracic cancer. Perhaps the most important changes were the new recommendations for following nodules less than 6 mm in diameter: If there were no risk factors for lung cancer, no follow-up was needed; if there were risk factors, follow-up was optional. The 2017 recommendations for patients with incidentally detected nodules are summarized in Table 41.1.

For patients with nodules measuring greater than 8 mm, the Fleischner Society recommends consideration of three options: surveillance chest CT at 3 months, PET/CT, or tissue sampling. Additional guidance regarding these three options is provided by evidence-based guidelines from the American College of Chest Physicians[33] (Fig. 41.2). These guidelines suggest using clinical intuition or a validated risk assessment model to make an initial assessment of the pretest probability of cancer. Based on the results of decision analytic models and related studies,[34–36] the guidelines suggest two approaches: When the probability of cancer is low (<5%), plan for CT surveillance at 3 to 6, 9 to 12, and 18 to 24 months; and when the probability of cancer is high (>65%), consider surgical diagnosis of approachable nodules in medically fit patients. For nodules with an intermediate probability of cancer (5–65%), the guidelines suggest either nonsurgical biopsy or PET/CT to characterize the nodule better. Nonsurgical biopsy is also suggested when a risk-averse patient wants confirmation of malignancy before surgery. Elicitation of patient preferences is critically important, in part because these are weak recommendations or suggestions based on low- or very low-quality evidence but also because patient preferences for either aggressive or conservative evaluation are likely to be strong.

Both the *American College of Radiology* (ACR) and the *National Comprehensive Cancer Network* (NCCN) have produced recommendations for the evaluation of screening-detected nodules. The ACR recommendations, newly updated in 2019, are embedded in the Lung-RADS classification system,

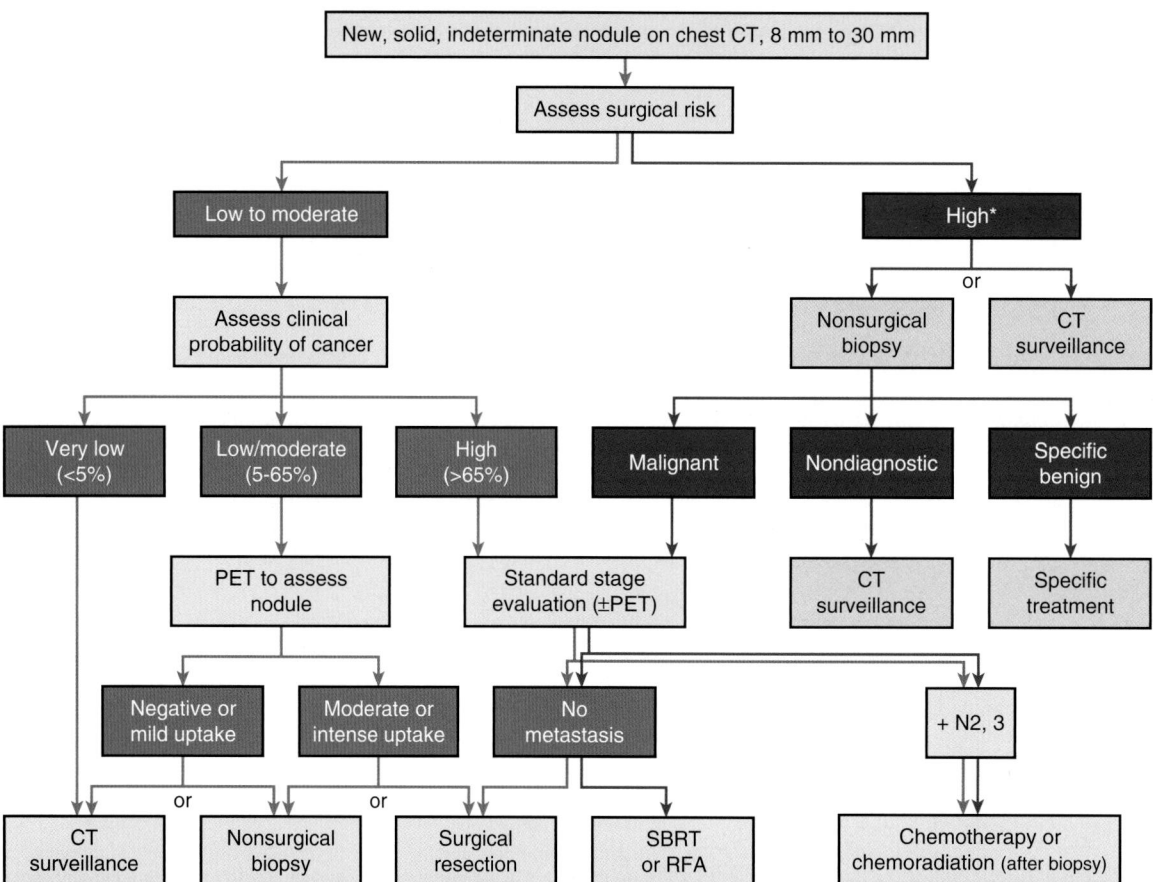

Figure 41.2 Management algorithm for individuals with solid nodules measuring 8 to 30 mm in diameter. *Among individuals at high risk for surgical complications, we recommend either nonsurgical biopsy, when the clinical probability of malignancy is moderate to high, or CT scan surveillance, when the clinical probability of malignancy is low to moderate. CT, computed tomography; PET, positron emission tomography; RFA, radiofrequency ablation; SBRT, stereotactic body radiotherapy. (From Gould MK, Donington J, Lynch WR, et al. Evaluation of individuals with pulmonary nodules: when is it lung cancer? Diagnosis and management of lung cancer, 3rd ed. American College of Chest Physicians Evidence-Based Clinical Practice Guidelines. *Chest.* 2013;143[suppl 5]:e93S–e120S.)

which categorizes nodules according to size, attenuation, and whether they are known to be new or growing.[10] A Lung-RADS category 1 finding of no nodules or a nodule with a benign pattern of calcification is considered to be negative. A category 2 finding of a small solid nodule (<6 mm), new solid nodule (<4 mm), part-solid nodule (<6 mm), nonsolid nodule (<30 mm), or a perifissural nodule (<10 mm) is considered to be a benign finding with a risk of cancer less than 1%. Patients with Lung-RADS category 1 or 2 findings should therefore return for annual screening. As nodule size increases, the risk of cancer increases from 1–2% in Lung-RADS category 3 nodules, to 5–15% in Lung-RADS category 4A nodules, to greater than 15% in Lung-RADS category 4B nodules. Thus, Lung-RADS recommends CT surveillance at 6 months or 3 months for category 3 or 4A findings, respectively, and short-interval chest CT, PET/CT, and/or tissue diagnosis for patients with category 4B findings, depending on the probability of cancer and whether the patient is fit to undergo surgery or nonsurgical biopsy. Additional details about the Lung-RADS classification system can be found in Figure 41.3. NCCN guidelines for lung cancer screening have been updated since their initial publication in 2011 and are largely consistent with Lung-RADS.[37]

Although not well known in North America, the *British Thoracic Society* (BTS) published guidelines for pulmonary nodule evaluation in 2015.[38] These guidelines were developed using rigorous methodology and an exhaustive series of systematic literature reviews. Distinctively, the BTS guidelines endorse CT surveillance for nodules with a risk of cancer less than 10% and the use of CT volumetric analysis at 3 months to check for growth of nodules measuring at least 6 mm in diameter (or 80 mm^3 in volume). Assessing the change in nodule size has traditionally been done by measuring the largest transverse cross-sectional diameter (Fig. 41.4). The volume doubling time of the nodule can then be estimated based on the change in size from baseline to follow-up CT scan. Volume doubling times can vary across histologic subtype of tumor and have been shown to be shorter in solid nodules compared to semisolid nodules or pure ground-glass nodules.[38] For solid nodules, the majority of nodules later determined to be malignant have a volume doubling time of less than 400 days.[39] This can be calculated manually using an exponential growth model that assumes uniform *three-dimensional* (3D) tumor growth. Alternatively, volumetric analysis can be conducted using semiautomated/automated software platforms. Studies comparing standard *two-dimensional* (2D) caliper measurements to semiautomated and automated 3D volumetric analysis have shown a better sensitivity for volumetric-calculated doubling time for malignancy.[40,41] Although these platforms are increasingly available, they are not always routinely used by all radiologists.

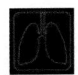

Lung-RADS® Version 1.1
Assessment Categories Release date: 2019

Category Descriptor	Lung-RADS Score	Findings	Management	Risk of Malignancy	Est. Population Prevalence
Incomplete	0	Prior chest CT examination(s) being located for comparison	Additional lung cancer screening CT images and/or comparison to prior chest CT examinations is needed	n/a	1%
		Part or all of lungs cannot be evaluated			
Negative No nodules and definitely benign nodules	1	No lung nodules			
		Nodule(s) with specific calcifications: complete, central, popcorn, concentric rings and fat containing nodules			
Benign Appearance or Behavior Nodules with a very low likelihood of becoming a clinically active cancer due to size or lack of growth	2	**Perifissural nodule(s)** *(See Footnote 11)* < 10 mm (524 mm³)	Continue annual screening with LDCT in 12 months	< 1%	90%
		Solid nodule(s): < 6 mm (< 113 mm³) new < 4 mm (< 34 mm³)			
		Part solid nodule(s): < 6 mm total diameter (< 113 mm³) on baseline screening			
		Non solid nodule(s) (GGN): < 30 mm (<14137 mm³) **OR** ≥ 30 mm (≥ 14137 mm³) and unchanged or slowly growing			
		Category 3 or 4 nodules unchanged for ≥ 3 months			
Probably Benign Probably benign finding(s) - short term follow up suggested; includes nodules with a low likelihood of becoming a clinically active cancer	3	**Solid nodule(s):** ≥ 6 to < 8 mm (≥ 113 to < 268 mm³) at baseline **OR** new 4 mm to < 6 mm (34 to < 113 mm³)	6 month LDCT	1-2%	5%
		Part solid nodule(s): ≥ 6 mm total diameter (≥ 113 mm³) with solid component < 6 mm (< 113 mm³) **OR** new < 6 mm total diameter (< 113 mm³)			
		Non solid nodule(s) (GGN) ≥ 30 mm (≥ 14137 mm³) on baseline CT or new			
Suspicious Findings for which additional diagnostic testing is recommended	4A	**Solid nodule(s):** ≥ 8 to < 15 mm (≥ 268 to < 1767 mm³) at baseline **OR** growing < 8 mm (< 268 mm³) **OR** new 6 to < 8 mm (113 to < 268 mm³)	3 month LDCT; PET/CT may be used when there is a ≥ 8 mm (≥ 268 mm³) solid component	5-15%	2%
		Part solid nodule(s): ≥ 6 mm (≥ 113 mm³) with solid component ≥ 6 mm to < 8 mm (≥ 113 to < 268 mm³) **OR** with a new or growing < 4 mm (< 34 mm³) solid component			
		Endobronchial nodule			
Very Suspicious Findings for which additional diagnostic testing and/or tissue sampling is recommended	4B	**Solid nodule(s)** ≥ 15 mm (≥ 1767 mm³) **OR** new or growing, and ≥ 8 mm (≥ 268 mm³)	Chest CT with or without contrast, PET/CT and/or tissue sampling depending on the *probability of malignancy and comorbidities. PET/CT may be used when there is a ≥ 8 mm (≥ 268 mm³) solid component. *For new large nodules that develop on an annual repeat screening CT, a 1 month LDCT may be recommended to address potentially infectious or inflammatory conditions*	> 15%	2%
		Part solid nodule(s) with: a solid component ≥ 8 mm (≥ 268 mm³) **OR** a new or growing ≥ 4 mm (≥ 34 mm³) solid component			
	4X	Category 3 or 4 nodules with additional features or imaging findings that increases the suspicion of malignancy			
Other Clinically Significant or Potentially Clinically Significant Findings (non lung cancer)	S	**Modifier - may add on to category 0-4 coding**	As appropriate to the specific finding	n/a	10%

IMPORTANT NOTES FOR USE:
1) Negative screen: does not mean that an individual does not have lung cancer
2) Size: To calculate nodule mean diameter, measure both the long and short axis to one decimal point, and report mean nodule diameter to one decimal point
3) Size Thresholds: apply to nodules at first detection, and that grow and reach a higher size category
4) Growth: an increase in size of > 1.5 mm (> 2mm³)
5) Exam Category: each exam should be coded 0-4 based on the nodule(s) with the highest degree of suspicion
6) Exam Modifiers: S modifier may be added to the 0-4 category
7) Lung Cancer Diagnosis: Once a patient is diagnosed with lung cancer, further management (including additional imaging such as PET/CT) may be performed for purposes of lung cancer staging; this is no longer screening
8) Practice audit definitions: a negative screen is defined as categories 1 and 2; a positive screen is defined as categories 3 and 4
9) Category 4B Management: this is predicated on the probability of malignancy based on patient evaluation, patient preference and risk of malignancy; radiologists are encouraged to use the McWilliams et al assessment tool when making recommendations
10) Category 4X: nodules with additional imaging findings that increase the suspicion of lung cancer, such as spiculation, GGN that doubles in size in 1 year, enlarged lymph nodes etc
11) Solid nodules with smooth margins, an oval, lentiform or triangular shape, and maximum diameter less than 10 mm or 524 mm³ (perifissural nodules) should be classified as category 2
12) Category 3 and 4A nodules that are unchanged on interval CT should be coded as category 2, and individuals returned to screening in 12 months
13) LDCT: low dose chest CT
Additional resources available at - https://www.acr.org/Clinical-Resources/Reporting-and-Data-Systems/Lung-Rads
Link to Lung-RADS calculator - https://brocku.ca/lung-cancer-screening-and-risk-prediction/risk-calculators/

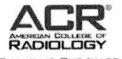

Figure 41.3 Lung Imaging Reporting and Data System (Lung-RADS) by the American College of Radiology. Version 1.1 Assessment Categories (2019 release): https://www.acr.org/Clinical-Resources/Reporting-and-Data-Systems/Lung-Rads.

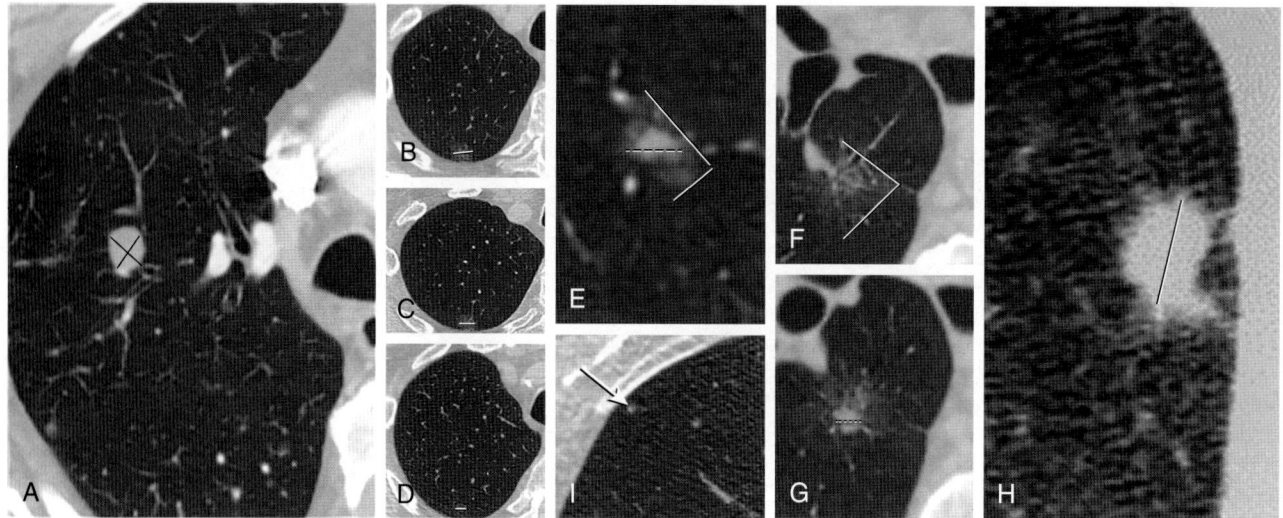

Figure 41.4 Appropriate measurement of lung nodules at chest *computed tomography* (CT). Measurements should be performed on thin-section CT images (reconstruction thickness ≤ 1.5 mm), displayed in lung windows, performed at full inspiration, and reconstructed with a high spatial frequency algorithm. Measurements are typically performed in the axial plane unless other planes, such as coronal or sagittal planes, better demonstrate the maximum nodule dimension. (A) Average of long-axis measurement and perpendicular maximal short-axis measurement *(lines)* of a nodule in the same plane. (B–D) For serial examinations, the current examination should be compared not only with the most recent examination but also with earlier examinations to determine more confidently if there has been nodule growth. In this example growth in the nodule *(line)* between the current (B) and most recent prior CT (C) is difficult to determine but is more clearly shown when the current examination (B) is compared to a more remote prior study (D). (E) For part-solid nodules, perform bidirectional measurements *(solid white lines)* through the largest dimension of nodule, including ground-glass and cystic components, if any, in whatever plane shows the longest dimension of the nodule, and then measure solid component of the nodule *(dashed white lines)* on the image in which the longest dimension is visualized. (F–G) In this example of another part-solid nodule, the solid core of the part-solid nodule *(dashed lines,* G) is at a different level than the longest dimension of the nodule *(solid white lines,* F). Note that it has been suggested by some that the size of the solid component of a part-solid nodule should be measured on soft tissue windows, but the Fleischner Society recommendations advise using thin-section lung windows reconstructed with a high spatial frequency algorithm for such measurements. (H) For spiculated nodules, measure only the solid core of the nodule *(line),* not the spiculations. (I) For nodules <3 mm *(arrow),* do not attempt to measure the nodule. Mark the nodule for reference, and refer to the nodule as a "micronodule." (Courtesy Michael B. Gotway, MD.)

Existing guidelines for pulmonary nodule evaluation provide a solid foundation for current clinical practice. However, there are several limitations, chiefly that they are not based on high-quality evidence from randomized, controlled trials or even from well-designed observational comparative effectiveness studies. In addition, whereas the use of longer-interval follow-up in nodules with a lower risk of cancer has the advantage of reducing unnecessary imaging for the large majority of individuals with benign nodules, a nodule with a low risk of cancer still has the potential to grow and spread if it is malignant. Thus there is a case to be made for short-interval (3-month) follow-up of all nodules. Last, existing guidelines are complicated, and this complexity may limit adherence by radiologists, providers, and patients. Further revision and refinement of existing guidelines should prioritize simplicity to maximize adherence.

COMMUNICATION

As with all diseases and conditions, it is important that clinicians communicate effectively and compassionately with patients with incidental and screen-detected nodules. The harms from procedural complications involved with nodule workup are important to consider,[42,43] but there are additional harms associated with inadequate communication. The harms that result from a "near cancer" diagnosis after a nodule is detected include physical harms plus psychological harms, such as distress, financial strain, and opportunity costs, which can further lead to nonadherence to suggested follow-up imaging and procedures.[44] In addition to harms, there are also benefits. Clinicians often consider diagnosis of

a nodule as an opportune time to discuss smoking cessation and try to communicate about it as a teachable moment. Communication strategies include many components and commonly focus on information exchange, patient-as-person by implicit or explicit consideration of the patients' values and preferences, and shared decision making where patients make decisions about their health care with as much or as little autonomy as desired. All these components are important, but they likely have differential effects on subsequent patient-centered outcomes.

There have been no randomized trials of different communication strategies for patients with nodules, but several observational studies can provide insights into high-quality communication techniques.[45] First, many patients suffer from distress as a result of pulmonary nodule detection, sometimes severely and for a prolonged period of time.[47–50] Although patients consistently report low levels of knowledge about their nodule,[48,50] communication strategies that emphasize consideration of the patents' values and preferences seems likely to assuage that distress.[47,51] Second, nonadherence to follow-up imaging surveillance is common.[52,53] Similar to communication strategies for reducing distress, techniques that consider the patients' values and preferences are associated with better adherence.[52] Third, most patients prefer to share decisions regarding nodule management with their clinicians,[54] a notion reflected in nodule evaluation guidelines.[33] Decision-making role concordance, when patients make decisions concordant with their preferences, is associated with medical care satisfaction.[54] Finally, as mentioned, nodule detection might be a teachable moment to facilitate positive smoking behavior changes. In the context of lung cancer screening, finding a pulmonary nodule is associated with smoking cessation, although the communication strategies that underlie this association are unknown, and this result was not confirmed in a small study among patients with incidentally detected nodules.[55,56]

Thus, it is important to share information with patients with nodules about the benefits and harms of different management strategies in a way that is respectful of their values and preferences and incorporates how they want to make decisions. Several organizations have developed educational materials to help patients with nodules understand the ramifications and likely follow-up procedures (e.g., http ://thoracic.org/patients/patient-resources/resources/lung-nodules-online.pdf). Patients and clinicians have also made suggestions for how to communicate effectively, which are included in Table 41.2.[45]

SOLID VERSUS SUBSOLID NODULES

Radiographically, nodules are often divided into solid versus subsolid, the latter further divided into nonsolid versus part-solid. With completely *nonsolid* nodules, the underlying lung parenchyma can still be visualized; these are often referred to as ground-glass opacities or nodules. *Part-solid* nodules have both solid and nonsolid components. These terms are sometimes used interchangeably and often ambiguously in both clinical and research settings. Thus, it is important for clinicians and researchers to exercise proper diligence when interpreting and reading individual images and when applying research findings in practice (see Chapter 20 and eFig. 20.47).

Compared to solid nodules, nonsolid nodules are more likely to have an indolent growth pattern. As a representative example, the investigators from the Multicenter Italian Lung Detection study of lung cancer screening using LDCT reported long-term findings of visually aided and *computer-aided diagnosis* (CAD)-detected nonsolid nodules.[57] Among 66 of 2303 subjects with visually detected nonsolid nodules, 9 subjects (14%) were ultimately diagnosed with lung cancer. Of importance, 30 of 389 (8%) subjects with a nonsolid nodule detected during screening were ultimately diagnosed as having lung cancer over 9.3 ± 1.2 years of follow-up. However, only 27% of these subjects' cancer arose from the original nonsolid nodule (e.g., the majority had cancer in a different nodule). In those who underwent surgical resection of a nonsolid nodule, the median surveillance period before surgery was 77 months, and pathology was adenocarcinoma in all cases. None of the subjects died of lung cancer originating in a nonsolid nodule. Overall, nonsolid nodules determined to be cancer have a very high rate of cure. In a systematic review of 712 lung cancers manifesting as ground-glass opacities, all were found to be stage I adenocarcinoma with a 5-year lung cancer–specific survival of 100%.[58]

Nonsolid nodules can have or can develop solid components. In the International Early Lung Cancer Action Program of lung cancer screening, 4% of subjects had at least one nonsolid nodule, of which only 3% were ultimately diagnosed with lung cancer.[59] Of the cancers, 26% developed a solid component. In general, the larger the solid component, the more likely the nodule is malignant. Table 41.3 shows the outcome of nonsolid nodules detected on a baseline lung cancer screening CT scan by size at detection.

Based on these and other similar findings, surveillance guidelines for nonsolid nodules usually recommend less frequent but longer duration of follow-up. The decision if and when to proceed to more invasive diagnostic procedures is often based on many factors, including the patient's comorbidities; preferences regarding diagnostic certainty; harms of diagnostic procedures, including inability to obtain a definitive diagnosis; and change in overall size or change in the solid component of a nodule.

FUTURE OF PULMONARY NODULE MANAGEMENT

MOLECULAR BIOMARKERS

Molecular biomarkers have the potential to add to nodule diagnostics, either alone or in combination with nodule prediction calculators and functional imaging. They can be tested in serum, blood, sputum, and airway epithelium. Currently, nodule biomarkers using proteomics, autoantibodies, circulating tumor DNA, circulating free DNA, mRNA, DNA methylation, and genomic signatures are in various stages of discovery, development, and validation. The goal is to expedite evaluation and treatment in malignant nodules while minimizing harms in those that are benign. Performance characteristics of the biomarker will depend on its design as a rule-in or rule-out test. A *rule-in test* would allow earlier diagnosis of malignancy without a significant increase in the number of invasive procedures done in patients with benign nodules. Alternatively, a *rule-out test* would result in a reduction of procedures performed on patients with benign nodules without delaying a cancer diagnosis in those with malignant nodules. The biomarker performance must allow clinicians to direct and/or alter management. The result must alter pretest probability of malignancy enough to shift management between categories of low risk and surveillance, intermediate risk and biopsy, and high risk and surgical intervention. Several phases are involved before testing for clinical utility, including biomarker discovery, analytic validation, and clinical validation.[60] There are a number of diagnostic biomarkers in various stages of development and validation with few entering into trials to determine clinical utility.

IMAGING BIOMARKERS AND DEEP MACHINE LEARNING

Radiographic features, including nodule size, contour, and growth, have traditionally been the main differentiators between benign and malignant nodules and are inputs into risk prediction calculators.[15,25,28] Nodule size, one of the strongest predictors of malignancy,[61] was traditionally assessed via measurement of the largest transverse diameter using a manual 2D caliper. More recently, however, screening trials and nodule management guidelines have recommended measurement of volume rather than diameter because it is more representative of a nodule's true size, has less interobserver and intraobserver variability, and is more sensitive to changes compared

Table 41.2 Suggestions to Improve Patient-Clinician Communication Regarding Pulmonary Nodules

PATIENT-AS-PERSON

1. Recognize that identifying a pulmonary nodule is often distressful although frequently underreported.
2. Discuss the nodule directly with the patient and provide a written summary. Examples:
   - Schedule an office or phone visit to discuss the nodule.
   - A written summary should:
      - Provide information about the nodule and address common concerns.
      - Avoid medical jargon or sending the CT report without further explanation.
3. Actively elicit patient feelings.
   - "It's common to be distressed after learning you have a pulmonary nodule. How are you feeling?"
   - "What's on your mind?"
   - "Some people with a nodule worry they have lung cancer… What have you been thinking?"
4. Provide reassurance and resources to decrease distress.
5. Make it easy for patients with persistent concerns to contact a knowledgeable clinician.
   - Provide phone number for nurse coordinator/manager.
   - Clarify ability to message clinician through the electronic health record.
6. Recognize that the nodule may be an important concern for patients and allow time for discussion of the patient's questions. Avoid minimizing or dismissive language.

INFORMATION EXCHANGE

Patient-Level Suggestions

1. Provide information about the causes of nodules, rationale for active surveillance rather than immediate biopsy, and follow-up plan details, including benefits and harms.
2. Report the semiquantitative risk of lung cancer and relevant nodule information that relates to risk prediction (e.g., lack of growth decreases malignancy risk).
3. Describe the follow-up plan in detail, including possible steps if the nodules change (e.g., biopsy or surgery for growing nodule).
4. Use pictures, summary tables, and plain, simple language.
5. Provide list of signs and symptoms that should prompt contact.
6. Outline key imaging dates and subsequent office visits or telephone calls, and provide a copy.
7. Provide written and/or online educational resources for obtaining further information. Examples:
   - Nodule risk calculator: http://reference.medscape.com/calculator/solitary-pulmonary-nodule-risk
   - Nodule patient education: http://www.thoracic.org/patients/patient-resources/resources/lung-nodules-online.pdf
8. Provide smoking cessation guidance if applicable, framed as a "teachable moment."

System-Level Suggestions

1. Health care systems can develop system-wide tools to increase patients' knowledge and understanding of the lung cancer evaluation process.
2. Health care systems should develop tools to monitor and ensure adherence to follow-up recommendations.

SHARED DECISION MAKING

1. Clarify that active surveillance is a decision that the patient can discuss and question.
   - "Let's talk together about what to do about your nodule."
2. Ask what role the patient prefers in the decision-making process.
   - "When we make this decision about what to do about your nodule, some patients want to make the decision on their own, some just want me to decide, and many want something in the middle. How about you?"
3. If the patient is comfortable with a shared approach, actively engage patients in decisions regarding the follow-up evaluation.
4. Take the patient's values and preferences into account before making a final decision.
   - "Some people are worried about getting lung cancer when thinking about nodule follow-up. What do you think?"
   - "I know you have worried about radiation exposure in the past, so let's talk about that before we decide on a plan."
   - "Most of the time the right decision is to watch the nodule over time, when we get another CT scan. But some people want to have an answer right away. How do you feel about waiting?"
   - "How would you like to get the results of your next CT scan?"

THERAPEUTIC ALLIANCE

1. Ask patients what they expect at the outset of the encounter to help define roles and prevent assumptions.
2. Evaluate patients' understanding of the concepts presented.
   - "To make sure I didn't forgot to tell you anything, can you repeat back to me when you're going to get your next CT scan? And what are you going to do if you have more questions or start to feel distressed?"

CT, computed tomography.

From Slatore CG, Wiener RS. Pulmonary nodules: a small problem for many, severe distress for some, and how to communicate about it. *Chest*. 2018;153:1004–1015.

Table 41.3   Frequency of Nonsolid Nodules and Diagnoses of Lung Cancer Identified in 2392 of 57,496 Participants at Baseline CT Screening According to Size of Largest Nonsolid Nodule

Parameter	<6 mm	6–9 mm	10–14 mm	15–30 mm	≥31 mm	Total
RESOLVED OR DECREASED	341	177	70	39	1	628
Lung cancer	0	0	0	0	0	0
STABLE OR GROWTH	1063	439	164	92	6	1764
Lung cancer	9	20	27	15	2	73
AAH, ABP	2	3	0	0	0	5
Nonmalignant diagnosis	1	1	1	1	0	4
Total	1404	616	234	131	7	2392

Data are numbers of nodules.
AAH, atypical adenomatous hyperplasia, a diagnosis made on histologic specimens; ABP, atypical bronchioloalveolar proliferation, a diagnosis made on cytologic specimens; CT, computed tomography.
From Yankelevitz DF, Yip R, Smith JP, et al. CT screening for lung cancer: nonsolid nodules in baseline and annual repeat rounds. *Radiology.* 2015;277:555–564.

to 2D measurements.[62] For volumetric measurements to be reliable, nodule segmentation (i.e., the delineation of a nodule boundary) must be accurate.[63] There are software packages that provide manual, semiautomated, and automated volumetrics. Although these provide repeat measurements that are reliable, there is variation between software packages that can make comparisons between images done at differing institutions difficult.[38] Volumetric measurements, while gaining traction, have not been widely adopted in the United States as standard practice for nodule evaluation.

There have previously been attempts to develop CAD algorithms to help radiologists distinguish benign from malignant nodules and improve diagnostic accuracy; however, these did not achieve widespread acceptance.[64] A new paradigm shift in computer-based diagnosis was seen after the introduction of *convolutional neural networks* (CNNs). This set of techniques allows computers to detect patterns beyond human perception, to classify imaging findings further. Research using CNNs to classify pulmonary nodules has demonstrated superiority to standard CAD techniques by reducing the number of false positives.[65–68] This form of deep machine learning has the ability to learn previously unknown features but requires large amounts of validated data. Unfortunately, there are few large validated imaging datasets with pathology-confirmed cancer available to allow training, tuning, and testing.[69] Efforts are underway to advance this technology for analysis of both incidental and screen-detected nodules. Ideally, much like clinician intuition or risk prediction calculators, deep machine learning would incorporate all available imaging, clinical, and biochemical data into determining likelihood for malignancy.

BRONCHOSCOPY

As discussed previously, guidelines recommend consideration of biopsy when pretest probability for malignancy is intermediate, after shared decision making with the patient. Biopsy can be performed using CT guidance with transthoracic needle aspiration with a diagnostic yield of approximately 90%.[70] The decision to pursue biopsy with flexible bronchoscopy hinges on the location of the lesion. Peripheral lesions are not visible beyond the segmental bronchi, whereas central lesions are visible and may have an endobronchial component. The sensitivity for bronchoscopy in central lesions is 88%.[70] The sensitivity for bronchoscopy in peripheral lesions varies depending on the number of transbronchial biopsies performed (six samples at 74% vs. 45% with one sample),[71] CT scan evidence of a bronchus extending to the lesion (60% vs. 25%),[72,73] and the size of the lesion (<2 cm [34%] vs. >2 cm [63%]).[70] Bronchoscopy guided beyond the camera image has seen a variety of advancements over the past 2 decades. These include radial *endobronchial ultrasound* (EBUS), guide sheaths to extend the bronchoscopy working channel, software platforms to assist with locating and planning a pathway to reach the lesion, electromagnetic navigation systems that link the CT plan and location of the tip of the bronchoscope and instruments at the time of bronchoscopy, and, most recently, robotic bronchoscopy.

There are data supporting the use of guided bronchoscopy. A meta-analysis of 39 studies, including studies of a combination of guided bronchoscopy (excluding robotic technology), showed a pooled diagnostic yield of 70%.[74] This study and others supported the guideline recommendations for the use of radial EBUS and/or electromagnetic navigational bronchoscopy in centers with technology and expertise for patients with peripheral lesions suspected to be lung cancer.[70] Results later published from the American College of Chest Physicians Quality Improvement Registry, Evaluation, and Education registry of bronchoscopy, however, demonstrated a lower yield for guided bronchoscopy than for standard bronchoscopy, suggesting that diagnostic outcomes in clinical practice may be different from that seen in large-volume single centers.[75] As new bronchoscopy technologies are evaluated, there is a need for well-designed large trials with clear definitions of what constitutes a diagnostic bronchoscopy to quantify diagnostic accuracy.

EXHALED BREATH ANALYSIS

Analysis of human breath has been described since the 1970s and has applications in other disease states. In patients with pulmonary nodules, analyzing breath to determine malignancy is desirable because of the noninvasive nature of the testing. Exhaled breath contains thousands of organic compounds; some are exogenous (from the environment) and others are endogenous (by-products from the body's biochemical processes). Although collection of breath is relatively easy, the optimal container for collection and modality for analysis vary. Analysis of breath has been performed by trained canines with sensitivities as high as 99% reported in various cancer types; however, recent studies have suggested outcomes may vary based on extent of training and the material used to carry the breath sample.[76] Volatile organic compounds are analyzed using a variety of techniques. Gas chromatography mass spectroscopy requires a level of skill to use, and careful calibration makes it both expensive and less practical in the clinical setting.[77] Smaller, more portable devices, such as the electronic nose, rely on sensors to detect volatile organic compound profiles. Research in exhaled breath analysis for characterization of pulmonary nodules is underway and has potential for assisting in management in the future.

Key Points

- The incidence of pulmonary nodules is increasing due to wide use of computed tomography imaging. The number of nodules detected will continue to rise with the implementation of lung cancer screening.
- Evaluation and management of pulmonary nodules starts with an assessment of pretest probability of malignancy.
- Pretest probability of malignancy incorporates radiographic features of the nodule (e.g., size, density, contour, and location) and patient level factors (e.g., age, smoking history, history of cancer). Assessment of pretest probability of malignancy can be determined by validated risk calculators or by clinician intuition.
- In solid nodules, those with a low pretest probability of malignancy should be monitored for growth with repeat imaging. Alternatively, those determined to be high risk should be considered for surgical resection if patient health status and nodule location are amenable to surgery. In an intermediate risk nodule, management options can include further evaluation with positron emission and/or computed tomography and/or biopsy, and decisions should include patient preferences.
- Nonsolid nodules, also known as pure ground-glass opacities, are less likely to be malignant and can be followed with less frequent but longer-duration surveillance imaging.
- Good-quality communication that incorporates patient values and beliefs is essential when making decisions surrounding nodule management.
- Biomarker testing to aid in nodule management must be clinically validated and demonstrate clinical utility before widespread implementation.
- The future of nodule management is likely to incorporate biomarkers, advanced bronchoscopic techniques, exhaled breath analysis, and deep machine learning.

Key Readings

Callister ME, Baldwin DR, Akram AR, et al. British Thoracic Society guidelines for the investigation and management of pulmonary nodules. *Thorax*. 2015;70(suppl 2):ii1–ii54.

Gould MK, Donington J, Lynch WR, et al. Evaluation of individuals with pulmonary nodules: when is it lung cancer? Diagnosis and management of lung cancer, 3rd ed: American College of Chest Physicians Evidence-Based Clinical Practice Guidelines. *Chest*. 2013;143(suppl 5):e93S–e120S.

Gould MK, Tang T, Liu IL, et al. Recent trends in the identification of incidental pulmonary nodules. *Am J Respir Crit Care Med*. 2015;192(10):1208–1214.

Huo J, Xu Y, Sheu T, Volk RJ, Shih YT. Complication rates and downstream medical costs associated with invasive diagnostic procedures for lung abnormalities in the community setting. *JAMA Intern Med*. 2019;179(3):324–332.

MacMahon H, Naidich DP, Goo JM, et al. Guidelines for management of incidental pulmonary nodules detected on CT images: from the Fleischner Society 2017. *Radiology*. 2017;284(1):228–243.

Rivera MP, Mehta AC, Wahidi MM. Establishing the diagnosis of lung cancer: diagnosis and management of lung cancer, 3rd ed: American College of Chest Physicians Evidence-Based Clinical Practice Guidelines. *Chest*. 2013;143(suppl 5):e142S–e165S.

Slatore CG, Golden SE, Ganzini L, Wiener RS, Au DH. Distress and patient-centered communication among veterans with incidental (not screen-detected) pulmonary nodules. a cohort study. *Ann Am Thorac Soc*. 2015;12(2):184–192.

Yankelevitz DF, Yip R, Smith JP, et al. CT Screening for lung cancer: nonsolid nodules in baseline and annual repeat rounds. *Radiology*. 2015;277(2):555–564.

Complete reference list available at ExpertConsult.com.

42

POSITIVE SCREENING TEST FOR TUBERCULOSIS

CHRISTINA YOON, MD, MPH, MAS

INTRODUCTION

Approximately 1.7 billion people (22% of the world's population) are estimated to have *latent tuberculosis infection* (LTBI).[1] This population represents a large reservoir of potential future disease because 5–10% of latently infected individuals will develop active disease if untreated.

Although treatment of individuals with active disease is the first priority of *tuberculosis* (TB) control, controlling and eventually eliminating TB also require identifying and treating individuals with LTBI. However, because there are no direct tests to diagnose LTBI definitively, latent TB remains a clinical diagnosis based on evidence of prior TB infection *and* exclusion of active disease. Currently, there are only two approaches available to identify individuals with asymptomatic TB infection: *tuberculosis skin testing* (TST) and *interferon-gamma* (IFN-γ) *release assays* (IGRAs).

INDICATIONS FOR TUBERCULIN SKIN TEST AND/OR INTERFERON GAMMA RELEASE ASSAYS

There are two indications for TST and/or IGRA testing: (1) to screen asymptomatic individuals for LTBI and (2) to guide decisions about empirical treatment for active TB among symptomatic individuals with negative microbiologic results. This chapter outlines the approach to screening individuals for LTBI. TST or/IGRA testing to guide decisions related to empirical treatment for active TB is discussed in Chapter 53.

SCREENING FOR LATENT TUBERCULOSIS INFECTION

In the United States and other low-burden countries, 80% or more of all TB cases are the result of reactivated latent infection,[2] and nearly all reactivated cases can be prevented by treatment of LTBI.[3] Therefore the goal of screening for LTBI is to identify *Mycobacterium tuberculosis (Mtb)*-infected individuals at increased risk of developing active TB. As such, only individuals who would benefit from treatment of LTBI should undergo screening.

Target Populations for Screening

Screening for LTBI should target individuals in two high-risk groups: (1) individuals with increased risk of *Mtb* infection (e.g., recent close contact with individuals with untreated pulmonary TB) and (2) individuals with certain clinical conditions (e.g., immunosuppression) associated with a high risk of reactivation (Table 42.1). Untargeted screening for LTBI (testing individuals without risk factors for infection or reactivation) should not be performed. Although untargeted screening and treatment of all individuals with LTBI would prevent most new cases of active disease, this approach is not cost-effective for settings with low TB incidence and would result in overtreatment because the specificity of current screening tests would yield more false-positive results than true-positive results.

Screening Individuals With Increased Risk of *Mycobacterium tuberculosis* Infection

Although most individuals exposed to *Mtb* lack evidence of sustained infection, approximately 30–50% will develop LTBI contained by host immune responses.[4] Although LTBI has the potential to progress to active TB at any time, risk

Table 42.1   Target Groups for Latent Tuberculosis Infection Screening

INDIVIDUALS WITH INCREASED RISK OF INFECTION

Contacts of individuals with untreated infectious active tuberculosis

Individuals who have immigrated to the United States within the past 5 years from tuberculosis endemic areas

Individuals who work and/or reside in high-risk congregate settings (e.g., hospitals, homeless shelters, prisons, nursing homes)

INDIVIDUALS WITH CONDITIONS ASSOCIATED WITH INCREASED RISK FOR REACTIVATION

High Risk for Reactivation (Risk of Reactivation Is at Least Six Times Higher Than for Healthy Individuals)

Human immunodeficiency virus infection

Severe immunosuppression (e.g., individuals receiving medication for solid-organ transplantation, chemotherapy, tumor necrosis factor-α inhibitors)

Certain malignancies (e.g., hematologic malignancies, head and neck cancers)

Silicosis

End-stage renal disease

Radiographic evidence of prior granulomatous disease (e.g., fibrotic lesions on chest imaging)

Children <5 years with a positive tuberculin skin test reaction

Moderate Risk for Reactivation (Risk of Reactivation Is Less Than Six Times Higher Than for Healthy Individuals)

Corticosteroid use (≥15 mg daily for ≥1 mo)

Diabetes mellitus

Underweight or malnourished individuals (includes malabsorptive conditions, such as gastrectomy, jejunoileal bypass surgeries)

Substance abuse (e.g., smoking, alcohol abuse, injection drug use)

Radiographic evidence of solitary or small granulomas

of developing active disease is greatest within 2 years of infection.[5–9] In a randomized controlled trial of TB vaccines given to children, 2550 unvaccinated children experienced TST conversion (≥10 mm increase in TST induration), of whom 121 (5%) developed active disease during 15-year follow-up.[10] Among those who developed active TB, 82% developed disease within 2 years of TST conversion. Thus individuals at risk for LTBI represent a high-priority group for screening.

Individuals with risk for *Mtb* infection include (1) recent close contacts of untreated individuals with infectious TB, (2) individuals who have recently immigrated from areas with high TB incidence, and (3) individuals who work and/or reside in congregate settings (e.g., hospitals, homeless shelters, prisons, nursing homes) with higher rates of active TB.

Close contacts are considered those sharing an enclosed space more than 4 hours per week.[11] These typically include individuals living in the same household, frequent visitors to the house, and individuals who work or attend school with the index case. *Mtb* transmission has also been documented among casual contacts of a highly infectious index case.[12] Casual contacts—individuals who spend fewer than 4 hours of contact per week with the index case—may include individuals who attend school, work, and/or reside in congregate settings with the index case. TB programs conducting contact investigations prioritize evaluation of close contacts and expand investigation to casual contacts if the index case

is deemed to be highly infectious (e.g., high acid-fast bacilli smear grade), evidence of transmission is found among close contacts, and/or the casual contact has risk factors for developing active disease (i.e., immunocompromise). All close and at-risk casual contacts should undergo TST or IGRA testing for LTBI screening, in addition to screening for active disease. If initial TST or IGRA testing is negative and initial testing was performed within 8 weeks of last exposure, testing should be repeated 8 to 10 weeks after last exposure because TB infection may have been so recent (within 3–8 weeks of initial testing) that delayed hypersensitivity has not yet developed (see later, "Approach to Individuals with Possible False-Negative TST or IGRA Results").

Individuals who have recently immigrated from areas with high TB incidence represent a high-priority population for latent TB screening and treatment. Although overall TB incidence among foreign-born persons is 13 times higher than among U.S.-born individuals,[13] the risk of developing active TB (reactivation of infection acquired in their country of origin) is highest within the first 5 years after immigration, with incidence decreasing over time to approach that of the U.S. population.[14] As such, all foreign-born individuals who immigrated to the United States from a high-burden country within the past 5 years should undergo LTBI screening in addition to screening for active disease. Although either TSTs or IGRAs may be used to screen individuals for LTBI, IGRA may be preferred as a more specific screening test for individuals with prior *bacillus Calmette-Guérin* (BCG) vaccination (see later, "Approach to TST-Positive Individuals With Prior Bacillus Calmette-Guérin").

Individuals who work and/or reside in congregate settings with higher rates of active TB are at increased risk of infection due to crowded conditions, which increases the likelihood of *Mtb* transmission. Although risk of infection varies greatly in such settings, serial LTBI screening is recommended for individuals with ongoing *Mtb* exposure risk, including selected groups of health care workers. In the United States, health care workers with high ongoing risk for occupational exposure to *Mtb* include emergency department staff, pulmonologists, and respiratory therapists. Although prior guidelines recommended annual screening for all U.S. health care workers,[15] recent data suggest that this is no longer necessary.[16] However, in the setting of a recognized exposure to *Mtb*, all exposed health care personnel with negative baseline TST or IGRA results should undergo screening for infection and, if TST or IGRA results are negative, testing should be repeated 8 to 10 weeks after last exposure.

Screening Individuals With Increased Risk of Reactivation

Risk of reactivation (i.e., progression of LTBI to active disease) is increased by certain clinical conditions, including immunodeficiency or immunosuppression, malignancy, and radiographic evidence of fibrotic lesions from prior TB (see Table 42.1). Among individuals with LTBI, *human immunodeficiency virus* (HIV) infection is the strongest known risk factor for progression to active disease. As such, all individuals newly diagnosed with HIV should be screened for LTBI. HIV-infected individuals who test negative for LTBI in the setting of advanced immunosuppression (i.e., CD4 cell counts less than 200 cells/μL) should undergo repeat testing after initiation of antiretroviral therapy,

Table 42.2 TST Cut-Point Used to Define a Positive TST Reaction

≥5 mm	≥10 mm	≥15 mm
People living with HIV	Recent immigrants (<5 years) from TB-endemic countries	Individuals with no known TB risk factors
Recent contacts of individuals with untreated infectious TB	Residents and employees of high-risk congregate settings (correctional facilities, homeless shelters, nursing homes, hospitals, other health care facilities)	
Individuals with fibrotic lesions on chest imaging	Mycobacteriology laboratory personnel	
Organ-transplant recipients	Children <5 years	
Individuals with other immunosuppressive conditions (e.g., individuals receiving chemotherapy, TNF-α inhibitors, corticosteroids ≥15 mg/daily for ≥1 month; individuals with certain malignancies)		

HIV, human immunodeficiency virus; TB, tuberculosis; TNF, tumor necrosis factor; TST, tuberculin skin test.

when CD4 cell counts increase to 200 cells/μL or greater, because of the higher rates of false-negative results associated with immunosuppression. TST- or IGRA-negative HIV-infected individuals with ongoing risk factors for *Mtb* exposure (e.g., work or reside in congregate settings) should undergo annual screening for LTBI.

Other populations at high risk for reactivation (at least six times higher than healthy individuals) for whom testing is recommended include individuals about to receive immunosuppressive therapy (e.g., chemotherapy, tumor necrosis factor-α antagonists); individuals with hematologic malignancies, head and neck cancers, and silicosis; and individuals with radiographic evidence of prior granulomatous disease (e.g., fibronodular changes). Populations with moderate risk for reactivation (less than six times higher than healthy individuals) include individuals receiving corticosteroids and individuals with malnutrition, diabetes mellitus, and/or radiographic evidence of small granulomas. Current U.S. guidelines recommend LTBI screening for populations with moderate or high risk for reactivation.[17]

SCREENING TESTS FOR LATENT TUBERCULOSIS INFECTION

Infection with *Mtb* produces a delayed-type hypersensitivity reaction to mycobacterial antigens; the cell-mediated immune response to such antigens can be measured by TST and IGRA, which serve as measurements of immunologic memory and as indirect evidence for the presence of mycobacteria.

TUBERCULIN SKIN TEST

Tuberculin Skin Test Placement and Interpretation

The TST consists of an intracutaneous injection on the inner surface of the forearm of tuberculin, a purified protein derivative from heat-killed cultures of *Mtb*.[18] Among individuals infected with *Mtb*, TST causes induration due to inflammatory cell infiltration at the injection site, beginning 5 to 6 hours after placement, peaking at 48 to 72 hours, then subsiding over several days. To read the test, the area of induration (not erythema) is measured along its transverse diameter (in millimeters) 48 to 72 hours after TST placement. If the TST cannot be read within 48 to 72 hours, repeat testing should be performed.

Based on the sensitivity and specificity of TST among populations with varying risk for active TB, three cut-points for induration are used to define a positive TST (≥5, ≥10, and ≥15 mm); the TST cut-point used to define a positive result is determined by the presence of certain TB risk factors.[17] Because sensitivity increases (and specificity decreases) as the cut-off for TST positivity decreases, the lowest cut-off (≥5 mm) is used for individuals with highest TB risk (e.g., HIV infection) to minimize the proportion of false negatives (i.e., *Mtb*-infected individuals missed by testing). Conversely, the highest TST cut-off (≥15 mm) is used for individuals with no TB risk factors to minimize the proportion of false positives (i.e., *Mtb*-uninfected individuals for whom latent TB treatment would be associated with unnecessary risk). Table 42.2 summarizes TST cut-points for populations undergoing testing for LTBI.

INTERFERON-GAMMA RELEASE ASSAYS

IGRAs are in vitro blood tests that measure IFN-γ released from memory T cells stimulated by previously encountered *Mtb* antigens: *early secreted antigenic target 6* (ESAT-6) and *culture filtrate protein 10* (CFP-10). ESAT-6 and CFP-10 are absent from all strains of BCG,[19,20] so IGRAs are more specific for *Mtb* than is TST, which uses a mixed purified protein derivative that contains more than 200 mycobacterial antigens, most of which are shared with BCG.[21–23]

Current Interferon-Gamma Release Assay Platforms

Two IGRA platforms using the ESAT-6 and CFP-10 antigens are currently available for commercial use: QuantiFERON-TB (QFT-TB) and T-SPOT.TB (Oxford Immunotec). Because IGRA testing requires more laboratory infrastructure than tuberculin skin testing, its use is generally limited to resource-rich settings.

The QFT-TB Gold In-tube and QFT-TB Plus assays use blood collection tubes coated with *Mtb* antigens ESAT-6 and CFP-10 and include a positive and negative control tube; the positive control contains a nonspecific T-cell stimulator, and the negative control tube contains no antigenic additives and no stimulator. Blood collected in the tubes is incubated overnight, and an enzyme-linked immunosorbent assay is used to measure the concentration of IFN-γ released by stimulated T cells, which is compared to the control tubes. Unlike TST, which requires two patient visits (one visit for placement and a second visit for interpretation), IGRAs require only one patient visit, and results may be available in 24 hours. Individuals are regarded as QFT positive if the IFN-γ concentration is above the test cut-point after subtracting the background IFN-γ response in the negative control.

Three IGRA assays using the QFT-TB platform have received U.S. Food and Drug Administration approval: QFT-TB Gold (QFT-Gold, Cellestis), Gold In-tube (QFT-GIT), and Gold Plus (QFT-Plus, Qiagen); however, only QFT-Gold and QFT-GIT have received endorsement by the *Centers for Disease Control and Prevention* (CDC) (validation studies for QFT-Plus are ongoing). The QFT-GIT assay includes a third *Mtb*-specific antigen (TB7.7), in addition to ESAT-6 and CFP-10, intended to improve test sensitivity beyond QFT-Gold. The QFT-Plus assay uses two antigen tubes: TB1 and TB2. Both TB1 and TB2 tubes are coated with ESAT-6 and CFP-10; however, TB2 tubes include shorter *Mtb* antigen peptides to stimulate a response from CD8+ T cells, in addition to CD4+ T cells. An individual is considered QFT-Plus positive if either tube is positive.

The T-SPOT.TB platform incubates isolated peripheral blood mononuclear cells with ESAT-6 and CFP-10 in microplate wells and uses an enzyme-linked immunospot (ELISPOT) assay to measure the number of IFN-γ–producing T cells (spots). Individuals are considered T-SPOT.TB positive if the spot counts in the antigen-containing wells exceed a certain threshold relative to negative control wells.

Interferon-Gamma Release Assay Interpretation

IGRA results are reported as both quantitative and qualitative (positive, negative, or uninterpretable) measurements. For QFT-based assays, a result is considered positive if the IFN-γ concentration is 0.35 *international units* (IU)/mL or more above the negative control. For the T-SPOT.TB assay, an individual is considered IGRA positive if there are eight or more spots above the negative control. Individuals are considered IGRA negative if IFN-γ concentrations are less than 0.35 IU/mL (after subtracting the background IFN-γ response in the negative control) for QFT-based assays and four spots or fewer are detected by T-SPOT.TB above the negative control. Uninterpretable results are possible with both QFT-based and T-SPOT.TB assays. For QFT-based assays, uninterpretable results are reported as "indeterminate" when there is an inappropriate response in the positive or negative control: insufficient response in the positive control or excessive response in the negative control (indicating a high level of spontaneous IFN-γ secretion despite the absence of antigen), respectively. For the T-SPOT.TB assay, uninterpretable results include "invalid" and "borderline" results. Invalid T-SPOT.TB results are equivalent to QFT indeterminates, seen when there is an inappropriate response in the positive or negative control. Borderline T-SPOT.TB results are reported when five to seven spots above the negative control are observed. Causes of uninterpretable IGRA results are discussed later.

Table 42.3 Current CDC Guidelines For TST, IGRA, or Dual Testing

SITUATIONS IN WHICH EITHER IGRA OR TST MAY BE USED WITHOUT PREFERENCE

All situations where TST is recommended

SITUATIONS IN WHICH TST IS PREFERRED BUT IGRA IS ACCEPTABLE

Children <5 years

SITUATIONS IN WHICH IGRA IS PREFERRED BUT TST IS ACCEPTABLE

Individuals who have received BCG (as a vaccine or for cancer treatment)

Individuals belonging to groups with low rates of returning to have TSTs read (e.g., homeless individuals, active drug users)

SITUATIONS IN WHICH DUAL IGRA AND TST TESTING MAY BE CONSIDERED

Situations Where the Initial Test Is Negative and Diagnostic Sensitivity Is Prioritized Over Specificity

Individuals with high risk for *Mtb* infection, disease progression, and poor outcomes (e.g., children younger than 5 years who were exposed to an individual with untreated active TB)

Individuals with suspected active TB for whom confirmation of *Mtb* infection is desired

Situations Where the Initial Test Is Positive, and

Additional evidence of *Mtb* infection is needed to encourage treatment acceptance and adherence (e.g., BCG-vaccinated individuals who believe their positive TST is due to prior BCG)

The individual has low risk of both infection and disease progression and additional evidence is desired to support the decision not to initiate treatment

BCG, bacillus Calmette-Guérin; CDC, Centers for Disease Control and Prevention; IGRA, interferon-gamma release assay; *Mtb, Mycobacterium tuberculosis;* TB, tuberculosis; TST, tuberculin skin test.

SELECTION OF TUBERCULOSIS SKIN TEST OR INTERFERON-GAMMA RELEASE ASSAYS FOR LATENT TUBERCULOSIS INFECTION SCREENING

Current CDC guidelines state that "IGRAs can be used in place of (but not in addition to) TST in all situations in which CDC recommends TST as an aid in diagnosing *Mtb* infection."[24] The following sections describe situations in which TST or IGRA is preferred and situations in which dual testing may be considered (Table 42.3).

SITUATIONS IN WHICH TUBERCULOSIS SKIN TEST IS PREFERRED

Children Younger Than 5 Years

TST is preferred but IGRA remains acceptable for testing children younger than 5 years. Although available data from high-quality studies of IGRAs suggest that sensitivity and specificity in children are comparable to estimates in adults, uninterpretable IGRA results appear to be more frequent in children (range, 0–17%). The rate of uninterpretable IGRA results also appears to be significantly higher (up to 40%) among children younger than 5 years,[25-27] the age group at highest risk for severe forms of active TB. Although the causes of uninterpretable IGRA results in children are not fully understood, children younger than 5 years have been shown to have lower IFN-γ response to *Mtb* antigens and mitogen (used in the positive control) than children 4 years or older,[26,28] suggesting that higher rates of uninterpretable IGRA results in this age group may be due to immunologic immaturity. Based on these results, current U.S. guidelines state that TST is preferred over IGRAs for children younger than 4 years.[24] In addition, some experts have recommended dual TST and IGRA testing for children younger than 4 years to maximize detection of *Mtb* infection, due to potential reduced sensitivity of both tests relative to adults.

SITUATIONS IN WHICH INTERFERON-GAMMA RELEASE ASSAY IS PREFERRED

Individuals With Prior Bacillus Calmette-Guérin

Situations in which IGRA is preferred but TST is acceptable include testing of individuals who have received BCG as a vaccine or as cancer treatment. For individuals who have received prior BCG, IGRAs can be expected to detect *Mtb* infection with greater specificity than can TST (see "Approach to Tuberculosis Skin Test–Positive Individuals With Prior Bacillus Calmette-Guérin"), limiting treatment to individuals most likely to have true *Mtb* infection.

Individuals at Risk of Being Lost to Follow-up

IGRA testing is also preferred for individuals belonging to groups with low rates of returning to have TSTs read (e.g., homeless persons, active drug users). For individuals belonging to groups with low rates of follow-up, IGRAs increase test completion rates, allowing health care providers to focus control efforts on those individuals most likely to benefit from treatment.

SITUATIONS IN WHICH DUAL TESTING MAY BE CONSIDERED

Although dual IGRA and TST testing is not routinely recommended, the CDC recognizes certain situations in which dual testing may be considered. For situations in which sensitivity is strongly prioritized over specificity, dual testing may be considered for individuals with a negative initial test result when (1) the risks for *Mtb* infection, for progression to active disease, and for poor outcomes are increased (e.g., immunosuppressed individuals, children <5 years) and (2) suspicion for active TB persists (based on clinical and/or radiographic assessment) despite negative microbiologic test results. Dual testing may also be considered for individuals with a positive initial test result when (1) additional evidence to support *Mtb* infection may facilitate treatment acceptance and adherence (e.g., BCG-vaccinated individuals who attribute their positive TST result to BCG) or (2) the initial test result is thought to be a false positive (e.g., individuals with low risk for *Mtb* infection) and additional evidence is desired to support the decision not to treat the individual for LTBI in the absence of other treatment indications (e.g., individuals with low risk for disease progression). Dual testing may also be considered for individuals with an uninterpretable IGRA result (on initial and/or repeat testing) and a reason for testing persists.

CLINICAL EVALUATION

Fig. 42.1 summarizes the approach to LTBI screening.

APPROACH TO TUBERCULOSIS SKIN TEST– OR INTERFERON-GAMMA RELEASE ASSAY– POSITIVE INDIVIDUALS

Before initiating treatment for LTBI, clinicians caring for TST- or IGRA-positive individuals should first assess the individual's risk for *Mtb* infection and risk for progression to active disease by obtaining a focused history that includes the following: country of origin and years since immigration, history of diagnosis and treatment for active disease or LTBI, contact with untreated individuals with known or suspected active TB, work and residential environment, and medical history and concomitant medications. If both risk of infection and of progression to active disease are determined to be low, the possibility of a false-positive TST or IGRA result should be considered and the benefits of latent TB treatment weighed against the risk of treatment-related adverse events.

Next, because individuals with *Mtb* infection are also at high risk for active disease, it is imperative to rule out active TB before initiating treatment for LTBI. The goal is to reduce the risk of acquired drug resistance that may develop when individuals with active TB are inadvertently treated for LTBI. Individuals should be screened for active TB by (1) assessing for the presence of symptoms (cough, fever, night sweats, and weight loss), (2) physical examination (abnormal lung examination findings, peripheral lymphadenopathy), and (3) chest radiographic imaging (see Chapter 53). Presence of any symptom, physical examination, and/or radiographic abnormality suggestive of active TB should be viewed as an indication for confirmatory TB testing. Furthermore, for immunosuppressed individuals with positive TST or IGRA results, thresholds for ordering confirmatory TB testing should be lowered because atypical presentation of active disease is more frequent in this population. For individuals with possible active TB, confirmatory TB testing should be performed. Confirmatory TB testing includes collection of at least two sputum specimens for acid-fast bacilli smear microscopy and mycobacterial culture and at least one sputum specimen collected for nucleic acid amplification testing (see Chapter 53). Only after excluding active TB by screening with or without confirmatory TB testing can treatment for LTBI be safely initiated.

APPROACH TO TUBERCULOSIS SKIN TEST– POSITIVE INDIVIDUALS WITH PRIOR BACILLUS CALMETTE-GUÉRIN

Although IGRAs are preferred for screening BCG-vaccinated individuals for LTBI, TST is also acceptable. If TST is performed, current U.S. guidelines state that BCG-vaccinated individuals with positive TST reactions should be regarded as true positives, without modification of the criteria used to define TST positivity.[17] Nonetheless, clinicians should be aware that cross reaction from BCG is a common cause of reduced TST specificity (i.e., false-positive TST reactions). In a meta-analysis of 11 studies of TST performance, pooled specificity of TST was lower among BCG-vaccinated individuals

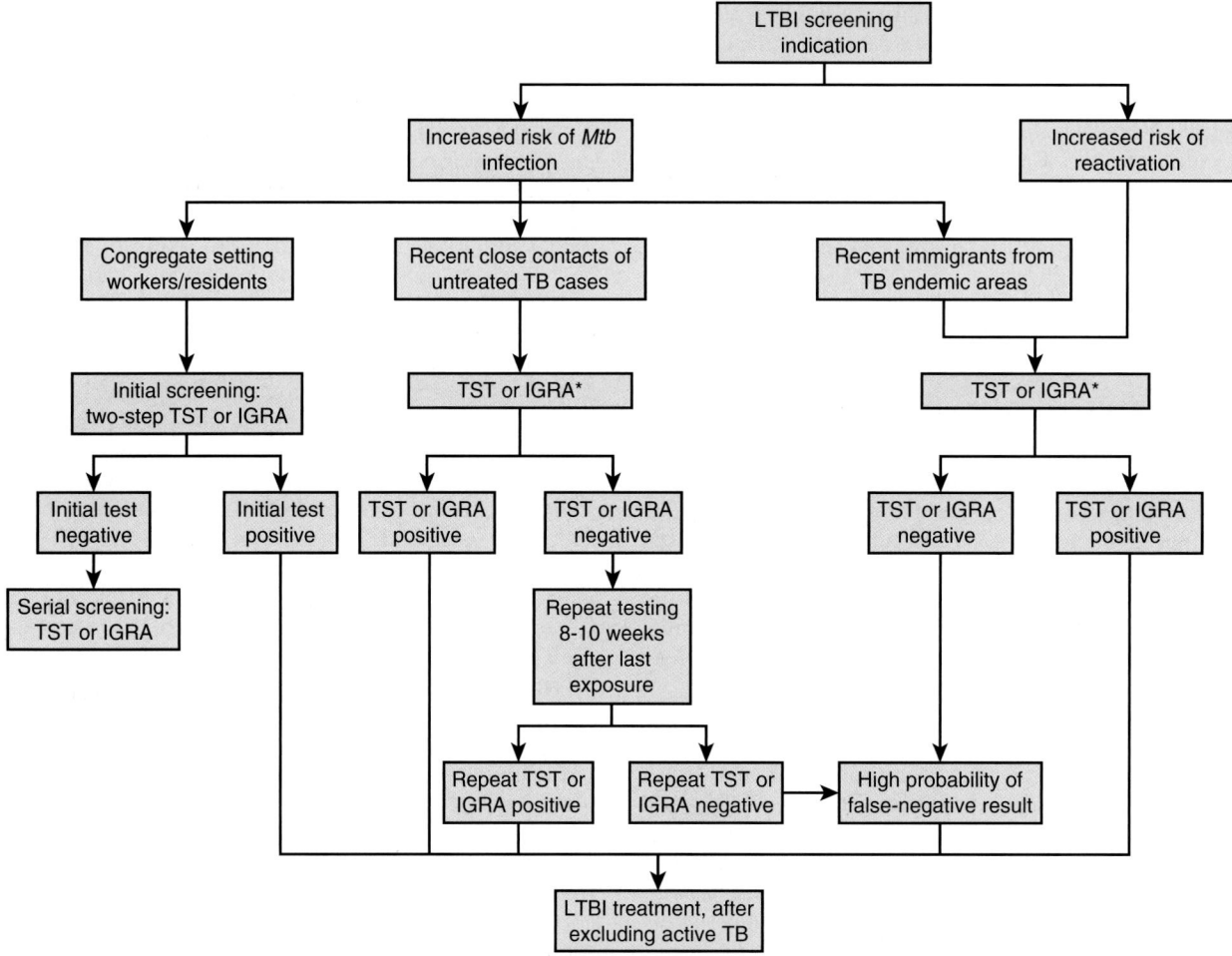

Figure 42.1 Latent tuberculosis infection screening algorithm. Individuals at high likelihood of having LTBI, due to demographic or specific exposure history or an untreated previously positive TST or IGRA, and a high probability of a presently false-negative result, due to immunodeficiency or immunosuppression, should be considered for treatment. *IGRA preferred for individuals with prior bacillus Calmette-Guérin and individuals at high risk for becoming lost to follow-up. TST preferred for children younger than 5 years. Dual testing (not shown) may be considered for certain situations. IGRA, interferon-gamma release assay; LTBI, latent tuberculosis infection; *Mtb, Mycobacterium tuberculosis;* TB, tuberculosis; TST, tuberculin skin test.

compared to unvaccinated individuals (59% vs. 97%).[29] In contrast, IGRA assays measure the T-cell response to antigens specific to *Mtb* and are thus not affected by prior BCG vaccination. A meta-analysis of 16 studies of IGRA performance among BCG-vaccinated and -unvaccinated patients found pooled specificity of QFT-based assays (QFT-Gold and QFT-GIT) and T-SPOT.TB to be similarly high (≥93% for all), regardless of BCG vaccination status.[29]

Among BCG-vaccinated individuals, an individual's age at vaccination and the time between vaccination and TST placement have also been shown to affect reactions to TST. If administered in the first year of life, BCG has been shown to have limited effect on TST specificity because the immune response to BCG given during infancy is less vigorous than the immune response to BCG given after 1 year of age.[30] As such, positive TST reactions among individuals vaccinated in infancy should not be attributed to BCG, whereas positive TST reactions among individuals vaccinated after infancy may be due to BCG or *Mtb* infection. Regardless of age at vaccination, tuberculin reactivity to BCG wanes over time so that positive TST reactions 10 or more years after vaccination should not be attributed to prior BCG.[31]

Although BCG-vaccinated individuals with positive TST reactions may be subsequently evaluated by IGRA, dual testing is not routinely recommended outside of certain situations (see "Situations in Which Dual Testing May Be Considered").

OTHER CAUSES OF FALSE-POSITIVE TUBERCULOSIS SKIN TESTING REACTIONS

Nontuberculous Mycobacterial Infection

Although nontuberculous mycobacterial infections are an uncommon cause of false-positive reactions to TST (responsible for 1–5% of all positive TST results), it is important to consider in areas with very low TB and high nontuberculous mycobacterial infection prevalence, such as in the southern United States. Clinical suspicion for nontuberculous mycobacterial infection as a cause of false-positive TST reactions may be prompted by the absence of *Mtb* infection risk factors (e.g., U.S. born, no known or possible contact with an untreated individual with active TB), presence of certain clinical conditions (e.g., chronic lung disease), and/or certain radiographic findings. However, nontuberculous mycobacterial infection and other potential causes of false-positive TST reactions should not influence treatment decisions for

LTBI for individuals with high risk for *Mtb* infection and/or progression to active TB.

For TST-positive individuals with suspected nontuberculous mycobacterial infection and both low risk for *Mtb* infection and disease progression, subsequent testing with IGRAs (i.e., dual testing) may be considered to support the decision not to initiate treatment for latent infection (see "Situations in Which Dual Testing May Be Considered"). Unlike TST, IGRA specificity is not affected by most nontuberculous mycobacteria, although specificity may be reduced among individuals infected with nontuberculous mycobacteria expressing ESAT-6 and/or CFP-10 (*Mycobacterium kansasii, M. szulgai, M. marinum,* and *M. flavescens*).[32]

Allergic Reaction to Tuberculin

Allergic (immediate hypersensitivity) reactions to tuberculin are also an uncommon cause of false-positive TST, seen in 2–3% of all individuals, more commonly among individuals with atopy.[33] Allergic reactions to tuberculin typically present as localized wheal-and-flare reactions within 6 to 12 hours of injection, but most reactions are immediate (within 20 minutes). Life-threatening systemic hypersensitivity reactions (anaphylaxis, angioedema, urticaria, and dyspnea) to tuberculin have also been reported but are rare; in the United States, 24 cases of life-threatening hypersensitivity reactions were reported over an 11-year period, during which time approximately 300 million tuberculin doses were administered (0.08 reported reactions per million doses of tuberculin).[34] Repeat TST is contraindicated for individuals with a prior allergic reaction to TST. If repeat *Mtb* infection testing is required for individuals with tuberculin allergy, IGRAs should be performed instead.

Tuberculin Skin Test Boosting

Although TST conversion (a positive TST result in a previously TST-negative individual) is considered to indicate new *Mtb* infection, some individuals with remote *Mtb* infection and negative reaction to initial TST (due to waned T-cell–mediated immunity) may have a positive TST reaction on repeat testing that may be misinterpreted as TST conversion. This phenomenon is referred to as "boosting" and is believed to result when tuberculin from the initial test stimulates T-cell memory, causing a positive or boosted reaction to tuberculin on repeat testing.[35] Other populations at risk for boosting include individuals with prior BCG[36,37] and nontuberculous mycobacterial infections[38,39] where cross reactions to tuberculin may be boosted with repeat testing.

The size of the boosted TST reaction is maximal if the interval between the initial and second TST is between 1 and 5 weeks.[6,35,40] However, the boosted reaction may persist 1 or more years after the initial negative TST. For this reason, two-step TST is recommended as the initial test for individuals for whom serial screening is recommended (e.g., health care workers). For such individuals, two-step TST is used to establish baseline LTBI status, thus reducing the risk that a future boosted reaction will be misinterpreted as recent *Mtb* infection. In two-step TST, if the first TST is negative, a second test is performed 1 to 3 weeks later. If the second TST is positive, the positive reaction is attributed to boosting, and the individual is classified as having LTBI after active disease has been ruled out. Of note, repeated administration of tuberculin with TST to *Mtb*-uninfected individuals is not associated with boosting.

CAUSES OF FALSE-POSITIVE INTERFERON-GAMMA RELEASE ASSAYS TESTING RESULTS

Interferon-Gamma Release Assay Boosting

Individuals undergoing a dual testing strategy inclusive of initial TST testing, followed by IGRA testing between 3 days to 3 months of initial TST, may experience IGRA boosting.[41–44] IGRA boosting refers to a phenomenon in which a positive IGRA result is seen in an *Mtb*-uninfected individual due to an increased T-cell response to *Mtb* antigens contained in tuberculin. To minimize the risk of false-positive IGRA results from IGRA boosting, blood for IGRA testing should be collected within 3 days of TST or 3 months after TST.

False Interferon-Gamma Release Assay Conversions

IGRAs have been shown to have poor reproducibility when repeat testing is performed. Poor reproducibility may be due to limitations inherent to IGRA testing (independent of the individual's risk of infection) or to fluctuations in an individual's IFN-γ response. The magnitude of change in quantitative IFN-γ response may be sufficient to cause qualitative changes from negative to positive (conversion) or from positive to negative (reversion). Relative to TST, IGRAs have substantially higher rates of both conversion and reversion.[45] In a study of 9153 U.S. health care workers undergoing serial IGRA screening, 4.4% of health care workers with a negative initial test result experienced conversion at 2 years (using the manufacturer's cut-point of ≤0.35 IU/mL), an 11-fold increase relative to that institution's historic TST conversion rate of 0.4% and expected incidence of LTBI.[46] Of interest, 65% of all converters in this study experienced reversion when IGRA was repeated within 60 days of the second test, suggesting that most IGRA conversions were false conversions.

Biologic causes of IGRA conversions and reversions remain unclear but are thought to represent clearance of *Mtb* infection or transitions within the spectrum of LTBI caused by changes in host immunity, resulting in periodic cycling between mycobacterial persistence, replication, and killing.[47] The clinical significance of conversions and reversions are also poorly understood. Data from longitudinal studies have shown higher TB incidence rates among IGRA converters and reverters, relative to individuals with persistently negative results and similar TB incidence rates among IGRA converters as among reverters.[48,49] However, substantial uncertainty remains regarding the use of IGRAs for serial screening and the use of current cut-points to define IGRA positivity, which are associated with higher conversion and reversion rates than TST.[49] More nuanced approaches to serial IGRA test interpretation have been proposed, including increasing the diagnostic threshold of the initial test (which reduces conversions but may also increase reversions), using more stringent criteria for defining IGRA conversion (e.g., change in IFN-γ values from <0.2 to >0.7 IU/mL), and using quantitative IGRA results to measure the absolute or percentage increase in IFN-γ values (or spot counts) over the initial test. Although such alternative approaches may reduce IGRA discordance and thus reduce the proportion of individuals referred for unnecessary preventive therapy, the optimal approach to serial IGRA interpretation has yet to be identified. Current U.S. guidelines define IGRA conversion as a qualitative change from negative to positive (using the manufacturer's cut-point) within 2 years, without any consideration of the magnitude of change in quantitative IFN-γ response.[24]

Technical Causes of False-Positive Interferon-Gamma Release Assay Results

Technical issues related to IGRA testing are more frequent causes of false-positive, false-negative, and uninterpretable results than are clinical causes. Potential technical causes of reduced IGRA specificity from false-positive or uninterpretable results include improper specimen collection (e.g., underfilling of tubes, filling positive control tubes before antigen tubes), improper specimen handling (e.g., overshaking of tubes), improper specimen processing (e.g., prolonged incubation time), test run errors, and manufacturing defects.[50] Technical causes of reduced IGRA specificity (and reduced IGRA sensitivity) are minimized by ensuring persons collecting and processing specimens are adequately trained and procedures for IGRA testing are standardized.

APPROACH TO INDIVIDUALS WITH POSSIBLE FALSE-NEGATIVE TUBERCULOSIS SKIN TEST OR INTERFERON-GAMMA RELEASE ASSAYS RESULTS

For individuals with a negative TST reaction or IGRA result, the possibility of a false-negative test should be considered by assessing for the presence of clinical conditions associated with diminished delayed-type hypersensitivity reactions to tuberculin and IGRA, including immunosuppression, very recent *Mtb* infection, recent live virus vaccination, natural waning of immunity, and overwhelming active TB.

False-negative results among immunosuppressed individuals (i.e., patients with HIV infection, patients receiving the equivalent of ≥15 mg/day of prednisone or tumor necrosis factor-α antagonists) are caused by decreased immunocompetence (TST and IGRA) or skin test anergy (TST). Relative to immunocompetent individuals, immunosuppressed individuals demonstrate a 20–30% lower sensitivity of both TST and IGRA.[51] Although current guidelines recommend the use of lower TST cut-points for immunosuppressed individuals to improve TST sensitivity, this strategy is less effective in severely immunosuppressed populations, in which anergy is prevalent. Because studies of HIV-infected individuals have demonstrated that the frequency of skin test anergy increases as risk for active TB increases (i.e., decreasing CD4 cell count),[52,53] severely immunosuppressed individuals should be considered for latent TB treatment despite negative TST reactions, after active TB has been effectively ruled out.

Although prior meta-analyses have found TST and IGRAs to have comparable sensitivity among immunosuppressed individuals,[51] sensitivity estimates of IGRA may be overestimated due to the higher proportion of uninterpretable results in this population. Furthermore, the frequency of uninterpretable IGRA results increases with increasing immunosuppression. A meta-analysis of IGRA performance among HIV-positive individuals found that the pooled proportion of uninterpretable IGRA results to be four times

higher among individuals with CD4 counts less than 200 cells/μL (12% vs. 3%).[54] These results suggest that *Mtb*-infected immunosuppressed individuals most in need of and most likely to benefit from treatment are also those individuals most likely to have an uninterpretable IGRA result.

Recent close contacts to untreated individuals with known or suspected TB have high risk of *Mtb* infection and of disease progression. As such, recent close contacts should be considered for empirical treatment for LTBI (after active disease has been excluded), despite negative TST or IGRA results. Individuals initiating empirical latent TB treatment should have TST or IGRA repeated 8 to 10 weeks after last exposure because delayed hypersensitivity reaction to *Mtb* antigens may take up to 10 weeks to develop.[12,35,55] If the second test is positive (i.e., conversion), latent TB treatment should be continued. If the second test is negative, treatment may be continued or discontinued, depending on the individual's risk for progression to active disease. Repeat testing to guide treatment continuation decisions is not warranted for individuals with negative TST or IGRA results caused by immunosuppression.

Technical Causes of False-Negative Tuberculosis Skin Test or Interferon-Gamma Release Assays

Technical problems associated with TST and IGRA testing may reduce test sensitivity. Technical causes of false-negative TST reactions include improper tuberculin storage and injection and improper TST interpretation, which are infrequent when TST is performed by experienced operators and settings. However, because IGRA testing is inherently more complex than tuberculin skin testing, the potential for reduced IGRA sensitivity (false-negative or uninterpretable results) from technical issues is higher than for TST. Reported technical causes of false-negative or uninterpretable IGRA results among individuals with true *Mtb* infection include improper specimen collection (e.g., overfilling of tubes; tubes filled out of standard order: negative control, antigen tube, positive control), improper specimen handling (e.g., insufficient shaking or differential shaking of tubes, delayed incubation), improper specimen processing (e.g., insufficient incubation time, inappropriate incubation temperature), test run errors, and manufacturing defects.[50] Technical causes of reduced IGRA sensitivity are minimized by ensuring persons collecting and processing specimens are adequately trained and procedures for IGRA testing are standardized. For individuals with uninterpretable IGRA results, repeat IGRA testing should be performed. Individuals with a positive or negative IGRA result on repeat testing should be managed in accordance with the repeat test result. Individuals with an uninterpretable IGRA result on repeat testing should undergo TST, and TST results should be used to inform subsequent management, including treatment decisions.

TREATMENT FOR LATENT TUBERCULOSIS INFECTION

Treatment for LTBI should be initiated for *Mtb*-infected individuals (based on TST/IGRA results or clinical suspicion) after active TB has been excluded by clinical history, physical examination, chest radiography, and confirmatory TB testing of respiratory specimens if indicated. Treatment regimens currently supported by the CDC include isoniazid

Table 42.4 Approved Treatment Regimens For Latent Tuberculosis Infection

Treatment Regimens	Duration	Frequency	Dose
INH-BASED REGIMENS			
INH	9 months*	Daily	Adult: 5 mg/kg Children: 10–20 mg/kg Maximum dose: 300 mg
		Twice weekly[†]	Adult: 15 mg/kg Children: 20–40 mg/kg Maximum dose: 900 mg
	6 months[‡]	Daily	Adult: 5 mg/kg Children: Not recommended Maximum dose: 300 mg
		Twice weekly[†]	Adult: 15 mg/kg Children: not recommended Maximum dose: 900 mg
RIFAMYCIN-BASED REGIMENS			
Rifampin	4 months	Daily	Adult: 10 mg/kg Children: 15–20 mg/kg Maximum dose: 600 mg
INH and RPT	3 months[§]	Weekly	Age >12 years: INH: 15 mg/kg rounding up to nearest 50 or 100 mg Maximum INH dose: 900 mg RPT: 300–900 mg, depending on weight Age 2–11 years: INH: 25 mg/kg Maximum INH dose: 900 mg RPT: 300–900 mg, depending on weight Age <2 years: not recommended
	1 month[¶]	Daily	HIV-infected individuals age ≥13 years: INH: 300 mg RPT: 300–600 mg, depending on weight

Shorter course regimens are preferred to facilitate treatment adherence and completion.

*Nine months of daily INH (daily or twice weekly) is the preferred regimen for pregnant women with high risk for progression to active disease (e.g., recent close contact).

[†]Twice weekly INH regimens must be administered via DOT.

[‡]Six months of daily INH is not recommended for immunosuppressed individuals (e.g., people living with HIV) or people with fibrotic lesions on chest imaging suggestive of untreated prior tuberculosis and children.

[§]Three months of daily INH and RPT can be administered via DOT or self-administered therapy.

[¶]1HP not yet approved by U.S. Centers for Disease Control and Prevention; data limited to HIV-infected individuals.

DOT, directly observed therapy; HIV, human immunodeficiency virus; INH, isoniazid; RPT, rifapentine.

monotherapy and rifamycin-based regimens (Table 42.4). All regimens have been shown to be effective, and no single treatment regimen has been shown to be superior to any other regimen. Therefore, regimen selection is based largely on the risk of adverse events by considering coexisting medical conditions and concomitant medications and the likelihood of treatment adherence and completion. To facilitate treatment adherence and completion, clinicians should consider shorter course regimens whenever possible.[56] Recently, the World Health Organization approved an ultrashort course treatment regimen for LTBI (*1 month of daily isoniazid and rifapentine* [1HP]) for both individuals with and without HIV,[57] although evidence to date has been limited to HIV-infected individuals. In a randomized trial among people living with HIV, 1HP was shown to have similar effectiveness and similar adverse event incidence as 9 months of daily isoniazid. However, the proportion of individuals completing treatment was significantly higher among those receiving 1HP (97% vs. 90%).[58] Based on these results, 1HP is anticipated to receive future CDC endorsement for HIV-infected individuals.

Although treatment regimens for LTBI are associated with hepatotoxicity, baseline liver function testing is not routinely indicated for all individuals before treatment initiation. Baseline liver function testing (serum aspartate aminotransferase, alanine aminotransferase, total bilirubin) is indicated for the following individuals belonging to groups with higher risk for adverse events: liver disease from any cause, risk factors for chronic liver disease, regular alcohol use, HIV infection, and pregnancy or less than 3 months postpartum.[56] Treatment for LTBI is contraindicated for asymptomatic individuals with aminotransferases greater than five times the upper limit of normal and symptomatic individuals with aminotransferases greater than three times the upper limit of normal. Those eligible for treatment who have abnormal baseline liver function tests should undergo repeat testing during LTBI treatment even if symptoms suggestive of acute hepatitis are absent. Similarly, individuals reporting symptoms suggestive of acute hepatitis during the course of treatment should have liver function testing performed, irrespective of their baseline risk for hepatotoxicity. Indications for withholding treatment include aminotransferases five or more times the upper limit of normal regardless of symptoms or three or more times the upper limit of normal with associated symptoms.

Key Points

- Targeted screening for *latent tuberculosis infection* (LTBI) is indicated for individuals with increased risk of infection and/or reactivation; individuals who test positive by *tuberculin skin testing* (TST) or *interferon-gamma release assays* (IGRAs) should be considered for treatment for LTBI after excluding active tuberculosis disease.
- Current U.S. guidelines support the use of IGRAs in all situations in which TST is recommended. However, TST or IGRAs may be preferred in certain situations, based on test performance and/or operational characteristics: TST is preferred for children younger than 5 years, IGRAs are preferred for individuals with prior *bacillus Calmette-Guérin* (BCG) vaccination and for individuals belonging to groups with low rates of returning to have TSTs read. Dual testing may be considered in certain situations.
- TST and IGRAs have comparable specificity for detecting *Mycobacterium tuberculosis* infection among non–BCG-vaccinated individuals. However, compared to TST, IGRAs have higher specificity among individuals with prior BCG and in settings with high prevalence of nontuberculosis mycobacterial infection.
- TST and IGRAs have comparable sensitivity for detecting *Mtb* infection, and sensitivity of both tests are reduced among individuals with compromised immune systems. Empirical treatment for LTBI should be considered for immunosuppressed individuals with negative TST or IGRA results.
- Before initiating treatment for LTBI, all individuals must be assessed for active disease because neither TST nor IGRAs are able to distinguish LTBI from active tuberculosis.

Key Readings

Andrews JR, Hatherill M, Mahomed H, et al. The dynamics of QuantiFERON-TB gold in-tube conversion and reversion in a cohort of South African adolescents. *Am J Res Crit Care Med.* 2015;191(5):584–591.

Dobler CC, Farah WH, Alsawas M, et al. Tuberculin skin test conversions and occupational exposure risk in US healthcare workers. *Clin Infect Dis.* 2018;66(5):706–711.

Farhat M, Greenaway C, Pai M, Menzies D. False-positive tuberculin skin tests: what is the absolute effect of BCG and non-tuberculous mycobacteria? *Intl J Tuberc Lung Dis.* 2006;10(11):1192–1204.

Mazurek GH, Jereb J, Vernon A, LoBue P, Goldberg S, Castro K. Updated guidelines for using interferon gamma release assays to detect *Mycobacterium tuberculosis* infection—United States, 2010. *MMWR Recomm Rep.* 2010;59(RR-5):1–24.

Menzies D. Interpretation of repeated tuberculin tests. Boosting, conversion, and reversion. *Am J Res Crit Care Med.* 1999;159(1):15–21.

Pai Madhukar, Denkinger Claudia M, Kik Sandra V, et al. Gamma interferon release assays for detection of *Mycobacterium tuberculosis* infection. *Clin Microbiol Rev.* 2014;27(1):3–20.

Pai M, Zwerling A, Menzies D. Systematic review: T-cell–based assays for the diagnosis of latent tuberculosis infection: an update. *Ann Intern Med.* 2008;149(3):177–184.

Slater ML, Welland G, Pai M, Parsonnet J, Banaei N. Challenges with QuantiFERON-TB gold assay for large-scale, routine screening of U.S. healthcare workers. *Am J Res Crit Care Med.* 2013;188(8):1005–1010.

Talwar A, Tsang CA, Price SF, et al. Tuberculosis—United States, 2018. *MMWR Morb Mortal Wkly Rep.* 2019;68(11):257–262.

Zuber PLF, McKenna MT, Binkin NJ, Onorato IM, Castro KG. Long-term risk of tuberculosis among foreign-born persons in the United States. *JAMA.* 1997;278(4):304–307.

Complete reference list available at ExpertConsult.com.

43 ASPIRATION

RUPAL J. SHAH, MD, MSCE • VYVY N. YOUNG, MD

INTRODUCTION

Aspiration is defined as the inhalation of fluid or solid material beyond the vocal cords and into the lower airways.[1] Aspiration is not always pathologic, and studies have shown that aspiration happens regularly in healthy adults. In one study nearly half of healthy adult male subjects had evidence of microaspiration during sleep.[2] However, aspiration is also associated with a wide range of pathology, ranging from bronchospasm to pneumonia. Aspiration leading to disease states is now thought to be a result of complex interactions between the host and the aspirated material.[3]

Aspiration happens as a result of impaired swallowing, leading to passage of oral or gastric contents into the respiratory tract. It is important to note that *gastroesophageal reflux disease* (GERD) can also contribute to aspiration syndromes. GERD has been associated with many pulmonary diseases, including asthma, chronic obstructive pulmonary disease, *interstitial lung disease* (ILD), and allograft health after lung transplant. The relationship between GERD and lung disease is thought to be related to aspiration or microaspiration of gastric contents as a result of reflux.

As our understanding of the pulmonary microbiome deepens, new hypotheses regarding how aspiration becomes pathologic have evolved. Historically, the lung was considered a sterile environment; however, it is now known there is a diverse range of microbiota throughout the respiratory tract (see also Chapter 17). The current understanding is that the lung microbiome is maintained by a complex relationship between migration of bacteria from the oropharynx and the upper respiratory tract, partly from microaspiration, and elimination of bacteria from host mucosal defense and mucociliary clearance.[4] Studies of healthy controls have found similar microbiota in the upper and lower airways; however, in subjects with respiratory diseases, there is a significant difference between the upper and lower airway microbiota.[5–7] This difference in microbiome may predispose certain subjects to pathology as a result of aspiration. Other possible contributing factors include ineffective host defense and large-volume aspiration that overwhelms clearance mechanisms. Noninfectious

injury from aspiration is related to aspiration of acid, pepsin, and bile acids, which cause inflammation, but there is also evidence to support the role of small nonacidified gastric particles in causing airway inflammation. Both acidic and nonacidic substances have been shown to trigger the inflammatory cascade with recruitment of neutrophils in the airways, leading to injury.[8]

Although the mechanisms of pathologic aspiration are still being elucidated, this chapter will cover the presentation, diagnosis, evaluation, and treatment of aspiration in adults, with a focus on manifestations in the pulmonary parenchyma.

EPIDEMIOLOGY AND PATHOGENESIS

The prevalence of aspiration is difficult to estimate because it can often be asymptomatic and requires a high degree of suspicion with appropriate testing for accurate detection. Prior studies have estimated that 5% to 15% of community-acquired pneumonias are related to aspiration.[9] A large Japanese study, in which they evaluated for aspiration in all patients hospitalized for community- or hospital-acquired pneumonia, found that 306 of 382 (80%) of patients 70 years of age and older had aspiration. The overall incidence of aspiration was 60% in community-acquired and 86.7% in hospital-acquired pneumonia.[10] In studies in which aspiration was studied outside of the presence of pneumonia, 70% of patients with depressed consciousness were found to aspirate, compared to 45% of healthy adults.[11] In addition, there have been associations between reflux and microaspiration with progression in ILD[12–14] and chronic rejection after lung transplant,[15,16] indicating that aspiration is relevant in many conditions outside of acute events.

Although aspiration is quite common, there is evidence that aspiration is underappreciated as an important clinical syndrome. For example, in a series of 59 patients who had evidence of aspiration on lung biopsy specimens, only 9% were suspected to have aspiration before biopsy.[17] As discussed later in this chapter, keeping aspiration at the forefront of the clinician's mind is essential in ensuring this potential contributing factor to the patient's presentation is not missed.

RISK FACTORS

Interruption of the normal function of many organ systems can increase the risk of aspiration (Fig. 43.1). Disease states that cause alteration of consciousness (such as stroke, dementia, or seizure), disorders of the spine, laryngeal abnormalities (including recent intubation or vocal fold paralysis), prior surgery or radiation, any esophageal disorder that causes difficulty with passage of food or saliva, and gastric motility disorders may lead to increased risk of aspiration.

PRESENTING CONDITIONS

The clinical presentation of aspiration is variable, and the clinician may encounter acute, subacute, and chronic forms of aspiration. It is also important to bear in mind that, although aspiration is often associated with cough, cough is not necessarily always present (so-called "silent aspiration"). In fact, patients may be completely asymptomatic. The presentation can include chronic cough, bronchospasm or worsening of asthma symptoms, foreign body aspiration, aspiration pneumonia, pneumonitis, lung abscess, bronchiectasis, bronchiolitis, lipoid pneumonia, ILD, and nontuberculous mycobacterial infection.[18,19]

VOCAL CORD DYSFUNCTION/PARADOXICAL VOCAL FOLD MOTION DISORDER

In *vocal cord dysfunction* (VCD), also known as *paradoxical vocal fold motion disorder* (PVFMD), the vocal folds intermittently adduct (close) with inhalation rather than the expected opening (abduction), which results in dyspnea and in severe cases, even stridor.[20–23] Many factors have been associated with VCD/PVFMD, including environmental irritants, stress, GERD, and *laryngopharyngeal reflux* (LPR), which refers to reflux of gastric contents up to the larynx/pharynx.[21–25] One hypothesis for the link between LPR/GERD and VCD/PVFMD is that repeated injury to the larynx results in an accentuation of the glottic closure reflex.[26] Although VCD/PVFMD often causes shortness of breath, its association with dysphagia (e.g., swallowing dysfunction) and aspiration risk remains unknown (see also Chapter 70).

FOREIGN BODY ASPIRATION

Foreign bodies are most commonly aspirated by children. It is unusual in adults, but its presentation can include wheezing, dyspnea, and chronic cough with or without hemoptysis. Radiographs may reveal radiopaque material with atelectasis, postobstructive or nonresolving pneumonia, or focal bronchiectasis. However, radiographs may also be unrevealing; therefore a high index of suspicion is important to ensure this diagnosis is not missed. Bronchoscopic extraction of a foreign body may be performed, with one large review demonstrating a 90% success rate for foreign body extraction via flexible bronchoscopy.[27] In rare cases, rigid bronchoscopy or surgical removal of a foreign body is necessary.

AIRWAYS DISEASE

Aspiration can cause myriad airway diseases, including cough, bronchospasm, and an asthma-like syndrome. It can also exacerbate asthma. In addition, aspiration can also

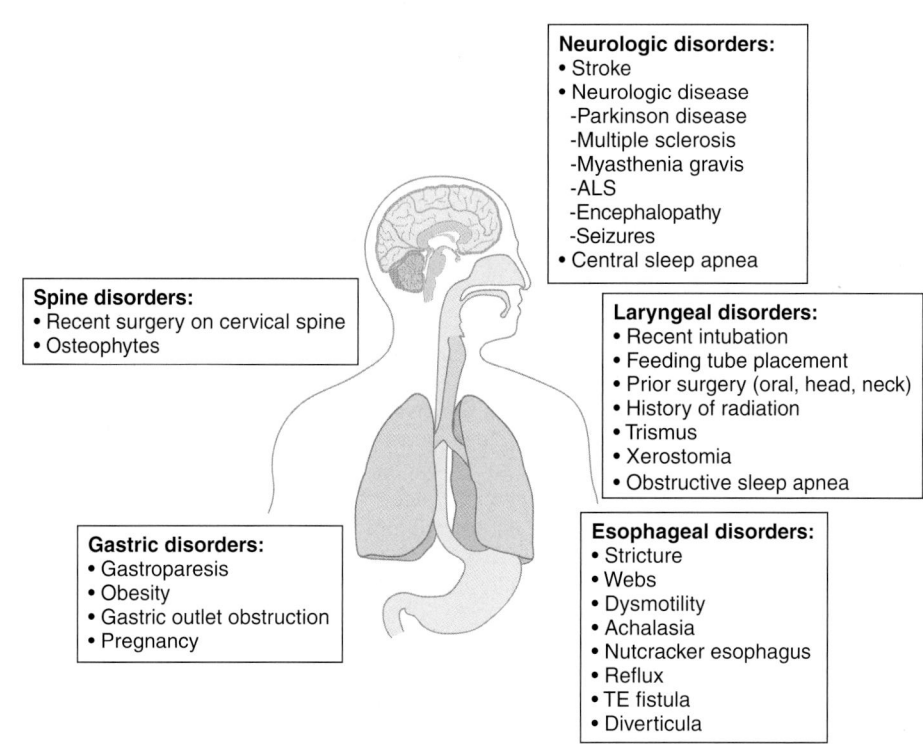

Figure 43.1 Risk factors for aspiration. ALS, amyotrophic lateral sclerosis; TE, tracheoesophageal.

Neurologic disorders:
• Stroke
• Neurologic disease
 -Parkinson disease
 -Multiple sclerosis
 -Myasthenia gravis
 -ALS
 -Encephalopathy
 -Seizures
• Central sleep apnea

Spine disorders:
• Recent surgery on cervical spine
• Osteophytes

Laryngeal disorders:
• Recent intubation
• Feeding tube placement
• Prior surgery (oral, head, neck)
• History of radiation
• Trismus
• Xerostomia
• Obstructive sleep apnea

Gastric disorders:
• Gastroparesis
• Obesity
• Gastric outlet obstruction
• Pregnancy

Esophageal disorders:
• Stricture
• Webs
• Dysmotility
• Achalasia
• Nutcracker esophagus
• Reflux
• TE fistula
• Diverticula

affect the lower airways, with manifestations ranging from bronchiolitis to bronchiectasis.

ASTHMA

There are conflicting reports on the role of aspiration, primarily related to uncontrolled GERD, in asthma exacerbations. There are several studies that report an association between GERD and decreased asthma control.[28,29] However, there are also data showing the relationship between GERD and asthma control may be overstated. In one study of 78 patients who underwent bronchoalveolar lavage, 59% had pepsin detected on bronchoalveolar lavage, but the presence of pepsin was not associated with disease severity, exacerbations, or lung function.[30] The most recent asthma management guidelines recommend evaluation for GERD in poorly controlled asthma, especially when there are nighttime symptoms, even in patients who do not present with typical symptoms of GERD.[31] The benefit of treating or evaluating for GERD in patients with mild-moderate asthma is not clear.

BRONCHIOLITIS AND BRONCHIECTASIS

Aspiration can manifest as bronchiolitis or inflammation in the small airways (bronchioles) of the lungs and bronchiectasis, which causes irreversible thickening and dilation of the airways. The term "diffuse aspiration bronchiolitis" was first coined by Matsuse and colleagues[32] based on autopsy results of patients at high risk for aspiration due to neurologic disorders. A larger series from the Mayo Clinic described 20 patients with diffuse aspiration bronchiolitis, where the majority were diagnosed by lung biopsy (either surgical or transbronchial).[33] The striking finding between these two series is that most of these patients were middle aged (between ages 40 and 50 years), which may be why biopsy was required, because aspiration, which is often thought of as a disease of the elderly, was not considered in this younger population. Typical high-resolution *computed tomography* (CT) findings of aspiration-induced bronchiolitis include micronodules with tree-in-bud changes, consistent with small airway inflammation (Fig. 43.2A). Pathology demonstrates bronchiolar inflammation and thickening with foreign matter. Pathology may also demonstrate foreign matter that displays birefringence under polarized light, although the absence of this finding does not exclude aspiration. Diagnosis can be made by documenting aspiration with typical CT features or by lung biopsy.

Aspiration-induced bronchiectasis is common in children and has been reported to account for about 10% of non–cystic fibrosis bronchiectasis in children.[34] In two large series identifying the etiology of bronchiectasis in adult patients, only 1% to 4% were thought to be related to aspiration, making this is a less common cause of bronchiectasis in adults.[35,36] Typical CT findings of aspiration-related bronchiectasis include lower lobe predominant bronchiectasis, dilated esophagus, or hiatal hernia.

PNEUMONITIS: ASPIRATION VERSUS CHEMICAL

There are two major manifestations of aspiration in the lung parenchyma: aspiration pneumonia, which is related to infection by specific microbes, and chemical pneumonitis, which is an inflammatory reaction in response to aspiration.[9] Aspiration pneumonia is indistinguishable in clinical presentation from non–aspiration pneumonia, which makes it challenging to diagnose. Risk factors for aspiration pneumonia include older age, lower body mass index, increased comorbidities, and decreased functional status. Aspiration pneumonia has a higher mortality, longer hospital length of stay, and higher risk of recurrence than community-acquired pneumonia, which makes it important to identify as an etiology for pneumonia.[37–39] CT findings that may raise suspicion for aspiration include posterior opacities and a pattern of focal, peripheral, or peribronchiolar consolidation involving one or more segments (compared to lobar pneumonia)[40] (see Fig. 43.2B). Aspiration can also result in lung abscess (see Fig. 43.2C) and empyema, as well as interlobular septal thickening and ground-glass opacities (see Fig. 43.2D). There is no evidence to suggest that patients with aspiration pneumonia should be treated with longer duration of antibiotics except in the case of lung abscess.[41] Pleural collections should be drained immediately and sent for routine studies, including culture. The pathology of aspiration pneumonia is illustrated in Fig. 43.3, with pulmonary alveolar septal thickening from type 2 pneumocyte hyperplasia, with increased numbers of macrophages and organizing pneumonia within airspaces. Vegetable matter may also be seen.

Oral hygiene may reduce the risk of aspiration pneumonia.[42,43] In one randomized controlled trial of nursing home residents, subjects with routine oral care and weekly care from dentists had a reduced risk of pneumonia compared to those without oral care. This was true regardless of presence of teeth, indicating oral care is important in edentulous patients as well.[44] However, a multicenter, cluster, randomized controlled trial of oral hygiene care (tooth brushing, chlorhexidine oral rinse twice a day, and upright positioning during meals) did not reduce the incidence of pneumonia in nursing home residents, a high-risk population for aspiration.[45] This is in line with data showing routine oral care in patients receiving mechanical ventilation may not prevent nosocomial pneumonia in certain patient populations.[46] Thus, oral care can be considered as one possible method to reduce risk of pneumonia but must be used in conjunction with other techniques, as discussed later in this chapter.

The classic teaching that aspiration is often associated with anaerobic infections is based on studies from the early 1900s linking bacteria found in lung abscess with gingival flora, and finding that those pathogens were anaerobic bacteria.[47] More recent data have been limited, given the challenges of culturing anaerobic bacteria in the laboratory. In one study using protected specimen brush sampling and minibronchoalveolar lavage in patients with aspiration pneumonia on a ventilator, only one anaerobic organism was isolated, with the rest being enteric gram-negative organisms, *Streptococcus pneumoniae*, and *Haemophilus influenzae*,[48] which calls into question the classic teaching of using anaerobic coverage for patients with suspected aspiration pneumonia. However, given the challenges of isolating anaerobes and the potential for significant pulmonary pathology with anaerobic infection, it is still recommended that anaerobic bacteria be covered empirically in the initial therapy for aspiration pneumonia.[49]

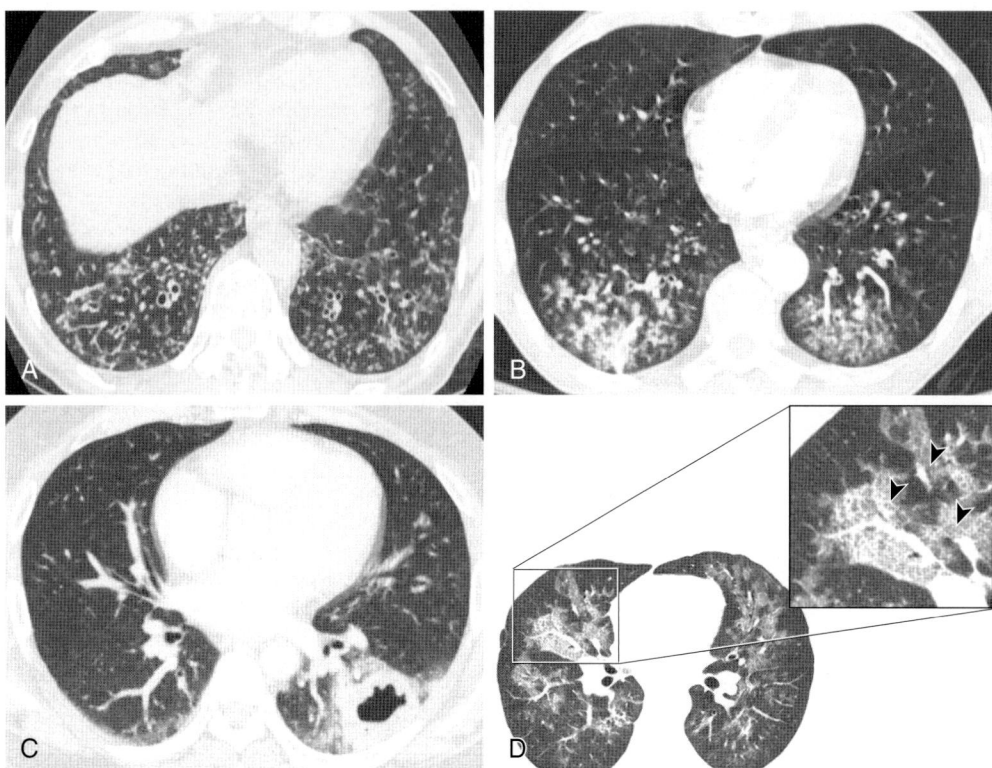

Figure 43.2 Computed tomography findings of aspiration. (A) Basilar predominant, patchy tree-in-bud opacities with mild bronchiectasis typical of recurrent aspiration. (B) Basilar predominant consolidation with tree-in-bud opacities consistent with aspiration-related bronchiolitis. (C) Cavitary lesion. (D) "Crazy paving" appearance in a patient with oil aspiration and lipoid pneumonia. Axial high-resolution computed tomographic image shows patchy, multifocal, geographically distributed ground-glass opacity associated with intralobular interstitial thickening and interlobular septal thickening, causing the reticular appearance in the regions of ground-glass opacity. The smooth interlobular septal thickening *(arrowheads)* is better appreciated in the magnified detail image. (Courtesy Michael B. Gotway, MD.)

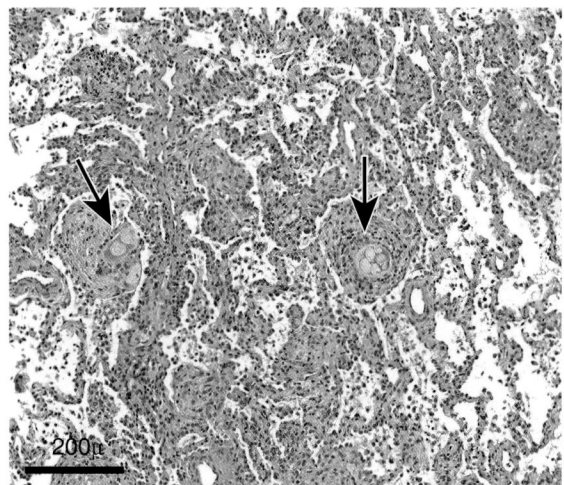

Figure 43.3 Histopathologic findings of aspiration pneumonia. The pulmonary alveolar septa are mildly thickened by type 2 pneumocyte hyperplasia, and there are increased numbers of macrophages and organizing pneumonia within airspaces. Two fragments of vegetable material are noted within the airspace organization *(arrows)*.

Chemical pneumonitis is related to macroaspiration of large-volume acidic fluid, also termed "massive aspiration." This entity is not typically seen after aspiration of tube feeds or blood, which has a higher pH than gastric acid. This is a noninfectious phenomenon whereby the acid recruits inflammatory cells to the lung.[50] This most commonly happens during anesthesia but has also been reported in drug overdose and in nursing home populations.[51] The incidence is low (<1%).[9] Emergency surgery increases the risk more than elective procedures. The clinical presentation can include shortness of breath, hypoxemia, tachycardia, and diffuse crackles or wheezes. Imaging is abnormal and can progress into an acute lung injury pattern. Lower respiratory tract cultures are typically sterile, and this has been used to differentiate pneumonitis from pneumonia.[41] The data do not support the routine use of antibiotics to prevent development of aspiration pneumonia,[41,52] although this may be considered in severely ill patients. Otherwise, management of chemical pneumonitis includes supportive care, including treatment of bronchospasm and edema, and reduction of the amount of acid exposure by aggressive suctioning or bronchoscopy. There is insufficient evidence to support the use of corticosteroids in this condition.

EXOGENOUS LIPOID PNEUMONIA

Aspiration of lipid-laden substances can result in accumulation of lipids in the lung parenchyma, which is known as lipoid pneumonia. Common inhalants include oil-based medications (such as laxatives or nasal instillation of oily substances to treat congestion), radiographic contrast material, or oil in foods.[53] Gagging during administration of oil-based medications, gastroesophageal reflux, or neurologic or psychiatric illness are predisposing factors for development of lipoid pneumonia.[54] Radiographic presentations can vary, and consolidation, ground-glass opacities, crazy paving (a pattern on CT defined by the combination of ground-glass attenuation, interlobular septal thickening, and intralobular lines, demonstrated in Fig. 43.2D), septal thickening, and mass-like lesions can all be presenting signs. Consolidations are often multilobar and bilateral. The hallmark of lipoid pneumonia is the presence of consolidations with areas of fat attenuation (typical range of −17 to −114 Hounsfield units).[55] Treatment of lipoid pneumonia is avoidance of the inhalant. Lipoid pneumonia can be asymptomatic but, in severe cases, can cause fibrosis. In addition, there can be secondary infections, such as with nontuberculous mycobacteria (described in detail later).

INTERSTITIAL LUNG DISEASE

Various forms of pulmonary fibrosis have been associated with aspiration. Organizing pneumonia, which is a pathologic pattern where plugs of granulation tissue are seen in the air spaces, has been associated with aspiration.[56–58] A careful history focused on dysphagia, swallowing, and reflux should be undertaken in any patient who presents with organizing pneumonia.

Microaspiration and GERD have been associated with *idiopathic pulmonary fibrosis* (IPF), a chronic, progressive fibrotic lung disease. In a study using ambulatory esophageal pH monitoring, 94% of patients with IPF had abnormal acid exposure compared to 50% of control subjects. Of note, only 4 of the 17 patients with IPF and abnormal acid exposure had symptoms.[59] Another large study of patients with IPF found that the use of GER medications was an independent predictor of longer survival time.[12] These data support the link between microaspiration and GER in pulmonary fibrosis, although the exact role is still being elucidated.

A study of laparoscopic fundoplication, an antireflux surgery, in patients with IPF and evidence of acidic GERD on pH monitoring showed that this procedure is safe and well tolerated. There was a nonstatistically significant reduction in exacerbation and death in the fundoplication arm.[60] More data are necessary to understand the utility of surgery in this population.

Esophageal dysmotility and reflux are common manifestations of connective tissue disorders. One study of patients with scleroderma with and without ILD found that reflux was more common in patients with ILD.[61] Whether the ILD makes the reflux worse or vice versa is still being evaluated. Fundoplication and other antireflux procedures are of unclear benefit, given the other gastrointestinal motility issues in this population.

NONTUBERCULOUS MYCOBACTERIAL INFECTION

There have been several case reports in the literature documenting a relationship between lipoid pneumonia and rapid growing mycobacterial infections (*Mycobacterium abscessus* and *M. fortuitum*).[19,62] In addition, patients with achalasia, an uncommon esophageal motility disorder characterized by the absence of esophageal peristalsis and impaired relaxation of the lower esophageal sphincter, are at higher risk for developing *nontuberculous mycobacterial* (NTM) infections.[18,63,64] Aspiration of lipid-laden contents

may create an environment for mycobacteria to grow. Patients are often misdiagnosed and have frequent courses of antibiotics, so it is important to consider NTM as an etiology in patients who do not respond to usual treatment with antibacterial therapy.

Aspiration has been implicated in a variety of pulmonary pathology. The exact mechanism between aspiration and disease is unclear but is likely a combination of both acid and non–acid-mediated injury accompanied by changes in the lung microbiome. Aspiration can be silent and is not limited to the elderly, so a high index of suspicion is required to ensure it is not missed. The following section will describe the evaluation and management of dysphagia and aspiration.

CLINICAL PRESENTATION

Swallowing difficulties (dysphagia) are an important risk factor for aspiration and should be evaluated and addressed, although it is important to note that rarely is dysphagia the *only* risk factor present.[65] Taking a comprehensive swallowing history is of critical importance in the identification of potential swallowing dysfunction and risk of aspiration. A simple open-ended question such as "How is your swallowing?" or "What are you eating these days?" can provide an opening for further discussion of this topic. A sample list of questions to be included in a comprehensive swallowing history is included in Table 43.1.[66] A screening questionnaire, such as the Eating Assessment Tool-10 (EAT-10), may help identify patients at risk for swallowing difficulties and aspiration.[67]

Clarification of the nature and type of swallowing difficulty is vital. Different consistencies (e.g., solids, liquids, or pills) may cause variable levels of difficulty; patients may have challenges with one type of oral intake but not others. Some patients may consciously or unconsciously use compensatory mechanisms (e.g., cutting pills in two or

Table 43.1 Pertinent Questions in Comprehensive Swallowing History

How is your swallowing?
What are you eating these days?
   ■ For instance, regular diet, soft foods only, liquids only
Are you avoiding any particular types of foods?
   ■ For instance, bread, meat, crackers, nuts
Have you had to change how you eat/drink?
   ■ For instance, adding more sauces/gravy, cutting food into smaller pieces, taking pills one (instead of a handful) at a time, taking pills with applesauce instead of water, sipping liquids instead of gulping/chugging
How long does it take you to eat a meal?
Are you coughing or choking with liquids?
Does it take effort to swallow?
Does it hurt to swallow?
Do you feel as if food/liquids/pills get "stuck"? If so, can you point to where you feel this?
Has your weight changed lately? How do your clothes fit?
Have you had pneumonia recently?
Have you ever needed the Heimlich maneuver?
Do you regurgitate? If so, is the material digested or undigested?
Do you experience heartburn, reflux, or indigestion?
What makes your swallowing worse?
What makes your swallowing better?

crushing them, adding more sauces/gravy, or cutting food into smaller pieces), which can mask the presence of underlying swallowing difficulties. A thorough history should elucidate these details; often family members or caregivers can provide additional insight. Although changes to swallowing function can be seen as a normal function of age,[68–73] the impact on a patient's ability to function and on his or her nutritional status and weight determines the degree to which any changes become a problem.

When obtaining a comprehensive swallowing history, it is important to note the duration of the symptoms and any precipitating events (e.g., stroke, intubation, acute illness, surgery, etc.). Identification of both aggravating and alleviating factors is also helpful. Many risk factors may contribute to swallowing difficulty and should be identified and addressed, when possible. These are summarized in Fig. 43.1.

Other symptoms, such as dysphonia (hoarseness), dyspnea, otalgia (ear pain), neck mass, dysarthria (slurred speech), globus (sensation of something in the throat), or reflux symptoms, may provide additional clues to identify the presence and/or etiology of concurrent dysphagia. In particular, reflux (either GERD or LPR) may result in swallowing difficulties. As noted earlier, there are multiple studies that suggest a link between LPR/GERD and microaspiration related to reflux, which can cause pulmonary disease. Reflux symptoms may include the traditional heartburn, indigestion, substernal pain, or burning sensation, but other symptoms that are potentially suggestive of reflux can include hoarseness, globus sensation, throat clearing, increased mucus, postnasal drip, chronic cough, bad or metallic taste in the mouth, or burning sensation in the mouth, throat, or chest.[74] The patient's tobacco, drug, and alcohol use history can also be potential risk factors for underlying disorders that can impact swallowing.

Among the many questions in a thorough history, it is particularly important to inquire about coughing or choking with liquids. These events raise a strong clinical suspicion of the potential for aspiration. However, it is vital to remember that aspiration may be taking place even in the absence of coughing (e.g., in the setting of changes in laryngotracheal sensation). This so-called "silent aspiration" can be even harder to identify; thus careful history taking, heightened awareness, and early identification are essential. Moreover, aspiration may not happen with every single swallow, but intermittent aspiration is not necessarily less harmful. In addition, worsening frequency or severity of coughing, choking, or dysphagic episodes can be worrisome signs.

It must be emphasized that choking or even coughing does not necessarily indicate aspiration. Furthermore, aspiration does not always result in pneumonia, and thus even the presence of frank aspiration should not automatically cause patients to be put on NPO status (nothing by mouth). Rather, the presence of choking, coughing, or any other symptoms or signs suggestive of aspiration should trigger a more comprehensive investigation of swallowing function.

EVALUATION AND TESTING

Evaluation of swallowing function is optimally performed in a multidisciplinary fashion with both an otolaryngologist and a speech-language pathologist. This multidisciplinary team should assess the patient's history, symptoms, and physical examination to determine the appropriate next step(s) for assessment. Simply watching patients swallow, even when performed by trained speech-language pathologists in what is commonly termed a "bedside swallow," is *inadequate* to identify the presence or absence of aspiration.[75]

A detailed physical examination of the head and neck should assess the status of all anatomic components that can impact swallowing function (Table 43.2). For example, the lips should be evaluated for masses, weakness, and oral competence (the ability to form a seal); the presence of drooling should be noted. The oral cavity and its mucous membranes should be examined for masses or dry mouth (xerostomia). Dental issues (e.g., presence or absence of teeth; condition of teeth; missing, broken, ill-fitting or unused dentures) can impair the patient's ability to masticate and form a bolus for swallowing. Gingival disease and dental caries provide a source of bacteria that, if aspirated, can provide a nidus of infection in the lung. The tongue should be examined for weakness, deviation to one side, presence of fasciculation, or postsurgical defects. Palatal asymmetry or velopharyngeal insufficiency (leading to nasal regurgitation) can also interfere with swallowing.

A thorough laryngoscopic examination is essential to identify abnormalities in the oropharynx, hypopharynx, larynx, and upper esophageal inlet. Endoscopic laryngeal examination can be performed using either a flexible or rigid laryngoscope. Because of its superior ability to assess neurologic function of the larynx (i.e., vocal fold motion and laryngeal sensation), flexible laryngoscopy is preferred for evaluation in patients with dysphagia complaints. Mirror laryngeal examination is of historical note and rarely used currently due to the advances in laryngoscopy (e.g., ease of use, enhanced quality of images obtained, and high tolerability). On flexible laryngoscopy, structural or anatomic changes (e.g., mass, tumor, surgical defect), vocal fold motion status, pooling of secretions, decreased or absent sensation, or presence of retained food particles are all noteworthy findings.

The flexible laryngoscope can also be used to observe some aspects of the swallowing function directly. This test, a *flexible endoscopic evaluation of swallowing* (FEES), allows direct observation of the nasopharynx and oropharynx before the swallow[76–78] (Videos 43.1 and 43.2). In addition, residual food materials that remain after the swallow

Table 43.2 Important Physical Examination Findings Potentially Related to Dysphagia

Lips: mass, weakness, oral competence (ability to form seal), presence of drooling

Teeth: presence or absence of teeth; condition of teeth; missing, broken, ill-fitting or unused dentures

Oral cavity: masses, xerostomia

Tongue: weakness, deviation, fasciculation, defect (postsurgical changes)

Palate: asymmetry, velopharyngeal insufficiency (leads to nasal regurgitation)

Larynx: unilateral or bilateral vocal fold paralysis, decreased sensation can be identified, and compensatory strategies may be tested at this time. However, because of the closure of the pharyngeal walls at the moment of swallowing (the so-called "whiteout" phase), direct visualization of vocal fold closure is obscured, and activity at this level during the actual swallow must be inferred. Frank aspiration may be readily visualized but can also be missed due to the whiteout phase. This disadvantage is offset by the advantages of FEES, including lack of radiation exposure and the high tolerance of this examination. During a FEES, the patient often tries to swallow materials of different consistencies. The exact protocol may differ between centers and is often guided by the patient's specific complaints and examination findings. A typical protocol may include thin liquids, thickened liquids (e.g., honey or nectar consistencies), pureed (e.g., applesauce), mixed consistency (solid and liquid together, e.g., fruit cocktail), and/or dry solid (e.g., cracker).

To evaluate swallowing function further, a *modified barium swallow* (MBS) is often pursued.[78] The MBS (also termed *video fluoroscopic swallow study* or *cookie test*) is performed in the fluoroscopy radiology suite in conjunction with a speech-language pathologist (Videos 43.3 and 43.4). This examination provides more detailed information about the oral, pharyngeal, and esophageal phases of swallowing and what can be observed at the level of the vocal folds in the midst of the swallow. Although an MBS does require a small degree of radiation exposure, this test also allows assessment of various consistencies and testing of concurrent compensatory strategies.[79] This test is distinguished from a *barium swallow* or esophagram, which only evaluates the propulsion of thin liquid barium through the esophagus to the stomach, focusing more on the evaluation of the esophageal anatomy. Although a barium swallow may identify gross aspiration, this test does not specifically assess swallowing function and thus is not typically considered sufficient as the sole method of evaluation of swallowing function.

Both FEES and MBS provide different types of information regarding a patient's swallowing function. These tests each have advantages and disadvantages and often provide complementary information about the patient's swallowing status. Thus it is not uncommon for patients to benefit from undergoing both types of evaluations, although both tests are not always required.[78] The comprehensive swallowing history and physical examination should guide decision making about the optimal test to identify the patient's underlying swallowing abnormality, the presence or absence of aspiration, and any potential compensatory strategies.

In situations of aspiration and dysphagia, the presence of reflux is important to note. However, the diagnosis of reflux can be quite challenging.[80] Often the diagnosis of GERD can be straightforward, particularly in patients with classic symptoms of heartburn and abdominal pain. GERD may be identified on esophagram (barium swallow) or endoscopy. By contrast, no gold standard has yet been established to make the diagnosis of LPR, wherein the stomach contents are thought to ascend the length of the esophagus and cause irritation or inflammation of the pharynx and potentially the larynx.[25] Frequently, a *clinical* diagnosis of LPR may be made based on the patient's symptoms and/or a clinical response to an empirical trial of antireflux treatment (often pharmacologic).[81]

A 24-hour dual-channel pH/impedance test, often performed with high-resolution manometry, may provide strong evidence for or even a definitive diagnosis of LPR, but there can be false-negative results as well.[81–83] In this test, a probe is inserted through the nose and left in place for a 24-hour period. During this time, patients note their symptoms (e.g., heartburn, indigestion, cough, regurgitation, throat clearing, globus) using a recording device. The test records the presence and number of reflux events, the pH of these events, how far proximally the events extend, and the correlation of these events with the patient's symptoms. Use of a dual-channel probe allows identification of proximal esophageal or pharyngeal events and is considered superior to a single-channel probe that would only assess distal esophageal events. Concurrent high-resolution manometry testing can provide additional information about the presence of esophageal dysmotility, which may also aggravate reflux symptoms.[84] Although pH/impedance testing with or without manometry may provide useful information about the presence or absence of LPR, it is important to understand that there may be false-negative results, and thus the gold standard for diagnosis of LPR remains elusive at present.[81–83]

TREATMENT

Management of dysphagia can be variable based on the underlying nature of the swallowing dysfunction. Treatment of penetration and aspiration, in particular, is based on the nature and timing of these events. All patients with swallowing difficulties should be monitored routinely for unintentional weight loss, development of lung infection (e.g., pneumonia), or progressive worsening of symptoms. In patients with known aspiration, meticulous oral care is of paramount importance. Patients at risk for aspiration should be counseled to brush their teeth every time after eating, to minimize the microbial load that may be aspirated into the lungs. Regular monitoring by their dentist to optimize dental care is imperative in these patients.

For any patient with swallowing symptoms, especially in the presence of weight loss, diet change, history of pneumonia, or reported coughing/choking when drinking liquids, formal multidisciplinary evaluation of swallowing dysfunction should be pursued, and treatment should be guided by the results of these assessments.

NIL PER OS STATUS

In circumstances of a sudden change in swallowing function, particularly if deemed likely to be temporary in nature (e.g., postsurgery), restricting a patient's oral intake may be indicated. If patients are NPO, then they should be given intravenous fluid hydration, enteral feeds (e.g., via nasogastric tube), or total parenteral nutrition. In cases of prolonged dysphagia and/or aspiration, a gastric (G-) or jejunal (J-) tube may need to be placed surgically. It is imperative to recall that enteral feeding via such tubes may not necessarily improve outcomes or quality of life, nor does it prevent aspiration.[85–87]

NPO status is not automatically required in cases of aspiration, and indeed, sometimes patients may choose to continue oral intake despite the presence of known aspiration. In this latter situation, patients and their families should be counseled about the risks of continued oral intake and the necessity of strict oral care so that they may make an informed decision about continuing oral intake in these circumstances.

COMPENSATORY STRATEGIES

Patients with dysphagia may be able to swallow safely with the use of various compensatory strategies. The specific strategy to use should be guided by the findings of the swallowing examination(s). Examples of helpful techniques can include changing the consistency of the diet, restricting bolus size to small sips and bites (e.g., cutting food into small pieces), and alternating solid and liquid consistencies. Other beneficial maneuvers can include hard (or consciously effortful) swallow, which improves posterior bolus propulsion and pharyngeal pressures to clear the bolus from the oropharynx; breath-hold during the swallow; or planned cough after swallowing, as well as certain positions, such as chin tuck, head turn, head tilt, or chin up. However, the utility of each of these strategies should be carefully assessed on a swallowing evaluation before clinical implementation.

SWALLOWING THERAPY

Swallowing therapy with a skilled speech-language pathologist may improve swallowing function, decrease dysphagia, and thus decrease the risk of aspiration. Again, the type and nature of swallowing therapy exercises should be determined by the specific findings of the swallowing evaluation, but overall these tend to focus on enhancing strength and coordination of the swallowing mechanism. Details regarding swallowing therapy are beyond the scope of this chapter but are briefly summarized as follows. Commonly used swallowing therapy exercises include the Masako (focused on holding the tongue to strengthen the propulsive ability of the base of tongue),[88,89] Shaker (lifting the head),[90,91] lingual resistance exercises,[92] and laryngeal elevation exercises. Examples of swallowing maneuvers that may improve dysphagia include effortful swallow,[88,93-95] Mendolsohn maneuver (targeting hyolaryngeal elevation, which helps to prolong cricopharyngeal opening during the swallow),[88,93] supraglottic swallow (breath-hold during swallow, followed by voluntary cough),[93] and super–supraglottic swallow (increased effort with supraglottic swallow).[93,96]

MEDICAL TREATMENT

Medical treatment of dysphagia should be directed at the underlying pathology. Addressing esophageal dysmotility (e.g., with prokinetic agents) can improve esophageal flow and decrease dysphagia. Salivary dysfunction (e.g., from postradiation xerostomia or rheumatologic disease) can also impair swallowing and should be addressed with aggressive hydration, sialogogues, artificial saliva, or other measures. Control of underlying rheumatologic disease (when applicable) is crucial.

Treatment of reflux may also be helpful in improving dysphagia and aspiration risk.[80,81] Management of reflux often relies on a combination of dietary and behavioral modifications with or without pharmacologic intervention. Patients should avoid, or at least minimize, specific foods known to trigger reflux, including, but not limited to, fried foods, high-fat content foods, spicy foods, tomato-based foods, dairy products, mint, citrus, caffeine, chocolate, and alcohol. Stress reduction, weight loss, and avoidance of late-night eating may also be beneficial. Use of a MediWedge or elevation of the head of the bed to 30 degrees is also recommended to reduce reflux. It is vital to note that the use of additional pillows to elevate the head alone is *not equivalent* to elevation of the entire head of the bed. The addition of pillows under the head results in increased bending at the stomach, which can increase intra-abdominal pressure and thus worsen reflux. In addition to these strategies, pharmacologic intervention, including proton pump inhibitors with or without histamine blockers may be pursued. For patients who are unwilling or unable to take or who remain symptomatic despite these medication(s), over-the-counter barrier medications (e.g., Gaviscon Advance [from outside the United States], Life Extension Esophageal Guardian, or Reflux Gourmet) may be an adjunctive or alternative option. Antacids may also be helpful in providing temporary symptom relief.

SURGERY

Surgery for dysphagia and aspiration should be targeted at addressing any anatomic changes or deficiencies that interfere with swallowing. A full description of the various surgical options for treatment of dysphagia is beyond the scope of this chapter; however, a brief overview of some common surgical treatments is included for initial reference. Surgery aimed at addressing dysphagia may decrease the risk for aspiration, *although it is important to note that the risk of aspiration cannot be eliminated entirely.*

In cases of incomplete vocal fold closure—often related to unilateral vocal fold paralysis, such as may be caused by thyroid or cervical spine surgery or after a stroke—a vocal fold augmentation procedure to restore vocal fold closure, particularly during the swallow, may be highly successful at improving dysphagia and eliminating aspiration. Vocal fold augmentation may be performed in a temporary or permanent fashion, via injection or open surgical placement of augmentation material, and potentially under local or general anesthesia, depending on the type of augmentation material.[97-100] Evaluation by an otolaryngologist, ideally in conjunction with a speech-language pathologist, will determine the optimal choice for such a procedure.

Cricopharyngeal dysfunction may improve with procedures targeted at the upper esophageal sphincter (e.g., dilation, botulinum toxin injection, or myotomy).[101-103] Velopharyngeal insufficiency may be addressed with a nasopharyngeal injection, if a palatal prosthesis was unsuccessful.[104] More aggressive surgical procedures are rarely performed except in cases of a completely nonfunctional larynx, typically with intractable aspiration and recurrent episodes of lung infection. Although laryngotracheal separation and total laryngectomy are options in these rare cases, they are complex procedures with a high degree of morbidity and should only be undertaken in highly selected cases, often as a last resort.[105-107]

Nissen fundoplication, or antireflux surgery, is a consideration for patients who have severe GERD that cannot be controlled by medical therapy or who have side effects or complications from medication. In this procedure, performed either laparoscopically or via open thoracotomy, a portion of the fundus of the stomach is wrapped around the lower esophageal sphincter. By "tightening" this sphincter function, the ability for gastric contents to come up (i.e., "reflux") into the esophagus is decreased.[108] There are some data to support its use in IPF and chronic lung allograft dysfunction after transplant.[60,109] Fundoplication is generally well tolerated and effective in preventing GERD, with common side effects, including dysphagia, bloating, and nausea.[110] The decision to pursue surgery should be made in careful collaboration with a gastroenterologist and surgeon on a case-by-case basis.

Key Points

- Aspiration can cause a wide variety of pulmonary manifestations, ranging from bronchospasm to lower respiratory tract infection.
- Knowledge of typical clinical, radiographic, and pathologic presentations, along with a high index of suspicion, is critically important because aspiration can be silent and is often missed.
- Detailed evaluation of dysphagia can identify patients at risk for aspiration.
- Taking a comprehensive history is fundamental, with the presence of coughing or choking with liquids raising concern for the potential for aspiration.
- The presence of aspiration does not mean that a patient must be made nil per os.
- Evaluation of swallowing function is optimally performed in a multidisciplinary fashion, including both an otolaryngologist and a speech-language pathologist.
- A flexible endoscopic evaluation of swallowing and a modified barium swallow provide complementary information regarding swallowing function; aspiration may be identified on either or both tests.
- Treatment for dysphagia and aspiration should be guided by the underlying pathology and the findings of the swallowing evaluation.
- Patients with dysphagia and risk of aspiration should be monitored regularly for unintentional weight loss, development of pneumonia, and progressive worsening of symptoms.

Key Readings

Brady S, Donzelli J. The modified barium swallow and the functional endoscopic evaluation of swallowing. *Otolaryngol Clin North Am.* 2013;46(6):1009–1022.

Christopher KL, Morris MJ. Vocal cord dysfunction, paradoxic vocal fold motion, or laryngomalacia? Our understanding requires an interdisciplinary approach. *Otolaryngol Clin North Am.* 2010;43(1):43–66, viii.

Hicks M, Brugman SM, Katial R. Vocal cord dysfunction/paradoxical vocal fold motion. *Prim Care.* 2008;35(1):81–103, vii.

ENThealth. American Academy of Otolaryngology-Head and Neck Surgery. Aspiration. https://www.enthealth.org/conditions/aspiration/.

ENThealth: American Academy of Otolaryngology-Head and Neck Surgery. Dysphagia. https://www.enthealth.org/conditions/dysphagia/.

Lascarrou JB, Lissonde F, Le Thuaut A, Bachoumas K, Colin G, Henry Lagarrigue M, et al. Antibiotic therapy in comatose mechanically ventilated patients following aspiration: differentiating pneumonia from pneumonitis. *Crit Care Med.* 2017;45(8):1268–1275.

Lee JS, Ryu JH, Elicker BM, Lydell CP, Jones KD, Wolters PJ, et al. Gastroesophageal reflux therapy is associated with longer survival in patients with idiopathic pulmonary fibrosis. *Am J Respir Crit Care Med.* 2011;184(12):1390–1394.

Mandell LA, Niederman MS. Aspiration pneumonia. *N Engl J Med.* 2019;380(7):651–663.

Raghu G, Pellegrini CA, Yow E, Flaherty KR, Meyer K, Noth I, et al. Laparoscopic anti-reflux surgery for the treatment of idiopathic pulmonary fibrosis (WRAP-IPF): a multicentre, randomised, controlled phase 2 trial. *Lancet Respir Med.* 2018;6(9):707–714.

Complete reference list available at ExpertConsult.com.

44 HYPOXEMIA

V. COURTNEY BROADDUS, MD • ANTONIO GOMEZ, MD

INTRODUCTION

Understanding hypoxemia is an important goal for every pulmonologist. Both in its acute and chronic presentations, hypoxemia reflects the functioning of the lung in its major role as a gas exchange organ. The physiologic mechanisms of hypoxemia are explained in Chapter 10. Aspects of hypoxemia are also discussed in several other chapters in this textbook. This new chapter has been introduced to amplify the understanding of the mechanisms of hypoxemia in the clinical context and to explore the practical aspects of this understanding and the approach to hypoxemia.

DEFINITION

It must first be clarified what hypoxemia is and what it is not. Hypoxemia is a low level of oxygen in the blood (-emia), defined as a low oxygen saturation or low *partial pressure of oxygen* (PO_2). The actual level used is somewhat arbitrary.[1] An arterial oxygen saturation less than 90% is a reasonable definition of hypoxemia; at this saturation, the arterial PO_2 is approximately 60 mm Hg (depending on the actual dissociation curve) (Figs. 44.1 and 10.12). At this level, the arterial PO_2 values approach the steep portion of the oxygen-hemoglobin dissociation curve, where small changes in arterial PO_2 have a large effect on saturation. However, investigators have defined hypoxemia at different points anywhere from 88–95% saturation,[1–3] thus emphasizing that the actual level has not been defined, either at rest or during exercise. One reason for the reluctance to set a single value for hypoxemia may be that arterial PO_2 varies significantly with age.[4] It has been pointed out that an arterial PO_2 of 66 mm Hg can be normal in an 80-year-old person.[5]

A key point is that hypoxemia is not the same as hypoxia, although these terms are often used interchangeably. Hypoxia is defined as an insufficient level of oxygen in the tissues (not the blood), and it is recognized by signs of ischemia, such as lactic acidosis, cardiac ischemia, or neurologic dysfunction. Hypoxemia, on the other hand, may not cause symptoms and may instead be detected incidentally, usually with pulse oximetry (see the later section on response).

MEASUREMENTS

Various measures are used to describe hypoxemia, including PO_2, oxygen saturation, *alveolar-arterial PO_2 difference* [(A–a)PO_2], and the *ratio of arterial PO_2 to the fractional concentration of oxygen in inspired gas* (FIO_2) (the P/F ratio).

Arterial PO_2: This is the partial pressure, or tension, of the oxygen in equilibrium with the arterial blood. The difference between the average alveolar partial pressure of oxygen and the arterial PO_2 is a measure of the efficiency of oxygenation, the (A–a)PO_2. Of note, it is the partial pressure that is detected by the carotid bodies. However, it is the saturation that indicates how much oxygen is carried in the blood.

Oxygen saturation: The relationship between the PO_2 (arterial PO_2) and the saturation of the blood is one of the most important relationships in medicine, as described by the oxygen-hemoglobin dissociation curve (also called the oxyhemoglobin dissociation curve) (see Figs. 44.1 and 10.12). This sigmoid relationship explains how oxygen loads and unloads rapidly onto the hemoglobin in the steep portion of the curve with small changes in arterial PO_2 and how, once fully loaded, the partial pressure can fall over a large range without much of a drop in the

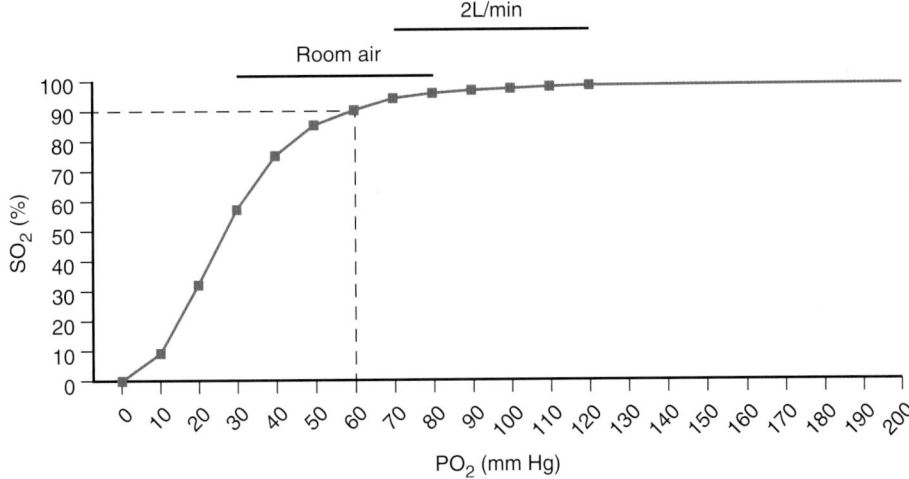

Figure 44.1 **The oxyhemoglobin dissociation curve.** The two bars show the range of arterial partial pressure of oxygen (PO_2) in a subject breathing room air and breathing supplemental oxygen at 2 L/min. With hypoventilation, the subject's arterial PO_2 decreases along the bar, moving to the left. On room air, the fall in partial pressure of oxygen due to hypoventilation will trigger a drop in saturation (SO_2) that can be detected by the pulse oximeter. On 2 L/min, the same fall in partial pressure of oxygen will remain on the flat portion of the curve and will not generate a low saturation and thus not be detected by the pulse oximeter (see also Table 44.1). The *dashed line* represents the defined level of hypoxemia (see text).

oxygen saturation. One can also appreciate that the arterial PO_2 can *increase* over a large range, as when high FIO_2 is given to patients, with almost no increase in oxygen saturation. The actual position of the curve is sensitive to systemic input; with fever or low pH, for example, the curve moves to the right, allowing more oxygen unloading at the same arterial PO_2 (see Fig. 10.12). It is the oxygen saturation that is measured by the pulse oximeter (see later).

(A–a)PO_2: It is important to state up front that this is a difference, not a gradient. Why? Because a gradient implies a difference between two points, from an alveolus to a pulmonary capillary, whereas the "*A*" indicates an average value for the alveoli in the lung and the "*a*" is not capillary blood, but arterial, and also represents something of an average value. The divergence of these two values comes from differences across the lung as a result of the heterogeneity of oxygenation; thus, the term "difference" is more apt than "gradient." At room air, the (A–a)PO_2 turns out to be an excellent measure of the efficiency of oxygen transfer. At a higher FIO_2, however, the difference increases and thus is affected by the FIO_2.[6] The P/F ratio was developed in part to address this problem (see below). The (A–a)PO_2 also widens with age[7,8]; a standard equation to correct the (A–a) PO_2 for the effect of age is (age/4) + 4. Finally, an abnormal (A–a)PO_2 is not specific for any single cause of hypoxemia; however, a normal value in the setting of hypoxemia is most compatible with hypoventilation.

P/F ratio: Compared with the (A–a)PO_2, the P/F ratio is more resistant to changes in FIO_2 but, even here, it has been shown to vary with the FIO_2.[9,10] Therefore, when monitoring changes over time, it is important to determine the P/F ratio when the FIO_2 has been set to the same level and after the lung has been maximally recruited.[11]

CONSEQUENCES

When is hypoxemia harmful? In healthy individuals, profound hypoxemia can be tolerated for short periods.[12] Most hypoxemia studies have been performed in the process of testing the function of pulse oximeters[12] or of measuring the ventilatory responses to hypoxemia.[13] No particular harm has been noted.[5]

Clearly, if the hypoxemia is low enough and prolonged enough, the heart and brain will fail. However, the pleasant surprise is how well the average person can tolerate hypoxemia for periods up to 30 minutes without noticeable injury. In the chronic ambulatory setting as well, hypoxemia may be tolerated. We know, however, that providing continuous oxygen to patients with COPD and an oxygen saturation of 88% or less (or arterial PO_2 ≤55 mm Hg) increases survival,[14] a finding implying that the low oxygen saturation or the consequence of it is harmful. The reasons for this increased survival are not clear but may involve various consequences of low oxygen saturation: (1) polycythemia, (2) hypoxic pulmonary vasoconstriction and increased pulmonary vascular resistance, (3) a reduced oxygen reserve for any interruption in breathing, especially during sleep, and (4) arrhythmias.

Acutely, if low enough, hypoxemia can cause hypoxic end-organ dysfunction and death. The rapidity of the drop may be important, as well as whether someone has developed physiologic adaptations to decreased oxygen, as shown by persons who can exercise at extremely high altitude.[15]

RESPONSE

Oxygen is sensed as the arterial PO_2 by the peripheral chemoreceptors, mainly the carotid bodies (and, to a lesser extent, the aortic chemoreceptors) (see Chapter 12). The ventilatory response to hypoxemia is hyperbolic and is activated at very low PO_2 levels; it has been likened to an emergency mechanism[16] (Fig. 44.2). In an early study,[16] healthy participants breathing low oxygen concentrations did not hyperventilate until the inspired oxygen concentration dropped to less than 8%. In a more recent study, similar patterns were found.[13] The other feature of the response to hypoxemia is the wide variability among healthy individuals. The response to hypoxemia is blunted in long-term residents at high altitude (see Fig. 44.2). The ventilatory response is also reduced with age and with coincident disease such as diabetes.[17] The ventilatory response is also dependent on the arterial *partial pressure of carbon dioxide* (PCO_2); if the arterial PCO_2 is low, the response to hypoxemia is lessened.[18] The sensation of

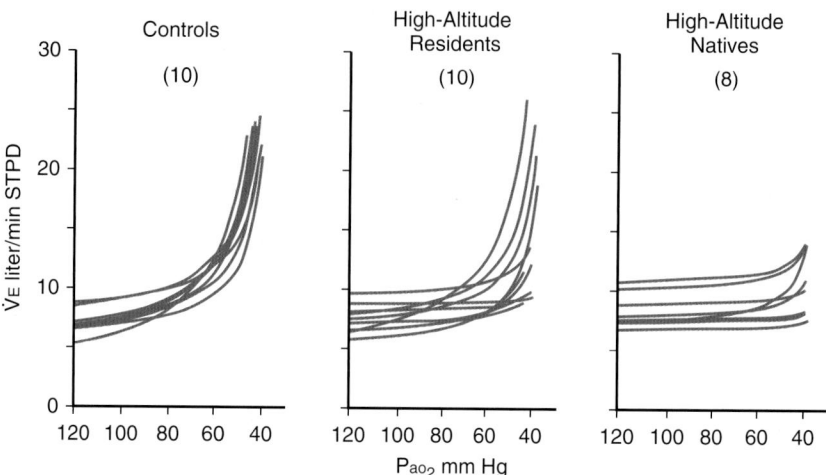

Figure 44.2 Response to hypoxemia in 10 control subjects, 10 who live in high altitude and 8 who are natives of high altitude. The normal response to hypoxemia is activated at low arterial partial pressure of oxygen (PaO$_2$) and serves as something of an emergency response to low oxygen tension. The more blunted responses after living at high altitude show that the response can be altered. Interestingly, persons who have lived all their lives at high altitude (Leadville, CO; elevation 3100 m) had almost no response at all. STPD, Standard temperature, standard pressure, and dry; V̇E, expired total ventilation. (From Weil JV, Byrne-Quinn E, Sodal IE, Filley GF, Grover RF. Acquired attenuation of chemoreceptor function in chronically hypoxic man at high altitude. *J Clin Invest.* 1971;50:186–195.)

Table 44.1 Hypoventilation Can Cause a Fall in Oxygen Saturation When a Patient Is Breathing Room Air But Not When Receiving Supplemental Oxygen*

	At Room Air			On 2 L/min	
PaCO$_2$	PaO$_2$	SaO$_2$		PaO$_2$	SaO$_2$
40	80	96		120	100
50	67.5	94		107.5	100
60	55	**88**		95	100
70	42.5	**84**		82.5	96
80	30	**60**		70	95

All values in mm Hg.
*According to the alveolar gas equation, if all else stays constant and the R = 0.8, for every rise in arterial PCO$_2$ of 10 mm Hg, the arterial PO$_2$ will fall by 12.5 mm Hg (see text under Hypoventilation). When the patient is breathing room air, the drop in arterial PO$_2$ will be at the steep portion of the oxyhemoglobin dissociation curve and can be detected as a drop in oxygen saturation (see abnormal saturations in the box); however, when the patient is receiving supplemental oxygen, the same relative fall in oxygen will be on the flat portion of the curve and will not trigger a noticeable fall in oxygen saturation. Thus, the pulse oximeter, by measuring oxygen saturation, cannot detect hypoventilation in a patient receiving supplemental oxygen (see also Fig. 44.1).
PaO$_2$, arterial partial pressure of oxygen; PaCO$_2$, arterial partial pressure of carbon dioxide; SaO$_2$, arterial oxygen saturation.

dyspnea appears to coincide with the initiation of the hypoxemic ventilatory response.[19]

In the recent era, many patients with coronavirus disease 2019 (COVID-19) have been noted to have strikingly low oxygen levels without any sensation of dyspnea. Although this phenomenon has not fully been explained, it is likely that this is a function of the insensitivity and variability described earlier. Older, diabetic patients can be expected to have a depressed ventilatory and dyspneic response to hypoxemia and, even without these factors, certain individuals have a lower sensitivity to hypoxemia as a result of normal variation.[5]

DETECTION

ARTERIAL BLOOD GAS

Obtaining a value for arterial PO$_2$ by analysis of an arterial blood gas is the gold standard for determining oxygenation.

With the measures of arterial PO$_2$ and PCO$_2$, one can calculate the (A–a)PO$_2$, as a useful assessment of the ability of the lung to oxygenate, and can exclude hypercarbia as a cause of the hypoxemia (see Chapter 10). One can also exclude interference by abnormal hemoglobins (e.g., carboxyhemoglobin, methemoglobin). For the assessment of acid-base and hypercarbia, see Chapters 12 and 45.

NONINVASIVE PULSE OXIMETER

The pulse oximeter enables detection of oxygen saturation. The reader is referred to excellent reviews of the technical aspects and applications of pulse oximetry.[20,21] In general, the technique depends on the detection of absorbance of two wavelengths selected to maximize the ability to distinguish oxyhemoglobin from deoxyhemoglobin and on the ability to separate pulsating (presumably arterial) blood from the background. Thus, without knowing any more, one can see that introduction in the blood of additional materials absorbing at either of these two wavelengths (e.g., carboxyhemoglobin, methemoglobin, methylene blue), interference with absorption (e.g., extraneous light, dark nail polish), or interference with detection of the arterial pulse (e.g., presence of venous pulsations, low cardiac output, an inflated blood pressure cuff) will interfere with the ability of the pulse oximeter to read the arterial saturation. (Pulse oximetry may also be affected by dark skin pigmentation; in a recent report, pulse oximetry was found to be more likely to overestimate oxygen saturation in Black individuals than in white individuals.[21a]) These technical points are important, but additional important errors in interpretation can arise even when the pulse oximeter is reading correctly.

What can go wrong even when the reading is correct? The main clinical problems come from the confounding of saturation with partial pressure. The sigmoid relationship of these two values means that the PO$_2$ can vary significantly without much change in the saturation. This behavior at the upper flat part of the dissociation curve is an advantage biologically because the hemoglobin can stay nearly fully saturated over a range of arterial PO$_2$, but it means that the pulse oximeter is insensitive to changes in PO$_2$ until a drop in saturation is detectable, often at a PO$_2$ below 60 mm Hg (see Fig. 44.1, room air). Because the rise in PCO$_2$ with hypoventilation is detected *indirectly* by a drop in PO$_2$, the insensitivity of the pulse oximeter to changes in P_{O_2} in this range can mean significant delays in detecting hypoventilation.

Importantly, the situation is worse in any patient receiving supplemental oxygen; in this situation, the pulse oximeter loses any ability to detect hypoventilation[22] (Table 44.1). Of all the messages to trainees in this chapter, this may be the most important. Supplemental oxygen moves the arterial P_{O_2} farther up onto the flat portion of the oxyhemoglobin dissociation curve (see Fig. 44.1, at 2 L/min), so that a similar rise in P_{CO_2} and fall in P_{O_2} cannot be detected by a drop in saturation. The inability of pulse oximetry to detect hypoventilation in a patient on supplemental oxygen has mandated the use of other methods to detect arterial P_{CO_2} *directly*, such as by capnography. In addition to pulse oximetry, capnography is now considered standard of care for monitoring during moderate sedation.[23]

A corollary point is worth emphasizing. If the patient does develop hypercarbia during supplemental oxygen administration, the removal of the oxygen, by a well-meaning clinician or by a confused patient, can lead to precipitous and profound hypoxemia (Table 44.2) (see later, under Hypoventilation). Thus, it is wise for the clinician to be aware that hypercarbia can develop silently in the background and, once hypercarbia is present, removal of the supplemental oxygen can be life-threatening. In this setting, prompt efforts to increase ventilation—by reversal of opioids, noninvasive ventilation, or invasive ventilation—are needed.

At very low oxygen saturations, pulse oximeter readings are not validated, basically because the readings have been determined by calibrating with human volunteers. Understandably, there has not been much calibration of saturations lower than 70% or so. The oximeter has been shown to underestimate the saturation at these low values,[24] a point raised recently in regard to some patients with COVID-19 who have extremely low saturations.

MECHANISMS OF HYPOXEMIA

Mechanisms of hypoxemia can be divided into those resulting from abnormalities of lung function (i.e., low ventilation-perfusion, shunting, and diffusion limitation) and those that do not depend on lung disease (i.e., pure hypoventilation and decreased inspired P_{O_2}) (Table 44.3). (Hypoventilation can, of course, be caused by lung disorders but, in this discussion, we consider hypoventilation as separate from lung disease.) The pathophysiology of these mechanisms is covered in Chapter 10 and in an excellent review.[25] Here we would like to explore their clinical relevance, keeping in mind that the mechanisms rarely exist in isolation. The major mechanisms generating hypoxemia clinically are low ventilation-perfusion, shunt, and hypoventilation. An approach to distinguishing these mechanisms clinically is proposed in Figure 44.3.

MECHANISMS WITH INCREASED ALVEOLAR-ARTERIAL PARTIAL PRESSURE OF OXYGEN DIFFERENCE

As mentioned, the first three mechanisms involve abnormality of the lung, as evidenced by an elevated $(A–a)P_{O_2}$ and venous admixture. Venous admixture is a measure of the amount of mixed venous blood that avoids oxygenation, whether because of low ventilation-perfusion, shunt, or diffusion limitation. With abnormal venous admixture, the mixed venous oxygen saturation contributes to hypoxemia and plays an increasing role as the venous admixture increases (see later).

Low Ventilation-Perfusion

Perfusion to areas with low *ventilation in relation to perfusion* (V/Q) is the most common cause of hypoxemia in clinical practice. Almost all lung diseases can worsen the matching of ventilation to perfusion. In fact, it is important to recall that even the normal lung has V/Q mismatching, leading

Table 44.2 The Danger of Undetected Hypoventilation When a Patient Is Receiving Supplemental Oxygen*

	Pa_{O_2}	Pa_{CO_2}
Room air	55	50
2 L/min	110	50
2 L/min	97.5	60
2 L/min	85	70
Room air	30	70

All values in mm Hg.

*In this patient receiving supplemental oxygen, the arterial P_{CO_2} starts to rise. With each 10 mm Hg rise, the arterial P_{O_2} falls 12.5 mm Hg (see text), although the arterial P_{O_2} (and oxygen saturation, not shown) never falls into a range to trigger the pulse oximeter. At the higher arterial P_{CO_2}, supplemental oxygen becomes a lifeline. The supplemental oxygen in effect allows the arterial P_{CO_2} to rise without detection of a drop in oxygen saturation by the pulse oximeter. Removing the oxygen when the Pa_{CO_2} has risen can lead to a precipitous fall in arterial P_{O_2} (the calculated value of 30). Pa_{CO_2}, arterial partial pressure of carbon dioxide; Pa_{O_2}, arterial partial pressure of oxygen.

Table 44.3 The Five Mechanisms of Hypoxemia and Their Effect on the Alveolar-Arterial Oxygen Tension Difference and Their Response to Moderate Increases in Fractional Concentration of Oxygen in Inspired Gas

Mechanism of Hypoxemia	$(A–a)P_{O_2}$	Response of Arterial P_{O_2} to Increase in F_{IO_2}
Low ventilation-perfusion	Increased	Improves
Shunt	Increased	Minimal improvement
Diffusion limitation	Increased	Improves
Hypercarbia	Normal	Improves
Decreased P_{IO_2}	Normal	Improves

$(A–a)P_{O_2}$, alveolar-arterial partial pressure of oxygen difference; F_{IO_2}, fractional concentration of oxygen in inspired gas; P_{IO_2}, partial pressure of inspired oxygen; P_{O_2}, partial pressure of oxygen.
Modified from Petersson J, Glenny RW. Gas exchange and ventilation-perfusion relationships in the lung. *Eur Respir J.* 2014;44:1023-1041.

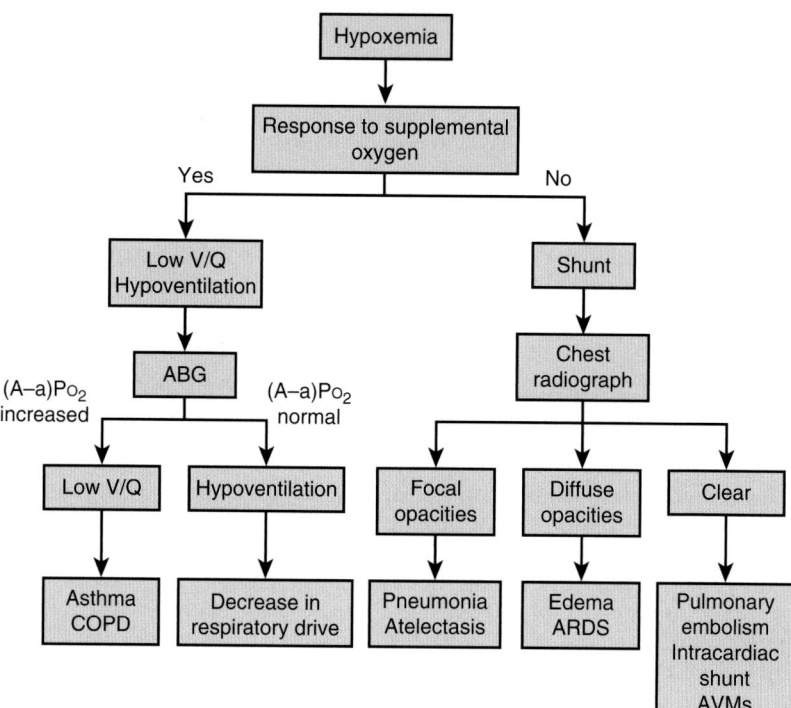

Figure 44.3 A simplified algorithm for distinguishing the major clinical causes of hypoxemia. Clinically, the most important first step is in knowing whether the patient responds well to supplemental oxygen. If the response is good, the likely mechanisms are low ventilation-perfusion (V/Q) or hypoventilation; if so, an arterial blood gas (ABG) determination will be the next step. If the response to oxygen is poor, one is likely dealing with a shunt. Imaging with chest radiography will help determine the likely cause and next steps, recognizing that the chest radiograph is not as sensitive as chest computed tomography. ARDS, acute respiratory distress syndrome; AVMs, arteriovenous malformations.

to variation from top to bottom mainly as a result of the effects of gravity on perfusion (which varies five- to sixfold) and ventilation (which varies three- to fourfold) (see Fig. 10.19). Lower V/Q exists at the base of the normal lung and may be clinically relevant with further decreases in lung volume and poor ventilation of the bases, as in obesity. It is the low V/Q areas that lead to hypoxemia, whereas high V/Q areas have no impact on hypoxemia but impair carbon dioxide elimination. Whenever there are areas in which ventilation is decreased relative to perfusion, as by airway disorders, the alveolar P_{O_2} and the capillary P_{O_2} in that area decrease. A similar low V/Q situation may be created when perfusion is *increased* relative to ventilation, as may happen in conditions such as pulmonary embolism that redirect the pulmonary circulation to other capillary beds.

The best clinical approach to hypoxemia due to the presence of low V/Q areas is to increase inspired oxygen. In those alveoli with at least some ventilation, the increase in $P_{I_{O_2}}$ will raise alveolar P_{O_2} and capillary P_{O_2}, leading to an overall improvement in arterial P_{O_2}. Most of these poorly ventilated alveoli are functioning on the steep portion of the oxyhemoglobin dissociation curve, and small increases in P_{O_2} can cause a large increase in oxygen saturation. Thus, this type of hypoxemia responds to small to moderate amounts of supplemental inspired oxygen. In fact, this response to small amounts of oxygen can be used clinically to identify low V/Q as the likely cause of hypoxemia (see Fig. 44.3).

Shunt

With shunt, mixed venous blood completely bypasses alveoli and is not exposed to alveolar P_{O_2}. The consequences can be profound because no amount of inspired oxygen can reach this shunted blood. A certain degree of shunting is normal; the physiologic shunt from post–pulmonary capillary entry of venous blood into the arterial system from bronchial veins and

thebesian veins is estimated at less than 7% of cardiac output. (Measurements of normal physiologic shunt vary by the technique used: 100% oxygen rebreathing detects these shunts, whereas the multiple inert gas technique does not [see later]).

Pathologic shunts can arise from intrapulmonary causes (e.g., complete consolidation resulting from lobar pneumonia or edema, pulmonary arteriovenous malformations) or intracardiac causes (e.g., right-to-left shunts through a patent ductus arteriosus or atrial septal defect). The intrapulmonary shunts can be divided further into two types: (1) those that arise from abnormal lung regions in which alveoli are collapsed or filled with fluid, called *parenchymal shunts;* and (2) those arising from vascular shunts within the lung, as from arteriovenous malformations or dilated pulmonary capillaries, called *vascular lung shunts.*[26] The value in dividing the intrapulmonary shunts into these two categories is that they act differently with regard to contrast echocardiography: the parenchymal shunt does not have the dilated abnormal vessels that allow bubbles to pass, whereas the vascular shunt does. Other differences have been described.[26] However, all types of shunt have a similar oxygenation defect in that the mixed venous blood flowing through the shunt fails to be oxygenated and dilutes and depresses the overall arterial oxygen saturation.

As shunt increases, the arterial P_{O_2} becomes less responsive to increases of $F_{I_{O_2}}$ (Fig. 44.4). In a patient with a large shunt, the main viable strategy for increasing arterial P_{O_2} is to decrease the shunt. In Figure 44.4, this would mean moving from one shunt line to one above it, which would increase the P_{O_2} at the same $F_{I_{O_2}}$. Means of decreasing shunt include *positive end-expiratory pressure* (PEEP) and moving the patient to a prone position, called proning. Once the shunt has been reduced as much as possible, the other major strategy for improving arterial oxygenation is to elevate the oxygen saturation of mixed venous blood (see later).

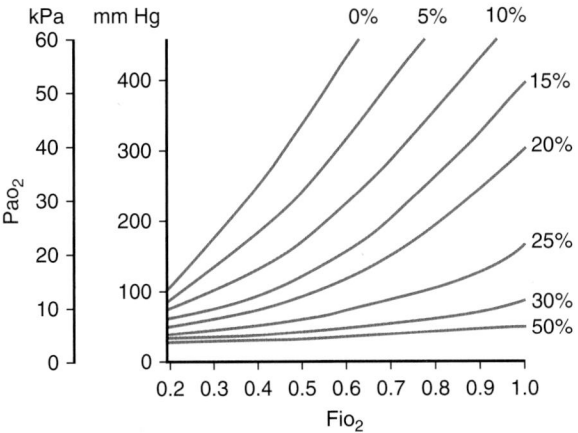

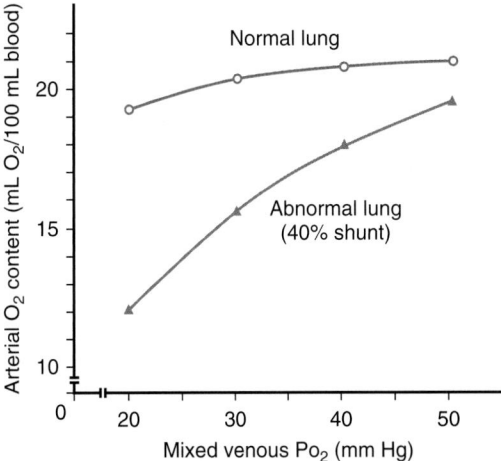

Figure 44.4 **The iso-shunt diagram showing the relationship between fractional concentration of oxygen in inspired gas and arterial partial pressure of oxygen at different levels of shunt.** With increasing shunt, the slope of the change in arterial partial pressure of oxygen (PaO_2) becomes increasingly flat so that a high fractional concentration of oxygen in inspired gas (FIO_2) has little effect on arterial PO_2. For shunts greater than 25% of cardiac output, even a fractional concentration of oxygen in inspired gas of 1.0 fails to raise the arterial PO_2 higher than 100 mm Hg. (From Petersson J, Glenny RW. Gas exchange and ventilation-perfusion relationships in the lung. *Eur Respir J.* 2014;44:1023-1041.)

Figure 44.5 **Effect of changes in mixed venous partial pressure of oxygen on arterial oxygen content in a normal lung and a lung with a 40% shunt.** In this model, the mixed venous partial pressure of oxygen (PO_2) was allowed to vary while the cardiac output and minute ventilation were held constant. In the normal lung, the arterial oxygen (O_2) content changes little over the range of mixed venous PO_2. With a 40% shunt, the arterial oxygen content becomes more sensitive to mixed venous PO_2 levels. (From Dantzker DR. Gas exchange in acute lung injury. In: Wiedemann HP, Matthay MA, Matthay RA, eds. *Critical Care Clinics: Acute Lung Injury.* Philadelphia: Saunders;1986:527-536.)

Diffusion Limitation

Diffusion limitation manifests when pulmonary capillary blood does not fully equilibrate with alveolar oxygen. This lack of equilibration means that there is some venous admixture, with some portion of the mixed venous blood reaching the arterial side. In the normal setting (see Fig. 10.16), capillary blood equilibrates fully and with a large reserve capacity. In certain circumstances, there is insufficient time for equilibration, generally when the capillary transit time is reduced, as with loss of capillaries in disease or with extreme exercise; when the alveolar PO_2 is low, as in high altitude; or when the mixed venous PO_2 is low, thereby increasing the gradient for diffusion.[27] Often, more than one mechanism is involved.

Mixed Venous Oxygen

Although not included as a direct mechanism of hypoxemia, a low mixed venous PO_2 is an important contributing mechanism when there is venous admixture. With venous admixture, in which some mixed venous blood reaches the arterial blood, a low mixed venous PO_2 can have a large effect on decreasing the arterial PO_2. (Venous admixture is calculated as the amount of mixed venous blood that would have to be added to the postcapillary blood to achieve the observed arterial PO_2). In the three mechanisms described earlier, the mixed venous blood that is not oxygenated drags down the PO_2 and oxygen saturation of the arterial blood. The mixed venous oxygen can significantly affect the arterial PO_2 even if the V/Q relationships are unchanged or improve (as often seen with exercise). The degree of its effect depends on the PO_2 of the mixed venous blood and the amount of venous admixture (Fig. 44.5). The role of mixed venous PO_2 in determining the arterial PO_2 is a reminder that decreases in arterial PO_2 may reflect systemic changes, such as increased muscle activity or dips in cardiac output, instead of decreases in lung function.[29]

MECHANISMS WITH NORMAL ALVEOLAR-ARTERIAL PARTIAL PRESSURE OF OXYGEN DIFFERENCE

The last two mechanisms of hypoxemia do not depend on an abnormality in the lung itself. Neither mechanism requires an increase in the $(A-a)PO_2$ or an increase in venous admixture.

Hypoventilation (see Chapters 45 and 132)

With a decrease in ventilation, there is a reduction in alveolar PO_2. Using the alveolar gas equation, one can calculate the change in PO_2 from the change in PCO_2 during pure hypoventilation or hyperventilation (i.e., without a change in venous admixture). In general, if the other factors of the alveolar gas equation remain constant (e.g., barometric pressure, FIO_2, the $(A-a)PO_2$), the change in PO_2 is reflected by a change (Δ) in PCO_2, as follows: $\Delta PO_2 = -\Delta PCO_2/R$. If the R is assumed to be 0.8, the equation can be written so that a change in PO_2 is equal but opposite to the change in $PCO_2 \times 1.25$. Thus, when all factors mentioned are constant, if the PCO_2 goes up by 10 mm Hg, the PO_2 goes down by 12.5 mm Hg (see also Fig. 132.2). This shortcut is used in Tables 44.1 and 44.2 to model the effect of changes in arterial PCO_2 on arterial PO_2.

As mentioned, supplemental oxygen can be given but, if the carbon dioxide should rise further, the patient will become increasingly dependent on the added inspired oxygen. As described in Chapters 45 and 132, an increase in inspired oxygen may lead to a rise in carbon dioxide because of a blunting of hypoxic pulmonary vasoconstriction that increases the inefficiency of ventilation, an overall decrease in ventilation, or the Haldane effect (in which oxygen decreases the affinity of hemoglobin for carbon dioxide).[30] If, by whatever mechanism, the PCO_2 does rise, removal of the supplemental oxygen can lead to a sudden and profound drop in Po_2 (see Table 44.2). Thus, once the Pco_2 starts to rise, the patient increasingly needs the higher Fio_2 to maintain arterial Po_2. The clinical response to this problem is not to remove the oxygen, but to increase ventilation.

Low Inspired Partial Pressure of Oxygen

A low inspired Po_2 and thus a low alveolar Po_2 will lead to a decrease in diffusion of oxygen and a lower arterial Po_2. This situation is usually an issue at high altitude, where the inspired Po_2 decreases significantly (see Table 105.1). However, at sea level, this situation can be created by the displacement of oxygen by other gases, such as nitrogen[31] or helium, accidentally or by intention. In addition, inspired Po_2 can drop and hypoxemia can develop when an increase in ventilation by a spontaneously breathing patient receiving supplemental oxygen leads to increased entrainment of room air.

MECHANISMS ACCOUNTING OF HYPOXEMIA IN RESPIRATORY DISEASES AND CONDITIONS

For most of the studies described in this section, the *multiple inert gas elimination technique* (MIGET) was essential in unraveling the various mechanisms of hypoxemia. Until the development of the MIGET, gas exchange abnormalities were of necessity lumped into three compartments of shunt, ideal, and dead space. This three-compartment model, as initially described by Riley, was a useful construct of gas exchange abnormalities,[32] but it was not possible to separate the presence of low V/Q units from shunt in determining the causes of hypoxemia. The MIGET, developed by Peter Wagner and colleagues in 1974,[33] enabled an almost continuous measurement of the V/Q ratios of the lung, thereby expanding the three compartments to almost 50. In effect, the black box of the lung could be illuminated by measuring how six inert gases with different solubilities were eliminated from the blood and then using computers to model those findings over the range of possible V/Q. The MIGET could also show whether shunt and V/Q abnormalities could fully explain the arterial Po_2 and, if not, could identify the residual contribution as due to diffusion limitation, the third possible cause of hypoxemia in an abnormal lung. The major limitation of MIGET is that it cannot localize the abnormalities in the lung. Newer techniques have been developed to visualize the heterogeneity of the diseased lung.[34] In the meantime, V/Q scanning has added some insights into the location of the abnormalities, as described later.

Of note, in the MIGET, healthy individuals have no calculated shunt.[33] Thus, this technique does not measure physiologic shunting from the bronchial and thebesian vessels, and any shunt measured by the MIGET is considered abnormal. The V/Q ratio considered to be low is usually less than 0.1.

PNEUMONIA

The mechanisms of hypoxemia in pneumonia involve an increase in perfusion both to shunt and to low V/Q units. In one study, the MIGET was used in patients with pneumonia of different severity.[35] In the 13 patients with mild to moderate hypoxemia who were spontaneously breathing (arterial Po_2 74 ± 6 mm Hg), there was an increase in the percentage of blood flow to shunt ($7.5 \pm 1.8\%$) and to low V/Q regions ($4.2 \pm 1.0\%$). These were shown to be sufficient to explain mild hypoxemia. In the same study, in 10 patients with severe pneumonia requiring mechanical ventilation and an elevated Fio_2 (0.46 ± 0.04), the percentage of blood going to shunt and to low V/Q regions was more than twice as high as in those patients with milder pneumonia (shunt, $21.9 \pm 4.5\%$; low V/Q, $10.9 \pm 4.6\%$). The likelihood is that, with increasing severity of pneumonia and increasing consolidation, both the shunt fraction and low V/Q areas increase. The response to supplemental oxygen depends on the degree of shunt.

PLEURAL EFFUSION

Pleural effusion can be associated with hypoxemia, generally mild. The effect of thoracentesis on the arterial Po_2 is inconsistent; sometimes arterial Po_2 increases, does not change, or actually decreases.[36] In one study,[37] MIGET was used in nine patients with effusions, with an arterial Po_2 of 82 ± 10 mm Hg, and with an elevated $(A-a)Po_2$ of 29 ± 10 mm Hg. The patients were shown to have a mildly elevated shunt ($6.9 \pm 6.7\%$). The increase in shunt with pleural effusions agrees with experimental data.[38] Interestingly, 30 minutes after removal of approximately 700 mL, the arterial Po_2, $(A-a)Po_2$, and shunt did not change significantly; the percentage of blood perfusing low V/Q regions actually increased slightly.[37] Another significant effect of pleural effusion, and one that is not often appreciated, is the effect on cardiac function, mainly on right ventricular filling. Echocardiographic studies have shown that large, mainly right-sided, effusions can have hemodynamic effects similar to that of tamponade[39,40] (see Chapter 14). Hypoxemia in this setting may be explained in part by low cardiac output and low mixed venous Po_2 in the setting of venous admixture. The proper approach consists of early recognition and thoracentesis.

PULMONARY EMBOLISM

Although hypoxemia is common in patients with *pulmonary embolism* (PE), it is not universal. In the Urokinase PE Trial, 12% of patients with PE had an arterial Po_2 greater than 80 mm Hg, and 5% had arterial Po_2 greater than 90 mm Hg. Even massive PE has been described without hypoxemia.[41] In addition, the $(A-a)Po_2$ can be normal in PE. One study reported that, in 3 of 64 patients with PE, the $(A-a)Po_2$ was normal for age.[42] Nonetheless, most patients exhibit hypoxemia.

The mechanism of the hypoxemia of PE has been something of a puzzle. After all, the direct effect of an embolus is to block perfusion to a segment of lung, thereby creating dead space, which would be expected to cause an increase in arterial Pco_2. However, most patients with PE respond to the elevation of Pco_2 and to other physical or chemical stimuli produced by the PE with a robust increase in ventilation, and they often present with hypocarbia, not hypercarbia. Nonetheless, it is important to keep in mind that, in patients who are unable to respond to the ventilatory stimulus, as in those paralyzed on a ventilator, with respiratory depression, or with underlying lung disease, or in those who have extensive pulmonary vascular obstruction, hypercarbia may be seen and should be recognized as a possible clue to a large PE.[43]

The finding of hypoxemia therefore has been somewhat mysterious and was attributed to many causes until the advent of the MIGET, which was able to untangle the contribution of low V/Q, shunt, and diffusion limitation. In one of the most comprehensive MIGET studies,[44] seven patients with large PEs were studied, with a pulmonary artery catheter to measure cardiac output and collect mixed venous blood. The patients were studied from 1 to 9 days after the PEs, which were large enough to occlude 35–65% of the pulmonary circulation. The mean arterial PO_2 was 67 ± 11 mm Hg (with all patients on room air except for two on FIO_2 0.3), and the PCO_2 was 30 ± 4 mm Hg. In the patients studied soon after the PE, the major oxygenation defect was an increase in perfusion to low V/Q units, without shunt. In the patients studied later, who at that time had opacities or atelectasis on chest radiographs, shunt had developed (from 3–17%). Nonetheless, the abnormalities identified were not large and, by themselves, were not thought sufficient to account for all the hypoxemia. The additional contribution was attributed to a low mixed venous PO_2 of 27 ± 5 mm Hg, associated with a depressed cardiac index (2.8 ± 0.9 L/min/m²). These investigators proposed that the low V/Q was created by redirection of perfusion to nonobstructed units, creating low V/Q areas by an increase in perfusion, although a decrease in ventilation from bronchoconstriction could also have participated. The shunt was seen when opacities or atelectasis appeared, likely reflecting the loss of surfactant. In addition, in the setting of the venous admixture caused by perfusion to low V/Q and shunt, mixed venous PO_2 became an important determinant of the arterial PO_2, as also emphasized in other studies.[45] Diffusion limitation was not found. As expected, dead space ventilation had doubled (from the calculated normal in these patients of 27% to an elevated 52%), but the ventilation had increased significantly (to 18 ± 7 L/min), thus accounting for the hypocarbia seen. Other studies, using MIGET in dogs with experimental emboli[46,47] and using quantitative V/Q scans in patients with PE,[48] have provided supporting evidence of the role of overperfusion of nonoccluded areas in generating low V/Q areas and hypoxemia in PE.

All the studies mentioned were in humans or animals with no known lung disease. In those with preexisting lung disease, the impact of PE is less well studied but likely to be more harmful. A presentation with severe hypoxemia also raises the possibility of an intracardiac shunt. Elevated pulmonary resistance and right-sided pressures can open a patent foramen ovale (PFO), leading to right-to-left shunting. A PFO can be identified in 9–24% of individuals.[49–51] Case reports have emphasized how a patient with PE can present with or develop profound hypoxemia resistant to increases in FIO_2, thereby leading to consideration of a PFO.[52–54] In these reports, efforts were directed to decrease pulmonary artery pressures by using inhaled nitric oxide, lytic agents, or surgical embolectomy. It is possible that, given the high prevalence of PFO, contribution by intracardiac shunting may also be a factor in less dramatic cases.

PNEUMOTHORAX

Hypoxemia is a common finding in pneumothorax, but the mechanism is still not well understood. In a study reported before the era of MIGET,[55] 12 patients were investigated. Nine of these patients had a PO_2 less than 80 mm Hg. In this study, the investigators estimated that the main mechanism of hypoxemia was shunt, which ranged from 2–27% and appeared to increase with the size of the pneumothorax.

ASTHMA OR COPD

Hypoxemia in these common airway diseases is mainly the result of low V/Q units. In asthma, hypoxemia is common,[56] and it can persist for up to 1 week or more after an acute attack.[57] As expected, the mild to moderate hypoxemia is usually responsive to small amounts of supplemental oxygen. In asthma, interestingly, the V/Q abnormalities do not correlate well with abnormalities in *forced expiratory volume in 1 second* (FEV₁), thus raising the suggestion that the low V/Q units are caused by abnormalities in small airways (e.g., resulting from mucus plugging), whereas the low FEV₁ reflects abnormalities in the medium to large airways (e.g., resulting from bronchoconstriction).[58,59] As support for this idea, bronchodilator therapy can improve the FEV₁ without improving the V/Q, which can stay the same or even worsen.[58,60]

In COPD, three different patterns of V/Q disturbance have been described[61] (see Chapter 10 and Fig. 10.21). Type A had predominantly high V/Q units, consistent with an emphysematous pattern and little if any hypoxemia. Type B, however, had increased perfusion to low V/Q units, most consistent with a chronic bronchitis pattern, and with significant hypoxemia. The third pattern had features of both types A and B. No shunt or diffusion abnormality was found, thus addressing controversies long held about the gas exchange abnormalities in COPD, especially because of the decreased single-breath diffusing capacity for carbon monoxide. As in asthma, the low V/Q did not correlate closely with the degree of airway obstruction.[62]

Even at rest, mixed venous PO_2 can have a large role on the arterial PO_2 in patients with COPD,[63] an effect that can be exacerbated with exercise[64] (see later). With exacerbations, gas exchange worsens, with increasing hypoxemia resulting from an increase in perfusion to low V/Q units in addition to a reduction in the mixed venous PO_2, primarily because of the increased work of the respiratory muscles.[65] Hypoventilation also depresses arterial PO_2 and should be considered as a possible mechanism for hypoxemia in patients with COPD. Again, no diffusion limitation has been identified.

INTERSTITIAL LUNG DISEASE OR IDIOPATHIC PULMONARY FIBROSIS

Hypoxemia in interstitial lung disease appears to be primarily the result of perfusion to low V/Q units, at least at rest. Although the restriction in the vascular bed reduces the transit time of erythrocytes through the capillaries, there is minimal to no diffusion limitation at rest. With exercise, the V/Q abnormalities do not change significantly, and the drop in arterial P_{O_2} is caused by both a drop in mixed venous P_{O_2} and a diffusion limitation created by the rapid transit and inability to recruit additional vessels.[28,66,67] This is one of the few lung diseases in which a diffusion limitation can be demonstrated at sea level.[68] The decrease in oxygenation with exercise is a reasonable marker of severity of disease.

ACUTE RESPIRATORY DISTRESS SYNDROME

In contrast to the conditions already discussed, *acute respiratory distress syndrome* (ARDS) is characterized by a large shunt. In an early MIGET study of ARDS,[69] 16 patients were shown to have shunt along with very low V/Q areas as a cause of the profound hypoxemia; only 52% of the cardiac output flowed to areas with normal V/Q. No diffusion limitation was present. The well-known consequence of this is that increases in inspired oxygen have little effect on the hypoxemia. Instead, the goal must be to decrease the shunt (see Fig. 44.4). In this same study, the effect of PEEP was studied, and PEEP was found to improve oxygenation by decreasing shunt. Later studies have confirmed these early findings.[70]

PEEP decreases shunt by opening and maintaining alveoli open, thereby transforming areas of shunt into areas with access to at least some ventilation (see Chapter 135). Other maneuvers, such as improving perfusion of ventilated areas by using inhaled vasodilators or decreasing perfusion to unventilated regions by using pulmonary vasoconstrictors, have been attempted to decrease shunting. Prone positioning often improves oxygenation (see later).

OBESITY

Hypoxemia is common in morbidly obese patients, and it is thought to result from the lower lung volumes and increased closing volume interfering with ventilation of the lung bases (see Chapters 10 and 131). One review[71] reported that the arterial P_{O_2} of 768 patients with an average body mass index of 48 kg/m^2 was 81 mm Hg (range, 50 to 95 mm Hg). With every 5 to 6 kg of weight loss, the arterial P_{O_2} rose by 1 mm Hg. In a study of 19 morbidly obese women (body mass index 45 kg/m^2), the average arterial P_{O_2} was 76 ± 2 mm Hg; when these women were studied again after bariatric surgery, with a drop in body mass index to 31 kg/m^2, the arterial P_{O_2} rose to 89 ± 2 mm Hg.[72] The MIGET identified a small shunt (4.3 ± 1.1%) and low V/Q areas as the major abnormalities, with improvement in both with weight loss. Interestingly, an earlier study using radioactive tracers for perfusion and ventilation showed that, in upright obese individuals with a low expiratory reserve volume, the ventilation tracer was reduced to the lower lobes, whereas the perfusion tracer was distributed predominantly to the lower lobes. Thus, it could be seen that the base of the lung of the upright obese person was an area of low V/Q or shunt.[73]

HEPATOPULMONARY SYNDROME

Hepatopulmonary syndrome is defined by an increased $(A-a)P_{O_2}$ in the setting of advanced liver disease or portal hypertension, and its severity is based on the level of arterial P_{O_2} (see Chapter 126).[74] Pulse oximetry has been shown to be insensitive, so arterial blood gas analysis is

needed to assess oxygenation.[75] The syndrome appears to involve primarily a loss of vasoregulation of pulmonary and systemic vasculature, with pulmonary capillary and precapillary dilation (see Fig. 126.1 and eFigs. 126.1 and 126.2). The role of vasoactivity is supported by the reversibility of abnormalities in V/Q and shunt with liver transplantation.[76]

The causes of the hypoxemia have been difficult to pin down, and all three mechanisms of the abnormal lung—low V/Q, shunt, and diffusion limitation—may participate and may vary with severity of disease. One source of confusion is that patients often have evidence of vascular shunting because of the transit of bubbles in contrast echocardiography, and yet they can respond to supplemental oxygen, which is not consistent with true shunt.

Low V/Q, most investigators agree, is the major mechanism of hypoxemia. This would explain the frequent response to supplemental oxygen. In patients with orthodeoxia, V/Q abnormalities have been shown to worsen with the upright position, because of increased perfusion at the bases.[77,78] In one MIGET study of patients with cirrhosis and a normal arterial P_{O_2}, increased perfusion of low V/Q units was confirmed.[79]

Diffusion limitation may contribute to hypoxemia. Due to both the vasodilation in certain areas and the high cardiac output seen with cirrhosis, the transit time of erythrocytes is reduced, and the distance from the alveolar gas to the erythrocytes, which tend to localize in the center of the flow in the dilated capillaries, is increased. MIGET studies have neither confirmed nor excluded this possibility.[78] A diffusion limitation would also be consistent with the response to oxygen in many patients.

Shunt may also be a feature, especially in patients with more severe hypoxemia. In a MIGET study of cirrhotic patients with severe hypoxemia (arterial P_{O_2} between 35 and 67 mm Hg upright), the major abnormality described was shunt.[78] Shunt is certainly suggested by the passage of bubbles or macroaggregated albumin through the lung but, even in these patients, there may be a response to 100% oxygen. This finding suggests that, at high inspired oxygen, the shunt can behave more like an area of low V/Q or diffusion limitation. Support for this concept has come from studies in which shunt measured by two methods was found to give different results. In one study of eight patients with hepatopulmonary syndrome and hypoxemia (arterial P_{O_2} 61.5 ± 4.5 mm Hg), the average shunt fraction measured by the transit of macroaggregates of technetium-99m–labeled albumin was 32%; however, the shunt fraction measured by the standard 100% oxygen technique was only 19%.[80] This finding indicated that there was some response to the 100% oxygen, thus reducing the calculation of shunt. There was heterogeneity, however; in some patients with cirrhosis, the shunt measurements were similar whereas, in others, they were quite different. Such variation suggests that the dilated vessels may differ either in size or location and may create either a pure shunt unresponsive to high F_{IO_2} or more of a low V/Q or diffusion limitation that can be overcome by high F_{IO_2}. This response to oxygen in areas thought to have shunt was also described in a patient with pulmonary telangiectasias; in this patient, the response to 100% oxygen led to an underestimation of shunt, when compared with the shunt measured by radionuclide studies.[81] Thus, in patients with either hepatopulmonary syndrome or telangiectasias, there may be a shunt-like mechanism of hypoxemia, in which vascular shunts can be detected by the transit of large particles through the lung, but they can also act as an area of low V/Q or diffusion limitation when they respond to high FIO_2.[81]

CORONAVIRUS DISEASE 2019

The novel coronavirus, severe acute respiratory syndrome coronavirus type 2, which causes COVID-19, can induce significant hypoxemia, sometimes without dyspnea or other respiratory symptoms. This can be a striking presentation, and it has been addressed recently by Tobin and colleagues.[5] The possible reasons for the lack of dyspnea in at least some patients include the following: (1) an insensitivity of the hypoxemic ventilatory response until arterial PO_2 drops to quite low values (see Fig. 44.2), (2) the large variability in response seen, even among healthy individuals, (3) the decrease of this ventilatory or dyspnea response with age and with diabetes, and (4) the blunting of the ventilatory response if the arterial PCO_2 is also low.

So, what is the cause of the hypoxemia? The reasons for the hypoxemia are currently unknown, and no MIGET study has yet been carried out. Clearly, shunt is a large component. It has been estimated at 50%, although the average fraction of consolidated lung is much less, at only 17%. This ratio of the degree of shunt to the apparent lung consolidation (approximately 3) is greater than that of ARDS (approximately 1.25).[82] The virus may cause pulmonary vasodilation in the nonaerated lung, either by a direct effect on the vessels or by an indirect interference with hypoxic pulmonary vasoconstriction. PEs may also develop[83] and redirect blood to poorly aerated regions. Suggestions have been put forward that there is pulmonary vasodilation seen on dual-energy computed tomography scanning[84] and that there is increased transit of bubbles through the lung[85] although, in a larger study of 60 critically ill patients, transpulmonary shunt was found in only 20% of patients.[86] The response to prone positioning suggests that the shunt behaves similarly to that of ARDS.

APPROACHES TO HYPOXEMIA

INCREASED INSPIRED OXYGEN

The first response of the clinician to hypoxemia is likely to provide supplemental oxygen. The response to that supplemental oxygen will guide the next steps (see Fig. 44.3). Noninvasive oxygen support can be provided from low-flow nasal prongs up to high-flow nasal cannulae (discussed in detail in Chapter 137). When shunts are large, intubation and mechanical ventilation may be necessary to decrease shunt, thus allowing FIO_2 to be given at safer levels (e.g., $FIO_2 \leq 0.6$) (discussed in Chapters 134 and 135).

LATERAL POSITIONING

Lateral positioning can improve oxygenation in several types of unilateral lung abnormalities, including pneumonia,[87] postthoracotomy status,[88] and pleural effusion.[89]

In a study of nine patients with atelectasis or opacities in one lung, the lateral "good lung down" position led to increases of arterial PO_2 from an average of 67 mm Hg in the supine position to 106 mm Hg.[87] The positional effect resolved when the underlying unilateral abnormality resolved. In nine patients with unilateral pleural effusions, the arterial PO_2 rose from 66.7 to 71.9 mm Hg when the patient was moved from the effusion side down to the normal side down.[89] The general conclusion of these studies is that having the normal lung down can increase arterial PO_2, presumably because of an increase in perfusion to better-ventilated areas. Few studies using MIGET have been applied to study this question: in one MIGET study of four patients undergoing mechanical ventilation with respiratory failure and unilateral opacities (three postoperative), improvements with the good lung down were the result of improved V/Q matching or decreased shunt, or both.[90]

PRONING

For patients with ARDS, the prone position increases the arterial PO_2, which remains elevated while the patient is prone (see also Chapters 133 to 135 and Fig. 134.7). Given that hypoxemia in patients with ARDS is predominantly the result of shunting, it has long been assumed that the prone position reduces shunt. Indeed, in one study using MIGET, patients with ARDS who responded to proning demonstrated a decrease in shunt of $11 \pm 5\%$, whereas patients who did not respond had no change in shunt.[90a] How is this accomplished? Most studies of patients and of animal models point to the following key benefits of the prone position: (1) a more even ventilation of the lung, with the sternum fixed and stiffened against the bed, with less compression by the heart on the left lower lobe, and with less effect of abdominal pressure; in combination with (2) a more even perfusion of the lung,[91] with continued perfusion of the dorsal region even in the prone position as a result of inherent geometric or other structural reasons[92] (Fig. 44.6). Novel imaging studies have confirmed that ventilation and perfusion are more evenly distributed, with less heterogeneity in the prone position (Fig. 44.6). The reasons for this are complicated but many studies concur that, in the prone position, there is a reduction in low V/Q areas and in shunt.[93] Although the reasons for the mortality benefit in patients with ARDS are not known, improved survival may not be related to the improved arterial PO_2 or lower FIO_2 but rather to the improved pulmonary mechanics.[93]

IMPROVING MIXED VENOUS PARTIAL PRESSURE OF OXYGEN

When efforts to improve V/Q matching and decrease shunt have been maximized, there is still another strategy to improve hypoxemia, that is, by improving mixed venous PO_2.[95] The greater the venous admixture, the more benefit any improvement of mixed venous PO_2 will have on the arterial PO_2. Options to improve mixed venous PO_2 are either to increase oxygen delivery (e.g., improve cardiac output, increase hematocrit) or to decrease oxygen utilization (e.g., sedate, paralyze, or cool the patient). As was pointed out, in settings of a large venous admixture,

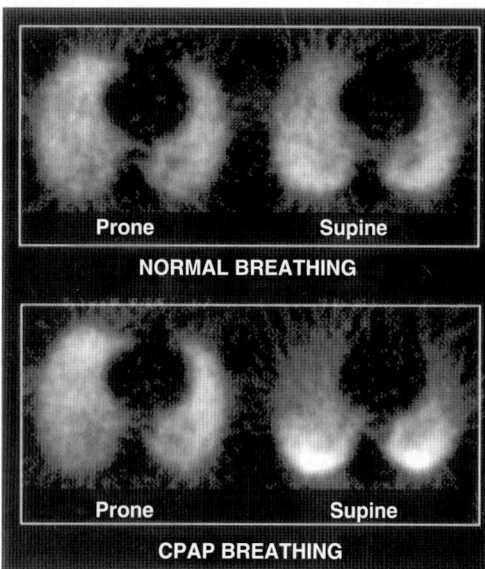

Figure 44.6 Images of single-photon emission computed tomography showing perfusion in prone and supine positions. This volunteer with healthy lungs lay supine or prone during infusion of macroaggregates of technetium-99m designed to lodge in the pulmonary capillaries. Then the subject was imaged in the supine position to detect where the macroaggregates had distributed. The image shows the heterogeneous perfusion of the lung in the supine position (normal breathing) that became more obvious during continuous positive airway pressure (CPAP) breathing. The perfusion was more homogeneous when the subject was in the prone position. (From Nyren S, Mure M, Jacobsson H, Larsson SA, Lindahl SG. Pulmonary perfusion is more uniform in the prone than in the supine position: scintigraphy in healthy humans. *J Applied Physiol.* 1999;86:1135-1141.)

sudden drops in arterial P_{O_2} may most likely be caused by sudden drops in mixed venous P_{O_2}.[29,95]

In patients with anemia, transfusion could be expected to improve oxygen delivery, mixed venous P_{O_2} and, in patients with venous admixture, arterial P_{O_2}. However, this has not been a consistent finding. In a study evaluating 29 patients with sepsis who were in the intensive care unit, transfusion of a mean of 1.4 units of packed red blood cells increased the hemoglobin from 8.1 to 9.4 g/dL; however, this increase in hemoglobin was not found to change the mixed venous oxygen saturation, thus indicating that the transfusion was not effective in improving arterial oxygenation.[96] The role of transfusion is still controversial, and may be limited by the high oxygen affinity of stored blood[96a] or may be better targeted, as for example to patients with lower central venous oxygen.[96b] Finally, the ultimate approach to raise the mixed venous P_{O_2} is with extracorporeal membrane oxygenation (see Chapter 138).

POSITIVE END-EXPIRATORY PRESSURE

As described earlier, PEEP has been shown by many studies to decrease shunt. PEEP is extensively discussed in Chapter 135.

Increases in PEEP can paradoxically act to decrease oxygenation.[97] A decrease in oxygenation may be caused by impairment in cardiac output and lowering of mixed venous P_{O_2}, by the redirecting of perfusion from more compliant areas to consolidated areas, by the advent of pneumothorax or other complication, or by the opening

of a PFO.[98] Shunting through a PFO has been found in 19.2% of patients with ARDS.[98] The opening of a large PFO would make lowering the pulmonary artery pressures a priority.

CLINICAL TESTS

EXERCISE

Exercise assesses the entire cardiovascular-pulmonary system and reveals abnormalities that may not be evident at rest. In patients with abnormal lungs, exercise may lead to hypoxemia, which is often used as a guide for oxygen therapy. The causes of this hypoxemia have been found to differ by the underlying disease.

In COPD, V/Q matching and shunt do not show consistent changes with exercise, at least in the patients with severe COPD who have been studied. No problems have been identified with diffusion limitation. Instead, two factors appear most important. The mixed venous P_{O_2}, which may be low in these patients even at rest,[63] falls further and is a large contributor to the ultimate fall in arterial oxygen.[64] This reduction, which can be seen in healthy individuals at the onset of exercise,[99] may account for a rapid drop in arterial P_{O_2} with exercise. In addition, hypoventilation may decrease alveolar and arterial P_{O_2}.

In fibrotic lung diseases, there are some similar findings in that the abnormalities in V/Q and shunt have not been shown to change with exercise. Unlike in COPD, hypoventilation is not a factor (at least until the fibrotic or restrictive disease is at the end stage). However, the fall in mixed venous P_{O_2} is an important factor. As mentioned, there is also evidence that a diffusion limitation contributes in that the diffusion of oxygen is not complete across the blood-gas barrier during exercise.[100]

CONTRAST ECHOCARDIOGRAPHY

Contrast echocardiography is used to evaluate for the presence of vascular shunts, either intracardiac or intrapulmonary (see Chapter 88). The use of a reflective particle, usually an air bubble (~30 μm diameter), allows detection of flow that bypasses the pulmonary capillaries (~7 μm diameter) and reaches the left ventricle.[101] The timing of the appearance may help to distinguish an intracardiac shunt (appearance with fewer than 3 beats) compared with an intrapulmonary vascular shunt (3 to 6 beats), although the accuracy of this distinction has been questioned.[101] This technique would detect the intrapulmonary vascular shunts coming from arteriovenous malformation, hepatopulmonary syndrome and, perhaps, COVID-19. However, it will not detect shunting in many conditions, such as ARDS and pneumonia, in which a normal pulmonary vasculature is supplying collapsed or fluid-filled alveoli, the so-called parenchymal shunting.[26]

BREATHING 100% OXYGEN

Breathing 100% oxygen until the nitrogen has been flushed from the alveoli creates a known alveolar P_{O_2} and enables the shunt to be calculated. With this technique, healthy individuals can be shown to have some amount of shunt, from less than 8.3%[102] to 9.5%.[103] This may be a slight overestimation because the oxygen may itself create microatelectasis by flushing out the nitrogen or may blunt hypoxic pulmonary vasoconstriction, or because of technical issues, such as tiny leaks. This test should be carried out in a controlled environment such as a pulmonary function laboratory, where any leaks can be scrupulously avoided and the procedure standardized.

As described earlier, the test may underestimate shunt in the setting of arteriovenous malformation, when compared with contrast echocardiography. In a study of patients with hereditary hemorrhagic telangiectasia, 210 patients underwent both contrast echocardiography and 100% oxygen breathing; the 100% oxygen shunt test detected only 51% of patients with arteriovenous malformation.[104] This finding may reflect the ability of oxygen to reach the blood in some of these abnormal vessels, as in the case of hepatopulmonary syndrome, and thus reduce the calculated shunt. Breathing 100% oxygen therefore has limitations when used for calculating intraparenchymal vascular shunts.

SLEEP

Hypoxemia is common during sleep. In healthy individuals, the decrease in ventilation with sleep rarely causes hypoxemia because the oxygen saturation is on the flat portion of the oxyhemoglobin dissociation curve (see Fig. 44.1). However, in persons who have an arterial P_{O_2} close to the steep portion of the curve, sleep, especially rapid eye movement sleep, can lead to a precipitous fall in oxygen saturation (see Chapters 117 and 119). Therefore, the changes during sleep may be of clinical significance for any patient with a lowered arterial P_{O_2}, no matter the underlying cause. Indeed, there may be value in screening patients for hypoxemia during sleep instead of during exercise, as, for example, in patients with COPD who do not meet criteria during wakefulness for supplemental oxygen.

Key Points

- Hypoxemia is generally considered a reduced level of oxygen saturation. It is not the same as hypoxia, which is an inadequate amount of oxygen at the tissues and recognized by elevations in lactate and end-organ ischemia.
- The ventilatory response to hypoxemia is hyperbolic, with a large response only at low arterial partial pressure of oxygen. This is also variable among individuals and reduced with age, thus making the response to hypoxemia insensitive and unpredictable.
- When a patient is receiving supplemental oxygen, the pulse oximeter becomes insensitive to hypoventilation.
- With a patient receiving supplemental oxygen, hypoventilation renders the patient increasingly dependent on the supplied oxygen; its removal can precipitate profound hypoxemia.

- Hypoxemia can be caused by five mechanisms: three are associated with abnormal lungs (low ventilation-perfusion, shunt, diffusion limitation), and two are associated with a low alveolar partial pressure of oxygen (hypoventilation, low inspired fractional concentration of oxygen in inspired gas).
- Hypoxemia in most lung diseases is due to perfusion of low ventilation-perfusion units, either because of decreases in ventilation to perfused units, as in asthma or COPD, or because of increases in perfusion to ventilated areas, as from redistribution of blood due to pulmonary embolism.
- In the initial approach to a patient with hypoxemia, the first step is to give added inspired oxygen; if the patient fails to respond, this likely indicates a major contribution of shunt.
- A large shunt has two clinical consequences: (1) hypoxemia will be resistant to inspired oxygen, and (2) arterial P_{O_2} will become increasingly dependent on the level of mixed venous P_{O_2}.
- Prone positioning acts to decrease shunt by reducing low ventilation-perfusion areas and shunt, by making both ventilation and perfusion more even from top to bottom.

Acknowledgment

We thank Dr. Nirav Bhakta for his careful review and suggestions.

Key Readings

Fu ES, Downs JB, Schweiger JW, Miguel RV, Smith RA. Supplemental oxygen impairs detection of hypoventilation by pulse oximetry. *Chest.* 2004;126(5):1552–1558.

Huet Y, Lemaire F, Brun-Buisson C, et al. Hypoxemia in acute pulmonary embolism. *Chest.* 1985;88(6):829–836.

Johnson NJ, Luks AM, Glenny RW. Gas exchange in the prone posture. *Respir Care.* 2017;62(8):1097–1110.

Petersson J, Glenny RW. Gas exchange and ventilation-perfusion relationships in the lung. *Eur Respir J.* 2014;44(4):1023–1041.

Schnapp LM, Cohen NH. Pulse oximetry. Uses and abuses. *Chest.* 1990;98(5):1244–1250.

Tobin MJ, Laghi F, Jubran A. Why COVID-19 silent hypoxemia is baffling to physicians. *Am J Respir Crit Care Med.* 2020;202(3):356–360.

Velthuis S, Vorselaars VM, Westermann CJ, Snijder RJ, Mager JJ, Post MC. Pulmonary shunt fraction measurement compared to contrast echocardiography in hereditary haemorrhagic telangiectasia patients: time to abandon the 100% oxygen method? *Respiration.* 2015;89(2):112–118.

Wagner PD, Laravuso RB, Uhl RR, West JB. Continuous distributions of ventilation-perfusion ratios in normal subjects breathing air and 100 per cent O2. *J Clin Invest.* 1974;54(1):54–68.

Walley KR. Use of central venous oxygen saturation to guide therapy. *Am J Respir Crit Care Med.* 2011;184(5):514–520.

Complete reference list available at ExpertConsult.com.

45 *HYPERCAPNIA*

BERNIE Y. SUNWOO, MBBS • BABAK MOKHLESI, MD, MSC

INTRODUCTION

Hypercapnia is defined as a *partial pressure of carbon dioxide in arterial blood* (arterial P_{CO_2}) greater than 45 mm Hg (6.0 kPa) at sea level. The lungs function to move oxygen from the air into the mixed venous blood and eliminate CO_2 from mixed venous blood back into the air. Hypercapnia results when there is a failure of this gas exchange function. Hypercapnia can appear acutely or develop gradually, typically first manifesting during sleep. This chapter discusses the causes of hypercapnia mechanistically, highlighting the complex interplay of the central respiratory controller, effectors, ventilation-perfusion relationship, and sensors in maintaining carbon dioxide homeostasis. Hypercapnia can affect multiple organ systems and timely recognition is important. The clinical manifestations of hypercapnia are discussed, focusing on a diagnostic approach to a patient with suspected hypercapnia. Finally, the chapter outlines an approach to the management of hypercapnia.

NORMAL CARBON DIOXIDE HOMEOSTASIS

Carbon dioxide is a by-product of aerobic cellular metabolism. It is estimated the human body contains 120 L of CO_2 and it is present in all fluids and tissues.[1,2] The partial pressure of carbon dioxide in arterial blood is proportional to the rate of CO_2 production and inversely proportional to the rate of CO_2 elimination as determined by alveolar ventilation. Alveolar ventilation is the component of expired minute ventilation that reaches perfused alveoli to participate in effective gas exchange and is equal to the minute ventilation minus dead space ventilation.

The alveolar ventilation equation:

$$P_{aCO_2} = \frac{k \cdot \dot{V}_{CO_2}}{\dot{V}_A}$$

$$= \frac{k \cdot \dot{V}_{CO_2}}{\dot{V}_E \times (1 - V_D/V_T)}$$

$$= \frac{k \cdot \dot{V}_{CO_2}}{(f)(V_T) \times (1 - V_D/V_T)}$$

where P_{aCO_2} is arterial P_{CO_2}, K is the proportionality constant, $\dot{V}_{CO_2}$ is CO_2 production (in L/min), $\dot{V}_A$ is alveolar ventilation (in L/min), $\dot{V}_E$ is minute ventilation (in L/min), f is breathing frequency (in breaths/min), V_T is tidal volume (in L), and V_D/V_T is dead space ratio. Normally, under steady-state conditions, the rate of CO_2 production equals CO_2 elimination via the respiratory system to maintain an arterial P_{CO_2} between 35 and 45 mm Hg.

MECHANISMS AND ETIOLOGIES

Mechanistically, hypercapnia results from loss of arterial P_{CO_2} homeostasis caused by:
1. Increased CO_2 production
2. Decreased minute ventilation from disorders of the central respiratory controller or respiratory system effectors
3. Increased dead space ventilation from increased anatomic dead space or ventilation-perfusion mismatch (increased physiologic dead space)

Often multiple mechanisms are involved, especially as hypercapnia progresses.

INCREASED CO_2 PRODUCTION

CO_2 is a product of cellular metabolism and, in adults, approximately 3 to 4 mL/kg/min of CO_2 is produced at rest. CO_2 production can rise with increased levels of activity, hypermetabolic states such as fever (13% increase in arterial P_{CO_2} for every 1°C increase in temperature above normal), thyrotoxicosis, increased catabolism such as sepsis and corticosteroids, metabolic acidosis, and carbohydrate loads or overfeeding.[3-5] Normally, however, ventilation can be increased to offset the increase in CO_2 production and maintain a normal arterial P_{CO_2}. Consequently, increased CO_2 production alone does not typically result in significant hypercapnia unless the individual has impaired ventilatory capacity that limits the ability to augment ventilation. Increased CO_2 production, however, can be a contributing factor to the development of hypercapnia.

DECREASED MINUTE VENTILATION

The respiratory system is a feedback system that consists of a central respiratory controller that processes afferent inputs from various sensors to generate signals to

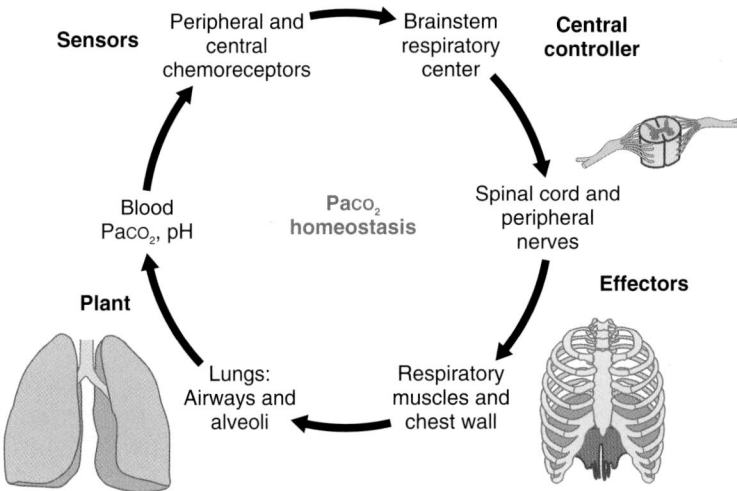

Sensors — Peripheral and central chemoreceptors → Brainstem respiratory center — **Central controller**

Pa_{CO_2} homeostasis

Spinal cord and peripheral nerves

Effectors

Blood Pa_{CO_2}, pH

Plant

Lungs: Airways and alveoli ← Respiratory muscles and chest wall

Figure 45.1 Homeostatic regulation of arterial P_{CO_2}. The respiratory feedback system consists of a central respiratory controller that processes afferent inputs from various sensors to generate signals to the effectors of the respiratory system, to maintain tight homeostatic regulation of arterial P_{CO_2} (Pa_{CO_2}). In a closed-loop system, the plant produces the signal (blood gases) sent to the sensors.

the effectors of the respiratory system, to maintain tight homeostatic regulation of arterial P_{CO_2} (Fig. 45.1). The central respiratory control center in the medulla and pons of the brainstem generates a respiratory rhythm. In particular, the pre-Botzinger complex in the ventrolateral region of the medulla appears to be crucial for the generation of this intrinsic rhythm. It is influenced by behavioral and cognitive inputs from the cortex. The central respiratory control center receives afferent signals from peripheral chemoreceptors at the carotid artery bifurcation and central chemoreceptors in the brain, close to the ventral surface of the medulla in the caudal region of the retrotrapezoid nucleus, to respond to changes in pH, arterial P_{CO_2}, and arterial P_{O_2}. The central respiratory center also receives input from the lungs and other receptors but, under normal conditions, the arterial P_{CO_2} is the most important factor in the control of ventilation. Hypercapnia stimulates neural output from the central respiratory control center within the brainstem to the effectors of the respiratory system: motor neurons in the spinal cord, motor nerves, neuromuscular junction, respiratory muscles, and chest wall. The diaphragm is the main muscle of inspiration and is innervated by the phrenic nerve supplied by cervical nerve roots C3 to C5. Contraction of the diaphragm expands the rib cage, causing the pleural and airway pressures to become more negative. Inspiratory airflow is generated resulting in the movement of gas into the lungs where gases can exchange at the alveolar-capillary membrane to eliminate CO_2.

Minute ventilation ($\dot{V}_E$) is the product of respiratory rate (f) and tidal volume (V_T) and it can be reduced by perturbation anywhere along this axis from the central respiratory control center in the brainstem to the respiratory muscles and chest wall. A reduction in total $\dot{V}_E$ with constant CO_2 production and dead space will lead to hypercapnia. Hypercapnia due to reduced minute ventilation can be associated with normal lungs and can mechanistically be divided into disorders of the central respiratory controller or disorders of the respiratory system effectors.

Disorders of the central respiratory controller are characterized by a reduced drive to breathe (i.e., "won't breathe"). Common causes of hypercapnia due to disorders of central respiratory control are outlined in Table 45.1.

Because the brainstem generates respiratory drive, pathologies involving the medulla and pons, such as stroke, encephalitis, neoplasm, and multiple sclerosis, can impair automatic respiratory rhythm and produce specific abnormal patterns of respiration. Medullary lesions have been associated with irregular breathing variable in rate and tidal volume or ataxic breathing, while lesions in the pons can cause sustained deep inspiration followed by brief expiration or apneustic breathing.[6] Similarly, pathologies involving the cerebral cortex can disrupt behavioral input to the control of respiration, thereby leading to hypercapnia.

The pre-Botzinger complex in the brainstem has also been identified as a major site of action mediating the respiratory depressive effects of opioids.[7,8] Opioids have been associated with central depression of the respiratory rate, amplitude, and reflex responses and reduced brain arousability.[8] Various abnormal breathing patterns, including ataxic breathing, Biot's breathing (high-frequency and regular tidal volume breathing interspersed with periods of apnea), Cheyne-Stokes respiration, and both central and obstructive sleep apnea have been described.[8] With the epidemic of opioid use, recognition of opioids and sedatives such as benzodiazepines as a cause for impaired central ventilatory drive and hypercapnia is important.

Congenital central hypoventilation syndrome (CCHS) is a rare disorder characterized by disordered respiratory control and diffuse *autonomic nervous system dysregulation* (ANSD). It is caused by a mutation in the paired-like homeobox 2B (*PHOX2B*) gene, which encodes for a transcription factor that plays a role in the development of the autonomic nervous system and regulation of neural crest cell migration.[9,10] A well-described relationship between *PHOX2B* genotype and CCHS phenotype exists. CCHS is a clinically heterogeneous disorder that can present with a spectrum of severity of hypoventilation and autonomic nervous system dysregulation. Hypoventilation is seen during non-REM sleep but, when more severe, can be present both during wakefulness and sleep. While typically diagnosed in newborns with episodes of cyanosis and apnea, patients can present as old as 35 years with late-onset CCHS, a variable presentation thought to reflect the variable penetrance of *PHOX2B* mutations.[11] Moreover, with advancements in knowledge and treatment, CCHS patients are now

Table 45.1   Causes of Hypercapnia Due to Decreased Minute Ventilation

Mechanism	Etiologies	
Decreased central respiratory drive (won't breathe)	Opioids and sedatives, brainstem and cerebral pathology (e.g., stroke, encephalitis, neoplasm, multiple sclerosis), congenital (e.g., congenital central alveolar hypoventilation), myxedema, metabolic alkalosis, hypothermia, obesity hypoventilation syndrome	
Disorders of the respiratory system effectors (can't breathe)	Spinal cord	Trauma, compressive (e.g., cervical spondylosis, herniated disc), vascular (e.g., infarction or hemorrhage), developmental (e.g., syringomyelia), inflammatory (e.g., transverse myelitis, multiple sclerosis), infectious, neoplasm
	Motor neurons/anterior horn cells	Motor neuron disease, spinal muscular atrophy, poliomyelitis, primary lateral sclerosis, hereditary biochemical, metabolic, toxins (e.g., lead)
	Peripheral nerves	Iatrogenic phrenic nerve injury (e.g., cardiothoracic or neck surgery), hereditary (e.g., Charcot-Marie-Tooth disease), inflammatory (e.g., Guillain-Barré syndrome, neuralgic amyotrophy or Parsonage-Turner syndrome, vasculitides), metabolic (e.g., porphyria, diabetes mellitus), critical-illness polyneuropathy, drugs, and toxins (e.g., organophosphates)
	NM junction	Myasthenia gravis, Lambert-Eaton myasthenic syndrome, botulism, drugs (e.g., paralytics)
	Respiratory muscles	Muscular dystrophies, inflammatory (e.g., polymyositis, dermatomyositis), congenital (e.g., nemaline myopathy), glycogen storage diseases (e.g., Pompe disease, McArdle disease, Tarui disease), mitochondrial myopathies, metabolic, drugs, and toxins (e.g., corticosteroids)
	Chest wall	Kyphoscoliosis, pectus excavatum, thoracoplasty, flail chest, ankylosing spondylitis, fibrothorax, obesity hypoventilation syndrome

surviving into adulthood. *Rapid-onset obesity with hypothalamic dysfunction, hypoventilation, and autonomic dysregulation* (ROHHAD) is another rare disorder that shares clinical similarities with CCHS but is a distinct entity. ROHHAD is characterized by dramatic weight gain, typically between ages 1.5 and 10 years, followed by hypothalamic dysfunction, central alveolar hypoventilation, and ANSD.[12]

Disorders of the respiratory system effectors are characterized by reduced ventilatory supply (i.e., "can't breathe"). Disruption at any level of the efferent arm, from the spinal cord to the muscles of respiration and the chest wall, can diminish minute ventilation causing hypercapnia. Causes of hypercapnia due to failure of the respiratory system effectors can be divided anatomically as shown in Table 45.1. See Chapters 130 and 131 for a more detailed discussion on the respiratory system and neuromuscular disease and chest wall diseases, respectively.

INCREASED DEAD SPACE

Following the movement of gas into the lungs, the arterial P_{CO_2} is ultimately determined by the diffusion of CO_2 from mixed venous blood at the alveolar-capillary membrane into alveolar gas, so-called gas exchange. Not all gas entering and leaving the lungs takes part in gas exchange. Minute ventilation participating in gas exchange is referred to as alveolar ventilation. Dead space ventilation reflects the amount of total ventilation that does not contribute to gas exchange and consists of anatomic and physiologic (or alveolar) dead space. Chapter 10 provides details regarding ventilation, blood flow, and gas exchange.

The anatomic dead space is the volume of gas that fills the conducting airways between the upper airways and terminal bronchioles and does not reach the alveolar-capillary membrane to partake in gas exchange. It is commonly expressed as a ratio of the tidal volume. In normal adults, the anatomic dead space is approximately 150 mL; with a tidal volume of approximately 500 mL, the dead space ratio would be approximately 0.3. An increase in the anatomic dead space can result in hypercapnia even when minute ventilation is maintained. It is commonly seen with any cause of rapid shallow breathing in which the anatomic dead space in the central conducting airways comprises a larger proportion of the smaller tidal volume, increasing the dead space to tidal volume ratio.

Even if gas does reach the alveolar-capillary membrane, effective gas exchange and CO_2 elimination requires the coordinated matching of perfusion with ventilation. CO_2 delivered by perfusion to the alveolar-capillary membrane diffuses into the alveolar gas and is removed from the lungs by ventilation. The partial pressure of oxygen and carbon dioxide in each alveolus is determined by its *ratio of ventilation to perfusion* (V/Q). When considering the simple lung model and one gas exchanging unit, ideally V/Q allows CO_2 and O_2 to be exchanged in a ratio equal to that of total lung CO_2 excretion to O_2 intake (respiratory quotient).[2] If an alveolus receives blood flow but no ventilation, V/Q is zero, O_2 cannot enter and CO_2 cannot leave the alveolus by ventilation, and the alveolar P_{O_2} and alveolar P_{CO_2} will be the same as the mixed venous blood, so-called intrapulmonary, right-to-left shunt. If ventilation is intact but perfusion is absent, V/Q is infinity, O_2 cannot leave and CO_2 cannot enter the alveolus from the blood, and the alveolar P_{O_2} and alveolar P_{CO_2} will be the same as in the conducting airways. Any V/Q ratio between zero and infinity can exist in the lung and will produce a unique alveolar P_{O_2} and alveolar P_{CO_2}. As V/Q increases, alveolar P_{CO_2} falls as ventilation removes more of the delivered CO_2; as V/Q decreases, alveolar P_{CO_2} rises and alveolar P_{O_2} falls.[2] Of note, lungs contain about 500 million alveoli with regional variations in ventilation and perfusion, leading to a distribution of V/Q ratios even in normal healthy lungs.[13]

Ventilation-perfusion inequality reduces the efficiency of gas exchange of the lungs. Those lung units with high ventilation-perfusion ratios, which are thus inefficient at eliminating CO_2, constitute a physiologic dead space. Increased physiologic dead space or V/Q mismatch is a common cause of hypercapnia. It is typically associated with abnormal lungs and concomitant hypoxemia. Etiologies include disorders of the pulmonary parenchyma, airways, and vasculature.

Ventilatory Supply and Demand

Typically, an increase in dead space stimulates minute ventilation in an attempt to normalize arterial P_{CO_2}. Normally, the available ventilatory supply significantly exceeds ventilatory demand. As a general rule, the maximum spontaneous ventilation that can be maintained without muscle fatigue (the maximum sustainable ventilation)[14] is approximately one-half the maximum voluntary ventilation.[15,16] Consequently, as ventilatory demand increases, the normally large ventilatory reserve means that hypercapnia does not develop unless fatigue of the respiratory muscles develops or there is reduced ventilatory drive to respond to the increased work of breathing.

Specific Diseases

While the causes of hypercapnia can be divided mechanistically as outlined above, more often than not, the hypercapnia observed in a given patient is multifactorial in etiology. This is highlighted in the following discussion of the more common disorders associated with hypercapnia.

COPD is a common, preventable, and treatable disease characterized by persistent respiratory symptoms and airflow limitation (postbronchodilator FEV_1/FVC <0.70) that is due to airway and/or alveolar abnormalities usually caused by significant exposure to noxious particles or gases. Hypercapnia is associated with a poor prognosis in COPD and can be seen both during acute exacerbations and chronically. Multiple mechanisms have been implicated in the development of hypercapnia in COPD, including ventilation-perfusion inequality and abnormalities in ventilatory control, respiratory muscle function, and pattern of breathing, but ventilation-perfusion mismatch predominates.[3] Airflow obstruction, destruction of the alveoli in emphysema, and reduced lung compliance at high lung volumes all contribute to ventilation-perfusion inequality. Hypercapnic COPD patients have been shown to have lower tidal volumes with unchanged or increased respiratory rate, resulting in normal or decreased total ventilation, increased dead space to tidal volume ratio, and ultimately reduced alveolar ventilation.[3] Whereas the work of breathing is increased, hyperinflation and the associated flattening of the diaphragm place this main muscle of inspiration at a mechanical disadvantage. This predisposes patients to fatigue and the development of hypercapnia.

Obesity hypoventilation syndrome (OHS) is characterized by the development of awake daytime hypercapnia in obese individuals (body mass index >30 kg/m^2) in the absence of other known causes of hypoventilation. The risk of developing OHS increases as body mass index increases. Additionally, the degree of hypercapnia seen in OHS appears to increase with weight. All OHS patients are obese but not all obese patients develop daytime hypercapnia. How and why only a subset of patients with obesity develops persistent daytime hypercapnia has been the subject of ongoing research. The mechanism is also thought to be multifactorial and a complex interplay between obesity-related changes in respiratory mechanics, sleep-disordered breathing, changes in central ventilatory drive, neurohormonal changes, and excessive CO_2 production.

Obesity imposes a mechanical load on the respiratory system resulting in reductions in lung volumes. There is a decrease in the functional residual capacity and expiratory reserve volume.[17-19] This is exacerbated in the supine body position where cephalic displacement of the diaphragm further reduces its mechanical efficiency. In addition, obese patients breathe at low lung volumes closer to the residual volume than do other patients. At these low lung volumes, both pulmonary and chest wall compliance are reduced and there is small airway closure, expiratory flow limitation, and air trapping, leading to an additional increase in the work of breathing and pulmonary ventilation-perfusion inequality. The chronic hypercapnia and hypoxemia seen in OHS has also been implicated in contributing to respiratory muscle impairment. With obesity, there is an approximate threefold increase in the work of breathing.[20-23] Normally the increased workload is offset by an increase in respiratory drive, but in OHS this drive is blunted. OHS has been associated with an acquired reduction in ventilatory responsiveness to hypoxia and hypercapnia.[24-26] Leptin resistance may be one mechanism for this reduced central respiratory drive. Leptin is an adipokine that acts on the hypothalamus both to produce satiety and to stimulate ventilation. In humans, a higher level of leptin is seen in obesity and, compared to weight-matched obese controls, even higher levels of leptin have been reported in OHS. As such, leptin resistance, possibly due to decreased CSF penetration, has been implicated in the development of daytime hypoventilation.[27-30]

Obesity is also a key risk factor for sleep-disordered breathing. Approximately 90% of OHS patients will have *obstructive sleep apnea* (OSA), with 70% having severe OSA defined by an apnea-hypopnea index greater than 30 events per hour of sleep. Studies have repeatedly identified severity of OSA as a risk factor for the development of daytime hypercapnia. A failure of compensation for nocturnal hypercapnia by either the lung or kidney has been proposed in OSA patients who go on to develop chronic daytime hypercapnia. Typically, obstructive apneas and hypopneas result in a transient increase in CO_2, but the obstructive respiratory events are usually followed by arousals and augmented ventilation to eliminate the accumulated CO_2 in order to maintain a steady-state arterial P_{CO_2}. Any imbalance between the duration of obstructive respiratory events and compensatory inter-apnea periods may lead to net CO_2 accumulation and daytime hypercapnia.[31-33] Kidney compensation also plays a role. CO_2 retention is partially offset by renal bicarbonate retention; however, if the excretion of bicarbonate is slow, the net retention of bicarbonate can result in further depression of ventilatory responsiveness to CO_2 during wakefulness. Thus, any compromise in the renal compensatory mechanisms may also contribute to the development of daytime hypercapnia.[23,34,35]

Table 45.2   Consequences of Hypercapnia

System	Effect
Cardiovascular	▪ Decreased cardiac contractility ▪ Decreased systemic vascular resistance ▪ Secondary effects due to sympathoadrenal activation ▪ Coronary vasodilation
Respiratory	▪ Rightward shift of oxyhemoglobin dissociation curve ▪ Pulmonary vasoconstriction (mild) ▪ Direct dilation of small airways ▪ Indirect constriction of large airways ▪ Increased lung compliance ▪ Impaired alveolar fluid reabsorption and alveolar epithelial repair[73]
Central nervous system	▪ Cerebral vasodilation and increased cerebral blood flow ▪ Increased intracranial pressure ▪ Increased cerebral oxygenation ▪ Biochemical changes (e.g., increased glutamine) ▪ Stimulation[39]
Metabolic	▪ Intracellular acidosis causing inhibition of glycolysis ▪ Increased renal bicarbonate resorption
Inflammation and Immunity	▪ Inhibition of neutrophil and macrophage migration and adhesion ▪ Decreased secretion of proinflammatory cytokines ▪ Decreased free radical generation

Data from Weinberger SE, Schwartzstein RM, Weiss JW. Hypercapnia. *N Engl J Med*. 321(18):1223–1231, 1989; and Curley GF KB, Laffey JG. Hypocapnia and hypercapnia. In Broaddus VC, Mason RJ, Ernst JD, et al, editors. *Murray & Nadel's Textbook of Respiratory Medicine*, 6 ed. Philadelphia: Elsevier; 2016.

CONSEQUENCES

The effects of hypercapnia vary depending on rate of development, severity, and duration. Hypercapnia leads to acidosis that suppresses most cellular functions affecting multiple organ systems, as summarized in Table 45.2.[35a]

CLINICAL MANIFESTATIONS AND EVALUATION

Given the consequences of hypercapnia, timely recognition of the symptoms and signs of hypercapnia is essential. History and physical examination should be directed at not only the clinical manifestations of hypercapnia but also its underlying cause.

At its most extreme, hypercapnia can present as respiratory failure, coma, and death. Hypercapnia reduces myocardial contractility, which can lead to progressive cardiovascular instability, arrhythmia, and cardiac arrest. At the other end of the spectrum, hypercapnia may be evident only during sleep.

Sleep is associated with changes in ventilation specific to the sleep stage, additionally described in Chapter 117. In healthy individuals, blunting of the drive to breathe, altered ventilatory response to hypoxia and hypercapnia, and increased upper airway resistance result in a decrease in ventilation in both non–rapid eye movement and rapid eye movement sleep when compared to

wakefulness.[36] Consequently, there is a small normal physiologic increase in the arterial P_{CO_2} of 4 to 6 mm Hg during sleep. This small increase in arterial P_{CO_2} during sleep is usually of little clinical consequence in healthy individuals; however, in patients with respiratory muscle weakness, altered respiratory mechanics, impaired gas exchange, and/or abnormal ventilatory drive, the patient may be especially likely to develop significant hypercapnia. Nocturnal hypoventilation usually precedes chronic daytime hypercapnia, but the extent to which sleep can elicit and exacerbate hypercapnia is often underappreciated. A detailed sleep history including symptoms of sleep-disordered breathing such as snoring, witnessed apneas, nocturnal gasping and choking, frequent awakenings, morning headaches, and excessive daytime sleepiness should be elicited in any clinical evaluation of hypercapnia.

Hypercapnia can lead to dyspnea and tachypnea, not only due to the underlying cause but also as a result of the initial compensatory increase in respiratory drive induced by the increased levels of arterial P_{CO_2} and associated acidemia. With progressive respiratory muscle fatigue or secondary to an underlying neuromuscular etiology, decreased diaphragmatic excursion and paradoxical thoracoabdominal movements may be seen, best observed supine. In the supine position, most breathing movements are abdominal, whereas in the upright position rib cage motion is greater.[37] Normally, as the diaphragm contracts, the abdominal wall is displaced outward but, as the diaphragm weakens, the fall in pleural pressure produced by contraction of the accessory muscles of inspiration is transmitted across the diaphragm to the abdomen to cause a fall in abdominal pressure and a paradoxical inward displacement of the abdomen.[38] Diaphragmatic fatigue may also cause alternate recruitment and derecruitment of the diaphragm and accessory inspiratory muscles, so that for a few breaths most of the inspiratory motion is abdominal, alternating with inspiratory movements that take place predominantly in the rib cage, so-called *respiratory alternans*.[37] Other symptoms and signs pointing to a neuromuscular disorder may be evident that vary depending on the level, laterality, degree of dysfunction, and associated comorbidities, including obesity. These include but are not limited to orthopnea, dyspnea when immersed in water, positional dyspnea, and difficulties with speech, swallowing, cough, and recurrent lower respiratory tract infections. Hypoventilation is also associated with hypoxemia. Normally, arterial P_{O_2} drops approximately in proportion to the rise in arterial P_{CO_2} as determined by the alveolar gas equation (see Chapter 44). Eventually ventilatory failure will lead to pulmonary hypertension and right heart dysfunction.

Hypercapnia is associated with cerebral vasodilation and increased cerebral blood flow, increased intracranial pressure, and biochemical changes in cerebrospinal fluid that can manifest as confusion, restlessness, asterixis, drowsiness, and loss of consciousness. An acute increase in arterial P_{CO_2}, however, has been shown in healthy volunteers to have *central nervous system* (CNS) stimulating effects, and the progressive CNS depression seen in hypercapnia is thought to be secondary to fatigue, aggravated by acidosis, rather than due to hypercapnia itself.[39] That is, the CNS depression seen in hypercapnia is likely a reflection of the

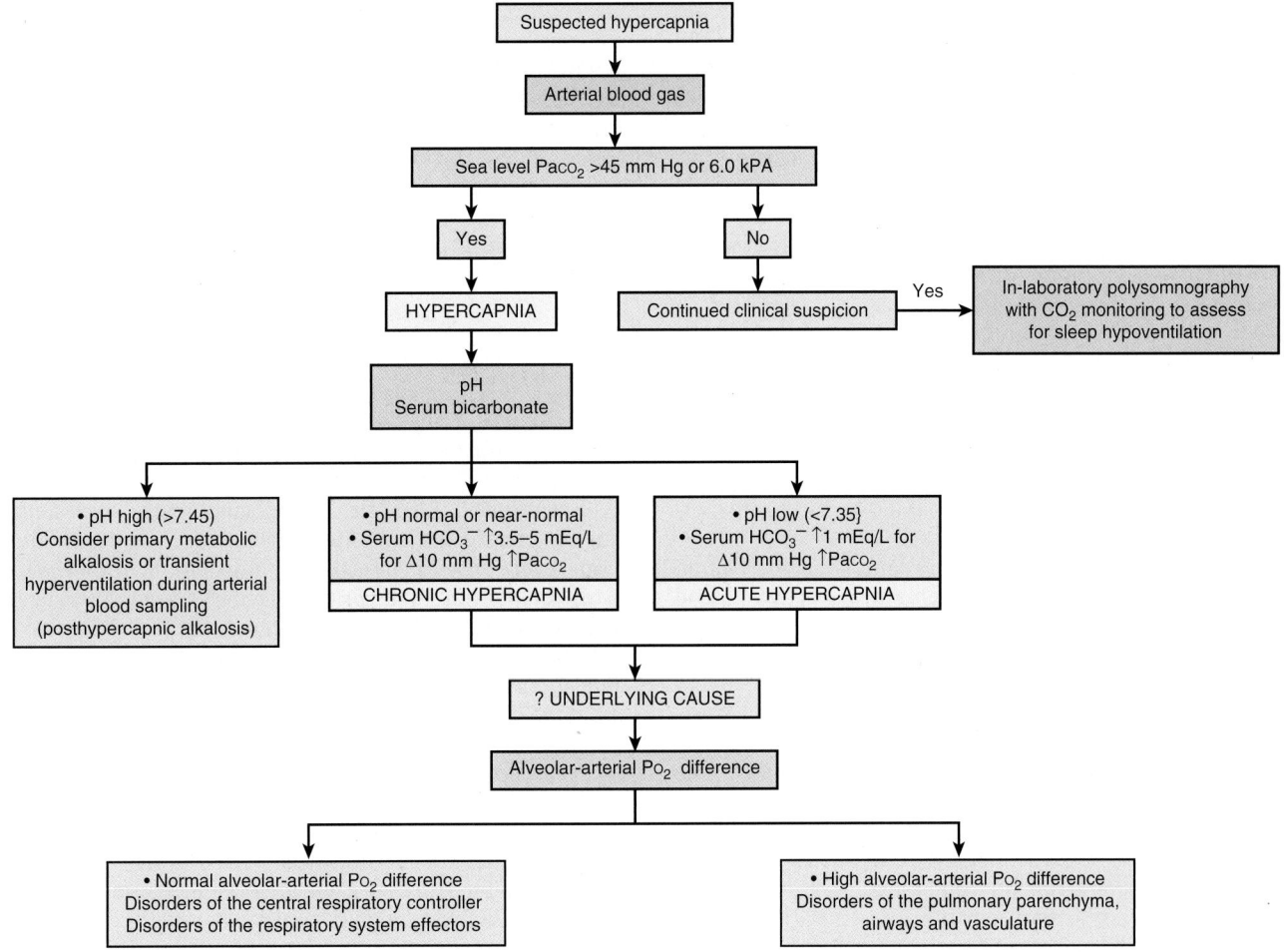

Figure 45.2 Algorithm demonstrating a diagnostic approach to a patient with suspected hypercapnia. PaO_2, alveolar PO_2; PaO_2, arterial PO_2; $PaCO_2$, alveolar PCO_2; $PaCO_2$, arterial PCO_2.

severity of respiratory failure and exhaustion. Normally, in acute hypercapnia, a depressed level of consciousness is not seen until the arterial PCO_2 is greater than 75 to 80 mm Hg, whereas, in chronic hypercapnia, symptoms and signs may not be evident until the arterial PCO_2 rises acutely to greater than 90 to 100 mm Hg.[5]

DIAGNOSTIC EVALUATION

When hypercapnia is suspected clinically, confirmation with arterial blood gas is required. Subsequent diagnostic testing is directed at finding the underlying etiology and assessing for potential complications and is influenced by the acuity and setting of clinical presentation (Fig. 45.2).

ARTERIAL BLOOD GAS

Arterial blood gas (ABG) allows for direct measurement of pH, arterial PCO_2, and arterial PO_2 and is the gold standard for assessing hypercapnia. The pH electrode measures the potential difference between a known solution within the measuring electrode and the sample solution at 37°C. The arterial PCO_2 electrode measures carbon dioxide tensions by allowing carbon dioxide to undergo a chemical reaction,

producing hydrogen ions. The hydrogen ion production causes a potential difference that is measured.[40] The serum bicarbonate HCO_3^- concentration is then calculated by using the Henderson-Hasselbalch equation. The normal pH is 7.35 to 7.45, arterial PCO_2 is 35 to 45 mm Hg (4.7-6.0 kPa), and HCO_3^- is 21 to 27 mEq/L. A common concern is whether the pain or anxiety induced by an arterial puncture leads to transient increase in respiratory rate and tidal volumes, which in turn normalizes arterial PCO_2 with a slightly alkalemic pH. However, one study demonstrated that, in the majority of patients, if local anesthesia with lidocaine was used, the degree of hyperventilation during arterial puncture was not significant.[41]

An arterial PCO_2 measurement greater than 45 mm Hg at sea level confirms hypercapnia. Hypercapnia is associated with predictable physiologic or secondary changes in pH and plasma bicarbonate, which help to differentiate acute from chronic and acute on chronic hypercapnia.[42,43] Acute hypercapnia is characterized by an elevated arterial PCO_2 greater than 45 mm Hg and a low pH less than 7.35. For every acute increase in arterial PCO_2 of 10 mm Hg above normal the pH falls by 0.08.[40] Initially, nonbicarbonate pH buffers present in all fluid compartments of the body give rise to a small increase in serum bicarbonate within 5 to 10 minutes.[44] This secondary response to acute respiratory acidosis increases the serum bicarbonate concentration by approximately 1 mEq/L for every 10 mm Hg (1.3 kPa) increase in the arterial P_{CO_2}.[43,44] As hypercapnia persists, renal compensation takes place. Over approximately 3 to 5 days, the kidneys increase reabsorption of proximal tubular bicarbonate, increase secretion of hydrogen ions, and increase ammonia production, and a new steady state emerges. Serum bicarbonate concentration increases and there is a rise in the systemic pH towards normal. Consequently, assuming normal renal function, chronic hypercapnia is characterized by an elevated arterial P_{CO_2} greater than 45 mm Hg and normal or near normal pH. Derived mainly from experiments on dogs and studies in hospitalized patients, when hypercapnia is chronic, every 10 mm Hg increase in arterial P_{CO_2} is accompanied by an increase in serum bicarbonate of 3.5 to 5 mEq/L.[42,44,45] A high arterial P_{CO_2} may also be caused by respiratory compensation for a primary metabolic alkalosis, but in this setting the pH will be abnormally high.

In addition to confirming the presence of hypercapnia and determining the rate of development, the arterial blood gas can also provide valuable information as to the possible cause. The *alveolar-arterial P_{O_2} difference* [$(A–a)P_{O_2}$] is defined as the alveolar P_{O_2} minus arterial P_{O_2}, where alveolar P_{O_2} is the alveolar pressure of oxygen and arterial P_{O_2} is the arterial pressure of oxygen. The normal $(A–a)P_{O_2}$ difference is approximately 10 mm Hg but varies with age.[46] The alveolar-arterial P_{O_2} difference helps to distinguish causes of hypercapnia with normal lungs from causes of hypercapnia due to lung disease, as discussed above. Hypercapnia with an alveolar-arterial P_{O_2} difference within the normal range suggests a reduced minute ventilation due to depressed central ventilatory drive or disorders of the respiratory system effectors, while hypercapnia in the setting of an abnormal alveolar-arterial P_{O_2} difference greater than 20 suggests underlying pulmonary disease may be contributing. $(A–a)P_{O_2}$, however, can be difficult to calculate in acute respiratory failure when supplemental oxygen is typically required.

SURROGATE ARTERIAL P_{CO_2} ESTIMATES

Arterial blood gas measurements require direct arterial puncture and, accordingly, there is interest in noninvasive measures to estimate the arterial P_{CO_2}, especially when frequent or continuous monitoring is desired.

The peripheral venous P_{CO_2} is a poor predictor of arterial P_{CO_2} and should not be relied on for assessing hypercapnia. A meta-analysis of 16 studies with a total of 1768 subjects that compared P_{CO_2} obtained from peripheral venous blood to arterial blood found poor agreement with sufficiently large differences to be of clinical significance.[47,48] However, a normal peripheral venous P_{CO_2} may have a role in excluding hypercapnia.[49,50] For pH, in contrast to P_{CO_2}, better agreement between peripheral venous and arterial values has been demonstrated. While the serum bicarbonate can increase with sustained hypercapnia, an elevated serum bicarbonate is not specific for hypercapnia and, despite being readily available, a serum bicarbonate alone should not be used as a surrogate for hypercapnia. In OHS, a serum bicarbonate level less than 27 mmol/L has been shown to have a high negative predictive value and

has been recommended to exclude the diagnosis of OHS in obese patients with sleep-disordered breathing when suspicion for OHS is not very high.[51] Even so, measurement of arterial blood gas is recommended in patients strongly suspected of having OHS. When compared to peripheral venous P_{CO_2}, the central venous P_{CO_2} allows more accurate estimation of arterial P_{CO_2}, differing from arterial P_{CO_2} by an amount described by the Fick principle.[52] As long as cardiac output is relatively normal, the central venous P_{CO_2} exceeds the arterial P_{CO_2} by approximately 4 mm Hg.[52]

SLEEP STUDIES

As discussed above, the sleep period is particularly vulnerable to the development of hypercapnia, and nocturnal hypoventilation usually precedes chronic daytime hypoventilation. Sleep studies utilizing appropriate signals can often detect hypercapnia before the development of more severe daytime hypercapnia and should be considered in any evaluation of hypercapnia.

In-laboratory *polysomnography* records multiple physiologic parameters including but not limited to airflow, chest and abdominal movements, and oxygen and is the gold standard diagnostic testing for sleep-disordered breathing. Measures of carbon dioxide can be added and are standard of care in pediatric sleep studies. Given the practical limitations of arterial blood gas monitoring during sleep, noninvasive methods for assessing arterial P_{CO_2} using end-tidal P_{CO_2} and *transcutaneous CO_2* ($tcCO_2$) monitoring have been used. These measures are also being increasingly explored in critically ill mechanically ventilated patients.

End-Tidal CO_2 Monitoring

End-tidal CO_2 devices sample exhaled air through a nasal cannula from the spontaneously breathing patient and provide continuous breath-to-breath analysis of CO_2 based on infrared absorption. In intubated and mechanically ventilated patients, the capnograph is placed between the endotracheal tube and the Y-connector of the ventilator circuit. The graphical display of end-tidal P_{CO_2} plotted against either time or exhaled volume is referred to as *time* or *volume capnography*, respectively. While end-tidal P_{CO_2} allows for continuous, breath-by-breath monitoring, its correlation with arterial P_{CO_2} depends on alveolar ventilation, cardiac output, ventilation-perfusion matching, and airflow obstruction.[2] Consequently, in critically ill patients, end-tidal P_{CO_2} can differ significantly from arterial P_{CO_2} and thus is not recommended to estimate arterial P_{CO_2} in this setting.[52] Similar inaccuracies with end-tidal CO_2 monitoring can be seen in the ambulatory setting, especially in specific disorders like COPD where rapid shallow breathing causes increased dead space and an inability to reach an end-tidal CO_2 plateau. In general, end-tidal CO_2 values tend to underestimate the arterial P_{CO_2} slightly.[52,53] End-tidal CO_2 monitoring can also have technical limitations including problems introduced by mouth breathing, which can entrain air and lower the end-tidal CO_2, and by obstruction of the sampling line. Thus, in general, end-tidal CO_2 monitoring should not be used as the sole mechanism in assessing arterial P_{CO_2}.

Transcutaneous CO_2 Monitoring

Compared to end-tidal CO_2 monitoring, $tcCO_2$ monitoring is more reliable and practical. $tcCO_2$ sensors heat the skin locally to increase blood flow and carbon dioxide diffusion. As CO_2 diffuses across the skin, it reacts with an electrolyte-containing solution to produce a measurable change in the pH that is then analyzed to measure $tcCO_2$.[52,53] There are a few considerations in using $tcCO_2$. For one, $tcCO_2$ values are approximately 4 to 5 mm Hg higher than arterial P_{CO_2} because the heat applied to the skin induces a local hypermetabolic state. For another, there is a lag in response to changes in arterial P_{CO_2} due to the time for CO_2 to diffuse across the skin. Nonetheless, $tcCO_2$ can provide an overall trend with respect to arterial P_{CO_2} changes. Practically, $tcCO_2$ is easy to apply and can be used in intubated patients as long as skin perfusion is not impaired. Calibration is required and $tcCO_2$ monitoring is currently expensive.

Because some hypoventilation during sleep is normal, pathologic hypoventilation during sleep has been difficult to define. The *American Academy of Sleep Medicine* (AASM) Sleep Apnea Definitions Task Force revised its scoring of hypoventilation during sleep in adults in 2012 to include two criteria: (1) an increase in arterial P_{CO_2} greater than 55 mm Hg for greater than 10 minutes or (2) an increase in arterial P_{CO_2} greater than 10 mm Hg during sleep in comparison to awake supine values to a value exceeding 50 mm Hg for greater than 10 minutes.[54] Although based on data that normal individuals rarely have an arterial P_{CO_2} greater than 55 mm Hg during sleep, the precise arterial P_{CO_2} level demarcating the transition from physiologic hypercapnia to pathologic hypoventilation remains unclear. Additionally, the duration of 10 minutes selected by the AASM Task Force was arbitrary and based on consensus with a lack of normative data on the amount of total sleep time at different arterial P_{CO_2} values in sleeping adults.

In addition to diagnosing sleep hypoventilation, polysomnography may also reveal a cause for the hypercapnia. OSA is characterized by repetitive reduction of airflow due to upper airway obstruction. It is seen in the majority of patients with OHS where it is typically severe and associated with significant hypoxemia. In contrast to OSA, in central sleep apnea, repetitive absent airflow is associated with absent respiratory effort. Central sleep apnea can be caused by a high or irregular drive to breathe, in which case the CO_2 is typically low or normal, or by a diminished drive to breathe, in which case the CO_2 is typically elevated.

Currently, home sleep apnea testing or portable unattended sleep apnea testing is not recommended for the evaluation of hypercapnia or sleep hypoventilation.[55] Portable monitoring devices differ in the numbers and types of signals recorded but record fewer physiologic variables when compared to polysomnography. Scoring of respiratory events, including obstructive and central apneas, is more challenging with fewer signals, especially in patients with underlying cardiopulmonary and neuromuscular disease prone to baseline hypoxemia or hypoventilation. For this reason, studies comparing an ambulatory management pathway using portable home sleep apnea testing and autotitrating continuous positive airway pressure to the traditional in-laboratory diagnostic and titration polysomnography have largely excluded patients with significant cardiac, pulmonary, and neuromuscular disorders where interpretation of limited channel recordings can be limited.[56] Similarly, continuous recording of oxygen saturation alone can have limitations in the evaluation of hypercapnia. Oxygen desaturation may be associated with hypoventilation but, because oxygen desaturation can also be seen with obstructive and central respiratory events, it cannot be relied on alone in diagnosing sleep hypoventilation.

DIAGNOSTIC TESTING FOR CAUSES OF HYPERCAPNIA

Additional diagnostic testing to try to find the underlying cause(s) is guided by the clinical history and physical examination.

If there is clinical suspicion for a disorder of central respiratory control, testing should be considered for the following: urine toxicology, thyroid function, basic metabolic function, liver function, and genetic associations, as well as CNS imaging including magnetic resonance imaging of the brainstem. If there is clinical suspicion for a disorder of the respiratory systems effectors, additional diagnostic testing is directed by the suspected level of efferent pathway involvement.

Physiologic measures of respiratory muscle function can help confirm respiratory muscle weakness and assess for severity (see also Chapter 130). Various measures of respiratory muscle function exist and combinations of measures may improve diagnostic precision.[57] Inspiratory muscle weakness is characterized by a reduction in *vital capacity* (VC) and *total lung capacity* (TLC). A *forced vital capacity* (FVC) less than 1 L is the best negative predictor of survival in patients with Duchenne muscular dystrophy and, in *amyotrophic lateral sclerosis*, the FVC has been linearly correlated with disease progression and survival.[58-60] In Guillain-Barré syndrome, progression to mechanical ventilation has been associated with a VC less than 20 mL/kg, a reduction of more than 30% in VC, *maximal inspiratory pressure* (MIP) less than 30 cm H_2O, and a *maximal expiratory pressure* (MEP) less than 40 cm H_2O. For these patients, placement in the intensive care unit is recommended when the VC declines rapidly or when it falls below approximately 18 mL/kg of body weight.[61,62] The supine FVC may be a better predictor of diaphragmatic weakness than the upright FVC.[63,64] Normally the VC declines less than 10% when going from upright to supine.[65] When the VC falls to this extent or less, clinically significant diaphragmatic weakness is unlikely, whereas a decrease in VC of 30–50% when supine supports a diagnosis of bilateral diaphragmatic paralysis.[38]

Respiratory muscle weakness can also be associated with reductions in the maximum voluntary ventilation and static MIP and MEP measured at the mouth. The MIP and MEP, when performed appropriately and with good patient effort, are sensitive and easily obtained measures of the strength of inspiratory and expiratory muscles of respiration, respectively; however, their utility is limited by the significant variation in normal reference values reported. MIP and MEP measurements are influenced by age, gender, posture, lung volume, and the type of mouthpiece used. A normal MIP is useful in excluding clinically important inspiratory respiratory muscle weakness, but an abnormal MIP can be difficult to interpret.[66] In patients with neuromuscular disorders involving the orofacial muscles, obtaining a tight seal around the mouthpiece for MIP and MEP measurements can be difficult. When a patient cannot use a mouthpiece, the *sniff nasal inspiratory pressure* (SNIP), which measures the nasal pressure in an occluded nostril as the patient sniffs through the contralateral unobstructed nostril, may provide a reasonable estimate of inspiratory muscle strength.[66] In amyotrophic lateral sclerosis, the SNIP has been shown to have greater predictive power for hypercapnia than either FVC or MIP.[67] The American Academy of Neurology has recommended consideration of noninvasive ventilation in amyotrophic lateral sclerosis if orthopnea is present, SNIP is less than 40 cm H_2O, FVC is less than 50% predicted, MIP is less than 60 cm H_2O, or when abnormal nocturnal oximetry is present.[67]

Again, depending on the suspected level of effector system involvement, imaging may be helpful. Hemidiaphragm paralysis can cause an elevated hemidiaphragm on chest radiograph. The chest radiograph has reasonable sensitivity in detecting unilateral diaphragmatic paralysis but low specificity (44%).[38,68] When suspected, fluoroscopy of the diaphragm with a sniff test can be used to evaluate diaphragmatic function. In the sniff test, the patient is asked to sniff forcefully while diaphragmatic movement is observed fluoroscopically. In unilateral diaphragmatic paralysis, there is a paradoxical cephalad movement of the paralyzed hemidiaphragm when compared to the descent of the normal contralateral hemidiaphragm (see Video 20.1). The test is not helpful in diagnosing bilateral diaphragmatic paralysis, leading to false-positive and false-negative results.[38] Ultrasonography may be considered in diagnosing both unilateral and bilateral diaphragmatic paralysis. Thickening of the diaphragm by ultrasound reflects diaphragmatic shortening, so that with diaphragmatic paralysis, there is a lack of thickening seen with inspiration. Once diaphragmatic paralysis is identified, computed tomography of the chest is required to evaluate the course of the ipsilateral phrenic nerve and exclude thoracic malignancies. Computed tomography of the chest can also be helpful in evaluating for chest wall deformities and parenchymal lung diseases.

Hypercapnia caused by increased dead space ventilation and disorders of alveolar ventilation is associated with abnormal pulmonary function testing. A decreased diffusion capacity can be seen with pathologies involving the alveolar-capillary membrane. Parenchymal lung diseases involving alveolar filling can also exhibit a decrease in diffusion capacity and restriction. Thus, chest imaging including chest radiographs and often computed tomography are indicated in the assessment of hypercapnia.

MANAGEMENT

Treatment priorities will vary depending on the acuity and severity of hypercapnia at presentation. In patients presenting with acute or acute on chronic hypercapnic respiratory failure, assessment and stabilization of the *airway, breathing, and circulation* (ABCs) take priority. Ventilatory support can be provided either noninvasively using a mask interface or invasively following endotracheal intubation, typically in the intensive care unit. Most ventilators now are positive-pressure devices that deliver pressurized gas to increase transpulmonary pressures and inflate the lungs, thereby augmenting ventilation. *Noninvasive ventilation* (NIV) should be considered in all patients in acute hypercapnic respiratory failure where mechanical ventilation is considered; however, success relies on both appropriate patient selection and proper application. Strong evidence now supports the use of NIV for acute exacerbations of COPD and cardiogenic pulmonary edema, to facilitate extubation in COPD patients, and in immunocompromised patients. An increasing number of studies are suggesting an ever-expanding role for NIV in hypercapnic respiratory failure. However, NIV should be avoided in hemodynamically unstable patients, patients at high risk of aspiration, and patients unlikely to tolerate a mask interface. Decreased mental status is not a contraindication to NIV, but inability to protect the airway (regardless of the mental status) is. NIV is not a substitute for endotracheal intubation when needed. See Chapters 135 and 136 for details on providing ventilatory support.

At the same time that ventilatory support is being provided, there should be efforts to identify the underlying cause(s) to target specific therapies directed at reversing the underlying cause. In chronic hypercapnia, because the patient is generally stable, identification and treatment of the underlying cause typically takes precedence, and the potential risks and benefits of chronic ventilatory support are weighed. Initiation of ventilatory support in the stable ambulatory patient typically starts noninvasively during sleep.

Hypercapnia often coexists with hypoxemia. The administration of supplemental oxygen in this setting has the potential to worsen hypercapnia by various mechanisms.[69] By increasing arterial Po_2, supplemental oxygen can inhibit hypoxic pulmonary vasoconstriction, an important mechanism that normally diverts pulmonary artery blood away from poorly ventilated regions; in this way, the supplemental oxygen can worsen ventilation-perfusion mismatch and reduce the efficiency of CO_2 elimination.[70] This appears to be the predominant mechanism for oxygen-induced hypercapnia. Supplemental oxygen can also worsen hypercapnia by the Haldane effect,[70-72] the phenomenon whereby increasing arterial Po_2 reduces the ability of the blood to store CO_2, thereby increasing arterial Pco_2. Additionally, supplemental oxygen may decrease stimuli from peripheral chemoreceptors to the central respiratory center and thereby decrease minute ventilation. Normally, an increase in the arterial Pco_2 can be offset by an increase in minute ventilation, but this may not be possible in significant lung disease. Knowing this, the application of supplemental oxygen in hypercapnia should be carefully titrated for a target Spo_2 of 90–93% with close monitoring.

Key Points

- Hypercapnia is defined as a partial pressure of carbon dioxide in arterial blood greater than 45 mm Hg at sea level. It is associated with predictable physiologic changes in pH and plasma bicarbonate, which help to differentiate acute from chronic hypercapnia.

- Hypercapnia results when alveolar ventilation is insufficient to meet the rate of CO_2 production due to a decrease in minute ventilation, an increase in dead space ventilation, or rarely an increase in CO_2 production. (A–a)Po_2 helps to distinguish causes of hypercapnia in the setting of normal lungs from those causes of hypercapnia due to lung disease.

- Hypercapnia caused by reduced total minute ventilation can mechanistically be divided into (1) disorders of the central respiratory controller characterized by a reduced drive to breathe (i.e., won't breathe) or (2) disorders of the respiratory system effectors due to disruption at any level of the efferent arm, from the spinal cord to the muscles of respiration and the chest wall, characterized by reduced ventilatory supply (i.e., can't breathe).

- Hypercapnia affects multiple organ systems and thus timely recognition is essential. Clinical assessment should be directed not only to the clinical manifestations of hypercapnia but also to its underlying cause.

- Sleep is associated with changes in ventilation specific to the stage of sleep and a normal physiologic 4 to 6 mm Hg increase in arterial Pco_2. Nocturnal hypoventilation usually precedes chronic daytime hypercapnia, and a sleep history should be elicited in the clinical evaluation of any patient with hypercapnia.

- Administration of supplemental oxygen has the potential to worsen hypercapnia by inhibiting hypoxic pulmonary vasoconstriction (and thereby worsening ventilation-perfusion inequality), by the Haldane effect, in which O_2 can displace CO_2 from hemoglobin, and by decreasing minute ventilation.

Key Readings

Gerdung CA, Adeleye A, Kirk VG. Noninvasive monitoring of CO_2 during polysomnography: a review of the recent literature. *Curr Opion Pulm Med.* 2015;22(6):527–534.

Kreit JW. Volume capnography in the intensive care unit: physiological principles, measurements and calculations. *Ann Am Thorac Soc.* 2018;16(3):291–300.

Nassar BS, Schmidt GA. Estimating arterial partial pressure of carbon dioxide in ventilated patients: how valid are surrogate measures? *Ann Am Thorac Soc.* 2017;14(6):1005–1014.

Weinberger SE, Schwartzstein RM, Weiss JW. Hypercapnia. *N Engl J Med.* 1989;321(18):1223–1231.

West JB. Causes of carbon dioxide retention in lung disease. *N Engl J Med.* 1971:1232–1236.

West JB, Luks AM. *West's Respiratory Physiology: The Essentials.* 10th ed. Philadelphia: Wolters Kluwer; 2016.

Complete reference list available at ExpertConsult.com.

INFECTIOUS DISEASES OF THE LUNGS

46 *COMMUNITY-ACQUIRED PNEUMONIA*

DAVID H. DOCKRELL, MD, FRCPI, FRCP(Glas), FACP • ANTONIA HO, MBCHB, PHD •
STEPHEN B. GORDON, MD, MA, FRCP, DTM&H

 An expanded version of this chapter is available at ExpertConsult.com.

INTRODUCTION

Community-acquired pneumonia (CAP) caused an estimated 2.4 million deaths worldwide in 2016.[1] In the United States, pneumonia accounted for approximately 900,000 hospitalizations in 2014 and one-third of episodes of sepsis.[2,3] Although many episodes are mild, CAP mortality in hospitalized patients is 5–10% and 20–50% for those admitted to the *intensive care unit* (ICU).

CAP implies the presence of lung inflammation of sufficient extent to lead to signs, symptoms, or radiologic features of an opacity with acute onset and community acquisition. An infectious etiology is inferred but is frequently not proven microbiologically,[4] and the condition must be distinguished from other conditions that present with similar features. CAP is distinguished from *hospital-acquired pneumonia* (HAP) by onset in the community or within 48 hours of hospitalization.[5] Its acute onset helps distinguish it in most cases from chronic infectious pneumonias caused by tuberculosis or fungi.

Diagnosis and management of pneumonia are challenging, especially in the growing number of individuals with multiple morbidities, immunocompromise or epidemiologic factors favoring antimicrobial resistance, or geographically restricted infections. Treatment is initially empirical, covering common bacterial or viral causes in the appropriate epidemiological setting but should be tailored by microbiological results and antimicrobial stewardship priorities.

PATHOPHYSIOLOGY AND PATHOGENESIS

As detailed in Chapter 17, the *lower respiratory tract* (LRT) was formerly thought to be sterile but more sensitive molecular techniques now demonstrate that a LRT low-density microbiome exists, with approximately 10^{2-3} bacteria per milliliter of *bronchoalveolar lavage* (BAL) fluid, as opposed to 10^6 bacteria/mL in the oropharynx.[6] The LRT microbiome in adults, although distinct from the upper airway, contains many of the same species. It is dominated by Firmicutes and Bacteroidetes, while the virome is dominated by *Anelloviridae* and bacteriophages.[6] The lung microbiome regulates local immune responses. For example, *Prevotella* species enhance *T helper 17 cells* (Th17) responses and reduce alveolar macrophage *toll-like receptor* (TLR) 4 responses.[7] Aspiration of oropharyngeal secretions is the main mechanism of microorganism translocation to the LRT in adults, while nasopharyngeal secretions also contribute in children. While a person is awake, glottal reflexes prevent aspiration; during sleep, 50% of normal persons aspirate small volumes of oropharyngeal secretions. Dysphagia and aspiration are more frequent in the elderly and in elderly patients with CAP compared to age-matched controls.[8,9] Dispersion along mucosal surfaces also contributes to colonization.

As an alternative to aspiration of bacteria colonizing the upper airways, *Mycoplasma pneumoniae*, *Chlamydophila* species, *Coxiella burnetii*, *Legionella* species, and viruses enter the LRT by direct inhalation. Inhalation pneumonia is most often due to microorganisms that survive suspended in the air for prolonged periods, are present in droplet nuclei smaller than 5 μm, and are able to evade innate immune responses.

The airway of healthy individuals is colonized by multiple microorganisms. These can promote health through limiting surface binding and nutrients, expressing antimicrobial bacteriocins, and promoting beneficial immune responses.[6,10,11] However, dynamic shifts in the population structure, such as by viral infection or exposure to pollutants, favor acquisition of *pathobionts*, that is, normally harmless organisms (i.e., symbionts) that can become pathologic.[6] Colonization is promoted by specific microbial adhesins interacting with cellular receptors. The *Streptococcus pneumoniae* capsule allows it to penetrate mucus so adhesins interact with receptors such as platelet-activating factor receptor on epithelial cells, an interaction enhanced by cigarette smoke, infection with respiratory viruses, and particulate air pollutants.[11–13] Likewise, *Staphylococcus aureus* express multiple adhesins that bind host extracellular matrix proteins.[14,15] Gram-negative bacteria such as *Klebsiella pneumoniae* utilize macromolecular structures, termed pili, to interact with extracellular matrix proteins.[16] Bacterial products or inflammatory responses including generation of reactive oxygen species also impair mucociliary function.[17]

The incidence of CAP is rare in comparison to the frequency of colonization with pathobionts such as *S. pneumoniae*, indicating that effective host defenses prevent CAP. Mucus and the bronchociliary escalator limit pathogen penetration to the distal airway and viral infections subvert bronchociliary function.[18] Respiratory epithelial cells and phagocytes synthesize antimicrobial peptides, termed defensins.[19] In the distal airways and alveoli, pulmonary surfactant proteins A and C can inhibit bacterial binding to host cells and also promote phagocytosis of selected bacteria.[20,21] The presence of complement and immunoglobulins (particularly *immunoglobulin A* [IgA]), also prevents colonization of the airway. Opsonic antibodies are crucial for phagocytosis of encapsulated bacteria, as illustrated for internalization of *S. pneumoniae* by alveolar macrophages.[22]

Inflammatory responses to bacteria and viruses are regulated by pattern recognition receptors (Chapter 15). These regulate production of cytokines and chemokines to activate resident cells and promote recruitment of other immune cells to control respiratory tract infection. In murine models, resident alveolar macrophages clear finite numbers from the alveolus, but their microbicidal responses are limited, and ultimately they undergo apoptosis to kill residual bacteria such as *S. pneumoniae*.[23] When their capacity for clearance is overwhelmed, neutrophils and CCR2$^+$ monocytes enhance pathogen clearance.[23,24] T cells are also key to responses during the escalation of inflammatory responses after alveolar macrophage responses are overwhelmed, but T cells must be regulated to prevent tissue injury.[25] Th17 responses, which are a key effector of mucosal immunity, facilitate macrophage and neutrophil recruitment to clear bacteria. In the upper airway, recruited macrophages control initial exposure to *S. pneumoniae*, while prior exposure promotes neutrophil-dependent clearance of *S. pneumoniae* in murine models.[26] Th17 cells are also increased in the BAL of patients with CAP.[27] The gut microbiota dampens CCR2$^+$ macrophage recruitment to the upper airway in infant mice; this has been suggested as a reason for prolonged colonization with pathobionts like *S. pneumoniae* in infants.[28] Type 1 interferon responses mediated by innate lymphoid cells are critical to promoting viral clearance from epithelial cells. Viral infection frequently modulates innate responses to bacteria by, for example, inhibiting macrophage phagocytosis via *interferon* (IFN)-γ–dependent mechanisms or by induction of apoptosis in key immune cells such as T cells.[29] Influenza virus enhances susceptibility to *S. pneumoniae* by neuraminidase release of sialic acid, which serves as a nutrient for *S. pneumoniae*,[30] or through increasing bacterial adherence to respiratory epithelial cells by exposing glycoconjugates previously capped by sialic acid[31] and/or through direct binding of influenza virus to *S. pneumoniae*.[32]

CAP results when the innate responses, including those of alveolar macrophages, are overwhelmed. Neutrophilic inflammation and activated T cells promote pathogen clearance, but at greater inflammatory cost than processes such as apoptosis-associated killing, and increase tissue injury. Immune responses designed to clear pathogens, such as production of reactive oxygen or nitrogen species and proteases, can promote tissue injury, and dysregulation of these responses impacts the outcome of CAP and can lead to excessive inflammatory responses such as *acute respiratory distress syndrome* (ARDS), a complication of 2% of cases of hospitalized CAP.[33] Viral infections such as influenza A virus can lead to excessive activation of immune cells, such as recruited CCR2$^+$ macrophages.[34] In many cases, CAP presents as a dysregulated acute inflammatory response rather than one of a failure of pathogen clearance. This may explain the inability to identify the causal pathogen in many cases. In other cases, the virulence of the pathogen or the kinetics of replication drive diffuse alveolar damage and extensive epithelial apoptosis; this is the case with many viral pneumonias, especially avian influenza and *Middle East respiratory syndrome coronavirus* (MERS-CoV).[35]

EPIDEMIOLOGY

The burden of CAP varies substantially across the world; the highest risks are associated with extremes of age; poverty; inadequate access to nutrition, sanitation, or vaccines; and immunocompromised status or medical comorbidities. The true incidence of CAP is uncertain because the illness is not reportable and only 20–50% of patients require hospitalization. Incidence estimates of CAP range from 6 to 34 cases per 1000 persons per year, with substantially higher rates in older adults.[36] In a study using active population-based

Table 46.1   Common Causes of Community-Acquired Pneumonia by Patient Location

Outpatient	Hospitalized	ICU
MOST FREQUENT		
Streptococcus pneumoniae	Streptococcus pneumoniae	Streptococcus pneumoniae
Mycoplasma pneumoniae	Mycoplasma pneumoniae	Viruses (e.g., influenza A virus)
Respiratory viruses	Respiratory viruses	
OTHER ORGANISMS OFTEN ISOLATED		
Chlamydophila pneumoniae	Haemophilus influenzae	Legionella species
Coxiella burnetii	Pseudomonas aeruginosa (and enteric gram-negative bacilli)	Staphylococcus aureus
Legionella species	Staphylococcus aureus	Pseudomonas aeruginosa (and enteric gram-negative bacilli)
Haemophilus influenzae	Legionella species	
	Aspiration pneumonia	

ICU, intensive care unit.
Modified from references 4, 40, 42–45.

surveillance, the incidence rate for CAP requiring hospitalization in adults was reported to be 2.5 per 1000 person-years.[4]

Although the severity of disease is influenced by the patient's age and the presence and type of coexisting conditions,[38–41] disease severity is also related to the pathogen. S. pneumoniae and respiratory viruses are common in all settings (Table 46.1).[4,40,42–45] The relative importance of different viruses as causes of pneumonia depends on season and patient age. During outbreaks, influenza virus accounts for more than 50% of viral pneumonia in adults. Additionally, rhinovirus, human metapneumovirus, respiratory syncytial virus (RSV), adenovirus, parainfluenza viruses, coronaviruses, and varicella virus cause pneumonia in healthy adults.[4] Other viruses continue to emerge in epidemics of severe acute pneumonitis, including hantavirus, coronaviruses (severe acute respiratory syndrome [SARS-1], MERS, and SARS-CoV-2), and avian influenza A viruses.

M. pneumoniae, C. pneumoniae, C. burnetii, and Haemophilus influenzae can cause pneumonia sufficiently severe to require hospitalization, though most cases are less severe. The most frequently identified pathogens causing severe CAP (i.e., CAP requiring ICU care) are S. pneumoniae, Pseudomonas aeruginosa, enteric gram-negative bacilli, S. aureus, Legionella pneumophila, and influenza viruses (Table 46.1).[40,42,44,46,47] Up to 20% of severe CAP episodes are caused by polymicrobial infection. The microbial etiology pathogen is not identified in up to 60% of patients with CAP, even with polymerase chain reaction (PCR)-based diagnostics.[4]

Pneumonia due to Legionella species is often associated with other cases in outbreaks from a common environmental source.[48] Gram-negative bacilli are more common causes in Asia and Southern Africa than in other regions, with K. pneumoniae most frequent, particularly in cases admitted to the ICU.[50,51] P. aeruginosa infection is uncommon in the absence of specific risk factors (recent antibiotic treatment, immunocompromise, and severe pulmonary comorbidity, especially bronchiectasis, cystic fibrosis, and severe COPD).[40,42,46] Methicillin-resistant S. aureus (MRSA), originally a nosocomial pathogen, has appeared in the community, where it is referred to as community-acquired MRSA [CA-MRSA]). CA-MRSA can lead to severe pulmonary infections, including necrotizing and hemorrhagic pneumonia.[49,52]

The contribution of M. pneumoniae and viral infections to CAP varies with the season. Influenza viruses, S. pneumoniae, and H. influenzae are more common in winter, while Legionella species causes infection predominantly in the summer and autumn.[53] Vaccination can also modify the prevalence of certain pathogens as causes of CAP. Pneumococcal conjugate vaccination in children is reducing the incidence of S. pneumoniae CAP, even in adults. In the Netherlands, use of the conjugate vaccine reduced S. pneumoniae CAP by 30% from 2004 to 2016,[54] although replacement with non-vaccine serotypes may modify this trend.

The etiology of severe CAP varies with age and medical comorbidities.[42,55-58]

AGE-RELATED FACTORS

Pneumonia is one of the major causes of morbidity in children. In children younger than 2 years, S. pneumoniae and RSV are the most frequent causes, whereas S. pneumoniae, viruses, and M. pneumoniae are common in older children and young adults.

In adults, increased age is associated with a change in the distribution of microbial causes and an increase in the frequency and severity of pneumonia.[59] The annual incidence of CAP in noninstitutionalized older adults is estimated to be between 18 and 44 per 1000 compared with 4.7 to 11.6 per 1000 in the general population.[36,59,60] Although older adults are particularly at risk for pneumococcal pneumonia, they also have increased rates of pneumonia due to H. influenzae, group B streptococci, Moraxella catarrhalis, L. pneumophila, gram-negative bacilli, C. pneumoniae, and polymicrobial infections.[36,46,61] The absolute rate of infection by M. pneumoniae does not decrease with age. However, this pathogen accounts for a smaller proportion of pneumonia in older adults than in younger populations. In patients older than 80 years, there is a higher incidence of aspiration pneumonia and lower incidence of infection with Legionella species than in younger patients.[62]

PERSONAL HABITS

Alcohol consumption is an important risk factor for CAP because of its potential to increase aspiration of oropharyngeal contents and to impair immune function. Alcoholism increases the rate and severity of pneumonia, especially pneumococcal CAP.[63,64] This predisposition persists several months after cessation of alcohol consumption.[63]

Smoking is one of the most important risk factors for CAP and is associated with an increased frequency of CAP due to S. pneumoniae, L. pneumophila, and influenza.[65,66] Smoking not only doubles the risk of CAP and is associated with approximately one-third of cases of CAP, but passive smoking in adults older than 65 years also increases CAP, making it potentially the most significant modifiable risk factor for CAP.[65,67] Cigarette smoke alters mucociliary transport and humoral and cellular defenses, affects epithelial cells, and increases adhesion of *S. pneumoniae* and *H. influenzae* to the oropharyngeal epithelium.[12]

COMORBIDITIES

The most frequent comorbidity associated with CAP is COPD (see Chapters 63 and 64). Patients with COPD have an increased risk for CAP due to alterations in mechanical and cellular defenses, including alveolar macrophage dysfunction, that increase bacterial colonization of the lower airways.[68,69] Patients with severe COPD (forced expiratory volume in 1 second <30% of predicted) and bronchiectasis have an increased risk for pneumonia caused by nontypeable *H. influenzae*, *P. aeruginosa*, and *S. aureus*.[66] However, a broad range of pathogens may cause CAP in this group, and many rarer etiologies of CAP have a predilection for patients with COPD. Despite this, *S. pneumoniae* remains a leading cause of CAP in COPD. In patients with COPD treated with oral corticosteroids for long periods, the risk for infection with *Aspergillus* species is increased.[70]

Pneumonia remains the major cause of morbidity and mortality in patients with cystic fibrosis. During the first decade of life, *S. aureus* and nontypeable *H. influenzae* are the most common pathogens, although *P. aeruginosa* is occasionally isolated in infants. By 18 years of age, 80% of patients with cystic fibrosis harbor *P. aeruginosa* and 3.5% harbor *Burkholderia cepacia*.[71] *Stenotrophomonas maltophilia*, *Achromobacter xylosoxidans*, and nontuberculous mycobacteria are emerging pathogens in this population.[72]

Other comorbidities associated with increased rates of CAP and consequent mortality include congestive heart failure, chronic kidney or liver disease, cancer, diabetes, dementia, cerebrovascular diseases, and immunodeficiencies (e.g., neutropenia, lymphoproliferative diseases, immunoglobulin deficiencies, and *human immunodeficiency virus* [HIV] infection).[73–75] Globally, HIV infection is a major risk factor for CAP and, whereas the widespread availability of antiretroviral therapy has decreased the risk of opportunistic infections, it has had a more modest impact on pneumococcal pneumonia, which remains the leading cause of CAP in this group.[76] High smoking rates and the increased incidence of COPD in people living with HIV compound the risk of CAP.[73,77]

While pneumococcal pneumonia remains the most common cause of CAP in most of these groups, other associations can increase the relative contribution of a particular etiologic agent in a specific comorbidity: liver disease with gram-negative bacteria and diabetes with *S. aureus*.[66] The contribution of proton pump inhibitor use as a CAP risk factor has been controversial; commencement of proton pump inhibitor in the previous 30 days increased CAP risk in a recent case control study, although some other studies including a meta-analysis have not shown an association.[78,78a] There have also been contradictory findings on the association between statin use and CAP; several observational studies have shown lower mortality with prior statin use[79,80] while others have not.[81]

VIRAL CAP IN IMMUNOCOMPROMISED HOSTS

Viral CAP can be an important problem for people with deficiencies in immunity as the result of cytotoxic chemotherapy,

immunosuppressive or biologic therapies for autoimmune diseases, organ transplantation, and HIV infection. The major respiratory viruses affecting persons with an intact immune system may also cause pneumonia in immunocompromised hosts; severe and prolonged pneumonias due to adenovirus, RSV, influenza, measles, or parainfluenza virus can develop in such patients. Immunocompromised patients can also shed respiratory viruses for prolonged periods and thus be responsible for extensive transmission of infection to others. Additionally, individuals with severe T cell immunodeficiency may develop pneumonia due to viruses, such as *cytomegalovirus* (CMV), that do not cause LRT infections in normal hosts. CMV causes severe primary viral pneumonia and predisposes patients to bacterial and fungal superinfections due to its immunosuppressive effects.[82] Varicella-zoster and herpes simplex virus pneumonias are relatively uncommon but cause serious infections in those with severe T cell or natural killer cell immunodeficiency.

GEOGRAPHIC AND OCCUPATIONAL CONSIDERATIONS

Geographic factors, seasonal timing, travel history, and occupational or unusual exposures modify the risk of various microbial etiologies of CAP. For example, an increased frequency of *S. pneumoniae* was found in barracked soldiers and South African gold miners, while painters and welders are at risk of developing a fulminant form of pneumococcal pneumonia with high mortality.[83] *Burkholderia pseudomallei* (melioidosis) is endemic in rural Asia.[84] Exposure to pet birds or work on a poultry (especially turkey) farm or processing plant increases the risk of psittacosis (*Chlamydia psittaci*),[85] while contact with horses or other large mammals including cattle, swine, sheep, goats, or deer increases exposure to *Rhodococcus equi*.[86] Rodent contact suggests the possibility of infection with *Yersinia pestis* (plague)[87,88] or hantavirus[89] in the rural southwestern United States, and *Francisella tularensis* (tularemia) in rural Arkansas or Nantucket, Massachusetts.[90,91] Exposure to sheep, dogs, and cats should prompt evaluation for *C. burnetii* (Q fever).[92] Pneumonia causing SARS due to a coronavirus emerged in epidemic form in Southeast Asia,[93,94] and another coronavirus causes MERS.[95] In late 2019 and 2020, the *coronavirus 2019* (COVID-19) pandemic was caused by another coronavirus, SARS-CoV-2. Finally, the infectious agents that cause anthrax, tularemia, and plague may be used for bioterrorism or biowarfare purposes and cause LRT infections.[96–98] Further information may be obtained from organizations such as the *U.S. Centers for Disease Control and Prevention* (CDC; www.cdc.gov), *Infectious Diseases Society of America* (IDSA; www.idsociety.org), and the *World Health Organization* (WHO; www.who.org) (see Chapter 59).

CLINICAL PRESENTATION

Pneumonia is characterized by the presence of fever, malaise, and respiratory symptoms, such as cough, sputum production, dyspnea, pleuritic pain, and hemoptysis. In older and immunocompromised patients, the signs and symptoms of pulmonary infection may be muted due to blunting of the signature inflammatory response and overshadowed by nonspecific complaints. Therefore, chest radiographs should be examined in these patients despite lack of classic signs and symptoms.

In older patients, especially those with multiple comorbidities, pneumonia may present with general weakness, decreased appetite, altered mental status, incontinence, or decompensation due to underlying disease. The presence of tachypnea may precede other signs of pneumonia by 1 to 2 days. Tachycardia is another common initial sign but is less frequent and specific than tachypnea. Fever is absent in 30–40% of older patients. Owing to the lack of specific symptoms, the diagnosis of CAP is frequently delayed in older adults.[36,61] Older patients with pneumonia who present with altered mental status without fever can have a delay in receiving antibiotics by more than 4 hours after arrival, a delay that increases mortality.[99]

Occasionally, there is a "classic" history, such as that of the patient with pneumococcal infection who presents with sudden onset of rigor followed by pleuritic chest pain, dyspnea, and cough with rusty sputum. Similarly, a patient with *Legionella* pneumonia may complain predominantly of diarrhea, fever, headache, confusion, and myalgia. For *M. pneumoniae* infection, extrapulmonary manifestations such as myringitis, encephalitis, uveitis, iritis, and myocarditis may be present. However, only rarely does the clinical history clearly suggest a specific etiology.

The clinical and radiographic features of sporadic cases of viral pneumonia are usually not sufficiently characteristic to permit specific viral diagnosis or differentiation from bacterial pneumonias on clinical grounds alone. Exceptions include measles (eFig. 46.1) and varicella pneumonia, in which the associated rash establishes the diagnosis. Some cases of viral pneumonia present as severe CAP and have a rapid and relentless fatal course, with generalized alveolar and interstitial opacities, development of ARDS, and progressive respiratory failure.

Information obtained from the clinical history and physical examination is insufficient to confirm the diagnosis of pneumonia. A definitive diagnosis requires the finding of a new opacity on the chest radiograph or *computed tomography* (CT) scan.

TYPICAL VERSUS ATYPICAL PNEUMONIA

CAP has been separated into typical and atypical pneumonia to help define pathogen etiology and empirical therapy.[38–41] Typical CAP was associated with *S. pneumoniae, H. influenzae,* and *K. pneumoniae.* The clinical features included an acute onset, with chill or rigors, cough productive of purulent or bloody sputum, pleuritic chest pain (especially with *S. pneumoniae*), and physical signs of pulmonary consolidation. Neutrophilia was common and chest radiography showed lobar consolidation with air bronchograms (Fig. 46.1A).

In contrast, atypical CAP was associated with *Legionella* sp, *M. pneumoniae, Chlamydia* sp, *C. burnetii,* and viruses. The clinical features included gradual onset of fever, nonproductive cough, and a relatively normal white blood cell count in the absence of culture of a pathogen. Frequently, systemic features predominated over pulmonary ones. However, several studies, including one that included patients with mild CAP treated on an outpatient basis, have found that neither the clinical symptoms nor the radiographic appearance are sensitive or specific enough to classify the etiology or to guide therapy.[100]

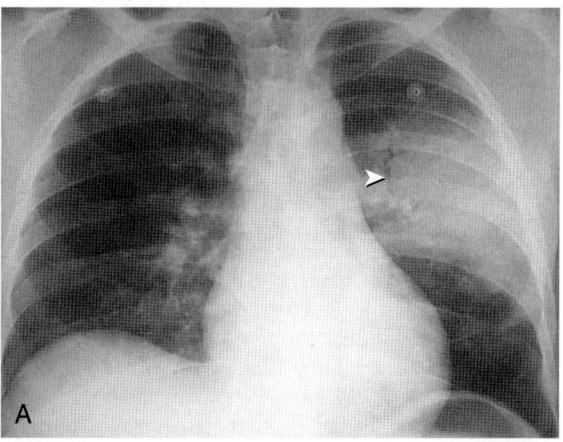

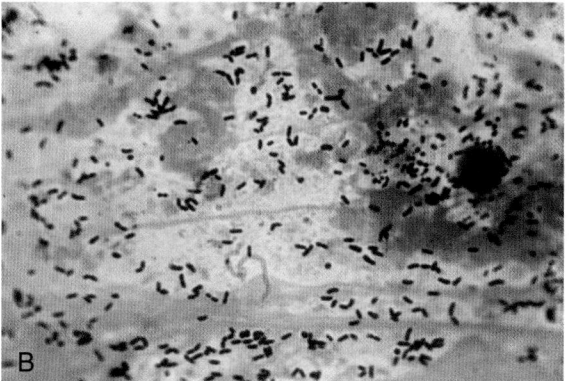

Figure 46.1 Pneumococcal pneumonia. (A) Frontal chest radiograph in a patient with pneumococcal pneumonia shows homogenous consolidation in the left upper lobe extending to the pleural surface. Note presence of air bronchograms (*arrowhead*). (B) Gram stain of sputum from a patient with pneumococcal pneumonia. The predominant organisms are gram-positive lancet-shaped diplococci. (A, Courtesy Michael B. Gotway, MD.)

PATIENT EVALUATION

Clinical Evaluation

The clinical findings that best differentiate CAP from other acute respiratory tract infections are cough, fever, tachycardia, and pulmonary crackles; CAP is present in 20–60% of persons who have all four factors, depending on the baseline prevalence of CAP.[101] Specific signs of pulmonary consolidation, including bronchial breath sounds, are present in only one-third of hospitalized patients and are less frequent in cases treated in the community. Early in disease, cough and physical abnormalities may be absent, and fever may be the only finding. In debilitated older patients, vague clinical presentations are common and undifferentiated fever with no apparent source, especially when accompanied by confusion or tachypnea, mandates a chest radiograph.

Clues to the etiologic diagnosis may lie outside the respiratory tract. Relative bradycardia (pulse should increase by 10 beats/min/°C of temperature elevation) has been associated with pneumonia due to *Legionella, C. psittaci, Mycoplasma,* or *F. tularensis. M. pneumoniae* infection may present with extrapulmonary manifestations, including arthralgia, cervical lymphadenopathy, bullous myringitis, diarrhea, myalgia, myocarditis, hepatitis, nausea, pericarditis, and vomiting.[102] Erythema multiforme or erythema nodosum may suggest *Mycoplasma* infection (as well as tuberculosis and endemic fungal infection or, for erythema multiforme, other pathogens associated with atypical pneumonia), whereas lesions of ecthyma gangrenosum are most often seen with *P. aeruginosa* infection. Complications such as pleural effusion, pericarditis, endocarditis, arthritis, and *central nervous system* (CNS) involvement may necessitate additional diagnostic procedures, drainage procedures for source control, or modification of antimicrobial selection and duration.[103]

In community settings or in *low- and middle-income countries*, clinical prediction rules are sometimes applied when radiology is not available or deemed nonessential. One example found that patients without alterations in specific vital or physical signs were unlikely to have CAP, and use of these criteria would miss only 5% cases of CAP and so could be applied to low-risk patients if patients could be readily followed up.[104]

Laboratory Evaluation

Patients being investigated for CAP should have pulse oximetry performed and, in those in whom hospital admission is being considered, blood cell counts, serum glucose and electrolyte measurements, and arterial blood gas assays should be performed to assess severity.[38-41] All patients with CAP should have an HIV test in view of the increased incidence of CAP in people living with HIV.

Marked leukocytosis is more often encountered with infections caused by *S. pneumoniae, S. aureus, H. influenzae,* and gram-negative bacilli than with atypical pneumonia or nonbacterial causes of pneumonia. Leukopenia may be seen with overwhelming Panton-Valentine leucocidin-producing *S. aureus* or gram-negative bacillary pneumonia. The serum level of *C-reactive protein* (CRP) and the erythrocyte sedimentation rate are increased to higher values with bacterial than with viral pneumonias. Thrombocytopenia and thrombocytosis are associated with a greater severity of pneumonia and higher mortality.[105]

Blood levels of *procalcitonin* (PCT), a precursor of calcitonin, are increased with bacterial infections, and PCT assays have been used to evaluate the severity, prognosis, and evolution of pneumonia.[106] Results of PCT assays have been used to deescalate antibiotics or to stop antibiotics in patients with severe bacterial infection, when the levels decrease to a certain cutoff point.[107] A randomized trial of a PCT-guided strategy compared with a guideline-based algorithm revealed equivalent primary outcomes of treatment of LRT infections, but the PCT-guided strategy resulted in reduced antibiotic exposure and duration, fewer adverse effects of antibiotic treatment, and shorter length of stay.[108] Despite this, the most recent ATS/IDSA CAP guidelines do not recommend basing initial decisions on whether to treat suspected CAP with antimicrobials on PCT values due to its variable sensitivity (38–91%) in the detection of bacterial infection.[109]

Radiologic Evaluation

Radiologic evaluation is usually required to establish the presence of pneumonia, because there is no combination of historical data, physical findings, or laboratory results that reliably confirms the diagnosis.[40,101,109,110] Limitations of chest radiography include interobserver variability

and suboptimal specificity, particularly in patients with ARDS.[40] Reported sensitivity ranges from 44–78%.[111,112] The sensitivity of the chest radiograph is decreased in (1) patients with emphysema, bullae, or structural abnormalities of the lung, who may present with delayed or subtle radiographic changes; (2) obese patients; and (3) patients with very early infection, severe dehydration, or profound granulocytopenia. CT of the chest provides a more sensitive means of detecting minor radiographic abnormalities.[101] It is, however, associated with higher cost and greater radiation exposure. Although high-resolution chest CT may be more sensitive at detecting opacities, it is not routinely recommended when the chest radiograph is negative.[38]

Although several radiographic patterns have been associated with pneumonia caused by specific microorganisms, the presence of a certain pattern is unreliable for diagnosing a specific pathogen.[113,114] Nonetheless, the presence of air bronchograms and a lobar (see Fig. 46.1A and eFig. 46.2) or segmental pattern is more characteristic of pneumococcal than other causes of pneumonia. In contrast, a mixed pattern (alveolar and interstitial disease) (eFig. 46.3) is more frequently observed with other pathogens. Pneumonia complicating aspiration (frequently from anaerobes) (eFig. 46.4) often involves the superior segment of the right lower lobe or posterior segment of the right upper lobe, or both, as well as the corresponding segments on the left. Infections developing from hematogenous seeding often appear as multiple rounded, small opacities, sometimes with cavities, with a basal predominance, where the distribution of blood flow is greatest. Necrotizing pneumonia, which can result in cavitation or a lung abscess (eFig. 46.5), suggests infection by anaerobes, *S. aureus, Streptococcus pyogenes*, gram-negative bacilli, or *Mycobacterium tuberculosis*. Pleural effusion frequently accompanies pneumonia; the size of the pleural effusion on the chest radiograph helps determine whether thoracentesis should be performed. Bedside ultrasound is a cheap and portable diagnostic aid that shows improved sensitivity over chest radiograph. It may be a useful adjunct to diagnosis of CAP in lower- and middle-income countries with sensitivity of 91–95% when compared to chest CT.[111,115]

Microbiologic Evaluation

Identification of the infecting microorganism facilitates the use of pathogen-directed therapy, limiting use of unnecessarily broad-spectrum antimicrobial agents and the collateral damage to the microbiome. Investigations that can establish the etiology of CAP are outlined in Table 46.2. Tests are indicated by clinical severity (eTable 46.1) or epidemiologic risk factors. PCR-based tests, particularly multiplex high-throughput systems, are increasingly available and are rapidly being adopted as the preferred diagnostic approach for pneumonia caused by viruses, by agents associated with atypical pneumonia, and increasingly by other bacteria[116] (see Chapter 19).

Sputum Examination

The current ATS/IDSA guidelines[109] recommend obtaining a sputum sample for Gram stain and culture in patients with CAP sufficiently severe to warrant hospitalization or in those who are believed to be at risk of MRSA or *P. aeruginosa* infection (eTable 46.2). Optimal culture results require that

Table 46.2 Recommended Microbiologic Evaluation in Patients With Community-Acquired Pneumonia

PATIENTS WHO DO NOT REQUIRE HOSPITALIZATION

None*

PATIENTS WHO REQUIRE HOSPITALIZATION

Two sets of blood cultures (obtained prior to antibiotics) in selected patients

Gram stain and culture of a valid sputum sample in selected patients

Urinary antigen test for detection of *Legionella pneumophila* (in endemic areas or during outbreaks)

Stain for acid-fast bacilli and culture of sputum (if tuberculosis is suggested by clinical history or radiologic findings)

Fungal stain and culture of sputum, and fungal serologies (if infection by an endemic fungus is suggested by the clinical history or radiologic findings)

Sputum examination for *Pneumocystis jirovecii* (if suggested by clinical history, HIV infection, or radiologic findings)

Nucleic acid amplification tests for *Mycoplasma pneumoniae*, *Chlamydophila pneumoniae*, *Chlamydophila psittaci*, *Coxiella burnetii*, *Legionella* species, respiratory viruses (in endemic areas or during outbreaks) and other agents (e.g., *Streptococcus pneumoniae*) if available

Culture and microscopic evaluation of pleural fluid (if significant fluid is present)

ADDITIONAL TESTS FOR PATIENTS WHO REQUIRE TREATMENT IN AN ICU

Gram stain and culture of endotracheal aspirate or bronchoscopically obtained specimens using a protected specimen brush or BAL

*Gram stain and culture should be strongly considered in patients with risk factors for infection by an antimicrobial-resistant organism or unusual pathogen.

BAL, bronchoalveolar lavage; ICU, intensive care unit.

specimens be obtained before initiation of antimicrobial therapy. Sputum samples must be carefully collected, transported, and processed to optimize the recovery of common bacterial pathogens. In many centers, however, sputum analysis, particularly Gram stain, is less often employed.

A valid expectorated sputum specimen can be obtained in about 40% of patients hospitalized with CAP. When interpreting sputum cultures, one must ensure that oropharyngeal contents do not unduly contaminate the specimens. The presence of greater than 10 squamous epithelial cells per low-power field (×100 magnification) indicates excessive oropharyngeal contamination and the specimen should be discarded.[38] A specimen with few or no squamous cells and abundant *polymorphonuclear leukocytes* (PMNs) (>25 cells/low-power field in a sample from a patient who is not granulocytopenic) is ideal. Gram-stained expectorated sputum specimens of acceptable quality should be carefully examined using ×1000 magnification (oil immersion objective). Specific fluorescent antibodies can be used to evaluate sputum or other respiratory tract specimens for the presence of *Legionella* and selected other pathogens (see Chapter 19).

When acceptable sputum is obtained, the specificity of the Gram stain for pneumococcal pneumonia is estimated to be greater than 80%.[117] Because the fastidious nature of *S. pneumoniae* and *H. influenzae* leads to the death of these organisms, the sensitivity of sputum culture may be lower than that of sputum Gram stain. In contrast, *S. aureus* and

gram-negative bacilli may dominate cultures even if they are not the cause of the patient's illness, because these bacteria are hardier and may proliferate during sample transport and processing. True pneumonia due to *S. aureus* or gram-negative bacilli is doubtful if the Gram stain of a valid sputum specimen does not corroborate the presence of these bacteria. In a good-quality Gram-stained sputum, the presence of a single or a preponderant morphotype of bacteria (≥90%) is considered diagnostic. In the absence of an informative Gram stain, the predictive value of sputum culture is very low.

Some bacterial agents of pneumonia cannot be cultivated on conventional laboratory media. For example, *Legionella* requires buffered charcoal yeast extract agar for isolation, whereas recovery of *Chlamydophila* species and *C. burnetii* requires culture in mammalian cell lines. When necessary, specimens can be sent to specialized or reference laboratories for appropriate procedures, including nucleic acid amplification assays (Chapter 19). Culture of certain agents of bacterial pneumonia poses major health risks to laboratory workers (e.g., *F. tularensis*, *Bacillus anthracis*, *C. burnetii*). Specimens suspected to harbor one of these agents should be dealt with carefully in a biologic safety hood, and isolation of the pathogens should be reserved for specialized laboratories.

Blood and Pleural Fluid Cultures

The latest IDSA/ATS guidelines[109] recommend obtaining blood cultures for hospitalized patients with the same clinical indications as are used to justify sputum collection (see eTable 46.2).

Although the overall yield of blood cultures is less than 20% in patients hospitalized for CAP, a positive culture of blood or pleural fluid can establish the etiologic diagnosis of pneumonia.[118] Unsurprisingly, the detected rate of bacteremia is lower in patients with mild CAP than in patients with severe CAP, especially those warranting ICU care. Prior antibiotic treatment decreases the yield of blood cultures.

A pleural effusion may be present in up to 40% of CAP cases. Although the specificity of pleural exudate cultures is very high, the sensitivity is very low because of the low incidence of pleural invasion. Diagnostic thoracentesis should be performed when a significant pleural effusion is present. Gram stain of pleural fluid may produce an indication of the infecting organisms within 1 hour, while culture identification may require 24 to 48 hours.

Antigen Detection

Commercial assays can be used to detect capsular polysaccharide antigens of *S. pneumoniae* or *L. pneumophila* serogroup 1 in urine, with results available in under an hour. The sensitivity of these tests is little affected by prior antibiotic treatment; indeed, results may remain positive several weeks after successful treatment. For *L. pneumophila* serogroup 1, the sensitivity is approximately 80% and the specificity is 99%.[119] Currently available tests detect *L. pneumophila* serogroup 1 antigen only. Nevertheless, this serogroup accounts for 80% of community-acquired *Legionella* disease.[120]

A meta-analysis estimated the sensitivity and specificity of *S. pneumoniae* urinary antigen for the diagnosis of *S. pneumoniae* infection in adult CAP to be 74% and 97%, respectively.[121] The degree of positivity for the *S. pneumoniae* urinary antigen test correlates with the Pneumonia Severity Index.[122] The *S. pneumoniae* antigen test may also be applied on pleural fluid with a sensitivity and specificity of almost 100%, but should be interpreted with caution in children due to low specificity caused by nasopharyngeal carriage.[123] Current IDSA/ATS guidelines[109] recommend *S. pneumoniae* and *L. pneumophila* urinary antigen detection with recent travel or exposure to *Legionella* outbreaks, or with severe CAP.

Antigens for many common respiratory viruses, including influenza virus, RSV, adenovirus, and parainfluenza viruses, can be detected by direct immunofluorescence or by enzyme-linked immunoassay. A rapid antigen detection test for influenza can provide an etiologic diagnosis within 15 to 30 minutes. Test performance varies according to the test used, viral strain, sample type, duration of illness, and patient age. Most show a sensitivity ranging from 50–70% and a specificity approaching 100% in adults. However, with the exception of RSV, rapid antigen tests have largely been superseded by nucleic acid amplification tests owing to their superior sensitivity (see Chapter 19).

Nucleic Acid Amplification Tests

Nucleic acid amplification tests are rapid and have much greater sensitivity than conventional methods in the diagnosis of respiratory viruses and atypical bacteria; some are now considered the gold standard.[124,125] The development of real-time multiplex PCR assays allowing detection of multiple respiratory viruses and atypical bacteria simultaneously can facilitate the rapid diagnosis of pneumonia, and has the potential to reduce the unnecessary use of antimicrobial treatment. Multiplex panels are expanding to include other bacterial causes of CAP such as *S. pneumoniae* and MRSA. Moreover, a number of rapid molecular tests primarily for the detection of influenza A and B viruses, RSV, and SARS-CoV-2 have been approved by the U.S. Food and Drug Administration. A result is available within 15 to 30 minutes and greater than 99% sensitivity and greater than 97% specificity are reported.[126]

Caution is necessary in the interpretation of viral PCR results because one or more respiratory viruses can be detected in up to 15% of healthy persons.[127] Detection of virus on nasopharyngeal or oropharyngeal samples may indicate upper respiratory tract infection or convalescent shedding rather than the causative pathogen of CAP. Furthermore, PCR-based methods can only detect targeted pathogens. (See Chapter 19 for detailed information on nucleic acid amplification tests for respiratory pathogens.)

Metagenomic Sequencing

Metagenomic *next-generation sequencing* is an emerging DNA technology that sequences multiple small DNA fragments in parallel. It allows unbiased detection of all microorganisms present, does not require preexisting knowledge of expected pathogens in the sample, and can provide detailed characterization of pathogen species and genomic sequences. Until recently, metagenomic next-generation sequencing of respiratory samples has been limited by poor sensitivity due to the relatively low abundance of pathogen nucleic acids compared to host and commensal nucleic acids (e.g., pathogen/host nucleic acid ratio $1/10^5$ in sputum).

Recent studies using hybridization-based sequence capture to enrich for respiratory viral detection,[128] as well as host DNA depletion and nanopore sequencing to detect bacteria and antibiotic resistance genes,[129] report improved sensitivity of greater than 95%. Nevertheless, high cost and the need for sequencing and computational expertise currently limits the use of metagenomic next-generation sequencing to research settings. (See Chapter 19 for detailed information on next-generation sequencing of respiratory pathogens.)

Serologic Evaluation

Before the development of nucleic acid amplification tests, serologic techniques were used to establish a microbiologic diagnosis for pneumonia caused by pathogens that cannot be readily cultured. Examples include common pathogens such as *M. pneumoniae*, *C. pneumoniae*, and *L. pneumophila* and less common causes of pneumonia such as those caused by the agents of tularemia, brucellosis, and psittacosis, and certain viruses. Diagnosis usually required that a convalescent specimen demonstrate a fourfold increase in IgG titer above that present in an acute specimen. These tests are unhelpful in initial patient management but are of utility in defining the epidemiology of the pertinent infectious agents. Because IgM antibodies appear earlier than IgG antibodies, the detection of pathogen-specific IgM in serum has been used for the early serologic diagnosis of certain acute infections.

Invasive Diagnostic Techniques

Invasive procedures may be necessary to obtain suitable material for microscopy and cultures in certain instances, such as in the management of patients with life-threatening CAP in whom diagnostic materials cannot otherwise be obtained, for patients with progressive pneumonia despite seemingly appropriate antimicrobial therapy, or for immunocompromised patients.[103]

Lower Airway Samples

Samples can also be obtained from the lower airway by bronchial wash obtained via an endotracheal tube or by BAL obtained by bronchoscopy. The reliability of bronchial sampling to determine the microbial etiology of pneumonia depends on the technique used and the organism sought. When compared with sputum cultures, optimally processed bronchial specimens demonstrate improved sensitivity and equal specificity for the culture of pathogenic fungi and mycobacteria but poor specificity for culture of bacteria that commonly cause CAP due to oropharyngeal contamination. Semiquantitative or quantitative cultures of materials obtained bronchoscopically with a protected sheath brush or through BAL and by direct lung aspiration have been successfully used for aerobic and anaerobic bacterial cultures.[130] For protected specimen brush cultures, a threshold of 10^3 cfu/mL has been recommended to distinguish colonization from infection. However, 14–40% of duplicate samples yield disparate quantitative results.

BAL fluid can be quantitatively cultured for bacteria and qualitatively cultured for fungi, mycobacteria, and viruses. A concentrate can be stained for cytochemical and fluorescence evaluation.[131] In one study, the threshold of 10^3 cfu/mL for diagnosing bacterial pneumonia correlated well with diagnoses based on protected sheath brush results and histologic examination of the lung.[132] BAL permits the immediate diagnosis of infection (i.e., intracellular bacteria in >2–5% of examined PMNs) and the exclusion of infection (i.e., the absence of bacterial pathogens in culture of BAL fluid, although sensitivity is reduced by prior antibiotic administration).[133]

In one ICU study, the use of quantitative cultures obtained by protected sheath brush and BAL, compared with qualitative cultures of endotracheal aspirates and clinical evaluation, was associated with lower 14-day mortality, earlier reversal of organ dysfunction, and less antibiotic use.[134] However, other randomized trials have not replicated these findings.[135,136]

Transthoracic Lung Aspiration

Transthoracic lung aspiration obtains specimens suitable for microbiologic and cytologic examination directly from lung parenchyma (eFig. 46.6). It is more widely used for diagnosing malignant pulmonary lesions than infections. In immunocompetent hosts, the diagnostic yield by transthoracic lung aspiration is approximately 50%. Its main utility has been in children, and it is less useful in adults. Serious complications of transthoracic lung aspiration include pneumothorax and hemoptysis, even when small-gauge needles are used.

Differential Diagnosis

Several diseases may present with fever and chest radiographic opacities and mimic CAP (eTable 46.3);[101] such diseases should be suspected when the radiographic resolution is unusually quick or when there is a lack of response to initial or subsequent antibiotic treatments.

THERAPEUTIC APPROACH TO PNEUMONIA

Once the diagnosis of pneumonia is made, the clinician must decide the appropriate treatment setting: outpatient, general hospital bed, or ICU. Applying prediction rules can facilitate this decision. The second key decision is the selection of initial antimicrobial therapy.

ASSESSMENT OF SEVERITY

The *Pneumonia Severity Index* (PSI) (Table 46.3) is a scoring system derived from a retrospective analysis of a cohort of 14,199 patients with CAP and prospectively validated in a separate cohort of 38,039 patients with CAP.[137] The PSI is heavily weighted by age, which means it is less useful at extremes of age and is not valid in children. Outpatient treatment is recommended for patients with a PSI score of 70 or less (class I or II). Patients with a PSI score of 71 to 90 (class III) may benefit from brief hospitalization, while inpatient care is appropriate for patients with a score greater than 90 (class IV and V). Prospective studies in both community and teaching hospitals demonstrate that hospital admission decisions based on PSI may be safely and effectively applied in clinical practice.[138–140] Additional studies have shown the use of the PSI increases the proportion of patients safely treated as outpatients.[141,142,143]

The British Thoracic Society validated the simpler CURB-65 score for admission triage decisions.[47] Their algorithm assigns 1 point for each of the following findings at presentation: (1) confusion; (2) urea greater than 7 mmol/L (equivalent to blood urea nitrogen >20 mg/dL); (3) respiratory rate of 30 breaths/min or greater; (4) low systolic (<90 mm Hg) or diastolic (≤60 mm Hg) blood pressure; and (5) age 65 years or greater. Outpatient treatment is recommended for 0 to 1 points, brief inpatient or supervised outpatient care is recommended for 2 points, and hospitalization is recommended for 3 or more points, with consideration of ICU care for patients with scores of 4 or 5.

Risk stratification for both PSI and CURB-65 was based on associated mortality. They are therefore not sensitive to logistic and social issues such as reliability of oral intake, including antibiotics, and home support. When compared to CURB-65, the PSI was a better predictor of short-term mortality and classified a larger number of patients as low risk.[144] Furthermore, recent studies in lower- and middle-income countries have demonstrated variable performance of CURB-65 in predicting mortality in adults with CAP, likely reflecting differences in demographics, comorbidities, and microbial etiology in these settings.[76,145] It has not proved particularly useful, for example, in sub-Saharan Africa.

Patients initially admitted to a general floor with subsequent transfer to the ICU have higher mortality than patients with equivalent severity of illness admitted directly to the ICU.[146] Neither PSI nor CURB-65 is accurate for determining need for ICU care in patients without an obvious indication, such as the need for mechanical ventilation or vasopressor support while still in the emergency department. Several scores have been developed for this critical decision.[147–150] These scores share many common risk factors and appear to be similarly effective.[151] Management of severe CAP using these guidelines has been associated with decreased mortality.[152–154] The optimal use of these scores is to identify at-risk patients who need additional evaluation or monitoring, even if not initially admitted to the ICU.

CORRECTION OF HOST ABNORMALITIES

Defects related to the host's immune system may impede recovery from pneumonia. Immunodeficiency may arise as a complication of age, cancer chemotherapy, immunosuppressive agents, or corticosteroid use; or it may result from a congenital (e.g., hypogammaglobulinemia) or acquired (e.g., HIV infection) immune defect. Many of these immune deficiencies are not remediable; however, drug-related immunosuppression may be improved by discontinuing the offending agent or reducing the dose when possible. Although reduction of immunosuppression may promote recovery from the active infection, it can also be complicated by enhanced inflammation due to immune reconstitution.[155]

Granulocytopenia (absolute granulocyte count <500 cells/mm^3) has been associated with fulminant, antibiotic-unresponsive pneumonia, and administration of *granulocyte colony-stimulating factor* (G-CSF) or *granulocyte-macrophage colony-stimulating factor* (GM-CSF) is effective in increasing the number of circulating neutrophils. Despite this effect on neutrophils, routine administration of G-CSF or GM-CSF has not been found

Table 46.3 Pneumonia Severity Index Scoring System for Determining Risk of Complications in Patients with Community-Acquired Pneumonia

Patient Characteristic	Points Assigned
DEMOGRAPHIC FACTORS	
Men	Age (yr)
Women	Age (yr) −10
Nursing home residents	Age (yr) +10
COMORBID ILLNESSES	
Neoplastic disease	+30
Liver disease	+20
Congestive heart failure	+10
Cerebrovascular disease	+10
Renal disease	+10
PHYSICAL EXAMINATION FINDINGS	
Altered mental status	+20
Respiratory rate ≥30 breaths/min	+20
Systolic blood pressure <90 mm Hg	+20
Temperature <35°C or ≥40°C	+15
Pulse ≥125 beats/min	+10
LABORATORY FINDINGS	
pH <7.35	+30
BUN ≥30 mg/dL (≥10.7 mmol/L)	+20
Sodium <130 mEq/L	+20
Glucose ≥250 mg/dL (≥13.9 mmol/L)	+10
Hematocrit <30%	+10
PaO_2 <60 mm Hg or O_2 saturation <90%	+10
Pleural effusion	+10

A risk score is obtained by summing the patient's age in years (age −10 for women) and the points for each applicable patient characteristic. Patients with a score <70 are candidates for outpatient treatment, whereas those with scores >90 warrant hospitalization. Proper management of patients with scores of 70 to 90 requires careful application of clinical judgment. BUN, blood urea nitrogen; PaO_2, arterial oxygen pressure.

Modified from Fine MJ, Auble TE, Yealy DM, et al. A prediction rule to identify low-risk patients with community-acquired pneumonia. *N Engl J Med.* 1997;336:243–250.

to improve survival from infections.[156] Because pneumonia is the infection most frequently associated with a poor clinical outcome in profoundly neutropenic patients, the use of G-CSF or GM-CSF in these patients may be justified even though a benefit has not been demonstrated.[157] GM-CSF has also been studied as an approach to correct the neutrophil phagocytosis defect in critically ill patients. In a small, multicenter randomized controlled trial, GM-CSF was safe and, although mean neutrophil phagocytosis was not increased, the proportion of patients with neutrophil phagocytosis was 50% or greater, suggesting GM-CSF could increase the proportion of patients with adequate phagocytosis.[158] Corticosteroid treatment has been investigated because of its suppressant effect on inflammatory responses; studies have yielded discordant findings without consistent benefits. Recent guidelines do not recommend corticosteroid therapy for CAP or influenza pneumonia, other than when indicated for refractory shock.[109]

SELECTION OF ANTIMICROBIAL AGENTS

Antimicrobial stewardship principles aim to select the most appropriate antimicrobial agent and optimize the dose and duration while minimizing the potential toxicity and emergence of antimicrobial resistance. Increasing rates of hospital-acquired infections such as MRSA and *Clostridioides* (formerly *Clostridium*) *difficile* infection also influence empiric antimicrobial prescribing. Whenever possible, treatment for pneumonia should use the antibiotic with the narrowest spectrum possible, selected on the basis of the underlying pathogen. However, pathogens are rarely identified at the time of presentation, especially when pneumonia is managed in the outpatient setting. Because optimal outcomes are associated with a rapid initiation of antibiotics, initial treatment for patients with pneumonia must be empirical. In selecting initial empirical antimicrobial therapy, physicians should consider the illness severity, presence of comorbidities and immunosuppression, recent antimicrobial therapy, and geographic and facility-specific epidemiology, such as the local and temporal prevalence of specific microorganisms (e.g., *C. burnetii*, *L. pneumophila*, endemic mycoses, and *multidrug-resistant* pathogens).

In patients being admitted to the hospital, specimens for culture should be obtained before treatment. A brief delay in starting therapy while performing diagnostic procedures is reasonable in patients who are not hypotensive. However, delays of more than 4 to 8 hours may increase the length of hospitalization and have been associated with increased mortality.[154,159]

It is important to recognize that all CAP treatment guidelines are based on broad epidemiologic considerations that may vary by location with respect to geographically restricted pathogens and antimicrobial resistance. Local incidence and susceptibility patterns guide empiric regimens to cover MRSA, gram-negative Enterobacteriaceae, or *P. aeruginosa*.[46,160]

Recent guidelines suggest use of amoxicillin, doxycycline, or macrolides for outpatient treatment of CAP (Table 46.4) in the absence of medical comorbidity; the guidelines no longer require routine coverage of atypical pneumonia.[109,161–163] Macrolides should not be used if local *S. pneumoniae* resistance exceeds 25%.[109] North American guidelines consider amoxicillin–clavulanic acid or oral cephalosporins combined with a macrolide or doxycycline, or a respiratory fluoroquinolone, for outpatient therapy in patients with medical comorbidity. This is to ensure coverage of additional pathogens, such as *H. influenzae*, that may produce a β-lactamase.[109] For inpatient therapy, a β-lactam is usually combined with an extended-spectrum macrolide (Table 46.5). The British Thoracic Society guidelines exclude the macrolide in mild disease and the European Respiratory Society/European Society of Clinical Microbiology and Infectious Diseases guidelines make it optional outside the ICU. North American guidelines recommend use of β-lactam/β-lactam inhibitors or cephalosporins for all hospitalized patients, while the British Thoracic Society guidelines only recommend these for more severe CAP, preferring amoxicillin or benzylpenicillin. The European Respiratory Society guidelines allow use of any of these β-lactams for mild to moderate CAP.

Table 46.4 Guidelines for Empirical Oral Outpatient Treatment of Immunocompetent Adults With Community-Acquired Pneumonia

ATS/IDSA[109]

No modifying factors[a]: amoxicillin,[b] doxycycline or advanced macrolide if *S. pneumoniae* macrolide resistance <25%[c,d]
Comorbidities[a]: β-lactam,[e] macrolide[f] or doxycycline,[d] or fluoroquinolone[g] alone

BTS[161,162]

Primary: amoxicillin
Alternatives: clarithromycin or doxycycline

ERS/ESCMID[163]

Amoxicillin or doxycycline with macrolide as alternative if low levels of resistance

DRSPTWG

Primary: amoxicillin, amoxicillin-clavulanate, cefuroxime, doxycycline, macrolide (if low rate of resistance)
Alternative: fluoroquinolone[h]

[a]American Thoracic Society/Infectious Disease Society of America comorbidities (modifying factors) include chronic heart, lung, liver or kidney disease, diabetes, asplenia, alcoholism, and malignancy.
[b]Amoxicillin 1 g q8h, doxycycline 100 mg q12h, azithromycin 500 mg on first day then 250 mg/day, clarithromycin 500 mg q8h, or clarithromycin extended release 1000 mg/day.
[c]Advanced macrolides are azithromycin and clarithromycin.
[d]Second-choice agent.
[e]Amoxicillin-clavulanate (500 mg amoxicillin plus 125 mg clavulanate q8h, 875 mg amoxicillin plus 125 mg clavulanate q12h or 2 g amoxicillin plus 125 mg clavulanic acid q12h), cefpodoxime, cefprozil, or cefuroxime.
[f]Because of increasing macrolide resistance, erythromycin cannot be relied upon to ensure coverage of β-lactamase–producing *Haemophilus influenzae*. A combination of a β-lactam/β-lactamase inhibitor is preferred.
[g]Antipneumococcal fluoroquinolones include levofloxacin, and moxifloxacin.
[h]Levofloxacin or moxifloxacin.
ATS/IDSA, American Thoracic Society/Infectious Diseases Society of America; BTS, British Thoracic Society; DRSPTWG, Drug-Resistant *Streptococcus pneumoniae* Therapeutic Working Group; ERS/ESCMID, European Respiratory Society and European Society for Clinical Microbiology and Infectious Diseases.

There is a differing emphasis on fluoroquinolones, with the North American guidelines considering them valid alternatives to the β-lactams plus macrolide combinations; however, European guidelines suggest they are less-preferred alternatives. This follows the European Medicines Evaluation Agency guidance that suggests they should be reserved for settings where other agents cannot be used or have failed. This reflects concerns about levels of hepatotoxicity, QT prolongation, fluoroquinolone-related musculoskeletal and neurologic adverse events, and propensity to contribute to *C. difficile* or MRSA infections.[163,164] Widespread fluoroquinolone use, especially in subtherapeutic doses, and use of ciprofloxacin have been associated with fluoroquinolone resistance in up to 13% of *S. pneumoniae* isolates in Hong Kong. Fluoroquinolone resistance and subsequent treatment failures are reported in pneumococcal CAP,[165–167] but this is less common with use of fluoroquinolones that have improved activity against respiratory pathogens. When tuberculosis is a possibility, fluoroquinolones should be avoided because as few as 10 days of fluoroquinolone administration is sufficient to select for fluoroquinolone-resistant *M. tuberculosis*.[168]

Retrospective studies suggest combination therapy for severe pneumococcal pneumonia and severe CAP in general is associated with lower mortality. A meta-analysis of observational data demonstrated reduced mortality with macrolide use in severe CAP.[169] In a large cohort of older patients with CAP needing hospitalization, antibiotic treatment including azithromycin was associated with a lower 90-day risk mortality compared with other antibiotics.[170] However, this has not been a uniform finding, as other studies have found no such benefit.[171]

In recent North American HAP/*ventilator-associated pneumonia* (VAP) guidelines, the former category of health care–associated pneumonia has been removed because patients previously fitting this category are generally infected with pathogens associated with CAP, which are not multidrug resistant.[172] Empiric coverage of MRSA or *P. aeruginosa* is reserved for hospitalized patients with prior evidence of the pathogens in the respiratory tract or for severe CAP in people who have been recently hospitalized and received parenteral antimicrobials, in addition to having locally validated risk factors for these pathogens.[109]

In most patients with normal immunity, supportive therapy of viral pneumonia is successful with early antimicrobial therapy of secondary bacterial infections, if present. Specific antiviral therapy may be beneficial and is discussed with the individual pathogens. Viral pneumonia with extensive involvement of lung tissue may require prolonged ventilatory assistance and pulmonary rehabilitation. Bacterial superinfections are common in influenza and RSV infections and should be sought and treated when a patient with one of these viral infections worsens clinically.

ADJUSTMENTS IN ANTIMICROBIAL THERAPY IN PATIENTS WHO ARE STABLE OR IMPROVING

If the etiologic agent of a patient's pneumonia has been identified, the initial antimicrobial regimen should be adjusted based on the results of in vitro susceptibility testing. The ideal drug for a known pathogen has the narrowest spectrum of activity and is the most efficacious, least toxic, and least costly. Recommendations for specific drug choices for specific microorganisms are discussed under the sections devoted to individual pathogens and are summarized in eTable 46.4. If a pathogen is not identified, reevaluation of the initial therapeutic regimen must take into account the patient's response to therapy. Change from parenteral to oral antimicrobial therapy can safely be made in hospitalized CAP patients when clinically stable and able to absorb oral antimicrobials[173,174]; this is often achieved within 2 to 3 days. In-hospital observation after switching from intravenous to oral antibiotics for CAP patients is not needed. Treatment duration is usually for as long as required to ensure clinical stabilization, as evidenced by normalization of clinical features such as vital signs and physiologic parameters such as pulse oximetry.[109] Treatment should be for a minimum of 5 days.[109]

Table 46.5   Guidelines for Empirical Parenteral Inpatient Treatment of Immunocompetent Adults With Community-Acquired Pneumonia

MILD TO MODERATE DISEASE

ATS/IDSA[109]

- Primary[c]: ampicillin and sulbactam, cefotaxime, ceftriaxone, or ceftaroline with azithromycin or clarithromycin
- Alternative: fluoroquinolone[a] alone or, if history of prior respiratory isolation of MRSA[d] or *Pseudomonas aeruginosa*,[e] treatment to cover these agents

BTS[161,162]

- Mild: oral amoxicillin. Alternatives parenteral amoxicillin or benzylpenicillin or clarithromycin
- Moderate: oral amoxicillin and clarithromycin (can consider clarithromycin monotherapy if prior therapy with amoxicillin)
- Alternative if unable to take oral medication: parenteral amoxicillin or benzylpenicillin plus clarithromycin (if intolerant of penicillin but able to take a cephalosporin parenteral second- or third-generation cephalosporin plus clarithromycin)
- Alternative: if unable to take penicillin or macrolide, oral doxycycline, or if not able to take any of these, a respiratory fluoroquinolone[a]

ERS/ESCMID[163]

- Aminopenicillin, aminopenicillin with β-lactamase inhibitor, penicillin, cefotaxime, ceftriaxone with or without macrolide
- Respiratory fluoroquinolone alone[a]

DRSPTWG

- Primary: cefuroxime, cefotaxime, ceftriaxone, or ampicillin-sulbactam; macrolide
- Alternative: fluoroquinolone[a]

SEVERE DISEASE

ATS/IDSA[109]

- Primary[c]: Ampicillin and sulbactam, cefotaxime, ceftriaxone, or ceftaroline with azithromycin or clarithromycin
- Alternative: broad-spectrum β-lactam as for primary with fluoroquinolone[a] or, if history of prior respiratory isolation or prior hospitalization with parenteral antimicrobials within 90 days in setting of locally validated risk factors for MRSA[d] or *P. aeruginosa*,[e] treatment to cover these agents

BTS[161,162]

- Primary: amoxicillin/clavulanate (or if penicillin intolerant cefuroxime, cefotaxime, or ceftriaxone) plus macrolide

ERS/ESCMID[163]

- Cefotaxime or ceftriaxone plus macrolide or respiratory fluoroquinolone
- Alternative: respiratory fluoroquinolone alone if no sepsis
- Alternative if risk factors for *P. aeruginosa*: piperacillin/tazobactam, anti-pseudomonal cephalosporin (ceftazidime[f] or cefepime) plus ciprofloxacin or plus macrolide and aminoglycoside[g]

DRSPTWG

- Primary: ceftriaxone or cefotaxime, macrolide; or ceftriaxone or cefotaxime, fluoroquinolone[a]
- Alternative (with caution): fluoroquinolone.[a]

[a]Antipneumococcal fluoroquinolones include levofloxacin 750 mg/day and moxifloxacin 400 mg/day.
[b]Advanced macrolides are azithromycin and clarithromycin.
[c]Ampicillin and sulbactam 1.5-3 g q6h, cefotaxime 1-2 g q8h, ceftriaxone 1-2 g/day, or ceftaroline 600 mg q12h and azithromycin 500 mg/day or 500 mg on day 1 and 250 mg once a day thereafter for mild disease) or clarithromycin 500 mg bid.
[d]Anti-staphylococcal treatments include vancomycin (15 mg/kg q12h, adjust based on levels) or linezolid (600 mg q12h).
[e]Antipseudomonal β-lactams include piperacillin-tazobactam (4.5 g q6h), cefepime (2 g q8h), ceftazidime (2 g q8h), imipenem (500 mg q6h), meropenem (1 g q8h), or aztreonam (2 g q8h).
[f]If ceftazidime used should be combined with penicillin to ensure coverage of pneumococci per ERS/ESCMID guideline.
[g]Recommendation to double cover *P. aeruginosa* with both a β-lactam and either ciprofloxacin or an aminoglycoside per ERS/ESCMID guideline.
ATS/IDSA, American Thoracic Society/Infectious Diseases Society of America; BTS, British Thoracic Society; DRSPTWG, Drug-Resistant *Streptococcus pneumoniae* Therapeutic Working Group; ERS/ESCMID, European Respiratory Society and European Society for Clinical Microbiology and Infectious Diseases.

ADJUSTMENTS IN ANTIMICROBIAL THERAPY IN PATIENTS WHO ARE DETERIORATING OR NOT IMPROVING

The optimal therapeutic approach to nonresolving pneumonia involves close monitoring, often transfer to a higher level of care, and optimization of the antibiotic regimen, including dosing.[175] The optimal time to make these changes is not defined, although it has been suggested to wait until at least 48 hours after treatment initiation except in the presence of severe clinical deterioration or dramatic radiologic progression.

In nonresponding CAP, new cultures should be obtained and empirical coverage for resistant *S. pneumoniae*, *P. aeruginosa*, MRSA, and anaerobes should be considered. Alternative diagnoses must also be considered, including fungal pneumonias in areas where endemic fungi are prevalent and tuberculosis in patients with a plausible history of exposure. The specific antimicrobial regimen chosen depends on patient risk factors, disease severity, and the local epidemiology of antimicrobial resistance. In CA-MRSA, antimicrobial regimens may include linezolid or clindamycin plus vancomycin, depending on results of susceptibility testing.[176] The increasing spread of virulent carbapenemase-producing *K. pneumoniae* also necessitates vigilance for these organisms that are especially challenging to treat.[177]

COMMON CAUSES OF PNEUMONIA

Individual pneumonia pathogens have unique epidemiology, diagnostic tests, and/or treatment. The sections that follow emphasize these unique aspects for selected pathogens (or groups).

MAJOR CAUSES OF PNEUMONIA

Streptococcus pneumoniae (Pneumococcal Pneumonia)

Epidemiology. S. pneumoniae is the most frequent cause of CAP among patients who require hospitalization.[40,41] The overall incidence of pneumococcal pneumonia is approximately 200 cases per 100,000 persons per year in the United States and other developed countries. This infection accounts for 40,000 deaths annually in the United States, with most deaths in the very young and the elderly. Risk factors, particularly in adults, include cigarette smoking, HIV infection (even with antiretroviral therapy and normal CD4 counts), heavy alcohol use, chronic liver disease, asthma and chronic lung disease, defects in host immunity, asplenia, and malnutrition.[178,179] Pneumococcal infections present predominantly in the winter and early spring and are often associated with prior infection by influenza or RSV.[180]

Use of the *pneumococcal conjugate vaccine* (PCV) has markedly decreased invasive pneumococcal infections in children, with a secondary reduction in adults in the United States.[181,182] This latter effect probably represents interruption of transmission because the conjugate vaccine reduces colonization.[183] However, widespread use of PCV in the United States has resulted in an increase in the number and proportion of cases of invasive pneumococcal disease due to non-vaccine serotypes.[184] Data from U.S. adults hospitalized with CAP in 2013 to 2016 show that, since a conjugate vaccine containing 13 capsular polysaccharide antigens was approved by the *U.S. Food and Drug Administration* (FDA) in 2012, approximately half of pneumococcal CAP is currently due to non-vaccine serotypes.[185]

Pathogenesis of *S. pneumoniae*. S. pneumoniae contains a core genome and a large number of noncore genes, promoting diversity.[186] The polysaccharide capsule exists in at least 92 antigenic types; because the polysaccharide capsule is the target of antibodies that provide protective immunity by promoting phagocytosis and intracellular killing, antigenic variation allows for repeated infections and promotes circulation of multiple antigenic types in a community.[187] Antigenic variation of the capsular polysaccharide also necessitates inclusion of multiple antigenic types in the currently available pneumococcal vaccines. The polysaccharide capsule also helps the pathogen avoid binding to mucus and inhibits recognition by phagocytes in the absence of specific antibodies. An additional virulence factor of S. pneumoniae is pneumolysin, a secreted toxin that inhibits ciliary function, limits complement opsonization, modulates reactive oxygen species generation, and promotes inflammation through cytokine production and T cell activation.[188] Pneumococcal surface proteins A and C inhibit opsonization with complement while an IgA protease inhibits IgA function, enabling colonization.[188] S. pneumoniae is an obligate extracellular pathogen because it is killed rapidly after being phagocytosed by neutrophils or macrophages. Therefore, its virulence strategies have principally evolved to evade phagocytosis.

Pneumococcal infection is preceded by colonization of the upper respiratory mucosa; bacteria that reach the distal airway are thought to be cleared by alveolar macrophages, especially if they are opsonized by anticapsular antibodies.[22,23] When alveolar macrophages are unable to clear the bacteria, neutrophils are recruited and become essential for bacterial clearance, although neutrophils depend on antibody opsonization of S. pneumoniae for optimal phagocytosis and killing.[23] Effective immune responses require a range of pattern recognition receptors, including TLR2, which recognizes lipopeptides, and *nucleotide oligomerization domain (NOD)-like receptor* (NLR) P3 inflammasomes activated by pneumolysin.[186,188] S. pneumoniae can also be cleared by apoptosis of bacteria-containing alveolar macrophages without triggering inflammation.[189]

Clinical Manifestations. The classic presentation of pneumococcal pneumonia consists of a rigor followed by sustained fever, cough, dyspnea, and production of rusty or mucoid sputum; gross hemoptysis is unusual. Pleuritic chest pain is common and may be severe. The typical radiographic appearance of pneumococcal pneumonia is lobar consolidation (see Fig. 46.1A and eFig. 46.2) or patchy bronchopneumonia (eFig. 46.7). Although pneumococci can cause necrotizing pneumonia, cavitation rarely develops.[178] Small, parapneumonic effusions are frequently present and can progress to frank empyema. Neutropenia may develop in patients with overwhelming infection and is associated with higher mortality.[190]

Microbiologic Diagnosis. A Gram stain of purulent sputum revealing numerous characteristic lancet-shaped diplococci with blunted ends (commonly seen in pairs and short chains) in the absence of other predominant flora is strongly suggestive of pneumococcal pneumonia (see Fig. 46.1B). However, a good-quality sputum specimen cannot always be obtained.[191] The organism is recovered from sputum culture in fewer than half of cases, and even a single dose of antibiotics can affect the yield of sputum cultures, which contributes to the discrepancy between sputum Gram stain and culture results. The frequency of positive blood cultures in hospitalized patients has decreased in the last few decades.[41] This decrease may reflect a greater percentage of blood cultures drawn after antibiotics due to the emphasis on prompt antibiotic dosing in the emergency department, de-emphasis on blood cultures in CAP in general, and/or a benefit of vaccination on invasive pneumococcal disease.[109]

The rapid urinary antigen S. pneumoniae test offers an alternative approach to the diagnosis of pneumococcal CAP and is becoming more widely used in diagnosis and in narrowing antibiotic therapy.[192–195] Despite satisfactory sensitivity and specificity, the urinary antigen test cannot provide information on antimicrobial susceptibility of the infecting organism.

Clinical Course. With an appropriate antibiotic, a clinical response is expected within 24 to 48 hours. The onset of suppurative complications, such as purulent pericarditis, meningitis, endocarditis, arthritis, and cellulitis after initiation of therapy is uncommon in the modern era. The exception is empyema, which appears to be increased due to serotype replacement in the vaccinated populations by serotypes more often associated with empyema.[196] Pneumococcal pneumonia remains a cause of septic shock and ARDS.[197]

Treatment. Antimicrobial resistance complicates treatment for *S. pneumoniae* in much of the world, including in the United States, with increasing rates of penicillin resistance, particularly in children in southern states.[198] For nonmeningeal isolates of *S. pneumoniae*, the redefinition of full susceptibility in 2002 as a *minimum inhibitory concentration* (MIC) of penicillin of 2 µg/mL or less and high-level resistance as MIC of 8 µg/mL or greater markedly changed the reported incidence of penicillin resistance.[199] This redefinition was driven by discordance between previous lower MIC breakpoints and clinical success rates. The rate of increase in the frequency of penicillin resistance may have stabilized, possibly as a consequence of the PCV and a shift in outpatient antibiotic prescription patterns away from β-lactams.[200]

Penicillin resistance in *S. pneumoniae* is due to alterations in penicillin-binding proteins rather than to β-lactamase production, and the anti-pneumococcal third- and fourth-generation cephalosporins (i.e., cefotaxime, ceftriaxone, and cefepime) retain activity against 75–95% of nonmeningeal isolates of *S. pneumoniae*.[201] By 2000, *S. pneumoniae* resistance rates to other antimicrobials in the United States had reached 30% for *trimethoprim-sulfamethoxazole* (TMP-SMX), 16% for tetracyclines, 26% for macrolides, and 9% for clindamycin.[198,200] High-level macrolide resistance (MIC >64 µg/mL) associated with the MLSB (macrolide, lincosamide, streptogramin B) phenotype is more common in Europe[202] and has been associated with in vitro resistance to clindamycin.[203] In the United States, PCV7 and PCV13 vaccination has been associated with reductions in macrolide resistance.[204] In contrast, 67% of pneumococcal isolates in adults with CAP or invasive pneumococcal disease in Asia between 2012 and 2017 had macrolide resistance with emergence of multidrug-resistant non-vaccine serotypes.[205] *S. pneumoniae* resistance to fluoroquinolones has also emerged with associated clinical treatment failures.[200,206] A contemporary study of global patterns of resistance in pneumococcal strains causing CAP in adults found overall resistance was low but most common for macrolides and penicillins and more common in Africa than other regions.[207] In keeping with this observation, African countries report high rates of antimicrobial resistance in pneumococci colonizing the nasopharynx in children; 22% penicillin, 77% TMP-SMX, and 50% doxycycline resistance was reported in Niger in 2014 to 2018.[208]

Recent exposure to an antibiotic increases the likelihood of the patient having a pneumococcal isolate resistant to that antibiotic (or class of antibiotics). Thus, it is important to avoid antibiotics that have been used in the prior 90 days when selecting a regimen for empirical treatment of a pneumococcal infection.[206] Some, but not all, retrospective and prospective observational studies have suggested

a benefit to treating severely ill patients with CAP or bacteremic pneumococcal infections with both a β-lactam and a macrolide.[209–211] Possible explanations for these results include nonbactericidal effects, such as inhibiting biofilm production, or an anti-inflammatory effect of the macrolide.

Legionella

Epidemiology. *L. pneumophila* causes outbreaks and sporadic infections; both patterns may be seen either in the community or in hospitals, and the incidence in the United States is increasing.[212] Outbreaks have been linked to contaminated potable water systems, ultrasonic mist devices, whirlpool baths, air-conditioning condensates, and water evaporation systems.[213] Recent stay in a hotel or travel on a cruise ship is also linked to infections,[214] and approximately 25% of cases are related to travel.[215] In 2015, approximately 20% of U.S.-reported cases were health care associated.[213] Person-to-person transmission has also been described.[216]

Unlike other pneumonia pathogens that colonize the upper respiratory mucosa prior to initiating pneumonia, *Legionella* is acquired through direct inhalation of contaminated aerosols. Sporadic cases of *L. pneumophila* pneumonia account for 2–6% of CAPs in immunocompetent hosts,[40] and *L. pneumophila* is one of the most common causes of severe CAP. Risk factors include exposure to contaminated water, immunosuppression, cigarette use, diabetes, chronic cardiac or respiratory conditions, cancer, end-stage renal disease, and alcohol use. In data from Germany, associations with heavy smoking, male sex, and diabetes only held for inpatients.[217] Infection with *L. pneumophila* is more common in specific geographic regions, such as the Mediterranean or the northeastern United States; warm and humid weather conditions increase the risk of pneumonia due to *Legionella*, also called Legionnaires' disease.[218] Effective water system management is a critical step in limiting the incidence of *Legionella* infections.[219]

In addition to *L. pneumophila*, 40 other *Legionella* species have been identified and account for less than 10% of sporadic cases.[217] Many, such as *Legionella micdadei* and *Legionella longbeachae*, produce a pneumonic illness indistinguishable from that of *L. pneumophila*. Much less is known about the epidemiology of non-pneumophila *Legionella* infections, but they also appear to be from water or soil-related sources; *L. longbeachae* has been associated with gardening and compost exposure.[220] Immunosuppression appears to be the major host risk for these species. Patients are less likely to be smokers and may present with severe disease.[221]

Pathogenesis of *Legionella* Infections. Unlike *S. pneumoniae*, legionellae are facultative intracellular pathogens and have evolved strategies to survive and replicate in host cells. In the environment, *Legionella pneumophila* is an intravacuolar resident of protozoa and it uses similar strategies for surviving in protozoa and in host macrophages.[222] Following inhalation of a *Legionella*-containing aerosol, the bacteria infect alveolar macrophages where they form *Legionella*-containing vacuoles that evade fusion with lysosomes and recruit endoplasmic reticulum; the latter supports replication of *Legionella*. Intracellular replication of *Legionella* requires a bacterial type IV secretion system that translocates over 300 proteins into the host cytosol to modulate host cell signaling.[223] The translocated bacterial proteins provide multiple functions that promote bacterial survival and replication. For example, bacterial replication is facilitated by MitF-mediated mitochondrial fission and a shift to glycolysis[224]; iron acquisition is facilitated by MavN, which inserts into the *Legionella*-containing vacuole to promote iron transport[225]; and the SidE family of effectors enables noncanonical ubiquitination of endoplasmic reticulum–associated Rab guanosine triphosphatases, modifying function and promoting formation of the *Legionella*-containing vacuole.[226] Replication also requires inhibition of host cell progression to S phase by depletion of the cyclin D1 cell-cycle regulator.[227] The secreted protein, RomA, is a methyltransferase that modifies histone H3 to suppress multiple genes, including innate immune responses.[228] By secreting these bacterial proteins into the host cell, *Legionella* optimize their intracellular replication and avoid elimination by innate immune mechanisms.

Legionella innate immune recognition involves TLR2, 5, and 9; the NLR Naip5; and the *cyclic guanosine monophosphate–adenosine monophosphate synthase–stimulator of interferon genes* (cGAS-STING) pathway.[229] An allele encoding reduced cGAS-STING function is associated with increased human susceptibility to *Legionella* species.[230] Flagellin is sensed by TLR5 and also by NLR Naip5, which activates the NLRC4 inflammasome and induces caspase-1–dependent pyroptosis to restrict pathogen replication in macrophages.[231] Neutrophils, recruited monocytes producing tumor necrosis factor-α and *interleukin* (IL)-12, and IFN-γ producing cells, including natural killer T cells and γδ T cells, all aid pathogen clearance.[229] As noted above, to survive and cause infection, *Legionella* utilizes multiple approaches to evade innate immunity. In addition, DNA from *Legionella* can be packaged into extracellular vesicles. These extracellular vesicles can stimulate the cGAS-STING pathway in bystander cells and inhibit T cell proliferation.[232]

Clinical Manifestations. The usual incubation period for *Legionella* pneumonia is 2 to 10 days but can be longer.[214] Lethargy, headache, fever, recurring rigors, anorexia, and myalgias are frequent early symptoms. After several days, cough becomes more pronounced, with thin watery sputum or purulent sputum in up to half of cases. Dyspnea is prominent in half of cases, and pleuritic chest pain may be present.[215] Extrapulmonary manifestations may overshadow respiratory complaints; gastrointestinal (watery diarrhea, nausea, vomiting, abdominal pain) and neurologic symptoms and signs (headache, confusion, obtundation, seizures, hallucinations) are particularly noteworthy. Patients may appear acutely ill and can develop rhabdomyolysis and acute kidney injury. Temperatures reach 40.5°C in one-third of patients, are typically sustained, and may be accompanied by relative bradycardia, a feature that distinguishes *Legionella* pneumonia and some other atypical pneumonias from pneumococcal CAP.[233] Physical findings are usually limited to the chest, including pleural friction rubs, but generalized abdominal tenderness, hepatomegaly, splenomegaly, cutaneous rash, nuchal rigidity, and focal neurologic deficits have all been described.

Hyponatremia and hypophosphatemia are present in more than half of severe cases. Mild elevations of serum creatinine, creatine phosphokinase, and liver enzymes are also common, as are hematuria and proteinuria, occasionally with rhabdomyolysis. There may be leukopenia and thrombocytopenia, especially in severely ill patients. Cold agglutinins may be present, as in infection due to *M. pneumoniae*. The presence of three or more clinical predictors (fever >102°F, erythrocyte sedimentation rate >90 mm/hr or CRP >180 ng/mL, ferritin >2 times normal, creatine phosphokinase >2 times normal, hypophosphatemia, and microscopic hematuria) and the absence of three or more eliminators (sore throat, severe myalgia, leukopenia, thrombocytopenia, negative chest radiograph) have been proposed as a scoring system to identify legionnaires disease as a cause of CAP.[234]

Chest radiographic findings typically lag behind the early clinical illness. Unilobar opacities are most common (Fig. 46.2).[215] Small pleural effusions may develop in up to 50% and may precede the parenchymal process. Multilobar opacities are also commonly seen (eFig. 46.8), particularly on chest CT. Frank cavitation is rare but can develop in immunocompromised hosts.[113] Lung abscesses are rare but can be associated with immunocompromised hosts with lymphopenia or with neutrophil recovery following neutropenia.[235]

Microbiologic Diagnosis. *Legionella* are obligatory aerobic, fastidious, gram-negative bacilli that stain poorly with Gram stain (see Chapter 19, Fig. 19.3). *L. micdadei* and

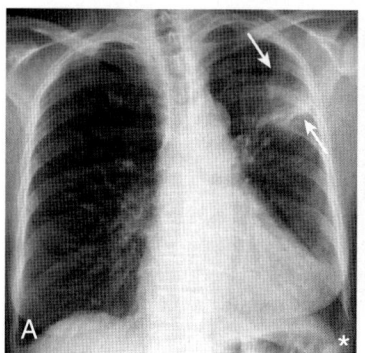
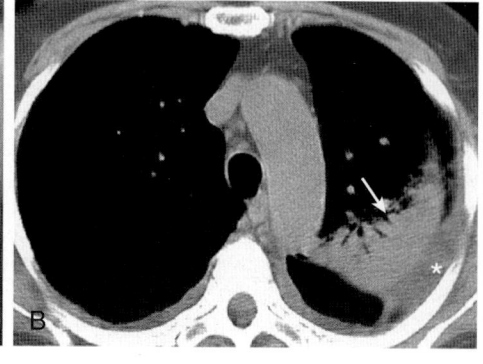

Figure 46.2 ***Legionella pneumophila* pneumonia: unilateral disease.** (A) Frontal chest radiograph shows subpleural left upper lobe consolidation (*arrows*). (B) Axial chest computed tomography displayed in soft tissue window confirms left upper lobe consolidation (*arrow*). A small left pleural effusion (*asterisk*) is present. (Courtesy Michael B. Gotway, MD.)

some other *Legionella* species may stain weakly acid-fast. Patients may not produce sputum and, early in the infection, even when sputum is available, it may contain few PMNs. Culture-based diagnosis is challenging, requires use of selective media, and has variable sensitivity (20–80%), in part reflecting difficulties in obtaining good-quality respiratory samples.[215]

The *Legionella* urinary antigen test is commonly used and has an overall sensitivity of 60–80%. It only reliably detects certain strains (mAb3/1) of the predominant serogroup 1.[214] However, it may detect other strains when antigen load is high, but with much lower sensitivity.[214] *Legionella* urinary antigen testing is recommended for all CAP that is severe, unresponsive to outpatient therapy, and associated with immunocompromised hosts or epidemiologic risk factors.[147] Direct fluorescent antibody staining of sputum is specific but has low sensitivity.[215] PCR-based assays for sputum are increasingly used and are becoming the preferred diagnostic test, allowing detection of a range of *Legionella* species.[214] Real-time PCR combined with urinary antigen had a 93% sensitivity and 98% specificity during a *L. pneumophila* outbreak, and *Legionella* species PCR can be combined with specific antibody detection to detect *L. longbeacheae*.[236] Adoption of PCR-based testing of respiratory samples enhances diagnosis of *Legionella* pneumonia.[237] Serologic testing with commercial kits has low positive predictive value of approximately 50%, limiting diagnostic utility outside specialist reference laboratories.[214] However, a significant rise in antibodies against serogroup 1 in the appropriate clinical setting can still support a diagnosis.

Clinical Course. A clinical response to appropriate antibiotic therapy is usually observed within 48 hours. In contrast, radiographic findings may continue to progress despite clinical improvement and may take months to resolve.[113] Acute renal failure and oliguria, often independent of shock and myoglobinuria, may develop in approximately 10% of patients, and dialysis may be required. Many patients note lingering fatigue and weakness for months following *Legionella* pneumonia.[215]

The mortality rate of community-acquired *Legionella* pneumonia is approximately 10%.[214] Poor clinical outcomes are associated with immunodeficiencies, comorbidities, delayed initiation of appropriate therapy, and the need for ventilatory support or dialysis.

Treatment. Azithromycin and fluoroquinolones are both superior to erythromycin or clarithromycin for treatment of *Legionella* infections and are associated with similar outcomes.[238] Doxycycline is recommended as an alternative therapy, but combinations with rifampicin are no longer recommended.[147] Durations are often recommended as 5 days for azithromycin and up to 10 days with levofloxacin.[215] Longer durations are recommended for severe or extra-pulmonary disease and immunocompromised hosts.[215] Prevention steps are key during outbreaks, and health care workers should always consider the possibility that one case is related to others. Biofilm formation in pipes and on surfaces limits the effectiveness of standard chlorination-based disinfection used in infection control measures.[239]

COMMON VIRAL CAUSES OF PNEUMONIA

The advent of molecular diagnostic tests has greatly improved the ability to detect and characterize the contribution of respiratory viruses to pneumonia. In contemporary pneumonia cohorts, viruses are the most frequently identified pathogens in CAP, detected in 27% of radiographically proven pneumonias in hospitalized adults[4] and 61–66% in hospitalized children.[240,241] These figures may overestimate the etiologic contribution of viruses to CAP because the diagnosis of viral pneumonia is usually performed on upper respiratory tract specimens (e.g., nasopharyngeal aspirate or swab). Detection of viruses from nasopharyngeal/oropharyngeal samples may represent coincidental upper respiratory tract infection or convalescent-phase shedding. Moreover, studies that have enrolled healthy controls have shown that the asymptomatic carriage of certain viruses (e.g., rhinovirus and adenovirus) is common.[127]

Influenza Virus

See Chapter 47 for a comprehensive review of influenza. This section solely focuses on selected aspects of influenza as a cause of CAP.

Clinical Manifestations. The most common of influenza-associated complications, influenza pneumonia can be categorized into primary viral pneumonia, secondary bacterial pneumonia, or mixed viral and bacterial pneumonia. Primary influenza viral pneumonia was first well documented in the 1957–58 pandemic.[242] The illness begins with typical influenza symptoms, followed by a rapid progression of fever, cough, dyspnea, and cyanosis. Typical radiographic changes include bilateral reticular or reticulonodular opacities (Fig. 46.3, eFigs. 46.9 and 46.10), sometimes suggestive of an acute lung injury pattern or ARDS (eFig. 46.11). Chest CT often shows multifocal areas of ground-glass opacities and peribronchovascular or subpleural consolidation (eFig. 46.12B–E).[243] Sputum cultures are negative for bacteria. Such patients do not respond to antibacterial drugs, and the mortality rate is high.[244]

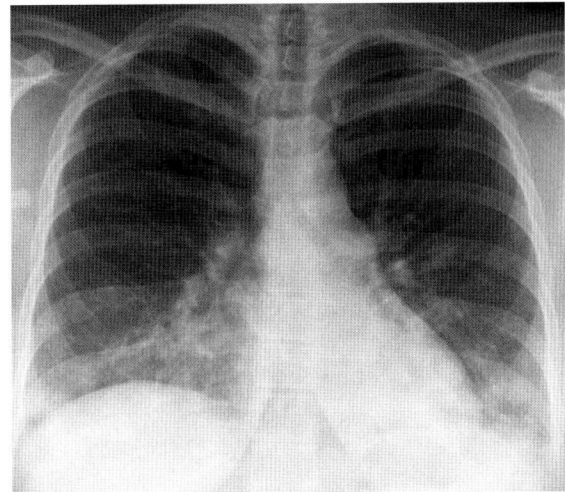

Figure 46.3 Seasonal influenza. Frontal chest radiograph shows multifocal, bilateral, perihilar, and lower lobe predominant bronchovascular thickening and somewhat nodular consolidation. (Courtesy Michael B. Gotway, MD.)

Secondary bacterial pneumonia is an important complication of influenza (eFig. 46.13). The classic description is of an influenza illness followed by a period of improvement, usually lasting 4 to 14 days. Recrudescence of fever is associated with symptoms and signs of bacterial pneumonia such as cough, sputum production, and an area of consolidation detected on physical examination and chest radiography. The most common bacteria implicated are *S. pneumoniae* and *S. aureus* (including MRSA), followed by *H. influenzae*, *S. pyogenes*, and gram-negative organisms including *K. pneumoniae* and *Escherichia coli*.[245] Mixed viral and bacterial pneumonia can also happen. Bacterial superinfections of influenza have been postulated as a major cause of death during the pandemic of 1918.[246]

Patients with a wide range of preexisting conditions are well recognized to be at higher risk for the development of pneumonia. During the 2009 pandemic, obese persons[247] and pregnant women[248,249] were noted to have increased risk of hospitalization or death due to influenza A H1N1pdm09, risks that had not been previously described.

Treatment. The CDC and IDSA recommend antiviral treatment for individuals at risk for more severe influenza or in individuals requiring hospitalization.[250,251] Treatment should be started as early as possible, but even delayed therapy can be of benefit in hospitalized patients. The antiviral agents of choice are neuraminidase inhibitors (oseltamivir, zanamivir, or peramivir) or a cap-dependent endonuclease inhibitor (baloxavir), with a recommended treatment duration of 5 days for oseltamivir and zanamivir and a single dose for peramivir and baloxavir.[251,252]

Combinations of antiviral agents have been evaluated in clinical trials,[253,254] but additional clinical benefit has not been demonstrated. Immunomodulatory agents have also been evaluated as adjuncts to antivirals, with variable results. Corticosteroid use in patients with severe influenza was associated with increased mortality in observational studies.[255] A randomized trial of clarithromycin, naproxen, and oseltamivir versus oseltamivir alone was associated with reduced mortality and length of hospital stay in the combination group.[256] Statins were associated with lower mortality in a U.S. surveillance study.[257] However, uncontrolled confounding is likely in this study.

Several antiviral agents are licensed for influenza treatment outside the United States and Europe (eTable 46.5). Additionally, a number of antiviral drugs with novel anti-influenza mechanisms have shown promise in animal models and/or early clinical studies, including sialidase,[258] polymerase inhibitors,[259,260] hemagglutinin inhibitor,[261] monoclonal antibodies,[262,263] and small interfering RNA.[264] Administration of convalescent plasma can also be valuable for treatment of influenza pneumonia, though it is only likely to be available in the later stages of an outbreak or pandemic because it must contain antibodies to the infecting strain of influenza virus.[265,266]

OTHER COMMON CAUSES OF PNEUMONIA

Haemophilus influenzae

Epidemiology. *H. influenzae* is a gram-negative coccobacillus and an obligate human pathogen. With the routine vaccination of children against *H. influenzae* type b, non-typeable *H. influenzae* has emerged as the leading cause of invasive disease and accounts for approximately 70% of cases of *H. influenzae* infections. Eighty percent of cases are seen in adults, and the overall incidence is 1 case per 100,000 adults annually in the United States.[267] Pneumonia and bacteremia are the most common presentations.[268] Advanced age, smoking, and medical comorbidity including structural lung disease are common associations.[269] In a Swedish study including real-time quantitative PCR for *H. influenzae*, and in which a microbiological diagnosis was established in approximately two-thirds of subjects, *H. influenzae* was detected in 5% of adult CAP cases[270] and, in a German study, accounted for 6% of CAP but 26% in patients with COPD.[269,271]

H. influenzae type f is now the leading capsulated cause of disease followed by type e, but these account for less than 10% of infections.[268] *H. influenzae* type b still causes a small amount of pneumonia in the elderly with medical comorbidity.[272] Type a has emerged as a cause of invasive *H. influenzae* in indigenous populations.[273]

Pathogenesis. *Haemophilus* species are a part of the respiratory microbiome, and *H. influenzae* quantity increases in patients with chronic lung disease, predominantly those with COPD.[274] Non-typeable strains may be able to persist inside epithelial cells and macrophages.[275,276] The pathogen can express a capsule to evade phagocytosis while IgA proteases and complement inhibitors prevent opsonization. Alveolar macrophages, neutrophils, and Th17 immune responses play key roles in host defense. Non-typeable strains demonstrate antigenic variation and lipo-oligosaccharides on the surface mimic host glycans to evade antibody generation. Recurrence of disease in children or in exacerbations of COPD can be associated with acquisition of new non-typeable strains, but Th17 responses can recognize conserved epitopes.[277] *H. influenzae* are potent activators of TLR and NODs and induce potent pro-inflammatory cytokine responses via nuclear factor κβ signaling pathways, which may contribute to the prominent neutrophilic inflammation, tissue damage, and pathogenic role in acute exacerbations of COPD.[276] Despite inducing neutrophilic inflammation, they may be able to withstand killing by *neutrophil extracellular traps* (NETs). Protein D and surface-expressed lipo-oligosaccharides promote ciliary disfunction, further contributing to lung dysfunction.

Clinical Manifestations. *Haemophilus* pneumonia is clinically indistinguishable from other bacterial pneumonias.[269] Leukocytosis and CRP greater than 100 mg/L are common. On radiographs, *Haemophilus* pneumonia may appear as a patchy bronchopneumonia or have areas of frank consolidation. Areas of fine nodular shadows on chest radiograph or tree-in-bud appearance on CT may suggest infectious bronchiolitis (eFig. 46.14). Multilobar opacities are seen in less than 15% and pleural effusions in less than 10%. Spherical radiographic opacities (so-called round pneumonia) have been described. Cavitation is uncommon.

Microbiologic Diagnosis. Diagnosing *H. influenzae* pneumonia by a Gram stain of sputum is difficult because the small, pleomorphic coccobacilli are easily overlooked. Culture of expectorated sputum reveals *H. influenzae* in only half of well-documented cases of *H. influenzae* pneumonia.[270] Asymptomatic colonization with non-typeable strains in patients with COPD complicates analysis of Gram stain and sputum cultures (eFig. 46.15). Bacteremia is infrequent.[267,271] Multiplex PCR-based diagnostics are increasingly used to diagnose *H. influenzae*.[236]

Clinical Course. The overall mortality rate of *H. influenzae* pneumonia is 2–7%, lower than for CAP in general, and ICU admission is also less frequent.[267,271] Bacteremia, medical comorbidity, and advanced age are associated with worse outcome.[267] Mortality of up to 20% is reported in bacteremic pneumonia, predominantly in elderly patients with comorbidity.[278]

Treatment. *H. influenzae* isolates produce β-lactamase in 20–50% of cases and are therefore often resistant to ampicillin. β-lactamase–negative ampicillin-resistant strains have emerged in Japan and some European countries that are also resistant to some cephalosporins, but these strains are still rare in the United States.[279] Increasing macrolide resistance also compromises empirical therapy with these agents, and azithromycin is the most active macrolide against these infections. Consequently, serious *H. influenzae* respiratory tract infections should be treated with a β-lactam/β-lactamase inhibitor while awaiting results of susceptibility testing. Due to antimicrobial stewardship considerations, second- or third-generation cephalosporin or fluoroquinolones are reserved as alternatives when other factors preclude a β-lactam/β-lactamase inhibitor. Serious infection in areas where β-lactamase–negative ampicillin-resistant strains are prevalent can be treated with ceftriaxone. Milder infections can commence treatment with amoxicillin/clavulanate if risk factors such as COPD make *H. influenzae* a potential pathogen and deescalate to amoxicillin if sensitivity is confirmed, with a macrolide as an alternative agent.

 Other infectious causes of CAP are detailed at ExpertConsult.com.

NONRESPONDING PNEUMONIA/ TREATMENT FAILURE

Two different clinical patterns of treatment failure in pneumonia have been described[175]: *progressive* pneumonia, in which there is clinical deterioration, even to the point of respiratory failure or septic shock, and *nonresponding* pneumonia, in which clinical improvement is not achieved (persistence of fever and clinical symptoms). Evaluation for response should be undertaken after 72 hours of antibiotic treatment.[175] In addition to clinical evaluation, reduction of PCT levels after 3 to 4 days of treatment correlates with clinical response.[106] Levels of certain biomarkers, in particular PCT, CRP, and IL-6, have also been found useful for predicting inadequate response. Elevated initial levels of PCT or CRP are independent predictors for inadequate response.[106]

The causes of nonresponding pneumonia are classified as infectious, noninfectious, and of unknown origin.[175]

eTable 46.6 lists common infectious and noninfectious causes. Reevaluation of the history and examination, chest CT, and consideration of bronchoscopy to obtain biopsy specimens and BAL for additional microbiological investigations guide diagnosis.

INFECTIOUS CAUSES

In patients hospitalized for CAP, specific infections are responsible for 40% of nonresponding cases. The most frequent microorganisms found are *S. pneumoniae*, *Legionella*, *P. aeruginosa*, and *S. aureus.*

Patients with CAP may fail to respond because of resistance to the empirical antibiotic regimen selected. *P. aeruginosa*, which is not covered by empirical therapy for CAP unless a fluoroquinolone is used, causes about 10% of cases of nonresponding CAP.[175] More unusual microorganisms include *Mycobacteria*, *Nocardia* species, anaerobes, fungi, *Pneumocystis jirovecii*, protozoa, and other organisms requiring antibiotics other than those recommended for CAP (see eFig. 46.61). Investigation of the etiology of nonresponding CAP to identify some of these microorganisms requires intensified microbiologic diagnostic testing as well as an exhaustive search for risk factors, including epidemiology (travel, occupational or animal exposures), personal habits, and environmental factors.

Local or metastatic infectious complications also contribute to treatment failure, as can bronchial obstruction by a tumor, foreign body, or teeth. Empyema (see eFig. 46.39) is one of the most frequent complications in pneumonia and is thus a cause of nonresponse that must be evaluated with thoracentesis when pleural effusion is present. Other causes of treatment failure are abscess formation (see eFig. 46.5) and necrotizing pneumonia (see eFigs. 46.36 and 46.37). Metastatic infections such as endocarditis, arthritis, pericarditis, meningitis, or peritonitis can contribute to treatment failure and are more common in bacteremic pneumonia. In approximately 30% of the cases, no specific cause for lack of response can be identified despite adequate antibiotic treatment. This may be due to the presence of comorbidities or to an exaggerated or diminished inflammatory response.[792]

NONINFECTIOUS CAUSES

Noninfectious diseases with acute involvement of the pulmonary parenchyma may simulate pneumonia. These include pulmonary infarction, pulmonary hemorrhage, organizing pneumonia, eosinophilic pneumonia, hypersensitivity pneumonitis, drug-induced lung disease, and neoplasms. Alveolar cell lung cancer (eFig. 46.62 and Video 46.2) may be particularly difficult to distinguish radiographically from pyogenic pneumonia. The frequency of noninfectious etiologies has been reported to be 22% in CAP.[175]

DIAGNOSTIC EVALUATION

The diagnostic approach to treatment failure requires a complete reevaluation of the history, physical examination, and laboratory studies, including factors that may be related to delayed response.[175,793] Reconsideration of the initial diagnosis is also an important component of the diagnostic approach. Important epidemiologic clues may suggest unusual microorganisms along with unexpected resistance to antimicrobials, or underlying immunodeficiency such as HIV infection.

MICROBIOLOGIC STUDIES

The microbiologic investigation of treatment failures requires comprehensive reexamination of initial microbiologic results, together with obtaining new samples for culture and other assays. A bronchoscopy to evaluate the airways for potential obstruction and obtain microbiologic samples from the LRT is recommended if not otherwise contraindicated. Both protected specimen brush and BAL sampling should be done during the same procedure for bacterial cultures, direct fluorescent antibody staining, and nucleic acid testing. Although culture results may be altered by the prior administration of antibiotics, the sensitivity of brush or BAL cultures approaches 40% in nonresponding CAP. In patients undergoing mechanical ventilation, the tracheal aspirate can provide diagnostic information. Gram stain of cytocentrifuged BAL fluid can rapidly identify intracellular microorganisms[794] and may guide decisions regarding changes in antimicrobial therapy. Comprehensive microbiologic studies should also be performed on samples from nonrespiratory sites (see Table 46.2). When present, pleural fluid should be obtained for culture, direct fluorescent antibody, and nucleic acid testing for likely pathogens. The role of transbronchial biopsy is not established, and its indication depends on the possible alternative diagnosis suspected.

IMAGING STUDIES

Chest radiographs may demonstrate complications such as pleural effusion, cavitation, or new opacities. Chest CT scans provide a more detailed study of the parenchyma, interstitium, pleura, and mediastinum, potentially suggesting specific microorganisms or alternative diagnoses. In a patient with applicable risk factors, the appearance of nodular opacities with the halo sign (i.e., a nodule surrounded by a halo of ground-glass attenuation, especially near the pleura) on CT scan is suggestive of pulmonary aspergillosis (eFigs. 46.63A and 46.64) or mucormycosis (eFig. 46.65).[795] Nodules of similar appearance have also been described in CMV infection (see eFig. 46.54), granulomatosis with polyangiitis, Kaposi sarcoma, and metastases with necrosis and/or hemorrhage. Ground-glass opacities consistent with interstitial pneumonia suggest *P. jirovecii* pneumonia. Nodules or multiple masses with or without cavitation are compatible with *Nocardia* species, *M. tuberculosis*, or Q fever. Diffuse or mixed interstitial and alveolar opacities may be due to viral infections or *M. pneumoniae*. Other imaging studies, such as chest CT pulmonary angiography, should be considered to evaluate the possibility of pulmonary

emboli and to exclude endobronchial lesions causing obstruction.

PREVENTION OF PNEUMONIA

VACCINES

The risk of pneumonia can be reduced by administering influenza and pneumococcal vaccines. Recommendations for administration of influenza[796] are included in Chapter 47. Recommendations for pneumococcal[797] vaccines are presented in eTable 46.7.

Inactivated influenza vaccination is recommended annually for all persons aged 6 months and older, including pregnant women. For those averse to injections, a live attenuated influenza vaccine can be given by intranasal administration to healthy persons 6 months to 49 years old. The live, attenuated vaccine must be avoided in pregnancy, in high-risk persons with chronic underlying diseases or immunodeficiencies, and in health care staff caring for immunosuppressed patients; it is not approved for use in those over 49 years. The standard-dose inactivated vaccine is less immunogenic and efficacious in individuals over 65 years[798]; thus high-dose (containing 60 μg hemagglutinin antigens compared to 15 μg in standard-dose vaccine) or adjuvanted preparations are recommended for this age group.[796] See Chapter 47 for further details on influenza vaccines.

Two pneumococcal vaccines are currently available. The purified polysaccharide vaccine (PPSV23) contains capsular antigens isolated from 23 of the most prevalent capsule types and is immunogenic in adults, although antibody levels decrease to prevaccination levels after 4 to 7 years. The pneumococcal conjugate vaccine (PCV13) contains polysaccharide antigens from 13 of the most prevalent capsule types, conjugated to a nontoxic mutant of diphtheria toxin protein, which generates T cell help and long-lived memory B cells specific for pneumococcal antigens. PPSV23 should be administered to all individuals 65 years of age and older as well as those aged 19 to 64 years with chronic conditions that increase the risk of invasive pneumococcal infection (e.g., diabetes; chronic lung, heart, or liver disease; cigarette smoking; or alcoholism). Patients aged 19 years and older with immunodeficiencies or other conditions that impose an especially high risk of invasive pneumococcal infection (asplenia, HIV or other congenital or acquired immunodeficiencies, myeloma, lymphoma, leukemia, chronic renal failure) should receive an initial dose of PCV13 followed at least 8 weeks later by PPSV23. eTable 46.7 lists the conditions and indications for which administration of each of the pneumococcal vaccines is currently recommended.[797] In 2014, the updated ACIP recommendations are that both PCV13 and PPSV23 should be administered in series to all adults 65 years and older. A dose of PCV13 should be received first followed by a dose of PPSV23 6 to 12 months later. Individuals previously vaccinated with PPSV23 should be given a dose of PCV13 after approximately 1 year.[797,799]

SMOKING CESSATION

Not only is smoking a risk factor for pneumococcal disease, quitting smoking reduces the risk.[179] IDSA/ATS recommend smoking cessation counseling and pneumococcal vaccination for smokers who are hospitalized with pneumonia.[39]

Key Points

- All patients with suspected pneumonia should have a chest radiograph. Gram stains of sputum and blood cultures should be obtained before treatment in all patients considered for hospitalization and in those with certain risk factors for methicillin-resistant *S. aureus* or *P. aeruginosa*. *S. pneumoniae* and *L. pneumophila* urinary antigens can make an etiologic diagnosis with reasonable sensitivity and specificity.
- Aspiration is the cause of infection with *S. pneumoniae*, *H. influenzae*, gram-negative bacilli, and other organisms, whereas aerosolization is the route of infection with intracellular bacteria: *Legionella* sp, *M. pneumoniae*, *Chlamydophila* sp, *C. burnetii*, and viruses such as influenza viruses.
- Nucleic acid amplification tests are increasingly used to diagnose viruses and fastidious bacteria, *M. pneumoniae*, *C. pneumoniae*, *L. pneumophila*, and *B. pertussis*, because culture procedures are too insensitive and too slow to guide treatment.
- In older and immunocompromised patients, the signs and symptoms of pneumonia may be muted and overshadowed by nonspecific complaints. Temperature greater than 38.5°C or accompanied by chills should never be attributed to bronchitis without examining a chest radiograph. Older patients with pneumonia who present with altered mental status without fever often have a delay in receiving antibiotics; this delay can increase mortality. Immunocompromised hosts may have a normal chest radiograph because signs of inflammation may be blunted. Computed tomography scans may be required to identify pneumonia.
- Treatment for pneumonia should be directed at a specific pathogen, but definitive identification of the patient's causal pathogen may be difficult. Therefore, disease severity, patient age, the presence of comorbidities and immunosuppression, previous antimicrobial therapy, and specific clinical and radiologic manifestations of the illness are used to select initial empirical antimicrobial therapy.
- If the etiologic agent has been identified, the antimicrobial regimen should be adjusted based on the results of in vitro susceptibility testing. The ideal drug for a known pathogen has the narrowest spectrum of activity and is the most efficacious, least toxic, and least costly.

Key Readings

Aliberti S, Blasi F. Clinical stability versus clinical failure in patients with community-acquired pneumonia. *Semin Respir Crit Care*. 2012;33:284–291.

Jain S, et al. Community-acquired pneumonia requiring hospitalization among U.S. adults. *N Engl J Med*. 2015;373:415–427.

Lim WS, et al. Defining community acquired pneumonia severity on presentation to hospital: an international derivation and validation study. *Thorax*. 2003;58:377–382.

Metlay JP, et al. Diagnosis and treatment of adults with community-acquired pneumonia. An official clinical practice guideline of the American Thoracic Society and Infectious Diseases Society of America. *Am J Respir Crit Care Med*. 2019;200:e45–e67.

Musher DM, Thorner AR. Community-acquired pneumonia. *N Engl J Med*. 2014;371(17):1619–1628.

Ruuskanen O, Lahti E, Jennings LC, Murdoch DR. Viral pneumonia. *Lancet*. 2011;377:1264–1275.

Welte T, Torres A, Nathwani P. Clinical and economical burden of community-acquired pneumonia among adults in Europe. *Thorax*. 2012;67:71–79.

Whitney CG, Farley MM, Hadler J, et al. Decline in invasive pneumococcal disease after the introduction of protein-polysaccharide conjugate vaccine. *N Engl J Med*. 2003;348:1737–1746.

Woodhead M, Blasi F, Ewig S, et al. Guidelines for the management of adult lower respiratory tract infections—full version. *Clin Microbiol Infect*. 2011;17(suppl 6):E1–E59.

Complete reference list available at ExpertConsult.com.

46a COVID-19

MONICA FUNG, MD • JENNIFER M. BABIK, MD, PHD • JOHN S. MUNGER, MD •
DAVID A. KAUFMAN, MD

INTRODUCTION

Coronaviruses are important human pathogens, and research into their behavior is nearly a century old.[1] In late 2019, a novel coronavirus emerged in Wuhan, China and spread worldwide. In February 2020, the World Health Organization designated COVID-19 (for coronavirus disease 2019) as the name of the human disease caused by *severe acute respiratory syndrome coronavirus 2* (SARS-CoV-2), which was previously known as 2019-nCoV.[2] Viral pneumonia is the most frequent serious clinical manifestation of COVID-19, prominently featuring fever, cough, dyspnea, hypoxemia, and bilateral opacities on chest radiography.[3–6] Severe hypoxemic respiratory failure consistent with the Berlin definition of *acute respiratory distress syndrome* (ARDS) develops in a significant proportion of patients with COVID-19 pneumonia.[7,8] Patients who require mechanical ventilation may have a high risk for death.[9] Since the outbreak, more than 22 million persons have been infected and more than 1 million have died. In the United States, as tracked by the Johns Hopkins Coronavirus Resource Center (https://coronavirus.jhu.edu/map.html), more than 28 million cases and more than 500,000 deaths were reported by March 2021.[10]

VIROLOGY

SARS-CoV-2 is a member of the Coronaviridae family of enveloped, single-stranded RNA viruses. Coronaviruses are so named because of the corona (crown) seen on electron micrographs that represents its densely packed membrane proteins.[11] SARS-CoV-2 is a novel virus related to, but distinct from, SARS-CoV and Middle East Respiratory Syndrome coronavirus.[12] SARS-CoV-2 is closely related to bat and pangolin coronaviruses, and it has been theorized that bats are the natural reservoir of the virus, whereas the pangolin, an endangered and commonly trafficked mammal, may have served as an intermediate host.[12,13] Although a market in Wuhan, China was initially thought to be the source of the outbreak, this has not been definitively proven.[13]

The life cycle of SARS-CoV-2 is believed to be similar to that of SARS-CoV and other coronaviruses (Fig. 46a.1). The spike protein on the virion surface binds to the *angiotensin-converting enzyme 2* (ACE2) protein, which acts as a receptor on host cells.[14] The virus is then internalized by endocytosis, which is mediated by spike protein cleavage by the transmembrane serine protease 2.[15] The viral genome is then translated by host machinery into a polyprotein that is cleaved by both host and viral proteases; a viral RNA-dependent RNA polymerase then amplifies the genome, and virions are assembled and then released by exocytosis.[11] It is notable that the ACE2 receptor has broad tissue distribution, including in the lungs (alveolar epithelial cells), upper airway, myocardium, gastrointestinal tract, kidneys, and vascular endothelial cells in most tissues.[16,17] This likely in part explains the broad clinical manifestations of COVID-19 (see later).

TRANSMISSION

Person-to-person spread by respiratory droplets is considered the predominant mode of transmission. Specifically, such transmission is thought to take place through respiratory droplets larger than 5 μm in diameter in close range (less than 6 feet, or 2 m). For example, when persons with SARS-CoV-2 infection cough, sneeze, or talk, their respiratory secretions may make direct contact with the mucous membranes of an uninfected individual. This is consistent with laboratory

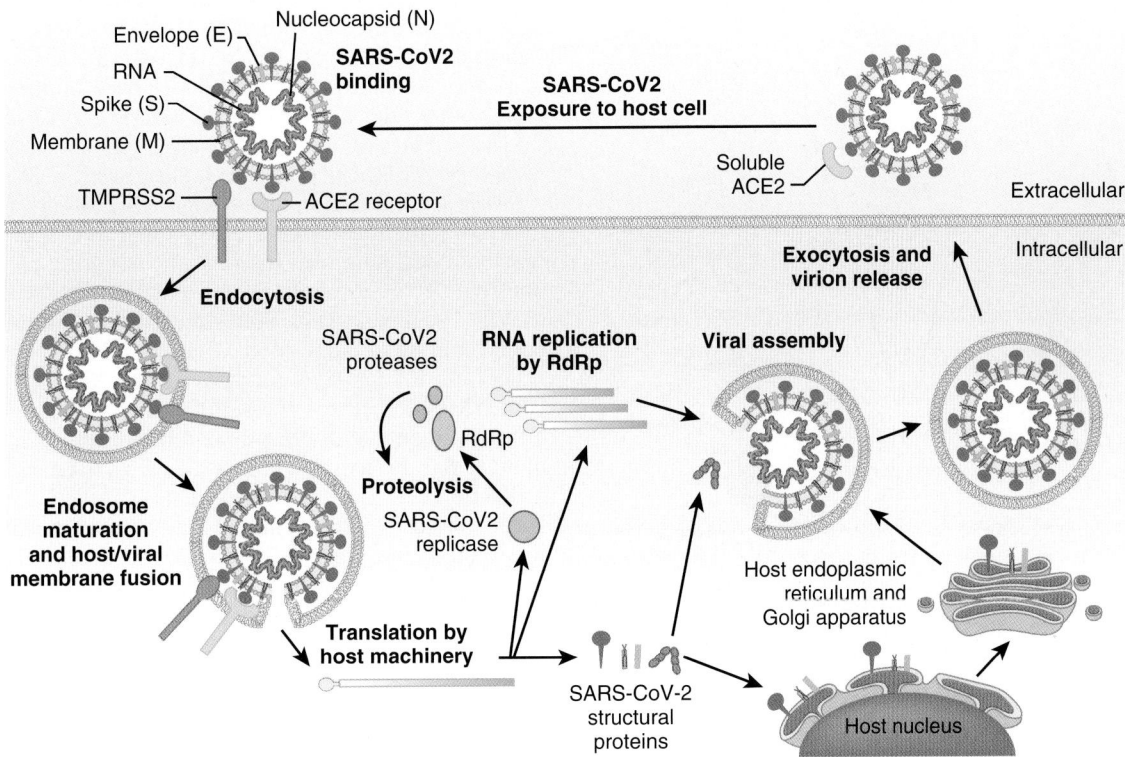

Figure 46a.1 Life cycle of *severe acute respiratory syndrome coronavirus 2* (SARS-CoV-2). SARS-CoV-2 binds to the *angiotensin-converting enzyme 2* (ACE2) receptor on the host cell membrane. After endocytosis, the membrane fuses between the mature endosome and virion with help from the *transmembrane serine protease 2* (TMPRSS2), followed by release of the SARS-CoV-2 RNA into the intracellular space. The RNA is translated by host machinery to produce the replicase and structural proteins. Host and SARS-CoV-2 proteases cleave the replicase into nonstructural proteins, including the RNA-dependent RNA polymerase (RdRp). RdRp mediates RNA replication and amplification. SARS-CoV-2 transmembrane proteins (spike [S], envelope [E], and membrane [M]) are shuttled through the endoplasmic reticulum and Golgi apparatus to the forming viral capsids. The virus is assembled with addition of the viral RNA and nucleocapsid (N) protein through association with the transmembrane viral proteins. Exocytosis results in release of the newly synthesized viral particles. (Modified from Atri D, Siddiqi HK, Lang JP, Nauffal V, Morrow DA, Bohula EA. COVID-19 for the cardiologist: basic virology, epidemiology, cardiac manifestations, and potential therapeutic strategies. *JACC Basic Transl Sci.* 2020;5:518–536.)

evidence of high levels of viral shedding in the upper respiratory tract of infected individuals (Fig. 46a.2).[18,19] For this reason, wearing masks in the community is considered a mainstay of SARS-CoV-2 prevention, with indirect evidence indicating efficacy.[20] For example, there was a 79% reduction among families in China who wore masks versus those that did not.[21]

Aerosol transmission plays a role, although its prominence is uncertain.[22] The importance of aerosolized virus (particles smaller than 5 μm in diameter that may remain suspended in the air) as a mode of transmission over distances greater than 2 m is controversial, but it likely contributes to some cases.[23] Evidence that supports aerosol transmission includes the following: (1) SARS-CoV-2 grown in tissue culture remained viable in aerosol for up to 3 hours; (2) SARS-CoV-2 RNA has been identified in ventilation systems of hospitals caring for patients with COVID-19; and (3) respiratory droplets generated by speaking have been shown to dehydrate into aerosols remaining airborne for extended periods.[24–27] More study is needed to clarify the relative contribution of aerosol transmission. Superspreading events, such as a choir practice where 88% of attendees were found to be infected, highlight the potential of airborne transmission.[28–30]

Fomite transmission, in which persons touch an infected surface and then touch their faces or mucous membranes,

has been documented as a source of infection with SARS-CoV-2. SARS-CoV-2 can persist on cardboard, steel, and plastic surfaces for days and can be detected in patients' rooms and on shoes of hospital staff.[25,31,32] Reassuringly, many types of disinfectants inactivate coronaviruses similar to SARS-CoV-2.[33]

Blood-borne or non–mucous membrane transmission is less likely to spread the virus. Although SARS-CoV-2 has been detected in nonrespiratory specimens, including stool, blood, semen, and even ocular fluid, extrapolating from experience with other respiratory viruses and with SARS-CoV and Middle East Respiratory Syndrome coronavirus, the likelihood of blood-borne or non–mucous membrane transmission appears to be low.[34–36] There is also no current conclusive evidence of vertical transmission.[37]

The precise duration of infectivity of a person with SARS-CoV-2 virus is not clear, but current evidence suggests that infected individuals may be infectious 2 to 3 days before the onset of symptoms, and that asymptomatic or presymptomatic infection plays a large role in disease transmission.[38] Viral RNA shedding is variable and potentially depends on the severity of illness; however, it is unclear whether RNA shedding correlates with the presence of infectious virus.[39,40] In a small study of nine patients with mild

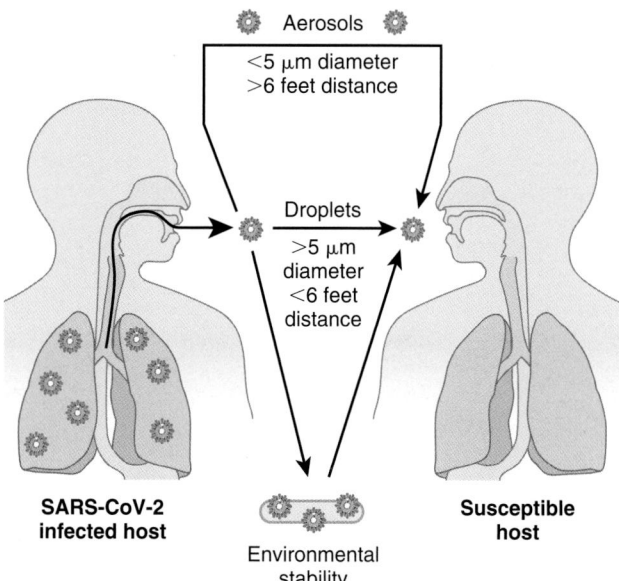

Figure 46a.2 Transmission of *severe acute respiratory syndrome coronavirus 2* (SARS-CoV-2) from person to person. The major mode of transmission is by droplets (>5 μm diameter), generated by coughing, sneezing, or talking, consistent with the known presence of virus in the upper respiratory tract. Aerosol transmission has been strongly suggested by certain spreading events, in which small particles (<5 μm) can spread more than 6 feet and remain suspended. Fomite transmission, by touching surfaces and spreading virus to the face, happens but appears to be a minor mode of transmission.

COVID-19, culturable virus was isolated from respiratory tract specimens only during the first 8 days of illness despite ongoing SARS-CoV-2 RNA detection beyond this period.[18]

With regard to presymptomatic transmission, a prospective study of patients with laboratory-confirmed COVID-19 cases and their close contacts found that the primary case transmitted the virus to secondary cases just before or within the first 6 days of symptom onset.[41] Another modeling study of transmission pairs in China suggested that individuals became more infective 2 to 3 days before symptom onset, with peak infectiveness 0.7 days before.[38] In a serial point-prevalence survey at a skilled nursing facility, 56% of 48 residents who tested positive for SARS-CoV-2 were asymptomatic at the time of testing, and the majority of these residents went on to develop symptoms as long as 6 days later.[42]

Transmission is also related to the type and duration of exposure, with prolonged close contact in closed indoor, crowded, or poorly ventilated settings conveying the highest risk.[43]

EPIDEMIOLOGY

Since the first reports of COVID-19 cases in Wuhan, China in late 2019, the SARS-CoV-2 virus has spread worldwide.[44,45] Within each country and community, the incidence of COVID-19 depends on population density, degree of testing, and timing of mitigation strategies such as social distancing. Multivariate models factoring in these variables have provided varying predictions of pandemic dynamics, although all predict at least 18 to 24 months of COVID-19 activity with periodic spikes or surges.[46,47]

Older patients and patients with comorbidities are at increased risk for severe illness and COVID-19 mortality.[4,6,48] Specifically, data from China,[49] Italy,[50] and the United States[51] have demonstrated incrementally higher rates of hospitalization and mortality from COVID-19 with increasing age. For instance, the Chinese Centers for Disease Control reported case-fatality rates of 8% and 15% among COVID-19 patients 70 to 79 years old and more than 80 years old, respectively, compared with the overall case-fatality rate of 2.3%.[8]

Other established epidemiologic risk factors for severe COVID-19 include chronic illness such as diabetes, hypertension, cardiovascular disease, chronic lung disease, and obesity.[4,6,48,52] Among 5700 patients hospitalized for COVID-19 in New York State, the median number of total comorbidities at admission was four.[53] In a prospective observational cohort of patients from 208 hospitals in the United Kingdom, there was significantly increased mortality among patients with chronic comorbidities, including cardiovascular disease (hazard ratio, 1.16), liver disease (hazard ratio, 1.51), obesity (hazard ratio, 1.33), and chronic kidney disease (hazard ratio, 1.33).[52] Immunosuppression has been a presumed risk factor for severe COVID-19, but data vary depending on the population studied. Specifically, patients with malignant disease and solid organ transplant recipients appear to be at increased risk of severe COVID-19 disease and death, whereas for persons with other types of immunocompromise, the evidence is less clear.[54]

Emerging evidence has also illustrated racial disparities in COVID-19 disease and death, with Black Americans accounting for a much larger proportion of COVID-19 deaths compared with the rest of the local population. For example, Black patients accounted for 81% of COVID-19 deaths in a 69% Black county in Georgia[55] and 73% of COVID-19 deaths in a 26% Black county in Wisconsin.[56] A subsequent analysis of the impact of COVID-19 on Black communities demonstrated that social conditions, structural racism, and other factors elevated risk for COVID-19 diagnoses and deaths in Black communities.[57,58] The burden of COVID-19 also appears to be higher in Hispanic, Native American, and Alaskan Native populations.[58]

CLINICAL PRESENTATION

It is currently estimated that approximately 40–45% of SARS-CoV-2 infections are asymptomatic.[59] The implications of this finding on the dynamics of SARS-CoV-2 transmission are significant, as previously discussed. For the remaining patients with symptomatic infection, data from China, Italy, and the United States indicate that approximately 80% of infections are mild (not requiring hospitalization), 15% are moderate to severe (requiring hospitalization), and 5% are critical (requiring intensive care unit care).[8,60–62] COVID-19 can involve almost every system in the body (Fig. 46a.3). For issues related to COVID-19 and pregnancy, see Chapter 129.

SYSTEMIC MANIFESTATIONS

The main systemic manifestations of COVID-19 are fever (>75%), myalgias (10–50%), and fatigue (20–40%).[4,48,53,62–64] Fever is present in the majority of

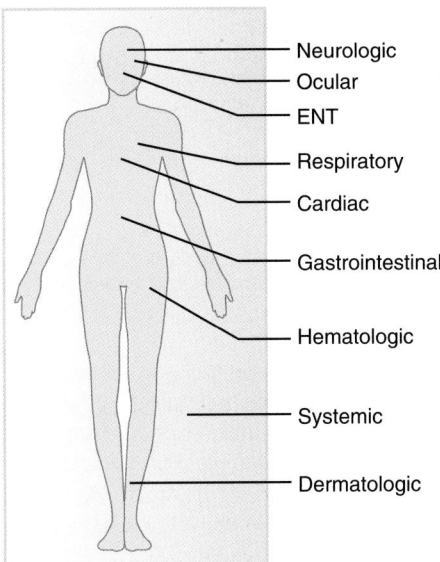

Figure 46a.3 Clinical manifestations of COVID-19. Neurologic manifestations are present in 36–57% of patients, with the most common findings of dizziness, headache, and impaired consciousness. The most common ocular manifestation is conjunctivitis. Disorders of taste and smell are very common *ear, nose, and throat* (ENT) manifestations, affecting as many as 89% of patients. Cough (45–80%) and dyspnea (20–55%) are common respiratory manifestations. Arrhythmias affect 7–17% of patients, and myocarditis is a cardiac manifestation described in several case reports. Gastrointestinal manifestations are less common (7–9% in meta-analyses), but they may be the only symptoms in some patients. Elevated D-dimer levels are a common hematologic disorder and likely confer an increased risk for thromboembolism. Rash may present as a dermatologic feature in up to 20% of patients with COVID-19, and these rashes may appear as erythema, urticaria, or vesicles. Fever, myalgias, and fatigue are common systematic symptoms in the influenza-like illness characteristic of COVID-19.

hospitalized patients, but it is present at the time of admission in only 25–50%. Therefore, the absence of fever does not exclude a diagnosis of COVID-19.

RESPIRATORY MANIFESTATIONS

Cough is a sign in 45–80% of patients (dry cough is more common than a productive cough); 20–55% of patients are dyspneic.[4,48,53,62–64] Headache and symptoms of upper respiratory tract infection (sore throat and rhinorrhea) are present in less than 20% of patients. In severely ill patients, hypoxemia is common (see Chapter 44). Among critically ill patients who require invasive mechanical ventilation, an increased ventilatory ratio (a surrogate for increased physiologic dead space) has been observed.[65–67] Abnormalities in ventilation-perfusion relationships attributed to vascular and endothelial damage have been revealed using dual-energy computed tomography.[68]

GASTROINTESTINAL MANIFESTATIONS

Nausea, vomiting, or diarrhea is present in up to 34% of patients with COVID-19 across different clinical studies.[4,48–53,62–64,69] However, two meta-analyses indicated that the pooled prevalence of nausea, vomiting, or diarrhea is lower, at 7–9%.[70,71] Gastrointestinal symptoms can be the only symptoms at presentation in up to 14% of patients.[72–74]

CARDIAC MANIFESTATIONS

There are multiple case reports of acute myocarditis associated with COVID-19.[75,76] Arrhythmias have been described in 7–17% of hospitalized patients.[5,63] One early small study of critically ill patients showed that one-third of patients (7 of 21) developed acute cardiomyopathy; however, this has not been observed in other studies of critically ill patients with COVID-19.[77,78] Finally, cardiac injury has been reported in 7–28% of patients and is associated with an increased risk of complications and death; a limitation of this finding, however, is that cardiac injury is defined largely by elevation of blood biomarker levels, which may be an unreliable method of diagnosing cardiac injury in acutely or critically ill patients.[5,79–81]

Because SARS-CoV-2 uses the ACE2 protein as its cell entry receptor (see the earlier section on virology), the effects of ACE inhibitors and angiotensin receptor blockers have been examined. These medications increase expression of ACE2, which raised the hypothetical possibility that their use could make patients more susceptible to SARS-CoV-2 infection or at risk for more severe COVID-19.[82] However, multiple studies have determined that there is no association between the use of these medications and the risk of SARS-CoV-2 infection or severe disease.[83–86]

EAR, NOSE, AND THROAT MANIFESTATIONS

Disorders of taste (dysgeusia, ageusia) and smell (hyposmia, anosmia) in COVID-19 are common, ranging from 34–89%.[87–89] These symptoms can manifest before other respiratory symptoms and can be present without nasal congestion. This latter finding raises the possibility that disorders of taste and smell may be in part direct effects of the virus rather than solely the results of nasal inflammation and obstruction.[88]

Symptoms related to taste and smell were rarely reported in early clinical studies from China; it is not clear whether this discrepancy is related to differences in symptom reporting or whether there is a true difference that may be mediated by variations in viral strain or ACE2 receptor density in the nasopharynx.[4,90]

OCULAR MANIFESTATIONS

Ocular symptoms have been described in 1–32% of patients.[91–95] The most common ocular finding is conjunctivitis, which appears to be more common in patients with severe disease.

NEUROLOGIC MANIFESTATIONS

Neurologic findings have been described in 36–57% of hospitalized patients.[96–98] The most common symptoms are dizziness, headache, and impaired consciousness; stroke has been observed in 2–3% of patients. A small but high-profile case series reported stroke in young patients with COVID-19, some of whom did not have clear vascular risk factors.[99] However, larger prospective studies are needed to clarify the risk of stroke in COVID-19, in particular among younger patients. It is unclear whether neurologic effects are related to a direct effect of the virus, to hypercoagulability or inflammation caused by the virus, or to the concurrent incidence of severe medical illness in patients with preexisting

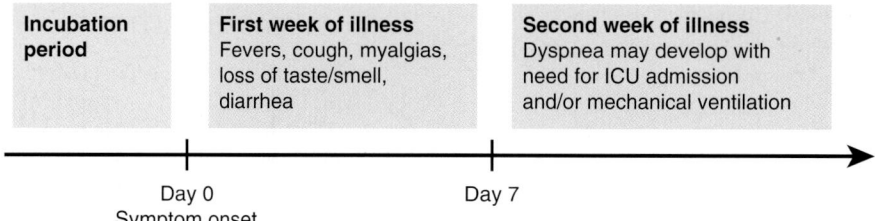

Figure 46a.4 Clinical course of COVID-19. The presymptomatic incubation period may last a median of 5 days. During the first week of illness, symptoms tend to be flulike, with the added symptoms of losses of taste and smell. Severe disease may develop in the second week, with dyspnea and the need for *intensive care unit* (ICU) treatment. Many patients remain asymptomatic during their illness.

vascular risk factors.[96,100] Several reports have also described Guillain–Barré syndrome in patients with COVID-19.[101–103]

HEMATOLOGIC MANIFESTATIONS

The incidence of venous thromboembolism (deep venous thrombosis or pulmonary embolism) in patients hospitalized with COVID-19 ranges from approximately 25–50%, and the risk appears to be higher in patients with elevated D-dimer levels.[104–109] The role of therapeutic anticoagulation in severe COVID-19 is controversial and, at present, limited data support anticoagulation in the absence of overt evidence of thromboembolism; the risks and benefits remain unclear, and prospective trials are needed.[110]

DERMATOLOGIC MANIFESTATIONS

Rash has been reported in less than 1% to 20% of patients.[4,111,112] The most common morphologic forms reported are erythematous, urticarial, and vesicular rashes. Chilblain-like lesions (known colloquially as "COVID toes") have been described commonly in patients during the COVID-19 pandemic, although a causal link to the virus has not yet been made.[113,114]

INFLAMMATORY SYNDROMES

The increased levels of inflammatory markers in patients with severe COVID-19 (discussed in detail later) have raised the possibility that critical illness in COVID-19 is a manifestation of an uncontrolled release of inflammatory mediators called a cytokine storm.[115] This concept underlies the rationale for trying to treat COVID-19 with anti-inflammatory medications (e.g., immunosuppression and steroids). Whether circulating inflammatory cytokines are higher in COVID-19 compared with other critical illnesses is uncertain at this time.[116] Another multisystemic inflammatory syndrome has been described in children; it has similarities to Kawasaki disease but is thought to be a distinct entity and is postulated to be immune system mediated.[117,118]

IMMUNOCOMPROMISED PATIENTS

Two questions with respect to immunocompromised patients are as follows: (1) Do they have atypical clinical manifestations? and (2) Are they at risk for more severe disease, or could immunosuppression actually be protective against deleterious inflammatory effects of COVID-19? Existing data indicate that immunocompromised patients have typical clinical manifestations of COVID-19.[54] Regarding risk for more severe disease, patients with cancer and solid organ

transplant recipients appear to be at higher risk for more severe disease and increased mortality, whereas patients taking biologic agents for inflammatory disorders do not appear to have increased risk.[54] Data on COVID-19 in persons with human immunodeficiency virus infection are conflicting, and the risk in this patient population is not yet clear.

CLINICAL COURSE

The median incubation period between infection and symptom onset is 5 days. Patients often do not manifest signs and symptoms of severe disease until the second week of illness (Fig. 46a.4).[48,119]

LABORATORY FINDINGS

Clinical studies have reported the results of both routine laboratory testing and biomarkers in hospitalized patients with COVID-19.[4,48,53,62–64] Patients with COVID-19 usually have a normal or low white blood cell count, with leukopenia in 15–45% of patients and leukocytosis seen in less than 25%. Lymphopenia is reported in 33–90% of patients. Platelet levels are usually normal, although they can be slightly low in up to one-third of patients. Transaminase levels are elevated in approximately 5–45% of patients, with two meta-analyses showing the pooled prevalence of transaminase elevation at 15–20%.[70,71]

Biomarkers of inflammation are commonly elevated in COVID-19, with C-reactive protein elevated in approximately 40–85% and lactate dehydrogenase in 30–75% of patients. Procalcitonin is elevated (using a cutoff of 0.5 ng/mL) in 5–17% of patients, although it is more commonly elevated in patients with severe disease or critical illness. High levels of inflammatory markers (including C-reactive protein, D-dimer, interleukin-6, ferritin) are associated with more severe disease and risk of death.[48]

Bacterial and viral coinfections are uncommon in patients presenting with COVID-19, with most studies indicating a coinfection rate less than 7%.[53,63,64,78] However, coinfections are clearly documented, and several studies show high rates of coinfections.[120] Therefore, the presence of another virus or bacterial infection does not exclude the possibility of COVID-19.

IMAGING

Chest radiographic findings are abnormal in 60% of patients hospitalized with COVID-19, whereas chest *computed tomography* (CT) scans are abnormal in 86%.[4] Two meta-analyses showed that the most common chest CT findings are ground-glass opacities (83–87%), which were usually bilateral (78–80%) and in a peripheral distribution

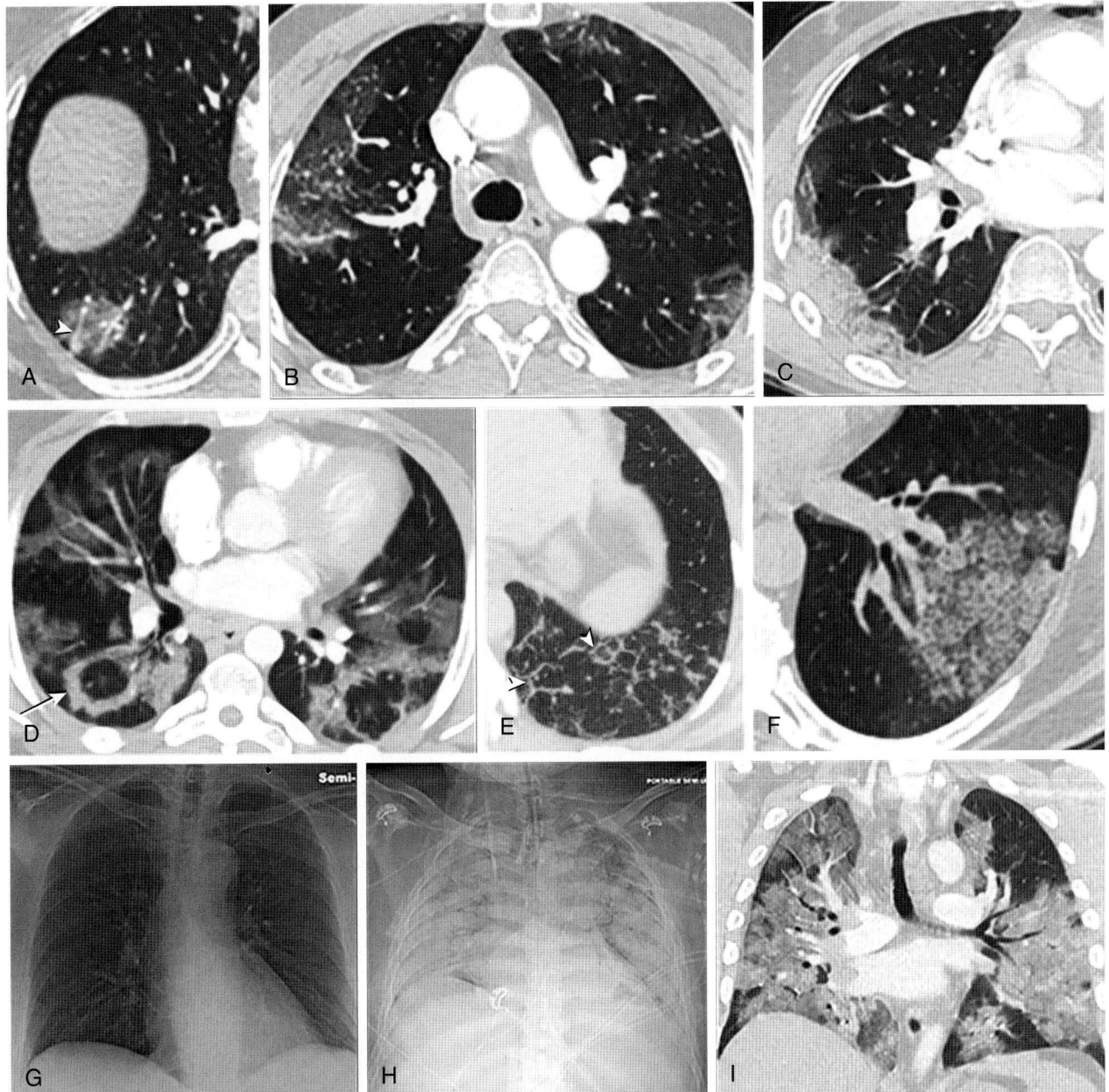

Figure 46a.5 COVID-19 pneumonia: chest radiographic spectrum and suggestive *computed tomography* (CT) findings. (A) Peripheral rounded ground-glass opacity. Note that the vessels (*arrowhead*) in the area of ground-glass opacity appear slightly larger than vessels in the unaffected lung, a feature that has been variously referred to as the "microvascular dilation" or "vascular dilation" signs. (B) Subpleural multifocal, bilateral ground-glass opacity. (C) Subpleural consolidation. Often, consolidation develops in areas previously affected by ground-glass opacity later in the disease course. (D–E) CT imaging features suggesting organizing pneumonia. (D) The "reverse [ground-glass opacity] halo" or "atoll sign": peripheral consolidation surrounding areas of central clearing (*arrow*). (E) Perilobular opacity: linear opacities outlining the secondary lobules (*arrowheads*), resembling interlobular septal thickening. (F) Crazy paving: ground-glass opacity associated with smooth interlobular septal thickening and intralobular interstitial thickening. (G) Essentially normal chest radiograph at presentation. Same patient as in the CT image in A, which was obtained 4 days after this chest radiograph. (H) Diffuse bilateral homogeneous opacities in a patient with respiratory failure who was undergoing extracorporeal membrane oxygenation. (I) CT in the same patient as in H, obtained at presentation and 6 days before the chest radiograph in H, shows multifocal bilateral ground-glass opacity–associated smooth interlobular septal thickening and intralobular interstitial thickening. (Courtesy Michael B. Gotway, MD.)

(75–77%).[121,122] Consolidations, septal thickening, and a crazy paving pattern are also considered typical in COVID-19 cases. Ground-glass opacities may evolve into a more consolidated appearance (eFig. 46a.1). Atypical findings have included pleural effusions, nodules, lymphadenopathy, tree-in-bud opacities, and pneumothorax. Abnormalities on plain chest radiographs or chest CT scans are similar to those found in other viral pneumonias. Typical CT findings are shown in Figure 46a.5.

DIAGNOSIS

The two major categories of SARS-CoV-2 diagnostic studies are tests for viral nucleic acid and tests for antibodies. The likelihood of detection of SARS-CoV-2 and the immune response to it depends on when the assay is performed relative to the time of exposure or infection (Fig. 46a.6).

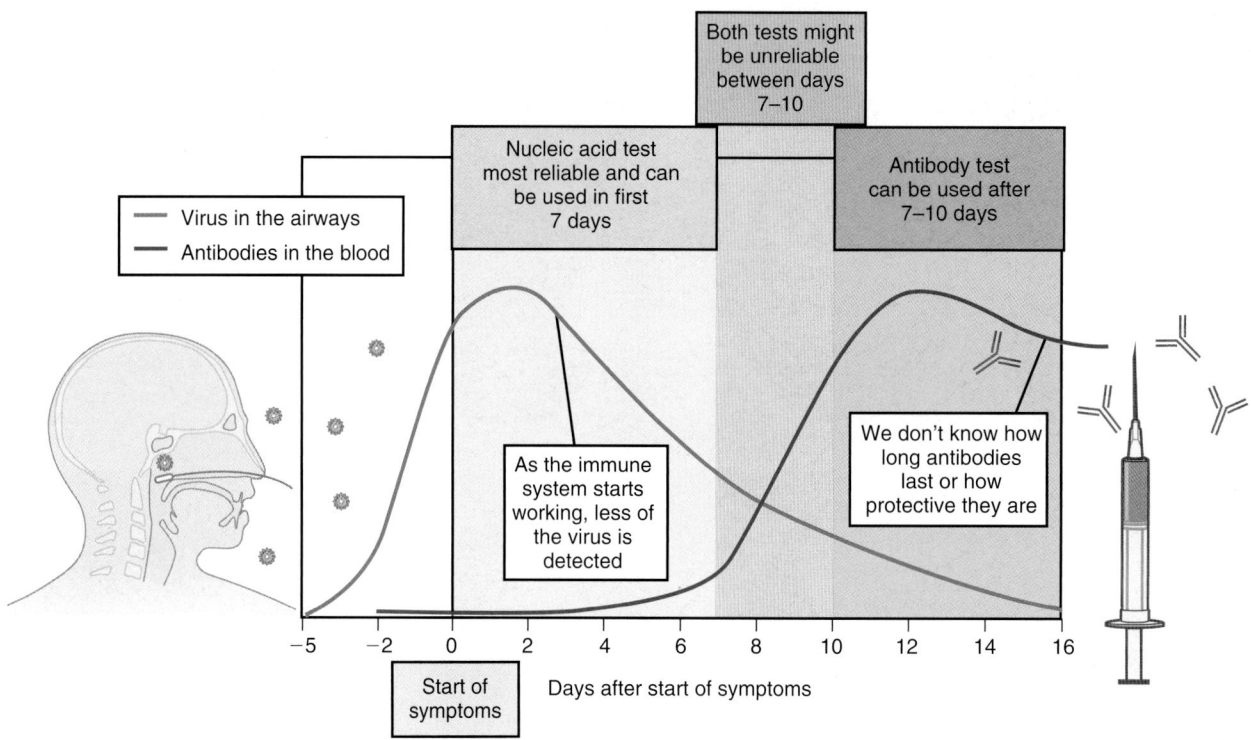

Figure 46a.6 Time course of viral exposure, clinical infection, and the results of clinical assays for severe acute respiratory syndrome coronavirus 2 and the immune response to it. Given the high virus counts, the patient may be most contagious in the few days before and after symptoms begin (see virus in airways, *blue line*). During the first week of symptoms, when virus is abundant, the nucleic acid tests are most reliable. With the onset of an immune response, virus numbers start to decline. By the second week, the immune system has been activated and, from 7 to 10 days after symptoms, the antibody test may be useful in detecting infection. Interestingly, both tests may be unreliable between the first and second weeks. (From UK Research and Innovation. What is the purpose of testing for COVID-19? 2020. **https://coronavirusexplained.ukri.org/en/article/vdt0006/.**)

SARS-COV-2 NUCLEIC ACID TESTING

Viral nucleic acid detection is the mainstay of testing for active infection. These *nucleic acid amplification tests* (NAATs) most commonly use reverse-transcriptase polymerase chain reaction technology, of which there are multiple kits that amplify and detect different regions of the SARS-CoV-2 genome (e.g., nucleocapsid gene, envelope gene, spike gene, open reading frame, RNA-dependent RNA polymerase gene).

The available NAATs are highly specific for SARS-CoV-2, but sensitivity can vary depending on the clinical scenario (Table 46a.1). Specifically, SARS-CoV-2 viral load in the upper respiratory tract is highest during the presymptomatic period or in the first week after symptom onset, whereas, later in the illness, the upper respiratory tract NAAT result may be negative even if lower respiratory tract involvement has developed.[36,123] In a retrospective study of patients in China with clinically diagnosed COVID-19 pneumonia, 12.5% of patients with an initial negative NAAT result were confirmed positive on a second test, a finding suggesting that the initial upper airway viral load was low.[124]

Beyond the issue of a low viral load, false-negative results may also arise because of improper sampling, sampling the wrong site, or viral mutations in the region targeted by the polymerase chain reaction. For this reason, among symptomatic patients who are either hospitalized or in high-risk settings such as congregate living, one or more negative NAAT results may not be sufficient to rule out COVID-19. Among patients with evidence of lower respiratory tract infection, polymerase chain reaction testing should be performed on a sample obtained from the lower respiratory tract while acknowledging that this approach may be limited by the transmission risk of the procedures.

SARS-COV-2 SEROLOGY TESTING

Serologic tests detect antibodies to SARS-CoV-2 in the blood. Multiple assays have been developed using different viral epitopes, and the available tests vary widely in their diagnostic performance (Table 46a.2).

In a study of 173 patients with COVID-19, the median time to antibody detection using an assay against the receptor-binding domain of the SARS-CoV-2 spike protein was 12 days for immunoglobulin M and 14 days for immunoglobulin G.[125] Because of this timeframe, current U.S. Centers for Disease Control and Prevention and World Health Organization guidelines recommend not using antibody tests to diagnose active SARS-CoV-2 infection where a false result may be caused by testing too early in the course of infection. Additionally, because there are limited data on whether certain antibodies confer immunity and on the duration of protection of neutralizing antibodies, SARS-CoV-2 serologic testing results should not be used to determine whether it is safe to return to work or to enter group living situations. Serologic testing has demonstrated value as a public health surveillance tool.

OTHER TESTS

Tests that identify SARS-CoV-2 antigen are under development and hold potential as rapid point-of-care assays. However, these assays are typically less sensitive than

Table 46a.1 The Sensitivity and Specificity of Nucleic Acid Amplification Tests for Severe Acute Respiratory Syndrome Coronavirus 2 Based on the Clinical Scenario

Test	Sensitivity, % (95% CI)	Specificity, % (95% CI)
SAMPLE LOCATION (3 STUDIES)		
Upper respiratory tract	76 (51–100)	100 (99–100)
Lower respiratory tract	89 (84–94)	100 (99–100)
UPPER RESPIRATORY TRACT SAMPLES (11 STUDIES)		
Oral	56 (35–77)	99 (99–100)
Nasal	76 (59–94)	100 (99–100)
Nasopharyngeal	97 (92–100)	100 (99–100)
Saliva	85 (69–94)	100 (99–100)
Midturbinate	100 (93–100)	100 (99–100)
REPEAT TESTING (WITH NP SWABS; 3 STUDIES)		
Single test	71 (65–77)	100 (99–100)
Repeat test	88 (80–96)	100 (99–100)

CI, confidence interval; NP, nasopharyngeal.
Modified from Hanson KE, Caliendo AM, Arias CA, et al. Infectious Diseases Society of America guidelines on the diagnosis of COVID-19: molecular diagnostic testing. *Infect Dis Soc Am*. 2020;Jan 22:ciab048.

Table 46a.2 Serologic Testing for Severe Acute Respiratory Syndrome Coronavirus 2

Type of Test	Time to Results	What It Tells Us	What It *Cannot* Tell Us
Rapid diagnostic test (RDT)	10–30 min	The presence or absence (qualitative) of antibodies against the virus present in patient serum	The amount of antibodies in the patient serum, or whether these antibodies are able to inhibit viral growth
Enzyme-linked immunosorbent assay (ELISA)	2–5 hr	The presence or absence (quantitative) of antibodies against the virus present in patient serum	Whether the antibodies are able to inhibit viral growth
Neutralization assay (plaque reduction neutralization test [PRNT])	3–5 days	The presence of active antibodies in patient serum able to inhibit viral growth ex vivo, in a cell culture system	May miss antibodies to viral proteins not involved in replication
Chemiluminescent immunoassay (CLIA)	1–2 hr	The presence or absence (quantitative) of antibodies against the virus present in the patient serum	Whether the antibodies are able to inhibit viral growth

Modified from Johns Hopkins University Center for Health Security. Serology-based tests for COVID-19. https://www.centerforhealthsecurity.org/resources/COVID-19/serology/Serology-based-tests-for-COVID-19.html.

NAATs. SARS-CoV-2 viral culture is performed only for research purposes.

PATHOLOGY AND PATHOMECHANISMS

PATHOLOGY OF COVID-19 PNEUMONIA

The main pathologic finding in SARS-CoV-2 lung infection is diffuse alveolar damage in the exudative or proliferative phase[126–132] (Fig. 46a.7). As in other forms of diffuse alveolar damage, there is alveolar epithelial cell desquamation, alveolar type 2 cell hyperplasia, and septal edema. Hyaline membranes contain viral antigen. Epithelium-derived syncytial cells, which form in response to the action of viral fusion proteins, are sometimes found in alveoli. Inflammatory infiltrates are either neutrophilic (particularly in the acute phase) or lymphocytic. A distinctive finding is the large burden of platelet-rich thrombi in the microvasculature.[132]

Medium and large vessels can also contain embolic thrombus. Megakaryocytes, normal cellular constituents of the lung, are present within alveolar capillaries in increased numbers.[133] SARS-CoV-2 virions or proteins can be detected in the epithelium of the airways, in the alveoli, and in alveolar macrophages. Some studies have detected SARS-CoV-2 virions within lung endothelial cells; however, other studies have not, and identification of virions is challenging as a result of virus-mimicking cellular structures.[129,132,134–138] In summary, the pathology of COVID-19 pneumonia falls within the spectrum of diffuse alveolar damage seen in other disorders; endothelial injury (endotheliitis) and microvascular thrombosis are distinctive, but not diagnostic, features.

IMMUNOPATHOLOGIC OBSERVATIONS IN COVID-19 PNEUMONIA

The immune response to SARS-CoV-2 pneumonia has been characterized by detailed analyses of cytokines and leukocytes in peripheral blood and in bronchoalveolar lavage

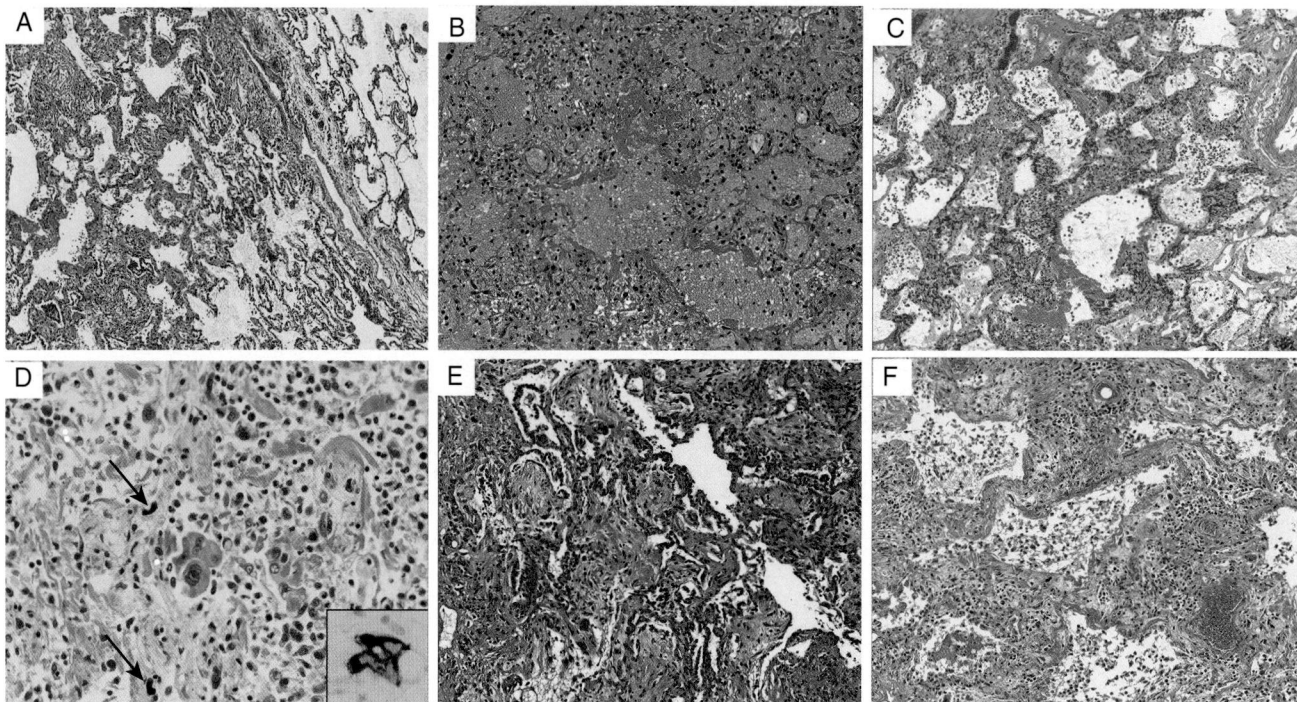

Figure 46a.7 Spectrum of diffuse alveolar damage seen in COVID-19 pneumonia. (A) All cases demonstrated diffuse alveolar damage, and seven of eight cases showed a component of acute phase diffuse alveolar damage. Note the demarcation between affected lung parenchyma with thickened alveolar septa and hyaline membranes (*lower left*) and the relatively preserved lung parenchyma (*upper right*) separated by a thickened edematous interlobular septum. (B) Edema of variable severity was seen in all cases and is marked in this example. Note also the conspicuous hyaline membranes. (C) The presence of interstitial neutrophilic infiltrates was seen in focal areas with acute diffuse alveolar damage. (D) Reactive alveolar type 2 epithelial cells within alveolar spaces showed abundant eosinophilic cytoplasm, irregular nuclear contours, occasional binucleation, vesicular condensed chromatin, and prominent macronucleoli. Intracapillary megakaryocytes (*arrows*) were also present within alveolar capillaries and were highlighted by CD61 immunohistochemistry (*inset*). (E) Lungs from six patients showed organizing phase diffuse alveolar damage alone or in combination with acute phase diffuse alveolar damage, with characteristic alveolar type 2 cell and fibroblastic proliferation within alveolar walls with focal intraluminal plugs of loose connective tissue. (F) Some areas within organizing diffuse alveolar damage showed interstitial chronic inflammation. (Modified from Sauter JL, Baine MK, Butnor KJ, et al. Insights into pathogenesis of fatal COVID-19 pneumonia from histopathology with immunohistochemical and viral RNA studies. *Histopathology*. 2020;77:915-925.)

fluid.[139–149] Lymphopenia is common, and its severity at an early stage correlates with the risk of severe disease and death.[150] CD4[+], CD8[+], and γδ T cells, T regulatory cells, and natural killer cells are decreased in peripheral blood, probably because of a combination of recruitment from the vasculature to lymphoid organs and to sites of infection and of cell death by mechanisms involving *interleukin-6* (IL-6) and Fas-Fas ligand signaling.[139] Numerous cytokines are elevated in blood; IL-6, IL-2, *interferon* (IFN)-γ, IL-8, IL-10, IP-10, macrophage chemotactic protein 3, and IL-1 receptor antagonist levels have been correlated with disease severity. Production of type I and III IFN, an antiviral response downstream of activation of pattern recognition receptors, can be impaired by viral mechanisms that block detection of viral RNA or inhibit downstream signaling responses.[139,151] The importance of an effective type I IFN response in controlling SARS-CoV-2 is provided by the findings that approximately 15% of patients with severe COVID-19 lack effective type I IFN responses because of genetic defects[152] or because of autoantibodies that neutralize type I IFNs.[153] Whether serum cytokine levels in COVID-19 represent a cytokine storm that is different from or more severe than in non-COVID ARDS is controversial.[116]

The phenotypes of mononuclear cells in blood and lung are altered.[139] Severely ill patients with COVID-19 have increased numbers of granulocyte-macrophage colony-stimulating factor–expressing CD4[+] T cells, which can secrete proinflammatory cytokines and may recruit inflammatory monocytes and macrophages.[139] Peripheral T cells, especially CD8[+] T cells, are activated in higher numbers than in control subjects, and they express markers suggestive of exhaustion (programmed cell death 1 and T cell immunoglobulin and mucin domain 3). Natural killer cells are functionally impaired, both in their ability to secrete chemokines and cytokines and in their expression of cytotoxic molecules. Natural killer cells from COVID-19 patients also express higher levels of immune checkpoint inhibitors. There are higher numbers of inflammatory monocytes in the peripheral blood of COVID-19 patients and, in the lung, there appears to be recruitment of inflammatory monocytes and monocyte-derived macrophages.[146]

Within 2 weeks of infection, CD4[+] and CD8[+] T cells with antigen receptors specific for SARS-CoV-2 antigens are detectable and, within 1 to 2 weeks, COVID-19 patients seroconvert.[139] Antibodies to the viral nucleocapsid and spike proteins are common. The receptor binding domain of the S protein is particularly immunogenic, and anti–receptor binding domain antibodies can be neutralizing. The relationship of circulating antibody levels to clinical disease is complex. Although increasing levels of anti-SARS-CoV-2 antibodies correlate with decreasing viral load, increasing titers of specific antibody can also correlate with increasing disease severity.[139] This finding suggests that viral clearance alone may not prevent severe disease or that differences in antibody targets or specific antibody functions influence the outcome of infection. Antibody-dependent enhancement, a process by which virus opsonized by antibody is able to access and activate macrophages in an Fc-receptor–dependent manner and thereby worsen disease, has been described in experimental models of SARS-CoV-1 infection, but there is no evidence yet of antibody-dependent enhancement in humans with SARS-CoV-2.[154,155] An antibody response may not be essential for recovery, however, because patients with X-linked agammaglobulinemia have recovered from COVID-19 after relatively mild illness.[156,157]

PATHOMECHANISMS OF COVID-19

The portals of entry for SARS-CoV-2 are ACE2-expressing epithelial cells in the upper and lower respiratory tract (eFig. 46a.2).[158] Viral loads in the upper airway peak sooner in SARS-CoV-2 infection than in SARS-CoV-1 infection.[19] The virus is also taken up by macrophages, which are probably unable to support SARS-CoV-2 replication.[134] Although macrophages likely contribute to viral clearance, virus-containing macrophages also amplify the inflammatory response and may act to spread viral infection within and outside the lung.[159] In an animal model of SARS-CoV-1 pneumonia, depletion of inflammatory monocyte-macrophages improved survival.[160]

Engagement of pattern recognition receptors during the initial stages of a viral infection triggers two general antiviral responses: release of types I and III IFNs, which induce expression of IFN-stimulated genes, and release of cytokines and leukocyte-recruiting chemokines, resulting in activation and recruitment of virus-clearing cells such as natural killer cells, inflammatory monocyte-macrophages, and neutrophils. In SARS-CoV-2 pneumonia, there may be a distinctive imbalance in these responses: the IFN-I or III response is blunted, at least in the early phase of infection, whereas release of other proinflammatory molecules is prominent.[161] The complexity of the response and the importance of timing are suggested by a SARS-CoV-1 animal model in which early IFN-I signaling is protective, whereas late signaling increases lethality,[162] as well as by observations that IFN-stimulated genes are up-regulated in bronchoalveolar lavage cells of COVID-19 patients in comparison with patients with SARS.[147] The type I IFN response may be more suppressed with a higher initial viral load and in older patients.[151] Recruited inflammatory monocyte-macrophages and activated resident macrophages likely become drivers of the hyperinflammatory response through release, in particular, of tumor necrosis factor-α and IL-6. The resulting response has similarities to a final common pathway of severe and systemic inflammation (in which macrophages, cytotoxic T cells, and natural killer cells drive tissue injury) also seen in disorders such as secondary hemophagocytic lymphohistiocytosis and the cytokine release syndrome seen with chimeric antibody receptor–T cell infusions.[163,164]

The endothelium is also a key contributor to COVID-19 lung pathology (eFig. 46a.3). In viral pneumonia, the endothelium regulates aspects of the inflammatory response, such as leukocyte egress, vascular leak, and the innate immune response.[165] In COVID-19 pneumonia, additional factors target the endothelium. ACE2 is down-regulated as a consequence of viral infection, and the resulting ACE-ACE2 imbalance may lead to an excess of angiotensin II signaling.[166,167] Angiotensin II induces endothelial injury, vasoconstriction, and thrombosis. Ace2 knockout mice develop more severe disease in lung injury models, and ACE2 has protective effects on lung beyond the epithelium, findings that support the idea that ACE-ACE2 imbalance is relevant to COVID-19.[166] In addition, endothelial cells may be directly infected by SARS-CoV-2, thus adding to endothelial cell injury and loss. Loss of endothelial cells and the resultant exposure of the basement membrane promote clot formation. The prominent microvascular thrombosis, as well as macroscopic thrombosis and thromboembolism, in COVID-19 is likely caused by a severe "immunothrombosis" state[168] resulting from endothelium dysfunction and loss, along with other prothrombotic phenomena (high levels of von Willebrand factor, factor VIII, fibrinogen, and possibly activation of complement[169] and formation of neutrophil extracellular traps).[170]

TREATMENT

At this time, treatment for COVID-19 is principally supportive. As of March 2021, the *U.S. Food and Drug Administration* (FDA) has issued emergency use authorizations for medical treatment (including remdesivir and convalescent plasma) and for medical devices in the care of COVID-19 patients. The best evidence for efficacy at the time of this publication is for remdesivir and dexamethasone (see later). We will discuss the evidence for the use of these treatments and refer the reader to updates here and elsewhere for the latest therapies.

Patients whose severity of illness does not warrant hospitalization should remain at home and as isolated as much as possible from uninfected close contacts. The duration of isolation depends on several factors. The U.S. Centers for Disease Control and Prevention make recommendations based on symptomatic versus asymptomatic infection.[171] Isolation should persist for 10 days after the resolution of symptoms *and* 24 hours after the resolution of fever (without the use of antipyretic agents). Hospitalized patients should wear surgical masks to limit droplet transmission whenever feasible, and they should be housed in negative-pressure isolation areas to limit nosocomial spread of SARS-CoV-2. Clinical care providers should wear personal protective equipment consisting of an impermeable clear face shield, an N-95 (or higher) respirator mask or a contained air-purifying respirator or powered air-purifying respirator, impermeable gloves, and an impermeable gown, as appropriate based on patient care activity.

For practical purposes, COVID-19 can be classified as mild, severe, or critical. In mild disease, patients have either no pneumonia or mild pneumonia, and they do not meet criteria for severe or critical illness.[8] Severe COVID-19 is defined as dyspnea, persistent tachypnea (respiratory rate ≥30/min), hypoxemia (oxyhemoglobin saturation <93%), a PaO_2/FIO_2 ratio less than 300, or an increase in lung opacities greater than 50% over 24 to 48 hours. Critical COVID-19 is characterized by respiratory failure, shock, or multiorgan dysfunction or failure.

Mild COVID-19 should be treated symptomatically, with measures taken to prevent contagion and monitor for clinical deterioration. The goals of treatment in severe or critical COVID-19 are supportive. Clinicians should provide measures required to reverse or prevent further clinical deterioration while avoiding overtreatment and the harms associated with it.[172–174]

RESPIRATORY CARE

Patients may be hypoxemic without other symptoms or signs of respiratory failure, such as dyspnea or use of accessory breathing muscles.[175,176] Despite their lack of dyspnea, patients with hypoxemia should receive supplemental oxygen. Clinicians often prescribe supplemental oxygen to achieve oxyhemoglobin saturations higher than a given threshold, often more than 90%. This goal may be difficult to achieve in some patients with severe COVID-19, for unknown reasons. Because the goal of supportive critical care is to provide sufficient arterial oxygen delivery to preserve or restore normal cellular metabolism, the therapeutic target for oxyhemoglobin saturation should focus on the value required to avoid or reverse anaerobic cellular metabolism, which may vary depending on individual patient characteristics.[176,177] Close monitoring for evidence of anaerobic metabolism (e.g., lactic acidosis) or incipient organ failure (e.g., altered mentation, myocardial injury) is advisable. Standard nasal cannulas, Venturi masks, and non-rebreather masks may supply enough oxygen to reverse critical hypoxemia in many patients, but severely ill patients may require additional therapy. High-flow or high-velocity nasal cannulas provide higher flows of oxygen and consequently a higher effective fractional concentration of oxygen in inspired gas. Furthermore, these devices may lower the work of breathing, rest the respiratory muscles, and limit oxygen consumption.[178] Noninvasive positive-pressure ventilation may be helpful in selected cases (when there is an imminently reversible cause of respiratory distress or when guided by advance directives), but because respiratory failure is often prolonged in patients with critical COVID-19 (median duration of mechanical ventilation in survivors >2 weeks), noninvasive ventilation should be used cautiously.[179] The use of high-flow nasal oxygen or noninvasive ventilation may increase the dissemination of SARS-CoV-2 and the risk of infecting health care personnel, so these treatments should take place in areas where appropriate isolation and environmental precautions and use of personal protective equipment by medical personnel are maintained. For patients with hypoxemia despite supplemental oxygen, prone positioning may improve oxygenation, but the results of limited preliminary reports involving small observational cohorts show mixed results. Many patients do not tolerate a prone position but, among those who do, improvements in oxygenation and respiratory rate are frequently, although not universally, observed. These improvements may not be durable.[180,181] More recommendations on the use of this intervention will require the results of ongoing clinical studies: at least 60 trials of prone positioning in COVID-19 were registered as of August 2020.[182] The use of inhaled selective pulmonary vasodilators is also an area of intense interest, and clinical trials of inhaled nitric oxide or inhaled prostacyclin are currently registered.[183,184]

The decision to proceed to endotracheal intubation and invasive positive-pressure ventilation for patients with severe COVID-19 is complicated. Some experts advocate early intubation and controlled ventilation to limit excessive patient breathing efforts that may damage already injured lungs.[185] Other experts advise caution and reserve intubation for frank respiratory failure only, by recognizing that a solid set of criteria for defining the need for intubation and ventilation remains elusive.[186,187] Without the results of clinical trials describing clinical benefit associated with a standardized set of criteria for progressing from supplemental oxygen and other noninvasive methods of respiratory support (see earlier) to intubation and mechanical ventilation, the decision will remain in the realm of clinical judgment. A small, retrospective, single-center study suggested that early intubation is not associated with a lower risk of death.[188] Because mechanical ventilation is often prolonged in patients with severe COVID-19, and because invasive mechanical ventilation is often accompanied by complications, clinicians should proceed carefully and use a broad evaluation to formulate a decision about whether to intubate and provide positive-pressure ventilation by assessing several parameters to determine whether an individual patient's work of breathing is too high to sustain.[189] Serial careful and consistent physical examinations are crucial, and patients who may require mechanical ventilation should undergo close monitoring with the highest level of care possible depending on the availability of resources. The most experienced and skilled clinician available should perform endotracheal intubation, and rapid sequence intubation with induction of anesthesia and neuromuscular blockade has been associated with increased intubation success.[190] The breathing circuit should contain a filter capable of trapping viral particles at all times to limit dispersion of SARS-CoV-2. Clinicians involved in intubation may have a high risk of exposure to SARS-CoV-2, even when they are wearing recommended personal protective equipment.[191]

Lung-protective ventilation to prevent alveolar overdistention and ventilator-associated lung injury is essential.[192] The targeted tidal volume should be based on the patient's predicted body weight, and tidal volumes between 6 and 8 mL/kg are advised, as long as the plateau airway pressure, driving pressure, or mechanical power (a summary variable including pressures, volumes, flows, and respiratory rate[193]) remains low. Either volume-controlled or pressure-controlled ventilation is acceptable, but clinicians should be aware that excessive patient efforts during pressure-controlled ventilation may result in excessive tidal volumes and in transalveolar pressures higher than the set inspiratory pressure target.[194] Patients who require mechanical ventilation for COVID-19 ARDS show heterogeneity of respiratory mechanics similar to the heterogeneity present in patients with ARDS from all other causes.[195] Clinicians should individualize ventilator settings, sedation, analgesia, and neuromuscular blockade to minimize the work of breathing when required, improve patient comfort and patient-ventilator coordination, and facilitate the earliest possible return to independent breathing, as long as airway pressures and gas exchange remain within safe ranges. The use of rescue therapies (lung recruitment, high positive end-expiratory pressure settings, inhaled selective pulmonary vasodilators, and extracorporeal gas exchange) remains undefined at present, although the results of large studies should guide practice in the near future.

Because the duration of mechanical ventilation may be prolonged, and because patients who undergo mechanical ventilation appear to be at high risk for death, clinicians should carefully discuss advance directives, goals of care, and surrogate decision making with their patients who have progressive respiratory failure. The need for timely and thorough conversations that elucidate patients' values and preferences regarding advanced medical interventions and end-of-life care is heightened by hospital infection-control policies that may severely limit visiting by families and loved ones. Clinicians and hospitals may choose to use technologies such as video conferencing to alleviate the isolation of hospitalized patients with COVID-19.

ANTIVIRAL AND ANTI-INFLAMMATORY THERAPIES

Remdesivir is an intravenous nucleotide prodrug that binds to the viral RNA-dependent RNA polymerase. inducing a premature termination of RNA transcription. On May 1, 2020, the FDA issued an emergency use authorization for the use of remdesivir for the treatment of COVID-19.[196] However, the evidence in support of remdesivir is still evolving. One single-center, prospective, double-blind, randomized controlled trial performed in Wuhan, China assessed the efficacy of remdesivir for COVID-19. The study enrolled 237 patients, and 158 of these patients received remdesivir. The primary end point of the study was time to clinical improvement, and no difference was observed between the placebo and remdesivir groups.[197] A larger multicenter, prospective, placebo-controlled, double-blind trial that enrolled 1062 patients, who were assigned 1:1 to receive remdesivir or placebo, with more than 98% adherence to remdesivir in the assigned group, found more favorable results. Time to recovery (as defined by an 8-point ordinal scale and assessed by log-rank analysis) was shorter, with a reduction of approximately 5 days in the duration of illness. This effect was more pronounced in the subgroup of patients with more severe disease, in whom the duration of illness was shortened by a median of 7 days. The remdesivir group had a lower number of deaths, and the effect on the risk of death was more pronounced in the group with severe respiratory illness. Remdesivir also appeared to reduce the risk of respiratory deterioration, such as a new requirement for supplemental oxygen or a new need for assisted ventilation, as well as a shorter duration of mechanical ventilation or extracorporeal membrane oxygenation, when used.[197] A single-center, open-label, prospective trial of combination lopinavir-ritonavir did not observe clinical benefit compared with placebo.[198]

Dexamethasone has been shown to have value in severely ill COVID-19 patients, supporting a pathogenic role for inflammation. An open-label randomized controlled trial of dexamethasone, 6 mg daily given either orally or intravenously, enrolled patients across 176 centers in the United Kingdom, with 2014 patients receiving dexamethasone and 4321 patients receiving usual care (RECOVERY). In the study, investigators observed an absolute reduction of 2.8% in the risk of 28-day mortality among all patients who received dexamethasone.[200] Among patients receiving supplemental oxygen at the time of randomization, the absolute risk reduction was 2.9% and, in patients undergoing mechanical ventilation at the time of randomization, the absolute risk reduction was 11.8%. Among patients neither receiving oxygen nor undergoing mechanical ventilation, mortality was 3.8% higher, although the 95% confidence interval for the risk ratio crossed 1.0. Dexamethasone was associated with a greater likelihood of reducing the risk for

28-day mortality among patients who had symptoms for 7 days or more before randomization. Dexamethasone was also associated with a lower risk of progressing to mechanical ventilation as well as a shorter duration of intensive care unit and hospital stay. The magnitude of mortality benefit among ventilated patients is similar to that found in a recently published trial of dexamethasone for patients with non–COVID-19 ARDS.[201]

The publication of the results of the RECOVERY trial resulted in a loss of equipoise and the cessation of several other studies of the effects of glucocorticoids in severe COVID-19.[202] The results of the CoDEX, CAPE COVID, and REMAP CAP trials were subsequently published despite early termination.[203–205] The World Health Organization, with the cooperation of several prospective trialists, carried out a prospective meta-analysis of seven ongoing randomized controlled trials that included RECOVERY, CoDEX, CAPE COVID, REMAP CAP, as well as three others that have not yet been published.[206] The meta-analysis included a total of 1703 patients, with 678 randomized to receive glucocorticoids and 1025 randomized to receive placebo. A total of 222 of 678 (33%) patients who received steroids died, whereas 425 of 1025 (42%) placebo-assigned patients died, thus resulting in a lower odds ratio for death among the glucocorticoid-treated group (odds ratio, 0.66; 95% confidence interval, 0.53 to 0.82). Glucocorticoids were associated with lower mortality among severely ill patients who were undergoing invasive mechanical ventilation at the time of randomization, as well as among severely ill patients who were not undergoing invasive ventilation. Glucocorticoids also appeared to be associated with more ventilator-free days. The meta-analysis found little heterogeneity among the seven studies, with little variation between the effects of hydrocortisone and dexamethasone; insufficient evidence was available about other formulations of glucocorticoids. Uncertainty persists about the dose, the duration of administration, and the timing of administration with respect to the onset of COVID-19 symptoms. Although the benefit of steroids appears to apply to severely ill patients who are not undergoing invasive mechanical ventilation, the exact level of severity at which an individual patient should receive steroids remains undefined.[202] A common approach is that severely ill COVID-19 patients with hypoxemic respiratory failure receive a minimum of hydrocortisone, 150 mg/day in divided doses, or dexamethasone, at a minimum dose of 6 mg daily, for at least 7 days, with a tapering schedule determined by the treating clinicians. Clinicians should weigh the risk-benefit balance carefully for patients with less severe disease.

Multiple investigations of additional anti-inflammatory or immunomodulating drugs are in progress at this time. Drugs under investigation include multiple formulations of glucocorticosteroids, immunotherapy with convalescent plasma or anti–SARS-CoV-2 monoclonal antibodies, intravenous immunoglobulin, and drugs that interrupt pathways involving various inflammatory molecules. A device that adsorbs circulating inflammatory mediators (CytoSorb, CytoSorbents Corp), which is approved in the European Union, received FDA emergency use authorization on April 10, 2020, for use in patients with established or imminent respiratory failure from COVID-19; data regarding the efficacy of this device remain preliminary.[199]

ANTICOAGULANT AND ANTITHROMBOTIC THERAPY

Multiple groups of investigators have observed an increased risk for arterial and venous thromboembolism and abnormal coagulation biomarkers in patients with COVID-19.[105,207–210] Abnormal coagulation may be associated with worse prognosis.[211] Although some reports associate therapeutic anticoagulation with improved outcomes, decisions about whom and when to treat remain uncertain.[212] Without more data to guide prescribing decisions, a common approach is to limit therapeutic anticoagulation with unfractionated heparin, low-molecular-weight heparin, or direct thrombin inhibitors to patients with overt evidence of venous or arterial thromboembolism. All hospitalized patients should receive thromboprophylaxis (in the absence of contraindications) according to current guidelines. Whether to commence therapeutic anticoagulation in response to suspected microthrombosis or severe abnormalities in coagulation biomarkers such as D-dimer levels remains uncertain.

FUTURE DEVELOPMENTS

Important advances are eagerly awaited in vaccine development, (with 3 vaccines now approved for emergency use by the FDA), as well as in other preventive approaches such as inhaled antibodies[213] or repurposed drugs to block the viral infection.[214] Further studies are in progress for rapid diagnostic tests and effective treatments. There is much to learn about the effects of SARS-CoV-2 on the lung, and studies are underway to ascertain the short-term and long-term effects of COVID-19.

This chapter will be updated frequently at ExpertConsult. com.

Key Points

- *Severe acute respiratory syndrome coronavirus 2* (SARS-2-CoV) is a member of the Coronaviridae family of enveloped, single-stranded, RNA viruses. It uses the angiotensin-converting enzyme 2 protein as its principal receptor to enter host cells.
- Person-to-person transmission through small respiratory droplets is probably the main means of spread, although aerosol transmission is also likely. Transmission by fomites may also happen. Asymptomatic carriage likely plays an important role in propagating viral spread.
- Approximately 40–45% of SARS-CoV-2 infections are asymptomatic. In the remainder, fever, fatigue, myalgias, and dry cough are common. Absence of fever does not preclude the diagnosis of COVID-19 because many infected patients do not manifest fever. Gastrointestinal symptoms are present in approximately one-third of patients. Neurologic or sensory manifestations are also common.
- Older patients with comorbidities such as diabetes mellitus, arterial hypertension, cardiovascular disease, chronic lung disease, and obesity have a higher risk for developing severe disease from SARS-COV-2 infection. Racial and ethnic disparities in risk for death exist in the United States, with members of Black, Hispanic, and Native American communities experiencing a high risk for death; the causes are likely related to disparities in social determinants of health.
- Hypoxemia is the most common severe manifestation of COVID-19, but evidence of renal, hepatic, and myocardial injury, as well as abnormal coagulation parameters, is also common. Chest radiography is abnormal in the majority of patients hospitalized with SARS-CoV-2 infection.
- The diagnosis of SARS-CoV-2 infection relies on nucleic acid amplification tests to detect the presence of virus in a suspected patient. These tests are highly specific, but sensitivity depends on factors including timing from symptom onset and sample type.
- The main pathologic finding in COVID-19 pneumonia is diffuse alveolar damage. Although no pathologic features of COVID-19 are diagnostic, COVID-19 pneumonia is characterized by an unusual degree of endothelial injury and microvascular thrombosis.
- Lung damage caused by SARS-CoV-2 results from direct viral injury and from the host immune response, with the latter likely more important in severe cases. The injurious immune response appears to consist of a markedly imbalanced immune response characterized by profound lymphopenia and lymphocyte exhaustion, hyperactivation of the innate immune response in monocyte-macrophages, and an aberrant interferon-I/III response.
- Hospital treatment is mainly focused on supportive care with supplemental oxygen and, if needed, mechanical ventilation. Patients with respiratory failure often meet criteria for acute respiratory distress syndrome, and mechanical ventilation for patients with respiratory failure caused by COVID-19 should be similar to that provided to patients with acute respiratory distress syndrome from other causes, with a focus on lung-protective ventilation.
- Thromboembolic complications are common in COVID-19, and therapeutic anticoagulation with unfractionated heparin or other drugs is advised when pathologic clots are detected. The utility of anticoagulation for patients with markedly abnormal coagulation parameters (but without clinical evidence of thromboembolism) is unknown.
- The antiviral agent remdesivir may be associated with earlier clinical improvement, but its effects on other important clinical end points remains unknown. Glucocorticoid administration is associated with a reduced risk for death among patients who require oxygen supplementation or mechanical ventilation.

Key Readings

Atri D, Siddiqi HK, Lang JP, Nauffal V, Morrow DA, Bohula EA. COVID-19 for the cardiologist: basic virology, epidemiology, cardiac manifestations, and potential therapeutic strategies. *JACC Basic Transl Sci.* 2020;5(5):518–536.

Beigel JH, Tomashek KM, Dodd LE, et al. Remdesivir for the treatment of Covid-19 - preliminary report. *N Engl J Med.* 2020;383:994.

Guan W, Ni Z, Hu Y, et al. Clinical characteristics of coronavirus disease 2019 in China. *N Engl J Med.* 2020;382(18):1708–1720.

He X, Lau EH, Wu P, et al. Temporal dynamics in viral shedding and transmissibility of COVID-19. *Nat Med.* 2020;26(5):672–675.

Oran DP, Topol EJ. Prevalence of asymptomatic SARS-CoV-2 infection. *Ann Intern Med.* 2020;173:362–367.

Richardson S, Hirsch JS, Narasimhan M, et al. Presenting characteristics, comorbidities, and outcomes among 5700 patients hospitalized with COVID-19 in the New York City area. *JAMA.* 2020;323(20):2052–2059.

Sauter JL, Baine MK, Butnor KJ, et al. Insights into pathogenesis of fatal COVID-19 pneumonia from histopathology with immunohistochemical and viral RNA studies. *Histopathology.* 2020;77:915–925.

Stokes EK. Coronavirus disease 2019 case surveillance—United States, January 22–May 30, 2020. *MMWR Morb Mortal Wkly Rep.* 2020;69:759–765.

Vabret N, Britton GJ, Gruber C, et al. Immunology of COVID-19: current state of the science. *Immunity.* 2020;52(6):910–941.

Wang W, Xu Y, Gao R, et al. Detection of SARS-CoV-2 in different types of clinical specimens. *JAMA.* 2020;323(18):1843–1844.

WHO Rapid Evidence Appraisal for COVID-19 Therapies (REACT) Working Group. Association between administration of systemic corticosteroids and mortality among critically ill patients with COVID-19: a meta-analysis. *JAMA.* 2020;324:1330–1341.

Wölfel R, Corman VM, Guggemos, et al. Virological assessment of hospitalized patients with COVID-2019. *Nature.* 2020;581(7809):465–469.

Wu Z, McGoogan JM. Characteristics of and important lessons from the coronavirus disease 2019 (COVID-19) outbreak in China: summary of a report of 72 314 cases from the Chinese Center for Disease Control and Prevention. *JAMA.* 2020;323:1239–1242.

Zhao J, Yuan Q, Wang H, et al. Antibody responses to SARS-CoV-2 in patients of novel coronavirus disease 2019. *Clin Infect Dis.* 2020;71:2027–2034.

Complete reference list available at ExpertConsult.com.

47 INFLUENZA

JUSTIN R. ORTIZ, MD, MS, FCCP • T. EOIN WEST, MD, MPH, FCCP

INTRODUCTION

Influenza viruses are respiratory pathogens transmitted mainly by droplets of respiratory secretions of infected persons.[1] Although most people with influenza illness experience mild, self-limited disease of the upper respiratory tract manifested by fever, cough, sore throat, myalgias, and/or malaise, complications are common and include primary influenza pneumonia, secondary bacterial pneumonia, exacerbations of underlying chronic diseases, and death. Influenza viruses circulate globally and cause seasonal epidemics in temperate regions and prolonged epidemics or year-round illness in tropical and subtropical regions.[2] The annual influenza attack rate is estimated to be 5–10% in adults and 20–30% in children.[1] Worldwide, seasonal influenza is responsible for an estimated 291,243 to 645,832 influenza-associated respiratory deaths each year,[3] with an increased risk of severe disease in children, older adults, and persons with chronic illness.[1,4]

CHARACTERISTICS OF INFLUENZA VIRUSES

Influenza viruses are members of the Orthomyxoviridae family of viruses. Three genera cause human disease: influenza A, influenza B, and influenza C.[5] Of these, influenza A and B are clinically most important. Although influenza A viruses infect many species of birds and mammals,[5] nonhuman influenza A virus strains occasionally infect humans and cause disease.[6] Influenza B viruses nearly exclusively infect humans.[7] Influenza A and B viruses continuously undergo mutations selected by immunologic pressure (called *antigenic drift*) that allow them to evade immune protection and to cause subsequent infections over the course of a lifetime.[8,9] Antigenic drift also accounts for the need to reformulate influenza vaccines up to twice annually to match the viral strains circulating globally.[10] Influenza A

virus strains can also undergo genetic reassortment within a common host, resulting in novel viruses to which a population may have little or no immunity (termed *antigenic shift*).[5]

An influenza pandemic can happen if novel influenza viruses emerge to which a population has little or no pre-existing immunity, the virus can spread efficiently from person to person, and the virus causes disease. The 1918 influenza pandemic killed 50 to 100 million people worldwide within 1 year, resulting in the deadliest single event in recorded human history.[11]

Formally, the full names of influenza virus strains follow a convention, for example, A/Brisbane/59/2007 (H1N1), describing the antigenic type (e.g., A, B, C); the host of origin (e.g., swine), although for human-origin viruses, no host of origin is given; the city or country of the initial isolate; and the strain number and year of isolation. Such nomenclature is typically not necessary for scientific communications unless a specific strain is being described; this chapter uses simplified nomenclature referencing virus type/subtype without further specification. For the virus that caused the 2009 influenza pandemic, the letters "pdm" follow the name (i.e., influenza A/H1N1pdm). For naming influenza A viruses, the *hemagglutinin* (H) and *neuraminidase* (N) antigens are further denoted, such as A/H1N1 or A/H3N2. The name is often shortened to refer only to the hemagglutinin and neuraminidase types.

The 1918 influenza pandemic was caused by an influenza A/H1N1 virus that spread directly from an avian reservoir to humans, without passage through another mammalian species, such as pigs.[12] The 1957 influenza A/H2N2 pandemic virus and the 1968 influenza A/H3N2 pandemic virus resulted from genetic reassortment between avian influenza viruses and seasonal influenza viruses.[12] The 2009 influenza A/H1N1pdm virus resulted from genetic reassortment between triple-reassortant North American swine influenza A/H1N1 (i.e., a virus containing genes from three different host sources: birds, humans, and swine) and a Eurasian swine influenza A virus.[12,13]

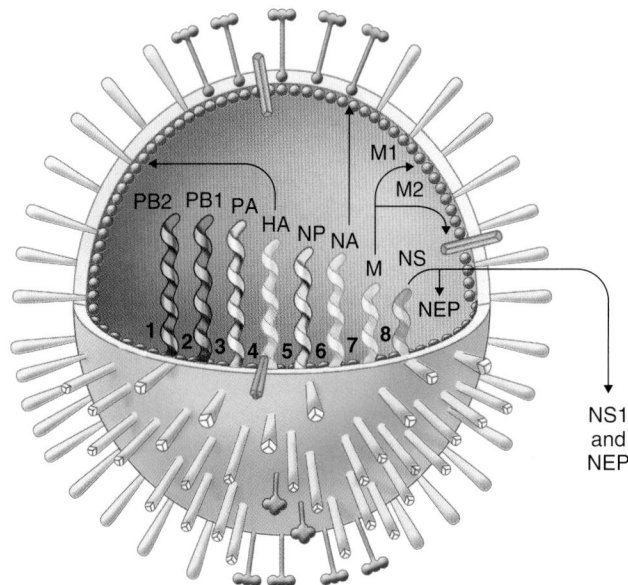

Figure 47.1 Influenza virus structure. Eight segments of viral RNA are contained within the lipid envelope and matrix (M1) shell. Each codes for one or more proteins that form the virus or regulate its intracellular replication. HA, hemagglutinin; M1, matrix; M2, proton channel; NA, neuraminidase; NP, nucleoprotein; NS1, nonstructural interferon antagonist; PB1, PB2, PA, polymerase proteins (1, 2, A); NEP, nuclear export protein. (Courtesy Dr. Robert G. Webster, St. Jude's Children's Research Hospital.)

Influenza viruses are enveloped, segmented, negative-strand RNA viruses.[5] The influenza A envelope consists of a lipid bilayer and three transmembrane proteins: *hemagglutinin* (HA), *neuraminidase* (NA), and a *proton channel* (M2). The eight RNA segments encode 11 proteins, including three RNA polymerase subunits, which have poor proofreading ability, leading to high mutation rates and antigenic drift; structural proteins (M1, a matrix protein, and M2, a proton channel protein needed for nuclear export and other functions), HA, and NA (Fig. 47.1).[14]

HA is responsible for binding to sialic acid, also known as neuraminic acid, the receptor on target cells.[5] HA comprises a globular head and stem (or stalk) regions. The receptor binding site lies in the globular head, the most variable region of the protein.[5] NA is less abundantly expressed than HA; it is responsible for release of new virus particles from infected cells by cleaving sialic acid moieties on cell membrane glycolipids and glycoproteins.[8,15] The NA is the target of the *NA inhibitor* (NAI) class of influenza antivirals.[16]

As of 2019, 18 different influenza HA glycoproteins and 11 different NA glycoproteins have been described.[17] The currently circulating influenza A virus subtypes in humans emerged from pandemics in 1968 (A/H3N1) and 2009 (A/H1N1pdm).[12] Two antigenically distinct influenza B virus lineages are cocirculating (B/Victoria and B/Yamagata).[5]

The titer of neutralizing antibodies to the HA glycoprotein correlates with protection against influenza after infection or vaccination.[18] From human challenge studies, an *HA inhibition* (HAI) titer of 40 or greater was associated with 50% protection of subjects from influenza illness, and higher HAI titers were associated with higher rates of protection.[19,20] A larger inoculum of influenza virus is required to cause infection in persons with higher HAI titers, and persons with higher HAI titers are less likely to develop clinical illness after influenza exposure.[21–23] *Inactivated influenza*

vaccines (IIVs) are designed to induce immunity to HA, and induction of HAI greater than or equal to 1:40 serves as the standard for IIV licensure.[9,18] More recent studies have shown the importance of other immune parameters, including antibodies to NA and the HA stalk, IgA, and T cell immunity, in protection from influenza.[24–29]

EPIDEMIOLOGY

In temperate regions, influenza viruses circulate in seasonal epidemics during the winter,[2] although summertime influenza illness may also happen.[30] In subtropical and tropical regions, influenza virus circulation may be prolonged or year round, with peak circulation typically during the cold or rainy season.[2] Influenza attack rates and severity differ from year to year, depending on circulating viruses and population immunity. Globally, seasonal influenza is estimated to cause more than 400,000 deaths annually from *lower respiratory tract infection* (LRTI).[3] This may be an underestimate of the total mortality due to influenza because approximately one-third of all influenza hospitalizations do not present as LRTI.[30] The economic costs of influenza, including work absenteeism and decreased productivity, associated costs of care, and disruptions in health care delivery during influenza epidemics, make seasonal influenza a major economic burden.[1] Influenza pandemics have an even greater health and economic impact.[1]

The highest influenza attack rates typically are seen in school-age children (from 5–20% annually) due to their limited preexisting immunity and extensive social mixing.[31] Although the risk of severe influenza is lower in this age group than in others, school-age children are thought to be the major drivers of influenza transmission within communities. As a result, rates of severe influenza illness in older persons typically increase 1 to 2 weeks after influenza is detected in children in a community. Influenza morbidity is greatest at the extremes of age and in persons with certain underlying morbidities. The *Centers for Disease Control and Prevention* (CDC) estimates that from 54,523 to 430,960 people in the United States have influenza-associated hospitalizations annually, with 9% of these in children younger than 5 years and 63% in persons older than 65 years.[32] The CDC also estimates that from 3349 to 48,614 people in the United States die from influenza each year.[33]

Persons with certain underlying medical conditions have a greater risk of severe influenza disease.[34] Among adults age 65 years and older, the risk of death is increased with an underlying lung disease (16-fold), heart disease (8-fold), and both lung and heart disease (21-fold) compared to persons without such conditions. A list of health factors and host factors associated with serious complications of influenza virus infection is in Table 47.1.[35]

INFECTION CONTROL

Influenza is primarily transmitted from person to person by large-particle respiratory droplets, generated by coughing and sneezing. Large-particle droplets generally travel only short distances through the air, requiring close contact for transmission. Indirect contact by touching virus-contaminated objects and then touching one's mucous

Table 47.1 Risk Factors for Serious Complications From Influenza Virus Infection

HEALTH RISK FACTORS

Asthma
Neurologic and neurodevelopment conditions
Blood disorders, such as sickle cell disease
Chronic lung disease, such as COPD and cystic fibrosis
Endocrine disorders, such as diabetes mellitus
Heart disease, such as congenital heart disease, congestive heart failure, and coronary artery disease
Kidney disorders
Liver disorders
Metabolic disorders, such as inherited metabolic disorders and mitochondrial disorders
Obesity with a body mass index of ≥40
Age <19 years on long-term aspirin- or salicylate-containing medications
A weakened immune system due to disease, such as people with HIV or AIDS, or some cancers, such as leukemia; taking medications, such as those receiving chemotherapy or radiation treatment for cancer; or persons with chronic conditions requiring chronic corticosteroids or other drugs that suppress the immune system

OTHER HIGH-RISK GROUPS

Adults ≥65 years
Children <2 years
Pregnant women and women up to 2 weeks after the end of pregnancy
Native Americans, including Alaska Natives
People who live in nursing homes and other long-term care facilities

AIDS, acquired immunodeficiency syndrome; HIV, human immunodeficiency virus.
Courtesy Centers for Disease Control and Prevention. People at high risk for flu complications; 2018. https://www.cdc.gov/flu/highrisk/index.htm.

membranes can also transmit influenza. The contribution of transmission by aerosol, a suspension of fine particles, to the overall influenza burden is uncertain, although it is likely low.[36] However, airborne precautions should be used during aerosol-generating procedures.

Influenza is moderately transmissible from person to person. The number of secondary cases produced by a single infection in a susceptible person has been estimated from contact tracing in outbreak investigations. On average, each person with seasonal influenza transmits the virus to one to two persons causing influenza illness,[37] although transmission depends on multiple viral, host, and environmental factors.[38]

Preventing transmission of influenza virus in health care settings requires multipronged strategies. The CDC core prevention strategies include (1) administration of annual seasonal influenza vaccine to all health care workers exposed to patients, (2) implementation of appropriate respiratory hygiene and cough etiquette to minimize potential exposures, (3) monitoring and management of ill health care workers to prevent or control nosocomial transmission, (4) adherence to standard and droplet precautions for all patient-care activities and respiratory precautions for aerosol- and droplet-generating procedures, and (5) environmental and engineering infection control measures.[39]

PATHOGENESIS

The incubation period from exposure to clinical illness is typically 2 to 3 days.[40] Virus shedding is maximal at the onset of illness and may continue for 5 to 7 days or longer in children.[41,42] Viral shedding precedes symptoms by 12 to 24 hours, although the viral load is typically low during this presymptomatic period.[41] In immunocompromised patients, especially recipients of solid-organ or hematopoietic stem-cell transplants, viral shedding can be prolonged for weeks to months.[24]

Influenza A viruses primarily infect epithelial cells of the airways.[43,44] The viral HA recognizes host cell glycoprotein and glycolipid sialic acid (also termed *neuraminic acid*) residues coupled to galactose by either α-2,3 or α-2,6 linkages. Human influenza virus strains preferentially bind α-2,6–linked sialic acid, which predominates in the upper respiratory tract but can also be found in the lower respiratory tract at lower abundance.[43] The human lower respiratory tract epithelium predominantly expresses α-2,3–linked sialic acid, in common with epithelial cells of birds, the natural reservoirs for most influenza viruses.[43] Animal influenza viruses that gain the ability to bind α-2,6–linked sialic acid can more efficiently be transmitted from human to human.[43] Viral attachment induces endocytosis, followed by acidification of the endosomes and a pH-dependent conformational change of the HA that enables fusion of the viral envelope with the endosome membrane and release of viral RNA into the cell cytoplasm for viral replication. The infection cycle is completed by NA-dependent release of new viral particles from the infected cells, allowing spread to neighboring cells for additional cycles of viral replication and amplification.[43] The influenza viral load in respiratory tract specimens generally correlates with levels of inflammatory mediators and with the severity of clinical illness. Mild influenza illness predominantly involves the upper respiratory tract and trachea, whereas severe influenza illness often involves the lower respiratory tract.[44]

Histologic changes due to influenza are nonspecific. Multifocal destruction and desquamation of the pseudostratified columnar epithelium of the upper respiratory tract and large airways are characteristic and can be found early in influenza illness.[44] Submucosal edema and congestion may be pronounced.[44,45] Influenza virus infection induces production of proinflammatory cytokines, including interleukin (IL)-1β, tumor necrosis factor, and IL-6, which activate epithelial and endothelial cells and increase their adhesion properties and permeability. Influenza virus also leads to production of CC motif chemokine ligand-2 and IL-8, which recruit monocytes and neutrophils, respectively.[45] Severe influenza pneumonia exhibits diffuse alveolar damage with hyaline membranes lining the alveoli; the alveolar air spaces contain edema fluid, strands of fibrin, desquamated epithelial cells, and inflammatory cells. The inflammatory state of influenza virus infection can activate inflammatory cells in atherosclerotic plaques and induce expression of genes linked to platelet activation, increasing the risk of influenza-associated myocardial infarction.[46] The pathophysiologic consequences of the respiratory tract damage and endothelial inflammation can persist after viral clearance and clinical resolution of the infection.[47,48]

Bronchoscopy of individuals with influenza may reveal diffuse inflammation of the larynx, trachea, and bronchi, as well as a range of histologic findings in biopsy samples, from vacuolization of columnar cells with cell loss to extensive desquamation of the ciliated columnar epithelium down to the basal layer of cells.[49–51] In influenza pneumonia, the tissue response becomes more prominent as one moves distally in the airway. Recovery is associated with rapid regeneration of the epithelial cell layer and pseudometaplasia.

Abnormal pulmonary function can be found in otherwise healthy, nonasthmatic young adults with uncomplicated influenza. Defects include diminished forced expiratory flow rates, increased total pulmonary resistance, and decreased forced expiratory flow rates consistent with generalized increased resistance in airways less than 2 mm in diameter[52,53] and increased responses to bronchoprovocation.[53] Abnormalities have also been found in the carbon monoxide diffusing capacity and the alveolar-arterial oxygen tension difference. Pulmonary function defects can persist for weeks after clinical recovery. Influenza in patients with asthma or COPD may result in acute declines in forced vital capacity and/or forced expiratory volume in 1 second. Individuals with acute influenza may be more susceptible to bronchoconstriction from air pollutants, such as nitrates,[52–54] or to bronchoprovocation.[53,55,56]

COPATHOGENESIS OF INFLUENZA WITH BACTERIA

The association between influenza and bacterial pneumonia is a well-established phenomenon, with recognition dating back to the 1918 pandemic, when most of the deaths likely resulted from secondary bacterial pneumonia.[57–59] Bacterial pneumonia is associated with contemporary pandemics and with seasonal influenza but is thought to cause less excess mortality than in the 1918 pandemic. Nonetheless, one-quarter to one-half of severely ill patients with 2009 A/H1N1pdm influenza had bacterial infections.[60–64] There is evidence that the incidence of secondary bacterial infection in critically ill patients with influenza is increasing, and that there is greater morbidity associated with secondary bacterial infection.[65,66]

The most common etiology of secondary infection is *Streptococcus pneumoniae*, but *Staphylococcus aureus* (including *methicillin-resistant S. aureus* [MRSA]) has become increasingly common, and *Streptococcus pyogenes* has also been reported.[61,67–74] Increasing age and immunosuppression may be risk factors for influenza-associated bacterial pneumonia.[65]

Animal models have shown that influenza virus infection enhances susceptibility to bacterial pneumonia.[69] The peak window of susceptibility is 1 to 2 weeks after influenza virus infection, although viral effects increasing susceptibility may persist for weeks to months.[75–78] The mechanisms leading to secondary bacterial pneumonia are complex. Influenza virus infection results in the compromise of natural physiologic barriers, such as the respiratory epithelium, with resulting exposure of attachment sites for invading bacteria; decreased mechanical clearance of bacteria due to impaired ciliary function; impairment in phagocyte, lymphocyte, and antimicrobial peptide function; depletion of alveolar macrophages; and reduced pathogen pattern recognition receptor sensing.[68,69,75] Interferons induced by influenza virus appear to be particularly important in

suppressing the host response to invading bacteria.[68,75] Influenza NA also releases free sialic acid, which can serve as a carbon source to promote growth of *S. pneumoniae*,[79] and there is evidence that influenza viruses can bind directly to *S. pneumoniae* or to *S. aureus* to promote bacterial binding to host epithelial cells.[80]

Susceptibility to pathogens after influenza virus infection may not be limited to bacteria because there have been several reports of influenza-associated pulmonary aspergillosis in severely ill patients.[81–86] Influenza-associated pulmonary aspergillosis has been found in both immunocompetent and immunocompromised patients, but at higher rates in the latter. One retrospective, multicenter cohort study found that 19% of adult influenza patients with acute respiratory failure admitted to the *intensive care unit* (ICU) had invasive pulmonary aspergillosis; the mortality rate exceeded 50%.[83] These studies suggest that influenza may be an independent risk factor for invasive pulmonary aspergillosis.

VACCINES

Two classes of influenza vaccines are currently available: IIVs and *live-attenuated influenza vaccines* (LAIVs). IIVs induce antibodies to the influenza virus HA glycoprotein as their primary mechanism of action.[5,18] They differ by production system (chicken eggs, cultured mammalian cells, or recombinant protein synthesized in cultured insect cells), manufacturing process, presence of adjuvants, dose and valence (number of strains), and age groups for which their use is approved (Table 47.2).[4,17] Recombinant vaccines, typically categorized with IIVs but more accurately called *nonreplicating influenza vaccines*, contain influenza antigens produced in noninfluenza virus systems but protect by the same mechanism of action as IIVs. Recombinant vaccines may be produced more rapidly than those produced in chicken eggs after identification of a new circulating virus type.

The major LAIV in use globally, FluMist (Fluenz in Europe), is licensed in the United States for use in persons 2 to 49 years of age. LAIVs were developed to mimic natural infection more closely by stimulating a broader immune response, resulting in more durable immunity than IIVs.[5] LAIVs are cold adapted so that they replicate optimally in nasal mucosa and are less able to replicate in the (warmer) lower respiratory tract. Early clinical trials found greater efficacy of LAIVs compared to IIVs in children, but subsequent observational vaccine effectiveness studies have not shown this benefit.[87] The presence of an underlying medical condition that can put people at higher risk of severe influenza complications (see Table 47.1) is considered a precaution to vaccination with LAIVs.[88]

In the United States, all persons age 6 months and older are recommended to receive annual influenza vaccination; no one vaccine product is currently prioritized for use.[4] However influenza vaccine policies differ among countries. Those with national influenza vaccine programs typically prioritize specific risk groups and may even prioritize certain vaccine products.[89] For example, the United Kingdom prioritizes LAIVs for children and adjuvanted or high-dose IIVs for older adults.[89,90]

Table 47.2 Influenza Vaccines: United States, 2019–20 Influenza Season

Trade Name	Age Indication	Antigen Amount per Vaccine Dose (HA Concentration in IIVs and RIV4) or Virus Count (LAIV4) (Each Vaccine Virus)	Production System	Adjuvant	Route
QUADRIVALENT* IIV (IIV4): STANDARD DOSE, CONTAINS INACTIVATED VIRUS					
Afluria Quadrivalent	≥6 mo	7.5 µg/0.25 mL (for <3 years) 15 µg/0.5 mL (for ≥3 years)	Egg	No	IM
Fluarix Quadrivalent	≥6 mo	15 µg/0.5 mL	Egg	No	IM
Flulaval Quadrivalent	≥6 mo	15 µg/0.5 mL	Egg	No	IM
Fluzone Quadrivalent	≥6 mo	7.5 µg/0.25 mL (for <3 yr) 15 µg/0.5 mL (for any age)	Egg	No	IM
Flucelvax Quadrivalent	≥4 yr	15 µg/0.5 mL	Cell culture	No	IM
TRIVALENT† IIV3: HIGH DOSE, CONTAINS INACTIVATED VIRUS					
Fluzone High Dose‡	≥65 yr	60 µg/0.5 mL	Egg	No	IM
TRIVALENT† IIV3: ADJUVANTED, CONTAINS INACTIVATED VIRUS					
Fluad‡	≥65 yr	15 µg/0.5 mL	Egg	Yes (MF59)	IM
QUADRIVALENT* RIV (RIV4): CONTAINS RECOMBINANT HA					
Flublok Quadrivalent	≥18 yr	45 µg/0.5 mL	Recombinant	No	IM
QUADRIVALENT* LAIV (LAIV4): CONTAINS LIVE, ATTENUATED, COLD-ADAPTED VIRUS					
FluMist Quadrivalent	2–49 yr	$10^{6.5-7.5}$ fluorescent focus units/0.2 mL	Egg	No	NAS

*Contain antigens from four viral strains, two to three from influenza A and one to two from influenza B.
†Contain antigens from three viral strains, usually two influenza A and one influenza B.
‡Licensed for those ≥65 years.
HA, hemagglutinin; IIV, inactivated influenza vaccine; IM, intramuscular; LAIV, live-attenuated influenza vaccine; NAS, intranasal; RIV, recombinant influenza vaccine.
From Grohskopf LA, Alyanak E, Broder KR, et al. Prevention and control of seasonal influenza with vaccines: recommendations of the Advisory Committee on Immunization Practices—United States, 2019–20 influenza season. *MMWR Recomm Rep.* 2019;68:1–21.

Although there is evidence that effectiveness of IIVs decreases over the course of the influenza season, potentially due to waning humoral immunity and/or drifting circulating virus strains, public health officials generally do not recommend delaying influenza vaccination once vaccines become available. The poor ability of the available IIVs to induce long-lived immunologic memory has led to efforts to develop new formulations of influenza vaccines that generate more durable protection.[91] Efforts to develop so-called "universal" influenza vaccines based on generation of broadly-neutralizing antibodies that recognize influenza antigens that do not mutate at high frequencies have shown promising results in preclinical studies.[92]

The effectiveness of influenza vaccines depends on many different factors, including the degree of antigenic match between the vaccine and circulating viruses, product differences, the age of the individual being vaccinated, and the outcome being measured. The CDC reports all-age vaccine effectiveness against medically attended, laboratory-confirmed influenza illness has ranged from 10–60% in recent years.[93] Observational studies have shown influenza vaccine effectiveness among persons with high-risk conditions,[94–101] and influenza vaccines are effective at preventing clinically important outcomes, such as hospitalizations,[95–98] critical illness,[94–98,102] and death.[103,104] A 2015 systematic review and meta-analysis found that in *randomized controlled trials* (RCTs) of influenza vaccine among persons with cardiovascular disease, vaccination significantly decreased the risk of all-cause cardiovascular deaths by 55%.[105] Influenza vaccination also reduces the

severity of *breakthrough* disease (infections that develop despite vaccination with the appropriate strain), including decreased in-hospital death, ICU length of stay, and hospital length of stay.[103,104]

Even with suboptimal vaccine effectiveness, the number of severe illnesses averted by vaccination programs is substantial. During the unusually severe 2017–18 influenza season, there were an estimated 953,000 hospitalizations and 79,400 deaths associated with influenza in the United States.[106] Although the seasonal influenza vaccine was only 38% effective that year, an estimated 109,000 hospitalizations and 8000 deaths were still averted by vaccination, mostly among persons age 50 years and older.[106]

Despite public health recommendations that all persons receive annual influenza vaccination, vaccine coverage remains suboptimal, particularly among groups at the highest risk of severe influenza complications (see Table 47.1). In the United States during 2012, only 45% of adults aged 18 to 64 years with at least one high-risk condition received the influenza vaccine, and coverage ranged from 44–53% among those with pulmonary diseases, diabetes, heart disease, and cancer.[107,108] White adults have about 10% greater influenza vaccine coverage than African Americans or Hispanics.[109] Behavioral studies have found that more adults would accept the influenza vaccine if it were recommended by a health care provider, if there were more opportunities for vaccination, and if systems were in place that bypassed the health care provider to determine patient vaccination status and to offer vaccination routinely.[110,111]

PATIENT MANAGEMENT

CLINICAL PRESENTATION

Influenza often presents with the sudden onset of symptoms, commonly fever, cough, and sore throat. Other symptoms associated with acute influenza illness include arthralgia, chest tightness, chills, conjunctivitis, nasal congestion, sinus congestion, coryza, decreased appetite, diarrhea, dry cough, dyspnea, fatigue/tiredness, headache, myalgia, nausea, rhinorrhea, and sweats.[112] No combination of clinical signs and symptoms is sufficiently predictive of influenza illness, necessitating laboratory testing to confirm influenza virus infection. Furthermore, research using highly sensitive and specific diagnostic tests has demonstrated great variability in presenting signs and symptoms among persons with influenza virus infection. In particular, very young, older, and immunocompromised patients may present with atypical symptoms, and hospital surveillance studies have shown that about 40% of hospitalized adults with confirmed influenza do not have a fever.[113] Contact testing in influenza outbreaks and controlled human infections with influenza have demonstrated that subclinical influenza virus infection can be common.[114]

The clinical practice guidelines prepared by the *Infectious Diseases Society of America* (IDSA) recommend that decisions to test patients for influenza should rely on consideration of the broader clinical and epidemiologic context, including the risk of patient exposure to circulating influenza,

the presence of high-risk conditions, the likelihood that antiviral treatment would be provided if there were a positive result, and whether a positive result would reduce the use of unnecessary antibacterial medicines.[34] An influenza testing algorithm adapted from the IDSA Clinical Practice Guidelines is shown in Fig. 47.2. This algorithm applies during periods of known influenza circulation. Although the risk of influenza illness substantially decreases outside of the traditional influenza season, summertime outbreaks and travel-related infections are observed.[115–117] The presence of sick contacts and travel-related exposures should be assessed when patients with influenza-like illness present outside of the usual influenza season. The differential diagnosis for influenza-like illness is broad, including other respiratory viruses, such as adenovirus, respiratory syncytial virus, metapneumovirus, coronavirus, rhinovirus, and parainfluenza virus; bacterial upper and lower respiratory tract infections; and systemic infections such as malaria. Therefore clinicians should also consider host factors, such as presence of high-risk conditions (see Table 47.1) or recent exposure to health care facilities and travel history or place of residence that may affect susceptibility or exposure to different pathogens, and should be prepared to treat sick patients presumptively for infection broadly and early as the diagnostic evaluation proceeds. The influenza vaccination status of the patient should not be considered when making testing decisions because vaccine failures are common.[93]

Not all hospitalized patients with influenza present with primary respiratory processes. Modeling studies

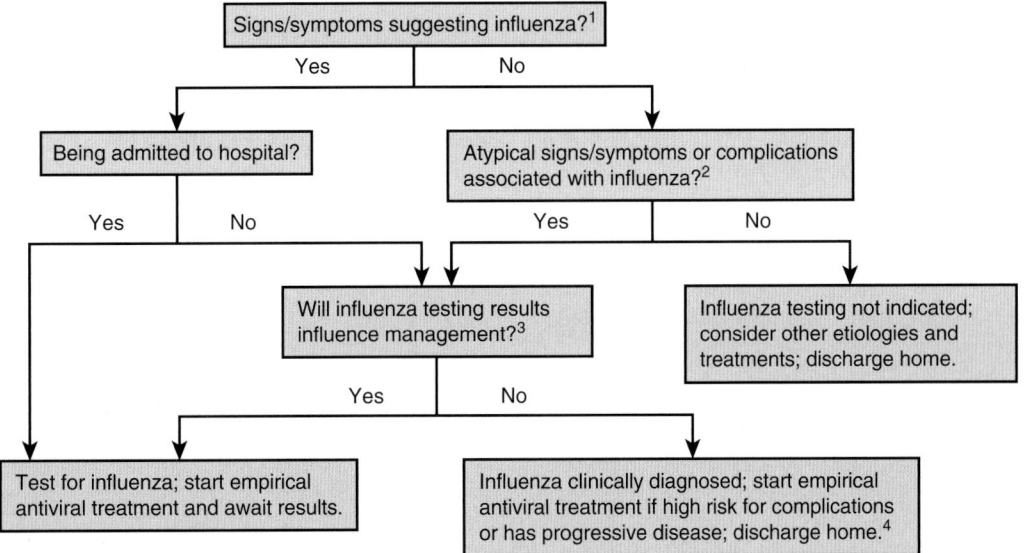

Figure 47.2 Algorithm for considering influenza testing during periods of known influenza circulation. *1,* Signs and symptoms may include fever with cough or other suggestive respiratory symptoms, often with myalgias or headache. Note that some individuals, especially older adults, infants, and immunocompromised, may have atypical presentations, including a lack of fever. *2,* Atypical signs and symptoms may include unexplained fever only or lack of fever with any respiratory symptoms, especially in immunocompromised or high-risk patients. Complications associated with influenza include pneumonia or exacerbation of chronic conditions, such as asthma, COPD, or heart failure. *3,* Influenza testing may be used to guide decisions on use of antibiotics or continuation of antiviral medication, on need for further diagnostic tests, on consideration for home care, or on recommendations for ill persons living with others who are at high risk for influenza complications. Influenza testing may be required to guide decisions on infection control practices. *4,* Antiviral treatment is recommended for outpatients with suspected influenza who are at high risk for complications from influenza or those with progressive disease not requiring hospital admission. Antiviral treatment of outpatients who are not at high risk for influenza complications can be considered based upon clinical judgment if presenting within 2 days of illness onset. (Modified from Uyeki TM, Bernstein HH, Bradley JS, et al. Clinical practice guidelines by the Infectious Diseases Society of America: 2018 update on diagnosis, treatment, chemoprophylaxis, and institutional outbreak management of seasonal influenza. *Clin Infect Dis.* 2019;68:895–902.)

suggest that one-third of hospitalized influenza cases may not have pneumonia but rather primary circulatory diagnoses, such as septic shock.[29] Influenza can exacerbate underlying conditions such as chronic lung disease or diabetes, or cause extrapulmonary complications, including encephalitis or myocarditis.[47,48] Influenza-triggered cardiovascular events, including myocardial infarction, heart failure, arrhythmias, and strokes, are increasingly recognized.[46,118,119] Patients presenting with symptoms suggestive of influenza should be evaluated to ensure identification of physiologic derangements such as hypoxemia, respiratory compromise, or hemodynamic instability.

DIAGNOSTIC TESTING

The definitive diagnosis of influenza requires laboratory testing. When influenza virus is circulating in the community, patients with influenza-like illness, pneumonia, or other nonspecific respiratory illness should be tested because these data will affect treatment, postexposure prophylaxis of close contacts, and infection control measures.

Specimens

Respiratory tract sampling is the optimal approach to influenza detection. For most patients, upper respiratory tract sampling is appropriate, preferably a nasopharyngeal swab. If nasopharyngeal specimens cannot be obtained, midturbinate nasal or combined nasal-throat swabs are acceptable. For patients with influenza-like illness undergoing mechanical ventilation, endotracheal aspirates should be obtained in parallel.[66,120–123] Invasive collection of respiratory specimens, such as by bronchoalveolar lavage, solely for the purpose of influenza testing is not recommended; however, such testing can be performed on these samples collected for other reasons.[124,125] Although viremia and detection of virus in other organs have been observed in severe influenza, there is no role for sampling of sites other than the respiratory tract in clinical practice.[126–128]

Rapid Antigen Detection Tests

Rapid antigen detection tests can be performed within 15 minutes and have low to moderate sensitivity but high specificity.[129–131] Use of these tests is not recommended if more sensitive, rapid molecular tests are available.

Immunofluorescence Assay

Immunofluorescence assay tests may be direct or indirect. They take 1 to 4 hours and have moderate sensitivity but high specificity.[132] Use of these tests is not recommended if more sensitive, rapid molecular tests are available.

Molecular Diagnostics

Molecular tests for influenza include *reverse-transcription polymerase chain reaction* (RT-PCR) and other nucleic acid amplification tests (see Chapter 19). Some rapid molecular tests can be performed within 30 minutes. All molecular tests are highly sensitive and specific.[130] Molecular tests may also indicate the subtype of influenza virus and can be combined in multiplex assays to detect other viruses. RT-PCR-based tests are the preferred diagnostic method for clinical decision making.[34]

Culture

Culture of virus takes several days but is sensitive and specific.[133] Unlike molecular diagnostics, only infectious (live) virus will be detected. Although culture is not recommended for routine use, this method has the advantage of furnishing virus for additional testing such as subtyping, antigenic identification, and antiviral drug susceptibility analyses.

Serology

Serologic diagnosis of influenza virus infection by HAI requires paired—acute and convalescent—sera tested at least 2 weeks apart demonstrating a fourfold or greater increase in antibody titer.[134] Serology cannot, therefore, be used for the timely diagnosis of influenza but may have a role for retrospective diagnosis or serologic epidemiology studies.

Summary

The IDSA Clinical Practice Guidelines recommend molecular influenza assays for testing outpatient and hospitalized patient specimens due to the high sensitivity and specificity, as well as the speed of these tests.[34] In hospitalized patients, the use of multiplex RT-PCR assays that identify a variety of respiratory pathogens should be considered; these multiplex assays are recommended in immunocompromised patients.[34]

RADIOGRAPHIC FINDINGS

The clinical manifestations of influenza virus infection may vary greatly and include severe influenza pneumonia and secondary bacterial pneumonia. Patients with clinical features suggesting pneumonia, such as dyspnea, hypoxemia, or hemodynamic instability, should undergo chest imaging. Radiographic findings in influenza pneumonia tend to be nonspecific in both immunocompetent and immunocompromised patients.[135,136] Chest radiographs may show bilateral abnormalities suggestive of pulmonary edema or multifocal pneumonia (Fig. 47.3 and eFig. 47.1), although unilateral consolidation is also reported.[135,137] Chest computed tomography scans in influenza pneumonia commonly demonstrate multifocal areas of ground-glass opacity and consolidation[138] (Fig. 47.4 and eFig. 47.2), although widely different patterns can be present (Fig. 47.5). Pleural effusions are uncommon. Point-of-care lung ultrasound may reveal evidence of interstitial syndrome, that is, the presence of B lines or lung consolidation.[139,140] Differentiating primary influenza pneumonia from influenza-associated bacterial pneumonia using chest imaging is difficult, although the presence of necrotizing pneumonia with cavitation or evidence of empyema suggest a bacterial etiology (eFig. 47.3).

ANTIVIRAL THERAPIES

Three classes of antiviral agents are currently approved in the United States for treatment and/or prevention of influenza: adamantanes (e.g., amantadine and rimantadine), which target the M2 ion channel protein of influenza A viruses; NAIs (e.g., oseltamivir, zanamivir, and

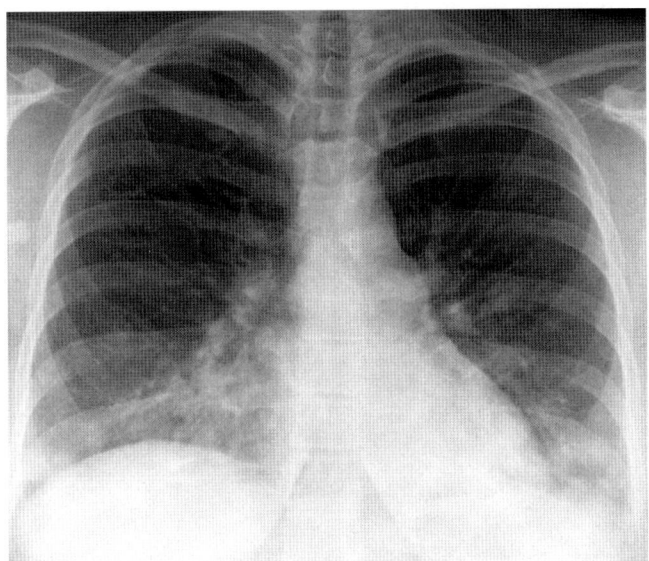

Figure 47.3 Influenza A virus infection. Frontal chest radiograph shows multifocal, bilateral, perihilar, and lower lobe predominant bronchovascular thickening and somewhat nodular consolidation. (Courtesy Michael B. Gotway, MD.)

peramivir), which block the viral NA enzyme of influenza A and B viruses; and the cap-dependent endonuclease inhibitor (baloxavir), which interferes with viral RNA transcription and viral replication in both influenza A and B viruses. Outside the United States three additional antiviral agents are available: laninamivir, an inhaled NAI; arbidol, an oral drug that interacts with HA to prevent membrane fusion; and favipiravir, an oral inhibitor of viral RNA-dependent RNA polymerase.[8]

Adamantanes

The M2 protein, the target of adamantanes, is located in the viral envelope, where it functions as a proton channel and is essential for viral entry into the host cell cytoplasm, where viral replication takes place. The M2-inhibiting adamantanes specifically block the ion channel function of the influenza A M2 protein and are not active against influenza B viruses. Resistance to these drugs emerges readily in treated individuals, particularly children, and there may be prolonged shedding of resistant viruses in immunocompromised patients.[141,142] For reasons that remain unclear, the first decade of this century has seen the emergence and spread of adamantane-resistant influenza A/H3N2 viruses;

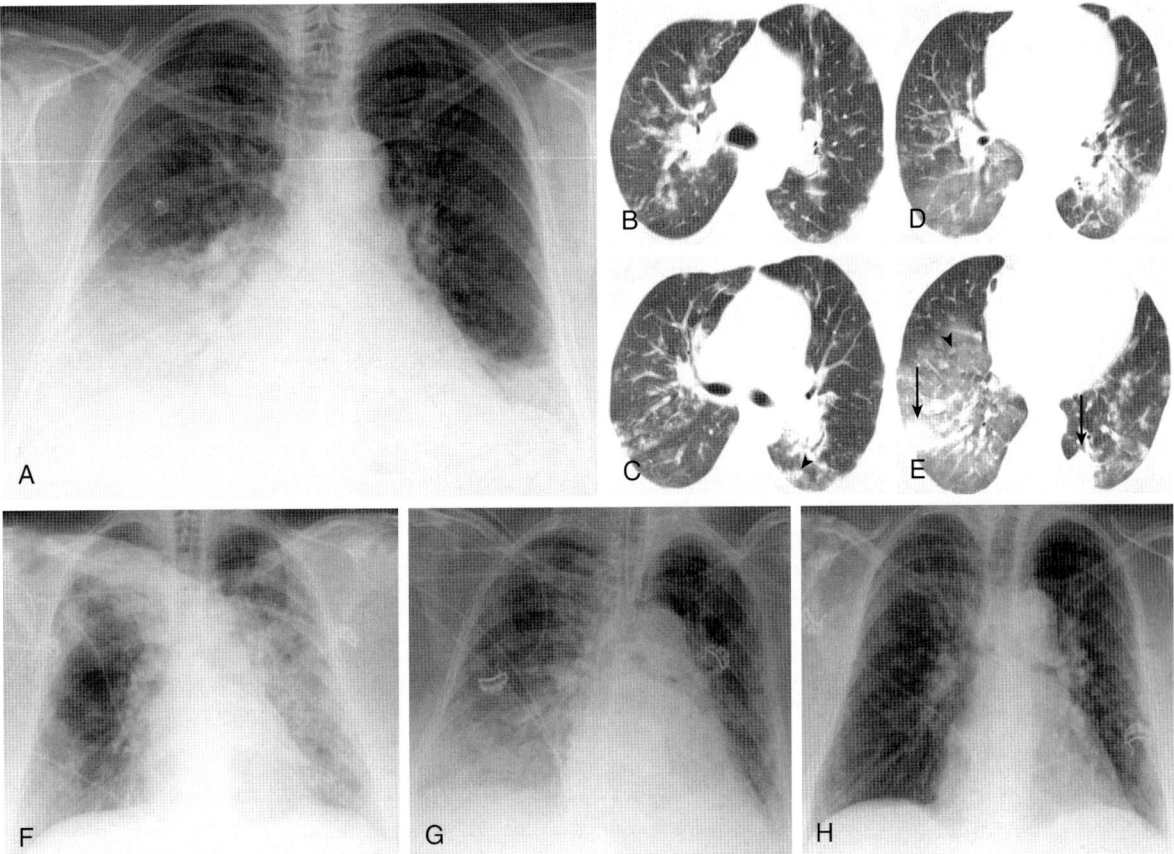

Figure 47.4 Influenza A/H1N1pdm virus infection: imaging findings. (A) Frontal chest radiograph in a patient subsequently diagnosed with A/H1N1pdm influenza during the 2009 pandemic shows multifocal basal predominant consolidation, consistent with bronchopneumonia but nonspecific. (B–E) Axial chest computed tomography displayed in lung windows shows nonspecific bilateral areas of ground-glass opacity, nodular subpleural consolidation (*arrows*), and other foci of patchy, peripheral, increased lung attenuation, and small nodules (*arrowheads*), some of which appear centrilobular. (F–H) Serial frontal chest radiographs obtained during the course of the disease show worsening of bilateral opacities associated with hypoxemic respiratory failure (F and G) but subsequent clearing of bilateral lung opacity after recovery (H). (Courtesy Michael B. Gotway, MD.)

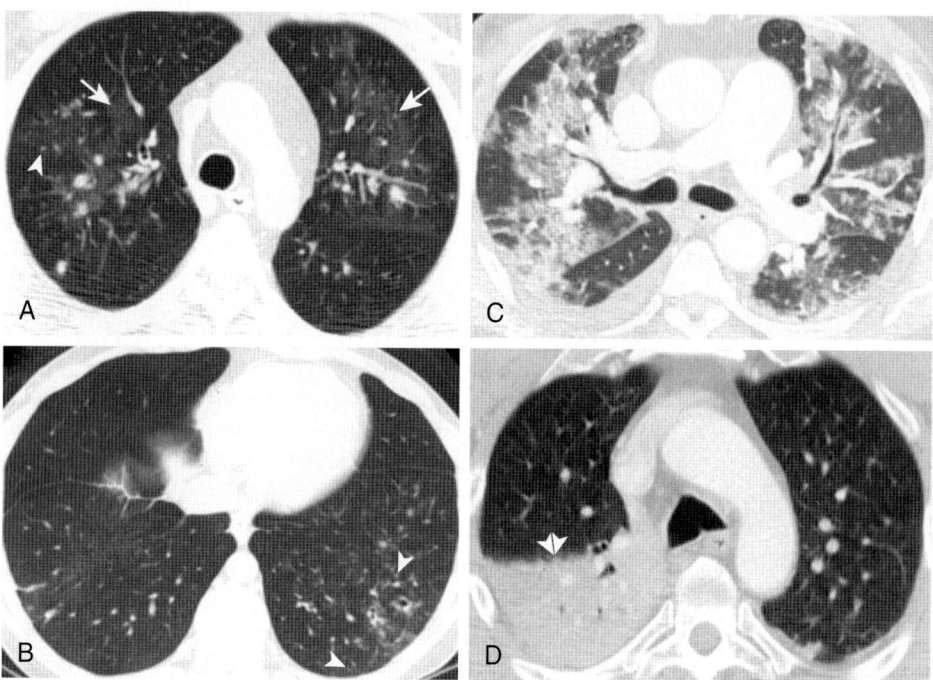

Figure 47.5 Influenza A/H1N1pdm virus infection in four different patients: strikingly different imaging findings at chest *computed tomography* **(CT).** (A–B) Axial chest CT displayed in lung windows shows patchy areas of upper lobe predominant ground-glass opacity *(arrows)* and small, solid, centrilobular nodules *(arrowheads)*. The opacity in the left lower lobe (B) appears somewhat segmental, suggestive of bronchopneumonia. (C) Axial chest CT shows multifocal, bilateral areas of ground-glass opacity associated with interlobular septal thickening and intralobular interstitial thickening but no clear zonal distribution; these findings are nonspecific and can be observed with numerous infections and noninfectious inflammatory pulmonary insults. (D) Axial chest CT shows right lower lobe superior segmental dense consolidation *(double arrowhead)*, suggestive of a lobar pneumonia pattern. (Courtesy Michael B. Gotway, MD.)

A/H1N1pdm viruses are also uniformly resistant.[143] Therefore the adamantane M2 inhibitor drugs do not have utility against current influenza viruses and are not presently recommended for use. They may have a role if susceptible strains emerge in the future.

Neuraminidase Inhibitors

NAIs are potent inhibitors of influenza virus in vitro and in vivo because NA activity is essential for viral release from infected cells, a necessary step for viral spread to other cells. Influenza B viruses are less sensitive to NAIs than influenza A viruses but are susceptible at clinically achievable concentrations. Oseltamivir phosphate is an orally bioavailable ethyl ester prodrug rapidly absorbed from the gastrointestinal tract and metabolized by hepatic esterases to the active metabolite, oseltamivir carboxylate. The metabolite is excreted unchanged in the urine by tubular secretion, with a serum half-life of 6 to 10 hours. The major adverse effects of oseltamivir are nausea and vomiting.[144,145] Oseltamivir is approved for treatment of adults and children and for prophylaxis in adults and children at least 3 months of age. Zanamivir is not orally bioavailable and is administered as a dry powder for inhalation. After inhalation, zanamivir concentrates in the respiratory tract, and systemic absorption is low.[146] Inhaled zanamivir may be associated with bronchospasm, particularly in those with underlying airways disease; this acute bronchospasm has sometimes been severe and has resulted in a recommendation that inhaled zanamivir not be given to patients with respiratory disease, such as asthma or COPD.[147] Zanamivir is approved for treatment of adults and children at least 7 years of age and

for prophylaxis in adults and children at least 5 years of age. Peramivir is the most recent NAI to become available in the United States, having been approved in 2014 for single-dose *intravenous* (IV) administration. Peramivir binds with greater affinity than oseltamivir to NA and has a half-life of 20 hours with renal clearance.[148] Peramivir is approved for the treatment of influenza in adults and children age at least 2 years of age but is not recommended for prophylaxis. All three NAIs are associated with risks of serious skin reactions and sporadic, transient neuropsychiatric events, mostly in children.

Cap-Dependent Endonuclease Inhibitor

Baloxavir marboxil is the newest antiviral agent available for use in the United States. Baloxavir marboxil is an oral prodrug of baloxavir acid that is a selective inhibitor of influenza cap-dependent endonuclease, thus preventing initiation of viral messenger RNA synthesis.[149] A phase III RCT found a significant reduction in time to alleviation of symptoms from 80.2 hours for individuals treated with placebo versus 53.7 hours for individuals treated with a single dose of baloxavir.[150] This was similar to oseltamivir. In addition, viral loads at 1 day were lower in patients treated with baloxavir compared to either placebo or oseltamivir.[150] To date, few adverse events have been associated with baloxavir.[151]

ANTIVIRAL RESISTANCE

The high mutation rate of influenza RNA polymerase can alter susceptibility to antiviral agents.[152,153] Although resistance to adamantanes is widespread, as of 2019, resistance to NAIs in circulating influenza viruses is uncommon.[143,154] For example, surveillance data through 2018 indicated that among seasonal influenza viruses, the frequency of oseltamivir resistance was less than 3.5%, and zanamivir resistance was less than 1%.[154] However, the emergence of resistance among seasonal influenza viruses has been observed, as for an H1N1 A/Brisbane/59/2007–like virus with a single amino-acid substitution that impaired oseltamivir binding. This strain rapidly became the predominant circulating strain globally, although it was subsequently replaced by the oseltamivir-sensitive A/H1N1pdm virus.[152] Therefore reemergence of influenza NAI resistance remains of great concern. Testing for resistance may be considered in patients who develop influenza while receiving prophylaxis with an NAI, in those who are immunocompromised, in those who have severe illness and continue to have evidence of viral replication or lack of improvement, and in those who received subtherapeutic treatment with NAIs with severe disease and evidence of viral replication.[34] In phase II and III trials of baloxavir, the emergence of viruses with mutations of the polymerase acidic protein (PA/I38X) was noted in 2.2–9.7% of baloxavir-treated patients.[150,153] These variant viruses were associated with increased infectious virus titers, prolonged shedding, delay in symptom alleviation, and symptom rebound.[153]

ANTIVIRAL TREATMENT DECISIONS

The efficacy of antiviral treatment depends on several factors, including the host's age, immune status and medical comorbidities, the virus type or subtype, and the timing of treatment initiation relative to the course of infection.[144,155–166] Several RCTs conducted primarily in outpatients indicate that NAIs, administered within 36 to 48 hours of illness onset, reduce the duration of fever and symptoms by 1 to 2 days.[157–159,167–170] Starting treatment within 6 hours of illness reduced symptoms by about 4 days.[164,171,172] Moreover, NAI treatment may decrease other complications, such as otitis media in children or need for antibiotic treatment for lower respiratory infection and hospitalization in adults.[144,145,173] A large individual patient-level meta-analysis of high-risk outpatients showed that NAI treatment reduced the likelihood of hospital admission.[174] There are limited RCT data of antiviral therapy in hospitalized patients to guide management of severe influenza. However, observational studies, individual patient-level meta-analyses, and meta-analyses suggest a clinical benefit of NAIs in hospitalized patients, even when therapy is delayed, although this may not include improvement in survival.[144,155–157,160,165,166,175–180] The CDC notes that prompt treatment with antivirals reduces the duration of symptoms and risk of some complications and may decrease mortality in high-risk groups,[181] and therefore clinical practice guidelines recommend the treatment of high-risk outpatients (see Table 47.1) and severely ill or hospitalized patients.[34] Treatment should be considered for symptomatic individuals who do not meet these criteria but who have been ill for less than 2 days or who are close contacts, including health care providers, of individuals at risk of complications from influenza, to prevent transmission to the latter. In these circumstances the CDC recommends initiating treatment for suspected influenza without awaiting laboratory confirmation.[151]

For nonhospitalized patients with uncomplicated influenza, any of the three NAIs (oral oseltamivir, inhaled zanamivir for 5 days, or a single dose of IV peramivir) or baloxavir is suggested. However, the CDC recommends prescribing oseltamivir for patients with severe, complicated, or progressive illness who are not hospitalized. For hospitalized patients, oseltamivir is the recommended NAI because there are limited or no data about the efficacy of inhaled zanamivir, IV peramivir, or oral baloxavir in patients with severe influenza. Oseltamivir is also preferred for pregnant women, and NAIs are generally considered safe in pregnancy.[151]

Clinicians should refer to clinical practice guidelines for further advice regarding influenza chemoprophylaxis and for further information regarding influenza diagnosis and treatment, particularly in special circumstances.[34,39,151]

PATIENTS WITH PNEUMONIA

Patients with influenza and radiographic evidence of pneumonia may have primary influenza pneumonia or bacterial pneumonia. Bacterial cultures of respiratory tract specimens and blood, and urinary antigen testing, should therefore be performed according to American Thoracic Society/ISDA guidelines.[182,183] Until the etiology of pneumonia is confirmed, empirical therapy for community-acquired or hospital-acquired pathogens should be administered as dictated by the patient's recent history of potential exposure to resistant pathogens.[182,183] In particular, antibiotics to cover common influenza-associated bacterial pathogens, especially *S. pneumoniae* and *S. aureus*, should be administered promptly. Due to the association of community-acquired MRSA pneumonia with influenza, severely ill patients should be given antibiotics active against MRSA.[34] Antibacterial treatment should be continued until bacterial infection is ruled out or adequately treated. Although several studies have evaluated the use of serum procalcitonin measurements to discriminate bacterial infection associated with influenza, a clear role for procalcitonin measurements in management of influenza patients has yet to be defined.[184,185]

CRITICALLY ILL PATIENTS

Seasonal influenza causes a substantial burden of disease worldwide.[3] As evidenced by the 2009 pandemic, influenza pandemics also place tremendous demands on critical care resources.[186–189] A 2019 review reported that among patients with influenza admitted to the ICU, A/H1N1pdm was the most common strain identified. Influenza pneumonia was present in 70%, secondary bacterial infection in 20%, and mortality associated with acute respiratory failure was 20%.[190] To reduce the risk of death, critically ill patients with suspected or diagnosed influenza illness should be given NAI therapy, preferably oseltamivir, without delay, even if symptoms have been present longer than 48 hours.[156] Appropriate concurrent antimicrobial coverage for bacterial respiratory pathogens is imperative. Oseltamivir administered via the enteral route yields adequate serum levels.[191] There does not appear to be a benefit of higher-dose oseltamivir.[192] The dose of oseltamivir should be reduced in patients receiving continuous renal replacement therapy but does not need adjustment during extracorporeal life support.[193–195] Zanamivir has a limited role in treatment of critically ill patients because the inhaler device is difficult to use effectively in individuals not breathing spontaneously and because the lactose powder formulation of zanamivir may cause ventilator filter obstruction in patients receiving mechanical ventilation.[196,197] Few studies guide the appropriate use of IV peramivir and, despite one study showing no benefit from peramivir in hospitalized patients, it remains an option if enteral administration of oseltamivir is not possible.[198] The optimal duration of antiviral therapy in critically ill patients with influenza is not known. Due to concern for prolonged viral replication and shedding in critically ill patients, longer courses of antiviral therapy may be considered.[121,199] In these cases repeat virologic testing may help guide therapy. Baloxavir has not been studied in severe illness, and combined antiviral therapy is not recommended.[34]

Clinicians should also be aware of the increased risk of myocardial infarction in the setting of influenza virus infection, and abnormal troponin levels should prompt further investigation of this possibility.[46] Among patients with influenza who have clinical indications for statins and aspirin, the medications should be continued or may be initiated if no contraindications are present.[46]

The inflammatory response induced by influenza, with or without secondary bacterial infection, can result in sepsis and multiorgan failure. Influenza-associated respiratory failure and *acute respiratory distress syndrome* (ARDS) are predominantly caused by influenza A viruses and are associated with high mortality.[60,200–204] Management of influenza-associated ARDS is similar to treatment of other etiologies of ARDS and should include lung protective ventilation and consideration of appropriate positive end-expiratory pressure, conservative fluid management, prone positioning, neuromuscular blockade, inhaled pulmonary vasodilators, and use of extracorporeal membrane oxygenation.[205,206]

OTHER THERAPIES

Corticosteroids are sometimes considered as adjunctive therapies of influenza because of studies suggesting possible benefit in sepsis and community-acquired pneumonia.[207,208] However, based on data from observational studies, corticosteroids may be associated with increased mortality.[166,209–217] This was confirmed by a recent Cochrane systematic review and meta-analysis, but the certainty of the evidence was very low due to concern about confounding by indication.[218] Corticosteroids are also associated with prolonged shedding, secondary infections, and development of antiviral resistance.[166,219–225] For these reasons, corticosteroids are not recommended for patients with severe influenza. However, corticosteroids should not be withheld if given for other indications, such as treatment of COPD exacerbation, refractory septic shock, or adrenal insufficiency.

Other therapies have been proposed to treat influenza, including passive immunotherapy with plasma or IV immunoglobulin, 3-hydroxy-3-methylglutaryl coenzyme A reductase inhibitors, and macrolide antibiotics.[179,226–229] There are insufficient data to recommend these therapies at present. Several additional therapeutics are currently being evaluated in preclinical or clinical

studies, including monoclonal antibodies to influenza proteins, and nitazoxanide, a thiazolide anti-infective that inhibits replication of influenza viruses by blocking maturation of HA.[230–234]

HUMAN INFECTION WITH NOVEL INFLUENZA VIRUSES

Numerous avian influenza A viruses have infected humans, including H5N1, H6N1, H7N2, H7N3, H7N7, H7N9, H9N2, H10N7, and H10N8 virus subtypes.[235] Avian influenza viruses are classified as *low pathogenic avian influenza* (LPAI) or *highly pathogenic avian influenza* (HPAI) on the basis of molecular and pathogenicity criteria in birds. The LPAI and HPAI classifications have no bearing on pathogenicity in humans. Clinical illness from human infection with avian influenza A viruses has ranged from asymptomatic infection to severe disease and death.[235] To date, none of these avian viruses has been able to sustain human-to-human transmission, but there is a risk that mutation or reassortment could allow the acquisition of this ability.[236] The CDC and the World Health Organization conduct routine risk assessments for the emergence of pandemic viruses, and two avian influenza viruses currently circulating in avian populations (A/H5N1 and A/H7N9) have caused human illness and are considered to have the greatest pandemic potential.[236]

A/H5N1

HPAI influenza A/H5N1 first emerged in wild birds in 1996 and was subsequently identified as the cause of a high-mortality outbreak in humans in Hong Kong in 1997. Since then, more than 800 human infections have been identified with Asian HPAI A/H5N1 viruses,[237] mostly in Southeast and East Asia, the Middle East, and Egypt. One case of human infection with A/H5N1 has been identified in the Americas in a traveler recently returned from China. As of 2019, A/H5N1 is enzootic in wild birds in six countries: Bangladesh, China, Egypt, India, Indonesia, and Vietnam.[238] Greater than 50% of human cases have been fatal. Transmission is thought to take place by inoculation of virus-contaminated poultry meat, blood, or feces on human mucous membranes. Risk factors for A/H5N1 infection in humans include close or direct contact with infected birds or infected sick contacts, visiting a live poultry market in endemic areas, or living in an area where A/H5N1 viruses are circulating among poultry.[238] Most patients with A/H5N1 virus infection present to the hospital with fever and features of lower respiratory tract infection. RT-PCR is the recommended diagnostic test; however, most clinical laboratories do not have the capacity to test specifically for A/H5N1, but they may identify influenza A virus that is unsubtypable, raising concerns of a novel influenza A virus infection and requiring confirmatory testing by a public health reference laboratory.[239] Oseltamivir, administered as early as possible, is the recommended antiviral treatment for suspected or confirmed A/H5N1 patients. Supportive care and specialized intensive care management are indicated for severe illness. Rapid implementation of infection control measures is recommended.[240]

A/H7N9

Asian lineage A/H7N9 is an avian influenza A virus that has caused five annual waves of high-mortality human epidemics focused in China since 2013.[241] Human infection is associated with exposure to infected poultry.[241] Until 2017, A/H7N9 from human and environmental samples was categorized as LPAI, with infections in birds causing only asymptomatic or mild illness.[242] Beginning in February 2017, a genetically similar HPAI A/H7N9 emerged in the same region, was found in environmental and bird samples, and has caused human illness.[242] Only sporadic cases were reported in 2018 and in early 2019.[240,241] The cumulative case-fatality of the detected cases is approximately 39%, with similar mortality seen with LPAI and HPAI infections in humans. Although limited cases of human-to-human transmission have been reported, there is no evidence of sustained transmission among persons.[240,241] As with A/H5N1, RT-PCR is the recommended diagnostic test for A/H7N9 cases, although, as with A/H5N1, most clinical laboratories may only detect it as influenza A virus that is unsubtypable, requiring confirmatory testing by specialty reference laboratories.[239] Oseltamivir therapy as early as possible, appropriate supportive therapies, and rapid implementation of infection control measures are recommended.[240]

Clinicians who suspect A/H5N1, A/H7N9, or other novel influenza viral illness should refer to public health recommendations for clinical guidance[240,243–246] and are encouraged to contact their local or state health department for further assistance.

Key Points

- Influenza is a high-burden disease. Persons at high risk of complications of influenza virus infection include children younger than 2 years; adults older than 65 years; pregnant women up to 2 weeks after the end of the pregnancy; people with certain underlying medical conditions, including obesity, kidney disease, heart disease, lung disease, and weakened immune systems; Native Americans, including Alaska Natives; and nursing home and other long-term care facility residents. Complications may include secondary infections, especially bacterial pneumonias,[247] and increased incidence of myocardial infarction.
- Influenza virus infection can cause a broad spectrum of nonspecific signs and symptoms of disease, including asymptomatic or subclinical illness, febrile acute respiratory infection, exacerbation of an underlying chronic disease, acute lower respiratory tract infection, and death. Infants, older adults, and the immunocompromised are more likely to have afebrile and atypical manifestations of influenza illness.
- Even with only moderate vaccine effectiveness, vaccines have a substantial public health impact, given the massive burden of influenza experienced annually.
- Patients are more likely to receive influenza vaccines if recommended by their health care providers. Even specialist physicians who do not provide immunization

services have an important role in increasing coverage in their vulnerable patients by inquiring about vaccination status, recommending vaccination, referring for vaccination, and documenting vaccine receipt.
- Clinicians should use rapid molecular assays to diagnose influenza, with reverse-transcription polymerase chain reaction–based assays for hospitalized patients to improve detection of influenza virus infection.
- Prompt treatment with antivirals reduces the duration of symptoms and risk of some complications and may decrease mortality in high-risk groups. Treatment decisions, particularly in high-acuity settings, should take into account the likelihood of influenza illness and the risk of severe outcomes.
- In institutional and inpatient settings, infection control measures (standard and droplet precautions) should be implemented as soon as possible when outbreaks are suspected, without waiting for results of influenza testing. Airborne precautions should be used during aerosol-generating procedures.
- Health care workers are at risk for infection by and transmission of influenza virus; therefore they should receive annual influenza vaccination and take additional precautions in the event of acute respiratory illness, such as influenza testing, not going to work, respiratory hygiene, face mask use, and/or potential reassignment when exposed to high-risk patients.

Key Readings

Centers for Disease Control and Prevention. *Avian Influenza: Information for Health Professionals and Laboratorians*; 2017. https://www.cdc.gov/flu/avianflu/healthprofessionals.htm.

Centers for Disease Control and Prevention. *CDC Seasonal Flu Vaccine Effectiveness Studies*; 2019. https://www.cdc.gov/flu/vaccines-work/effectiveness-studies.htm.

Centers for Disease Control and Prevention. *Influenza Antiviral Medications: Summary for Clinicians*; 2018. https://www.cdc.gov/flu/professionals/antivirals/summary-clinicians.htm.

Centers for Disease Control and Prevention. Prevention strategies for seasonal influenza in healthcare settings: guidelines and recommendations. https://www.cdc.gov/flu/professionals/infectioncontrol/healthcaresettings.htm.

European Centre for Disease Prevention and Control. Expert opinion on neuraminidase inhibitors for the prevention and treatment of influenza—review of recent systematic reviews and meta-analyses. ECDC. https://ecdc.europa.eu/sites/portal/files/documents/Scientific-advice-neuraminidase-inhibitors-2017.pdf.

Grohskopf LA, Sokolow LZ, Broder KR, Walter EB, Fry AM, Jernigan DB. Prevention and control of seasonal influenza with vaccines: recommendations of the advisory committee on immunization practices—United States, 2018-19 influenza season. *MMWR Recomm Rep.* 2018;67(3):1–20.

Hayden FG, Sugaya N, Hirotsu N, et al. Baloxavir marboxil for uncomplicated influenza in adults and adolescents. *N Engl J Med.* 2018;379(10):913–923.

Memoli MJ, Athota R, Reed S, et al. The natural history of influenza infection in the severely immunocompromised vs nonimmunocompromised hosts. *Clin Infect Dis.* 2014;58(2):214–224.

Uyeki TM, Bernstein HH, Bradley JS, et al. Clinical practice guidelines by the Infectious Diseases Society of America: 2018 update on diagnosis, treatment, chemoprophylaxis, and institutional outbreak management of seasonal influenza. *Clin Infect Dis.* 2019;68(6):895–902.

Complete reference list available at ExpertConsult.com.

48 *HOSPITAL-ACQUIRED PNEUMONIA*

MARK L. METERSKY, MD • ANDRE C. KALIL, MD, MPH

INTRODUCTION

Hospital-acquired pneumonia (HAP) is one of the most common hospital-acquired infections.[1] Substantial evidence links HAP to poorer patient outcomes due to increased mortality, morbidity, including admission to the ICU, need for mechanical ventilation, hospital length of stay, and cost.[2,3]

Despite its high prevalence, HAP is likely overdiagnosed because other respiratory complications in hospitalized patients can mimic it. Unlike patients with *ventilator-associated pneumonia* (VAP) in whom lower respiratory secretions can easily be sampled, obtaining samples in nonintubated patients is more difficult. Consequently, in most patients with HAP, adequate cultures of respiratory tract secretions are not obtained. In addition to necessitating the use of empirical antibiotic therapy without the benefit of confirmatory cultures, this factor adds to the difficulty in diagnosing HAP and limits our understanding of its epidemiology and microbiology.

To standardize the terminology surrounding this condition, the 2016 Infectious Diseases Society of America/American Thoracic Society (IDSA/ATS) HAP/VAP guidelines defined HAP and VAP as mutually exclusive entities.[4] HAP was defined as pneumonia in a nonventilated patient becoming apparent more than 48 hours after admission to the hospital. Postoperative pneumonia, therefore, is a subcategory of HAP. Pneumonias in patients living in non–acute care facilities such as nursing homes and rehabilitation centers were not considered to be HAP. VAP was defined as pneumonia in a patient receiving mechanical ventilation for more than 48 hours and is addressed in Chapter 49.

PATHOGENESIS

HAP, like most other pneumonias, develops when oropharyngeal secretions contaminated with pathogenic bacteria are aspirated into the lung in sufficient amounts to evade local host defenses and replicate. Less common mechanisms that can lead to HAP include large volume gastric aspiration or hematogenous spread of infection. An additional cause of HAP is inhalation of contaminated aerosols; this is the most common cause of HAP due to *Legionella*.[5]

Normal individuals have multiple mechanisms to protect the lungs from infection. The larynx protects against aspiration and coughing expels aspirated material. When these mechanisms fail, mucociliary clearance and the immune system come into play. In addition to the physical action of the cilia moving bacteria trapped in the mucus, numerous substances in the mucus layer assist in preventing infection. These include secretory immunoglobulin A and proteins such as lysozyme and lactoferrin. The airways and alveolar spaces possess numerous other immune mechanisms, including both cellular and humoral immune function, phagocytosis by resident macrophages and recruited neutrophils, and antimicrobial activity of surfactant proteins.[6]

Hospitalized patients are at greater risk than normal individuals of aspirating secretions contaminated with pathogenic bacteria due to two major factors. The first factor is that hospitalized patients develop oropharyngeal colonization with pathogenic bacteria, most commonly with gram-negative bacilli.[7,8] While the mechanisms resulting in this colonization are not known, alterations in mucosal cell surface carbohydrates may facilitate bacterial adherence.[9] A second factor is that hospitalized patients are at increased risk of aspiration of oropharyngeal secretions. This is due to impairment of consciousness related to anesthesia, opioids, and other sedating medications, as well as underlying acute and chronic neurologic comorbidities that impair level of consciousness and swallowing function. Other patient-level risk factors for HAP common in hospitalized patients include impairment of cough due to pain or sedation, and immune defects due to malnutrition, iatrogenic causes and, in the elderly, immune senescence.

EPIDEMIOLOGY

INCIDENCE

A point prevalence survey performed in U.S. hospitals in 2011 found that HAP was the third most prevalent hospital-acquired infection after surgical-site infection and gastrointestinal infection.[1] The authors' extrapolations suggested that approximately 96,000 patients develop HAP each year in the United States; a follow-up study using similar methods estimated approximately 110,000 per year.[10] Notably, HAP is two- to threefold more frequent than VAP in these and other studies.[11] These point prevalence studies demonstrated that approximately 0.6% of hospitalized nonventilated patients have HAP at any time. Other studies report that approximately 0.5–2% of hospitalized patients will develop HAP.[12–14] The risk for HAP varies greatly depending upon the underlying acute illness and comorbidities, with certain conditions resulting in markedly increased risk. Approximately 13% of non–*intensive care unit* (ICU) stroke patients develop HAP.[15] Among surgical patients overall, approximately 1% develop postoperative pneumonia,[16] with large variation depending on the type of surgery. Among patients undergoing lobar pulmonary resection, the postoperative pneumonia rate has been reported as high as 5.8%[17] but is decreased by at least one-third in patients who undergo video-assisted thoracic resection as compared to open resection.[18] Approximately 3% of patients undergoing major abdominal surgery develop postoperative pneumonia.[19] Overall, cardiothoracic and abdominal surgeries (especially upper abdominal) increase the risk of postoperative pneumonia more than surgeries involving other parts of the body,[20] likely due to impairment of deep breathing and cough related to direct and indirect effects of the surgical manipulation, including pain.

Numerous other risk factors for HAP have been identified. Predictive tools have been developed for patients hospitalized for common conditions, including various types of surgery.[20–22] COPD predisposes to HAP in both medical and surgical patients,[23,24] as does the presence of a higher comorbidity index[25] and of measures of acute severity of illness.[14] Other than COPD, comorbidities that appear to increase the risk of postoperative pneumonia include advanced age, diabetes, malnutrition, cerebrovascular disease, and dysphagia.[2,19,26,27] Preoperative oropharyngeal colonization or bronchial colonization/infection with pathogenic organisms has been reported to increase the risk of postoperative pneumonia in patients undergoing surgery.[28,29] Gastric acid suppression with proton-pump inhibitors is also a risk for HAP in non-ICU patients,[30] although this was not found in patients undergoing elective surgery.[31]

IMPACT ON OUTCOMES

Patients who develop HAP have significantly worse outcomes compared to similar patients who do not. They are at increased risk of mortality, ICU admission, subsequent need for mechanical ventilation, and prolonged hospital length of stay. No study has rigorously quantified the attributable mortality associated with HAP, but case-control studies have found excess mortality rates of between 2% and 14%.[2,12] Excess hospital length of stay has been estimated as 2.5 days to 15.9 days and excess cost approximately $30,000 to $40,000 per case.[12]

ETIOLOGIC AGENTS

Studies of the microbiology of HAP are hindered by several factors that make the relevant data less robust and less reliable compared to the extensive data available for VAP. First, it is often difficult to obtain adequate samples of respiratory secretions in patients with HAP because these patients frequently have impaired cough due to mental status changes, debility, and pain from surgical incisions. This is in contrast to VAP, in which an endotracheal tube provides direct access to the lower airways. In as many as 50–90% of patients with HAP, no pathogens are isolated,[2,32] either because respiratory samples are not obtained[33] or because they are inadequate or obtained after antibiotics are started. Second, because of the difficulty in obtaining respiratory secretions, the studies reporting microbiology are likely biased by more rigorous attempts to obtain respiratory secretions in higher risk or more severely ill patients, with these patients more likely to be infected with high-risk, antibiotic-resistant pathogens. Indeed, a retrospective study of HAP limited to ICU patients found that 84% of patients had a respiratory sample cultured, much higher than studies not limited to the ICU. In that study, there was a higher prevalence of *Pseudomonas aeruginosa* and *methicillin-resistant Staphylococcus aureus* (MRSA) than in studies of HAP not limited to the ICU.[34] Finally, respiratory secretions may be contaminated with oral flora, which in hospitalized patients often contain potentially pathogenic bacteria but may not represent the etiology of the pneumonia.

These factors notwithstanding, those bacteria causing HAP are more similar to those causing VAP than to *community-acquired pneumonia* (CAP). Gram-negative bacilli account for approximately 35% of isolates. These include nonfermenting organisms (approximately 20%) such as *P. aeruginosa*, *Stenotrophomonas maltophilia*, and *Acinetobacter* sp, and enteric gram-negative bacilli (approximately 15%) such as *Escherichia coli*, *Klebsiella* sp, *Proteus* sp, and *Enterobacter* sp. *S. aureus* causes about 15% of HAP. In the meta-analysis reported in the 2016 IDSA/ATS HAP-VAP guidelines,[4] *P. aeruginosa* accounted for 13% of HAP, *Acinetobacter* sp 4%, enteric gram-negative bacilli 16%, methicillin-sensitive *S. aureus* 10%, and MRSA 6%. These rates are similar to the rates seen in VAP but are generally slightly lower. *Acinetobacter* has been increasing in frequency as a cause of HAP but is less common in the United States than the 4% figure obtained in the meta-analysis. Most cases of bacterial HAP not caused by the above organisms are caused by *Streptococcus* sp. and *Hemophilus influenzae* or by organisms that could not be identified. *Legionella pneumophila* may cause clusters of HAP because of contamination of the hospital water supply,[35] but overall it is a rare cause of HAP. HAP can also be caused by nonbacterial pathogens. Respiratory viruses can be identified in over 20% of patients with HAP, often with bacterial coinfection, especially in immunocompromised patients.[2,36] The most common viruses detected in the largest study were rhinovirus, influenza, and parainfluenza. In severely immunocompromised patients, HAP may be caused by fungi, most commonly *Aspergillus* sp. Although *Candida* sp may rarely

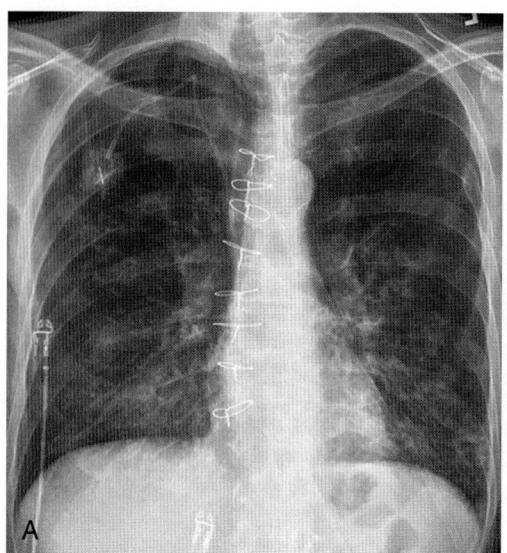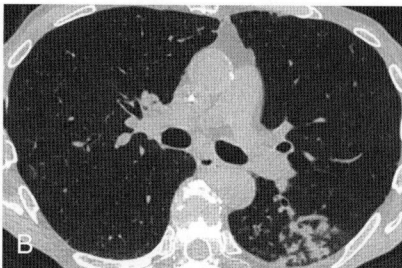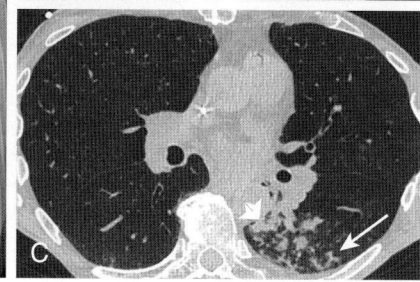

Figure 48.1 Hospital-acquired broncho-pneumonia. (A) Frontal chest radiograph shows patchy, faintly nodular opacity with a segmental distribution in the left lower lobe. (B–C) Axial chest computed tomography displayed in lung windows shows left lower lobe small, branching nodules *(arrow)* and small foci of consolidation *(arrowheads)* consistent with bronchopneumonia.

cause pneumonia in critically ill ventilated patients, there is no evidence to suggest that it causes pneumonia in nonventilated patients. The etiologic agents of HAP in patients with specific underlying conditions such as stroke[37] or postoperative pneumonia do not differ greatly from those of HAP patients overall.

Risk factors for developing HAP caused by antibiotic-resistant organisms have not been studied as extensively in HAP as in CAP and VAP; however, similar to these other entities, recent exposure to intravenous antibiotics within 90 days is a significant risk factor for HAP.[38–40]

DIAGNOSIS

ESTABLISHING A CLINICAL DIAGNOSIS

The 2016 IDSA/ATS guidelines[4] defined HAP as pneumonia appearing more than 48 hours after admission in a nonventilated hospitalized patient. These same guidelines adopted the definition of pneumonia stated in the 2005 guidelines, the presence of a "new lung infiltrate plus clinical evidence that the infiltrate is of an infectious origin, which include the new onset of fever, purulent sputum, leukocytosis, and decline in oxygenation."[41] At the bedside, clinical manifestations are those commonly associated with bacterial pneumonia, including cough, sputum, dyspnea, fever, and a decline in mental status, such as lethargy or delirium. Common signs include worsening oxygenation, manifesting as a decreased oxygen saturation or requirement for higher levels of oxygen supplementation, tachypnea, and abnormal lung exam. Laboratory findings of sputum purulence and an elevated white blood cell or band form count also support the diagnosis. The presence of some of these signs and symptoms, in combination with a new or worsening pulmonary opacity seen on chest radiograph (Fig. 48.1A) or chest *computed tomography* (CT) scanning (Fig. 48.1B–C) leads to a clinical diagnosis of HAP.

Most published studies use a similar definition that requires the presence of a new or progressive pulmonary opacity and at least two of the following: fever or hypothermia, leukocytosis or leukopenia, dyspnea, signs of

consolidation on respiratory exam, and purulent respiratory secretions.[2,14,34] However, there is no consensus about which or how many of these signs and symptoms must be present to confirm a diagnosis of HAP, nor have any studies tested the accuracy of these criteria for the diagnosis of HAP. A recent review of HAP diagnosis demonstrated that each of 10 cohort studies of HAP used different criteria for inclusion in the HAP cohort.[42]

The clinical diagnosis of HAP may be inaccurate. Many patients will manifest some of the common clinical findings associated with HAP for reasons other than pneumonia; they may demonstrate fever due to noninfectious causes or to other hospital-acquired infections, abnormal lung sounds due to impaired secretion clearance or heart failure, or abnormal chest imaging due to atelectasis, heart failure, or pleural effusions. In one study, 35% of patients diagnosed with HAP did not have radiographic findings consistent with pneumonia, and these patients had lesser elevations of inflammatory markers than in patients with chest imaging suggestive of pneumonia.[33] In another study of ICU patients with pneumonia, mostly HAP and VAP, chest radiography showed poor sensitivity and specificity compared to CT (Fig. 48.2) and ultrasound.[43] Due to the inaccuracy of chest radiography and the nonspecific nature of many of the signs and symptoms associated with HAP, there is a common belief among experts that HAP is overdiagnosed. To maximize the accuracy of a clinical diagnosis of HAP, clinicians should carefully consider other explanations for the clinical findings that prompt the evaluation for HAP. Furthermore, a good quality frontal and lateral chest radiograph provides more accurate information than a portable film alone (Fig. 48.3), so if the patient is stable enough to be sent to the radiology suite, doing so is preferable. If doubt persists, a chest CT is the most sensitive for detecting opacities.

In addition to the usual clinical criteria, other modalities have been explored for their use in the diagnosis of HAP. Biomarkers such as procalcitonin and C-reactive protein, which have been extensively investigated as aids to the diagnosis of CAP and VAP, have also been investigated in HAP, although there are much less data available[44-46] so

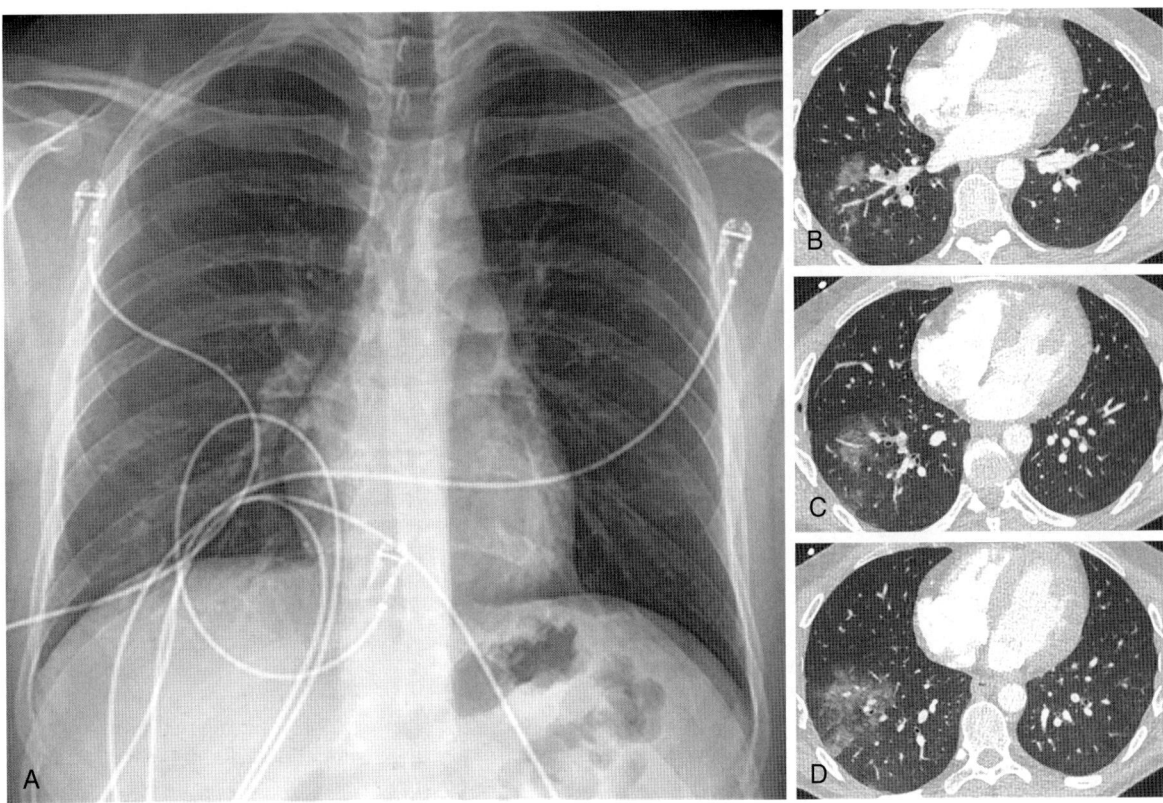

Figure 48.2 Detection of subradiographic pneumonia using computed tomography. (A) Frontal chest radiograph in a recently hospitalized patient re-presenting with fever and cough shows no clear findings to suggest pneumonia. (B–D) Axial chest computed tomography displayed in lung windows shows poorly defined lobular ground-glass opacity in the right lower lobe consistent with bronchopneumonia. The abnormalities are difficult to visualize at chest radiography and were overlooked prospectively.

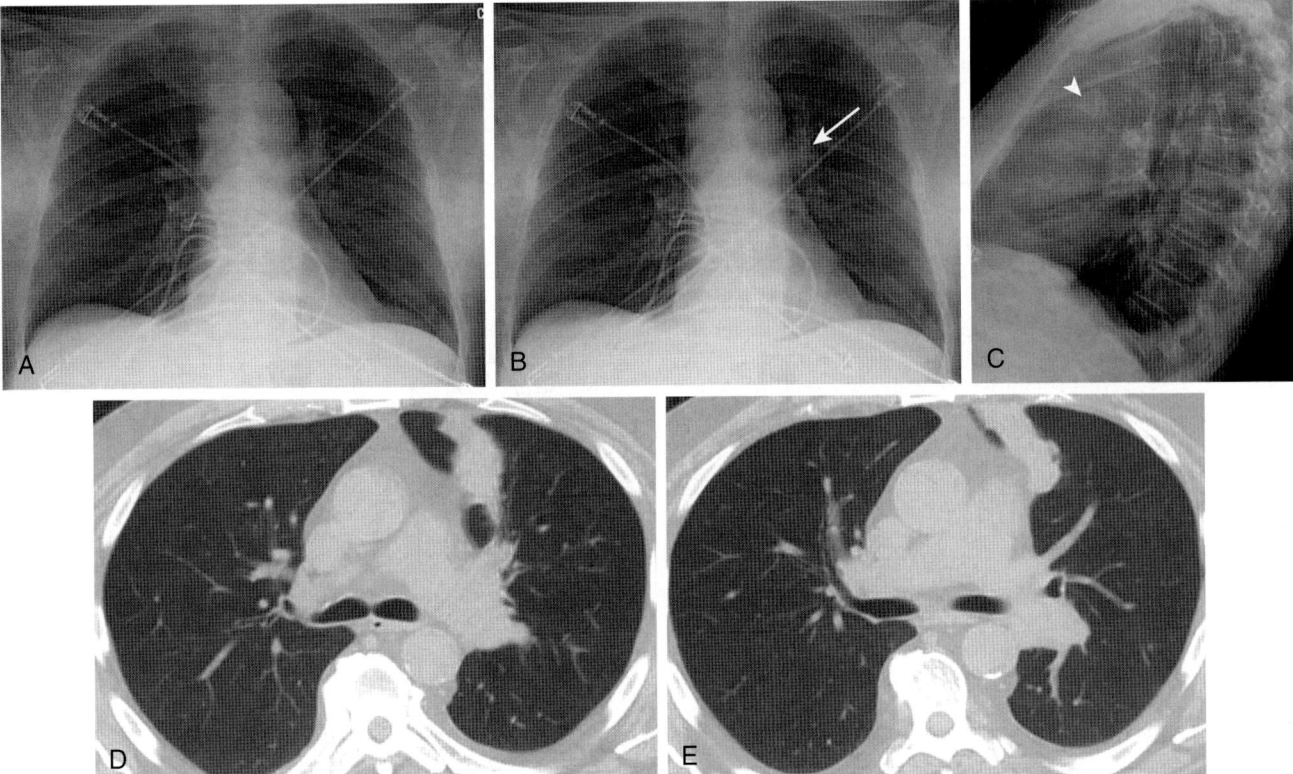

Figure 48.3 Value of frontal and lateral chest radiography over portable radiography for pneumonia detection. (A) Frontal portable chest radiography in a patient with new fever and cough shows no specific abnormalities. (B–C) Frontal and lateral chest radiography performed shortly following the portable chest radiograph shows increased opacity overlying the left hilum *(arrow)* corresponding to a nodular focus on the lateral projection *(arrowhead)*. (D–E) Axial chest computed tomography displayed in lung windows confirmed left upper lobe consolidation, representing pneumonia, as the cause of the frontal and lateral chest radiographic findings.

neither of these is currently recommended for identifying HAP.

The *clinical pulmonary infection score* (CPIS) is a set of six criteria (temperature, white blood cell count, volume and purulence of respiratory secretions, oxygenation, chest radiograph findings, and semiquantitative culture of respiratory secretions) used by some clinicians to determine the need for antibiotic treatment in ventilated patients with suspected VAP.[47] However, the 2016 IDSA/ATS HAP/VAP guidelines did not recommend utilization of the CPIS for patients with VAP.[40] The CPIS has not been studied with respect to its performance characteristics for the diagnosis of HAP.

Pulmonary ultrasound has been shown to be highly sensitive and specific for the diagnosis of CAP in expert hands[48] and has also been used for VAP.[49] Although there are limited data for HAP, ultrasound may have similar value in diagnosing HAP (see Chapter 23).

DETERMINING THE ETIOLOGIC AGENT

Because of the high prevalence of potentially *multidrug-resistant* (MDR) pathogens as the causative agents of HAP, guidelines recommend an attempt to identify the pathogen by culturing respiratory secretions.[50,51] Doing so provides three potential advantages. First, the Gram stain of an adequate quality respiratory sample may allow more accurate targeting of empirical antibiotic therapy. Second, accurate culture results with accompanying antimicrobial susceptibility data could ensure accurate, narrower-spectrum antibiotic therapy. Finally, a negative culture of an adequate quality respiratory sample could allow discontinuation of broad-spectrum antibiotics targeting MDR pathogens (especially if obtained prior to antibiotic treatment). Despite these potential advantages, there is little evidence specific to HAP to support the recommendation to obtain a culture of respiratory secretions or to support the three rationales above. Instead, the recommendation is based on the inherent logic that it is helpful to know the pathogen causing a serious infection when there is likelihood that MDR could result in inadequate empirical therapy or need for prolonged broad-spectrum empirical therapy. Inadequate initial empirical therapy has been associated with increased mortality in HAP.[52] Early studies found high rates of inadequate initial empirical therapy in HAP,[53,54] but it is unknown if this continues in the era of widely disseminated guidelines for broad-spectrum initial empirical therapy for HAP.

Some of the reasoning in favor of obtaining culture data is extrapolated from the experience with CAP and VAP. In CAP, the Gram stain of a good quality sputum is considered reliable in identifying the class of pathogen (gram-positive vs. gram-negative) when a predominant morphotype is found. In VAP patients, cultures of tracheal aspirates accurately predict the pathogen obtained from invasive modalities. However, these cultures may prompt overtreatment because pathogens present in low numbers may represent colonization and may not need to be treated with antibiotics or might need only a very short course of antibiotics. There are data in HAP patients that the culture of expectorated sputum usually correlates with the results of invasive sampling using bronchoscopy, supporting the use of expectorated sputum results to guide antibiotic therapy.[55]

Despite low sensitivity, blood cultures are also suggested in patients with suspected HAP, since a positive blood culture can identify the etiologic source of HAP and direct antibiotic therapy.[50] In sum, samples for cultures of sputum and blood should be obtained and the results should be used to guide antibiotic therapy in HAP.

The published guidelines on HAP have considered whether noninvasive or invasive modalities should be employed to obtain a sample of respiratory secretions.[4] The noninvasive modality most commonly used is spontaneously expectorated sputum, occasionally nasotracheally suctioned sputum in patients unable to cough effectively, or endotracheal aspirate culture in a patient with HAP who subsequently requires invasive mechanical ventilation. Bronchoscopy with bronchoalveolar lavage is the most frequently used invasive modality to obtain respiratory samples. The potential advantages of using bronchoscopy include the ability to obtain samples in the 50% or more of patients with suspected HAP who cannot produce an adequate sample and to obtain a sample less likely to be contaminated with oropharyngeal flora. The potential risks of bronchoscopy are adverse events related to sedation and worsening gas exchange due to instillation of lavage fluid into the lungs, increasing the risk of respiratory deterioration and requirement for respiratory support.

There are few studies specifically designed to investigate the optimal approach to identifying the etiologic agent of HAP. This is in contrast to VAP, in which an invasive approach, usually with bronchoalveolar lavage and quantitative cultures, has been promulgated as a method to decrease inappropriate antibiotic use. In patients with suspected VAP who have a negative culture or a positive culture but with low numbers of organisms, antibiotics can be safely withheld. Given the likely frequent overdiagnosis of HAP, the same logic might apply. However, bronchoscopy is more difficult and carries greater risk in a patient suffering from respiratory distress who is not already intubated. For these reasons, few studies have investigated invasive diagnosis of HAP. One randomized controlled trial investigated an invasive strategy for HAP and found that patients randomized to bronchoscopy with protected specimen brushing had no improvement in outcomes relative to patients receiving empirical treatment.[56] However, this study was underpowered to detect a difference in most important outcomes. In a larger retrospective observational study of ICU-acquired HAP, the diagnostic yield and patient outcomes were compared among those who had noninvasive and invasive sampling. Approximately 60% of patients had bronchoscopic sampling, often after intubation. Among patients who were never intubated, about 50% produced a sputum sample, of which about 30% were positive, a yield similar to bronchoscopy (34%) in patients who were not intubated. While patient outcomes stratified by sampling methodology were not reported, there was a higher rate of antibiotic de-escalation in patients who had invasive sampling.[55] Other studies have reported diagnosing the etiologic agent of HAP with sputum culture in 13–50% of patients,[32,33] although, in the study reporting the lowest yield, sputum samples were obtained as late as 7 days after diagnosis, by which time antibiotic therapy would be expected to decrease the yield of sputum culture significantly.[32]

The use of nasal MRSA screening for pneumonia has been assessed in several studies and two meta-analyses.[57,58] These studies included patients with CAP/*health care–associated pneumonia* (HCAP)/HAP and VAP. Specificity was low because many patients have nasal colonization with MRSA but have other etiologies of pneumonia. Sensitivity for all types of MRSA pneumonia was 70–80%, while the sensitivity for HAP was not provided. Despite this low sensitivity, the negative predictive value is over 90% due to the low prevalence of MRSA as a cause of HAP. As expected, the accuracy in predicting MRSA pneumonia diminishes the longer the time between the performance of the MRSA screening test and the clinical suspicion of pneumonia. This is important in the case of HAP because in many hospitals MRSA screening is performed routinely at the time of admission, but not subsequently. Because *polymerase chain reaction* (PCR)-based MRSA screening has a rapid turnaround time, a negative screen, especially if performed at the time that pneumonia is suspected, may allow safe withholding or rapid discontinuation of anti-MRSA antibiotic therapy.[57]

Culture-independent methods are available for diagnosis of infectious diseases and detection of resistance genes (see Chapter 19). Multiplex PCR platforms for rapid detection of respiratory viruses, bacteria, and antimicrobial resistance genes are widely implemented by hospitals for use in patients with community-acquired respiratory tract infections, although evidence of improved outcomes or decreased antibiotic utilization (if a virus is detected) are limited. Other methods include mass spectrometry, exhaled breath biomarkers, and fluorescence microscopy. In many of these, differentiating colonization from infection can be difficult due to the ability of these techniques to detect low numbers of organisms. Data using these platforms in the setting of HAP are limited,[59] so none of these techniques can be recommended for routine use. However, it is likely that these platforms will find a role for more rapid pathogen and antibiotic susceptibility identification. Given the prevalence of viruses as a cause of HAP, detection of a virus, perhaps in the setting of a normal serum inflammatory biomarker, may allow the avoidance of unnecessary antibiotic therapy.

In summary, because of the prevalence of MDR pathogens in HAP and the potential usefulness of positive cultures to allow targeted therapy and antibiotic de-escalation, guidelines recommend an attempt to obtain and culture a noninvasive sample of respiratory secretions from patients with suspected HAP.[4] Invasive sampling is not generally recommended given the potential risks and the lack of evidence that doing so improves patient outcomes. In certain patients, invasive sampling should be considered, such as in a patient who is not improving despite antibiotic therapy or in a patient at risk for unusual or opportunistic infections. Although not recommended by any guidelines, because of the prevalence of influenza in HAP,[2,36] consideration should be given to testing for influenza in patients with suspected HAP who have a suggestive clinical presentation at a time when influenza is circulating in the community. The use of PCR-based MRSA screening may allow anti-MRSA therapy to be withheld safely, although definitive data are lacking. There is limited experience with multiplex PCR platforms in the setting of HAP, but there is a potential for these modalities to establish a rapid identification of specific bacteria, respiratory viruses, and genes conferring antibiotic resistance.

TREATMENT

The optimal treatment of HAP requires consideration of all evidence available, including epidemiologic, clinical, laboratory, radiologic, and microbiologic data.[4,40,50,51] At the patient's initial evaluation, it is rare to have definitive microbiologic information to guide antibiotic therapy; thus the choice of initial antibiotic therapy is mostly based on empirical evidence, while completion of treatment should be with targeted therapy selected according to results of cultures and antibiotic susceptibilities.

EMPIRICAL TREATMENT APPROACH

The choice of the empirical antibiotic regimen requires balancing the competing goals of ensuring the most effective coverage while avoiding the use of unnecessary antibiotics. The time to HAP onset (i.e., early onset versus late onset) cannot reliably determine the risk of MDR infection[60-64]; thus, information on the time to onset should not be used alone to guide empirical antibiotics. To maximize the efficacy of the empirical regimen, a combination of three factors must be evaluated for the risk of MDR HAP[4]:

1. *History of intravenous antibiotic use*: the use of intravenous antibiotics within 90 days prior to current hospitalization puts patients at higher risk for MDR infections.
2. *Local antibiogram*: an antibiogram is a summary of the percentage of individual bacterial pathogens cultured at that location, with their antimicrobial susceptibility information. The antibiogram should be based on data collected in the hospital unit where the patient is currently located but, if this is not available for specific units due to the small size of the hospital, an institutional antibiogram could also guide the empirical therapy. There are concrete benefits to be gained from the antibiogram; the knowledge of the prevalence of respiratory microorganisms can provide the relevant information as to whether specific antibiotic coverage is necessary (or not) for the empirical treatment of patients with HAP. For example, if only 2% of all HAPs are due to *P. aeruginosa* based on the hospital antibiogram, then 98% of all patients with HAP would not benefit from the empirical use of antibiotics against *P. aeruginosa*. The frequency of specific MDR patterns in the hospital antibiogram can help to direct the empirical coverage for MDR HAP. For example, in a hospital where 40% of all gram-negative isolates are resistant to multiple broad-spectrum antibiotics, the use of empirical antibiotics to cover MDR organisms should be part of the routine standard of care.
3. *Disease severity*: if the patient with HAP requires intubation due to the infection, or develops septic shock, it is more likely that the HAP could be secondary to MDR microorganisms, so the empirical coverage should be broader.[50,51]

In clinical practice, the empirical approach for HAP falls within three treatment categories: (1) low disease severity and no risk factors for MRSA (antibiotic monotherapy with anti-pseudomonal activity), (2) low disease severity and presence of risk factors for MRSA (one anti-pseudomonal plus one anti-MRSA antibiotic), and (3) high disease severity (either septic shock or need for intubation due to HAP dual anti-pseudomonal plus anti-MRSA antibiotics). Once the antibiotic susceptibility is known, then the combination

Table 48.1   Recommended Initial Empirical Antibiotic Therapy for Hospital-Acquired Pneumonia (Non–Ventilator-Associated Pneumonia)

Not At High Risk of Mortality* and no Factors Increasing the Likelihood of MRSA[†‡]	Not At High Risk of Mortality* but with Factors Increasing the Likelihood of MRSA[†‡]	High Risk of Mortality or Receipt of Intravenous Antibiotics During the Prior 90 Days*[‡]
One of the following:	**One of the following:**	**Two of the following (avoid 2 β-lactams):**
Piperacillin-tazobactam[§] 4.5 g IV q6h *or* Cefepime[§] 2 g IV q8h *or* Ceftazidime/avibactam 2.5 g IV q8h *or* Ceftolozane/tazobactam 3 g IV q8h	Piperacillin-tazobactam[§] 4.5 g IV q6h *or* Cefepime[§] or ceftazidime[§] 2 g IV q8h *or* Ceftazidime/avibactam 2.5 g IV q8h *or* Ceftolozane/tazobactam 3 g IV q8h	Piperacillin-tazobactam[§] 4.5 g q6h *or* Cefepime[§] or ceftazidime[§] 2 g q8h *or* Ceftazidime/avibactam 2.5 g q8h *or* Ceftolozane/tazobactam 3 g q8h
Levofloxacin 750 mg IV daily	Levofloxacin 750 mg IV daily *or* Ciprofloxacin or 400 mg IV q8h	Levofloxacin 750 mg IV daily *or* Ciprofloxacin 400 mg IV q8h
Imipenem 500 mg IV q6h *or* Meropenem[§] 1 g IV q8h	Imipenem[§] 500 mg IV q6h *or* Meropenem[§] 1 g IV q8h	Imipenem[§] 500 mg IV q6h *or* Meropenem[§] 1 g IV q8h
	Aztreonam 2g IV q8h	Aztreonam[¶] 2 g IV q8h
		Amikacin 15–20 mg/kg IV daily *or* Gentamicin 5–7 mg/kg IV daily *or* Tobramycin 5–7 mg/kg IV daily *or*
	Plus: Vancomycin 15 mg/kg IV q8 –12h with goal to target 15–20 mg/mL (trough level) (consider a loading dose of 25–30 mg/kg × 1 for severe illness), *or* Linezolid 600 mg IV q12h	**Plus:** Vancomycin 15 mg/kg IV q8 –12h with goal to target 15 to 20 mg/mL (trough level) (consider a loading dose of 25–30 mg/kg × 1 for severe illness), *or* Linezolid 600 mg IV q12h
If patient has severe penicillin allergy and aztreonam is going to be used instead of any β-lactam-based antibiotic, include coverage for MSSA. Options include levofloxacin, clindamycin.		If MRSA coverage is not going to be used, include coverage for MSSA. Options include piperacillin-tazobactam, cefepime, levofloxacin, imipenem, and meropenem Oxacillin, nafcillin, and cefazolin are preferred for the definitive treatment of MSSA, but would ordinarily not be used in an empirical regimen for HAP.

*Risk factors for mortality include intensive care unit admission, need for ventilatory support due to pneumonia, septic shock, and markedly elevated procalcitonin.

[†]Indications for MRSA coverage include prior detection of MRSA culture or nonculture screening, antibiotic treatment during the prior 90 days, and treatment in a unit where the prevalence of MRSA among *S. aureus* isolates is not known or is >20%. The 20% threshold was chosen to balance the need for effective initial antibiotic therapy against the risks of excessive antibiotic use; hence individual units can elect to adjust the threshold in accordance with local values and preferences. If MRSA coverage is omitted, the antibiotic regimen should include coverage for MSSA.

[‡]If patient has factors increasing the likelihood of gram-negative infection, two anti-pseudomonal agents are recommended. If patient has structural lung disease increasing the risk of gram-negative infection (i.e. bronchiectasis or cystic fibrosis), two anti-pseudomonal agents are recommended. A high-quality Gram stain from a respiratory specimen with numerous and predominant gram-negative bacilli provides further support for the diagnosis of a gram-negative pneumonia, including fermenting and non–glucose fermenting microorganisms.

[§]Extended infusions may be appropriate.

[¶]In the absence of other options, it is acceptable to use aztreonam as an adjunctive agent with another β-lactam based agent because it has different targets within the bacterial cell wall.

HAP, hospital-acquired pneumonia; MRSA, methicillin-resistant *Staphylococcus aureus*; MSSA, methicillin-sensitive *Staphylococcus aureus*.

Modified from Kalil AC, Metersky ML, Klompas M, et al. Management of adults with hospital-acquired and ventilator-associated pneumonia: 2016 clinical practice guidelines by the Infectious Diseases Society of America and the American Thoracic Society. *Clin Infect Dis.* 2016;63(5):e61-e111.

therapy can be safely changed to monotherapy. The specific selection of initial empirical antibiotics according to the patient's risk profile can be seen in Table 48.1. These antibiotic recommendations are based on the 2016 IDSA/ATS HAP/VAP guidelines, with some additional antibiotics that became available after these guidelines were written.[65,66] These recommendations will not apply to all situations. For example, in a hospital with very low rates of gram-negative resistance to a certain antibiotic, single gram-negative coverage with this agent may be appropriate, even in critically ill patients at risk for gram-negative infection.

There is accumulating evidence that a negative nasal MRSA screen by PCR performed at the time of diagnosis of respiratory infection is associated with a very high negative predictive value for MRSA pneumonia, with some of the evidence in patients with HAP but most in CAP.[57] While not supported by prospective controlled studies, many clinicians will withhold or discontinue MRSA coverage in HAP and CAP patients with a negative MRSA screen, a practice supported by expert opinion and small retrospective studies in which outcomes in patients in whom anti-MRSA therapy was withheld or discontinued had similar outcomes as those treated for MRSA.[67]

TARGETED TREATMENT APPROACH

Once the etiology of HAP becomes known through culture results of respiratory or, less commonly, blood specimens, the empirical therapy can be safely changed to targeted therapy, with the goal to focus the treatment on the causal microorganism as well as to avoid the continuation of unnecessary antibiotics. The selection of targeted antibiotics is based on the susceptibility results from the final culture of respiratory or blood specimens. Antibiotics that can be used for the treatment of HAP are provided in Table 48.1. As a general rule, vancomycin and linezolid can be used to treat HAP due to MRSA. (Telavancin can be used as a backup option but generally only if the patient does not respond to vancomycin and cannot receive linezolid, because there were safety concerns in a telavancin clinical trial.[68]) Daptomycin should never be used for a pulmonary infection because it is inactivated due to binding to pulmonary surfactant.[69] For HAP due to *methicillin-sensitive S. aureus* (MSSA), cefazolin, oxacillin, and nafcillin are the preferred choices but, if the patient also needs gram-negative coverage, cefepime, piperacillin-tazobactam, levofloxacin, imipenem, or meropenem can also cover MSSA. For HAP due to *P. aeruginosa*, piperacillin-tazobactam, levofloxacin, cefepime, ceftazidime, ceftazidime-avibactam, ceftolozane-tazobactam, imipenem, meropenem, and aztreonam are options. For HAP due to lactose-fermenting organisms (e.g., enterics), piperacillin-tazobactam, levofloxacin, ciprofloxacin, ceftriaxone, cefepime, ceftazidime-avibactam, and ceftolozane-tazobactam are appropriate choices. Ceftaroline is not FDA approved for the treatment of HAP, while ceftobiprole is approved for the treatment of HAP caused by a small number of specific organisms, but not for empiric therapy.

PHARMACOKINETIC/PHARMACODYNAMIC ANTIBIOTIC DOSING

One of the important goals for the treatment of severe respiratory infections such as HAP is to maximize the antibiotic delivery to the source of infection (i.e., lungs) while minimizing the toxicity risk of antibiotic overexposure. One way to achieve these goals is through use of *pharmacokinetic/pharmacodynamic* (PK/PD) principles to optimize the dosing of antibiotics. The PK/PD optimization methods include measurement and targeting of serum antibiotic concentrations, extended and continuous infusion, and weight-based dosing of specific antibiotics. While the use of PK/PD has been controversial in the past, there is growing and consistent evidence that the use of PK/PD for the antibiotic treatment of HAP is associated with survival benefits. The 2016 IDSA/ATS guideline performed several meta-analyses on PK/PD studies and found improvements in mortality, clinical cure, and ICU length of stay.[4] In addition, other studies published after the guideline provided further support for these PK/PD benefits.[70-72]

INHALED ANTIBIOTICS

There is an intuitive biologic rationale for inhaled antibiotics to be among the therapeutic choices for treatment of HAP due to their high peak concentration and low systemic exposure, which in turn could lead to less selective pressure and less frequent development of bacterial resistance than intravenous antibiotics.[73] However, there is no strong evidence supporting the use of inhaled antibiotics as either monotherapy or adjunctive therapy of HAP. If there will be a role for inhaled antibiotics in the future, the optimal antibiotic chemical properties and the best device delivery method still need to be determined. Hence, intravenous antibiotics remain the mainstream approach to treat HAP. However, there is one exception:

patients who develop HAP due to MDR gram-negative microorganisms sensitive only to aminoglycosides or polymyxins. In this situation, there is evidence supporting the use of inhaled antibiotics in conjunction with intravenous antibiotics.[4]

ANTIBIOTIC DE-ESCALATION AND DURATION OF TREATMENT

When culture and susceptibility results are available, antibiotic de-escalation from empirical to targeted therapy should be performed by selecting the antibiotics to which the isolated bacteria are susceptible, and then making the final antibiotic choice based on its PK/PD properties to achieve optimal lung parenchyma penetration. De-escalation is more complex when there is no identified bacterial etiology for HAP, which is common. In this case, a thorough evaluation of the clinical, laboratory, and radiologic picture at regular intervals will determine the direction of patients' progression while receiving the empirical treatment. If patients' clinical symptoms are resolving; fever, white blood count, and inflammatory markers are decreasing; and imaging is improving, consideration for narrowing antibiotic coverage can be made in an individual basis. If anti-MRSA coverage is still being provided, a negative MRSA screen supports the discontinuation of such coverage.

Another tool that can guide antibiotic de-escalation is the assay of inflammatory biomarkers. One of these biomarkers, procalcitonin, has been evaluated in randomized trials and meta-analyses of patients with HAP and has been shown to be an effective adjunct tool to de-escalate antibiotics safely.[74-78] Antibiotic de-escalation has been shown to be safe[79] and may have potential beneficial survival outcomes in patients with sepsis and VAP.[80,81] There are no systematic data assessing the safety of antibiotic de-escalation in HAP patients in whom there are no culture data. In HAP patients with a negative culture of an adequate quality respiratory sample obtained before the start of antibiotics, some experts believe de-escalation to a single broad-spectrum antibiotic is safe, especially if a nasal MRSA screen is negative, but data supporting this practice are limited.

The recommended duration of antibiotic therapy for pneumonia has varied substantially in the past. However, more recent studies (observational and randomized) and meta-analyses have demonstrated that short courses (7 days) are as effective as longer courses (8–15 days) of antibiotics.[82-87] One of the previous concerns with short courses was the potential for recurrence of HAP, especially due to *P. aeruginosa*. However, a new analysis with updated evidence performed by the IDSA/ATS guideline panel demonstrated that, even in HAP caused by nonfermenting gram-negative bacteria, there were no significant differences between short course and longer course therapy regarding mortality, clinical cure, recurrent pneumonia, or mechanical ventilation duration.[4] Thus, based on current evidence, 7 days of antibiotic therapy is recommended for most patients with HAP. In some patients, treatment can be shorter or longer, depending on the individual patient progression with respect to clinical, radiologic, and laboratory parameters.[50,51]

PREVENTION

Since bacterial HAP is commonly caused by aspiration of pathogens from the oropharynx into the lower airways, HAP prevention strategies are comprised of two fundamental approaches: minimizing colonization of the oropharynx with pathogenic bacteria and minimizing the opportunity for resident pathogens to reach the lower airways.

MINIMIZING OROPHARYNGEAL COLONIZATION

Several modalities of oral care interventions have been studied for their efficacy in preventing HAP, presumably by decreasing the intensity of oropharyngeal colonization with pathogenic bacteria. These include mechanical interventions such as professional dental care, toothbrushing, and the use of antimicrobial agents such as chlorhexidine and povidine-iodine.[88,89] Meta-analyses of these studies have found statistically significant reductions in HAP rates associated with these interventions; however, when only high-quality studies were considered, the benefit was less apparent. Furthermore, chlorhexidine can cause oral irritation, allergic reactions and, if aspirated into the lungs, acute lung injury. Increasing the concern regarding potential toxicity of chlorhexidine, accumulating evidence, including a recent meta-analysis and observational study, have demonstrated increased risk of mortality associated with the use of chlorhexidine oral hygiene.[90,91]

While mechanical oral care such as toothbrushing would seem to have little risk of harm, the evidence of benefit of this modality in isolation is limited and, even in combination with other modalities, the results have been mixed with respect to prevention of pneumonia. A multicomponent intervention including toothbrushing twice daily and chlorhexidine rinse failed to prevent pneumonia in a large-cluster randomized study of at-risk nursing home patients.[92]

Gastric acid suppression increases the reservoir of potentially pathogenic bacteria residing in the stomach and is associated with increased risk of HAP in a general non-ICU hospitalized population[93] and in specific patient populations such as stroke[30] and hematology/oncology.[94] To the extent that gastric acid–suppressing medications predispose to HAP, avoiding their use in patients who do not need them may reduce the risk of HAP and of other complications such as *Clostridioides difficile* colitis.

Vaccines targeting common pathogens in HAP, including *P. aeruginosa* and *S. aureus*, are under investigation for VAP but have not yet been studied in patients at risk for HAP. The pneumococcal vaccines prevent morbidity from *S. pneumoniae* and should be provided to individuals for whom they are indicated, but they have not been studied specifically in the context of HAP. Similarly, because viruses, including influenza, cause a substantial percentage of HAP episodes, influenza vaccination should be provided to all individuals in whom there is no contraindication and to all health care workers who have direct patient contact. A large matched cohort study demonstrated lower rates of postoperative pneumonia and mortality in elderly patients who had preoperative influenza vaccine than in those who did not.[95]

PREVENTING ASPIRATION

Dysphagia is common among hospitalized patients and increases the risk for aspiration and pneumonia. Its causes are numerous, including neurologic conditions, frailty, sedating medications, prolonged intubation, and oropharyngeal and laryngeal anatomic abnormalities. Patients at risk should be promptly evaluated for dysphagia. In patients with dysphagia, interventions including diet modification, swallowing training and nonoral feeding may reduce the frequency of HAP, although the evidence is derived mostly from observational studies, predominantly in stroke patients. While a meta-analysis of RCTs failed to find decreased rates of HAP associated with dysphagia screening and treatment, a subsequent pre-post study did.[96,97] In patients with dysphagia, it is not clear whether nasogastric or percutaneous gastric tube feedings decrease the risk of pneumonia compared to oral feedings, although there is evidence supporting this practice.

Sedating medications such as opioids and benzodiazepines increase the risk of aspiration and, in adults living in the community, both opioid and benzodiazepine use have been associated with an increased risk of pneumonia. The contribution of opioid-induced immunosuppression to this increased risk is unclear. There is much more limited evidence regarding this issue in hospitalized patients, but one study found an increased risk of postoperative respiratory complications, including an increased risk of pneumonia, in patients who received higher doses of fentanyl intraoperatively.[98] Other studies have found decreased risk for postoperative respiratory complications overall (pneumonia rates not specified) with the use of multimodality postoperative pain control versus opioid-only pain control.[99] Taken together, these data suggest that minimizing the use of sedating medications, especially opioids, may reduce the risk of HAP.

AIRWAY CLEARANCE, EARLY MOBILIZATION, PAIN CONTROL

In hospitalized patients, factors including sedation, physical inactivity and, in postoperative patients, pain, decrease the clearance of respiratory secretions. This has led to the use of various modalities designed to improve respiratory secretion clearance. One frequently used device is the incentive spirometer, which is provided to postoperative patients in many hospitals. Meta-analyses and systematic reviews have concluded that there is low-quality evidence demonstrating lack of benefit in preventing postoperative pulmonary complications, including pneumonia.[100] Pain control is a challenge with respect to postoperative pulmonary complications, including pneumonia. Inadequate pain control can increase the risk of pulmonary complications by preventing mobilization, cough, and deep breathing, while excessive sedation can increase the same complications. Epidural pain control may decrease the risk of these complications, including pneumonia, after cardiac surgery, high-risk abdominal surgery, and vascular surgery, but meta-analysis results were mixed.[101-103] Intercostal nerve blocks for postoperative pain after upper abdominal surgery reduced pulmonary complications in patients undergoing biliary surgery via a subcostal incision but increased the risk in patients who had an upper abdominal incision.[104]

PROPHYLACTIC ANTIBIOTICS

Some studies have demonstrated an increased risk of postoperative pneumonia in patients who have respiratory tract colonization with potentially pathogenic bacteria at the time of surgery.[105,106] Based in part on this knowledge, prophylactic antibiotic treatment beyond the 24 hours typically given for surgical site infection prevention has been studied to prevent postoperative pneumonia. Most studies demonstrated no improvement,[105,107] while one observational study found lower rates of postoperative pneumonia in lung cancer resection patients who received antibiotics for 3 days after the surgery. However, the control group in this study had a very high rate of pneumonia (16%), limiting the interpretation of the results.[108]

MULTIPRONGED INTERVENTIONS

There have been several reports of multipronged interventions to reduce postoperative pulmonary complications, including postoperative pneumonia. All had a quasi-experimental/pre-post intervention design without a concurrent control or randomization. Interventions included incentive spirometry, coughing and deep breathing, oral care, patient and family education, early mobilization, and head-of-bed elevation.[109-111] These reports described successful reductions in postoperative pulmonary complication rates, including pneumonia. But, given the imprecise nature of HAP diagnosis, the lack of high-quality evidence supporting any of the individual interventions, and the lack of a concurrent control group, higher-quality evidence is needed before recommending widespread adoption of these multipronged interventions.

In summary, numerous strategies have been recommended to prevent HAP, but high-quality evidence regarding the effectiveness of these strategies is lacking. Therefore, no major guidelines provide specific recommendations for HAP prevention. There is some evidence in support of oral care to minimize bacterial colonization as well as evaluation and intervention for dysphagia, particularly in stroke patients. There is reason to believe that employing best practices with regard to several processes of care, including minimization of sedating medications, optimizing pain control, avoidance of proton pump inhibitors in patients for whom they are not indicated, and early mobilization might improve patient outcomes through mechanisms that include a reduction in HAP rates. Standard infection prevention practices, including hand hygiene and isolation of patients with communicable infectious diseases should be adhered to, although evidence of benefit for HAP prevention is lacking.

Key Points

- *Hospital-acquired pneumonia* (HAP) is the third most common hospital-acquired infection after surgical site infection and gastrointestinal infections. Approximately 100,000 people develop HAP in the United States each year, representing over 0.5% of hospitalized patients.
- HAP is associated with excess mortality, hospital length of stay, and cost.
- HAP is most commonly caused by aspiration of oropharyngeal secretions contaminated with pathogenic bacteria. Risk factors include numerous comorbidities, impairment of swallowing, and altered mental status.
- The pathogens responsible for HAP include *P. aeruginosa*, *Staphylococcus aureus*, enteric gram-negative bacilli, *Streptococcus* sp, and less frequently *S. pneumoniae* and *H. influenzae*. Respiratory viruses, including influenza, may cause up to 20% of hospital-acquired pneumonia episodes.
- Attempts to diagnose the etiologic agent should be made to allow accurate antibiotic therapy; use of expectorated sputum is recommended in most cases.
- Initial treatment is usually empirical and should target potentially resistant organisms such as methicillin-resistant *S. aureus* and *P. aeruginosa* unless there is evidence that the patient has low risk for these organisms, or the hospital antibiogram shows low prevalence of multidrug-resistant organisms. When a definitive culture returns, antibiotics should be de-escalated to a narrow-spectrum agent targeting the pathogen identified.
- For most patients, a 7-day course of antibiotics is recommended.
- There are no preventive measures supported by high-quality evidence, but there may be a benefit of optimal oral hygiene and assessment and intervention for risk of aspiration.

Key Readings

Chastre J, Wolff M, Fagon JY, et al. Comparison of 8 vs 15 days of antibiotic therapy for ventilator-associated pneumonia in adults: a randomized trial. *JAMA*. 2003;290:2588–2598.

Esperatti M, Ferrer M, Theessen A, et al. Nosocomial pneumonia in the intensive care unit acquired by mechanically ventilated versus nonventilated patients. *Am J Respir Crit Care Med*. 2010;182:1533–1539.

Herer B, Fuhrman C, Gazevic Z, Cabrit R, Chouaid C. Management of nosocomial pneumonia on a medical ward: a comparative study of outcomes and costs of invasive procedures. *Clin Microbiol Infect*. 2009;15:165–172.

Johanson WG, Pierce AK, Sanford JP. Changing pharyngeal bacterial flora of hospitalized patients. emergence of gram-negative bacilli. *N Engl J Med*. 1969;281:1137–1140.

Kalil AC, Metersky ML, Klompas M, et al. Management of adults with hospital-acquired and ventilator-associated pneumonia: 2016 clinical practice guidelines by the Infectious Diseases Society of America and the American Thoracic Society. *Clin Infect Dis*. 2016;63:e61–e111.

Kaneoka A, Pisegna JM, Miloro KV, et al. Prevention of healthcare-associated pneumonia with oral care in individuals without mechanical ventilation: a systematic review and meta-analysis of randomized controlled trials. *Infect Control Hosp Epidemiol.* 2015;36:899–906.

Magill SS, O'Leary E, Janelle SJ, et al. Changes in prevalence of health care-associated infections in U.S. hospitals. *N Engl J Med.* 2018;379:1732–1744.

Micek ST, Chew B, Hampton N, Kollef MH. A case-control study assessing the impact of nonventilated hospital-acquired pneumonia on patient outcomes. *Chest.* 2016;150:1008–1014.

Mitchell BG, Russo PL, Cheng AC, et al. Strategies to reduce non-ventilator-associated hospital-acquired pneumonia: a systematic review. *Infect Dis Health.* 2019;24(4):229–239.

Naidus EL, Lasalvia MT, Marcantonio ER, Herzig SJ. The diagnostic yield of noninvasive microbiologic sputum sampling in a cohort of patients with clinically diagnosed hospital-acquired pneumonia. *J Hosp Med.* 2018;13:34–37.

Ranzani OT, De Pascale G, Park M. Diagnosis of nonventilated hospital-acquired pneumonia: how much do we know? *Curr Opin Crit Care.* 2018;24:339–346.

Ranzani OT, Senussi T, Idone F, et al. Invasive and non-invasive diagnostic approaches for microbiological diagnosis of hospital-acquired pneumonia. *Crit Care.* 2019;23:51.

Russell CD, Koch O, Laurenson IF, O'Shea DT, Sutherland R, Mackintosh CL. Diagnosis and features of hospital-acquired pneumonia: a retrospective cohort study. *J Hosp Infect.* 2016;92:273–279.

Sopena N, Sabria M, Neunos Study G. Multicenter study of hospital-acquired pneumonia in non-ICU patients. *Chest.* 2005;127:213–219.

Torres A, Niederman MS, Chastre J, et al. International ERS/ESICM/ESCMID/ALAT guidelines for the management of hospital-acquired pneumonia and ventilator-associated pneumonia: Guidelines for the management of hospital-acquired pneumonia (HAP)/ventilator-associated pneumonia (VAP) of the European Respiratory Society (ERS), European Society of Intensive Care Medicine (ESICM), European Society of Clinical Microbiology and Infectious Diseases (ESCMID) and Asociacion Latinoamericana del Torax (ALAT). *Eur Respir J.* 2017;50:1700582.

Complete reference list available at ExpertConsult.com.

49 VENTILATOR-ASSOCIATED PNEUMONIA

JEAN CHASTRE, MD • CHARLES-EDOUARD LUYT, MD, PHD

INTRODUCTION

Ventilator-associated pneumonia (VAP) is the most frequent *intensive care unit* (ICU)–acquired infection among patients who are treated with mechanical ventilation.[1,2] In contrast to infections of other organs (e.g., urinary tract and skin), for which mortality ranges from 1–4%, the mortality rate for VAP, defined as pneumonia developing more than 48 hours after the onset of mechanical ventilation, ranges from 20–50%, and can even be higher when lung infection is caused by high-risk pathogens.[3] Although the attributable mortality rate for VAP is still debated, good evidence indicates that VAP prolongs the duration of mechanical ventilation and of the ICU stay.[2,3] Approximately 50% of all antibiotics prescribed in an ICU are administered for true or supposed respiratory tract infections.[4] Because several studies have shown that appropriate antimicrobial treatment of patients with VAP significantly improves outcome, rapid identification of infected patients and accurate selection of antimicrobial agents are important clinical goals.[3] Agreement is lacking, however, about the appropriate diagnostic, therapeutic, and preventive strategies for VAP.

PATHOGENESIS

Multiple defense mechanisms protect the normal human respiratory tract from infection. Examples include anatomic barriers, such as the glottis and larynx; cough reflexes; constituents of tracheobronchial secretions; mucociliary clearance; epithelial lining fluid and surfactant components; cell-mediated and humoral immunity; a phagocytic system that involves alveolar macrophages and recruited neutrophils; and both humoral and cell-mediated adaptive immunity. When these coordinated components function properly, invading microbes are eliminated and clinical disease is avoided. When these defenses are impaired, or if they are overcome by a high inoculum of organisms or organisms of unusual virulence, pneumonitis results.[5,6]

As suggested by the infrequent association of VAP with bacteremia, most of these infections appear to result from aspiration of potential pathogens that have colonized the mucosal surfaces of the oropharyngeal airways, the dental plaque, and/or the paranasal sinuses. Endotracheal intubation not only compromises the natural barrier between the oropharynx and trachea, it also facilitates the entry of bacteria into the lungs by pooling and leakage of contaminated secretions around the endotracheal tube cuff from the subglottic area to below the true vocal cords. Contaminated secretions leak into the lungs of most intubated patients and may be facilitated by the supine position. Moreover, biofilm formation on the inner and outer surfaces of the endotracheal tube provides a protected environment for pathogens. Bacterial aggregates in biofilm dislodged during suctioning are dangerous for the lung because they are difficult to clear by host immune defenses and difficult to eradicate with antibiotics.[3,6]

Tracheobronchial colonization with *gram-negative bacilli* (GNB) usually precedes the onset of VAP. Risk factors for tracheobronchial colonization appear to be the same as those that favor pneumonia, and include advanced age, more severe illness, longer hospitalization, prior or concomitant use of antibiotics, malnutrition, endotracheal intubation, depressed level of consciousness, immune suppression from disease or medication, azotemia, underlying pulmonary disease, and longer duration of mechanical ventilation.[7,8] Experimental studies have linked some of these risk factors with changes in adherence of GNB to respiratory epithelial cells. Although formerly attributed to protease-induced changes in epithelial cell surface proteins, these changes in adherence also reflect alterations of cell surface carbohydrates. Bacterial adhesins and prior antimicrobial therapy appear to facilitate the process. Interestingly, Enterobacteriaceae usually appear first in the oropharynx, whereas *Pseudomonas aeruginosa* more often appear first in the trachea.[9]

Although the stomach can be a reservoir for potential pneumonia pathogens, the gastropulmonary route of infection is not the primary route of infection in most critically ill patients.[10] Progression of colonization from the stomach to the upper respiratory tract with subsequent episodes of VAP could not be demonstrated in several studies, and efforts to eliminate the gastric reservoir with antimicrobial therapy without decontaminating the oropharyngeal cavity have generally failed to prevent VAP.[10] In fact, there is more than one potential pathway for colonization of the oropharynx and trachea in such a setting, including cross infection from the hands of health care personnel and contaminated respiratory therapy equipment. Patient care activities, such as bathing, oral care, tracheal suctioning, enteral feeding, and tube manipulations, provide many opportunities for transmission of pathogens when meticulous infection control practices are not followed.

EPIDEMIOLOGY

INCIDENCE

The exact incidence of VAP varies widely depending on the case definition of pneumonia and the population being evaluated. For example, the incidence of VAP may be up to two times greater in patients when the diagnosis is made by qualitative or semiquantitative sputum cultures rather than by quantitative cultures of lower respiratory tract secretions. However, studies have confirmed that nosocomial pneumonia is considerably more frequent in ventilated patients than in other ICU patients, with the incidence being as much as 6-fold to 20-fold higher in ventilated patients than in nonventilated patients.[3,11] VAP manifests in 9–27% of all intubated patients, and its incidence increases with duration of intubation. The risk of VAP is highest early in the course of the hospital stay—estimated to be 3% per day during the first 5 days of intubation, 2% per day during days 5 to 10 of intubation, and 1% per day after day 10.[7] Because most mechanical ventilation is short term, approximately half of all episodes of VAP develop within the first 4 days of mechanical ventilation. In a large epidemiologic study, independent predictors of VAP determined by multivariate analysis were: primary admitting diagnosis of burns, trauma, central nervous system disease, respiratory disease, or cardiac disease; mechanical ventilation during the preceding 24 hours; witnessed aspiration; and use of paralytic agents.[7] Exposure to antibiotics conferred protection, but this effect was attenuated over time. According to four studies, the VAP rate was higher in patients with *acute respiratory distress syndrome* (ARDS) than in other ventilated patients, affecting between 34% and more than 70% of patients with ARDS and often leading to the development of sepsis, multiple organ failure, and death.[12,13]

Attributable Mortality, Morbidity, and Costs

In mechanically ventilated patients in the ICU, those with VAP appear to have a 2-fold to 10-fold higher risk of death than those without pneumonia. Although these statistics indicate that VAP can be lethal, previous studies have not clearly demonstrated that pneumonia is responsible for the higher mortality rate of these patients. It is often difficult to determine whether ICU patients with severe underlying illness would have survived if they had not developed VAP. VAP, however, has been recognized in several case-control

studies or studies using multivariate analysis as an important prognostic factor for different groups of critically ill patients.[14-18] Based on a multistate progressive disability model that appropriately handled VAP as a time-dependent event in a high-quality database of 2873 mechanically ventilated patients, VAP-attributable mortality was found to be 8.1% overall.[19] These results are consistent with those obtained in other observational studies using also multistate models and causal analysis, detecting a relatively limited mortality attributable to VAP.[20]

Other factors beyond the simple development of VAP, such as the severity of the disease, the adequacy of antimicrobial therapy, or the responsible pathogens, may be more important determinants of outcome for patients in whom pneumonia develops. Indeed, it may be that VAP increases mortality only in the subset of patients with intermediate severity of illness,[21] in those for whom initial treatment is inappropriate,[22] and/or in patients with VAP caused by high-risk pathogens, such as *P. aeruginosa*.[23] Patients with very low severity and early-onset pneumonia caused by organisms such as *Haemophilus influenzae* or *Streptococcus pneumoniae* have excellent prognoses with or without VAP, whereas very ill patients with late-onset VAP would be unlikely to survive.

Studies have clearly shown that patients with VAP have prolonged duration of mechanical ventilation and lengthened ICU and hospital stay than do patients who do not have VAP.[1,3] Summarizing available data, VAP appears to extend the ICU stay by at least 4 days, with the attributable ICU length of stay being longer for medical than surgical patients and for patients infected with high-risk rather than low-risk organisms.[24] The prolonged hospitalization of patients with VAP underscores the considerable financial burden imposed on the health care system by the development of VAP.[24,25]

Etiologic Agents

Microorganisms responsible for VAP differ according to geographic areas, characteristics of the ICU patients, durations of hospital and ICU stays before onset of the disease, and risk factors for *multidrug-resistant* (MDR) pathogens.[26,27] However, multiple studies have shown that GNB—particularly *P. aeruginosa* and Enterobacteriaceae—cause many of the respiratory infections in this setting, with relatively minor changes in the distribution of the pathogens during the last decade.[28,29] Although VAP typically involves infection with a single pathogen, polymicrobial infections are also common.[30]

Until recently, MDR pathogens were isolated more frequently in late-onset VAP cases than in early-onset (within 4 days of hospital admission) cases, mostly reflecting prior use of broad-spectrum antibiotics in these patients.[31] However, several later studies found similar rates of etiologies in patients with early- and late-onset VAP, emphasizing that the local ICU ecology is the most important risk factor for acquiring MDR pathogens, irrespective of the length of intubation.[32,33]

Extended-spectrum β-lactamase–producing Enterobacteriaceae (ESBL-PE) are increasingly encountered in patients with hospital-acquired infections, including VAP, with additional mortality and cost.[34] They now represent 19–61% of the episodes caused by Enterobacteriaceae, varying according to species and to countries. Systematic screening of ESBL-PE fecal carriage may help to guide initial therapy in patients with VAP when cultures are negative because they have a very good negative predictive value for subsequent ESBL-PE infections. Conversely, a positive specimen only has a predictive value from 35–40% and thus does not imply that initial antimicrobial therapy should systematically cover this pathogen.

Tracheal colonization with *P. aeruginosa* increases with increased length of hospitalization, prior antibiotic use, and severity of illness and is an important risk factor for VAP caused by this microorganism. In one study, the odds of developing *P. aeruginosa* VAP were eight times higher in patients with prior *P. aeruginosa* colonization than in noncolonized patients, confirming that screening for *P. aeruginosa* tracheal colonization by biweekly active surveillance cultures could reliably exclude the need for targeting this microorganism when cultures are negative for this microorganism.[35] *Acinetobacter baumannii* is also a common cause of ICU-acquired infection, accounting for 8–14% of VAP in the United States and Europe, but much higher rates (19% to >50%) in Asia, Latin America, and some Middle Eastern countries.[36,37] Importantly, many isolates are now resistant to all antimicrobials except colistin (polymyxin E) and tigecycline, and some infections are resistant to these antimicrobial agents as well.[38]

The emergence of infections caused by *carbapenem-resistant Enterobacteriaceae* (CRE) worldwide represents another alarming problem, although the prevalence of such infections is highly variable across different countries.[39] Prior use of carbapenems and prior hospitalization in a country where CRE is highly prevalent have been reported as independent risk factors for the acquisition of carbapenemase-producing Enterobacteriaceae and other CRE.

Legionella sp, anaerobes, fungi, viruses, and even *Pneumocystis jirovecii* are also potential causative agents, but these microbes are not commonly found when pneumonia is acquired during mechanical ventilation. Several of these causative agents, including viruses, might be more common than reported because they are difficult to identify.[40,41] Isolation of fungi, most frequently *Candida* sp, poses interpretative problems. Invasive disease has been reported in VAP, but yeasts are isolated frequently from respiratory tract specimens in the absence of apparent disease. The use of the commonly available respiratory sampling methods (bronchoscopic or nonbronchoscopic) in ventilated patients is not sufficient to make the diagnosis of *Candida* pneumonia, and evidence of lung tissue invasion is also needed.[42-45]

DIAGNOSIS

VAP is typically identified at the bedside by combining three criteria: (1) clinical observations suggesting infection, such as the new onset of fever, purulent sputum, leukocytosis, increased minute ventilation, arterial oxygenation decline, and/or the need for increased vasopressor infusion to maintain blood pressure; (2) new or progressive persistent radiographic opacities; and (3) "positive" microbiologic culture results for a potentially pathogenic microorganism isolated from tracheal aspirates, *bronchoalveolar lavage* (BAL) fluid,

pleural fluid, and/or blood.[1,3] However, this definition of VAP is frequently inaccurate and leaves room for subjective interpretation.[46–48] Because a new pulmonary opacity is the only criterion confirming involvement of the intra-alveolar pulmonary spaces by the infectious process, it is considered a prerequisite for the diagnosis of VAP. However, most of the time it is not present, with the infection remaining confined to an already abnormal region of the lung. Thus, it is mandatory to consider the diagnosis of VAP in patients who deteriorate clinically, and/or in whom vasopressors need to be increased in order to maintain blood pressure, even in the absence of a clear-cut progression of radiographic abnormalities.

The presence of a pathogen at the level of the proximal airways does not suffice for making the diagnosis of VAP because most ventilated patients are colonized with pathogens very early after the initiation of mechanical ventilation. Even deciding which threshold should be applied to define a "positive" culture when using semiquantitative or quantitative tracheal aspirate or BAL fluid cultures can be challenging, especially for specimens obtained after starting new antibiotics.[3] Thus, the absence of indisputable reference standards continues to fuel controversy about the adequacy and relevance of many studies in this field and has led investigators to describe other types of lower respiratory tract infection, such as ventilator-associated tracheobronchitis, or even to abandon the concept of VAP and replace it by a new construct that comprises different levels of ventilator-associated events, including infection-related ventilator-associated condition.[49-52]

In practice, either of two conceptually different diagnostic strategies can be used when VAP is suspected.[3] Current evidence is insufficient to favor either approach to diagnosis of VAP regarding clinical outcomes, although evidence indicates that the second (invasive) approach can reduce use of antibiotics.

The first strategy is to treat every patient clinically suspected of having a pulmonary infection with new antibiotics, even when the likelihood of infection is low, arguing that several studies showed that immediate initiation of appropriate antibiotics is associated with reduced mortality.

The second strategy is to use an invasive diagnostic approach based on quantitative cultures of distal *lower respiratory tract* (LRT) specimens obtained using bronchoscopic or nonbronchoscopic techniques, such as BAL or a protected specimen brush, to improve the identification of patients with true VAP and facilitate decisions about whether or not to treat with antibiotics.[53] Although no consensus exists on the best diagnostic strategy for patients clinically suspected of having VAP, the goal of each strategy is to institute early appropriate antibiotic therapy in patients with true VAP and to withhold it in others.[54]

THE CLINICAL DIAGNOSTIC STRATEGY

With the clinical strategy, all patients suspected of having VAP are treated with antibiotics that they have not received recently. The selection of appropriate empirical therapy is based on risk factors and local microbiologic and resistance patterns and involves qualitative testing to identify possible pathogens. The initial antimicrobial therapy is adjusted

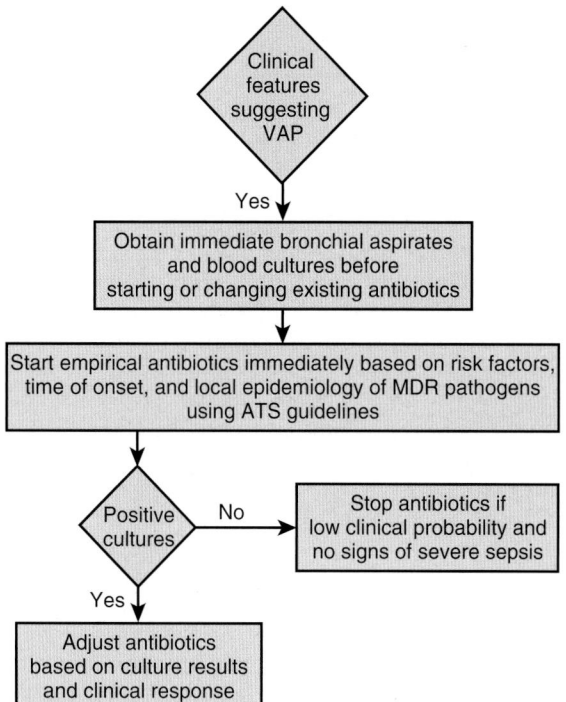

Figure 49.1 The clinical diagnostic strategy. Diagnostic and therapeutic algorithms applied to patients with a clinical suspicion of *ventilator-associated pneumonia* (VAP) managed with the clinical strategy. ATS, American Thoracic Society; MDR, multidrug resistant.

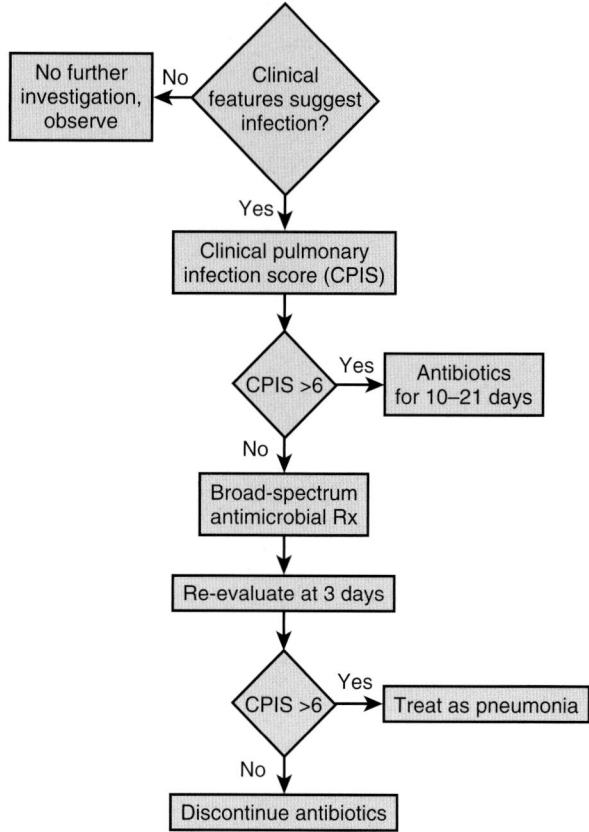

Figure 49.2 The clinical diagnostic strategy guided by a clinical score. Diagnostic and therapeutic strategy applied to patients managed with a clinical strategy guided by the *Clinical Pulmonary Infection Score* (CPIS).[57]

according to culture results or clinical response (Fig. 49.1). Antimicrobial treatment is discontinued only if the following three criteria are fulfilled on day 3: (1) clinical diagnosis of VAP is unlikely (there are no definite opacities found on chest radiography at follow-up and no more than one of the three following findings is present [temperature greater than 38.3°C, leukocytosis or leukopenia, and purulent tracheobronchial secretions]) or an alternative noninfectious diagnosis is confirmed, (2) tracheobronchial aspirate culture results are nonsignificant, and (3) severe sepsis or shock is not present.[55]

This clinical approach has two undisputable advantages: first, no invasive and/or specialized diagnostic procedures, such as fiberoptic bronchoscopy, BAL, and quantitative microbiologic techniques are required and, second, the risk of missing a patient who needs antibiotic treatment is minimal when all suspected patients are treated with new antibiotics. The disadvantages include the potential sampling errors inherent in specimens obtained from the proximal airways and lower specificity) for distinguishing airway colonization from true pneumonia.

Slightly different variants of the clinical approach including the use of quantitative or semiquantitative cultures of endotracheal aspirates for defining a positive result have been described to increase specificity and avoid undue prolongation of antibiotic therapy. While the simple qualitative culture of tracheal aspirates is a technique with a high percentage of false-positive results, several studies suggest that the diagnostic accuracy of quantitative cultures is similar to the accuracy of more invasive techniques, limiting the risk of overusing antibiotics in patients with colonized proximal airways and/or a mild form of tracheobronchitis

but no true pneumonia.[56] Another option when using the clinical approach is to follow the strategy described by Singh and colleagues, in which decisions regarding initial antibiotic therapy are based on a clinical score constructed from seven variables, the *Clinical Pulmonary Infection Score* (CPIS).[57] Patients with a CPIS greater than 6 are considered to have VAP and are treated with antibiotics for 10 to 21 days; if the CPIS score is 6 or less, antibiotics are discontinued after 3 days (Fig. 49.2). Such an approach avoids prolonged treatment of patients who have a low likelihood of infection while allowing immediate treatment of patients who are more likely to have VAP. Antibiotics can also be stopped very early in patients with suspected VAP but minimal and stable ventilator settings. These patients may not have pneumonia at all or they may have comparatively mild pneumonias that can be adequately treated with very short courses of antibiotics (1 to 3 days).[58]

THE INVASIVE DIAGNOSTIC STRATEGY

With the invasive strategy, direct microscopic examination and quantitative cultures of LRT secretions obtained using BAL (performed with or without a bronchoscope) are used to define both the presence of pneumonia and the etiologic pathogen.[3,59] Growth above a threshold concentration is required to make a diagnosis of VAP and determine the causative microorganisms. Growth below the threshold is assumed to be due to colonization or contamination. Using this strategy, therapeutic decisions are made according to

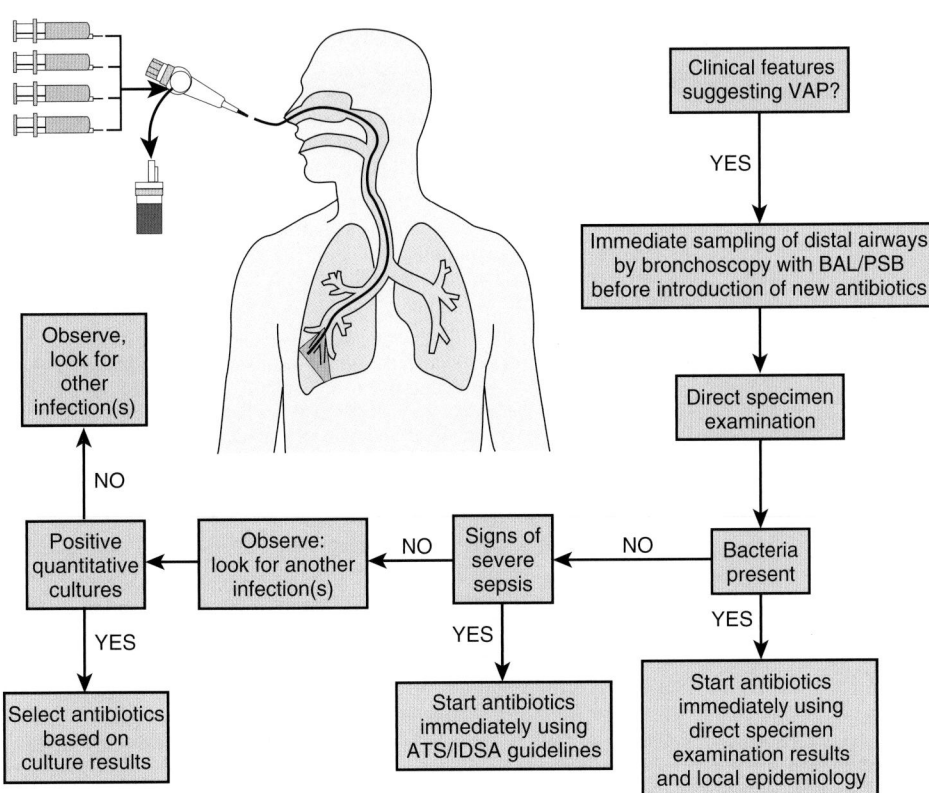

Figure 49.3 **The invasive diagnostic strategy.** Diagnostic and therapeutic strategy applied to patients with a clinical suspicion of *ventilator-associated pneumonia* (VAP) managed according to the invasive strategy. ATS, American Thoracic Society; BAL, bronchoalveolar lavage; IDSA, Infectious Diseases Society of America; PSB, protected specimen brush.

a strict protocol, using the results of direct examination of distal pulmonary samples and results of quantitative cultures in deciding whether to start antibiotic therapy, which pathogens are responsible for infection, which antimicrobial agents to use, and whether to continue therapy (Fig. 49.3).

Quantitative cultures of BAL specimens consistently yield a lower frequency of positive results (based on a quantity of microorganisms above the diagnostic threshold) than are obtained when only qualitative cultures of tracheal aspirates are used. Thus, when therapeutic decisions are based on these data, fewer patients are treated with antibiotics and a potentially narrower spectrum of therapy is used than when using the clinical approach, thereby limiting the emergence and dissemination of drug-resistant strains and antibiotic toxicity.

Another compelling argument in favor of the invasive strategy is that this approach directs attention away from the lungs as the source of fever when BAL quantitative culture results are negative. Many ICU patients with negative bronchoscopic cultures have other sites of infection, such as wounds, the urinary tract, or intravascular catheters that need to be identified to avoid delays in initiating appropriate treatment.

The accuracy of quantitative cultures of LRT secretions obtained using BAL is questionable in patients who have received prior antibiotics, particularly when new antibiotics are introduced after the onset of the symptoms suggestive of nosocomial pneumonia and before pulmonary secretions are collected. In that case, the newly initiated antibiotics can increase the number of false-negative results, regardless of the way in which the secretions are obtained.[60]

One major technical problem with all bronchoscopic techniques is proper selection of the sampling area in the tracheobronchial tree. The sampling area is usually selected based on the location of the radiographic opacity or on the bronchoscopic identification of a pulmonary segment that has purulent secretions. In patients with diffuse pulmonary opacities or minimal new changes in a previously abnormal chest radiograph, determining the correct segment to sample can be difficult. In such cases, sampling should be directed to the area where endobronchial abnormalities are maximal. Because autopsy studies indicate that VAP frequently involves the posterior portion of the right lower lobe, this area should probably be given priority for sampling.

SUMMARY OF THE EVIDENCE

Aside from decision-analysis studies and a single retrospective study, five trials to date have used a randomized scheme to assess the effect of a diagnostic strategy on antibiotic use and outcome in patients suspected of having VAP.[53,61-64] No differences in mortality and duration of mechanical ventilation were apparent by analysis of pooled data.[65] However, in a randomized study of 413 patients, those managed with an invasive strategy that combined quantitative cultures of BAL specimens with an algorithm for treatment de-escalation had a significant increase in antibiotic-free days at day 14 (5.0 vs. 2.2) and day 28 (11.5 vs. 7.5) compared with noninvasive methods using qualitative cultures, clearly indicating a decrease in antibiotic exposure.[53] Several prospective studies have also concluded that antibiotics can be stopped in patients with negative quantitative cultures, without adversely affecting the recurrence of pneumonia and mortality.[66-69]

Although no consensus has yet been reached on appropriate diagnostic strategies for VAP, the authors of the recent European guidelines on HAP/VAP suggest obtaining

Table 49.1   Proposed Strategy for Managing Antimicrobial Therapy in Patients with Ventilator-Associated Pneumonia

Proposed Strategy	Rationale
Step 1: Start therapy using broad-spectrum antibiotics	Due to the emergence of multiresistant GNB, such as *P. aeruginosa* and ESBL-producing GNB, and the increasing role of MRSA, empirical treatment with broad-spectrum antibiotics is justified in most patients with a clinical suspicion of VAP (see Fig. 49.4).
Step 2: Stop therapy if the diagnosis of infection becomes unlikely	The goal is to ensure that ICU patients with true bacterial infection receive immediate appropriate treatment. However, this can result in more patients receiving antimicrobial therapy than necessary because clinical signs of infection are nonspecific.
Step 3: Use narrower spectrum antibiotics once the etiologic agent is identified	For many patients with VAP, including those with late-onset infection, therapy can be narrowed once the results of respiratory tract and blood cultures are available, either because an anticipated organism (e.g., *P. aeruginosa* and *Acinetobacter* sp or MRSA) was not recovered, or because the organism isolated is sensitive to a more narrow-spectrum antibiotic than used in the initial regimen.[118,119]
Step 4: Use pharmacokinetic-pharmacodynamic data to optimize treatment	Clinical and bacteriologic outcomes can be improved by optimizing the therapeutic regimen according to pharmacokinetic and pharmacodynamic properties of the agents selected for treatment.
Step 5: Switch to monotherapy on days 3 to 5	There are no clinical benefits to using a regimen combining two antibiotics for more than days 3 to 5, provided that initial therapy was appropriate, the clinical course appears favorable, and microbiologic data do not point to a very difficult-to-treat microorganism.
Step 6: Shorten the duration of therapy	Reducing duration of therapy in patients with VAP has led to good outcomes with less antibiotic use. Prolonged therapy leads to colonization with antibiotic-resistant bacteria, which may precede a recurrent episode of VAP.

ESBL, extended-spectrum β-lactamase; GNB, gram-negative bacteria; ICU, intensive care unit; MRSA, methicillin-resistant *Staphylococcus aureus;* VAP, ventilator-associated pneumonia.

LRT quantitative samples (prior to any antibiotic treatment) to reduce antibiotic exposure in stable patients with suspected VAP and to improve the accuracy of the results (weak recommendation, low quality of evidence).[1] Because BAL removes cells (approximately 1 million) and secretions from a large lung area and samples can be examined microscopically immediately after the procedure to verify the presence or absence of intracellular or extracellular bacteria in the lower respiratory tract, this examination is particularly useful and well adapted to allow rapid identification of an infection having reached the distal bronchioles and the intra-alveolar spaces. As such, our own position is to recommend the use of a strategy based on systematically performing BAL in all patients clinically suspected of having VAP.[46] If BAL performed with or without a bronchoscope is not available, results of tracheal aspirate quantitative cultures can be used as an acceptable substitute, provided that a sufficiently high threshold (i.e., $\geq 10^5$ CFU/mL) is applied, to avoid overusing antibiotics in patients with only proximal airway colonization.

Whether the diagnosis of VAP can be improved by lung ultrasonography and/or new methods for identifying and quantifying the bacterial burden present in the lower respiratory tract warrant investigation. A growing number of rapid diagnostic techniques using biomolecular approaches, including quantitative and multiplex polymerase chain reaction, *matrix-assisted laser desorption ionization time-of-flight mass spectrometry* (MALDI-TOF MS), peptide nucleic acid fluorescence in-situ hybridization, and morphokinetic cellular analysis using advanced optics microscopy, are available that allow early pathogen identification and determination of antimicrobial susceptibility.[70,71] These new technologies, when coupled with strong antibiotic stewardship programs, are expected to reduce the time to appropriate antimicrobial therapy in patients infected with MDR pathogens, as well as avoiding broad-spectrum regimens when the infection can be treated by a narrow-spectrum antibiotic, but these assays remain susceptible to the problems of contamination and colonization.

TREATMENT

Antimicrobial therapy of patients with VAP is a two-stage process. The *first* stage involves administering broad-spectrum antibiotics to avoid inadequate treatment of patients with true bacterial pneumonia. The second stage focuses on achieving this objective without overusing or abusing antibiotics. In general, the first stage can be accomplished by rapidly identifying patients with pneumonia and starting therapy with an empirical regimen likely to treat the most common etiologic agents in a particular institution. This requires that the initial antibiotic choice be driven by knowledge of the likely etiologic pathogens and the local patterns of antimicrobial resistance. The *second* stage involves stopping therapy in patients with a low probability of VAP, focusing and narrowing treatment once the etiologic agent is known, switching to monotherapy after day 3 whenever possible, and shortening the duration of therapy to 7 to 8 days in most patients, as determined by the patient's clinical response and information about the bacteriology (Table 49.1).[1,3,72]

INITIAL TREATMENT

Optimal treatment of VAP implies that the initial antimicrobial agents could be selected based on an accurate prediction of the responsible pathogens and of their susceptibility patterns, to avoid both ineffective therapy when

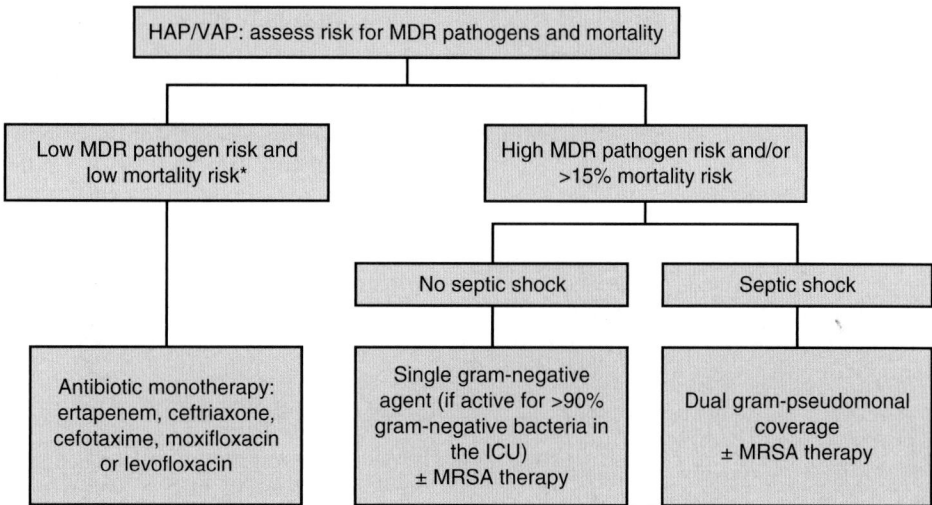

Figure 49.4 Empirical antibiotic treatment algorithm. The algorithm follows the European Guidelines for hospital-acquired pneumonia/ventilator-associated pneumonia (HAP/VAP) in selecting initial empiric use of antibiotics.*Low risk for mortality is defined as a ≤15% chance of dying, a mortality rate that has been associated with better outcomes using monotherapy than combination therapy when treating serious infection. ICU, intensive care unit; MDR, multidrug-resistant; MRSA, methicillin-resistant *Staphylococcus aureus*. (From Torres A, Niederman MS, Chastre J, et al. International ERS/ESICM/ESCMID/ALAT guidelines for the management of hospital-acquired pneumonia and ventilator-associated pneumonia. *Eur Respir J* 50[3]:2017.)

the pathogen is highly resistant to antibiotics and excessive antibiotic use when it can be covered by a narrow-spectrum agent. Failure to initiate prompt appropriate therapy (i.e., using an agent to which the etiologic organism is sensitive, with the optimal dose and route of administration) has been consistently linked with increased mortality in patients with VAP.[73] Due to the emergence of multiresistant GNB, such as *P. aeruginosa*, ESBL Enterobacteriaceae, and carbapenemase-producing *Klebsiella pneumoniae*, and the still-important role of gram-positive bacteria, such as *methicillin-resistant Staphylococcus aureus* (MRSA), empirical treatment with broad-spectrum antibiotics is justified in most patients with a clinical suspicion of VAP.[1,2] The choice of agents should be based on local patterns of antimicrobial susceptibility and anticipated side effects, and should take into account the antibiotics that the patients have received within the prior 2 weeks, striving not to use the same antimicrobial classes, if possible. Having current knowledge about local bacteriologic patterns can increase the likelihood that appropriate initial antibiotic treatment will be prescribed. A suggested approach for the selection of the initial treatment, as proposed in the European Guidelines for HAP/VAP, is summarized in Figure 49.4. Only patients with a low mortality risk and low MDR pathogen risk, such as those without prolonged duration of hospitalization, admission from a health care–related facility, or recent prolonged antibiotic therapy, can be treated with a relatively narrow-spectrum drug, such as a nonpseudomonal third-generation cephalosporin.[1]

Several published reports have demonstrated the need to adjust the target dose of antimicrobial agents used in treating severe VAP to the individual patient's pharmacokinetics and the putative bacterial pathogens' susceptibilities.[74,75] Most investigators distinguish between antimicrobial agents that kill by a concentration-dependent mechanism (e.g., aminoglycosides and fluoroquinolones) and those that kill by a time-dependent mechanism (e.g., β-lactams

and vancomycin). Altered pharmacokinetics secondary to an increase in the volume of distribution in critically ill patients can result in insufficient serum β-lactam concentrations when standard doses are administered, emphasizing the need to monitor peak and trough levels of antibiotics carefully when treating resistant pathogens.[74] Regimens with higher doses than those usually recommended and/or a prolonged duration of infusion are frequently needed in such circumstances. Development of dosing algorithms based on minimal inhibitory concentrations, patient creatinine clearance and weight, and a clinician-specified area under the inhibitory curve target, as well as therapeutic drug monitoring, might be a valid way to improve treatment of these patients, leading to a more precise approach than provided by current antimicrobial guidelines.

AVOIDING OVERUSE OF ANTIBIOTICS

The need to ensure that ICU patients with true bacterial infections promptly receive an appropriate antibiotic regimen can lead to many more patients receiving antimicrobial therapy than is actually necessary, because clinical signs of infection are nonspecific. Thus, when a clinical approach to VAP is used, it is important to perform serial clinical and microbiologic evaluations, and to reevaluate therapy after 48 to 72 hours so that it can be stopped if infection is unlikely. To accomplish this, all diagnostic strategies designed for managing patients with a clinical suspicion of VAP should make explicit the decision tree used to identify patients with a low probability of infection, in whom therapy can be stopped when infection appears improbable.

For many patients with VAP, including those with late-onset infection, therapy can be narrowed once the results of respiratory tract and blood cultures are available, if no resistant organism (e.g., *P. aeruginosa*, *Acinetobacter* sp, or MRSA) is recovered or if the isolated organism is sensitive to a narrower spectrum antibiotic. For example, vancomycin and linezolid should be stopped if MRSA is not identified, unless the patient is allergic to β-lactams and has an infection caused by a gram-positive microorganism. Very-broad-spectrum agents, such as carbapenems, piperacillin-tazobactam, and/or cefepime, should be restricted to patients with infection caused by pathogens only susceptible to these agents. Clinicians must be aware that the emergence of resistant variants may lead to treatment failure when third-generation cephalosporins are chosen to treat infections caused by *Enterobacter, Citrobacter, Morganella morganii*, indole-positive *Proteus*, and *Serratia* sp due to the presence of inducible β-lactamases, even if the isolate is initially characterized as susceptible.

The most common reason to use combination therapy in initial management of patients with VAP is to achieve synergy in treating *P. aeruginosa* or other difficult-to-treat GNB. However, antibiotic synergy has been shown to be valuable only in vitro and in patients with neutropenia or bacteremic infection, which is uncommon in VAP. A meta-analysis evaluated all prospective randomized trials of β-lactam monotherapy compared with β-lactam/aminoglycoside combination regimens in 7586 patients with sepsis, of whom at least 1200 patients had VAP.[76] The clinical success rates were similar with monotherapy versus combination therapy, and combination therapy had no advantage in the treatment of *P. aeruginosa* infections. Importantly, combination therapy did not prevent the emergence of antimicrobial resistance during treatment, but it was associated with a significantly higher rate of nephrotoxicity. Based on these data, therapy can be switched to monotherapy in most patients after 3 or 5 days, as long as initial therapy is appropriate, the clinical course is favorable, and microbiologic data do not identify a difficult-to-treat microorganism with a high in vitro minimal inhibitory concentration, as is found with some lactose-nonfermenting GNB.

Efforts to reduce the duration of therapy for VAP are justified by studies of the natural history of the response to therapy. Most patients with VAP who receive appropriate antimicrobial therapy have a good clinical response within the first 6 days.[77] Prolonged therapy promotes colonization with antibiotic-resistant bacteria, which may lead to a recurrent episode of VAP. A multicenter randomized controlled trial of 401 patients with microbiologically proven VAP showed that the clinical outcomes of patients who received appropriate empirical therapy for 8 days were similar to those of patients who received therapy for 15 days.[78] A trend to greater rates of relapse for short-duration therapy was seen when the etiologic agent was *P. aeruginosa* or *Acinetobacter* sp, but the clinical outcomes were indistinguishable. These results were confirmed in two later studies, including a prospective randomized trial of 290 patients evaluating an antibiotic discontinuation policy.[79,80] Patients for whom a shorter duration of therapy may not be appropriate include immunosuppressed patients, those whose pneumonia was complicated by empyema and/or pulmonary abscess, those whose initial antimicrobial treatment was not appropriate for the causative microorganisms, and those whose infection was caused by nonfermenting GNB and who had no improvement in clinical signs of infection.

Many clinicians remain hesitant about prescribing antibiotics for fewer days for patients with VAP, and they prefer to customize antibiotic duration based on the clinical course of the disease and/or using serial determinations of a biomarker such as procalcitonin. The rationale for using a biomarker to tailor antibiotic treatment duration relies on evidence that the inflammatory response is often proportional to infection severity. When that response is absent or low, it might be logical to discontinue antibiotics earlier. Thus, adapting antimicrobial treatment duration to procalcitonin kinetics seems reasonable and has been demonstrated as useful in several randomized trials targeting patients with acute respiratory infection, including five trials conducted in the ICU.[81,82]

AEROSOLIZED THERAPY

The recent development of vibrating-mesh nebulizers has renewed interest in antibiotic aerosolization in patients with VAP. Their use allows very high concentrations of antimicrobial agents to be achieved in respiratory secretions, including the fluid lining the alveolar compartment, far above those achievable using the intravenous route.[83] However, data in critically ill patients with pneumonia are limited; most reported experiences are case reports, descriptive studies, or literature review. Moreover, aerosols are likely to reach only ventilated regions of the lungs, and not consolidated areas involved with pneumonia. According to systematic reviews and meta-analyses results, administration of aerosolized antibiotics might increase the likelihood of clinical resolution, particularly in VAP caused by MDR pathogens.[84] However, no significant improvements in important outcomes such as mortality or duration of mechanical ventilation have been consistently documented, and results of a double-blinded, placebo-controlled, randomized trial failed to demonstrate superiority of adjunctive aerosolized antibiotics versus standard of care in any clinically relevant end point.[85] Thus, although promising, the widespread use of aerosolized antibiotics to treat pneumonia in the ICU setting cannot be recommended.[84] It should be restricted to the treatment of extensively resistant gram-negative pneumonia susceptible only to antibiotics with limited efficacy and high toxicity when given by the IV route (i.e., aminoglycosides and colistin), or in patients who are not responding to IV antibiotics alone, as a last resort therapy, whether the infecting organism is or is not MDR.[2] In these cases, the use of a vibrating-mesh nebulizer seems to be more efficient, but specific settings and conditions are required to improve lung delivery.[86]

PREVENTION

Because VAP is associated with increased morbidity, longer hospital stay, increased health care costs, and higher mortality rates, prevention is an important goal.

CONVENTIONAL INFECTION CONTROL APPROACHES

The design of the ICU has a direct effect on the potential for nosocomial infections. Adequate space and lighting, properly functioning ventilation systems, and appropriate handwashing facilities all lead to lower infection rates.[87] It is important to note, however, that upgrading the physical environment does not reduce the infection rate unless the attitudes and practices of health care personnel are also optimized. In any ICU, one of the most important factors is the health care staff, including the number, quality, and motivation of medical, nursing, and ancillary members. The team should include a sufficient number of nurses to minimize their movement from one patient to another and to avoid having them work under constant pressure.[88] The importance of personal cleanliness and attention to aseptic procedures must be emphasized at every opportunity. It is clear that careful monitoring, decontamination, and compliance with guidelines for the use of respiratory equipment all reduce the incidence of nosocomial pneumonia.[89] Handwashing and hand rubbing with alcohol-based solutions remain the most important components of effective infection control practices in the ICU.[90]

Environmental and patient-oriented microbiologic monitoring facilitates the early recognition of colonization and infection and has been associated with significant reductions in nosocomial infection rates. The focal point for infection control activities in the ICU is a surveillance system designed to establish and maintain a database that identifies endemic rates of nosocomial infections. This information facilitates the recognition of outbreaks, when infection rates rise above the endemic threshold for a specific type of nosocomial infection.

An antibiotic policy that restricts the prescription of broad-spectrum agents and inappropriate antibiotics is of major importance. Better use of antibiotics in the ICU can be achieved by implementing strict guidelines, avoiding the treatment of patients who do not have bacterial infections, using narrow-spectrum antibiotics whenever possible, and reducing the duration of treatment.[91,92] Similarly, transfusion of red blood cells and other allogenic blood products should follow a strict policy because several studies have identified exposure to allogenic blood products as a risk factor for postoperative infection and pneumonia.[93]

SPECIFIC PROPHYLAXIS AGAINST VENTILATOR-ASSOCIATED PNEUMONIA

Specific strategies aimed at reducing the duration of mechanical ventilation (a major risk factor for VAP), such as improved methods of sedation, use of protocols to facilitate and accelerate weaning, mobilizing patients as soon as possible, and using low tidal volume with adequate levels of positive end-expiratory pressure, are integral parts of any VAP prevention program.[94-97] All are based on the application of strict protocols. Similarly, noninvasive positive-pressure ventilation using a face mask should be used whenever possible.[98]

Some very simple, safe, inexpensive, and logical measures may have beneficial effects on the frequency of VAP in mechanically ventilated patients. These include avoiding nasal insertion of endotracheal and gastric tubes, maintaining the endotracheal tube cuff pressure above 20 cm H_2O to prevent leakage of bacteria around the cuff into the lower respiratory tract, promptly reintubating patients who are likely to fail extubation, keeping patients in the semirecumbent position when enteral nutrition is used, removing tubing condensate, and providing adequate oral hygiene with sterile water alone, even though the level of evidence for the efficacy of these measures is low.[89,99,100]

Continuous or intermittent suctioning of oropharyngeal secretions has been proposed as a means to avoid chronic aspiration of secretions through the tracheal cuff of intubated patients. However, an updated meta-analysis of subglottic secretion drainage reported no impact on duration of mechanical ventilation, ICU length of stay, or mortality, casting some doubt on the efficacy of such a measure.[101] Investigators have also proposed a number of innovations in endotracheal tube cuff materials, shape, and design, as well as more consistent and frequent cuff pressure monitoring, in order to prevent microaspirations of microbe-laden secretions along the vertical microfolds that develop along the endotracheal tube cuff. Unfortunately, none of these innovations have thus far been proven to prevent VAP or improve objective patient outcomes.[102-104]

Gastric colonization by potentially pathogenic organisms increases with decreasing gastric acidity. Thus, medications that decrease gastric acidity (antacids, histamine 2 blockers) can increase the gastric bacterial burden and increase the risk of VAP. However, whether stress ulcer prophylaxis increases VAP incidence is still debated. Krag and colleagues randomized 3298 patients in 33 European ICUs to daily intravenous pantoprazole versus placebo.[105] Patients randomized to pantoprazole had a lower rate of clinically notable gastrointestinal bleeding (2.5% vs. 4.2%) but no difference in the rates of red blood cell transfusions, pneumonia, *Clostridioides difficile* infections, or 90-day mortality. While this trial somewhat tempers the concern that stress ulcer prophylaxis may increase the risk of pneumonia in critically ill patients, it simultaneously fails to provide clear evidence that stress ulcer prophylaxis improves objective patient outcomes.

Oral care with chlorhexidine was considered until recently as an important measure for preventing VAP; however, new data have questioned its true efficacy and safety. While meta-analyses of randomized trials have reported that oral care with chlorhexidine lowers VAP rates by about 30%, this signal is only evident in open-label studies. If one restricts the meta-analysis to double-blind studies, the signal is diminished and no longer significant. Furthermore, no benefit in duration of mechanical ventilation or mortality has ever been demonstrated.[106] There are also some concerns regarding a possible increased risk of mortality and ventilator-associated events, as noted on meta-analyses of randomized trials and several observational studies.[106,107]

Selective decontamination of the digestive tract (SDD) includes a short course of systemic antibiotic therapy, such as cefotaxime, trimethoprim, or a fluoroquinolone, and topical administration of nonabsorbable antibiotics (usually an aminoglycoside, polymyxin E, and amphotericin) to the mouth and stomach, to eradicate potentially pathogenic bacteria and yeast that may cause infections. Since the original study published by Stoutenbeek and coworkers in 1984, which demonstrated a decrease of the overall infection rate in patients receiving the SDD regimen, more than 40 randomized controlled trials and eight meta-analyses have been published.[108,109] All eight meta-analyses reported a significant reduction in the risk of VAP, and four reported a significant reduction in mortality. Several prospective, randomized, controlled trials, all performed in ICUs with low rates of antibiotic resistance, that were large enough to show a significant survival benefit in SDD-treated patients have been published.[110-113] All were in favor of treatment with SDD, the largest and most recent one demonstrating a relative decrease in 28-day mortality rate (odds ratio, 0.83; 95% confidence interval, 0.72 to 0.97) and an absolute survival benefit of 3.5%.[112] Even so, widespread use of SDD in ICU patients remains controversial. The major concern with use of SDD is that it can promote the emergence of resistant bacteria, particularly gram-positive bacteria such as MRSA. This is likely to be an even greater problem in ICUs with a high baseline rate of resistance. In contrast to what was expected, most studies that have evaluated this issue showed a lower incidence of colonization with resistant bacteria in SDD-treated patients than in control patients, even after many years of utilization, possibly because decontamination prevents some infections and thus saves some patients from needing treatment with intravenous antibiotics.[109,114] Nonetheless, active surveillance for resistant pathogens among all ICU patients (not just those receiving digestive or oral decontamination) suggests that SDD is associated with small but significant and sustained increases in the unit-wide prevalence of antibiotic-resistant organisms.[110,113] The most recent European guidelines on the management of HAP and VAP issued a weak recommendation in favor of selective oral decontamination alone, not SDD, and only for settings with low rates of antibiotic-resistant bacteria and low rates of antibiotic consumption.[1] The recent publication of a trial that assessed the value of oral care with 2% chlorhexidine versus selective oral decontamination versus SDD, each compared with standard of care, in a cluster randomized crossover trial among 13 European ICUs with moderate to high rates of antibiotic resistance at baseline supports this recommendation, having found no differences between arms in either ICU-acquired bloodstream infections with resistant organisms or 28-day mortality.[111]

IMPLEMENTING A STRUCTURED PREVENTION POLICY

The application of consistent evidence-based interventions to prevent VAP has been highly variable from one ICU to another and is often suboptimal. Furthermore, no single preventive measure can succeed alone, emphasizing the need to use multifaceted and multidisciplinary programs to prevent VAP. Such programs are frequently referred to as *care bundles*. A care bundle is a set of readily implementable interventions required to be undertaken for each patient on a regular basis. The goal is for every intervention to be implemented for every patient on every day of his or her stay in the ICU. Compliance is assessed for the bundle as a whole, so failure to complete even a single intervention means failure of the whole bundle. The interventions need to be packaged in such a way that compliance is readily assessed, which usually means that no more than five interventions are included in each care bundle. The performance goal is to achieve over 95% compliance routinely. Care bundles make it possible to introduce evidence-based

preventive measures, including achieving appropriate nurse staffing levels, avoiding intubation, and initiating specific strategies aimed at reducing the duration of mechanical ventilation, as described above. Several studies using quasi-experimental design have confirmed the usefulness of this strategy for preventing VAP in the ICU.[115,116]

The lack of methodologic rigor of the reported studies, however, precludes any conclusive statements about "care bundle" effectiveness or cost-effectiveness. The exact set of key interventions that should be part of the VAP-prevention bundle is also not currently known, nor are factors contributing to its success. Successful VAP prevention requires an interdisciplinary team, educational interventions, system innovations, process indicator evaluation, and feedback to health care workers. As shown in a recent study, simply having a checklist available for reference without consideration of a robust implementation and adherence strategy is unlikely to maximize patient outcomes.[117]

In the United States, the Centers for Medicare and Medicaid Services has proposed ending hospital reimbursements for care made necessary by preventable complications, including nosocomial infections, aiming for a zero VAP rate. Although this plan may have the desirable consequences of improving the quality of care, it also may penalize hospitals that admit high-risk patients and inadvertently encourage institutions to underreport VAP or to overuse antibiotics, thereby favoring dissemination of MDR microorganisms. This possibility further underscores the need to evaluate all new strategies potentially aimed at preventing VAP by comparing them to current best clinical practices.

Key Points

- *Ventilator-associated pneumonia* (VAP) is associated with mortality in excess of that caused by the underlying disease alone, particularly in the case of infection due to high-risk pathogens, such as *P. aeruginosa* and methicillin-resistant *S. aureus*, and/or when the initial therapy is inappropriate.
- The predominant organisms responsible for infection are *P. aeruginosa*, *S. aureus*, and Enterobacteriaceae, but etiologic agents differ widely according to the population of hospital patients, the duration of hospital stay, and prior antimicrobial therapy.
- Because even a few doses of an antimicrobial agent can negate results of microbiologic cultures, pulmonary secretions in patients suspected of having developed VAP should always be obtained before new antibiotics are administered.
- The initial approach to antimicrobial therapy involves administering broad-spectrum antibiotics to avoid inadequate treatment in patients with true bacterial pneumonia.
- The management of antibiotic therapy for VAP should optimize care without overusing and abusing antibiotics by stopping therapy in patients with a low probability of VAP, streamlining treatment once the etiologic agent is known, switching to monotherapy after days 3 to 5, and shortening duration of therapy

to 7 to 8 days, as dictated by the patient's clinical response to therapy and information about the bacteriology of the infection.

- Evidence-based preventive measures include staffing nurses at appropriate levels, avoiding intubation by using noninvasive ventilation whenever possible in suitable populations, and reducing the duration of ventilation by maintaining low tidal volume ventilation and sedating at minimal levels coupled with paired daily spontaneous awakening and breathing trials.
- Current evidence is insufficient to favor either a clinical or invasive approach to diagnosis of VAP regarding clinical outcomes, although evidence indicates that the invasive approach can reduce use of antibiotics.

Key Readings

Chastre J, Fagon JY. Ventilator-associated pneumonia. *Am J Respir Crit Care Med.* 2002;165:867–903.

Chastre J, Wolff M, Fagon JY, et al. Comparison of 8 vs 15 days of antibiotic therapy for ventilator-associated pneumonia in adults: a randomized trial. *JAMA.* 2003;290:2588–2598.

Fagon JY, Chastre J, Wolff M, et al. Invasive and noninvasive strategies for management of suspected ventilator-associated pneumonia. A randomized trial. *Ann Intern Med.* 2000;132:621–630.

Heyland D, Dodek P, Muscedere J, et al. A randomized trial of diagnostic techniques for ventilator-associated pneumonia. *N Engl J Med.* 2006;355:2619–2630.

Kalil AC, Metersky ML, Klompas M, et al. Management of adults with hospital-acquired and ventilator-associated pneumonia: 2016 clinical practice guidelines by the infectious diseases society of America and the American thoracic society. *Clin Infect Dis.* 2016;63:e61–e111.

Klompas M, Branson R, Eichenwald EC, et al. Strategies to prevent ventilator-associated pneumonia in acute care hospitals: 2014 update. *Infect Control Hosp Epidemiol.* 2014;35(8):915–936.

Melsen WG, Rovers MM, Groenwold RH, et al. Attributable mortality of ventilator-associated pneumonia: a meta-analysis of individual patient data from randomised prevention studies. *Lancet Infect Dis.* 2013;13:665–671.

Roberts JA, Abdul-Aziz MH, Lipman J, et al. Individualised antibiotic dosing for patients who are critically ill: Challenges and potential solutions. *Lancet Infect Dis.* 2014;14:498–509.

Schuetz P, Briel M, Christ-Crain M, et al. Procalcitonin to guide initiation and duration of antibiotic treatment in acute respiratory infections: an individual patient data meta-analysis. *Clin Infect Dis.* 2012;55:651–662.

Torres A, Niederman MS, Chastre J, et al. International ERS/ESICM/ESCMID/ALAT guidelines for the management of hospital-acquired pneumonia and ventilator-associated pneumonia. *Eur Respir J.* 2017;50(3).

Complete reference list available at ExpertConsult.com.

50 | *LUNG ABSCESS*

NISHA H. GIDWANI, MD

INTRODUCTION	**RADIOGRAPHIC FEATURES**	Antimicrobial Therapy
DEFINITION	**DIAGNOSTIC STUDIES**	Surgical Intervention
PATHOPHYSIOLOGY	**MICROBIOLOGY**	Percutaneous Tube Drainage
CLINICAL MANIFESTATIONS	**COMPLICATIONS**	Endoscopic Drainage
DIFFERENTIAL DIAGNOSIS	**TREATMENT**	**KEY POINTS**

INTRODUCTION

A lung abscess forms as a result of lung tissue necrosis, most commonly due to a polymicrobial infection creating a cavity. Organisms originating in the oral cavity are usually responsible for causing lung abscesses; however, other organisms may be involved in certain contexts, such as in patients with immunodeficiency. This chapter discusses the clinical manifestations, differential diagnosis, diagnostic studies, and therapeutic options for lung abscesses.

DEFINITION

A lung abscess can be defined by chronicity or by the isolation of a specific organism. For example, if symptoms have been present for more than 1 month prior to seeking medical attention, the abscess is considered chronic. If an organism is isolated on culture, the lung abscess can be defined by the organism (e.g., a *Pseudomonas* lung abscess). As detailed later, isolation of anaerobic organisms requires specialized culture conditions and, if a sample is not handled rapidly and properly, cultures may be negative even if organisms are apparent on Gram-stained specimens. If no pathogen is identified, it is termed a nonspecific lung abscess.

A lung abscess can also be described as primary or secondary. Primary lung abscesses develop in immunocompetent individuals most commonly due to large-volume or frequent, small-volume aspiration. Secondary lung abscesses are associated with an underlying pulmonary parenchymal condition or immunodeficiency.

PATHOPHYSIOLOGY

Most lung abscesses are thought to be caused by aspiration of anaerobic bacteria from the oral cavity, primarily from the gingival crevices. Periodontal disease is a major risk factor for the development of anaerobic pleuropulmonary infections.[1] Individuals with teeth or dentures have an increased incidence of oropharyngeal colonization by respiratory pathogens compared to edentulous patients.

Aspiration may be secondary to dysphagia or a reduced level of consciousness from alcohol, sedating drugs, head trauma, seizures, or general anesthesia. With a decreased level of consciousness and a defective cough reflex, patients cannot clear the bacteria from their lungs. Pneumonitis can develop over 7 to 14 days and, in certain circumstances, necrosis may follow. Apart from primary lung infection, pulmonary cavities may develop due to many noninfectious causes (see later), which may mimic infectious lung abscesses. A small subset of lung abscesses are due to complications from bronchoscopic procedures, including from transbronchial forceps biopsy, endobronchial ultrasound-guided mediastinal biopsy, and transbronchial lung cryobiopsy.[3,4]

CLINICAL MANIFESTATIONS

In lung abscesses caused by anaerobic bacteria, symptoms are usually indolent. Fever, cough, and sputum production can develop over weeks to months. Symptoms can also include night sweats and weight loss, especially when an underlying systemic process exists. Occasionally, patients report pleuritic chest pain, hemoptysis, and foul-smelling sputum. The physical examination is often nonspecific. Findings may include fever, a decreased level of consciousness, and poor dentition. Lung exam may reveal crackles, egophony, and/or dullness to percussion if a pleural effusion is present.

DIFFERENTIAL DIAGNOSIS

Bacterial organisms are the leading cause of tissue necrosis and lung abscess formation; however, fungi and parasites must also be kept in the differential diagnosis. The cavity appearance on imaging is not specific for the type of organism (Figs. 50.1 and 50.2). Noninfectious causes of pulmonary cavities include septic emboli, vasculitis (e.g., granulomatosis with polyangiitis), malignancy, bronchiectasis, and bronchostenosis caused by a foreign body or an obstructing mass (Figs. 50.3 and 50.4).

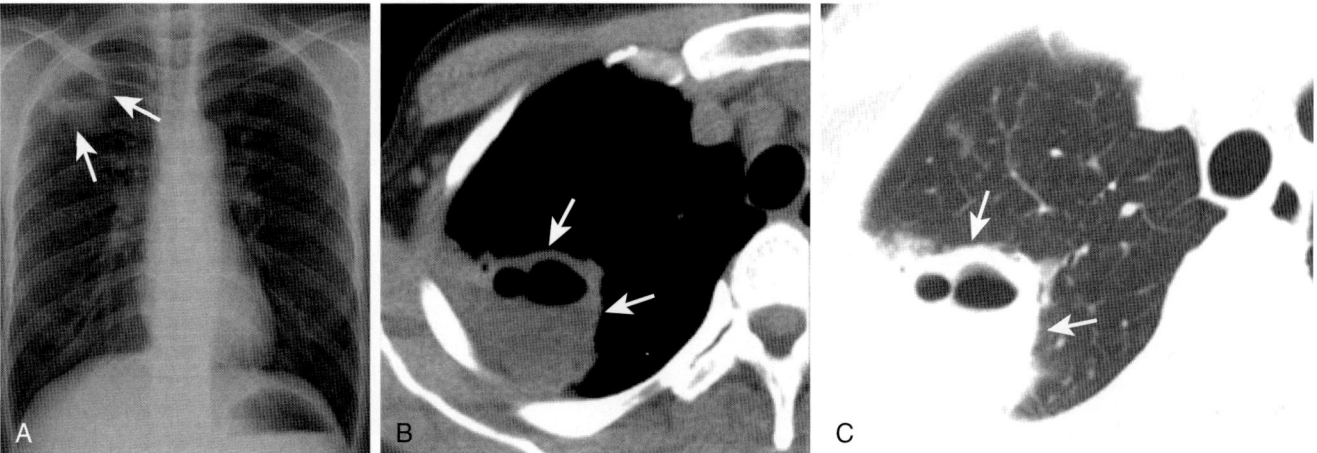

Figure 50.1 *Klebsiella pneumoniae* lung abscess. (A) Frontal chest radiograph shows a subpleural right apical cavity (*arrows*) with an air-fluid level consistent with a pulmonary abscess. Axial thoracic computed tomography displayed in soft tissue (B) and lung (C) windows shows a nonspecific cavity (*arrows*) consistent with a pulmonary abscess. (Courtesy Michael B. Gotway, MD.)

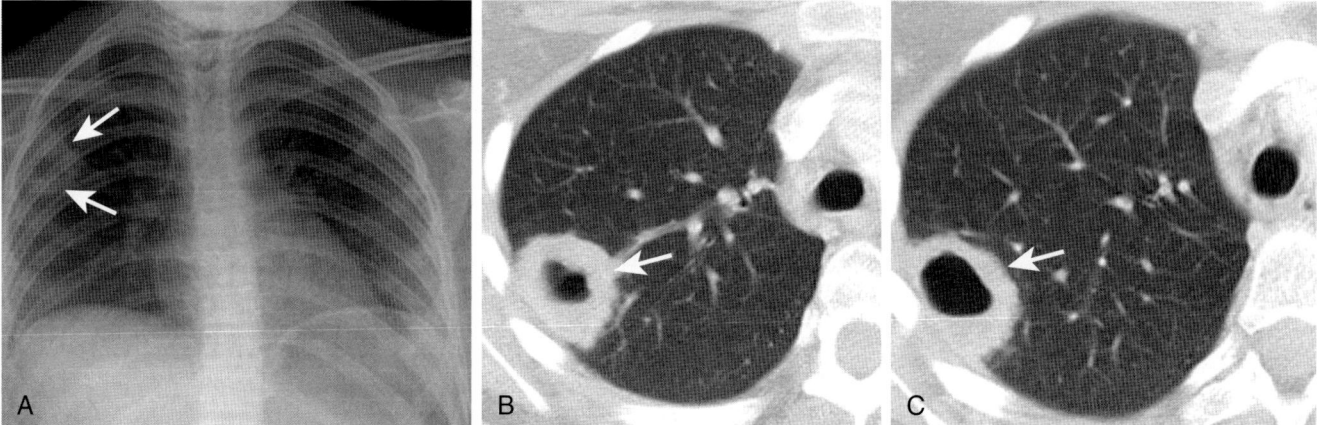

Figure 50.2 *Nocardia asteroides* lung abscess. (A) Frontal chest radiograph shows a poorly defined opacity (*arrows*) in the subpleural right upper lobe. (B–C) Axial thoracic computed tomography displayed in lung windows shows a subpleural right upper lobe cavity (*arrows*) containing an air-fluid level. This lesion is nonspecific in appearance and could be the result of a number of infections, but *Nocardia asteroides* was recovered at biopsy. (Courtesy Michael B. Gotway, MD.)

RADIOGRAPHIC FEATURES

Chest imaging allows the practitioner to confirm a diagnosis of lung abscess. Chest radiographs may demonstrate a cavity with an air-fluid level and a surrounding infiltrate (Fig. 50.5). The abnormality is commonly noted in the posterior segment of the upper lobes or the superior segment of the lower lobes, areas most dependent in a supine person and thus most susceptible to aspiration. Because the right main bronchus is shorter, larger in diameter, and more vertical than the left bronchus, aspiration tends to favor the right lung.[5] If there is uncertainty in the diagnosis based on chest radiographs, *computed tomography* (CT) of the chest can be obtained. Chest CT can also be helpful in evaluating secondary causes of lung abscess.

Features on CT imaging may help to distinguish a pulmonary abscess from a benign cavity, a malignant lesion, septic emboli, or an empyema. Benign cavities tend to have a thin wall without surrounding abnormalities such as ground-glass opacities or a consolidation. Although data are limited, features that favor a lung abscess include an air-fluid level, a surrounding parenchymal opacity such as ground-glass opacity or consolidation, and an irregular ("shaggy") inner wall. Characteristics that suggest a malignant lesion include a more nodular inner wall and a wall thickness of 16 mm or greater, although this can vary depending on the type of malignancy (see Fig. 50.3).[6] Lymphadenopathy and a pleural effusion may also favor a malignant process. In contrast, septic emboli in the lung usually manifest as multiple, distinct nodules (1 to 3 cm in diameter) with cavities in different stages. They also cause subpleural wedge-shaped infiltrates.[7] A pleural empyema is often oblong in appearance, has a smooth lining, and compresses the surrounding lung, whereas a pulmonary abscess is typically round (a similar dimension in different views), has a ragged inner lining, and does not compress the adjacent lung because it primarily causes necrosis of the lung parenchyma (see Fig. 108.2). Additional nodules and cavities in the lung strongly suggest embolization or a noninfectious inflammatory disorder, such as vasculitis (see Fig. 50.4).

DIAGNOSTIC STUDIES

When a pulmonary abscess is suspected, expectorated sputum should be sent for Gram stain and aerobic culture. Because many anaerobic bacteria are rapidly killed by exposure to atmospheric oxygen, accurate results from anaerobic cultures require rapid transport and handling by the microbiology

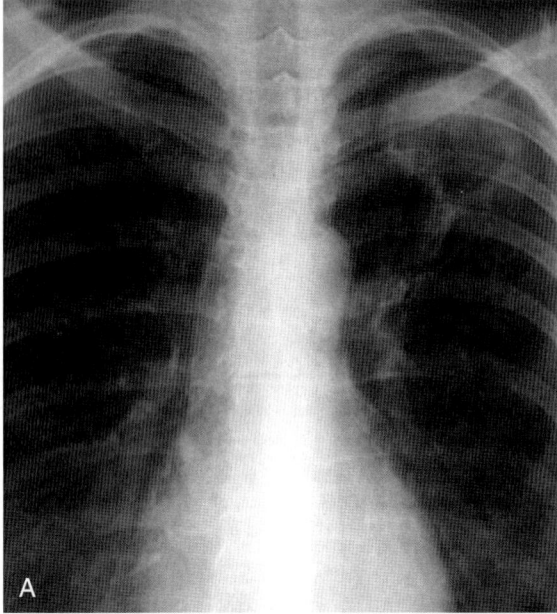

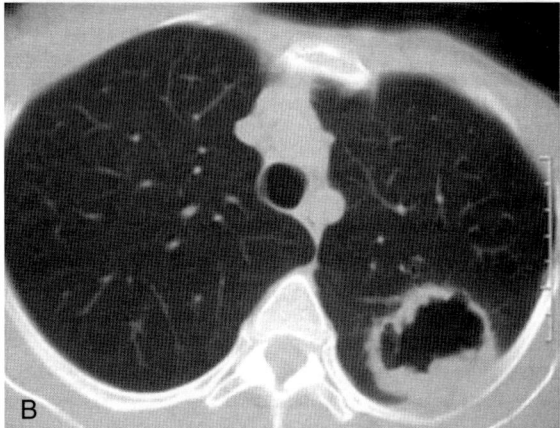

Figure 50.3 Lung abscess mimics: squamous cell carcinoma of the lung. (A) Frontal chest radiography shows a left apical cavitary lesion. The patient had poor dentition with a history of alcoholism and presented with fever; aspiration pneumonia and abscess were considered. Follow-up chest radiography 2 weeks later following broad-spectrum antibiotic therapy showed no change in the lesion, which prompted *computed tomography* (CT). (B) Axial CT displayed in lung windows shows that the cavitary left apical lesion has an irregularly thick posterior wall (>15 mm) with a grossly nodular appearance. The asymmetric wall thickening and nodularity suggest a malignant etiology for the cavity. (Courtesy Michael B. Gotway, MD.)

laboratory. Even with appropriate handling, samples may be contaminated by bacteria from the oral cavity. Whether metagenomic sequencing can be useful in diagnosis and treatment decisions remains to be determined.[8] For optimal results, samples should be obtained and submitted to the microbiology laboratory prior to initiation of antibiotic therapy.

Procedures such as thoracentesis, bronchoscopy, and transthoracic needle aspiration may be warranted, especially if an individual is not improving with antibiotic therapy. A thoracentesis should be performed if a pleural effusion exists because it provides an uncontaminated specimen that may represent the etiologic agent of an adjacent abscess. If the abscess is anaerobic, bronchoscopy with bronchoalveolar lavage or quantitative brush catheter cultures may not recover the causative organism, because there are only a limited number of cases in which anaerobic organisms have been isolated.[9] Nonetheless, efforts should be made to recover a causative organism, and bronchoalveolar lavage samples should be sent for bacterial, mycobacterial, and fungal cultures. Outside of obtaining cultures, bronchoscopy can be used to evaluate the airways, biopsy a mass, or remove a foreign body if present. Bronchoscopy with bronchoalveolar lavage is often considered early in immunocompromised patients, for whom evaluating opportunistic infections is a high priority.

Transthoracic needle aspiration can provide a clean specimen for culture. It can also be helpful for drainage of abscesses that do not openly communicate with a bronchus. The procedure should be considered early in those with an abscess greater than 4 cm because they have a higher risk of not responding to antibiotic therapy.[10]

If a vasculitis is suspected (see Fig. 50.4), serum markers (e.g., *antineutrophil cytoplasmic antibodies* [ANCAs]) should be obtained. Blood cultures are not routinely recommended in those who do not have sepsis or septic shock. However, when septic emboli are a possibility, especially in the setting of multiple abscesses, blood cultures and a transthoracic echocardiogram to evaluate for vegetations should be obtained.

MICROBIOLOGY[5,11–13]

Most infectious causes of a lung abscess are due to anaerobes and facultative anaerobes that colonize the oral cavity. Lung abscesses are usually polymicrobial, with the most common organisms being *Peptostreptococcus,*

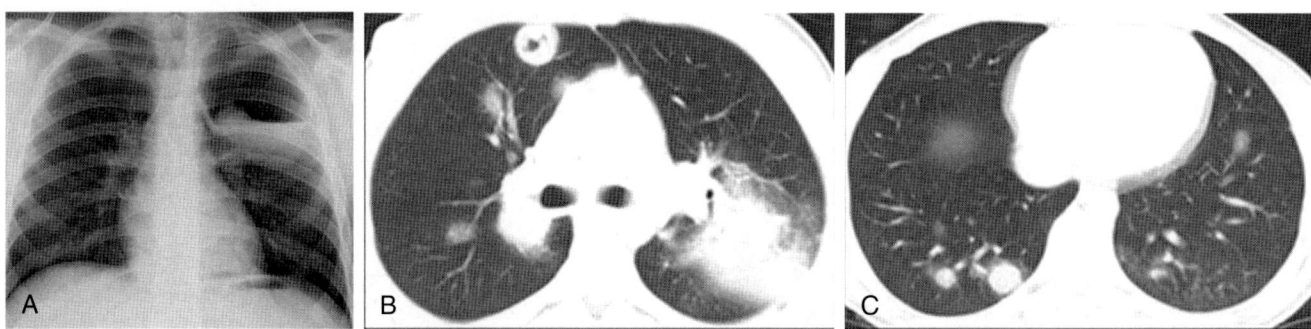

Figure 50.4 Lung abscess mimics granulomatosis with polyangiitis. (A) Frontal chest radiography shows a large left upper lobe cavity with a gas-fluid level resembling a pulmonary abscess. (B–C) Axial computed tomography through the mid and lower lungs demonstrates additional nodules and cavities in the right lung. This strongly favors either systemic embolization or a noninfectious inflammatory disorder, such as vasculitis, over a pulmonary abscess. (Courtesy Michael B. Gotway, MD.)

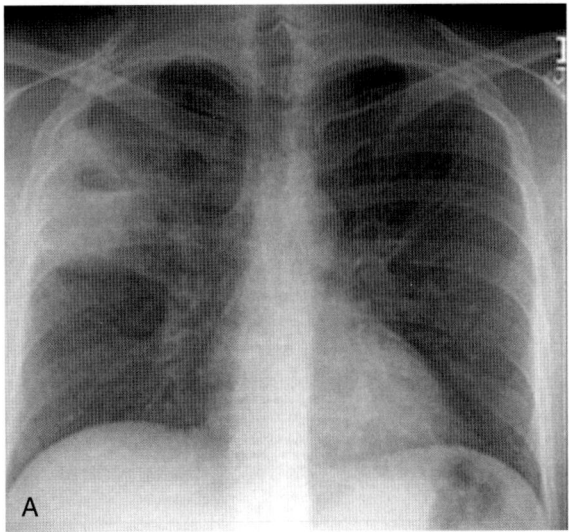

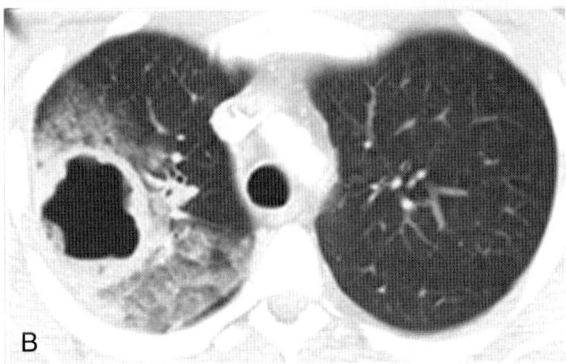

Figure 50.5 **Pyogenic lung abscess.** (A) Frontal chest radiography shows a subpleural right upper lobe cavitary lesion with a gas-fluid level. (B) Axial computed tomography displayed in lung windows shows a mildly thick-walled cavitary lesion with a lobulated internal border and surrounding ground-glass opacity located within the subpleural right apex. (Courtesy Michael B. Gotway, MD.)

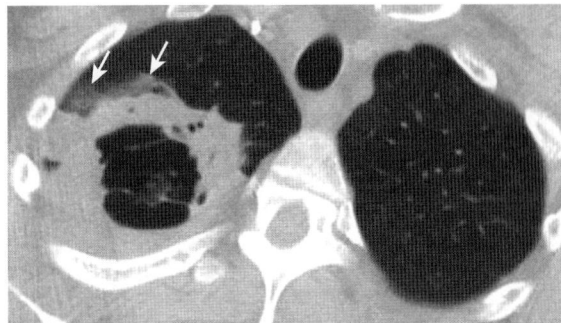

Figure 50.6 **Lung abscess with hemoptysis.** Axial chest computed tomography displayed in lung windows shows a complex, thick-walled right apical cavity consistent with a pyogenic abscess. Ground-glass opacity (*arrows*) surrounds the anterior margin of the cavity, consistent with hemorrhage given the history of hemoptysis, although the imaging appearance is nonspecific. (Courtesy Michael B. Gotway, MD.)

intervention in attempts to drain a lung abscess. With bronchoscopic drainage, pus can also spill from the abscess to other areas of the lung.[18,19]

The bronchial arteries are responsible for supplying blood to a lung abscess and are the major source of hemoptysis.[22] Minor hemoptysis may be seen with a lung abscess (Fig. 50.6). Although rare, life-threatening hemoptysis can also be a complication of abscess[20,21] and may require emergent pulmonary resection of the lesion to allow for hemostasis.[23]

Central nervous system complications, such as stroke[24] and brain abscess, are recognized consequences of lung abscess. These may arise because clots and bacteria can bypass the filtering action of the lung to reach the systemic circulation. In a population-based, nested case-control study of more than 1300 patients with brain abscess, lung abscess or bronchiectasis was associated with brain abscess by an adjusted odds ratio of 8.2 (95% confidence interval, 3.6 to 18.5).[25]

Fusobacterium, *Prevotella*, and *Bacteroides* species (usually not *B. fragilis*).[14–16] Monomicrobial abscesses can be caused by *Staphylococcus aureus*, *Streptococcus pyogenes*, *Klebsiella pneumoniae*, *Pseudomonas aeruginosa*, and other gram-negative bacilli. Multidrug-resistant *K. pneumoniae* has been isolated from lung abscesses of patients in Taiwan, suggesting a possible shift in the bacteriology of abscesses or a different prevalence based on region.[17] Fungi, parasites, and mycobacteria may also cause pulmonary abscesses. These organisms must be considered, especially if a patient is not responding to antimicrobial therapy or is immunocompromised.

Some organisms have unique characteristics. *S. aureus* is known to cause a secondary infection with cavity formation in patients with underlying influenza virus. *Pneumocystis jirovecii* can cause cysts in the lung mimicking cavities.

COMPLICATIONS

Complications of a lung abscess can include hemoptysis, bronchopleural fistula, empyema, and mediastinitis. The latter three complications can be seen after surgical

TREATMENT

In a landmark paper in 1936 (pre-antibiotic era), 2114 cases of pyogenic lung abscesses were divided between conservative management, drainage by bronchoscopy or posturing, and surgery. For all three therapies, the mortality rate was between 32% and 34%.[26,27] With the advent of antibiotics, the mortality from lung abscess has decreased to 15–20%. In immunocompromised patients, those with bronchial obstruction, or large abscesses (>6 cm), mortality may be as high as 75% despite appropriate therapy.[28,29]

ANTIMICROBIAL THERAPY

Empirical therapy must include antibiotics to cover strict anaerobes and facultative anaerobic streptococci. Recommended therapy is a combination of a β-lactam plus β-lactamase inhibitor or clindamycin.[30] Clindamycin is a good option if a patient has a β-lactam allergy; however, it is generally avoided due to the concern for developing *Clostridium difficile* infection. A carbapenem with good bioavailability in the lung parenchyma is another option;

however, monotherapy with meropenem does not have activity against streptococci and hence should be avoided.

Monomicrobial *S. aureus* abscesses are a known complication of influenza.[31] For methicillin-susceptible *S. aureus*, choice of antibiotic includes cefazolin, nafcillin, or oxacillin. For methicillin-resistant *S. aureus* infection, the drug of choice is linezolid with the alternative being vancomycin. Of note, daptomycin has poor bioavailability in the lungs and should not be used.

With empirical antibiotic therapy, clinical improvement should be apparent within 3 to 4 days, with defervescence in 7 to 10 days. If clinical improvement is not apparent, one must consider reasons for a delayed response, such as an obstruction (foreign body vs. neoplasm), resistant bacteria, mycobacteria or fungus, large cavity size (>6 cm in diameter), or empyema. Vasculitis and septic emboli should also be reconsidered and evaluated based on clinical suspicion.

Duration of antibiotic therapy averages between 4 and 6 weeks. This largely depends on radiographic improvement. If the patient is worsening clinically or new symptoms develop, imaging should be obtained sooner. On chest radiographs or CT, the abscess should completely resolve or reduce in size to a stable lesion prior to the discontinuation of antibiotics. This can usually be achieved with an oral antibiotic regimen.

SURGICAL INTERVENTION

Surgical resection of an abscess is needed in approximately 10% of cases.[32] Indications for surgical intervention include hemoptysis, bronchopleural fistula, empyema, large cavity size (>6 cm), an obstructed bronchus, or lack of response to 12 weeks of antibiotic therapy. Lobectomy is preferred to segmentectomy due to concern for incomplete removal of the abscess and necrotic tissue with risk of reinfection.[33] Video-assisted thoracoscopy is preferred if the lung abscess is peripherally located and there are no pleural adhesions. A double-lumen endotracheal tube is often used to avoid spillage of contents into the unaffected lung. Other less invasive alternatives to surgery include percutaneous and endoscopic drainage of the lung abscess.

PERCUTANEOUS TUBE DRAINAGE

Percutaneous tube drainage is largely considered in those who cannot tolerate surgery; however, it is becoming more commonly used when available.[34,35] First described in 1938, it was initially used to drain cavities caused by tuberculosis. It grew to be used for the management of all lung abscesses prior to the antibiotic era (see eFig. 21.9). Indications for this intervention include abscess size of greater than 4 cm, peripherally located lesions, and lack of adequate spontaneous drainage.[36,37] Evaluation with bronchoscopy is important in ruling out a bronchial obstruction because this would be an indication for surgery instead. Percutaneous tube drainage can be used for palliation in septic patients with lung abscess and underlying lung cancer.[38]

The procedure is usually performed under CT guidance but can be performed at the bedside with ultrasound guidance.[39] The affected lung is placed down to minimize spillage into the unaffected lung. Once the catheter is in place, the fluid is aspirated. Gentle irrigation with normal saline is performed daily. The value of placing fibrinolytic agents into the abscess is unknown but is not recommended due to concern for complications.[40] A reduction in the size of the abscess with clinical improvement and no evidence of purulent drainage for 3 days is one measure used to determine the appropriate time to remove the catheter.

Complications of percutaneous tube drainage include hemoptysis, pneumothorax, hemothorax, and obstruction of the catheter. A bronchopleural fistula may also develop and cause contamination of the pleural space resulting in an empyema.

ENDOSCOPIC DRAINAGE

Endoscopic drainage is considered when medical therapy has failed and percutaneous tube drainage is not an option. An endoscopic approach typically is used when the location of the abscess is central, if there is concern for an endobronchial obstruction, or in patients with coagulopathies.[41]

Bronchoscopy is performed by the nasal approach with a flexible bronchoscope, after which a guidewire is placed into the cavity under fluoroscopic guidance. The bronchoscope is then removed and a pigtail catheter is placed over the guidewire. With the use of contrast through the pigtail catheter, the appropriate positioning is confirmed. The guidewire is then removed and the catheter secured to the nose. In one study, the catheter was kept open to gravity and flushed with a mixture of gentamycin and normal saline twice a day. The primary concern of doing this procedure is spillage of abscess contents to unaffected portions of the lung.[18]

Endoscopic drainage using laser to access the cavity has also been reported. The pigtail catheter is introduced via bronchoscopy and the laser is used to puncture the abscess to create a path to insert the catheter. Catheters were kept in for 4 to 6 days with both clinical and radiographic improvement.[19]

Key Points

- Most lung abscesses are caused by aspiration of anaerobic bacteria from the oral cavity.
- Patients typically present with indolent symptoms such as fever, cough, and sputum production over weeks to months.
- Symptoms, duration of symptoms, and chest imaging (chest radiography or computed tomography) with findings of a cavity and often an air-fluid level lead to the diagnosis.
- Routine Gram stain and culture (including mycobacterial and fungal) should be sent, although false-negative cultures are common due to the prevalence of anaerobic bacteria. Coverage of anaerobic bacteria is crucial when choosing antibiotic therapy.
- If a pleural effusion exists, a thoracentesis should be performed to obtain an uncontaminated specimen and evaluate for an empyema.

- If a patient is not improving clinically, it is important to consider other conditions such as bronchial obstruction, cancer, vasculitis, resistant organisms, or other organisms such as mycobacterium and fungi not adequately covered by the current antibiotic regimen.
- Duration of antibiotic therapy ranges from weeks to months, depending on clinical and radiographic improvement. Close clinical monitoring with a low threshold for repeat radiographic imaging is imperative.
- If a patient is not responding to antibiotic therapy, surgery, percutaneous transthoracic tube drainage, or endoscopic drainage may be warranted.

Key Readings

Bartlett JG, Finegold SM. Anaerobic infections of the lung and pleural space. *Am Rev Respir Dis.* 1974;110:56.

Bartlett JG, Gorbach SL, Tally FP, Finegold SM. Bacteriology and treatment of primary lung abscess. *Am Rev Respir Dis.* 1974;109:510.

Hirshberg B, Sklair-Levi M, Nir-Paz R, et al. Factors predicting mortality of patients with lung abscess. *Chest.* 1999;115:746.

Kuhajda I, Zarogoulidis K, Tsirgogianni K, et al. Lung abscess-etiology, diagnostic and treatment options. *Ann Transl Med.* 2015;3(13):183.

Yazbeck MF, Dahdel M, Kalra A, Browne AS, Pratter MR. Lung abscess: update on microbiology and management. *Am J Ther.* 2014;21(3):217–221.

Wang J-L, Chen K-y, Fang C-T, et al. Changing bacteriology of adult community-acquired lung abscess in Taiwan: Klebsiella pneumoniae versus anaerobes. *Clin Infect Dis.* 2005;40:915–922.

Complete reference list available at ExpertConsult.com.

51 TUBERCULOSIS: EPIDEMIOLOGY AND PREVENTION

PHILIP C. HOPEWELL, MD • MIDORI KATO-MAEDA, MD, MS

INTRODUCTION
EPIDEMIOLOGY OF TUBERCULOSIS
TRANSMISSION OF *M. TUBERCULOSIS*
Source Case
Environmental Factors
Circumstances of Exposure
Host Factors

Lessons from genotyping *M. Tuberculosis*
Risk Factors for Disease
PREVENTION OF TUBERCULOSIS
Prompt Diagnosis and Effective
Treatment
Infection Control Measures to Reduce
Transmission of *M. Tuberculosis*

Treatment of Latent Tuberculosis
Infection
Immunization with Bacille
Calmette-Guérin
New Tuberculosis Vaccines
KEY POINTS

INTRODUCTION

Tuberculosis (TB) has been recognized as a scourge of humanity since antiquity. TB was considered the "captain of all these men of death," according to John Bunyan—a plague that seemingly carried away the young and talented members of society. TB continues to ravage much of the developing world and is still the single most common infection causing death.[1]

TB is caused by any one of three mycobacterial pathogens that are part of the *Mycobacterium tuberculosis* complex: *Mycobacterium tuberculosis*, *Mycobacterium bovis*, and *Mycobacterium africanum*. *M. bovis* and *M. africanum* produce relatively few cases of human TB and *M. africanum* is restricted to specific regions of Africa or people from those regions. *Mycobacterium canettii* is not part of the *M. tuberculosis* complex, but has been identified as a cause of TB in a small number of patients from or with connection to East Africa.[2]

The *M. tuberculosis* phylogenetic tree has a geographic structure from which the initial *M. tuberculosis* major lineage names were derived: Indo-Oceanic (lineage 1), East-Asian (lineage 2), Indian and East-African (lineage 3), Euro-American (lineage 4), West-African 1 (lineage 5), West-African 2 (lineage 6), and Ethiopian (lineage 7).[3] The two West-African lineages together comprise *M. africanum*.[4] Studies have suggested that different lineages of *M. tuberculosis* may be associated with different degrees of pathogenicity, as reflected in differing rates of *tuberculin skin test* (TST) conversion, rates of TB following exposure, genotypic clustering, and virulence in guinea pigs.[5-13]

EPIDEMIOLOGY OF TUBERCULOSIS

Infection with *M. tuberculosis* is prevalent throughout the world. It is estimated that one-fourth of the world population (1.7 billion people in 2014) is infected with *M. tuberculosis*, although the distribution is heterogeneous.[14,15] TB infection and disease are found in all countries regardless of their state of development, and the movements of people from and to areas of high prevalence influences the incidence of TB everywhere. For this reason, TB has been declared by the *World Health Organization* (WHO) as a global public health emergency to be addressed by global strategies and initiatives, the most recent being a United Nations high-level meeting on TB in 2018, in which heads of state endorsed a commitment to end TB by 2030.[16]

For most of recorded history, TB has been a problem of enormous dimensions worldwide—and it still is. Although both the number of new cases of TB and the number of deaths has been decreasing in the last 15 years, the annual reduction trend will not be sufficient to reach the goal of 90% reduction in TB incidence (relative to 2015) by 2035.[17,18] In 2018, there were an estimated 10 million new TB cases, of which only 7.0 million were reported to national public health authorities, leaving an estimated 3 million unaccounted for.[17] In the same year, there were 1.2 million deaths due to TB[17] with a case fatality rate of 15%.[18] Relative to 2017, in 2018 there was no decline in the number of new cases, but there was a decline of 9% in the number of deaths.[18] The epidemiology of TB varies widely around the world. In 2018, 86% of the cases were identified in the WHO regions of Southeast Asia (44%) (incidence 220 per 100,000 persons), Africa (24%) (incidence 231 per 100,000 persons), and the Western Pacific (18%) (incidence 96 per 100,000).[17] Most of the high-income countries have an incidence of less than 10 new cases per 100,000 population,[17] and TB elimination is an achievable goal.

The prevalence of the *human immunodeficiency virus* (HIV) infection is an important determinant of TB epidemiology.[18] *People living with HIV* (PLHIV) are 20 to 30 times more likely to develop TB than those without HIV.[19]

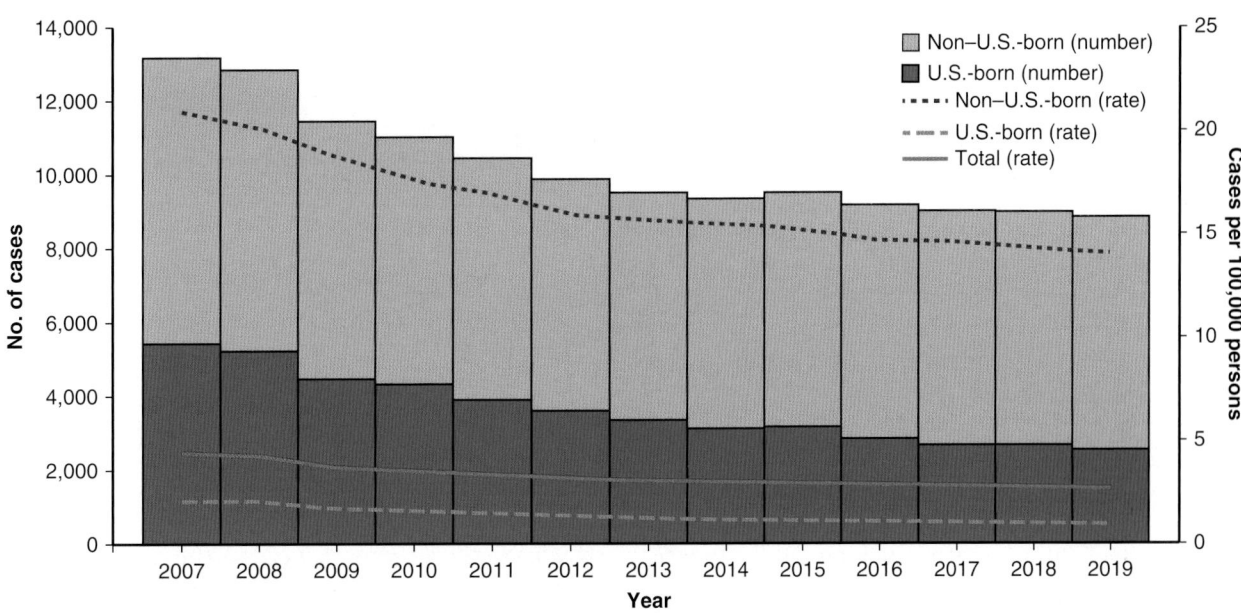

* Number of cases with unknown national origin not shown (range = 2–60 per year; median = 7). Total rate includes cases with unknown national origin.

†Rates for non–U.S.-born and U.S.-born persons were calculated using Current Population Survey estimates. Total rate was calculated using U.S. Census Bureau population estimates.

Figure 51.1 Tuberculosis case counts and rates by national origin, United States: 2007–19. The number of cases with unknown national origin is not shown (range, 2–60 per year; median = 7). Total rate includes cases with unknown national origin. Rates for non-U.S.-born and U.S.-born persons were calculated using Current Population Survey estimates. Total rate was calculated using U.S. Census Bureau population estimates. (From Schwartz NG, Price SF, Pratt RH, Langer AJ. Tuberculosis—United States, 2019. *MMWR Morb Mortal Wkly Rep.* 2020;69:286–289.)

In 2018, 8.6% of all TB cases were among persons with HIV infection. TB causes one in three HIV deaths.[20] Most of the cases of HIV-TB and deaths were in Africa, where 70% of the 37 million people living with HIV live.[20]

Diabetes mellitus triples the risk for TB and increases the likelihood of poor treatment outcomes. In 2017, there were an estimated 425 million people living with diabetes and it is predicted that it will increase by 48% to 629 million in 2045, which will likely make achievement of the global TB targets even more difficult. The biggest increases will be in Africa and Asia, where most of the TB burden is located.[21,22] In patients with TB worldwide, the prevalence of diabetes was 15.3% and varied from 0.1% in Latvia to 45.2% in Marshall Islands.[21]

Poverty is a powerful determinant of TB. Although it is not possible to quantify the number of TB cases directly associated with poverty, crowded and poorly ventilated living spaces, malnutrition, and lack of empowerment to act on health issues, all of which are associated with poverty, are important risk factors for TB and TB transmission.[23]

Drug-resistant TB is challenging global control efforts and is an important component of the TB epidemic. Despite the reduction in the number of cases of TB worldwide, progress is threatened by *multidrug-resistant* (MDR) TB (caused by organisms resistant to at least isoniazid and rifampin) and *extensively drug-resistant* (XDR) TB (MDR organisms also resistant to at least one fluoroquinolone and to at least one injectable second-line agent).[24] It is estimated that in 2018, 500,000 people developed TB resistant to rifampicin, the most effective first-line anti-TB drug, 78% of whom had MDR-TB.[17] Almost half of

the rifampin-resistant/MDR-TB cases were seen in people from three countries: India (24%), China (13%), and Russia (10%).[17] In 2006, XDR TB was reported for the first time[25,26] and, by the end of 2018, XDR-TB had been reported by 131 WHO member states.[17] In 2017, 6.2% of MDR TB cases had XDR-TB.[17] In 2018, only 32% of patients with MDR TB received second-line treatment and cure rates were far lower than those with drug-susceptible TB (56% vs. 85%, respectively).[17] Since 2000, WHO has implemented programs to increase access to drugs and to increase quality care for persons with drug-resistant TB. In spite of these efforts, a mathematical model forecasted that drug-resistant TB will increase in the four countries studied, reaching 12.4% among incident cases in India, 8.9% in the Philippines, 32.5% in Russia, and 4.7% in South Africa.[24] This increase will be driven by transmission of resistant strains rather than acquisition of resistance during treatment.[24]

In the United States following the introduction of effective chemotherapy, rates of TB decreased at an average annual rate of approximately 5%. However, from 1984 to 1992, the number of TB cases increased by 20%, because of the epidemic of infection with HIV and the deterioration of public health systems.[27] This resurgence clearly made the point that, no matter how successful the fight against TB seems to be, the guard cannot be let down. Interacting with and amplifying these two major factors were socioeconomic conditions, particularly homelessness that led to crowding, and immigration of persons from countries with high prevalence of TB.[27,28] With renewed effort and increased funding, case rates began to decline in 1993 (Fig. 51.1).[29] However, since 2012, the rate of decline has slowed to −1.5% per year, which is not sufficient to achieve TB elimination in the United States.[29]

In 2019 in the United States, 8920 cases (2.7 cases per 100,000 persons) were reported, the lowest number since systematic national reporting began in 1953; 71% of the cases were reported in non-U.S.-born persons. While the incidence of TB decreased overall by 71% from 1993 to 2019, the reduction was seen disproportionately among the U.S.-born population (86% reduction vs. 57% among non-U.S.-born persons).[29a]

TRANSMISSION OF *M. TUBERCULOSIS*

The key to elimination of TB is halting transmission of *M. tuberculosis*. Knowledge of the factors that govern transmission from a potentially infectious source and of the sequence by which the disease develops in a new host is vital for devising strategies for TB control and for evaluating the risk of a person becoming infected after exposure.[30]

The determinants of TB epidemiology differ in high-burden and low-burden settings.[31] In high-burden settings, ongoing transmission with rapid (within 1–2 years) progression to disease is the driving force.[32] In low-burden settings, TB more commonly results from reactivation of latent infection acquired earlier. However, both pathogenic sequences are seen in high- and low-burden settings.

The infectiousness of patients with TB is very heterogeneous. Transmission of *M. tuberculosis* is influenced by features of the source case, particularly the bacillary load, by the closeness of the potential recipient of the organism to the source, and by the circumstances of the exposure. A possible additional factor is the infectivity of the organism—the degree to which *M. tuberculosis* is able to establish itself within the lung or other sites in the new host. However, even taking these factors into account, there is substantial unexplained variability in the degree to which persons with untreated TB transmit the infection to persons to whom they are exposed.[33]

SOURCE CASE

TB is an airborne infection.[34] In nearly all instances infection is acquired by inhalation of *M. tuberculosis* contained in airborne particles (1 to 5 μm) that reach the alveoli. For a person with TB to be infectious, the organisms must access the environmental air and be aerosolized. *M. tuberculosis* expelled from the lungs in small droplets may remain suspended in the air for several hours.[35,36] Generally, only patients with pulmonary TB are infectious. Rarely, however, aerosols may be generated from other sources (e.g., irrigation of a tuberculous abscess).[37] There are at least four key factors determining infectiousness of a source case (Table 51.1).

The first factor determining infectiousness is the ability of the source case to generate aerosols containing droplets. Coughing is the most effective mechanism for generating aerosols that include droplet nuclei, but it is not the only way. Forced expiratory maneuvers, such

Table 51.1 Factors Influencing Infectiousness of the Source Case

Severity of coughing
Bacillary population
Antituberculosis therapy
Strain of *M. tuberculosis*

as sneezing, yelling, singing, and loud talking can also generate infectious droplets. In general, the greater the volume of respiratory secretions, the greater the number of potentially infectious droplets will be present. Studies have demonstrated marked variability in the infectious potential of TB patients that, in part, could be related to the severity of coughing.[38,39] Simple maneuvers, such as covering the mouth while coughing, can reduce formation of droplet nuclei by deflecting droplets from the air stream. Similarly, a mask worn by the patient is effective because particles are trapped while they are still large, before the water content has evaporated. For exposed persons, especially health care personnel, properly fitting N95 masks (disposable particulate respirators) are very efficient in removing respirable particles that may contain *M. tuberculosis*.[40]

The infectiousness of HIV-infected patients with TB is very heterogeneous. In an HIV-TB hospital ward, 90% of the infections in guinea pigs exposed to air exhausted from the ward were caused by 10 of 97 hospitalized patients.[41] Likewise, in a study of household contacts of TB patients, the likelihood of transmission was lower if the source case was HIV-infected and had a CD4 T cell count lower than 250/μL.[42]

A second factor determining infectiousness of the source case is the bacillary population in the lungs. This can be inferred from the extent and morphology of the disease, as determined by the chest radiograph and more directly estimated by microscopic examination of sputum. The bacillary population of tuberculous lesions depends on the morphology of the lesion.[43] The number of bacilli in solid nodular lesions ranges from 10^2 to 10^4 organisms, whereas in cavitary lesions, populations are on the order of 10^7 to 10^9 bacilli.[43] The prevalence of tuberculin reactors among contacts of patients with TB increases as the radiographic extent of involvement increases.[39] Thus, in TB control, the contacts of persons with more-extensive TB should be accorded a higher priority for evaluation than the contacts of persons with less-severe disease.

Another means of estimating bacillary population is microscopic examination of stained sputum smears. An average viable bacillary population of 5000 to 10,000 organisms per milliliter of sputum is required for the organisms to be seen in an acid-fast-stained sputum smear.[44] The contacts of patients who have organisms detected in sputum smears have a much higher prevalence of infection than do contacts of patients with negative smears and either positive or negative cultures.[45-48] However, the contacts of sputum smear-negative patients may still acquire tuberculous infection and develop TB.[49] Surprisingly, in a study of contact investigation conducted in the United States, neither smear positivity nor cavitation on the chest radiograph of the index case was a risk factor for incident TB among contacts.[50] However, the investigators did not examine incident infections (TST or *interferon-γ release assay* [IGRA] conversion from negative to positive). Other studies have shown that infectiousness was associated with the presence of cultivable organisms in coughed aerosols, which did not correlate with sputum smear results.[51]

A third important factor in determining the infectiousness of a source case is the use of antituberculous chemotherapy. Patients who had positive sputum smears but who were receiving antituberculosis drugs were much less infectious for guinea pigs than were untreated patients.[38,52] The relative infectiousness of untreated patients in comparison with treated patients was estimated at 50:1.[38,41,52] Consistent with these observations, clinical data indicate that, once treatment is begun to which the organisms are susceptible, transmission of *M. tuberculosis* decreases quickly and the major factor associated with persistent culture-positive aerosols is lack of effective treatment.[51] The most important mechanism by which anti-TB chemotherapy reduces infectiousness is the direct effect of the drug on the bacillary population in the lungs. There is a reduction in colony counts of nearly 2 $\log_{10}$ per milliliter of sputum in the first 2 days of treatment[53]; overall, in the initial 2 weeks of treatment there is a reduction of 99.9% in colony counts.[44] In addition to reducing the number of viable bacilli, anti-TB chemotherapy also promptly decreases coughing by 40% after 1 week of treatment and by 65% after 2 weeks.[39] The sum of these effects is that, once a patient with TB is placed on effective therapy, transmission of tubercle bacilli ceases to be a concern.

A final factor in the infectiousness of the source case is the particular strain of *M. tuberculosis*. Different strains of *M. tuberculosis* have different degrees of infectiousness. Estimates for the relative fitness of drug-resistant *M. tuberculosis* are heterogeneous, but overall showed a decrease in the ability to cause secondary cases, lower growth rate in vitro,[54] less progression to disease in guinea pigs,[55] or less transmissible and less able to progress to disease in modelling studies.[56] For example, strains of *M. tuberculosis* resistant to isoniazid caused fewer secondary cases than fully susceptible organisms.[57,58] However, even if there is lesser pathogenicity, this effect can easily be offset by a prolonged period of infectiousness, as might be expected with ineffective treatment or with exposure of an immunocompromised host.[41] In fact, outbreaks of TB caused by MDR and XDR strains of tubercle bacilli have taken place in hospitals or correctional facilities and disproportionately involve HIV-infected persons, although immunocompetent persons have also been involved.[25]

ENVIRONMENTAL FACTORS

The physical laws that apply to aerosolized particles dictate that droplet nuclei essentially become part of the environmental air; thus, environmental factors are of extreme importance in influencing transmission. In a study, under standard conditions of temperature and humidity indoors, 60% to 71% of aerosolized *M. tuberculosis* organisms survived for 3 hours, 48% to 56% for 6 hours, and 28% to 32% for 9 hours.[59] The influence of the concentration of

organisms in the environmental air in transmission of *M. tuberculosis* is exemplified by the outbreak that took place aboard a U.S. Navy vessel with a closed, recirculating ventilation system.[60] The index case had a positive sputum smear and a brisk cough, and infected 53 of 60 persons (88%) in his berth compartment, of whom six developed TB. In a second compartment connected to the same ventilation system, 43 of 81 persons (53%) became infected and one developed TB. Environmental factors may be manipulated to decrease the concentration of tubercle bacilli, mainly removing them by effective filtration, killing them with ultraviolet light, or both.[61] Since early in the twentieth century, it has been known that exposure to ultraviolet radiation kills tubercle bacilli.[38] The major usefulness of ultraviolet lights is for providing ultraviolet irradiation of room air, for example, by using appropriately shielded lamps on the upper walls in hospital areas or clinics where patients with untreated TB are likely to be encountered, such as waiting rooms.[62]

CIRCUMSTANCES OF EXPOSURE

The circumstances of exposure have a major influence on the number of infectious particles inhaled. If the exposure is of long duration and takes place under conditions that would be associated with a high concentration of droplet nuclei in the air inhaled by the contact, there is a greater likelihood of transmission.[63] This is reflected in data from the United States showing that rates of both clinical TB and tuberculin reactivity are much higher among close (generally household) than among nonclose (generally out-of-household) contacts. In general, the rate of TB is in the range of 15 per 1000 close contacts and 3 per 1000 nonclose contacts. Of close contacts, approximately 50% are infected, in comparison with approximately 15% of nonclose contacts.[64] Because the risk of TB is higher among close contacts, they should be screened and considered for preventive therapy. In the United States, treatment of *latent TB infection* (LTBI) among infected contacts reduced the rate of TB from 9.8% to 0.2% among contacts who completed a full course of treatment.[50] However, studies using molecular epidemiology to track transmission dynamics have shown that substantial transmission may take place outside the household, especially in areas with a high burden of TB.[65-68]

HOST FACTORS

There is substantial evidence that susceptibility to acquisition of infection with *M. tuberculosis* is highly variable. Not all individuals exposed to *M. tuberculosis* will become infected. In San Francisco, only 11% of household contacts and 3.8% of nonhousehold contacts developed new infection as reflected by conversion from negative to positive of the TST or IGRA.[68] Although variations in the intensity of exposure contribute to the likelihood of becoming infected, variations in host susceptibility are also likely to contribute. Strong evidence for variable susceptibility to acquisition of infection with *M. tuberculosis* was provided by a prospective study of student nurses in a TB hospital in Philadelphia in the era before anti-TB chemotherapy.[69] In that study, in which student nurses were assigned to rotations on the same TB wards, 30% remained uninfected (TST unreactive) after 2 years of nursing school, indicating that despite repeated exposure, some of the student nurses were less susceptible to infection. However, by the end of the third year of nursing school, 100% of the students had become infected, indicating that resistance to infection is quantitative, not absolute, and can be overcome by sufficient exposure.

Studies suggest that human genetic variability contributes to susceptibility or resistance to *M. tuberculosis* infection and in regulating both the establishment and the progression of the infection.[70,71] Both twins are more likely to develop TB if they are monozygotic than dizygotic (66.7% vs. 23%).[72] More recently, a review of host genetic studies concluded that, "the involvement of a human genetic component in susceptibility to infection with *M. tuberculosis* and progression to active disease is incontestable."[73] Several studies have demonstrated mutations associated with resistance or susceptibility to TB. However, there is little overlap in the loci identified in the individual studies.

LESSONS FROM GENOTYPING *M. TUBERCULOSIS*

Since the early 1990s, genotyping of *M. tuberculosis* has been used to determine if TB develops from exogenous or endogenous infection. *M. tuberculosis* DNA fingerprinting derived from different genotyping markers and methods has been used to track specific isolates of *M. tuberculosis* in a community.[74] Patients with TB with similar or identical genotypes are considered to be part of the same transmission chain.[75] In such situations, TB can be assumed to be due to a recent exogenous infection with rapid progression to TB. In contrast, patients with a unique DNA fingerprint are considered to have TB due to reactivation of latent infection acquired previously.

Genotyping can similarly be used to differentiate relapse from reinfection in a patient with recurrent TB: a patient with relapse will have a similar *M. tuberculosis* DNA fingerprint in both episodes while a patient with reinfection will have different strains.[76] Since the early 1990s, these markers have also enabled TB control programs, mainly in high-income settings, to track specific isolates of *M. tuberculosis* in a community to determine population-level risk factors for transmission, establish tailored public health strategies, and gauge the success of control measures.[77,78]

The genetic markers used to track strains in the community are sufficiently polymorphic to distinguish among unrelated isolates yet stable enough to recognize isolates that are part of the chain of transmission.[79] Genotyping using CRISPR (also known as spoligotypes)[80] and MIRU-VNTR (MIRU-type)[81] are currently widely used to track a strain in the community. More recently, the availability of high-throughput sequencing technology and the dramatic decrease in costs have enabled the use of whole genome sequencing to study transmission of *M. tuberculosis*.[82] Whole genome sequencing resolves transmission clusters with greater precision.[83] It also allows the identification of microevolutionary events (i.e., at the level of single nucleotide polymorphisms) within a chain of transmission, which can be used to determine the directionality of the transmission events.[84,85]

RISK FACTORS FOR DISEASE

After acquiring an infection, not all persons are at equal risk of developing TB.[86] Many conditions increase the likelihood of TB and serve as markers of increased risk. In healthy populations, the risk of developing TB is highest during the first year after infection; from 3–10% of newly infected persons develop TB during this period. The three factors presumably involved are the pathogenicity of the bacterial strain, the dose of bacilli implanted in the lungs, and the adequacy of the host response in countering the invasion. The "inoculum effect" (in which the likelihood of infection is directly related to the dose of bacteria) has not been clearly demonstrated in humans but is strongly suggested by results of animal experiments.[38] It is currently assumed that beyond the first year after infection has taken place, the immune response has fully developed, the number of organisms has been substantially reduced, and the remaining bacterial population has shifted to a state of persistence and slow replication. Understanding how this latent infection can shift to disease is critical in controlling TB.

Age is another risk factor. Among persons with TB infection, case rates vary markedly with age. Rates are considerably increased in infants and relatively increased in adolescents and young adults.[87] The reasons for the variations are not fully understood but are likely to relate to age-dependent influences on the effectiveness of the immune response.[88]

HIV infection is by far the most potent risk factor for TB worldwide. In the era before effective antiviral therapy, the TB case rate for persons who were infected with both HIV and *M. tuberculosis* was 7.9 per 100 person-years, which exceeds the rate in a population with LTBI without HIV infection.[89] It also appears that the risk of rapid progression to TB among persons who are infected with HIV and who then become infected with *M. tuberculosis* is tremendously increased, as has been demonstrated in descriptions of two such outbreaks.[90,91] The reported rates of TB in cohorts of persons with HIV infection vary widely and depend on the prevalence of TB in the environment, particularly the presence of infectious cases; the frequency with which treatment for LTBI is used; the severity of immune compromise within the HIV-infected group; and whether dually infected persons are receiving antiretroviral therapy, which substantially reduces the risk.[92,93]

Antiretroviral treatment of HIV markedly reduces the incidence of TB, although the effect is not complete. A meta-analysis revealed that antiretroviral treatment and reconstitution of CD4+ T cell counts reduces the incidence of TB as much as sixfold.[93] However, despite immune reconstitution to CD4 T cell counts greater than 700 cells/μL, the incidence of TB in antiretroviral-treated HIV-infected people remains 4.4-fold higher than in HIV-uninfected people in the same community.[94]

In persons with both HIV and LTBI, antiretroviral therapy and preventive treatment with isoniazid substantially decrease the incidence of TB. In Ivory Coast, a randomized trial demonstrated that a 6-month regimen of isoniazid preventive therapy in patients with HIV (median CD4+ T cell count of 463) receiving early or delayed antiretroviral therapy resulted in significantly fewer TB events than those assigned to no isoniazid preventive therapy.

Results showed a significant adjusted hazard ratio (aHR) of 0.43 in individuals with positive IGRA and a non-significant aHR among those with a negative IGRA. In this trial, isoniazid lowered the incidence of TB by 56% (31–72%) during the first 2.5 years of follow-up and lowered mortality by 37% (3–59%) after 4.9 years (median) of follow-up.[95,96] In South Africa, another randomized study demonstrated that 12 months of isoniazid resulted in 37% (6–59%) reduction in the hazard of TB over a median follow-up time of 2.5 years.[97] A mathematical model, using the data from South Africa, estimated that the use of antiretroviral therapy and isoniazid preventive therapy for 12 months will lower the incidence of TB by 23% among people receiving antiretroviral therapy and by 5.2% in the total population because of the impact on transmission.[98]

Inhibition of *tumor necrosis factor* (TNF) is another well-characterized risk factor for TB. TNF can be antagonized by treatment with a biologic agent, either with a monoclonal antibody to TNF itself or soluble receptor analogues that block the interaction of TNF with its receptor.[99] TNF plays a major role in the initial and long-term control of TB. The mechanisms by which this cytokine contributes to the control of *M. tuberculosis* infection are multiple (see Chapter 52). Patients treated with TNF antagonists have up to a 25-fold higher risk of TB.[100] Screening patients by TST or IGRA, followed by treatment of LTBI before initiating TNF antagonists, reduces the risk of TB in this setting.[101,102]

Other conditions or therapies that interfere with cell-mediated immunity also increase the risk of TB. These relationships, although well described and generally accepted, are poorly quantified. Examples of these disorders include hematologic malignancies and cancer chemotherapy. In addition, conditions such as diabetes mellitus and uremia are thought to fit into this general category of risk-enhancing diseases, although the basis for this effect is not established.[103] The risk of TB is also increased considerably in persons with silicosis, presumably owing to the effect of silica on both the innate and adaptive immunity.[104,105]

As mentioned earlier, genetic factors have been associated with both infection and disease. Genetic differences are also suggested by the pattern of TB noted among Filipinos in the U.S. Navy, whose rate of disease increased with duration of enlistment, in contrast to the decrease observed in African Americans and whites.[106]

Undernutrition is known to interfere with cell-mediated responses and thus is thought to account for the increased frequency of TB in malnourished persons.[107,108] Vitamin D deficiency has also been linked to TB. Studies on several continents have documented a higher frequency of vitamin D deficiency in patients with active TB than in control subjects. Moreover, a study in South Africa revealed reciprocal seasonal variations in serum vitamin D levels and TB notification rates: During the winter, vitamin D levels were lowest and TB notifications were highest, whereas the converse was true in the summer.[109] Because in vitro studies have revealed a role for vitamin D in regulating macrophage expression of antimicrobial peptides that restrict intracellular growth of *M. tuberculosis*, it is likely that vitamin D deficiency

Table 51.2   Approaches for Prevention

Prompt diagnosis and effective treatment
Infection control
Treatment of latent TB infection
- Persons with HIV
- Close contacts
- Persons with recent infection
- Persons with stable radiographic findings consistent with prior TB
- Persons with other conditions
Vaccination with BCG in children

BCG, bacille Calmette-Guérin; HIV, human immunodeficiency virus; TB, tuberculosis.

increases the risk of TB, rather than that vitamin D deficiency is a consequence of TB.

Despite the number of risk factors for TB that have been identified, the majority of cases have no identified immunologic or physiologic abnormality.

PREVENTION OF TUBERCULOSIS

There are four approaches to the prevention of TB: Prompt diagnosis and effective treatment (see Chapters 53 and 54) to reduce the bacillary population rapidly in persons with the disease, infection control measures to prevent transmission of *M. tuberculosis* in health care and congregate living settings, treatment of LTBI to prevent progression from infection to active TB, and administration of *bacille Calmette-Guérin* (BCG) vaccine that decreases severity of TB in infants and children, although it has inconsistent protective effects in adults (see Table 51.2).

PROMPT DIAGNOSIS AND EFFECTIVE TREATMENT

In regions with a low TB burden and adequate resources, a pillar of TB control consists of evaluating contacts of active cases of pulmonary TB, and treating the contacts with the highest risk of infection and progression to disease.[110] This approach has not been widely applied in high-burden regions because of a lack of evidence of effectiveness. However, a recent cluster-randomized trial in a high-burden country (Vietnam) demonstrated that active surveillance of household contacts (with symptom screen, physical examination, and chest radiograph at baseline, 6, 12, and 24 months after diagnosis of the index case) was effective, because it identified 2.5-fold more cases of TB than did passive case finding.[111] Moreover, a cluster-randomized study of community-wide screening using Xpert TB/RIF to assay sputum in community members, regardless of symptoms, compared the prevalence of TB in the screened versus the control communities after 3 years of community screening.[112] This revealed that, in the screened communities, TB prevalence was reduced by 44% compared with that in the control communities (126 vs. 226 per 100,000). In addition, the rate of TB infection (IGRA positivity) in children 3 to 10 years of age was 50% lower in the screened compared with the control communities, consistent with a reduction in TB transmission due to sputum screening of adults irrespective of symptoms.

Together, these studies provide evidence of feasibility and effectiveness of enhanced TB screening in preventing TB transmission.

INFECTION CONTROL MEASURES TO REDUCE TRANSMISSION OF *M. TUBERCULOSIS*

Measures to reduce transmission of *M. tuberculosis* fall into four main categories: clinician awareness and prompt, appropriate responses; administrative controls; environmental controls; and personal protective equipment.[113] Together, these measures protect health care workers and patients.

Clinician Awareness

Clinical suspicion of TB generally varies inversely with the frequency of the disease in the population served by the facility or provider. However, TB may appear in almost anyone at any time. Given the frequency of comorbidities in persons with TB, clinical presentations are commonly confusing, thus, maintaining a heightened index of suspicion and obtaining appropriate diagnostic tests is critical to early diagnosis and treatment. Ideally a rapid molecular test should be available as per current guidelines.[114] A rapid and specific diagnosis will minimize unnecessary time in isolation for the patient,[115] and an effective treatment will rapidly reduce the infectious potential; thus, this is an effective preventive measure.

Administrative Controls (Policies)

Prompt respiratory isolation of persons with or suspected of having TB which, in some facilities, may be triggered automatically by the act of ordering a sputum examination for mycobacteria, serves to reduce exposure of health care workers and other patients to a person with potentially infectious TB. Patients should wear disposable surgical masks when being transported within the facility.

Environmental Controls

Engineering features such as a specified number of air exchanges per hour and ventilation features that create pressure gradients that exhaust the air to the outside augment other preventive measures.[116] Upper room germicidal irradiation may also be used as a highly effective disinfectant.[117]

Personal Respiratory Protection

N95 respirators (defined as a mask that, properly fitted, blocks out 95% of particles as small as 0.3 microns) should be worn by staff and visitors entering a respiratory isolation room.[118] In some circumstances, such as bronchoscopy on a highly infectious patient, personal air-purifying respirators should be used.

TREATMENT OF LATENT TUBERCULOSIS INFECTION

LTBI is defined by WHO as a state of persistent immune response to stimulation by *M. tuberculosis* antigens with no evidence of clinically manifest active TB.[119] Several large U.S. Public Health Service studies involving approximately 70,000 participants demonstrated the effectiveness

of isoniazid in preventing TB. The findings were remarkably similar in all groups who had a variety of risk factors for TB. Participants given isoniazid had a reduction of approximately 80% in the incidence of TB during the year the medication was given, in comparison with those given placebo. The protective effect decreased during subsequent years, but the treated groups still showed approximately 50% less TB than did the control groups each year after the medication year through 10 to 12 years of observation. Overall, isoniazid reduced the incidence of TB by approximately 60%.[120]

The effectiveness of antituberculosis drugs in preventing TB is presumably a result of the reduction of the viable bacilli population in inactive or radiographically invisible lesions in the lungs and elsewhere. However, on occasion, treatment may be given to persons who have been exposed to TB but do not have a positive tuberculin reaction or IGRA. In this situation, treatment is assumed to prevent the establishment of infection with *M. tuberculosis*, an example of "primary prophylaxis."

Indications for Treating Latent TB Infection

The recommendations for testing for and treatment of LTBI reflect the concept that only persons who are at increased risk of TB should be tested for latent infection: persons who are either known or presumed to have been recently infected with *M. tuberculosis* and persons who have clinical conditions that increase the risk of progressing from latent infection to active TB. Any person who is tested and is found to have a positive test should be considered for treatment.[121,122] The specific groups in which treatment is indicated are as follows (in order of decreasing degree of risk for developing TB).

Persons with HIV Infection. The rates of TB among persons who are infected with both *M. tuberculosis* and HIV are extremely high, ranging from 3–16% per year.[123,124] It is estimated that people living with HIV are 21 times more likely to develop active TB than those without HIV infection.[125] Moreover, TB is the leading cause of death in PLHIV.[17] In a Cochrane review, preventive therapy (any anti-TB drug) versus placebo was associated with a lower incidence of active TB with a relative risk (RR) of 0.68. The benefit was greater in individuals with a positive tuberculin skin test (RR, 0.38) than in those who had a negative test (RR, 0.89). The efficacy was similar for all regimens, regardless of drug type, frequency, or duration of treatment.[126] More recent studies have shown that the benefit persists in persons receiving antiretroviral therapy.[119]

Currently, WHO recommends that all PLHIV who do not have evidence of active TB should receive preventive therapy, regardless of the tuberculin skin test or IGRA result.[119] (See screening approaches to exclude TB in Chapter 53.) Some data suggest that a 36-month treatment duration further reduces the risk of TB in persons with HIV infection in a high TB incidence country, perhaps by reducing reinfection with *M. tuberculosis*.[127] This duration of treatment is conditionally recommended by WHO.[119]

Close Contacts of New TB Cases. Two percent to 4% of persons in close contact with a person with infectious TB develop TB in the year after exposure.[128-130] In young children and adolescents, the risk is perhaps twice that in adults. Because the tuberculin reaction or IGRA result may be negative if infection is recent, all close contacts should be treated. Those with a reaction of 5 mm or more should be considered to be infected and should receive a full course of preventive therapy. Close contacts who have negative tuberculin reactions should be retested 2 to 3 months after the index case is no longer infectious or after contact has been broken. If the tuberculin reaction at that time is less than 5 mm or the IGRA has not converted, treatment can be discontinued and, if the reaction is 5 mm or more or an IGRA has converted from negative or indeterminate to positive, treatment should be continued for a full course. Contacts who are known to be HIV-infected should be treated even if the tuberculin test result is negative.[119]

Persons With Recent Infection. Because the risk of developing TB is greatest during the initial 1 to 2 years after acquisition of the infection, any person who is documented to have had a conversion of the skin test reaction or an IGRA from negative to positive should be considered newly infected and receive treatment. A skin test conversion is defined as an increase in reaction size of 10 mm or more within a 2-year period for persons younger than 35 years and a 15 mm or more increase for persons older than 35 years. Tuberculin skin test reactors younger than 5 years should be accorded a high priority for preventive therapy; because they obviously have been infected relatively recently, the risk of infections is high[131] and there is a potential for severe disease in this age group. There is no consensus on the change in the IGRA result that defines a conversion.

Persons with Stable Radiographic Findings Consistent with Previous Tuberculosis. This group includes persons with a history of TB who never received anti-TB chemotherapy or who were not treated adequately, and persons with no known history of the disease. The rate at which new episodes of TB develop in these groups ranges from approximately 0.4–3.5% per year.[132-134] The risk is lowest in persons with small lesions that have been stable for a long period. In persons with radiographic abnormalities, it is essential that current TB be excluded by a careful clinical and bacteriologic evaluation. Because exclusion of active TB might not be feasible or possible at the initiation of therapy, an alternative approach is to begin therapy with multiple drugs: isoniazid, rifampin, and pyrazinamide, sometimes with ethambutol. If active disease is present as determined by a positive culture or by radiographic improvement, therapy should be continued for 6 months. If there is no suggestion of active disease, therapy can be stopped after 4 months, and the course of treatment will be sufficient for preventive purposes.

Persons with Other Conditions That Increase the Risk of Tuberculosis. Although the risk of TB is not always quantifiable, there is sufficient evidence to warrant preventive therapy in certain situations: silicosis or coal worker's pneumoconiosis; prolonged therapy with corticosteroids (usually 15–20 mg or more of prednisone daily,

or its equivalent, for more than 2 to 3 weeks); immunosuppressive therapy; hematologic or reticuloendothelial malignancies, and perhaps certain solid tumors; end-stage renal disease; clinical conditions associated with rapid weight loss (including intestinal bypass for obesity and inadequate nutritional intake); after gastrectomy; and before treatment with TNF antagonists.[135] In addition, even in the absence of any of these risk factors, persons in the following circumstances who have tuberculin skin test readings of 10 mm or more should be considered for preventive therapy: foreign-born persons from areas of high TB prevalence; medically underserved, low-income populations, including high-risk racial and ethnic groups; residents of long-term care facilities (e.g., correctional institutions and nursing homes); and other groups that, on the basis of local epidemiologic patterns, have been shown to have a high incidence of TB (e.g., migrant workers, homeless persons).[121]

Current Treatment Regimens

For many years the only regimen available for treating latent infection was isoniazid given for 6, 9, or 12 months; but as a result of several clinical trials, three preferred regimens and two alternative regimens were released in February 2020.[136] These regimens apply to persons infected with *M. tuberculosis* that is presumed to be susceptible to isoniazid or rifampin.

Preferred Regimens

1. Three months of once-weekly isoniazid and rifapentine for a total of 12 doses. In a controlled clinical trial, the 12-dose regimen was demonstrated to be non-inferior to isoniazid alone given for 9 months.[137] A subsequent systematic review and meta-analysis concluded that this regimen achieved substantially higher treatment completion rates.[138] This regimen is recommended for adults and children older than 2 years of age with or without HIV infection. Disadvantages include the cost, the possibility of an influenza-like syndrome that can include syncope and hypotension, and potential drug interactions. The recommended doses for individuals 12 years of age and older are isoniazid 15 mg/kg rounded up to the nearest 50 or 100 mg (900 mg maximum) and rifapentine 300 mg (weight 10–14 kg), 450 mg (14.1–25 kg), 600 mg (25.1–32 kg), 750 mg (32.1–49.9), or 900 mg (>50 kg). For children aged 2 to 11 years, the recommended doses are isoniazid 25 mg/kg (900 mg maximum) and rifapentine as described for older children.[136]
2. Four months of daily rifampin. Rifampin alone given in a daily single dose of 10 mg/kg for adults and 15 to 20 mg/kg for children with a maximum dose of 600 mg is the preferred treatment for individuals not infected with HIV.[139] Caution should be taken due to the many drug interactions.
3. Three months of daily isoniazid plus rifampin. This regimen is conditionally recommended for adults and children with or without HIV infection. The recommended doses for adults are isoniazid 5 mg/kg (300 mg maximum) and rifampin 10 mg/kg (600 mg maximum). For children, the doses are isoniazid 10 to 20 mg/kg (300 mg maximum) and rifampin 15 to 20 mg/kg (600 mg maximum).[136]

Alternative Regimens. The alternative regimen is 6 or 9 months of daily isoniazid. The 6-month regimen is strongly recommended for HIV-negative adults and children of all ages and conditionally recommended for HIV-positive adults and children of all ages. The 9-month regimen is conditionally recommended for adults and children of all ages, both HIV negative and HIV positive. Isoniazid is given in a single daily dose of 5 mg/kg for adults and 10 to 20 mg/kg for children up to 300 mg/day. It may also be given at 15 mg/kg for adults and 20 to 40 mg/kg for children up to 900 mg twice weekly to facilitate direct observation of treatment.

Treatment of latent tuberculous infection with isoniazid or a rifamycin should not be undertaken in persons who have active, unstable liver disease. Stable chronic liver disease is not a contraindication, but such patients deserve careful consideration regarding the indications and need close attention during the course of treatment. Other persons who should be monitored especially closely during the administration of preventive therapy include persons older than 35 years; those taking other medications with which there may be interactions (such as phenytoin, disulfuram, or antiretroviral drugs); and persons with other disorders such as alcoholism, diabetes mellitus, or renal insufficiency that may increase the risk of adverse reactions, mainly hepatitis and peripheral neuropathy.

Pregnancy is not a contraindication to isoniazid; however, in view of the concern with elective administration of any drug during the course of pregnancy, it is generally prudent to wait until after delivery to give isoniazid. The exceptions to this are women who have a documented tuberculin conversion during pregnancy or who are HIV-infected and have a positive tuberculin reaction. However, a recent randomized trial in HIV-infected pregnant women revealed a higher rate of adverse pregnancy outcomes in those that received daily isoniazid in the immediate period (during pregnancy) compared to the deferred period (initiated 12 weeks postdelivery).[140] In both groups, a high rate (~6 per 100 person-years) of postpartum hepatotoxicity was observed, indicating that especially close monitoring is necessary in this patient population.

Management of Exposure to Drug-Resistant Organisms

The treatment of contacts exposed to MDR-TB or LTBI with *M. tuberculosis* that is presumed to be resistant to isoniazid and rifampin is based on limited data, and expert consultation should be obtained. The guidelines published in 2019 suggest offering treatment for LTBI versus following with observation. For treatment of MDR LTBI (conditional recommendation, very low certainty in the evidence), the regimens include 6 to 12 months of a later-generation fluoroquinolone alone or with a second drug on the basis of drug susceptibility of the source case *M. tuberculosis* isolate. Because of the toxicity, pyrazinamide should not be used as the second drug. If fluoroquinolone resistance is suspected, pyrazinamide/ethambutol (if source case isolate drug susceptibility testing shows susceptibility to these drugs) can be used.

Monitoring for Adverse Reactions

Adverse reactions have been associated with all drugs used in preventive therapy regimens, although most reactions are minor (see Chapter 54). Patients receiving treatment for LTBI should be seen by a provider at regular intervals (depending on the regimen) and questioned regarding possible symptoms of adverse reactions.[119] Patients receiving treatment should be advised to contact a provider promptly should symptoms develop that are suggestive of hepatotoxicity such as anorexia, nausea, vomiting, abdominal discomfort, persistent fatigue or weakness, dark urine, pale stools, or jaundice. If a health care provider is not available, the patient should be instructed to stop treatment immediately. There is insufficient evidence to support baseline testing of liver function. Baseline testing is, however, strongly encouraged for patients with a history of liver disease, regular use of alcohol, chronic liver disease, HIV infection, age older than 35 years, and pregnancy or in the immediate postpartum period (within 3 months of delivery). For individuals with abnormal baseline test results, clinical judgment is required to ensure that the benefit of treatment outweighs the risks, and liver function should be tested at subsequent visits. Liver function testing should also be performed for patients who develop symptoms while on treatment. Persons at risk for peripheral neuropathy, such as those with malnutrition, alcohol use disorder, HIV infection, renal failure or diabetes, or who are pregnant or breastfeeding, should receive vitamin B_6 supplements when taking isoniazid-containing regimens.

IMMUNIZATION WITH BACILLE CALMETTE-GUÉRIN

BCG is an attenuated *M. bovis* that was found to protect a variety of animal species against TB. It was first used in humans in 1921 and has since become the most widely used vaccine in the world: up to 80% of infants in developing countries receive BCG immunizations, yet no vaccine has been the subject of greater controversy.[141] In children, BCG has been demonstrated to reduce both the frequency and severity of disseminated TB and TB meningitis.[142,143] In addition to the ameliorating effects on severe forms of TB, a meta-analysis of studies using IGRAs to detect new infection in children given BCG compared with control cohorts found that BCG provided protection against tuberculous infection.[144,145]

In adults, the results of BCG vaccination are less clear; in controlled clinical trials of BCG vaccination against pulmonary TB in adults, protection has ranged from 0–77%.[141,146] No protection was seen in the South Indian Trial of more than 200,000 people monitored for 15 years, although all patients who developed TB had developed TST positivity following administration of the vaccine.[147] In contrast, BCG was effective in studies performed in the United Kingdom.[146] It is unclear why BCG appears to be effective in some parts of the world and not in others (a finding that is also evident in protection against leprosy).[143]

There are many variables that potentially could account for the discordant results.[148] These include host genetic factors, variations in pathogenicity of tubercle bacilli, variations in potency of the strains of BCG used, technique of administration, handling of the vaccine, and prevalence of infection with nontuberculous mycobacteria, which may confer some degree of protection.[143,149] Partly because of these factors, it is now generally accepted that BCG is not a tool that can be used to decrease the overall incidence of TB in a population. However, it appears that BCG reduces the likelihood of the more severe forms of the disease in children, and it is with this goal in mind that it continues to be a component of WHO immunization recommendations for developing countries. Due to the widespread acceptance and use of BCG and its benefits to young children, it is not likely that new vaccines for TB will immediately replace BCG. Instead, they will likely be used initially to boost responses after an initial dose of BCG, in an effort to induce responses that reliably protect adults against pulmonary TB.

In the United States, BCG has limited applicability. It is recommended only for TST-negative persons who are repeatedly exposed to potentially infectious patients who are being ineffectively treated. In general, the recommendation is limited to children. As a live vaccine, BCG should not be given to immunocompromised persons, including those with HIV infection, or to pregnant women.

NEW TUBERCULOSIS VACCINES

New approaches to vaccination are being shown to protect against TB. A prevention of infection trial in HIV-infected, IGRA-negative adolescents at high risk of infection compared placebo, revaccination with BCG, and an adjuvanted protein vaccine called H4:IC31.[150] Although neither vaccine regimen reduced the rate of IGRA conversion from negative to positive (interpreted as initial infection), revaccination with BCG significantly increased the frequency of IGRA reversion to negative after initial conversion (interpreted as prevention of sustained infection); the effect of H4:IC31 was not statistically significant. Another prevention of disease trial in HIV-uninfected, IGRA-positive adults compared M72/AS01E, an adjuvanted protein vaccine, to placebo and revealed an overall efficacy of 54% for the vaccine in preventing bacteriologically confirmed active pulmonary TB.[151] Initial analyses of this trial revealed substantial variation in efficacy depending on age and gender; subsequent analyses after longer follow-up determined that the vaccine efficacy of approximately 50% was maintained for 3 years, and there was no difference in efficacy dependent on age or gender.[152] Moreover, antibody and CD4 T cell responses were maintained through the third year of follow-up. These results provide evidence for proof of principle that an adjuvanted subunit vaccine can be efficacious in preventing TB disease and indicate that studies in additional populations are warranted. More recently, when delivery by the intravenous route was compared to intradermal or aerosol routes, the intravenous administration of BCG showed better protection against *M. tuberculosis* infection in a highly susceptible rhesus macaque model. The intravenous immunization induced systemic and CD4

and CD8 T cell responses, especially in the peripheral blood mononuclear cells and lung, which may facilitate the elimination of *M. tuberculosis*.[153]

Key Points

- Although tuberculosis cases and case rates are consistently declining in high- and most middle-income countries, the disease continues to be highly prevalent in low- and some middle-income countries.
- The epidemic of HIV infection, especially in sub-Saharan Africa, is leading to extremely high tuberculosis case rates.
- Both HIV infection and resistance to antituberculosis drugs, especially multidrug resistance and extensive drug resistance, present major problems in worldwide tuberculosis control.
- Adequate treatment for tuberculosis, both drug susceptible and drug resistant, is the major intervention for decreasing transmission of *M. tuberculosis*.
- Newer, shorter regimens are available for treatment of latent TB infection and wide implementation of latent TB infection treatment will be necessary to reach the goals of a 90% reduction in new cases and 95% reduction in deaths by 2035.
- New TB vaccines are in development and in clinical trials and have the potential to make a large impact on the global TB epidemic.

Key Readings

Borisov AS, Bamrah Morris S, Njie GJ, et al. Update of recommendations for use of once-weekly isoniazid-rifapentine regimen to treat latent mycobacterium tuberculosis infection. *MMWR Morb Mortal Wkly Rep.* 2018;67(25):723–726.

Houben RM, Dodd PJ. The global burden of latent tuberculosis infection: a re-estimation using mathematical modelling. *PLoS Med.* 2016;13(10):e1002152.

Kato-Maeda M, Choi JC, Jarlsberg LG, et al. Magnitude of *Mycobacterium tuberculosis* transmission among household and non-household contacts of TB patients. *Int J Tuberc Lung Dis.* 2019;23(4):433–440.

Kendall EA, Azman AS, Maartens G, et al. Projected population-wide impact of antiretroviral therapy-linked isoniazid preventive therapy in a high-burden setting. *AIDS.* 2019;33(3):525–536.

MacNeil A, Glaziou P, Sismanidis C, Maloney S, Floyd K. Global epidemiology of tuberculosis and progress toward achieving global targets—2017. *MMWR Morb Mortal Wkly Rep.* 2019;68(11):263–266.

Mathema B, Andrews JR, Cohen T, et al. Drivers of tuberculosis transmission. *J Infect Dis.* 2017;216(suppl 6):S644-s53.

Sharma A, Hill A, Kurbatova E, et al. Estimating the future burden of multidrug-resistant and extensively drug-resistant tuberculosis in India, the Philippines, Russia, and South Africa: a mathematical modelling study. *Lancet Infect Dis.* 2017;17(7):707–715.

Complete reference list available at ExpertConsult.com.

52

TUBERCULOSIS: PATHOGENESIS AND IMMUNITY

JENNIFER A. PHILIPS, MD, PHD • JOEL D. ERNST, MD

INTRODUCTION

Despite its discovery in 1882 as the cause of tuberculosis, the mechanisms of *Mycobacterium tuberculosis* pathogenesis and protective host immunity were not elucidated until the twenty-first century. Although the understanding of *tuberculosis* (TB) pathogenesis is far from complete, it is now known that complex biologically active lipids and certain secreted proteins account for several of the mechanisms that allow *M. tuberculosis* to evade macrophage microbicidal mechanisms and use host cells as survival and replication niches. Likewise, while multiple mechanisms of innate and adaptive immunity have been discovered to contribute to protection against TB disease, it remains unclear what immune mechanisms can be targeted by vaccines to prevent infection, disease, and transmission.

M. TUBERCULOSIS AND THE *M. TUBERCULOSIS* COMPLEX

Tuberculosis is caused by several species of the *Mycobacterium tuberculosis* complex (MTBC), including *M. tuberculosis*, *M. africanum*, *M. bovis*, and rarely by other animal-adapted species. The rod-shaped bacteria grow slowly, and are characterized by their acid-fastness (they retain chemical dyes after washing with solutions of strong acid in alcohol), which in turn is attributable to a bacterial envelope composed of mycolic acids with acyl chains up to 90 carbons in length, with diverse structural characteristics including cyclopropane rings, methyl branches, ketones, and methoxy groups.[1] Although *M. tuberculosis* can infect and cause disease in many mammalian species, humans are the only significant reservoir and, with rare exceptions, infected humans are the source of transmission.

The genome of the MTBC consists of approximately 4.4 × 10^6 nucleotides in a single circular chromosome and is guanine-cytosine rich (overall 65.6%). The genome of the reference strain H37Rv (isolated from a patient in 1905)

encodes 4006 proteins and 50 RNA species[2]; there is also experimental evidence for noncoding RNAs with regulatory functions.[3]

Much of the MTBC genome contains genes in common with other bacteria, including those whose products function in metabolism, cell wall synthesis, membrane transport, cell division, RNA synthesis, and adaptation to environmental conditions. The MTBC genome encodes at least three distinct protein secretion systems. Of these, the type VII secretion system, which is also present in certain gram-positive bacteria, consists of five loci, termed Esx loci due to the initial discovery of the locus that secretes *early secreted antigenic target of 6 kD* (ESAT-6). Of these, ESX-1 is responsible for secreting proteins (ESAT-6 and CFP-10), which are important for virulence and are also targets of recognition by host immune responses (see later and Fig. 52.1). ESX-3 secretes the substrate EsxH, implicated in impeding phagosome maturation and MHC class II antigen presentation,[4,5] and essential for bacterial iron acquisition.[6,7] ESX-5 is required for secretion of PE and PPE proteins (described later) that contribute to regulation of virulence and immunity. The functions of ESX-2 and ESX-4 are not yet defined.

The genome of the MTBC includes several multigene families, including the *proline-glutamate (pe)* and *proline-proline-glutamate (ppe)* genes, named for proline-glutamic acid or proline-proline-glutamic acid motifs, near the amino termini of their protein products. These gene families are unique to mycobacteria and are markedly expanded in pathogenic mycobacteria (e.g., 99 *pe* and 69 *ppe* genes in *M. tuberculosis* H37Rv).[8] Although the functions of the *pe* and *ppe* genes are poorly understood, the individual members of these gene families are under markedly different evolutionary selection pressures, indicating that they do not serve redundant functions,[9] despite their sequence and structural similarities.

Comparative genomic studies have established that the MTBC comprises a phylogenetic structure with seven major branches, with each branch having a geographic association, indicating that the MTBC coevolved with humans after major human population migrations transported ancestral MTBC strains from their origin in East Africa,[10] followed by differentiation and expansion coincident with the human populations in the respective regions (Fig. 52.2). The significance of the phylogenetic diversity of the MTBC remains a topic of investigation, although there is evidence that strains in a given lineage may be especially well adapted to humans in the ethnic groups in which the corresponding lineages coevolved.[11,12]

INNATE IMMUNITY

Innate immunity serves as a front-line defense against microbes (see Chapter 15). Although innate immune responses undoubtedly play an important role in tuberculosis, studies in individuals with *human immunodeficiency virus* (HIV) and in animal models demonstrate that innate immunity is insufficient to control *M. tuberculosis* infection. Normally, during an effective immune response, macrophages and neutrophils kill and clear bacteria, and dendritic cells promote development of adaptive immune responses. An important aspect of *M. tuberculosis* pathogenesis is its ability to undermine the function of these innate immune cells. Indeed, instead of killing *M. tuberculosis*, these cells serve as niches for bacterial replication.

CELLULAR NICHES AND GRANULOMAS

M. tuberculosis is transmitted by aerosolized respiratory secretions and infects numerous innate immune cell types in the lung, including macrophages, neutrophils, and dendritic cells.[13] After inhalation, *M. tuberculosis* first infects alveolar macrophages,[14] a macrophage population adapted to minimize lung injury,[15] which makes it poorly equipped to control *M. tuberculosis*.[15,16] Over time, monocyte-derived and interstitial macrophages also become infected by *M. tuberculosis*; however, prior to the onset of adaptive immunity, they confer only modest control over bacterial replication. Numerous phagocytic receptors can mediate uptake of *M. tuberculosis* into macrophages.[17,18] The particular phagocytic receptors that *M. tuberculosis* engages may influence the subsequent ability of macrophages to control infection,[19] and mycobacteria may selectively parasitize more permissive macrophages.[20] Neutrophils are recruited to the lung in the first two weeks of infection and, rather

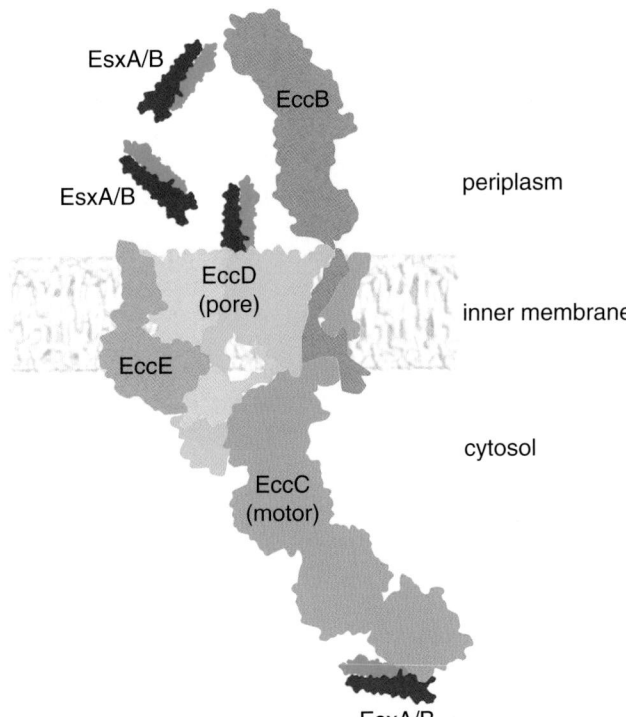

Figure 52.1 Structural model of the ESX-1 type VII secretion system based on cryo-EM analysis of the purified intact ESX-3 complex of *M. smegmatis*. Substrates shown here, dimers of *EsxA/B* (also termed ESAT-6 and CFP-10, respectively) are selected by interaction with ATPase 3 of *EccC* in the bacterial cytoplasm and transported via the upper cytoplasmic gate to the *EccD* translocon pore for secretion to the bacterial periplasm and extrabacterial space, using the energy generated by hydrolysis of ATP. The other ESX type VII secretion systems are thought to function similarly, to export distinct substrates (such as EsxG/EsxH, by ESX-3). (Courtesy Oren Rosenberg, MD, PhD, University of California San Francisco.)

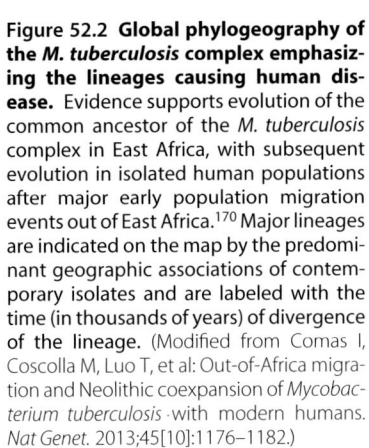

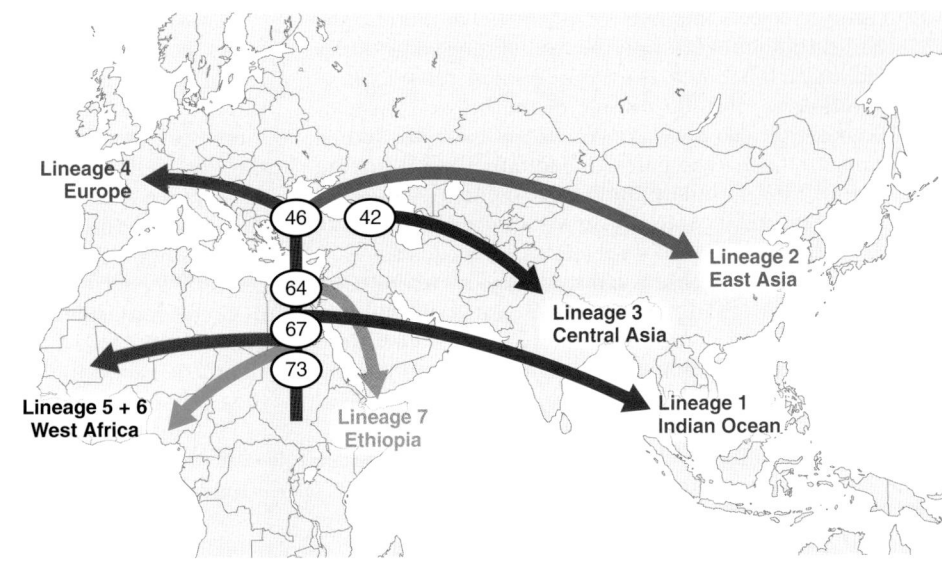

Figure 52.2 Global phylogeography of the *M. tuberculosis* complex emphasizing the lineages causing human disease. Evidence supports evolution of the common ancestor of the *M. tuberculosis* complex in East Africa, with subsequent evolution in isolated human populations after major early population migration events out of East Africa.[170] Major lineages are indicated on the map by the predominant geographic associations of contemporary isolates and are labeled with the time (in thousands of years) of divergence of the lineage. (Modified from Comas I, Coscolla M, Luo T, et al: Out-of-Africa migration and Neolithic coexpansion of *Mycobacterium tuberculosis* with modern humans. *Nat Genet*. 2013;45[10]:1176–1182.)

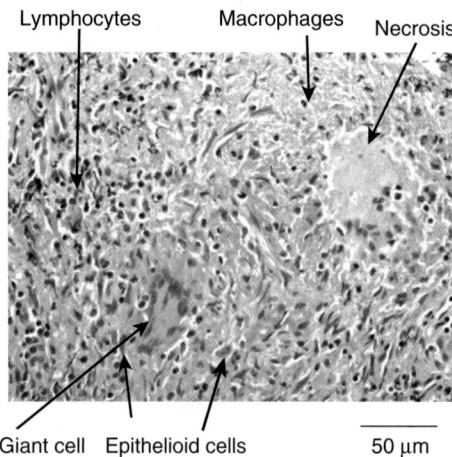

Lymphocytes   Macrophages   Necrosis

Giant cell   Epithelioid cells   50 μm

Figure 52.3 Representative granuloma from a human patient with tuberculosis. The granuloma consists of dense aggregates of macrophages, accompanied by variable numbers of lymphocytes. Some macrophages fuse to form multinucleated giant cells, while others undergo transitions to epithelioid cells, and some die by necrosis. While most lymphocytes in granulomas are T cells (predominantly CD4 T cells), B cells can also be found in and adjacent to granulomas. Dendritic cells and variable numbers of neutrophils can also be detected in tuberculous granulomas. The hematoxylin and eosin staining procedure does not visualize the bacteria. (Courtesy Stephen Nishimura, MD, University of California San Francisco.)

than restricting infection, overly exuberant neutrophil recruitment can create a nutrient-rich environment that supports *M. tuberculosis* replication.[21,22]

As the infection progresses, the cellular response is characterized by an organized collection of cells termed a granuloma, including macrophages, neutrophils, and lymphocytes. Macrophages aggregate, and some undergo an epithelioid transformation or form multinucleated giant cells (Fig. 52.3). Granulomas can undergo necrosis and cavitation, where *M. tuberculosis* can replicate to high numbers extracellularly. A characteristic feature of these granulomas is *caseating* necrosis, in which there is loss of tissue structure until the texture resembles soft cheese. (The term *caseating* derives from the Latin word *caseum*, meaning cheese.) The granuloma was long thought to serve a host-protective function in restricting dissemination of *M. tuberculosis*. This is supported by the observation that patients with immune defects imposed by HIV or *tumor necrosis factor* (TNF)-α inhibitors fail to form well-organized granulomas and, in such patients, there is also an increased risk of dissemination of infection outside of the lungs. However, granulomas can also facilitate cell-to-cell bacterial spread within macrophage aggregates. In addition, the granuloma architecture may stimulate the bacilli to enter a nonreplicating, drug-tolerant state and may also block access of adaptive immune cells and antibiotics to the bacteria.[23–25] Indeed, progressive disease is characterized by an increase in granuloma size and number; the increased infiltration in immune cells leads to increasing tissue damage rather than to effective microbial killing. Even within a given person, there are differences in the rate of progression of individual granulomas, and the mechanisms that account for this heterogeneity are not well understood. In conclusion, the initial innate immune cells that encounter *M. tuberculosis* are unable to control bacterial replication and, whereas the organized collection of cells in granulomas may benefit the host in certain stages of infection, it also appears that the pathogen is adapted to use the granulomatous response to its advantage. The bacilli are able to respond to and adapt to distinct host environments through two component systems, such as DosS/DosT, and PhoP/PhoR, as well as sigma factors. These enable the bacteria to detect and respond to altered levels of oxygen, nitric oxide, and carbon monoxide.

MACROPHAGE SUBCELLULAR NICHES

Once *M. tuberculosis* is ingested by host phagocytes, it resides in distinct subcellular environments and perturbs the normal function of these cells.[26,27] Considerable work has explored how *M. tuberculosis* impacts macrophage biology. Seminal studies by Armstrong and Hart and colleagues revealed that pathogenic mycobacteria survive and replicate in macrophages by perturbing the maturation of the *phagosome*. Normally, after microbial ingestion, the phagosome acidifies, acquires lysosomal hydrolases and antimicrobial peptides, and restricts essential nutrients such as iron.[28–30] The NADPH oxidase is also recruited to the phagosome where it generates *reactive oxygen species* (ROS) that can kill invading microbes and also promote a phagosome maturation pathway called microtubule-associated protein *light chain 3* (LC3)-associated phagocytosis.[31,32] *M. tuberculosis* and related species such as *M. marinum* prevent these normal maturation events. Instead of maturing to a phagolysosome, the mycobacterial vacuole retains early endosomal markers normally cleared from the maturing phagosomal surface, while the NADPH oxidase, LC3, and numerous late endosomal and lysosomal markers are diminished or absent.[33] There are numerous protein and lipid effectors that have been identified that enable *M. tuberculosis* to impair phagosome maturation,[34] thereby avoiding the degradative environment of the lysosome. However, this is not the only intracellular niche inhabited by *M. tuberculosis*. Some bacilli are delivered to lysosomes, where they are able to survive by resisting mechanisms of lysosomal killing, using enzymes that protect against redox stress, including catalase, *superoxide dismutase* (SOD), and alkyl hydroperoxidase, while the membrane protein Rv3671c maintains a neutral bacterial pH in the face of a low pH environment.[35,36]

Central to the pathogenesis of *M. tuberculosis* is its ability to perforate the phagosome membrane.[37] Perforating the phagosome allows *M. tuberculosis* to deliver effectors to the cytosol and access host nutrients and, over time, with increasing membrane damage, bacteria can translocate to the host cell cytosol.[38–40] When the phagosomal contents are exposed to the cytosol, they also provoke a host response, as discussed in more detail later. Phagosomal damage depends upon the ESX-1 type VII secretion system. ESX-1 is essential for virulence of *M. tuberculosis* and it is missing in BCG, the nonvirulent strain of *M. bovis* used as a tuberculosis vaccine.[41–43] ESX-1–deficient bacteria do not perforate efficiently or escape the phagosome into the cytosol,[38,40,44] and they do not stimulate the host signaling pathways, which have sensing mechanisms in the cytoplasm.[45,46] Recent work shows that the mycobacterial lipid *phthiocerol dimycocerosate* (PDIM) works in concert with ESX-1 in mediating phagosomal damage.[47–49] Like mutants defective in ESX-1, PDIM mutants are attenuated, and they fail to promote host cell death or induce type I interferon responses that are correlated with phagosomal damage. The host detects and repairs minor damage to membranes with a multiprotein system called the *endosomal sorting complex required for transport* (ESCRT).[50,51] ESCRT responds to mycobacterial-induced phagosomal damage.[52,53] However, the *M. tuberculosis* EsxH protein, which is secreted by the ESX-3 type VII secretion system, interferes with ESCRT.[4,52] Thus two important virulence systems of *M. tuberculosis* are involved in modulating the integrity of the phagosomal membrane: ESX-1 causes damage, and ESX-3 interferes with host repair of the damage.

Disruption of phagosome membrane integrity also activates host signaling pathways (type I interferon signaling and the inflammasome, discussed later) and a lysosomal trafficking pathway called macroautophagy (hereafter, autophagy). The autophagy system, originally characterized for its role in degradation of endogenous cellular proteins and organelles, recognizes damaged phagosomes and bacilli that have escaped into the cytosol. *Autophagy-related proteins* (ATG) coordinate the formation of a double-membrane compartment, the autophagosome, which can sequester the microbe, and fuse with lysosomes.[54] *Interferon-gamma* (IFN-γ) and small molecules that augment autophagy promote *M. tuberculosis* clearance, while under basal conditions, autophagy makes a limited contribution to controlling *M. tuberculosis*.[21,44,55,56] The limited efficacy of autophagy in clearing *M. tuberculosis* points to evasion mechanisms on the part of the bacilli.[57,58] *M. tuberculosis* inhibits expression of *ATG* genes and secretes protein effectors such as PE_PGRS47, a member of the *pe* family described earlier, to interfere with autophagy.[59–61]

In addition to altering intracellular trafficking pathways of macrophages, *M. tuberculosis* induces profound changes in the metabolic state of the cells it infects. *M. tuberculosis* alters macrophage metabolism by inducing the Warburg effect,[62–64] a shift from oxidative phosphorylation to glycolysis, initially described in cancer cells. *M. tuberculosis* also modulates host lipid metabolism and induces the formation of lipid-droplet-filled or "foamy" macrophages.[65–67] Foamy macrophages are found within the inner layers of granulomas, and the bacilli themselves can be found in close approximation to intracellular lipid droplets. It is thought that lipid bodies serve as a source of nutrients for the bacilli in the form of cholesterol esters and fatty acids.[67–73] The relationship between these host metabolic changes and *M. tuberculosis* pathogenesis is an active area of investigation, and a number of host-directed therapies under investigation for TB, such as statins and metformin, modulate host metabolism.[74,75]

CYTOKINE RESPONSES

In addition to phagocytosing *M. tuberculosis*, innate immune cells respond to microbial challenge by initiating signaling pathways that result in secretion of proinflammatory and anti-inflammatory cytokines. These signaling pathways are initiated when cells detect bacterial components that activate *pathogen-recognition receptors* (PRRs). *M. tuberculosis* has numerous pathogen-associated molecular patterns that activate *toll-like receptors* (TLR2, 4, and 9) and C-type lectin receptors (DC-SIGN, Dectin-1, Mincle, and MCL).[76] Because *M. tuberculosis* bacilli perforate the phagosome,

they also activate cytosolic sensors, including *nucleotide-binding and oligomerization domain* (NOD) 2, cGAS-STING, and the inflammasome (discussed later).

In response to activation of these PRRs, macrophages and dendritic cells secrete cytokines that contribute to control of infection and regulate specific aspects of immunity. Of the cytokines induced by *M. tuberculosis*, TNF is especially well characterized as essential for immunity to tuberculosis in humans. Patients with rheumatoid arthritis and other conditions treated with agents that block TNF activity have up to a 25-fold higher risk of tuberculosis than control populations[77] and are more likely to have disseminated infection.[78] TNF contributes to immunity to tuberculosis by activating microbicidal activities of macrophages and by enhancing the death of infected cells.[79–81] In addition, infliximab, one of the antibodies used to block TNF, increases the risk of tuberculosis by depleting a specific subset of CD8 T cells containing membrane-bound TNF that may contribute to killing intracellular *M. tuberculosis*.[82]

IFN-γ plays an essential role in immune control of tuberculosis. IFN-γ–deficient[83,84] or IFN-γ receptor–deficient [85] mice succumb to rapidly progressive *M. tuberculosis* infection and, in patients with IFN-γ receptor mutations, tuberculosis is especially severe, with a greater likelihood of disseminated and/or recurrent disease.[86] IFN-γ is believed to contribute to immune control of tuberculosis through activating the microbicidal activities of macrophages, including the production of nitric oxide and enhancement of autophagy,[55,56,87,88] and by modulating inflammation at the site of infection.[85,89] Although multiple cell types can be sources of IFN-γ, the principal cellular sources are lymphocytes, including innate lymphoid cells, as well as adaptive CD4 and CD8 T cells.

Interleukin (IL)-12 is another innate cytokine essential for immunity to tuberculosis. The best-characterized role of IL-12 is in directing differentiation of CD4 T cells into type 1 T helper cells that secrete IFN-γ and other cytokines and contribute to control of tuberculosis (see later). Evidence that IL-12 is essential for control of tuberculosis is provided by experiments in IL-12-deficient mice[90,91] and by observations that children with mutations in the IL-12 receptor beta-1 chain are susceptible to tuberculosis and other mycobacterial infections.[92]

Other cytokines can enhance *M. tuberculosis* pathogenesis. One important aspect of tuberculosis pathogenesis is the induction of type I IFN (IFN-α and/or IFN-β) secretion. Production of type I IFN depends upon ESX-1 secretion, the lipid PDIM, and phagosome permeabilization, as discussed earlier. Mycobacterial DNA and mitochondrial DNA that enter the cytosol trigger the cGAS-STING pathway, leading to IFN production.[44,93–96] The importance of type I IFN in human infection was revealed by whole blood transcriptome analysis of human genes that are differentially expressed in tuberculosis, which revealed a transcriptional signature dominated by IFN-responsive genes[97–100] that correlated with the extent of disease.[101] Whether type I IFN plays a pathogenic role or is a secondary effect of active tuberculosis in humans remains to be defined, although humans with a hypofunctional mutant type I INF receptor have a lower frequency of tuberculosis.[102] In mice, type I IFNs play a pathogenic role,[103] at least partially by enhancing recruitment of mononuclear cells that support intracellular bacterial replication.[104,105] In addition, type I IFNs limit expression of IL-1β, a cytokine that is essential for control of *M. tuberculosis* (see later).[106,107] There are strain-dependent differences, including those related to drug resistance, that result in differences in the production of type I IFN and IL-1-β production and their importance during infection.[96,108] Despite the growing evidence for a detrimental role of type I IFNs in tuberculosis, therapeutic administration of type I IFN for multiple sclerosis or hepatitis C has not been accompanied by a noticeable increase in the frequency of active tuberculosis.

M. tuberculosis activates another cytosolic immune sensor called the inflammasome, leading to IL-1β and IL-18 secretion. The inflammasome is composed of *NOD-like receptors* (NLRs), apoptosis-associated speck-like protein containing a caspase recruiting domain, and the caspase-1 protease. There are many NLRs that can activate the inflammasome in response to distinct stimuli. During *M. tuberculosis* infection of macrophages, the NLRP3-inflammasome is activated in response to phagosomal damage,[109,110] and there is evidence that *M. tuberculosis* blocks activation of the AIM2-inflammasome.[111,112] The inflammasome processes IL-1β and IL-18 to their mature forms and triggers a distinct cell death pathway termed pyroptosis. IL-1β and IL-18 are important cytokines for host immune defense against *M. tuberculosis*.[106,113,114] In addition, they can contribute to exuberant inflammation and tissue damage.[115-117] Thus the activation of the inflammasome can be beneficial or detrimental.

VITAMIN D

Vitamin D (whose active form is 1,25-dihydroxyvitamin D) has extensive associations with tuberculosis (reviewed by Martineau[118]). Vitamin D deficiency is commonly found in humans at the time of TB diagnosis, and exposure to sunlight (which activates synthesis of vitamin D in the skin) was thought to be valuable as a component of TB treatment in sanatoria in the prechemotherapy era. Moreover, in some populations, but not all, polymorphisms in the genes encoding the vitamin D receptor and vitamin D binding protein have been associated with the risk of active TB.

Vitamin D acts through a nuclear receptor to regulate specific genes, including genes whose products relate to TB immunity. Treatment of cultured human macrophages with 1,25-dihydroxyvitamin D induces expression of the antimicrobial peptide cathelicidin LL37, which has direct antimycobacterial activity and also enhances autophagy; production of reactive oxygen and nitrogen intermediates is also increased.

Considering the evidence for a role of vitamin D in immune control of TB, multiple clinical trials have been performed to determine whether vitamin D supplementation is a useful adjunct to drug treatment of TB. A recent meta-analysis concluded that addition of vitamin D does not accelerate sputum clearance in cases of drug-susceptible TB, although a beneficial effect has been more consistently observed in cases of multidrug-resistant TB.[119] Despite the modest impact on bacterial clearance, vitamin D supplementation has been found to accelerate resolution of inflammation during treatment of TB.[120]

CELL DEATH PATHWAYS

Infection can cause host phagocytes to undergo a variety of different types of cell death, which influences the infection outcome.[121] *M. tuberculosis* promotes necrotic cell death while limiting apoptosis (programmed cell death). This is a strategy that appears to favor the bacilli, because apoptosis minimizes inflammation, and *M. tuberculosis*–infected macrophages that undergo apoptosis can be rapidly ingested by neighboring uninfected macrophages and the bacilli killed, through a process called efferocytosis.[122] In addition, by inhibiting uptake of apoptotic cells, *M. tuberculosis* limits cross-presentation to CD8 T cells that would otherwise result from bacterial antigens associated with apoptotic cell fragments.[123] The ability of *M. tuberculosis* to cause necrosis depends upon the ESX-1 secretion system and the NAD+ glycohydrolase, tuberculosis necrotizing toxin, which induces necrotic cell death by depleting NAD+.[124] *M. tuberculosis* also potentiates necrosis by causing mitochondrial inner membrane disruption[125] and inhibiting plasma membrane repair.[126] Many bacterial factors have been shown to limit apoptosis,[34] some of which appear to work by limiting host ROS, including mycobacterial proteins NuoG, a subunit of the type I NADH dehydrogenase, and SodA, superoxide dismutase.[127-130] Evidence that inhibition of apoptosis is a virulence mechanism is provided by the findings that proapoptotic mutants of *M. tuberculosis* are less pathogenic in vivo in animal models.[131]

ADAPTIVE IMMUNITY

CLASSICAL T CELLS

The term *classical T cells* refers to CD4 and CD8 T cells that express *T cell antigen receptors* (TCRs) consisting of an α- and β-chain, and that recognize peptides bound to HLA class II or class I molecules, respectively.

Considerable evidence supports an essential role for CD4 T cells in control of *M. tuberculosis*. In mice, developmental absence or antibody depletion of CD4 T cells leads to rapid progression and accelerated mortality with high burdens of *M. tuberculosis*.[132] In humans, HIV infection with CD4 T cell depletion markedly increases susceptibility to active tuberculosis.[133] CD4 T cells recognize a vast range of peptide epitopes derived from several hundred *M. tuberculosis* proteins, though it is currently unknown whether CD4 T cell responses to certain antigens are better able to provide protective immunity than are responses to other antigens. In mice, CD8 T cells also contribute to control of *M. tuberculosis*, although the impact of their absence is less striking than the absence of CD4 T cells.[132] The contributions of CD8 T cells to protective immunity to *M. tuberculosis* in humans are less clear, principally due to a lack of evidence.

T cells can provide protective immunity through secretion of cytokines, expression of membrane effector molecules, and cytolytic activity targeting *M. tuberculosis*–infected cells. Of the cytokines produced by T cells, IFN-γ, TNF, IL-17, and granulocyte-macrophage colony-stimulating factor have each been implicated in contributing to immune control of *M. tuberculosis* in mice; genetic unresponsiveness to IFN-γ[134,135] and therapeutic blockade of TNF[136] have established the importance of these cytokines for immunity to *M. tuberculosis* in humans (as discussed earlier). Recent evidence in mice, nonhuman primates, and humans indicates that a CD4 T cell membrane effector molecule in the TNF superfamily (TNFSF8, also known as CD153) contributes to control of *M. tuberculosis* infection.[137] Although each of these effector mechanisms is implicated in immune protection, it is currently unclear which ones should be prioritized as goals of TB vaccine development (see later).

The importance of T cell recognition of specific *M. tuberculosis* antigens is the topic of active investigation, to identify those antigens whose recognition by T cells (or antibodies) makes the greatest contributions to protective immunity. *M. tuberculosis* differs from other pathogens in that its antigens do not vary at high frequency as a mechanism of immune escape.[138,139] Current efforts focus on antigens expressed by actively replicating bacteria, by "dormant" bacteria, or during resuscitation from dormancy, with the goal of providing protective immunity during all stages of *M. tuberculosis* infection.

NONCLASSICAL T CELLS

T cells that express antigen receptors consisting of γ and δ (instead of α and β) chains do not recognize peptide fragments and do not depend on HLA class I or II molecules as the basis for their target recognition. A specific subset of γδ T cells characterized by TCRs containing the Vγ9 and Vδ2 chains respond to isoprenyl pyrophosphates and other phosphorylated small molecules,[140] and are activated by *M. tuberculosis*–infected macrophages.[141]

Mucosal-associated innate-like T cells (MAITs) share certain properties with γδ T cells, but their TCRs recognize low-molecular-weight microbial metabolites, including intermediates in vitamin biosynthesis, bound to the HLA class I–like molecule, MR-1.[142] Although γδ T cells and MAITs are enriched at mucosal surfaces and can be activated by *M. tuberculosis*–infected cells, their contributions to immune control of *M. tuberculosis* remain unclear.[143,144]

Another subset of T cells expresses TCR αβ chains that recognize specific complex mycobacterial lipids (for example, glucose monomycolate, dideoxymycobactin, and phosphomycoketide) bound to the HLA class I–like molecules CD1a, CD1b, or CD1c.[145] Although the contributions of CD1-restricted lipid antigen-specific T cells to protective immunity remains to be determined, there is evidence that these cells are expanded in persons with active TB,[146] and a polyporphism in the *CD1a* gene is associated with increased susceptibility to TB.[147]

OTHER MECHANISMS OF IMMUNITY

Although antibodies were thought unlikely to contribute to protective immunity to TB, recent investigations have provided evidence that some individuals exposed to *M. tuberculosis* who remain well produce antibodies with protective activity in vitro and upon passive transfer to mice.[148] Moreover, *M. tuberculosis*–reactive antibodies isolated from human subjects with active TB exhibit distinct properties compared with those from humans that remain healthy, including differential glycosylation of the Fc domains and isotype prevalence.[149] These and other studies (reviewed in [150]) have intensified investigation of the value of developing TB vaccines that induce protective antibodies.

Aside from the contributions of adaptive (T and B) lymphocytes, functionally similar *innate lymphoid cells* (ILCs) can contribute to early responses to pathogens, including *M. tuberculosis*. Analogous to subsets of T cells, there are three major subsets of ILCs, categorized by their lineage-defining transcription factors and functional responses. ILC1s express T-bet and produce IFN-γ; ILC2s express GATA-3 and produce IL-4, IL-5, and IL-13; and ILC3s express Rorγt and secrete IL-17 and/or IL-22. Unlike B or T cells, ILCs lack antigen receptors, and are activated by cytokines and other stimuli produced by mucosal epithelial and mononuclear cells. ILC3s have been found to contribute to immunity to *M. tuberculosis* by expanding, accumulating in the lungs of humans with active TB, and controlling bacterial growth in the lungs of infected mice.[151]

EVASION OF ADAPTIVE IMMUNITY

A characteristic of immunity to *M. tuberculosis* is that it is often incomplete and unable to eliminate the bacteria reliably. As a consequence, a proportion (5–10%) of individuals can develop progressive or reactivation disease. Incomplete immunity may also underlie the necessity for prolonged antimicrobial therapy for active TB. Multiple mechanisms have been discovered that contribute to *M. tuberculosis* manipulating, evading, or exploiting immune responses to survive and to be transmitted. As discussed earlier, numerous bacterial proteins and lipids are implicated in evading the innate immune response. Similarly, to limit the efficacy of CD4 T cells in immunity to *M. tuberculosis*, the bacteria employ multiple mechanisms for evading CD4 T cell recognition of infected cells. Since the bacteria reside prominently in antigen-presenting cells (macrophages and dendritic cells), they are well-positioned to limit the activities of CD4 T cells by modulating antigen presentation. At least three mechanisms contribute to *M. tuberculosis* manipulation of antigen presentation. The ESX-3 effector protein, EsxH, directly interacts with the host protein hepatocyte growth factor–regulated tyrosine kinase substrate, and interferes with MHC/HLA class II antigen presentation to CD4 T cells by limiting antigen processing.[5] An additional *M. tuberculosis* protein, PE_PGRS47, inhibits autophagy and antigen presentation to CD4 T cells,[152] and *M. tuberculosis*–infected cells divert bacterial antigens from the class II antigen presentation pathway and export them to the extracellular space.[153] As another mechanism for evasion of T cells, *M. tuberculosis* dynamically regulates expression of the genes encoding certain immunodominant antigens such as Ag85B. Ag85B is expressed early after infection, allowing priming and expansion of Ag85B-specific CD4 T cells, but markedly downregulates Ag85B expression later in infection, thereby avoiding the effects of Ag85B-specific T cells.[154] Together, these results indicate that *M. tuberculosis* employs multiple mechanisms to manipulate antigen presentation and recognition of infected cells by CD4 T cells. Evidence for the functional importance of limiting antigen presentation is the finding that *M. bovis* BCG-infected cells present the same antigen more effectively than do *M. tuberculosis*–infected cells, and yet *M. bovis* BCG can be eliminated from mouse lungs in a T cell–dependent manner.[155]

In addition to manipulating CD4 T cell activation and recognition of infected cells, M. tuberculosis possesses mechanisms to counter T cell effector mechanisms such as the effects of the cytokine IFNγ. One antimicrobial IFNγ-induced gene encodes the enzyme indoleamine-2,3-dioxygenase, which catalyzes the essential amino acid tryptophan to kynurenine; tryptophan depletion is lethal to many pathogens, but M. tuberculosis responds by synthesizing tryptophan, allowing the bacteria to survive and replicate despite the effects of IFNγ.[156]

LATENCY/DORMANCY AND REACTIVATION

Although for clinical and public health purposes, latent TB infection is considered to represent persistent infection contained in most individuals by effective immune responses, the biologic state of latent TB infection is likely to be more complex, and has been suggested to comprise a spectrum of bacterial and immune states.[157,158] Because existing assays of TB infection depend on T cell responses to selected M. tuberculosis antigens and thereby reflect immunologic memory rather than persistent infection, the spectrum may include at one extreme, elimination of the bacteria, and at the other extreme, a state of subclinical active infection with bacterial replication uncontained by host immunity. The importance of latent TB infection is that, in 5–10% of individuals, it progresses to active, transmissible TB, so it can contribute to sustaining the TB epidemic,[159] although an alternative perspective recently has been provided.[160]

Diverse risk factors, such as age, nutritional state, diabetes, malignancy, and smoking, are associated with higher rates of progression from latent to active TB, but only two, HIV and TNF blockade, have clear immunologic mechanisms.[161] While the contributions from the other risk factors may be related to waning or fluctuating immunity, bacterial factors may also contribute to progression from latent to active TB, as exemplified by specific mechanisms used by M. tuberculosis to adapt to and manipulate the host environment. Among these are regulatory mechanisms that promote adaptation of M. tuberculosis to hypoxic environments and allow the bacteria to recover from hypoxia and to resume growth.[162,163] M. tuberculosis also expresses "resuscitation promoting factors" that act on bacterial cell wall peptidoglycan to promote growth during recovery from dormancy.[164,165] Together, these findings suggest that, under some circumstances, M. tuberculosis may itself drive reactivation of latent TB infection, in the absence of identifiable host immune deficits.

An additional topic of current investigation is identification of the tissue and cellular sites of M. tuberculosis during latent infection. Although early studies identified viable bacteria in lung and lymphoid tissues of individuals with latent TB infection, recent studies have reported evidence for residence of dormant bacteria in adipose tissue, lymphatic endothelial cells, and mesenchymal and hematopoietic stem cells (reviewed in Mayito et al.[166]).

NEW TUBERCULOSIS VACCINES

Two recent clinical trials provide optimism for the development of TB vaccines that are more efficacious than the widely used intradermal BCG vaccine.

A novel prevention of infection trial compared BCG revaccination or an adjuvanted protein subunit vaccine (termed H4:IC31) to placebo in adolescents at high risk but no evidence of prior M. tuberculosis infection (as reflected by a negative result on an interferon gamma release assay [IGRA]). While neither BCG revaccination nor H4:IC31 prevented initial infection as indicated by conversion from IGRA-negative to positive, BCG revaccination but not H4:IC31 prevented "sustained" infection (IGRA conversion from negative to positive, without reversion to negative) with approximately 45% efficacy.[167] Although the significance of IGRA reversion is uncertain, it may reflect clearance of infection.

A prevention of disease trial at multiple sites in Africa compared another adjuvanted protein subunit vaccine termed M72:AS01$_E$ and placebo, given to IGRA-positive, HIV-negative adults who had previously been vaccinated with BCG. When participants were followed for 2 years, the M72:AS01$_E$ vaccine exhibited overall efficacy of 54% in preventing progression to definite pulmonary TB compared with the control.[168] The efficacy was age dependent and may have been more efficacious in men than in women.

In addition to these human trials, a study in nonhuman primates using a vaccine consisting of recombinant rhesus cytomegalovirus expressing M. tuberculosis antigens exhibited dramatic protection with sterile immunity following M. tuberculosis challenge.[169] Additional studies in nonhuman primates revealed that intrapulmonary mucosal[171] or intravenous administration of BCG provided a high level of protection, including sterile immunity, after inhalational challenge with virulent M tuberculosis.[172]

Together, the results of these studies provide substantial evidence for the feasibility of developing efficacious TB vaccines, though more studies are needed to determine the optimal target populations and strategies for vaccine implementation.

Key Points

- M. tuberculosis is evolutionarily ancient and has coevolved with humans.
- M. tuberculosis employs multiple mechanisms of pathogenesis, using specific lipid and protein virulence factors to survive intracellularly, predominantly in mononuclear phagocytes.
- Human immunity protects most individuals from active tuberculosis disease. Immunity requires CD4 T cells; other mechanisms of immunity, including antibodies, may also contribute to protection against progression of tuberculosis.
- M. tuberculosis employs multiple mechanisms to evade CD4 T cell recognition, resulting in partial immunity and, in some people, lifelong infection.
- Novel tuberculosis vaccines are in development, and initial results of clinical trials provide optimism for the development of effective tuberculosis vaccines.

Key Readings

Armstrong JA, Hart PD. Response of cultured macrophages to Mycobacterium tuberculosis, with observations on fusion of lysosomes with phagosomes. J Exp Med. 1971;134(3 Pt 1):713–740.

Berry MP, et al. An interferon-inducible neutrophil-driven blood transcriptional signature in human tuberculosis. *Nature.* 2010;466(7309):973–977.

Comas I, et al. Out-of-Africa migration and Neolithic coexpansion of *Mycobacterium tuberculosis* with modern humans. *Nat Genet.* 2013;45(10):1176–1182.

Li H, Javid B. Antibodies and tuberculosis: finally coming of age? *Nat Rev Immunol.* 2018;18(9):591–596.

Li H, et al. Latently and uninfected healthcare workers exposed to TB make protective antibodies against *Mycobacterium tuberculosis. Proc Natl Acad Sci U S A.* 2017;114(19):5023–5028.

Martin CJ, et al. Efferocytosis is an innate antibacterial mechanism. *Cell Host Microbe.* 2012;12(3):289–300.

Mayer-Barber KD, et al. Innate and adaptive interferons suppress IL-1α and IL-1β production by distinct pulmonary myeloid subsets during *Mycobacterium tuberculosis* infection. *Immunity.* 2011;35(6):1023–1034.

Mehra A, et al. *Mycobacterium tuberculosis* type VII secreted effector EsxH targets host ESCRT to impair trafficking. *PLoS Pathog.* 2013;9(10):e1003734.

Philips JA, Ernst JD. Tuberculosis pathogenesis and immunity. *Annu Rev Pathol.* 2012;7:353–384.

Portal-Celhay C, et al. *Mycobacterium tuberculosis* EsxH inhibits ESCRT-dependent CD4(+) T-cell activation. *Nat Microbiol.* 2016;2:16232.

Pym AS, et al. Loss of RD1 contributed to the attenuation of the live tuberculosis vaccines *Mycobacterium bovis* BCG and *Mycobacterium microti. Mol Microbiol.* 2002;46(3):709–717.

Quigley J, et al. The cell wall lipid PDIM contributes to phagosomal escape and host cell exit of. *Mycobacterium tuberculosis. MBio.* 2017;8(2).

Saini NK, et al. Suppression of autophagy and antigen presentation by *Mycobacterium tuberculosis* PE_PGRS47. *Nat Microbiol.* 2016;1(9):16133.

Shi L, et al. Infection with *Mycobacterium tuberculosis* induces the Warburg effect in mouse lungs. *Sci Rep.* 2015;5:18176.

Singhal A, et al. Metformin as adjunct antituberculosis therapy. *Sci Transl Med.* 2014;6(263):263ra159.

Srivastava S, Ernst JD, Desvignes L. Beyond macrophages: the diversity of mononuclear cells in tuberculosis. *Immunol Rev.* 2014;262(1):179–192.

Upadhyay S, Mittal E, Philips JA. Tuberculosis and the art of macrophage manipulation. *Pathog Dis.* 2018;76(4).

van der Wel N, et al. *M. tuberculosis* and *M. leprae* translocate from the phagolysosome to the cytosol in myeloid cells. *Cell.* 2007;129(7):1287–1298.

Wong KW. The role of ESX-1 in *Mycobacterium tuberculosis* pathogenesis. *Microbiol Spectr.* 2017;5(3).

Complete reference list available at ExpertConsult.com.

53 TUBERCULOSIS: CLINICAL MANIFESTATIONS AND DIAGNOSIS

PRIYA B. SHETE, MD, MPH • ADITHYA CATTAMANCHI, MD, MAS • CHRISTINA YOON, MD, MPH, MAS

INTRODUCTION

Tuberculosis (TB) continues to be a global public health threat, with more than 10 million people developing the disease and an estimated 1.2 million deaths each year.[1] Early diagnosis followed by linkage to appropriate treatment remains essential for improving patient outcomes and reducing transmission. This chapter reviews the general approach to evaluating persons who may have TB and the available diagnostic tests.

DIAGNOSIS OF PULMONARY TUBERCULOSIS

DIAGNOSTIC EVALUATION

Clinicians must recognize that, in evaluating persons who may have TB, they are both providing care to an individual patient and assuming an essential public health function. Early and accurate diagnosis is critically important to TB care and control.[2] Despite dramatically improved access to high-quality TB services worldwide during the past 2 decades, there is substantial evidence that failure to identify and treat cases early is a major weakness in efforts to ensure optimal outcomes for the patient and to control the disease. Diagnostic delays result in ongoing transmission in the community and more severe, progressive disease in the affected person.

Globally, there are three main reasons for delays in diagnosing TB: the affected person not seeking or not having access to care; the provider not suspecting the disease; and the lack of sensitivity of the most commonly available diagnostic test, smear microscopy of sputum (or other specimen).[3,4] Approaches to reducing these delays are, obviously,

quite different. Reducing delays on the part of the affected person entails providing accessible health care facilities, enhancing community and individual awareness, and pursuing active case finding in high-risk populations. Reducing delay by the provider is best approached by increasing provider awareness of the risks for and symptoms of TB and by enhancing the availability and use of appropriate diagnostic tests. Rapid molecular tests that increase both the speed and the sensitivity for identifying *Mycobacterium tuberculosis* are increasingly available and now recommended by the *World Health Organization* (WHO) as the initial diagnostic test for *M. tuberculosis* where available.[5,6]

PATIENT HISTORY

There must be a clinical suspicion of TB before proper diagnostic tests are ordered. Clinical suspicion is prompted largely by the presence of symptoms and by awareness of comorbidities and epidemiologic circumstances that increase the risk of TB in an individual patient. These risks are summarized in the WHO guidelines for screening for TB.[7] The most commonly reported symptom of pulmonary TB is persistent cough that generally, but not always, is productive of mucus and sometimes blood. In persons with TB, cough is often accompanied by systemic symptoms, such as fever, night sweats, and weight loss. In addition, findings such as lymphadenopathy, consistent with concurrent extrapulmonary TB, may be noted, especially in patients with *human immunodeficiency virus* (HIV) infection. However, chronic cough with sputum production is not always present, even among persons with sputum smears showing acid-fast bacilli. Data from several TB prevalence surveys in countries with a high incidence of the disease show that many persons with active TB do not have cough of 2 or more weeks' duration, a criterion that, conventionally, has been used to define suspected TB.[8,9] In these studies, 10–25% of patients with bacteriologically confirmed TB do not report cough.[10,11] These data suggest that evaluation for TB using a symptom review that includes *cough of any duration, fever, night sweats, or weight loss* may be indicated in selected risk groups, especially in areas where there is a high prevalence of the disease and in high-risk populations and individuals with increased susceptibility, such as persons with HIV infection. Use of this broadened set of questions in a population of persons with HIV infection was found to have a negative predictive value of 97.7% for TB.[12] The presence of any one of the symptoms should be viewed as an indication for an evaluation for TB in high-risk groups or in high-incidence areas.

Hemoptysis is usually seen with more extensive involvement but does not necessarily indicate an active tuberculous process. Hemoptysis may also result from inactive TB, as from bronchiectasis left as a residual of healed TB; from rupture of a dilated vessel in the wall of an old cavity (*Rasmussen aneurysm*); from bacterial or fungal infection (especially in the form of a fungus ball [*aspergilloma or mycetoma*]) in an old residual cavity (eFig. 53.1); or from erosion of calcified lesions into the lumen of an airway (*broncholithiasis*).

The systemic features of TB include fever in approximately 35–80%, malaise, and weight loss; there may be a variety of hematologic abnormalities, especially leukocytosis and anemia.[13–15]

PHYSICAL EXAMINATION

In most cases, physical findings are not specific for pulmonary TB. Crackles may be heard in the area of involvement, along with bronchial breath sounds, when lung consolidation is close to the chest wall. Amphoric breath sounds (like the low sound produced by blowing across the top of an open bottle), if present, may be indicative of a cavity. Findings such as lymph node enlargement, suggestive of extrapulmonary TB, may also indicate concurrent pulmonary involvement.

RADIOGRAPHIC FEATURES

Radiographic examination of the chest is commonly the first diagnostic study undertaken, after the history and physical examination.[16,17] However, in resource-limited settings, a chest radiograph is not necessarily included as part of the routine evaluation because of cost, complexity, and nonspecificity of the findings.[18]

Pulmonary TB nearly always causes detectable abnormalities on the chest radiograph, although, in patients with HIV infection, a chest radiograph may be normal in up to 11% of patients with positive sputum cultures, and the chest radiograph may be normal in laryngeal TB.

In *primary* TB, resulting from recent infection, the process is generally seen as a middle or lower lung zone opacity, often associated with ipsilateral hilar adenopathy (Fig. 53.1). Atelectasis may result from compression of airways by enlarged lymph nodes. If the primary process persists beyond the time when specific cell-mediated immunity develops, cavities may form (so-called progressive primary TB).

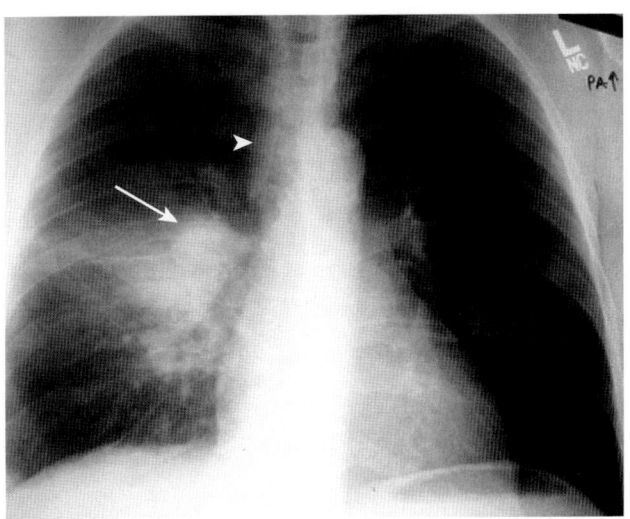

Figure 53.1 Primary tuberculosis. Frontal chest radiograph in a young adult shows superior segment right lower lobe consolidation associated with right hilar lymphadenopathy (*arrow*) due to primary *Mycobacterium tuberculosis* infection. Mild right paratracheal lymph node enlargement (*arrowhead*) is also visible. (Courtesy Michael B. Gotway, MD.)

In *reactivation* TB, developing at a time remote from the original infection, one sees involvement of the upper lobes of one or both lungs. Cavitation is common in this form of TB. The most frequent sites are the apical and posterior segments of the right upper lobe (Fig. 53.2) and the apical-posterior segment of the left upper lobe. Healing of the tuberculous lesions usually results in development of a fibrotic scar with shrinkage of the lung parenchyma and, often, calcification. Involvement of the anterior segments alone is unusual. In the immunocompetent adult with TB, intrathoracic adenopathy is uncommon. When the disease progresses, infected material may be spread via the airways (i.e., "bronchogenic" spread) into the lower portions of the involved lung or to the other lung. Erosion of a parenchymal focus of TB into a blood or lymph vessel may result in dissemination of the organism and a miliary pattern on chest imaging (Fig. 53.3; see Fig. 20.21). Radiographic findings in HIV-infected patients are affected by the degree of immunosuppression. As further explained and illustrated in Chapter 123, TB early in the course of HIV infection—before profound depletion of CD4 T cells—tends to produce typical radiographic findings with predominantly upper lobe infiltration and cavitation.[20] With more advanced HIV disease and CD4 T-cell deficiency, the radiographic findings become more "atypical": cavitation is uncommon, and lower lung zone or diffuse opacities and intrathoracic adenopathy are frequent (Fig. 53.4). Surprisingly, a substantial number of HIV-infected patients with pulmonary TB have normal radiographs at the end of their course of treatment.[21]

The activity of a presumed tuberculous process cannot be determined simply from a single chest radiograph, although new imaging modalities may assist with making this distinction (see below). A cavity might be a sterile residual of an old infection, whereas a fibrotic-appearing lesion may be active. Conversely, not all radiographic worsening of the residua of prior tuberculous lesions can be ascribed to reactivation of the disease, although such worsening

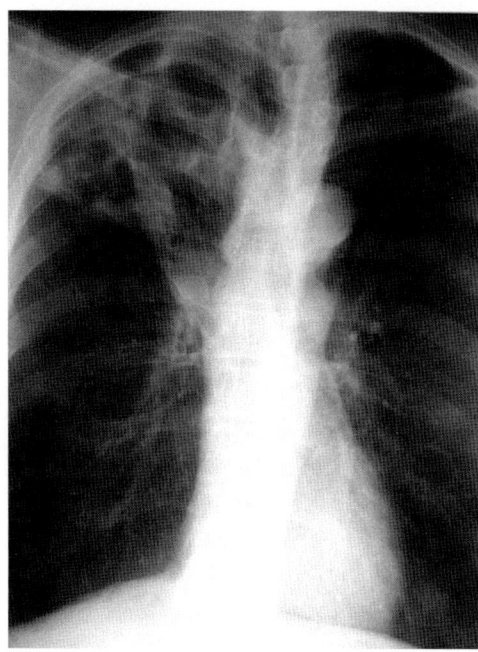

Figure 53.2 Cavitary tuberculosis. Frontal chest radiograph in a patient with tuberculosis shows extensive right upper lobe cavitation. (Courtesy Michael B. Gotway, MD.)

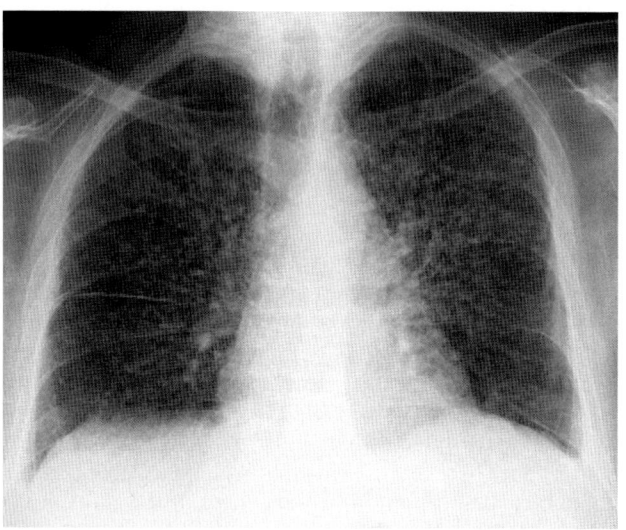

Figure 53.3 Disseminated tuberculosis. Frontal chest radiograph in a patient with disseminated tuberculosis shows numerous small, randomly distributed nodules bilaterally, representing the miliary pattern. (Courtesy Michael B. Gotway, MD.)

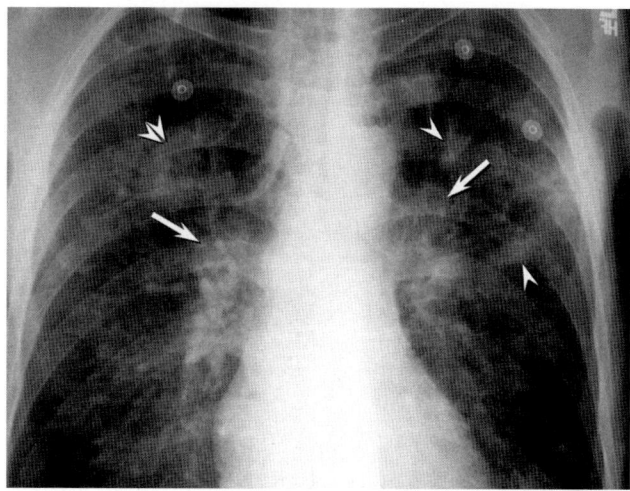

Figure 53.4 Tuberculosis in an patient with human immunodeficiency virus. Frontal chest radiograph in a patient with tuberculosis shows bilateral hilar lymph node enlargement (*arrows*) associated with poorly defined parenchymal nodular opacities (*arrowheads*) and nodular areas of consolidation (*double arrowheads*). (Courtesy Michael B. Gotway, MD.)

should always be of concern. Superimposed infections with other organisms or bleeding from bronchiectasis or from residual cavities may cause new infiltrations to appear. In addition, carcinomas may arise from within the area of scarring (so-called scar carcinomas) and can be the cause of radiographic changes.[22]

Chest radiography in most settings remains a central component of radiographic evaluation of pulmonary TB, particularly of primary pulmonary TB. However, emerging evidence describes the potential role of other imaging modalities such as *computed tomography* (CT), *magnetic resonance imaging* (MRI), and *positron emission tomography* (PET) scan, especially for nonparenchymal changes and to characterize post–primary TB. Chest CT, for example, is more sensitive at detecting lymphadenopathy than is chest radiography and is better at demonstrating bronchogenic spread characteristic of TB caused by reactivation.[23] In addition, CT has higher sensitivity of predicting active TB compared to chest radiography, with a sensitivity of 96% compared to 48%.[24] This is primarily because CT scans can demonstrate radiographic findings more associated with highly infectious progressive primary TB disease, including consolidation involving the lung apices, consolidation involving the superior segments of the lower lobes, cavitary lesions, and characteristics of nodules, including clusters.[25]

Although CT increasingly is being used for the diagnosis and characterization of progressive primary pulmonary TB, alternative imaging methods without ionizing radiation are also being adapted, including MRI. Traditionally, MRI has not been used to evaluate for pulmonary diseases due to the concern of poor image quality caused by low proton density in the lung, rapid signal decay due to high magnetic susceptibility at the air-tissue interface, and intrinsic motion artifacts from respiratory motion.[26] With new motion-correcting protocols, MRI may be better than CT for evaluation of pleural involvement including pleural effusion and to characterize the presence of caseous necrosis and liquefaction. MRI has been shown to be comparable to CT in describing lymphadenopathy and consolidations, although sensitivity for pulmonary nodules is lower.[27] Thus, radiographic surveillance with MRI as opposed to CT should be considered in vulnerable populations in whom the use of ionizing radiation is of concern, such as pregnant women and children.[28] Finally, there is growing evidence for the additional role that fluorodeoxyglucose-PET/CT may have in monitoring treatment response and differentiating active pulmonary TB from old or inactive disease,[29] with sensitivity and specificity reported to be 100% when using a maximal standardized uptake value threshold of at least 1.05. Additional research is needed to establish standardized uptake value thresholds that predict disease activity in specific populations.

Consideration should be given to the extensive resources that CT, MRI, and PET/CT may require in most settings.

Because primary TB infection can result in parenchymal disease, lymphadenopathy, pleural effusion, or miliary disease, the differential diagnosis of radiographic abnormalities that may be consistent with TB is still broad. Parenchymal disease with or without associated cavitation can mimic a variety of bacterial or fungal pneumonias. Nodules with or without concomitant ground glass may be consistent with other infections or with malignancy, and bronchiectasis may be consistent with *nontuberculous mycobacterial* (NTM) disease. Therefore, a nondiagnostic microbiologic evaluation should prompt a careful assessment for other causes of the radiographic abnormality. From this discussion, it should be obvious that the radiologic findings, although extremely valuable, cannot provide a definitive diagnosis of TB. Because of the radiographic similarities among the other disorders in the differential diagnosis, and because of the uncertainties in assessing disease activity and in determining the reasons for progressive radiographic changes, careful microbiologic evaluation is always indicated.

LABORATORY DIAGNOSTIC EVALUATION

Testing for Suspected Pulmonary Tuberculosis

All adults and children who are suspected of having active pulmonary TB should have at least two sputum specimens collected for *acid-fast bacilli* (AFB) smear microscopy and mycobacterial culture and at least one sputum specimen collected for *nucleic acid amplification testing* (NAAT). Although collecting more than two sputum specimens increases the yield only slightly, in the United States, collection of three sputum specimens for AFB smear microscopy and culture is considered routine practice and is strongly recommended to improve sensitivity by the Centers for Disease Control and Prevention, American Thoracic Society, and Infectious Disease Society of America.[30] NAAT is recommended for the initial sputum specimen in the United States and other low-incidence countries; however, NAAT results should be interpreted in conjunction with AFB smear microscopy results. For AFB smear–positive persons, a positive NAAT result offers rapid confirmation of TB diagnosis. A negative result may suggest another etiology, such as NTM, because NAATs are able to distinguish *M. tuberculosis* from nontuberculous mycobacteria. For AFB smear–negative persons with intermediate to high probability of disease, a positive NAAT result is used as presumptive evidence of TB. For AFB smear–negative persons with low probability of disease, a positive NAAT result should be interpreted with caution because of the higher probability of false positives in this population. For AFB smear–negative persons with suspected pulmonary TB, a negative NAAT result does not exclude active disease; current NAATs do not possess sufficient sensitivity to replace mycobacterial culture.

In most countries with a high incidence of TB, culture is not routinely performed in the evaluation of persons with suspected pulmonary TB because culturing mycobacteria from clinical specimens requires costly laboratory infrastructure and biosafety conditions not available in many low-resource settings. As such, TB diagnosis in high-incidence settings relies primarily on AFB smear microscopy and increasingly, Xpert MTB/RIF (Cepheid), an automated, self-contained real-time NAAT that detects *M. tuberculosis* complex and rifampin resistance in 90 minutes. Although U.S. policymakers recommend using NAATs including Xpert MTB/RIF as an adjunct test to AFB smear microscopy, the WHO recommends Xpert MTB/RIF as the preferred initial test for suspected pulmonary TB cases with HIV infection, risk factors for multidrug-resistance, and serious illness.[31] In addition, the WHO recommends that, where feasible, Xpert MTB/RIF testing can be used as the initial test in place of two specimens submitted for smear microscopy for all adults and children with suspected TB. However, individuals diagnosed with active TB by Xpert MTB/RIF testing should submit additional sputum for AFB smear microscopy and culture (if rifampin resistance is detected) because conventional microscopy remains essential for monitoring treatment response and culture is required for phenotypic drug susceptibility testing.

Specimen Collection

As noted previously, a definitive diagnosis of TB can be established only by isolation of tubercle bacilli in culture or by identification of specific nucleic acid sequences. When the lung is involved, sputum is the initial specimen of choice. Two sputum specimens should be collected, which can be obtained on the same day because the sensitivity of tests using same-day specimens is similar to tests using specimens collected on different days.[32] The collection of the sputum on one day allows results to be available the same day, thereby increasing the efficiency of sputum smear microscopy.[32] The strategies for same-day microscopy include the preparation of two or three slides from sputum samples obtained the first day the patient is assessed. Collecting more than two sputum specimens increases the yield only slightly.[33]

There are several options for obtaining specimens from patients who are not producing sputum. The first and most useful in terms of yield and avoidance of patient discomfort is *sputum induction,* in which sputum production is enhanced by the inhalation of a hypertonic (3–5%) saline mist generated by an ultrasonic nebulizer. Sputum induced by this technique is clear and resembles saliva; thus, it must be properly labeled or it may be discarded by the laboratory. This is a benign and well-tolerated procedure, although bronchospasm may be precipitated in asthmatic patients.

Sampling of gastric contents via a nasogastric tube has a lower yield than sputum induction and is more complicated and uncomfortable for the patient. However, in children and some adults, gastric contents may be the only specimen that can be obtained. Gastric lavage should be performed early in the morning before the patient has gotten out of bed, eaten, or performed dental hygiene. Once the specimen is obtained, the specimen should be sent to the laboratory and processed the same day. To prolong the viability of the bacteria, neutralization of gastric acid with an equal volume of sterile 1% sodium bicarbonate is recommended when the specimen is not processed immediately.[34,35]

Depending on the clinical circumstances, if the sputum is negative or cannot be obtained, the next diagnostic step is usually fiberoptic bronchoscopy with bronchoalveolar lavage and, in some instances, transbronchial lung biopsy. The yield of bronchoscopy is high in miliary TB and in focal disease as well. Bronchoscopic procedures have been especially helpful in the diagnostic evaluations of patients with HIV infection with negative sputum smear microscopy.[36] Needle aspiration-biopsy may also provide specimens from which mycobacteria are isolated, but the technique is especially suited to the evaluation of peripheral nodular lesions for which there is a suspicion of malignancy.

A diagnosis of TB can also be made by an appropriate response to antituberculosis therapy. For example, in some situations, a trial of antituberculosis chemotherapy may be indicated before more invasive studies are undertaken. For example, when there is a radiographic abnormality consistent with TB in a person younger than 40 years, a nonsmoker, and from a country with a high prevalence of TB, either current or past TB is much more likely than a neoplasm, even in the presence of negative smears and cultures of sputum. In such a patient, improvement in the chest radiograph concomitant with antituberculosis treatment would be sufficient reason for making a diagnosis of TB and continuing with a full course of therapy. A response should be seen within 2 months of starting treatment. If no improvement is noted, the abnormality must be the result of either old TB or another process. An algorithm illustrating this approach is shown in Figure 53.5. However, for individuals with risk factors for drug-resistant TB (e.g., prior TB, high prevalence of drug-resistant TB in the country of origin), empiric trials of antituberculosis chemotherapy should be avoided and microbiologic confirmation should be aggressively pursued for drug susceptibility testing whenever possible.

Because of the potentially disastrous consequences of delays in diagnosis of TB, it is essential that tests for *M. tuberculosis* be performed rapidly and the results be reported promptly. Waiting days for the results of AFB smear microscopy and NAAT, weeks for culture results, and months for speciation and susceptibility studies is not acceptable.

Acid-Fast Staining

Historically, the first step in the diagnostic sequence consisted of staining and examining readily available specimens for AFB. Current recommendations now support both AFB smear microscopy and NAAT on the initial respiratory specimen (see below for recommendations for use of rapid molecular tests in the initial evaluation). Finding AFB is generally specific for mycobacteria but provides no information about species. However, the sensitivity of microscopic examination is relatively low; the level of detection is approximately 10,000 bacilli/mL of secretions if 100 oil immersion microscopic fields are examined. The sensitivity of sputum smear microscopy can be increased by concentrating the sample either by centrifugation or sedimentation after chemical processing.[37] Sensitivity can also be increased by about 10% using a fluorochrome staining procedure with auramine O, a fluorescent stain.[38] This procedure requires use of a fluorescent microscope, which requires an excitation light source. There are two types of light sources. The first one is the short-arc mercury vapor lamp, which has a limited lifespan (200 to 300 hours), is costly, requires high maintenance, and is potentially toxic due to its mercury content. The second is the light-emitting diode, which has a life span of more than 50,000 hours, is less expensive, and has a performance similar to the MVP-based microscopy.[39] Fluorochrome-based procedures are faster than acid-fast staining because the intensity and contrast of the fluorescent signal on a dark background enables slides to be scanned at lower magnification.

Smears are generally interpreted as negative or, if positive, are reported as rare (3 to 9 organisms per slide), few (10 or more per slide), or numerous (1 or more per high-power oil immersion field). In most situations in which acid-fast organisms are detected by microscopy, they should be assumed to be *M. tuberculosis* until proven otherwise. Assuming the patient has TB will trigger the appropriate prompt responses from the physicians responsible for treatment and from public health agencies. In practice, the sensitivity of sputum smears varies widely: 20–80% of patients with *M. tuberculosis* isolated in culture have positive smears.[37]

Mycobacterial Culture

Culture in liquid media is considered the current diagnostic gold standard and can detect as few as 10 to 1000 viable mycobacteria/mL of sputum. Culture is a necessary step for diagnosis and is essential for phenotypic drug susceptibility testing. Culture of sputum usually involves digestion, decontamination, and concentration of the specimen before inoculation of media. This process decreases bacterial overgrowth and, when solid media are used, enables more uniform plating of the specimen. For specimens other than sputum, digestion and decontamination are not required. At a minimum, laboratories performing culture should be able to identify *M. tuberculosis* by phenotypic or molecular methods (see below). Isolates that are not *M. tuberculosis* or are of questionable identity should then be sent to a more specialized laboratory for definitive speciation.

Culture can be performed in solid or liquid media. Solid media are usually less expensive and allow the morphologic examination of the colonies to be used for presumptive species identification. However, results on solid media are delayed due to the slow growth of mycobacteria and, in some settings, the delayed culture results may have limited or no impact on patient management.[40] The solid media can be based on egg such as Lowenstein-Jensen media or on agar such as Middlebrook 7H10 or 7H11 media. *M. tuberculosis* colonies appear in 2 to 8 weeks, and cultures without growth at 8 weeks are reported as negative, although they are generally kept for another 2 to 4 weeks before being discarded because some strains grow more slowly than the average.

Liquid media are more sensitive and increase the yield by 10%. They enable *M. tuberculosis* growth to be detected in 10 to 14 days. However, liquid media also have a higher rate of contamination with other bacteria or fungi.[41] The growth of *M. tuberculosis* in liquid media produces fluorimetric or colorimetric reactions, detected using manual or automated systems. The automated systems permit a higher throughput and should be used in settings with high workloads, especially for drug susceptibility testing. The manual systems are less expensive and are used in areas with limited resources.

***M. tuberculosis* Identification.** The methods to identify *M. tuberculosis* can be classified as (1) phenotypic methods including biochemical tests and specific cell and colony characteristics and (2) molecular methods targeting *M. tuberculosis complex*–specific nucleic acids or proteins.

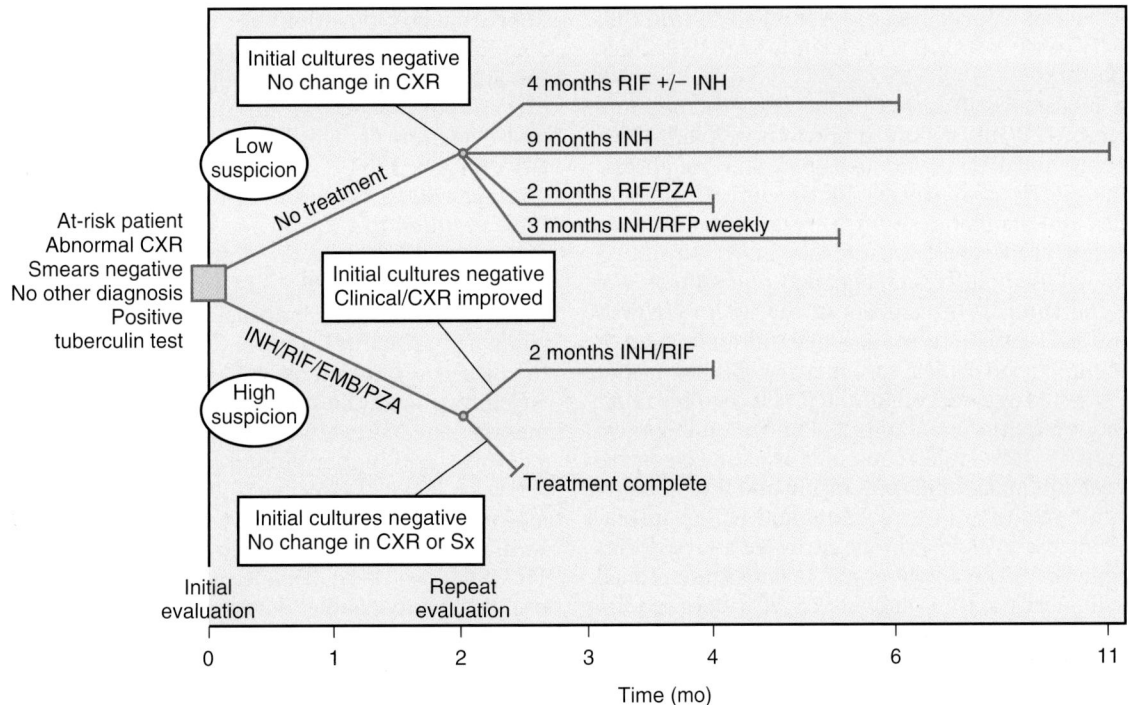

Figure 53.5 Approach to diagnosis and treatment for active, culture-negative pulmonary tuberculosis and inactive tuberculosis. The decision to begin treatment for a patient with sputum smears that are negative depends on the degree of suspicion that the patient has tuberculosis. If the clinical suspicion is high (lower portion of figure), then multidrug therapy should be initiated before acid-fast smear/culture results are known. If the diagnosis is confirmed by a positive culture, treatment can be continued to complete a standard course of therapy. If initial cultures remain negative and treatment has been with multiple drugs for 2 months, then there are two options depending on repeat evaluation at 2 months (lower portion of figure). In option 1, if the patient demonstrates symptomatic or radiographic improvement without another apparent diagnosis, then a diagnosis of culture-negative tuberculosis can be inferred. Treatment should be continued with isoniazid and rifampin for an additional 2 months. In option 2, if the patient demonstrates neither symptomatic nor radiographic improvement, then tuberculosis is unlikely and treatment can be stopped. In low-suspicion patients not initially on treatment (upper portion of figure), if cultures remain negative, the patient has no symptoms, and the chest radiograph is unchanged at 2 to 3 months, there are four treatment options: (1) isoniazid for 9 months; (2) rifampin with or without isoniazid for 4 months; (3) rifampin and pyrazinamide for 2 months; or (4) isoniazide and rifapentine weekly for 3 months. (See discussion of latent tuberculous infection.) CXR, chest radiograph; EMB, ethambutol; INH, isoniazid; PZA, pyrazinamide; RIF, rifampin; RFP, rifapentine; Sx, symptoms. (From Blumberg HM, Burman WJ, Chaisson RE, et al, for the American Thoracic Society/Centers for Disease Control and Prevention/Infectious Diseases Society of America. Treatment of tuberculosis. *Am J Respir Crit Care Med.* 2003;167:603–662.)

PHENOTYPE-BASED IDENTIFICATION METHODS. The classical phenotype-based methods to identify *M. tuberculosis* complex require a positive culture for mycobacteria. These tests include niacin production, nitrate reduction, and inactivation of catalase at 68°C. The tests also use the time to growth, usually 12 to 42 days in solid media; the presence of rough, cauliflower-like, and colorless colonies; and the presence of organisms that are tangled and form corded masses when observed by microscopy.

The *microscopic observation of drug susceptibility* (MODS) assay is a culture-based method that discriminates between *M. tuberculosis* complex and NTM and determines the drug susceptibility to rifampin and isoniazid at the same time. MODS incorporates the antituberculosis drugs in the culture media at the beginning of the assay. The method uses a sealed 24-well tissue-culture plate with liquid culture media containing different antibiotics and controls that are examined periodically under an inverted light microscope. *M. tuberculosis* can be identified by the observation of a tangled or corded mass of organisms and by a time to detection (including susceptibility test), typically less than 2 weeks. The overall sensitivity of MODS to detect *M. tuberculosis* growth was 92% and the specificity was 96% compared with conventional culture. The mean time from receipt of specimen to results was 9.2 days, and contamination was

present in 7%.[42] There is currently a MODS kit commercially available, and its use is recommended by the WHO in laboratories where genotypic or automated liquid culture and drug-susceptibility testing capacity are being developed.[43]

MOLECULAR IDENTIFICATION METHODS. Several molecular methods are available to identify *M. tuberculosis* directly on the specimen or in mycobacterial culture. They are based on nucleic acid amplification technologies in which as few as 1 to 10 copies of DNA or ribonucleic acid specific to *M. tuberculosis* complex are amplified to detectable levels. Other targets include proteins specific to *M. tuberculosis*. All these tests identify the presence of *M. tuberculosis* complex and can rule out the presence of NTM. Importantly, some NAATs are able to identify the presence of *M. tuberculosis* complex and drug resistance–associated mutations in the same test. There are several commercial technologies, although only two, Xpert MTB/RIF and GenProbe Amplified *M. tuberculosis* Direct test, are available in the United States. The current recommendation by the Centers for Disease Control and Prevention is to use a NAAT on at least one specimen, preferably the first diagnostic specimen from each patient in whom a TB diagnosis is being considered.[44] The recommended interpretation algorithm includes the use of clinical judgment when the NAAT is negative. This limitation has been applied because it has been found that the sensitivity of the tests is not sufficiently high to exclude *M. tuberculosis*.[44,45]

A major breakthrough in NAAT has been the development of Xpert MTB/RIF. As noted previously, Xpert MTB/RIF is an automated, self-contained, real-time *polymerase chain reaction* (PCR) assay capable of detecting *M. tuberculosis* complex and rifampin resistance–associated mutations directly in clinical specimens with results in 90 minutes.[46] This system is based on the amplification of a sequence of the *rpoB* gene specific to members of the *M. tuberculosis* complex and the rifampin resistance–determining region. It can be used directly on clinical specimens or specimens that have been digested and decontaminated.[47] It requires minimal biosafety measures[48] and minimal hands-on technical time.[49] It consists of two main components: (1) a disposable cartridge that contains sample processing and the *M. tuberculosis*-specific real-time PCR reagents and (2) an instrument that controls the fluidics in the cartridge and performs the PCR analysis.[46] The operational challenges are related to the specific needs of the components: cartridges require a temperature below 28°C and have a 12-month shelf-life, and the instrument requires a stable electrical power supply and an ambient temperature below 30°C.[49] A meta-analysis showed that, as an initial test replacing smear microscopy, Xpert MTB/RIF pooled sensitivity was 89% and pooled specificity 99%.[50] As an add-on test following a negative smear microscopy result, Xpert MTB/RIF pooled sensitivity was 67% and specificity 99%. For smear-positive, culture-positive TB, Xpert MTB/RIF pooled sensitivity was 98%. For people with HIV infection, Xpert MTB/RIF pooled sensitivity was 79% and, for people without HIV infection, it was 86%. The pooled sensitivity to detect rifampin resistance was 95%, and the pooled specificity was 98%.[50] This assay has a median time to detection of *M. tuberculosis* of hours compared with 1 day for microscopy, 16 days for culture in liquid media, and 30 days for culture on solid media. The median time to detection of rifampin resistance with the automated and self-contained real-time PCR assay was 1 day compared with 106 days for phenotypic tests.[51] More importantly, Xpert MTB/RIF reduced the median time to treatment of patients with sputum smear-negative TB from 56 days to 5 days.[51] On the basis of its diagnostic accuracy, WHO endorsed the Xpert MTB/RIF for the diagnosis of TB in 2010.[52,53] WHO recommends that, for all patients (including children) who are suspected of having pulmonary TB and are capable of producing sputum, a single specimen submitted for Xpert MTB/RIF testing can be used as the initial test in place of two specimens submitted for smear microscopy. In addition, WHO recommends that Xpert MTB/RIF should be used as the preferred initial test for patients who are at risk for drug resistance, who have HIV risks, or who are seriously ill; because of the speed of diagnosis, the test is also preferred for use with *cerebrospinal fluid* (CSF) in patients suspected of having tuberculous meningitis.

WHO recommendations for the use of Xpert MTB/RIF now also apply to the use of Xpert MTB/RIF Ultra,[54] Cepheid's next-generation assay developed to improve sensitivity of TB diagnosis, as the initial test for all adults and children with suspected pulmonary TB and in the testing of selected extrapulmonary specimens (e.g., CSF, lymph nodes, and tissue specimens). Key modifications to improve assay sensitivity for the detection of *M. tuberculosis* include a larger DNA reaction chamber that doubles the amount of purified DNA delivered to the PCR reaction (50 μL PCR reaction in Ultra vs. 25 μL in Xpert MTB/RIF) and detection of two different multicopy *M. tuberculosis* DNA targets (IS6110 and IS1081) instead of a single-copy *M. tuberculosis* DNA target (*rpoB*). These modifications have resulted in the Ultra assay having a lower limit of detection (16 bacterial colony forming units/mL) compared to Xpert MTB/RIF (114 colony forming units/mL). A multicenter noninferiority diagnostic accuracy study comparing the Ultra assay to Xpert MTB/RIF in reference to culture found that overall sensitivity of the Ultra assay was higher than the standard assay (88% vs. 83%), higher among smear-negative culture-positive TB cases (63% vs. 46%), and higher among people with HIV coinfection (90% vs. 77%).[55] However, overall specificity of the Ultra assay was lower compared to the Xpert MTB/RIF (96% vs. 98%) and lower among individuals with a history of TB (93% vs. 98%) because the increased sensitivity of the Ultra assay enables detection of nonreplicating or nonviable bacilli present in individuals with a recent history of TB, reducing the overall specificity of Ultra in high-incidence settings. The Xpert MTB/RIF Ultra assay is not yet available in the United States for clinical use.

Other commercially available molecular methods can be used directly on clinical samples (smear-positive specimens) or mycobacterial cultures for identification of the *M. tuberculosis* complex and drug resistance–associated mutations on the same day the specimen is received.[56] However, because of the higher risk of exposure to TB, these technologies require more technical expertise and a more complex laboratory infrastructure (separate rooms for DNA extraction, preamplification procedures, and amplification/postamplification procedures; unidirectional workflow, stringent cleaning protocols, and restricted access to avoid contamination; and biosafety level 3 laboratories if performed using culture specimens).

The line probe assay uses a DNA strip-based test that allows the simultaneous identification of *M. tuberculosis* and common genetic mutations causing resistance to isoniazid and rifampin from smear-positive sputum samples or from positive cultures. Line probe assays determine the drug resistance profile of a strain by the pattern of binding of amplified DNA to probes on the strip. When one of the known mutation resistance genes is amplified in the TB strain, a line or band appears on the strip. Currently, four line probe assays exist: the INNO-LiPARif.TB assay (Fujirubio),[57] which is available for research use only for the detection of *M. tuberculosis* and rifampin resistance, Genoscholar NTM+MDRTBII (Nipro) and two versions of the GenoTypeMTBDR assay (Hain LifeScience). Genoscholar NTM+MDRTB II and the GenoTypeMTBDRplus detect *M. tuberculosis* and rifampin and isoniazid resistance,[58] and the GenoTypeMTBDR*sl* detects the most common mutations in the *gyrA* gene for fluoroquinolone resistance; in the *rrs* gene for amikacin, capreomycin, and kanamycin resistance; and in the *embB* gene for ethambutol resistance.[59] Of these, the GenoTypeMTBDR assays have been the most widely studied and used at reference laboratories in low- and middle-income countries following WHO endorsement initially in 2008[60] and updated in 2016.[58]

The gene targets and sensitivity and specificity data for the commercial line probe assays approved for clinical use are summarized in eTable 53.1.

Non–Sputum-Based Tests

Urine Tests. Recently, tests based on the detection of *lipoarabinomannan* (LAM) antigen in urine have emerged as novel tests for TB diagnosis. LAM is a lipopolysaccharide present in mycobacterial cell walls released from metabolically active or degenerating bacterial cells from people with active TB disease. Detecting LAM in urine for TB diagnosis has several advantages relative to conventional sputum-based diagnostics: urine is easily accessible, thus facilitating TB testing for adults and children unable to produce sputum; collection and processing of urine specimens for TB testing requires minimal biosafety measures; and detection of LAM is amenable to inexpensive point-of-care platforms. However, the only commercially available urine LAM assay (Determine TB LAM Ag; Alere) has been shown to have suboptimal sensitivity for active TB. However, unlike traditional tests, sensitivity was higher among people living with HIV and further increased as CD4 cell count decreased.[61] The higher sensitivity of urine LAM in those settings may be explained by a higher mycobacterial burden, increased likelihood of extrapulmonary TB (i.e., genitourinary TB), and increased glomerular permeability associated with HIV-related immunosuppression.[62]

A meta-analysis evaluating the diagnostic accuracy of Determine TB LAM Ag among people living with HIV showed a pooled sensitivity of 42% and a pooled specificity of 91%.[63] Pooled sensitivity and specificity significantly varied by testing indication (e.g., whether by targeted testing of patients presenting with TB symptoms vs. screening of unselected patients irrespective of symptoms), health care setting (e.g., hospitalized patients vs. outpatients), and degree of HIV-associated immunosuppression (i.e., CD4 cell counts). Pooled sensitivity was higher (and pooled specificity generally lower) for (1) symptomatic patients than unselected patients (pooled sensitivity 42% vs. 35%), (2) symptomatic inpatients than symptomatic outpatients (pooled sensitivity 62% vs. 31%), and (3) symptomatic patients with CD4 cell counts less than 200 cells/μL than symptomatic patients with CD4 cell counts 200 cells/μL or greater (pooled sensitivity 45% vs. 16%). A meta-analysis evaluating the incremental change in sensitivity and specificity when combined with smear or Xpert MTB/RIF found that when Determine TB LAM Ag was combined with sputum smear microscopy (i.e., using any positive test), pooled sensitivity was 59% (a 19% increase relative to smear microscopy alone) and pooled specificity was 92% (a 6% decrease relative to smear microscopy alone).[64] When Determine TB LAM Ag was combined with sputum Xpert MTB/RIF, pooled sensitivity was 75% (a 13% increase relative to Xpert MTB/RIF alone) and pooled specificity was 93% (a 4% decrease relative to Xpert MTB/RIF alone). Based on these results, the Determine TB LAM Ag test is recommended by the WHO as the initial test for all HIV-infected inpatients and outpatients with TB symptoms, irrespective of CD4 cell count and irrespective of symptoms if CD4 cell count less than 200 cells/μL (inpatients) or CD4 cell count less than 100 cells/μL (outpatients),[65] although this test is not currently available in the United States.

Because urine LAM has a high potential for use as a point-of-care assay for TB diagnosis, development of next-generation highly sensitive and specific urine LAM assays is a current area of active research. Possible methods for improving urine LAM sensitivity include novel approaches to concentrating LAM antigen in urine,[66] removal of inhibitors in urine,[67] and pairing high-affinity monoclonal antibodies to target LAM epitopes.[68] The FujiLAM assay (FujiFilm), which combines pairing high-affinity monoclonal antibodies to target LAM epitopes and a silver-based amplification step that increases the visibility of test and control lines of a lateral flow assay, has been shown in studies using stored specimens to increase sensitivity substantially among HIV-infected inpatients (70% vs. 42%) and outpatients (68% vs. 45%), relative to Determine TB LAM.[63,69] FujiLAM is currently available for research use only; prospective evaluations are currently ongoing.

Serologic Tests. Several antigens, including highly purified and recombinant antigens specific for *M. tuberculosis* complex, have been used in serologic antibody tests with variable results. A systematic review found that the results of serologic tests are highly variable and not better than sputum smear microscopy.[70,71] On the basis of these results, WHO has strongly recommended against the use of serologic tests for the diagnosis of pulmonary and extrapulmonary TB.[72]

Tuberculin Skin Test or Interferon-γ Release Assays to Guide Empiric Treatment Decisions for Active Tuberculosis. Clinicians caring for suspected TB cases with negative smear and NAAT results are often faced with the dilemma of whether to initiate empiric treatment for individuals for active disease or to wait up to 8 weeks for final culture results. Although smear- and NAAT-negative patients are less infectious than smear and/or NAAT-positive patients, patients with paucibacillary TB are still capable of transmitting infection, with a relative transmission rate of smear-negative cases compared to smear-positive cases estimated to be 24%.[73] Furthermore, because half of all TB cases are smear negative, the population-level contribution of paucibacillary TB cases to overall disease transmission is substantial, with molecular studies estimating smear-negative cases to be responsible for 13–17% of all TB transmission.[73-75] While early initiation of antituberculosis chemotherapy for all patients with active disease is necessary to reduce disease transmission and individual morbidity and mortality risk, careful selection of patients for empiric treatment is required to minimize medication toxicity for individuals without active disease.

Decisions regarding initiation of empiric treatment are based on clinical presentation, radiographic findings, presence of TB risk factors, and exclusion of other non-TB diseases. Assessing for the presence of TB risk factors should include *tuberculin skin testing* (TST) or *interferon-γ release assay* (IGRA) testing to identify individuals with *Mtb* infection. If TST or IGRA results are positive, suspicion for active disease is increased because a positive TST or IGRA result has been shown consistently to be a strong predictor of a positive culture result among smear-negative individuals with suspected TB.[76,77] However, the suboptimal sensitivity of both TST and IGRAs for *Mtb* infection precludes decisions to withhold empiric therapy based on negative test results alone; empiric therapy may still be warranted despite negative TST and IGRA results if suspicion for active disease is sufficiently high.

Drug Susceptibility Testing

Determination of susceptibility to antimicrobial agents is of considerable clinical importance. Because of concerns regarding TB caused by drug-resistant organisms, drug susceptibility testing is recommended for all initial *M. tuberculosis* isolates. Unfortunately, due to lack of resources, drug susceptibility testing is not done in most high-burden areas or is limited to *M. tuberculosis* strains isolated from patients at high risk of having drug-resistant TB. There are two general methods for determining resistance: phenotypic and genotypic.[78] Some of the methods are designed to identify *M. tuberculosis* and determine the drug susceptibility in the same test, such as MODS, Xpert MTB/RIF, and line probe assays, all of which are described in the preceding section on *M. tuberculosis* identification.

The *phenotypic methods* are based on culture of *M. tuberculosis.* There are two methods: absolute and proportional. These can be done in liquid or solid media. The reference standard is the proportional method, and it is recommended in liquid media. The proportional methods involve inoculating one or more dilutions of cultured mycobacteria on drug-free media and on media containing appropriate concentrations of antituberculosis drugs. Resistance is generally considered to be present when the growth on the drug-containing medium is 1% or more of the control growth on the drug-free media.

There are several approaches to detect mycobacterial growth.[79] The colorimetric method is based on the reduction of an oxidation-reduction indicator (i.e., alamarBlue, resazurin, or tetrazolium) added to the culture media after the cells of *M. tuberculosis* are exposed to the antibiotic. Resistance to antibiotics is identified by the presence of a change in color in the media due to the oxidation/reduction process by viable mycobacteria. This method is highly sensitive and specific for the detection of rifampin and isoniazid resistance (98% and 97% sensitive, respectively; 99% and 98% specific, respectively) when compared with conventional culture-based drug susceptibility methods.[78,80] The nitrate reductase assay is based on the ability of *M. tuberculosis* to reduce nitrate to nitrite, also detected by a color reaction. The sensitivity of the test was 97%, and the specificity was 100% for the detection of rifampin resistance and 97% and 99%, respectively, for detection of isoniazid resistance.[78,80]

Testing for susceptibility to isoniazid and rifampin is accurate,[80] and resistance to rifampin has been used as an indicator for multidrug-resistant TB.[81] Testing for susceptibility to streptomycin, ethambutol, and pyrazinamide is less reliable and reproducible.[80] Testing for second-line drugs is generally performed in reference laboratories and is recommended mainly for *multidrug-resistant* strains. Critical drug concentrations have been established and resistance testing is recommended preferably using automated liquid culture systems for all WHO group A drugs (moxifloxacin, levofloxacin, bedaquiline, and linezolid), the WHO group B drug clofazimine, and the group C drugs (amikacin,

delamanid, and pyrazinamide[82]). However, pyrazinamide resistance testing can lead to high rates of false-positive results without appropriate quality assurance. Testing for resistance to the other recommended second-line drugs (group B: cycloserine, terizidone; group C: ethambutol, ethionamide, prothionamide, para-aminosalicylic acid, imipenem-cilastatin, meropenem) is not standardized and not currently recommended.[82]

The *genotypic methods* to identify drug resistance are integrated with the *M. tuberculosis* identification methods; therefore, these methods are faster than culture-based tests. The genotypic methods are based on the detection of drug resistance–associated mutations: mutations in the *rpoB* rifampin resistance–determining region are present in 96% of rifampin-resistant strains,[83] mutations in *katG* or *inhA* in 65–75% of isoniazid-resistant strains,[83] and mutations in *gyrA* and *gyrB* in 42–85% of quinolone-resistant strains.[83,84]

In addition to PCR-based genotypic methods, *next-generation sequencing* is increasingly being used to provide comprehensive drug resistance profiles. Next-generation sequencing can provide rapid and comprehensive sequence information for whole genomes or all gene regions of interest, overcoming the limitations of PCR-based genotypic methods. There are at least two commercial targeted next-generation sequencing assays. The Deeplex Myc-TB assay (GenoScreen) identifies mutations in 18 main MTB drug resistance–associated gene targets to detect resistance to 13 anti-TB drugs/drug classes including all first- and most second-line drugs (i.e., injectables, fluoroquinolones, bedaquiline, clofazimine, linezolid, and ethionamide). DeepChek-TB (Advanced Biological Laboratories) identifies the established high- and medium-confidence drug resistance targets for the same 13 anti-TB drugs/drug classes as the Deeplex Myc-TB assay. Both assays can be performed directly on clinical specimens and provide results within 48 hours. Both also include applications for rapid and automated analysis of raw sequence data, user-friendly interpretation, and reporting.[85–90]

A common limitation of all genotypic methods is the inability to detect drug-resistant strains that do not harbor the common mutations. Therefore, it is essential to use conventional phenotypic methods to exclude drug-resistant TB.

EXTRAPULMONARY TUBERCULOSIS

Extrapulmonary TB presents more of a diagnostic problem than does pulmonary TB. In part this relates to its being less common and therefore less familiar to most clinicians.[91,92] In addition, extrapulmonary TB involves relatively inaccessible sites and often, because of the vulnerability of the areas involved, much greater damage can be caused by fewer bacilli. The combination of small numbers of bacilli in inaccessible sites makes bacteriologic confirmation of a diagnosis more difficult, and invasive procedures are frequently necessary to establish a diagnosis. In addition to the need for invasive diagnostic procedures, surgery may be an important component of management.

PLEURAL TUBERCULOSIS

Although the pleural space is within the thorax, for reporting purposes, it is considered an extrapulmonary site of TB. The difference in pathogenesis of pleural TB results in different clinical presentations, approaches to diagnosis, treatment, and sequelae. TB pleuritis may present as either acute or subacute syndromes, likely due to early pathogenesis and host response to infection. The first mechanism manifests early in the course of a tuberculous infection—a few tubercle bacilli may gain access to the pleural space and, in the presence of cell-mediated immunity, can cause an inflammatory response.[93,94] This form of tuberculous pleuritis commonly goes unnoticed, and the process may resolve spontaneously; those with resolved tuberculous pleuritis, however, have a high likelihood of developing active TB in the next 2 years,[95] so tuberculous pleuritis should be considered and treated if found. In some patients, the tuberculous involvement of the pleura is manifested as an acute illness with fever, cough, pleuritic pain, and occasionally dyspnea and weight loss.[96,97] If the effusion is large, it may cause dyspnea, although the effusions are generally small and rarely bilateral.

The diagnosis of pleural TB is generally established by analysis of pleural fluid and by a pleural biopsy with concomitant sputum evaluation. In a patient with a pleural effusion that might be tuberculous, a diagnostic thoracentesis should be performed. Sufficient fluid should be obtained for cell count, cytologic examination, biochemical analysis, and microbiologic evaluation, but enough fluid should be left to allow a needle biopsy to be performed if the original specimen proves to be exudative and no diagnosis is evident. Diagnosis of TB pleuritis requires identification of the bacilli in either fluid or pleural tissue using microscopy, GeneXpert, or culture; or by visualization of caseating granulomas in pleural tissue biopsy. The fluid is nearly always straw colored, although it may be slightly bloody. Leukocyte counts are usually in the range of 100 to 5000 cells/μL.[98] Early in the course of the process, polymorphonuclear leukocytes may predominate, but subsequent influx of lymphocytes causes them to predominate later. The fluid is exudative, with a protein concentration greater than 50% of the serum protein concentration, and the glucose level may be normal to low. Therefore lymphocyte to neutrophil ratio for exudative effusions is typically greater than 0.75, which reflects a later stage in the course of an effusion, when lymphocytes predominate.[99]

The second variety of tuberculous involvement of the pleura, which is much less common than tuberculous pleurisy with effusion, is a true empyema that follows the spilling into the pleural space of a large number of organisms, usually from rupture of a cavity or an adjacent parenchymal focus via a bronchopleural fistula.[100] Tuberculous empyema is usually associated with evident pulmonary parenchymal disease on chest films. In this situation, the fluid generally is thick and cloudy and may contain cholesterol, which causes the fluid to look like chyle. The fluid is exudative and usually has a relatively high white blood cell count, nearly all of which are lymphocytes. In TB empyema, acid-fast smears and mycobacterial cultures are usually positive, making pleural biopsy unnecessary.

Diagnosis of non-empyematous pleural TB, a paucibacillary disease, remains challenging. Because few organisms are present in the pleural space, acid-fast smears of pleural fluid are rarely positive, and M. tuberculosis is isolated by culture in only 20–40% of patients with proven tuberculous pleuritis.[96,101] A single closed-needle biopsy of the pleura with a Cope or an Abrams needle, with collection of three or four specimens for histologic examination, acid-fast staining, and culture of the tissue, confirms the diagnosis in approximately 65–75% of patients in whom tuberculous pleuritis is ultimately diagnosed. NAATs such as Xpert MTB/RIF have variable sensitivity in pleural fluid, likely due to the paucibacillary nature of the disease. But in pleural tissue, Xpert MTB/RIF, for example, has a sensitivity of 90% and a specificity of 90–100%.[102] A second set of specimens in patients whose initial biopsy is negative increases the yield to 80–90%.[101] The results of thoracoscopy are nearly always diagnostic, but the procedure is invasive, costly, and not always available. In a patient with an exudative lymphocytic pleural effusion that remains undiagnosed after a full evaluation, including pleural biopsy, and who has a positive tuberculin reaction or IGRA result, antituberculosis treatment should be initiated.

Challenges with diagnosis have led to increased interest in biomarkers to assist in clinical decision making and diagnosis of pleural TB. Adenosine deaminase (ADA) is a T-lymphocyte enzyme that has been shown to have high sensitivity (93%) and specificity (92%) for diagnosing pleural TB[103] when present at greater than 35 U/L in pleural fluid. The effect of variability in laboratory techniques for measuring ADA has not been shown to affect diagnostic accuracy.[104] A significant exception to the utility of ADA has been in diagnosing TB pleuritis in HIV-infected patients and others with acquired or induced immunosuppression, including the elderly who have fewer functional lymphocytes.[105] Individuals with parapneumonic effusions and empyemas as well as lymphomas may test as false positives for pleural TB based on their high ADA levels. Two additional biomarkers, interferon (IFN)-γ and interleukin (IL)-27, have been considered for the diagnosis of pleural TB and have been reported to have both high specificity in HIV-infected and HIV-uninfected patients. However, sensitivity is considerably lower than for ADA (sensitivity of 89% and 94%, in IFN-γ and IL-27, respectively).[106,107] In addition, unlike with ADA, there are no established guidelines for IFN-γ and IL-27 thresholds most predictive of pleural TB, and testing is too costly for routine health care settings.[108] The evidence concerning ADA test characteristics for the general population (not HIV-infected or immunosuppressed individuals) suggests that, even in settings with low to medium incidence of TB, pleural fluid ADA should be used to rule out suspected TB and should be performed before considering more invasive and potentially morbid procedures such as closed pleural biopsies.[108]

DISSEMINATED TUBERCULOSIS

Miliary TB, although it nearly always involves the lungs, is considered extrapulmonary because of the multiplicity of organs affected. The term *miliary* is derived from the similarity of the lesions to millet seeds. Grossly, these lesions are 1- to 2-mm yellowish nodules that are granulomas on histologic examination.

Because of the multisystem involvement in disseminated TB, the clinical manifestations are protean. Initial screening laboratory studies are not particularly helpful. The chest radiograph, however, is abnormal in most but not all patients with disseminated TB: the frequency of a classic miliary pattern has ranged from 50–90% (See Fig. 53.3). Overall, it appears that, at the time of diagnosis, approximately 85% of patients have the diffuse tiny nodules characteristic of miliary TB.[109] Other abnormalities may be present as well. These include upper lobe opacities with or without cavitation, pleural effusion, and pericardial effusion. As noted previously, HIV-infected patients may not be able to form granulomas; thus, they may have a diffuse uniform pattern of opacification instead of discrete individual lesions.

Autopsy series have shown the liver, lungs, bone marrow, kidneys, adrenal glands, and spleen to be the organs most frequently involved in miliary TB, although any organ can be the site of disease.[110] Because of the multiplicity of sites involved, there are many potential sources of material to provide a diagnosis. Acid-fast smears of sputum are positive in 20–25% of patients (even when the patient is not spontaneously coughing), and cultures of sputum are positive in 30–65%.[111–113] In a patient with an abnormal chest radiograph and negative sputum examinations, bronchoscopy should be the next step, with appropriate biosafety protections for the medical staff. Combinations of bronchoalveolar lavage culture and PCR in combination with transbronchial biopsy can increase the diagnostic rate of culture-positive, smear-negative, and PCR-negative TB to 92%.[114,115] Other potential sites for biopsy include liver and bone marrow, each of which has a high likelihood of showing granulomas (70–80%), but only a 25–40% chance of providing bacteriologic confirmation; urine cultures may be positive in up to 25% of patients.[112,113] Selection of other potential sources of diagnostic material should be guided by specific findings.

The role of rapid NAATs for identification of *M. tuberculosis* in patients with miliary TB has not been defined, and neither of the two tests licensed by the U.S. Food and Drug Administration is approved for nonrespiratory specimens, although the WHO recommends Xpert MTB/RIF for use with specimens from extrapulmonary sites.[116] The reported data are difficult to interpret because, often, the results of specimens from different sites are combined, patients are selected by a variety of criteria, and test performance varies.[117–119] In contrast, several studies have shown that Xpert MTB/RIF can provide rapid molecular diagnostic assessment when extrapulmonary TB is suspected. The growing body of literature, including two large studies, demonstrated a sensitivity of 81% and specificity of 99%.[120–122]

Before the era of chemotherapy, disseminated TB was uniformly fatal. With recognition and treatment, however, the reported case-fatality rates range from 29–64%.[113] Meningeal involvement increases mortality and, when it is present, the duration of standard chemotherapy should be

extended from 6 to 9 or 12 months, and corticosteroids may be useful to reduce mortality.[123]

LYMPHATIC TUBERCULOSIS

Tuberculous lymphadenitis usually presents as painless swelling of one or more lymph nodes. The nodes most commonly involved are those of the cervical chain or supraclavicular fossa. Frequently the process is bilateral, and other noncontiguous groups of nodes can be involved. At least initially, the nodes are discrete and the overlying skin is normal. With ongoing disease, the nodes may become matted and the overlying skin inflamed. Rupture of the node can result in formation of a sinus tract, which may persist for years. Although cervical lymphadenopathy (i.e., scrofula) is one of the most common forms of extrapulmonary TB, there may also be axillary and inguinal TB lymphadenopathy. Intrathoracic adenopathy, with or without concomitant pulmonary TB, can cause compression of bronchi and atelectasis, thereby leading to lung infection and perhaps bronchiectasis. Although rare, upper airway obstruction may result from cervical node enlargement. Chylothorax and chylous ascites have resulted from intrathoracic or abdominal node involvement with obstruction of the thoracic duct or retroperitoneal lymphatics. Epidemiologically, TB lymphadenitis is rarely associated with pulmonary TB but is associated with HIV infection and is slightly more likely to affect women than men.[124] TB lymphadenitis may also appear or worsen as a manifestation of immune reconstitution inflammatory syndrome among HIV-infected individuals (Fig. 53.6). Finally, TB lymphadenitis has historically been more prevalent in children than adults; however, increasing evidence suggests that the prevalence is actually higher in adolescents and young adults than in children.[125]

The diagnosis of tuberculous lymphadenopathy is established by lymph node biopsy or aspiration with histologic examination, including stains for acid-fast organisms, and culture of the material. Smears show acid-fast organisms in approximately 25–50% of biopsy specimens, and *M. tuberculosis* is isolated in approximately 70% of instances in which the final diagnosis is considered to be TB.[126] Caseating granulomas are seen in nearly all biopsy specimens from immunocompetent patients. In immunodeficiency states, granulomas may be poorly formed or absent.[127]

GENITOURINARY TUBERCULOSIS

Genitourinary TB is a common form of extrapulmonary TB, accounting for 15–40% of all extrapulmonary TB cases.[128] In patients with genitourinary TB, local symptoms predominate and systemic symptoms are less common.[129,130] Delayed diagnosis and care can lead to serious sequelae, including renal failure and death. Delays in diagnosis typically happen because of subtle initial symptoms such as dysuria and increased urinary frequency that later can progress to hematuria, flank pain, and ultimately renal failure.[131] However, in general the symptoms are subtle, and often there is advanced destruction of the kidneys by the time a diagnosis is established.[132] Whereas it is suspected that genitourinary TB predominantly affects females, the

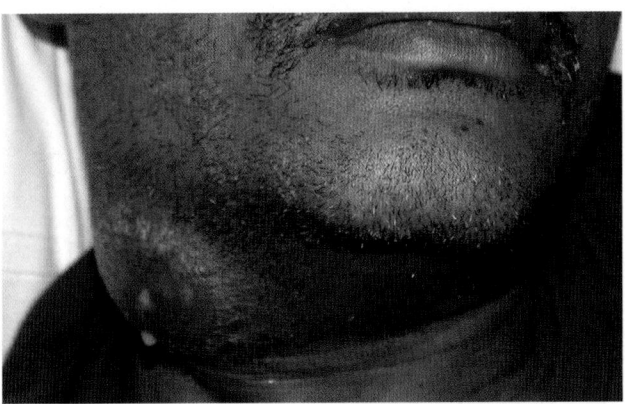

Figure 53.6 Tuberculous lymphadenitis in a patient with immune reconstitution inflammatory syndrome after initiation of antiretroviral therapy. With development of immune reconstitution inflammatory syndrome, there was swelling of an anterior cervical node and onset of purulent drainage from the node. (Courtesy Dr. Henry M. Blumberg, Emory University.)

true burden of disease in women is likely underreported. In women, genital involvement is more common than in men and may cause pelvic pain, menstrual irregularities, and infertility as presenting complaints; however, these symptoms are likely indolent, underreported, and receive TB evaluation only after infertility is noted.[130,133] In men, a painless or only slightly painful scrotal mass is probably the most common presenting symptom of genital involvement, but symptoms of prostatitis, orchitis, or epididymitis may also exist.[129] A substantial number of patients with any form of genitourinary TB are asymptomatic, and the disease is detected because of an evaluation for an abnormal urinalysis. In patients with renal or genital TB, urinalyses are abnormal in more than 90%; the main findings are pyuria, hematuria, or mixed pyuria and hematuria. Pyuria in an acidic urine with no organisms isolated from a routine urine culture should prompt an evaluation for TB. Occasionally, when there is an isolated genital focus of disease or when a tuberculous kidney is blocked by a ureteral stricture, the urinalysis may be normal and cultures may be sterile.

The suspicion of genitourinary TB should be heightened by the presence of abnormalities on the chest film. In most series, 50–75% of patients have chest radiographic abnormalities, although many of these may be the result of previous, not current, pulmonary TB.[129,130] When genitourinary TB is suspected, at least three first-voided early morning urine specimens should be collected and stained for AFB and cultured for mycobacteria. In settings with heightened risk of drug-resistant TB, drug susceptibility testing should be conducted. In men, saprophytic *Mycobacterium smegmatis* may cause a positive smear. However, in the presence of abnormalities suggesting TB, the finding of a positive smear should be interpreted as confirming the diagnosis of genitourinary TB until the results of cultures are known. *M. tuberculosis* is isolated from the urine in 80–95% of cases of genitourinary TB.[129,130] Diagnosis of isolated genital lesions usually requires biopsy because the differential diagnosis often includes neoplasia as well as other infectious processes. There are advances being made in the diagnosis of genitourinary TB. For example, one multicenter evaluation of Xpert MTB/RIF for detecting urinary tract TB from urine samples demonstrated a sensitivity of 94% and specificity

of 89% in comparison to the gold standard of liquid culture.[134] Additional studies are required to evaluate the utility of Xpert testing for rapid diagnosis of genitourinary TB.

Positive urine cultures may manifest in the absence of any clinical, laboratory, or radiographic findings, which suggests concomitant genitourinary TB in patients with other forms of TB. Bentz and colleagues[135] found unanticipated positive urine cultures in 21% of patients with other extrapulmonary forms of TB and in 5% of those with pulmonary TB alone.

Renal TB, at least as indicated by a positive urine culture, may develop in patients with HIV infection. In one series, positive urine cultures were found in 12 (71%) of 17 cultures submitted in patients with TB and advanced HIV infection, although this was not a systematic sampling.[136]

BONE AND JOINT TUBERCULOSIS

It is presumed that most osteoarticular TB results from endogenous reactivation of foci of infection seeded during the initial bacillemia, although spread from paravertebral lymph nodes has been postulated to account for the common localization of spinal TB to the lower thoracic and upper lumbar vertebrae. It is also postulated that the predilection for TB to localize in the metaphyses of long bones is due to the relatively rich blood supply and scarcity of phagocytic cells in this portion of the bone.[137] After beginning in the subchondral region of the bone, the infection spreads to involve the cartilage, synovium, and joint space. This produces the typical findings of metaphyseal erosion and cysts and loss of cartilage with narrowing of the joint space. Typically, in the spine, these changes involve two adjacent vertebrae and the intervertebral disc (Fig. 53.7). An "atypical" form of spondylitis without evidence of disc involvement may be seen and may account for more than half of the patients.[138–140] Paravertebral or other para-articular abscesses may develop with occasional formation of sinus tracts. Although weight-bearing joints are the most common sites for skeletal TB, any bone or joint may be involved.[137] In most series of osteoarticular TB, TB of the spine (Pott disease) makes up 50–70% of the cases reported.[141,142] In adults, the lower thoracic and upper lumbar vertebrae are most commonly involved, whereas in children the upper thoracic spine is the most frequent site. The hip or knee is involved in 15–20% of cases, and shoulders, elbows, ankles, wrists, and other bones or joints also make up 15–20%. Usually only one bone or joint is involved, but occasionally the process may be multifocal. Evidence of either previous or current pulmonary TB is found in approximately half the reported patients, and other extrapulmonary sites may be involved as well.

The first diagnostic test undertaken is usually a radiograph of the involved area. Early in the process, the only abnormality noted may be soft tissue swelling. MRI of the spine is considerably more sensitive than routine radiographs and should be obtained when there is a high index of suspicion of an infectious process. MRI can diagnose a tuberculous bone lesion with 100% sensitivity and 88% specificity, allowing for diagnosis before deformity develops.[143] Findings on MRI consistent with osteoarticular TB include disease of the vertebral bodies, disk destruction,

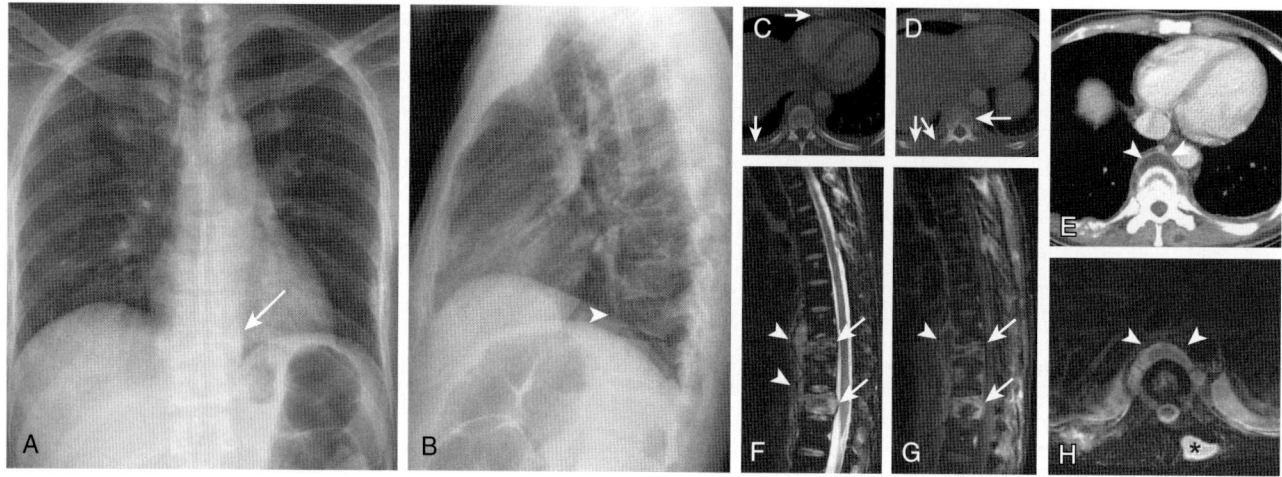

Figure 53.7 Tuberculosis involving the spine. (A) Frontal and (B) lateral chest radiographs show left inferior paraspinous line displacement (*arrow,* A) consistent with a posterior mediastinal mass. The lateral chest radiograph shows loss of height of a thoracic vertebral body (*arrowhead*) at this level, but the adjacent intervertebral disc spaces are maintained. Contrast-enhanced axial chest computed tomography displayed in bone (C–D) and soft tissue (E) windows shows lytic vertebral body destruction (*long arrows,* D) at the level of vertebral body loss of height seen on the lateral chest radiograph (B). Osseous lytic foci are also present in the sternum (*short arrows,* C) and posterior ribs (*short arrows,* C–D). A paraspinous fluid collection with peripheral enhancement, consistent with an abscess (*arrowhead,* E) is seen anterior to the involved thoracic vertebral body. Sagittal T2-weighted (F) and contrast-enhanced T1-weighted (G) and axial T2-weighted (H) magnetic resonance images show the anterior paraspinous abscesses (*arrowhead*), typical of subligamentous spread. Note the extensive high signal within the vertebral bodies (*arrows,* F) representing bone marrow edema. The clear vertebral body enhancement (*arrows,* G) indicates the presence of osteomyelitis. Note the relative sparing of the intervertebral disc spaces, typical of granulomatous infections and distinct from the common appearance of other causes of bacterial osteomyelitis. Extensive fluid collections are seen in the left erector spinae muscle (*asterisk*) and involve the adjacent right posterior rib as well. These findings were all the result of tuberculosis. (Courtesy Michael B. Gotway, MD.)

cold abscess, vertebral collapse, and presence of vertebral column deformities.[144]

The differential diagnosis of vertebral TB includes brucellar spondylitis, pyogenic spondylitis, sarcoidosis, osteoporosis, and metastatic disease, including lymphoma and multiple myeloma.[145] Confirmation of the diagnosis is obtained by aspiration of joint fluid or periarticular abscesses or by biopsy of bone or synovium with histologic and microbiologic evaluation of the material obtained. Acid-fast stains are positive in 20–25% of samples of joint fluid, and *M. tuberculosis* is isolated in approximately 60–80% of them.[137] Biopsy specimens of synovium or bone have a higher yield and enable histologic examination as well. More recently, the use of Xpert MTB/RIF for diagnosis of bone and joint TB demonstrates good diagnostic accuracy irrespective of the type of specimen sampled.[146] The pooled sensitivity and specificity of Xpert MTB/RIF were 81% and 99% compared to a composite reference standard, respectively, and 96% and 85% compared to culture, respectively. Evidence of granulomatous inflammation even in the absence of bacteriologic proof of the diagnosis is sufficient evidence of TB to begin therapy unless another cause is found.

CENTRAL NERVOUS SYSTEM TUBERCULOSIS

Central nervous system (CNS) manifestations of TB and their sequelae can be challenging to diagnose because the symptoms and imaging studies of CNS TB are often indistinguishable from those of other diseases. The most common CNS manifestations of TB include TB meningitis and intracranial tuberculomas.

TB meningitis is the most lethal form of TB. If left untreated, TB meningitis is fatal, with a median time to death from symptom onset of 19 days.[147] Among adults, HIV is the single most important epidemiologic driver of disease, likely due to impaired host response to the pathogen, particularly in the CSF.[148] Despite this, evidence is equivocal on whether HIV-infected individuals have different symptomatology from TB meningitis than HIV-noninfected persons; however, it is more lethal, with a mortality rate approaching 50% for treated patients with HIV.[149] While TB meningitis represents approximately 1% of TB cases among adults, incidence rates are as high as 10% in children.[148] Meningitis is thought to result from direct meningeal seeding and proliferation during a tuberculous bacillemia either at the time of initial infection or reactivation of an old pulmonary focus, or it can also result from reactivation of an old parameningeal focus with rupture into the subarachnoid space.[150] The consequences of subarachnoid space contamination include diffuse meningitis, a localized arteritis, encephalitis, and myelitis. The symptoms depend primarily on which of these processes predominates. With meningitis, the process is primarily located at the base of the brain.[151] Symptoms therefore include those related to cranial nerve involvement in addition to headache, decreased level of consciousness, and neck stiffness.[148] The duration of illness before diagnosis is variable. In a large series of patients, the average duration of illness was 12 days, although the range between symptom onset and presentation is between 5 and 30 days and does not vary based on comorbid conditions including HIV coinfection.[152] Although symptom duration less than 5 days has been used to distinguish between bacterial meningitis and TB meningitis in children and immunosuppressed individuals, it is important to note that subacute symptoms (>5 days) can also be consistent with cryptococcal meningitis.[153] In most series, more than 50% of patients with meningitis have abnormalities on chest radiograph consistent with an old or current tuberculous process, often miliary TB. At autopsy, disseminated disease is found in a high percentage of patients with meningitis.

In patients with tuberculous meningitis, sputum cultures have been positive in 40–50%; thus, a substantial number of patients have pulmonary and systemic symptoms in addition to those referable to the CNS. Patients in whom arteritis is the predominant manifestation of meningitis can present with a variety of focal CNS ischemic syndromes in addition to the symptoms already described.

In tuberculous meningitis, the lumbar puncture usually shows increased opening pressure, and the CSF usually contains between 10 and 1000 cells/μL.[91,152] In approximately 65–75% of patients, lymphocytes predominate, whereas polymorphonuclear leukocytes predominate in the remainder, generally early in the course of the illness.[154] More recently, specific genotypes for *leukotriene A4 hydrolase* have been identified that are linked to either inadequate inflammatory response or hyperinflammation in response to mycobacterial infection.[155] While routine genotyping of individuals with TB meningitis is not currently clinically feasible in most contexts, it is important to note that different outcomes to adjuvant use of corticosteroids in the treatment of TB meningitis may be linked to these leukotriene A4 hydrolase genotypes. A recent systematic review and meta-analysis, however, showed that use of corticosteroids as adjuvant therapy for TB meningitis drastically reduced mortality by 25%.[156] The CSF protein concentration is elevated in nearly all patients. Very high protein concentrations have been associated with a poor prognosis; the glucose concentration in CSF is usually low, but not as low as that often found in pyogenic bacterial meningitis.[152,157] Acid-fast organisms are seen on smears of CSF in only 10–20% of patients, and the rate of culture positivity varies from 25–80% but is generally in the lower end of the range.[152] In a substantial number of patients, *M. tuberculosis* is isolated from other sources, which, in the presence of compatible CSF findings, is sufficient to diagnose tuberculous meningitis. Additional potential CSF biomarkers include CSF ADA, which may be considered as a rule-in test for levels greater than 8 U/L or a rule-out test for levels less than 4 U/L.[158] However, CSF ADA cannot distinguish between bacterial meningitis and TB meningitis. CSF tryptophan may be a useful metabolite for diagnosing TB meningitis. In one observational study, it was differentially detected in patients with TB meningitis as compared to those without disease, and had a substantially higher level in patients who died from TB meningitis than in those who survived.[157] In view of the severity of TB meningitis, a presumptive diagnosis justifies empirical treatment if no other diagnosis can be established promptly. Because of the difficulty in establishing a diagnosis of TB meningitis by bacteriologic methods, a consensus case definition has been proposed by Marais and colleagues[159] that supports a scoring system based on clinical manifestations, CSF studies, CNS radiographic findings, and findings of TB elsewhere as well as the exclusion of other explanatory diagnoses (Table 53.1).

A meta-analysis of 14 studies of NAATs for the diagnosis of tuberculous meningitis found a combined sensitivity of 56% and a specificity of 98%.[117] Thus, when a NAAT is positive, one can assume that the etiology is TB, but a negative result does not exclude the diagnosis and should be treated with caution.

The other major CNS form of TB, the tuberculoma, presents a more subtle clinical picture than does TB

meningitis.[160] The usual presentation is that of a slowly growing focal lesion, although a few patients have increased intracranial pressure and no focal findings. The CSF is usually normal, and the diagnosis is established by CT or MRI and subsequent resection, biopsy, or aspiration of any ring-enhancing lesion.

Table 53.1 Diagnostic Criteria for Classification of Definite, Probable, Possible, and Nontuberculous Meningitis[159]

	Diagnostic Score
CLINICAL CRITERIA (MAXIMUM 6 POINTS)	
Symptom duration >5 days	4
Systemic symptoms suggestive of tuberculosis (one or more of the following): weight loss (or poor weight gain in children), night sweats, or persistent cough for >2 weeks	2
History of recent (within past year) close contact with an individual with pulmonary tuberculosis or a positive TST or IGRA (only in children <10 years)	2
Focal neurologic deficit	1
Cranial nerve palsy	1
Altered consciousness	1
IMAGING CRITERIA (MAXIMUM 6 POINTS)	
Hydrocephalus	1
Basal meningeal enhancement	2
Tuberculoma	2
Infarct	1
Precontrast basal hyperdensity	2
CSF CRITERIA (MAXIMUM 4 POINTS)	
Clear appearance	1
Cells: 10–500 per μL	1
Lymphocytic predominance (>50%)	1
Protein concentration greater than 1 g/L	1
CSF to plasma glucose ratio of <50% or an absolute CSF glucose concentration <2.2 mmol/L	1
EVIDENCE OF TUBERCULOSIS ELSEWHERE (MAXIMUM 4 POINTS)	
Chest radiograph suggestive of active tuberculosis: signs of tuberculosis = 2; miliary tuberculosis = 4	2/4
CT/MRI/ultrasound evidence for tuberculosis outside the CNS	2
AFB identified or *Mycobacterium tuberculosis* cultured from another source (i.e., sputum, lymph node, gastric washing, urine, blood culture)	4
Positive commercial *M. tuberculosis* NAAT from extraneural specimen	4

A definite diagnosis is considered *M. tuberculosis* culture and/or NAAT positivity. When imaging is not available, a probable diagnosis is considered with a score ≥10 (out of 20); possible, 6–9; and other than TB, <6.
AFB, acid-fast bacilli; CNS, central nervous system; CSF, cerebrospinal fluid; CT, computed tomography; IGRA, interferon-γ release assay; MRI, magnetic resonance imaging; NAAT, nucleic acid amplification testing; TST, tuberculin skin test.
From Marais M, Thwaites G, Schoerman J, et al. Tuberculous meningitis: a uniform case definition for use in clinical research. *Lancet Infect Dis.* 2010;10:803–812.

INTESTINAL TUBERCULOSIS

The clinical manifestations of intestinal TB depend on the areas of involvement. In the gut itself, TB may be in any location from the mouth to the anus, although lesions proximal to the terminal ileum are unusual. The most common sites of involvement are the terminal ileum and cecum; other portions of the colon and the rectum are involved less frequently.[161] In the terminal ileum or cecum, the most common manifestations are pain (which may lead to a misdiagnosis of appendicitis) and intestinal obstruction. A palpable mass may be noted that, together with its radiographic appearance, can easily be mistaken as a carcinoma. Rectal lesions usually present as anal fissures or fistulas or perirectal abscesses. In addition to carcinoma, the differential diagnosis of these findings includes inflammatory bowel disease. Because of the concern regarding carcinoma, the diagnosis often is made surgically.[162] The similarities in symptoms between intestinal TB and inflammatory bowel disease are likely responsible for delays in starting antituberculosis treatment for patients with intestinal TB.[163] Symptoms include abdominal pain, weight loss, nausea, change in bowel habits, and fever. Imaging with abdominal CT scan may be helpful at raising suspicion for intestinal TB. While some findings, such as bowel wall thickening, are relatively nonspecific, other findings, such as lymphadenopathy with central necrosis, are likely to distinguish intestinal TB from inflammatory bowel disease.[164] In addition, colonoscopic evaluation may be particularly helpful both for visualizing intestinal lesions and for obtaining biopsies for histopathologic evaluation. Colonoscopic findings that point towards a diagnosis of intestinal TB include terminal ileitis with ulceration, pseudodiverticulae, and atrophic mucosa.[165] In case series, histopathology provided a diagnosis of intestinal TB in 40–55% of specimens, whereas yield from culture alone was 20–50%.[164,166,167] Finally, histopathology and culture are important in distinguishing intestinal TB from infections caused by *M. bovis* or *M. fortuitum*, which are both linked to consumption of unpasteurized dairy products and can also present with abdominal pain, appendicitis, and peritonitis.[168]

PERITONEAL TUBERCULOSIS

Tuberculous peritonitis commonly causes pain as its presenting manifestation, often accompanied by abdominal swelling. Fever, weight loss, and anorexia are also common. Active pulmonary TB is uncommon in patients with tuberculous peritonitis. Because the process frequently coexists with other disorders, especially cirrhosis with ascites, the symptoms of TB may be obscured. The combination of fever and abdominal tenderness in a person with ascites should always prompt an evaluation for intra-abdominal infection, and paracentesis should be performed. Ascitic fluid in tuberculous peritonitis is exudative and contains between 50 and 10,000 leukocytes/μL, the majority of which are lymphocytes, although polymorphonuclear leukocytes occasionally predominate.[169] Acid-fast organisms are rarely seen on smears of the fluid, and cultures are positive in only approximately 50%, although the yield increases if a large volume of fluid is submitted for culture. Ascitic fluid ADA has a high sensitivity and specificity for tuberculous peritonitis (93%

and 96%, respectively).[170] Because of the generally low yield from culture of the ascitic fluid, laparoscopic biopsy is often necessary to confirm the diagnosis using histopathology.

PERICARDIAL TUBERCULOSIS

The most common form or stage of tuberculous pericarditis is characterized by pericardial effusion with little pericardial thickening or epicardial involvement. Because in most instances the fluid accumulates slowly, the pericardium can expand to accommodate large volumes (2 to 4 L) with little apparent hemodynamic compromise. Symptoms of cardiopulmonary origin tend to manifest later and include cough, dyspnea, orthopnea, ankle swelling, and chest pain.[171] The chest pain may occasionally mimic angina but usually is described as being dull, aching, and often affected by position and inspiration.

The pericardial fluid itself is usually serosanguineous or occasionally grossly bloody, is exudative, and has a white blood cell count ranging from 500 to 50,000 cells/μL, with an average of 5000 to 7000 cells/μL.[172] The cells are predominantly mononuclear, although polymorphonuclear leukocytes occasionally predominate. Tubercle bacilli have been identified in pericardial fluid in approximately 40–60% of cases (with higher yield when combined with culture).[172] Biopsy of the pericardium with both histologic and bacteriologic evaluation is much more likely to provide a diagnosis, although a nonspecific histologic pattern and failure to recover the organisms do not exclude a tuberculous cause. Because TB pericarditis represents a disseminated form of TB, chest radiography as well as evaluation of sputum for AFB, TB PCR, and culture should be performed because 30–80% of patients with pericardial TB also have pulmonary TB.[173] Finally, elevated ADA levels in the context of a lymphocytic pericardial exudate are sufficient for a clinical diagnosis, where ADA has a sensitivity of 87% and specificity of 89%. A composite scoring system including pericardial ADA, lymphocyte/neutrophil ratio, peripheral leukocyte count, and HIV status reported a sensitivity of 96% and specificity of 97% for diagnosing tuberculous pericarditis even in the absence of biopsy.[172] Like other forms of extrapulmonary TB, the utility of PCR such as GeneXpert for diagnosis of pericardial TB is equivocal, especially in nonendemic settings. Sensitivity of the test on pericardial fluid has been reported as low as 52% and thus should be included as part of a complete workup but not as a stand-alone diagnostic test.[174]

Chronic fibrotic pericarditis may develop in 30–60% of patients with or without antituberculosis therapy or steroids.[175] Before the advent of antituberculosis therapy, 88% of one series of patients who had tuberculous pericarditis showed evidence of chronic constriction.[176] Constriction has also been observed to develop during the course of antituberculosis chemotherapy, although this appears to be uncommon in patients who have had symptoms for less than 3 months; it is frequent in patients who have had symptoms for more than 6 months. The fibrotic reaction progresses to complete fusion of visceral and parietal pericardium and encasement of the heart in a rigid scar that often becomes calcified. Impairment of coronary circulation is common. At this point the histologic pattern is usually nonspecific; thus, confirmation of a tuberculous etiology is infrequent.

The HIV epidemic has increased the burden of tuberculous pericarditis in endemic settings and is a major consideration in understanding the natural history, clinical manifestations, and treatment of this disease. In contrast to the slowly developing effusion in immunocompetent patients with TB pericarditis, TB pericarditis develops quickly in HIV-infected individuals in whom TB represents the cause of pericarditis 85% of the time.[177] In addition, myocardial damage, or myopericarditis as measured by ST segment changes on electrocardiogram, presents more frequently in HIV-infected patients, and correlates with lower CD4 counts.[178] HIV-infected patients are less likely to develop constrictive pericarditis.[179] Finally, mortality from TB pericarditis is higher in HIV-infected patients than in immunocompetent patients.

The definitive diagnosis of tuberculous pericarditis requires identification of tubercle bacilli in pericardial fluid or tissue. Although not conclusive, demonstration of caseating granulomata in the pericardium and consistent clinical circumstances provide convincing evidence of a tuberculous etiology. Less conclusive but still persuasive evidence is the finding of another form of TB in a patient with pericarditis of undetermined cause. Approximately 25–50% of patients with tuberculous pericarditis have evidence of other organ involvement, particularly pleuritis, at the time pericarditis is diagnosed.[180] Still less direct and more circumstantial evidence of a tuberculous etiology is the combination of a positive intermediate-strength TST or IGRA reaction and pericarditis of unproved cause.

Key Points

- Clinical suspicion for *tuberculosis* (TB) should remain high in endemic settings, or in settings in which patient risk factors and local epidemiology suggest a high risk of infection.
- All patients suspected of having pulmonary TB should have at least two sputum samples collected for acid-fast bacilli smear microscopy and mycobacterial culture and at least one sputum specimen collected for nucleic acid amplification testing.
- Tuberculin skin tests and interferon-γ release assays have no role in the diagnosis of active pulmonary TB but can increase suspicion for active disease among smear-negative individuals with suspected TB.
- Therapeutic trials of antituberculosis chemotherapy may be indicated even if testing of sputum or other specimens is negative, especially when high clinical suspicion remains. However, empirically treated patients require close follow-up to assess for clinical and radiographic improvement.
- Phenotypic drug susceptibility testing is recommended for all initial *M. tuberculosis* isolates; drug resistance is increasingly detected by molecular genotyping assays.
- Extrapulmonary TB should be diagnosed using tissue or fluid sampling from the suspected site of disease, although yield is variable depending on the specimen type, and recommended tests in addition to smear and culture are evolving.

Key Readings

Behr MA, Warren SA, Salamon H, et al. Transmission of *Mycobacterium tuberculosis* from patients' smear-negative for acid-fast bacilli. *Lancet.* 1999;353(9151):444–449.

Berry MP, Graham CM, McNab FW, et al. An interferon-inducible neutrophil-driven blood transcriptional signature in human tuberculosis. *Nature.* 2010;466(7309):973–977.

Caws M, Thwaites G, Dunstan S, et al. The influence of host and bacterial genotype on the development of disseminated disease with *Mycobacterium tuberculosis.* PLoS Pathog. 2008;4(3):e1000034.

Coussens AK, Wilkinson RJ, Hanifa Y, et al. Vitamin D accelerates resolution of inflammatory responses during tuberculosis treatment. *Proc Natl Acad Sci U S A.* 2012;109(38):15449–15454.

Dheda K, Gumbo T, Maartens G, et al. The Lancet Respiratory Medicine Commission: 2019 update: epidemiology, pathogenesis, transmission, diagnosis, and management of multidrug-resistant and incurable tuberculosis. *Lancet Respir Med.* 2019;7(9):820–826.

Dooley KE, Savic R, Gupte A, et al. Once-weekly rifapentine and isoniazid for tuberculosis prevention in patients with HIV taking dolutegravir-based antiretroviral therapy: a phase 1/2 trial. *Lancet HIV.* 2020;7(6):e401–e409.

Hamada Y, Lujan J, Schenkel K, Ford N, Getahun H. Sensitivity and specificity of WHO's recommended four-symptom screening rule for tuberculosis in people living with HIV: a systematic review and meta-analysis. *Lancet HIV.* 2018;5(9):e515–e523.

Huang CC, Tchetgen ET, Becerra MC, et al. The effect of HIV-related immunosuppression on the risk of tuberculosis transmission to household contacts. *Clin Infect Dis.* 2014;58(6):765–774.

Kato-Maeda M, Ho C, Passarelli B, et al. Use of whole genome sequencing to determine the microevolution of *Mycobacterium tuberculosis* during an outbreak. PLoS One. 2013;8(3):e58235.

Keshavjee S, Amanullah F, Cattamanchi A, et al. Moving toward tuberculosis elimination. Critical issues for research in diagnostics and therapeutics for tuberculosis infection. *Am J Respir Crit Care Med.* 2019;199(5):564–571.

Lewinsohn DM, Leonard MK, LoBue PA, et al. Official American Thoracic Society/Infectious Diseases Society of America/Centers for Disease Control and Prevention clinical practice guidelines: diagnosis of tuberculosis in adults and children. *Clin Infect Diss.* 2017;64(2):e1–e33.

Marks GB, Nguyen NV, Nguyen PTB, et al. Community-wide screening for tuberculosis in a high-prevalence setting. *N Engl J Med.* 2019;381(14):1347–1357.

Philips JA, Ernst JD. Tuberculosis pathogenesis and immunity. *Annu Rev Pathol.* 2012;7:353–384.

Reid MJA, Arinaminpathy N, Bloom A, et al. Building a tuberculosis-free world: the Lancet Commission on tuberculosis. *Lancet.* 2019;393(10178):1331–1384.

The CRyPTIC Consortium and the 100,000 Genomes Project. Prediction of susceptibility to first-line tuberculosis drugs by DNA sequencing. *N Engl J Med.* 2018;379:1403–1415.

Thillai M, Pollock K, Pareek M, et al. Interferon-gamma release assays for tuberculosis: current and future applications. *Expert Rev Respir Med.* 2014;8(1):67–78.

Uplekar M, Weil D, Lonnroth K, et al. WHO's new end TB strategy. *Lancet.* 2015;385(9979):1799–1801.

World Health Organization. *Policy Update: Automated Real-Time Nucleic Acid Amplification Technology For Rapid And Simultaneous Detection Of Tuberculosis And Rifampicin Resistance: Xpert Mtb/Rif System.* Geneva: World Health Organization; 2020.

Xie YL, Chakravorty S, Armstrong DT, et al. Evaluation of a rapid molecular drug-susceptibility test for tuberculosis. *N Engl J Med.* 2017;377:1043–1054.

Yoon C, Semitala FC, Atuhumuza E, et al. Point-of-care C-reactive protein-based tuberculosis screening for people living with HIV: a diagnostic accuracy study. *Lancet Infect Dis.* 2017;17(12):1285–1292.

Complete reference list available at ExpertConsult.com.

54 TUBERCULOSIS: TREATMENT OF DRUG-SUSCEPTIBLE AND DRUG-RESISTANT

DAVID J. HORNE, MD, MPH • PAYAM NAHID, MD, MPH

INTRODUCTION

BACKGROUND

Before the availability of effective chemotherapy, tuberculosis was often fatal. Among individuals with smear-positive pulmonary *tuberculosis* (TB), the case-fatality rate was approximately 70%.[1] The era of effective antituberculosis chemotherapy was launched in 1946 with the introduction of streptomycin.[2] In a landmark study considered the first randomized trial in medicine,[3] streptomycin resulted in clinical responses and improved short-term mortality but showed little benefit over 5 years of follow-up due to the emergence of streptomycin-resistant *Mycobacterium tuberculosis*. The use of a two-drug regimen that included *p*-aminosalicylic acid resulted in a significantly decreased risk of streptomycin resistance.[4] This lesson resonates today. Treatment of TB disease requires a combination of drugs because treatment with a single drug fails by selecting for resistant bacteria. TB treatment was greatly enhanced by the introduction of *isoniazid* (INH) in 1952, a drug that is bactericidal and less toxic than the other antituberculous medications of that era. Further studies in the 1960s identified the importance of *rifampin* (RIF) as a sterilizing agent and the advantage of *pyrazinamide* (PZA) for the first 2 months in allowing shorter courses of curative therapy.[4] Studies in multiple international settings led to the regimen that remains the cornerstone of therapy for drug-susceptible TB. Subsequent efforts have sought shorter treatment regimens and new medications for treatment of drug-resistant TB. Governmental and nongovernmental organizations have been essential to the support of research and development of new drugs and regimens.[5] These include not-for-profit product development partnerships such as the Global Alliance for TB Drug Development and the TB Drug Accelerator. The U.S. *Centers for Disease Control and Prevention* (CDC) and National Institutes of Health–supported consortia, including the TB Trials Consortium and *Acquired Immunodeficiency Syndrome* (AIDS) Clinical Trials Group, have performed critical multicenter international trials of novel treatment regimens. Information on drugs in development is available at the Stop TB Partnership's Working Group for New TB drugs site (https://www.newtbdrugs.org/pipeline/clinical).

PRINCIPLES OF TREATMENT

The treatment of TB benefits the individual by limiting organ damage and preventing death and benefits the community by interrupting transmission. Treatment regimens are chosen based on their success in curing the patient of TB disease while minimizing relapse rates, drug toxicity, selection of resistant bacteria, and medication nonadherence.[2,4] The success of drug treatment depends upon many factors, and studies have found an increased risk of relapse among patients with signs of more extensive disease (e.g., cavitation, more diseased lung on chest radiograph, or higher bacterial burdens),[6–10] and/or slower response to treatment (e.g., delayed culture conversion at 2 or 3 months).[2,7,11,12] More recently, an analysis of data from several contemporary *randomized controlled trials* (RCTs) demonstrated additional risk factors for poor treatment outcomes, including submaximal treatment adherence, *human immunodeficiency virus* (HIV) infection, and low body mass index.[13]

RCTs have supported the use of an initial intensive phase of treatment followed by a continuation phase. Effective, uninterrupted treatment is more important in the *intensive phase* of therapy when the bacillary population is highest and the chance of selecting drug-resistant mutants greatest. During the *continuation phase*, the number of bacilli is much lower, and the goal of therapy is to kill persisting organisms. The preferred regimen for treating adults with TB caused by organisms not known or suspected to be drug resistant consists of an intensive phase of 2 months of INH, RIF, PZA, and *ethambutol* (EMB), followed by a continuation phase of 4 months of INH and RIF (Tables 54.1 and 54.2).[4,14,15] INH and RIF are currently the most important drugs for the treatment of drug-susceptible TB because they are key to effective short-course treatment.

The "three-populations" model of chemotherapy hypothesizes the presence of different populations of *M. tuberculosis* (MTB) bacilli with differing levels of metabolic activity.[16,17] These bacillary populations consist of (1) an actively multiplying extracellular population, (2) a slowly multiplying population present in acidic compartments, and (3) a sporadically multiplying population. The composition of the standard regimen for drug-susceptible TB can be explained by referencing this model.[2,17] INH exhibits the greatest early bactericidal effect (i.e., bacillary death within the first 48 hours of drug action), which greatly reduces the population of extracellular actively multiplying bacilli.[18,19] PZA has high sterilization capacity, and its unique effectiveness against bacilli in acidic environments allows the overall treatment length to be shortened from 9 to 6 months. RIF has excellent sterilizing activity resulting in greater killing of both slowly and sporadically multiplying bacilli.[20] Due to the proportion of new TB cases worldwide caused by organisms resistant to INH, EMB is included in the intensive phase of treatment to protect against the emergence of RIF-resistant bacteria because PZA is not considered protective against the emergence of resistance to other antituberculosis drugs.[16]

See the Appendix on ExpertConsult.com for a detailed description of antituberculous chemotherapeutic drugs.

MECHANISMS AND PHARMACOLOGY OF DRUGS USED TO TREAT DRUG-SUSCEPTIBLE TUBERCULOSIS

INH is a prodrug activated by the mycobacterial enzyme KatG, which exerts its concentration-dependent bactericidal activity by inhibiting mycolic acid synthesis. INH is metabolized by *N-acetyltransferase 2* (NAT2), a hepatic phase II drug-metabolizing enzyme with a trimodal phenotypic distribution,[21] which varies in frequency by ethnicity.[22]

- *Rifampin* (also termed *rifampicin*, [RIF]) is a semisynthetic rifamycin derivative that inhibits bacterial DNA-dependent RNA polymerase and suppresses the early elongation of the nucleotide chain in RNA synthesis. RIF's bactericidal activity is concentration dependent.[20]
- *Pyrazinamide* (PZA) is a prodrug activated by mycobacterial pyrazinamidase to *pyrazinoic acid* (POA). The mechanism of action of POA is incompletely understood and likely relies on multiple targets for effect, including inhibition of fatty acid synthesis.[23] PZA is generally considered bacteriostatic against MTB.
- *Ethambutol* (EMB) inhibits synthesis of arabinogalactan of the mycobacterial cell wall and is bacteriostatic at usual doses.[24]

The *pharmacokinetics* (PKs) of antituberculosis drugs vary in different individuals (see Table 54.3).[18] This is a concern for clinicians because cure of TB is predicated on achieving adequate drug exposure. The use of *pharmacokinetic/pharmacodynamic* (PK/PD) data allows for the most effective use of antimicrobials by achieving maximal pathogen killing in the shortest time.[18] PK thresholds associated with treatment failure in the first-line treatment of drug-susceptible TB have been reported[25] and underscore the wide variability seen in drug exposures, especially in those with HIV, renal, and hepatic disease (see "Therapeutic Drug Monitoring" later).

TB treatment is often straightforward, but it can be complicated. Drug-resistant TB, adverse drug effects, HIV and other comorbidities, and complex drug-drug interactions are some of the situations in which expert consultation should be obtained. Consultation support for TB diagnosis and management is available through local health department TB control programs and/or regional CDC-supported TB Centers of Excellence for Training, Education, and Medical Consultation (http://www.cdc.gov/tb/education/rtmc/default.htm) (Fig. 54.1).

TREATMENT

TREATMENT INITIATION

The decision to initiate antituberculous chemotherapy is based on clinical, radiographic, laboratory, patient, and public health factors. The decision is clear in patients with a positive culture for *M. tuberculosis* or a positive rapid molecular test, but the decision to initiate treatment often must be made before microbiologic confirmation is available. In the presence of clinical evidence of TB, a positive *acid-fast bacillus* (AFB) smear provides strong support for treatment initiation. If the diagnosis is confirmed by isolation of *M. tuberculosis* or a positive rapid molecular test, or is inferred from clinical or radiographic improvement consistent with a response to TB treatment, the regimen is continued to complete a standard course of therapy.

In patients with a positive AFB smear but a negative rapid molecular test,[26,27] it is unlikely that the positive smear is due to *M. tuberculosis*, particularly if molecular testing of a second smear-positive specimen fails to detect *M. tuberculosis*.[28] In these situations, which are suggestive of infection

Table 54.1   Drug Regimens for Microbiologically Confirmed Pulmonary Tuberculosis Caused by Drug-Susceptible Organisms

Regimen	INTENSIVE PHASE		CONTINUATION PHASE		Total Doses	Comments[‡§]	Regimen Effectiveness
	Drugs*	Interval and Doses[†] (Minimum Duration)	Drugs	Interval and Doses[†‡] (Minimum Duration)			
1	INH RIF PZA EMB	7 days/wk for 56 doses (8 wk) *or* 5 days/wk for 40 doses (8 wk)	INH RIF	7 days/wk for 126 doses (18 wk) *or* 5 days/wk for 90 doses (18 wk)	130–182	This is the preferred regimen for patients with newly diagnosed pulmonary tuberculosis.	Greater
2	INH RIF PZA EMB	7 days/wk for 56 doses (8 wk) *or* 5 days/wk for 40 doses (8 wk)	INH RIF	Three times weekly for 54 doses (18 wk)	94–110	Preferred alternative regimen in situations in which more frequent DOT during continuation phase is difficult to achieve.	
3	INH RIF PZA EMB	Three times weekly for 24 doses (8 wk)	INH RIF	Three times weekly for 54 doses (18 wk)	78	Use regimen with caution in patients with HIV and/or cavitary disease. Missed doses can lead to treatment failure, relapse, and acquired drug resistance.	
4	INH RIF PZA EMB	7 days/wk for 14 doses then twice weekly for 12 doses[‖]	INH RIF	Twice weekly for 36 doses (18 wk)	62	Do not use twice-weekly regimens in HIV-infected patients or patients with smear positive and/or cavitary disease. If doses are missed then therapy is equivalent to once weekly, which is inferior.	Lesser

*Other combinations may be appropriate in certain circumstances; additional details are provided in section "Recommended Treatment Regimens for Drug-Susceptible Tuberculosis."

[†]When DOT is used, drugs may be given 5 days/wk and the necessary number of doses adjusted accordingly. Although there are no studies that compare five with seven daily doses, extensive experience indicates this would be an effective practice. DOT should be used when drugs are administered for fewer than 7 days/wk.

[‡]Based on expert opinion, patients with cavitation on initial chest radiograph and positive cultures at completion of 2 months of therapy should receive a 7-month (31 wk) continuation phase.

[§]Pyridoxine (vitamin B₆), 25–50 mg/day, is given with INH to all persons at risk of neuropathy (e.g., pregnant women; breastfeeding infants; persons with HIV; patients with diabetes, alcoholism, malnutrition, chronic renal failure, or with advanced age). For patients with peripheral neuropathy, experts recommend increasing pyridoxine dose to 100 mg/day.

[‖]See reference 206. Alternatively, some U.S. tuberculosis control programs have administered intensive-phase regimens 5 days/wk for 15 doses (3 wk) then twice weekly for 12 doses.

DOT, directly observed therapy; EMB, ethambutol; HIV, human immunodeficiency virus; INH, isoniazid; PZA, pyrazinamide; RIF, rifampin.

From Nahid P, Dorman SE, et al. Official American Thoracic Society/Centers for Disease Control and Prevention/Infectious Diseases Society of America clinical practice guidelines: treatment of drug-susceptible tuberculosis. *Clin Infect Dis*. 2016;63:e147–e195.

Table 54.2   Doses of Drugs for Treatment of Adults and Children with Drug-Susceptible Tuberculosis

Medication	Administration	Dose*	Notes
INH	Oral: tablets (50/100/300 mg), elixir Intravenous Intramuscular	Daily: 5 mg/kg (max 300 mg), tiw: 15 mg/kg (max 900 mg), biw: 15 mg/kg (max 900 mg)	Avoid taking with fatty foods because absorption is decreased up to 50% No dosing adjustments for renal impairment
RIF	Oral: capsules (150/300 mg) Intravenous	Adults: daily/biw/tiw: 10 mg/kg (max 600 mg) Children[†]: daily/biw/tiw: 10–20 mg/kg (max 600 mg)	Avoid taking with fatty foods because absorption is decreased No dosing adjustments for renal impairment
PZA	Oral: tablets (500 mg)	40–55 kg: 1000 mg (daily), 1500 mg (tiw), 2000 mg (biw) 56–75 kg: 1500 mg (daily), 2500 mg (tiw), 3000 mg (biw) 76–90 kg: 2000 mg (daily), 3000 mg (tiw), 4000 mg (biw) <40 kg: 30–40 mg/kg (daily), 50 mg/kg (tiw/biw)	If CrCl < 30 mL/min, reduce dose to 25–35 mg/kg tiw Consider not using if patient has gout
EMB	Oral: tablets (100/400 mg)	40–55 kg: 800 mg (daily), 1200 mg (tiw), 2000 mg (biw) 56–75 kg: 1200 mg (daily), 2000 mg (tiw), 2800 mg (biw) 76–90 kg: 1600 mg (daily), 2400 mg (tiw), 4000 mg (biw) <40 kg: 20 mg/kg (daily), 50 mg/kg (tiw/biw)	If CrCl < 30 mL/min, reduce dose to 20–25 mg/kg tiw Avoid antacids within 2 hours of EMB administration

*Dosing based on actual weight is acceptable in patients who are not obese. For obese patients (>20% above ideal body weight), dosing based on ideal body weight may be preferred for initial doses.

[†]Adult dosing begins at 15 years of age or weight >40 kg in younger children.

biw; twice weekly; CrCl, creatinine clearance; EMB, ethambutol; HIV, human immunodeficiency virus; INH, isoniazid; max, maximum; PZA, pyrazinamide; RIF, rifampin; tiw, three times weekly.

From Nahid P, Dorman SE, et al. Official American Thoracic Society/Centers for Disease Control and Prevention/Infectious Diseases Society of America clinical practice guidelines: treatment of drug-susceptible tuberculosis. *Clin Infect Dis*. 2016;63:e147–e195.

Table 54.3 Pharmacology and Adverse Effects of Antituberculosis Medications

Drug	Pharmacology	Adverse Effects
INH	Prodrug, activated by bacterial catalase/peroxidase, KatG Peak plasma concentration: 1–2 hr after ingestion C_{max}: 3–5 µg/mL Half-life: 2–5 hr (slow acetylators), 0.5–2 hr (fast acetylators) Metabolism: hepatic acetylation (NAT2 enzyme) and excreted in urine	Liver injury Peripheral neuropathy due to pyridoxine deficiency; give pyridoxine (25–50 mg) with each INH dose if at risk (patients with diabetes, HIV, renal disease, alcohol abuse, malnutrition, pregnancy) or if neuropathy develops CNS toxicity: headache, poor concentration, depression, seizures, optic neuritis Rash Hematologic abnormalities INH inhibition of cytochrome P-450 causes increases in serum concentrations of certain medications including phenytoin, carbamazepine, valproic acid, clopidogrel, warfarin, theophylline, ketoconazole
RIF	Peak plasma concentration: 1–4 hr after ingestion C_{max}: 8–24 µg/mL Half-life: 2–3 hr; prolonged with liver disease Metabolism: hepatic deacetylation to enterohepatically recirculated active metabolite	Liver injury: usually cholestatic pattern of injury GI upset Hypersensitivity (flulike syndrome); symptoms include fever, headache, malaise, myalgias that start 1–2 hr postadministration; may resolve with change from intermittent to daily RIF therapy Rash Hematologic abnormalities Discoloration of body fluids (e.g., urine, feces, tears) Cytochrome P-450 induction causes decrease in serum concentrations of many medications, including antiretrovirals, anticonvulsants, anticoagulation, immunosuppressants, chemotherapy, methadone, oral contraceptives, levothyroxine, and antihypertensives
PZA	Prodrug, activated by bacterial pyrazinamidase enzymes Peak plasma concentration: 1–4 hr after ingestion C_{max}: 20–40 µg/mL Half-life: 10 hr Metabolism: hydrolyzed by liver, excreted in urine	Liver injury Arthralgias, gout: consider avoiding in patients with gout GI upset Rash Photosensitivity
EMB	Peak plasma concentration: 2–4 hr after ingestion C_{max}: 2–6 µg/mL Half-life: 3–4 hr Primarily excreted through kidneys in unchanged form Reduce dose in patients with impaired renal function	Optic neuritis: perform patient education, baseline and monthly assessment of visual acuity, and color discrimination while receiving EMB Rash GI upset
Levofloxacin	Peak plasma concentration: 1–2 hr postingestion C_{max}: 8–12 µg/mL Half-life: 6–8 hr Primarily excreted through kidneys in unchanged form; if CrCl < 30 mL/min, administer tiw (not daily)	GI: nausea, vomiting, diarrhea, abdominal pain CNS toxicity: headache, insomnia, dizziness, tremulousness QT prolongation Tendon effects: tendonitis, tendon rupture (more common in elderly) Arthralgias Peripheral neuropathy Rash
Moxifloxacin	Peak plasma concentration: 1–3 hr postingestion C_{max}: 3–5 µg/mL Half-life: 11–13 hr Hepatic metabolism via glucuronide and sulfate conjugation; approximately 45% excreted unchanged in urine and feces	GI: nausea, vomiting, diarrhea, abdominal pain CNS toxicity: dizziness, headache, insomnia, tremulousness, confusion QT prolongation Tendon effects: tendonitis, tendon rupture (more common in elderly) Arthralgias Peripheral neuropathy Rash Liver injury (rare)
Bedaquiline	Peak plasma concentration: 5 hr after ingestion (should be taken with food which increases bioavailability) C_{max}: 2.7 µg/mL (200 mg dose) Half-life: ~5.5 mo Hepatic metabolism via CYP3A4, excreted in feces	Nausea QT prolongation Headache Rash Arthralgia Transaminitis
Linezolid	Peak plasma concentration: 1–2 hr after ingestion C_{max}: 12–24 µg/mL Half-life: 5 hr Hepatic metabolism, urinary excretion	Peripheral neuropathy Hematologic: thrombocytopenia, leukopenia, anemia GI: diarrhea, nausea Optic neuropathy Serotonin syndrome: risk increased in presence of other serotonergic medications

Table 54.3 Pharmacology and Adverse Effects of Antituberculosis Medications—cont'd

Drug	Pharmacology	Adverse Effects
Clofazimine	Peak plasma concentration: 4–8 hr if taken with food (take with food to improve absorption and tolerability) C_{max}: 0.5–2.0 µg/mL Half-life: 70 days Hepatic metabolism, excretion unknown	Skin discoloration (reversible) in 75–100% of patients Photosensitivity GI: abdominal pain, nausea, splenic infarction Dry skin QT prolongation
Cycloserine	Peak plasma concentration: 2–4 hr after ingestion, C_{max}: 20–35 µg/mL Half-life: 12 hr Hepatic metabolism; approximately 65% excreted unchanged in urine	CNS toxicity: lethargy, difficulty with concentration, depression, confusion, psychosis, seizures; pyridoxine may prevent/treat symptoms Peripheral neuropathy Rash
Delamanid	Prodrug, activated by bacterial nitroreductase Peak plasma concentration: 4 hr after ingestion (take with food, which increases bioavailability threefold) C_{max}: 0.37 µg/mL Half-life: 30–38 hr Metabolized by plasma albumin, excreted in feces	GI: nausea, vomiting, abdominal pain Headache, insomnia, dizziness, tinnitus QT prolongation Palpitations
Pretomanid	Prodrug, activated by bacterial nitroreductase Peak plasma concentration: 4–5 hr after ingestion (take with food, which increases bioavailability 75%) C_{max}: 2 µg/mL Half-life: 16–20 hr No single major metabolic pathway identified, although CYP3A4 contributes ~20% to metabolism; excreted in urine and feces	Adverse effects reported based on combination treatment with bedaquiline and linezolid: peripheral and optic neuropathy, QT prolongation Myelosuppression: hematologic: thrombocytopenia, leukopenia, anemia Transaminitis, hepatic toxicity Lactic acidosis GI: diarrhea, nausea Rash Headache

C_{max}, maximum concentration; CNS, central nervous system; CrCl, creatinine clearance; CYP3A4, cytochrome P-450 enzyme; EMB, ethambutol; GI, gastrointestinal; HIV, human immunodeficiency virus; INH, isoniazid; NAT2, N-acetyltransferase 2; RIF, rifampin; PZA, pyrazinamide; tiw, three times weekly.

with nontuberculous mycobacteria, it is reasonable to withhold TB treatment pending culture results.

A failure to isolate *M. tuberculosis* from specimens in persons suspected of having pulmonary TB on the basis of clinical and/or radiographic findings does not exclude a diagnosis of active TB. Low bacillary populations, inadequate sputum specimens, temporal variations in the number of expelled bacilli, overgrowth of cultures with other microorganisms, and errors in specimen processing can lead to false-negative results.[28a] Whereas in resource-limited settings empirical initiation of TB treatment is uncommon, U.S. guidelines recommend that empirical treatment with a standard regimen be initiated promptly in patients with a high likelihood of having TB or in those seriously ill with a disorder suspicious for TB, even before AFB smear microscopy, molecular tests, and mycobacterial culture results are known.[29] Use of molecular tests directly on clinical samples has been shown to shorten time to diagnosis,[28,30] and some tests (GeneXpert MTB/RIF, Xpert MTB/RIF Ultra [Cepheid])[31] provide information on drug susceptibility. The decision to treat empirically is based on the risk versus benefits of TB regimens. Severely ill individuals, especially those suspected to have *central nervous system* (CNS) and/or disseminated TB, or those at risk of becoming severely ill, particularly young children (<5 years) and immunocompromised individuals, will benefit from initiation of empirical antituberculosis treatment. The initiation of empirical treatment may enable earlier release from contact isolation, allowing patients to return sooner to work, school, and other social settings while the diagnosis of TB is being further evaluated. Given the low risk of serious adverse effects related to TB medications early in the course of treatment,

especially in patients younger than 60 years,[32] the benefits of empirical treatment outweigh treatment-related risks in patients considered to have moderate to high risk for TB.

If empirical treatment is started and adhered to, and serial cultures throughout are negative, patients who show clinical and radiographic improvements at 2 months may be diagnosed with culture-negative TB (discussed later). In patients without a clinical and radiographic response to treatment despite full adherence, treatment for TB may be discontinued and alternative diagnoses should be pursued. If the patient has evidence of latent TB infection (i.e., positive interferon gamma release assay or tuberculin skin test), then consideration of TB preventive therapy is warranted (see Chapters 42 and 51).

RECOMMENDED TREATMENT REGIMENS FOR DRUG-SUSCEPTIBLE TUBERCULOSIS

Recommended treatment regimens for drug-susceptible TB are listed in Tables 54.1 and 54.2. If therapy is being initiated after drug susceptibility test results are known and the patient's isolate is susceptible to both INH and RIF, EMB is not necessary and the intensive phase can consist of INH, RIF, and PZA only. EMB can be discontinued as soon as the results of drug susceptibility studies demonstrate that the isolate is susceptible to INH and RIF.

DOSING FREQUENCY AND TREATMENT ADHERENCE

The most recent *American Thoracic Society/CDC/Infectious Diseases Society of America* (ATS/CDC/IDSA) guidelines recommend that, resources permitting, daily therapy in both

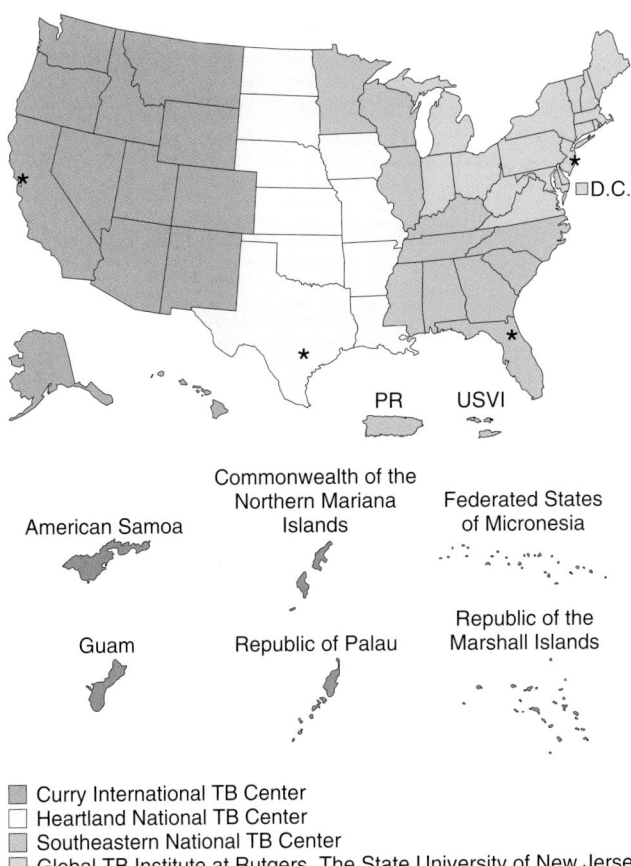

- Curry International TB Center
- Heartland National TB Center
- Southeastern National TB Center
- Global TB Institute at Rutgers, The State University of New Jersey
- Jointly served by all 4 TB centers
★ Center location

Figure 54.1 Centers for Disease Control and Prevention–funded TB Centers of Excellence for Training, Education, and Medical Consultation. These centers support domestic *tuberculosis* (TB) control and prevention efforts with a focus on increasing knowledge, skills, and abilities for TB prevention and control through communication, education, and training activities (https://sntc.medicine.ufl.edu/rtmccproducts.aspx) and on improving sustainable evidence-based TB clinical practices and patient care through the provision of expert medical consultation. PR, Puerto Rico; USVI, U.S. Virgin Islands. (Courtesy the Centers for Disease Control and Prevention, Atlanta, GA.)

the intensive and continuation phases be used.[29] Since the guidelines were published, a patient-level analysis of several RCTs that evaluated TB treatment regimens has provided new information on adherence, dosing frequency, and outcomes that adds evidence to this recommendation.[13] In that analysis, even minimal nonadherence to a standard treatment regimen was associated with an increased risk of poor treatment outcomes. Greater than 90% (but less than perfect) adherence was associated with a *hazard ratio* (HR) of 2.4 (95% *confidence interval* [CI], 1.6 to 3.6), and 90% or less adherence was associated with an HR of 5.9 (95% CI, 3.3 to 10.5) for poor treatment outcomes. Similarly, a dosing schedule of 5 or 6 out of 7 days was associated with poor treatment outcomes compared to 7 days per week administration.[13] These results support a strict dosing of TB treatment of 7 days per week through the intensive and continuation phases.[13]

PATIENT-CENTERED CARE

It is crucial that the patient be involved in making decisions concerning treatment supervision and overall care for TB.

In most public health settings, a patient with TB is assigned a case manager who assesses patient needs and barriers that may interfere with treatment adherence.[33] Together, the case manager and the patient develop an individualized case management plan with interventions to address the identified needs and barriers.[34–36] The plan is reviewed periodically and revised as needed.

DIRECTLY OBSERVED THERAPY

Given the critical importance of chemotherapy for the patient and for public health, ensuring adherence to the treatment regimen is a major focus of the management plan. Management strategies should use a broad range of approaches to maximize treatment completion.[29] Among these, *directly observed therapy* (DOT), the practice of observing the patient swallow the antituberculosis medications, has been widely used as the standard of practice in many programs and deserves special emphasis. DOT, compared to *self-administered therapy*, is associated with improved treatment success (the sum of patients cured and patients completing treatment) and with decreased time-to-sputum smear conversion, but not with significant differences in mortality, treatment completion, and relapse.[29,37] Because DOT is a multifaceted public health intervention that may not be amenable to conventional clinical trial approaches, and because participation in DOT can be advantageous for early recognition of adverse drug reactions and treatment irregularities and for allowing providers to establish rapport with the patient, DOT remains the standard of practice in the majority of TB programs in the United States[38–40] and Europe.[41] DOT decisions about protecting privacy and other concerns must be made in concert with the patient,[41–43] including the location for medication administration. Many TB programs use Internet-based video and mobile phones as less resource-intensive forms of DOT, especially in patients who have demonstrated good adherence with traditional DOT.

PATIENT EVALUATION

Recommended baseline and follow-up evaluations for patients suspected of having TB and treated with first-line medications are summarized in eFig. 54.1. At a minimum, a sputum specimen for AFB smear and culture is obtained at monthly intervals until two consecutive specimens are negative on culture. For patients who had positive AFB smears at the time of diagnosis, follow-up smears may be obtained at more frequent intervals (e.g., every 1–2 weeks until two consecutive specimens are negative) to provide an early assessment of the response to treatment, especially for patients who are awaiting release from isolation.

Susceptibility testing for INH, RIF, EMB, and PZA is performed on an initial positive culture. A rapid molecular test for drug resistance, which identifies mutations associated with resistance to first- and/or second-line antituberculosis medications, is performed in patients at risk for drug-resistant TB.[41,44] Second-line drug susceptibility testing should be done only in reference laboratories and is limited to specimens from patients who have had prior therapy, have been in contact with a patient with known drug-resistant TB, have suspected or demonstrated resistance to RIF and/or other first-line drugs, are unable to tolerate RIF, have positive cultures after more than 3 months of treatment, or are from a region or population with high rates of *multidrug-resistant* (MDR)-TB.[41,44]

Additional indicated testing includes the following:

- Chest radiograph at baseline for all patients. An end-of-treatment chest radiograph is optional, but it serves as a new baseline reference if the patient develops future respiratory symptoms, including those suggesting TB recurrence. For patients treated for culture-negative TB, a chest radiograph should be obtained at 2 months to assess treatment response.
- Liver function tests at baseline for all patients. Further monitoring of liver function is indicated if there are baseline abnormalities or as clinically indicated. In the presence of baseline abnormalities and/or ongoing risk factors (e.g., alcohol use disorder), liver function may be tested more frequently than monthly.
- Creatinine at baseline for all patients, with further monitoring if there are baseline abnormalities or as clinically indicated.
- HIV testing in all patients.
- Monitor weight monthly to assess response to treatment; adjust medication doses if there are changes in weight.
- While receiving EMB, baseline visual acuity (Snellen test) and color discrimination tests, followed by monthly testing.[45]
- Patients with hepatitis B or C risk factors, such as injection drug use, birth in Asia or Africa, or HIV infection, should have screening tests for these infections.
- Fasting glucose or hemoglobin A1c for patients with risk factors for diabetes, according to the American Diabetes Association, including age older than 45 years, body mass index greater than 25, first-degree relative with diabetes, and race/ethnicity of African American, Asian, Hispanic, Native American/Alaskan Native, or Hawaiian Native/Pacific Islander.

PATIENT RESPONSE TO TREATMENT

BACKGROUND

The overall rate of failure or relapse in patients with drug-susceptible TB receiving DOT with a standard rifamycin-based regimen is low.[46–48] In patients receiving 6-month regimens who have drug-susceptible organisms, the estimated failure rate is less than 1% and the relapse rate is 4%.[14] Studies from low-burden settings, where reinfection with *M. tuberculosis* is uncommon, have identified relapse and recurrence rates that are even lower.[49–51] Although current TB regimens are highly effective, their generalized use means that some patients are overtreated, whereas other patients may be undertreated and at greater risk for poor outcomes.[13] The most effective means of decreasing the likelihood of relapse for patients at risk has not yet been determined by clinical trials; however, indirect evidence from a controlled clinical trial and an observational

study among patients with pulmonary TB in Hong Kong showed that prolonging treatment decreased the rate of relapse.[52,53] It has also been reported that for patients at high risk of relapse, prolongation of the once-weekly INH/rifapentine continuation phase from 4 to 7 months resulted in a decreased relapse rate.[54]

IDENTIFYING PATIENTS AT RISK FOR POOR OUTCOMES

Certain baseline and on-treatment characteristics may identify patients who might benefit from treatment prolongation. The result of a sputum culture obtained at completion of the intensive phase of treatment (2 months) correlates with the likelihood of relapse, albeit with low sensitivity.[10,55–57] Cavitation has also been shown to be a risk factor for relapse.[10,53] Having both cavitation and a positive culture at completion of 2 months of therapy is associated with relapse rates of approximately 20%, compared with 2% among patients with neither factor, after a 6-month treatment regimen.[10,57] Therefore, for patients who have cavitation on the initial chest radiograph and a positive culture at completion of 2 months of therapy, the continuation phase with INH and RIF is extended an additional 3 months (i.e., a continuation phase of 7 months, corresponding to a total of 9 months of therapy).[29]

Because patients who had either cavitation or a positive culture at 2 months have increased relapse rates,[10,57] patients with one of these risk factors are followed more closely, and consideration is given to extending treatment duration (i.e., 9 months of total treatment) if there is evidence of a poor response. Additional factors to be considered in prolonging treatment in patients with either cavitation or a positive culture at 2 months include being more than 10% underweight (especially with poor weight gain during the intensive phase of treatment); being a smoker; having diabetes, HIV infection, or other immunocompromising condition; or having extensive disease on chest radiograph.[13,56,58–62] Poor adherence, particularly if less than 90% of the intended doses are ingested, is also associated with poor treatment outcomes.[13]

POOR TREATMENT RESPONSE AND TREATMENT FAILURE

Treatment failure is defined as continuously or recurrently positive cultures after four (United States) or five (European and *World Health Organization* [WHO])[63] months of treatment in a patient receiving appropriate chemotherapy. Among patients with drug-susceptible pulmonary TB, even with extensive lung cavitation, 90–95% will be culture negative after 3 months of treatment with a regimen that contains INH and RIF. During this time, most patients show clinical improvement. Patients with persistently positive cultures after 3 months of chemotherapy should be evaluated to determine the cause of delayed response.

Multiple reasons for poor treatment response and treatment failure exist. For patients not receiving DOT, non-adherence should be considered as an explanation. Other potential reasons include unrecognized drug resistance (drug susceptibility testing not done, misreported, or misinterpreted; reinfection with a drug-resistant strain), malabsorption (diarrhea, prior *gastrointestinal* [GI] resection, or taking TB medications with antacids or other drugs/substances that interfere with drug absorption), or diabetes mellitus.[64-72] Some experts use therapeutic drug monitoring (see later) to evaluate poor drug exposure as a contributing factor to treatment failure.[73] Laboratory error (e.g., cross contamination or mislabeling of specimens) is a possible reason for a positive culture in a patient who is doing well clinically.[74]

On occasion, patients have smear-positive sputum samples with no growth on culture. Culture conversion before smear conversion is thought to represent the presence of nonviable or dead bacilli.[75] The reappearance of smear-positive sputum samples in a patient with multiple negative prior smears and cultures may also be due to this phenomenon. These findings are more common in patients with high-burden (e.g., initial 4+ smear positivity) pulmonary TB.[76]

Patients treated for TB may experience transient clinical or radiographic worsening (paradoxical reactions) despite appropriate therapy. Examples of this include ongoing inflammation at sites of lymphadenitis, worsening symptoms in CNS TB, or the new appearance of pleural effusions. Such paradoxical worsening can be seen in patients with or without HIV infection. The diagnosis of a paradoxical reaction is made only after a thorough evaluation for other etiologies, including the emergence of drug resistance.[77-79]

For patients who meet criteria for treatment failure, the possible reasons listed earlier should be addressed promptly. The patient's recent mycobacterial isolates should be sent to a reference laboratory for susceptibility testing with first- and second-line drugs. Clinicians not familiar with the management of drug-resistant TB should consult with a specialty center immediately. If treatment failure is suspected to be due to drug resistance and the patient is seriously ill or has a positive sputum AFB smear, an empirical regimen for drug-resistant TB is started immediately and continued until susceptibility tests are available to guide therapy. However, if the patient's clinical presentation is not severe, one may either initiate an empirical treatment regimen or wait for drug susceptibility results from a recent isolate. Of note, patients who are not on the correct regimen remain infectious.[80,81] A single new drug should *never* be added to a failing regimen because it can lead to amplification of drug resistance, including acquired resistance to the newly added drug.[82] To lessen the likelihood of increasing resistance, it is prudent to add two to three new drugs to which susceptibility could be inferred (e.g., using regional drug-resistance surveillance data and the patient's history of medication use). When drug susceptibility results are available, the regimen is adjusted accordingly.

CASE MANAGEMENT

ADVERSE EFFECTS

In a single-center study, approximately 9% of patients treated for TB experienced major adverse effects requiring permanent discontinuation of the offending drug, with higher risk in patients older than 60 years, women, people living with HIV, and Asian-born patients.[32] PZA was responsible for most of the major adverse effects. Patients should be advised in advance about the possible adverse effects of the medications in their regimen (listed in Table 54.3) and that they must stop taking their medications and inform their health care team immediately if problems arise. Informing patients in advance will also increase their investment in finding a well-tolerated regimen.

Mild adverse effects usually can be managed with treatment directed at controlling the symptoms. For more severe adverse effects known to be attributable to a single drug in the regimen, that medication may be stopped, and a replacement drug, typically from a different drug class, may be included in the regimen.

The following suggested practices for handling common adverse effects during treatment are based on expert opinion.

Hepatotoxicity

Drug-induced hepatitis is the most frequent serious adverse reaction to first-line drugs; INH, RIF, and PZA can all cause liver injury.[83] Given its greater specificity, *alanine aminotransferase* (ALT) is preferred over *aspartate aminotransferase* (AST) for diagnosing drug-induced liver injury. An asymptomatic increase in ALT concentration may be observed in nearly 20% of patients treated with the standard four-drug regimen and is frequently due to INH through a process called hepatic adaptation, which resolves despite continuation of treatment.[84,85] Therapy should not be altered because of modest asymptomatic elevations of ALT, but the frequency of clinical and laboratory monitoring should be increased. However, if ALT levels are more than five times the *upper limit of normal* ([ULN], with or without symptoms) or more than three times normal in the presence of symptoms, hepatotoxic drugs must be stopped and the patient evaluated. Other causes of abnormal liver tests (e.g., viral hepatitis, biliary tract disease, alcohol use, other hepatotoxic drugs) must be excluded before diagnosing drug-induced hepatotoxicity. Serum ALT and prothrombin time or international normalized ratio levels should be followed until they return to baseline. The clinician should consult a liver specialist if the patient's clinical or laboratory status continues to worsen. Liver injury that produces transaminitis only is more likely to be due to INH or PZA. Similarly, a significant increase in bilirubin and/or alkaline phosphatase is cause for a prompt evaluation; disproportionate increases in bilirubin and alkaline phosphatase (compared to increases in serum ALT) may be seen with RIF hepatotoxicity.[83]

Whether to initiate a "liver-sparing regimen" while awaiting normalization of aminotransferases depends on the patient's infectiousness, severity of disease, and treatment phase. A liver-sparing regimen typically includes EMB, a fluoroquinolone such as *levofloxacin* (LFX), and an aminoglycoside. If a patient is advanced in treatment and/or has a low bacillary burden, it is reasonable to hold all TB treatment while awaiting normalization of liver function.

Once the ALT returns to less than two times the ULN, antituberculosis medications are restarted individually.[83] In patients with elevated baseline ALT from pre-existing liver disease, drugs are restarted when the ALT returns to near baseline levels. The optimal approach to reintroducing TB treatment after hepatotoxicity is not known.[86,87] However, most TB programs use sequential reintroduction of drugs. If symptoms recur or ALT increases, the last drug added should be stopped. Because RIF is much less likely to cause hepatotoxicity than INH or PZA, it is restarted first (with or without EMB, depending on the treatment phase). If there is no increase in ALT after 3 to 7 days, INH may be restarted. The decision to restart PZA (3–7 days after INH) depends on the treatment phase and the severity of liver injury. A prolonged (several weeks) time course to normalization of aminotransferases supports PZA as the responsible medication.[83] If RIF and INH are tolerated and hepatitis was severe, PZA can be assumed to be responsible and is discontinued. In this last circumstance, depending on the number of doses of PZA taken, severity of disease, and bacteriologic status, the total duration of therapy may be extended to 9 months.

Gastrointestinal Symptoms

GI reactions, including nausea, vomiting, poor appetite, and abdominal pain, are the most common adverse effects seen early in treatment.[88] Aminotransferases and bilirubin should be checked to ensure that GI symptoms are not due to hepatotoxicity. If applicable, pregnancy should be considered as an etiology of the patient's symptoms.

- To minimize symptoms, patients receiving self-administered or video-observed therapy may take the medication that is causing symptoms at bedtime.
- GI intolerance can be treated with antacids, including proton pump inhibitors.[89]
- A light snack (low-fat food) before taking medications may decrease symptoms.
- Nausea may be treated by giving antiemetics 30 minutes before TB medications. Options include ondansetron, promethazine, and metoclopramide.

Rash

All first-line antituberculosis drugs can cause rashes, the severity of which determines management.[90] If a rash is mainly itchy without mucous membrane involvement or systemic signs, such as fever or mucosal involvement, treatment is symptomatic with antihistamines with or without corticosteroid creams. Specific types of dermatologic adverse effects require different responses:

- Photosensitivity may be due to PZA and may persist for weeks after stopping PZA. Patients should avoid sun exposure and use sunscreen.
- A petechial rash is concerning for thrombocytopenia, which may be caused by RIF.[91] If the platelet count is low, RIF should be stopped. When the platelet counts have recovered, *rifabutin* (RFB) may be considered as a replacement for RIF.[92]
- Involvement of mucous membranes and/or fever suggests Stevens-Johnson syndrome or toxic epidermal necrosis. Rash with eosinophilia, lymphadenitis, fever, and/or other organ system involvement is consistent with *drug rash with eosinophilia and systemic symptoms* (DRESS) syndrome. A dermatologist should be consulted in addition to a TB expert for these syndromes.

When the rash has improved, medications can be reintroduced serially at intervals of 2 to 3 days. If the rash recurs, the last drug added is stopped.

Neurotoxicity

Neurotoxic effects of antituberculosis medications include peripheral neuropathy, headaches, drowsiness, and problems with concentration and irritability. INH causes a functional deficiency of pyridoxine (vitamin B_6) that is usually clinically significant only in high-risk patients. Pyridoxine (25–50 mg) is given with each INH dose to all persons at risk of neuropathy, including patients with diabetes, HIV, renal disease, alcohol abuse, or malnutrition; pregnant or breastfeeding mothers, or those with chronic renal failure or of advanced age.[93,94] Some experts routinely provide pyridoxine supplementation to all patients receiving INH. For patients who develop neuropathy while on pyridoxine, doses may be increased to 100 mg daily; pyridoxine supplementation above this dose is unlikely to be helpful. The other listed neurotoxic adverse effects typically resolve with continuation of TB medications and are best addressed with supportive methods. Seizures, including status epilepticus, may develop as a result of INH toxicity, including overdoses; patients should be immediately hospitalized and treated with intravenous pyridoxine and antiepileptic drugs.[95,96]

Optic Neuritis

EMB-related visual impairment during treatment of active TB has been estimated to happen in 19 of 1000 persons receiving EMB at 27.5 mg/kg/day or less for 2 to 9 months' duration.[97] The onset of optic neuritis is usually more than 1 month after treatment initiation but can happen within days.[98,99] To avoid permanent deficits, EMB is promptly discontinued if visual abnormalities are found, and ophthalmologic consultation should be obtained. Recovery of vision takes 3 months on average.[97]

THERAPEUTIC DRUG MONITORING

Therapeutic drug monitoring (TDM) consists of measurements of drug concentrations in serum specimens, usually collected 2 and 6 hours after a dose of a drug. No prospective randomized trials clearly define the role of TDM for antituberculosis drugs, and opinions vary regarding its utility. TDM should be reserved for specific indications because the majority of patients will not require it. TDM may be helpful in situations in which drug malabsorption, drug underdosing, or clinically important drug-drug interactions are suspected. Situations in which TDM may be indicated include (1) patients with delayed sputum conversion or treatment failure not explained by nonadherence or drug resistance, (2) patients with medical conditions (e.g., malabsorption or reduced renal function) suspected of leading to subtherapeutic or toxic drug concentrations, and (3) patients undergoing treatment for drug-resistant TB. Practical considerations in obtaining TDM include the following:

- Blood should be obtained after the patient has been on a stable dose of the medication for approximately 1 week to ensure a steady state.

- For INH, RIF, EMB, and PZA levels, blood should be collected 2 and 6 hours after ingestion of the medication. The 2-hour blood draw captures peak concentration and is usually higher than the 6-hour sample.
- If the 6-hour level is higher than the 2-hour level, this is consistent with delayed absorption.
- If both the 2-hour and 6-hour levels are low, then malabsorption may be present.
- Laboratories with extensive experience in analyzing TB drug levels may be found at the University of Florida, Gainesville (http://idpl.pharmacy.ufl.edu) and National Jewish Health, Denver (http://njlabs.org). Results from these laboratories include target serum drug levels.
- If drug concentrations are lower than the targeted range, then the dose of that medication should be increased.

INTERRUPTIONS IN THERAPY

Interruptions in therapy are common in the treatment of TB. When therapy is interrupted, the person responsible for supervision must decide whether to restart a complete course of treatment or to continue as originally intended. In general, the earlier the break in therapy and the longer its duration, the greater the need to restart treatment from the beginning. Continuous treatment is more important in the intensive phase of therapy, when the bacillary population is highest and the chance of developing drug resistance is greatest. During the continuation phase, the number of bacilli is much lower, and the goal of therapy is to kill persisting organisms. The duration of the interruption and the bacteriologic status of the patient before and after the interruption are also important considerations. The approach summarized in Table 54.4 is presented as an example.[100]

CULTURE-NEGATIVE TUBERCULOSIS

Patients who have negative cultures but are presumed to have pulmonary TB should have thorough clinical and radiographic follow-up after 2 months of therapy. The most recent CDC guidelines recommend that a 4-month treatment regimen is adequate for HIV-uninfected adults with culture-negative pulmonary TB.[29] Treatment is initiated with the intensive phase of daily INH, RIF, PZA, and EMB. If all cultures on adequate samples are negative and there is clinical or radiographic response after 2 months of intensive phase therapy, the continuation phase with INH and RIF can be shortened to 2 months. Clinical and radiographic response, assessed at the end of treatment, is used to determine whether an extension in treatment to a full standard 6-month regimen is needed. The local health department should be notified of individuals with culture-negative TB.

EXTRAPULMONARY TUBERCULOSIS

With the exceptions of CNS and bone and joint TB, treatment of patients with extrapulmonary TB is similar to that of patients with pulmonary TB.[29] The preferred frequency of dosing for extrapulmonary TB is once daily for both the intensive and continuation phases. In extrapulmonary TB, response to treatment is often judged on the basis of clinical and radiographic findings because of the difficulty in obtaining samples for follow-up cultures.[29]

Table 54.4 Management of Treatment Interruptions*

Time Point of Interruption	Details of Interruption	Approach
During intensive phase	Lapse is <14 days in duration	Continue treatment to complete planned total number of doses (as long as all doses are completed within 3 mo)
	Lapse is ≥14 days in duration	Restart treatment from the beginning
During continuation phase	Received ≥80% of doses and sputum was AFB smear negative on initial testing	Further therapy may not be necessary
	Received ≥80% of doses and sputum was AFB smear positive on initial testing	Continue therapy until all doses are completed
	Received <80% of doses and accumulative lapse is <3 mo in duration	Continue therapy until all doses are completed (full course), unless consecutive lapse is >2 mo If treatment cannot be completed within recommended time frame for regimen, restart therapy from the beginning (i.e., restart intensive phase, to be followed by continuation phase)[†]
	Received <80% of doses and lapse is ≥3 mo in duration	Restart therapy from the beginning, new intensive and continuation phases (i.e., restart intensive phase, to be followed by continuation phase)

*According to expert opinion, patients who are lost to follow-up (on treatment) and brought back to therapy, with interim treatment interruption, should have sputum resent for AFB smear, culture and drug susceptibility testing.
†The recommended time frame for regimen, in tuberculosis control programs in the United States and in several European countries, is to administer all of the specified number of doses for the intensive phase within 3 mo and those for the 4-mo continuation phase within 6 mo so that the 6-mo regimen is completed within 9 mo.
Modified from Bureau of Tuberculosis Control. *Clinical Policies and Protocols*, 4th ed. New York City Department of Health and Mental Hygiene; 2008.
AFB, acid-fast bacillus.

CENTRAL NERVOUS SYSTEM

CNS TB may present with meningitis or intracranial tuberculomas. Tuberculous meningitis remains a potentially devastating disease associated with death rates of 18–40%[101] and disabling neurologic deficits in 10–30% of survivors[101,102] despite prompt initiation of appropriate chemotherapy.[103] Current U.S. guidelines recommend an intensive phase that includes INH, RIF, PZA, and EMB, with a continuation phase of INH and RIF.[29] However, the continuation phase should be extended to 7 to 10 months for 9 to 12 months of total treatment.

In children with tuberculous meningitis, the *American Academy of Pediatrics* (AAP) lists an initial four-drug regimen of INH, RIF, PZA, and ethionamide or an aminoglycoside for 2 months (in place of EMB), followed by 7 to 10 months of INH and RIF,[104] although there are no data from controlled trials to guide selection of EMB versus an injectable or ethionamide as the fourth drug for TB meningitis.[105] A trial of TB meningitis treatment regimens that evaluated LFX and higher-dose RIF did not detect a difference in outcomes compared to standard treatment.[102] There are several studies of alternative regimens (e.g., high-dose RIF, adding linezolid; http://clinicaltrials.gov) or host-directed therapeutics[106] to improve outcomes in patients with TB meningitis.

Based on expert opinion, repeated lumbar punctures should be considered to monitor changes in cerebrospinal fluid cell count, glucose, and protein, especially early in the course of therapy. As a closed-space infection, an overly robust inflammatory response may worsen patient outcomes, and TB meningitis is one of the few infections where high-quality evidence supports the clinical use of corticosteroids,[101] although the benefit may be limited to subsets of patients with greater inflammatory responses.[107] An updated systematic review that informed the current CDC guidelines found a mortality benefit from the use of adjuvant corticosteroids, which may be administered as dexamethasone. Whereas the CDC guidelines do not make dexamethasone dosage recommendations, based on contemporary trials, the following dosages of corticosteroids can be considered: adults (>14 years) should receive dexamethasone 0.4 mg/kg/24 hr with a reducing course over 6 weeks (some experts extend to 8 weeks). Children (<14 years) should receive prednisolone 4 mg/kg/24 hr (or equivalent dose of dexamethasone: 0.6 mg/kg/24 hr) for 4 weeks, followed by a reducing course over 2 to 4 weeks.[29,105]

Cerebral tuberculomas may be present in patients with and without TB meningitis, and antituberculosis treatment may lead to a paradoxical worsening in tuberculoma size and symptoms. Adjunctive corticosteroids may decrease tuberculoma size and improve symptom control.[105] Selected complications of tuberculous meningitis warranting neurosurgical intervention include hydrocephalus, tuberculous cerebral abscess, and paraparesis.[105]

BONE AND JOINT

Guidelines recommend 6 to 9 months of treatment for bone and joint TB (i.e., extending the continuation phase by an additional 3 months).[108] In the setting of extensive orthopedic hardware involvement, some experts extend treatment to 12 months. Several trials found no additional benefit of surgical débridement in combination with chemotherapy compared with chemotherapy alone for spinal TB.[109–113] Uncomplicated cases of spinal TB are managed with medical rather than surgical treatment. Surgery should be considered when (1) there is poor response to chemotherapy with evidence of ongoing infection or clinical deterioration, (2) relief of cord compression is needed, or (3) there is instability of the spine.[114]

PERICARDIAL

Previously, corticosteroids were recommended as adjunctive therapy for tuberculous pericarditis.[115–117] However, a large RCT did not find a difference in outcomes between study arms, although subgroup analysis suggested a benefit in preventing constrictive pericarditis.[118] The current U.S. guidelines recommend that adjunctive corticosteroids should not be used routinely in the treatment of patients with pericardial TB.[108] There may be a role for the selective use of corticosteroids in patients at the highest risk for inflammatory complications, such as those with large pericardial effusions, high levels of inflammatory cells or markers in pericardial fluid, or signs of constriction.[119]

LYMPH NODE

A 6-month regimen is adequate for treatment of drug-susceptible tuberculous lymphadenitis,[120–125] although responses may be slower than in pulmonary TB. Paradoxical upgrading reactions, defined as enlarging or new nodes or a new draining sinus in patients who have received at least 10 days of treatment, develop in more than 20% of patients with lymph node TB regardless of HIV status.[126] These paradoxical reactions are not indicative of treatment failure, although drainage or fine-needle aspirate may be obtained for culture and to ensure drug susceptibility. Some experts use corticosteroids to decrease inflammation.[127] Incision and drainage techniques applied to cervical lymphadenitis, however, have been reported to be associated with prolonged wound discharge and scarring.[128]

SPECIAL POPULATIONS

PEOPLE LIVING WITH HUMAN IMMUNODEFICIENCY VIRUS

The principles of treatment of TB in patients living with HIV and receiving antiretroviral therapy are similar to those in patients who are HIV negative. However, there are important differences in people living with HIV, including interactions between antiretroviral drugs and rifamycins, which are potent inducers of *cytochrome P-450* (CYP) enzymes and thus accelerate metabolism of many drugs. *Cytochrome P-450 3A4* (CYP3A4) is especially relevant because it is involved in metabolism of multiple classes of antiretroviral drugs.

Other considerations are the *immune reconstitution inflammatory syndrome* (IRIS) and increased risk for poor treatment outcomes. HIV infection in the presence of TB increases the risk of TB relapse[129–131] and death.[132] In addition, intermittent TB treatment regimens in people living with HIV are associated with the emergence of drug resistance.[10,133,134] Use of a thrice-weekly RIF-based regimen during the intensive and continuation phases of treatment was associated with higher relapse rates and rifamycin resistance in people living with HIV not receiving antiretrovirals, compared with antiretroviral-treated people living with HIV or patients without HIV infection.[135]

U.S. guidelines make the following recommendations[29]:

- For antiretroviral-treated people living with HIV, the standard 6-month daily regimen consisting of an intensive phase of 2 months of INH, RIF, PZA, and EMB, followed by a continuation phase of 4 months of INH and RIF, for the treatment of drug-susceptible pulmonary TB is appropriate.
- For people living with HIV who are *not* receiving antiretrovirals, the continuation phase should be extended for an additional 3 months (i.e., a continuation phase of 7 months in duration for a total of 9 months of therapy).
- Treatment should be given daily in both the intensive and continuation phases to avoid recurrent disease and the emergence of rifamycin resistance.

IRIS in association with TB treatment is the worsening of symptoms in a patient receiving appropriate treatment and may include high fevers, worsening respiratory symptoms, increase in size and inflammation of involved lymph nodes, new lymphadenopathy, expanding CNS lesions, worsening of pulmonary parenchymal infiltrations, new or increasing pleural effusions, and development of intra-abdominal or retroperitoneal abscesses.[136] IRIS is more common in patients with severe immunosuppression at baseline (CD4-cell counts < 50 cells/mm^3) and antiretroviral-naive individuals who initiate antiretrovirals earlier in the TB treatment course.[137] The diagnosis of IRIS is made only after excluding other possible causes. Management of IRIS is symptomatic. For most patients with mild IRIS, TB and antiretroviral therapies can be continued with the addition of nonsteroidal anti-inflammatory drugs.[29] For patients with worsening pleural effusions or abscesses, drainage may be necessary. In severe cases of IRIS, treatment with corticosteroids may be required.[138] Prednisone may be given at a dose of 1.25 mg/kg/day (50–80 mg/day) for 2 to 4 weeks, with tapering over a period of 6 to 12 weeks or longer. In an RCT, prednisone (40 mg/day for 14 days, followed by 20 mg/day for 14 days), given to TB/HIV coinfected individuals (CD4 cell counts < 100 cells/mm^3) who were initiating antiretroviral therapy within 30 days of starting antituberculosis therapy resulted in a lower incidence of IRIS compared to placebo.[139]

Through induction of CYP3A4 and other P-450 cytochromes, rifamycins accelerate the metabolism of many antiretroviral agents, potentially leading to subtherapeutic levels. *Integrase strand transfer inhibitor* (INSTI)-based regimens are the first-line regimens for treatment of HIV infection in the United States and Europe and were endorsed by the WHO as the preferred regimen.[140] Trough concentrations of the INSTIs raltegravir and dolutegravir are significantly reduced by concomitant use of RIF.[141,142] The REFLATE TB trial showed that RIF-based antituberculosis treatment and raltegravir at 400 mg or 800 mg twice daily was associated with similar antiviral effectiveness; both raltegravir doses were more effective than efavirenz 600 mg daily.[141] However, PK data favor increasing the raltegravir dose to 800 mg twice daily, and expert opinion in the United

States favors this strategy.[143] PK studies demonstrate that coadministration of RIF and dolutegravir at a dosage of 50 mg twice daily results in adequate trough concentrations of dolutegravir.[142] RIF is contraindicated in patients receiving tenofovir alafenamide–containing formulations, protease inhibitors, PK boosters (e.g., cobicistat, ritonavir), and most non-nucleoside reverse transcriptase inhibitors other than efavirenz.

RFB is a less potent inducer of CYP3A4 and may be used in patients receiving non-nucleoside reverse transcriptase inhibitors and boosted protease inhibitors, as well as dolutegravir or raltegravir (400 mg twice daily). RFB itself is metabolized by CYP3A enzymes, and the antiretroviral agent ritonavir (used to boost protease inhibitor levels) inhibits CYP3A enzymes, resulting in increased concentrations of RFB. High concentrations of RFB are associated with an increased risk of uveitis and other toxicities, so dose adjustment of the standard RFB dosage of 300 mg daily is necessary.[144] Expert opinion is to use RFB at a dose of 150 mg/day or 300 mg every other day as part of a combination antituberculosis regimen for patients receiving ritonavir-boosted protease inhibitors.[145] In patients receiving dose-adjusted RFB because of concomitant protease inhibitor use, frequent assessment of adherence to both medicines is prudent because discontinuation of the protease inhibitor while continuing dose-adjusted RFB (i.e., in the context of DOT TB therapy but self-administered antiretrovirals) may result in subtherapeutic concentrations of rifamycin. These complicated interactions underscore the importance of expert consultation in treating individuals with concurrent HIV and TB. For situations involving complex drug-drug interactions, some clinicians prefer to measure the concentrations of the interacting drugs and to dose these drugs based upon individualized data.[73]

For people living with HIV who are receiving antiretroviral therapy and are diagnosed with TB, the antiretroviral regimen may need modifications to allow use of a rifamycin (RIF or RFB). Useful sources regarding drug interactions (TB/HIV and other) are available through the following organizations: AIDSinfo, CDC, University of California San Francisco, University of Liverpool, and Indiana University. For individuals with TB who are not receiving antiretrovirals, there are guidelines on when to initiate antiretroviral therapy[146]:

- Individuals with CD4 count less than 50 cells/mm^3: Start antiretrovirals within the first 2 weeks of TB treatment; this has been shown to reduce morbidity and mortality.[147–149]
- Individuals with CD4 counts greater than or equal to 50 cells/mm^3: Start antiretrovirals within the first 8 weeks of TB treatment.
- People living with HIV with TB meningitis: Use caution with early initiation of antiretroviral therapy because a study from Vietnam demonstrated a higher rate of severe IRIS events in participants randomized to immediate antiretrovirals compared to those started on antiretroviral therapy at month 2 of TB treatment.[150]

HEPATIC DISEASE

TB treatment in patients with liver disease poses challenges because the likelihood of drug-induced hepatitis is increased with advanced liver disease,[151] liver transplant,[152] or viral hepatitis.[83,153,154] Abnormal baseline aminotransferases alone are an independent risk factor for drug-induced liver injury.[151,155] Hepatic TB may also cause elevated aminotransferases, which improve with effective TB treatment.[156]

PZA, INH, and RIF may all cause hepatic injury. Regimens with fewer potentially hepatotoxic agents are selected in patients with advanced liver disease or whose serum ALT is more than three times the ULN at baseline (and thought not to be caused by TB). The importance of INH and RIF warrant their use, if at all possible, even in the face of preexisting liver disease. Expert consultation is advisable, and adjustments during treatment may be necessary. Alternative regimens for use in patients with hepatic disease (i.e., ALT > 3 × ULN) include the following[83]:

- Treatment without PZA: PZA has often been implicated in drug-induced liver injury. A potential regimen could be INH and RIF for 9 months with EMB given for the first 2 months, or until susceptibility to INH and RIF is determined.[157,158]
- Treatment without INH and PZA: For advanced liver disease patients, RIF and EMB with a fluoroquinolone (injectable), or cycloserine for 12 to 18 months, depending on the extent of the disease and response.[159]
- Regimens with little or no potential hepatotoxicity: For severe, unstable liver disease patients, EMB combined with a fluoroquinolone, cycloserine, and second-line injectable for 18 to 24 months (similar to an MDR-TB regimen) can be considered.[160] Some experts avoid aminoglycosides in patients with severe, unstable liver disease due to concerns about renal insufficiency or bleeding from the site of injected medication due to thrombocytopenia and/or coagulopathy.

Clinical monitoring and patient education for manifestations of liver injury are warranted for all patients.[83] In patients with known hepatic disease, serum aminotransferases and total bilirubin concentrations should be assessed at baseline and every 1 to 4 weeks for at least the first 2 to 3 months of treatment. The international normalized ratio may also be periodically followed for patients with severe hepatic impairment.[83,161,162] Reintroduction of antituberculosis treatment may entail rechallenge and/or substitution of agents, and strategies have been published.[83] Whenever feasible, management of TB in the setting of severe hepatic disease should include expert consultation.

KIDNEY DISEASE

TB patients with chronic renal failure have worse clinical outcomes than those without renal failure, and experts recommend close monitoring during TB treatment.[163] The PKs of antituberculosis drugs are altered because some are cleared by the kidneys and/or removed via hemodialysis.[164,165] RIF and INH are metabolized by the liver, and conventional dosing can be used in the setting of renal insufficiency. PZA is also metabolized by the liver, but its metabolites may accumulate in patients with renal insufficiency. Approximately 80% of EMB clearance is by the kidneys and may accumulate in patients with renal insufficiency. For patients with a creatinine clearance of less than

30 mL/min and those receiving hemodialysis, guidelines recommend maintaining the dosage of PZA and EMB but decreasing the frequency of administration (i.e., changing from daily to three times weekly).[29,73,166] Postdialysis administration of all antituberculosis medications is preferred to facilitate DOT and to avoid premature clearance of drugs. Monitoring serum drug concentrations, along with careful clinical and pharmacologic assessment, in patients with end-stage renal disease may be necessary. For patients receiving peritoneal dialysis, there is a paucity of PK and dosing data, and the appropriate dosages are not known. Such patients may require close monitoring for toxicity, and measurements of the serum concentrations of antituberculosis drugs before and after peritoneal dialysis should be considered.

OLDER PATIENTS

By age, the highest TB rates in the United States are among individuals 65 years and older.[167] The treatment of TB in older populations may be complicated by comorbidities, polypharmacy, and frailty, which can result in undesirable treatment outcomes, including increased rates of medication-related adverse reactions.[168] Because PZA is the most common cause of severe adverse effects,[32,169,170] the benefits of including PZA in the initial regimen for elderly patients with modest disease and low risk of drug resistance have been questioned, and some experts avoid the use of PZA during the intensive phase among patients older than 75 years.[29] However, recent studies have not demonstrated higher rates of PZA-related adverse effects in the elderly compared to younger patients,[170] or among elderly patients, based on the inclusion of PZA in TB treatment regimens.[171] If PZA is not used during the intensive phase, the total duration of TB treatment should be extended to at least 9 months. When elderly patients have TB with high bacillary burden, the benefits and risks of keeping PZA or adding a fluoroquinolone versus no fourth drug should be carefully considered. The frequency of drug interactions is increased in the elderly, and dose adjustments or use of alternative regimens may be necessary.

CHILDREN

The diagnosis of TB in children is challenging due to the paucibacillary nature of the disease, and sputum specimens for bacteriologic evaluations cannot usually be obtained in younger children,[172] so drug susceptibility or resistance often must be inferred from results from the presumed source case. When drug resistance is suspected or no source case isolate is available, attempts to isolate organisms are critical; approaches including obtaining three early morning *gastric* aspirations (optimally during hospitalization), sputum induction,[173] bronchoalveolar lavage,[174] or tissue biopsy must be considered.[29]

Because TB in infants and children younger than 4 years is more likely to disseminate, empirical treatment must be started as soon as the diagnosis is suspected, and particular care is given to drug dosage selection as an important component of achieving adequate concentrations of bactericidal drugs in body fluids, including cerebrospinal fluid.[175]

Several controlled and multiple observational trials of 6-month therapy in children with known or presumed drug-susceptible pulmonary TB have been published.[176] The AAP[177] and WHO[178,179] list a four-drug regimen (INH, RIF, PZA, and EMB) for 2 months, followed by a two-drug (INH and RIF) regimen for 4 months, as the preferred regimen for children with suspected or confirmed pulmonary TB. When feasible, daily dosing is preferred[177,179,180]; however, twice- or thrice-weekly dosing has also been endorsed during the continuation phase of treatment for HIV-uninfected children in settings where DOT is well established.[177] The AAP recommends that children receiving EMB should be monitored monthly for visual acuity and color discrimination if they are old enough to cooperate. The decision to use EMB in young children whose visual acuity cannot be monitored requires consideration of risks and benefits, but it can be used to treat TB disease in infants and children unless otherwise contraindicated.[177] Some clinicians use a three-drug regimen (INH, RIF, and PZA) in the initial 2 months of treatment for children who are HIV uninfected, have no prior TB treatment history, are living in an area of low prevalence of drug-resistant TB, and have no exposure to an individual from an area of high prevalence of drug-resistant TB. However, because the prevalence of and risk for drug-resistant TB can be difficult to determine, the AAP and most experts include EMB as part of the intensive phase regimen for children with TB.

Most forms of extrapulmonary TB in children can be treated with the same regimens as are used in adults.[29] For tuberculous meningitis, the AAP lists an initial four-drug regimen of INH, RIF, PZA, and an aminoglycoside or ethionamide for 2 months, followed by 7 to 10 months of INH and RIF. For patients who may have acquired TB in regions where resistance to streptomycin is common, amikacin is used instead of streptomycin.[177] In the United States, DOT is the default programmatic approach to treating children with TB.[181] Parents should not supervise DOT for their children.[29]

PREGNANCY AND BREASTFEEDING

Untreated active TB poses a far greater hazard to a pregnant woman and her fetus than does treatment for the disease.[182] Although antituberculosis drugs cross the placenta, they do not appear to have teratogenic effects in humans.[183–186] Due to limited data, the inclusion of PZA in the treatment regimen for pregnant women is controversial in the United States, and the CDC has recommended against its use during pregnancy. However, PZA has been used extensively in high-burden countries for many years and is recommended by the WHO for TB in pregnancy as part of the standard treatment regimen.[63] Expert opinion is that in pregnant women with TB and HIV, extrapulmonary or severe TB, it is more beneficial to include PZA in the treatment regimen than to not include PZA. Discussions regarding the risks and benefits of the different treatment regimens will support the patient in making an informed decision, recognizing that for all first-line drugs, risk cannot be ruled out as there are no adequate and well-controlled studies in humans. If a decision is made to exclude PZA from the regimen, a minimum of 9 months of INH, RIF, and EMB is required.

Breastfeeding is encouraged for women who are noninfectious and are being treated with first-line agents. The low concentrations of antituberculosis drugs measured in breast milk neither present a risk to the infant[177] nor reach adequate concentrations to be considered effective treatment for active TB in a nursing infant. Whenever INH is given to a pregnant or nursing woman, supplementary pyridoxine, 25 to 50 mg/day, is prescribed.[93,94,187,188] According to the AAP, supplementary pyridoxine (1–2 mg/kg/day) is also prescribed to exclusively breastfed infants, even those not receiving INH,[177,189] although liquid formulations may be difficult to obtain.

DRUG-RESISTANT TUBERCULOSIS

Drug-resistant TB is due to *M. tuberculosis* isolates resistant to any of the first-line drugs. Due to the importance of INH and RIF in the treatment of drug-susceptible TB, disease caused by isolates resistant to both these drugs defines MDR-TB. MDR-TB that is resistant to a fluoroquinolone or a second-line injectable drug (amikacin, kanamycin, or capreomycin) is termed *pre-extensively drug-resistant TB* (pre–XDR-TB) and if resistant to both classes of drugs is termed *extensively drug-resistant TB* (XDR-TB). For an in-depth discussion of this complicated and evolving topic, guidelines should be consulted.[45,190,191]

INITIATING EMPIRICAL TREATMENT FOR DRUG-RESISTANT TUBERCULOSIS

In patients who are being treated for TB and had drug susceptibility results at the start of treatment that demonstrated susceptibility to the standard first-line regimen, drug-resistant TB should be suspected when there is lack of culture conversion by months 3 to 4 (especially if the initial AFB smear results were less than 4+)[76] and/or when there is lack of improvement or worsening of TB symptoms or imaging.[45] Suspicion for the emergence of drug resistance should be heightened when the patient has been receiving treatment without DOT.

In patients with a history of treated TB who present with a strong suspicion or new diagnosis of TB, the following are situations in which drug-resistant TB should be suspected:

- Patients with a history of treatment for drug-resistant TB
- Patients who did not receive DOT throughout the course of their TB treatment
- Patients who were treated with a nonstandard or inappropriate regimen
- Patients who did not complete the entire recommended duration of treatment (e.g., 6 months of treatment for uncomplicated drug-susceptible pulmonary TB)
- People living with HIV who received an intermittent regimen[133,134]

Efforts should be made to obtain past treatment records whether the patient was treated within or outside the United States.

For patients without a history of treated TB who present with a new diagnosis of TB or are strongly suspected of having TB, the following are situations in which drug-resistant TB should be suspected:

- Close contact with an individual with drug-resistant pulmonary TB
- Origin in a country with high rates of drug-resistant TB, such as countries formerly part of the Soviet Union

In all the above situations, rapid testing for drug resistance should be performed. GeneXpert MTB/RIF can simultaneously detect *M. tuberculosis* and RIF resistance, and results are available 2 hours after processing (see Chapters 19 and 53). The CDC provides a Molecular Detection of Drug Resistance Service to identify mutations that are most frequently associated with INH and RIF resistance; testing is also available for mutations associated with resistance to second-line drugs (https://www.cdc.gov/tb/topic/laboratory/default.htm). Results of rapid testing should be confirmed with culture-based drug-susceptibility testing. When resistance to RIF or more than one first-line drug is identified, drug susceptibility testing should be requested for the second-line drugs.[45] Resistance to fluoroquinolones should be evaluated whenever INH resistance is found.

KEY PRINCIPLES OF TREATING DRUG-RESISTANT TUBERCULOSIS

For patients being evaluated and treated for any form of drug-resistant TB, the following principles apply[191]:

- Consultation should be requested with a TB expert. In the United States, TB experts can be found through CDC-supported TB Centers of Excellence for Training, Education, and Medical Consultation (http://www.cdc.gov/tb/education/rtmc/default.htm).
- Regimens should include only drugs to which the patient's *M. tuberculosis* isolate has documented or high likelihood of susceptibility. Drugs known to be ineffective based on in vitro growth-based or molecular resistance should *not* be used.
- Never add a single new drug to a "failing" regimen; this will likely select for resistance to the new drug. Rather, multiple new drugs must be initiated.
- Treatment response should be monitored clinically, radiographically, and bacteriologically, with cultures obtained at least monthly for pulmonary TB. When cultures remain positive after 3 months of treatment, susceptibility tests for drugs should be repeated.

MECHANISMS AND PHARMACOLOGY OF DRUGS USED TO TREAT DRUG-RESISTANT TUBERCULOSIS

- Fluoroquinolones: Fluoroquinolones, which exhibit concentration dependent killing, are bactericidal through inhibition of bacterial DNA gyrases, preventing DNA synthesis. LFX and moxifloxacin are the preferred fluoroquinolones for treatment of TB because they have greater activity against MTB than ciprofloxacin or ofloxacin.[192] Fluoroquinolones should not be given within 2 hours of ingestion of milk-based products or antacids because absorption is impaired. LFX is primarily excreted through urine in an unchanged form;

for this reason, dosing is thrice weekly (not daily) in patients with creatinine clearance less than 30 mL/min.

- Bedaquiline is a diarylquinolone with strong bactericidal activity against MTB through inhibition of mycobacterial ATP synthase and is active against both replicating and nonreplicating bacilli.
- Linezolid is an oxazolidinone that blocks bacterial ribosomal protein synthesis through binding to the 50S bacterial ribosomal subunit. Linezolid has modest early bactericidal activity against rapidly growing bacilli[193] and sterilizing activity.[194] Linezolid exhibits time-dependent killing, in which the 24-hour area under the curve to minimum inhibitory concentration ratio is predictive of bacillary eradication. Because discontinuation of linezolid due to adverse effects is common, some experts recommend monitoring trough levels after 2 weeks of therapy and minimizing toxicity by maintaining levels less than 2 µg/mL.
- Clofazimine is an *r*-iminophenazone pigment used to treat leprosy. The mechanism of clofazimine's bactericidal activity against MTB is incompletely understood, although it likely involves respiratory inhibition and production of reactive oxidant species.[195] Obtaining clofazimine requires the submission of an Investigational New Drug application to the *U.S. Food and Drug Administration* (FDA) and accessing the medication through the manufacturer (Novartis).
- Cycloserine is an analog of an amino acid, D-alanine, that impairs bacterial cell wall synthesis through competitive inhibition of two enzymes. Depending on tissue concentrations, cycloserine may be bacteriostatic or bactericidal. Cycloserine may cause adverse psychiatric effects including depression, psychosis, and suicidal ideation and should be avoided in patients with a history of psychiatric illness. Concomitant provision of pyridoxine may ameliorate these effects and should be given at 50 mg per 250 mg of cycloserine.[45] Adverse effects may be reduced by monitoring cycloserine levels to maintain peak concentration less than 35 µg/mL.
- Delamanid, a nitrodihydroimidazooxazole, is a prodrug bioactivated by mycobacterial nitroreductase.[196] Delamanid has bactericidal activity through inhibition of mycolic acid synthesis and is effective against actively and sporadically multiplying bacilli. Although approved for use in Europe, it has not yet been approved by the FDA.
- Pretomanid, like delamanid, is a nitroimidazole that inhibits mycolic acid synthesis and is bactericidal against actively and sporadically multiplying bacilli.[197] Pretomanid was approved by the FDA in 2019 for inclusion in a regimen for treatment of XDR-TB and resistant/intolerant MDR-TB (see later).

EMPIRICAL EXPANDED REGIMENS

There are situations in which an expanded empirical regimen is initiated for suspected drug-resistant TB, even before having results from rapid or phenotypic drug susceptibility testing. This decision is based on the probability that the patient has drug-resistant TB and on the severity of the patient's illness. An expanded regimen includes first-line drugs (INH, RIF, PZA, EMB) because the patient may have drug-susceptible TB and two or more new drugs for possible drug-resistant TB. An expanded regimen may include a fluoroquinolone, linezolid, and/or amikacin, in addition to the first-line drugs (Table 54.5).

EMPIRICAL REGIMENS FOR MULTIDRUG-RESISTANT TUBERCULOSIS

If drug susceptibility testing reveals RIF (±INH) resistance, an empirical MDR-TB treatment regimen should be prescribed. Guidelines on the treatment of drug-resistant TB encourage the use of all oral regimens whenever possible.[190,191] A recent patient-level meta-analysis investigated associations between treatment outcomes in MDR-TB and the specific drugs in a regimen, the number of drugs in the regimen, and the duration of the different phases of treatment.[198] Treatment success was most likely when five or more effective drugs were included in the intensive phase. For the continuation phase, four drugs were associated with the greatest success.[198] Table 54.5 shows the recommended algorithm for building an empirical MDR-TB treatment regimen. The hierarchy of drug selection is based on treatment success associated with the different second-line agents

and the adverse effect profiles of these medications.[198] If drug-susceptibility testing subsequently identifies resistance to any of the medications in the treatment regimen, the drug to which the isolate is resistant should be replaced with an effective medication. The final choice of drugs depends on patient preferences, harms and benefits associated with the agents, the capacity to monitor for significant adverse effects, consideration of drug-drug interactions, comorbidities, and drug availability. The doses of the drugs for treating adults and children with MDR-TB are provided in eTable 54.1.

TREATMENT DURATION

Similar to drug-susceptible TB, treatment of drug-resistant TB is composed of an initial intensive phase that uses more medications when the bacillary burden is highest and a continuation phase with fewer medications. Unlike the treatment of drug-susceptible TB, the duration of the intensive phase in MDR-TB is based on the timing of culture conversion. Based on findings from a patient-level meta-analysis,[198] guidelines recommend an intensive-phase treatment of between 5 and 7 months *after* culture conversion in patients

Table 54.5 Clinical Strategy to Build an Individualized Treatment Regimen for MDR-TB

Build a regimen *using five or more drugs to which the isolate is susceptible* (or has low likelihood of resistance), preferably with drugs that have not been used to treat the patient previously.
Choice of drugs is contingent upon capacity to monitor appropriately for significant adverse effects, patient comorbidities, and preferences/values (choices therefore subject to program and patient safety limitations).
In children with TB who are contacts of infectious MDR-TB source cases, the isolate from the source case can be used for drug susceptibility testing if an isolate is not obtained from the child. TB expert medical consultation is recommended (ungraded good practice statement).

Step	Action	Drug
1	Choose one later-generation fluoroquinolone	Levofloxacin Moxifloxacin
2	Choose both of these drugs	Bedaquiline Linezolid
3	Choose both of these drugs	Clofazimine Cycloserine
4	If a regimen cannot be assembled with five effective oral drugs, *and the isolate is susceptible*, use one of these injectable agents*	Amikacin Streptomycin
5	If needed or if oral agents are preferred over injectable agents in Step 4, use the following drugs†	Delamanid‡ Pyrazinamide Ethambutol
6	If limited options and cannot assemble a regimen of five effective drugs, consider use of the following drugs	Ethionamide or prothionamide§ Imipenem-cilastin/clavulanate *or* meropenam/clavulanate¶ *p*-Aminosalicylic acid‖ High-dose isoniazid**

*Amikacin and streptomycin should be used only when the patient's isolate is susceptible to these drugs. Because of their toxicity, these drugs should be used only when more effective or less toxic therapies cannot be assembled to achieve a total of five effective drugs.
†Patient preferences in terms of the harms and benefits associated with injectables (the use of which is no longer obligatory), the capacity to appropriately monitor for significant adverse effects, consideration of drug-drug interactions, and patient comorbidities should be considered in selecting step 5 agents over injectables. Ethambutol and pyrazinamide had mixed/marginal performance on outcomes assessed in the IPDMA; however, some experts may prefer these drugs over injectable agents to build a regimen of at least 5 effective oral drugs. Use pyrazinamide and ethambutol only when the isolate is documented to be susceptible.
‡Data on dosing and safety of delamanid are available in children down to 3 years of age.
§Mutations in the *inhA* region of *Mycobacterium tuberculosis* can confer resistance to ethionamide/prothionamide as well as to INH. In this situation, ethionamide/prothionamide may not be a good choice unless the isolate is shown to be susceptible with in vitro testing.
¶Divided daily intravenous dosing limits feasibility. Optimal duration of use not defined.
‖Fair/poor tolerability and low performance. Adverse effects reported to be less common in children.
**Data not reviewed in the IPDMA, but high-dose isoniazid can be considered despite low-level isoniazid resistance, but not with high-level INH resistance.
The following drugs are no longer recommended for inclusion in MDR-TB regimens: capreomycin and kanamycin, amoxicillin/clavulanate (when used without a carbapenem), azithromycin and clarithromycin.
INH; isoniazid; IPDMA, individual participant data meta-analysis; MDR-TB, multidrug-resistant tuberculosis.
Data from Nahid P, Mase SR, Migliori GB, et al. Treatment of drug-resistant tuberculosis. An official ATS/CDC/ERS/IDSA clinical practice guideline. *Am J Respir Crit Care Med.* 2019;200:e93–e142.

with MDR-TB.[191] The optimal duration for the continuation phase was 15 to 18 months.[198] The ATS/CDC/IDSA guidelines recommend that MDR-TB treatment be continued for 15 to 21 months after culture conversion (5–7 months of which include the intensive phase).[191]

NEW REGIMEN FOR EXTENSIVELY DRUG-RESISTANT TUBERCULOSIS OR TREATMENT-INTOLERANT OR NONRESPONSIVE MULTIDRUG-RESISTANT TUBERCULOSIS

The efficacy, safety, and tolerability of an all-oral 6-month regimen comprising bedaquiline, pretomanid (a nitroimidazooxazine), and linezolid (BPaL [bedaquiline + pretomanid + linezolid] regimen) was recently evaluated in a single-arm trial enrolling patients with highly-resistant TB (Nix-TB Trial, ClinicalTrials.gov identifier: NCT02333799). The three-drug, all-oral, 6-month regimen stably converted sputum cultures to negative with a median time of less than 6 weeks, with 90% of the 109 patients enrolled in the study achieving relapse-free cure. In August 2019, the FDA approved the BPaL regimen for the treatment of a specific limited population of adults with pulmonary XDR-TB or treatment-intolerant or nonresponsive MDR-TB.[2,141] Additional trials that include diverse patient populations will be essential to understand optimal use of the regimen, including the best approaches to minimizing toxicities. Neuropathy and other linezolid-associated adverse events caused more than 60% patients to interrupt treatment at least once in the trial.

ISONIAZID MONORESISTANCE

Monoresistance to INH is frequent, with an estimated global prevalence of 8% of TB cases.[199] INH monoresistance has been reported in up to 20% of non–U.S.-born residents from high-risk Asian countries.[200,201]

A meta-analysis found that the treatment of INH-monoresistant TB with first-line drugs, including the previously recommended regimen of RIF, EMB, and PZA for 6 months,[202] was associated with poorer treatment outcomes compared to drug-susceptible TB.[203] For this reason, current guidelines make the following recommendations for the treatment of INH-resistant TB[191]:

- A later-generation fluoroquinolone (i.e., moxifloxacin or LFX) should be added to a regimen of RIF, EMB, and PZA, all given daily for 6 months.
- PZA may be included for only the first 2 months of treatment in situations when the initial disease burden is low (e.g., noncavitary pulmonary TB) and/or when there are PZA-related adverse events.

Recommendations are available on treatment regimens for other drug-resistance patterns and special situations.[45]

SURGERY

Surgery was one of the first therapeutic approaches for TB, but since effective chemotherapy became available, surgery has been relegated to specific situations. For the management of MDR-TB, there appears to be a benefit from an elective partial lung resection (e.g., lobectomy or wedge resection) when offered together with a recommended MDR/XDR-TB regimen compared to medical therapy alone.[191] Specifically, surgery may be indicated when clinical judgment, supported by bacteriologic and radiographic data, suggest a strong risk of treatment failure or relapse with medical therapy alone.[204,205]

Key Points

- *Tuberculosis* (TB) treatment should be administered through directly observed therapy, and this is particularly important when treating patients living with HIV infection, on intermittent therapy, or with drug-resistant TB.
- Adequate treatment for TB is the major intervention needed for decreasing transmission of *M. tuberculosis*, both for drug-susceptible and drug-resistant strains. Treatment consists of an initial *intensive* phase to eliminate actively replicating bacteria, followed by a *continuation* phase to eliminate the persisting organisms.
- Assuming an adequate regimen, patient adherence is the critical factor that determines the success of treatment.
- When drug resistance is suspected or identified during treatment, two or more new drugs active against the patient's isolate must be added. A single drug should *never* be added to a failing regimen.
- The treatment of extrapulmonary TB is largely the same as the treatment of pulmonary TB. The exceptions are central nervous system TB and TB involving bones and joints, in which treatment of longer duration is recommended.
- Expert consultation should be obtained when treating patients with drug-resistant TB, those who develop medication-related adverse effects, and patients with TB/HIV coinfection or underlying liver disease. In the United States, TB experts can be found through local health department TB control programs and/or regional Centers for Disease Control and Prevention-supported TB Centers of Excellence for Training, Education, and Medical Consultation (http://www.cdc.gov/tb/education/rtmc/default.htm).

Key Readings

Ahmad N, Ahuja SD, Akkerman OW, et al. Treatment correlates of successful outcomes in pulmonary multidrug-resistant tuberculosis: an individual patient data meta-analysis. *Lancet.* 2018;392(10150):821–834.

Curry International Tuberculosis Center and California Department of Public Health. *Drug-Resistant Tuberculosis: A Survival Guide for Clinicians.* 3rd ed.; 2016. http://www.currytbcenter.ucsf.edu/products/drug-resistant-tuberculosis-survival-guide-clinicians-3rd-edition.

Nahid P, et al. Executive summary: official American Thoracic Society/Centers for Disease Control and Prevention/Infectious Diseases Society of America clinical practice guidelines: treatment of drug-susceptible tuberculosis. *Clin Infect Dis.* 2016;63(7):853–867.

Nahid P, Mase SR, Migliori GB, et al. Treatment of drug-resistant tuberculosis. an official ATS/CDC/ERS/IDSA clinical practice guideline. *Am J Respir Crit Care Med.* 2019;200:e93–e142.

WHO Consolidated Guidelines on Drug-Resistant Tuberculosis Treatment. Geneva: 2019. https://www.who.int/tb/publications/2019/consolidated-guidelines-drug-resistant-TB-treatment/en/.

Complete reference list available at ExpertConsult.com.

55 NONTUBERCULOUS MYCOBACTERIAL INFECTIONS

CHARLES L. DALEY, MD • KEVIN L. WINTHROP, MD, MPH •
DAVID E. GRIFFITH, MD

INTRODUCTION

Soon after the discovery of *Mycobacterium tuberculosis* in 1882 by Robert Koch, several other species of mycobacteria were described. It was not until half a century later, however, that these mycobacteria were recognized to cause disease in humans and, by the 1980s, they were known to cause a broad spectrum of disease.[1] Over the years, these organisms have gone by many names, including mycobacteria other than tuberculosis, environmental mycobacteria, anonymous or atypical mycobacteria, and *nontuberculous mycobacteria* (NTM), which is the preferred term.[2-4] The epidemic of the *human immunodeficiency virus* (HIV) heralded a new awareness of NTM infections because of the high rates of disseminated infections due to *Mycobacterium avium complex* (MAC)[5] and other species.[6] On the one hand, disseminated NTM infections have declined significantly in HIV-infected populations after the advent of antiretroviral drugs; on the other hand, rates of NTM disease in those without HIV are increasing.

NTM represent a broad array of organisms ubiquitous in the environment. They have been isolated from natural and municipal (tap) waters and from soil, and exposure to these reservoirs is thought to be the primary source of human infection. Approximately 200 species and subspecies of NTM have been identified (http://www.bacterio.net/mycobacterium.html), and many of these have been reported to cause disease in both immunocompetent and immunocompromised patients. Unlike *M. tuberculosis*, NTM do not appear to be transmitted from human to human in the absence of extraordinary circumstances; they vary greatly in their ability to cause disease; and they do not show evidence for latency. Unfortunately, NTM are difficult to treat because of high levels of resistance to antimicrobial drugs, which require long courses of therapy with relatively poor outcomes when compared to *tuberculosis* (TB). Not surprisingly, these factors result in a treatment cost comparable to other chronic infectious diseases, such as HIV/*acquired immunodeficiency syndrome* (AIDS).[7] To date, our lack of understanding of the transmission and pathogenesis of these increasingly important infections has limited our ability to develop public health measures aimed at preventing infection.

MICROBIOLOGY AND TAXONOMY

The genus *Mycobacterium* has traditionally consisted of organisms within the *M. tuberculosis* complex, *Mycobacterium leprae*, and NTM. The latter were classified in 1959 by Runyon into groups based on pigmentation in the presence or absence of light (photochromogens, scotochromogens, nonchromogenic) and growth characteristics (slow vs. rapid).[8] Recently, investigators proposed that the genus *Mycobacterium* be divided into five genera, including four new genera: *Mycobacteroides*, *Mycolicibacter*, *Mycolicibacterium*, and *Mycolicibacillus*.[9] The proposed new genera are based on genomic analysis, but the taxonomy is controversial and has not been widely adopted.[10] The proposed genera do not replace the traditional taxonomy used by microbiologists, scientists, and clinicians for the past century. This chapter uses the traditional genus and species designations.

All mycobacteria are characterized by their relatively slow growth rate when compared with other bacterial species. NTM can be divided into rapidly growing and slowly growing organisms: Rapid growers can be distinguished by growth in subculture in less than 7 days. NTM, like all mycobacteria, are also characterized by a thin peptidoglycan layer surrounded by a thick lipid-rich outer membrane.[11] The lipid-rich outer membrane results in a number of properties that allow the organisms to survive in diverse and ostensibly hostile environments. For example, the hydrophobic cell surface allows surface attachment, resistance to disinfectants and antibiotics, slow growth, and tolerance to heat.[12] Additional important properties that allow survival in the environment are the ability to grow in low carbon concentrations (i.e., oligotrophic) and low oxygen concentrations.

The availability of molecular methods for NTM species identification has rendered the Runyon classification obsolete for clinical purposes and resulted in a marked increase in the identification of new NTM species. In 1997, approximately 50 species of NTM had been identified, with only 13 described as respiratory pathogens. Currently, there are approximately 200 identified NTM species and subspecies with at least 80 associated with lung disease, although for most, only rarely (http://www.bacterio.net/mycobacterium.html) (Table 55.1).

The primary explanation for the increase in NTM species can be found in the mycobacteriology laboratory. Before the era of DNA sequencing for organism identification, NTM were identified based on their morphologic and biochemical characteristics and in vitro susceptibility patterns. The inadequacy or insensitivity of these techniques was reflected in the number of organisms grouped as complexes, such as the *Mycobacterium fortuitum* complex, which previously included multiple rapidly growing species, such as *M. fortuitum, Mycobacterium chelonae,* and *Mycobacterium abscessus.* Although, it was apparent that multiple species were present with similar growth and morphologic properties, standard laboratory techniques were not adequate to distinguish them at the species level.

The revolutionary change in NTM identification was due to the advent of readily available DNA sequencing, especially the sequencing of the 16S ribosomal RNA gene, which is highly conserved so that 1% or greater differences in this gene sequence can define an NTM species. Publicly available databases of 16S ribosomal RNA gene sequences allow relatively easy comparison of mycobacterial isolates to identify the species or to determine whether a new NTM species is present. Alternatively, sequences of the heat shock protein 65 (*hsp65*), *rpoB*, and *secA* genes, or the entire genomic DNA sequence of an NTM species, can be compared to other publicly available gene sequence databases. Although the molecular methods are quite appealing, no method is flawless and applicable in all circumstances. For instance, even with *whole-genome sequencing* (WGS), controversy exists about criteria to define species and subspecies designations. It is also increasingly clear that organisms can appropriate genetic material from other organisms, further blurring the lines between species.

The expansion of new NTM species in the past 20 years is therefore primarily a consequence of more sensitive identification techniques capable of separating closely

Table 55.1   Nontuberculous Mycobacteria Reported to Cause Pulmonary Disease

SLOWLY GROWING MYCOBACTERIA		RAPIDLY GROWING MYCOBACTERIA	
M. alsense	M. malmoense	M. abscessus*	M. immunogenum
M. arosiense	M. marseillense	M. alvei	M. iranicum
M. arupense	M. nebraskense	M. aubagnense	M. goodii
M. asiaticum	M. nonchromogenicum	M. boenickei	M. holsaticum
M. avium	M. palustre	M. brisbanense	M. houstonense
M. bouchedurhonense	M. paraense	M. brumae	M. llatzerense
M. branderi	M. paraffinicum	M. canariasense	M. mageritense
M. chimaera	M. parascrofulaceum	M. celeriflavum	M. monacense
M. celatum	M. persicum	M. chelonae	M. moriokaense
M. colombiense	M. phlei	M. chubuense	M. mucogenicum
M. conspicuum	M. riyadhense	M. conceptionense	M. novocastrense
M. europaeum	M. saskatchewanse	M. confluentis	M. peregrinum
M. florentinum	M. scrofulaceum	M. cosmeticum	M. phocaicum
M. fragae	M. seoulense	M. elephantis	M. porcinum
M. gastri	M. senuense	M. fortuitum	M. rhodesiae
M. gordonae	M. sherrisii	M. houstonense	M. septicum
M. haemophilum	M. shimodei		M. thermoresistible
M. heckeshornense	M. shinjukuense		
M. heidelbergense	M. simiae		
M. genavense	M. szulgai		
M. interjectum	M. talmoniae		
M. intermedium	M. timonense		
M. intracellulare	M. triviale		
M. kansasii	M. triplex		
M. kubicae	M. tusciae		
M. kyorinense	M. xenopi		
M. lentiflavum	M. yongonense		

*Including *Mycobacterium abscessus* subsp. *abscessus, massiliense,* and *bolletii.*
From *List of Prokaryotic Names With Standing in Nomenclature.* http://www.bacterio.net/mycobacterium.html.

related NTM species. Predictably, many of these newly identified species have microbiologic properties very similar to other closely related NTM so that identification of the new NTM species may not be associated with any new or surprising clinical properties. It remains to be seen if this revolution in NTM species identification will have an equally profound impact on clinical NTM disease. What is certain, however, is that clinicians will need to become familiar with many more NTM species names as new NTM species are identified.

EPIDEMIOLOGY

INCIDENCE AND PREVALENCE

The epidemiology of NTM disease has been difficult to determine because reporting of NTM pulmonary disease is not mandatory in most countries, including most of the United States. Our lack of understanding of early disease presentation and the difficulty differentiating between *infection* (i.e., NTM isolation without clinical or radiographic evidence of progression) and *disease* presents even more formidable epidemiologic obstacles, especially for determining disease incidence. The prevalence of NTM infections has varied significantly across studies, partially because the studies have used different methodologies and studied different populations.[13] Data suggest that the prevalence of NTM infections is increasing in many areas.

Delayed-type hypersensitivity reactions to subcutaneously injected mycobacterial antigens (i.e., skin test reactivity to NTM) have been reported in 11–33.5% of the population in the United States.[14–16] One study used data from the *National Health and Nutritional Examination Survey* (NHANES) cohort to describe skin reactivity to *purified protein derivative-B* (PPD-B, or the Battey antigen), believed to be indicative of exposure to *M. avium* complex, during two time periods. For the years 1971–72 and 1999–2000, rates of a positive skin test were 11.2% and 16.6%, respectively.[16] Skin test reactivity was noted to increase between the two time periods in foreign-born but not in U.S.-born individuals, suggesting either a higher rate of exposure and infection in the foreign-born individuals or possibly cross-reactivity to infection with *M. tuberculosis*.

Early laboratory-based studies used consecutive isolates from a well-defined catchment area to estimate the frequency of infection. Survey data from state laboratories in the United States in the early 1980s estimated a prevalence of NTM infection of 1 to 2 cases per 100,000 population.[17] A similar follow-up survey from 1993–96 reported an annual case rate of 7 to 8 per 100,000, documenting an increase in NTM isolation when compared to the previous survey.[18] More recent laboratory-based surveys have demonstrated higher prevalences, including a large laboratory-based study from Japan that reported that, of 26,059 patients who tested positive for NTM at least once, 27.5% of these patients met *American Thoracic Society/Infectious Diseases Society of America* (ATS/IDSA) criteria for disease, giving a 2-year prevalence of 24.0 per 100,000.[19]

Studies using clinical isolates from many countries, including Czechoslovakia,[20] England and Wales,[21–23] Ireland,[24] Australia,[25–27] Korea,[28,29] Taiwan,[30] Canada,[31,32] and the United States,[33] have reported increases in prevalence. In some reports, the increase in the rate of NTM infection was associated with a decline in the rate of TB.[34] For example, in Japan from 1971–84, the incidence of pulmonary TB decreased from 133.1 to 46.3 per 100,000, whereas the incidence of NTM pulmonary disease increased from 0.9 to 2.2.[35] Similarly, in Switzerland, the incidence of pulmonary TB decreased from 16.2 to 13.2 per 100,000 over 6 years, whereas the incidence of pulmonary NTM increased from 0.4 to 0.9 per 100,000.[36] The frequencies of *M. tuberculosis* and NTM isolates also showed a reciprocal trend in Taiwan from 2002–07, with NTM isolates increasing 2.6-fold.[37]

Perhaps the most significant increases in NTM prevalence have been reported from North America. Marras and coworkers[31] reported an increase in the number of pulmonary NTM isolates (isolation prevalence) in Ontario from 9.1 per 100,000 in 1997 to 14.1 per 100,000 in 2003; during this same time period, the rate of TB declined. In a subsequent analysis of these data, Iseman and Marras[38] noted that the prevalence was likely to be in the range of 14 to 35 per 100,000, far exceeding the prevalence of TB in Ontario. A study from the United States reported a significant increase in the annual prevalence of NTM pulmonary disease in patients hospitalized in 11 states between 1998 and 2005.[39] Annual prevalence increased among men and women in Florida (3.2%/yr and 6.5%/yr, respectively) and among women in New York (4.6%/yr), but there was no significant increase in California. The annual prevalence of NTM pulmonary disease in U.S. Medicare beneficiaries (all ≥65 years of age) increased from 20 per 100,000 in 1997 to 47 per 100,000 in 2007.[40] The annual percentage change for women was 9.1%, which was significantly higher than that for men (6.4%). In a study from Oregon, clinical and radiographic data from patients with NTM respiratory isolates were evaluated. This study found an overall prevalence of 8.6 per 100,000 persons and 20.4 per 100,000 in those at least 50 years of age.[41] Although not all studies have documented an increase in NTM prevalence,[42] the preponderance of evidence suggests that pulmonary disease due to NTM is increasing.

The lack of reporting of NTM cases in the United States has made it difficult to determine the incidence of NTM. Investigators in Oregon contacted all laboratories in the state and collected demographic and specimen information for patients with NTM isolated during 2007–12.[33] They were able to determine that the incidence of NTM pulmonary disease increased from 4.8 per 100,000 in 2007 to 5.6 per 100,000 in 2012. Incidence increased with age to more than 25 per 100,000 in those 80 years of age or older. Using a large managed care database in the United States, investigators reported that the annual incidence of NTM pulmonary disease increased from 3.1 per 100,000 person-years in 2008 to 4.7 per 100,000 in

2015, and the prevalence increased from 6.8 to 11.7 per 100,000 person-years[43] (Fig. 55.1). The increases were particularly notable among women and those older than 65 years.

The reasons for the increase in incidence and prevalence have not been explained, although increased clinician awareness of the disease and improved diagnostic techniques, especially the widespread application of high-resolution chest *computed tomography* (CT) scanning, could be factors. Once diagnosed with NTM pulmonary disease, patients are more refractory to treatment than TB patients, which means they accumulate or persist, thereby augmenting prevalence figures. A true increase in incidence could be related to changes in the host,

such as an aging population, an increased prevalence of chronic lung disease, or an increase in the number of immunocompromised individuals. The observation of a decreased incidence of pulmonary TB and an increased incidence of pulmonary NTM, as noted previously, could be explained by cross-immunity between mycobacterial species. An increase in the prevalence or virulence of environmental organisms or changes in human behavior leading to increased exposure to organisms could be contributing factors.

NTM pulmonary disease is associated with a high mortality, although most patients die as a result of causes other than NTM infection. A systematic review reported an all-cause 5-year mortality for MAC pulmonary

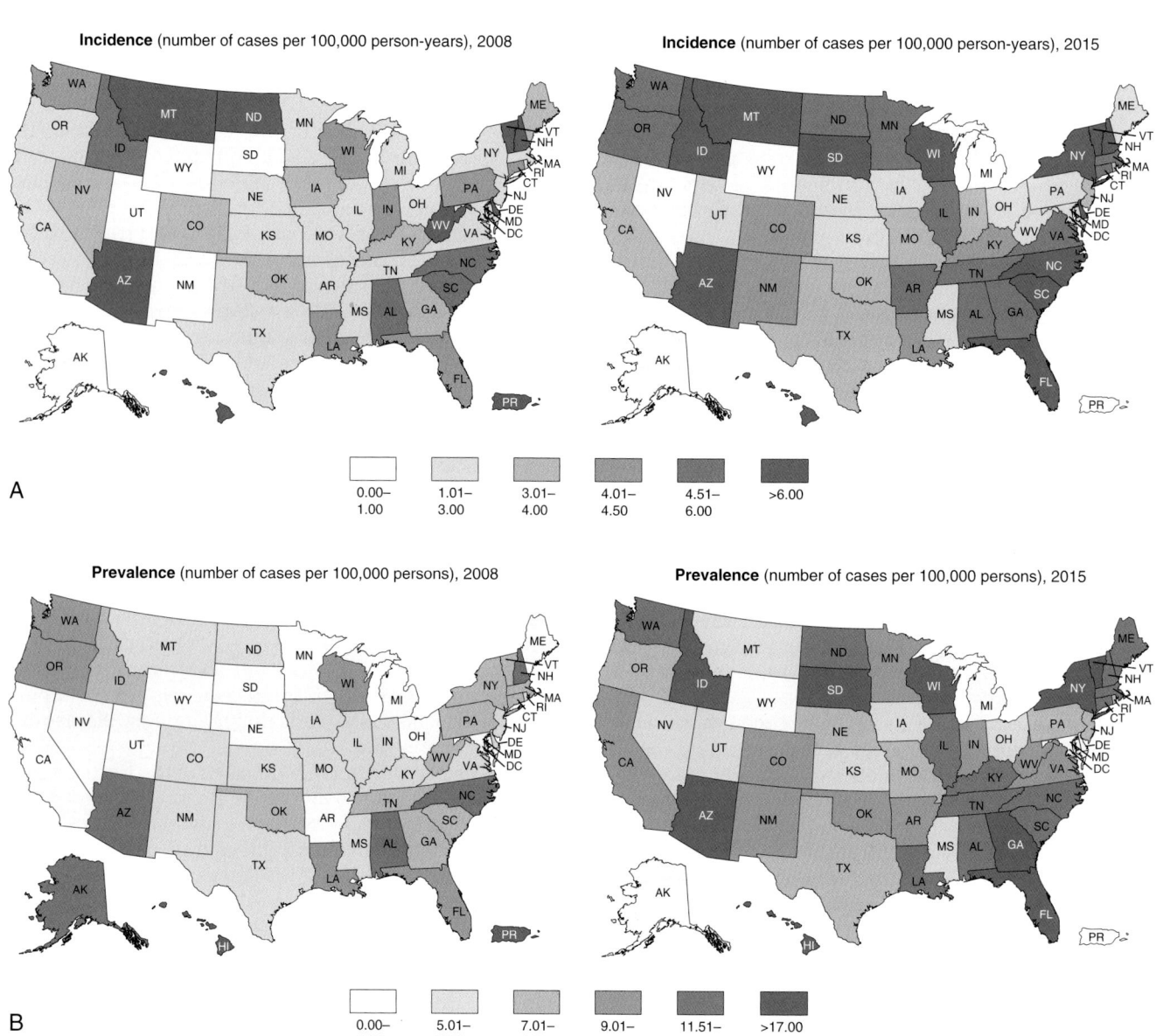

Figure 55.1 Incidence (A) and prevalence (B) of *nontuberculous mycobacteria* (NTM) pulmonary disease in the United States, by state, in 2008 and 2015. (From Winthrop KL, Marras TK, Adjemian J, et al. Incidence and prevalence of nontuberculous mycobacterial lung disease in a large U.S. managed care health plan, 2008–2015. *Ann Am Thorac Soc.* 2020;17:178–185.)

disease of 27%, ranging from 10–48%.[44] In Oregon, 35% of patients with NTM pulmonary disease (84% with MAC) died within 5 years of isolating NTM from a respiratory specimen.[45] Patients with NTM pulmonary disease (per ATS/IDSA criteria) had a slightly higher risk of death compared with those who had infection only. In a population-based study from Ontario, Canada, both NTM pulmonary disease and pulmonary infection had a higher mortality than "unexposed" matched individuals, and those with disease had a higher rate of death than those with only infection.[46] A recent study from Korea described prognostic factors associated with long-term mortality among patients with NTM pulmonary disease.[47] Among 1445 treatment-naive patients, the 5-, 10-, and 15-year cumulative mortality rates were 12.4%, 24.0%, and 36.4%, respectively. In these studies, factors associated with mortality included older age, male gender, low body mass index, chronic pulmonary aspergillosis, malignancy, chronic heart or liver disease, and elevated erythrocyte sedimentation rate.[44,47] Mortality was also associated with the infecting species (e.g., infection with *Mycobacterium intracellulare* and *M. abscessus* was associated with a worse prognosis than with *M. avium*) and radiographic presentation (e.g., cavitary disease had a worse prognosis than noncavitary).[47]

GEOGRAPHIC DISTRIBUTION AND VARIATION

NTM have been reported to cause pulmonary disease around the globe, although there is marked variation in the prevalence of disease and in the species that predominates.[48] In the United States, the southeastern region (southern Atlantic and Gulf coasts) has traditionally been considered to have the highest rates of infection.[13,49,50] NTM have been recovered with higher frequency from water samples in the southeastern than in the northern United States, so exposure is likely higher in these regions.[51] However, a recent study reported that, among Medicare patients, the states with the highest period prevalences of pulmonary NTM were Hawaii (396 per 100,000), followed by California (191 per 100,000).[40] Florida, Louisiana, and Mississippi also had high period prevalences ranging from 151 to 200 per 100,000. Another study that used a large managed care database also documented important geographic variations in both incidence and prevalence of NTM pulmonary disease, including marked increases in both the incidence and prevalence of NTM pulmonary disease in Florida and adjacent states.[52] Among *cystic fibrosis* (CF) patients in the United States, the prevalence of NTM isolation varied geographically; for MAC, the highest prevalences were in Nevada (24%), Kansas (21%), Hawaii (20%), and Arizona (20%) and, for *M. abscessus*, the highest prevalences were in Hawaii (50%), Florida (17%), and Louisiana (16%)[53] (Fig. 55.2).

The reasons for such geographic variation are not well understood. Pulmonary NTM cases were identified from a nationally representative sample of Medicare Part B beneficiaries, and their counties of residence were divided into low- and high-risk counties to identify potential sociodemographic and environmental

risk factors.[54] The investigators identified seven clusters of pulmonary NTM cases and compared them to five low-risk areas. Counties in the high-risk areas were larger and had greater population densities, higher education, and income levels than the low-risk counties. In addition, high-risk counties had a higher mean daily potential for evapotranspiration (combination of *evaporation* [transfer of water from land to atmosphere] and *transpiration* [transfer of water from plants to atmosphere]) and greater percentages of their area covered by surface water. Thus, specific environmental factors appear to correlate with the rates of pulmonary NTM infection.

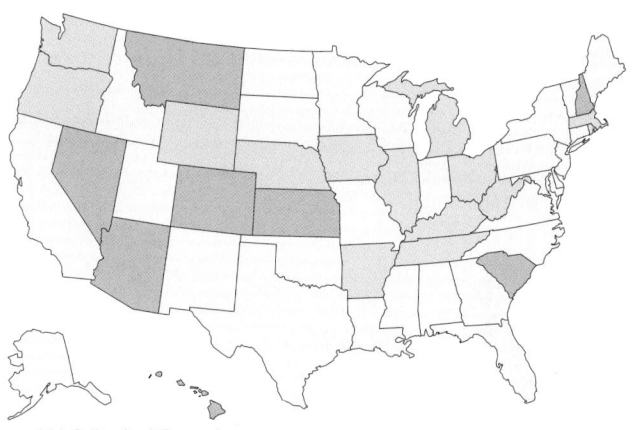

MAC Period Prevalence
☐ 5–10%
☐ >10–15%
■ >15%
A

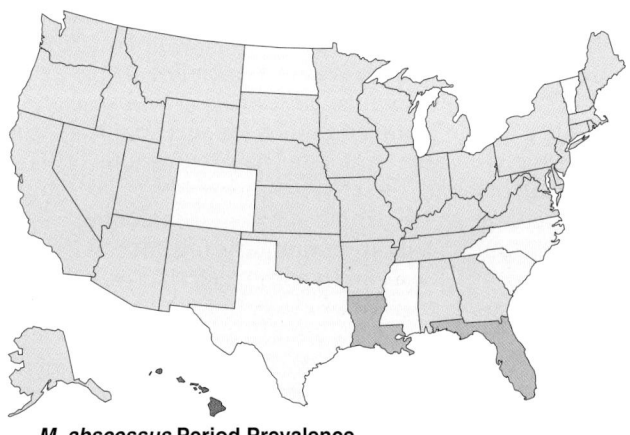

M. abscessus **Period Prevalence**
☐ 0–10%
☐ >10–15%
■ >15–20%
■ >20%
B

Figure 55.2 Geographic distribution of *nontuberculous mycobacteria* (NTM). The distribution is shown as prevalence of NTM cultured from patients with cystic fibrosis during the period 2010–14 by U.S. state for (A) *Mycobacterium avium* complex (MAC) and (B) *Mycobacterium abscessus*. (From Adjemian J, Olivier KN, Prevots DR. Epidemiology of pulmonary nontuberculous mycobacterial sputum positivity in patients with cystic fibrosis in the United States, 2010–2014. *Ann Am Thorac Soc.* 2018;15:817–825.)

The predominant species causing pulmonary disease in North America is MAC. Data from a national hospitalization database, including more than 5 million patients, demonstrated that MAC was the most common species causing disease, ranging from 61–91%, with the highest frequency in the southern and northeastern regions.[55] *M. abscessus*/*M. chelonae* ranged from 2–18% and was more common in the western region. Other NTM, such as *M. fortuitum* and *Mycobacterium kansasii*, ranged from 7–26% and again were more common in the West. MAC has also been reported as the predominant species in Central and South America, Europe, and Asia.[13] Which species of MAC predominates also varies from region to region. In some areas, such as Europe and South America, *M. avium* is the predominant species whereas, in Australia and South Africa, *M. intracellulare* in the most common MAC isolate. A large laboratory study from Japan reported that *M. avium* pulmonary disease was more common in northeastern Japan, whereas *M. intracellulare* was more common in southwestern Japan.[19] *Mycobacterium xenopi* is common in Europe and Canada, whereas *Mycobacterium malmoense* is more common in Northern than Southern Europe. Populations of miners in Czechoslovakia[20] and South Africa[56,57] have been reported to have high rates of *M. kansasii* infection.

TRANSMISSION AND PATHOGENESIS

TRANSMISSION

NTM are ubiquitous in the environment and have been found in natural and drinking waters, biofilms, soil, and aerosols.[12,58,59] The presumed source of infection is exposure to these environmental reservoirs because human-to-human transmission has only been documented under extraordinary circumstances.[60–62] Studies using genotyping techniques, such as *pulsed field gel electrophoresis* (PFGE), variable number tandem repeat analysis, and WGS have been able to isolate the same strains of NTM from patients and their environments.[63–65] Although the mechanism by which an environmental exposure eventually leads to pulmonary infection is poorly understood,[66] it has been hypothesized that exposure to infected aerosols can lead to infection and possibly disease. To determine whether household plumbing could serve as a source for NTM infection, 394 water samples were obtained from 37 households across the United States.[67] Seventeen (46%) of the households yielded one or more mycobacterial isolate of the same species found in the patient, and in seven patients the isolate had the same genotype. In a study from Philadelphia, Pennsylvania, variable number tandem repeat genotyping and WGS with core genome single-nucleotide polymorphism analysis were used to compare *M. avium* from household plumbing biofilms with *M. avium* isolates from patient respiratory specimens. *M. avium* was recovered from 30 (81.1%) of 37 households, including 19 (90.5%) of 21 *M. avium* patient households. For 11

(52.4%) of 21 patients with *M. avium* disease, isolates recovered from their respiratory and household samples were of the same genotype. Within the same community, 18 (85.7%) of 21 *M. avium* respiratory isolates genotypically matched household plumbing isolates.[68] In a report from Australia, 35% of patients with NTM pulmonary disease had the same species isolated from their home water supply.[69]

A study conducted in Oregon and Washington used interviews to evaluate aerosol-generating activities and water supply features in the homes and gardens of patients with MAC pulmonary disease compared with controls and found that that these activities and factors seemed not to be risk factors for MAC pulmonary disease in HIV-negative adults.[70] Prior lung disease and immunosuppressing drugs were associated with susceptibility. Although it appears that underlying host susceptibility is the major risk for developing NTM pulmonary disease, exposure to NTM is still required for infection. A subsequent case-control study using the same subjects reported that NTM were isolated from shower aerosols more often than in control subjects.[71] Other home environmental samples, such as tap water and soil, were not associated with NTM disease.

Until recently, human-to-human transmission was considered an unlikely mode of transmission.[72] However, several studies have described possible transmission from human to human in CF clinics.[60–62] The first report described a potential outbreak of *M. abscessus* subsp. *massiliense* in a CF clinic in Seattle.[60] It is presumed that a smear-positive patient transmitted infection to four other CF patients at the same clinic because the infecting strain was indistinguishable by PFGE and polymerase chain reaction analysis. In a retrospective study using WGS from Papworth hospital in the United Kingdom, there were genomically highly similar clusters of *M. abscessus* subsp. *massiliense* among 31 adult CF patients, some of whom had opportunities for cross-infection.[61] The authors noted that direct person-to-person transmission was unlikely but that cross-infection (i.e., transfer of infection between patients through physical contact or shared environmental source, such as spirometric or bronchoscopic equipment) in the hospital setting was likely. A study from the Great Ormond Street hospital in the United Kingdom used a similar approach, focusing on *M. abscessus* subsp. *abscessus* isolates in 20 pediatric CF patients.[73] Although high genetic similarity was noted among four patients, no epidemiologic connections were made except for a sibling pair living in the same household.[73] A study from Italy analyzed 162 *M. abscessus* isolates from 48 patients across four geographically diverse CF centers.[74] They identified genetically similar isolates across all three subspecies with seven possible transmission episodes; however, in only three was there epidemiologic evidence of potential cross-infection. Moreover, the authors were unable to identify any significant outbreaks over a 12-year period at the centers, suggesting minimal risk for person-to-person transmission. A study that sequenced 145 isolates of *M. abscessus* from 62 patients at four hospitals in two countries over a 16-year period was able to identify only one episode of possible transmission in a sibling pair.[75] Further evidence for potential transmission comes from a study that performed WGS on more than a 1000 isolates of *M. abscessus* from 510 CF patients across Europe, the United States, and Australia.[62] The study identified three dominant circulating clones among all CF clinics and countries studied. These same clones were identified in non-CF populations[76] and in a nationwide outbreak of soft tissue infections in Brazil.[77] *M. abscessus* appears to be a highly genomically conserved organism, and the widespread geographic presence of these dominant clones associated with disease makes it difficult to use molecular methods to identify suspected transmission events either between patients or the environment.[78] Whether the widespread geographic presence of these clones in patients with CF is due to person-to-person transmission or to resident genotypes more fit for human infection is not known.

Extrapulmonary NTM infections involving soft tissue or bone and joints are usually the result of a puncture wound or surgery. A recent outbreak of skin and soft tissue infections due to *M. abscessus* subsp. *massiliense* involved more than 2000 patients who had undergone invasive procedures, such as laparoscopic, arthroscopic, plastic, or cosmetic surgery.[79] Since 2013, at least 52 patients from nine states have been diagnosed with skin and soft tissue infections after undergoing cosmetic surgery in the Dominican Republic.[80–82] There is even potential for an NTM, specifically *Mycobacterium chimaera*, to cause disease intraoperatively without direct inoculation but rather after aerosolization and subsequent deposition onto vulnerable tissue.[83–85]

FACTORS ASSOCIATED WITH INFECTION

A prospective study using skin testing data from Palm Beach, Florida, reported that 32.9% of 447 participants in a population-based random household survey had a positive reaction to *M. avium* sensitin.[86] (*Sensitin* is the standardized antigenic material used for delayed-type hypersensitivity skin testing for *M. avium*, analogous to tuberculin for *M. tuberculosis*).[87] Independent predictors of a positive reaction included Black race, birth outside the United States, and more than 6 years' cumulative exposure to soil. Exposure to water, food, or pets was not associated with skin test reactivity. Using NHANES data, investigators reported similar findings with regard to sensitization to *M. intracellulare*[16]: male sex, non-Hispanic Black race, and birth outside the United States were each independently associated with sensitization. The highest rate of skin test reactivity was in persons who were 20 to 39 years of age. These two studies are interesting in that skin test reactivity to either *M. avium* or *M. intracellulare* sensitin was associated with likely soil exposure and was more common in men and foreign-born individuals. However, in contrast to skin reactivity, disease seems to be more common in older women and in U.S.-born individuals. In addition, the source for *M. avium* infection, frequently associated with nodular bronchiectatic MAC pulmonary disease, appears to be primarily municipal (tap) water in the United States, whereas *M. intracellulare* infection is acquired through some other source, likely soil.[88]

Pathophysiologically, it is still not clear what positive skin test reactions to mycobacterial sensitin signify. For tuberculin skin test reactors, it is assumed a positive test reflects "latent" infection; however, a latent state has not yet been demonstrated for NTM pathogens. In that context, it is possible that positive skin test responses to NTM sensitins reflect subclinical infection and therefore that the risk factors for infection are different from those associated with disease.

FACTORS ASSOCIATED WITH DISEASE

Most NTM are significantly less pathogenic than *M. tuberculosis* and likely require some degree of host impairment to establish infection. A number of risk factors for disease have been described, which can be subdivided broadly into three groups: (1) factors leading to impaired local (lung) immunity (e.g., lung disease), (2) factors impairing host immunity, and (3) factors relating to the infecting species. These factors can be reduced further into the "susceptible person" model and the "unusual dose" model.[89] In the susceptible person model, it is assumed that some susceptibility is necessary for infection whereas, in the unusual dose model, it is postulated infection happens because of an unusually large exposure to NTM. It is likely that, in most patients, both models of pathogenesis are at play to varying degrees.

Chronic pulmonary disease is perhaps the most important risk factor for the development of NTM pulmonary disease. NTM disease has been described in association with bronchiectasis (with or without CF), COPD (including alpha$_1$-antitrypsin deficiency), cavitary lung disease, pneumoconiosis, prior TB, and pulmonary alveolar proteinosis.[90] Studies have documented a high prevalence of NTM in sputum cultures from patients with CF, with estimates ranging from 6.6–13.7%.[91–93] Among 16,153 persons with CF in the United States from 2010–14, risk factors for NTM isolation included having a diagnosis of CF at an older age, having a lower body mass index, higher *forced expiratory volume in 1 second* (FEV$_1$)% predicted, and fewer years on chronic macrolide therapy.[94]

Gastroesophageal reflux disease (GERD) or other esophageal disorders are often found in patients with NTM pulmonary disease. Historically, it has been reported that patients with *rapidly growing mycobacteria* (RGM) often have associated esophageal disorders[95–97]; recent reports have also described a high frequency of GERD in patients with MAC pulmonary disease.[98,99] In a report from South Korea using pH probes to diagnose GERD, the authors reported that the prevalence of GERD in patients with NTM lung disease was 26%; those with GERD were more likely to have smear-positive sputum and more extensive disease than those without GERD. Of interest, a minority of those with GERD (27%) had symptoms of GERD.[98]

Postmenopausal women make up one of the most interesting patient populations to develop NTM pulmonary disease. These women often have characteristic morphologic features, including pectus excavatum, scoliosis, thin body habitus, and mitral valve prolapse. This constellation was first described by Prince and colleagues[100] in 1989 and subsequently by Iseman and others.[101] Recently, investigators reported that women with pulmonary NTM disease were taller and thinner and weighed less than matched control subjects[102] (Fig. 55.3); 51% had scoliosis, 11% had pectus excavatum, and 9% had mitral valve prolapse, all significantly more common than in reference populations. Another interesting feature of this syndrome is the predilection for right middle lobe and lingular bronchiectasis. To date, extensive evaluation of the immune system of these patients has shown mixed results, but mutations in the *cystic fibrosis transmembrane regulator* (CFTR) gene are common.[102–104] Among 103 women with pulmonary NTM, the normal relationship between the adipokines and body fat was lost compared with uninfected control subjects.[104] In addition, in one study, interferon-γ (IFN-γ) and *interleukin-10* (IL-10) levels were significantly suppressed in stimulated whole blood of patients with pulmonary NTM.[104] However, it remains uncertain if these findings are clinically significant.

Impairment in host immunity is also a risk factor for NTM disease but, in this setting, it often leads to disseminated disease or skin and soft tissue involvement rather than pulmonary disease. In AIDS, NTM most commonly cause disseminated disease that presents with nonspecific symptoms, such as fever, night sweats, diarrhea, abdominal pain, and lymphadenopathy, with *M. avium* being the most frequently isolated NTM.[105] The incidence of disseminated MAC can be as high as 20–40% in people with HIV and advanced immunosuppression in the absence of effective antiretroviral therapy (ART) or chemoprophylaxis.[105,106] Fortunately, the incidence of disseminated MAC has continued to decline in the modern ART era to fewer than two cases of MAC per 1000 person-years.[107] Factors associated with MAC disease include CD4 cell counts less than 50 cells/mm³, plasma HIV RNA levels greater than 1000 copies/mL, ongoing viral replication despite ART, previous or concurrent opportunistic infections, and reduced in vitro lymphoproliferative immune response to *M. avium* antigens.[108–110] Despite the fact that MAC is isolated from the sputum in up to 10% of AIDS patients with CD4 T cell counts less than 50 cells/μL, pulmonary disease due to MAC is uncommon.[111] Pulmonary disease has been reported in 2.5–8% of patients with disseminated MAC[112] and, rarely, has also been reported in the absence of dissemination.[113] Patients with pulmonary disease tend to have higher CD4 counts and focal alveolar opacities, which rarely cavitate. *M. kansasii* can also cause disease in patients with HIV and AIDS. In one study, the risk for infection with *M. kansasii* was increased 150-fold in HIV-infected patients and 900-fold in those with AIDS.[114] In contrast to MAC, *M. kansasii* only rarely causes indolent disease and should almost always be treated as a pathogen.[115]

Other immunocompromised populations, including transplant recipients, have been noted to develop pulmonary disease due to NTM. Rates may be as high as 6.5% after heart or lung transplantation[116] and 2.9% after bone marrow transplantation,[117] but are probably much lower in patients after liver or kidney transplantation.[118,119]

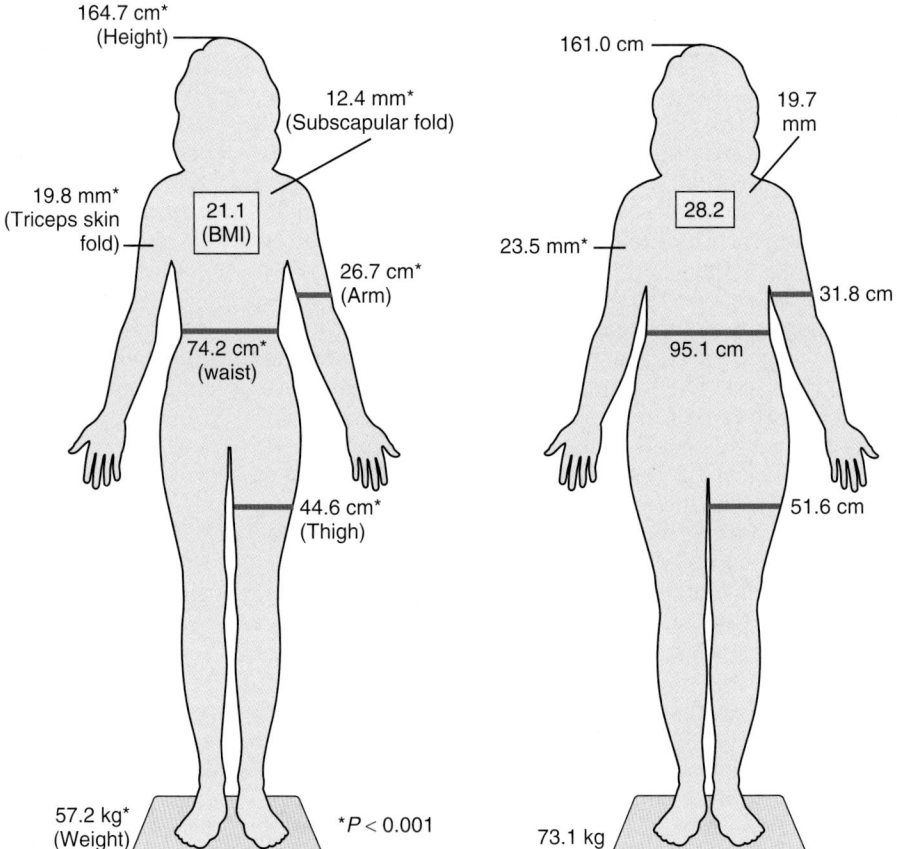

Figure 55.3 Schematic depiction of the anthropometrics of women with pulmonary nontuberculous mycobacterial disease (*n* = 60) (*left*) compared with National Health and Nutrition Examination Survey age-, sex-, and race-matched control subjects (*right*). BMI, body mass index. (From Kim RD, Greenberg DE, Ehrmantraut ME, et al. Pulmonary nontuberculous mycobacterial disease: prospective study of a distinct preexisting syndrome. *Am J Respir Crit Care Med.* 2008;178:1006–1074.)

M. abscessus infection in patients with CF who have undergone lung transplantation has sometimes been associated with severe and sometimes fatal disease.[120–122] Patients with rheumatoid arthritis are more likely to develop NTM disease than individuals without rheumatoid arthritis.[123,124]

Cytokine or certain cellular defects may predispose to NTM infection, including pulmonary disease. Multiple cytokines are necessary for granuloma formation and eventual containment of mycobacterial infections. The most important among these are interferon-γ, IL-12, and tumor necrosis factor-α. Patients with defects in each cytokine are susceptible to infection with NTM. Mutations in the *IFN-γ receptor 1* (IFN-γR1), IFN-γR2, IL-12 p40, and the IL-12 receptor are all associated with human disease.[125] The dominant and recessive IFN-γR1 deficiencies have distinct clinical presentations. Adult-onset immunodeficiency can result from the development of autoantibodies against IFN-γ; this condition is associated with severe disseminated opportunistic infections, including NTM.[126] Mutations in a transcription factor involved in stem cell maintenance, GATA2, are associated with autosomal dominant and sporadic monocytopenia and disseminated mycobacterial infections called the monoMAC syndrome.[127]

Inhibitors of tumor necrosis factor-α and of other cytokines are now routinely given therapeutically to large numbers of patients with inflammatory bowel disease, rheumatoid arthritis, or psoriatic arthritis. Although initially demonstrated to predispose to TB,[128] recent reports have linked these therapies to NTM infections as well.[129–131] Patients with suspected or known mycobacterial infections should not receive these medications without proper antimycobacterial therapy. Corticosteroids, including inhaled corticosteroids, have been associated with an increased risk of developing NTM disease,[70,132,133] with a strong dose-response relationship between incident NTM pulmonary disease and cumulative inhaled corticosteroid dose over 1 year.[132]

Microbial factors are also likely to be important in explaining NTM disease. A population-based assessment of the clinical significance of NTM in a region of The Netherlands demonstrated a wide range of pathogenicity among different NTM species.[134] Studies have identified isolates and phenotypes associated with increased virulence with in vitro models.[135–137] For example, *M. abscessus* is known to exist in a smooth (colonizing) and rough (invasive) phenotype. The presence of glycopeptidolipids on the smooth strains appears to mask the underlying antigenic cell wall lipids, allowing the smooth organisms to evade the immune response, colonize, and form biofilms in the lung airways.[135] When the organism switches to a rough phenotype, the glycopeptidolipids are lost, and the rough strain now elicits an innate immune response. Limited clinical data suggest that the rough phenotype may be more virulent than the smooth variety.[138,139]

DIAGNOSIS AND MANAGEMENT OF SPECIFIC PATHOGENS

Approximately 80% of patients with NTM infection present with pulmonary disease, which can have diverse

manifestations (Table 55.2).[33,140] This chapter focuses on the most common clinical presentations in the immunocompetent host—chiefly, TB-like (cavitary) disease and disease associated with nodules and bronchiectasis (nodular bronchiectatic disease). However, it is important to recognize that there is a great deal of overlap between these two phenotypes. The diagnostic evaluation usually consists of (1) assessment for the presence of one or more compatible symptoms, which are usually insidious in onset (cough, sputum production, fatigue, weight loss, fever, hemoptysis); (2) radiographic evaluation, which frequently includes CT scans of the chest; and (3) microbiologic evaluation, which consists of three or more sputum specimens for microscopy and mycobacterial culture and/or bronchoscopic specimens. The most important diagnosis to exclude is TB. Additional laboratory evaluation aimed at identifying potential reasons for underlying lung disease, specifically bronchiectasis, that might predispose to NTM infection may include testing for CF, alpha₁-antitrypsin deficiency, primary ciliary dyskinesia, or esophageal disorders in patients with pulmonary disease.

Making the diagnosis of NTM pulmonary disease can be challenging. Unlike pulmonary TB, in which a single positive culture of a sputum or bronchoscopic specimen establishes the diagnosis (barring laboratory contamination), confirmation of the diagnosis of NTM pulmonary disease usually requires repeated isolation of a particular NTM species. Diagnostic criteria have been developed to aid the clinician in the evaluation of persons suspected of having pulmonary NTM disease.[2,4] The NTM diagnostic criteria outlined in Table 55.3 are based on experience with common and well-described respiratory pathogens, such as MAC, *M. kansasii*, and *M. abscessus*. However, it is important to note that, because of the varying pathogenicity among the many NTM species, no single diagnostic approach will work for all cases. Diagnostic criteria that are too sensitive promote overdiagnosis and the unnecessary exposure of patients to potentially toxic antimicrobial medications. By contrast, diagnostic criteria that are overly rigid put patients at risk for undertreatment and progressive NTM disease. Fortunately, NTM lung disease is usually sufficiently indolent that there is enough time for a careful patient assessment to determine with confidence the presence or absence of significant disease.

Table 55.2 Diversity of Nontuberculous Mycobacteria Pulmonary Disease

Tuberculosis-like (cavitary) disease

Disease associated with nodules/bronchiectasis

Disease associated with genetic airway abnormalities and abnormal airway clearance (cystic fibrosis, primary ciliary dyskinesia, alpha₁-antitrypsin deficiency)

Hypersensitivity-like lung disease

Disease associated with esophageal motility disorders

Disease associated with disseminated disease and immune suppression
- HIV/AIDS
- Defects in interferon-γ and interleukin-12 pathways
- Tumor necrosis factor-α antagonists

AIDS, acquired immunodeficiency syndrome; HIV, human immunodeficiency disease.

Table 55.3 Microbiologic Criteria for Diagnosis of Nontuberculous Mycobacteria Lung Disease

Specimen	Results
At least three sputum results available *or*	Two positive cultures* regardless of the results of AFB smear
Single available bronchial wash or lavage *or*	One positive culture regardless of the results of AFB smear
Tissue biopsy	Compatible histopathology (granulomatous inflammation) and a positive biopsy culture for NTM Compatible histopathology (granulomatous inflammation) and a positive sputum or bronchial wash or lavage culture for NTM

*Two positive cultures isolating the same species or subspecies in the case of *Mycobacterium abscessus.*
AFB, acid-fast bacilli; NTM, nontuberculous mycobacteria.
Data from Daley CL, Iaccarino JM, Lange C, et al. Treatment of nontuberculous mycobacterial pulmonary disease: an official ATS/ERS/ESCMID/IDSA clinical practice guideline. *Clin Infect Dis.* 2020;71(4):905–913.

The difficulty in determining the clinical significance of an NTM respiratory isolate results from several factors. NTM isolates can contaminate clinical specimens, usually from environmental sources. Many NTM species, such as *Mycobacterium gordonae*, are generally nonpathogenic and almost invariably represent specimen contamination rather than true infection. NTM can be found in potable (municipal or tap) water, such as *M. kansasii*, MAC, *Mycobacterium simiae*, *M. abscessus*, and *M. xenopi*, so that their presence in a clinical specimen can be due to waterborne contamination of the specimen, even though the isolated species is sometimes associated with significant clinical disease. Sometimes, the recovery of even potentially virulent and pathogenic NTM may not be associated with active or progressive disease for reasons that are not understood. Unfortunately, no easily applied algorithm addresses all NTM species in all clinical circumstances. The clinician must have not only some knowledge of the disease-producing potential of NTM species but also an awareness of the circumstances associated with the isolation of the NTM species.

A single positive sputum culture for NTM is usually regarded as indeterminate for the diagnosis of NTM pulmonary disease. In contrast, when two or more sputum cultures are positive, the diagnosis of disease is more likely. For example, in a study from Japan, 98% of patients with two or more positive sputum cultures for MAC had evidence of progressive disease during follow-up.[141] Unlike sputum, a single positive NTM culture from bronchoscopy can be diagnostic for disease (see Table 55.3). However, the clinician must keep in mind NTM species that are usually respiratory contaminants (especially *M. gordonae*) and NTM species that can be found in tap water (discussed earlier), which may result in pseudo-outbreaks of NTM disease if the bronchoscopic equipment has been inappropriately rinsed with tap water.[142] The criterion that a single positive culture from bronchoscopy is diagnostic does not mean that bronchoscopy has a better yield for detection of NTM than expectorated (induced) sputum, but rather that it would be inappropriate to subject a patient to multiple bronchoscopic procedures simply to obtain multiple respiratory specimens. In fact, in the largest study comparing bronchial washing cultures with sputum cultures, the yields were equivalent.[143] Patients who are suspected of having NTM lung disease but do not meet the diagnostic criteria should be followed clinically until the diagnosis is either firmly established or excluded, a process that can take months to years.

Even among those who meet ATS/IDSA diagnostic criteria, progressive disease does not inevitably follow, at least in short-term follow-up. In two studies from Korea that included almost 1000 patients who met ATS/IDSA diagnostic criteria for MAC pulmonary disease, 24–41% were stable without antimicrobial treatment over a period of at least 3 years.[144,145] In both studies, approximately 50% of the stable patients spontaneously converted cultures to negative with airway clearance measures alone. In another study from Korea, 45% of 1012 patients with noncavitary NTM pulmonary disease did not initiate treatment over a median follow-up period of 3.6 years; 34% spontaneously converted, but 17% redeveloped NTM pulmonary disease with a species different from the original species.[146]

Diagnosis of NTM pulmonary disease does not necessitate the institution of therapy, which is a decision based on potential risks and benefits of therapy for individual patients. Factors that might influence the decision to treat NTM pulmonary disease include the virulence of the NTM pathogen and the potential for disease progression, the severity (or lack of severity) of symptoms and radiographic findings, the presence of known indolent disease, and the presence of advanced age and/or severe comorbid conditions (with limited life expectancy). Another factor is the inability to tolerate the prolonged and sometimes toxic antimicrobial regimens for NTM disease. Again, there is no substitute for physician familiarity with NTM pathogens and the individual patient for optimal management of NTM pulmonary disease.

Other clinical manifestations of NTM infection include lymphadenitis; disseminated disease; and skin, soft tissue, and bone disease. Lymphadenitis is the most common NTM disease manifestation in children and is usually due to MAC or, less commonly, *Mycobacterium haemophilum* or *Mycobacterium scrofulaceum*.[147] The most important differential diagnosis is TB lymphadenitis, although NTM account for approximately 90% of mycobacterial lymphadenitis in American children (but only 10% in adults).[148] Symptoms are usually minimal, with frequent unilateral involvement of submandibular, submaxillary, preauricular, or cervical lymph nodes. Skin and soft tissue infections are usually due to the RGM—*M. abscessus, M. fortuitum, M. chelonae,* or *Mycobacterium marinum*—and are the result of direct inoculation after either trauma or surgery.[2,149] Dissemination of NTM pathogens is most often associated with the severe immunosuppression of advanced AIDS and is caused by MAC.[105,150–152] NTM infections can disseminate in other immunocompromised states, such as organ transplantation, or in association with indwelling foreign bodies, such as venous catheters, dialysis catheters, or other prosthetic devices.[153–156]

LABORATORY DIAGNOSIS

Diagnosis of NTM disease is based on isolation of these organisms from clinical specimens. Cultures should include both solid and broth media for detection of mycobacteria, with a semiquantitative reporting of colony counts.[2] A meta-analysis of nine studies showed a 15% increase in the sensitivity of culture for NTM if a solid medium was incubated along with a liquid culture system.[157] Despite the increased yield with inoculation of both solid and liquid media, most referral laboratories in the United States use liquid media only.

The optimal temperature for growth of most NTM species is between 28°C and 37°C, although some species require either higher or lower temperatures for optimal growth, and some species require special supplementation for recovery from culture. The Clinical and Laboratory Standards Initiative has suggested incubation temperatures of 36 ± 1°C for slow growers and 28 ± 2°C for rapid growers.[158] Most NTM grow within 2 to 3 weeks of subculture, but the group of rapidly growing NTM appear within 7 days of subculture.

Speciation can be based on phenotypic characteristics, analysis of biochemical and lipid profiles, *mass-assisted laser desorption/ionization–time of flight mass spectrometry* (MALDI-TOF MS), and molecular methods. NTM can be categorized phenotypically by their growth rate and pigmentation, although these characteristics are not specific enough for final speciation. Biochemical testing, such as niacin production and nitrate reduction tests, often is not sufficient to differentiate all NTM, particularly some of the newly identified species. High-pressure liquid chromatography, which analyzes the chromatographic profile of the mycolic acids extracted from the bacterial cell wall, can be used to speciate a large number of NTM.[159] However, high-pressure liquid chromatography is unable to differentiate all species, and of importance, it cannot differentiate the subspecies of *M. abscessus*. MALDI-TOF MS is based on disruption of bacterial cells by laser and ionization of proteins and can provide a cheaper alternative to sequencing but remains less discriminatory for subspeciation of *M. abscessus*. Although MALDI-TOF MS works well on pure cultures, its performance on newly positive respiratory specimens is less robust.[160,161] In a small study from The Netherlands, only 12 (22%) of 54 respiratory isolates were identified directly from liquid culture.[160] A recent study evaluated two commercially available systems and reported that 92–95% of the NTM strains tested were able to identify to the complex/group level.[162] However, both systems had difficulty differentiating between members of *M. abscessus*, *M. fortuitum*, *Mycobacterium mucogenicum*, *M. avium*, and *Mycobacterium terrae* complexes/groups.

Molecular methods for speciation include nucleic acid probes, polymerase chain reaction and other amplification methods, and nucleic acid sequencing.[163–168] Identification of mycobacteria by 16S ribosomal DNA sequencing[163,164] provides more accurate determination of the species, although 16S ribosomal DNA sequencing cannot differentiate all species of NTM. The commercially available AccuProbe technology (Gen-Probe) is currently recommended for identification of *M. tuberculosis* complex, *M. avium* complex (as well as *M. avium* and *M. intracellulare* separately), *M. kansasii,* and *M. gordonae*. Given the varying pathogenicity of the many NTM species and variation in treatment outcomes by species and, in the case of *M. abscessus* subsp., additional methods of speciation are

needed. Partial gene sequencing targeting *rpoB*, *hsp65*, and *secA* can provide high degrees of discrimination but are costly and are only feasible in laboratories with sequencing capabilities.[169,170] Multilocus sequencing can increase the discriminatory power to the level of subspecies for *M. abscessus*.[171,172] Line probe assays can identify more common species and provide rapid detection of resistance mutations for macrolides and amikacin.[173] In addition, line probe assays can identify the normal or truncated *erythromycin resistance methylase (erm)* gene, *erm(41)*, and the presence of C28T mutations that can render the *erm(41)* gene nonfunctional.

Antimicrobial susceptibility testing has unclear value for the management of patients with NTM disease because in vitro results do not correlate well with clinical outcomes for some drugs.[4] For MAC, the Clinical and Laboratory Standards Initiative recommends broth microdilution for antimicrobial testing against clarithromycin and amikacin only.[174] Seeking guidance from in vitro susceptibility results for other antibiotics is unreliable and often misleading. Initial isolates should be tested for response to clarithromycin and amikacin, as should isolates from patients with treatment failures and relapses, patients who have taken macrolides previously, and AIDS patients who develop bacteremia on macrolide prophylaxis. For clarithromycin, a *minimal inhibitory concentration* (MIC) of 32 or greater is considered resistant.[174] For amikacin, an MIC of 64 or greater and an MIC of 128 or greater are considered resistant for parenteral and liposomal inhaled, respectively. For *M. kansasii*, isolates should be tested for response to rifampin (rifampicin) because resistance to rifampin is associated with treatment failure or relapse.[175] For rifampin, the cutoff for resistance is an MIC of 2 or greater.[174] If rifampin resistance is documented, additional drugs, including clarithromycin and moxifloxacin, should be tested. For RGM, broth microdilution MIC determination for susceptibility testing is recommended.[175] In general, for most species, antimicrobial susceptibility testing should be used to guide selection of antibiotics to be used in the treatment regimen recognizing the limitations of such testing.

SLOWLY GROWING MYCOBACTERIA

Although there are slightly fewer species of slowly growing NTM than rapidly growing species, the slow growers are more common causes of pulmonary disease (see Table 55.1). The slow growers include approximately 90 species (http://www.bacterio.net/mycobacterium.html), with a wide range of pathogenicity, from organisms such as *M. kansasii,* which are probably second only to *M. tuberculosis* in terms of disease-producing capability, to *M. gordonae,* which rarely causes disease.[4]

Mycobacterium avium Complex

MAC includes 12 species, of which *M. avium, M. intracellulare,* and *M. chimaera* are the most common to cause pulmonary disease.[176] Differentiation of the separate MAC species is not possible with routine laboratory techniques, although DNA probes can identify *M. avium* and *M. intracellulare*. In most circumstances, the differentiation of *M. avium* and *M. intracellulare* does not likely make a significant

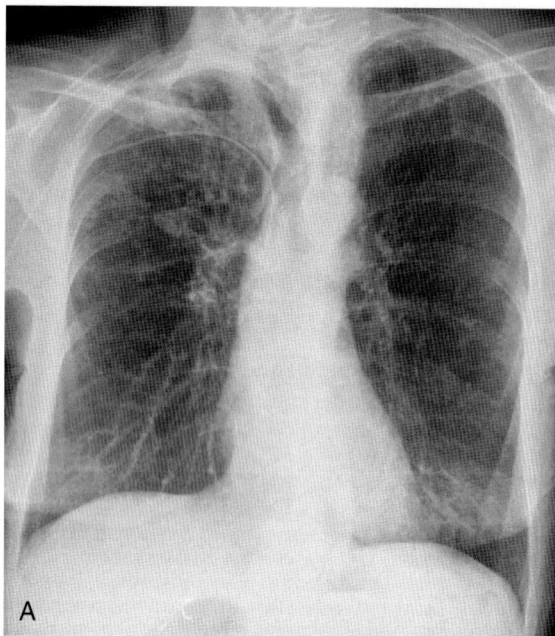
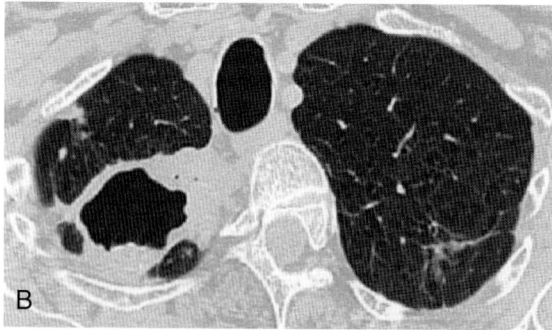

Figure 55.4 Cavitary *Mycobacterium avium* complex (MAC) pulmonary disease. A 63-year-old woman with smoking history with cavitary MAC lung disease. The patient, who presented with cough, fatigue, weight loss, and intermittent hemoptysis, was diagnosed with MAC in 2004. She did not respond to two courses of multidrug therapy, and her sputum remained strongly culture positive for MAC. (A) Chest radiograph showing cavitary consolidation in the right apex and scattered nodular and reticulonodular opacities in both lungs. (B) Computed tomography scan showing large cavity in right apex.

difference clinically or therapeutically, although recent data from South Korea suggest that *M. intracellulare* may be more virulent than *M. avium;* patients with *M. intracellulare* presented with more severe disease and had a worse prognosis.[177,178]

The traditionally recognized presentation of MAC pulmonary disease has been as apical fibrocavitary disease similar to TB, sometimes with large cavities, usually in men but also in women; patients generally are in their fifth or sixth decade of life and have a history of cigarette smoking and alcohol abuse (Fig. 55.4). If left untreated, this form of disease is generally progressive, can result in extensive cavitary lung destruction, and is associated with increased mortality compared with noncavitary MAC lung disease.[179–181] The necessity for initiation of therapy with cavitary MAC pulmonary disease is clearly much more pressing than with noncavitary MAC disease.

MAC pulmonary disease also presents with nodular opacities associated with bronchiectasis, which frequently involve the right middle lobe or lingula, predominantly in postmenopausal nonsmoking white women (Fig. 55.5). This form of disease, termed nodular bronchiectatic disease, tends to have a much slower progression than cavitary disease so that long-term follow-up may be necessary to demonstrate clinical or radiographic changes. Even with this more indolent form of disease, however, death may result from progressive disease.[100] Nodular bronchiectatic MAC pulmonary disease is radiographically characterized by CT findings that include multiple small peripheral pulmonary nodules and cylindrical bronchiectasis (see Fig. 55.5). The CT pattern of these predominantly peripheral small nodular densities has been described as tree-in-bud and reflects inflammatory changes including bronchiolitis (eFig. 55.1).

Patients with nodular bronchiectatic MAC pulmonary disease often have additional coinfections associated with bronchiectasis, including respiratory cultures positive for *Pseudomonas aeruginosa; Nocardia* sp; fungal species, such as *Aspergillus*; and occasionally other NTM, such as *M. abscessus*. Nonmycobacterial exacerbations of bronchiectasis often complicate the assessment and management of MAC disease and strategies aimed at treatment of the bronchiectasis may improve patients' symptoms.

Therapy of *Mycobacterium avium* Complex Pulmonary Disease. Several aspects of treatment for MAC pulmonary disease are difficult to explain and are even counterintuitive. The greatest misunderstanding about treatment regimens for NTM pathogens is the expectation that all NTM infections should respond in a predictable manner to antimicrobial therapy, as does *M. tuberculosis* infection. In reality, when treatment regimens are based on in vitro susceptibility testing, the NTM pathogen very often does not respond to antimicrobial agents as predicted. A frustrating aspect of NTM therapy for many clinicians is the lack of a clear association between the in vitro susceptibility results and the clinical (in vivo) response. For many NTM, including MAC, laboratory cutoffs for "susceptible" and "resistant" do not have a demonstrable clinical correlate and have not been confirmed to be clinically meaningful. For disease caused by MAC, response to treatment correlates primarily with in vitro susceptibility to macrolides (clarithromycin and azithromycin) and amikacin but not to other antimicrobial agents.[182–190] Several other NTM species (*M. abscessus, M. simiae, M. malmoense, M. xenopi,* etc.) lack established correlation between in vitro susceptibilities and in vivo responsiveness to any antimicrobial agent. The explanations for the dichotomy between laboratory susceptibility testing results and clinical benefit for many NTM are currently not known. In accordance, clinicians must use in vitro susceptibility data for many NTM with the awareness that, unlike for TB, the results are an imperfect guide to treatment outcome. Three comprehensive reviews summarize the multiple and complicated factors that likely account for this troubling aspect of NTM disease therapy.[191–193]

There is another difficult-to-explain phenomenon associated with MAC drug therapy. Patients who have not responded to prior MAC therapy, with or without a macrolide, have lower sputum conversion rates with macrolide-containing treatment regimens, even with macrolide-susceptible MAC isolates, than do patients with no prior therapy.[183,186,194,195]

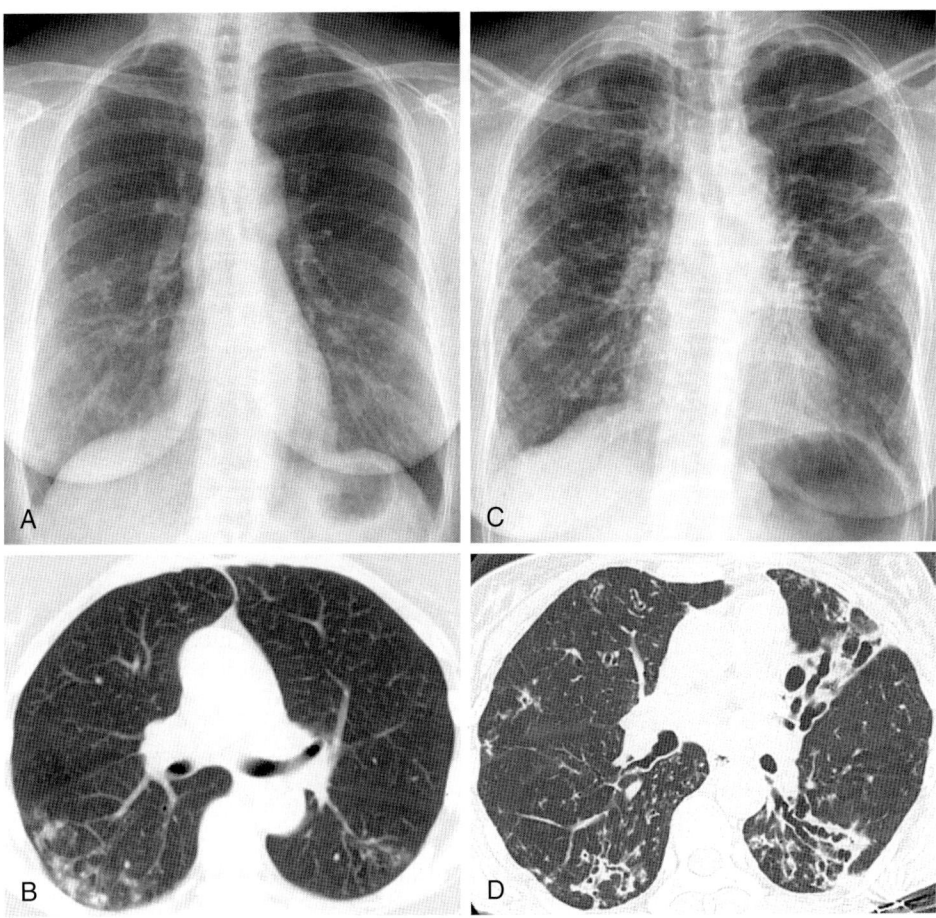

Figure 55.5 Nodular bronchiectatic *Mycobacterium avium* complex (MAC) pulmonary disease in two patients. (A) Posteroanterior chest radiograph from a 60-year-old nonsmoking woman with several years of chronic cough and recurrent "pneumonia." Sputum was acid-fast bacilli smear positive and culture positive for MAC at the time of the radiograph and on multiple subsequent collections. Chest radiograph shows primarily middle and lower lung nodular and reticulonodular abnormalities. (B) High-resolution chest computed tomography from this patient showing bilateral bronchiectasis with variable-sized nodular and reticulonodular opacities in a tree-in-bud pattern. (C) Posteroanterior chest radiograph from a 74-year-old woman with more than 20 years of cough with sputum production, recurrent "pneumonia," severe fatigue, and weight loss. Sputum was strongly acid-fast bacilli smear positive and culture-positive for MAC on multiple collections. (D) High-resolution chest computed tomography from this patient showing extensive, severe, multilobar bronchiectasis.

Although the explanation for this observation is not clear, it is evident that the best chance for treatment success in MAC pulmonary disease is the first treatment effort. Finally, patients who are successfully treated for nodular bronchiectatic MAC disease can be reinfected by new MAC strains, sometimes with renewal of progressive disease.[196–198]

The recommended regimen for the treatment of MAC pulmonary disease includes a macrolide (azithromycin or clarithromycin), ethambutol, and a rifamycin (rifampin or rifabutin).[4] The regimen can be administered three times weekly in patients with nodular bronchiectatic disease but should be administered daily in those with cavitary disease. For those with cavitary or otherwise extensive radiographic disease or with macrolide-resistant disease (see later), a parenteral aminoglycoside (amikacin or streptomycin) should be considered.[4]

Because the macrolides azithromycin and clarithromycin are the principal and most important antimicrobial agents for which there is a demonstrated correlation between in vitro susceptibility and in vivo response for MAC pulmonary disease, these agents, partnered with ethambutol, serve as the cornerstones of MAC therapy (Table 55.4). Azithromycin is preferred over clarithromycin because it is associated with fewer drug interactions and has improved tolerance, lower pill burden, and once-daily dosing. Addition of a third drug, such as a rifamycin, may

Table 55.4 Treatment of *Mycobacterium avium* Complex Pulmonary Disease

Type of Disease	Regimen
Nodular/bronchiectatic disease	1. Clarithromycin 1000 mg tiw or azithromycin 500–600 mg tiw *and* 2. Ethambutol 25 mg/kg tiw *and* 3. Rifampin 600 mg tiw
Cavitary disease	1. Clarithromycin 500–1000 mg/day or azithromycin 250–300 mg/day *and* 2. Ethambutol 15 mg/kg daily *and* 3. Rifampin 450–600 mg daily *and* 4. Include streptomycin or amikacin 15 mg/kg tiw for first 2–3 months
Advanced or previously treated disease	1. Clarithromycin 500–1000 mg/day or azithromycin 250–300 mg/day *and* 2. Ethambutol 15 mg/kg daily *and* 3. Rifabutin 150–300 mg daily or rifampin 450–600 mg daily *and* 4. Include streptomycin or amikacin 15 mg/kg tiw for first 2–3 months
Treatment-refractory disease	1. Add amikacin liposome inhalation suspension 590 mg once daily

tiw, three times per week.
From Daley CL, Iaccarino JM, Lange C, et al. Treatment of nontuberculous mycobacterial pulmonary disease: an official ATS/ERS/ESCMID/IDSA clinical practice guideline. *Clin Infect Dis.* 2020;71(4):905–913.

reinforce the regimen and possibly prevent the emergence of macrolide-resistant MAC isolates. Macrolides should *never* be used as monotherapy for treatment of MAC disease, either pulmonary or disseminated.[199]

For some patients who are taking clarithromycin, the doses may need to be split (e.g., 500 mg twice daily) because of gastrointestinal intolerance. For patients of low body weight (<50 kg) or older age, the clarithromycin dose for daily regimens may need to be reduced to 500 mg/day because of gastrointestinal intolerance. However, it should be noted that in a small (*n* = 34) three-arm retrospective study from Japan, a dose of 400 mg daily was associated with a lower sputum conversion rate at 18 months than a daily dose of 800 mg.[200] Patients receiving clarithromycin and rifabutin should be carefully monitored for rifabutin-related toxicity, especially hematologic (leukopenia) and ocular (uveitis). For some patients, especially those with nodular bronchiectatic MAC disease, intermittent or thrice-weekly therapy may facilitate tolerance of the multidrug treatment regimen.

MAC pulmonary disease should be treated until there are 12 months of sputum culture negativity,[2] a goal that requires patients to have sputum collected for mycobacterial culture on a regular basis throughout the course of treatment. The optimum duration of a parenteral aminoglycoside is unknown, but a retrospective study from Korea reported that patients with cavitary MAC pulmonary disease who received 3 or more months of an aminoglycoside showed higher treatment success rates than those treated for less than 3 months.[201]

Treatment outcomes for MAC pulmonary disease have varied significantly across studies but are better when macrolide-based regimens are used. A systematic review reported sustained sputum culture conversion in 54% (191 of 356) of patients on macrolide-containing regimens versus 32% (38 of 120) for macrolide-free regimens.[202] Another systematic review reported overall treatment success using macrolide-containing regimens was 52.3% (95% confidence interval [CI], 44.7–59.9%), and success increased to 61.4% if treated with an ATS/IDSA three-drug regimen, and to 65.7% if further treated for at least 12 months.[203]

Some patients do not respond to therapy despite administration of an appropriate regimen. A definition for treatment failure was proposed to be the reemergence of multiple positive cultures or the persistence of positive cultures with the causative species from respiratory samples after 12 or more months of antimycobacterial treatment while the patient is on treatment.[204] However, detection of treatment failure at an earlier time point is likely to be beneficial to the patient. In a study reporting the treatment outcomes of patients with MAC pulmonary disease, 83% of patients had their first negative culture within 6 months of starting therapy, and the change in semiquantitative culture scores as early as 2 to 3 months was predictive of culture status at 12 months.[205] In a study from Korea, culture conversion by 6 months was predictive of culture status at 12 months.[206] In a randomized clinical trial evaluating the efficacy and safety of *amikacin liposome inhalation suspension* (ALIS) in patients with treatment-refractory MAC pulmonary disease, cultures converted by 6 months in only 9% of patients who continued to receive *guideline-based therapy*

(GBT) alone (the control arm).[189] Based on these studies, lack of culture conversion after 6 months of therapy may be a better time point at which to determine treatment failure.

For patients with treatment-refractory MAC pulmonary disease, ALIS should be added to GBT.[4] ALIS was introduced as a way to increase amikacin uptake into alveolar macrophages, allow biofilm penetration, and limit systemic exposure.[189] In a phase II controlled trial, treatment-refractory patients (e.g., with culture positivity after at least 6 months of GBT that included a macrolide) with MAC (*n* = 57) or *M. abscessus* (*n* = 32) pulmonary disease were kept on their multidrug regimen and randomized to investigational ALIS (*n* = 44) versus placebo (empty liposomes, *n* = 45).[190] Although the primary end point of reduction in semiquantitative mycobacterial culture growth from baseline was not achieved, significantly more patients who received ALIS achieved culture conversion by day 84 and had greater improvement in distance achieved on the 6-minute walk test. In a recent randomized controlled phase III trial, ALIS, when added to GBT for treatment-refractory MAC pulmonary disease, was associated with a higher proportion of patients with negative cultures at 6 months compared to those who continued to take the standard regimen only.[189] Culture conversion was achieved by 29.0% (65 of 224) of patients treated with ALIS plus GBT compared with 8.9% (10 of 112) with GBT alone. Adverse reactions were reported in 10% or more of patients in the ALIS plus GBT arm, including dysphonia, cough, hemoptysis, dyspnea, fatigue, diarrhea, nausea, and oropharyngeal pain. These events infrequently led to early discontinuation of ALIS or withdrawal from the study. Based on the phase II and III trial results, ALIS was approved by the U.S. Food and Drug Administration for treatment of MAC pulmonary disease in patients who have not responded to therapy after at least 6 months of GBT.

Other treatment options include addition of parenteral amikacin (or streptomycin), oral clofazimine, bedaquiline, or moxifloxacin. Parenteral amikacin has been associated with improved culture conversion in patients with treatment-naive disease[207] and improved treatment outcomes in patients with macrolide-resistant disease (see later).[199,208] Clofazimine has been reported to be associated with culture conversion in patients with MAC pulmonary disease also receiving a macrolide and ethambutol,[209] with relatively good tolerance.[209,210] Bedaquiline was used in treatment-refractory disease, and again the drug was well tolerated; although some patients demonstrated microbiologic improvement, few converted over the 6 months of therapy.[211] In Korea, addition of moxifloxacin to treatment-refractory patients with MAC pulmonary disease was associated with culture conversion in approximately 30% of patients, although that has not been our experience.

Disease recurrence is common and often due to reinfection. Studies have reported recurrence rates of 25–50%, of which 50–75% have been reinfected as determined by either PFGE or repetitive element palindromic polymerase chain reaction.[197,198,212] Microbiologic recurrence was twice as common among patients with nodular bronchiectatic disease compared with cavitary disease, so lifelong follow-up is particularly important is this patient population.[198]

Macrolide-resistant MAC pulmonary disease is associated with a poor prognosis.[199,208,213] The two major risk factors for macrolide-resistant MAC disease are macrolide monotherapy or macrolide therapy with inadequate companion medications.[199,208] The treatment strategy associated with the most success for macrolide-resistant MAC pulmonary disease includes both the use of a multidrug regimen, including a parenteral aminoglycoside (amikacin or streptomycin), and surgical resection (debulking) of diseased lung.[199,208] The optimal drug regimen for treating macrolide-resistant strains is unknown, but some experts recommend ethambutol, rifabutin, a parenteral aminoglycoside, and possibly another oral drug, such as clofazimine or bedaquiline. The role for ALIS in this setting has yet to be determined. The continuation of a macrolide or addition of moxifloxacin has not been shown to improve outcomes.[208,214]

Therapy of Disseminated *Mycobacterium avium* Complex Disease. Successful treatment of disseminated MAC in persons with AIDS is based on treatment of both the mycobacterial and HIV infections. ART should be started as soon as possible after the diagnosis of MAC disease.[107] Clinicians must therefore be aware of the drug-drug interactions between the antimycobacterial and antiretroviral medications. Current guidelines for the use of antimycobacterial drugs together with HIV therapies can be found at https://clinicalinfo.hiv.gov/en/guidelines/adult-and-adolescent-arv/whats-new-guidelines.

Patients with disseminated MAC disease should be treated with clarithromycin, 1000 mg/day or 500 mg twice daily (or, as an alternative, azithromycin at a dose of 500 mg daily), and ethambutol at a dose of 15 mg/kg daily.[215–217] A third drug, such as rifabutin, may be added because one clinical trial reported that the addition of rifabutin to a regimen of clarithromycin and ethambutol was associated with improved survival and, in two randomized trials, this approach reduced the emergence of resistance.[215,218] It should be noted that the combination of clarithromycin and rifabutin may lead to increased risk of drug toxicity to rifabutin, so azithromycin may be a better companion macrolide. As with macrolide-resistant MAC pulmonary disease, patients with disseminated disease from macrolide-resistant strains are far less likely to be treated successfully.[219] Treatment of MAC in patients with AIDS should be considered lifelong, unless immune restoration is achieved by ART. MAC treatment may be stopped for patients who are asymptomatic, have completed 12 months or more of therapy, and have maintained a CD4+ T cell count greater than 100 cells/mm³ for at least 6 months after initiation of ART.[107]

Primary prophylaxis (e.g., prevention of the first infection) against disseminated MAC disease is not recommended for adults and adolescents who immediately initiate ART.[107] However, patients who are not receiving ART or who remain viremic should receive prophylaxis if they have CD4 counts less than 50 CD4+ cells/mm³. Several operational cohorts have demonstrated that the overall incidence of MAC disease is very low and not different between those who did and did not take MAC prophylaxis while on ART.[109,220,221] Plasma HIV RNA level greater than 1000 copies/mL was the main risk factor for developing MAC disease regardless of MAC prophylaxis.[109,221] If primary prophylaxis was previously initiated, it should be discontinued in those who are continuing on a fully suppressive ART regimen.[107] Two randomized, placebo-controlled trials and observational data have demonstrated that patients can discontinue primary prophylaxis safely.[222–226]

Based on efficacy and ease of use, azithromycin—given as 1200 mg once weekly—is the preferred agent for primary prophylaxis.[227] Clarithromycin is also effective; however, it is considered an alternative agent because it must be given twice daily, and the risk of breakthrough with macrolide-resistant strains is higher with daily clarithromycin than with weekly azithromycin. Rifabutin is also effective but should only be used when a macrolide cannot be tolerated. Primary MAC prophylaxis should be discontinued among adult and adolescent patients who are continuing on a fully suppressive ART regimen.[107] Primary prophylaxis should be reintroduced if the CD4+ T lymphocyte count decreases to less than 50 to 100 cells/mm³.

Secondary prophylaxis (i.e., prevention of reinfection) should be provided to those patients in whom a fully suppressive ART regimen is not possible and who have a decline in their CD4 count to levels to below 100 cells/mm³.

Therapy of *Mycobacterium avium* Complex Lymphadenopathy. The treatment of choice for MAC lymphadenopathy and localized lymphadenopathy due to most NTM pathogens is complete surgical resection of the involved lymph nodes.[147,148,228,229] When complete surgical resection is not possible due to, for instance, nerve impingement or encasement by infected nodes, then chemotherapy with MAC treatment regimens similar to those for lung and disseminated disease is effective.[230] Some studies have also suggested that a conservative, "wait and see" approach is also as effective as either surgery or antibiotic therapy for the majority of children with this process.[231–233] Clearly, expert evaluation is advisable for optimal management of these children.

Mycobacterium kansasii

M. kansasii is the second most common cause of pulmonary disease caused by a slow grower in the United States but has also been reported in Europe, Asia, and Africa. So far, municipal tap water is the only known reservoir for *M. kansasii*.[234–236] *M. kansasii* lung disease most closely parallels the clinical course of *M. tuberculosis*, including radiographic abnormalities (Fig. 55.6, eFig. 55.2). Although most patients with *M. kansasii* pulmonary disease have upper lobe fibrocavitary findings, some patients have been reported with nodular bronchiectatic radiographic abnormalities. In HIV-infected patients, *M. kansasii* can present with essentially any pattern of radiographic abnormality.[237]

Therapy of *Mycobacterium kansasii* Pulmonary Disease. *M. kansasii* is susceptible to a broad array of antimicrobial agents, including rifamycins, macrolides, fluoroquinolones, clofazimine, ethambutol, isoniazid, trimethoprim-sulfamethoxazole, and aminoglycosides. Newer agents, such as bedaquiline and delamanid, have in vitro activity also.[238] Initially, a regimen including isoniazid was used, but treatment success was unsatisfactory[239] until the introduction of rifampin.[240,241] The recommended regimen for treating pulmonary *M. kansasii* disease has traditionally included daily rifampin (600 mg/day), isoniazid

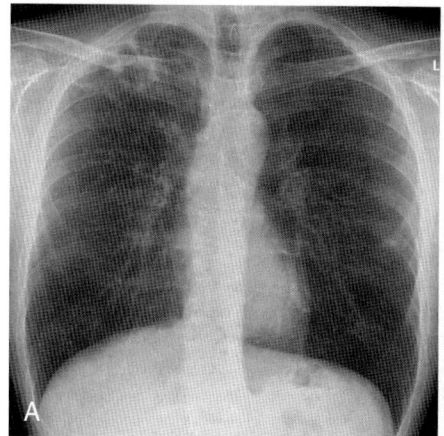
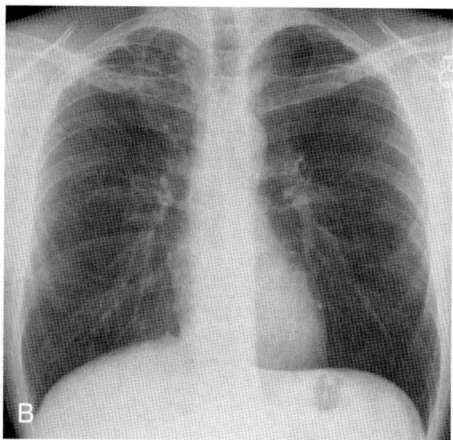

Figure 55.6 *Mycobacterium kansasii.* A 46-year-old man with smoking history with *M. kansasii* lung disease. The patient presented with cough and weight loss. He was treated as a tuberculosis suspect initially, but his sputum specimen was strongly culture positive for *M. kansasii.* (A) Chest radiograph showing right upper lobe cavitary consolidation. (B) Chest radiograph with improvement in abnormalities after completing therapy.

(300 mg/day), and ethambutol (15 mg/kg/day) for at least 12 months.[2,3] Sputum cultures convert in approximately 90% of patients with this regimen[242] and in nearly 100% in patients who complete therapy.[241,243–246] Limited data suggest that therapy with rifampin, ethambutol, and clarithromycin for *M. kansasii* disease can also be successful,[247,248] including when taken as intermittent therapy.[249] Based on the in vitro activity of macrolides against *M. kansasii,* and the two studies that demonstrated good treatment outcomes when clarithromycin was substituted for isoniazid, either isoniazid or a macrolide can be used in combination with rifampicin and ethambutol.[4] Expert opinion favors inclusion of a macrolide over isoniazid. Parenteral aminoglycosides are seldom needed in the treatment of *M. kansasii.*

In patients treated with rifampin, ethambutol, and a macrolide, treatment can be administered either daily or three times a week.[4] However, for those with cavitary disease, daily treatment is recommended instead of intermittent administration. For patients treated with an isoniazid, ethambutol, and rifampicin regimen, daily therapy is also recommended because data regarding intermittent administration of this regimen are lacking. Treatment should continue for at least 12 months.[4] A study that evaluated a two-drug (rifampin, ethambutol) regimen given for 9 months was associated with a culture conversion of 89%, but the recurrence rate was high at 10%.[243]

When *M. kansasii* isolates have become resistant to rifampin as a result of previous therapy, patients have been treated successfully with a regimen that consists of high-dose daily isoniazid (900 mg), high-dose ethambutol (25 mg/kg/day), and sulfamethoxazole (1.0 g three times/day) combined with several months of streptomycin or amikacin.[250] The excellent in vitro activity of clarithromycin and moxifloxacin against *M. kansasii* suggests that multidrug regimens containing these agents and at least one other agent, such as ethambutol or sulfamethoxazole, based on in vitro susceptibilities, are likely to be even more effective for treatment of a patient with rifampin-resistant *M. kansasii* disease.

Therapy of Disseminated *Mycobacterium kansasii* Disease. The treatment regimen for disseminated disease, as usually observed in patients with AIDS, should be the same as for pulmonary disease.[2] Because of the critically important role of rifamycins in the treatment of *M. kansasii* disease, it is important to construct *M. kansasii* and antiretroviral treatment regimens that are compatible (see https://clinicalinfo.hiv.gov/en/guidelines/adult-and-adolescent-arv/whats-new-guidelines). An option for treating HIV-infected patients who receive an antiretroviral regimen not compatible with rifamycins is to substitute a macrolide or moxifloxacin for the rifamycin. There is no recommended prophylaxis regimen for disseminated *M. kansasii* disease.

Mycobacterium xenopi

M. xenopi is a thermophile that survives in hot water systems and natural hot water reservoirs. Its survival in flowing water systems and resistance to common disinfectants enable *M. xenopi* to contaminate laboratory samples and medical devices, such as bronchoscopes, thus causing health care–acquired disease (pseudoinfections) and laboratory contamination of specimens. Clusters of isolates related to pseudoinfections from contamination of bronchoscopes have been reported from the United States and Europe.[251] Because of its environmental presence, the differentiation of true clinical infection from pseudoinfection may be difficult but is of paramount importance. Among 40 patients in The Netherlands who met NTM pulmonary disease criteria, at least half were thought to have disease related to the isolate.[252]

M. xenopi is rarely isolated in the United States; however, it is the second most common cause of NTM lung disease in Canada, the United Kingdom, and some parts of Europe.[252] Pulmonary *M. xenopi* infections are most common, but extrapulmonary and disseminated infections have been reported. Impaired immunity, either local (i.e., preexisting pulmonary disease) or systemic (i.e., HIV, immunosuppressive medications) appear to predispose to *M. xenopi* infections. Radiographic findings with *M. xenopi* pulmonary disease are variable but most often include upper lobe cavitary abnormalities compatible with TB.

Treatment outcomes have been reported as variable. A systematic review that examined 48 studies, including 1255 subjects, described that, among 188 subjects who received at least 6 months of therapy, 65% had a sustained disease-free outcome, with better long-term success in those who received fluoroquinolones.[253] However, another systematic review reported sputum culture conversion, after subtracting recurrence, in only 32% of patients.[242]

Mortality is high. In one report describing treatment outcomes for *M. xenopi* infections, overall mortality was 68% and mostly unrelated to *M. xenopi* disease; the response to chemotherapy was not correlated with in vitro susceptibility results.[254] *M. xenopi* isolates demonstrated favorable in vitro sensitivities to isoniazid, rifampin, and ethambutol.[252] In this study, even with variable treatment regimens, antimicrobial treatment cured 58% of patients who met ATS/IDSA criteria for *M. xenopi* pulmonary disease. There was no correlation between failure or treatment relapse and in vitro susceptibility results. In a randomized controlled trial, a regimen of clarithromycin, rifampin, and ethambutol was compared to ciprofloxacin, rifampin, and ethambutol; treatment success, failure, or relapse did not differ between the two groups.[255] All-cause mortality was again relatively high and higher in the ciprofloxacin, rifampin, and ethambutol arm (47%) than the clarithromycin-containing arm (29%). A combination of ethambutol and rifampin with either clarithromycin or moxifloxacin was shown to be bactericidal in vitro and ex vivo.[256] In a mouse model, amikacin-containing regimens were the most effective.[256] Although the optimal pharmacologic management has yet to be determined, a regimen is recommended consisting of a macrolide (or moxifloxacin), rifampin, and ethambutol, administered for a duration of therapy that includes 12 months of sputum culture negativity.[4] In patients with cavitary or advanced/severe bronchiectatic *M. xenopi* pulmonary disease, parenteral amikacin should be added to the regimen. The unusually high overall mortality is likely a reflection of the comorbidities of the patients with *M. xenopi* disease.

Mycobacterium malmoense

M. malmoense is considered the second most serious pathogen after MAC in Northern Europe.[257] The clinical relevance (i.e., met ATS/IDSA diagnostic criteria for disease) of *M. malmoense* isolates has been described as 70–80% in Europe, although isolates in the United States are infrequently deemed clinically significant.[258] Patients with *M. malmoense* pulmonary disease frequently have preexisting obstructive lung disease. Not surprisingly, *M. malmoense* pulmonary disease often presents in a manner similar to that of other cavitary NTM disease pathogens. Overall, treatment response does not correlate with in vitro susceptibility to antimicrobial agents. A recent systematic review[242] reported a weighted average proportion of treatment success of 54.4% (95% CI, 34.7–73.4%); however, this estimate is limited by the high all-cause mortality in the studies. In a randomized controlled trial, clarithromycin, rifampin, and ethambutol were compared to a regimen consisting of ciprofloxacin, rifampin, and ethambutol.[259] Although a more favorable response to therapy was attained with the macrolide-containing regimen, overall mortality did not differ between the two regimens. The optimal antimicrobial management of *M. malmoense* has yet to be determined, although treatment should probably include at least three agents guided by in vitro susceptibility: azithromycin 250 to 500 mg/day, rifampin 600

mg/day, and ethambutol 15 mg/kg/day. Amikacin 10 to 15 mg/kg/day *intravenous* (IV) or 15 to 25 mg/kg three times a week should be considered for cavitary/severe disease. Moxifloxacin 400 mg/day or clofazimine 100 mg/day may be used as alternative drugs. Although the optimal treatment duration is not known, experts have recommended that treatment continue for 12 months beyond the date of culture conversion.[2]

Mycobacterium simiae

M. simiae has been recovered from clinical specimens in several geographic regions, including Israel, Cuba, Réunion Island, and the southwestern United States.[2,260] The organism is most often isolated as a single positive culture from a patient who is smear negative and without clinical disease. Several pseudo-outbreaks have been reported in which the organisms were recovered from the local tap water.[261–263] In most published series, the majority of *M. simiae* isolates have been judged not to be clinically significant.[264,265] When *M. simiae* is a significant pathogen, it is most often associated with pulmonary disease or, in immunocompromised hosts, with disseminated disease.

As with other NTM, there is no established correlation between in vitro susceptibility of the organism and clinical response to antimicrobial agents, nor is there an established, predictably reliable treatment regimen for *M. simiae* disease. In a study from Israel,[265] there were no recurrences reported in 102 patients with *M. simiae* pulmonary disease after treatment with rifampin, ethambutol, and clarithromycin given daily for at least 12 months of negative sputum cultures. These results are in sharp contrast to the experience of many expert consultants in the United States who find *M. simiae* to be among the most difficult to treat of the pulmonary NTM pathogens. Some experts suggest using macrolide-based regimens with other agents, such as amikacin, fluoroquinolones, sulfamethoxazole, and linezolid.[2] A reasonable regimen would include at least three of the following drugs: azithromycin 250 to 500 mg/day, moxifloxacin 400 mg/day, trimethoprim-sulfamethoxazole 800 or 160 mg twice a day, linezolid 600 mg/day, and amikacin 10 to 15 mg/kg/day IV or 15 to 25 mg/kg three times a week. Optimal treatment duration is unknown, and experts consider treating at least 12 months after culture conversion.[2]

Mycobacterium szulgai

M. szulgai is characterized primarily by cavitary disease in patients with underlying chronic pulmonary disease that resembles disease due to *M. tuberculosis*. As with other NTM pathogens, it can also be associated with nodular bronchiectatic disease. The organism is often susceptible in vitro to most anti-TB drugs and to the fluoroquinolones and macrolides.[266–270] Most respiratory isolates of *M. szulgai* are associated with significant lung disease: 73% (11 of 15) of patients in The Netherlands who grew *M. szulgai* from their sputum met current ATS/IDSA criteria for disease.[271] In vitro susceptibilities demonstrate susceptibility to rifampin, isoniazid, ethambutol, and clarithromycin. Regimens containing rifamycin, ethambutol, and clarithromycin, with or without a fluoroquinolone administered for approximately 12 months, have almost 100% treatment success.[271] Unlike many other NTM pathogens, susceptibility on in vitro testing for *M. szulgai* appears to predict favorable treatment response.

RAPIDLY GROWING MYCOBACTERIA

RGM are distinguished by growth in subculture in less than 7 days and comprise approximately 100 distinct species (http://www.bacterio.net/mycobacterium.html), at least 30 of which have been associated with lung disease, although rarely (see Table 35.1). Because many RGM are not pathogenic in humans, it is important to subclassify organisms within this group to the species, and even subspecies level in the case of *M. abscessus*, because this affects both treatment and prognosis. Although RGM can produce pulmonary disease, they have a propensity to produce skin and soft tissue infections.

Mycobacterium abscessus

M. abscessus causes at least 80% of pulmonary infections due to RGM in the United States.[95] Genomic sequencing has determined that *M. abscessus* can be divided into three subspecies: *M. abscessus abscessus*, *M. abscessus bolletii*, and *M. abscessus massiliense*.[272] Most patients with pulmonary disease due to *M. abscessus* are nonsmoking white women older than 60 years who have no predisposing conditions, a similar patient population as seen with nodular bronchiectatic MAC pulmonary disease.[95] The usual clinical presentation is similar to that of other NTM pulmonary infections and includes cough and easy fatigability. For most patients with no predisposing conditions, the disease is slowly progressive; however, more fulminant, rapidly progressive disease has been seen in patients with gastroesophageal disorders and CF. The chest radiograph usually shows multilobar, patchy, reticulonodular, or mixed reticulonodular-alveolar opacities (Fig. 55.7). High-resolution CT findings include the presence of cylindrical bronchiectasis with multiple small nodules, similar to the findings in MAC pulmonary disease.[95,273,274] Cavitation has been reported in 10–20% of patients.

Therapy of *Mycobacterium abscessus* Pulmonary Disease. *M. abscessus* is typically resistant in vitro to most of the medications used to treat TB and has demonstrated in vitro activity to only a few antimicrobial agents. Cure can be elusive for many patients with *M. abscessus* disease. Among 65 patients from South Korea with *M. abscessus* pulmonary disease treated with a standardized regimen, including 4 weeks of IV amikacin and cefoxitin, along with oral ciprofloxacin, clarithromycin, and doxycycline for a total duration of 24 months, 58% of patients had sputum conversion with maintenance of negative sputum cultures for more than 12 months.[275] In a study from the United States, 107 patients were treated with individualized therapy that included IV imipenem (or cefoxitin) and amikacin along with various oral and inhaled combinations of therapy.[276] Results showed that 48% converted and maintained negative cultures for at least 12 months.

Current guidelines recommend that therapy usually consists of 2 to 4 months of IV agents, such as imipenem, cefoxitin, tigecycline plus amikacin given daily or three times weekly.[4] Oral agents demonstrating in vitro activity should be included in the treatment regimen. Although

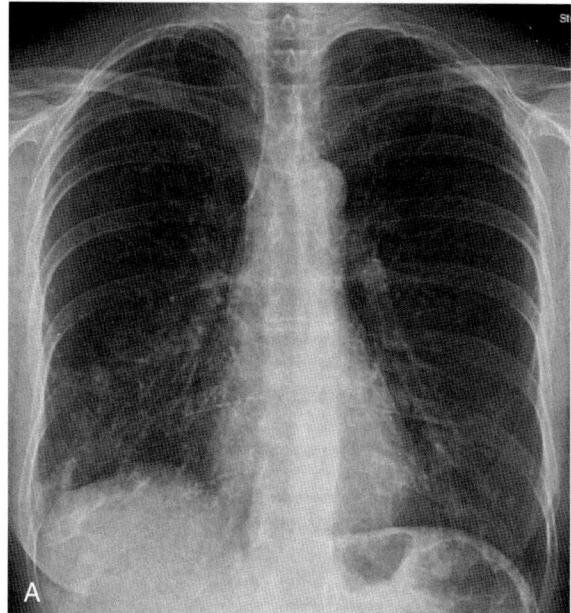

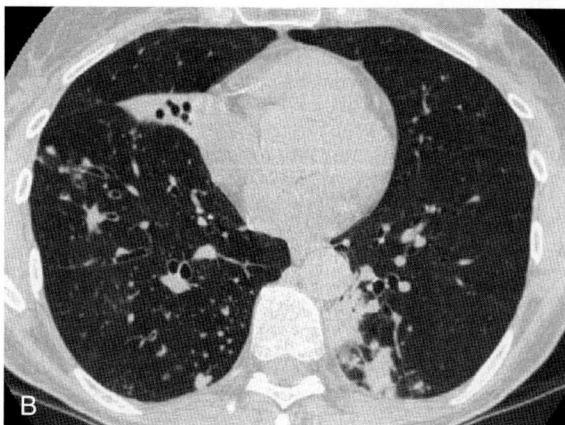

Figure 55.7 *Mycobacterium abscessus.* A 68-year-old nonsmoking woman with several-year history of cough, fatigue, and weight loss. Her sputum cultures were consistently positive for *M. abscessus*. (A) Chest radiograph showing middle and lower lung zone nodular opacities and bronchiectasis. (B) Chest computed tomography scan showing right middle lobe atelectasis and bronchiectasis with bilateral lower lobe bronchiectasis and nodular opacities. Note the left lower lobe air space opacity in this patient with severe reflux and probable chronic aspiration.

macrolides have traditionally been used in this role, recent studies have questioned the importance of macrolides in the treatment of *M. abscessus* subsp. *abscessus* because approximately 80–90% of strains contain a functional *erm(41)* gene[277–279]; when the organism is incubated in the presence of clarithromycin, the gene is induced and the organism rapidly acquires macrolide resistance. (Approximately 15% of strains of *M. abscessus* subsp. *abscessus* have a T to C mutation at position 28 that renders the *erm(41)* gene nonfunctional.) In contrast, *M. massiliense* has a truncated, nonfunctional copy of the gene, so macrolide resistance is not induced in the presence of clarithromycin.[279] In a study from South Korea, patients infected with *M. massiliense* were more likely to improve clinically, radiographically, and bacteriologically than those with *M. abscessus*: Eighty-eight percent of those with *M. massiliense* converted sputum cultures to negative, compared to 25% with *M. abscessus*.[279]

In a recent systematic review and meta-analysis, sustained culture conversion was reported in 54% of those with subsp. *massiliense* compared to only 34% of patients with subsp. *abscessus*.[280] Similarly, an individual patient data meta-analysis noted treatment success in 57% of patients with subsp. *massiliense*, compared to only 33% of patients with subsp. *abscessus*.[281] Limited data suggest that azithromycin may be more effective against *M. abscessus* than is clarithromycin.[281-283]

Species identification discriminating between subsp. *abscessus* and subsp. *massiliense* would inform clinicians about the likely presence of an active *erm(41)* gene and the best presumptive antibiotic choices but is frequently not available from hospital or reference laboratories. However, the presence of an active *erm(41)* gene can be ascertained in most specialized mycobacteriology laboratories in a relatively short time frame and is the critical information needed by the clinician to guide antibiotic therapy for isolates initially identified as *M. abscessus*.

Linezolid, an oxazolidinone, is active against some strains of *M. abscessus* but is frequently associated with significant hematologic toxicity and peripheral neuropathy, particularly at higher doses.[284-286] Tedizolid, another oxazolidinone, has greater in vitro activity than linezolid, but clinical data are lacking.[287,288] Tigecycline has significant in vitro activity against *M. abscessus* but is available only as an IV preparation and is associated with significant nausea and vomiting.[289,290] Eravacycline and omadacycline are two recently released cyclines with similar activity to that of tigecycline and may be better tolerated.[288] Clofazimine has in vitro activity against *M. abscessus* and synergistic activity with amikacin,[291] but its role in the management of these patients remains to be defined. Studies that included clofazimine in treatment regimens in patients with *M. avium* complex and also *M. abscessus* have demonstrated modest improvement in patients with refractory disease.[210,292]

Once the patient has demonstrated a clinical response to therapy, there are several possible choices for continued treatment: (1) stop therapy after 2 to 4 months and follow the patient for signs of progression of disease and, if present, periodically reinstitute treatment; (2) stop the aminoglycoside and continue the cefoxitin or imipenem for a longer period along with oral agent(s); or (3) continue the oral agent(s) and institute inhaled amikacin. The studies published to date reported experiences with options 2 and 3. However, the optimum choice is not known; ultimately, treatment decisions therefore will need to be individualized, and often some form of therapy will be given periodically on a lifelong basis. Expert consultation is strongly recommended.

A combination of surgical resection and chemotherapy may increase the chance of cure in patients who have focal lung disease and who can tolerate resection.[275,276] If resection is planned, patients should be treated with an initial period of antimicrobial drug therapy before surgery to lessen the bacillary load. In three studies, patients who underwent surgical resection in addition to antimicrobial chemotherapy had improved microbiologic outcomes compared with those who received chemotherapy alone.[95,275,276] As with MAC pulmonary disease, surgery should be performed by thoracic surgeons experienced in performing this type of surgery.[293]

Therapy of *Mycobacterium abscessus* Skin, Soft tissue, and Bone Infections. Serious infections should be treated with a regimen similar to that used for pulmonary disease. Skin and soft tissue infections should be treated for a minimum of 4 months and bone infections for a minimum of 6 months.[2] Surgery is generally indicated for extensive disease, abscess formation, or when drug therapy is difficult. Foreign bodies, such as prosthetic joints, percutaneous catheters, and breast implants, should be removed and the patient treated with a prolonged antimicrobial treatment regimen.

Mycobacterium chelonae

M. chelonae is more likely to produce skin, soft tissue, and bone infections than pulmonary disease.[149] Keratitis due to *M. chelonae* has been associated with wearing contact lenses and with ocular surgery, such as *laser-assisted in situ keratomileusis* (LASIK).[294,295] Disseminated disease has been reported in immunocompromised patients and usually presents with characteristic cutaneous lesions.[296] The clinical and radiographic presentation of *M. chelonae* pulmonary disease is similar to that of other RGM.

Isolates of *M. chelonae* are usually susceptible to tobramycin, macrolides, linezolid, and imipenem.[155,297,298] The *M. chelonae* genome does not include an active *erm* gene, so macrolides should be considered active.[277] Other active drugs may include amikacin, clofazimine, doxycycline, and the fluoroquinolones. *M. chelonae* isolates are uniformly resistant to cefoxitin. Treatment of *M. chelonae* infections should be based on in vitro susceptibility results. Administration of clarithromycin 500 mg twice daily for 6 months was reported to have a high cure rate in patients with cutaneous lesions associated with disseminated disease.[299] However, one patient who relapsed did so with a macrolide-resistant strain, so multidrug regimens are recommended. Patients have also responded to linezolid with or without clarithromycin.[300,301] Patients with serious skin, soft tissue, and bone infections should be treated with two or more drugs similar to those used in *M. abscessus* disease. For corneal infections, both topical and oral agents are often used, and many patients may require corneal transplants for recovery of vision or cure.

Mycobacterium fortuitum Complex

Mycobacterium fortuitum complex consists of 12 species,[302-304] of which *M. fortuitum* is the most common in respiratory specimens.[305] *M. fortuitum* is responsible for at most 15% of RGM infections in the United States but is a relatively uncommon cause of pulmonary disease except in patients with disorders associated with chronic aspiration.[95] Among 26 patients in the Republic of Korea with two or more positive cultures for *M. fortuitum*, only one was treated, and none of the 25 untreated patients showed progression over a median of 12.5 months of follow-up.[306] The clinical and radiographic presentation of patients with pulmonary disease is similar to that of other RGM. Application of current diagnostic guidelines must be used with caution and even some skepticism when evaluating patients with *M. fortuitum* respiratory isolates. Skin, soft tissue, and bone infections are more common than pulmonary disease. Both sporadic and clustered outbreaks of furunculosis due to *M. fortuitum* (and other RGM) have been reported after exposure to contaminated water during pedicures.[307–309]

In contrast to *M. abscessus*, *M. fortuitum* demonstrates broader in vitro susceptibility to both oral and IV antimicrobial drugs, including the newer macrolides, the fluoroquinolones, doxycycline, minocycline, the sulfonamides, and two IV drugs—imipenem and cefoxitin.[2] Although most isolates of *M. fortuitum* are susceptible in vitro to the macrolides, these drugs should be used with caution because of the presence of an inducible erythromycin methylase (*erm*) gene, *erm(39)*.[310] Greater than 80% of *M. fortuitum*, *Mycobacterium porcinum*, and *Mycobacterium septicum* are inducibly resistant to clarithromycin, in contrast to *Mycobacterium peregrinum*, which is inducibly resistant in about one-third of isolates.[305]

M. fortuitum lung disease should be treated with at least two drugs to which in vitro susceptibility has been demonstrated.[2] As with other NTM pulmonary infections, treatment should be continued for at least 12 months of negative sputum cultures. Skin, soft tissue, and bone infections should be treated similarly to *M. abscessus* infections, although more effective oral agents are usually available.

CYSTIC FIBROSIS AND NONTUBERCULOUS MYCOBACTERIA

Individuals with CF have particularly high rates of NTM pulmonary disease, which appear to be increasing. The true rate of NTM infection is difficult to determine due to variability in screening practices, culture techniques, and data collection.[78] Estimates of the prevalence of NTM isolation in people with CF have ranged from a low of 1.3% in the earliest study from 1984[311] to as high as 50% in individuals older than 40 years seen at an adult CF clinic in Colorado.[312] Some of the largest studies, including more than 1000 patients each, reported isolation prevalences ranging from 6.6–13.7%.[91–93] More recent longitudinal data from the U.S. CF Patient Care Registry reported that, of 16,153 persons with CF, 20% had a least one pathogenic NTM species isolated over a 5-year period, although this varied geographically (see Fig. 55.2).[94]

As with NTM disease in non-CF patients, the prevalence appears to be increasing in persons with CF. Among individuals younger than 16 years, the prevalence of an NTM-positive respiratory culture increased from 1.3% in 2010 to 3.8% in 2015. In a study from Israel the NTM prevalence increased threefold from 5% in 2003 to 14.5% in 2011.[313] Using data from the U.S. CF Patient Care Registry, NTM disease prevalence showed a significant relative increase of 5% per year from 11.0% in 2010 to 13.4% in 2014.[94]

The most common NTM to cause pulmonary disease in people with CF are MAC and *M. abscessus*. Their relative importance varies by geographic area and age. For example, in Europe, *M. abscessus* is isolated in 40–60% of cases compared with 15–25% in the United States.[314] And, in the United States, MAC, on the other hand, has been isolated in up to 70% of people with CF who have NTM isolated. Of importance, approximately 25% of patients have another NTM isolated in 5 years and 36% at 10 years, so reinfection is common.[315] *M. abscessus* affects patients at a younger age than MAC, with one study from France reporting that 90% of people with CF acquired *M. abscessus* by 10 years of age.[316]

A number of risk factors have been associated with acquisition of NTM infection. Studies from both the United States and Europe have described increasing NTM prevalence with increasing age.[91,317] For example, data from the European CF Registry showed that for every decade increase in life, the risk of acquiring NTM increased by 17.5%.[317] In Denver, Colorado, among adults with CF who were older than 40 years, 32.7% had positive NTM cultures.[312] Other risk factors for NTM infection have included concurrent allergic bronchopulmonary aspergillosis, chronic *Pseudomonas* infection, and use of inhaled steroids.[314] Proximity to water and high amounts of atmospheric water content have been associated with an increased risk of NTM infection. In one study in the United States, for every one-unit increase in saturated water vapor pressure, the risk of NTM infection increased by 6%.[53]

Chronic azithromycin has been shown to decrease pulmonary exacerbations and improve lung function in people with CF and chronic *Pseudomonas* infection.[318] Concern has been raised about the potential of azithromycin monotherapy leading to development of macrolide-resistant NTM infections. A nested-case control study using data from the U.S. Cystic Fibrosis Foundation Patient Registry found that long-term azithromycin use was associated with a decreased risk of acquiring NTM (MAC or *M. abscessus*) in adolescents and adults with CF.[319] A study of adults with CF in France reported similar findings, but one *M. avium* isolate acquired macrolide resistance.[320] The development of macrolide-resistant NTM remains a concern, so individuals with CF should be screened for evidence of NTM pulmonary infection before initiation of macrolide monotherapy and periodically while on therapy.

As noted previously (see "Transmission and Pathogenesis"), several studies have described possible transmission of *M. abscessus* from human to human in CF clinics,[60–62] whereas other studies have been unable to confirm transmission despite high degrees of genomic similarity between strains of *M. abscessus*.[73–75] Although WGS has provided a powerful tool to improve our understanding of transmission of NTM, the sequencing information will need to be paired with rigorous environmental assessments and epidemiology to explain the transmission dynamics of NTM in CF populations.

The U.S. CF Foundation and European Cystic Fibrosis Society have published guidelines for the diagnosis and treatment of NTM infections in people with CF.[321] Cultures for NTM are recommended annually in spontaneously expectorating individuals even when stable. ATS/IDSA diagnostic criteria (see Table 55.3) are recommended, but, because of the high rate of concurrent bacterial and fungal infections and universally abnormal radiographs, application of the criteria is often more challenging than in a non-CF bronchiectasis population. Approximately 50–60% of those with CF who have an NTM isolated from respiratory specimens will convert cultures to negative without antimicrobial therapy.[315,322] In retrospective studies of children and adults with CF, approximately 60–70% of patients had evidence of transient or stable NTM disease.[315,323] As in non-CF bronchiectasis, isolation of NTM from a respiratory specimen does not necessarily mean that progressive disease will follow. Ultimately, the decision to treat will be based on whether the patient is responding to treatment of other copathogens (e.g., *Pseudomonas*), the virulence of the infecting species, evidence of radiographic progression, loss of lung function over time, and bacterial load (e.g., acid-fast bacilli smear status).

Treatment of NTM pulmonary disease uses the same general approach as is used in non-CF patients. A three-drug macrolide-containing regimen is administered for macrolide-susceptible MAC pulmonary disease; however, unlike with non-CF bronchiectatic disease, intermittent therapy is not recommended because of the concern for inadequate drug absorption and lung penetration.[321] As in non-CF patients, azithromycin is the preferred macrolide. With the widespread use of CFTR-modulating drugs, rifamycins have become difficult to use because of drug interactions through the CYP3A4/5 system. Rifamycins are strong inducers of this enzyme system, and ivacaftor is metabolized through this system, resulting in low serum concentrations when coadministered with a rifamycin.[324] Currently, rifamycins are not recommended to be used with CFTR modulators.

Treatment outcome data are very limited but tend to mirror those in non-CF patients with NTM pulmonary disease. In a retrospective review of CF patients from Colorado, the rate of culture conversion in response to treatment for MAC was 60%.[315] Eradication of *M. abscessus* in children and adults with CF has been reported in 20–50% of patients using GBT.[325-328] In a retrospective study, including 37 CF patients with *M. abscessus* pulmonary disease, of whom most were treated with a multidrug GBT regimen, only 10 patients experienced sustained culture conversion.[325] In a retrospective review of CF patients from Colorado, the rate of culture conversion in response to treatment for *M. abscessus* (not subspeciated) was 45%.[315] However, lung function improved, demonstrating a treatment benefit. In another study reporting treatment outcomes in patients with NTM pulmonary disease, treatment was associated with a reversal of the pretreatment decline in FEV_1% predicted.[315] As in non-CF patients with *M. abscessus* pulmonary disease, treatment outcomes for *M. abscessus* subsp. *massiliense* are much better than for subsp. *abscessus*, with cultures converting in greater than 80% of patients with subsp. *abscessus* compared with 25% of those with subsp. *abscessus*.[93]

CF is the most common indication for lung transplantation in children and the third most common condition leading to lung transplantation in adults.[329,330] The U.S. CF Foundation and European Cystic Fibrosis Society recommend that all individuals with CF being considered for lung transplantation should be evaluated for NTM pulmonary disease and that the presence of NTM should not preclude individuals from being evaluated for transplant.[321] In the largest CF-specific cases series from the University of North Carolina, approximately 20% of people with CF referred for lung transplantation had NTM isolated from respiratory specimens.[331] In a study of CF and non-CF transplants, NTM was isolated after transplantation in 22.4% (53 of 237 individuals), of whom two fulfilled ATS/IDSA diagnostic criteria for disease.[332] Although morbidity after transplant can be significant, mortality has varied between studies.

M. abscessus pulmonary disease has been considered by some to be a relative contraindication for lung transplantation in CF patients[122,333]; however, recent reports suggest that lung transplantation for CF patients with *M. abscessus* infection can be accomplished with success rates comparable to CF patients without infection.[334-337] For patients with isolation of *M. abscessus* before transplantation, treatment with a multidrug regimen before and after transplantation has been successful even when the organism could not be eradicated pretransplantation.[336,337] In one report, patients infected with *M. abscessus* subsp. *massiliense* did better than those with subsp. *abscessus*.[338] Nevertheless, *M. abscessus* infection in patients with CF who have undergone lung transplantation can have significant posttransplant infections that can be severe and sometimes fatal.[120-122] Current guidelines do not recognize infection with NTM, including *M. abscessus*, as a contraindication for lung transplant.[321]

SURGICAL RESECTION

Patients with NTM pulmonary disease whose disease is predominantly localized to one lung and who can tolerate resectional surgery should be considered for surgery under the following conditions: (1) poor response to drug therapy, (2) development of macrolide-resistant MAC disease, or (3) presence of significant disease-related complications, such as hemoptysis. Outcomes of surgery have generally been good, with greater than 80% culture conversion documented postoperatively.[4,293,339,340] Operative mortality has been low, and complications (e.g., bronchopleural fistula, prolonged air leak, and pneumonia) have been reported in 7–35% of cases.[4] In a study reporting the outcomes of 134 patients undergoing video-assisted thoracoscopic surgery, there were no deaths, the complication rate was 7%, and cultures converted in 84% of the patients.[340] Whenever possible, surgery should be performed by thoracic surgeons who have had considerable experience with resectional lung surgery for mycobacterial disease.[293] Surgery for NTM pulmonary disease can be technically difficult due to pleural adhesions, fibrotic lung tissue, fused fissures, and hypertrophied bronchial circulation.[341]

THERAPEUTIC DRUG MONITORING

The role of therapeutic drug monitoring remains unclear. Low serum concentrations of clarithromycin have been reported when the drug is given in combination with rifampin.[342,343] A study that examined the pharmacokinetic and pharmacodynamic relationships in 481 patients with MAC pulmonary disease reported that peak serum concentrations were below the target range for ethambutol (48%), clarithromycin (56%), and azithromycin (35%).[343] Concurrent administration of rifampin reduced the serum concentration of clarithromycin by 68% and that of azithromycin by 23%. Pharmacodynamic indices were seldom met for rifampicin, clarithromycin, amikacin, and moxifloxacin. This study did not examine a possible correlation between clinical outcome and the poor pharmacodynamics indices. A study from South Korea reported that peak plasma concentrations of clarithromycin were lower in MAC patients who received daily or intermittent therapy when in conjunction with rifampicin compared with *M. abscessus* patients who received clarithromycin without rifampicin.[344] In this study, treatment outcomes were not associated with plasma drug concentrations; however, no attempt was made to increase the dosage in patients with low concentrations to see if outcomes would have improved. In a subsequent study, a higher maximum azithromycin serum concentration was associated with favorable microbiologic responses in patients who received daily therapy but not in those who received intermittent therapy.[345] Therapeutic drug monitoring should be considered in patients who are not responding to therapy, have end-stage renal disease, are receiving aminoglycosides, or are taking medications known to cause drug interactions.[2]

HYPERSENSITIVITY PNEUMONITIS–LIKE NONTUBERCULOUS MYCOBACTERIA PULMONARY DISEASE

Most reports describing the development of a typical pattern of hypersensitivity pneumonitis-like pulmonary disease have been in patients associated with hot tub exposure, although similar clinical presentations have been associated with other indoor standing water sources and exposures.[64,346,347] In the cases of exposure to hot tubs, MAC has been isolated from sputum, bronchoalveolar lavage, tissue, and hot tub water. Furthermore, when assessed by genotyping methods, MAC isolates from both the hot tub water and the lung specimens have demonstrated identical patterns. Controversy still exists, however, as to whether hot tub lung is an infectious process, inflammatory process, or a combination.

Patients with hypersensitivity pneumonitis-like lung disease tend to be young and without preexisting lung disease. The clinical presentation varies from mild respiratory symptoms to respiratory failure requiring mechanical ventilatory support.[348] Key elements to the diagnosis of MAC hypersensitivity-like lung disease include a compatible clinical history (subacute onset of respiratory symptoms, hot tub exposure); characteristic radiographic findings (diffuse centrilobular nodules and ground-glass opacities) (eFig. 55.3); and MAC isolates in sputum, bronchoalveolar lavage, tissue, and hot tub water (and compatible histopathology when available).

Patient prognosis is generally excellent independent of severity on presentation.[346] The most benefit is gained by simply removing the patient from further antigen exposure. In the case of hot tub lung, removal from antigen exposure generally involves drainage of hot tub water and complete avoidance of hot tub use. Whether continued exposure to ambient environmental MAC organisms can propagate the hypersensitivity pulmonary reaction is uncertain. For selected patients with hypersensitivity pneumonitis-like lung disease, use of systemic corticosteroids may be of benefit and hasten recovery of pulmonary symptoms, gas-exchange abnormalities, and radiographic abnormalities. Likewise, antimycobacterial therapy, with the same medications as for standard pulmonary MAC lung disease, may be required in some patients but for shorter durations of therapy, usually 3 to 6 months. Most patients can be expected to have nearly complete resolution of respiratory symptoms and of pulmonary function and radiographic abnormalities.

PREVENTION OF NONTUBERCULOUS MYCOBACTERIA INFECTIONS

NTM are ubiquitous in the environment, so complete avoidance is difficult, if not impossible. The organisms generally have very low virulence for humans compared with *M. tuberculosis*, so NTM disease may be more of a problem with host susceptibility than with organism virulence. With some notable exceptions previously discussed, the specific susceptibility of an individual patient to NTM infection may be impossible to determine at this point; in accordance, disease prevention remains problematic. The question remains, however, should patients with known vulnerabilities to NTM infection be advised to avoid known environmental sources of NTM? For instance, should vulnerable patients be advised not to take showers, which are known to be colonized with NTM?[63,64,349,350] Currently the answer is unknown, and prevention of most environmentally acquired NTM infection remains a challenge.

HEALTH CARE–ASSOCIATED NONTUBERCULOUS MYCOBACTERIA DISEASE

Transmission of NTM disease in the health care setting has most frequently been linked to tap (municipal) water exposure.[142] Since 2013, there has been a global outbreak of disseminated disease due to *M. chimaera* related to exposure to heater-cooler units during various cardiac surgeries.[83–85] The infections were eventually tracked to water contamination at the factory.[351,352] Although various NTM species, including MAC, *M. kansasii*, *M. xenopi*, and *M. simiae*, have been isolated from municipal water supplies, *M. fortuitum* and *M. abscessus* have been most often implicated in health care–associated NTM disease. Even with use of potent disinfectants, including organomercurials, chlorine, bromine, 2% formaldehyde, and glutaraldehyde, NTM organisms may persist on equipment or devices after tap water exposure. The large outbreak of *M. massiliense* in Brazil involved a single clone tolerant to 2% glutaraldehyde.[79] The inability to eliminate these organisms underscores the importance of avoidance of tap water for preventing health care–associated NTM diseases, such as those after median sternotomy; cosmetic surgery procedures; liposuction; LASIK; dialysis; and the implantation of long-term central IV catheters, tympanostomy tubes and prosthetic devices, such as heart valves, knee and hip joints, lens implants, and metal rod bone stabilizers.[2] Pseudo-outbreaks have involved bronchoscopes contaminated with *M. abscessus*, *M. simiae*, and *M. immunogenum*. Documented outbreaks of *M. fortuitum* and *M. mageritense* furunculosis in association with use of contaminated whirlpool footbaths have been described in nail salons.[307–309,353]

As a result of the increased understanding of environmental NTM reservoirs and reports linking the use of tap water to health care–associated NTM infections (and pseudoinfections), it is recommended that tap water never be used in preparation of surgical procedures, prosthetics, intravascular catheters, in cleaning fiberoptic endoscopes, or in rinsing the mouth out before collecting expectorated sputum samples. Moreover, recognition that alternative medicines or unapproved substances for injection may also be at risk of contamination by NTM warrants caution against use of these products as well.

- Treatment of rapidly growing mycobacterial infections should be based on the results of in vitro drug susceptibility testing, but the clinical outcome varies significantly depending on the causative species and presence of a functional erythromycin resistance methylase (41) gene.
- Health care–associated infections have been linked to the use of tap water, a reservoir for certain NTM. Tap water should never be used to wash surgical instruments, clean fiberoptic endoscopes, or rinse out the mouth before collecting sputum samples.

Key Points

- *Nontuberculous mycobacteria* (NTM) comprise approximately 200 different species and subspecies that are ubiquitous in our environment. Members of the *Mycobacterium avium* complex (MAC) are the most common causes of NTM pulmonary disease.
- Infection follows exposure to NTM in the environment: Human-to-human transmission is exceptionally uncommon, except perhaps in the setting of cystic fibrosis.
- Epidemiologic studies suggest that the prevalence of NTM infections is increasing in some areas of the world, including the United States.
- Risk factors for pulmonary NTM disease include underlying chronic lung diseases, such as bronchiectasis, chronic obstructive pulmonary diseases, cystic fibrosis, alpha$_1$-antitrypsin deficiency, and prior tuberculosis.
- Diagnosis of NTM pulmonary infections is often challenging and requires that the patient meet certain clinical, radiographic, and microbiologic criteria.
- The recommended treatment for MAC pulmonary disease is a macrolide, plus ethambutol and a rifamycin, with or without an aminoglycoside administered for at least 12 months of culture negativity. Macrolides should *never* be used as monotherapy for treatment of MAC disease, either pulmonary or disseminated.
- For treatment-refractory MAC, amikacin liposome inhalational suspension should be added to guideline-based therapy.
- The recommended treatment for *Mycobacterium kansasii* pulmonary disease is a macrolide (or isoniazid), a rifamycin, and ethambutol administered for at least 12 months.
- Resectional surgery should be considered for patients with focal disease and (1) poor response to drug therapy, (2) development of macrolide-resistant MAC disease, or (3) presence of significant disease-related complications, such as hemoptysis.

Key Readings

Adjemian J, Olivier KN, Seitz AE, Holland SM, Prevots DR. Prevalence of nontuberculous mycobacterial lung disease in U.S. Medicare beneficiaries. *Am J Respir Crit Care Med.* 2012;185:881–886.

Brown-Elliott BA, Woods GL. Antimycobacterial susceptibility testing of nontuberculous mycobacteria. *J Clin Microbiol.* 2019;57(10). e00834-19.

Bryant JM, Grogono DM, Greaves D, et al. Whole-genome sequencing to identify transmission of *Mycobacterium abscessus* between patients with cystic fibrosis: a retrospective cohort study. *Lancet.* 2013;381:1551–1560.

Daley CL, Iaccarino JM, Lange C, et al. Treatment of nontuberculous mycobacterial pulmonary disease: an official ATS/ERS/ESCMID/IDSA clinical practice guideline: executive summary. *Clin Infect Dis.* 2020;71(4):905–913.

Falkinham 3rd JO. Nontuberculous mycobacteria from household plumbing of patients with nontuberculous mycobacteria disease. *Emerg Infect Dis.* 2011;17:419–424.

Griffith DE, Aksamit T, Brown-Elliott BA, et al. An official ATS/IDSA statement: diagnosis, treatment, and prevention of nontuberculous mycobacterial diseases. *Am J Respir Crit Care Med.* 2007;175:367–416.

Griffith DE, Eagel G, Thomson R, et al. Amikacin liposome inhalation suspension for treatment-refractory lung disease caused by *Mycobacterium avium* complex (CONVERT). A prospective, open-label, randomized study. *Am J Respir Crit Care Med.* 2018;198:1559–1569.

Haworth CS, Banks J, Capstick T, et al. British Thoracic Society guidelines for the management of non-tuberculous mycobacterial pulmonary disease (NTM-PD). *Thorax.* 2017;72:ii1–ii64.

Kim RD, Greenberg DE, Ehrmantraut ME, et al. Pulmonary nontuberculous mycobacterial disease: prospective study of a distinct preexisting syndrome. *Am J Respir Crit Care Med.* 2008;178:1066–1074.

Koh WJ, Jeon K, Lee NY, et al. Clinical significance of differentiation of *Mycobacterium massiliense* from *Mycobacterium abscessus. Am J Respir Crit Care Med.* 2011;183:405–410.

van Ingen J, Boeree MJ, van Soolingen D, Mouton JW. Resistance mechanisms and drug susceptibility testing of nontuberculous mycobacteria. *Drug Resist Updat.* 2012;15:149–161.

van Ingen J, Egelund EF, Levin A, et al. The pharmacokinetics and pharmacodynamics of pulmonary *Mycobacterium avium* complex disease treatment. *Am J Respir Crit Care Med.* 2012;186:559–565.

Winthrop KL, Marras TK, Adjemian J, Zhang H, Wang P, Zhang Q. Incidence and prevalence of nontuberculous mycobacterial lung disease in a large U.S. managed care health plan, 2008-2015. *Ann Am Thorac Soc.* 2020;17:178–185.

Complete reference list available at ExpertConsult.com.

56 FUNGAL INFECTIONS: ENDEMIC

JOSHUA D. NOSANCHUK, MD • GEORGE R. THOMPSON III, MD

Note: Antifungal drugs and their use are included in Chapter 57.

INTRODUCTION

Geographically restricted (or endemic) mycoses include histoplasmosis, coccidioidomycosis, blastomycosis, paracoccidioidomycosis, sporotrichosis, talaromycosis (formerly penicilliosis), and emergomycosis (Fig. 56.1). These are *dimorphic* pathogens because they grow as two forms: as mycelium in nature and as yeasts (or spherules) upon acquisition by humans. *Mycelium*, the vegetative part of a fungus, consists of branching structures called hyphae and represents the mold form of the fungus. *Yeasts* are single-celled forms of the fungus and represent the major pathogenic form. These phases can be achieved in the laboratory by cultivation of the fungi at lower ($\approx 25^\circ$C, mycelial) or higher (37°C, yeast) temperatures. Hence these fungi are termed thermally dimorphic. Acquisition is typically via inhalation of spores or mycelial fragments, although sporotrichosis is most commonly acquired by direct inoculation through the skin. The severity of clinical illness is linked to the quantity of the inoculum as well as to the immunologic status of the individual. Defects in cellular immunity are especially associated with more severe disease. Latent infections can reactivate in individuals whose immune responses have been compromised, such as by corticosteroid therapy, receipt of *tumor necrosis factor* (TNF) inhibitors or other immune-modulating agents, chemotherapy, or *human immunodeficiency virus* (HIV). The geographically restricted mycoses are often overlooked as etiologies of infectious syndromes, including as causes of community-acquired pneumonia.[1] In part this happens when clinical disease manifests in individuals outside of the geographic territories historically linked to endemicity of the pathogens.

Diagnosis is frequently delayed, and treatment of these diseases requires several months to more than 1 year. Because the forms that exist in tissues differ from the forms transmitted in the environment, these pathogens are not transmitted between humans.

HISTOPLASMA

HISTORY AND EPIDEMIOLOGY

Histoplasma is a dimorphic fungus primarily acquired via respiratory exposure that is responsible for approximately 500,000 infections annually in the United States, which makes it the most prevalent cause of fungal pulmonary disease.[2] Similarly, these calculations also indicate that nearly 50 million Americans are latently infected with the fungus. The fungus can be found worldwide, although there are areas with a high incidence of disease. The Ohio and Mississippi River valleys are highly endemic regions, and skin testing has shown that up to 90% of adults in these regions have been exposed to the fungus.[3,4] High endemicity areas are also present in Latin America, particularly in Brazil, Venezuela, Ecuador, Paraguay, Uruguay, and Argentina.[5]

The most recent data on rates of clinically significant disease in the United States are from an analysis conducted by the Centers for Disease Control and Prevention between 2011 and 2014.[6] This report relied on surveillance data available from state health departments and did not include two states with a high incidence of histoplasmosis (Missouri and Tennessee). Even with this limitation, 3409 symptomatic cases were reported. The median age of patients was 49 years and 61% of patients ($n = 1273$) were male; 57% were hospitalized and 7% died. The incidence rates varied markedly between and within states, and the majority of cases were observed in counties abutting the Mississippi

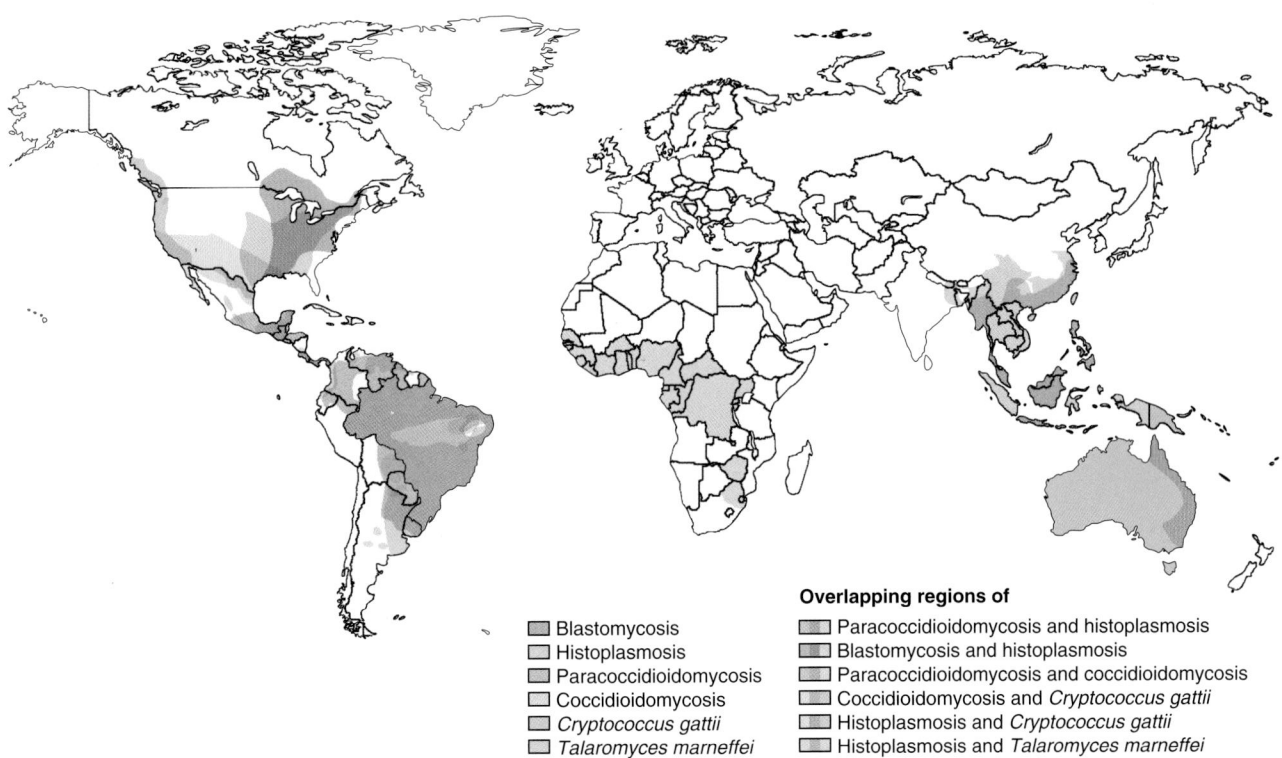

Figure 56.1 Global distribution of the endemic fungi. Although there is geographic restriction of the specific fungi, there is also overlap in the geographic ranges, and the differential diagnosis in those overlapping regions is more challenging. (From Schwartz S, Kontoyiannis DP, Harrison T, Ruhnke M: Advances in the diagnosis and treatment of fungal infections of the CNS. *Lancet Neurol* 2018;17[4]:362–372.)

River. The high hospitalization rate suggests that histoplasmosis surveillance underestimates the true number of cases. A similar male predominance has been observed in other studies of histoplasmosis and for patients with other fungal infections, including coccidioidomycosis and blastomycosis.[7–9] The reasons for this gender disparity are not clear, although differences in recreational or occupational exposure have been proposed.[10]

The genus *Histoplasma* was designated in 1906 by Samuel Darling, who described the fungus in the lungs, liver, spleen, and lymph nodes of a carpenter from Martinique working on the Panama Canal.[11] Darling incorrectly characterized the 1- to 4-μm intracellular ovoid yeast as protozoa, similar to *Leishmania* sp. A genome-wide population genetic study suggested that the genus *Histoplasma* contains at least four species that are genetically isolated, although these taxonomic changes have not been uniformly accepted.[12]

PATHOGENESIS

Histoplasma exists in either a mycelial or yeast form, depending mainly on temperature and nutritional conditions.[13] In the environment and at ambient temperatures, *Histoplasma* is mycelial. This saprophytic mold grows particularly well in soils enriched with organic nitrogen sources, such as soil contaminated with bird or bat droppings. Hyphal elements are 1.25 to 2.0 μm in diameter, and they produce two types of conidia: thick-walled macroconidia (8–15 μm diameter) and microconidia (2–5 μm). Both conidial forms are produced singly at the tips of narrow, short conidiophores that branch at right angles to vegetative hyphae. The microconidia are believed to be the infectious form because their size is most effective for aerosolization and inhalation and deposition into distal lung structures. Environmental disturbances, especially construction or tree removal, are associated with aerosolization of *Histoplasma* and have been associated with outbreaks.[7] At 37°C or in humans, the yeast form predominates. Yeast cells have thin walls and are oval with diameters of 2 to 5 μm. The cells reproduce by polar budding with a narrow bridge between the mother and daughter cells. Rarely it is possible to find both yeast and mycelial forms in lung tissues[14] as well as on endovascular devices,[15] so the presence of mycelial forms should not rule out histoplasmosis.

Histoplasmosis is initiated by inhalation and deposition of microconidia within alveoli. This event is followed by conversion of microconidia to the yeast form,[16] which begins within several hours to days.[17] Morphogenesis is initiated by the shift in temperature and availability of nutrients. Notably, despite Darling including "capsulatum" in the fungi's name based on a mistaken observation of encapsulation, the cells lack a capsule. During primary infection, the yeast cells are phagocytosed into the endosomal compartment of phagocytes, and these infected host cells then migrate to hilar and mediastinal lymph nodes and subsequently disseminate hematogenously, distributing the fungus into diverse tissues. In fact, autopsy studies have found that approximately 70% of individuals with history of histoplasmosis have splenic granulomas.[18] The incubation period for disease manifestations is typically 8 to 17 days, though heavy exposure may result in disease in as few as three days.[19]

Effective immune control of histoplasmosis requires activation of cellular immunity in concert with innate responses because, when cellular immunity is compromised, the infection can disseminate.[20] Additionally, impairment of cellular immunity in latently infected individuals can result in reactivation of previously controlled foci of infection. Although less common in the current era of effective antiretroviral therapy, individuals with *acquired immunodeficiency syndrome* (AIDS) are at high risk for reactivation disease. Reactivation histoplasmosis has increasingly been seen in patients receiving anticytokine therapies.[21] Reactivation disease has also been documented in liver transplant recipients with disease originating from latent infections in the transplanted organs,[22] and disease is associated with a high incidence of graft loss and mortality.

Neutrophils are considered the primary responders to *Histoplasma* in the lung[23]; however, in a murine model, the majority of yeast are found within immature dendritic cells on the first day after experimental pulmonary infection. In the same murine model, neutrophils predominate for several days thereafter. Human neutrophils effectively inhibit the fungus, and azurophilic granules are responsible for this fungistatic effect.[24] After experimental infection, resident and inflammatory macrophages contain yeast cells by 3 days, and inflammatory macrophages contain most of the yeast cells by the end of the first week. Although experimental systems have shown that murine dendritic cells and macrophages fail to control replication and facilitate dissemination, human dendritic cells and macrophages, especially activated macrophages, can kill *Histoplasma* yeast cells.[25] Moreover, human dendritic cells can inhibit conidial germination,[26] which can modify subsequent disease progression by presenting fungal antigens to CD8+ T cells. Several experimental studies have suggested that CD8+ T cells are instrumental in initial clearance of *Histoplasma* yeast cells, whereas CD4+ T cells are required for survival.[20] The role of antibodies in histoplasmosis is controversial, although administration of monoclonal antibodies can modify the course of disease.[27,28] Consistent with an immunoregulatory role for B cells in histoplasmosis is the finding that depletion of B cells significantly enhances the severity of disease.[29]

Among the many innate elements engaged in protective immunity to *Histoplasma* are several cytokines, including interleukin-12 and -17, TNF-α, granulocyte-macrophage colony-stimulating factor, and interferon-γ.[20] The ability of lymphocytes and phagocytes to produce these cytokines constitutes a major effector mechanism of host resistance. The critical role of TNF is underscored by the association of inhibition of this cytokine and the development of severe histoplasmosis. In the setting of intact immunity, granuloma formation can be caseating and indistinguishable from that caused by *Mycobacterium tuberculosis*. Also similar to tuberculosis, healing of granulomas can result in calcification, especially in lymph nodes and the liver and spleen.[18]

CLINICAL MANIFESTATIONS

The severity of histoplasmosis is closely linked to the number of spores inhaled, the virulence of the infecting strain, and the immunologic status of the exposed individual.[30] The most common presentation is pneumonia, though the disease can also manifest as a fulminant life-threatening disseminated sepsis that may involve virtually any tissue. Low inoculum infection leads to asymptomatic disease in 99%, with 1% of individuals developing self-limiting disease.[31] In contrast, high inoculum infection leads to symptomatic disease in 50–100% of exposures.[32] In general, infection usually results in a mild, often asymptomatic respiratory illness, but may progress to life-threatening systemic disease, particularly in immunocompromised individuals. In the setting of HIV infection, disseminated histoplasmosis has been considered an AIDS-defining illness, although the prevalence of histoplasmosis in individuals with HIV has been markedly reduced with the widespread use of antiretroviral drugs.

Acute Histoplasmosis

The most common outcome after exposure to *Histoplasma* is asymptomatic infection. However, in some individuals, symptomatic acute disease manifests 1 to 3 weeks after exposure.[33] Symptomatic histoplasmosis typically presents as a flulike illness with the rapid onset of fever, chills, headache, myalgia, nonproductive cough, and chest pain. Chest radiographs are generally unrevealing, although mediastinal lymphadenopathy with or without opacities may be seen (Fig. 56.2A). Approximately 1 in 2000 exposed adults will develop acute progressive pneumonia,[34] often associated with a heavy exposure to *Histoplasma*.[35] In acute disease, approximately 10% of patients have rheumatologic symptoms, such as arthritis or severe arthralgia accompanied by erythema nodosum.[36] Pericarditis can develop in approximately 10% of patients with acute disease,[37] although pericarditis is typically a late manifestation or can manifest after the resolution of pulmonary symptoms.

Histoplasmosis has a propensity to involve the mediastinal lymph nodes (see Chapter 116). Clinical disease may include mediastinal adenitis (eFig. 116.7), an acute presentation that may respond to antifungal agents, and two late presentations, mediastinal granuloma and fibrosing mediastinitis, which appear to be inflammatory and fibrotic reactions to fungal components. Mediastinal granuloma is thought to arise from a conglomeration of lymph nodes that expand and compress mediastinal structures (Figs. 116.6 and 116.7, eFigs. 116.8 and 116.9). Surgery may be warranted to drain the inflammatory semiliquid material to relieve pressure; of note, antifungal agents or anti-inflammatory agents may not be particularly effective (see Chapter 116). Fibrosing mediastinitis, a rare but serious postinfectious complication, is a fibrosing process in the mediastinum that may compress and occlude vital mediastinal structures, including airways and vessels[38] (Fig. 116.5, eFig. 56.1). Fibrosing mediastinitis is thought to be due to an abnormal inflammatory response to residual *Histoplasma* proinflammatory components.[39] Steroids or antifungal agents are not useful in combating fibrosing mediastinitis, and surgery has not proven to be effective, although endovascular stenting has been reported to alleviate vascular complications[40] (see Chapter 116).

The majority of patients with acute pulmonary histoplasmosis recover over several weeks without sequelae, though occasional patients complain of fatigue persisting for months. Subsequent radiographs may appear normal or demonstrate a single calcified (eFig. 56.2) or noncalcified nodule or "coin" lesion or a miliary pattern of calcified granulomas indistinguishable from that found in certain tuberculosis patients[19] (Fig. 56.3). The miliary appearance

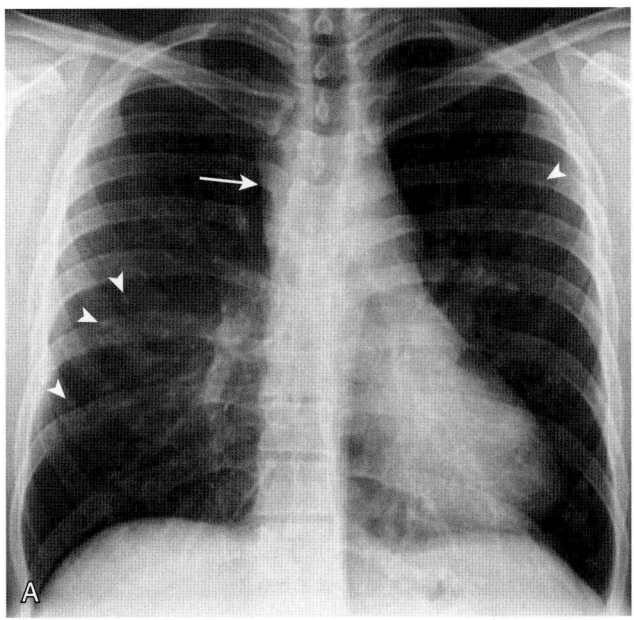

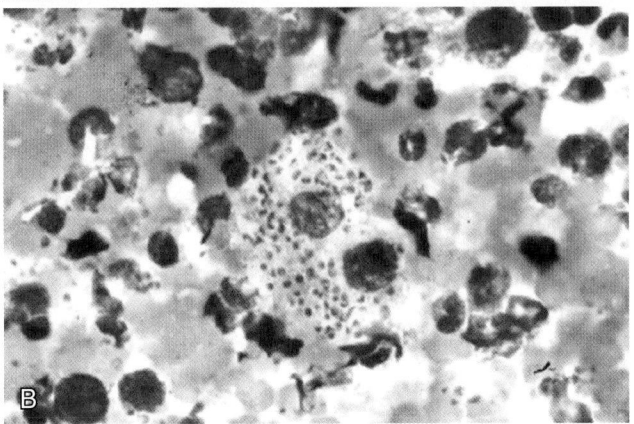

Figure 56.2 Acute histoplasmosis. (A) Frontal chest radiograph in a patient with acute histoplasmosis shows numerous bilateral small nodules *(arrowheads)* and right paratracheal lymphadenopathy *(arrow)*. (B) Photomicrograph of bone marrow biopsy specimen shows abundant small yeast in macrophages. There were no well-formed granulomas. (Wright stain; ×450 original magnification.) (A, Courtesy Michael B. Gotway, MD.)

is more common after a high inoculum exposure or in immunocompromised patients. Although it is well recognized that pulmonary coin lesions can be sequelae of histoplasmosis, surgical resections continue to be performed due to suspicion of neoplasm.[41] Positron emission tomography scans are not helpful in distinguishing infection from tumor because they can display enhanced uptake in histoplasmosis nodules.[42]

Disseminated Histoplasmosis

H. capsulatum can rapidly spread throughout an infected host as the fungus is transported intracellularly by phagocytes from the lungs via the hilar lymphatics into the systemic circulation.[23] Although the majority of infected patients control this process, systemic histoplasmosis develops in approximately 0.05% of individuals after exposure.[34] Disease most commonly disseminates in individuals with preexisting immunosuppression, largely due to malignancy, corticosteroid use, or HIV (eFig. 56.3). Clinical manifestations of disseminated histoplasmosis can vary from indolent

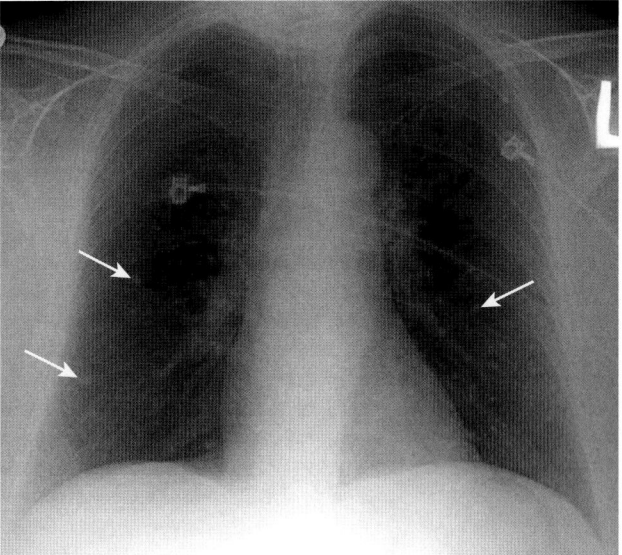

Figure 56.3 Multiple calcified pulmonary granulomas due to histoplasmosis. Frontal chest radiograph shows numerous small calcified nodules *(arrows)* bilaterally due to previous disseminated histoplasmosis. (Courtesy Michael B. Gotway, MD.)

to fulminant disease. Patients typically present with fever, weight loss, and respiratory symptoms with hepatomegaly and/or splenomegaly. Cutaneous and mucous membrane lesions are not uncommon, and patients should be considered to have disseminated disease if *Histoplasma* is isolated from these sites. Patients with acute disease often have anemia, thrombocytopenia, leukopenia, and abnormal liver function tests as well as coagulopathies.[43] The majority of patients have diffuse pulmonary opacities, but chest radiographs can be unrevealing in approximately 30% of patients.[44] The central nervous system can be involved in 10–20% of cases.[45] Endovascular disease is not common; interestingly, in patients with endovascular prostheses, mycelial and yeast forms have both been found in the vegetations.[15] Adrenal dysfunction, including bilateral adrenal masses, may develop in approximately 50% of patients with disseminated histoplasmosis, although adrenal insufficiency is uncommon.[46] Mucocutaneous involvement is uncommon in immunologically normal individuals, but typically presents as one or more ulcers of the skin, oral mucosa, and gastrointestinal tract. Acute progressive disease is lethal without treatment.

Chronic Pulmonary Histoplasmosis

Individuals with long-standing lung diseases, particularly emphysema or COPD, can develop a chronic respiratory illness after acquiring *Histoplasma*. The disease can manifest after acute infection or after reactivation of previously latent infection. Chronic histoplasmosis is characterized by indolent, progressive lung opacities, fibrosis, and cavitation[47] (Fig. 56.4). Bullae are most frequently located in the apices. The majority of patients present with fever, weight loss, increasingly severe cough, and dyspnea. This disease manifestation is clinically and radiologically similar to that of cavitary tuberculosis.[48] Without therapy, progression of disease develops in approximately 50% of affected individuals.[47] It is not uncommon for these patients to receive several

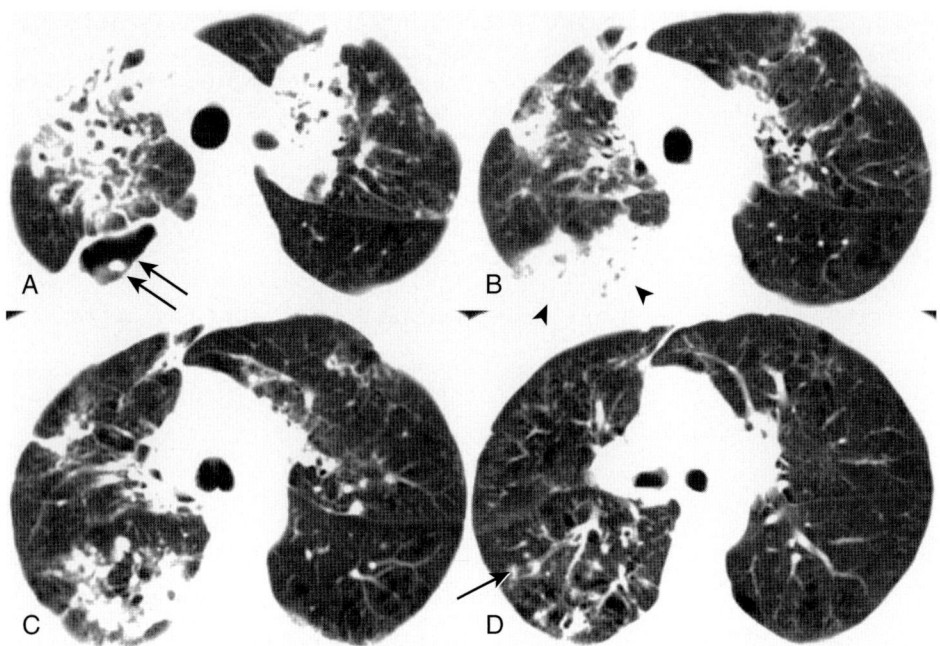

Figure 56.4 **Chronic histoplasmosis.** (A–D) Axial chest computed tomography shows upper lobe bronchovascular thickening with architectural distortion and areas of consolidation (*arrowheads*, B). Small nodules (*single arrow*, D) are also present. A cavity (*double arrows*, A) is present within the right upper lobe. The appearance closely resembles postprimary tuberculosis. (Courtesy Michael B. Gotway, MD.)

courses of antibacterial antibiotics for suspected anaerobic infections prior to consideration of histoplasmosis.[49]

Transmissibility

In general, *Histoplasma* is not contagious via the person-to-person route.[50] However, transmission has been reported in the setting of organ transplant with reactivation of *H. capsulatum* in the implanted organ.[51] The risk of reactivation of endogenous infection during immunosuppression is very low (<0.5%), even in high-risk groups such as renal or bone marrow transplant patients.[52] The mycelial phase of *H. capsulatum* is extremely hazardous to laboratory workers, and the ability to disperse large numbers of spores makes this organism a potential biological weapon. Biosafety level 3 precautions are indicated when processing *H. capsulatum* mold cultures, soil, or other material potentially contaminated with conidia. In the laboratory, biosafety 2 precautions are appropriate for the yeastlike form.

DIAGNOSIS

The gold standard for diagnosis is culture of *Histoplasma*; however, this process takes a minimum of 1 week and growth may not be detected for approximately 1 month. Moreover, respiratory cultures are positive in less than 50% of patients with acute pulmonary histoplasmosis.[53] In contrast, cultures are positive in 65–85% of patients with chronic pulmonary histoplasmosis. These data are complicated by the fact that studies have not critically examined the relative worth of different respiratory samples, although bronchoscopy with biopsy may provide the most effective testing mechanism because it can allow rapid visualization of the fungus in tissue. Direct observation of the fungus in respiratory secretions has a high specificity, but low sensitivity. In disseminated disease, the fungus is usually detectable in bone marrow aspirates[54] (Fig. 56.2B), and can even be identified in peripheral blood, especially in a buffy coat.[55] (see Chapter 19).

In the absence of positive cultures, serologic techniques such as immunodiffusion,[56] complement fixation,[57] enzyme immunoassay,[58] and radioimmunoassay[59] have been used to provide immunologic evidence of *Histoplasma* infection. These serologic tests for the detection of either antibodies and/or antigen in clinical specimens (such as serum or urine) offer a rapid alternative methodology for the diagnosis of histoplasmosis. Notably, there are issues with each of these methodologies and cross reactivity with other geographic fungi. Although promising, polymerase chain reaction or mass spectroscopy methodologies for detecting *Histoplasma* are not yet well-developed enough for routine use.

In the United States, antigen detection is commonly used in diagnosis of histoplasmosis. Polysaccharide *H. capsulatum* antigen can be detected in the urine of 92% of patients with disseminated histoplasmosis, 83% with acute disease, and 88% with chronic pulmonary histoplasmosis.[53] Additionally, antigen can frequently be detected in the serum of patients with disseminated disease, suggesting that testing of both urine and blood will increase the sensitivity of testing. Antigen testing of bronchoalveolar lavage fluid or cerebrospinal fluid can lead to the diagnosis of pulmonary or meningeal histoplasmosis, respectively. The assay is useful for following response to therapy and evaluating for disease relapse. The current *Infectious Diseases Society of America* (IDSA) guidelines recommend following antigen levels during and after treatment of histoplasmosis.[60] However, this and other antigen assays have significant cross reactivity with other endemic fungi.[61]

At present, the aforementioned tests are costly and frequently impractical for use in less economically developed countries. A mainstay of diagnosis in many regions is an immunodiffusion test for detection of H and M precipitin bands utilizing *histoplasmin* (HMIN) as the antigen; HMIN is a well-characterized antigen obtained from *Histoplasma* mycelia.[62] The H antigen is a β-glucosidase[63] and the M antigen is a catalase.[64] These antigens can be detected by approximately 1 month after infection. The M band is detectable in approximately 75% of patients and can persist for years, whereas the H antigen can be identified in less than 25% of patients and is absent within 6 months.[65] Complement fixation tests utilize both HMIN and intact yeast cells; this reaction is positive by approximately 3 weeks of disease and can persist for months to years.[66] A titer of 1:32 or greater is strongly suggestive of acute disease, though a titer of 1:8 in a patient with a high suspicion of histoplasmosis is consistent with disease. Titers are negative in approximately 30% of patients with acute histoplasmosis and in 50% with disseminated disease. Most laboratories perform both the immunodiffusion and complement fixation tests concurrently for increased sensitivity. Immunocompromised patients with histoplasmosis frequently fail to mount an effective antibody response and specific antibodies to the disease cannot be routinely detected, which complicates and delays diagnosis.[67]

Enzyme-linked immunsorbent assay (ELISA) has been reported for the detection of antibodies in sera using HMIN, and deglycosylated or metaperiodate-treated HMIN to improve sensitivity and reduce cross reactivity. ELISAs using HMIN compared to deglycosylated HMIN have sensitivities and specificities of 57% and 93% versus 92% and 96%, respectively.[58,68] Treatment of purified HMIN with metaperiodate further improved the ELISA resulting in an overall specificity of 96% with sensitivities of 100%, 90%, 89%, 86%, and 100% in acute disease, chronic disease, disseminated infection in individuals without HIV infection, disseminated disease in the setting of HIV infection, and mediastinal histoplasmosis, respectively.[69]

TREATMENT

Comprehensive treatment recommendations for histoplasmosis have been made by the *American Thoracic Society* (ATS) in 2011[70] and the IDSA in 2007.[60] The majority of individuals who acquire histoplasmosis are either asymptomatic or have a mild, self-limited flulike illness. Unless the patient is immunocompromised, there is no need to administer antifungal agents under these conditions.[71]

Mild to Moderate Acute Pulmonary Histoplasmosis

If a patient has been symptomatic for more than 3 weeks or if a patient has moderate disease, itraconazole is appropriate. Itraconazole should be given as a loading dose of 200 mg three times daily for 3 days followed by 200 mg twice daily for 6 to 12 weeks. Ketoconazole should not be used as a systemic antifungal and fluconazole is less effective than itraconazole. Voriconazole and posaconazole can be considered for use in patients not responding to itraconazole.[72–74] Echinocandins should not be used to treat *Histoplasma* because of intrinsic resistance of *Histoplasma* to this class of drugs.[75]

Moderately Severe to Severe Acute Pulmonary Histoplasmosis

Liposomal amphotericin is more effective than itraconazole in clearance of *Histoplasma* in experimental histoplasmosis.[76] Liposomal amphotericin is favored over the conventional deoxycholate formulations because the liposomal amphotericin has an improved toxicity profile and may provide a survival benefit.[77] Liposomal amphotericin should be administered at 3 to 5 mg/kg daily for 1 to 2 weeks, followed by itraconazole 200 mg three times daily for 3 days and then 200 mg twice daily for 12 weeks. If liposomal amphotericin is not available or if the patient is at low risk for nephrotoxicity, 0.7 to 1 mg/kg deoxycholate amphotericin should be used. In patients with hypoxemia or significant respiratory distress, corticosteroids should be considered, particularly in HIV-infected individuals receiving antiretroviral therapy at risk for immune reconstitution syndromes.[78] Methylprednisolone 0.5 to 1 mg/kg can be intravenously administered for the first 1 to 2 weeks adjunctively with antifungals. Alternatively, oral prednisone 40 to 60 mg/day can be used.

Chronic Cavitary Histoplasmosis

Itraconazole should be given as a loading dose of 200 mg three times daily for 3 days, followed by 200 mg twice daily for a minimum of 1 year. Extending treatment to 18 to 24 months may reduce the likelihood of relapse, which otherwise can be expected in approximately 15% of patients. Critically ill patients may benefit from initial treatment with amphotericin.[79]

Disseminated Histoplasmosis

Treatment should be initiated with liposomal amphotericin, if available, for 1 to 2 weeks, followed by itraconazole. Treatment should be continued for a minimum of 1 year.[62] Occasionally, disseminated disease can be diagnosed in patients who have only mild to moderate symptoms. In immunocompetent individuals, itraconazole can be considered for initial therapy.

Immunocompromised Patients

Therapy with itraconazole 200 mg once or twice daily should be continued indefinitely in immunocompromised patients whose immunosuppression cannot be discontinued.[62] In patients with HIV, therapy should be continued lifelong unless CD4 counts can be restored to levels greater than 200/μL. Patients on maintenance itraconazole should have *Histoplasma* antigen testing performed each year.

Drug Monitoring

Serum levels of itraconazole should be measured at 2 weeks of therapy and then every 3 to 6 months while on therapy.[80] Similarly, if voriconazole or posaconazole are being used as salvage, serum drug levels should be monitored.[81]

Management of Complications

Pericarditis is generally managed with administration of nonsteroidal medications. Pericardiocentesis should be performed if hemodynamic compromise is present. In patients with hemodynamic compromise or persistent symptoms despite nonsteroidal therapy, prednisone should be administered with a taper performed over approximately 2 weeks. Patients treated with steroids should receive itraconazole treatment for 6 to 12 weeks. Broncholithiasis (eFig. 56.4) is an uncommon condition in which patients experience wheezing, dyspnea, or hemoptysis after erosion of a calcified lymph node into the airway. If the patient fails to expectorate the broncholith, bronchoscopic removal may be required[82]; rarely, surgery is necessary for severe obstruction, fistualization, or massive hemoptysis.[83] No antifungal treatment should be administered for patients with broncholithiasis in the absence of other findings.

Of the different types of mediastinal involvement, mediastinal adenitis usually does not require treatment, but severe disease with compression complications should receive steroids and itraconazole. Mediastinal granuloma may warrant surgery to drain the caseous material pressing on structures. As noted above, there is no effective medical treatment for fibrosing mediastinitis. However, if it is unclear whether a patient has fibrosing mediastinitis, mediastinal granuloma, or mediastinal adenitis due to *Histoplasma*, then itraconazole should be administered at 200 mg/kg orally once or twice a day for 12 weeks (see Chapter 116).

Rheumatologic syndromes are also generally managed with nonsteroidal therapy. However, if symptoms do not remit, prednisone and itraconazole should be given. No antimicrobial therapy should be administered when biopsy of a nodule incidentally shows *Histoplasma* in an asymptomatic individual, especially when the fungus cannot be cultured.

COCCIDIOIDES

HISTORY AND EPIDEMIOLOGY

Coccidioidomycosis is a primary pulmonary infection caused by two species of *Coccidioides*, *C. posadasii*, and *C. immitis*, endemic to Arizona, New Mexico, western Texas, the Central Valley of California, central Washington state, and in sections of Central and South America where there are arid to semiarid life zones. Coccidioidomycosis is also known as San Joaquin Valley Fever or simply Valley Fever since the San Joaquin Valley of California is a historic hot spot for the microbe. In the United States, it is estimated that there are approximately 150,000 infections annually and that approximately 50,000 of these develop symptomatic disease.[84] California and Arizona actively track cases of coccidioidomycosis, and both states have reported increases in disease rates over the past decade,[84] with California now having more cases yearly than Arizona. In 1995, the annual incidence was 1.9 per 100,000; in 2009, it increased to 8.4 per 100,000; in 2016, it further increased to 13.7 per 100,000.[85] A nationwide analysis found an estimated 3000 hospitalizations per year, with a mortality rate of 1–5%.[86]

Disturbances of the soil are highly associated with acquisition of the fungus. Hyphae grow in moist soil and, during dry periods, viable arthroconidia can survive for protracted periods. The organism is thought to grow in soil to a depth of approximately 8 inches and is frequently isolated from rodent burrows. Arthroconidia are frequently aerosolized due to agricultural activity, excavation, or construction, and individuals participating in these activities are at high risk for coccidioidomycosis in endemic regions. Additionally, soldiers marching behind tanks or other vehicles are at risk for inhalation of arthroconidia. Individuals with advanced HIV infection or patients on corticosteroids or other immunosuppressants are at increased risk for severe disease, as are women in their third trimester of pregnancy and individuals of African or Filipino descent.[87]

Disease is indistinguishable between the two species of *Coccidioides*. The separation into the species was possible due to phylogenic studies demonstrating divergence between the historically well-described species, *C. immitis*, and the newer named species, *C. posadasii*.[88] There are phenotypic differences, such as differential growth rates under stress conditions, but they are morphologically indistinguishable and routine laboratory testing does not separate the species. Initially, *C. immitis* was thought to be limited to the San Joaquin Valley in California and in Washington state, whereas *C. posadasii* was thought to be present throughout the endemic regions detailed for the fungus, but more recent data suggest that there is significant overlap in the distribution of the two species.[89,90]

Coccidioidomycosis was first described in 1892 by Alejandro Posadas in an Argentinian soldier.[91] The organism was initially thought to be a protozoan of the order Coccidia, leading to its name. *Coccidioides* was not confirmed to be a fungus until 1900.[92]

PATHOGENESIS

The specialized environmental structures, arthroconidia, arise from hyphae and form chains of cells. The arthroconidia are 2 to 4 μm × 5 to 6 μm ovoid cells, and the chain usually consists of an intact multinucleate arthroconidium alternating with a degenerated cell (disjunctor cells). The thinner wall of the degenerated cell is readily disrupted when the chain is disturbed, such as during a wind storm or construction, and individual or small collections of arthroconidia can then be aerosolized and subsequently inhaled.[93] The arthroconidia undergo morphogenesis in humans or under specialized laboratory conditions at 37°C into a unique structure, a spherule. Arthroconidia convert to a spherule over approximately 2 to 4 days. The arthroconidia first develops into a round cell and then the spherule forms by successive growth and segmentation into an oval structure of 20 to 150 μm in diameter that contains dozens to hundreds of 2 to 4 μm endospores (Fig. 56.5A). Rupture of mature spherules leads to the release of endospores that, in the absence of effective host immunity, can develop locally into spherules or disseminate through hematogenous or lymphatic routes to other tissues. Notably, arthroconidia and septate hyphae can be identified in some patients with chronic disease, especially diabetes, in which there is low oxygen tension and tissue necrosis.

Coccidioides causes disease in immunocompetent or immunocompromised individuals, with disease severity typically being worse in immunocompromised patients.[94] Initial host responses to arthroconidia include influx of macrophages and neutrophils. Interestingly, neutrophils may stimulate arthroconidia to convert into spherules,[95] yet they can impede morphogenesis after the induction of antibody and with activated complement.[96] Phagocytosis is augmented in the presence of antibody to *Coccidioides* antigens. The oxidative burst is effective against arthroconidia and immature, but not mature, spherules. Additionally, after conversion to a spherule, the sheer size of this form precludes its phagocytosis by neutrophils or macrophages.[97] In tissues, organized necrotizing granulomatous inflammation predominates, with significant numbers of T and B cells present at the margins of the lesions.

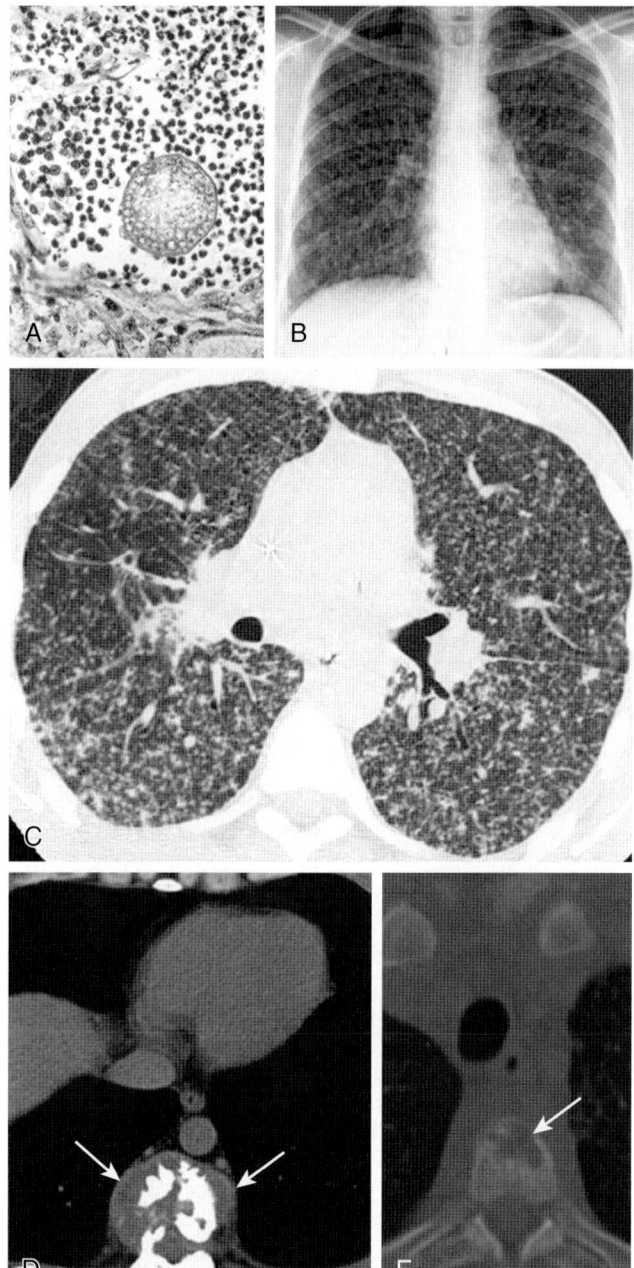

Figure 56.5 Disseminated coccidioidomycosis in an immunosuppressed patient. (A) Photomicrograph shows a characteristic giant spherule of coccidioidomycosis in a lung biopsy. (Hematoxylin and eosin stain; ×450 original magnification.) (B) Frontal chest radiograph shows numerous, randomly disseminated nodules bilaterally consistent with a miliary pattern. (C) Chest computed tomography (CT) shown in lung windows confirms the miliary pattern. Axial chest CT shown in soft tissue (D) and bone (E) windows demonstrates bilateral paraspinous masses *(arrows)* associated with vertebral body destruction. The CT image shown in bone windows (E) reveals the vertebral body destruction *(arrow)* to advantage. (Courtesy Michael B. Gotway, MD.)

T lymphocyte responses are critical for protection against *Coccidioides*. Moreover, Th1 responses are protective, whereas Th2 responses are less effective. Consistent with this, cytokines such as interferon-γ are associated with resistance whereas interleukin-4 is linked to susceptibility.[98] Consistent with the importance of CD4+ T lymphocytes, disease is often more severe in patients with advanced HIV

infection. Additionally, individuals with delayed-type hypersensitivity responses to *Coccidioides* antigens generally have improved outcomes relative to those who do not react.

Individuals with prior symptomatic infection are generally protected against reinfection with either species of *Coccidioides*. However, waning immunity, such as in advanced HIV, or treatment with immunosuppressants can lead to reactivation of latent lesions or abolish protection against reinfection.

CLINICAL MANIFESTATIONS

Disease manifestations can range from asymptomatic infection to pneumonia, cavitary pulmonary disease, and disseminated infection that can involve skin, bone, central nervous system, and visceral organs.[99] Approximately 60% of individuals infected with *Coccidioides* are either asymptomatic or have only mild respiratory symptoms.[100] However, 1 to 4 weeks after inhalation of the arthroconidia, approximately 40% develop moderate to severe respiratory symptoms. Although the majority of these patients resolve without sequelae, approximately 5% have persistent or progressive pulmonary disease (eFig. 56.5). Furthermore, approximately 1% will have disseminated disease, which is more common in immunocompromised patients[94] (Fig. 56.5B–E).

Pulmonary Coccidioidomycosis (Valley Fever or Primary Coccidioidal Infection)

Primary symptomatic infection is typically a subacute pulmonary disease. The initial symptoms are flulike, with patients commonly presenting with fever, cough, dyspnea, fatigue, headaches, myalgias, and arthralgias. Patients who progress to pneumonia typically have segmental or lobar disease, and mediastinal and/or hilar lymphadenopathy is characteristic (eFig. 56.6). In areas with high endemicity, up to 15–30% of cases of community-acquired pneumonia are due to *Coccidioides*.[101] Dermatologic immunologic manifestations such as erythema nodosum or erythema multiforme may develop, and are associated with a favorable host response to the fungus. Pleural effusions complicate 5–15% of patients, though the presence of an effusion does not correspond to increased severity of disease. The pleural fluid can be either transudative or exudative, and lymphocytes and eosinophils predominate.[102] In approximately 20% of those with effusions, coccidioidal empyema can develop, requiring aggressive intervention (Fig. 56.6A).

Acute Respiratory Failure and Acute Respiratory Distress Syndrome

Fortunately, the presentations of acute respiratory failure or *acute respiratory distress syndrome* (ARDS) are uncommon; they can accompany advanced immunosuppression. However, massive exposures to arthroconidia during construction or archeological excavation can lead to rapidly progressive respiratory failure. Mortality rates for ARDS due to disseminated coccidioidomycosis approach 100% (eFig. 56.7).

Disseminated Coccidioidomycosis

The presentation of disseminated disease may be acute or chronic. Disease may be multifocal or restricted to a

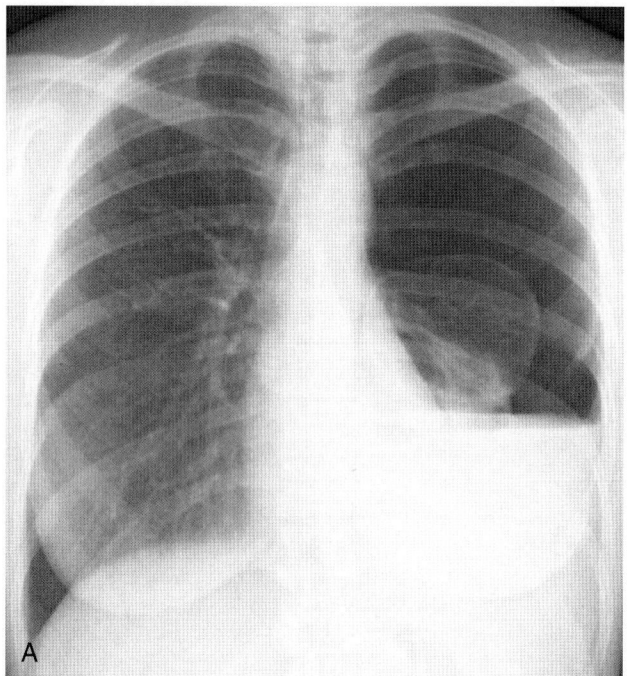

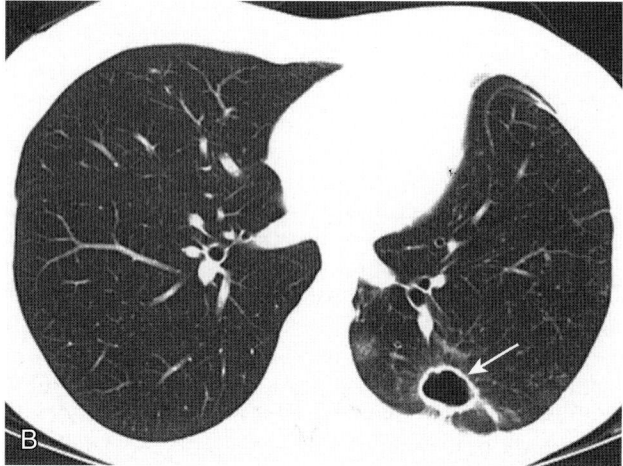

Figure 56.6 Coccidioidomycosis peripheral cavity with rupture into pleural space and empyema and bronchopleural fistula. (A) Frontal chest radiograph shows a large left hydropneumothorax; note air-fluid level. The patient was treated with extended tube thoracostomy, antifungal therapy, and eventually video-assisted thoracoscopic pleural space débridement. *Coccidioides* spherules were recovered from the left pleural space. (B) One year later, the chest computed tomography shows a uniformly thin-walled, peripheral cavity *(arrow)* characteristic of prior *Coccidioides immitis* pulmonary infection. (Courtesy Michael B. Gotway, MD.)

single extrapulmonary site. Prognosis of the single extrapulmonary lesion is typically better than multifocal disease, except in the case of meningitis (eFig. 56.8). Multifocal disease has a mortality rate of approximately 50%. Meningitis is frequently progressive, and shunts are often required to manage increased intracranial pressures. As mentioned, immunosuppression is a risk factor for disseminated disease as are advanced age, male gender, pregnancy, and being of Filipino and African descent.[103]

Miliary coccidioidomycosis is an unusual presentation in which numerous small granulomas develop throughout the lungs and other organs. Radiographs depict 3 to 4 mm nodules (eFig. 56.9) throughout the lung fields,

indistinguishable in appearance from miliary tuberculosis. Notably, this presentation is a risk factor for the development of ARDS.

Pulmonary Nodule (Coccidioidoma)

A coccidioidoma typically is a single nodule (eFigs. 56.10 and 56.11A) in the peripheral lung tissue. Coccidioidomas are frequently misdiagnosed as a possible malignancy, leading to invasive procedures being performed. It is difficult to distinguish a coccidioidoma from other lesions without histopathologic or culture evidence.[104]

Cavitary Coccidioides

Although uncommon, thick- or thin-walled cavities (Fig. 56.6B, eFig. 56.11B–D) may develop during resolution of coccidioidomycosis. Cavities likely form as a consequence of infarction or necrosis. If the cavities are peripheral, there are risks for fistula formation and/or pneumothorax. Surgical resection may be considered for large cavities to prevent cavity rupture. Smaller cavities can be monitored radiographically (see eFig. 56.11B–D) and do not always close. Another cavitary disease process is a chronic fibrocavitary pneumonia (eFig. 56.12) characterized by multilobar opacities and cavities. This disease is more common in people with diabetes, and fever, chills, night sweats, and weight loss are typical symptoms.

Transmissibility

Person-to-person transmission is rare and almost exclusively seen in donor-derived organ transplant infections.[105,106] The infectivity of *Coccidioides* from the environment or culture is quite high, making this organism a potential biological weapon. There is significant risk of *Coccidioides* for laboratory workers, and these fungi have been associated with severe infections due to exposures.[107] In fact, Valley Fever was first associated with *Coccidioides* in 1929 when a medical student at Stanford, Harold Chope, opened a petri dish with mycelial *Coccidioides* and subsequently developed classic symptoms of Valley Fever. *Coccidioides* should only be handled under biosafety level 3 conditions.

DIAGNOSIS

The gold standard for diagnosis remains isolation of *Coccidioides* from infected tissues; however, patients frequently do not produce sputum, and cultures may take a minimum of a week to several weeks to grow. Direct examination of sputum is not sensitive. The majority of testing utilizes serologic methodologies. However, antibody responses may lag behind clinical symptoms, especially in immunocompromised individuals, and provide only a presumptive diagnosis. Hence, negative antibody testing in such patients does not exclude infection with *Coccidioides*. Immunodiffusion assays for *immunoglobulin* (Ig) M and IgG antibodies have been commonly used because they are considered to be highly specific. Commercial enzyme-linked immunoassays can detect IgM and IgG antibodies to *Coccidioides*, and are more sensitive but less specific than immunodiffusion assays.[108] A complement-fixing antibody method in which the major antigen is a chitinase detects IgG antibodies to *Coccidioides* and is useful to follow response to therapy.[109] Notably, both immunodiffusion and complement fixation can be used to monitor responses to treatment. An antigen test has become available and can be used in selected circumstances and may be of use in the highly immunocompromised population.[110] Molecular methodologies have only recently been validated for coccidioidomycosis but are not in wide use.[102,111]

TREATMENT

Comprehensive treatment recommendations for coccidioidomycosis have been made by the ATS in 2011[70] and the IDSA in 2016.[84] An update in recommendations is currently in progress by the IDSA.

Uncomplicated Acute Pneumonia

Mild to moderate pulmonary disease in an immunocompetent individual is not an indication for treatment.[112] However, patients with HIV, pregnant women, or otherwise immunosuppressed patients are typically treated. In immunocompetent individuals, treatment is recommended if symptoms persist for more than 8 weeks or if the patient has lost more than 10% total body weight, has night sweats for more than 3 weeks, or if disease is present in more than half of a single lung, is multilobar, or is associated with persistent hilar lymphadenopathy. Additionally, complement fixation titers of greater than 1:16 often prompt treatment. If antifungal therapy is initiated for mild to moderate disease, it is generally administered for 3 to 6 months. If disease progresses to chronic fibrocavitary pneumonia, a minimum of one year of antifungal therapy is recommended. Long-term azole therapy should be considered for severely immunocompromised individuals.

Treatment is usually with either oral fluconazole (400 to 800 mg/day) or itraconazole (200 mg two or three times daily), with the higher doses used in more severe cases of *Coccidioides*.[113] Drug levels for itraconazole should be obtained after 2 weeks of therapy.[80] In more severe disease, liposomal amphotericin B (2.0 to 5.0 mg/kg/day) or deoxycholate amphotericin B (0.5 to 1.5 mg/kg/day) can be administered. Although promising, there are insufficient data to evaluate the efficacy of voriconazole and posaconazole for coccidioidomycosis, although utility in refractory cases has been demonstrated.[114,115] Echinocandins are not recommended because of intrinsic resistance in dimorphic fungi such as *Coccidioides*. Even in the absence of treatment, patients should be monitored every 3 to 6 months to document resolution of radiologic evidence of disease and confirm the absence of pulmonary or other complications.

Complicated Pneumonia With or Without Dissemination

Diffuse disease, particularly reticulonodular pneumonia or miliary opacities, is treated initially with an amphotericin formulation (followed with fluconazole) or high-dose fluconazole. If dissemination is present, especially if the patient has meningitis, treatment with fluconazole is preferred. Steroid therapy may be useful in patients with severe pulmonary coccidioidomycosis with ARDS using approaches validated for *Pneumocystis jirovecii*: prednisone 40 mg two times daily for 5 days, then 40 mg/day, and then 20 mg/day for 11 days. For complicated pneumonia, recovery

is frequently slow, with symptoms resolving over weeks. Treatment is for a minimum of 1 year.

Pulmonary Nodule

If a solitary nodule is identified as being due to *Coccidioides* after a biopsy, there is no need to administer antifungal therapy or to resect the lesion. If the nodule was excised, no additional treatment is necessary. Treatment with an azole should be considered in a patient with a nodule if the patient becomes immunocompromised.

Pulmonary Cavity

Asymptomatic cavities should be followed clinically and radiographically (see eFig. 56.11). If a patient is symptomatic or has an elevated antibody titer, treatment with an azole for 3 to 6 months should be considered, although 12 to 18 months may be necessary for immunocompromised individuals. Larger cavities are often resected after 2 or more years if they have not resolved. Bacterial superinfection is a complication that requires aggressive antimicrobial treatment, and subsequent resection of the cavity is prudent. Cavity rupture is rare, but can lead to pyopneumothorax (see Fig. 56.6A–B) requiring antifungal therapy and decortication.

BLASTOMYCES

HISTORY AND EPIDEMIOLOGY

Blastomyces sp, dimorphic fungi endemic to North America, are the causative agents of blastomycosis. Genomic evaluation has identified numerous novel species of *Blastomyces* including *B. gilchristii*, *B. helicus*, *B. parvus*, and *B. silverae*. Most *Blastomyces* are soil-based fungi associated with riverbanks along the Mississippi, Ohio, and St. Lawrence rivers as well as in regions adjacent to the Great Lakes.[116] *B. helices*, however, has been found primarily in the Rocky Mountain region of North America.[117] Risk factors for acquisition of the fungus include exposures to waterways, soils, or woods. Interestingly, approximately 30% of forestry workers in endemic areas of Minnesota and Wisconsin have serologic evidence of prior infection.[118] Infection with *Blastomyces* is thought to follow inhalation of aerosolized conidia, and the common clinical manifestations include pneumonia, skin and bone lesions, and involvement of the genitourinary tract.

The rates of disease significantly vary with regions, even within the same state. For example, a 1992 study of 11 years of laboratory-confirmed blastomycosis showed that the rate of disease in Wisconsin was approximately 1.4 cases per 100,000, but there were regions with approximately 40 cases per 100,000.[119] Most cases are sporadic, but outbreaks have been observed. In 2003, there were 771 patients hospitalized with a diagnosis of blastomycosis, with a 6% mortality rate in adults.[120] A later analysis has shown an increasing rate of hospitalizations for blastomycosis, with 64% of hospitalizations among men.[121]

Thomas Gilchrist described blastomycosis in 1894,[122] and blastomycosis is also referred to as Gilchrist disease. Gilchrist misidentified the fungus as a protozoan but later corrected this error. Early descriptions emphasized the cutaneous manifestations, so blastomycosis was initially considered primarily as a localized dermatologic condition rather than a systemic infection.

PATHOGENESIS

Blastomyces exists as a mycelial form in the environment or under laboratory conditions at approximately 25°C. Inhalation of conidia or cultivation at 37°C results in their transformation into yeast cells (8 to 12 μm in diameter) that bud with a broad-based connection between the mother and daughter cells (Fig. 56.7A and Fig. 19.4B–C). In tissue, yeast forms of 25 to 40 μm in diameter can also be found. After inhalation, conidia are engaged by neutrophils and macrophages, which can kill the cells and/or inhibit conidial morphogenesis.[123] The yeast form is more resistant to killing, especially by neutrophils,[124] and conidia have been reported to inhibit the enzymatic activity of macrophage-inducible nitric oxide synthase.[125] The yeast cells can disseminate from the lungs via the bloodstream or lymphatics to any tissue. In tissues, neutrophilic infiltrates appear early in disease followed by a granulomatous response characterized by multinucleated giant cells and noncaseating granulomas. Activation of effective cell-mediated responses is required to halt disease.[126] *Blastomyces* adhesin-1, an essential virulence factor of *B. dermatitidis*, suppresses host inflammatory response by inhibiting TNF-α.[127] The outcome of this dynamic between host and pathogen responses dictates disease manifestations.

CLINICAL MANIFESTATIONS

Pulmonary infection with *Blastomyces* leads to asymptomatic infection, acute or chronic pneumonia, or disseminated disease. Patients are asymptomatic in approximately 50% of infections[118,128]; when disease develops, it is usually after an incubation period of 4 to 8 weeks. Some studies suggest a seasonality to blastomycosis, which corresponds to outdoor activities in the endemic regions, resulting in mild, self-limited pulmonary infections at the end of summer into early fall, with these individuals subsequently presenting with extrapulmonary disease in the next year.[129] The initial mild presentations manifest with influenza-like symptoms, including fever, cough, myalgias, and arthralgias.[130]

Acute Pulmonary Blastomycosis

The diagnosis of pulmonary blastomycosis is often delayed because the manifestations are nonspecific and not different from those of community-acquired pneumonia. In addition to fever and cough, mild hemoptysis may be present.[131] Radiologic findings can vary in acute disease and similar manifestations can be present in chronic disease. The most common presentation is focal (Fig. 56.7B) or diffuse airspace consolidations,[44,132] and the upper lobes are most frequently involved. However, even asymptomatic patients can have masslike lesions, cavities (eFig. 56.13), or single or multiple (eFig. 56.14) nodules. Acute progressive blastomycosis is infrequent, but pulmonary disease can progress to ARDS, which is associated with mortality rates of approximately 75%.[133] Progressive disease can manifest as diffuse multilobar opacities, endobronchial infection, or miliary blastomycosis. Approximately half of the patients with severe disease are immunosuppressed,[134] including

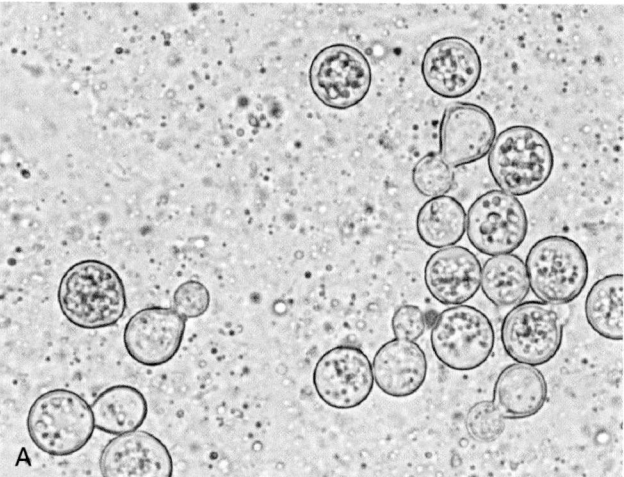

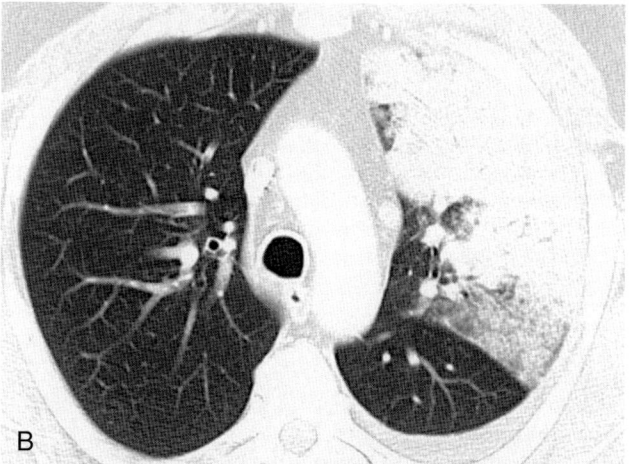

Figure 56.7 Focal pulmonary blastomycosis. (A) Micrograph shows *Blastomyces dermatitidis* in fresh sputum after 10% potassium hydroxide digestion. Note the broad neck of attachment, the double refractile cell wall, and the multiple nuclei. (×1000 original magnification.) (B) Axial chest computed tomography shows a lobar left upper lobe consolidation pattern. (B, Courtesy Jeff Kanne, MD, Associate Professor, Thoracic Imaging, Department of Radiology University of Wisconsin School of Medicine and Public Health.)

cancer patients, transplant recipients (eFig. 56.15), patients on TNF-inhibitors, or individuals with advanced HIV infection.[135]

Chronic Pulmonary Blastomycosis

Similar to histoplasmosis and coccidioidomycosis, blastomycosis can present as a chronic pneumonia clinically indistinguishable from tuberculosis or as a pulmonary malignancy. Patients with chronic blastomycosis frequently report being ill for more than 2 months, with fever, weight loss, night sweats, cough, and chest pains.[128,136] The most frequent radiographic findings include consolidations, mass lesions, and interstitial fibronodular opacities.[132] Cavitation is uncommon, though small pulmonary effusions may be present.

Extrapulmonary Disease

The reported incidence of extrapulmonary disease has been approximately 20–75% of cases, with the upper range being present in patients with chronic blastomycosis.[119,128] More recently, overall rates of disseminated disease are closer to 25–40%.[137] The most frequent site to manifest disseminated lesions is the skin, seen in 40–80% of cases of extrapulmonary disease. The typical presentation is a crusting verrucous lesion with a central draining micro-abscess (or microabscesses) (Fig. 56.8), although nodular, pustular or ulcerative lesions can be present.[138] Multiple lesions are typical, and mucous membranes can also be involved. Cutaneous lesions can overlay osteomyelitis with sinus tracts to the skin. *Blastomyces* can infect the bone in approximately 5–50% of patients with extrapulmonary disease, although approximately 75% of patients with osseous disease have concomitant active pulmonary involvement.[9] Bone radiographs typically reveal focal osteolytic lesions without periosteal reactivity, though lesions can be highly destructive. The third most frequent site of extrapulmonary disease is the genitourinary tract, seen in 10–30% of cases. The incidence is higher in men in whom disease frequently manifests in the prostate, testicle, or epididymis. Although *Blastomyces* can affect any tissue, the most formidable disease is that of the central nervous system, which is found in up to 10% of extrapulmonary blastomycosis, generally in immunosuppressed patients. Prior to the availability of effective combination antiretroviral therapy, 40% of individuals with AIDS developed central nervous system disease resulting in approximately 40% mortality.[139] Risk factors for severe or extrapulmonary disease and increased mortality include cellular immunodeficiencies, older age, and Aboriginal or Hmong ethnicity.[136]

Transmissibility

B. dermatitidis is generally not transmissible from person to person. However, there have been rare cases of presumed conjugal transmission as well as acquisition in utero. Dogs are at high risk for blastomycosis in endemic areas; a vaccine utilizing the *Blastomyces* adhesin-1 protein has recently been shown to be protective in canines[140] and may be a candidate for use as a human vaccine. Bites from infected dogs have led to cutaneous blastomycosis in humans.

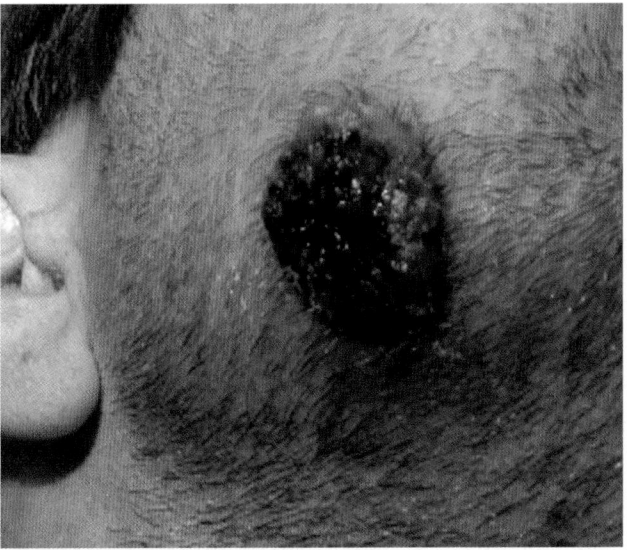

Figure 56.8 Cutaneous lesion of blastomycosis. (Courtesy Bruce Klein, MD, University of Wisconsin Departments of Pediatrics and Medical Microbiology and Immunology.)

DIAGNOSIS

The gold standard for diagnosing blastomycosis is culture.[9] Growth can be detected after several days to weeks on mycologic medium. However, cultures are not a perfect test because, even with specimens obtained by bronchoscopy, the rate of positivity is less than 70%. Direct observation is the most rapid method for diagnosis. Sputum, other fluids, or skin scrapings treated with potassium hydroxide should be examined by microscopy; similar assessment of respiratory specimens can reveal *Blastomyces* yeast forms (see Fig. 56.7A and Fig. 19.4B–C) in up to 46% of patients. Cytologic evaluation with Papanicolaou or other stains can detect *Blastomyces* in up to 71% of patients with pulmonary disease. Histologic examination can also be helpful, with identification of the yeast as described above.

A commercial enzyme immunoassay for *Blastomyces* antigen, similar to the *Histoplasma* antigen assay, has an overall sensitivity of approximately 93%.[141] Antigenuria can be detected in patients with pulmonary or extrapulmonary disease, and testing can also be performed on serum, plasma, cerebrospinal fluid, bronchoalveolar lavage fluid, or other sterile fluids. The test is also reportedly useful to follow response to treatment or assess for relapse. However, there is substantial cross reactivity with *H. capsulatum* and other dimorphic fungi. Although commercial antibody tests are available, they lack clinical utility given the cross reactivity with other endemic mycoses. Molecular testing of patient samples for *Blastomyces* is promising, although its utility has not been confirmed.

TREATMENT

Comprehensive treatment recommendations for *Blastomyces* were made by the ATS in 2011[70] and the IDSA in 2008.[142] It is important to note that, in immunocompetent individuals, acute disease is often mild and resolves without antifungal therapy. Nevertheless, expert opinion is that treatment should be administered because it is not currently possible to identify individuals with a negligible risk of dissemination, and triazole therapies are effective and well tolerated.

Mild to Moderate Blastomycosis

Current consensus is that mild to moderately ill patients with pulmonary blastomycosis should receive itraconazole (200 mg twice daily) for 6 months. Levels of itraconazole should be verified after 2 weeks of administration and periodically during treatment.[80] Therapy for mild to moderate pulmonary blastomycosis is not altered if there is nonmeningeal dissemination, except in the setting of bone disease, for which therapy is extended to 1 year.

Moderately Severe to Severe Blastomycosis

Patients with moderately severe to life-threatening pulmonary blastomycosis, including those with ARDS, are initially treated with liposomal amphotericin B (5 mg/kg/day) or amphotericin deoxycholate (0.7 to 1.0 mg/kg/day) until clinical improvement is evident (usually 1 to 2 weeks) and then switched to itraconazole (200 mg twice daily for 6 to 12 months). Though there are limited data to support the use of corticosteroids, administration of steroids in the setting of extensive disease with hypoxemia may be efficacious. In patients with meningitis, amphotericin with or without fluconazole (800 mg daily) or itraconazole (200 mg twice daily) is used initially (typically for 4 to 6 weeks) followed by 6 to 12 months of treatment with an azole, with many experts favoring a minimum of 12 months. Voriconazole may be considered for use in refractory disease. Echinocandins should not be used because *Blastomyces* and other dimorphic fungi are intrinsically resistant. If the patient is immunocompromised, treatment should be a minimum of 12 months or continued indefinitely.

PARACOCCIDIOIDES

EPIDEMIOLOGY

Paracoccidioides sp, the causative agent of paracoccidioidomycosis, is a dimorphic, soil-based fungus that is endemic in southern Mexico, Central America, and South America. *Paracoccidioides* has recently been split into two closely related species (*P. brasiliensis* and *P. lutzii*).[143] However, to date, the diseases caused by these species are indistinguishable. *Paracoccidioides* is the major causative agent of systemic mycosis in Latin America,[144] and it is a leading cause of disability and death among young adult rural workers.[145] A 2001 analysis estimated that approximately 10 million people were infected with *Paracoccidioides* sp.[146] However, only approximately 1–2% develop symptomatic disease, with pulmonary disease the most common form. An epidemiologic study in Brazil reported a mean incidence of 2.7 cases per 100,000 inhabitants per year, a stable incidence from 1960 to 1999.[147]

PATHOGENESIS

In the environment or under laboratory conditions at less than 28°C, *Paracoccidioides* grows as a mycelium that produces chlamydoconidia, terminal conidia, and arthroconidia, the purported infectious form. In tissues or at greater than 37°C, yeast forms predominate, which typically are a 5- to 30-µm diameter ovoid mother cell displaying several blastoconidia (forming a "pilot's wheel") (Fig. 56.9) or with two larger buds (reminiscent of Mickey Mouse's head).

Interestingly, the ratios of clinical disease in men to women average approximately 13:1, but can be as high as 150:1. Perhaps women have less clinical disease because

Paracoccidioides expresses β-estradiol receptors on the conidial cell membrane; binding to these receptors inhibits morphogenesis to the yeast form, blocking disease progression.[148] Women are not protected against infection, but clinical disease is less likely.

Disease is more severe in the setting of immunosuppression. The initial host response to *Paracoccidioides* predominantly consists of neutrophils followed by recruitment of macrophages and granuloma formation. This process is highly regulated by cellular responses; Th1 responses are protective, whereas Th2 responses are common in patients unable to control their disease.[149,150] The impact of cellular immunity is further underscored by the increased incidence of disseminated disease in patients with AIDS. A review of mortality due to systemic mycoses in 3583 AIDS patients in Brazil from 1996 to 2006 revealed that paracoccidioidomycosis was responsible for approximately 50% of deaths.[151] Individuals on steroids, receiving chemotherapy, or status post–organ transplant are also at increased risk for severe disease.

CLINICAL MANIFESTATIONS

The majority of infections are asymptomatic, and individuals are believed to acquire the infection in childhood. There are two patterns of disease manifestation: the acute or subacute form (also called juvenile type) and the chronic form (or adult type). The juvenile type, which accounts for less than 10% of cases, most frequently develops in prepubescent teenagers to adults younger than 30 years. Patients are acutely ill, often presenting with fever, weight loss, and lymphadenopathy. Additionally, patients can have hepatosplenomegaly, intestinal lesions, and bone disease with or without bone marrow dysfunction. In contrast, the chronic form involves the lungs in approximately 90% of patients; this is believed to be due to reactivation of latent disease. However, new acquisition of the fungus is possible. Disease is localized to the lung in approximately 25% of patients, with the remainder presenting with multifocal disease, including dissemination to mucous membranes, lymph nodes, skin, adrenals, and other organs. Importantly, disease manifestations can mimic tuberculosis, which can also coinfect approximately 10% of these patients.[152]

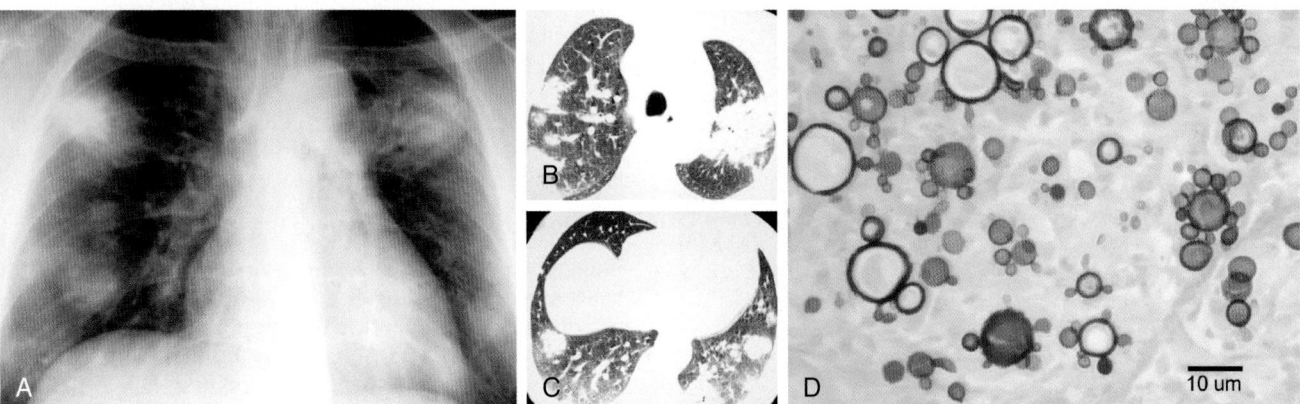

Figure 56.9 Pulmonary paracoccidioidomycosis. (A) Frontal chest radiograph shows bilateral poorly defined masses. (B–C) Axial chest computed tomography images confirm the presence of bilateral nodules, masses, and masslike areas of consolidation. Percutaneous transthoracic needle biopsy subsequently proved paracoccidioidomycosis. (D) *Paracoccidioides braziliensis* yeast forms. Several large mother cells with associated blastoconidia (forming a "pilot's wheel") are present. (Gomori methenamine silver stain.) (A–C, Courtesy Michael B. Gotway, MD; D, courtesy Dr. Carlos Taborda, PhD, University of São Paulo, Brazil.)

Radiologic findings are nonspecific and range from diffuse opacities to masses (see Fig. 56.9) and cavities (eFig. 56.16). Lymphadenopathy is often prominent. More than 50% of patients with significant chronic pulmonary disease develop long-term complications, most often impaired respiratory function due to fibrosis (eFig. 56.17). The development of right heart dysfunction is common in these patients. Additionally, compression of structures, such as the trachea, can develop. Single residual nodules without calcification are common.

DIAGNOSIS

Culture and microscopy are generally used for diagnosis. As noted, the yeast form has distinct shapes that can be identified in approximately 60–70% of sputum samples from patients with chronic paracoccidioidomycosis (see Fig. 56.9D). Culture remains a problem because the fungus routinely takes approximately 30 days to grow on mycologic agar. Diagnosis can also be supported by results of serologic testing. The major diagnostic antigen is a 43 kDa glycoprotein of *P. brasiliensis* (gp 43, a laminin-binding molecule), identified in approximately 90% of patients in the plasma, urine, or saliva.[153,154] An immunodiffusion test with antigen from the culture filtrate of yeast is highly specific and is positive in 65–100% of cases of acute or chronic pulmonary infection or disseminated paracoccidioidomycosis. A complement fixation test using the antigen from yeast culture filtrate is less specific than the immunodiffusion test, and cross reactions are observed with histoplasmosis. However, complement fixation titers of 1:8 or more are considered presumptive evidence of paracoccidioidomycosis[155] and, where the complement fixation test is available, it can be useful in following responses to treatment, which are accompanied by decreases in the titer.

TREATMENT

Optimal treatment regimens for paracoccidioides have not been formally validated.[70,152] In severely ill patients with dissemination, amphotericin therapy is usually initiated, often with deoxycholate formulations due to cost constraints in the endemic countries. Amphotericin is either continued until approximately a 2-g total dose or until the patient improves and is switched to an oral drug. Ketoconazole (200 to 400 mg/day) or itraconazole (200 to 400 mg/day) are the most commonly utilized azoles for paracoccidioidomycosis. Voriconazole and posaconazole may also have utility but have not been extensively studied. In patients with less severe disease, primary azole therapy is administered. Interestingly, in addition to amphotericin and azole drugs, sulfonamide derivatives have potent activity against the fungus.[156,157] Typical regimens for mild to moderate paracoccidioides with sulfonamide derivatives include sulfadiazine (4 to 6 g/day) or trimethoprim/sulfamethoxazole (160 mg/800 mg two or three times daily). Azole regimens usually range in duration from 6 to 18 months, whereas sulfa-based regimens range from 18 to 24 more months.

SPOROTHRIX

Sporotrichosis is principally caused by the dimorphic fungus *Sporothrix schenckii*, which is globally ubiquitous and grows in decaying vegetation, sphagnum moss, soil, and other environmental niches. The vast majority of infections follow cutaneous inoculation of the fungus, though pulmonary disease is increasingly recognized.[158] Such cases of pulmonary disease are primarily seen in men of middle age; risk factors include COPD and alcoholism. Radiographically, pulmonary sporotrichosis appears as cavitary and fibronodular disease.[159] Disseminated disease is rare and is primarily in severely immunocompromised individuals, especially in individuals with advanced HIV infection. Hence diagnosis of sporotrichosis in a patient with AIDS should lead to an assessment for dissemination.

The standard for diagnosis of invasive sporotrichosis is culture. However, culture results generally take 1 to 4 weeks. Biopsy material is often unrevealing of the organism, largely due to the small number of organisms that are needed to cause disease. The ovoid yeast cells are 3 to 5 μm in diameter, and eosinophilic projections from the yeast may be present, representing the "asteroid body" associated with *S. schenckii*. Severe to life-threatening pulmonary sporotrichosis should be initially treated with amphotericin B (liposomal amphotericin 3 to 5 mg/kg/day or deoxycholate amphotericin 0.7–1.0 mg/kg).[160] Once the patient's condition has stabilized, typically within 2 weeks, itraconazole (200 mg twice daily) can be administered for at least 1 year of total antifungal therapy. Adjunctive surgery may be especially useful in the setting of severe focal disease. If the disease is less severe at the outset, itraconazole can be used as initial therapy.[159] Serum levels of itraconazole should be verified after 2 weeks of administration and periodically thereafter. Treatment is generally from 3 to 6 months. Importantly, antifungals used for other manifestations of sporotrichosis, such as terbinafine, saturated solution of potassium iodide, or fluconazole, are not effective for pulmonary disease. Voriconazole is not effective and experience with posaconazole is limited.

TALAROMYCES

Talaromyces marneffei (formerly *Penicillium marneffei*), is a dimorphic fungus responsible for a systemic mycosis geographically restricted to southeast Asia, India, and southern China, especially in individuals with HIV.[161] In the environment, *T. marneffei* exists as a mycelial form whereas, in tissues, it is in a yeastlike form (arthroconidium) that is notable for replicating by fission. Talaromycosis is the third most common opportunistic infection in individuals with HIV in parts of tropical Asia, after tuberculosis and cryptococcosis. Although the majority of cases take place in the setting of advanced HIV infection, disease also presents in patients with immunosuppression due to malignancy or medical therapies as well as in patients with underlying lung disease. Patients with disseminated disease develop fever, weight loss, generalized lymphadenopathy, skin lesions (frequently papules with central necrosis), and hepatomegaly. The pathobiology of *T. marneffei* is comparable to that of histoplasmosis because *T. marneffei* survives in macrophages and manifests a similar spectrum of disease. Diagnosis is typically by culture and microscopy. The simplest approach is biopsy of skin lesions or lymph nodes with histologic assessment for fission arthroconidium. *T. marneffei* can also be visualized in peripheral blood smears in patients with fulminant disease. Initial therapy with amphotericin B has been proven superior to itraconazole.[162]

EMERGOMYCES

Emergomyces (formerly *Emmonsia*) is a newly described genus first identified as a cause of disseminated disease in AIDS patients within South Africa (*Es. africanus*).[163] This dimorphic fungus is the most common endemic mycosis in South Africa. Presenting symptoms are most frequently fever, weight loss, elevated liver enzymes, and radiographic findings of the chest are similar to those of tuberculosis. Skin disease is also common and presents concurrently with other clinical findings. Subsequent investigation has identified other *Emergomyces* sp, including *Es. orientalis*, *Es. canadensis*, *Es. europaeus*, and *Es. pasteurianus*.[164,165] Isolates are frequently misidentified as *Blastomyces* and sequencing is often necessary to differentiate these organisms. Treatment of this infection has yet to be refined; however, initial therapy with amphotericin B is recommended until clinical improvement is observed, followed by itraconazole, voriconazole, or posaconazole.[166]

Key Points

- Endemic mycoses are able to infect and cause disease in previously healthy immunocompetent hosts.
- Exposure may be unavoidable with travel or residence within the endemic region because of the high density of the fungi in certain environments.
- Clinical manifestations may be nonspecific, but respiratory symptoms are common at early and late stages of infection.
- The fungi that cause endemic mycoses have specific morphologic features in tissue samples and when cultured in the laboratory.
- Noninvasive testing (antigen testing and serology) are available for the majority of these infections.
- Many infected individuals resolve endemic fungal infections without treatment but, in some individuals, severe pulmonary and disseminated infections develop and can be life-threatening.

Key Readings

Andes D, Pascual A, Marchetti O. Antifungal therapeutic drug monitoring: established and emerging indications. *Antimicrob Agents Chemother.* 2009;53(1):24–34.

Baddley JW, Winthrop KL, Patkar NM, et al. Geographic distribution of endemic fungal infections among older persons, United States. *Emerg Infect Dis.* 2011;17(9):1664–1669.

Benedict K, Mody RK. Epidemiology of histoplasmosis outbreaks, United States, 1938–2013. *Emerg Infect Dis.* 2016;22(3):370–378.

Brown J, Benedict K, Park BJ, Thompson 3rd GR. Coccidioidomycosis: epidemiology. *Clin Epidemiol.* 2013;5:185–197.

Cooksey GS, Nguyen A, Knutson K, et al. Notes from the field: increase in coccidioidomycosis—California, 2016. *MMWR Morb Mortal Wkly Rep.* 2017;66(31):833–834.

Engelthaler DM, Roe CC, Hepp CM, et al. Local population structure and patterns of Western Hemisphere dispersal for *Coccidioides* spp., the fungal cause of valley fever. *mBio.* 2016;7(2):e00550-e00516.

Galgiani JN, Ampel NM, Blair JE, et al. Coccidioidomycosis. *Clin Infect Dis.* 2005;41(9):1217–1223.

Grim SA, Proia L, Miller R, et al. A multicenter study of histoplasmosis and blastomycosis after solid organ transplantation. *Transpl Infect Dis.* 2012;14(1):17–23.

Heidari A, Quinlan M, Benjamin DJ, et al. Isavuconazole in the treatment of coccidioidal meningitis. *Antimicrob Agents Chemother.* 2019;63(3).

Le T, Thwaites G, Wolbers M. Itraconazole or amphotericin B for talaromycosis. *N Engl J Med.* 2017;377(14):1403.

Limper AH, Knox KS, Sarosi GA, et al. An official American thoracic society statement: treatment of fungal infections in adult pulmonary and critical care patients. *Am J Respir Crit Care Med.* 2011;183(1):96–128.

Sathapatayavongs B, Batteiger BE, Wheat J, Slama TG, Wass JL. Clinical and laboratory features of disseminated histoplasmosis during two large urban outbreaks. *Medicine (Baltim).* 1983;62(5):263–270.

Seitz AE, Younes N, Steiner CA, Prevots DR. Incidence and trends of blastomycosis-associated hospitalizations in the United States. *PLOS One.* 2014;9(8):e105466.

Teixeira Mde M, Patane JS, Taylor ML, et al. Worldwide phylogenetic distributions and population dynamics of the genus *Histoplasma*. *PLOS Negl Trop Dis.* 2016;10(6):e0004732.

Thompson 3rd GR, Barker BM, Wiederhold NP. Large-scale evaluation of in vitro amphotericin b, triazole, and echinocandin activity against *Coccidioides* species from U.S. institutions. *Antimicrob Agents Chemother.* 2017;61(4).

Thompson 3rd GR, Lewis 2nd JS, Nix DE, Patterson TF. Current concepts and future directions in the pharmacology and treatment of coccidioidomycosis. *Medical Mycol.* 2019;57(suppl 1):S76–S84.

Complete reference list available at ExpertConsult.com.

57 | *FUNGAL INFECTIONS: OPPORTUNISTIC*

JENNIFER L. SAULLO, MD, PHARMD • BARBARA D. ALEXANDER, MD, MHS

INTRODUCTION

The epidemiology of opportunistic mycoses is evolving. In certain populations, the frequency of opportunistic mycoses is increasing due to expanding use of immunomodulating therapies, a higher frequency of invasive procedures and devices, and changes in climate and regional environments. In other populations, the frequency of opportunistic mycoses is decreasing due to antifungal prophylaxis in high-risk patients and reconstitution of immunity with antiretroviral therapy for *human immunodeficiency virus* (HIV) infection. Heightened clinical awareness of fungal infections and the availability of improved diagnostics contribute to their increased recognition, and the availability of newer antifungal drugs provides broader therapeutic options.

Fungi are eukaryotic microorganisms that grow as yeasts or molds. Yeasts are unicellular fungi and exist as single rounded or elongated cells and reproduce primarily by budding. The primary opportunistic yeasts reviewed here are *Candida* and *Cryptococcus*. In contrast, molds are multicellular filamentous fungi composed of hyphae that grow by branching with extension at the hyphal apices. Clinically relevant opportunistic molds are often categorized on the basis of their hyphae. Aseptate (or sparsely septate) hyphae infrequently demonstrate cross walls that divide the hyphae into compartments, whereas septate do contain these cross walls. This distinction can be used in identifying molds in respiratory samples and tissue histopathology. Aseptate (or sparsely septate) hyphae are seen in mucormycosis, caused by molds such as *Mucor* and *Rhizopus* (historically referred to as *Zygomycetes*). Septate hyphae are found in opportunistic molds that are further subdivided as hyaline or dematiaceous molds. Hyaline molds produce colorless or lightly pigmented hyphae in tissue and infections are referred to as *hyalohyphomycoses*. Dematiaceous or black molds are septate molds that contain melanin in their cell walls, resulting in brown pigmentation, which can be seen in histopathology specimens and under direct microscopic examination. Infections with the dematiaceous molds are referred to as *phaeohyphomycoses*. Endemic fungi such as *Blastomyces dermatitidis* and *Histoplasma capsulatum*, reviewed in Chapter 56, are considered dimorphic fungi, growing as molds at room temperature and yeast or yeastlike forms at body temperature.

This chapter discusses the most common opportunistic mycoses of the respiratory tract and their epidemiology, clinical characteristics, diagnosis, and treatment. Although *Pneumocystis jirovecii* (previously *P. carinii*) is an opportunistic yeastlike fungus, it is discussed in Chapters 123 and 125 because of its distinctive biology and approaches to therapy.

ANTIFUNGAL THERAPY

Rapid initiation of antifungal therapy is essential in the management of *invasive fungal infections* (IFIs). The primary classes of antifungal agents target either the plasma membrane or the cell wall. *Amphotericin B* (AmB) was previously the primary antifungal agent for IFIs; however, newer antifungals, including the extended-spectrum azoles and echinocandins, have broadened the therapeutic options, and lipid formulations of AmB have less toxicity. In addition, combination therapy should be considered in certain IFIs. The following section is a broad overview of the major antifungal agents. eTables 57.1 and 57.2 summarize details of the available agents, including their spectrum of activity, primary toxicities, interactions, recommendations for therapeutic drug monitoring, and the *U.S. Food and Drug Administration* (FDA)–approved indications.

763

POLYENES

The polyenes include nystatin and AmB. AmB binds to ergosterol, an essential component of the fungal cell membrane. AmB binding increases membrane permeability and causes fungal cell death.[1] AmB also induces proinflammatory cytokines by activating toll-like receptor 2, which contributes to the acute side effects of fever and myalgias, and may augment host responses to fungal infection.[2] AmB has activity against multiple fungal pathogens including *Aspergillus*, *Candida*, the endemic mycoses (e.g., blastomycosis, coccidioidomycosis, cryptococcosis, histoplasmosis), and mucormycosis.[3] However, certain fungi, including *Aspergillus terreus*, *Candida lusitaniae*, *Lomentospora* (previously *Scedosporium*) *prolificans*, and *Trichosporon beigelii*, may be intrinsically resistant to AmB, and other pathogens, such as *Fusarium* species and select dematiaceous molds, may have high *minimal inhibitory concentrations* (MICs) to AmB.[4]

The lipid formulations of AmB were introduced to reduce nephrotoxicity seen with conventional amphotericin, called *amphotericin B deoxycholate* (AmB-d). The lipid formulations of AmB are now often used as first-line therapy, particularly in patients with renal dysfunction or on concurrent nephrotoxic medications. Lipid formulations include *liposomal AmB* (LAmB) and *AmB lipid complex* (ABLC). Encochleated AmB, MAT2033, the first orally administered polyene formulation, is a suspension of AmB carried in cochleates (stable multilayered phospholipid-cation precipitates) to facilitate oral absorption. It has demonstrated activity in animal models of candidiasis and aspergillosis with multiple phase I and II clinical trials either planned or ongoing.[5]

AZOLES

Triazoles (i.e., "azoles") have emerged as a primary class of antifungals for treatment and prevention of IFIs. The most widely used azoles are fluconazole, itraconazole, isavuconazole, posaconazole, and voriconazole. These agents act on the fungal cell membrane by inhibiting the cytochrome P-450–dependent 14-α-demethylase, a critical enzyme in the conversion of lanosterol to ergosterol. This is encoded in yeasts and molds by *ERG11* and *cyp51*, respectively.[6] The azoles are fungistatic or fungicidal, depending on the specific azole and fungal species.[7] Immunomodulating effects have been described with azoles and may contribute to their efficacy.[2] While earlier azoles, such as fluconazole, are only active against yeasts, the extended-spectrum azoles, including itraconazole, voriconazole, isavuconazole, and posaconazole, are active against yeasts and molds. Fluconazole is active against *Cryptococcus* and *Candida* and has variable activity against endemic fungi, including *Coccidioides*. *Candida krusei* is intrinsically resistant to fluconazole and high-level resistance has emerged among some non-*albicans Candida* species, including *Candida glabrata*. Itraconazole has little role in treatment of most opportunistic fungal infections; its principal indications are treatment of indolent, non–*central nervous system* (CNS) blastomycosis or histoplasmosis and as an alternative to fluconazole for treatment of indolent non-CNS coccidioidomycosis. Itraconazole is also indicated in treatment of allergic bronchopulmonary aspergillosis and some forms of chronic pulmonary aspergillosis. Itraconazole exhibits highly variable absorption and pharmacokinetics; therapeutic drug monitoring is essential to guide optimal dosing for an individual patient.

The extended-spectrum azoles have activity against many molds, including *Aspergillus*, non-*Aspergillus* hyaline hyphomycetes such as *Fusarium*, *Scedosporium*, *Lomentospora*, and *Paecilomyces*, and some dematiaceous molds. Voriconazole is the drug of choice for the treatment of invasive *Aspergillus* infections. Isavuconazole, the newest of the extended-spectrum azoles, is also FDA approved for the treatment of *invasive aspergillosis* (IA) as well as mucormycosis.[8] Isavuconazole is a water-soluble prodrug and, unlike other extended-spectrum azoles such as voriconazole and posaconazole, the intravenous formulation is devoid of the solubilizing moiety cyclodextrin, which can accumulate in patients with renal dysfunction. In contrast to other azoles that can prolong the QT interval, isavuconazole has been shown to shorten the QT interval, though the full clinical significance of this remains unclear.[8] Among the azoles, only posaconazole and isavuconazole have significant activity against the agents of mucormycosis.

ECHINOCANDINS

The echinocandins, including caspofungin, micafungin, and anidulafungin, are increasingly used given their efficacy, tolerability, lack of drug interactions, and the prevalence of azole-resistant *Candida* species. Unlike AmB and the azoles, the echinocandins act on the fungal cell wall via noncompetitive binding to the catalytic subunits of (1→3)-β-D-glucan synthase, thereby inhibiting production of (1→3)-β-D-glucan (β-D-glucan), an essential component of the fungal cell wall. Echinocandins are fungicidal against multiple *Candida* species, including *C. albicans*, *C. dubliniensis*, *C. glabrata*, and *C. krusei*; however, certain *Candida* species, such as *C. guilliermondii* and *C. parapsilosis*, typically have higher MICs. The echinocandins are fungistatic, rather than fungicidal, against filamentous fungi such as *Aspergillus* species because their activity is restricted to sites where the fungal cell wall is actively growing (i.e., hyphal tips and branching junctional cells) but not on subapical hyphal cells.[9] Echinocandins lack significant activity against other fungal pathogens such as *Cryptococcus*, *Mucorales*, and *Trichosporon* species and the endemic fungi.[10] Immunostimulatory effects of echinocandins on monocytes and monocyte-derived macrophages may be of particular importance against *Aspergillus*.[11,12]

A novel, next-generation echinocandin, rezafungin (CD101), is a structural analog of anidulafungin with a long half-life allowing for once-weekly intravenous dosing. Rezafungin is currently under investigation in phase III clinical trials for treatment of candidemia and/or invasive candidiasis as well as for prophylaxis of *Aspergillus*, *Candida*, and *Pneumocystis* in high-risk allogeneic *hematopoietic cell transplant* (HCT) recipients. Ibrexafungerp (SCY-078), the first member of a new glucan synthase inhibitor subclass that also targets (1→3)-β-D-glucan, is available as an oral formulation. Ibrexafungerp has activity similar to echinocandins but also offers promise for use with some echinocandin-resistant fungal pathogens including *Candida auris*.[13] In vitro activity against some non-*Aspergillus* molds such as *Paecilomyces variotti* and the often multidrug-resistant *Lomentospora prolificans* has also been demonstrated, although the clinical applicability against such non-*Aspergillus* molds remains to be determined.[5,14]

FLUCYTOSINE

Flucytosine (5-FC) is an antimetabolite that inhibits fungal DNA and protein synthesis. It is used in combination with other antifungal agents given the high frequency of emergence of resistance with monotherapy.[15] It is fungistatic or fungicidal, depending upon the organism, and is most often used in combination with AmB against *Cryptococcus*[16] and in severe *Candida* infections such as endocarditis and CNS infections.[17]

TERBINAFINE

Terbinafine is a synthetic allylamine that exerts its antifungal effects via inhibition of fungal squalene epoxidase, an enzyme involved in ergosterol formation. Terbinafine is fungicidal and is used most commonly for dermatophyte infections and the treatment of chromoblastomycosis.[18] In vitro synergy data have led to its use in combination, most often with extended-spectrum azoles and AmB, for the management of severe or refractory mold infections such as *Lomentospora*,[19] *Fusarium*,[20] and other hyaline and dematiaceous molds.[18]

CRYPTOCOCCOSIS

EPIDEMIOLOGY

Cryptococcosis is an invasive fungal infection caused primarily by *Cryptococcus neoformans* and *C. gattii*. *C. neoformans* is most common and has a global distribution and can be isolated from the soil and excreta of birds such as pigeons. *C. neoformans* var. *grubii* is the predominant pathogen worldwide; however, infections with *C. neoformans* var. *neoformans* are prevalent in Northern Europe.[21] *C. gattii* was originally found in tropical and subtropical regions including Australia, Southeast Asia, and Central Africa. However, serious infections with *C. gattii* have also been recognized in Vancouver, British Columbia, and in the Pacific Northwest United States.[22,23] With advances in molecular diagnostics, the genetic diversity of cryptococcosis is increasingly recognized. New taxonomy has been proposed to divide *C. neoformans* further into *C. neoformans* and *C. deneoformans*, and *C. gattii* into five distinct species.[24] While infections with *C. gattii* can develop in immunocompetent hosts, most cryptococcal infections are seen in immunocompromised hosts, including patients with advanced HIV infection,[25] malignancies,[26] *solid organ transplants* (SOTs),[27] and other conditions.[28] Cryptococcosis is one of the most common life-threatening fungal infections in HIV-infected patients,[29] and it is the third most common invasive fungal pathogen (after *Candida* and *Aspergillus*) in SOT recipients in whom it causes 8% of IFIs.[30] *Cryptococcus* affects HCT patients less often, causing 0.6% of IFIs.[31]

PATHOGENESIS

Infections with *Cryptococcus* are typically initiated by inhalation of small yeast or spores. Once in the alveoli, the outcome is determined by the virulence of the infecting strain, host genetic polymorphisms, innate and adaptive immune responses, and the presence of comorbidities. The virulence of *Cryptococcus* is related to its polysaccharide capsule as well as the presence of specific enzymes, including laccase, phospholipase B, and inositol phosphosphingolipid-phospholipase.[32] In the lungs, the *Cryptococcus* capsule protects against phagocytosis and impairs host immune response by interfering with macrophage antigen presentation to T cells, reducing cytokine production, depleting complement components, and reducing leukocyte migration.[33] Successfully phagocytosed cryptococci reside and replicate in mature phagolysosomes and subsequently spread to other cells using multiple mechanisms.[34]

The innate immune response to *Cryptococcus* results in cytokine production and a Th1 CD4$^+$ T cell response.[35] CD4$^+$ cells are necessary to prevent dissemination from the lungs; both CD4$^+$ and CD8$^+$ cells are required for clearance of infection in mice.[36] Although antibody-mediated immunity contributes to control of cryptococci in mice,[35,37] defects in humoral immunity are less commonly associated with cryptococcal infections in humans than are defects in cellular immunity.[38] The presence of autoantibodies to granulocyte-macrophage colony-stimulating factors may predispose otherwise immunocompetent individuals to infection with *C. gattii*.[39]

CLINICAL MANIFESTATIONS

The clinical presentation of cryptococcal infection is determined by the immune status of the host, the *Cryptococcus* species, and the site of infection. The lungs are the most commonly involved primary site; the CNS is the most common site of dissemination. *Cryptococcus* is also believed to cause latent infection in the lung and reactivate in the setting of depressed immunity. In fact, most infections may represent reactivation, and transfer of infection with donor organs may contribute to infection in SOT recipients.[40] Dissemination may develop during primary infection or reactivation. Most pulmonary infections are asymptomatic or mildly symptomatic in immunocompetent hosts and may be discovered incidentally on radiographic imaging. Acute infection in the immunocompetent host may manifest with fever, fatigue, cough, and sputum production. In immunocompromised patients, severe symptoms, including fever, cough, and shortness of breath, can rapidly progress to respiratory failure and acute respiratory distress syndrome. In a prospective multicenter international study of 111 SOT recipients, cryptococcal infections were diagnosed a median of 21 months after transplant, and pulmonary (60%) and CNS (58%) involvement predominated.[41] In patients with advanced HIV infection, meningoencephalitis is the predominant presentation.[42]

The radiographic findings in cryptococcal pulmonary infections commonly include focal or diffuse pulmonary nodules or patchy airspace consolidation (eFig. 57.1). However, other findings include cavitation (see Fig. 57.1A, eFig. 123.21), mass lesions (i.e., cryptococcomas

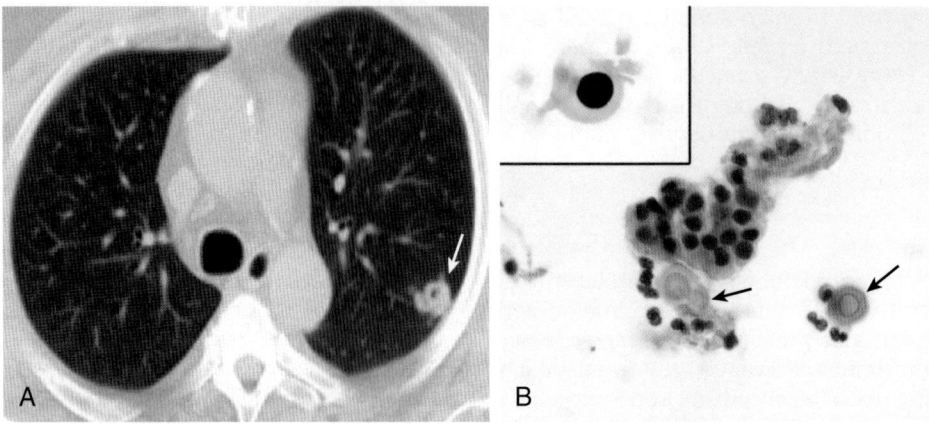

Figure 57.1 Cryptococcosis. Pulmonary infection with *Cryptococcus* in an asymptomatic cardiac transplant patient on chronic immunosuppression with new, bilateral pulmonary nodules. (A) Axial chest computed tomography (CT) demonstrates a cavitary nodule (*arrow*) with small surrounding satellite nodules. (B) CT-guided fine-needle aspiration of the pulmonary nodule shows encapsulated yeast (*arrows*), with the typical morphology of *Cryptococcus neoformans*. (Papanicolaou stain; ×400 original magnification.) *Inset*, Yeast showing mucin capsule with organism staining positive. (Methenamine silver stain; ×400 original magnification.) (B, Courtesy Dr. Thomas Sporn, Duke University Medical Center, NC.)

[see eFig. 123.23]), reticulonodular patterns, ground-glass attenuation (see eFig. 123.21), and associated effusions or lymphadenopathy (see eFig. 123.24A–B).[43,44] In a study of *computed tomography* (CT) radiographic findings of cryptococcosis, immunocompromised patients had more extensive pulmonary involvement with cavitation and parenchymal consolidation than did immunocompetent hosts—a finding that contrasts with that in tuberculosis.[43] Cryptococcomas in both the CNS and in the lungs are seen more commonly with *C. gattii* than with *C. neoformans* infection, and they are more common in immunocompetent hosts.[45]

DIAGNOSIS

The diagnosis of pulmonary cryptococcosis is based on symptoms, chest radiography, culture, histopathologic findings (Fig. 57.1B), and *cryptococcal antigen* (CrAg) testing. *Cryptococcus* can be cultured from respiratory specimens, including sputum and *bronchoalveolar lavage* (BAL), lung biopsy tissue specimens, and from pleural cultures in cases associated with pleural involvement. Blood cultures are typically only positive in disseminated infections. *Cryptococcus* is easily identified under the microscope as 5- to 10-μm, spherical to oval yeast cells with a surrounding capsule, although capsule-deficient variants do exist. Biochemical testing can be used to confirm the identification.[46] In tissue samples, specialized stains such as Mayer's mucicarmine, which stains mucin within the polysaccharide capsule, are also helpful in establishing a diagnosis.[46] *Matrix-assisted laser desorption ionization–time of flight mass spectrometry* (MALDI-TOF MS) and molecular methods such as the *polymerase chain reaction* (PCR) are increasingly utilized by clinical laboratories as a less labor-intensive means of rapid identification of cryptococci.[47,48]

Commercial assays available for detection of the CrAg in clinical specimens (e.g., serum, *cerebrospinal fluid* [CSF]) include the latex agglutination test, enzyme-linked immunosorbent assay, and the *lateral flow assay* (LFA). The latter was more recently introduced as a rapid, inexpensive point-of-care diagnostic and is ideally suited for resource-limited settings. While the serum CrAg assays have high sensitivity and specificity in disseminated infection and cryptococcal meningoencephalitis, they can be negative in patients with isolated pulmonary infection. In a study of patients undergoing SOT, serum CrAg was detectable in 73% of patients (22 of 30) with isolated pulmonary involvement and was more likely to be negative with solitary pulmonary nodules than with multiple nodules and more extensive pulmonary disease. Titers of serum CrAg were higher in those patients with concurrent extrapulmonary infection.[49] False-negative results related to a prozone phenomenon[50] in samples containing a large burden of antigen as well as false-positive results due to cross reaction with other pathogens (e.g., *Trichosporon*,[51] *Ustilago maydis*,[52] and *Stomatococcus*[53]) and disinfectants[54] have also been reported.

Determining the presence of disseminated infection and extent of organ involvement is crucial to the selection of appropriate therapy. Thus, CSF evaluation (e.g., cell count, fungal culture, CrAg) should be performed in all immunosuppressed patients with pulmonary cryptococcosis. Multiplex PCR testing platforms have also been applied to CSF specimens but may not reliably rule out cryptococcal CNS infection.[55] Whether CSF analysis is essential in immunocompetent patients with pulmonary cryptococcosis is less clear. Factors associated with higher likelihood of disseminated disease and the need for CSF analysis include neurologic findings, signs of systemic infection, such as fever and weight loss, and serum CrAg titer of at least 1:64.[56]

TREATMENT

The choice of therapy depends on the immune status of the host and the presence of extrapulmonary infection; current treatment recommendations are available from both the *American Thoracic Society* (ATS)[57] and *Infectious Diseases Society of America* (IDSA).[16] For cryptococcosis in patients with evidence of disseminated infection, CNS involvement, or severe pneumonia, treatment is separated into induction, consolidation, and maintenance regimens (Fig. 57.2). The choices of antifungals, doses, and duration are dependent on the patient's underlying risk group (e.g., organ transplant recipient, HIV infected, or non–HIV infected,

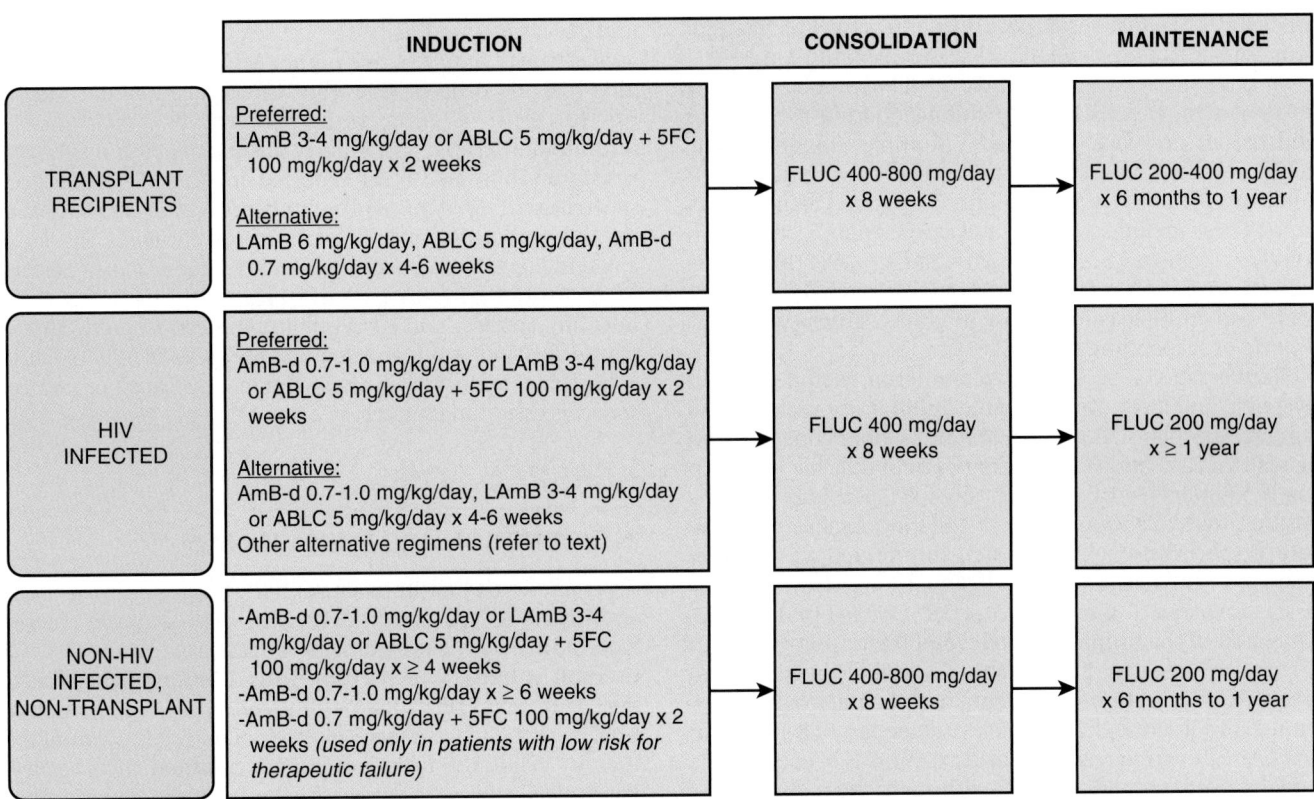

	INDUCTION	CONSOLIDATION	MAINTENANCE
TRANSPLANT RECIPIENTS	<u>Preferred:</u> LAmB 3-4 mg/kg/day or ABLC 5 mg/kg/day + 5FC 100 mg/kg/day x 2 weeks <u>Alternative:</u> LAmB 6 mg/kg/day, ABLC 5 mg/kg/day, AmB-d 0.7 mg/kg/day x 4-6 weeks	FLUC 400-800 mg/day x 8 weeks	FLUC 200-400 mg/day x 6 months to 1 year
HIV INFECTED	<u>Preferred:</u> AmB-d 0.7-1.0 mg/kg/day or LAmB 3-4 mg/kg/day or ABLC 5 mg/kg/day + 5FC 100 mg/kg/day x 2 weeks <u>Alternative:</u> AmB-d 0.7-1.0 mg/kg/day, LAmB 3-4 mg/kg/day or ABLC 5 mg/kg/day x 4-6 weeks Other alternative regimens (refer to text)	FLUC 400 mg/day x 8 weeks	FLUC 200 mg/day x ≥ 1 year
NON-HIV INFECTED, NON-TRANSPLANT	-AmB-d 0.7-1.0 mg/kg/day or LAmB 3-4 mg/kg/day or ABLC 5 mg/kg/day + 5FC 100 mg/kg/day x ≥ 4 weeks -AmB-d 0.7-1.0 mg/kg/day x ≥ 6 weeks -AmB-d 0.7 mg/kg/day + 5FC 100 mg/kg/day x 2 weeks *(used only in patients with low risk for therapeutic failure)*	FLUC 400-800 mg/day x 8 weeks	FLUC 200 mg/day x 6 months to 1 year

Figure 57.2 Treatment of cryptococcosis in patients with evidence of disseminated infection, central nervous system involvement, or severe pneumonia. ABLC, amphotericin B lipid complex; AmB-d, amphotericin B deoxycholate; FLUC, fluconazole; HIV, human immunodeficiency virus; LAmB, liposomal amphotericin B; 5FC, flucytosine. (Data from Perfect JR, Dismukes WE, Dromer F, et al: Clinical practice guidelines for the management of cryptococcal disease: 2010 update by the Infectious Diseases Society of America. *Clin Infect Dis* 2010;50[3]:291–322.)

non-transplant recipient).[16] In HIV-infected patients with cryptococcal meningoencephalitis in resource-limited settings, data have emerged demonstrating comparable efficacy with induction courses consisting of one week of AmB or 2 weeks of high-dose fluconazole (1200 mg/day), each in combination with 5-FC.[58] Mild-to-moderate infection isolated to the lungs is treated with fluconazole 400 mg/day for a minimum of 6 to 12 months. Some experts maintain that asymptomatic patients with resected solitary nodules, undetectable serum CrAg, and no evidence of extrapulmonary infection may be observed closely without specific antifungal therapy.[16] Infections with *C. gattii* have been associated with delayed clinical response to antifungal therapy; potential explanations include high in vitro antifungal MICs, particularly with fluconazole, and a higher incidence of pulmonary and cerebral cryptococcomas with decreased drug penetration to these lesions.[16,59,60]

Immune reconstitution inflammatory syndrome (IRIS) may complicate treatment of any opportunistic mycosis but is most common in cryptococcosis. IRIS is usually characterized by worsening of clinical signs and symptoms of the original infection, which can be misinterpreted as progressive infection.[16,61] IRIS arises most commonly with initiation of antiretroviral therapy in HIV infection and with abrupt reduction of immunosuppression in SOT recipients. IRIS can also manifest in patients with hematologic malignancies during neutrophil and monocyte recovery following myeloablative chemotherapy[62] and with lymphocyte recovery after receipt of monoclonal antibodies such as alemtuzumab.[63] Manifestations of IRIS in pulmonary

disease may be severe and include acute respiratory distress syndrome. Transplant recipients developing IRIS also have increased potential for allograft loss.[64] While nonsteroidal anti-inflammatory drugs may be sufficient to ameliorate the symptoms of IRIS, high-dose corticosteroids may also be required, and treatment of IRIS in transplant recipients includes careful adjustment of immunosuppressive drugs.[16] (See also Chapter 123.)

CANDIDIASIS

The epidemiology of invasive *Candida* infections has evolved substantially in recent decades and depends on a multitude of factors including patient-specific risks and geography.[65–71] Non-*albicans Candida* species including *C. glabrata*, *C. parapsilosis*, *C. tropicalis*, and *C. krusei* account for an increasing proportion of infections.[17,67,71,72] *C. auris*, which can be multidrug-resistant and associated with poor clinical outcomes, was first identified clinically in 2009[73] and subsequently emerged as a global threat, associated with horizontal transmission seen in large outbreaks in health care facilities.[74–77]

Candida infections of the thorax include empyema, tracheobronchial and mediastinal infection, and pneumonia. *Candida* pneumonia is rare and is most often found in the setting of candidemia with dissemination to the lung in immunocompromised patients.[78,79] Rarely, primary pneumonia develops due to aspiration of oropharyngeal contents.[78,80,81] Mediastinitis may complicate thoracic surgical procedures,[82] and pleural space infection, as well as tracheo-bronchial infection, can follow lung transplantation.[83,84]

Candida species have multiple virulence determinants; virulent strains consistently exhibit adherence to devices and tissues and form biofilms.[66] Multiple human genetic polymorphisms have been identified that contribute heightened susceptibility to mucosal and invasive *Candida* infections. These include common and rare sequence variants in toll-like receptors 1, 2, and 4, cytokine signaling (*interleukin* [IL]-10, and the shared subunit of IL-12 and IL-23 receptors), and multiple genes whose products contribute to generating or responding to IL-17.[85,86]

Manifestations of *Candida* pneumonia include cough, dyspnea, and fever. Radiographic findings are variable and can include lobar (eFig. 57.2) and multilobar consolidation as well as cavitation.[79] The diagnosis of *Candida* pneumonia is complicated by the generally low specificity and low *positive predictive value* (PPV) of isolating *Candida* in respiratory specimens, which is often interpreted as colonization.[78,79,87,88] Consequently, histopathologic evidence of tissue invasion is required to prove *Candida* pneumonia. Detection of the fungal cell wall component β-D-glucan in serum may assist in distinguishing colonization from invasive *Candida* infection. In patients with hematologic malignancy and in critically ill patients, detection of β-D-glucan has been shown to result in earlier diagnosis of candidemia and invasive candidiasis,[89,90] although the specificity of this test is limited by multiple sources for false-positive tests and cross reactivity due to synthesis of β-D-glucan by other fungi, and low PPV. Blood cultures have an overall low sensitivity for detection of invasive candidiasis along with slow turnaround times due to the extended period required for organism growth and identification.[91] MALDI-TOF MS[92] and molecular techniques including peptide nucleic acid fluorescence in situ hybridization[93,94] and multiplex PCR[95] are currently used to expedite the identification of *Candida* species but still require growth in culture. *C. auris* is often misidentified using commercial identification platforms including MALDI-TOF MS; a national effort to improve recognition/identification of this particular pathogen by clinical laboratories is being led by the Centers for Disease Control and Prevention.[96] Culture-independent methods to expedite the diagnosis of invasive candidiasis include T2Candida (T2 Biosystems), which utilizes PCR and T2 magnetic resonance to detect nanoparticle-labeled probes for five *Candida* species, namely *C. albicans*, *C. glabrata*, *C. parapsilosis*, *C. tropicalis*, and *C. krusei*, directly in whole blood.[97,98] While other molecular methods for invasive candidiasis have been developed, to date none are FDA approved for clinical use.[99,100]

Given the increasing number of infections with non-*albicans Candida* species and the potential for infection with azole cross-resistant strains,[101–104] echinocandins are typically preferred for initial therapy while awaiting species identification and susceptibility testing. Lipid formulations of AmB should be considered in patients with extensive prior echinocandin exposure; *C. glabrata* in particular has demonstrated resistance to echinocandins with associated poor outcomes, most often in the context of prior echinocandin exposure and *FKS1* and *FKS2* gene alterations.[105–108] *C. lusitaniae* is often resistant to AmB, and *C. tropicalis* has shown increasing acquired resistance to azoles

and to echinocandins.[105,106,109,110] *C. parapsilosis* and *C. guilliermondii* tend to have higher MICs for the echinocandins than do other species, but the clinical significance is unclear.[111–113] *C. auris* can harbor or develop resistance to antifungal therapy, particularly fluconazole, but multidrug resistance has also been reported inclusive of extended-spectrum azoles, AmB, and echinocandins.[114] These observations underscore the importance of knowing the local epidemiology and resistance patterns for *Candida* within an institution and the patient's prior antifungal exposure, infecting species, and susceptibility pattern to guide therapeutic decision making. Adequate drainage of infected fluid collections, including those in the mediastinum or pleural space, is essential for cure.

ASPERGILLOSIS

INTRODUCTION AND EPIDEMIOLOGY

Aspergillus is a ubiquitous saprophytic fungus found indoors and outdoors in association with soil, organic debris, food, and water. *Aspergillus* produces large numbers of 2 to 3 μm conidia, which easily enter the lungs via inhalation. Outbreaks often follow renovation and construction, activities that place a large number of *Aspergillus* conidia in the air. While the lung is the most common site of entry, *Aspergillus* may gain access to the host via other routes, including direct cutaneous inoculation. Among *Aspergillus* species, *A. fumigatus* is the most common pathogen, in part due to specific virulence factors,[115] but non-*fumigatus* species, including *A. flavus*, *A. niger*, and *A. terreus*, also cause human disease.[30,31,116] *A. terreus* is notable for intrinsic AmB resistance.[117,118] Application of azole prophylaxis has also led to the emergence of breakthrough infections with *A. ustus* complex, which tends to have high MICs to the mold-active azoles.[119] In addition, *A. nidulans*, an otherwise rare pathogen, is uniquely associated with chronic granulomatous disease, second only to *A. fumigatus* as the most common mold infections in this population.[120]

Aspergillus is a hyaline hyphomycete characterized by septate, narrow (3 to 6 μm) hyphae with acute angle (45 degrees) branching (Fig. 57.3) in respiratory secretions and tissue specimens. The non-*Aspergillus* hyaline hyphomycetes, discussed later, have a similar appearance in clinical specimens and are differentiated from *Aspergillus* in culture based on the morphologic characteristics of their reproductive structures. Aspergillosis most commonly presents as infection limited to the lung but may also present as a skin/soft tissue, ocular, gastrointestinal, cardiac, sinus, CNS, or disseminated infection.[121]

Two major forms of pulmonary aspergillosis are addressed in this chapter: *invasive pulmonary aspergillosis* (IPA), and *chronic pulmonary aspergillosis* (CPA). *Allergic bronchopulmonary aspergillosis* (ABPA), a saprophytic, noninvasive form of aspergillosis, caused by hypersensitivity to *Aspergillus* antigens is covered in detail in Chapter 96.

PATHOGENESIS

Although *Aspergillus* species are not obligate pathogens, their evolution to survive in decomposing organic matter has provided them with mechanisms that contribute

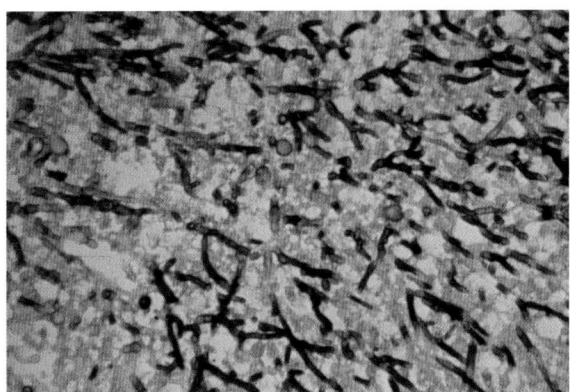

Figure 57.3 Invasive aspergillosis. Micrograph shows findings of invasive *Aspergillus* infection represented by septate hyphae with finger-like branching at acute angles. (Methenamine silver stain; ×450 original magnification.)

to virulence in humans and other mammals. *Aspergillus* possesses multiple defenses against reactive oxygen intermediates; some of these defenses include melanin,[122] catalases,[123] superoxide dismutases,[124] and glutathione transferases.[125] *Aspergillus* is also able to survive in hypoxic environments, which may confer a survival advantage when it renders tissues hypoxic by invading blood vessel walls. Other mechanisms that may contribute to pathogenesis include production of diverse toxins, including gliotoxin and fumagillin, and secretion of elastase, which may promote tissue invasion.[126]

Work in humans and in murine models has provided considerable insight into the elements and mechanisms of innate and adaptive immune responses that provide protection against invasive *Aspergillus* infections (see Chapters 15 and 16).[127–130] *Aspergillus* spores possess a hydrophobic protein coat made up of rod-shaped structures (rodlets), which mask the cell wall and prevent recognition by innate immune receptors.[131] This allows individuals to inhale millions of fungal spores every day without induction of an inflammatory response. Spores that swell and germinate before being killed expose the fungal cell wall that contains multiple pathogen-associated molecular patterns recognized by innate immune cells. In particular, β-D-glucan is recognized by host dectin-1, which initiates production of proinflammatory cytokines and chemokines, and modulates differentiation of CD4+ T cells. The importance of specific pathways of innate immune recognition has been demonstrated by finding that HCT recipients who receive donor cells that possess sequence variants of toll-like receptor 4 or dectin-1 are at increased risk for invasive *Aspergillus* infections.[132–134] Other important elements of innate immunity have been identified by finding that polymorphisms of mannose-binding lectin,[135,136] chemokine (C-X-C motif) ligand 10 (CXCL-10),[137] tumor necrosis factor,[138,139] plasminogen,[140] and others[141,142] are associated with increased susceptibility to ABPA or IA in certain populations. In humans and mice, CD4+ T cells also contribute to defense against IA; both Th1 and Th17 cells contribute to optimal immunity. In contrast, excessive Th2 responses contribute to the pathogenesis of ABPA.

INFECTION TYPES

Invasive Pulmonary Aspergillosis

Epidemiology and Pathogenesis. IPA is the most severe form of pulmonary aspergillosis and is a major cause of fungal morbidity and mortality. It is seen most commonly in immunocompromised hosts, including transplant recipients and those with advanced HIV infection, primary immunodeficiency diseases including chronic granulomatous disease, and hematologic malignancies. In a retrospective Italian cohort of nearly 12,000 patients with hematologic malignancies, more than half of the 538 proven or probable IFIs were due to molds, primarily *Aspergillus*, and patients with acute myelogenous leukemia were most commonly affected.[143] The elevated risk in this population is primarily driven by prolonged neutropenia induced by cytotoxic chemotherapy.[144] The application of targeted immunomodulating therapies is changing the epidemiologic landscape of IFIs, including IPA, in hematologic malignancy as well as other patient populations. For example, historically lower risk groups for IFIs, such as patients with chronic lymphoproliferative disorders, are increasingly diagnosed with IFIs with pathogens such as *Aspergillus*, including disseminated infections to the CNS, when treated with ibrutinib, an irreversible inhibitor of Bruton tyrosine kinase.[145] Multicenter, prospectively obtained epidemiologic data confirm *Aspergillus* as the most common cause of invasive mold infection in both HCT and SOT recipients.[30,31] In HCT recipients, *Aspergillus* is the most common IFI overall, predominantly seen during two periods: (1) early after transplantation during neutropenia, and (2) after engraftment, in the setting of graft-versus-host disease. Of the SOT patients, lung transplant recipients are at highest risk for IPA. IPA has also been described in critically ill patients in the intensive care unit lacking "traditional" risks but with underlying comorbidities including renal failure, diabetes, COPD, and cirrhosis[146–148] and in association with severe influenza infections.[149,150]

IPA is characterized by tissue invasion, frequently involving blood vessels. Hyphae within the alveoli penetrate the respiratory mucosa and alveolar capillaries into endothelial cells and pulmonary arterioles. Cell injury and inflammation contribute to intravascular thrombosis, local hypoxia, and necrosis. Angioinvasive disease is accompanied by tissue infarction and coagulative necrosis, whereas nonangioinvasive disease is more commonly associated with pyogranulomatous inflammation and inflammatory necrosis.[151]

Clinical Presentation and Diagnosis. The clinical presentation of IPA typically involves fever, cough, hemoptysis, and pleuritic chest pain. Angioinvasive IPA is seen predominantly in the setting of neutropenia during which progression can be rapid, with clinical deterioration over hours to days. Patients with disseminated disease may have additional symptoms related to other sites of infection. *Aspergillus* can extend directly to surrounding areas, including the chest wall (see eFig. 123.27),[152] mediastinum, and great vessels.[153]

Early diagnosis of IPA is essential for prompt initiation of therapy, which has been associated with improved survival.[154] However, multiple factors make the diagnosis

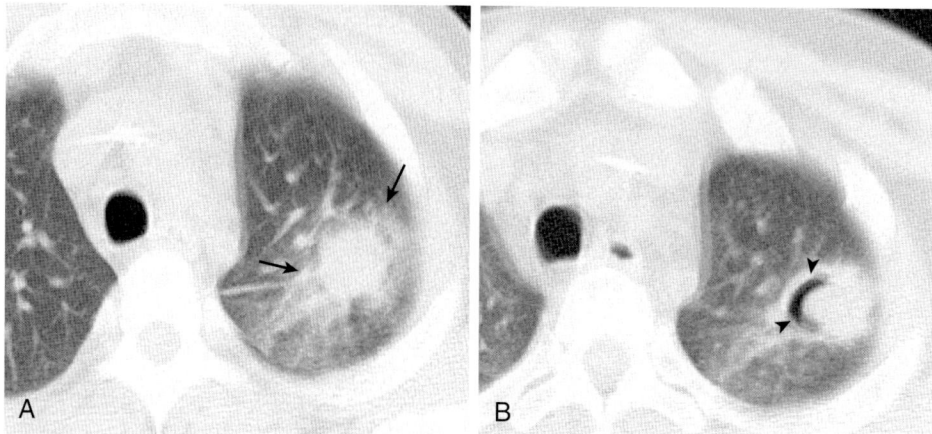

Figure 57.4 Invasive pulmonary aspergillosis. (A) Axial chest computed tomography displayed in lung windows performed in a hematopoietic cell transplant recipient during profound neutropenia demonstrates a poorly defined nodule with surrounding ground-glass opacity (*arrows*) representing the halo sign. (B) The nodule has become cavitary (*arrowheads*), representing the air crescent sign. (Courtesy Michael B. Gotway, MD.)

difficult, including the lack of symptoms early in the course of illness, challenges in obtaining appropriate tissue for histopathology and culture in critically ill or cytopenic hosts, and the variable sensitivity and specificity of many of the available diagnostic tests. Imaging findings associated with IPA are often nonspecific, including nodules (see eFig. 123.27B), consolidation (see eFig. 125.3), cavitation (see eFigs. 123.26A–B and 123.27), and effusions (see eFig. 125.3). The halo sign, demonstrated by ground-glass opacities surrounding a pulmonary nodule, is the result of alveolar hemorrhage around an infarcted area of the lung (Fig. 57.4A, see eFig. 125.3) and is typically seen early in the course of infection.[155] The halo sign has a high specificity for IPA in neutropenic patients.[156] The air crescent sign tends to be seen later in the course of infection (typically with recovery of neutrophils in the neutropenic host) and represents air that has filled the space between necrotic and healthy lung tissue (see Fig. 57.4B).[157]

Direct microscopy of sputum or BAL lacks both sensitivity and specificity.[158] Histopathologic evaluation of tissue specimens using standard hematoxylin and eosin, periodic acid–Schiff, and/or Gomori's methenamine silver staining with demonstration of characteristic hyphae supports the diagnosis of IPA (see Fig. 57.3), but culture is required to confirm the identity of the pathogen. Furthermore, in up to 70% of tissues with evidence of invasive septate hyphae, *Aspergillus* fails to grow in culture.[159] When positive, cultures for most *Aspergillus* species typically grow within 48 to 72 hours.[160] The application of molecular assays directly to fresh or formalin-fixed paraffin-embedded tissue specimens has also been employed in the diagnosis of *Aspergillus*, though this testing lacks standardization and is not currently approved by the FDA for clinical use.

Other primary diagnostic modalities for *Aspergillus* include assays for fungal *galactomannan* (GM) and β-D-glucan. GM is a heteropolysaccharide component of the cell wall of *Aspergillus* and other fungi released during hyphal growth. Platelia *Aspergillus* EIA (Bio-Rad Laboratories) is an FDA-approved, commercially available test for detecting GM in serum and in BAL specimens from patients with hematologic malignancies and recipients of HCT. The positive cutoff value is an *optical density index* (ODI) of 0.5. A meta-analysis of 27 studies using surveillance

serum GM in immunocompromised hosts with invasive *Aspergillus* reported an overall sensitivity and specificity of 71% and 89%, respectively.[161] Subgroup analysis showed that test performance was higher in patients with hematologic malignancy (sensitivity, 70%; specificity, 92%) and in HCT recipients (sensitivity, 82%; specificity, 86%) compared to SOT recipients (sensitivity, 22%; specificity, 84%). The poor performance of serum GM testing in the SOT population resulted in the recommendation that it not be used in cardiothoracic organ transplant recipients in guidelines from the *International Society for Heart and Lung Transplantation* (ISHLT).[162] Better performance in patients with hematologic malignancies and in those undergoing HCT may be related to the higher likelihood of neutropenia and angioinvasion in these populations, which, in turn, is associated with increased GM release into the circulation.[163] Other factors that influence the utility of the GM assay include cross reactivity with other fungi (e.g., *Alternaria, Fusarium, Geotrichum, Histoplasma, Paecilomyces,* and *Penicillium*), false-positive results secondary to the presence of GM in antimicrobials[164] and nutritional supplements,[165] and lower sensitivity with the concomitant administration of antifungal therapy.[166,167] The magnitude of GM and/or trend with serial testing may predict clinical outcomes.[168,169]

Assaying BAL specimens for GM complements testing of serum, particularly in a non-neutropenic host with IPA who may lack a positive serum GM. A meta-analysis of 30 studies evaluating BAL GM using a cutoff ODI of 0.5 for proven and probable IA found an overall sensitivity of 87% and specificity of 89%. Compared to serum GM, BAL GM had a higher sensitivity but a lower specificity.[170] Increasing the positive ODI cutoff value from 0.5 to 1.0 improved specificity, albeit with some compromise to sensitivity (from 88–78% based on a more contemporary meta-analysis of 17 studies).[171] The ideal ODI cutoff in BAL specimens remains uncertain. In the lung transplant population, high rates of colonization with molds such as *Aspergillus* and *Penicillium* can result in false-positive tests for BAL GM, thereby limiting application in this population.[172] However, the BAL GM is considered an acceptable diagnostic modality for cardiothoracic organ recipients in the current ISHLT guidelines.[162] Standardization of the process of GM testing in BAL is also imperative because certain factors, such as the volume of BAL collected, have been shown to impact results significantly.[167]

Assays of β-D-glucan, another fungal cell wall component, may detect many medically relevant fungal pathogens, including *Aspergillus*, *Candida*, and *Pneumocystis*, based on the abundance of β-D-glucan in their cell wall. Noted exceptions include *Cryptococcus* and the agents of mucormycosis.[173] The FDA-approved assay, the Fungitell test, has a positive cutoff value of 80 pg/mL or more (sensitivity, 64%; specificity, 92%) for patients with proven or probable IA.[174] Compared to GM, β-D-glucan may be detectable earlier in the course of IA.[175] False-positive β-D-glucan results happen, associated with cellulose membranes used in hemodialysis,[176] intravenous immunoglobulin and other blood products,[177,178] and bacterial bloodstream infections.[173,179] In a study to assess the utility of serial monitoring in lung transplant recipients with the β-D-glucan assay, 90% of subjects without an IFI had at least one positive β-D-glucan result (≥80 pg/mL), leading to a low PPV (9%).[175] Similar issues were encountered when β-D-glucan assays were used to monitor for invasive candidiasis in an intensive care unit setting; 45% of subjects had false-positive results ultimately attributed to receipt of intravenous immunoglobulin and hemodialysis.[90] These issues resulted in ISHLT guidelines not recommending β-D-glucan testing in the cardiothoracic populations.[162]

Nucleic acid-based tests (NATs), including real-time PCR, have the potential for specificity to the genus and species level and, while many laboratory-developed and commercial *Aspergillus* NAT tests exist, there is currently no FDA-approved *Aspergillus* NAT for testing clinical specimens. The European *Aspergillus* PCR initiative was established to standardize PCR testing for clinical use and has defined methods for specimen processing and nucleic acid extraction so that PCR testing will be included in the new *Mycoses Study Group/European Organization for Research and Treatment of Cancer* (MSG/EORTC) definitions for IA.[180] However, the kinetics of *Aspergillus* nucleic acid circulation in the systemic circulation are incompletely understood and may be intermittent and/or influenced by angioinvasion and receipt of prophylactic antifungals, as is also seen with GM. Accordingly, performance of a NAT test will likely have different performance characteristics in different patient populations and with different specimen types. White et al[181] found the sensitivity of PCR was higher while the specificity was lower than that of GM and β-D-glucan, with an overall high negative predictive value. A meta-analysis evaluating PCR testing in blood, primarily in high-risk patients with hematologic malignancy and/or undergoing HCT, found lower sensitivity (58%) but improved specificity (96.2%) by requiring two consecutive positive test results.[182] A combined monitoring strategy in high-risk hematologic malignancy and HCT patients utilizing serum GM and *Aspergillus* PCR was associated with an earlier diagnosis of IA, suggesting these blood tests may be used to complement, rather than replace, one another.[183] Regarding BAL testing, studies of a commercially available *Aspergillus* PCR assay in BAL collected from lung transplant recipients suggested the assay performs more as a detection test for the presence of *Aspergillus* rather than as a diagnostic test for invasive disease. Accordingly, BAL PCR results should be used as a diagnostic test only in combination with other tests (e.g., radiology, culture).[184] Avni and associates[185] found improved sensitivity with stable specificity when BAL PCR and BAL GM were used together, suggesting an advantage to combination testing.

Newer diagnostic tests, including LFAs to detect antigens secreted during the growth of *Aspergillus* species, may provide rapid and inexpensive point-of-care testing.[186] Data evaluating the application of LFAs to urine,[187] serum,[188] and BAL[189] in comparison to and in combination with other diagnostic tests, including GM and PCR, are promising.

Diagnostic criteria for IPA have been proposed by the MSG/EORTC and include proven, probable, and possible IA.[190] A diagnosis of proven IPA requires microscopic evidence of *Aspergillus* tissue invasion or a positive culture from a normally sterile site. A diagnosis of probable IPA requires an at-risk host, corroborating radiographic findings, and direct or indirect mycologic evidence. An updated revision of these definitions is forthcoming.[191] Other clinical algorithms continue to be introduced to assist in differentiating *Aspergillus* colonization from true IPA in critically ill intensive care unit patients without clear predisposing host factors (as identified by MSG/EORTC) but with positive respiratory specimens and/or clinical concern for IPA.[192]

Treatment. As with other IFIs, management of IPA may involve a combination of surgical, pharmacologic, and other adjunctive interventions. Attempts to restore host immunity should be made wherever feasible, being mindful of the risk for IRIS.[193] Indications for surgical intervention include life-threatening hemoptysis, presence of lesions contiguous to the great vessels and/or pericardium, and invasion of the chest wall, as well as presence of isolated lesions in patients with impending intensive chemotherapy or HCT.[121] Based on recommendations from both IDSA[121] and ATS[57] and data from a large prospective randomized trial of IA that demonstrated significantly better response and overall survival in those treated with voriconazole than those treated with AmB-d, the drug of choice for IPA is voriconazole.[194] Therapy is typically administered intravenously in critically ill patients and in patients otherwise not tolerating oral therapy, with transition to the oral route once patients stabilize and can tolerate oral medications. While most patients are treated for a minimum of 6 to 12 weeks, the total duration of therapy for IPA is not clearly defined and is dependent upon the immune status of the host and clinical response to treatment (eFig. 57.3).

Isavuconazole, the newest extended-spectrum azole, is also FDA approved for first-line treatment of IA. This approval was based on a randomized controlled trial in 527 patients with suspected IFI wherein isavuconazole demonstrated noninferiority to voriconazole on the basis of the primary end point of 42-day all-cause mortality in the intent-to-treat population (19% with isavuconazole, 20% with voriconazole).[195] Significantly fewer patients in the isavuconazole treatment arm reported drug-related adverse events (109 [42%] vs. 155 [60%]; $P < 0.001$), including fewer hepatobiliary, eye, and skin disorders. In subgroup analysis, voriconazole had greater success among patients with unresolved neutropenia.[196] This latter finding may prove significant given reports of breakthrough IA and other IFIs when applying isavuconazole as prophylaxis in high-risk hematologic malignancy and HCT patients.[197] However, clinical trials demonstrating isavuconazole efficacy in the prophylactic setting are lacking and breakthrough reports remain limited to retrospective, single-center experiences.[197–199]

Posaconazole may be an effective alternative to voriconazole or isavuconazole, although it has not been studied as primary treatment. In patients with IA who are refractory to or intolerant of other antifungal therapies, response to posaconazole was superior (45 of 107; 42%) compared with the external control group (22 of 86; 26%), the latter primarily treated with AmB or itraconazole.[200] Other researchers have also shown success with posaconazole as salvage therapy in patients receiving prior voriconazole.[201,202]

The emergence of azole resistance among fungal pathogens, including *Aspergillus*, is an important clinical concern. Resistance acquisition is typically dependent on scenarios of prolonged azole exposure, such as in treatment for CPA.[203] However, it is more commonly described in association with environmental exposure and broad application of azoles as fungicides in agricultural settings[204] for which the mechanism of resistance involves mutations (TR34/L98H or TR46/Y121F/T289A) in *cyp51A*, which encodes the azole target, 14-α-demethylase.[205] Importantly, the TR34/L89H mutation confers resistance to all mold-active azoles, and clinical infections with isolates carrying these mutations have been associated with poor outcomes.[206] A prospective international surveillance study reported this acquired azole resistance in *A. fumigatus* to be widespread in Europe, detected in 3.2% of *A. fumigatus* clinical isolates recovered in 11 of 17 European centers in nine countries,[207] but with a prevalence as high as 30% in one HCT center in Germany.[208] Based on passive surveillance data accrued since 2011 in the United States, seven such isolates have been recovered from clinical specimens in three states in the United States, and notably, four of the seven patients had no known previous exposure to antifungal medications.[209] The emergence of such resistant isolates emphasizes the importance of susceptibility testing as a tool for informing clinical care. The Clinical Laboratory Standards Institute[210] has standardized methods for performing antifungal susceptibility testing on fungi. Although Clinical Laboratory Standards Institute interpretive breakpoints defining clinical resistance are limited to those for *A. fumigatus* to voriconazole, epidemiologic cutoff values (the upper limit of the wild-type MIC distribution range) are useful for detecting isolates with potential resistance mutations (i.e., if the isolate's MIC is greater than the epidemiologic cutoff value, then the isolate may harbor a resistance mutation).[211] IDSA clinical practice guidelines[121] currently recommend antifungal susceptibility testing for *Aspergillus* species only in cases of suspected azole resistance, including for patients who are unresponsive to therapy; however, other international experts advocate screening in all patients requiring antifungal therapy in regions where the prevalence of azole resistance is high.[212]

Polyenes are used for the treatment of IPA in patients refractory to or intolerant of azoles. The lipid formulations of AmB are currently preferred because of their reduced nephrotoxicity compared with that of AmB-d. Currently, the IDSA recommends ABLC 5 mg/kg/day or LAmB 3 to 5 mg/kg/day for the treatment of IPA.[121] LAmB 3 mg/kg/day was

compared with LAmB 10 mg/kg/day in a double-blind trial of patients with proven or probable IA to assess whether higher doses would improve response; there was no clinical advantage with the higher dose, but there was significantly more hypokalemia and nephrotoxicity.[213]

Echinocandins are an appealing option for IA given their favorable toxicity profile and lack of significant drug interactions. However, echinocandins are static against *Aspergillus*, and use is typically limited to patients who are refractory to or intolerant of other first-line therapies or in combination regimens. Randomized controlled trials evaluating echinocandins as primary therapy for IA are lacking. Maertens et al[214] evaluated 83 adults with proven or probable IA refractory to or intolerant of standard anti-*Aspergillus* therapy, including 64 with IPA, who were treated with caspofungin; 45% (50% of those with IPA) obtained a complete or partial response. Based on these data, caspofungin was cleared by the FDA as salvage therapy for IA. For micafungin, a large report from Japan indicated a 71% (90 of 130) clinical response rate in patients with IA treated with micafungin monotherapy (doses ranged from 50 to 300 mg/day)[215] but, in other reports, response rates ranged from 38–44%.[216,217] To date, minimal data exist for anidulafungin as monotherapy in the treatment of IA.

Given the high mortality associated with IPA and emerging concerns for azole-resistant *Aspergillus* isolates, combination therapy is often considered. While in vitro and in vivo data support a role for combination therapy,[218,219] it is not recommended first line in all patients with IA due to the lack of significant supporting data from randomized controlled trials. When combination therapy is used, echinocandins are most often paired with polyenes or azoles based on their activity at a different site: the echinocandins act on the fungal cell wall while the azoles and polyenes act on the fungal membrane. A large randomized controlled trial comparing voriconazole monotherapy with combination voriconazole plus anidulafungin for IA in high-risk patients with hematologic malignancy or HCT failed to show significant benefit with the combination in 6-week mortality.[220] However, subgroup analysis showed a significant reduction in 6-week mortality in patients diagnosed with probable IA based on the combination of radiographic imaging and serum or BAL GM testing, possibly reflecting earlier disease. On the basis of available data, current IDSA guidelines suggest use of combination therapy with echinocandins and voriconazole in severe disease, particularly in patients with hematologic malignancy and/or prolonged neutropenia.[121] Other expert consensus supports combination therapy in regions with high prevalence of azole resistance (defined as >10%) until susceptibility can be confirmed.[212] Additional adjunctive measures used to optimize outcomes of IPA include granulocyte or granulocyte-macrophage colony-stimulating factor, interferon-gamma, and granulocyte infusions.[121]

Invasive Tracheobronchial Aspergillosis

Epidemiology and Pathogenesis. While there can be saprophytic, allergic, and invasive forms of *tracheobronchial aspergillosis* (TBA), this section focuses on invasive TBA. TBA can be seen alone or with IPA and should be considered as a spectrum, including mild tracheobronchitis and obstructive, ulcerative, and pseudomembranous TBA, often with more than one form present concurrently.[221] Mild tracheo-bronchitis demonstrates only superficial mucosal inflammation; obstructive, ulcerative, and pseudomembranous forms may be superficial or progress to involve the entire bronchial wall with necrotizing tracheobronchitis and invasion of the surrounding tissue.[222] A rare form of IPA, TBA is most commonly encountered in lung and heart-lung transplant recipients,[223,224] although it has been reported in other patient populations including those with advanced HIV,[225] diabetes,[226] COPD,[227,228] and hematologic malignancies, and those undergoing HCT.[229,230]

Clinical Manifestations, Diagnosis, and Treatment.

In lung and heart-lung transplant recipients, TBA is often discovered early in the posttransplant period when patients may have asymptomatic ulceration and/or pseudomembrane formation at the bronchial anastomotic site visible by bronchoscopy (Fig. 57.5).[231] In contrast, patients with hematologic malignancies are typically symptomatic at the time of discovery, with productive cough, dyspnea, fever, wheezing, stridor, hemoptysis, and respiratory failure.[221,228] Early diagnosis is crucial given the potential for progressive symptoms and disseminated infection and complications, including bronchial obstruction, anastomotic rupture, and bronchopleural or bronchoarterial fistulas.[223,232] While chest imaging may demonstrate bronchial wall thickening, luminal narrowing, and/or endobronchial lesions (eFig. 57.4),[228,233] the findings are not diagnostic. Serum GM is often of limited value for isolated tracheobronchial aspergillosis.[234] Diagnosis is made via bronchoscopy with visualization of plaques, ulceration, pseudomembranes, and obstructive mucous plugs and/or masses (Fig. 57.6) together with pathologic and microbiologic findings.

Treatment of TBA is similar to that for other forms of IPA.[121] Voriconazole is the preferred first-line therapy; other antifungals, including isavuconazole, posaconazole, AmB, and echinocandins, may be used. Systemic therapy has also been combined with aerosolized and topical endobronchial application of AmB in severe TBA in lung transplant recipients.[235] In addition to pharmacologic therapy, bronchoscopic débridement with removal of obstructive lesions may be necessary but can be associated with significant bleeding.[236,237] Other adjunctive approaches, including serial dilation and airway stenting in cases of pseudomembranous TBA with airway obstruction, have been described.[238]

Chronic Pulmonary Aspergillosis

Epidemiology and Definitions. CPA, based on consensus definitions,[239] is an overlapping spectrum of clinical entities differentiated by the affected host, clinical presentation, and radiographic findings. It includes *Aspergillus* nodule(s), aspergilloma, *chronic cavitary pulmonary aspergillosis* (CCPA), *chronic fibrosing pulmonary aspergillosis* (CFPA), and *subacute invasive pulmonary aspergillosis* (SIPA), the latter formerly called chronic necrotizing pulmonary

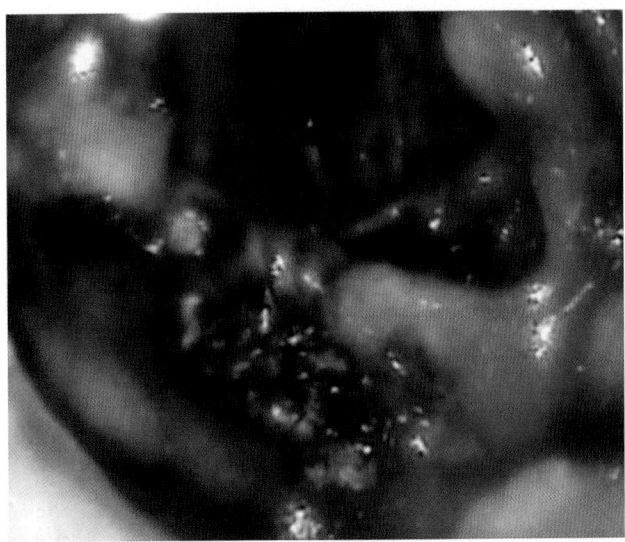

Figure 57.5 Tracheobronchial aspergillosis. Bronchoscopic visualization of the right mainstem bronchus in a lung transplant recipient demonstrates tracheobronchial aspergillosis with *Aspergillus fumigatus*. Stenosis and extensive necrotic pseudomembranes and debris are seen at the anastomotic site. (Courtesy Dr. Scott Shofer, Duke University Medical Center, NC.)

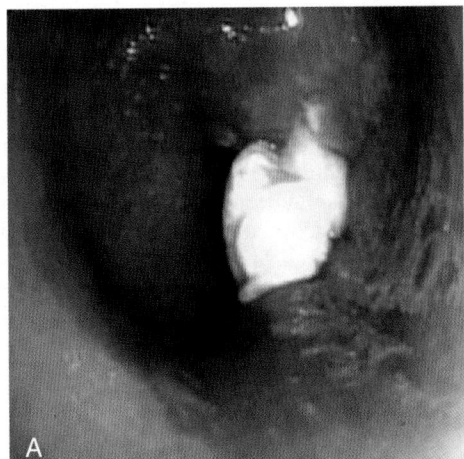
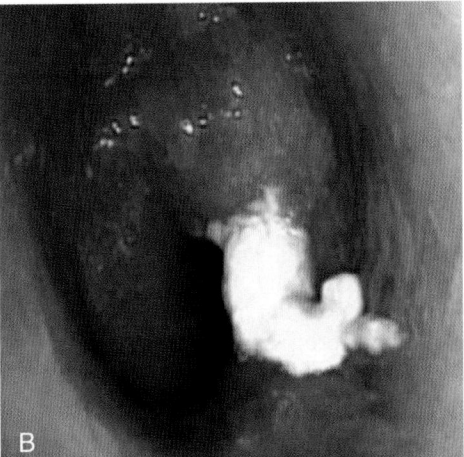

Figure 57.6 Tracheobronchial aspergillosis. Subglottic mass in a patient with a hematologic malignancy and prolonged neutropenia with histopathologic and culture data consistent with *Aspergillus fumigatus* tracheobronchial aspergillosis. (A) Bronchoscopic visualization beyond the vocal cords revealing a friable subglottic tracheal mass with surrounding mucosal edema resulting in approximately 50% obstruction. (B) Movement of the mass with breathing creating a ball-valve, extrathoracic obstruction. (A, closing partially with inspiration; B, opening partially with expiration.) (Courtesy Kamran Mahmood, MD, MPH, Duke University Medical Center, NC.)

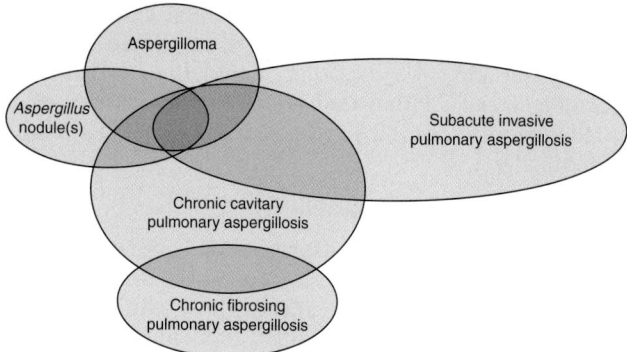

Figure 57.7 The overlapping spectrum of chronic pulmonary aspergillosis. (From Denning DW, Cadranel J, Beigelman-Aubry C, et al: European Society for Clinical Microbiology and Infectious Diseases and European Respiratory Society. Chronic pulmonary aspergillosis: rationale and clinical guidelines for diagnosis and management. *Eur Respir J.* 2016;47[1]:45–68.)

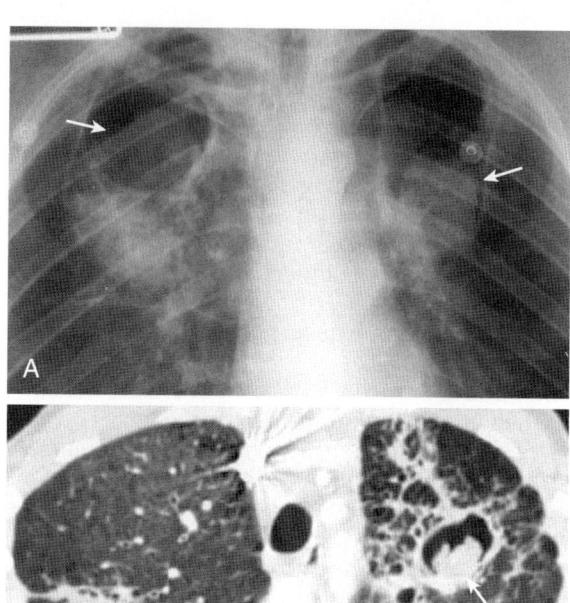

Figure 57.8 Aspergillomas in sarcoidosis cavities. (A) Frontal chest radiograph in a patient with sarcoidosis demonstrates biapical thin-walled cavities containing rounded intracavitary opacities (*arrows*) that represent aspergillomas. (B) Axial chest computed tomography displayed in lung windows performed in another patient with sarcoidosis demonstrates biapical aspergillomas (*arrows*). The background bronchovascular thickening and subpleural nodularity reflects sarcoidosis. (Modified from Gotway MB, Dawn SK, Caoili EM, et al: The radiologic spectrum of pulmonary *Aspergillus* infections. *J Comput Assist Tomogr.* 2002;26:159–173.)

aspergillosis (Fig. 57.7). It affects at least three million individuals worldwide.[240] Aspergillus nodule(s), a rare form of CPA, is characterized by one or more nodules, with or without cavitation, and without an invasive component.[241] This generally benign entity is often diagnosed when a nodule is removed due to concerns for malignancy. An aspergilloma (or fungus ball) develops within a preexisting pulmonary cavity; it is a tangled mass of fungal hyphae, cellular debris, mucus, and fibrin that may or may not adhere to the cavity wall. It can be seen in all forms of CPA except *Aspergillus* nodules. CCPA, the most common form of CPA, is characterized by multiple cavities, with or without intracavitary aspergillomas, alongside pulmonary and systemic symptoms demonstrated over at least a 3-month period.[242] Progression of untreated CCPA can result in expanding cavitation, pericavitary opacities, and even pleural involvement. Further, CCPA can progress to CFPA, defined by marked fibrosis and irreversible fibrotic destruction of at least two lobes of the lung.

Most subtypes of CPA are found in apparently immunocompetent individuals with structural lung disease due to prior or concomitant etiologies such as infections with mycobacteria[243] and other fungi,[244,245] sarcoidosis, lung cancer, cystic fibrosis, COPD, or asthma.[242] In contrast, SIPA is a subtype of CPA that is invasive and spans the boundaries of both IPA and CPA in patients with variable degrees of immunosuppression and/or comorbidities including diabetes, alcoholism, and advanced HIV.[246,247] SIPA is associated with more rapid progression than CCPA. Further, this notion of a reasonably "immunocompetent" host in most subtypes of CPA is continually challenged as underlying immune defects and genetic polymorphisms associated with CPA are increasingly understood.[135,136,248]

CPA is most commonly caused by *A. fumigatus* but can be seen with non-*fumigatus Aspergillus* molds. It can be confused with other infectious processes, including chronic lung infections due to mycobacteria or other fungal pathogens such as endemic fungi and non-*Aspergillus* molds,[249–252] as well as lung cancer.

Clinical Presentation and Diagnosis. Patients with *Aspergillus* nodules and aspergillomas are often asymptomatic, with lesions discovered incidentally on chest imaging. Aspergillomas may remain stable and asymptomatic

over long periods, regress, spontaneously resolve, or progressively enlarge.[253] Symptoms, when present, are most commonly cough, shortness of breath, and hemoptysis; hemoptysis may develop in up to of 85% of cases and ranges from mild to life-threatening.[253,254] Systemic symptoms, including fever, fatigue, weight loss, and night sweats, are more commonly seen in CCPA, CFPA, and SIPA.

Radiographically, *Aspergillus* nodules may be single or multiple cavitary or noncavitary nodules (eFig. 57.5). Aspergillomas are typically found in the upper lung fields and classically appear as a solid rounded mass within a cavity (Fig. 57.8). The mass may be mobile (eFig. 57.6) or adherent to the cavity wall; peripheral lesions may be associated with pleural thickening. Imaging findings with CCPA and SIPA show cavities of variable wall thickness (eFig. 57.7), consolidation, and pericavitary opacities often with varying degrees of associated pleural thickening.[239,242] Overlap between these two entities exists, and differentiation is often made based on the clinical presentation and radiographic progression, which are both typically more indolent in CCPA compared with SIPA.[255] CFPA is demonstrated by the development of extensive concomitant pulmonary fibrosis.

Diagnostic criteria for CPA have been proposed by the *European Society of Clinical Microbiology and Infectious Disease and European Respiratory Society* (ESCMID/ERS)[242] and the IDSA[121]; however, differences exist in these criteria, particularly in the types of direct or indirect evidence for *Aspergillus* accepted for definitive diagnosis.[256] In general, diagnosis requires incorporation of patient history and clinical presentation, characteristic radiographic imaging findings across time, and evidence of *Aspergillus* infection or an immunologic response to *Aspergillus* antigens. Further, to be classified as CPA, disease must be present for a minimum of 3 months. *Aspergillus* IgG or precipitins are detectable in serum of nearly all patients (>90%) with an aspergilloma[239,242] though *Aspergillus* IgG testing is preferred because it is a more sensitive and overall superior test compared to *Aspergillus* precipitins in diagnosing CPA.[240] Respiratory cultures and biopsy specimens may be positive for *Aspergillus*, and other diagnostic tests such as a positive serum and/or BAL GM or PCR as well as elevated erythrocyte sedimentation rate or C-reactive protein further support the diagnosis. Histopathologic findings of resected pulmonary lesions demonstrate chronic inflammation with hyphae within the cavities, with or without granulomas. The presence of invasion into surrounding tissues or vasculature signals the presence of either SIPA or IPA and should not be seen with the other forms of CPA.

Treatment. The goals in treatment of CPA include symptom reduction and prevention of disease progression. Due to the overall rarity of disease, optimal treatment has not been defined and is based in large part on expert opinion and data derived from cohort studies and case reports.[121,242] For aspergillomas in asymptomatic patients with stable lesions, monitoring alone is sufficient. In symptomatic patients, particularly with hemoptysis or progressing lesions, the primary curative approach is surgical resection. However, surgical resection remains a high-risk intervention in individuals with lung disease and poor pulmonary reserve. Potential complications include contamination of the pleural space and *Aspergillus* empyema, persistent hemorrhage, and death.[257] Application of pre-, peri-, and postoperative antifungal therapy is recommended in cases wherein spillage and pleural contamination are possible.[121,257] Bronchial artery embolization may be used as a temporizing measure in the setting of acute bleeding. Nonsurgical interventions in symptomatic patients include direct intracavitary instillation of antifungal agents such as AmB, nystatin, natamycin, and itraconazole via endobronchial and percutaneous CT-guided approaches; they may further reduce fungal burden and the risk of recurrent bleeding but are not curative.[258–260]

The primary treatment of selected cases of aspergilloma and the remaining types of CPA is systemic antifungal therapy. Indications for surgical intervention in CPA outside of aspergilloma include persistent hemoptysis or other evidence of refractory disease, including azole-resistant *Aspergillus*.[121,242] Azoles are most commonly used, and the preponderance of data are with oral itraconazole, which is considered first-line therapy.[261–265] The only randomized controlled trial of itraconazole in CPA compared itraconazole (*n* = 17) to supportive care (*n* = 14) and demonstrated higher overall response rates (defined as a composite of clinical and radiographic response) in the itraconazole group compared with the control group (76.5% vs 35.7%, respectively; *P* = 0.02). Voriconazole[266–271] is now considered a first-line therapy, and posaconazole[271–274] is also utilized in this setting. Major concerns with long-term azole administration are the emergence of resistance and

toxicities. Toxicities of particular concern with extended use of voriconazole include the development of skin cancers.[203,271,275,276] Isavuconazole demonstrated improved overall tolerability in patients treated for CPA compared with voriconazole.[277] Intravenous agents such as LAmB and echinocandins are typically reserved for patients refractory to or intolerant of azoles, including those with azole-resistant *Aspergillus* infections and/or severe disease.[242] Duration of therapy is a minimum of 4 to 6 months; however, in responders, therapy is often continued indefinitely.

MUCORMYCOSIS

EPIDEMIOLOGY

Mucormycosis is caused by molds in the order Mucorales in the subphylum Mucormycotina.[278] *Rhizopus* and *Mucor* are the genera most commonly associated with infections although *Lichtheimia, Apophysomyces, Cunninghamella, Rhizomucor, Saksenaea* complex, *Syncephalastrum*, and others also cause disease.[279–286] These are ubiquitous molds found in soil and decaying plant material that gain access to the host via inhalation, skin penetration, or, less commonly, ingestion. Infection sites include skin and soft tissue, rhino-orbital-cerebral, gastrointestinal, and lower respiratory tract, as well as disseminated infection with multiorgan involvement.[279,283,286,287] Mortality rates are as high as 96% in patients with disseminated disease.[286] In a comprehensive review and meta-analysis of 851 cases of mucormycosis from 2000 to 2017, the most commonly affected patients had diabetes (340 of 851; 40%), and the most frequent presentation was sinus involvement, including rhino-orbital-cerebral infections.[279] Hematologic malignancy was the second most common underlying condition (275 of 851; 32%), most often acute myeloid leukemia (116 of 275; 42%), and pulmonary infection predominated. Based on a prospectively maintained database across multiple centers, mucormycosis is the third most common IFI in the HCT population, representing 8% of IFIs[31] compared with 2% of IFIs in SOT recipients.[30] Surveillance data suggest an increasing incidence of mucormycosis.[31,286,288,289] Further, there are multiple reports of "breakthrough" mucormycosis in patients receiving azole therapy, most notably voriconazole, which lacks activity for Mucorales species,[290–293] although reports are also emerging with isavuconazole,[197,198] which has activity against some species. These reports raise the question of whether the antifungal therapies pose a unique risk, perhaps by increasing pathogen virulence as suggested in fly and murine models.[294,295] However, this association is likely multifactorial, including changes in immunosuppression and improved patient survival across time, and not solely attributable to the antifungal therapies.

PATHOGENESIS

After fungal spores gain access to the host, mononuclear and polymorphonuclear phagocytes normally serve as a primary host defense against invasion.[296] However, hyperglycemia and acidosis in people with poorly controlled diabetes impair phagocyte function.[297] Moreover, growth of pathogenic Mucorales is enhanced by free iron; thus iron overload and treatment with deferoxamine, which behaves as a siderophore that increases iron availability to the fungus, are associated with mucormycosis. Likewise, systemic acidosis increases free iron by decreasing iron binding to transferrin.[287] Similar to *Aspergillus* and certain other pathogenic molds, mucormycosis is angioinvasive, resulting in thrombosis, infarction, and tissue necrosis, with risk for dissemination to other sites. One mechanism that may promote angioinvasion by *Rhizopus arrhizus* (also called *R. oryzae*) is glucose- and iron-induced expression of glucose-regulated protein 78 by vascular endothelial cells, which promotes binding of *Rhizopus* to endothelial cells in vitro and in vivo.[298]

CLINICAL MANIFESTATIONS

Pulmonary mucormycosis is often acute and severe, particularly in neutropenic patients, with fever, cough, dyspnea, pleuritic chest pain, and hemoptysis.[299,300] In patients with diabetes, the course may be more subacute.[301] Pulmonary involvement may also be associated with life-threatening hemoptysis due to vascular invasion by the fungus, and the infection may disseminate or expand locally to involve contiguous structures, including the mediastinum and chest wall.[299] Although uncommon, bronchopleural, bronchocutaneous, and bronchoarterial fistulas have been reported.[299,302] Tracheobronchial infections present rarely in diabetics and in patients with chronic lung disease as well as those with underlying hematologic malignancies and transplant recipients. Endoscopic findings include luminal narrowing or obstruction with pseudomembranes and necrosis.

Pulmonary mucormycosis may present radiographically similar to IPA, including with nodular (eFig. 57.8) and mass (eFigs. 57.9 and 57.10) lesions, ground-glass opacities, and consolidative and cavitary (see eFig. 125.5) lesions. The presence of multiple (10 or more) pulmonary nodules and pleural effusions favors the diagnosis of mucormycosis over IPA, although this is not absolute.[300] Both the halo sign and the reversed halo sign (i.e., a ground-glass opacity surrounded by either a ring or a crescent of consolidation; Fig. 57.9) may be seen,[156] but the reversed halo appears to be more common in mucormycosis.[303,304] However, this CT finding has been noted less frequently in non-neutropenic than neutropenic patients, an important distinction to keep in mind when considering this diagnosis.[305]

DIAGNOSIS

Timely diagnosis is essential to optimizing outcomes in mucormycosis because mortality increases with delays in diagnosis and in initiation of therapy.[306,307] The diagnosis is typically made based on a combination of clinical, imaging, culture, and histopathologic findings. Currently available noninvasive tests (i.e., serum β-D-glucan and serum GM) are not helpful in the diagnosis of mucormycosis because Mucorales species lack significant quantities of these components in their cell walls. Direct examination of sputum and BAL specimens may show the characteristic broad 10- to 20-μm, ribbon-like, irregularly branching hyphae. Potassium hydroxide wet mounts enhanced with calcofluor (which stains chitin) may assist in detecting the fungus in fresh specimens; periodic acid–Schiff and/or

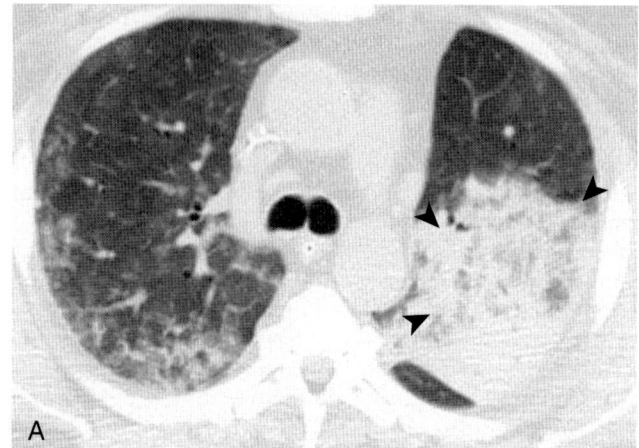

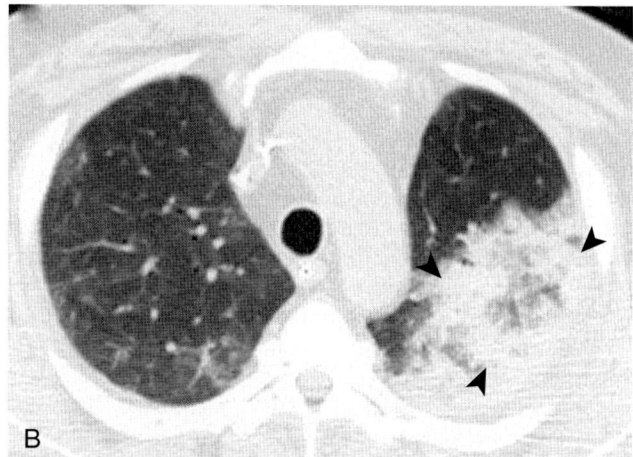

Figure 57.9 Mucormycosis. (A–B) Axial chest computed tomography displayed in lung windows performed in a hematopoietic stem cell transplant patient demonstrates left upper lobe consolidation (*arrowheads*) with surrounding ground-glass opacity consistent with the reversed halo sign. (Courtesy Michael B. Gotway, MD.)

Gomori's methenamine silver staining are used to visualize the fungi in tissue samples.[308] Prior receipt of mold-active therapy may alter the characteristic morphology in fresh specimens. In addition, although organisms may be visualized in tissue or respiratory specimens, cultures can be negative in up to one-third of cases.[309] Mucorales species may also be identified directly from culture and tissue specimens via molecular methods such as sequencing.

TREATMENT

Treatment of invasive mucormycosis includes pharmacologic therapy, nonpharmacologic intervention (e.g., reducing immunosuppression, correcting metabolic acidosis, and optimizing control of diabetes; eFigs. 57.11 and 57.12), and often surgery. Surgery, when feasible, is useful for debulking infection and preventing spread to contiguous structures, and is associated with decreased mortality compared to medical treatment alone.[310–313] Controlled trials to guide antifungal selection for mucormycosis are lacking given the rarity of infection, so recommendations are based on information gained through in vitro testing, animal models, and clinical observations. Guidelines for management of mucormycosis have been proposed based on consensus recommendations.[314,315] The use of susceptibility testing to guide antifungal therapy is controversial given the lack of established clinical breakpoints (i.e., the selected levels of the antifungal concentrations used to define susceptibility). Thus therapy is currently recommended by consensus guidelines, particularly because the activity of antifungal therapy varies depending on the drug and species of the infecting pathogen.[316,317]

Polyenes appear to be the most active agents and remain the agents of choice in the empiric management of mucormycosis. AmB-d has largely been replaced by lipid formulations; LAmB is considered by many to be the preferred agent, due to reduced nephrotoxicity, superior activity in murine models of infection,[318] retrospective clinical data,[319] and rabbit models showing improved CNS penetration compared to both AMB-d and ABLC.[320] LAmB is typically initiated at a dosage of 5 mg/kg/day but has been increased to 10 to 15 mg/kg/day in severe infections that fail to respond.[321] Despite the lack of approved clinical breakpoints, in a limited dataset wherein AmB was used as first-line therapy for proven and probable IFIs with non-*Aspergillus* molds, including mucormycosis (representing 8 of 10 cases), the 6-week response was significantly better when the pathogen MIC was 0.5 µg/mL or less versus more than 0.5 µg/mL (83% vs 0%, $P = 0.05$).[322]

Azoles are typically utilized for step-down therapy or as a component of salvage regimens in patients refractory to or intolerant of AmB. Among the azoles active against molds, posaconazole, and isavuconazole have in vitro activity against mucormycosis. Among 91 cases of mucormycosis in which posaconazole was used for salvage therapy (either alone or in combination), 60% showed complete or partial response at 12 weeks.[323] Similar responses were reported in another retrospective review of 96 cases of mucormycosis.[324] Posaconazole delayed-release tablets were approved by the FDA in late 2013, and the intravenous formulation was approved in 2014. Available data suggest improved overall bioavailability with the delayed-release tablets compared with the original posaconazole suspension.[325-328] Therapeutic drug monitoring is recommended with therapy to maintain trough concentrations of at least 1.0 mg/L. Isavuconazole was evaluated for treatment of mucormycosis in a single-arm open-label trial of 37 patients with proven or probable mucormycosis who received primary isavuconazole therapy and were compared to external controls receiving AmB.[329] Day 42 crude all-cause mortality was 33% (7 of 21) in the isavuconazole primary treatment group compared to 39% (13 of 33) in the AmB-treated controls ($P = 0.595$). Whereas isavuconazole was FDA approved for the treatment of mucormycosis, because of the overall small sample size in this open-label trial and the lack of abundant clinical experience, isavuconazole cannot be recommended as first-line therapy.

Echinocandins do not have significant in vitro activity against agents of mucormycosis and should not be used as monotherapy in the treatment of these infections. However, there may be a role for polyene-echinocandin combination therapy. Animal studies have shown improved survival with caspofungin compared with no treatment in mice[330] and with polyene-echinocandin combination therapy.[331,332] Combination azole (isavuconazole) and echinocandin (micafungin) did not demonstrate synergy in a mouse model.[333] Clinical data for combination therapy including any combination of a polyene, echinocandin, or azole are limited and mixed. A small retrospective study from two centers evaluated 41 patients, most of whom had diabetes (83%) with rhino-orbital and rhino-orbital-cerebral mucormycosis, and found that polyene-caspofungin combination therapy improved outcomes compared to polyene monotherapy.[334] However, the benefit of combination therapy was not demonstrated in a 20-year retrospective evaluation of mucormycosis in 106 high-risk patients with hematologic malignancy including HCT recipients. In that population, there was no benefit in propensity score–adjusted probability of 6-week survival—60% versus 56% ($P = 0.71$) for patients receiving combination therapy.[335]

The duration of therapy for invasive mucormycosis is not well defined and is determined on a case-by-case basis and is dependent on multiple factors including extent of infection, clinical response, and immune reconstitution. In patients receiving up-front AmB therapy, transition to azole step-down therapy is typically done after patients have demonstrated clear-cut improvement and clinical stability. Although adjunctive therapy with the iron chelator deferasirox showed promise in both murine models and a small clinical trial,[336,337] a multicenter clinical trial comparing LAmB-deferasirox to LAmB-placebo found a significantly higher 90-day mortality in those receiving deferasirox.[338] The increased mortality may have been related to an unbalanced enrollment, because more patients in the deferasirox treatment group had hematologic malignancies and neutropenia, which are associated with poorer outcomes. Nonetheless, its use is not currently recommended. Other adjunctive agents that have been used include hyperbaric oxygen, granulocyte colony-stimulating factors, and interferon-γ.[314,339]

NON-*ASPERGILLUS* HYALINE HYPHOMYCETES

EPIDEMIOLOGY AND PATHOGENESIS

Hyalohyphomycosis refers to infections caused by septate molds with colorless or lightly pigmented hyphae. *Aspergillus* is the most common of the hyaline molds; however, non-*Aspergillus* hyphomycetes, including *Acremonium*,[340,341] *Fusarium*,[342] *Paecilomyces/Purpureocilium*,[343,344] *Rasamsonia* (previously *Geosmithia*),[345,346] *Scedosporium/Lomentospora*,[347] and *Trichoderma*,[348] among others, are increasingly reported.[119,288,349,350] These pathogens can cause infection in immunocompetent or immunocompromised hosts. *Fusarium* and *Scedosporium/Lomentospora* are the most common causes of infection from this group in SOT and HCT recipients.[288]

The majority of these molds are ubiquitous in nature and can be recovered from clinical specimens as nonpathogens/colonizers. Invasive infections can be associated with local inoculation of nails, eyes, skin, and soft tissues. Inhalation of airborne conidia can lead to sinopulmonary infections ranging from mild allergic sinusitis and *allergic bronchopulmonary mycosis* (ABPM) to severe and invasive sinopulmonary infections. Many of these pathogens are uniquely capable of sporulating in infected tissue, a process called *adventitious sporulation*, which, when coupled with endovascular invasion, results in fungemia. Although fungemia is uncommon in *Aspergillus* infections, it has been reported in more than 50% of patients with disseminated *Fusarium* infections.[351] Adventitious sporulation has also been described with *Acremonium*,[352] *Paecilomyces/Purpureocilium*,[352] *Scedo-*

sporium/Lomentospora,[353] and *Trichoderma.*[348] Mycotoxin production and adherence factors that promote colonization and infection may contribute to the pathogenicity of these molds.[354]

Localized skin, soft tissue, ocular, and sinopulmonary infections are seen in immunocompetent hosts, and chronic colonization can be present in patients with chronic lung diseases (e.g., cystic fibrosis, pulmonary fibrosis). Fungemia and invasive infections develop predominantly in patients with impaired cellular and/or humoral immunity. In these patients, dissemination from the lungs or local spread from the sinuses can lead to extension to the CNS and brain abscess formation. Severe invasive infection is typically limited to immunodeficient patients with one notable exception: in immunocompetent near-drowning victims, CNS and sinopulmonary infections have been described with pathogens including *Scedosporium,* presumably because the submersion in water resulted in alveolar damage with fungal penetration and severe fungal pneumonia.[355–357]

CLINICAL PRESENTATION AND DIAGNOSIS

The respiratory presentation of non-*Aspergillus* hyalohyphomycosis resembles that of IA and includes sinusitis, ABPM, tracheobronchial disease, pneumonia, and pleuropulmonary infections. Patients may present with fever, sinus congestion and pain, cough, purulent sputum, and hemoptysis (eFig. 57.13). In patients with disseminated infection, depending on the pathogen, skin manifestations may be an early clue. Skin lesions are typically painful, erythematous, nodular eruptions that rapidly develop central pallor and necrosis (Fig. 57.10).

The diagnosis of infection with one of these pathogens is challenging due to difficulties in differentiating between fungal colonization and true infection, and in obtaining appropriate tissue specimens for evaluation. Furthermore, while histopathologic, cytopathologic, or direct microscopic examination from affected tissue is critical in making the diagnosis, these findings do not discriminate among the hyaline molds; culture data are required for definitive identification and diagnosis. Radiographic findings (e.g., pulmonary nodules, cavitation, and halo, reversed halo, and air-crescent signs) provide further support for infection but are not specific.[358] Noninvasive diagnostic testing such as serum or BAL GM, used primarily for the diagnosis of IA, may cross-react with the non-*Aspergillus* hyaline molds including *Fusarium,*[359] *Paecilomyces/Purpureocilium,* and *Penicillium,*[360] but lack both sensitivity and specificity in diagnosing these infections; the same applies to β-D-glucan.[361] The role of other molecular diagnostic tests such as sequence-based identification[362,363] and MALDI-TOF MS[364] continues to be defined.

TREATMENT

Treatment of these infections is multimodal. Immunosuppression should be reduced whenever feasible, and augmentation of host responses with growth factors and granulocyte transfusions should be considered. Removal of foreign devices and surgical intervention/débridement, particularly in localized disease, are also critical in management. Many of these pathogens are intrinsically resistant

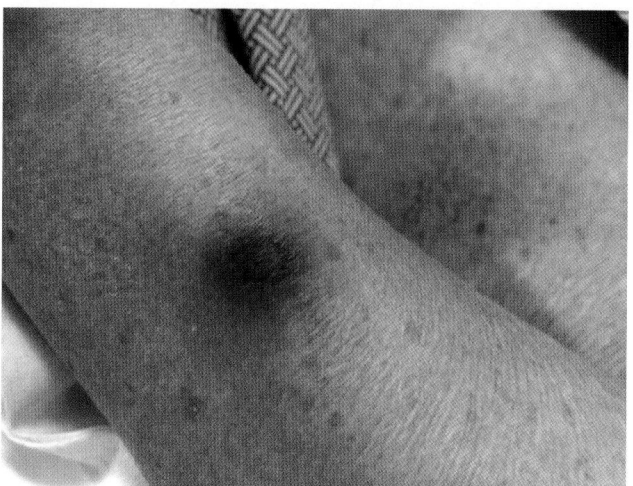

Figure 57.10 Disseminated *Fusarium* infection. Skin lesions in a patient with disseminated *Fusarium* infection demonstrating central necrosis with surrounding erythema.

to conventional antifungal therapies and/or have species-dependent variability in MICs to antifungal drugs; identification to the species level is imperative. While clinical breakpoints need to be defined, in many cases susceptibility testing can provide additional guidance in drug selection.

Exemplifying the complexity of managing infections with non-*Aspergillus* mold infections, *Fusarium*[365,366] and *Scedosporium/Lomentospora*[367,368] species exhibit variable levels of resistance to most antifungals. *F. solani,* the most common of the clinical isolates, is also often azole-resistant, with high MICs to voriconazole and posaconazole.[342,365] Therefore, the optimal antifungal regimen for fusariosis is not clear; single-agent lipid formulations of AmB or voriconazole may be applied up front, though initial combination therapy may be employed, particularly in severe infections while awaiting MIC data.[366] ABLC treatment of invasive *Fusarium* infections in patients with hematologic malignancy or undergoing HCT resulted in improvement or cure of infection in 46% of patients evaluated.[369] Pooled analysis of 21 patients with invasive *Fusarium* infections treated with voriconazole showed similar success in 43%, resulting in FDA approval of voriconazole for refractory infections or intolerance to other therapies.[370] While it is not FDA approved for this indication, posaconazole has been used as salvage therapy in patients with hematologic malignancies and invasive fusariosis.[371] *Fusarium* species are intrinsically resistant to echinocandins; however, in combination therapy with AmB, synergy has been demonstrated in vitro and in vivo.[372–374] Other combinations including lipid formulations of AmB and voriconazole[375] have been used with clinical success, as have combinations that include terbinafine.[376]

Lomentospora (formerly *Scedosporium*) *prolificans* often demonstrates high-level resistance to all antifungals and is associated with poor clinical outcomes.[377] In contrast, *S. apiospermum* tends to be more susceptible to antifungals, particularly extended-spectrum azoles such as voriconazole.[378] Successful responses to voriconazole were demonstrated in 63% (15 of 24) of patients with *S. apiospermum* infections resulting in FDA approval for this specific *Scedosporium* species. A compilation of 107 cases of scedosporiosis managed with voriconazole derived from the voriconazole clinical trials database (maintained by Pfizer) reported a successful therapeutic response in 57% (61 of 107) of patients with overall higher success in *S. apiospermum* (45 of 70; 64%) compared with *S. prolificans* (16 of 36; 44%) infections (*P* = 0.052).[378] Combination therapies of voriconazole with terbinafine[379,380] or with an echinocandin with or without AmB,[381] particularly in multidrug-resistant infections, may be effective.

Finally, there are important considerations when managing infections due to *P. variotti* and *P. lilacinum* given differing antifungal susceptibility patterns. AmB has poor activity against *P. lilacinum* but is highly active against *P. variotti.*[382] In addition, while voriconazole demonstrates low MICs with *P. lilacinum*, MIC ranges are notably higher for the *P. variotti* species complex so that posaconazole is the preferred extended-spectrum azole for this group.[383,384]

DEMATIACEOUS (MELANIZED) HYPHOMYCETES

The dematiaceous fungi, the agents of phaeohyphomycoses, represent an assorted group of molds with more than 70 genera and 150 species.[385] The overall burden of infection is underrepresented because their presence in culture is often dismissed as contamination; however, invasive infection can be seen in immunodeficient and immunocompetent hosts. Dematiaceous fungi contain melanin in their cell walls, which contributes to their pathogenicity and accounts for the dark brown color seen in culture and/or histopathology.[386] These fungi are found in soil and vegetation worldwide and can enter the host via inhalation or the cutaneous route. They are responsible for an array of infections, including skin and soft tissue infections, allergic and invasive sinopulmonary disease, ocular, CNS, and disseminated infections. Isolated skin and soft tissue infections are more common in immunocompetent hosts, whereas pulmonary and disseminated infections are predominantly seen in immunosuppressed patients. Among a prospective transplant cohort inclusive of SOT and HCT recipients, of 2191 invasive fungal infections, 2.6% represented phaeohyphomycoses.[387]

Alternaria, Bipolaris, Cladophialophora, Curvularia, Exophiala, Exserohilum, Ochroconis (previously *Dactylaria*), *Phialemonium,* and *Phialophora* are some of the more common black molds associated with infection. Intrathecal injection of corticosteroids contaminated with *Exserohilum* led to a large outbreak of fungal meningitis in immunocompetent patients in the United States.[388,389] Accurate identification is important because molds within this group may have a particular tropism that is important to consider when determining the sites of infection. *Bipolaris* and *Curvularia* are often associated with allergic and chronic inflammatory diseases, including allergic fungal sinusitis and ABPM.[390] *Cladophialophora bantiana,*[391,392] *Rhinocladiella mackenziei,*[393,394] *Exophiala (Wangiella) dermatitidis,*[395] and *Ochroconis gallopava*[396] have a predilection for dissemination to the brain and can cause severe disease in immunocompetent and immunosuppressed patients.[397] Disseminated infections with dematiaceous molds have been associated with mortality rates of up to 80%.[398]

Sinopulmonary manifestations with the dematiaceous molds include allergic fungal sinusitis, ABPM, and asymptomatic pulmonary nodules, as well as invasive sinus and pulmonary infections. The latter two entities more commonly affect immunocompromised hosts and those with preexisting lung disease. CT findings are nonspecific (eFig. 57.14) and consistent with findings described with the other invasive pulmonary mycoses. Fungal elements seen on direct microscopy from clinical specimens can be associated with either colonization or contamination; documentation of tissue invasion is essential for diagnosis. Pigmented hyphae can be seen on standard hematoxylin and eosin stains. However, the Fontana-Masson stain is often preferred to ensure that those with decreased amounts of pigmentation are not misidentified as hyaline molds.[399] Other diagnostic methods including sequence-based identification and MALDI-TOF MS continue to evolve.[400]

As with other invasive molds, treatment includes reduction of immunosuppression and surgical debulking (when feasible) to augment antifungal therapies. Clinical breakpoints for antifungal susceptibility are not defined for the dematiaceous molds. Although resistance to AmB has been seen,[401] AmB demonstrates good in vitro activity against most of the dematiaceous molds. However, the extended-spectrum azoles, including voriconazole and posaconazole, have demonstrated in vitro activity against the majority of dematiaceous molds[385,401,402] and are used more frequently given their improved toxicity profile. Data with isavuconazole are sparse, with variable MICs dependent on the pathogen; however, clinical success with isavuconazole therapy has been demonstrated, suggesting this may represent a viable treatment option.[403] Combination therapies including azoles, AmB, terbinafine, and echinocandins have been employed for severe disease; however, an optimal regimen has not been defined.[399]

Key Points

- Invasive pulmonary aspergillosis may have a clinical presentation similar to that of other angioinvasive molds such as mucormycosis and the non-*Aspergillus* hyphomycetes such as *Fusarium* and *Scedosporium* and dematiaceous molds, such as *Exophiala.*
- Galactomannan is a component of the cell wall of some but not all fungi and can be a useful noninvasive diagnostic aid in serum or bronchoalveolar lavage.
- Voriconazole is the treatment of choice for invasive pulmonary aspergillosis. The total duration of therapy depends on the immune status of the host and clinical and radiographic response to infection. However, patients are treated for a minimum of 6 to 12 weeks.
- Although mucormycosis can be associated with a multitude of clinical manifestations with multiorgan involvement, the most common presentations include rhino-orbital-cerebral and pulmonary infections, particularly in those with poorly controlled diabetes and in immunodeficient patients, especially those with hematologic malignancies.
- *Candida* pneumonia is rare and develops most often following candidemia and dissemination to the lung in immunocompromised populations.
- Combination antifungal therapy may offer benefit in infections due to drug-resistant fungi.

Key Readings

de Heer K, Gerritsen MG, Visser CE, Leeflang MM. Galactomannan detection in broncho-alveolar lavage fluid for invasive aspergillosis in immunocompromised patients. *Cochrane Database Syst Rev.* 2019;5:Cd012399.

Denning DW, Cadranel J, Beigelman-Aubry C, et al. Chronic pulmonary aspergillosis: rationale and clinical guidelines for diagnosis and management. *Eur Respir J.* 2016;47(1):45–68.

Herbrecht R, Denning DW, Patterson TF, et al. Voriconazole versus amphotericin B for primary therapy of invasive aspergillosis. *New Engl J Med.* 2002;347(6):408–415.

Limper AH, Knox KS, Sarosi GA, et al. An official American Thoracic Society statement: treatment of fungal infections in adult pulmonary and critical care patients. *Am J Respir Crit Care Med.* 2011;183(1):96–128.

Pappas PG, Kauffman CA, Andes DR, et al. Executive summary: clinical practice guideline for the management of candidiasis: 2016 update by the Infectious Diseases Society of America. *Clin Infect Dis.* 2016;62(4):409–417.

Patterson TF, Thompson 3rd GR, Denning DW, et al. Executive summary: practice guidelines for the diagnosis and management of aspergillosis: 2016 update by the Infectious Diseases Society of America. *Clin Infect Dis.* 2016;63(4):433–442.

Patterson TF, Donnelly JP. New concepts in diagnostics for invasive mycoses: non-culture-based methodologies. *J Fungi (Basel, Switzerland).* 2019;5(1):e9.

Perfect JR, Dismukes WE, Dromer F, et al. Clinical practice guidelines for the management of cryptococcal disease: 2010 update by the Infectious Diseases Society of America. *Clin Infect Dis.* 2010;50(3):291–322.

Vallabhaneni S, Kallen A, Tsay S, et al. Investigation of the first seven reported cases of *Candida auris*, a globally emerging invasive, multidrug-resistant fungus—United States, May 2013-August 2016. *Am J Transplant.* 2017;17(1):296–299.

Wong EH, Revankar SG. Dematiaceous molds. *Infect Dis Clin North Am.* 2016;30(1):165–178.

Complete reference list available at ExpertConsult.com.

58 PARASITIC INFECTIONS

KAMI KIM, MD • LOUIS M. WEISS, MD, MPH

INTRODUCTION

Parasitic infections that involve the lungs include both multicellular helminths and unicellular protozoa. *Paragonimus*, the lung fluke, specifically targets the lung, but several other parasitic infections that primarily target other organs commonly present with pulmonary manifestations. Helminths, for example, migrate through the lungs en route to the gastrointestinal tract and, during migration, cause pulmonary disease (e.g., eosinophilic pneumonia). Many parasites that affect the lungs more commonly infect the gastrointestinal tract (e.g., *Entamoeba*, *Echinococcus*); others involve the lungs as part of a generalized systemic infection (e.g., *Toxoplasma*, *Plasmodium*) (Table 58.1).

Although these infections classically have been associated with tropical and subtropical regions, they also have been seen in temperate and arctic regions. Furthermore, travel and immigration have led to the globalization of many of these formerly geographically restricted infectious diseases. The increased population of immunosuppressed patients living with *human immunodeficiency virus* (HIV) and *acquired immunodeficiency syndrome* (AIDS) or being treated with immune-modulating therapy used in organ transplantation, rheumatologic diseases, and cancer has resulted in the expansion of populations vulnerable to opportunistic parasitic diseases. Moreover, climate change and ecologic perturbations have affected the transmission and geographic range of certain human parasites. These factors necessitate greater familiarity of all physicians with parasitic infections previously seen only by specialists in tropical medicine.

This chapter reviews the pulmonary complications of parasitic infections that exhibit four major patterns: (1) parasites that primarily involve the lungs, (2) parasites that involve the lungs as a transient event in their life cycles, (3) parasites that involve the lungs less often than they involve other organs such as those of the gastrointestinal tract, and (4) parasites that involve the lungs during widespread, systemic infections (see Table 58.1). Specific aspects of certain parasitic infections are also discussed in Chapter 123 on the pulmonary complications of HIV and Chapter 96 on eosinophilic lung diseases.

INITIAL EVALUATION OF A PATIENT WITH POSSIBLE PARASITIC INFECTION OF THE LUNGS

Because parasitic infections differ in their geographic distribution, to arrive at a differential diagnosis, clinicians must consider the diseases found in areas where a patient has traveled or resided. Parasites can have complex life cycles with numerous hosts; many are vector borne and others are acquired by exposures to contaminated soil or water. Many emerging parasitic infections are zoonoses, in which the disease is spread from nonhuman animals to humans. It is therefore important to obtain a detailed travel and contact history with information on foods and liquids consumed, swimming or wading, insect bites, animal exposures, and medications taken.

In developing a differential diagnosis for respiratory complaints that may have a parasitic etiology, knowledge of the geographic distribution of various parasites, potential vectors, and potential sources of environmental contamination is essential. The interval between the time of travel or emigration and the onset of symptoms may provide clues: enteric protozoa or helminthic infections typically present more than 2 weeks after exposure and some parasites such as *Strongyloides*, *Plasmodium vivax* or *ovale*, and *Entamoeba histolytica* can present years after exposure.

Laboratory tests that may be helpful in initial evaluations include a complete blood count with differential, liver function tests, and a basic metabolic panel; in some contexts, examination of the sputum and/or stool samples is essential. Peripheral eosinophilia suggests a potential parasitic cause of pulmonary disease, but most protozoan infections are not associated with eosinophilia, and a lack of eosinophilia does not exclude parasitic infection. Diagnosis of intestinal parasites often depends on microscopic exams that require adequate specimens and experienced lab personnel. Depending on the parasite suspected, stool antigen tests (*E. histolytica*), microscopic examination of blood smears (malaria and babesiosis), or collection of respiratory samples including sputum or *bronchoalveolar lavage* (BAL), or serologic tests (*Strongyloides enzyme-linked immunosorbent assay* [ELISA]) may be warranted.[1,2] Specialized laboratories are able to

Table 58.1   Characteristics of the Most Common Parasites Causing Pulmonary Pathology

Parasite	Distribution	Pulmonary Manifestation	Extent of Lung involvement*	Diagnosis	Treatment
HELMINTHS					
Nematodes (Roundworms)					
Ascariasis: *Ascaris lumbricoides*	Worldwide, but widely in tropics	Loeffler syndrome, usually 9–12 days after exposure to eggs; cough, substernal discomfort, rales and wheezing, transient opacities	Transient	Examination of sputum; eosinophilia during larval migration; stool ova and parasite, usually positive after pulmonary symptoms resolved; serology	Albendazole Mebendazole
Dirofilariasis (dog heartworm): *Dirofilaria immitis* and *D. repens*	Worldwide (associated with dogs)	Pulmonary nodule	Primary	Usually requires biopsy to rule out other causes	None (benign, so no treatment necessary)
Hookworm: *Ancylostoma duodenale* and *A. ceylanicum*; *Necator americanis* and *N. brasiliense*	Worldwide, especially tropics	Loeffler syndrome; transient opacities	Transient	Eosinophilia during larval migration	Albendazole Mebendazole
Strongyloidiasis (also a hookworm, but unique due to autoinfection cycles): *Strongyloides stercolasis* (and sometimes other *Strongyloides* sp)	Worldwide but particularly in tropic or subtropical regions	Loeffler syndrome; chronic cough; pneumonia or sepsis in hyperinfection	Systemic (rarely primary)	Sputum examination; eosinophilia during larval migration; stool ova and parasite; serology (cannot discriminate acute vs. past)	Ivermectin (may need longer doses for immuno-compromised hosts); due to risk of hyperinfection, consider treating all seropositives, screening all patients receiving immune modulating agents
Trichinosis (also a hookworm but encysts): *Trichinella spirallis*	Worldwide zoonosis	Respiratory distress, radiographic appearance variable	Transient	Muscle biopsy	Albendazole
Tropical pulmonary eosinophilia (lymphatic filariasis): *Wucharia bancrofti* and *Brugia malayi*	Tropics, particularly South Asia	Tropical eosinophilic pneumonia with interstitial opacities, chronic cough	Systemic	Circulating antigen, serology, BAL, eosinophilia	Diethylcarbamazine Doxycycline (treats endosymbiont)
Visceral larval migrans (nonhuman ascarid): *Toxocara canis* and *T. cati*	Worldwide	Interstitial opacities with eosinophilic pneumonia	Transient	Serology, eosinophils in blood and sputum	May not be needed; Albendazole (or ivermectin) in severe cases
Trematodes (Flukes)					
Paragonimiasis (lung flukes): *Paragonimus westermani, P. africanus, P. caliensis, P. kellicotti* (U.S.)	Southeast Asia, Central and South America, Africa; United States	Pulmonary parenchymal invasion (larvae mature in lung) with cavitary lesions; hemoptysis	Primary	Eosinophilia; eggs in sputum or stool; serology	Praziquantel
Schistosomiasis: *Schistosoma mansoni, S. haematobium, S. japonicum, S. intercalatum*	Asia, South America, Africa	Hematogenous seeding with heavy infection; pulmonary hypertension	Systemic	Eosinophilia; serology; stool ova and parasite	Praziquantel
Cestodes (Tapeworms)					
Hydatid cyst: *Echinococcus granulosus* and *E. multilocularis*	Worldwide (especially in sheep-rearing locales)	Pulmonary cyst; second most common site after liver; hemoptysis	Other organs (usually liver)	Serology, eosinophilia rare	Surgical, albendazole

Table 58.1   Characteristics of the Most Common Parasites Causing Pulmonary Pathology—cont'd

Parasite	Distribution	Pulmonary Manifestation	Extent of Lung involvement*	Diagnosis	Treatment
PROTOZOA					
Amebiasis: *Entamoeba histolytica*	Worldwide; mostly tropical	Abscess; lungs second most common extraintestinal site after the liver, hemoptysis	Systemic or secondary extension	Percutaneous aspiration, serology, antigen, PCR	Metronidazole Tinidazole
Malaria: *Plasmodium* sp (*falciparum, vivax, ovale, malariae, knowlesi*)	Africa, Asia, Central and South America	Interstitial opacities; ARDS	Systemic	Blood smear, RDT; PCR	Antimalarial treatment, specifics depend on species and geographic distribution of drug resistance
Toxoplasmosis: *Toxoplasma gondii*	Worldwide; most common in immunocompromised especially, HIV-infected with CD4 < 100	Interstitial pneumonia usually associated with disseminated disease	Systemic	Smear of BAL, PCR; serology (cannot discriminate acute from past)	Pyrimethamine/sulfadiazine Pyrimethamine/clindamycin
Rarer Protozoan Pulmonary Parasite Syndromes					
Free-living ameba: *Acanthamoeba castellani* or *A. polyphagia, Balamuthia mandrillaris, Naeglaria fowleri*	Worldwide	Rare, usually immunocompromised; more frequently seen as CNS disease	Systemic	Smear/tissue section	No highly effective treatment Treatment varies according to species involved in the infection
Babesiosis: *Babesia microti, B. divergens*	U.S., Europe	Interstitial opacities: ARDS	Systemic	Blood smear; PCR	Quinine/clindamycin Atovaquone/azithromycin
Cryptosporidiosis: *Cryptosporidium parvum* and *C. hominus*	Worldwide	Primarily gastrointestinal; respiratory syndrome and transmission proposed	Primary (rare)	Smear of BAL or sputum; stool ova and parasite; PCR	No highly effective treatment (nitizoxinide approved for children with diarrhea)
Leishmaniasis: *Leishmania donovani*	Africa, Central and South America	Interstitial pneumonia usually associated with disseminated disease	Systemic	Smear or histopathology of tissue, PCR	Pentavalent antimonials, amphotericin B, miltefosine
Microsporidiosis (related to fungi): Many species	Worldwide; especially in immunocompromised	Interstial pneumonia, tracheobronchitis	Primary or systemic	Stains of sputum, smears or tissue, PCR	Albendazole, fumagillin
American trypanosomiasis: *Trypanosoma cruzi*	Central and South America	Interstitial pneumonia usually associated with disseminated disease	Systemic	Serology, blood smear, PCR	Nifurtimox, benznidazole

Serologic testing can be performed by enzyme-linked immunosorbent assay (ELISA also often abbreviated EIA), immunofluorescence (IFA), or Western blot. In general ELISA is most common because there are standardized cutoff points and less operator variability. Antigen tests can be performed by Western blot or ELISA designed to detect the antigen of choice. For gastrointestinal pathogens and blood pathogens, PCR is increasingly available or being incorporated into multipathogen panels. These tests may be available at the CDC or state public health laboratories.
*Extent of lung involvement: (1) *primary:* parasites that primarily involve the lungs, (2) *transient:* parasites that involve the lungs as a transient event in their life cycles, (3) *systemic:* parasites that involve the lungs during widespread systemic infection as part of dissemination of the infection, and (4) *secondary extension:* parasites that form an abscess or other collection that can rupture through the diaphragm infecting the lung.
ARDS, acute respiratory distress syndrome; BAL, bronchoalveolar lavage; CNS, central nervous system; HIV, human immunodeficiency virus; PCR, polymerase chain reaction; RDT, rapid diagnostic test.

perform polymerase chain reaction tests or other nucleic acid–based tests for specific parasites. Several recently available molecular gastrointestinal panels (e.g., BioFire Film array) include pathogenic protozoa (e.g., *E. histolytica, Cyclospora, Cryptosporidia,* and *Giardia*),[3] but they do not include pathogenic metazoa (e.g., helminths, cestodes). Rapid antigen tests for the diagnosis of malaria are approved and widely available. In some cases, specialized testing is available at the *US Centers for Disease Control and Prevention* (CDC); the CDC website provides useful resources for diagnostic testing (http://dpd.cdc.gov/dpdx/Default.htm), and the CDC provides access for certain antiparasitic medications not routinely available in the United States.

HELMINTHS

Helminths are common parasites divided into two major phyla: (1) nematodes (roundworms), which include the major intestinal worms and the filarial worms that cause lymphatic filariasis and onchocerciasis, and (2) platyhelminths (flatworms), which include flukes (or trematodes), such as *Schistosoma*, and tapeworms (or cestodes).[4] These parasites are most common in areas of poverty, particularly in rural environments. Disease is proportional to worm burden, as assessed by the number of eggs per gram of feces. With the exception of *Strongyloides*, these infections do not have significant autoinfective cycles in the host.

NEMATODES

Infection with helminths is an important etiology of eosinophilic pneumonia, which can be caused by several infectious and noninfectious syndromes (see Chapter 96).[5] The parasitic nematodes (roundworms) of humans that cause ascariasis, hookworm disease, trichinosis, and strongyloidiasis have a respiratory phase as part of their life cycles.[6] In each, larvae migrate through the lungs in transit to the gastrointestinal tract. In most cases, this migratory phase is asymptomatic, but cough, substernal discomfort, and wheezing may be accompanied by transient opacities and eosinophilia (Loeffler syndrome). This is often accompanied by peripheral eosinophilia, bronchospasm, and elevated serum IgE levels. If the burden of infection is high, the eosinophilic pneumonia may result in an asthma-like syndrome or in pulmonary damage due to release of cytotoxic, cationic proteins from eosinophil granules.[7] After larvae migrate through the lungs, they move up the respiratory tree and are swallowed, thereby reaching the gastrointestinal tract where they mature into adult worms. During acute infection and migration, stool ova and parasite examinations are often negative because adult worms often are not yet present in the gastrointestinal tract.

Ascariasis

Ascariasis, caused by the nematode *Ascaris lumbricoides*, is the most common human helminth infection and is estimated to infect almost 1 billion people.[4,6] Although highly prevalent, ascariasis is associated with chronic disability rather than death. It has a worldwide distribution, being most common in tropical and semitropical regions. An estimated 4 million people in the United States are infected,[8] primarily children in rural areas of the southern United States. Humans are the only known host of *Ascaris lumbricoides*, although the pig species *A. suum* is very similar biochemically and morphologically. Eggs (ova) shed in the stool mature in moist environments; humans are infected by swallowing eggs that contaminate water, food, or soil. The eggs bear noninfective, first-stage rhabditiform larvae that hatch in the intestine. The resulting larvae burrow through the intestinal wall, enter the hepatic circulation via capillaries and lymphatics, and migrate via the right side of the heart into the lungs. The worms migrate up the bronchial tree, are swallowed, and make their way to the duodenum, where they mature into adults after several months. They can live as adults in the intestine for 1 to 2 years. Once the worms reach the intestines, patients may have nausea, vomiting, abdominal pain, and anorexia, reflecting high worm burdens that can lead to obstruction or chronic malnutrition.[8]

Clinical Features. Infected individuals are typically asymptomatic. The most common symptoms are nonspecific abdominal complaints. Some patients experience malaise and fever with or without respiratory symptoms such as cough, chest pain, dyspnea, bronchospasm, and hemoptysis. Pulmonary symptoms can develop 9 to 12 days after ingestion of eggs and can persist 2 to 3 weeks. This stage of the infection can be associated with leukocytosis and eosinophilia. Rarely, acute eosinophilic pneumonia can cause respiratory distress requiring intubation.[9,10] Pneumonitis can be seen seasonally in geographic regions where climate conditions favor seasonal transmission of ascariasis.[11]

Diagnosis. Thoracic imaging during the initial stage of infection may reveal transient unilateral or bilateral opacities (eFig. 58.1). The diagnosis is difficult to confirm during acute infection because ova do not appear in the stool until 2 to 3 months following initial infection. Peripheral eosinophilia may be detected, and larvae, eosinophils, or Charcot-Leyden crystals may be found in sputum or gastric contents.

Treatment. The treatment of choice for ascariasis is albendazole, although mebendazole and ivermectin are also efficacious against adult worms. Although the pulmonary phase is self-limiting, the persistent gastrointestinal phase warrants treatment to relieve symptoms and reduce transmission.

Hookworm Disease

Hookworm disease is caused by *Ancylostoma duodenale*, *A. ceylanicum*, or *Necator americanus*. These helminths infect at least 500 million people worldwide,[4,6] primarily in tropical and subtropical regions. They reside in the small intestine where they attach to the mucosa and feed on blood and host tissue, causing iron deficiency anemia as their major morbidity. Unlike the case with other helminths, hookworm prevalence increases with age, and there is no protective immunity.

Clinical Features. Hookworm ova are passed in the stools of an infected person, which then hatch into rhabditiform larvae that molt and become filariform larvae in contaminated soil. Filariform larvae then penetrate the skin, classically on the feet. This is often associated with a pruritic rash. The larvae then enter lymphatics or venules and ultimately reach the pulmonary circulation where they break through capillaries and enter the alveolar spaces. This stage can be associated with cough, bronchospasm, and transient pulmonary opacities with or without fever.[12,13] Peripheral and pulmonary eosinophilia are common during this stage of infection. The larvae then migrate up the tracheobronchial tree and are swallowed. Once the worms reach the intestine, an individual may have nonspecific gastrointestinal symptoms, including nausea and abdominal pain. Iron-deficiency anemia is the most important consequence of hookworm infection and can lead to cognitive problems. Malnutrition and hypoproteinemia can also complicate hookworm infection.

Diagnosis and Treatment. Stool examination will reveal hookworm ova 2 to 3 months after pulmonary symptoms but, in cases of light infection, concentration of stool may be necessary to detect the ova. Diagnosis during the pulmonary phase is difficult and relies upon identification of larvae in respiratory secretions, BAL fluid, or gastric secretions. The treatment of choice is albendazole (single dose) or mebendazole (twice daily for 3 days). These drugs kill the adult worms but are not effective against the pulmonary larval stages. Patients should be screened for ova in stools 1 month after treatment; if ova are still present, retreatment is indicated to eliminate adults that developed after the initial treatment.

Strongyloidiasis

Although there are more than 50 species of *Strongyloides*, *Strongyloides stercoralis* is the species seen in most human infections. *S. stercoralis* is present in most geographic environments. It is endemic in Latin America, South Asia, sub-Saharan Africa, the United States (especially the southern states and Appalachia), Europe, and Australia.[14] At least 100 million people are estimated to be infected,[15] and many experts believe that the prevalence of infection is significantly higher.[16] Due to lack of awareness among clinicians and its prevalence in people in resource-poor settings, *Strongyloides* infection is often undiagnosed.

Strongyloides has a complex life cycle consisting of free-living and parasitic forms. Humans are the primary reservoir and acquire infection from soil or vegetation contaminated with human feces. Similar to hookworm infection, strongyloidiasis is initiated by penetration of the skin by infective filariform larvae, frequently through the soles of the feet. Unlike hookworm, *Strongyloides* sp are capable of an autoinfective life cycle, in which rhabditiform larvae may molt into filariform larvae while still in the small bowel and then invade the mucosa of the colon or the perianal area, recapitulating the early migratory phase.[17,18] After penetration of the infective filariform larvae through the skin or gut mucosa, they are carried via the circulation to the lungs and penetrate into alveoli and then ascend the tracheobronchial tree. The larvae are swallowed and reside in the small intestine where they ultimately develop into adult worms. Ova are released and hatch into rhabditiform larvae, which are passed in feces. These larvae can transform into filariform larvae, some of which can cause autoinfection. The larvae can also molt and transform into free-living adults in soil, where they may transform into infective filariform larvae.

Infection with *Strongyloides* results in a variety of clinical syndromes ranging from a mild disease to the hyperinfection syndrome seen in immunocompromised hosts.[19,20] Cell-mediated immunity that develops after primary infection limits the extent of autoinfection, so larvae and adult worms largely remain confined to the intestine, where they can survive for decades in immunocompetent individuals. With immunosuppression, especially caused by steroids, and other immunodeficient states, especially infection with *human T-lymphotropic virus-1* (HTLV-1),[21] autoinfection can become pronounced and lead to hyperinfection.

Clinical Features. The clinical manifestations of strongyloidiasis depend on the intensity of infection and immunologic status of the individual. Acute infection is rarely symptomatic, but pneumonitis can develop during the larval migration phase. More than 50% of patients with chronic infections are asymptomatic. Up to 75% of symptomatic patients have peripheral eosinophilia and elevated serum IgE levels; strongyloidiasis should be in the differential diagnosis of any person who presents with persistent eosinophilia. Patients can present with abdominal pain, diarrhea, and weight loss.[15] Dermatologic symptoms include pruritis, urticaria, and skin eruptions, including larva currens, manifest as linear streaks that can be seen on the trunk, thighs, and buttocks due to migrating larvae (Fig. 58.1). Reactive arthritis, nephrotic syndrome, chronic malabsorption, duodenal obstruction, and hepatic lesions have also been associated with chronic strongyloidiasis.

The common pulmonary manifestations in immunocompetent individuals are transient pulmonary opacities with productive cough, dyspnea, and bronchospasm. Chest radiographs range from being normal to showing bilateral nonspecific opacities. Strongyloidiasis may cause asthma, and improvement may follow eradication of the infection. Patients from highly endemic areas who have asthma or COPD with eosinophilia should always be screened for *Strongyloides* infection before instituting steroid therapy in order to avoid hyperinfection.

The *Strongyloides* hyperinfection syndrome develops due to accelerated autoinfection. Hyperinfection is usually observed in the setting of immunosuppression, especially when caused by high-dose corticosteroids,[19,21–24] although other immunosuppressive drugs and radiation therapy have also been implicated. Infection with HTLV-1 markedly predisposes to hyperinfection; this is thought to be secondary to deficiency of Th2 cells that normally contribute to control of helminths.[19,25] In addition, immunosuppression associated with lymphoma, leukemia, malnutrition, organ transplantation, and HIV/AIDS predisposes to *Strongyloides* hyperinfection (see eFig. 123.29), although some studies indicate the risk is not increased by HIV.[19,26] Hyperinfection is characterized by prominent gastrointestinal symptoms, including abdominal pain, nausea, vomiting, diarrhea, and ileus.

The lung is also an important target in hyperinfection. One study found that 15 of 16 cases with severe infection had pulmonary symptoms, with 13 cases having detectable organisms in respiratory secretions.[27] As filariform larvae migrate through the lungs, they cause pneumonitis with cough, hemoptysis, and respiratory failure. As the larvae leave the lumen of the gastrointestinal tract and invade the intestinal mucosa, they may carry bacteria from the gastrointestinal

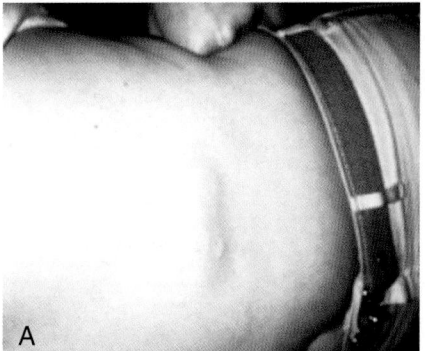
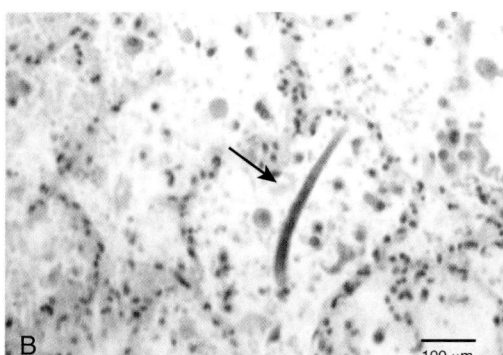
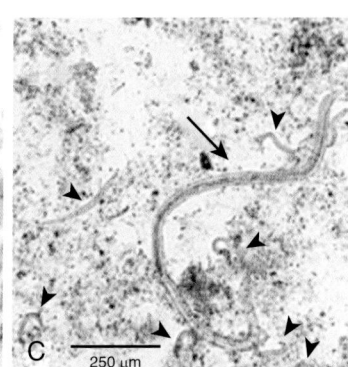

Figure 58.1 Strongyloidiasis. (A) Larva currens in a patient with chronic strongyloidiasis. (B) Filariform larva (*arrow*) in a pulmonary biopsy specimen. (C) Filariform (*arrow*) and rhabditiform (*arrowheads*) larval stages of *Strongyloides stercoralis* in the stool from a patient with hyperinfection syndrome. These were also found in the sputum. (A–B, From Zaiman H. A Pictorial Presentation of Parasites. https://www.astmh.org/education-resources/zaiman-slide-library. Courtesy American Society of Tropical Medicine and Hygiene.)

tract resulting in polymicrobial bacteremia, bacterial pneumonia, ARDS, and gram-negative bacillary meningitis.[27,28] *Strongyloides* hyperinfection has also been reported to mimic accelerated idiopathic pulmonary fibrosis.[29] Mortality of disseminated strongyloidiasis can be as high as 90%.

Diagnosis. In *Strongyloides* hyperinfection, larvae, ova, and adult worms may be observed in sputum, urine, BAL fluid, and other body fluids (see Fig. 58.1 and eFig. 123.29C). Diagnosis of *Strongyloides* infection may be difficult if the parasite load is low because the most common diagnostic test is based on detection of *Strongyloides* ova in stool samples (see Fig. 58.1). Serology assays use ELISA or immunofluorescence to detect serum antibodies to *Strongyloides*. Although ELISA is more sensitive than detecting ova in stool, the specificity of this test is suboptimal in regions where other nematodes such are filariae are endemic, because cross-reactive antibodies are common.[30] *Polymerase chain reaction* (PCR) tests exist for diagnosis but are not commercially available. It is not known how long DNA persists in the stool after successful treatment. Eosinophilia is common during hyperinfection; lack of eosinophilia is associated with a poor prognosis.[19,25]

Treatment. Ivermectin is the treatment of choice, eliminates the worm in over 90% of subjects,[16] and is more effective than albendazole.[32] All patients with *S. stercoralis* infection should be treated because of the risk of autoinfection and dissemination. For routine infection, a 2-day course of ivermectin is sufficient; however, treatment for hyperinfection is usually extended and individualized to ensure eradication.[19] Elimination or reduction of immunosuppression is important in achieving cure in the hyperinfection syndrome. HTLV-1 coinfection is associated with a higher rate of treatment failure,[33] and some patients may require additional therapy to prevent recurrence. Combination treatment with ivermectin and albendazole has also been proposed in severe cases or in chronic infections with HTLV-1 coinfection when ivermectin alone has failed. In hyperinfection cases where oral treatment cannot be absorbed or tolerated, the veterinary preparation of ivermectin has been administered subcutaneously.[34–36] There is no reliable test to monitor for cure, but many individuals have reversion or decline of IgG serologies with successful treatment.[30]

Most experts recommend that patients from highly endemic areas have a screening serology for strongyloidiasis before (or at the time of) starting steroids or organ transplantation; if they are seropositive, treatment is indicated to prevent the hyperinfection syndrome.

Tropical Pulmonary Eosinophilia

Tropical pulmonary eosinophilia (TPE) is a distinct clinical syndrome in patients from tropical areas endemic for lymphatic filariasis such as *Wuchereria bancrofti* or *Brugia malayi*.[37] Most cases have been described in India, Pakistan, Sri Lanka, Southeast Asia, parts of the African continent, and South America, especially Brazil and Guyana. TPE is now recognized in nonendemic areas, predominantly in immigrants; TPE is not thought to be a significant risk during a brief visit to an endemic area.

Clinical Features. Filariae have five morphologic stages. Humans are infected with third-stage larvae transmitted by mosquitoes. Infective larvae molt twice and develop into adults that survive in a human host for up to 20 years. The first-stage larvae, or microfilariae, are released into the circulation by female adult worms. *Wucheria* and *Brugia* microfilariae circulate in the blood in a temporal pattern that coincides with the feeding habits of their mosquito vectors. TPE is seen predominantly (80%) in men, usually in middle age. The major clinical features of TPE include nocturnal paroxysmal cough and bronchospasm, low-grade fever, weight loss, and lymphadenopathy; some patients also have hepatosplenomegaly. Leukocytosis, marked peripheral eosinophilia, and elevated serum IgE levels are common, and sputum or BAL specimens often contain eosinophils. Pulmonary function tests reveal both restrictive and obstructive defects. Although TPE is caused by filaria, patients with TPE do not have detectable microfilaremia. The pathogenesis of TPE is poorly understood but is believed to represent a response to microfilariae trapped in the lungs.[38,39]

Diagnosis. The diagnosis of TPE is based on the combination of clinical, radiologic, epidemiologic, and laboratory data, without the need for lung biopsy. Patients have nocturnal dyspnea with eosinophilia, elevated serum IgE, and a positive serologic test (ELISA) for antibodies to filarial antigens. Because the specificity of filarial serology tests is compromised by cross-reactivity with other helminths, other data are important for an accurate diagnosis.[1,40] Chest radiographs usually reveal increased bilateral bronchovascular markings and reticulonodular opacities or diffuse miliary lesions, or opacities in the middle and lower lung fields

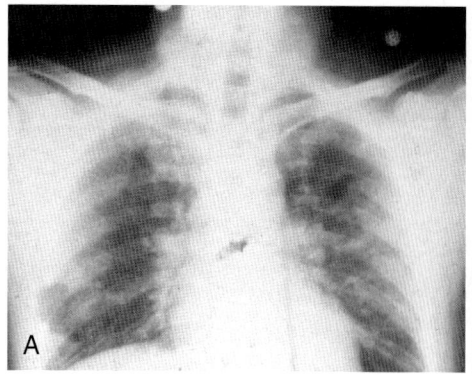
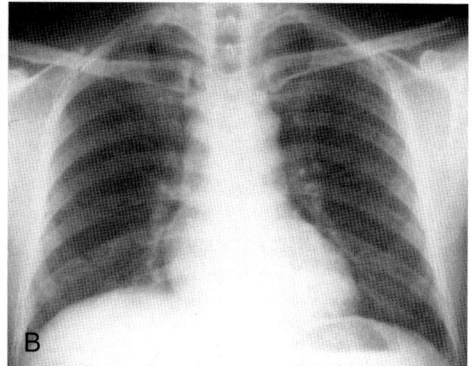

Figure 58.2 Tropical pulmonary eosinophilia. (A) Chest radiograph of a patient from Sri Lanka with confirmed tropical pulmonary eosinophilia shows subpleural right lung consolidation, subpleural left midlung opacity, and bilateral perihilar interstitial thickening. (B) Chest radiograph of the same patient after treatment with diethylcarbamazine. Note the improved opacities.

(Fig. 58.2, eFig. 58.2). Cavitation, bronchiectasis, and pleural effusion have been reported but are uncommon; chest radiographs may also be normal. When pathologic specimens have been obtained, eosinophilic infiltration of the interstitial and perivascular areas, eosinophilic abscess formation, and eosinophilic granulomas can be observed, and worm fragments are occasionally found.[41] Electron microscopic examination of the lung has demonstrated degranulation of the eosinophils, implying that tissue destruction may be mediated by cytotoxic granule proteins released by these cells. Fibrosis may be present if the course of the disease has been prolonged.

Treatment. All patients should be treated because TPE can progress to chronic restrictive lung disease. Administration of diethylcarbamazine, an antifilarial drug, results in improvement in the signs and symptoms of TPE, with reduced eosinophilia and serum IgE levels. The optimal duration of therapy is not established, but most guidelines recommend 3 weeks of diethylcarbamazine, although response may be incomplete or some patients may relapse.[42] Some experts have suggested ivermectin therapy either alone or in combination with diethylcarbamazine, although ivermectin has little effect on adult filariae and some patients require retreatment, regardless of the regimen. Steroid therapy should be administered with caution because TPE and pulmonary strongyloidiasis have similar presentations and steroids may enhance the morbidity and mortality of strongyloidiasis.

Wolbachia, a bacterial endosymbiont of *W. bancrofti*, is thought to play an importat role in the survival and the pathogenesis of *Wuchereria*. Doxycycline, which eliminates *Wolbachia*, has been shown to be effective in the treatment of filariasis.[43] *Wolbachia* is proving a valuable target for many of the filarial diseases, especially because it can be targeted with doxycycline, which is better tolerated than diethylcarbamazine, but no trials have compared the efficacy of short versus long courses of diethylcarbamazine with diethylcarbamazine with doxycycline.

Visceral Larva Migrans

Visceral larva migrans (VLM) is a clinical syndrome caused by human zoonotic infection with *Toxocara canis* (from dogs) or *Toxocara cati* (from cats).[44] Infection is acquired by ingesting eggs in contaminated soil or sandbox contents; a history of pica is common in infected children.[45] Although VLM usually afflicts children, adults have also been described with VLM. A VLM-like syndrome has also been reported as a result of infection with *A. suum*, the parasite of pigs,[46] and *Baylisascaris procyonis*, the raccoon ascarid.[47,48] The hatched larvae cannot mature into adults in humans (which are dead-end hosts), and the larvae migrate throughout the visceral organs of humans causing an acute eosinophilic syndrome.

Clinical Features. VLM affects multiple organs.[49] Pulmonary manifestations are found in 80% of cases and include cough, shortness of breath, and wheezing, resembling asthma.[50] Although symptoms are usually mild, severe respiratory symptoms have been reported.[51,52] VLM damages the lung due to immune responses to migrating larvae.[53] Other manifestations that can be seen are urticaria, lymphadenopathy, hepatosplenomegaly, seizures and other CNS involvement,[54–56] ocular disease, and myocardial disease.[57,58]

Diagnosis and Treatment. The radiographic appearance in VLM is variable and includes bilateral or segmental and patchy opacities, which can be migratory; subpleural opacities may be detected by *computed tomography* (CT). Laboratory evaluation may reveal leukocytosis, marked eosinophilia, elevated anti-A or anti-B isohemagglutinin titers, and abnormal liver function tests; IgE levels are frequently elevated. The diagnosis is made by ELISA and immunoblot testing. Because larvae do not mature to adults in humans, there are no ova in the stool. Because VLM is a self-limited syndrome, antiparasitic drugs may not be required. However, if the symptoms are moderate or severe, albendazole is the drug of choice; diethylcarbamazine is an alternative therapy. In severe cases, adjunctive steroids may accelerate symptom resolution. Preventive measures include control of soil contamination, curbing pica, and regular deworming of dogs and cats.

Dirofilariasis

Dirofilaria immitis, the dog heartworm, is an important cause of morbidity and mortality in dogs.[59] It is transmitted by mosquitoes, but humans are dead-end hosts. In the United States, most cases have been described in the Southeast. The worms migrate via the venous circulation and right heart where they reach the pulmonary arteries. In humans, the filariae are vascular parasites in the pulmonary artery, inducing vasculitis and formation of a pulmonary nodule upon death of the parasite (Fig. 58.3).[59] The majority of cases are asymptomatic, although some individuals may have cough and pneumonitis.[60] Eosinophilia

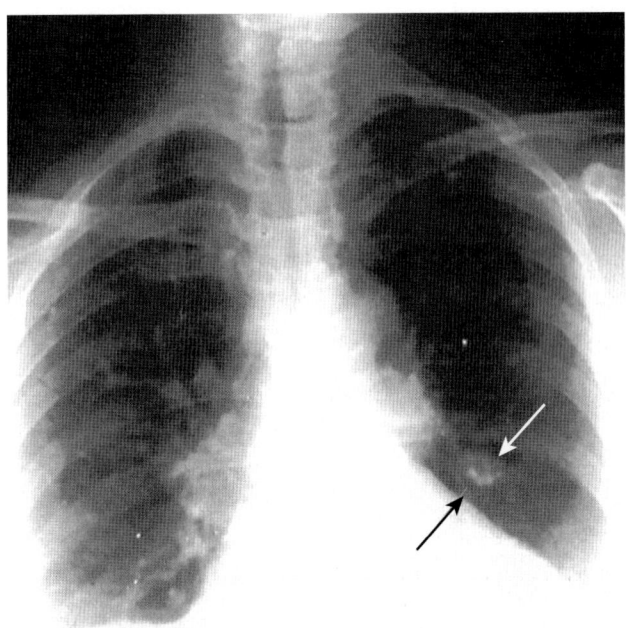

Figure 58.3 *Dirofilaria immitis.* Chest radiograph showing a solitary nodule (*arrows*) in the lung from a patient with confirmed *Dirofilaria immitis.* (From McCall GW, Genchi C, Kramer LH, et al. Heartworm disease in animals and humans. *Adv Parasitol.* 2008;66:193–285.)

is absent. Chest radiographs usually reveal a well-defined homogeneous spherical or oval coin lesion with smooth edges. Because there is no reliable noninvasive test for *Dirofilaria* infection, nearly all cases require biopsy to establish the diagnosis. Surgery is both diagnostic and curative.

Trichinosis

Trichinosis is caused by the parasites of the genus *Trichinella*, especially *T. spiralis*. These nematodes are found intracellularly in striated muscle. Humans usually acquire the infection by ingesting cysts containing the coiled larvae in raw or partially cooked pork, pork products, or game such as wild boar.

Clinical Features. Larvae emerge in the gastrointestinal tract from contaminated meat and invade the small intestine and disseminate throughout the body. This enteral stage may be either asymptomatic or may be accompanied by signs and symptoms of gastroenteritis. During dissemination, the larvae enter the bloodstream and circulate to various organs. Larvae encyst in peripheral skeletal muscle, forming the "nurse cell," consisting of an infected myocyte fed by vessels formed by neoangiogenesis. Most symptoms are due to inflammation associated with the invasion of larvae through the intestine and with influx of eosinophils and mast cells in the region of nurse cells. During the acute stage of infection, common symptoms include malaise, abdominal pain, fever, nausea, vomiting, myalgias, and muscle weakness with facial and generalized edema. Respiratory tract involvement is uncommon but, in severe cases, there may be dyspnea and transient pulmonary opacities. Dyspnea may result from larval invasion of the diaphragm and the accessory muscles of respiration[61]; however, lung inflammation may also play a role.[62]

Diagnosis and Treatment. Trichinosis is diagnosed based on its clinical presentation, epidemiology, eosinophilia, and a positive ELISA.[1] Muscle biopsy is definitive but has a low sensitivity. Treatment is with albendazole; corticosteroids may be added in severe cases, especially those with pneumonitis, myocarditis, or meningoencephalitis. It is unclear whether treatment alters the course of infection, particularly because it does not appear to affect worms after they have already encysted. Trichinosis is prevented by consuming meats fully cooked to a temperature of 140°F.

Gnathostomiasis

Gnathostomiasis is caused by helminths of the genus *Gnathostoma* and is endemic in South Asia and Southeast Asia, China, and Latin America, especially in cultures in which uncooked fish is consumed.[63,64] *Gnathostoma spinigerum* is the most common agent of human infection with this zoonotic pathogen. *G. spinigerum* has a complex life cycle involving two intermediate hosts; its definitive hosts are cats and dogs.[65] Humans usually become infected with third-stage larvae by ingesting raw or inadequately cooked freshwater fish or other intermediate hosts such as snakes, frogs, and chickens. Alternative routes of infection are ingestion of water containing infected copepods and penetration of the skin of food handlers by third-stage larvae from infected meat.[64] Larvae migrate from the gastrointestinal tract to the liver and abdominal cavity and then return

to the stomach, where they embed in the wall, resembling a tumor with an aperture communicating with the lumen to release eggs.[66] The mechanical damage of migrating larvae has been cited as the primary cause of symptoms. Migration of larvae through tissues results in characteristic hemorrhagic tracts, surrounded by eosinophilic infiltration. When the lungs are involved, patients present with cough, pleuritic chest pain, hemoptysis, lobar consolidation, lobar collapse, pleural effusion, pneumothorax, or hydrothorax. Subcutaneous swellings, unexplained eosinophilic pleural effusion, and peripheral eosinophilia are considered a clinical triad and should prompt consideration of gnathostomiasis.

Diagnosis and Treatment. Diagnosis is based on the presence of eosinophilia, migratory inflammation, and history of exposure risk. The diagnosis can be confirmed by identification of the worm in tissue or by serology. The treatment of choice is albendazole or ivermectin.

TREMATODES

Paragonimiasis

The lung flukes of the genus *Paragonimus* encompass several species important in human disease.[67] *Paragonimus westermani* is found in humans and animals in Asia, Africa, and South America. More than 90% of cases are seen in Asia and *P. westermani* is rarely contracted in the United States.[68] Most cases of paragonimiasis acquired in the United States are due to *Paragonimus kellicotti*[65,69] from the ingestion of crayfish. This parasite has a complex life cycle involving freshwater snails, crustaceans, and mammals. Humans become infected by ingesting raw, partially cooked, or pickled crustaceans such as crab or crayfish containing an encysted larval form called a *metacercaria*, which excyst in the duodenum and penetrate the intestinal wall to enter the peritoneal cavity. Larval forms penetrate the diaphragm and enter the pleural cavity and lung parenchyma where they mature to adult worms. Pairs of adult worms live in cystic cavities near bronchial passages (Fig. 58.4) and produce eggs. Cystic cavities eventually rupture into a bronchiole, allowing eggs to be expectorated or swallowed and passed in feces.

Clinical Features. Although most acute infections are asymptomatic, some individuals present with abdominal pain, diarrhea, fever, chest pain, cough, urticaria, peripheral eosinophilia, and elevated levels of IgE.[70] These symptoms and signs usually manifest 2 weeks after ingestion of the metacercaria. Following acute infection, clinical disease has an insidious onset with clinical manifestations 5 to 10 years following exposure. These late clinical symptoms include cough productive of thick, rusty-colored or bloody sputum with Charcot-Leyden crystals, with or without pleuritic chest pain.[71] There may be frank hemoptysis resembling that in tuberculosis[72] (see Fig. 58.4). Fever and eosinophilia are often absent. A common finding is an abnormal chest radiograph in an asymptomatic patient. Pneumonia, bronchiectasis, and vasculitis may be present.

Diagnosis. Chest radiographs demonstrate a variety of lesions including focal involvement or consolidation.

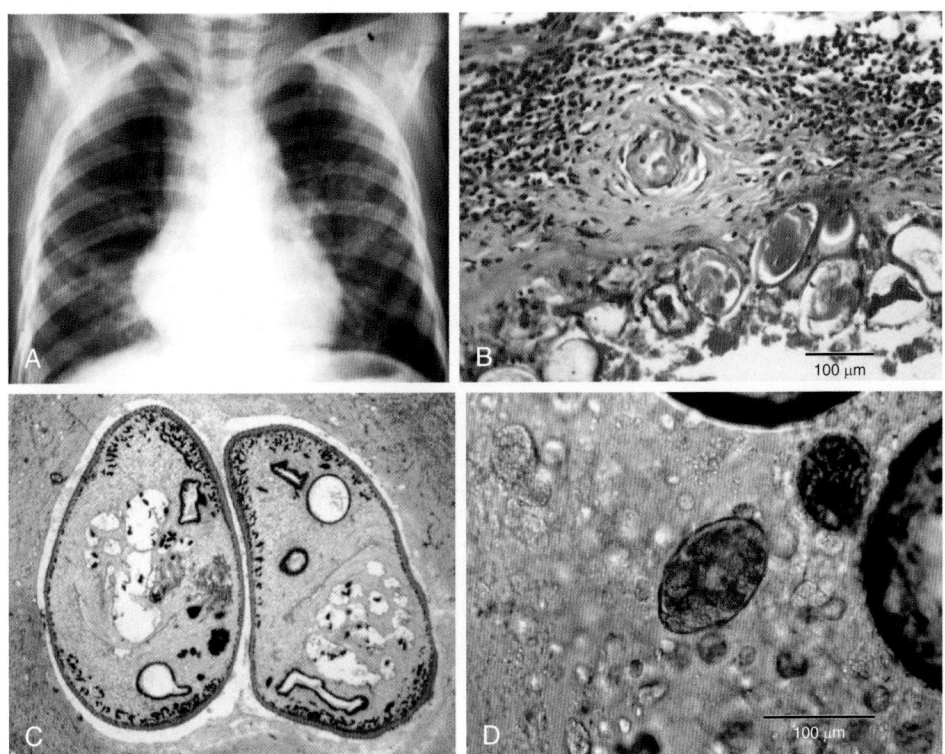

Figure 58.4 *Paragonimus westermani.* (A) Chest radiograph of a patient who presented with hemoptysis shows minimal perihilar left and right infrahilar linear and reticular opacities. (B) Granuloma surrounding ova. (C) Cross section of a pair of adults in the lung. (D) Ovum in the sputum.

Cavitary lesions may measure up to 4 cm in diameter; small cysts and calcified or noncalcified nodules (eFig. 58.3) may be present. Pleural effusion, pneumothorax, and pleural thickening may develop in a minority of patients.[71–73] The pleural fluid characteristically contains leukocytes, many eosinophils, elevated concentrations of protein and lactate dehydrogenase, and low concentrations of glucose. Histopathologic examination of the lung reveals adult worms within fibrous cysts communicating with bronchi or bronchioles; granulomas may contain eggs at the center (see Fig. 58.4B). Acute and chronic pathologic changes may coexist within the same pulmonary lesions.

When the diagnosis of paragonimiasis is suspected, it can be confirmed by finding morphologically characteristic eggs in sputum, stool, gastric aspirates, or tissue (see Fig. 58.4D). Bloody sputum is the most likely to yield positive results. ELISA and immunoblot assays that detect antibodies to *Paragonimus* antigens are useful for diagnosis.

Treatment. Praziquantel is the drug of choice. Untreated pulmonary paragonimiasis may resolve within 5 to 10 years (the life span of the adult worms), but chronic infection may be accompanied by extensive fibrosis. Paragonimiasis can be prevented by avoiding eating uncooked crabs and crayfish.

Schistosomiasis

Schistosomiasis is found in tropical and subtropical areas of the world including South America, Africa, the Middle East, and East Asia, including the Philippines.[74] The World Health Organization estimates that more than 200 million people are infected worldwide.[75] Five species of schistosomes cause human disease: *Schistosoma hematobium*, *S. mansoni*, *S. japonicum*, *S. mekongi*, and *S. intercalatum*. Infection is acquired when the free-swimming larval forms

called *cercariae* penetrate the skin during contact with fresh water while the person is bathing, wading, or doing laundry. After penetrating the skin, the cercariae lose their tails and quickly transform into juvenile forms (schistosomula) that migrate to the lung and liver. These transform into adults that mate and then travel to their tissue destination. *S. hematobium* are found in the venous plexus of the urinary bladder while *S. mansoni* and *S. japonicum* reside in mesenteric veins. Female worms lay eggs that are excreted either in the urine (*S. hematobium*) or feces (*S. mansoni*, *S. japonicum*). Adult schistosomes may live and produce eggs for as long as 30 years.

Clinical Features. A rash consisting of erythematous raised 1- to 3-cm lesions may develop within hours (and as late as 1 week) after cercarial penetration of skin (especially in those infected for the first time). Symptoms usually develop between 4 and 8 weeks after exposure, which coincides with maturation of adults and the beginning of egg laying. In acute infection, in naive hosts, "Katayama fever" can develop after heavy exposure to *S. japonicum* or *S. mansoni*.[76,77] Katayama fever is characterized by urticaria, fever, chills, cough, wheezing, headaches, lymphadenopathy, hepatosplenomegaly, peripheral eosinophilia, and elevated serum IgE levels. The symptoms usually resolve within several weeks but can lead to death in rare instances. The major pathologic finding in schistosomiasis is that of granulomas surrounding eggs.[78] Chronic pulmonary schistosomiasis is the result of deposition of eggs in pulmonary vessels followed by granuloma formation and obstruction of blood flow.[79] Vasospasm and inflammation also contribute to the pulmonary findings in chronic pulmonary schistosomiasis.[80] Pulmonary hypertension develops in approximately 5% of patients with hepatosplenic schistosomiasis, usually after many years of untreated infection.[81,82]

Figure 58.5 Schistosomiasis. (A) Computed tomography scan of the lung showing macronodules with ground-glass halo *(arrow)*. (B) Granuloma in the lung surrounding a *Schistosoma* ovum. (A, From Weber-Donat G, Donat N, Margery J. Acute pulmonary schistosomiasis: computed tomography (CT) findings. *Am J Trop Med Hyg.* 82:364, 2010. B, From Zaiman H. A Pictorial Presentation of Parasites. https://www.astmh.org/education-resources/zaiman-slide-library. Courtesy American Society of Tropical Medicine and Hygiene.)

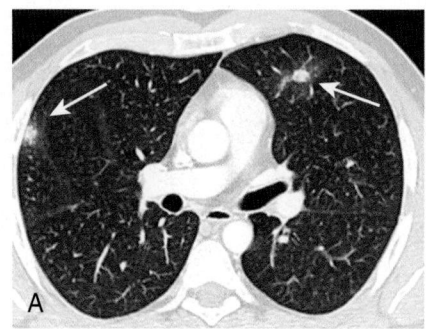
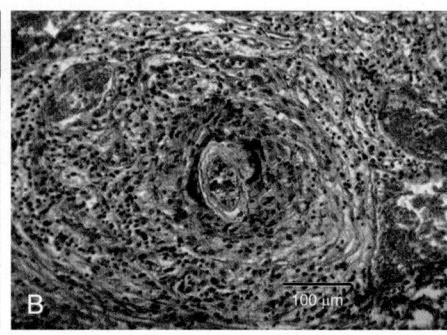

Diagnosis and Treatment. Chest radiographs of patients with Katayama fever often demonstrate diffuse pulmonary opacities or nodules with indistinct borders, which may have a ground-glass "halo" appearance on CT (Fig. 58.5A).[83] Pleural effusions and thoracic lymphadenopathy may also be present. In chronic pulmonary schistosomiasis, imaging demonstrates nodules, miliary lesions, and cavitary lesions as well as signs of pulmonary hypertension.

Diagnosis is made by stool or urine examination or rectal biopsy, although shedding of eggs usually does not commence until 6 weeks after exposure.[84] Nearly all patients with Katayama fever have eosinophilia and elevated serum IgE levels. ELISA and immunoblot assays that detect antibodies to schistosomal antigens are available, but these tests may be negative in acute infection and may remain positive years after treatment. Lung biopsies may reveal the granulomas surrounding eggs (Fig. 58.5B).

The treatment of choice for schistosomiasis is praziquantel. Praziquantel kills adult worms but may not kill immature parasites. In some cases, symptoms can transiently worsen after treatment; this is presumed to be due to release of proinflammatory components of dead parasites. Pulmonary hypertension due to schistosomiasis can also worsen with antiparasitic treatment.

CESTODES

Echinococcosis

Echinococcus granulosus, the dog tapeworm, has a scattered worldwide distribution.[85] It remains an important public health problem in the Mediterranean basin where it is especially common in Italy, Spain, Albania, and the countries of the former Yugoslavia. It is also found throughout Central America and South America and in scattered areas of sub-Saharan Africa, China, Russia, and the countries of the former Soviet Union. *Echinococcus multilocularis*, the fox tapeworm, is endemic in Canada, parts of the United States, central Europe, the countries of the former Soviet Union, China, and northern parts of Japan.[85–88]

E. granulosus (Fig. 58.6) usually infects canines and sheds millions of eggs in feces. Intermediate hosts, including sheep and humans, become infected when they ingest the ova in contaminated food or water. Larvae are released from ova after ingestion and migrate via the bloodstream or lymphatics to various organs, usually the liver and lung, but kidney, bone, and brain may also be involved. The larvae mature into cysts, called echinococcal or hydatid cysts. The *E. granulosus* cyst is fluid filled and unilocular, consisting of an inner germinal layer and an outer acellular laminated layer. Daughter cysts may arise from the inner layer,

the endocyst. There is also an outer layer, the pericyst, composed of fibrous tissue, which is host derived.

Clinical Features. The lungs are involved in 20–40% and the liver in 50–70% of cases of cystic echinococcosis.[85,89] Infection usually presents as a solitary cyst involving one organ; 10–15% of individuals have more than one organ involved. In children, the lungs are involved more often than the liver.[90] Pulmonary echinococcosis is commonly discovered as an incidental finding on chest imaging (eFig. 58.4). In symptomatic patients, the clinical manifestations of pulmonary echinococcosis are most often the consequence of cyst rupture; less frequently, symptoms are due to compression by an enlarging cyst. Rupture of a hydatid cyst into a bronchus results in fever and cough, which can have an abrupt onset. In some patients, the sputum can contain macroscopic fragments of the parasite. Ruptured cysts that communicate with an airway can become secondarily infected by bacteria and/or fungi. Rupture of a hydatid cyst into the pleural space can be associated with hypersensitivity responses, including fever, urticaria, and wheezing; frank anaphylaxis can also develop, but is rarely fatal. Rupture into the pleural space can also cause empyema, with or without bacterial superinfection. Cysts that enlarge without rupturing may erode into adjacent structures and cause bone pain, hemorrhage, or airway compression.[91]

Diagnosis and Treatment. Diagnosis depends on the combination of imaging, serology, and microscopy. On chest radiographs, uncomplicated (unruptured) hydatid cysts appear as homogeneous oval or round masses 1 to 20 cm in diameter with smooth borders and normal adjacent lung tissue (see Fig. 58.6C and eFig. 58.4). If a cyst ruptures into a large airway, partial discharge of the cyst contents results in an air-fluid level. If the cyst ruptures, cyst fragments, especially the rigid mouthparts (scolices) of the parasite, may be detected by microscopic examination of sputum or pleural fluid. A hydatid cyst completely emptied of liquid contents and collapsed can exhibit a "water lily" sign (see Fig. 58.6D), which is pathognomonic of a collapsed cyst but is rare. The water lily sign is created when air enters the cyst, allowing detachment of the inner endocyst from the outer pericyst, so that the endocyst collapses to float on the fluid in the partially filled pericyst, creating the appearance of a water lily floating on a pond. CT scans may allow distinction of hydatid cysts from other pulmonary cysts by revealing the presence of daughter cysts within a larger cyst. Other complications, such as cardiac echinococcosis and pulmonary embolization of organisms are rare (eFig. 58.5).

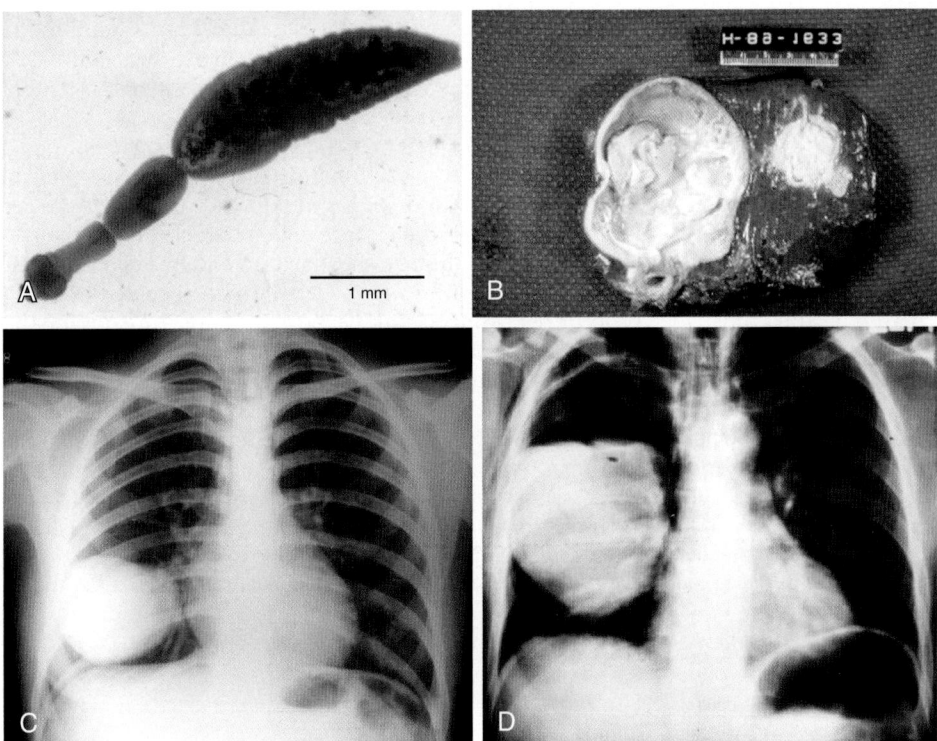

Figure 58.6 **Echinococcal cysts.** (A) Adult *Echinococcus granulosis*. (B) *Echinococcus* cyst of the liver near the diaphragm. (C) *Echinococcus* cyst of the lung. (D) Ruptured *Echinococcus* cyst of the lung with the "water lily" sign. (A and D, From Zaiman H. A Pictorial Presentation of Parasites. https://www.astmh.org/education-resources/zaiman-slide-library. Courtesy American Society of Tropical Medicine and Hygiene. C, Courtesy Dr. Saul Santivanez, Lima, Peru.)

Serologic testing consists of an ELISA that detects antibodies to a cyst antigen. Although the assay is quite sensitive in patients with hepatic involvement, the sensitivity in patients with pulmonary echinococcosis is only about 50%, so serology is confirmatory rather than diagnostic. The current ELISA also has cross-reactivity to cysticercosis.

Treatment. Surgical removal is the principal therapeutic approach in patients who can tolerate the procedure.[85] Surgery must be planned to minimize the likelihood of intraoperative cyst rupture, because rupture can result in anaphylaxis and parasite dissemination with subsequent relapse. Preoperative administration of albendazole can reduce the consequences of dissemination.[91] Praziquantel is added to albendazole, particularly if the cyst has ruptured, because it has a scolicidal effect. Intraoperative administration of a helminthicide agent such as hypertonic saline or 1% formaldehyde, left in place in the cyst lumen for 15 minutes or more before further manipulation, is also thought to minimize the consequences of spillage of cyst contents.[91–93] In patients with symptomatic or complicated echinococcal cysts who cannot tolerate a thoracic surgical procedure, prolonged treatment with albendazole may improve symptoms, but is curative in only a minority of cases. Praziquantel also has activity, and a combination of albendazole and praziquantel may have greater efficacy than either drug alone. Monitoring responses to drug treatment must be based on clinical findings and imaging procedures; serial serologic assays have been found to be without value.

Echinococcus multilocularis

Alveolar echinococcosis caused by *E. multilocularis* is a rare but potentially fatal disease. Wild canines are the definitive hosts and small animals are the intermediate hosts. The liver is the initial target of this parasite and the incubation period can be exceedingly long. It can spread to the lung as a result of metastatic dissemination or by direct extension through the diaphragm of a liver cyst with rupture into the thorax. *E. multilocularis* can involve the bronchial tree, pleural cavity, and mediastinal structures. The diagnosis is made by serology and biopsy. The only cure is radical resection followed by long-term therapy with albendazole. If not amenable to surgery, life-long treatment with albendazole may be beneficial.

PROTOZOA

Protozoa are unicellular eukaryotic organisms. They are usually acquired either by ingestion or by the bite of a vector. Gastrointestinal or systemic symptoms generally predominate in protozoal infections, although pulmonary symptoms can develop.

AMEBIASIS

Amebiasis, caused by *E. histolytica*, predominantly affects individuals who live in Mexico, Central and South America, Africa, and the Indian subcontinent; however, travel and immigration have globalized this infection. *Entamoeba* are estimated to cause 40,000 to 100,000 deaths yearly[94] and infect 500 million people,[94] although more recent data suggest many of these are infected with the nonpathogenic *Entamoeba dispar* rather than pathogenic *E. histolytica*.[95] *E. histolytica* does not involve intermediate hosts and has a simple life cycle, alternating between environmentally hardy cysts and invasive trophozoites. Cysts have a chitinous cell wall that enables them to persist in the environment for weeks to months and to infect subsequent hosts that ingest contaminated food or water. In 4–10% of individuals infected with *E. histolytica*, trophozoites invade the intestinal mucosa to cause intestinal disease. In others, the trophozoites enter the bloodstream and can establish infection in the liver, brain, or lungs.[96,97]

Clinical Features. Intestinal amebiasis is associated with abdominal pain, tenesmus (constant urge to defecate), and diarrhea, which may be bloody, mucoid, or watery. Fever may be present. Symptoms can last several weeks. Fulminant infection with ileus and intestinal perforation can also develop. The most common site for extraintestinal amebiasis is the liver (eFig. 58.6); a smaller proportion of cases affect the lungs, and amebic brain abscesses are uncommon. The typical patient with an amebic liver abscess is an adult man who has acquired the infection in an endemic area and presents with fever and right upper quadrant pain without intestinal symptoms. Amebic liver abscesses are approximately 10-fold more common in men than women; the reason for this sex difference is unknown but it is not due to differences in rates of infection.[98] Mouse models of amebiasis also demonstrate differences in host immune response between male and female mice.[99] Many patients presenting with extraintestinal amebiasis do not have cysts or trophozoites in the stool. A prior amebic abscess or amebiasis does not confer immunity to recurrence. Extraintestinal manifestations of amebiasis can present years after leaving an endemic area.[94]

The lung is the second most common extraintestinal site of *E. histolytica* infection and usually results from the extension of a right lobe hepatic abscess, so patients may have right upper quadrant abdominal pain as well as pulmonary symptoms. Pleuropulmonary amebiasis complicates amebic liver abscess in 7–20% of cases,[4] although the chest radiograph is abnormal in nearly 50% of cases. Although any lobe of the lungs can be affected, the right lower lobe is most commonly involved,[100] and pulmonary amebiasis can be confused with bacterial pneumonia (see eFig. 46.61).[94] Findings include an elevated right hemidiaphragm, right pleural effusion, right lobe atelectasis, pulmonary consolidation with abscess formation, and hepatic-bronchial fistulas. An empyema may develop from rupture of a liver abscess into the pleural space.[101] Patients can present with shortness of breath[102] or rarely with respiratory failure[103] or the expectoration of "anchovy-paste" sputum, which represents the contents of an amebic abscess.[104] Rarely, pulmonary amebiasis results from hematogenous spread without liver abscess. Hepatic abscesses can also rupture into the pericardium and cause cardiac tamponade.[101,105,106]

Diagnosis. *Entamoeba* infections can result from either *E. histolytica* or the nonpathogenic *E. dispar*. *E. histolytica* and *E. dispar* trophozoites are indistinguishable; however, antigen and PCR assays can differentiate these species.[107] Serology tests are highly sensitive for the diagnosis of extraintestinal amebiasis, but can remain positive for years after an infection. Therefore, serology cannot distinguish current and past infection. In cases of suspected pulmonary involvement in amebiasis, CT scanning of the lung and adjacent liver should be used to define the extent of involvement and presence of fistulae (see eFig. 46.61).[108]

Treatment. Because of the potential for asymptomatic infection to develop into dysentery or extraintestinal disease, or to be transmitted, all *E. histolytica* infections should be treated.

Patients with liver abscesses can usually be managed medically without percutaneous aspiration, but pleural or pericardial effusions[101] should be drained and larger lesions (>300 mL) may improve more quickly if drained.[109] Metronidazole is highly effective and can be used orally or systemically. Monitoring responses with repeated imaging procedures is not useful, because it is not unusual for the radiographic appearance to worsen before improvement.[108] Another nitroimidazole, tinidazole, is an alternative and has efficacy and toxicity similar to that of metronidazole. Agents such as paromomycin and diloxanide furoate that kill cysts in the intestine are not effective against extraintestinal amebiasis. After tissue-invasive amebiasis has been treated with metronidazole or tinidazole, a cysticidal agent is usually used (e.g., paromomycin or diloxanide) to decrease the possibility of relapse or transmission of infection.[94]

MALARIA

Human malaria is caused by *P. falciparum*, *P. vivax*, *P. malariae*, *P. ovale*, or *P. knowlesi*. *P. knowlesi*, a simian malaria seen in Southeast Asia, has been associated with zoonotic malaria infections in humans.[110] Because this species resembles *P. malariae* morphologically, the parasite was mistaken for *P. malariae*, but *P. knowlesi* malaria has a more virulent course that can result in death. The World Health Organization estimates in 2017 there were 219 million malaria cases and approximately 435,000 deaths due to malaria, primarily in children infected with *P. falciparum* in sub-Saharan Africa. Severe malaria, including cerebral malaria, is seen in many areas of the tropical and subtropical world and among travelers and immigrants in nonendemic areas. Severe malaria can include anemia, coma, and respiratory failure; these are most frequent with *P. falciparum* infection. Most fatalities in the developed world are due to delayed diagnosis because patients and clinicians are unaware of the risk of severe malaria.

Plasmodium species are transmitted by the bite of the female *Anopheles* mosquito. Sporozoites injected into the bloodstream traffic to the liver and initiate the clinically silent hepatic phase, which results in the release of thousands of merozoites that infect erythrocytes. The erythrocytic stages are responsible for clinical disease. The pathogenesis of severe malaria is not completely understood, but is thought to be caused by inflammatory mediators such as cytokines and chemokines and by vascular leukocyte adhesion molecules. *P. falciparum* elaborates a family of variant antigens that enables infected erythrocytes to adhere to microvascular endothelium.[111] Sequestration of infected erythrocytes in tissue microvessels is thought to be critical for pathogenesis of the most severe manifestations of malaria including cerebral malaria.[112] There is no sterile immunity (i.e., resulting in the elimination of all organisms) to malaria, and malaria has exerted a profound selective pressure upon human evolution. Nearly all genetic erythrocyte defects, including sickle cell anemia, thalassemia, and pyruvate kinase deficiency, are most prevalent in regions of the world with high malaria prevalence and some, including heterozygous HbS, protect from severe malaria.[113]

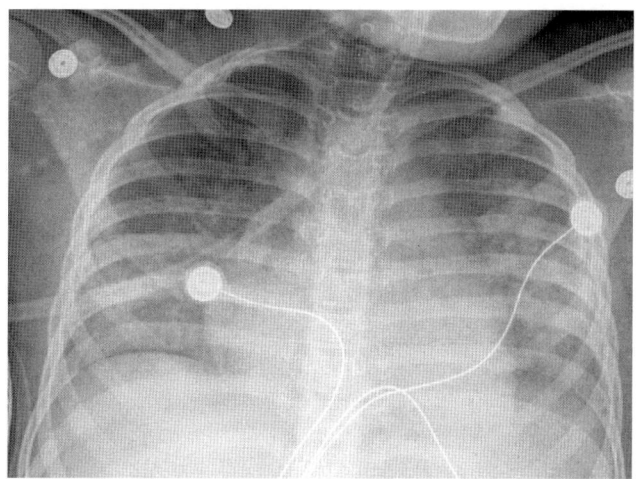

Figure 58.7 Malaria. Diffuse bilateral symmetric lung opacities resembling pulmonary edema in a child with malaria.

Clinical Features. Severe malaria is associated with fever, chills, anemia, thrombocytopenia, jaundice, and renal failure. *P. falciparum* malaria can progress within days to cause multiorgan failure, especially in nonimmune patients. Fever is associated with the lysis of infected erythrocytes, and is classically periodic (every day for *P. knowlesi*, every 2 days for *P. falciparum*, *P. vivax*, and *P. ovale*; every 3 days for *P. malariae*) and nocturnal. However, this is not a reliable clinical sign, particularly for *P. falciparum*.

Patients with malaria may present with cough and minimal involvement of the lung or with severe symptoms and signs of acute lung injury and acute respiratory distress syndrome.[114] Children, pregnant women, and nonimmune travelers to endemic areas are most susceptible to pulmonary complications (Fig. 58.7). Chest radiographs may reveal bilateral opacities and lobar consolidation and pleural effusions, and alveolar macrophages may contain hemozoin, a brown degradation product of hemoglobin produced by the parasite. Bronchiolitis and pneumonia have been reported in the setting of *P. vivax* infection.[115] Patients in coma as a result of cerebral malaria may be susceptible to aspiration pneumonia, and may require antibiotic therapy.

Noncardiogenic pulmonary edema may develop in patients with severe malaria with any species of *Plasmodium*, even after several days of antimalarial therapy. The pathogenesis of the noncardiogenic pulmonary edema is unclear. Increased permeability of the alveolar capillaries appears to be an important mechanism by which the liquid fills the alveolar space, and pulmonary edema may be aggravated by fluid overload. The mortality rate of severe falciparum malaria is high.

Diagnosis. Diagnosis is made by rapid diagnostic test or examination of a blood smear, although PCR may be available from some reference labs. Thick blood smears are used to determine whether parasites are present, while thin blood smears are used by experienced technicians to identify the *Plasmodium* species by morphology. For *P. falciparum*, only the immature ring forms are detectable in the peripheral blood, so initial malaria smears may be negative. Mature intraerythrocytic forms of *P. falciparum* cause infected cells to adhere to the microvasculature and are thus rarely evident in peripheral blood. The presence of mature *P. falciparum* forms in the blood and high parasitemia (>10% of erythrocytes containing parasites) are signs of severe disease. *P. vivax* infects only reticulocytes, so parasitemias are lower than with *P. falciparum*. Because initial malaria smears may be negative, a smear should be repeated after 8 hours, and empirical treatment begun if the patient is seriously ill.

Rapid diagnostic tests for *P. falciparum* and *P. vivax* malaria antigens are available as point-of-care diagnostic tests and are often the only test used in malaria endemic settings. Because antigen can persist, these tests do not reliably discriminate current from very recent infection. PCR tests are not currently commercially available.

Treatment. All travelers to malaria endemic regions are advised to take antimalarial prophylaxis and use insecticide-treated bed nets to prevent malaria, but a history of malarial prophylaxis does not rule out malaria and some travelers who have taken prophylaxis either had subtherapeutic levels of drug or acquired resistant organisms.

Supportive care, in addition to specific antimalarial therapy, is extremely important, especially in the case of noncardiogenic pulmonary edema. The treatment of malaria is dependent on the species and the geographic area of the world where it was contracted. Although *P. vivax*, *P. ovale*, *P. malariae*, and *P. knowlesi* can be treated with chloroquine, *P. falciparum* is nearly universally resistant to chloroquine. Intravenous (IV) artesunate is the treatment of choice for patients with pulmonary manifestations of malaria, which usually signifies severe malaria.[116] IV quinidine or quinine is no longer available in the United States; as of March 2019, severe malaria must be treated with IV artesunate, available by contacting the toll-free CDC Malaria Hotline (855-856-4713). Outside business hours, providers should call 770-488-7100 and ask to speak with a CDC malaria expert. IV quinidine is still approved and available outside the United States.

Artesunate resistance has been detected in *P. falciparum* with increasing frequency, especially in Southeast Asia, and is manifested by slower clearance of parasitemia, thus requiring a longer duration of treatment to achieve cure.[117] Careful attention to fluid balance is required to maintain adequate end-organ perfusion and prevent respiratory insufficiency due to fluid overload. Correction of hypoglycemia and attention to oxygenation are critical. The CDC no longer recommends exchange transfusion in patients with high parasitemias (>10%) because the clinical benefit of exchange transfusion has not been established. Severe malaria may also be complicated by concurrent pneumonia or bacterial sepsis that must be managed with appropriate antibiotics.

Clinicians seeking help for diagnosis or treatment of malaria should consult www.cdc.gov/malaria/, or call the phone numbers given previously. Once the patient improves, there are a variety of choices for oral treatment. *P. vivax* and *P. ovale* treatment regimens should include primaquine to eliminate hypnozoite forms within the liver after determining the patient's glucose-6-phosphate dehydrogenase status.

TOXOPLASMOSIS

Toxoplasma gondii is a ubiquitous Apicomplexa protozoan parasite of mammals and birds. *T. gondii* can propagate clonally in its intermediate hosts via tissue cysts, which can initiate infection in hosts that ingest these cysts in raw or undercooked meat. Cats are the definitive hosts and oocysts shed in cat feces are highly infectious, providing a source for contamination of food and water. In humans, infection can transmit vertically to the fetus in a serologically naive mother, leading to congenital toxoplasmosis.[118] The prevalence of infection, as assayed by seropositivity, varies with geography and ranges from 10–90%. *T. gondii* can cause opportunistic infections in immunocompromised hosts, including individuals with AIDS (see Chapter 123).[119] *T. gondii* has a predilection for the central nervous system, where it causes necrotizing encephalitis, and for the eye, where it causes retinochoroiditis. The development of clinically apparent toxoplasmosis is usually a consequence of reactivation of slowly replicating bradyzoites found within tissue cysts into actively replicating, morphologically distinct tachyzoites.[120–122]

Clinical Features. In most cases of pulmonary toxoplasmosis, pulmonary disease is part of multisystem disease in an immunocompromised host such as in persons with HIV/AIDS (CD4 T cells < 50/μL[123–126]), in patients with hematologic malignancies, and in organ transplant recipients.[127–130] Pulmonary toxoplasmosis may rarely develop in immunocompetent persons where it may resemble atypical pneumonia.[131] Clinical symptoms include fever, cough, and shortness of breath.[123–125] A more fulminant pneumonia associated with acute toxoplasmosis has been seen in South America where highly virulent strains of *T. gondii* have caused "Amazonian toxoplasmosis," presenting as severe disseminated systemic disease.[132]

Diagnosis. Chest radiographs reveal bilateral diffuse opacities and/or nodular bilateral opacities that may be confused with *Pneumocystis* pneumonia.[123–125] Examination of the sputum or fluid from BAL may reveal organisms that stain with Giemsa.[133] Pleural fluid, if present, may contain tachyzoites.[134] PCR-based molecular techniques are also available if the parasite is suspected but cannot be found by staining. At autopsy, the lungs are congested and hemorrhagic with areas of consolidation. Histopathologic examination reveals an interstitial pneumonitis and alveolar damage. A frank necrotizing pneumonia may also be observed, with many extracellular and intracellular tachyzoites. Nearly all patients with toxoplasmosis are seropositive, and a negative serologic test suggests another diagnosis. Rarely, primary infection can present as disseminated disease, and serologies may be negative.

Treatment. The treatment of choice for toxoplasmosis is pyrimethamine and sulfadiazine with leucovorin to prevent bone marrow toxicity, but there are several alternatives, including pyrimethamine and clindamycin with leucovorin. Although pyrimethamine and sulfadiazine are considered the treatment of choice, trimethoprim-sulfamethoxazole is active against *T. gondii* and has been suggested as primary therapy in resource-poor areas due to its low cost.[135]

OTHER PROTOZOA

Several other protozoa have been reported to be associated with pulmonary manifestations. Some of the more common parasites that can occasionally present with pulmonary disease are discussed here. Many of these have been increasingly reported, presenting as disseminated disease involving multiple organs, including the lungs, in association with HIV infection or other immunocompromised states.[136] In addition, *Cyclospora cayetanensis*, *Trichomonas vaginalis*, *Trichomonas tenax*, *Trichomonas hominis*, and *Balantidium coli* have been reported to present with pulmonary disease.[136]

Babesiosis

Babesia are intraerythrocytic protozoan parasites.[137–139] *Babesia microti* is transmitted by the tick *Ixodes scapularis*, the Lyme disease tick vector, and has been described in infections in Massachusetts, New York, Rhode Island, Connecticut, New Jersey, and the upper Midwest. Other *Babesia* species have been described in California, Oregon, and Washington. In Europe, babesiosis is rarer but more frequently lethal, and is associated with *Babesia divergens*. Blood transfusion is another mode of transmission. The onset is usually gradual with malaise, fever, chills, sweats, and myalgias. Nausea, vomiting, headache, and psychiatric problems are also reported. There may be splenomegaly, anemia, thrombocytopenia, a normal or low white blood cell count, mild elevation of hepatic enzymes, and evidence of hemolysis. Asplenic and immunocompromised patients often have more severe disease, including jaundice, renal failure, pancytopenia, high-level parasitemia, shock, and disseminated intravascular coagulation. The major pulmonary complication is noncardiogenic pulmonary edema.[140,141] As in malaria, the etiology of noncardiogenic pulmonary edema is not well understood.

Diagnosis. The diagnosis of babesiosis is made by identification of the parasitized erythrocytes on blood smears or by PCR. Immunofluorescence antibody-based serologic tests for *Babesia* have also been developed, but the high rate of seroprevalence in endemic regions limits the usefulness of these tests. Blood can be injected into a hamster for verification of active infection, and PCR-based diagnostic tests may be deployed for blood screening.[142] *B. microti* is treated with quinine and clindamycin or azithromycin and atovaquone.[143] There have been reports of immunocompromised persons developing possible resistance to azithromycin and atovaquone after multiple treatments.[144]

Cryptosporidiosis

The genus *Cryptosporidium* contains several species widely distributed in animals including birds, cattle, and sheep. *C. parvum*, *C. hominis*, and *C. meleagridis* most commonly infect humans and are acquired by the ingestion of oocysts via water or food. The most common clinical manifestation of cryptosporidiosis is watery diarrhea, which is self-limiting in immunocompetent hosts but chronic in immunocompromised hosts. In patients with HIV/AIDS, diarrhea may be persistent, and may be massive and fatal.[145] Extraintestinal manifestations of cryptosporidiosis have been observed. *Cryptosporidium* involvement of the lower respiratory tract is most common in patients with HIV/AIDS but can also develop in patients with other conditions.[146–148] Common symptoms include cough, fever, and shortness of breath; there may also be respiratory insufficiency.

Although the mechanism by which *Cryptosporidium* colonizes the respiratory tract is not clear, aspiration and hematogenous spread from the intestinal tract have both been suggested.[149] Chest radiographs are consistent with interstitial pneumonitis. Alveolar damage and interstitial fibrosis and hyperplasia of alveolar epithelial type 2 cells have been found at autopsy of patients with pulmonary cryptosporidia.[149]A study of HIV-negative Ugandan children with *Cryptosporidium* diarrhea and cough or other respiratory symptoms revealed that 17 of 48 (35.4%) had *Cryptosporidium* in their sputum,[150] suggesting that *Cryptosporidium* may cause more pulmonary disease than previously suspected and that respiratory transmission is possible.

Diagnosis. *Cryptosporidia* can be detected in stool or respiratory samples by a modified acid-fast stain or by immunofluorescence, although PCR is now emerging as the test of choice as part of multipathogen panels.

Treatment. Treatment in immunocompromised individuals has been suboptimal. Nitazoxanide is approved for treatment of cryptosporidiosis in immunocompetent children and adults.[151–153] Nitazoxanide is not efficacious in immunodeficient individuals. Although azithromycin and paromomycin have been associated with improvement in some patients, clinical trials have not confirmed their efficacy in immunodeficient adults.

Free-Living Ameba

Four genera of free-living ameba infect humans: *Naegleria*, *Acanthamoeba*, *Balamuthia*, and *Sappinia*.[154] Infections with these species are rare but worldwide. *Naegleria* and *Acanthamoeba* are commonly found in lakes, swimming pools, tap water, and air conditioning units. *Acanthamoeba* sp are usually associated with granulomatous skin lesions and corneal ulcers. In immunocompromised patients, *Acanthamoeba* sp and *Balamuthia mandrillaris* may cause subacute or chronic granulomatous encephalitis accompanied by respiratory symptoms, nodular opacities, consolidation, and respiratory failure. In those patients, parasites have been recovered from BAL; organisms can also be detected in lung tissue (Fig. 58.8). *Naegleria fowleri* is associated with primary amebic meningoencephalitis that is acute and usually lethal. A PCR-based assay to identify ameba species in clinical samples is available from the CDC.[155] The mortality of these infections is high. Based on case reports, miltefosine is currently used for therapy.

Leishmaniasis

Leishmania sp are found in Asia, Africa, Central and South America, and regions of Europe that border the Mediterranean.[156] Transmission of *Leishmania* sp is through the bites of sand flies, and three clinical syndromes are recognized: cutaneous, mucocutaneous, and visceral. Cutaneous and mucocutaneous forms may also be observed in the viscera in immunocompromised individuals. Visceral leishmaniasis caused by *Leishmania donovani*, *L. infantum*, and *L. chagasi* is characterized by fever, abdominal pain, and hepatosplenomegaly, often accompanied by anemia, thrombocytopenia, leukopenia, and generalized bone marrow suppression. In immunocompromised patients such as those with HIV/AIDS,[157] intracellular forms (amastigotes) may be observed in macrophages of many organs. In the respiratory tract, amastigotes have been observed in the mucosa of the larynx and in the lung and pleura.[158–163] Interstitial pneumonitis, granulomatous inflammation of the bronchial mucosa, and mediastinal lymphadenopathy have all been described in patients with visceral leishmaniasis.[164]

Diagnosis and Treatment. Identification of the parasite by microscopy is the most commonly used method of diagnosis. Culture and molecular techniques such as PCR with *Leishmania* species-specific primers are also available. *Leishmania* amastigotes can be found in samples obtained by BAL, thoracentesis, or transbronchial biopsy.[165] Therapy of leishmaniasis includes pentavalent antimony compounds and amphotericin B formulations.[157] Miltefosine, an oral agent, has also been approved for the treatment of leishmaniasis.[166]

Microsporidiosis

Microsporidia are ubiquitous intracellular parasites found in invertebrate and vertebrate hosts and are related to the Cryptomycota (i.e., fungi). The phylum contains more than 200 genera and over 1500 species. Microsporidia infect nearly all animal phyla. They predominantly infect the digestive tract, but infections of almost all organ systems are documented. The microsporidia that cause human

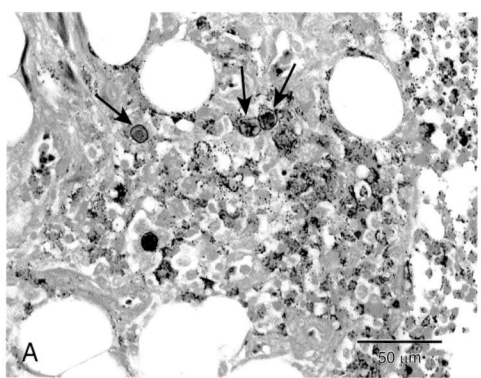
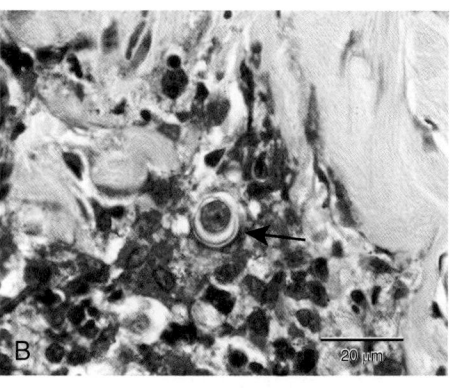

Figure 58.8 *Acanthamoeba*. (A) Silver stain showing *Acanthamoeba (arrow)*. (B) Periodic acid–Schiff stain showing the organism *(arrow)*. (A, From Zaiman H. A Pictorial Presentation of Parasites. https://www.astmh.org/education-resources/zaiman-slide-library. Courtesy American Society of Tropical Medicine and Hygiene. B, Courtesy Dr. Govinda S. Visvesvara.)

disease are zoonotic and/or water borne. *Enterocytozoon bieneusi* and *Encephalitozoon intestinalis* are the most common human pathogens, followed by *Encephalitozoon cuniculi* and *Encephalitozoon hellem*. In immunocompromised hosts, particularly in patients with advanced AIDS, these organisms have been associated with a diarrheal and chronic wasting syndrome. Other risk factors for infection include treatment with anti–tumor necrosis factor-α antibodies, chemotherapy, other immune-modulating drugs, and organ transplantation. Immune restoration by antiretroviral therapy has markedly reduced the incidence of microsporidiosis in HIV infection.[135]

Clinical Features. Involvement of the respiratory tract and the sinuses by microsporidia can cause rhinitis, sinusitis, and nasal polyposis.[167–173] Involvement of the lower respiratory tract has been observed in the setting of disseminated disease and presents as an interstitial pneumonitis. *E. hellem* infection has been reported to involve the entire length of the respiratory tract, with manifestations including erosive tracheitis and bronchiolitis. There are case reports of *E. cuniculi*, *E. hellem*, and *E. intestinalis* causing bronchiolitis with and without pneumonia. Respiratory tract infection due to *E. bieneusi* has also been reported.[174] *Tubulonosema acridophagus* infection with respiratory failure and pulmonary opacities has been described in which spores of the organism were recovered by BAL.[175]

Diagnosis and Treatment. Diagnosis of this infection can be made by finding microsporidian spores in clinical samples by microscopy; PCR-based molecular techniques are also available. Treatment depends on the species identified. In general, albendazole combined with immune reconstitution is the treatment of choice, although albendazole is not recommended for *E. bieneusi* or *Vittaforma corneae* infection due to intrinsic resistance.[135] Fumagillin, an agent with a broader anti-microsporidian activity, is another option.[176]

Trypanosomiasis

Trypanosoma cruzi is the cause of Chagas disease, which is found in areas of Mexico and in Central and South America.[177] It is transmitted by Triatominae bugs (e.g., bloodsucking insects also called kissing bugs) or by blood transfusion, organ transplantation, ingestion of contaminated food and fluids, or vertical transmission (mother to child). Babies born with congenital Chagas disease have a variety of manifestations including pneumonia and, in these cases, amastigotes have been reported in the lung.[178] Pneumonitis and acute pulmonary edema may be seen in acute Chagas disease. Congenital and acute disease are treated with either nifurtimox or benznidazole.[179]

Patients with chronic Chagasic cardiomyopathy may have congestive heart failure and thromboembolic events. Chronic Chagasic patients with megaesophagus may have a variety of pulmonary complications including aspiration pneumonia, bronchiectasis, and lung abscess.

Key Points

- Helminthic parasites often migrate through the lungs en route to another organ, particularly the gastrointestinal tract. Migration is often associated with eosinophilia or eosinophilic pneumonia.
- Tropical pulmonary eosinophilia is in the differential diagnosis of eosinophilic pneumonias, and should be considered in any patient from an endemic area of filarial infections and who presents with eosinophilia and pulmonary opacities.
- Paragonimiasis, echinococcosis, and dirofilariasis can be symptomatic or asymptomatic, and present as pulmonary nodules or mass lesions.
- Pulmonary paragonimiasis is commonly associated with hemoptysis. Because tuberculosis and paragonimiasis often coexist in the same geographic areas of the world, it is important to consider the diagnosis of paragonimiasis in a TB suspect and, if indicated, to examine the sputum and stools for ova and to perform a serologic test for this parasite.
- Schistosomiasis can cause pulmonary hypertension, usually after many years of untreated infection, which is thought to be due to deposition of eggs in pulmonary vessels, granuloma formation, and obstruction to blood flow.
- Strongyloidiasis is unique in that there is chronic infection with autoinfection that can result in a potentially lethal hyperinfection syndrome, particularly in patients given glucocorticoids.
- Protozoan parasites usually do not preferentially infect the lungs but, because many are highly prevalent in human populations, pulmonary disease may be seen, particularly as part of a disseminated infection.

IN MEMORIAM

This chapter is dedicated to Dr. Herbert B. Tanowitz, an exceptional physician and scientist, whose contributions significantly enhanced our understanding of parasitic infections and the pathophysiology of these important diseases.

Key Readings

Jourdan PM, Lamberton PHL, Fenwick A, Addiss DG. Soil-transmitted helminth infections. *Lancet.* 2018;391:252–265.

Krolewiecki A, Nutman TB. Strongyloidiasis: a neglected tropical disease. *Infect Dis Clin North Am.* 2019;33:135–151.

Martinez-Giron R, et al. Protozoa in respiratory pathology: a review. *Eur Respir J.* 2008;32(5):1354–1370.

Nabeya D, Haranaga S, Parrott GL, et al. Pulmonary strongyloidiasis: assessment between manifestation and radiological findings in 16 severe strongyloidiasis cases. *BMC Infect Dis.* 2017;17:320.

Stanley Jr SL. Amoebiasis. *Lancet.* 2003;361(9362):1025–1034.

Taylor WR, et al. Respiratory manifestations of malaria. *Chest.* 2012;142(2):492–502.

Complete reference list available at ExpertConsult.com.

59 OUTBREAKS, PANDEMICS, AND BIOTERRORISM

WILLIAM A. FISCHER II, MD • DAVID A. WOHL, MD •
DAVID J. WEBER, MD, MPH • NICOLE LURIE, MD, MSPH

INTRODUCTION	Reporting	Leadership
CLINICAL PRESENTATIONS	Supportive Care	Communication
Awareness and Recognition	Diagnostics	**PREPAREDNESS**
MANAGEMENT	Therapeutics	**KEY POINTS**
Infection Prevention and Control	**COORDINATION**	

INTRODUCTION

The U.S. *Centers for Disease Control and Prevention* (CDC) lists 27 bacteria, natural toxins, and viral families that are potential agents of bioterror; seven are listed as high priorities given their lethality, relative ease of production, hardiness, and suitability for airborne dissemination.[1] Intentional release of such agents is not hypothetical. In 2001, spores of anthrax were mailed to U.S. lawmakers and journalists. In total, 22 people contracted anthrax, five of whom died. Ricin, a toxin found in castor beans, was mailed in a similar attack on U.S. officials. In addition, naturally occurring outbreaks of known and novel pathogens have long been a feature of human existence but are now almost routine. Examples include the global influenza pandemic of the early twentieth century and the spread of human immunodeficiency virus from a small region of West Africa to all inhabited parts of the world. More recently, there have been recurrent outbreaks of viral hemorrhagic fevers, particularly Ebola; the resurgence of arthropod-borne infections such as Dengue, Chikungunya, and Zika; and ongoing outbreaks of measles, including in the United States. The ongoing pandemic of COVID-19, caused by *severe acute respiratory syndrome–associated coronavirus 2* (SARS-CoV-2), demonstrates the dramatic worldwide impact of a serious viral disease readily transmitted by the respiratory route. Whether naturally occurring or the result of a laboratory accident or deliberate attack, additional future outbreaks are increasingly likely given geopolitical and climate-related upheavals and the emergence of synthetic biology. Although the circumstances of an outbreak will vary, in any such event many of those affected will likely require intensive care, highlighting the unique and important roles for the pulmonary critical care clinician.

This chapter first reviews the major roles that the critical care clinician can expect to play during a consequential bioterrorism event or outbreak. Foremost, it is the clinician who may be among the first to notice unusual signs and symptoms or atypical manifestations of a disease process in the severely ill that signal suspicion of an outbreak. As the course of the public health emergency unfolds, the critical care physician may be called upon to play roles beyond that of the bedside clinician, such as adapting frameworks and triggers for patient triage when intensive care capacity is overwhelmed and when population-based critical care is needed; advising on allocation of scarce resources (e.g., ventilators, dialysis machines); supporting optimal infection prevention and control measures; and setting hospital policies and procedures. They may also be expected to participate in data collection efforts aimed at tracking and controlling the event, understanding the natural history of a disease, or developing and testing treatments. Finally, the involved intensivist is often a trusted source of information in crises and can be called upon to explain the situation to hospital staff or, through media, to the broader community. Responding to such events therefore requires not only clinical acumen, but also a readiness to act in a variety of ways that may be unfamiliar to the critical care clinician.

Next, major clinical syndromes that may signal a consequential event and their treatment are outlined. Although pandemic influenza is the infectious agent most likely to cause a worldwide crisis (see Chapter 47 for a full discussion of influenza), and the ongoing pandemic of COVID-19 (see Chapter 46a), which demonstrates the large impact of other respiratory viruses, this chapter focuses on the recognition of other dangerous pathogens that may be less familiar to most clinicians and the countermeasures available to prevent or treat them. Attacks involving chemicals, trauma, or nuclear weapons/radiation (see Chapters 103 and 104) are beyond the scope of this review, although there are commonalities in the critical care clinician's roles in response to biologic and nonbiologic catastrophic events.

CLINICAL PRESENTATIONS

AWARENESS AND RECOGNITION

Like a mass shooting, chemical attack, earthquake, or severe weather event, a novel virulent infection incident may first present without warning. More likely, however, an outbreak of a consequential pathogen, such as a novel influenza virus or the coronaviruses responsible for the SARS

Table 59.1   Clues of an Emerging Outbreak or Bioterror Attack

EPIDEMIOLOGIC CLUES

- A rapidly increasing disease incidence
- Unusual clustering of disease for the geographic area
- Disease outside of the normal transmission season
- Simultaneous outbreaks of different infectious diseases
- Disease outbreak in humans after recognition of disease in animals
- Unexplained number of dead animals or birds
- Disease requiring a transmission vector previously not seen in the area
- Rapid emergence of genetically identical pathogens from different geographic areas

MEDICAL CLUES

- Unusual route of infection
- Unusual age distribution or clinical presentation of common disease
- More severe disease and higher fatality rate than expected
- Unusual variants of organisms
- Unusual antimicrobial susceptibility patterns
- Uncommon disease with bioterrorism potential

and COVID-19, will emerge and spread more slowly, quietly smoldering before it is recognized. The clinical manifestations of some public health emergencies are pathognomonic, but particularly when an unexpected, highly communicable disease presents with syndromic symptoms only, the clinical diagnosis will not be immediately recognized.

While public health agencies continually monitor patterns of illness or health care utilization (especially emergency department visits and hospitalizations) for signals that could portend significant outbreaks, the astute clinician is often the first to recognize and report an unusual case or illness cluster (Table 59.1). The storied recognition of *Legionella pneumophilia* in 1976 is attributed to a Bloomsburg, Pennsylvania, physician who noted that three men under his care died unexpectedly in rapid succession shortly after attending a convention in Philadelphia.[2] One of the first men to die was presumed to have suffered a myocardial infarction and, even when scores became ill, swine flu was initially believed to be the culprit. The physician's report to state health authorities helped to trigger an investigation that ultimately resulted in the identification of the pathogen and its transmission via a hotel air conditioning system. Likewise, the 2001 anthrax attack was first suspected by a clinician who noted box-car shaped bacilli on a Gram stain from the cerebrospinal fluid of a patient who presented to the emergency department and rapidly deteriorated.[3] The 2015 Zika outbreak was initially recognized when a practicing obstetrician noted an unusual cluster of cases of neonatal microcephaly in northeastern Brazil.[4]

In each of these examples, observant clinicians noted suspicious patterns that led to the recognition of an emerging event. However, an awareness of emerging events can also help the clinician to recognize suspected cases. Growth in global travel coupled with decreases in flight times mean that within a day, a contagious traveler can be almost anywhere on the planet. Given this relatively recent connectivity of humanity, the critical care clinician needs to maintain a general awareness of major outbreaks developing around the world.

The necessity of such a perspective was dramatically highlighted during the 2014 to 2015 West Africa Ebola outbreak, when an asymptomatic man boarded a flight to the United States four days after helping transport a symptomatic pregnant woman to an Ebola treatment unit in Liberia.[5] He became ill after arriving in Texas, presenting to a health care facility with fever, abdominal pain, nausea, and headache. A travel history was not noted and, diagnosed with sinusitis, he was sent home with antibiotics. Only when his condition deteriorated and he returned to the emergency department was a travel history obtained, revealing his recent travel to Liberia during its raging Ebola outbreak. A diagnosis of Ebola virus disease was ultimately made late in the clinical course; the patient died, and two nurses involved in his care were infected. Alerts about emerging infections and outbreaks from trusted sources are readily available and can be subscribed to for automated email delivery. Electronic health records can be programmed to incorporate such alerts. Epidemiologic reports issued by state public health authorities should be reviewed regularly by all potential health care first responders, including intensivists, and relevant threats shared with staff.

Classical Syndromes and High-Consequence Pathogens

Central to the detection of any emerging outbreak or biologic threat is making a diagnosis. Illness caused by natural or human-produced threats can range in severity from mild to severe and present with subtle signs and symptoms that could be mistaken for routine illnesses. They can also present with highly unusual, often pathognomonic manifestations. Clusters of three common symptom complexes—typically accompanied by fever—should raise the suspicion of a potentially serious outbreak: rash, respiratory distress, and hemorrhage.

Dermatologic Syndromes

Rash accompanied by fever can be caused by a number of common infectious and noninfectious etiologies but, when the skin manifestations are atypical or when observed in a cluster of patients, they should raise concern about novel infections. Anthrax, tularemia, smallpox, measles, and a host of other potentially epidemic diseases can present foremost with skin lesions, but the pathognomonic presentation of each of these pathogens is different[1,6-9] (Fig. 59.1).

Skin lesions following exposure to anthrax are typically small and blister-like, often located in groups on the face, neck, or upper extremities. They are painless, with a central black eschar. Tularemia, caused by infection with the bacterium *Francisella tularensis*, can also cause an ulcerative skin lesion but one that is painful, with associated swelling of regional lymph nodes and high fever.

Although smallpox was eradicated in 1980, stocks of the virus exist in U.S. and Russian government laboratories, and there are concerns about its release as a bioterror agent or during a laboratory accident.[10] The viral exanthem associated with smallpox is a centrifugally spread vesicular rash with all lesions at the same stage of development appearing first in the mouth, then spreading to the face and the extremities followed by the trunk, palms, and soles. Over time the vesicles fill with fluid and grow before forming a

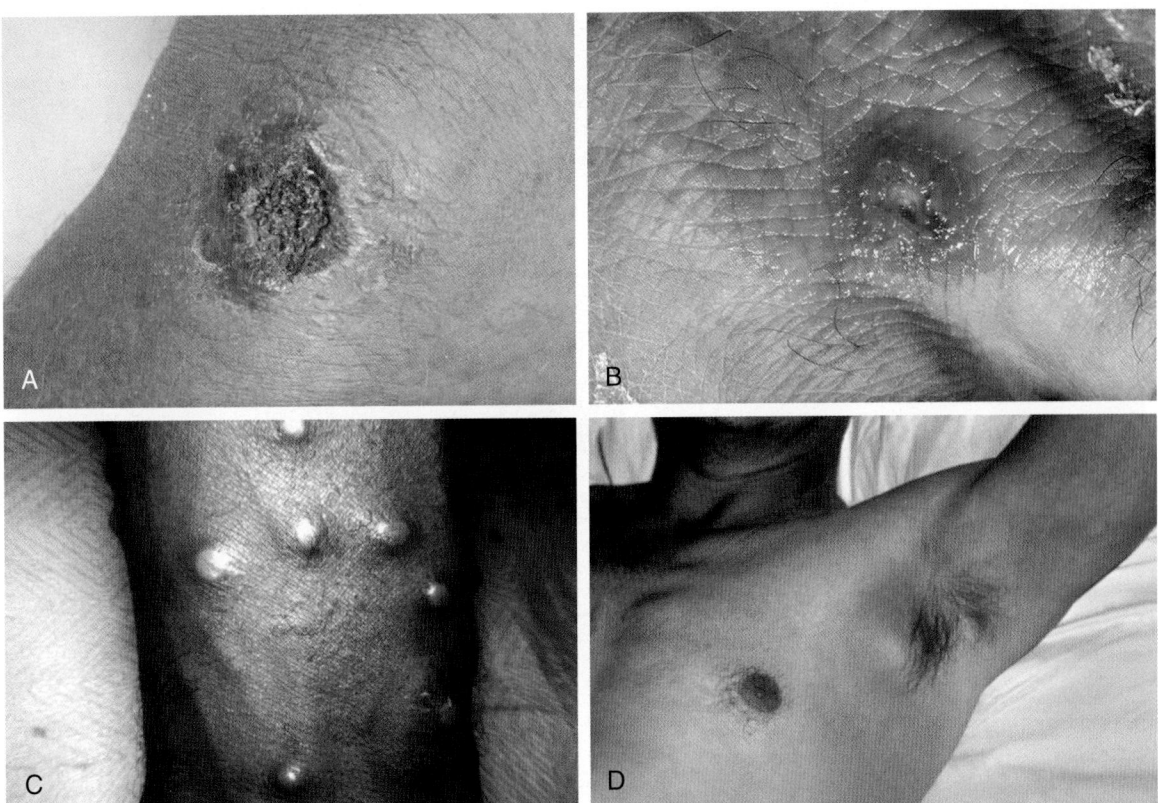

Figure 59.1 Anthrax, tularemia, smallpox, and plague. (A) The anthrax lesion on the skin of the forearm is caused by the bacterium *Bacillus anthracis*. The cutaneous ulceration has begun to turn black, hence the origin of the name "anthrax," after the Greek word for coal. (B) A tularemia lesion is shown on the dorsal skin of the right hand caused by the bacterium *Francisella tularensis*. (C) The maculopapular lesions on this patient's arm were caused by the smallpox virus, variola major. These lesions were in their pustular phase of development. (D) An axillary bubo and edema exhibited by a patient with plague. (Courtesy Centers for Disease Control and Prevention, Public Health Image Library. A, #2033, James H. Steele. B, #2032, Dr. Brachman. C, #10495, Dr. John Noble Jr. D, #2061, Margaret Parsons and Dr. Karl F. Meyer.)

crust and then a scab that eventually falls off. Again, fever accompanies the rash.

Measles (rubeola), noted here because of its preventable worldwide reemergence in 2019,[11] is associated with a morbilliform rash that initially appears on the face at the hairline and spreads downward to the neck, trunk, arms, legs, and feet, often described as centripetal spread. The presence of Koplik spots (small mouth lesions that appear like white grains of sand surrounded by a red ring, often on the buccal mucosa) and patchy erythema with central pallor on buccal mucosa should arouse a high level of clinical suspicion for measles, especially in the unvaccinated or under-vaccinated.

Pulmonary Syndromes

The pneumonic form of many high-consequence infections, including anthrax, plague, avian influenza, tularemia, and coronavirus-associated infections (e.g., SARS, Middle East respiratory syndrome, COVID-19), is clinically indistinguishable from the clinical presentation of pneumonia due to other bacterial and viral etiologies; thus clinical suspicion is driven by clustering or by exposure and travel history.[1]

Anthrax spores, considered by the CDC to be the most likely bioterror agent to be used in an attack,[12] can be inhaled and then germinate in the mediastinal lymph nodes, where released toxins cause hemorrhagic necrosis. Mediastinitis ensues, producing the classic widened mediastinum on chest imaging, sometimes with necrotizing pneumonia

(Fig. 59.2). The course is biphasic; prodromal symptoms are nonspecific and can easily be mistaken for influenza. Nausea, odynophagia, chest pain, and hemoptysis are distinguishing features of the presentation that should raise suspicion for a diagnosis other than influenza. Unrecognized and untreated, the respiratory status deteriorates to a fulminant phase that is typically fatal even if antibacterial therapy is initiated. Monoclonal antibodies to the anthrax lethal toxin have been approved by the U.S. *Food and Drug Administration* (FDA) for treatment of inhalational anthrax (see later).

Pneumonic plague, caused by *Yersinia pestis*, can arise naturally but, like anthrax, is rare in the United States.[13] It is a rapidly progressive illness that begins acutely and is often fatal if antibacterial therapy is not instituted on the first day. The tempo of the illness and often the presence of hemoptysis may be clues, along with any that are epidemiologic, such as travel to an endemic area, such as the southwest United States, or clustering of similar cases.

Hemorrhagic Fevers

Viral hemorrhagic fevers (VHFs), including Ebola virus disease, Marburg virus disease, and Lassa fever, often present with nonspecific symptoms that evolve into a sepsis phenotype that is difficult to distinguish from other sepsis etiologies.[14-17] Despite their being labeled hemorrhagic, most patients infected with these viruses do not have evidence of significant bleeding. However, the recent outbreaks of Ebola in West Africa and the Democratic Republic

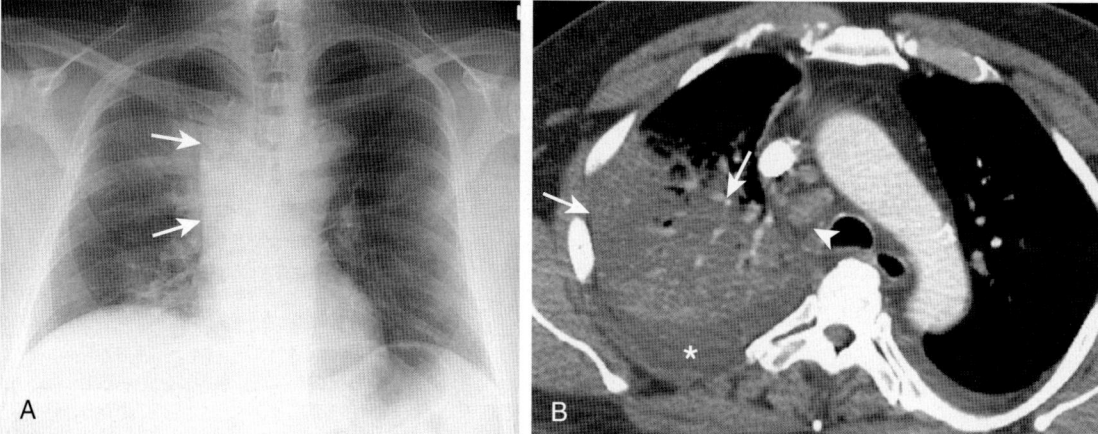

Figure 59.2 Imaging findings in inhalation anthrax: chest radiography. (A) Frontal chest radiograph in a 61-year-old man with a 3-day history of productive cough, fever, and exertional dyspnea shows poorly defined medial right upper lobe ground-glass opacity associated with a markedly widened right mediastinum (*arrows*). During recent travel through parks in the western United States, he had been exposed to animal antlers and hides, wild bison, and donkeys. (B) Axial enhanced chest computed tomography scan displayed in soft tissue windows shows right upper lobe consolidation (*arrows*) and a small right pleural effusion (*asterisk*) and trace left pleural liquid associated with right paratracheal lymphadenopathy (*arrowhead*). *Bacillus anthracis* was isolated from blood culture. (Courtesy Mark D. Sprenkle, MD, Pulmonary and Critical Care Medicine, Hennepin County Medical Center, Minneapolis, MN. From Sprenkle MD, Griffith J, Marinelli W, et. Al. Lethal factor and anti-protective antigen IgG levels associated with inhalation anthrax, Minnesota, USA. *Emerg Infect Dis.* 2014;20:310–314.)

of the Congo have sensitized many clinicians to the hemorrhagic manifestations of VHFs and, in endemic areas, gastrointestinal bleeding or continued ooze from venipuncture sites can trigger concern for a VHF. In those with advanced VHFs, petechiae, ecchymosis, and gastrointestinal and vaginal bleeding can accompany late stages of the disease.

Other Syndromes

Outbreak pathogens can present in myriad ways in addition to the most common syndromes noted earlier.[1] Botulism, for instance, produced by the toxin of *Clostridium botulinum* bacteria, produces profound neurologic symptoms starting with bilateral cranial neuropathies and symmetrical descending weakness in the absence of fever. Patients are responsive with slow to normal heart rates, are normotensive, and have no sensory deficits other than blurred vision. Ricin toxin, in contrast, can produce less-specific symptomatology that can be predominantly pulmonary or gastrointestinal depending on the route of exposure.

MANAGEMENT

INFECTION PREVENTION AND CONTROL

When a suspected outbreak or exposure is identified, immediately implementing infection prevention and control procedures (including isolation of the patient, use of appropriate personal protective equipment) and informing local health authorities are paramount.

The critical care clinician, along with the hospital infection prevention team, has an obligation to ensure that staff and unaffected patients are protected from exposure. Therefore, appropriate infection prevention measures should be implemented as soon as a potentially transmissible disease is suspected, even before a diagnosis is confirmed. Such procedures are routine in hospital settings, such as in the case of suspected tuberculosis, *Clostridioides difficile* colitis, or varicella. The type of isolation followed (e.g., respiratory, droplet, contact) and protective equipment

used depends on the nature of the transmission of the suspected or confirmed pathogen. Hospital infection prevention staff should be involved immediately so that protective approaches can be coordinated in all areas and for all staff of potential relevance (i.e., laboratories, radiology). While the critical care clinician will likely not be responsible for implementing infection and control procedures, all clinicians should recognize that infection prevention involves much more than use of personal protective equipment, be familiar with the tiered nature of infection control practices, and advocate for their full implementation in their institutions.

For pathogens for which there are preventive vaccines, it is also important to incorporate immunization into response plans. Vaccination for routine infections like influenza may need to be augmented to include pathogens with a potential to become epidemic or be used as biologic weapons. First responders and health care personnel are priority groups for vaccination during influenza and coronavirus pandemics to reduce the likelihood that they themselves would become ill and to reduce transmission to other patients and staff. Licensed vaccines are available to prevent anthrax and smallpox, and health care personnel would likely be prioritized to receive vaccination in the setting of an emergency involving one of these pathogens. Vaccines for other consequential pathogens such as Q fever, agents of viral encephalitis, and Ebola Zaire may be available from the CDC.

REPORTING

Each state has requirements for the reporting of certain pathogens, and these policies need to be followed to ensure centralized data collection and epidemiologic surveillance. Clearly, not all biologic threats are included on lists of reportable pathogens; therefore, critical care clinicians should work with hospital infection control staff to communicate suspicions regarding a pathogen of consequence to health authorities, who in turn may alert federal public health entities. In the United States, state health departments as well as the CDC are available every hour of every day of the year. For many infectious and noninfectious public health threats, specialized testing of biospecimens and/or environmental samples may be available only at state or national public health laboratories.

SUPPORTIVE CARE

Because the precise etiology of disease may not be immediately apparent, supportive care represents the foundation of patient management. Effective supportive care involves close patient monitoring with frequent clinical assessments and intervention as needed; intravenous and oral fluid resuscitation accompanied by monitoring and correction of metabolic, glycemic, and electrolyte abnormalities; identification and treatment of coinfections and comorbidities; management of advanced organ-supportive care such as renal replacement therapy and mechanical ventilation; and the support for essential organ function until either the body's endogenous immune response or pathogen-specific therapy can control the infection.

Data from the West African Ebola outbreak highlight the value of supportive care even in the setting of this progressive and highly lethal VHF.[15,18] Among the 27 expatriate patients transported back to the United States or Europe, the case fatality rate was 19% compared to over 60% for those managed in West Africa. Investigational therapeutics were administered to most of the repatriated patients, but it was the advanced supportive care, including laboratory monitoring, fluid resuscitation, and mechanical organ function support, that is considered to have been most consequential.[18]

Important considerations during the management of any serious systemic illness are sepsis, septic shock, and *acute respiratory distress syndrome* (ARDS); often these are the final common pathways for infections with high-consequence pathogens. For example, sepsis has been recognized as a cause of rapid deterioration in patients with Ebola virus disease, and bacterial pneumonia with methicillin-resistant *Staphylococcus aureus* is a common complication of ARDS, including from pandemic influenza.[19,20] Patients with these diseases experience better rates of survival when cared for in centers with more resources, lower provider-to-patient ratios, and greater clinical experience.[21] For diseases of outbreak potential, the rapid recognition of both the source of infection and the severity of illness will also help to reduce community and nosocomial transmission through the transfer of that patient to a designated area prepared for high-consequence or highly transmissible pathogens.

The Surviving Sepsis campaign has prioritized the use of *Quick Sepsis-Related Organ Failure Assessment* (qSOFA) scoring using altered mental status (Glasgow Coma Scale score of <15), respiratory rate (≥22 breaths/min), and hypotension (systolic blood pressure ≤100 mm Hg) to identify patients with sepsis rapidly in order to institute lifesaving supportive care.[22,22a] The Surviving Sepsis Hour-1 bundle targets the measurement of serum lactate and the collection of blood cultures prior to initiation of antibiotics. The administration of broad-spectrum antibiotics, initiation of intravenous crystalloid resuscitation for mean arterial pressures less than 65 mm Hg or a lactate level greater than 4 mmol/L, and infusion of vasopressors in the presence of hypotension during or after fluid resuscitation are considered key interventions to reduce sepsis and septic shock–associated morbidity and mortality.

Anthrax, tularemia, plague, avian or pandemic influenza, Middle East respiratory syndrome, SARS, and COVID-19 can all present with pneumonia-associated respiratory failure.[1] In the absence of controlled studies demonstrating the efficacy of one supportive intervention over another, the management of these illnesses follows recommendations created for ARDS. Data from the ARDS literature suggest improved mortality with the use of low tidal volume ventilation; conservative fluid management once there is no evidence of shock for 12 hours; avoidance of high-dose systemic corticosteroids in the context of most viral pneumonias unless needed for adrenal insufficiency, refractory hypotension, or obstructive lung disease; prone ventilation for severe ARDS; and the consideration of extracorporeal membrane oxygenation in the setting of refractory hypoxia.[23,24] A notable exception to the avoidance of corticosteroids is in the management of COVID-19, because administration of dexamethasone has been shown to provide a survival advantage to patients who require oxygen, with or without mechanical ventilation.[24a] Current guidelines recommend targeting lower tidal volumes of 4 to 8 mL/kg per breath calculated using predicted body weight to reduce volutrauma, targeting a lower plateau pressure of less than 30 cm H_2O to limit barotrauma, and the use of prone positioning for at least 12 hours a day in patients with severe ARDS (PaO_2/FIO_2 ratio <100 mm Hg).[25]

DIAGNOSTICS

Appropriate diagnostic tests should be directed by clinical presentations, physical exam findings, and epidemiologic links. Appropriate specimens (e.g., plasma, serum, upper and lower respiratory secretions, cerebrospinal fluid, skin lesion swabs) should be collected early and empiric treatment begun, pending laboratory analyses. Stains and cultures of blood or involved tissues or fluids can confirm the diagnosis of some bacterial pathogens of outbreak potential, including anthrax, botulism, pneumonic plague, and tularemia. Molecular techniques are increasingly able to detect consequential viruses rapidly, including SARS-CoV-2, many VHFs, and smallpox. Fluorescent antibody testing can also play a role, such as for the diagnosis of tularemia.

Coordination with state health officials and the CDC can facilitate the transfer of appropriate samples to state or regional reference labs for relevant diagnostic testing. At present, each U.S. state public health laboratory has the ability to respond to a biologic terrorism emergency, either individually or through a regional reference lab.[26] Laboratories (state or local) should be made aware when highly communicable pathogens are being considered in the differential diagnosis so that protective measures can be implemented to safeguard laboratory staff.

THERAPEUTICS

Direct treatment of an outbreak pathogen, when available, is often administered empirically given the severity of the disease on presentation and potential delays in confirmation of the diagnosis. For bacterial pathogens such as anthrax, tularemia, and plague, antibacterials with activity against these infections exist (Table 59.2).[1,26] Antitoxins can be used to neutralize toxins associated with anthrax, botulism, and ricin.[27] Immune globulin directed against botulinum

Table 59.2 Clinical Features and Management of Biothreat Agents

Disease	Signs and Symptoms	Incubation Time (Range)	Person-to-Person Transmission	Isolation	Diagnosis*	Postexposure Prophylaxis	Treatment†
Anthrax (*Bacillus anthracis*)							
Inhalation	Flu-like symptoms including fever and chills, shortness of breath, cough, sweats, fatigue, and myalgias. May also have confusion, headache, nausea, vomiting or stomach pain	1–43 days (range, up to 60 days)	None	Standard	CXR with widened mediastinum; cultures of sputum and blood	Antibiotics, vaccine	Antibiotics, antitoxin
Cutaneous	Initially a group of small blisters or bumps that may itch. Swelling may develop around the sore; blisters develop into a painless skin sore (ulcer) with a necrotic (black) center; lesions most commonly on face, neck, arms, or hands	5–7 days (range, 1–12 days)	Rarely	Contact	Cultures of blood and lesion (swab)		
Gastrointestinal	Fever and chills, lymphadenopathy (neck), pharyngitis, dysphagia, nausea and vomiting (may be bloody), diarrhea, headache, abdominal pain, and flushing and conjunctivitis	1–6 days	None	Standard	Cultures of blood and stool		
Botulism (*Clostridium botulinum* toxin) via inhalation	Double or blurred vision, ptosis, dysarthria, dysphagia, dysphonia, shortness of breath, dry mouth, muscle weakness; ascending flaccid paralysis. Suggested by absence of fever, symmetrical neurologic deficits, patient responsive, normal or slow heart rate with normal blood pressure, and no sensory deficits with exception of blurred vision	12–72 hours (2 hours to 8 days)	None	Standard	Presumptive based on clinical findings. Identification of toxin in serum, stool, or vomitus. Culture of stool, wound, or food source	None	Antitoxin, botulinum immune globulin
Pneumonic plague (*Yersinia pestis*)	Fever, headache, weakness, and a rapidly developing pneumonia with shortness of breath, chest pain, cough, and sometimes bloody or watery mucus. Septicemic plague may develop	1–4 days	Via respiratory droplets	Droplet	Cultures of blood (usually positive), sputum, bronchial washings	Antibiotics	Antibiotics

Table 59.2 Clinical Features and Management of Biothreat Agents—cont'd

Disease	Signs and Symptoms	Incubation Time (Range)	Person-to-Person Transmission	Isolation	Diagnosis*	Postexposure Prophylaxis	Treatment†
Smallpox (Variola)	Initial stage (2–4 days): high fever, prostration, myalgias, vomiting Rash: starts as small red spots on tongue and in mouth, changes to sores that rupture, then rash on face that spreads to arms and legs, and then to hands and feet	10–14 days (range, 7–19 days)	Via airborne spread	Contact, airborne (special precautions required)†	PCR of clinical specimens (i.e., skin lesions, NP swab, blood), isolation of small virus, serology**	Vaccine	Vaccine, tecovirimat
Pneumonic tularemia (*Francisella tularensis*)	Cough, chest pain, shortness of breath	3–5 days (range, 1–14 days)	None	Standard	Culture of skin lesions (swab or scrapings), lymph node (aspirate or biopsy), pharynx (swab), or sputum	Antibiotics	Antibiotics
VHF§: Ebola virus	Fever, severe headache, myalgias, weakness, fatigue, diarrhea, vomiting, abdominal pain, unexplained hemorrhage (bleeding or bruising)	8–10 days (range, 2–21 days)	Via direct or indirect contact	Contact (special precautions required)†	PCR of clinical specimens (blood)**	Vaccine‡	Supportive, monoclonal antibodies for Ebola Zaire
VHF§: Marburg	Sudden onset of fever, chills, headache, myalgias Around fifth day after onset of symptoms, maculopapular rash on trunk; then nausea, vomiting, chest pain, pharyngitis, abdominal pain, diarrhea May progress with jaundice, delirium, shock, liver failure, massive hemorrhage, and multiorgan dysfunction	5–10 days	Via direct or indirect contact	Contact (special precautions required)†	PCR of blood or tissue, ELISA and IgM-capture ELISA**	None	Supportive
VHF§: Lassa	Mild disease: slight fever, malaise, weakness and headache Serious disease: hemorrhage (gums, eyes, nose), respiratory distress, vomiting, pain in chest and abdomen, and shock	6–21 days	Via direct or indirect contact	Contact (special precautions required)†	ELISA (IgM, IgG), RT-PCR of clinical specimens, viral culture**	Antivirals	Ribavirin

*Always alert lab before sending specimens for diagnosis.
†Consult infectious disease physician, infection prevention personnel, health department; review current guidelines (e.g., CDC, WHO).
‡Investigational (contact state health department, Food and Drug Administration).
§Other viral hemorrhagic fevers could be used as a biothreat agent and present with similar findings such as Junin (Argentine hemorrhagic fever) and Machupo virus (Bolivian hemorrhagic fever).
¶Alert lab if patient has meningeal symptoms; obtain spinal fluid culture.
**Alert lab, Public Health Department, and CDC as soon as diagnosis suspected.
CXR, chest radiograph; CDC, Centers for Disease Control and Prevention; ELISA, enzyme-linked immunosorbent assay; NP, nasopharyngeal; PCR, polymerase chain reaction; VHF, viral hemorrhagic fever; WHO, World Health Organization.
Modified from Centers for Disease Control and Prevention. Control of Communicable Diseases Manual, 20th edition, 2015.

toxin is also available, and two monoclonal antibodies that neutralize *Bacillus anthracis* toxin, raxibacumab and obiltoxaximab, are approved by the FDA for the prevention and treatment of inhalational anthrax.[28] Viral infections present a greater therapeutic challenge because there are fewer antivirals available and most have not been tested against these rarer pathogens. For smallpox, tecovirimat is FDA approved based on studies in nonhuman primates but is available only via the U.S. Government's Strategic National Stockpile.[29] Ribavirin is routinely used to treat Lassa fever, although its efficacy is questionable. Two monoclonal antibody products have recently shown promise for treating Ebola Zaire,[30] and monoclonal antibodies are in clinical trials for SARS-CoV-2.

Chemoprophylaxis may also play a role in an outbreak. Antimicrobials can be administered to prevent disease in those potentially exposed to anthrax, plague, tularemia, brucellosis, and Q fever.[26] Oseltamivir prophylaxis is a part of almost every pandemic influenza plan, although it will be important to establish that the virus is susceptible to the drug.

COORDINATION

LEADERSHIP

Critical care clinicians may be looked to not only for the medical management of individual patients but also for leadership of the response within a facility or health care network. As the steward of the units where intensive care is delivered, the critical care clinician will almost always need to supervise the coordination of the intensive care unit response, including triage, staffing, resource management and supplies, and care plans. Although many critical care clinicians have worked in hospitals that have experienced shortages of intravenous fluids or essential medicines, an outbreak can present a much graver situation. While most will be involved in bedside care, their duty to care for an individual patient may conflict with the need to provide population-based care, including allocation of scarce resources. The National Academy of Medicine has promoted guidelines for avoiding such situations and recommends that triage and allocation decisions be made by experts not directly involved in bedside care.[31]

Working with infection prevention experts, the critical care clinician will also implement policies to reduce intrafacility transmission of infection or contamination. Depending on the scale of an event, the clinician may also work to coordinate with counterparts at other medical centers such as those nearby or where special expertise or resources are located. In the United States, almost all hospitals have an incident command system and participate in local or regional health care coalitions, and the critical care clinician must be prepared to be part of such a system, because it will be responsible for handling the crisis.

COMMUNICATION

Epidemics of infectious diseases are often accompanied by secondary epidemics of fear. Communication among health care providers and patients, patients' family members, and affected communities ensures that sound scientific advice is shared and disseminated and that rumors do not interfere with the rapid identification, isolation, and initiation of care for suspect and confirmed patients. Delays in identification, isolation, and care of severe progressive infections can have profound effects on outcomes and may also perpetuate community transmission. Community engagement and communication strategies, when effective, can crowdsource surveillance efforts that will ultimately accelerate the identification, isolation, and initiation of care for suspect patients.

By being directly involved in the care of affected patients, the critical care clinician may also be asked to serve as a public face for communications with other patients in the hospital as well as with the media and the public. Updates on the status of affected patients, on system responses to meet treatment and infection control needs, and on the event itself may fall to the critical care clinician. Coordination of messaging with other stakeholders inside and outside of the facility, such as emergency department providers and other clinicians (including those in neighboring facilities), infection prevention staff, public health authorities, community leaders, elected officials, and security (police, military), will be critical, albeit often difficult in the dynamic situation of such events. Clarity regarding communications with the public should be established early through the local public information officer, followed closely, and revised as necessary by those leading the response.

PREPAREDNESS

The best response is built on strong day-to-day systems and begins prior to an outbreak with preparedness. Because the critical care clinician is often at the front line of care in a public health emergency, he or she will want to ensure that the hospital, as well as other facilities in the community, is fully prepared for such an event. Although outbreaks and other consequential public health events typically appear with little or no warning, measures can be taken to prepare for such emergencies by developing relevant procedures and policies, conducting training and drills, and stocking supplies, equipment, and medications. Crucial aspects of preparedness include rostering of essential staff, establishing a safe and effective health care structure, optimizing systems such as predeveloped care protocols and checklists, ensuring adequate infection prevention and control and biosecurity, and knowing other facility plans, as outlined in Table 59.3.

The critical care clinician has a stake in the development of hospital policy for determining who will and will not be expected to care for infected patients. In the setting of an outbreak, there may be a need for surge capacity to attend to a growing number of suspected and confirmed cases, all the while maintaining routine medical care to others to the extent possible. At the same time, health care providers and/or their family members may become ill and therefore may be unavailable. In addition, restrictions regarding who is eligible to be part of the care team

Table 59.3   Preparedness for Managing a Highly Communicable Emerging Infectious Disease

GENERAL

- Ensure the facility has a comprehensive plan for managing a highly communicable emerging infectious disease. This should be contained within the general disaster plan.
- Base the plan on the route(s) of transmission for the infectious agent.
- Learn the basics of the hospital incident command structure and ensure it is part of the plan.
- Periodically train key personnel on the plan.
- Ensure plan includes care of single patients (e.g., Ebola) as well as management of a large number of patients in an epidemic (e.g., novel influenza).
- Incorporate communications with local and state health department officials.
- Develop a plan for prophylaxis of health care workers and facility staff.
- Develop a plan with neighboring health care facilities, ideally through a regional health care coalition, to coordinate patient distribution for highly pathogenic respiratory viruses and other highly transmissible infections when tertiary care facilities or designated facilities are not available.

SCREENING AND SIGNAGE (WHEN APPROPRIATE BASED ON THE THREAT OF A HIGHLY COMMUNICABLE DISEASE)

- Place signs at every entrance to the hospital and clinics that include the following: epidemiologic clues to possible disease exposure (i.e., travel locations), signs and symptoms of infection, and whom to notify if the patient or visitor has both exposure and appropriate signs and/or symptoms.
- Include messaging about the signs and symptoms of the concerning disease in all telephone contacts with the patient (e.g., reminders about appointments) and who to contact prior to arrival at the health care facility.
- Screen all patients immediately at the time of all health care visits.
- Include screening in the electronic medical record (also have alerts in the medical record that require screening).
- Place an appropriate isolation sign on the door of all patients being isolated due to the possibility of a highly communicable disease.
- Emphasize respiratory hygiene for diseases transmitted via the droplet or airborne routes (i.e., immediate use of a mask and proper disposal of tissues) as well as proper hand hygiene.
- Ensure all messaging is in appropriate languages for the region.

TRIAGE

- Train front-line personnel in all clinics and the emergency department in appropriate use of personal protective equipment.
- Identify and make appropriate personal protective equipment available. Use dedicated equipment during the patient evaluation.
- Have a designated location in the emergency department and all clinics in which to place the patient (a private room; ideally with access to a sink and toilet and, if possible, one that meets standards for a disease transmitted by the airborne route [i.e., negative pressure, out exhausted air, >12 air exchanges per hour]) if applicable. For diseases transmitted by the airborne route and when an airborne isolation room is not available, ideally place a portable high-efficiency particulate air machine in the room.
- Have a well-defined process for alerting key health care facility officials about the presence of a patient with a possible highly communicable disease (e.g., disaster manager, infection control preventionist).
- Avoid blood tests or other procedures that may place the laboratory staff or other health care personnel at risk.
- Have a well-defined and safe method for transporting a patient either to a properly equipped emergency department or to a hospital facility able to care for a patient safely.

INPATIENT CARE

- Have a well-defined plan for the inpatient location that will provide care to a patient with a highly communicable disease (or a plan for transporting such a patient to facility that can provide such care).
- Designate areas that are "hot" (i.e., potentially contaminated) and "cold" (i.e., areas that are not contaminated), and monitor compliance with that designation as appropriate.
- Develop appropriate staffing models based on the infectious agent and anticipated patient acuity.
- Have a preidentified, multidisciplinary, and well-trained medical care team. For highly communicable diseases (e.g., Lassa, Ebola), ideally provide three-step training: (1) Individual training, including demonstration of competencies, on personal protective equipment donning and doffing (including how to manage contamination of the environment from a spill and a breach of the personal protective equipment). Such training should be individualized to the specialty of the health care providers (i.e., physician, nurse, respiratory therapist, etc.). (2) Team training using mannequins. (3) Team training in the designated containment unit.
- Train team personnel on donning and doffing using an explicit written list of all donning and doffing steps.
- Screen and exclude health care personnel unable to wear the proper personal protective equipment. Consider excluding from the care team personnel at high risk for disease acquisition and/or more severe illness such as persons with nonintact skin, pregnancy, and immunocompromise. Consider excluding trainees from providing care.
- Store an adequate supply of personal protective equipment.
- Have dedicated point of care laboratory equipment.
- Develop a method to dispose of solid and liquid wastes safely.
- Restrict visitors (if indicated) and maintain a log for all visitors.
- Maintain a log of all health care personnel providing care.
- Develop a plan for monitoring symptoms among health care workers providing care.
- Develop a plan for managing health care personnel with unprotected exposure to the infectious agent (e.g., needlestick).
- Develop a plan for decedent management.
- Ensure that care team members receive proper rest and psychological first aid as needed.
- Develop specific protocols for special populations, such as pediatric and obstetric patients.

should be considered, such as exclusion of pregnant care providers or less-experienced staff (e.g., medical and nursing students, physicians in training such as residents). Critical care clinicians supervising intensive care units may be expected to care for patients with highly communicable diseases; arguably there is a duty to care for such

patients. However, for other staff, participation in the care of patients with serious communicable infections may be considered voluntary. Steps to ensure a safe care environment and to address fear among staff and their families are essential. In some centers, clinical staff, including physicians, nurses, respiratory therapists, and others, may volunteer as first-line providers; a roster of those willing to care for such patients can facilitate adequate staffing. The critical care clinician will also want to ensure that staffing is available to provide laboratory and radiologic and other services, including environmental services and security. Being involved in the establishment of plans and criteria before an outbreak situation is preferable to developing these during an evolving crisis.

Key Points

- A novel infectious agent, whether related to an emerging infectious disease or to bioterrorism, can present without warning.
- Early recognition of an emerging infection or a bioterrorism agent almost always relies on the astute clinician.
- High-consequence pathogens may present with signs and symptoms that may be mistaken for other illnesses. Clusters of common symptom complexes should raise the suspicion of a potentially serious outbreak: fever, rash, respiratory distress, and hemorrhage.
- In addition to providing clinical care, the critical care clinician may be expected, and should thus be prepared, to play other roles in the hospital or community, including provision of population-based critical care.
- Hospital infection prevention and control staff and public health authorities should be alerted immediately if a novel infectious disease or bioterror agent is suspected, in order to protect other patients, health care workers, and the community.
- Aggressive supportive care, including frequent monitoring, fluid management, and early recognition and treatment of sepsis and acute respiratory distress syndrome, are the mainstays of critical care.
- Licensed vaccines and/or therapeutics are now available to prevent and treat key bioterror agents, including smallpox, anthrax, botulism, plague, and tularemia. Approved vaccines and therapeutics for Ebola Zaire are available, and clinical trials are ongoing for COVID-19 vaccines and therapeutics, many of which have received Emergency Use Authorization by the U.S. Federal Drug Administration at the time of this printing.

Key Readings

Adalja AA, Toner E, Inglesby TV. Clinical management of potential bioterrorism-related conditions. *N Engl J Med.* 2015;372:954.

Feldmann H, Sprecher A, Geisbert TW. Ebola. *N Engl J Med.* 2020;382(19):1832–1842.

Heymann DL. *Control of Communicable Diseases Manual.* 20th ed. Washington, DC: American Public Health Association; 2015.

Hunt L, Gupta-Wright A, Simms V, et al. Clinical presentation, biochemical, and haematological parameters and their association with outcome in patients with Ebola virus disease: an observational cohort study. *Lancet Infect Dis.* 2015;15:1292.

Moss WJ. Measles. *Lancet.* 2017;390:2490.

Mulangu S, Dodd LE, Davey RT Jr, et al. A randomized, controlled trial of Ebola virus disease therapeutics. *N Engl J Med.* 2019;381(24):2293–2303.

Prentice MB, Rahalison L. Plague. *Lancet.* 2007;369:1196.

Society of Critical Care Medicine. Surviving sepsis campaign. https://www.sccm.org/SurvivingSepsisCampaign/Home.

U.S. Centers for Disease Control and Prevention. Anthrax: the threat. https://www.cdc.gov/anthrax/bioterrorism/threat.html.

U.S. Centers for Disease Control and Prevention. Bioterrorism agents/diseases. https://emergency.cdc.gov/agent/agentlist-category.asp.

Uyeki TM, Mehta AK, Davey Jr RT, Working Group of the U.S.–European Clinical Network on Clinical Management of Ebola Virus Disease Patients in the U.S. and Europe, et al. Clinical management of Ebola virus disease in the United States and Europe. *N Engl J Med.* 2016;374(7):636–646.

World Health Organization. Clinical management of severe acute respiratory infection when Middle East Respiratory Syndrome Coronavirus (MERS-CoV) infection is suspected: interim guidance. https://www.who.int/csr/disease/coronavirus_infections/case-management-ipc/en/.

Complete reference list available at ExpertConsult.com.

OBSTRUCTIVE DISEASES

ASTHMA: PATHOGENESIS AND PHENOTYPES

60

PRESCOTT G. WOODRUFF, MD, MPH • NIRAV R. BHAKTA, MD, PHD •
VICTOR ENRIQUE ORTEGA, MD, PHD • BART N. LAMBRECHT, MD, PHD •
JOHN V. FAHY, MD, MSC

INTRODUCTION

Asthma is a common disease with a prevalence that has increased throughout the world for several decades. Studies of the epidemiology, natural history, and pathogenesis have clearly demonstrated that asthma is a heterogeneous disease, with multiple etiologies and contributing cofactors, complex pathobiologic mechanisms, and diverse molecular phenotypes. Understanding these differences is critically important for developing therapeutic strategies that will be effective for the various phenotypes of asthma.

EPIDEMIOLOGY

PREVALENCE

In the United States, the overall prevalence of asthma has risen since 1980, even after accounting for changes in the definition of current asthma in National Health Interview Survey questionnaires (Fig. 60.1). In 2017 (the most recent data), the overall current prevalence of asthma in the United States was 7.9%. There are marked and persistent differences in asthma prevalence across specific subgroups of the U.S.

population, making asthma extremely common in certain vulnerable populations (Fig. 60.2). In 2017, current asthma prevalence was very high in Black non-Hispanics (10.6%), those of Puerto Rican heritage (12.8%), and among those living below the poverty threshold (11.7%). Current asthma prevalence was higher in children (age <18 years; 8.4%) than adults (age 18+ years; 7.7%) and was higher among females (9.3%) than males (6.4%) overall, although the female/male balance changes with age so that asthma is less common in females than males during childhood (<18 years, 7.3% vs. 9.5%, respectively) but more common in females than males during adulthood (≥18+ years, 9.8% vs. 5.4%, respectively). These imbalances in prevalence between women and men, adults and children, ethnic groups, and across poverty levels have not changed since 2001.

The global burden of asthma in 2017–18 was assessed by the Global Asthma Network in 135 countries using standardized methods (similar to the International Study of Asthma and Allergies in Childhood study). They found that asthma affects approximately 339 million people, causes approximately 1000 deaths per day, and is in the top 20 causes of years of life with disability.[1] As in the United States, the international prevalence has increased over time,[2] although this increase may have plateaued in some high-income countries.[3] Two large multinational studies have systematically assessed the worldwide prevalence of asthma: the European Community Respiratory Health Survey in adults[4] and the *International Study of Asthma and Allergies in Childhood in Children* [ISAAC].[5] ISAAC phase I studied 156 centers in 56 countries cross-sectionally during the period 1992–96[6,7] and confirmed the great geographic variability in asthma prevalence inferred from prior smaller studies. However, it also found that some low- and middle-income countries had a prevalence of asthma symptoms similar to those in western, developed countries. Thus, the geographic trends are not absolute.

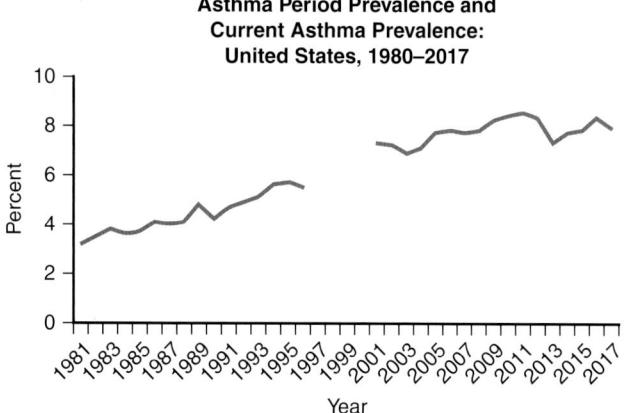

Figure 60.1 **Prevalence of current asthma in the United States.** Data are based on the National Health Interview Survey over two periods that used different case definitions (1980–96 and 2001–17). (Data from the U.S. Centers for Disease Control and Prevention, https://www.cdc.gov/asthma/asthma_stats/default.htm, compiled Aug 26, 2019.)

ISAAC confirmed the overall increase in asthma prevalence from phase I (1992–96) to phase III (2000–03). However, these time trends in asthma symptom prevalence showed different regional patterns.[8] With the exception of India, all of the countries with very low symptom prevalence rates at first evaluation reported increases in prevalence. However, in English-speaking, developed countries, in which asthma prevalence was already high, there was little further increase. The *European Community Respiratory Health Survey* (ECRHS) studied representative samples of 20- to 44-year-old men and women in 48 centers, predominantly in Western Europe.[9] Although ECRHS included data from fewer countries than ISAAC, there was relatively good agreement between ISAAC and ECHRS with respect to the prevalence of asthma symptoms across the 17 countries that both studies sampled.[10]

MORTALITY

Although death from asthma was once thought to be uncommon,[11] data from the World Health Organization in 2007 suggested that there are 250,000 asthma-related deaths each year worldwide.[12] The countries with the highest death rates in the World Health Association report were not necessarily those with the highest prevalence, suggesting that poor access to care and medications are contributing factors to mortality. In specific instances, asthma medications may have contributed to increased mortality. For example, there was an abrupt increase in asthma deaths in the 1960s in the British Isles, Australia, New Zealand, and Norway.[13] This increase was attributed to a high-dose preparation of a potent, nonselective inhaled β-agonist, isoproterenol, and mortality fell following the preparation's withdrawal. A second, even more dramatic increase in

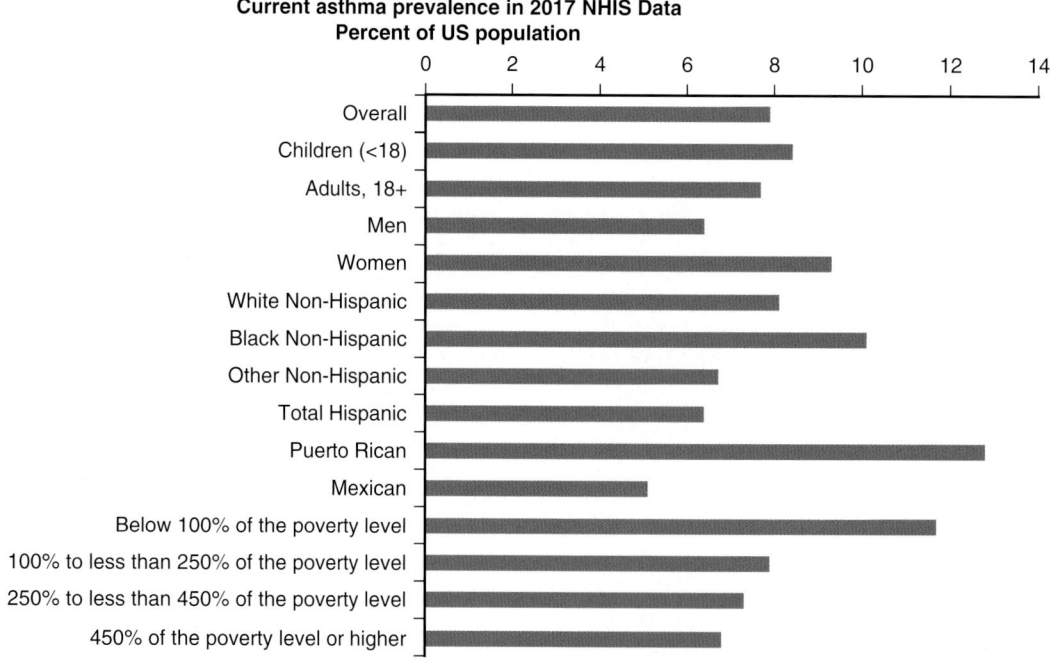

Figure 60.2 **Current asthma prevalence in the United States by age, gender, ethnic group, and income.** Asthma prevalence is highest in certain vulnerable populations, including children, Puerto Ricans, non-Hispanic Blacks, and those living below the poverty level. NHIS, National Health Interview Survey. (Data from the U.S. Centers for Disease Control and Prevention, https://www.cdc.gov/asthma/most_recent_national_asthma_data.htm, compiled Aug 26, 2019.)

asthma mortality in New Zealand in the 1970s was again attributed to sales of a particular β-agonist, fenoterol.[14] The increased asthma mortality observed with inhaled isoproterenol and fenoterol may relate to their increased potential for extrapulmonary effects (inotropy and hypokalemia).[15]

In 2017, the U.S. death rate attributable to asthma was 9.9 per 1 million population. As is true for asthma prevalence, asthma mortality disproportionately affects certain segments of American society such as Black non-Hispanics (22.7 per 1 million persons).[16] This excess mortality in Black Americans may be due to both biologic factors and societal factors such as access to health care, insurance coverage, access to medication or asthma education, environmental exposures, and racism.

RISK FACTORS

Allergy

The strongest risk factor for asthma is a family history of atopic disease,[17,18] which increases the risk of developing asthma by threefold to fourfold.[19] In children 3 to 14 years old, both positive skin tests and higher total serum *immunoglobulin* (Ig) E are strongly associated with asthma.[20,21] Serum IgE also correlates strongly with bronchial hyperresponsiveness.[22] In adults, the odds of having asthma increases with the number of positive skin tests to common allergens.[23]

Because much allergic asthma is associated with sensitivity to indoor allergens, and because western styles of housing favor greater exposure to indoor allergens, attention initially focused on increased exposure to these allergens in infancy and early childhood as a primary cause of the rise in asthma. Specific allergens of interest include house dust mites,[24,25] dog and cat dander,[26] and cockroach allergen,[27] especially in the inner city. These and other observations support the hypothesis that allergen controls should be valuable in the treatment or prevention of asthma.[28,29] However, even after more than 50 individual studies of allergen control have been completed, the conclusions drawn from those studies via meta-analyses and expert review have been at odds and hotly debated.[30,31] One alternative hypothesis is that appropriate exposure to allergens early in life could induce tolerance and decrease both sensitization to these allergens and the development of allergic disease. Recent experience in the prevention of peanut-related food allergy through controlled exposure to peanut allergens early in life support this alternative hypothesis.[32]

The Hygiene Hypothesis

The *hygiene hypothesis* holds that the rise in allergies in children is an unintended consequence of the success of domestic hygiene in reducing the rate of infections or exposure to bacterial products in early childhood. This hypothesis was proposed to explain the inverse relationship between hay fever and family size[33] and was cited later when children raised in West Germany were found to have significantly higher rates of asthma and hay fever than those raised in East Germany[34] despite the more severe air pollution in East Germany.[35] In these studies, children living on farms had a lower prevalence of hay fever and asthma than their nonagrarian peers. The risk reduction was greater for children living on a full-time farm, and risk was even lower if the farm housed livestock.[36,37] Long-term exposure to stables until age 5 years was associated with very low rates

of asthma (0.8%), hay fever (0.8%), and atopic sensitization (8.2%).[38] Follow-up studies of the protective effects of farm life have shown that endotoxin levels in the home were inversely related to the development of hay fever, atopic asthma, and atopic sensitization.[39] Another study employing two cohorts found that farm children had lower prevalences of asthma and atopy, were exposed to a greater variety of environmental microorganisms than the children in the reference groups, and that the diversity of microbial exposure was inversely related to the risk of asthma.[40]

The Human Microbiome

One potential link between changes in hygiene and allergic disease is the effect that "improved" hygiene may have on our indigenous microbiota and the role this microbiota may play in shaping our immune system.[41–45] The biologic model most commonly cited to explain this association is that early life exposure to factors that promote *type 1* (T1) immunity are necessary to blunt exuberant *type 2* (T2) immunity. Animal studies provide some support for this model[46–54] (see also Chapter 17).

Respiratory Viral Infections

Viral respiratory tract infections appear to play an important role in the development of asthma.[55,56] Children who have lower respiratory tract infections caused by respiratory syncytial virus (are at a three- to fourfold risk of subsequent wheezing during early school-years.[57–60] The presence of *rhinovirus* during wheezing episodes is an even stronger predictor of subsequent asthma.[61,62] Some studies suggest that viral lower respiratory tract infections interact with concurrent atopic disease in conferring subsequent asthma risk.[61]

Longitudinal studies of the natural history of wheezing illnesses have identified complex and, at times, inconsistent relationships between early wheezing phenotypes and the ultimate development of asthma. Briefly, some children who have wheezing illnesses at younger than 3 years of age continue to wheeze at age 6 years. However, not all children fit this "persistent wheezer" pattern. Similarly, there are children who wheeze at age 6 who never had wheezing illnesses before age 3 years. Thus, a propensity for wheezing can be transient and the causes may be different at different ages. Factors associated with wheezing before age 3 years include small airway caliber and maternal smoking, whereas factors associated with wheezing after age 3 include elevated serum IgE and a maternal history of asthma.[63] Furthermore, viral lower respiratory tract infections may unmask a predisposition to predominant T2-like responses already present at the time of the infection[64] and that manifest later as asthma.

Atypical Bacterial Infections

Although typical bacterial infections are not thought to cause asthma, at least two bacterial causes of "atypical" pneumonia have been implicated in the development of chronic wheezing illnesses, *Chlamydia pneumoniae* and *Mycoplasma pneumoniae*.[65] These atypical infections may be associated with asthma exacerbations.[66] Despite this evidence, a randomized trial of clarithromycin for the treatment of suboptimally controlled asthma showed no improvement in asthma control, whether or not *M. pneumoniae* or *C. pneumoniae* was detected by PCR in endobronchial biopsies.[67]

Air Pollution

Air pollution is associated with both the development of asthma and exacerbation of preexisting asthma.[68,69] In principle, exposure of the lung to air pollution could increase local oxidative stress, induce or modify local inflammation, enhance sensitization to allergens, impair lung development, or injure small airways. Several studies have focused specifically on asthma incidence and prevalence by proximity to heavy automobile traffic and suggest that exposure to respirable particulate matter and nitrogen dioxide in this setting are both associated with the future development of asthma[69–75] (see also Chapter 102).

Other Early Life Factors

Intrauterine risk factors include growth rates (both high and low),[76,77] dietary vitamin D and E,[78,79] exposure to microbial products,[80] parental smoking,[81] and parental stress.[82] Perinatal risk factors associated with asthma include prematurity[83] and chorioamnionitis.[84] Finally, early childhood risk factors associated with asthma include a shorter period of breastfeeding,[85,86] obesity,[76] absence of older siblings or daycare attendance,[87] bacterial colonization of the airways in early childhood,[88] antibiotic use,[89] and acetaminophen use.[90]

Occupational Exposures

Finally, occupational exposures constitute an important risk factor for a specific subset of patients. Asthma induced by occupational exposure accounts for as much as 17% of all adult-onset asthma.[91] A full description of the occupational exposures that can cause asthma is beyond the scope of this chapter because the known exposures number in the hundreds. However, in general, occupational asthma can either result from immunologically mediated sensitization to occupational agents (i.e., *sensitizer-induced asthma*) or from exposure to high concentrations of irritant compounds (i.e., *irritant-induced asthma*) (see Chapter 100).

NATURAL HISTORY

Neonatal Period

A predisposition to asthma may begin as early as the neonatal period. The immunologic milieu at the fetal-maternal interface is skewed towards a T2 phenotype, and this immune bias is carried into neonatal life.[92] Unless the pattern of immune response in the airways is "reprogrammed" towards a T1 pattern, the infant may have a prolonged high-risk window for allergic sensitization to aeroallergens.[93]

Childhood

Although asthma is the most prevalent chronic disease in children, it is difficult to diagnose in infants and preschoolers. Recurrent wheezing is the most common early symptom associated with asthma; however, only a minority of preschoolers with recurrent wheezing still have "asthma" at the age of 6 years. Patterns of wheezing in early childhood have been intensively studied in longitudinal cohorts such as the Tucson Children's Respiratory Health Study[63] and the British Avon Longitudinal Study of Parents and Children.[94] The Tucson Children's Respiratory Health Study found that 48% of children had at least one wheezing illness at some point in the first 6 years of life, 34% had at least one wheezing illness before age 3 years (defined as

early wheezing), and approximately half of these children continued to have wheezing at age 6 years. In the remainder of children with wheezing episodes before age 3 years, these episodes were transient and resolved before the age of 6 years. Finally, approximately 15% of children presented with late-onset wheezing, defined as wheezing illnesses after age 6 years. Most of the early wheezing illnesses (before age 3 years) can be ascribed to viral respiratory infections such as respiratory syncytial virus or rhinovirus and do not necessarily reflect atopy.[95] In addition, transient early wheeze is associated with maternal smoking. However, wheezing at and after age 6 years (persistent and late-onset wheeze, respectively) is more strongly associated with atopy. Furthermore, children who had either persistent or late-onset wheeze were more likely to go on to wheeze later in life and be diagnosed with asthma. The risk for continued wheeze after age 6 years appears to be associated with severity of airflow obstruction and the degree of allergen sensitization.[96] The British Avon Longitudinal Study of Parents and Children provided some additional granularity to the categories of childhood wheezing illnesses by defining intermediate-onset wheeze (onset of symptoms after 18 months of age) and early prolonged wheeze (onset in the first year of life but with remission at 69 months of age).[94]

Atopic or Allergic March

The terms *atopic march* and *allergic march* are synonyms referring to a characteristic pattern of atopic disease development during infancy and childhood.[97,98] The most common pattern begins with atopic dermatitis or eczema in the first year of life, sometimes associated with food intolerance or food allergy, followed by rhinoconjunctivitis and/or wheezing illnesses that are ultimately diagnosed as asthma. Thus, the natural history of atopic disease may more generally follow a specific pattern of organ-specific development, which suggests a stereotyped set of underlying cellular and molecular mechanisms.[99]

Teenage Years

After puberty, the demographics of patients with prevalent asthma switches from a male predominance to a female predominance, which suggests a change in the nature of incident cases of asthma. One straightforward inference would be that some incident cases of asthma in girls during teenage years relate specifically to hormonal factors. This is a compelling hypothesis and some data provide clues to potential mechanisms, including possible protective effects of androgens and deleterious effects of estrogens and progesterone.[100,101]

Remission

In long-term follow-up of a population-based birth cohort evaluated annually to age 26 years,[102] just over half (51%) reported wheezing at more than one assessment. In this cohort, wheezing persisted until adulthood in 15%, whereas wheezing remitted in 27%. This remission was often temporary, however, because wheezing recurred by age 26 years in nearly half of those in whom it had remitted. This finding echoes those of 15 earlier studies of the natural history of asthma, showing that about 50% of adults who recall having childhood asthma continue to have symptoms.[103] Risk factors associated with persistence into adulthood include house dust mite sensitization, lower forced expiratory volume in 1 second, airway hyperresponsiveness, female gender, and smoking.[102] Whether "spontaneous remission" truly reflects the disappearance of airway T2 inflammation in asthma is unknown. Even in patients with complete absence of symptoms and medications, exhaled *nitric oxide* (NO) is elevated, airway responsiveness is increased, and bronchial biopsies show increases in eosinophils, T cells and mast cells, and subepithelial fibrosis.[104,105]

Progressive Airflow Obstruction

Some people with asthma have accelerated rates of decline in pulmonary function, and asthmatic smokers have greater rates of decline than healthy smokers.[106,107] Furthermore, many nonsmoking asthmatics develop severe, irreversible airflow obstruction.[108,109] One possibility is that progressive narrowing of the airways in chronic asthma results from airway remodeling, which is a summary term for the deposition of collagen and accumulation of blood vessels, smooth muscle, secretory cells, and glands in the asthmatic airway.[110,111] Nonetheless, it is not possible to prove that airway remodeling is the cause of progressive airflow obstruction in asthma.

Adulthood

Even though many adults with asthma had asthma during childhood, adult asthma is particularly heterogeneous. The female predominance that first appears in teenage years continues in adult asthma. Alternatively, asthma symptoms can begin de novo in an adult, and not all patients have atopic features. In some instances, the onset of wheezing is attributed to a specific acute respiratory illness that became persistent. In others, it is possible that atopy and wheezing illness as a child were modest and subclinical.

Asthma in the Elderly

If asthma is present in an adult, it will often remain as the adult ages. Surprisingly, new-onset asthma can also present in the elderly.[112] In this age group, misdiagnosis of asthma (often as COPD) and under-treatment appear to be common.[113,114] Furthermore, elderly patients with asthma are more likely to have fixed airway obstruction.[115] The term *intrinsic asthma*, often used to describe nonatopic reversible bronchoconstriction, has traditionally been associated with asthma in the elderly,[116] and more than 60% of elderly patients in one study reported the first onset of asthma symptoms following an upper respiratory infection.[112] However, at least one study has shown positive skin reactivity to one or more common allergens in almost two-thirds of elderly asthmatic patients.[117] In addition, a subset of adult-onset asthmatics have high blood eosinophils, poor asthma control, and high exacerbation rates despite the use of inhaled corticosteroids, a distinct clinical entity now termed *adult-onset eosinophilic asthma*.[118]

GENETICS OF ASTHMA

EARLY EVIDENCE THAT ASTHMA IS HERITABLE

The genetic basis for asthma was described in 1860 by Henry Salter, who reported that asthma showed "distinct traces of inheritance" among related individuals.[119] Genetic variation influences asthma susceptibility through the cumulative effects of many different genes that are polymorphic (contain gene variants or polymorphisms) or

interact with multiple potential environmental exposures to cause asthma. The first genetic studies for asthma susceptibility were early family-based genome-wide linkage studies that used genetic variants equally spaced throughout the genome to identify chromosomal susceptibility regions for asthma and associated phenotypes (bronchial hyperresponsiveness, serum IgE levels, etc.).[120–130] These studies identified evidence for linkage with asthma and related phenotypes in multiple different chromosomal regions (chromosomes 5q, 6p, 7q, 11q, 12q, 14q, and 16q), which have subsequently been studied to identify specific genes.[121,128,130–143] These studies also demonstrated gene-gene interactions in asthma susceptibility between chromosomes 5q31, 8p23, 12q22, and 15q13 and evidence for gene-by-environment interactions with passive cigarette smoking at chromosomes 1p, 5q, and 9q, and 17q21.[122,127,144–146]

The first novel gene for asthma susceptibility identified using family-based linkage approaches was the *a disintegrin and metalloprotease-33* (*ADAM33*) gene on chromosome 20p13.[125] *ADAM33* is among the most replicated genes from linkage analysis for asthma and affects lung growth, morphogenesis, and airway remodeling while also being implicated in longitudinal progression of airflow obstruction.[147–155] Several other asthma susceptibility genes have been identified using fine mapping or positional cloning techniques and include the genes encoding *protocadherin-1* (*PCDH1*), HLA-G, *neuropeptide S receptor-1* (*GPRA*), *PHD finger protein-11* (*PHF11*), and *peptidase-10* (*DPP10*), a locus identified in a subsequent genome-wide association study of African Americans and African Caribbeans.[121,141,156–161]

CANDIDATE GENE ASSOCIATION STUDIES

Case-control association studies compare the frequency of the alleles of a gene variant between unrelated cases and controls, typically leveraging *single nucleotide polymorphisms* (SNP, denoted by a reference sequence number). Over 100 biologic candidate genes have been examined in candidate gene studies based on plausible biologic mechanisms and chromosomal regions linked to asthma. Before genome-wide association studies, the most replicated candidate genes were in the broad categories of lung development (*ADAM33*), T2 inflammation (*IL4*, *IL13*, *IL4R*, *FCER1B*), innate immunity (*HLA-DRB1*, *HLA-DQB1*, *CD14*), and cellular inflammation (*TNF*, *DPP10*).[121,125,156,157,161–171]

GENOME-WIDE ASSOCIATION STUDIES

In 2007, the first asthma *genome-wide association study* (GWAS) was performed by the *Multidisciplinary Study to Identify the Genetic and Environmental Causes of Asthma in the European Community* (GABRIEL) consortium in a European cohort. This study found asthma-associated SNPs in the *orosomucoid 1-like 3* gene (*ORMDL3*) region on chromosome 17q12; a second larger GWAS by the GABRIEL consortium found additional susceptibility loci in the neighboring *gasdermin-like* genes (*GSDMB* and *GSDMA*).[120,172] The 17q12 locus is the most frequently replicated asthma risk locus with the highest statistical significance across studies in individuals of European descent, including Puerto Ricans (eTable 60.1).[173–182] Variation in this locus regulates the mRNA expression of both *ORMDL3* and *GSDMB*, but the precise mechanisms through which these genes contribute to asthma pathogenesis remains unclear.[183–185] The second GABRIEL GWAS was among the first of many to identify additional novel risk loci, including the genes coding for *thymic stromal lymphopoietin (TSLP)*, *IL1RL1/IL18RL1* (between the IL-1 and IL-18 receptor genes), *HLA-DQ*, *IL33*, and *SMAD3* (see eTable 60.1).[172,178] These associations are both highly significant and reproducible associations across independent cohorts.

Asthma in Diverse Ethnic Groups

Only a few GWASs have been performed in multiethnic populations including Hispanic and African American subjects. This is of particular importance because African Americans and Puerto Ricans have a greater asthma incidence, morbidity, and mortality compared to whites and other Hispanic groups (i.e., Mexican Americans).[186,187] GWASs in these groups have been substantially less frequent with smaller sample sizes compared to whites, but have identified both overlapping and unique asthma risk loci (see eTable 60.1). A GWAS from the EVE consortium was the first large-scale, multiethnic study representing Americans of European descent, African Americans, African Caribbeans, and Hispanics (Mexican Americans and Puerto Ricans) and identified significant associations in the 17q12 locus, *IL1RL1*, *TSLP*, and *IL33*, confirming their importance as asthma risk loci in ethnically diverse populations.[120,172,178] The 17q21 locus has been replicated in African descent multiethnic cohorts that included Puerto Ricans, and in Puerto Ricans alone, but has not been replicated in African Americans alone who have, on average, higher African and lower European ancestry compared to Puerto Ricans.[156,173,180,188] Another large multiracial GWAS identified SNPs in the *pyrin and HIN domain family member 1 (PYHIN1)* gene that were only associated with asthma in African Americans and African Caribbeans.[178] Additional GWASs of populations from a primarily African ancestry have identified additional novel, race-specific susceptibility loci including the *DPP10* locus and the gene encoding *patched domain-containing protein-3 (PTCHD3)*, which is related to the hedgehog signaling pathway implicated as a genetic determinant of lung function.[121,156,157,188–194] These ancestry-specific differences in asthma risk loci have been recapitulated in larger multiethnic GWASs of asthma, but the number of GWASs consisting of African Americans and Hispanics remains relatively small.[189,195]

Severe Asthma and Disease Severity

GWASs of cohorts enriched for severe asthma have confirmed prior asthma genes and identified novel risk loci including multiple SNPs in *RAD50* adjacent to *IL13*, *HLA-DQB1*, and between *HLA-DQB1* and *HLA-DQA2*.[128,143,170,196–198] A GWAS of children with severe asthma identified four previously identified susceptibility loci in *GSDMB*, *IL33*, *RAD50*, and *ILRL1* and a novel SNP in the gene encoding *cadherin-related family member-3 (CDHR3)*, which was subsequently confirmed in an independent asthma GWAS and found to function as a receptor for rhinovirus C.[199–201] A recent large GWAS for moderate-to-severe asthma based on the U.K. Biobank population confirmed 21 risk loci including novel variants in genes encoding a GATA binding protein

(*GATA3*) and *MUC5AC*, a gene that encodes for an asthma-relevant secreted mucin glycoprotein.[202]

GWASs in asthma cohorts have identified loci associated with lung function, a fundamental determinant of asthma severity. A GWAS of lung function in a U.S. non-Hispanic white cohort enriched for severe asthma identified novel variants associated with lung function and asthma severity in T1 immunity pathway genes that regulate the inflammatory response associated with viral and bacterial infections (*IL12A*, *IL12RB1*, *STAT4*, *IRF2*).[203] In addition, GWASs of lung function in a general population have found SNPs in *HHIP* (hedgehog-interacting protein) and *PTCH1*, which are cumulatively associated with lower lung function across different ethnic groups with asthma.[193,194,204] These findings suggest that gene variants that determine asthma severity can be different from those that determine risk. As one exception, variants in the IL-6 receptor gene (*IL6R*) were associated both with asthma risk and with lung function in two, independent GWASs.[175,205] Another strongly linked coding variant in *IL6R*, Asp[358]Ala, is also associated with lung function and with bronchial responsiveness in individuals with asthma.[206]

Lessons Learned

To date, GWASs have discovered more than 73 loci associated with asthma susceptibility, most of which are in regulatory or noncoding regions due either to the fact that most of the human genome is noncoding or the fact that identified GWAS SNPs potentially tag for variation that could be within coding exons. Highly replicated asthma susceptibility loci identified through GWASs are presented in eTable 60.1. These GWASs have revealed several lessons about the genetic factors that underlie asthma risk. First, asthma risk loci span multiple genes from biologic pathways related to (1) epithelial responses triggered by allergens or infection (*IL1RL1*, *IL33*, *CDHR3*); (2) airway inflammation, remodeling, and hyperresponsiveness in response to tobacco smoke, lipopolysaccharides, allergens, or alterations in sphingolipid biosynthesis (*ORMDL3*, *GSDMB*); (3) T2 inflammation (*TSLP*, *IL13*, *GATA3*, *DENND1B*); (4) innate immunity (*TLR1*, *MICB*, *IL2RB*, HLA locus); and (5) cellular inflammation (*TNFSF4*, *TNIP1*, *IL6R*). Second, the genetic determinants of asthma risk vary across ethnic groups from different ancestral backgrounds, and GWASs in diverse multiethnic cohorts have identified ethnic-specific loci (*PTCHD3*, *PYHIN1*, *ADRAB1*, *PTGES*) not found in whites of European descent.[156,178,188,189] Finally, identified variants have weak effects and cumulatively account for a small proportion of the observed heritability of asthma.[189,200] This "missing heritability" of asthma is related, at least in part, to the challenges of objectively diagnosing asthma in large cohorts and to gene-gene and gene-by-environment interactions.[207]

EPIGENETIC STUDIES FOR ASTHMA SUSCEPTIBILITY AND SEVERITY

Environmental exposures may trigger epigenetic modifications and therefore contribute to asthma pathogenesis in ways not detectable using traditional genetic approaches. The epigenome can be regulated through DNA methylation, altered histone binding, and chromatin condensation at gene promoters, which alter gene transcription without changes in the DNA code. Some asthma susceptibility genes from early linkage studies and GWASs have been evaluated with epigenetic approaches. For example, a small epigenetic study of the 17q21 locus in peripheral blood leukocytes from European pediatric asthma cases and controls identified differences in methylation across CpG sites at *ORMDL3* that associated with *ORMDL3* mRNA expression and asthma, independent of adjacent risk SNP loci.[208] *Epigenome-wide association studies* have been relatively small and limited by the availability of whole-blood DNA or asthma-relevant tissues but have provided some insight into how environmental exposures interact with genes to influence asthma risk.[209–211] Epigenome-wide association studies of whole blood inflammatory cell and nasal epithelial cell tissue DNA from an inner city cohort have identified multiple sites of differential CpG methylation near genes within biologic pathways relevant to nitric oxide synthesis (*CAT, KLF6*), immunity (*HLA-DPA1, TNFSF13, IFNGR2, EXOC2*), T2 inflammation (*IL4, IL13, POSTN, ALOX15, CAPN14*), collagen, and the extracellular matrix (*COL16A, COL5A2, COL5A3, HAS3, MMP14*).[212,213] An epigenome-wide association study of cord blood mononuclear cell DNA from infants identified *SMAD3*, a gene from prior GWASs, as a gene with increased methylation associated with childhood asthma risk.[172,200,214,215] The genes and biologic pathways associated with asthma through GWASs and epigenome-wide association studies seem to overlap, but larger studies in cohorts with available tissue will be needed to characterize the epigenetic mechanisms that contribute to the missing heritability of asthma.

MOLECULAR AND CELLULAR BASIS OF ASTHMA

HISTOPATHOLOGY OF ASTHMA

Asthma is a disease of the airways characterized by pathologic changes in both the epithelium and the submucosa (Fig. 60.3). These changes, often summarized by the term airway remodeling, include abnormal deposition of collagen in the subepithelium and changes in structural cells such as goblet cells, submucosal gland cells, smooth muscle cells, and blood vessel cells. Goblet cell metaplasia and hyperplasia increase the amount of stored gel-forming mucins in the airway epithelium.[216] Desquamation of epithelial cells can be seen in acute severe asthma exacerbations but not in chronic stable asthma.[217] Deposition of collagen types I, III, and IV and of fibronectin and tenascin in the subepithelium immediately under the true basement membrane is most prominently seen in T2 asthma,[218–220] even in early-onset disease. Myofibroblasts are increased in number in asthma and are an important cellular source of matrix protein deposition in the subepithelium. Hyperplasia of airway smooth muscle is easy to demonstrate by morphometric measurements, even in mild forms of asthma, whereas true airway smooth muscle hypertrophy is found in more severe subtypes of asthma.[221,222] By contrast, inherent smooth muscle dysfunction and hypercontractility, which are modeled in vitro, are more difficult to demonstrate in vivo in asthmatics.[221] Measurements of isometric tension in airway smooth muscle tissue from asthmatic subjects have not shown consistent evidence for enhanced force generation but have shown increased shortening.[223] Such increases in isotonic shortening in airway smooth muscle could result not only from alterations in the contractile apparatus,[224] but also from alterations in the biophysical properties of the extracellular matrix.[225] Bronchial blood vessel number and size are increased in asthma, and these vessels may have an important role in regulating airway caliber because an increase in vascular volume may swell the mucosa and narrow the airway lumen.[226–228] Many inflammatory mediators cause vasodilation, which may be accompanied by increased permeability at the postcapillary venule, plasma extravasation, and airway mucosal edema. Histologic analyses of lungs from patients who die from acute severe asthma show extensive mucus plugging of airways, airway wall thickening, smooth muscle hypertrophy, and submucosal gland hypertrophy.[229] Silicone rubber casts of autopsy lungs from patients with asthma show marked airway truncation from mucus plugs and also reveal longitudinal ridges and horizontal corrugations corresponding to elastic bundles and smooth muscle hypertrophy.[229]

NERVES AND NERVE RECEPTORS IN ASTHMA

The neurologic "wiring" of the airway includes innervation of airway smooth muscle by sympathetic and parasympathetic nerves. When activated, airway nerves can markedly constrict airways or dilate contracted airways. The nervous system is therefore an important regulator of airway caliber. A key detail is that the predominant contractile innervation of airway smooth muscle is parasympathetic and cholinergic in nature, while the primary relaxant innervation of the airways is comprised of noncholinergic (nitric oxide synthase– and vasoactive intestinal peptide–containing) parasympathetic nerves.[230,231] These anatomically and physiologically distinct parasympathetic nerves are differentially regulated by reflexes. Perhaps surprisingly, given the clinical utility of adrenergic agonists as bronchodilators, sympathetic-adrenergic nerves have only minor physiologic roles in regulation of airway smooth muscle tone.[232]

The term neurogenic inflammation refers to the inflammatory responses caused by tachykinins, which are peptidergic neurotransmitters that activate specific receptors as part of the *nonadrenergic noncholinergic* system.[233] Excitatory nonadrenergic noncholinergic effects are mediated by release of tachykinins such as neurokinin A and substance P acting on *neurokinin-1 and -2 receptors*. In general, neurokinin-1 receptor mediates gland secretion, plasma extravasation, vasodilation, and leukocyte adhesion, whereas neurokinin-2 receptor mediates contraction of airway smooth muscle. Inhibitory nonadrenergic noncholinergic effects are thought to be mediated principally by vasoactive intestinal peptide and nitric oxide. Evidence for an operative nonadrenergic noncholinergic system in asthma comes from studies showing that asthmatic subjects develop bronchoconstriction after inhaling neurokinin A or substance P.[234] Although a neurokinin-1 and -2 receptor antagonist protected against

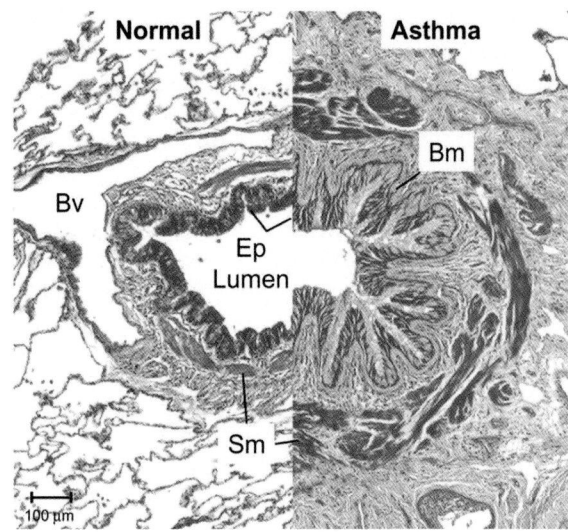

Figure 60.3 Airway pathology in asthma. Photomicrograph illustrating pathologic differences in a medium-sized airway from a nonasthmatic patient (*left*) and a patient with asthma (*right*). The stain is a Movat pentachrome stain. The airways in asthma show significant structural remodeling. The epithelium in asthma shows goblet cell hyperplasia, subepithelial fibrosis, and increased smooth muscle (Sm) volume. Scale bar 100 μm. Bm, basement membrane; Bv, blood vessel; Ep, epithelium. (From Wadsworth S, Sin D, Dorscheid D. Clinical update on the use of biomarkers of airway inflammation in the management of asthma. *J Asthma Allergy.* 2011;4:7786.)

bradykinin-induced bronchoconstriction in asthmatic subjects, a selective neurokinin-1 receptor antagonist did not protect against hypertonic saline-induced cough or bronchoconstriction.[235]

Cholinergic nerves innervate airway smooth muscle, and hyperresponsiveness of airway smooth muscle is a central pathophysiologic feature of asthma. The mechanism of this hyperresponsiveness is complex and not fully understood. Past concepts that the hyperresponsiveness reflects an imbalance in neural signals that constrict or dilate airways have been difficult to prove in human studies and are likely to underestimate the role of non-neural mechanisms. Parasympathetic nerves also innervate submucosal glands and regulate mucin secretion from submucosal gland cells. Notably, inflammatory cells in the airway all express parasympathetic receptors, so that these cells may be under parasympathetic nerve control. These nerves produce and release inflammatory mediators and can contribute to the recruitment and activation of leukocytes. These leukocytes can then alter production and release of neurotransmitters from nerves. In this way, crosstalk between airway nerves and leukocytes may help maintain chronic inflammation in asthma. Consequently, anticholinergic treatment should benefit patients with asthma not just because of bronchodilator effects. Indeed, it is known that vagotomy decreases inflammation in the lungs of asthmatic patients and that treating patients with uncontrolled asthma with a long-acting anticholinergic drug (tiotropium bromide) improves asthma control.[238]

Transient receptor potential vanilloid 4 (TRPV4) is a broadly expressed, polymodally gated ion channel highly expressed in airways.[239] It is an osmosensor and thermosensor activated by temperature or by endogenous or exogenous chemical stimuli. TRPV4-mediated activation of airway afferents is a putative mechanism of cough and bronchoconstriction,

and pharmacologic inhibitors of TRPV4 are being considered as novel asthma treatments.[240]

OVERVIEW OF MOLECULAR IMMUNOLOGY OF ASTHMA

Asthma is a clinical diagnosis that results from heterogeneous immune disorders of the airways. These disorders include aberrant T2 (allergic) immune responses that underlie the dominant T2-high subtype of asthma and non-allergic immune responses that underlie disease in smaller subsets of patients (T2-low forms of asthma).

T2-high asthma is characterized by T2 immune responses. T2 immune responses include prominent eosinophil infiltration of tissues, driven by T2 cytokines (IL-4, IL-5, and IL-13) secreted by multiple immune cell types, including the Th2 subset of CD4+ T cells, group 2 *innate lymphoid cells* (ILCs), mast cells, and basophils. To perform key functions in T2 immunity, mast cells and basophils are armed with IgE derived from B cells under the influence of IL-4. T2 immune responses usually arise in response to helminth and parasite infections, where eosinophils undergo cytolysis and release toxic granules to kill the parasite, and epithelial cells overproduce mucus to encapsulate the helminths and facilitate expulsion from the gastrointestinal tract. In response to insect and snake bites, mast cell and basophil proteases usually function to neutralize extracellular toxins. If all of this fails, a fibrosis program is initiated as a barrier against the parasite or toxins. T2 immune responses can also be inappropriately mounted against innocuous environmental antigens (allergens) resulting in allergy and asthma. Specifically, an excess of T2 cytokines in the lower airway in patients with T2-high asthma will promote IgE-mediated hypersensitivity, activate epithelial cell mucus production, mediate inflammatory eosinophil-rich cell influx to the airway, cause remodeling responses in the epithelium and subepithelial matrix, and promote alterations in smooth muscle reactivity leading to bronchial hyperreactivity. The sensitivity of T2 inflammation to corticosteroids explains why T2-high asthma is usually responsive to corticosteroid treatment.[220]

T2-low forms of asthma represent a more heterogeneous and less well-understood group, yet the prevalence is high. In patients with less severe asthma, the prevalence of patients who lack airway eosinophilia or other markers of T2 inflammation is 60–70%; in those with more severe asthma, the lack of T2 inflammation may be seen in 40–50%.[241-244] Although analyses of inflammation in airway specimens collected from patients with asthma have shown a lack of airway inflammation in a subset of patients (paucigranulocytic asthma),[245] other subsets of patients show signals for activation of pathways related to T1 or *type 3* (T3) immunity or for neutrophilic inflammation independent of T3 immunity.[246] T1 immunity consists of interferon-γ–producing cells (group 1 ILCs, CD8+ cytotoxic T cells, and CD4+ Th1 cells), which normally protect against intracellular microbes through activation of mononuclear phagocytes but which can be co-opted to drive chronic inflammatory disease. T3 immunity is mediated by group 3 ILCs and Th17 cells producing IL-17, IL-22, or both, which activate mononuclear phagocytes but also recruit neutrophils and induce epithelial antimicrobial responses, thus protecting against extracellular bacteria and fungi. Although T1 and T3

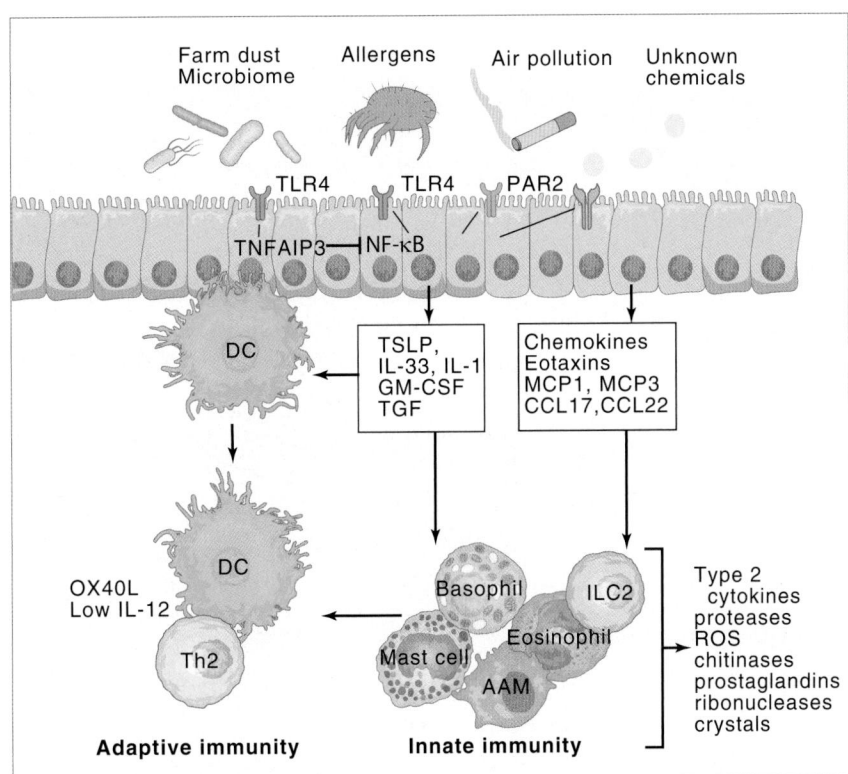

Figure 60.4 Early innate immune response driving asthma. Most allergens and many air pollutants trigger epithelial cell production of cytokines and chemokines through activation of toll-like receptors (TLRs) or protease-activated receptors. This leads to activation of dendritic cells (DCs) that migrate to draining lymph nodes. DCs in lymph nodes will promote Th2 development in the presence of OX40 ligand (OX40L) and when interleukin (IL)-12 levels are relatively low. In addition, epithelial cell production of cytokines leads to activation of innate immune cells that are recruited to the airways and produce mediators that contribute to airway inflammation. Cytokines like thymic stromal lymphopoietin (TSLP), IL-33, and granulocyte-macrophage colony-stimulating factor (GM-CSF) and chemokines such as monocyte chemokine proteins, eotaxins, and C-C chemokines (CCL17- and CCL22) are all potential drug targets for new biologics. Some environmental exposures such as chronic exposure to farm dust can suppress the airway epithelial response to allergens because these induce expression of a negative regulator of nuclear factor-κB (NF-κB) activation called tumor necrosis factor-α induced protein-3 (TNFAIP3). AAM, alternatively activated macrophages; ILC2, innate lymphoid cell 2; MCP, monocyte chemoattractant protein; PAR2, proteinase activated receptor 2; ROS, reactive oxygen species; ILC2, innate lymphoid cell 2; TGF, transforming growth factor.

immunity are usually implicated in autoimmune diseases, there are data to implicate these responses as a disease mechanism in subgroups of asthma patients. In addition, subsets of patients have systemic inflammation and metabolic dysfunction,[241] and asthma in these patients may represent airway dysfunction caused by inflammatory stimuli that arise outside the lung.

MOLECULAR IMMUNOLOGY OF T2-HIGH ASTHMA

Airway epithelial cell crosstalk with immune cells in the underlying submucosa is a fundamental mechanism of T2-high asthma (Fig. 60.4).[247,248] Inhaled insults, including microbes, aeroallergens, and oxidants (cigarette smoke, car exhaust pollutants) activate airway epithelial cells through multiple pattern recognition receptors that detect and respond to danger signals. These receptors include toll-like receptors and receptors for alarmins such as uric acid and adenosine triphosphate. Other exposures such as farm dust can suppress airway epithelial response to allergens via increased expression of *tumor necrosis factor* (TNF)-α induced protein-3, a negative regulator of nuclear factor-κB activation (see Fig 60.4). Activated epithelial cells release TSLP, IL-33, IL-1β, and *granulocyte-macrophage colony-stimulating factor* (GM-CSF). These cytokines and chemokines recruit *dendritic cells* (DCs) from the bone marrow to

the airway epithelium where the DCs sample inhaled antigens, process them to linear peptides, and present them on their cell surface as part of the class II major histocompatibility heterodimer complex to naive T cells in the draining lymph nodes, thus initiating allergic T2 sensitization upon first exposure to allergens. Upon repeated encounter with an allergen, DCs can also stimulate effector and memory T cells to orchestrate inflammation locally in the airways. Full-blown effector differentiation of CD4+ T cells initiated in draining lymph nodes is completed following exposure of CD4+ Th2 cells to IL-33 and TSLP in the epithelial and subepithelial space[249] (Fig. 60.5). The epithelial cytokines also activate cells of the innate immune system, including mast cells, basophils, and ILC2s, that work together with CD4+ Th2 effector cells to produce IL-13 and IL-5. IL-5 promotes the development and activation of eosinophils. IL-13 activates airway epithelial cell programs that increase expression of chemokines, mucins, and inducible nitric oxide synthase. Chemokines such as eotaxins and stem cell factor recruit eosinophils and mast cells, and mucins are secreted apically to create an adherent and stiff mucus gel. Nitric oxide, produced from L-arginine by inducible nitric oxide synthase activity, is a potent mediator of vascular permeability, and exhaled nitric oxide is a useful biomarker of IL-13 activation of the airway epithelium. Other less well-understood products of IL-13-activated epithelial cells have roles in promoting smooth muscle pathology in asthma and

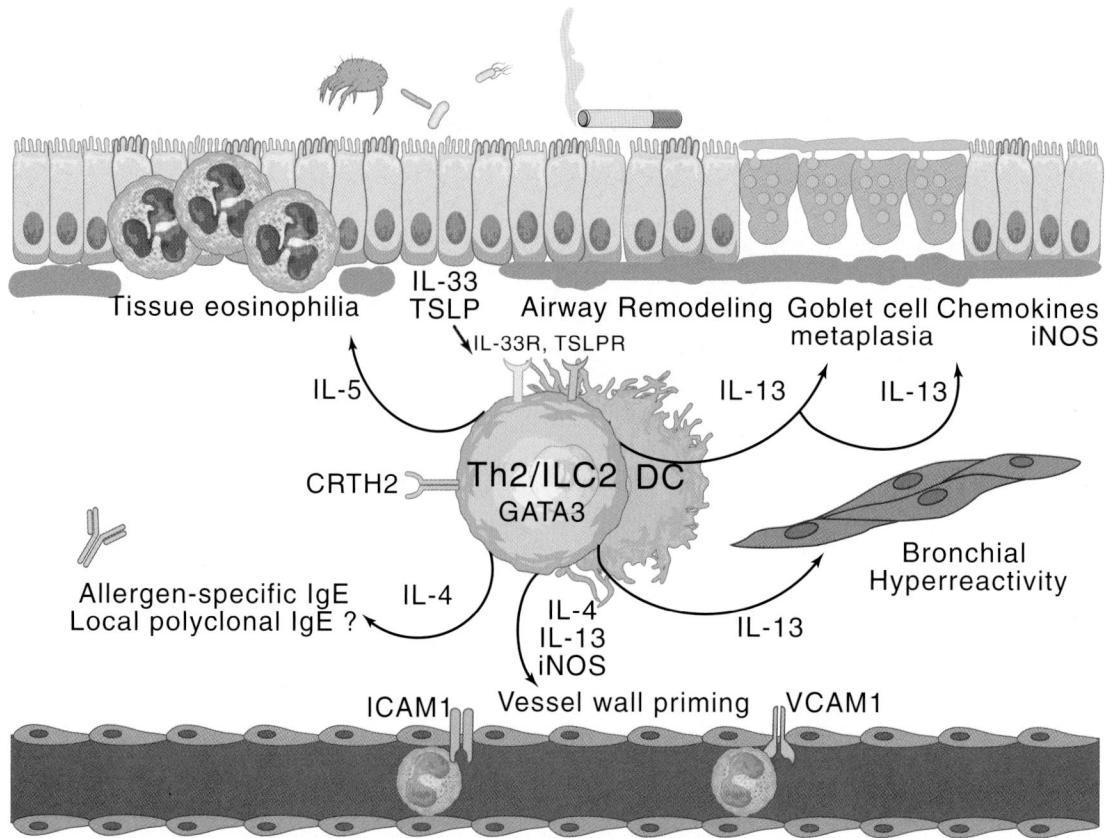

Figure 60.5 Central role of type 2 (T2) and innate lymphocytes in controlling key features of T2-high asthma. T2-high asthma is marked by airway eosinophils and by nitric oxide in exhaled air (iNOS). It is often accompanied by goblet cell metaplasia and high-level production of the airway mucin MUC5AC. T2 memory lymphocytes are restimulated by dendritic cells (DC) upon allergen recognition and produce interleukin (IL)-4, IL-5, and IL-13. In some patients with T2-high asthma, group 2 innate lymphoid cells (ILC2) are activated directly by epithelial cytokines such as thymic stromal lymphopoietin (TSLP) and IL-33 to produce IL-5 and IL-13. Th2 cells and ILC2s share many features such as expression of cytokine receptors, transcription factor GATA-binding protein 3 (GATA3), and chemokine receptor expressed by Th2 cells (CRTH2). IL-5 drives the development and activation of airway eosinophils. IL-13 drives iNOS production in airway epithelial cells, goblet cell metaplasia, and bronchial hyperreactivity. IL-4 promotes immunoglobulin E (IgE) synthesis (allergen specific in the case of allergic asthma) and primes the vessel wall for extravasation of eosinophils through induction of vascular cell adhesion molecule (VCAM-1) and intercellular adhesion molecule (ICAM-1) by acting on IL-4R. The *brown lines* beneath the airway epithelium signify excess subepithelial collagen.

in driving subepithelial cell collagen deposition, a hallmark of T2-high asthma.

T2-high forms of asthma can develop in childhood or in adulthood. In childhood, T2-high asthma typically presents as a lung manifestation of atopy. Adult-onset T2-high asthma is more typically associated with upper airway disease (chronic rhinosinusitis with nasal polyps) and sensitivity to aspirin. The relative roles of CD4+ Th2 cells, ILC2s, mast cells, and basophils as cellular sources of T2 cytokines in childhood versus adult-onset T2 asthma is an area of active research.

Mast cells are considered central effector cells in T2-high forms of asthma (Fig. 60.6). Mast cells constitutively express multiple receptors on their cell surface, including the *high affinity IgE receptor* (FcεRI), the IL-33 receptor (ST2), and Siglec8. Basophils are circulating granulocytes that also express FcεRI, the prostaglandin D2 receptor (*chemokine receptor expressed by Th2 cells* [CRTH2]), ST2, and the *IL-5 receptor* (IL-5R). Antigen-induced cross-linking of IgE leads to aggregation of IgE-FcεRI complexes, which stimulate mast cells and basophils to release autocoids (histamine, serotonin), proteases (tryptase, chymase, carboxypeptidase

A3), proteoglycans (heparin and/or chondroitin sulfates), lipid-derived mediators (*prostaglandin D2* [PGD$_2$], leukotriene B$_4$, leukotriene C$_4$, leukotriene D$_4$, and leukotriene E$_4$), and T2 cytokines. The aggregate response to mediators released shortly after mast cell and basophil degranulation is called an immediate hypersensitivity (or early phase) reaction and includes airway smooth muscle contraction, heightened bronchovascular permeability, and increases in mucin secretion. The physiologic consequence is a decrease in airflow but, in extreme cases, also includes hypotension and anaphylaxis if the response is systemic. Although the inflammation and functional changes associated with early phase responses resolve within 1 to 3 hours, a second late phase reaction can develop in some asthmatics, typically beginning 2 to 6 hours after exposure and lasting for 24 to 48 hours, accompanied by influx of more DCs, CD4 T cells, eosinophils, and basophils. Late-phase responders are often studied in proof-of-concept studies of novel controller medications for asthma because a drug's ability to inhibit late phase responses to inhaled allergen in these studies is a good predictor of its efficacy in improving asthma control outcomes in clinical trials.[250]

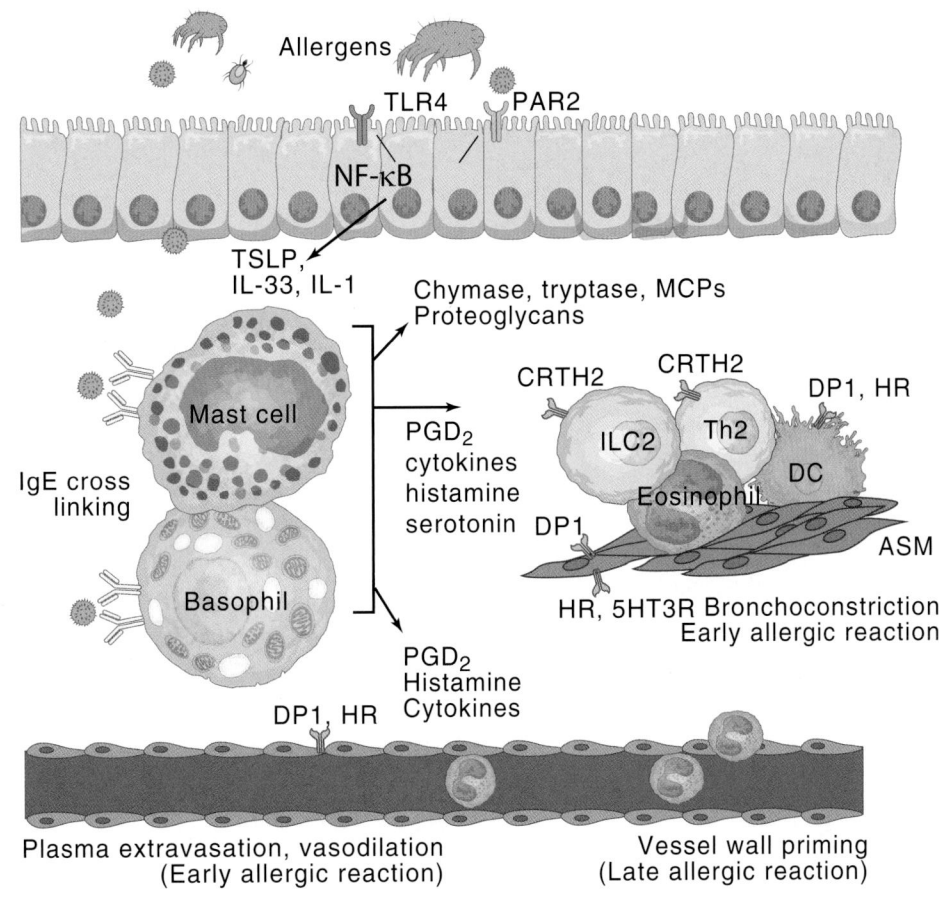

Figure 60.6 Role of mast cells and basophils in asthma. Aeroallergens may be sensed by protease-activated receptors on airway epithelial cells leading to secretion of multiple epithelial cell cytokines, including thymic stromal lymphopoietin (TSLP), interleukin (IL)-33, and IL-1. In addition, aeroallergens (*in green*) cross-link allergen-specific immunoglobulin E (IgE) on mast cells and basophils leading to immediate degranulation and release of many mediators such as prostaglandin D2 (PGD$_2$), which can act on the type 1 prostaglandin D1 receptor (DP1) or the chemokine receptor expressed by Th2 cells (CRTH2) to cause inflammation and immediate bronchoconstriction (early allergic reaction). Histamine will also cause bronchoconstriction and plasma leakage from nearby vessels. Cytokines released with PGD$_2$ will prepare the vessel wall for later extravasation of leukocytes (late allergic reaction). ASM, airway smooth muscle; HR, histamine receptor; 5HT3R, human serotonin 3 receptor; MCPs, monocyte chemoattractant proteins; NF-κB, nuclear factor-κB.

Eosinophils are major effectors of T2 asthma and act through release of toxic granules containing eosinophil peroxidase, cationic proteins, and eosinophil-derived neurotoxins.[251] Major basic protein can cause bronchial hyperreactivity by interfering with bronchoconstricting muscarinic receptors.[236] Eosinophil degranulation can alter the characteristics of airway mucus gels in asthma (Fig. 60.7). For example, *eosinophil peroxidase* catalyzes oxidation of thiocyanate (transported from the blood compartment to the airway lumen by SLC26A4 transporter/pendrin, an epithelial cell transporter) by hydrogen peroxide to generate oxidants that cross-link mucin polymers and stiffen mucus gels.[252] In addition, eosinophil-derived Charcot-Leyden crystals can stimulate mucin production, and the presence of these crystals within the mucus plugs could plausibly alter the biophysical properties in ways that decrease mucus clearance.[253] Although eosinophils are very corticosteroid sensitive in vitro by undergoing apoptosis, corticosteroid-induced apoptosis in vivo is less common. When corticosteroids reduce eosinophil numbers, therefore, they may do so via suppression of upstream cytokine networks, such as suppression of the eosinopoietins IL-5 and GM-CSF or prevention of activation of the cells producing these cytokines. Because IL-5 and GM-CSF are produced by corticosteroid-sensitive CD4+ Th2 cells in many asthmatics, corticosteroids reduce eosinophilia in most T2-high asthmatics. In patients with alternative sources of IL-5, such as ILC2s producing IL-5 in severe asthmatics with nasal polyposis, corticosteroids are not as effective, perhaps because ILC2s are more corticosteroid resistant. These patients benefit much more from therapeutic proteins that block the action of IL-5 directly or cytotoxic antibodies that directly deplete eosinophils by targeting IL-5R (and potentially Siglec8).

A consistent feature of T2-high forms of asthma in childhood and adulthood is the persistence of aberrant T2 immunity over long periods of time. Recent advances in understanding the molecular basis of "trained immunity" provide a framework to explain this persistence.[254,255] *Trained immunity* results when innate immune cells, adaptive immune cells, or epithelial stem cells display long-term changes in their functional program through metabolic and epigenetic programming. Although such memory is a mechanism of adaptive host protection, it can also be a mechanism

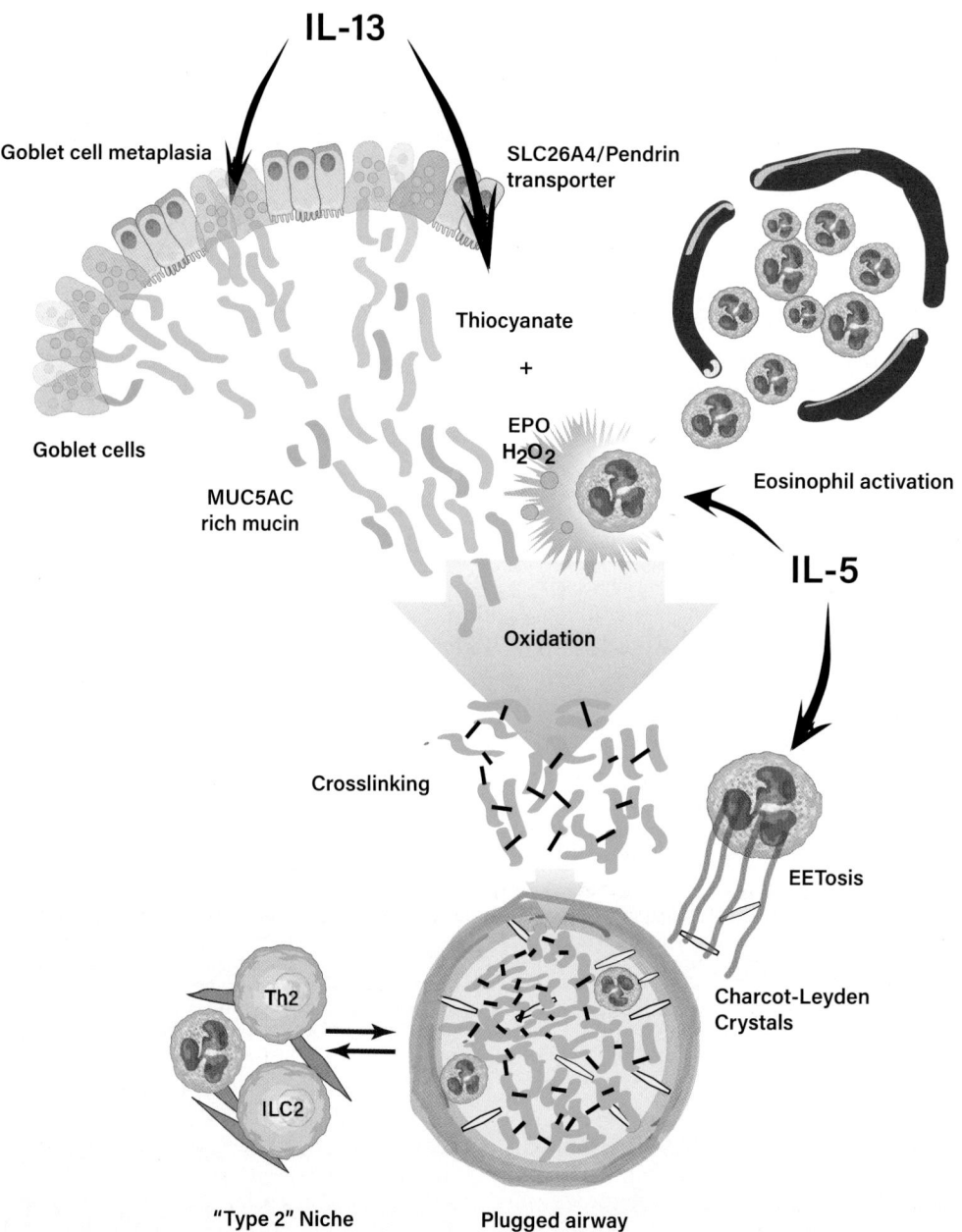

Figure 60.7 Contribution of type 2 immunity and the eosinophil to mucus plugging of the airways. Interleukin (IL)-13 from Th2 cells and from group 2 innate lymphoid cells (ILC2s) drive goblet cell metaplasia and overproduction of MUC5AC-rich mucin. IL-13 also drives expression of pendrin, a transporter protein that carries thiocyanate into the airway lining fluid. IL-5 from Th2 cells and ILC2s drives the activation of eosinophils that release eosinophil peroxidase (EPO). In the presence of H_2O_2 and thiocyanate, airway mucins get cross-linked, stiffening the elastic mucus gel and inhibiting expectoration. Profound eosinophil activation leads to eosinophilic extracellular trap cell death (EETosis), the release of DNA nets and granules coated with galectin-10, which can form Charcot-Leyden crystals (mainly observed in mucus plugs in severe acute asthma and in allergic bronchopulmonary aspergillosis). Regions with mucus plugging have intense type 2 inflammation; the remodeled airway tissue around a chronic mucus plug may form a niche for eosinophils and persistent activation of type 2 lymphocytes. MUC5AC, mucin gene 5AC; SLC26A4, solute carrier family 26, member 24.

of immune dysregulation including chronic T2 inflammation. Trained immunity can be demonstrated in vitro. For example, ex vivo cultured basal cells from the upper airways in patients with chronic rhinosinusitis with nasal polyps are known to retain intrinsic memory of IL-4/IL-13 exposure,[256] and lung epithelial cells can continue to produce GM-CSF even after prolonged culture in vitro. Thus, it is possible that

aberrant T2 immune programs in the airway in childhood-onset T2-high asthma become fixed because they are established during critical time windows in early life when the immune system and lung epithelium is plastic and susceptible to epigenetic changes. A second window may open in later life, perhaps the result of immune senescence and other age-related failures in normal immune regulation.

Because epigenetic changes persist in dividing cells, they provide a mechanism for environmental factors to cause stable alterations in phenotype without changes in genotype. The epigenome may not change uniformly in all the airways of an individual patient. For example, airway mucus plugs are a feature of T2-high asthma and have been observed in specific airways within a patient, persisting in the same airways over many years.[252] These mucus plugs mark airways with intense T2 inflammation and represent an inflammatory niche (T2 airway niche). The biology of immune niches is just beginning to be understood, but it is likely that genomic or metabolic reprogramming of airway epithelial cells, immune cells, and neuronal pathways renders T2 airway niches self-sustaining because of feed-forward reinforcing signals between the key cellular players. As understanding of this biology improves, it may be possible to provide treatments that interrupt persistent T2 inflammation in T2-high forms of asthma.

MOLECULAR ASPECTS OF T2-LOW FORMS OF ASTHMA

Many patients with asthma do not have an excess of airway eosinophils or other markers of T2 inflammation.[241–244] Because T2 inflammation is decreased by corticosteroid treatment, the common use of corticosteroids in patients with more severe forms of asthma may lead to underestimation of T2-high disease in these patients. Despite this possibility, there is consensus now that non-T2 mechanisms of disease exist in all forms of asthma and account for poor corticosteroid responsiveness and disease control in many patients. The cellular and molecular drivers of T2-low forms of asthma are uncertain, but research to date has identified a subset of patients with no inflammation signals (paucigranulocytic asthma) and other subsets with signals for T1 immunity, T3 immunity, airway neutrophilia, or systemic inflammation.

Paucigranulocytic Asthma

Granulocytes such as neutrophils and eosinophils are not always present in excess in airway secretions or tissues from patients with asthma.[257] Similarly, transcriptomic analyses of airway biopsies do not always show signals for specific pathology.[258] The lack of airway inflammation in some patients with asthma is puzzling, and it may mean that chronic inflammation is not needed for expression of phenotypic features of asthma, including smooth muscle dysfunction. In general, patients with paucigranulocytic asthma have less severe forms of asthma.

Type 1 Immunity in Asthma

T1 immunity is an important mechanism for host defense against intracellular microorganisms. By secreting *interferon* (IFN)-γ and TNF-α, the CD4+ Th1 cells, CD8+ cytotoxic T cells, and group 1 ILCs activate mononuclear phagocytes to convert them to potent effector cells. T1 immunity also plays pathogenic roles in autoimmune organ-specific disorders and may be a disease mechanism in subgroups of asthma patients as well. For example, pathway analysis of epithelial cell transcripts in mild asthma shows increased expression of IFN-stimulated genes, and there is an inverse

association between expression of these genes and reduced lung function.[259] In addition, other studies have shown that airway IFN-γ+ CD4+ T cells (Th1 cells) are more prevalent in severe asthma than in mild-to-moderate asthma.[260] Despite these findings, the role of T1 immunity as a molecular subtype of asthma and the potential for treatment of any T1 immune dysfunction to improve asthma control in targeted population has not yet been established.

Type 3 Immunity in Asthma

T3 immunity is devoted to protection against extracellular bacteria and fungi and relies on lymphocytes that produce IL-17 and/or IL-22 as signature cytokines. These lymphocytes include CD4+ Th17 cells, CD8+ Tc17 cells, and group 3 ILCs. The cooperative activity of IL-17 and IL-22 leads to upregulation of chemokines and growth factors in epithelial cells and endothelial cells, which recruit and sustain neutrophils. IL-17–mediated upregulation of proteases and growth factors in fibroblasts and other stromal cells also enhances access of neutrophils to tissues and further promotes neutrophilia. Although beneficial in combatting infection, IL-17–mediated recruitment of neutrophils and immune cells is also a mechanism of chronic inflammation and autoimmunity, and it has been implicated in the pathophysiology of diseases such as rheumatoid arthritis, psoriasis, and inflammatory bowel disease. Although data for upregulation of IL-17 in asthma are not as robust, some studies have identified subsets of asthma patients with increases in IL-17 gene signatures in airway specimens.[261] However, a clinical trial of therapeutic antibody targeting IL-17 in patients with asthma was negative,[262] casting doubt on the role of IL-17 as an important mediator of T2-low forms of asthma. It remains possible that improved selection for patients with elevated levels of IL-17 will result in better clinical trial results.

Neutrophils and Asthma

Independent of any putative role for T3 immunity in asthma, neutrophilic inflammation is considered a possible mechanism of T2-low forms of asthma. Neutrophils are an abundant cell type in airway secretions in both healthy subjects and asthmatic subjects, reflecting important roles in host defense.[263,264] The relatively large numbers of airway neutrophils even in health can make it difficult to determine when neutrophils are contributing to disease severity. In large asthma datasets, it is possible to find correlations between airway neutrophils and measures of airflow obstruction,[265,266] but other analyses that rely on neutrophil cutoffs have had less consistent results. One lesson from these studies is that the activation state of neutrophils rather than their number may be a more important indicator of the contribution of neutrophils and their products to disease severity. Possible mechanisms by which activated neutrophils could impair lung function in asthma include neutrophil-mediated oxidative stress, neutrophil protease-mediated activation of airway epithelial cells, or neutrophil protease-mediated goblet cell degranulation. In addition, *neutrophil extracellular traps* mediate inflammasome activation and IL-1β secretion from monocytes and cause airway epithelial cell injury. Indeed, high extracellular DNA concentration in sputum has been found to mark a subset of patients with more severe asthma.[267] Despite a plausible mechanism by which neutrophils can injure airways, a clinical trial targeting neutrophils did not show clinical benefit in patients with asthma.[268] It is possible that this trial was negative because it relied on neutrophil counts rather than neutrophil activation biomarkers, but it remains the case that definitive evidence linking neutrophilic inflammation to the pathogenesis of chronic asthma is lacking. Relevant here is the consistent finding of a subset of patients who have both airway eosinophilia and airway neutrophilia.[269,270] These patients are notable for having more severe disease. The mechanism for sustained combined eosinophilic and neutrophilic granulocytic inflammation is poorly understood.

Systemic Inflammation and Metabolic Dysfunction

Analyses of clinical traits in asthma cohorts show that the clusters of patients with more severe asthma typically include those who are older and those who are obese.[271] This association with age and obesity raises the possibility that systemic inflammation—common in obesity because of increased production of IL-1, IL-6, or TNF-α by white adipose tissue—could have consequences for airway function in asthma. Evidence for this possibility comes from studies showing that patients with asthma who have high plasma IL-6 levels have more severe asthma than those with normal IL-6 levels,[241] IL-6 is regulated by IL-1β so that increased IL-6 in these studies may be marking increased IL-1β activity as well. Circulating IL-1β could plausibly cause airway epithelial cell dysfunction. Studies in mice and human bronchial epithelial air-liquid interface cultures have shown that IL-1β triggers a cytokine response in epithelial cells leading to production of IL-33, TSLP, and GM-CSF.[272] The importance of systemic inflammation as a driver of organ dysfunction and cancer has recently been highlighted by successful clinical trials of IL-1β inhibition in patients at risk for cardiovascular disease and selected on the basis of high circulating IL-6. In these trials, inhibiting IL-1β using a monoclonal antibody, canakinumab, not only reduced the risk of cardiovascular events,[273] it also reduced rates of lung cancer.[273] Efforts are now underway to initiate clinical trials of IL-1β or IL-6 inhibitors in patients with asthma selected for having biomarkers of systemic inflammation. This effort marks formal acknowledgement that T2 axis cytokines are not the only cytokines that should be considered therapeutic targets in asthma.

LIPID MEDIATORS

The *cysteinyl leukotrienes* (cys-LTs) are peptide-conjugated arachidonic acid-derived inflammatory mediators generated by multiple cells, including eosinophils, basophils, mast cells, macrophages, and type 2 DCs.[274] Cys-LTs are generated in the lipid bilayer of the cell membrane when arachidonic acid is oxidized by 5-lipoxygenase in successive enzymatic conversions to generate leukotriene C_4, LTD_4, and LTE_4.[274] There are two main receptors for Cys-LTs: Cys-LT1R and Cys-LT2R. Cys-LT1R is expressed on airway smooth muscle cells and Cys-LT1R and Cys-LT2R are coexpressed on inflammatory cells, airway epithelial cells, and vascular endothelial cells. Activation of Cys-LT1Rs on smooth muscle cells induces muscle contraction, whereas

activation of Cys-LT1R and Cys-LT2R on endothelial cells increases vascular permeability. Medications targeting this pathway, including zileuton (a 5-lipoxygenase inhibitor) and montelukast/zafirlukast (selective antagonists of Cys-LT1R), are effective in asthma, especially in patients with aspirin sensitivity and Samter triad (i.e., aspirin sensitivity, nasal polyps, and asthma).[275] When these patients ingest cyclooxygenase-1 inhibitors, such as aspirin or other nonsteroid anti-inflammatory drugs, arachidonic acid metabolism is diverted away from prostanoid metabolites of arachidonate and towards excessive generation of cys-LTs. Consequently, urinary LTE_4 levels are especially high in aspirin-sensitive patients.[276]

Prostaglandins are generated by metabolism of arachidonic acid by prostaglandin synthase enzymes and cyclooxygenase. PGD_2 is the prostanoid most relevant to asthma pathogenesis. Mast cells are the most important cellular source of PGD_2, but Th2 cells, DCs, and airway epithelial cells also produce PGD_2 at relatively low levels.[277,278] There is good evidence that PGD_2 participates in airway responses to inhaled allergen in asthmatics. Allergen challenge in asthmatic patients leads to rapid and large increases in PGD_2 in bronchoalveolar lavage fluid,[279] and PGD_2 inhalation challenge causes bronchoconstriction and airway eosinophilia.[280] PGD_2 exerts its biologic effects via two receptors—*prostaglandin D1 and D2 receptors* (DP1/DP and DP2/CRTH2)—that collectively are expressed on a wide range of cells, including hematopoietic cells, DCs, epithelial cells, goblet cells, endothelial cells, and platelets.[278] Small molecule inhibitors of CRTH2 are currently in clinical trials as treatments for asthma, atopic dermatitis, and allergic rhinitis and are showing some promise.

Lipoxins are also enzyme-derived products of arachidonic acid metabolism with putative but less well-established roles in asthma. Lipoxins are derived from arachidonic acid and omega-3 fatty acids; they are counter-regulatory lipid mediators that inhibit inflammation and are rapidly inactivated.[281] Their anti-inflammatory actions include inhibition of granulocyte activation and locomotion, promotion of monocyte-derived macrophage phagocytosis of apoptotic granulocytes, blockade of T lymphocyte cytokine release, and epithelial proinflammatory cytokine and chemokine release. Lipoxin A_4 also prevents PGD_2-stimulated release of IL-13 from ILC2s.[282]

ASTHMA EXACERBATIONS AND INTERFERON BIOLOGY IN THE AIRWAY

Asthma exacerbations represent an acute worsening of airflow obstruction in the setting of chronic disease, due to worsening of airway smooth muscle contraction, airway wall edema, and luminal obstruction with mucus.[283] The mucus plug pathology reflects formation of pathologic mucus gels characterized by increases in the elastic behavior of the mucus gels with consequences including poor clearance from the airway. As a result, the airways become occluded with mucus plugs. Autopsy studies indicate that mucus-plugged airways are especially prominent in fatal and near fatal asthma.[284] Common upper respiratory tract viruses, especially rhinoviruses, are the most common and important cause of exacerbations in both children and adults.[285,286] Airway mucosal remodeling increases susceptibility to this acute reduction in airflow in asthmatics. Changes in the epithelium that increase mucin stores in airway smooth muscle that render it more hyper-reactive and in blood vessels that render them more leaky, predispose many asthmatics to exaggerated airway responses to inhaled environmental insults, such as viruses, allergens, or pollutants.[283] Asthmatic airways are hyperreactive in several ways; concentric smooth muscle contraction from hyperresponsiveness is one element, but mucosal edema from vascular permeability and excess mucus from mucin hypersecretion are others. The efficacy of corticosteroids in preventing exacerbations likely relates to their effects not only in reducing inflammatory cell numbers (especially eosinophils) but also through improvements in pathologic changes to goblet cells, smooth muscle cells, and blood vessels.

Viral infections are among the most important of the environmental stimuli implicated in asthma initiation. Airway epithelial cells are considered active sentinels and master coordinators of antiviral responses in the lung, usually mediated by IFNs. There are three distinct IFN families.[287] The type I IFN family mainly comprises IFN-α subtypes and IFN-β. The type II IFN family consists of just IFN-γ. The type III IFN family comprises IFN-λ subtypes with similar functions to type I IFN cytokines but restricted activity because their receptor is restricted to epithelial cell surfaces. Type I IFNs are important for host defense against viruses, and it has been hypothesized that dysregulation of IFNs in the airway may promote virus-induced exacerbations. Indeed, it has been shown that rhinovirus-induced IFN-λ induction is deficient in epithelial cells and alveolar macrophages from asthmatics.[288,289] However, it is not clear whether these impaired IFN responses represent a feature of asthma or an effect of treatment. For example, corticosteroids—frequently used to treat asthma—impair IFN responses,[290] and suppression of IFNs by corticosteroids during virus-induced exacerbations of airway disease may be a mechanism of infection and exacerbation risk. Also, mice deficient in the type I IFN-α/β receptor have suppressed antimicrobial peptide and enhanced mucin responses to rhinovirus infection.[290] These data have provided rationale for inhaled IFN-β therapy to prevent exacerbations, but preliminary reports of the efficacy of this approach in asthma have not been encouraging. Much more encouraging have been the beneficial effects of therapeutic proteins targeting T2 immunity (IgE, IL-4Rα, and IL-5 pathways) on asthma exacerbation rates. Notably, genetic polymorphisms in *IL4RA* are associated with a history of severe asthma exacerbations.[291] Potential mechanistic explanations include reversal of the inhibitory effect of T2 cytokines on production of type I IFNs, or improvement of inflammatory and remodeling features of asthma that render asthmatics more susceptible to viral infection, or exacerbations in general. Related to this, mice infected with influenza and mild asthmatics experimentally infected with rhinovirus produce IL-33 that subsequently suppresses production of type I IFN and antiviral immunity.[292] Omalizumab reverses the inhibitory effect that IgE has on production of type I IFNs by plasmacytoid DCs, a mechanism that may explain how it reduces exacerbation frequency.[293]

PHENOTYPING

ASTHMA HETEROGENEITY

By definition, all asthmatics manifest either airflow limitation on spirometry with a significant response to bronchodilators or airway hyperresponsiveness to specific or nonspecific challenge, as well as symptoms that include shortness of breath, chest tightness, wheeze, and cough. Nonetheless, patients with asthma can have a great deal of heterogeneity with respect to severity of airflow limitation, symptoms, degree of reversibility, and therapeutic response. In up to 45% of asthmatics, lung function does not improve with high doses of *inhaled corticosteroids* (ICS).[294,295] Furthermore, there is significant heterogeneity in asthma triggers, the frequency and severity of exacerbations, and long-term outcomes such as progressive loss of lung function.

Several approaches have been taken to assign asthmatics to distinct sub-phenotypes. Simple categories based on degree of airway obstruction on spirometry or frequency of symptoms and rescue medication use have been in national guidelines for asthma classification and care,[296] but these categories do not provide insight into molecular or cellular mechanisms. These guidelines have been instrumental in public health efforts to improve asthma education and care through the promotion of ICS use, but a better appreciation of disease heterogeneity at a molecular and cellular level will be important in treating severe asthma and in the clinical application of emerging asthma therapies.

CELLULAR PHENOTYPES

Analyses of sputum, bronchoalveolar lavage, and endobronchial biopsy specimens from living asthmatics and postmortem samples from those who died with asthma have found that the majority of asthmatics have elevated eosinophils.[297] However, not all asthmatics have eosinophils in their sputum and, based on analysis of induced sputum samples, non-eosinophilic asthma may be seen in up to 73% of asthmatics not on treatment and 50% of those on treatment[298] Non-eosinophilic asthma responds poorly to ICS.[244,299–301] Furthermore, non-eosinophilic asthma is seen across a range of asthma severity and, in those with severe asthma, has been associated with fewer mast cells, and less sub-epithelial fibrosis (i.e., airway remodeling).[302] These observations and others have led to a cellular classification of asthma based on induced sputum cytologic analysis with four categories: (1) eosinophilic (often defined as >2–3% in induced sputum), (2) neutrophilic (>60–75%), (3) mixed eosinophilic and neutrophilic, and (4) paucigranulocytic asthma, which lacks observable inflammatory cells.[269,298,303,304] Eosinophilia is most commonly seen in classic atopic asthma with allergen-induced inflammation. Patients with eosinophilia, except for severe cases, generally respond well to ICSs with reduced eosinophils, airway obstruction, and symptoms.[298,305–307] Neutrophilia has been noted in asthmatics with acute and chronic infection, obesity, smoking, and irritant exposure such as pollutants,[298] in subsets of patients with severe asthma,[302] and during acute asthma exacerbations.[263] Neutrophilia is also associated with reduced forced expiratory volume in 1

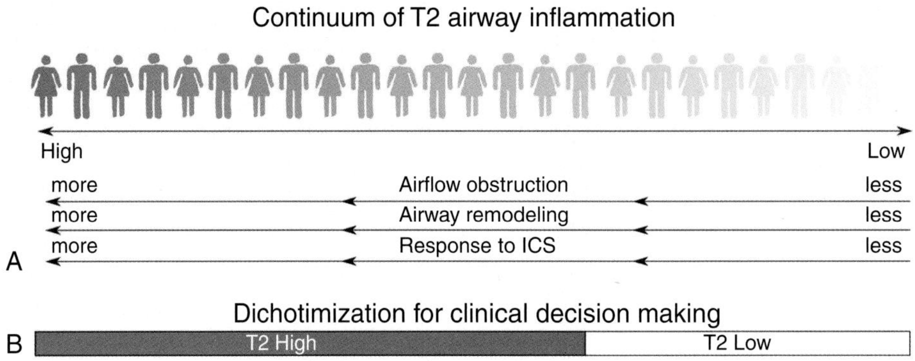

Continuum of T2 airway inflammation

Figure 60.8 **Molecular phenotypes (endotypes) in asthma.** (A) Type 2 (T2)-driven inflammation is a dominant inflammatory signal in asthma. Nonetheless, across individuals, there is a continuum of T2 inflammation ranging from high levels of T2 inflammation to very low levels, approaching the baseline activity found in healthy controls. Higher T2 inflammation is associated with greater airflow obstruction and airway remodeling, and a greater improvement in lung function with inhaled corticosteroids. The long-term temporal stability of these phenotypes is not yet known. (B) The level of T2 inflammation can guide the use of targeted therapies by dichotomizing individuals to either T2-high or T2-low groups.

second, independent of the presence of eosinophils.[266,308] Mixed neutrophilia and eosinophilia have been reported in refractory asthma. One study found that subjects with mixed neutrophilia and eosinophilia had the lowest lung function, highest frequency of daily wheeze, and highest health care utilization.[269]

MOLECULAR PHENOTYPES (ENDOTYPES)

Subgrouping asthma based on the activity of specific molecular pathways has the advantage of pointing to specific pharmaceutical targets and biomarkers for clinical trials of targeted pharmaceuticals. Subgroups of patients who share an underlying disease biology have been named *endotypes*.

T2-High Endotype

One such endotype emerged from a study that analyzed the expression levels of three epithelial genes that serve as surrogate markers of inflammation associated with T2 cytokines, especially IL-13.[220] These three genes, *periostin, CLCA1,* and *serpinB2*, were identified using genome-wide profiling of airway epithelial brushing obtained at bronchoscopy.[309] In this study, nearly half of subjects with mild to moderate asthma were indistinguishable from healthy controls based upon the expression of these three genes in epithelial brushings. This suggested that this population of asthmatics was heterogeneous; some had T2-high inflammation and others T2-low inflammation. In subsequent analyses, T2-high asthma showed exaggerated airway hyperresponsiveness (based on the PC_{20} methacholine test), serum IgE levels, and both blood and especially bronchoalveolar lavage eosinophilia.[220] T2-high subjects also had greater sub-epithelial fibrosis, differences in epithelial mucin gene expression (higher *MUC5AC/MUC5B* ratio), and higher numbers of intra-epithelial mast cells.[310] In a randomized placebo-controlled trial of ICS in this same study, those in the T2-high endotype showed improved lung function with ICS, whereas those in the T2-low endotype did not. Although these analyses suggest distinct endotypes of asthma based on degree of T2 inflammation and dichotomous classification of subjects can be clinically useful, the degree of T2 inflammation present in subjects with asthma can alternatively be seen as a continuum (Fig. 60.8).

Across a range of asthma studies and severity, the group of individuals with high levels of T2 cytokines represents 30–70% of asthmatics and is enriched for chronic rhinosinusitis with nasal polyps, atopic dermatitis, more bronchodilator reversibility, and airway mucus plugging as seen on chest computed tomography scans.[252,311,312] Aspirin-exacerbated asthma as well as allergic bronchopulmonary aspergillosis are also associated with high levels of T2 inflammation. Eosinophils are usually present in the blood and sputum of those with elevated levels of T2 inflammation in the airways, a process driven by IL-5. These eosinophils likely contribute to many of the clinical associations, including mucus plugs. An increased level of T2 inflammation can be found across the age spectrum and, when it persists despite high doses of ICS or systemic corticosteroids, it is associated with older age and more airflow obstruction and exacerbations.[312] Thus, although T2 airway inflammation is generally associated with a favorable response to corticosteroids, a number of patients with severe asthma on adequate corticosteroid treatment have persistent, or refractory, T2 inflammation.

The many clinical implications of the T2 endotype have led to the study of potential noninvasive biomarkers. Sputum eosinophils have the best performance, which may be better with repeated determinations.[244,312,313] However, sputum induction and the accurate quantification of eosinophils is limited to specialized centers, and not all patients can produce an acceptable sample for analysis. Fortunately, although blood eosinophil levels are not in perfect correlation with sputum measures, they track well enough with eosinophilic airway inflammation to be a clinically useful biomarker in a number of trials of ICSs and monoclonal antibodies targeting T2 cytokines.[244,314,315] Generally, the number of eosinophils per microliter of blood has been studied. Although blood eosinophil count tracks with airway inflammation and treatment response in a continuous manner, a large range of cutoffs has been proposed to guide clinical management. For example, large treatment trials of monoclonal antibodies targeting the IL-5 pathway used blood eosinophil cutoffs ranging from 150 to 400/μL.[314,316,317] In morbidly obese individuals, blood eosinophils may not accurately reflect airway T2 inflammation.[312] Serum IgE levels poorly reflect airway

T2 inflammation, though they may have value in younger patients.[311,312,318]

Measurement of the *fraction of nitric oxide in exhaled breath* (FeNO) is an alternative noninvasive biomarker of T2 airway inflammation in asthma. FeNO levels are increased in asthma[319,320] and are highly reproducible.[321] In the setting of T2 cytokine-driven airway inflammation, cells such as eosinophils and epithelial cells can increase NO production in part through increased transcription of inducible NO synthase. Although there is a strong rationale for the use of FeNO as an asthma biomarker, the results of clinical trials that apply FeNO to guide treatment have been mixed. Possible reasons for the mixed performance of FeNO in these clinical studies include high sensitivity but poor specificity for eosinophilic inflammation based on the cutoff selected in specific studies,[322] the existence of non-eosinophilic T2-high asthma, the use of fixed rather than age and sex-adjusted cutoffs, and confounding by comorbidities that influence FeNO such as nasal polyps.[323]

T2-Low Asthma

Individuals with asthma but without elevated T2 airway inflammation have poor response to existing therapies and represent a major unmet need. In general, T2-low asthma is associated with less severe airflow obstruction and exacerbation frequency compared to T2-high asthma. However, these patients often have symptoms that are refractory to treatment. Mechanisms for T2-low asthma may be unique to T2-low asthma or may be present across a spectrum of T2 inflammation (see Fig. 60.8). Some of these mechanisms may reflect a consequence of corticosteroid treatment. Therefore, the study of non-T2 mechanisms has the potential to produce novel therapies that also help patients with T2-high asthma, particularly those resistant to existing T2-directed treatments.

Although specific molecular mechanisms of T2-low asthma remain elusive, some clues have emerged from studies of gene transcripts and immune cells in airway biospecimens from patients with T2-low asthma. In T2-low asthma, gene expression studies of cells obtained from induced sputum have revealed gene signatures indicative of mitochondrial oxidative stress, inflammasome-activation (with increased sputum IL-1β), and reduced CD8+ T cell cytotoxicity.[324–326] IL-17 and other cytokines such as IL-6 may also be important. Bronchoalveolar lavage samples from patients with asthma and uncharacterized T2 status have shown increased numbers of IL-17A-producing cells[327–330]; there was evidence of Th17 activity through identification of specific Th17 cells, and IL-17A/F was found in human airway tissue.[331–335] In general, higher levels of IL-17 are associated with more airway neutrophilia. However, transcriptional profiling of epithelial brushings and induced sputum cells has not consistently shown more IL-17–related inflammation in asthma compared to health.[336–338] These findings, the absence of IL-17–driven signatures in other studies, and a negative clinical trial of an anti–IL-17 receptor monoclonal antibody—albeit in a population not selected for high biomarker levels—make the relevance of this pathway in asthma uncertain.[262] Elevated plasma IL-6 is present in both T2-low and -high asthma, probably reflects systemic inflammation, and is associated with obesity.[241] Heightened IL-6-mediated signaling in epithelial cells was associated with more barrier dysfunction, airway inflammation, and more exacerbations.[339] Other studies have suggested a role for Th1 cells and IFN-driven inflammation,

dysbiosis, and neutrophil extracellular traps.[260,267,340–342] Impaired resolution of inflammation by natural killer cells may also contribute to airway inflammation across the spectrum of T2 airway inflammation.[343] The transition of these potential non-T2 pathways into asthma endotypes awaits successful coupling to targeted therapies.

Noninflammatory mechanisms may also contribute to T2-low endotypes of asthma (see Fig. 60.8).[327–335,344–354] Airway hyperresponsiveness is in part the result of an abnormal airway smooth muscle response to mediators of contraction such as histamine and acetylcholine. Although a proinflammatory cytokine milieu and infiltration of smooth muscle with inflammatory cells are likely a major influence on abnormal airway smooth muscle contraction, intrinsic abnormalities in the signal transduction or contractile functions of smooth muscle cells in human asthma are relatively less well studied. Because a role for airway smooth muscle hyperplasia or hypertrophy has been demonstrated in patients with asthma,[221,355] abnormal accumulation of smooth muscle and increased airway narrowing on that basis represents another possible noninflammatory mechanism for increased airway hyperresponsiveness in asthma. Epithelial barrier dysfunction, neuronal abnormalities, and underlying disturbances in mucin production and characteristics may also interact with inflammation or smooth muscle pathology to contribute to an asthma phenotype.

Key Points

- Asthma is a common disease, and its prevalence has increased throughout the world for the past several decades.
- Studies of the epidemiology, natural history, and pathogenesis demonstrate that asthma is a heterogeneous disease, with multiple etiologies and contributing cofactors, complex pathobiologic mechanisms, and diverse molecular phenotypes.
- Genetic variation has major effects on asthma susceptibility and represents the effects of many different genes that are polymorphic or undergo epigenetic regulation.
- Family-based studies provided the first clues about the polygenic nature of asthma; however, subsequent biologic candidate gene studies and larger genome-wide association studies have resulted in discoveries of important susceptibility and disease-modifying loci.
- The clinical heterogeneity of asthma may be explained by different underlying mechanisms. For example, *type 2* (T2) inflammation is associated with eosinophils, greater airflow obstruction, and airway remodeling including mucus plugging. However, the degree of T2 inflammation varies across individuals, ranging from high levels (T2-high asthma) to low or absent levels (T2-low asthma).
- The recognition that asthma is heterogeneous and comprises molecular phenotypes, or endotypes, has led to the development of targeted therapies and of biomarkers that can identify those who will respond to these treatments. Nonetheless, T2-low asthma does not respond well to existing therapies and non-T2 mechanisms are an important focus of research.

Key Readings

Bush A. Pathophysiological mechanisms of asthma. *Front Pediatr.* 2019;7:68.

Carr TF, Kraft M. Use of biomarkers to identify phenotypes and endotypes of severe asthma. *Ann Allergy Asthma Immunol.* 2018;121(4): 414–420.

Daya M, Rafaels N, Brunetti TM, et al. Association study in African-admixed populations across the Americas recapitulates asthma risk loci in non-African populations. *Nature Commun.* 2019;10:880.

Fahy JV. Type 2 inflammation in asthma--present in most, absent in many. *Nat Rev Immunol.* 2015;15(1):57–65.

Global Asthma Network. *The Global Asthma Report;* 2018. http://www.globalasthmareport.org/.

Lambrecht BN, Hammad H, Fahy JV. The cytokines of asthma. *Immunity.* 2019;50(4):975–991.

Moffatt MF, Kabesch M, Liang L, et al. Genetic variants regulating ORMDL3 expression contribute to the risk of childhood asthma. *Nature.* 2007;448:470–473.

Ober C. Asthma genetics in the post-GWAS era. *Ann Am Thorac Soc.* 2016;13(suppl 1):S85–90.

Ortega VE, Meyers DA. Pharmacogenetics: implications of race and ethnicity on defining genetic profiles for personalized medicine. *J Allergy Clin Immunol.* 2014;133:16–26.

Shrine N, Portelli MA, John C, et al. Moderate-to-severe asthma in individuals of european ancestry: a genome-wide association study. *Lancet Respir Med.* 2019;7:20–34.

Strachan DP. Hay fever, hygiene, and household size. *BMJ.* 1989;299(6710):1259–1260.

Torgerson DG, Ampleford EJ, Chiu GY, et al. Meta-analysis of genome-wide association studies of asthma in ethnically diverse North American populations. *Nat Genet.* 2011;43:887–892.

von Mutius E, Martinez FD, Fritzsch C, Nicolai T, Roell G, Thiemann HH. Prevalence of asthma and atopy in two areas of West and East Germany. *Am J Respir Crit Care Med.* 1994;149(2 Pt 1):358–364.

Woodruff PG, Modrek B, Choy DF, Jia G, Abbas AR, Ellwanger A, Koth LL, Arron JR, Fahy JV. T-helper type 2-driven inflammation defines major subphenotypes of asthma. *Am J Respir Crit Care Med.* 2009;180(5):388–395. Erratum in: Am J Respir Crit Care Med. 2009;15;180(8):796.

Complete reference list available at ExpertConsult.com.

61 ASTHMA AND OBESITY

ANNE E. DIXON, MA, BM, BCH • MICHAEL C. PETERS, MD, MAS

INTRODUCTION

Obesity is a growing global epidemic. The obesity epidemic has fundamentally shifted the burden of chronic disease in the developed world, and being overweight or obese is now the fifth leading risk factor for death worldwide.[1,2] Obesity, defined as a *body mass index* (BMI) measurement greater than 30 kg/m^2, is particularly common in the United States, where 40% of adults and 21% of adolescents are obese.[3]

Obesity is remarkably common in patients with asthma,[4–6] raising the possibility that obesity plays an important role in the development and pathobiology of asthma. The observation that obesity and asthma are common comorbidities was initially described in a cohort study of nurses in the United States. Camargo et al. found that obese women ages 26 to 46 years had a threefold increased risk of developing asthma over 4 years compared with lean women.[4] These findings were confirmed in a large meta-analysis demonstrating that asthma incidence increased by 50% in overweight/obese individuals compared to normal-weight individuals.[7] Similar data have been reported in children; obese children have an 18–38% increased risk of developing asthma when compared to healthy weight children. These findings suggest that up to 25% of new asthma cases in children are related to obesity.[8]

This increased asthma incidence in obese patients results in an asthma prevalence significantly higher in people with obesity than in those with normal weight. In the United States, the prevalence of asthma in lean, overweight, and obese adults is 7.1%, 7.8%, and 11.1%, respectively.[9] The association between BMI and asthma is remarkably pronounced in patients with severe obesity; the frequency of asthma in patients with a BMI greater than 60 may be greater than 30%.[10]

There is a sex disparity in the prevalence of asthma between obese men and women. Asthma rates are higher in overweight (9.1%) and obese (14.6%) women compared to lean women (7.9%). However, in men, these differences in asthma prevalence across obese subgroups may be less pronounced; obese men suffer from asthma at a frequency (7.1%) only slightly higher than lean men (6.1%).[9] This observation that the interaction between obesity and asthma is more pronounced in female patients has been observed in some, but not all, asthma studies[7,10–12] and has led to the hypothesis that obese female patients exhibit a unique asthma phenotype.[11]

The relationship between obesity and asthma is bidirectional; obesity is a risk factor for the development of asthma, and asthma is also a risk factor for the development of obesity. Studies in children with early-onset allergic asthma show that asthma at the age of 4 years approximately doubles the risk of developing obesity by the age of 8 years.[13] Thus obesity likely causes asthma in some patients and is a complication associated with asthma in others. These epidemiologic links between asthma and obesity are striking; the reasons for the association are multifactorial.

PATHOPHYSIOLOGY

The excessive accumulation of visceral adipose tissue results in two important metabolic derangements collectively called *metabolic dysfunction* (Fig. 61.1). The first is a state of chronic low-grade systemic inflammation (meta-inflammation) characterized by increased blood levels of a variety of pro-inflammatory cytokines, including *interleukin* (IL)-6, IL-1, tumor necrosis factor-α, and leptin.[14] The second is insulin resistance seen when cells in muscle, fat, and liver tissue fail to respond appropriately to insulin.[15] This impaired insulin sensitivity requires the pancreas to secrete additional insulin to enable glucose uptake into cells. This cycle leads to higher levels of insulin and glucose in the systemic circulation, which, if unchecked, progresses to diabetes.[16] These two principal features of metabolic dysfunction are established risk factors for the development of cardiovascular disease, neurovascular disease, renal failure, and certain types of cancer.[14] Until recently, the association between features of metabolic dysfunction and asthma was poorly understood (see Fig. 61.1). Lately, studies measuring systemic IL-6 protein levels in asthma have repeatedly demonstrated that increases in systemic IL-6 are associated with features of more severe asthma, including lower lung function,

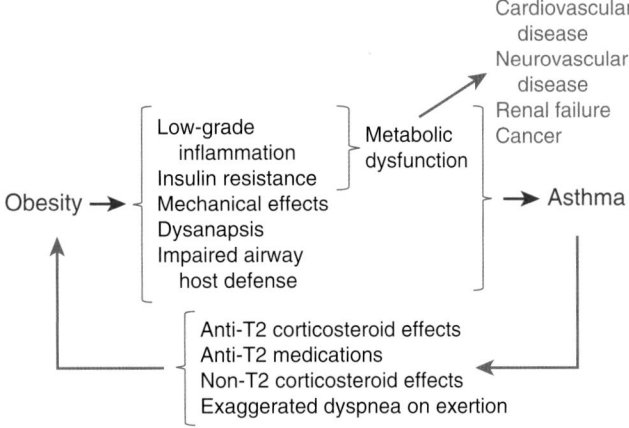

Figure 61.1 The interaction of obesity and asthma. Excessive visceral adipose tissue deposition leads to both chronic low-grade systemic inflammation and insulin resistance, characteristic of metabolic dysfunction. The various effects of obesity lead to multiple disease states and are now appreciated as risk factors for asthma. In turn, asthma and its therapies are recognized to increase the risk for obesity.

worse asthma symptoms, and higher asthma exacerbation rates.[17,18] These patients with high plasma IL-6 levels are also characterized by other features of metabolic dysfunction, including high rates of hypertension, diabetes, and increased BMI, suggesting that asthma and airway disease are made worse by the associated metabolic dysfunction.[17] However, whereas this association between metabolic dysfunction and more severe asthma is now well established, the principal pathologic abnormality linking metabolic dysfunction to asthma severity remains unknown.

OBESITY AND INHIBITION OF TYPE 2 INFLAMMATION

Increases in airway *type 2* (T2) inflammation is the most well-established pathobiologic mechanism in asthma.[19] One of the essential functions of the T2 immune response is to control parasitic infections, but this response is also increasingly recognized as an important regulator of organism homeostasis and metabolism. For example, IL-33 promotes adipose tissue T2 innate lymphoid cells to secrete IL-5, which in turn leads to adipose tissue eosinophilia and activation of alternatively activated macrophages.[20,21] Classically activated macrophages play key roles in the recognition and elimination of microbes.[22] However, in the presence of eosinophils and the canonical T2 cytokines IL-4 and IL-13, macrophages shift to an alternatively activated macrophage phenotype.[20,23] Alternatively activated macrophages are important in eliminating parasitic infections, but they also function to maintain visceral adipose tissue homeostasis via lipolysis, maintenance of insulin sensitivity, and induction of thermogenesis.[20,24,25] Thus, immune cells responsible for orchestrating the T2 immune response are also protective against the development of obesity. Conversely, obesity leads to a shift in adipose tissue macrophages from an alternatively activated macrophage to classically activated macrophage phenotype.[20,26] This transition results in the chronic low-grade systemic inflammation associated with obesity and metabolic dysfunction. Furthermore, the role of the IL-33/innate lymphoid cell-2 axis and metabolism is not limited to the effect of IL-33 in

adipose tissue. It is now known that IL-33 impacts whole body metabolism by induction of nonshivering thermogenesis, an increase in metabolic heat production not caused by muscle activity and thought to be a mechanism opposing obesity. Treatment with IL-33 promotes pancreatic insulin production and glucose clearance.[21,24] These findings demonstrate a pivotal role of the T2 immune system in maintaining visceral tissue homeostasis and suggest that medications that inhibit T2 inflammation (such as corticosteroids or new anti-T2 biologic agents) might lead to increases in obesity and metabolic dysfunction. Thus, one potential mechanistic link between obesity and asthma is by treatment with asthma drugs. Principally, medications that reduce airway T2 inflammation might promote obesity and metabolic dysfunction by decreasing the homeostatic role of T2 inflammation in adipose tissue (eFig. 61.1).

OBESITY AND NON–TYPE 2 MECHANISMS OF ASTHMA

In addition to the potential link between the inhibition of T2 inflammation and obesity, it is likely that obesity impacts airway immunity via non-T2 pathways. In fact, human studies investigating the association between biomarkers of T2 inflammation and obesity conclude that T2 biomarkers are either no different or lower in obese asthma subjects compared to nonobese asthma subjects.[11,12,27] These findings suggest that both T2 and non-T2 mechanisms contribute to disease in patients with obese asthma.

Unfortunately, non-T2 mechanisms of asthma remain poorly understood, and thus a thorough understanding of how non-T2 inflammation alters obese asthma remains an area of significant uncertainty. However, one of the more intriguing possibilities is that obesity and metabolic dysfunction lead to impairments of airway host defense. This hypothesis is substantiated by the recent observation that metabolic dysfunction increases the risk of developing severe respiratory viral illnesses such as COVID-19 and influenza.[28,29] Recent work suggests a similar susceptibility in asthma in which obesity and metabolic dysfunction increase the risk of developing exacerbation-prone asthma.[31,32] The molecular underpinning for why obesity leads to more severe or more frequent viral illness is unclear, but multiple immune cells involved in initiating adaptive immune responses are impaired in obesity. Specifically, cytotoxic T lymphocytes (natural killer cells and CD8+ T cells) are essential for identifying and eliminating cells infected by virus or cells that have undergone malignant transformation.[33–35] Obesity can result in cytotoxic T cell dysfunction and an impaired ability of these cells to eliminate infected cells or cells that have undergone malignant transformation.[35] This dysfunction of cytotoxic T lymphocytes increases susceptibility to viral infections and encourages tumor progression.[35,36] This impairment has been demonstrated in asthma and, compared to lean asthmatics, obese asthmatics have alterations in natural killer cell function and decreases in airway gene expression signals for cytotoxic T lymphocytes.[27,37] Further work is needed to confirm the role of cytotoxic T lymphocytes in the obese asthma phenotype, but it is possible that impairments in host immune defense could explain the increase in asthma exacerbation rates in obese asthma patients and their increased susceptibility to viral upper respiratory infections[31,32] (see eFig. 61.1).

IMPACT OF OBESITY ON PULMONARY AND ASTHMA PHYSIOLOGY

Obese patients breathe at decreased lung volumes because mechanical loading of the chest wall and abdomen with adipose tissue decreases *functional residual capacity* (FRC), the point at which elastic outward recoil of the chest wall is in equilibrium with the inward recoil of the lungs[38] (Fig. 61.2; see also Chapter 131 and Fig. 131.12). At low lung volumes, airway diameter is smaller; thus, breathing at low lung volumes means an increased work of breathing. Obese individuals can have the sensation of dyspnea even without increased airway responsiveness. Because of increased airway closure at the bases, obese individuals may direct more of the initial breath to the apices (see Chapter 10). Such differences in air distribution can affect the regional delivery of methacholine for testing and the delivery of inhaled medications.

Studies in normal volunteers suggest that breathing at low lung volumes (without taking deep breaths) may increase airway reactivity,[39] leading to speculation that breathing at low lung volumes instigates airway reactivity in patients with obesity.[40] However, many obese people with a decreased FRC do not have asthma. Also, in studies in mice, increased airway reactivity in obese compared with lean mice is independent of lung volume.[41] Furthermore, while the negative association with FRC and BMI is uniform in obese people, the relationship between BMI and airway reactivity is significantly more heterogeneous.[42] Thus, whereas reduced lung volume may modulate airway reactivity, it does not completely account for the relationship between asthma and obesity.[43,44]

Obese patients with asthma demonstrate unique physiologic characteristics. These unique traits suggest that the physiology of asthma in obesity differs from that in lean individuals. For example, weight loss in obese patients with asthma is associated with improvements in peripheral lung compliance, suggesting that obese asthma patients have predominantly small airway disease.[45] The physiologic characteristics of airway reactivity itself differ in obese compared with lean patients; obese patients develop greater dynamic hyperinflation (air trapping) than lean patients during bronchoconstriction. This air trapping suggests that small airway closure limits exhalation to produce progressive air trapping and increased work of breathing in obese patients.[46] In addition, the closing index—the degree of airway closure relative to airway narrowing during induced bronchoconstriction—increases in patients with obesity[47,48] and, related to this, sensitivity to airway closure (measured by the dose of methacholine required to produce a given amount of closure) improves significantly with weight loss surgery.[49] Asthma in obese adults affects peripheral airway function, increasing the tendency towards airway closure and air trapping during bronchoconstriction.

Superimposed upon altered airway function may be anomalies related to altered growth patterns in those with childhood-onset obesity. Obesity in children is associated with an increase in FVC relative to *forced expiratory volume in 1 second* (FEV$_1$) (a phenomenon known as *dysanapsis*, or a discrepancy in size due to a greater growth of the lungs than of the airways). This growth pattern produces a decrease in the FEV$_1$/FVC ratio and contributes to the development of airflow limitation.[50,51] How abnormalities in airway growth related to obesity affect airway function in adults with lifelong obesity is not yet known, but will require longitudinal studies to address this question.

CLINICAL FEATURES

Asthma in obese patients tends to be more severe than asthma in lean patients.[11] Studies in the United States of patients with severe asthma report that nearly 60% of people with severe asthma are obese.[52] One manifestation of this is the increased risk of asthma exacerbations in obese compared with lean patients,[53] and the twofold to fourfold risk of requiring hospitalization.[54,55] Among those hospitalized for asthma, obese patients have a higher risk of requiring mechanical ventilation or noninvasive ventilation for respiratory support, and a longer hospital stay.[56] Obese asthma patients frequently have increased asthma

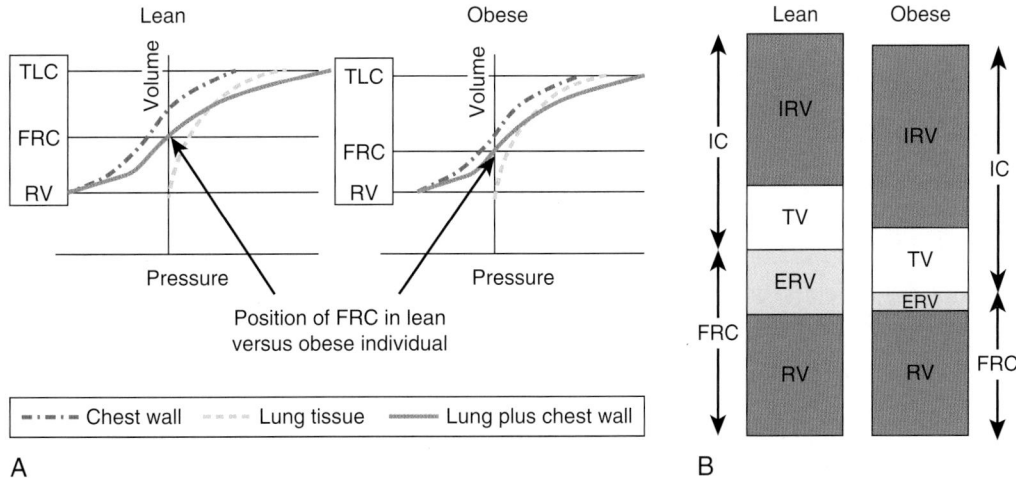

Figure 61.2 **Mechanics of the thorax in lean and obese state.** (A) Pressure-volume relationship of chest wall and lung in the lean and obese states. The volume of the lung within the chest *(brown line)* is determined by the balance between the recoil pressure of the chest wall *(blue dotted line)* and that of the lung tissue *(green dotted line)*. In the obese state, the chest wall is weighted with adipose tissue, and this reduces the resting volume of the lung (the *functional residual capacity* [FRC], *arrows*). (B) Overall effect of pressure-volume relationship on lung volumes in lean and obese state. In the obese state, *expiratory reserve volume* (ERV) and FRC are particularly decreased. IC, inspiratory capacity; IRV, inspiratory reserve volume; RV, residual volume; TLC, total lung capacity; TV, tidal volume.

Table 61.1   Factors Contributing to Increased Asthma Severity in Obese Patients

Altered physiology (e.g., decreased functional residual capacity, dysanapsis)

Lower baseline lung function

Increased risk of infection

Altered response to infection

Impaired response to medications

Comorbidities

Table 61.2   Comorbidities That May Contribute to Asthma Severity in Obese Patients

Gastroesophageal reflux

Obstructive sleep apnea

Depression

Nasal polyposis

Table 61.3   Treatment of Asthma in Obesity

Standard asthma medications*

Treatment of comorbidities

Dietary intervention

Lifestyle weight loss interventions (including exercise)

Bariatric surgery

*Note that response to bronchodilators and inhaled corticosteroids may be decreased. Systemic steroids should be avoided if at all possible. Also note that anti-T2 therapies may worsen obesity.

symptoms and worse asthma control; obese patients have increased asthma symptoms during both the day and night and increased rescue use of short-acting β-agonists compared to nonobese people with asthma.[57]

Many factors likely contribute to increased severity and worse control (Table 61.1). One factor may be that, at baseline, obese patients have reduced lung function[47] compared to lean patients. This decrease in lung function results in less pulmonary reserve during illness. However, as previously discussed, these spirometric decrements in lung function are unlikely to explain the entire role of obesity as a mechanism for asthma severity.

Another important factor may be the increased risk of—and worse outcomes related to—respiratory infections, as previously mentioned.[58] For example, compared to lean individuals, obese individuals are more likely to develop influenza infection despite vaccination and have worse outcomes following influenza infection.[59,60] This may explain why obese adults with asthma who experience a respiratory tract infection are nearly three times more likely to require systemic corticosteroids than lean patients.[31] Furthermore, obese asthma patients demonstrate labile asthma control and are more likely to self-report viruses as the cause of their asthma exacerbations.[32] Interestingly, obese children do not appear to have the same susceptibility to more severe asthma during respiratory tract infections, suggesting that a factor related to aging as well as obesity may explain the predilection to worse outcomes in adults with asthma and respiratory tract infections.[31]

Other factors possibly contributing to increased severity and worse control are altered responses to medications and the presence of comorbidities, which are discussed in detail below.

DIAGNOSTIC EVALUATION

PHARMACEUTICAL INTERVENTIONS

The general pharmacologic approach to patients with asthma is similar whether they are obese or not, and many obese asthma patients can be managed according to conventional asthma medication algorithms. Some obese patients may not respond as well as lean patients to medications[61,62]; this impaired response likely reflects slightly lower rates of T2 inflammation in patient populations with obesity[11] and perhaps some intrinsic biologic differences in obese patients. However, overall differences in treatment response rates are relatively small and generally should not alter the initial treatment approach.

Comorbidities may be particularly important in obese patients (Table 61.2). Many obese patients have comorbid conditions related to obesity, including gastroesophageal reflux, obstructive sleep apnea, and depression, as well as comorbidities seen in lean severe asthma patients, such as nasal polyposis. Treating underlying comorbid conditions is particularly important in effective management of the obese asthma patient (Table 61.3).

MEDICATION RESPONSE TO CONVENTIONAL ASTHMA MEDICATIONS IN OBESE ASTHMA PATIENTS

Rescue medications are important in asthma management, but obese asthma patients may be less likely to respond appropriately to bronchodilator treatment. Obese Black and Hispanic children with asthma are less likely to respond to bronchodilators than their lean counterparts,[63] and obese adults with asthma have smaller improvements in FEV$_1$ with short-acting β-agonists than lean adults.[64]

Many studies report impaired responses both to inhaled corticosteroids and to combination therapy with inhaled corticosteroids and long-acting β-agonists in older children and adults who are obese.[62,65–68] Response to long-acting muscarinic antagonists, at least in terms of lung function, appears to be similar in lean and obese patients with asthma.[66] However, effects of long-acting muscarinic antagonists on asthma control and asthma exacerbations in obese individuals with asthma have not been reported. One intriguing finding is that, for unclear reasons, obese patients can have a paradoxical response to theophylline, with increased exacerbations in obese patients on theophylline compared with placebo.[70] Thus, the response rate to conventional controller medications may be slightly altered in the setting of obesity.

These differences in treatment effects are similar to differences observed between individuals with T2-high and

T2-low asthma phenotypes—fewer obese patients may be responsive because fewer obese patients have T2-high disease.[11,12] Other factors that might decrease response rates to traditional asthma medications include differences in deposition of inhaled medication due to altered ventilatory patterns,[71] changes in medication pharmacokinetics,[72] and impaired induction of anti-inflammatory pathways in response to corticosteroids.[67]

MEDICATION RESPONSE TO ASTHMA BIOLOGICS IN OBESE ASTHMA PATIENTS

Treatment of obese patients with anti-T2 biologic agents has not been directly assessed in randomized clinical trials, but some retrospective studies have evaluated the effectiveness of this class of medications in obese asthma patients. One complicating factor in evaluating T2 inflammation and response is that obesity may alter traditional T2 biomarkers, including eosinophils and exhaled nitric oxide. Because eosinophils play key roles in metabolism, circulating blood eosinophils could reflect changes in metabolism or nutritional status[20,21,73,74] and thus change the performance characteristics of blood eosinophils as a biomarker of airway T2 inflammation. Indeed, blood eosinophil cell counts, while a useful biomarker of airway T2 inflammation in normal-weight individuals with asthma, have been shown to perform poorly as a biomarker of airway T2 inflammation in obese patients.[12,75] The fraction of exhaled nitric oxide might also be altered in obese individuals, and some studies have reported alterations in exhaled nitric oxide based upon age of asthma onset in obesity.[76] This alteration in the performance characteristics of T2 biomarkers in obesity complicates the evaluation of T2 biologic inhibitors responses in obese asthma patients because many trials stratify treatment response or enrollment by blood eosinophil cell counts.[77,78] Few publications have compared responses to biologics in lean and obese patients, and the limited available data show conflicting results. One study suggested a similar response to the anti-immunoglobulin E therapeutic, omalizumab,[79] while another study suggested differing responses.[80] Weight-based dosing also precludes the use of omalizumab in severely obese patients. The role of anti-T2 biologic agents, and also the assessment of T2 inflammation in obese individuals with asthma, is not yet clear.

One intriguing and as yet unstudied potential side effect of T2 inhibitors is their potential to worsen obesity and metabolic disease. Clearly, murine models have demonstrated a role for T2 immunity in preventing obesity, and blocking these important cytokines could potentially worsen obesity in some patients.[20,24] Further work is needed to address this possibility, but it is important that clinicians are aware of this potential complication. Similarly, other medications such as intermittent or chronic systemic or inhaled corticosteroids that suppress T2 inflammation could have similar unwanted side effects. Furthermore, corticosteroids worsen obesity and metabolic dysfunction via direct effects on cortisol and the hypothalamic-pituitary-adrenal axis.[81] Thus, it is of paramount importance to limit overall exposure to systemic corticosteroids in asthma patients with obesity. Use of as-needed inhaled corticosteroid regimens in patients with mild to moderate persistent asthma[82] might be a strategy to limit total corticosteroid exposure. Finally, prior to escalating therapy, treatment of comorbidities and lifestyle interventions should be attempted.

COMORBIDITIES

Obese patients with asthma have increased comorbidities related to their obesity compared with lean patients, some of which can significantly impact asthma (see Table 61.2). Pertinent comorbidities include gastroesophageal reflux disease, obstructive sleep apnea, and depression.

Gastroesophageal reflux disease (GERD) may contribute to poorly controlled asthma in some patients, but there are no compelling data that this is the case in obese patients with asthma. In a study of obese adults with asthma without symptomatic GERD requiring active treatment, acid reflux was not associated with worse asthma control or lower lung function, suggesting that treatment of asymptomatic acid reflux is unlikely to be helpful in this patient population.[83] A similar study in children found that GERD symptoms were associated with worse asthma control but better lung function, and the authors speculated that perhaps symptoms of GERD were being misattributed to asthma.[84] The available data do not suggest that acid reflux contributes to poor asthma control in obesity, but perhaps that GERD symptoms may be misattributed to asthma.

Obstructive sleep apnea (OSA) is more prevalent in obesity. In fact, asthma itself may also predispose to the development of OSA.[85] Some studies suggest OSA is associated with poor asthma control and worse asthma outcomes.[83,86] OSA is also associated with altered airway inflammation, in particular with increased sputum neutrophils.[87] There are some small studies suggesting that treatment of OSA might improve some outcomes related to asthma,[88] but there are no definitive studies of the efficacy of treating OSA on asthma outcomes. Because OSA should be treated for its own sake and is associated with poor asthma control and increased neutrophilic airway inflammation, it seems reasonable to screen for OSA in obese patients with poorly controlled asthma and treat when appropriate with some expectation that it might improve asthma control.

Depression is another comorbidity increased in obese people with a possible effect on asthma. Epidemiologic studies show an increased prevalence of depression in obese people.[89] Some studies have also shown that depression in obese patients with asthma is associated with poor asthma control.[90,91] There are no prospective studies addressing whether treatment of depression might affect asthma control in obese patients but, because uncontrolled depression is a serious comorbidity, assessing and treating this condition is reasonable in obese patients with asthma.

Obese patients with asthma commonly also have comorbidities found in lean asthma patients, such as nasal polyposis. We are not aware of any data that obesity worsens nasal polyposis but, as with lean asthma patients, these comorbidities need to be addressed.

DIET, EXERCISE, AND WEIGHT LOSS INTERVENTIONS

Prospective studies suggest that losing at least 5% of body weight is associated with improvement in asthma control,[92] and that addition of exercise might also be beneficial.[93] Weight loss is also an effective treatment for many comorbidities and is therefore a desirable goal for a patient's overall health. While weight loss is likely to improve asthma control, simply stating a need to lose weight is only modestly effective.[94] A more effective intervention is enrollment into a structured weight loss program.[95]

Losing weight is challenging for anyone and, for those with asthma, the challenge is greater due to the additional anxiety of shortness of breath and bronchoconstriction during exercise. Thus, improving diet quality is an important weight loss intervention in addition to efforts focused on exercise. Obesity is often associated with poor dietary quality—a diet high in processed foods and sugars and low in fiber, fruit, and vegetables. Despite limited data, some studies suggest a beneficial role for dietary interventions in asthma, apart from effects on obesity.[93] Poor dietary quality might affect airway inflammation and decrease bronchodilator responsiveness,[96] and a diet high in fruit and vegetables might decrease asthma exacerbations.[97] Given the beneficial effects of improving dietary quality, and the small studies suggesting dietary quality might affect outcomes relevant to asthma, it seems reasonable to focus on improving dietary quality in obese patients with asthma.[96]

Because weight loss is difficult, diet and exercise may be inadequate interventions in many patients with morbid obesity. Bariatric surgery is a reasonable approach in morbidly obese patients. Bariatric surgery improves other comorbid conditions associated with obesity and has been shown to improve asthma control.[43,98,99] In one retrospective study, there was a significant reduction in asthma exacerbations in the 2 years after bariatric surgery compared with the 2 years before bariatric surgery.[99] While patients with uncontrolled asthma likely are at increased risk related to surgery, laparoscopic approaches are well tolerated and minimize surgical risks. Therefore, bariatric surgery is a reasonable intervention in some obese patients with asthma who have not responded to nonsurgical approaches. This surgery should only be considered after carefully discussing the risks and benefits with the patient.

Key Points

- Obesity is associated with severe, difficult-to-control asthma.
- Obesity is a risk factor for the development of asthma, and asthma is also associated with an increased risk of developing obesity.
- The immune cells responsible for initiating airway *type 2* (T2) inflammation also play key roles in adipose tissue homeostasis. Thus, medications inhibiting T2 inflammation may worsen metabolic dysfunction and contribute to weight gain.
- Patients with obesity and metabolic dysfunction demonstrate deficiencies in immune cells responsible for host defenses against viral and bacterial pathogens. This defect in host defense may predispose obese asthma patients to the development of viral upper respiratory tract infections.

- Both T2-high and T2-low phenotypes of asthma can be seen in obese individuals, though performance characteristics of biomarkers for type 2 disease are altered in obese individuals.
- Airway disease in obesity is related to multiple factors, including altered lung mechanics, poor diet, immune dysfunction, and metabolic dysfunction.
- Obese patients do not respond as well to standard therapies and likely need an approach that includes consideration of treatment of lifestyle factors and comorbidities as well.

Key Readings

Camargo Jr CA, Weiss ST, Zhang S, Willett WC, Speizer FE. Prospective study of body mass index, weight change, and risk of adult-onset asthma in women. *Arch Intern Med.* 1999;159:2582–2588.

Dixon AE, Pratley RE, Forgione PM, et al. Effects of obesity and bariatric surgery on airway hyperresponsiveness, asthma control, and inflammation. *J Allergy Clin Immunol.* 2011;128:508–515. e501–502.

Duvall MG, Barnig C, Cernadas M, et al. Natural killer cell–mediated inflammation resolution is disabled in severe asthma. *Sci Immunol.* 2017;2(9):5446.

Freitas PD, Ferreira PG, Silva AG, et al. The role of exercise in a weight-loss program on clinical control in obese adults with asthma. A randomized controlled trial. *Am J Respir Crit Care Med.* 2017;195:32–42.

Hasegawa K, Tsugawa Y, Chang Y, Camargo Jr CA. Risk of an asthma exacerbation after bariatric surgery in adults. *J Allergy Clin Immunol.* 2015;136:288–294.

Lugogo N, Green CL, Agada N, et al. Obesity's effect on asthma extends to diagnostic criteria. *J Allergy Clin Immunol.* 2018;141:1096–1104.

Michelet X, Dyck L, Hogan A, et al. Metabolic reprogramming of natural killer cells in obesity limits antitumor responses. *Nat Immunol.* 2018;19(12):1330–1340.

Molofsky AB, Nussbaum JC, Liang H-E, et al. Innate lymphoid type 2 cells sustain visceral adipose tissue eosinophils and alternatively activated macrophages. *J Exp Med.* 2013;210(3):535–549.

Peters MC, Kerr S, Dunican EM, et al. Refractory airway type 2 inflammation in a large subgroup of asthmatic patients treated with inhaled corticosteroids. *J Allergy Clin Immunol.* 2019;143(1):104–113. e14.

Peters MC, McGrath KW, Hawkins GA, et al. Plasma interleukin-6 concentrations, metabolic dysfunction, and asthma severity: a cross-sectional analysis of two cohorts. *Lancet Respir Med.* 2016;4(7):574–584.

Peters MC, Ringel L, Dyjack N, et al. A transcriptomic method to determine airway immune dysfunction in T2-high and T2-low asthma. *Am J Respir Crit Care Med.* 2018. Oct 29.

Wang Z, Aguilar EG, Luna JI, et al. Paradoxical effects of obesity on T cell function during tumor progression and PD-1 checkpoint blockade. *Nat Med.* 2019;25(1):141.

Wood LG, Garg ML, Gibson PG. A high-fat challenge increases airway inflammation and impairs bronchodilator recovery in asthma. *J Allergy Clin Immunol.* 2011;127:1133–1140.

Wu D, Molofsky AB, Liang H-E, Ricardo-Gonzalez RR, Jouihan HA, Bando JK, et al. Eosinophils sustain adipose alternatively activated macrophages associated with glucose homeostasis. *Science.* 2011;332(6026):243–247.

Complete reference list available at ExpertConsult.com.

62 ASTHMA: DIAGNOSIS AND MANAGEMENT

NJIRA LUGOGO, MD • LORETTA G. QUE, MD • TARA F. CARR, MD • MONICA KRAFT, MD

INTRODUCTION

Asthma is a common chronic heterogeneous disease of the airways. Asthma affects 8% of the U.S. population, which is more than 26 million Americans, including 7 million children.[1] In 2010, 1.8 million people sought emergency department attention for asthma, and almost 500,000 required hospitalization due to an asthma attack.[1] Between 1980 and 2010, childhood asthma prevalence almost tripled.[1,2] In response to this public health concern, asthma has attracted a tremendous scope of biomedical investigation, from evaluation of endotype-defining inflammatory pathways at the gene transcription level to studies of novel biologic pharmaceuticals for severe asthma. These studies continue to refine the scientific understanding of asthma and promote novel approaches to primary prevention and treatment. This chapter reviews the foundational clinical knowledge of asthma and incorporates some high-impact, transformative scientific achievements informing our approach to diagnosis and treatment. This chapter builds on Chapter 60, which explores the pathogenesis and phenotypes of asthma, and Chapter 61, which focuses on the phenotype of obesity and asthma.

DEFINITION

Asthma has been more often described than defined. The earliest feature described was the labored, rapid breathing typical of asthmatic attacks; the word "asthma" is derived from the ancient Greek word for "panting." As knowledge about asthma has grown, the features described as characteristic of asthma have expanded. Measurement of maximal expiratory flow led to recognition of *reversible airflow obstruction* as a characteristic feature; measurement of changes in airflow after inhalation of chemical or physical irritants led to the definition of *bronchial hyperresponsiveness*. In addition, studies of bronchial biopsies added a description of characteristic pathologic features including *chronic inflammation*.

This evolution in the understanding of asthma is summarized in the definition offered in the 2019 *Global Initiative for Asthma* (GINA) guidelines (http://ginasthma.org): "Asthma is a heterogeneous disease, usually characterized by chronic airway inflammation. It is defined by the history of respiratory symptoms such as wheeze, shortness of breath, chest tightness, and cough that vary over time and in intensity, together with variable expiratory airflow limitation."

This consensus conference "definition" of asthma serves well as a description of the major features of asthma but does not hold up as a precise definition. No feature is unique to asthma, and no feature is universal in patients with the condition. Thus, the modern approach to asthma diagnosis, assessment, and treatment has changed in response to the recognition that asthma is a heterogeneous disease that encompasses many phenotypes with variable responses to therapy. For example, focusing a clinical trial on a certain asthma phenotype, characterized by observed characteristics such as the presence of eosinophilic inflammation, allergy, or chronic airflow limitation, has improved our ability to identify targeted therapeutics for individuals with these characteristics. This recognition of asthma as a complex, multifactorial disorder has led to a greater focus on the individual and is advancing the field toward more precise understanding of asthma pathogenesis and treatment.

CLINICAL DIAGNOSIS

The diagnosis of asthma is often made in the ambulatory care setting and is based on a careful personal history, physical examination, and lung function testing (Fig. 62.1). A number of different diseases can mimic asthma and cause some or all of the symptoms of asthma. These include vocal cord dysfunction, COPD, cystic fibrosis, bronchiectasis, congestive heart failure, sleep apnea, pneumonia, sarcoidosis, and psychosomatic diseases and should be considered when making the diagnosis of asthma.

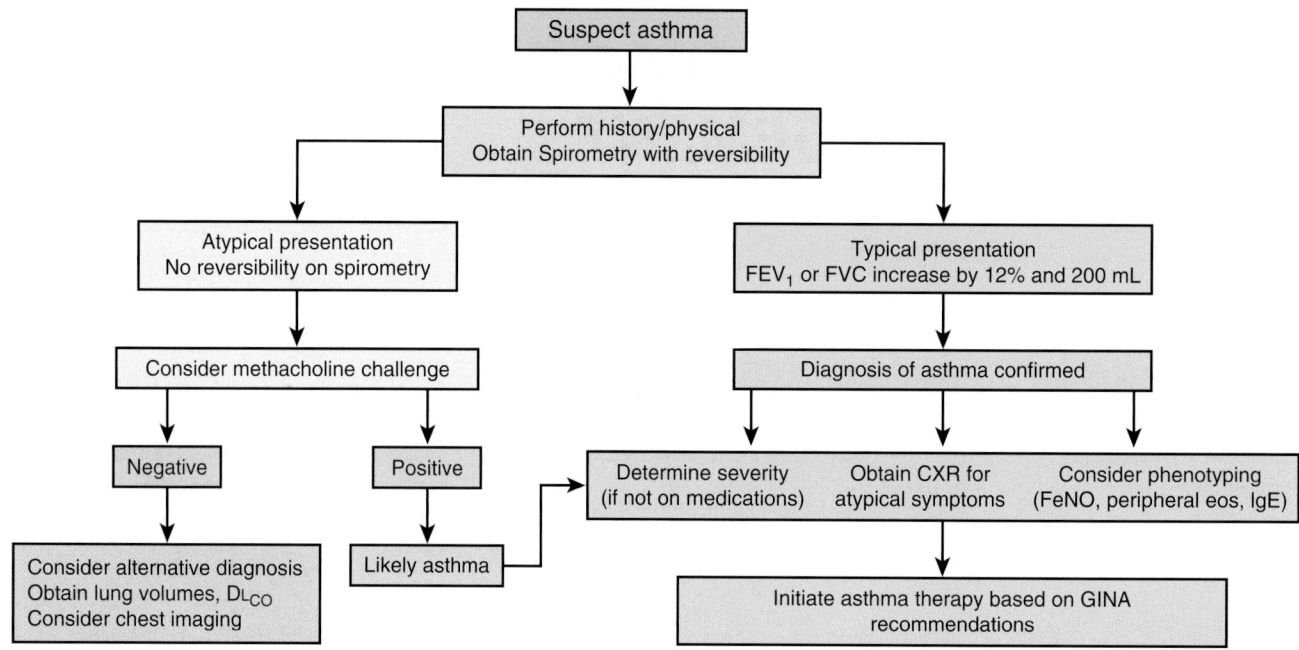

Fig. 62.1 Algorithm for diagnosing asthma in adults. The diagnosis of asthma is based on a careful personal history, physical examination, and lung function testing. Spirometry should be obtained in every patient in whom asthma is suspected. Other tests are useful when clinical features are atypical, and to determine severity and asthma phenotype. CXR, chest radiograph; DL_{CO}, diffusing capacity for carbon monoxide; eos, eosinophils; FeNO, fraction of exhaled nitric oxide; FEV_1, forced expiratory volume in 1 second; FVC, forced vital capacity; IgE, immunoglobulin E; GINA, Global Initiative for Asthma.

PERSONAL HISTORY

Asthma can arise at any age but often presents for the first time in childhood.[2] Risk factors for childhood asthma include a family history of asthma and a personal or family history of atopy (e.g., atopic dermatitis, seasonal allergic rhinitis, conjunctivitis).[3] In addition, asthma can develop in individuals sensitive to aspirin or exposed to chemical toxins.[4]

A comprehensive history for symptoms suggestive of the reversible airflow obstruction and *airway hyperresponsiveness* (AHR) characteristic of asthma is essential for the assessment of the asthmatic patient. Most patients with asthma report intermittent symptoms including cough, shortness of breath, chest tightness or heaviness, and/or wheezing, often described as a high-pitched musical whistling, heard usually at the end of expiration but may also be heard in both inspiratory and expiratory phases. They often experience periods of symptom-free normal breathing interrupted by periods of difficulty breathing. Asthma symptoms can last for a few minutes or days. Cough is a frequent complaint in asthma; the cough may or may not be accompanied by sputum production, may worsen at night or with activity, and may develop after exposure to allergens.[5,6] Shortness of breath and wheezing manifest during an exacerbation and can be triggered by infection, cold air, exercise, exposure to chemical fumes or other airborne irritants, pet dander, molds, house dust mites, or other allergens.[7] In contrast, wheezing heard predominantly during inspiration may be a sign of stridor. Complaints of sharp stabbing or knifelike pain would be unusual in asthma and should direct the clinician to alternative diagnoses (see Chapter 39).

Asthma guidelines support applying characteristics of these asthma symptoms toward determining a patient's asthma severity, as indicated by degree of impairment or risk of exacerbations.[8] For example, the frequency with which an individual experiences asthma symptoms can differentiate between someone with mild or severe disease. Similarly, an individual for whom the asthma symptoms markedly impair daily activities and function would likely indicate requirement for therapy for more severe disease than an individual for whom the same symptoms had little effect on function. Patients may report one or many prior diagnoses of "bronchitis" treated with systemic steroids and short-acting bronchodilators, which could be interpreted as exacerbations of asthma.

WORK HISTORY

Symptoms that improve on weekends and vacations and worsen at work should raise the suspicion of occupational and/or work-exacerbated asthma. Occupational asthma is new-onset asthma due to causes and conditions attributable to a particular occupational environment, whereas work-exacerbated asthma is defined as exacerbation of known asthma by the work environment.[9] Indeed, up to 15% of all adult asthma can be attributed to occupation.[10,11] The work exposure history should focus on identifying agents present at the time of asthma diagnosis or when asthma symptoms worsened. There are two major types of occupational asthma: sensitizer-induced asthma and irritant-induced asthma. Sensitizers are often further classified into low-molecular-weight (small chemicals) and high-molecular-weight (usually protein) agents.[4] *Reactive airway dysfunction syndrome*, the best-defined form of irritant-induced asthma, results from a single high-dose exposure to irritants. (For a more detailed discussion of

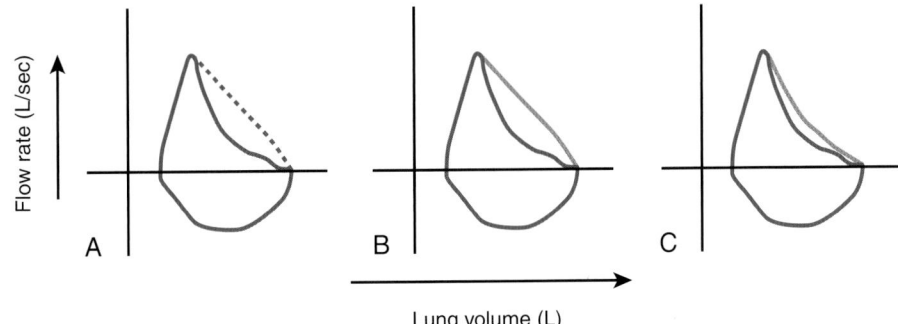

Fig. 62.2 Flow-volume loops in asthma. (A) The typical scooped appearance of the flow-volume loop in asthma is shown as the *solid blue line*. The predicted normal flow-volume loop is shown by the *dashed line*. (B) The scooped appearance of the initial flow-volume loop (*blue line*) may show complete reversal following use of a bronchodilator (*brown line*). (C) In some cases, the reversal of the scooped appearance following use of a bronchodilator is incomplete (*brown line*). (From Sameer KM. Asthma: diagnosis and management. *Med Clin North Am.* 2006;90:39–60.)

reactive airway dysfunction syndrome and occupational asthma, see Chapter 100.)

PHYSICAL EXAMINATION

The physical examination should focus on the head and neck, chest, and skin. The physical examination is often normal, particularly for patients who are asymptomatic at the time of examination; however, findings such as wheezing during normal breathing and/or a prolonged expiratory phase may suggest asthma. Forced exhalation, a maneuver to enhance wheezing, is not specific for asthma and suggests airway obstruction or collapse.[12] In addition to breathing abnormalities, subjects with asthma often have concomitant signs of associated allergic conditions and evidence of upper respiratory tract inflammation and obstruction with inflamed nasal passages and/or nasal polyps or large tonsils. The findings of eczema, hives, or atopic dermatitis on skin examination are supportive of an atopic asthma diagnosis.[8]

Objective measurements of lung function support an asthma diagnosis when the clinical history is suspicious for asthma (Fig. 62.2). Commonly available tests for measurement of airflow obstruction include spirometry and *peak expiratory flow* (PEF) measurement. Comparison of results before and after treatment with a bronchodilator will assess for reversibility of obstruction. Finally, AHR can be determined through inhalational or exercise challenges. Application of these tests is described in the following sections.

PHYSIOLOGY OF AIRFLOW LIMITATION

As understanding of the pathogenesis of asthma improves and strategies for treatment evolve, it is important to recognize that the link between the pathophysiology and the treatment of asthma is functional, involving variable limitation of airflow. These two cardinal manifestations of asthma, limitation of airflow and variability of symptoms in response to environmental factors, are crucial to making the diagnosis of asthma and distinguishing asthma from other obstructive lung diseases.

During asthma exacerbations, diffuse narrowing of the airways results in profound physiologic consequences. This narrowing has been thought to take place disproportionately in the small bronchi,[13] resulting in abnormal lung function tests with an increase in airway resistance and a

decline in maximal expiratory flow. Airway narrowing also prevents the lungs from completely emptying (air trapping) due to resistance to expiratory flow and bronchial closure at higher than normal lung volumes. The breath-to-breath variability of asthmatic obstruction and air trapping can lead to dynamic hyperinflation,[14] a situation in which patients breathe at higher total lung volumes (i.e., increased residual volume).[15] Despite elevated total lung volumes, asthmatics typically have reduced tidal ventilation.

At high lung volumes, flow limitation due to bronchial narrowing is offset somewhat by increased circumferential traction on the bronchial airways due to "tethering" of airways to inflated alveoli,[16] thereby reducing airway resistance. However, the diaphragm and intercostal muscles become overloaded due to thoracic hyperinflation and are mechanically disadvantaged due to suboptimal positioning on their length-tension curves.[17] As a result, accessory muscles of respiration, including the abdominal muscles and the sternocleidomastoids, are recruited.[18] Overall, due to the mechanical disadvantage of the respiratory muscles and recruitment of additional muscle groups, the work of breathing at higher lung volumes is increased.

The airway obstruction and closure in asthma is nonuniform, with significant regional variability.[19,20] Ventilation-perfusion mismatching leads to a widened alveolar-arterial oxygen tension difference that tracks with increasing asthma severity.[21,22] Arterial carbon dioxide tension initially falls as alveolar ventilation increases because carbon dioxide elimination is less impaired by ventilation-perfusion mismatching than is oxygen uptake.[23] As respiratory muscles fatigue, carbon dioxide tension increases, so a normal or elevated partial pressure of carbon dioxide during an asthma exacerbation suggests impending respiratory failure.[24]

PULMONARY FUNCTION TESTING

In ambulatory patients, decreased expiratory flow can be easily and reproducibly detected with a peak flowmeter; PEF measurements attempt to correlate physiologic function with the clinical severity of asthma. However, peak flow measurements are not standardized and do not correlate well with other measures of lung function.[25] PEF as a percentage of its predicted value is 10% higher than the percent predicted of the *forced expiratory volume in 1 second* (FEV$_1$) on average, with a great deal of variability between measurements.[26] Currently, the recommended use of PEF measurement is for the daily monitoring of ambulatory patients with difficult-to-manage asthma.

Spirometry

The most standardized test of airflow obstruction is FEV_1. FEV_1 may be normal or near-normal between asthma flares. It has the advantage of being an objective, non-patient-reported measurement of lung function. Improvement in FEV_1 of greater than 12% and 200 mL after bronchodilator treatment indicates reversible airflow obstruction and is suggestive, but not diagnostic, of asthma.[27]

Accurate measurement requires stopping *long-acting β_2-agonists* (LABAs) for at least 12 hours and short-acting bronchodilators for at least 6 hours. The absolute value of the FEV_1 is dependent on the *forced vital capacity* (FVC). Interpretation of FEV_1 therefore requires simultaneous FVC measurement. In asthma, the relative reduction in FEV_1 is typically greater than the reduction in the FVC. As a result, the FEV_1/FVC ratio in asthma is usually less than 70%. However, in severe asthma, this ratio may actually increase as air trapping increases residual volume and reduces the FVC. A 20% and 200 mL increase in the FVC after bronchodilator is also suggestive of asthma.[27]

An alternative measure of airflow obstruction is the mid-expiratory flow, measured between 25% and 75% of the FVC (*forced expiratory flow* $[FEF]_{25\%-75\%}$). Measured at lower lung volumes than FEV_1, reductions in the $FEF_{25\%-75\%}$ may be more sensitive for identifying obstruction in small airways.[28] However, the clinical utility of the $FEF_{25\%-75\%}$ is limited by the lack of acceptable standardized values and poor reproducibility.[29] High numbers of false-positive and false-negative results are seen when 80% of predicted $FEF_{25\%-75\%}$ is used to define normal.[30]

Single-breath diffusing capacity is a marker of carbon monoxide gas transfer in the lungs. In asthma, the diffusing capacity is normal or elevated if airflow obstruction is not severe; this finding can be useful in distinguishing asthma from other obstructive lung diseases.[31] Elevated diffusing capacity in asthma has been attributed to increased perfusion of the upper lung zones and is associated with large lung volumes. The unexpected finding of an increase in diffusing capacity should raise the possibility of undiagnosed asthma, whereas decreased diffusing capacity in a suspected asthmatic is suggestive of an alternative diagnosis or coexisting condition.[32]

Provocative Challenges and Airway Hyperresponsiveness

Airway Hyperresponsiveness. AHR to environmental stimuli is a hallmark of asthma. Patients suspected of having asthma despite normal lung function testing usually develop bronchoconstriction in response to a provocative stimulus. Direct stimulation with methacholine inhaled into the airways is the most widely used method of assessing bronchial hyperresponsiveness. Nebulized methacholine is delivered in doubling concentrations until FEV_1 falls by more than 20%, referred to as the PC_{20} (provocative concentration resulting in 20% fall in the FEV_1). The PC_{20} can be used to quantify the degree of AHR. A PC_{20} less than 16 mg/mL is consistent with mild AHR, less than 4 mg/mL is consistent with moderate AHR, and less than 1 mg/mL

with severe AHR,[33] with lower PC_{20} levels generally corresponding to more severe asthma[34] (see Chapter 31).

Impulse Oscillometry. Impulse oscillometry is a form of forced oscillometry testing, a noninvasive technique to characterize the airway through the superimposition of sound waves on normal tidal breathing.[35] The disturbances in flow and pressure caused by the sound waves are used to calculate resistance to airflow at frequencies of 5 Hz (R5) and at 20 Hz (R20) and reactance, the energy generated by the lungs' recoil against that pressure wave at 5 Hz (X5). These measurements allow calculation of the force necessary to propagate this pressure wave through the respiratory system, known as impedance. The site of airway disease can also be localized because lower-frequency oscillations tend to travel to the lung periphery and higher-frequency ones reach only the most proximal airways.

Measurements are recorded during normal passive tidal breathing and require little training. Not surprisingly, the majority of impulse oscillometry studies in asthma have been in children. Significant correlations between FEV_1 and FVC by spirometry and impedance and resistance by impulse oscillometry have been described.[36] A decrease in R5 by 30–35% in children is considered to be a positive bronchodilator response.[37,38] In another study of children, a 50% decrease in X5 was found to be roughly equivalent to a 20% decrease in FEV_1.[39] Most impressively, impulse oscillometry has outperformed spirometry in sensitivity and specificity for the diagnosis of asthma in young children when compared to a methacholine challenge and validated clinical questionnaire.[38,40] Despite increasing acceptance in the pediatric population, experience in adult patients remains limited.[41]

EVALUATION AND TREATMENT OF ASTHMA

INTRODUCTION

The *National Heart Lung and Blood Institute* (NHLBI) *Expert Panel Report* (EPR) Guidelines for the Diagnosis and Management of Asthma and GINA documents have provided clinicians with a reliable framework for evidence-based management of patients with asthma.[1,8] These guidelines emphasize maintaining long-term control of symptoms through attention to environmental and social components of asthma and using treatment regimens tailored to the severity of each patient's symptoms. Crucial components of management as recommended by the EPR and GINA guidelines include initial evaluation of control (Table 62.1)[41a]; determination of severity by "step" of treatment required to control symptoms (Table 62.2); appropriate pharmacologic therapy to reverse bronchoconstriction and ameliorate inflammation; identification and control of environmental factors that worsen symptoms or trigger exacerbations; and creation of a partnership between the patient and the health care professional to ensure that therapy is tailored to each patient's needs. Modern approaches to therapy also recognize that heterogeneity of asthma pathobiology will lead to variability in each individual's clinical response to each therapy, and therefore incorporate

Table 62.1   Classification of Asthma Control in Adults and Adolescents >11 Years per GINA Guidelines

Asthma Symptom Control	Yes	No
In the past 4 weeks, has the patient had: ■ Daytime asthma symptoms more than twice per week? ■ Any night waking due to asthma? ■ Reliever needed for symptoms more than twice per week? ■ Any activity limitation due to asthma?		

Total:

Level of asthma symptom control is based on total number of "yes" responses:
■ If 0, asthma is well controlled
■ If 1–2 of these, asthma is partly controlled
■ If 3–4 of these, asthma is uncontrolled

Risk factors for poor asthma outcomes: ■ Uncontrolled symptoms ■ Medication challenges (frequent short-acting bronchodilator use, poor adherence, incorrect technique, not on inhaled corticosteroid) ■ Comorbidities (obesity, chronic rhinosinusitis, GERD, pregnancy) ■ Exposures (smoking, allergens, air pollution) ■ Low lung function (FEV_1 <60% predicted) or highly reversible bronchoconstriction ■ Psychological or socioeconomic factors ■ History of severe exacerbation	Any of these risk factors increases the patient's risk of exacerbations even if they have few asthma symptoms

FEV_1, forced expiratory volume in 1 second; GERD, gastroesophageal reflux disease; GINA, Global Initiative for Asthma.
Courtesy GINA, www.ginasthma.org.

Table 62.2   Classification of Asthma Severity (GINA 2019)

ASSESS SYMPTOM CONTROL WHEN PATIENT HAS BEEN ON REGULAR CONTROLLER TREATMENT FOR SEVERAL MONTHS	
Mild asthma	Well controlled with step 1 or step 2
Moderate asthma	Well controlled with step 3
Severe asthma	Requires step 4 or step 5 to prevent it from being uncontrolled, or is still uncontrolled despite this therapy

Steps are levels of treatment, as defined in Fig. 62.3.
Uncontrolled asthma is defined by the International European Respiratory Society/American Thoracic Society Guidelines for Severe Asthma as described later.
FEV_1, forced expiratory volume in 1 second; GINA, Global Initiative for Asthma.
Courtesy GINA, www.ginasthma.org.

biomarker and phenotype assessments to optimize treatment decisions.

ASSESSMENT

Asthma Impairment and Risk

The assessment of patients with asthma involves two essential steps: determining the current degree of *impairment* from asthma based on symptoms, reliever medication use, recent exacerbations, and lung function; and evaluating the *risk of future adverse outcomes* including exacerbations, lung function decline, and adverse medication outcomes. With this in mind, the NHLBI updated guidelines and GINA offer a parallel scheme for asthma assessment based on expert opinion[1,8] (see Tables 62.1 and 62.2). The NHLBI and GINA classifications represent categorical interval variables with threshold values to determine severity and control. The importance of control indices is underscored by the relationship between poor asthma control and substantial degrees of physical impairment and diminished quality of life, even after taking the baseline severity of asthma into account.[42]

Several different validated instruments exist for assessing asthma within this framework, including the Asthma Control Questionnaire, Asthma Control Test, Asthma Therapy Assessment Questionnaire, and Asthma Control Scoring System.[43–46] All are useful because they direct history taking, provide goals for the management of symptoms, and guide adjustments in treatment.[47]

While the NHLBI guidelines suggest that asthma severity is to be determined initially based on the severity of symptoms—both impairment and risk domains—at the time of diagnosis, the GINA guidelines recommend defining severity by the amount of medication required to control asthma symptoms (see Table 62.2). While guidelines provide recommendations for starting therapy at each severity level (Fig. 62.3), providers must reassess every patient to ensure adequate asthma control. Importantly, in determining severity, guidelines also take into account the amount of treatment necessary to maintain control of asthma.

Lung Function

Lung function testing is an important part of assessing asthma, both for making the initial diagnosis and as a means of evaluating the response to therapy. Although the FEV_1, FEV_1/FVC ratio, and PEF are useful in the diagnosis and monitoring of asthma, the utility of these measurements in improving the outcome of asthma remains incompletely defined. However, a low FEV_1 is a strong predictor of decline in asthma control and of increased risk of needing acute care.[48] In mild asthma, however, FEV_1 is often normal or near-normal and thus may not show significant bronchodilator response. PEF measurement is a standard method to correlate physiologic function with asthma severity and has been used as a marker of asthma control in many clinical trials. However, individual PEF measurements are highly variable and the *variability* in peak flow has a greater predictive value for future exacerbations than individual PEF measurements themselves.[48] The clinical usefulness of

	Step 1	Step 2	Step 3	Step 4	Step 5
Preferred Controller *To prevent exacerbations and control symptoms*	As-needed low-dose ICS-formoterol*	Low-dose ICS, *or* as-needed ICS-formoterol*	Low-dose ICS-LABA	Medium-dose ICS-LABA	High-dose ICS-LABA Refer for phenotypic assessment ± add-on therapy (e.g., tiotropium, anti-IgE, anti-IL5/5R, anti-IL4R)
Other controller options	Low-dose ICS taken whenever SABA is taken†	LTRA or low-dose ICS taken whenever SABA is taken†	Medium-dose ICS, *or* low-dose ICS+LTRA‡	High-dose ICS, add-on tiotropium, *or* add-on LTRA‡	Add low-dose oral corticosteroids, but consider side effects
Preferred Reliever	As-needed low-dose ICS-formoterol*				
Other reliever option	As-needed SABA				

At all levels:	Assess	Adjust	Review Response
	Confirmation of diagnosis Symptom control & modifiable risk factors (including lung function) Comorbidities Inhaler technique & adherence Patient goals	*Treatment of modifiable risk factors & comorbidities Non-pharmacological strategies Education & skills training Asthma medications*	*Symptoms Exacerbations Side effects Lung function Patient satisfaction*

Fig. 62.3 Medication recommendations for control of asthma in adults and children older than 12 years. Controller medications should be initiated and subsequently adjusted up or down in a stepwise approach with a goal of achieving good control of symptoms and minimizing future risk of exacerbations, airflow obstruction, and adverse effects from medications. At onset of treatment and every 2 to 3 months thereafter, assess clinical factors, adjust medications, and review response. *Off-label; data only available for budesonide-formoterol. †Off-label; separate or combination ICS and SABA inhalers. ‡Consider adding house dust mite sublingual immunotherapy for sensitized patients with allergic rhinitis and FEV$_1$ >70% predicted. ICS, inhaled corticosteroid; Ig, immunoglobulin; IL, interleukin; LTRA, leukotriene receptor antagonist; LABA, long-acting β$_2$-agonist; SABA, short-acting β$_2$-agonist. (Modified from GINA 2019 Guidelines, www.ginasthma.org.)

PEF measurements is also limited by patient resistance to home monitoring and difficulty with consistently maintaining peak flow records.

Imaging

Although traditionally thoracic imaging has been used to rule out alternative pathologies, recent advances in imaging offer additional noninvasive techniques to support the diagnosis of asthma. The chest radiograph is most commonly normal in stable asthmatics, although nonspecific findings such as hyperinflation and bronchial wall thickening can be appreciated.[49] In patients admitted with status asthmaticus, pneumothorax and pneumomediastinum identified on chest radiograph have been reported in 0.5–2.5% of patients, respectively.[50] The primary role of the plain chest radiograph remains to rule out asthma mimics in those with atypical symptoms and to evaluate difficult-to-control symptoms.

Clinically, chest *computed tomography* in asthma is used to evaluate chest radiographic abnormalities, diagnose complications of associated conditions (i.e., pneumothorax and pneumomediastinum), and identify mimics less apparent on plain chest radiographs (i.e., bronchiolitis, bronchiectasis, tracheobronchomalacia, endobronchial lesions, and vascular anomalies).[49,51] Increasingly, high-resolution chest computed tomography techniques offer a useful tool to assess large and small airway pathology. Nonspecific

findings such as bronchial wall thickening, airway dilation, bronchiectasis, mucoid impaction, and mosaic lung attenuation consistent with air trapping are described in studies of asthmatic subjects.[52]

Asthma Phenotypes, Endotypes, and Biomarkers

The identification of asthma *phenotypes*, which are collections of clinical characteristics that define a particular type of asthma, and their *endotypes*, which are defined by particular biologic pathways, has now moved into center stage when evaluating the patient with asthma, particularly severe asthma.[53]

The endotypes associated with *type 2* (T2) inflammation characterized by T2 cytokines such as *interleukin* (IL)-4, IL-5, and IL-13 include early-onset allergic asthma with or without obesity, aspirin-sensitive asthma and late-onset eosinophilic asthma, exacerbation prone asthma, and exercise-induced asthma. Clinical phenotypes of asthma not associated with T2 inflammation (T2-low), and for which the pathobiologic pathways are not yet defined, include patients with obesity-related late-onset asthma, asthma with fixed airflow obstruction and very little inflammation (paucigranulocytic), and asthma associated with neutrophilia. Other T2-low clinical phenotypes that are less well defined but that may share similar endotypes include smoking-related

Table 62.3 Asthma Biomarkers and Associated Phenotypes as Predictors of Response to Specific Therapies

Biomarker	Asthma Phenotype	Predicts
Elevated exhaled nitric oxide (>50 ppb in adults, >35 ppb in children)	T2-high	Response to inhaled steroids
Sputum eosinophils >3%	T2-high	Response to inhaled steroids
Peripheral blood eosinophils (>0.3 × 10⁹/L or 300/μL)	T2-high	Response to anti-IL-5 therapy
Elevated total IgE >30 IU	Allergic/T2	Response to omalizumab
Allergy skin tests and elevated specific IgE	Allergic/T2	Response to immunotherapy, omalizumab
Lack of elevated peripheral and sputum eosinophils and low FeNO	T2-low	Response to tiotropium and macrolides (likely to be poor responders to steroids)

FeNO, fraction of exhaled nitric oxide; IgE, immunoglobulin E; T2, type 2.

asthma, occupational asthma due to low-molecular-weight agents[54] or environmental pollution,[55] and respiratory infections.[56]

Biomarkers. The emergence of an increased body of literature to support the presence of asthma phenotypes and endotypes has made it imperative that we have tools at our disposal for identification of these patient cohorts. *Biomarkers* are measurable characteristics of an individual that relate to a disease, such as an elevated level of blood eosinophils. Applying biomarkers to identify phenotypes and endotypes of severe asthma may have a variety of purposes. For example, the currently recognized and published phenotypes and endotypes of severe asthma are largely defined by observable and measurable characteristics of the disease or patient and not yet by specific diagnostic biomarkers[53] (Table 62.3). For example, early-onset, allergic asthma is characterized by the presence of allergen-specific *immunoglobulin E* (IgE), and late-onset, hypereosinophilic asthma is characterized by elevated peripheral blood and sputum eosinophils. Eosinophil and IgE levels can be used as diagnostic biomarkers for these phenotypes. However, blood eosinophils are commonly present in patients with early-onset allergic asthma, and allergen-specific IgE may be present in patients with late-onset, hypereosinophilic asthma. Although these commonly used biomarkers may give clues as to the phenotype or endotype of a severe asthmatic patient, they are not pathognomonic or mutually exclusive and do not necessarily address the molecular mechanisms underlying each endotype. Notably, asthma endotypes are not yet well described and mechanisms are not well defined, perhaps contributing to these limitations. Combinations of biomarkers may be more helpful to characterize patients into one of these categories, and novel biomarkers in development may provide improved specificity for one or multiple phenotypes. Furthermore, these biomarkers could be applied as diagnostic of a phenotype, as predictive of a response to therapy, and as useful dynamic markers of a response to therapy. These varied applications of biomarkers may be useful to drive therapy with targeted biologic agents, which is discussed in more detail in the section on treatment of asthma.

Eosinophils and Eosinophil-Related Biomarkers.
Eosinophils may be detected in one or multiple compartments, including the peripheral blood, the airway submucosa, and the airway lumen. The presence of eosinophilia is not always consistent in these compartments.[57,58] Eosinophils are primarily tissue-dwelling leukocytes, and therefore blood counts may not necessarily indicate the extent of eosinophil involvement in the affected tissues.[58,59] A systematic review and meta-analysis of blood biomarkers found that peripheral blood eosinophil counts had a sensitivity of 71% and specificity of 77% for detecting sputum eosinophils of greater than 3%.[60] The extremes of blood eosinophil levels may be more sensitive and specific for identifying sputum eosinophils.[61–63] For example, patients with blood eosinophil counts of less than 90 eosinophils/μL are highly unlikely to have airway eosinophilia; alternatively, almost all patients with more than 400 eosinophils/μL of blood can be expected to have significant sputum eosinophilia.[64] Reference values for sputum eosinophil percentages have been determined through epidemiologic studies of healthy patients.[65,66] In general, sputum eosinophil levels of greater than 2–3% and blood eosinophil counts of greater than 300/μL may be used to define eosinophilic disease.[63,67]

Similarly, sputum eosinophilia can identify patients who will likely have a clinical response to systemic and inhaled corticosteroids.[68,69] However, measurement of sputum eosinophils in the clinical arena requires specialized expertise that is not widely available.

A limitation of the eosinophil number as a predictive biomarker for diagnosis or treatment of asthma may include the failure to identify eosinophil functional stimulation and activity related to severe asthma. Markers of eosinophil activation may be more pathophysiologically relevant as diagnostic and predictive biomarkers for response to therapy or other disease characteristics. For example, eosinophil peroxidase is one of the major granule contents released by eosinophils on activation.[70] In sputum, eosinophil peroxidase is highly correlated with sputum eosinophil levels, increases with allergen challenge, and is specific for those with eosinophilic disease.[71] Eosinophil peroxidase is also readily detected in nasal and pharyngeal swabs, and values at both sites are highly correlated with sputum eosinophils in patients with poorly controlled eosinophilic asthma.[72]

Bromotyrosine is an oxidation product of eosinophil peroxidase. Elevated levels of bromotyrosine can be identified in the airway of clinically stable patients with asthma[73] and can be induced by airway allergen challenge.[74] Bromotyrosine is a stable compound excreted in the urine[75] where it can be measured noninvasively. Elevated urinary levels of bromotyrosine strongly correlate with uncontrolled asthma and risk of asthma exacerbations in children.[76] As might be expected, urinary bromotyrosine also can be used as a predictor of clinical response to *inhaled corticosteroids* (ICSs) in asthma,[77] further emphasizing the distinction between the pathobiologic contribution of total eosinophil counts compared to measures of activated eosinophils.

Fraction of Exhaled Nitric Oxide. *Nitric oxide* (NO) and related compounds are generated by various resident and inflammatory airway cells and have a broad variety of functions as inflammatory mediators, vasodilators, bronchodilators, and neurotransmitters.[78] In the asthmatic airway, NO exhibits a paradoxical response by enhancing airway dilation at low concentrations but propagating inflammatory responses at higher concentrations.

The measurement of the *fraction of exhaled NO* (FeNO) is used clinically as a biomarker of airway inflammation related to IL-4– and IL-13–mediated pathways. This relationship is supported by the observation that FeNO levels decline with IL-4 and IL-13 inhibition.[79–81] Higher levels of FeNO are related to severe, early-onset, allergic, and eosinophilic asthma and therefore can help to identify patients with these phenotypes.[82] More recent studies show that not only is FeNO a strong predictor of sputum eosinophils, it predicts sputum eosinophilia better than serum eosinophils do and also predicts response to ICSs and long-acting muscarinic antagonists.[83]

Noninvasive measurements of FeNO have been standardized for clinical use and may serve as a complementary tool in asthma diagnosis and management. In 2011, guidelines for interpretation of clinical use of FeNO in the diagnosis and management of asthma were published by the *American Thoracic Society* (ATS); however, a *European Respiratory Society* (ERS)/ATS task force later recommended against routine use of FeNO to diagnose asthma and to monitor therapy in patients with severe disease.[84] More recently, Essat et al.[85] and the Agency for Healthcare Research and Quality[86] advocated for additional research to establish a role for FeNO in asthma management.

FeNO has some advantages in detecting eosinophilic asthma and monitoring asthma control compared with counting the number of sputum eosinophils. FeNO can be measured rapidly in a primary care setting, requires less technical expertise, and provides real-time objective physiologic data. Major limitations of using FeNO to confirm the diagnosis of asthma include the relatively high prevalence of noneosinophilic phenotypes characterized by a lack of increased FeNO and the difficulty with clinical interpretation of values obtained in the setting of concomitant steroid use that may lead to false-negative results.[78] However, there is still a role for FeNO in phenotyping patients by identifying those with a Th2 high/eosinophilic phenotype, regardless of asthma severity.

Immunoglobulin E. IgE is an important marker of airway inflammation and may play a key role in allergic asthma. The presence of allergen-specific IgE is required to define the phenotype of early-onset allergic asthma, with panels of clinically relevant aeroallergen skin testing or specific

IgE serology functioning as essential biomarkers. In addition, it may be present and relevant in adult-onset asthma. The *National Institutes of Health* (NIH) Asthma Outcomes Workshop suggested that total and specific serum IgE be considered important outcomes for interventional and observational studies of asthma.[59] Independent of specific aeroallergen sensitization, total IgE is a marker of asthma risk.[87] Both specific aeroallergen sensitization and elicitation of symptoms on exposure to that specific aeroallergen should be present in the clinical syndrome of allergic asthma. This requires clinician assessment of exposure-related symptoms in addition to specific IgE testing through percutaneous skin testing or specific IgE serum assays.

IgE levels are informative and diagnostic in the setting of allergic bronchopulmonary aspergillosis or, as more generally called, *allergic bronchopulmonary mycosis*, which is an endotype of severe asthma. Pathognomonic diagnostic and dynamic biomarkers of allergic bronchopulmonary mycosis include markedly elevated serum total IgE and specific IgE to molds (detected by percutaneous skin testing or serum analysis, most commonly to *Aspergillus fumigatus*) in the setting of severe asthma, mucus plugging, and often central bronchiectasis.

Blood Neutrophils. A significant proportion of patients with severe asthma will have airway granulocytes, including neutrophils and eosinophils.[88] Those with significant proportions of airway neutrophils (ranging from 40–76% of total sputum cells) but lacking significant airway eosinophils are considered to have the neutrophilic phenotype of severe asthma. Therefore, sputum granulocyte counts can be used as a diagnostic biomarker for this severe asthma phenotype. However, the use of systemic or ICSs at the time of sputum collection, because these treatments induce neutrophilia, could make interpretation of this finding more challenging. This phenotype is not well understood but may be driven by chronic infection, such as with atypical bacteria or occupational/environmental exposures.[89]

Imaging as a Biomarker. There is increased interest in using quantitative computed tomography to evaluate disease severity in asthma.[90] In 123 subjects enrolled in the NIH Severe Asthma Research Program, airway percentage wall thickness (wall thickness divided by outer airway diameter) was higher in subjects with severe asthma than in those with mild asthma or no disease. Percentage wall thickness also inversely correlated with baseline FEV_1% and positively correlated with change in FEV_1% with bronchodilator challenge. Similar results for the percent airway wall area (airway wall area divided by the total area of the airway) and the percent airway lumen area (airway lumen area divided by the total area of the airway) were also seen.[91] These studies and others support a further relationship between asthma severity and measured airway thickness.[91–93]

Also gaining in acceptance are research tools for investigating regional lung structure and function using high spatial resolution ventilation images with hyperpolarized gas (helium-3 and xenon-129) magnetic resonance imaging.[90,94–96] Moreover, the ability of magnetic resonance imaging to measure regional variation in ventilation may be particularly useful for severe asthmatics for whom bronchial thermoplasty is considered.

ASTHMA TREATMENT APPROACHES

Overview

Current guidelines recommend adjusting therapy in a stepwise fashion to reduce daily symptoms and risk of exacerbations while minimizing the use of medications (see Fig. 62.3).[1,8] The hierarchy of treatment recommendations is based on the available literature about efficacy and safety and provides a prominent role for controller medications at all levels of asthma treatment. In general, the strategy and recommendations in adults and children are similar, with differences attributable to lack of clinical trials in pediatric populations.

Specific Pharmacologic Agents

β_2**-Agonists.** The bronchodilatory effect and tolerability of selective β_2-agonists have cemented these drugs as the cornerstone of asthma therapy.[97] β_2-agonist activity is primarily mediated by binding to a specific G-coupled transmembrane receptor found in high abundance on airway smooth muscle. Receptor binding leads to increased intracellular cyclic adenosine monophosphate and relaxation of airway smooth muscle.[98] Notably, β_2-receptors are also found on other resident airway cells, including airway epithelial cells and circulating immune cells, and binding to these sites may reduce vascular permeability and inflammatory mediator release.[99] One concern raised about the chronic use of β_2-agonists is that of receptor desensitization.[100] As with most signaling receptors, repeated exposure to β_2-agonists can lead to decreased responsiveness of membrane receptors through receptor down-regulation via receptor endocytosis and uncoupling of receptors from downstream transduction pathways. However, clinical data suggest that "as-needed" versus scheduled *short-acting β_2-agonist* (SABA) treatment is associated with improved physiology[101–103] and fewer, less-severe exacerbations.[104] Therefore, the risk of receptor desensitization may be most pronounced when albuterol is overused for asthma management.

β_2-selective agonists are usually administered by aerosol, which maximizes delivery to target tissue while minimizing the exposure of nontarget tissues.[105] SABAs and LABAs are available, and the onset and duration of action are primarily related to lipophilicity.[105] SABAs are used for rescue or emergent treatment, whereas LABAs are used in combination with ICSs for chronic management of asthma.

A number of highly selective SABA preparations are now available, and all have a rapid onset of action with peak action between 60 and 90 minutes. Because they are inhaled directly into the airways, systemic side effects are minimal, even at high doses. Standard albuterol is racemic, that is, it contains two enantiomers: R- (levalbuterol) and S-. A β_2-agonist preparation containing only levalbuterol was developed in an attempt to minimize side effects due to unwanted activation of β_2-receptors in nonpulmonary tissue. Cardiac stimulation causes tachycardia and arrhythmias, whereas skeletal muscle stimulation causes tremors and hypokalemia. However, clinical trials have not shown significant differences in outcome or tolerability compared with standard (racemic) albuterol.[106]

On the basis of current guidelines, SABAs should be used to treat patients with symptoms despite a regimen of long-acting controller agents. Increased frequency of SABA use is a sign of inadequate control of symptoms or overreliance on rescue medication. Patients requiring more than two SABA doses per week should be considered for a step up in therapy.[1,8] LABAs have minimal utility for treating acute asthmatic symptoms because of their delayed onset of action. However, in patients with inadequately controlled asthma, they can be added to ICSs to improve symptoms and efficacy of the ICS. Multiple LABA preparations are available with differential properties. Of these, formoterol has a shorter onset of action, whereas the ultra-LABA preparations may be administered once daily. Each has been shown to improve lung function, reduce symptoms, and reduce the frequency of exacerbations.[107] Although LABAs are effective at improving symptoms and lung function, a study of salmeterol (LABA) monotherapy versus triamcinolone (ICS) monotherapy demonstrated significantly more treatment failures in the salmeterol group.[108] For this reason, LABA monotherapy for asthma is not recommended. In addition, adverse events with LABAs have been of concern, specifically related to the increased risk of death in African American subjects in the Salmeterol Multicenter Asthma Research Trial,[109] which was attributed in part to overall poorer control of symptoms at baseline (with more exacerbations and hospitalizations) and a lower rate of ICS use than in the white patients.[109] This further supports the recommendation against LABA monotherapy for asthma. Importantly, the use of LABAs with ICSs in the same metered-dose inhaler has since been shown to be safe and effective in adults and children.[110–112] Commonly used inhaled steroid-LABA combination inhalers are summarized in eTable 62.1.

Several studies have explored the relationship between polymorphisms in the β_2-receptor and responses to β-agonist therapy. Specifically, in patients treated with scheduled albuterol, the presence of the Arg/Arg polymorphism at the codon 16 locus (B16) was associated with lower PEF and FEV_1, increased symptoms, and more rescue inhaler use compared with patients who were Arg/Gly or homozygous Gly/Gly. All of these symptoms improved when regular albuterol was withdrawn.[101,103,113] Use of LABAs (with and without ICSs) has been shown to worsen physiologic markers of respiratory function in Arg/Arg patients in some studies, although these findings are not consistent.[114,115] The LARGE study demonstrated beneficial effects of LABAs in combination with ICS irrespective of B16 genotype, and the authors recommended against alterations in the current use of LABAs.[116] Further research is required; however, thus far there are no indications that use of LABAs in the Arg/Arg genotype is associated with undue risk. Additional genetic studies are examining potential mechanisms by which β-adrenergic receptor polymorphisms may contribute to the risk of LABA therapy in some patients with asthma.[117]

Anticholinergics. Anticholinergic agents act as bronchodilators by competing with acetylcholine at neuromuscular junctions, thereby blocking transmission of bronchoconstrictor reflexes.[118] The short-acting anticholinergic ipratropium bromide is effective in patients with COPD but is considered a second-line agent for treating asthma, most likely because cholinergic tone contributes less to bronchoconstriction in asthma. While short-acting anticholinergics and SABAs both provide bronchodilation,[119,120] randomized trials studying the addition of anticholinergics to β-agonists do not show any additional benefit in patients with chronic asthma.[121] However, specific asthma phenotypes might be more likely to respond to anticholinergic treatment, including patients with fixed airflow obstruction, advanced age,[122] or longer duration of disease.[123] Furthermore, anticholinergics may be an acceptable alternative for certain subgroups of patients who do not tolerate β-agonist treatment or for patients with the Arg/Arg B16 genotype, although this has not been studied directly.

Tiotropium, a long-acting anticholinergic agent, was approved by the U.S. *Food and Drug Administration* (FDA) for treatment of asthma after multiple randomized controlled trials indicated a role for tiotropium as add-on therapy to both ICS and ICS/LABA combination therapy in patients with moderate to severe asthma.[124–126] Bronchodilator responsiveness to albuterol, higher resting cholinergic tone (defined by a lower resting heart rate), and increased airway obstruction (defined by a lower FEV_1/FVC ratio) are predictors of response to tiotropium.[127] The Steroids in Eosinophil Negative Asthma study by the NHLBI AsthmaNet group compared the relative benefit of ICSs and tiotropium in mild asthma with low sputum eosinophils (<2%).[83] In this clinical trial, among those with low eosinophils, there was no significant difference in treatment response in this group, suggesting tiotropium may be a reasonable alternative for mild asthma control in this phenotype.

Inhaled Corticosteroids. With recognition of the central role of inflammation in the pathophysiology of asthma, contemporary treatment strategies emphasize ICSs for long-term control of symptoms. Corticosteroids suppress inflammatory responses by broadly influencing signal transduction and gene expression pathways. Corticosteroids bind to a specific cytoplasmic receptor that translocates to the nucleus, where it modulates expression of inflammatory genes through inhibition of histone acetyltransferases and recruitment of histone deacetylases, two classes of histone modifiers that control DNA unwinding and gene expression epigenetically.[128,129] Corticosteroids thereby reduce airway inflammatory cell influx and markers of airway inflammation in asthma.[130,131]

Systemic corticosteroids have been used in the treatment of asthma since the 1940s and continue to be a cornerstone of the management of acute exacerbations. However, systemically administered corticosteroids are associated with a variety of undesirable side effects. The introduction of ICSs in the 1970s ushered in a new era in the treatment of asthma. As with bronchodilators, delivery of drug directly into the lungs through the use of inhaled preparations minimizes systemic toxicity and improves therapeutic benefit.

The use of ICSs improves all aspects of asthma control. ICSs reduce asthmatic symptoms, improve lung function, decrease airway inflammation, and control AHR.[132,133] A large meta-analysis showed that ICSs reduce asthma exacerbations by 55% when compared with placebo[134] and reduce the risk of hospitalization by 50% when compared with use of as-needed β-agonists alone.[135] Furthermore,

ICSs reduce the risk of death from asthma in a dose-response manner.[136] As a result, ICS are considered to be first-line therapy for all patients requiring more than twice-weekly β-agonist use.[1,8] Predictors of response to ICSs include FeNO level greater than 47 ppb,[137] reversibility to albuterol and a decreased FEV_1,[138] and the presence of increased sputum eosinophils (>2–3%).[139] Interestingly, a large proportion of asthma patients are persistently noneosinophilic and unlikely to respond to therapy with ICSs, supporting the need for standard phenotyping of asthma with subsequent personalized therapy.[139–141]

The initial recommendations regarding the use of ICSs in patients with mild to moderate persistent asthma emphasized their use on a daily to twice-daily basis. Recently, there has been increased evidence that ICSs can be efficacious at reducing asthma symptoms and achieving asthma control when used intermittently in both children and adults, and the GINA guidelines now recommend that mild asthma be treated with intermittent budesonide/formoterol or that intermittent ICSs be taken every time rescue therapy is used.[8,142–145]

There are multiple different ICS preparations and delivery devices on the market (see eTable 62.1). The inhalers differ in particle size, ranging from a mass median aerodynamic diameter of about 1 μm to those with large particles 2 to 5 μm in size. The delivery devices include dry powder inhalers and metered-dose inhalers. The choice of ICS is based on the physician's discretion about the patient's needs and often rests on cost, convenience of dosing, and reduction of side effects. Some patients with very severe obstruction may be unable to generate the high inspiratory flows required for dry powder inhalers and may therefore do better with metered-dose inhalers (see also Chapter 13).

One key factor that warrants consideration is the role of small airway inflammation and associated obstruction as a key component of asthma pathophysiology. The presence of preserved FEV_1 with decreased mid expiratory flow and increased distal resistance is indicative of a small airway phenotype.[146] Targeted therapies to help modulate small airway inflammation are important, and there are several small particle size inhalers that have improved deposition into the distal lung.[147] Utilization of these inhalers may result in improvements in lung function measurements and asthma control.[147,148] In spite of the increased evidence that small particle size inhalers are efficacious, superiority comparisons with large particle size inhalers are lacking, and specific recommendations to help guide clinicians on choice of ICS for any particular patient therefore cannot be made at this time.[149]

The risk of systemic toxicity from steroids is diminished with the use of ICSs, particularly at doses less than 400 μg budesonide daily or the equivalent, but the risk is not absent. Data are conflicting about the risk of bone demineralization from ICSs; although a small observational study suggested increased risk,[150,151] a meta-analysis of several randomized controlled trials did not corroborate this finding.[151,152] The risks of cataract formation[152] and glaucoma[153] are slightly increased, whereas hypothalamic-pituitary axis suppression, gastrointestinal bleeding, and other complications of systemic steroids are not associated with inhaled preparations. The Towards a Revolution in COPD Health trial of the use of ICSs for COPD showed an increased risk of pneumonia, but this has not been demonstrated in patients with asthma.[154] The use of ICSs in the pediatric population has raised concerns about growth suppression. However, available data show only a small and transient decrease in growth trajectory that does not translate into a reduction in adult height.[133,140,155]

Leukotriene Modifiers. *Leukotrienes* (LTs) are derived from cell membrane arachidonic acid metabolism. LT receptors on airway smooth muscle and macrophages mediate bronchoconstriction, mucus hypersecretion, and mucosal edema.[156] As a result, the LT pathway is a primary target for the development of asthma controller medications. Commercially available *leukotriene modifiers* (LTMs) work in one of two places in the LT pathway. Zileuton inhibits the activity of 5-lipoxygenase, the enzyme that converts arachidonic acid to leukotriene A_4, which is the first step in LT synthesis. Montelukast, zafirlukast, and pranlukast are all cysteinyl leukotriene-1–receptor antagonists, blocking the final step in the LT pathway. All are taken orally as either once-daily or twice-daily doses.

LTMs have a modest bronchodilator effect and may improve asthma symptoms and exacerbation rates.[157] Physiologic benefits have also been seen, with improvements in spirometry and measures of airway inflammation.[158] Whereas the subpopulation of patients with aspirin-sensitive asthma may derive great benefit from LTMs,[159] data also suggest that LTMs are adequate as single agents in mild persistent asthma.[160,161] Although LTMs treat multiple asthma symptoms, they are less effective than low-dose ICSs. LTMs can be used as monotherapy in exercise-induced asthma and in patients with relatively mild asthma symptoms that do not require therapy with ICSs, and can be combined with ICSs as a step up in therapy.[161] The addition of LTMs may lead to a reduction in the required corticosteroid dose or an improvement in asthma control.[162,163] In general, LTMs are less effective than LABAs as adjunctive therapy and do not seem to confer added benefits when added to a regimen that includes an ICS and a LABA.[164,165]

Overall, LTMs are well tolerated. Initial reports suggested a link between LTMs and eosinophilic granulomatosis with polyangiitis, but this is now thought more likely to be due to an unmasking of the syndrome by a reduction in corticosteroid dose with the introduction of an LTM.[166] LTMs have been linked to mood changes and suicidal ideation, particularly in children; therefore, monitoring of these symptoms is prudent.[167] Zileuton is metabolized by the cytochrome P-450 system and has been associated with reports of hepatotoxicity. As a result, liver function should be monitored during its use. At present, zileuton is reserved for patients with refractory asthma or who have an asthmatic phenotype suggesting benefit from the use of a leukotriene modifier.[168]

Phosphodiesterase Inhibitors. Theophylline is a well-established phosphodiesterase inhibitor that has mild anti-inflammatory properties. Because of its narrow therapeutic index, theophylline is not widely used in treating asthma. However, the discovery of additional anti-inflammatory properties, likely mediated by histone deacetylation, has led to a resurgence of interest.[169] Although no longer a recommended therapy and not recommended for use in children, theophylline is sometimes used in low doses as adjunctive treatment for moderate to severe asthma difficult to control with steroids alone.[8,170] The addition of theophylline to an existing drug regimen for poorly controlled asthma improves markers of control (e.g., less rescue inhaler use, better lung function) to a greater extent than LTMs.[171] Dose-related side effects, such as anorexia, palpitations, dysrhythmias, and seizures, require careful clinical and laboratory monitoring. Newer specific phosphodiesterase type 4 inhibitor drugs have been developed, and their safety profile is better than that of theophylline. Roflumilast has demonstrated efficacy in improving FEV_1 in asthma.[172,173] Although roflumilast is not approved for asthma, it has bronchodilating and anti-inflammatory properties that may be beneficial in asthma.

Macrolides and Asthma. Macrolides were initially shown to be effective in a subset of asthma patients who had evidence of mycoplasma in their airways by polymerase chain reaction.[174,175] These positive results generated interest in a broader use of macrolides for poorly controlled asthma. Subsequent clinical trials demonstrated variable effects on improving asthma symptoms or exacerbation risk.[176–178] In a recent clinical trial, azithromycin 500 mg 3 times weekly was associated with fewer exacerbations in both eosinophilic and noneosinophilic phenotypes and was well tolerated.[179] Additional studies to identify phenotypic or endotypic markers of response to therapy will help drive the most appropriate use of this intervention.

Targeted Biologic Agents. Over the past 5 years, there has been a significant increase in the number of biologics approved for the treatment of asthma. The era of personalized therapy in asthma is slowly being realized, making it imperative for clinicians to understand each individual patient's asthma phenotype as detailed in the biomarkers section of this chapter. The latter is especially important in those with severe asthma and is essential in identifying those more likely to respond to biologic therapies. At this time, there are five FDA-approved biologics for the treatment of asthma: omalizumab (Xolair), mepolizumab (Nucala), reslizumab (Cinqair), benralizumab (Fasenra), and dupilumab (Dupixent) (Table 62.4).

IMMUNOGLOBULIN E TARGETED THERAPIES. Omalizumab was the first FDA-approved monoclonal antibody for asthma and is now also indicated for the treatment of idiopathic urticaria. Omalizumab targets the FCεRI receptor–binding portion of IgE, preventing it from interacting with immune cells to cause degranulation.[180] Treatment with omalizumab reduces unbound IgE capable of binding to its receptor by 90–95%.[181] It must be administered subcutaneously, and the dose is based on IgE levels and body surface area. The addition of omalizumab to ICSs in poorly controlled allergic asthmatics is associated with improved asthma control and fewer exacerbations.[182] Omalizumab is generally well tolerated, but rare reports of anaphylaxis have been reported.[183] The importance of utilizing biomarkers to identify potential responders to omalizumab was highlighted by the EXTRA study, which demonstrated significantly decreased numbers of exacerbations in subjects with high FeNO, high serum eosinophils, and elevated serum

Table 62.4   Summary of FDA-Approved Biologics for Treatment of Moderate to Severe Asthma

Biologic Agent	MOA	Patient Selection	Dosing	Notes
Omalizumab (Xolair) FDA approved in 2003	Humanized IgG1 antibody that binds to the Cε3 domain of free IgE and prevents it from binding to FcεR1	■ Age ≥6 years in the U.S. (≥12 years in the UK) ■ IgE: 30-700 IU/mL ■ Allergic sensitization by skin prick or specific IgE testing	75–375 mg SC per IU every 2-4 weeks based on age, weight and IgE levels	■ Highest efficacy in T2-high patients ■ Efficacy not based on IgE level or eosinophil count ■ Data from real-world studies demonstrate efficacy when dosed outside accepted weight and IgE levels ■ Indicated for *moderate to severe* allergic asthma
Mepolizumab (Nucala) FDA approved in 2015	Humanized IgG1 antibody that inhibits IL-5 from binding to the α-subunit of the IL-5 receptor complex on eosinophils	■ ≥12 years ■ Blood AEC of ≥150 cells/μL at the time of testing or ≥300 cells/μL in the previous year ■ ≥300 cells/μL only in the UK	■ 100 mg SC every 4 weeks ■ 300 mg SC every 4 weeks for EGPA	■ Approved for home administration via the auto injector ■ In clinic dosing using the lyophilized powder ■ Only biologic currently approved for EGPA ■ Demonstrated OCS-sparing effects ■ Indicated for severe eosinophilic asthma
Reslizumab (Cinqair) FDA approved in 2016	Humanized IgG4 antibody that inhibits IL-5 from binding to the α-subunit of the IL-5 receptor complex expressed on eosinophils	■ Age ≥18 years ■ Blood AEC ≥400 cells/μL in the previous year	3 mg/kg IV infusion every 4 weeks	■ Response is better with higher eosinophil counts ■ No data on OCS-sparing effects; SC OCS dosing study was negative ■ Indicated for severe eosinophilic asthma
Benralizumab (Fasenra) FDA approved in 2017	Humanized recombinant IgG1 antibody that binds with high affinity to the α-subunit of the IL-5 receptor	■ Age ≥12 years ■ Blood AEC ≥300 cells/μL in the previous year	30 mg SC every 4 weeks for the first 3 doses then every 8 weeks	■ Available for prefilled auto injector ■ Results in total depletion of eosinophils ■ Demonstrated OCS-sparing effects ■ Indicated for severe eosinophilic asthma
Dupilumab (Dupixent) FDA approved in 2018	Fully human monoclonal antibody to the α-unit of IL-4 receptor; blocks IL-4 and IL-13	■ Age ≥12 years ■ Moderate to severe asthma ■ Blood AEC ≥300 cells/μL in the previous year ■ FeNO >25 ppb	■ 200 mg or 300 mg SC every 2 weeks after initial loading dose. No loading dose required for nasal polyps ■ 200 mg for moderate to severe persistent asthma, 300 mg for atopic dermatitis, nasal polyps and oral steroid-dependent asthma	■ Home administration only ■ Antidrug antibody in 2–5% patients ■ Indicated for nasal polyps, atopic dermatitis, and asthma (*moderate to severe* persistent eosinophilic asthma or oral steroid–dependent asthma regardless of T2 markers) ■ Demonstrated OCS-sparing effects ■ Exercise caution in patients with baseline eosinophils >1500 cells/μL due to transient elevation of eosinophils for 4 months post initiation of therapy

AEC, absolute eosinophil count; OCS, oral corticosteroid; EGPA, eosinophilic granulomatosis with polyangiitis; FDA, Food and Drug Administration; FeNO, fraction of exhaled nitric oxide; Ig, immunoglobulin; IL, interleukin; IU, international units; IV, intravenous; SC, subcutaneous.

periostin compared with subjects with low biomarker levels.[184] Interestingly, the recently published PROSPERO real-world study demonstrated that peripheral eosinophils and FeNO levels at baseline had variable impacts on asthma outcomes. For instance, high eosinophils and FeNO had no impact on the response to omalizumab with regard to exacerbations and hospitalizations but were associated with more significant improvements in FEV_1 and mean change in Asthma Control Test scores from baseline.[185] Furthermore, this study demonstrated that patients outside the approved dosing tables on the basis of either IgE level or weight had similar improvements in Asthma Control Test scores to those dosed within the recommended levels, further supporting the assertion that baseline IgE level is a poor predictor of clinical response to omalizumab and should be interpreted with caution. In addition, it is imperative to note that IgE levels should not be used in isolation. Clinicians must identify evidence of allergic sensitization using specific IgE measurements or skin prick testing to identify individuals most likely to respond to omalizumab therapy. In addition, clinical evidence of allergic disease is necessary, and a history of allergic rhinitis, seasonal variability in exacerbations, allergic conjunctivitis, eczema, and urticaria should be sought to understand the impact of allergic disease on the patient's asthma.

INTERLEUKIN-5 TARGETED THERAPIES. There are currently two anti–IL-5 antibodies (mepolizumab and reslizumab) and one anti–IL-5 receptor antibody (benralizumab) approved for use in the United States. Mepolizumab, a humanized monoclonal antibody to IL-5 approved by the FDA in 2015, has demonstrated efficacy in reducing exacerbations in patients with severe asthma and is dosed as a once-monthly subcutaneous injection.[186,187] The anti–IL-5 antibody significantly decreases eosinophil differentiation, maturation, and migration.[188] Mepolizumab significantly decreases exacerbations[189] and oral corticosteroid dose in oral corticosteroid–dependent asthma.[189] Mepolizumab results in modest improvements in FEV_1, asthma control, and quality of life.[189] In long-term safety studies, continued use of mepolizumab persistently reduces exacerbations.[190] No significant safety issues have been identified.[191] The safety profile of the medication led to its approval for home dosing via an auto-injector device by the FDA in 2019. Mepolizumab is indicated as add-on maintenance therapy for patients older than 12 years with severe eosinophilic asthma. In clinical trials, patients were required to demonstrate eosinophils greater than 150 cells/μL at baseline or greater than 300 cells/μL within the past year. Adverse reactions including hypersensitivity may be seen within hours of administration of the medication but are rare overall. There is a warning regarding herpes zoster infection based on the presence of two cases of zoster in the registration trials. It remains unclear if this was associated with the medication. Vaccination for zoster is recommended if possible prior to initiation of therapy.

Reslizumab was approved by the FDA in 2016 for use in asthma. It is a humanized IgG4 antibody that inhibits IL-5 from binding the α-subunit of the IL-5 receptor complex expressed on eosinophils. Reslizumab improves FEV_1, asthma control, quality of life, and exacerbation rates.[192] Patients with high blood eosinophils and frequent exacerbations had the greatest benefit in terms of exacerbation reduction and improvement in FEV_1.[193,194] Reslizumab is indicated as add-on maintenance therapy for patients with severe eosinophilic asthma; the clinical trials required peripheral eosinophils 400 cells/μL or greater. Reslizumab is administered at a dose of 3 mg/kg by intravenous infusion over 20 to 50 minutes every 4 weeks. Hypersensitivity reactions including anaphylaxis are rare and, in general, reslizumab is well tolerated. Long-term efficacy was demonstrated in an open-label study.[195]

Benralizumab was approved by the FDA in 2017 and is a humanized recombinant IgG1 antibody that has high affinity binding to the α-subunit of the IL-5 receptor, resulting in inhibition of proliferation and activation of eosinophils. Benralizumab also mediates apoptosis of eosinophils,

leading to peripheral eosinopenia.[196] In Phase III trials, benralizumab demonstrated a significant reduction in exacerbation rates and improvements in FEV_1 similar with every 4-week and every 8-week dosing.[197,198] In addition, benralizumab resulted in a significant reduction in oral steroid dose while maintaining a concomitant reduction in exacerbations in patients with oral steroid–dependent asthma.[199] Benralizumab is indicated as add-on maintenance therapy for patients with severe eosinophilic asthma, and the best results were noted in those with eosinophil counts greater than 300 cells/μL. It is administered subcutaneously at 30 mg once a month for 3 months (loading phase) and then every 2 months thereafter. Adverse reactions include a low rate of hypersensitivity reactions (3%), which is slightly higher than those reported with mepolizumab and reslizumab. Benralizumab results in total depletion of eosinophils in the airway, blood, and bone marrow.[200] Long-term safety concerns of total depletion of eosinophils remain, but thus far no significant issues have been identified.[201] Post hoc analysis identified clinical markers that predict a more robust response to benralizumab including adult-onset asthma, decreased FVC, presence of nasal polyps, and oral steroid–dependent disease.[202]

IL-4 TARGETED THERAPIES. Dupilumab is a fully human monoclonal IgG4 antibody to the α-subunit of the IL-4 receptor. The IL-4 receptor binds both IL-4 and IL-13, two key cytokines produced by T cells and by type 2 innate lymphoid cells, and results in downstream up-regulation of IgE production (mediated by IL-4) and mucus hypersecretion and AHR (mediated by IL-13). Dupilumab was approved by the FDA in 2018 and is indicated for atopic dermatitis, moderate to severe persistent eosinophilic asthma, oral steroid–dependent asthma, and chronic rhinosinusitis with nasal polyposis. Dupilumab resulted in a significant reduction in exacerbations, particularly in patients with an elevated FeNO and/or elevated blood eosinophil count (>300 cells/μL).[203] In oral steroid–dependent asthma, patients responded to dupilumab regardless of eosinophil count or FeNO level with improvements in FEV_1 and a reduction in oral steroid dose.[204] It is approved for home dosing exclusively and is available in two formulations in a prefilled syringe (200 mg and 300 mg) for administration subcutaneously every 2 weeks. The higher doses were studied in atopic dermatitis, nasal polyposis, and oral steroid–dependent asthma. In asthma, dupilumab is approved for patients older than 12 years. Patients with asthma receive a loading dose (2 injections of the formulation prescribed) followed by every-2-week dosing. Dupilumab results in transient elevations in peripheral eosinophils over the initial 4 months of therapy; therefore caution must be exercised in prescribing the drug to patients with peripheral eosinophil counts greater than 1500 cells/μL. Hypersensitivity reactions are rare. Local skin reactions are seen more frequently in those receiving the higher dose of medication, although these are not common.

BIOLOGIC THERAPY: PATIENT SELECTION, RESPONSE, AND SWITCHING. The increased availability of biologic therapies for asthma has led to the need for a paradigm shift in the manner in which clinicians manage severe asthma. Clinical decision making surrounding which therapy to initiate first, how to monitor patients for response, how to define response, and whether or not to switch therapies has become increasingly complex and warrants a systematic approach. GINA guidelines now include a pocket guide for the management of severe asthma that aims to address these challenges by providing algorithms that clinicians can follow while managing patients with severe asthma. Biologics should be considered early in the course of therapy for patients with severe asthma who are adherent to conventional inhaled therapies but continue to have poorly controlled disease. Poor control can be recognized by at least one of the following: frequent exacerbations, decreased lung function, poor quality of life and, in the most extreme cases, dependence on oral corticosteroids. A suggested algorithm for when to consider initiating a biologic agent is shown in Figure 62.4.

The selection of initial biologic therapies should be based on the clinical features and baseline biomarkers. For instance, allergic sensitization and the presence of uncontrolled allergic asthma may prompt initiation of anti-IgE targeted therapies. Comorbid conditions such as nasal polyps, atopic dermatitis, and idiopathic urticaria that require concomitant therapy will likely alter the initial therapy selected. Concomitant eosinophilic diseases such as eosinophilic granulomatosis with polyangiitis, hypereosinophilic syndrome, and other eosinophilic disorders should be considered as well. Baseline biomarkers are important for making therapeutic decisions, but the limitations of these biomarkers should always be taken into consideration. Peripheral eosinophils are highly variable and affected by steroid therapy; therefore, caution should be exercised with interpretation of single values, and the clinical context must be taken into consideration. Repeating biomarkers is recommended in the current GINA guidelines.[8] FeNO and eosinophils may be less reliable in obese patients.[205,206] The majority of severe asthma patients will have overlapping T2 biomarkers, making the clinical characteristics and comorbid conditions associated with each individual's asthma more important in selecting a biologic therapy. Shared decision making regarding the biologic to initiate is essential in severe asthma, particularly given the prevalence of many different dosing schedules, drug delivery mechanisms, and the options for home dosing (with two of the available biologics). Patient preference is key because all the biologics appear to have similar safety and efficacy profiles overall. Biologics are costly medications and a commitment to adhere to therapy is essential, particularly when embarking on home-dosing regimens. We propose the algorithm shown in Figure 62.5 for initiating T2 biologic therapy based on biomarkers and clinical characteristics.

It is imperative to determine which markers of response will be monitored in advance of initiation of biologic therapies and to allow a sufficient amount of time to assess response. The responses in the following domains should be measured and recorded consistently to allow for consideration when switching between available therapies. Biologic therapies can improve some or all of these outcomes in patients. The degree to which one responds in each of these areas can be used to identify partial as well as complete response to therapy.

1. Exacerbation reduction by a factor of between 30% and 50% compared to baseline.
2. Oral corticosteroid use reduction. Remember that not all biologics have been shown to reduce oral corticosteroid dose.

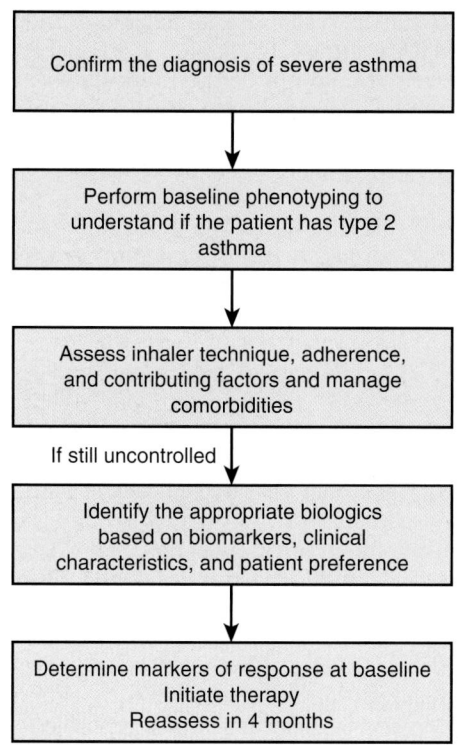

Fig. 62.4 Recommended process toward initiating biologic therapy. A diagnosis of severe asthma should be confirmed using objective measures of lung function, and evidence for type 2 asthma should be assessed. Before initiating biologic therapy, evaluate for comorbid conditions, alternative diagnoses, and poor inhaler technique or adherence. Measurement of type 2 biomarkers will help select initial therapy. Reassess for clinical response in 4 months.

3. Asthma control improvement. The Asthma Control Questionnaire or Asthma Control Test should be measured consistently. Improvements are often modest and usually at the minimally clinically important level.
4. Lung function improvement. Not all patients experience increases in FEV_1 and improvements are often delayed, with a change of between 120 to 300 mL in general.
5. Rescue bronchodilator use reduction.
6. Adequate safety and tolerability.
7. A positive overall impression of the patient regarding response to therapy and satisfaction with the changes. It is important to identify what the patient's expectations are up front and to follow the response with regard to patient expectations.

Response can be identified in three ways. A small proportion of patients, the complete responders, experience a remarkable response to biologics with complete amelioration of all the factors described above. Most patients, the partial responders, experience meaningful improvements in some, but not all, the parameters. About 10–15% of patients, the nonresponders, show no response despite careful patient selection and an expectation that response should be more robust. In these patients, attention should be paid to compliance with background therapy, optimization of comorbid conditions, and adherence to biologics. Alternative diagnoses and contributing factors should also be considered. These patients likely have multiple inflammatory pathways causing asthma symptoms and will benefit from either switching to other biologic therapies or, in

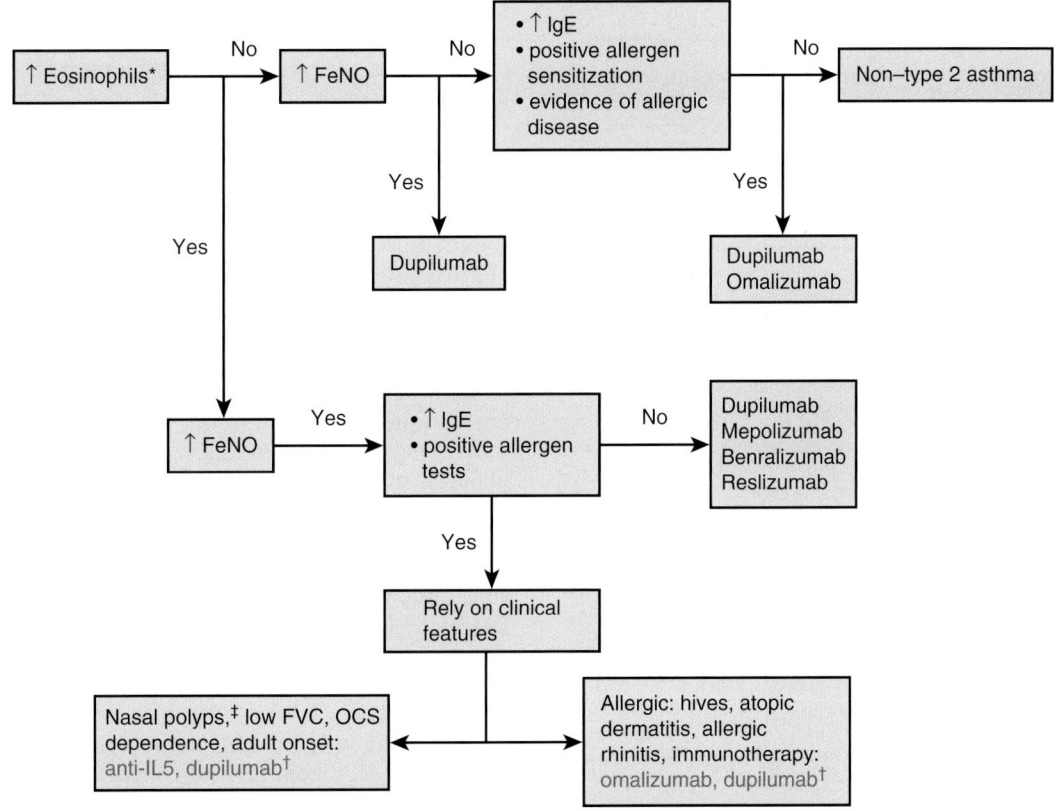

Fig. 62.5 Decision tree for selecting initial biologic therapy for severe asthma in patients with type 2 features. This algorithm is guided by high-quality evidence from clinical trials and supporting data. Medications are listed alphabetically, not in order of preference. Patients should have regular assessment of clinical benefit, and treatment should be adjusted until asthma control is achieved. *Increased eosinophils is defined by blood eosinophil counts >150–300/μL. Dupilumab should not be used for patients with >1500 eosinophils/μL. †At the time of publication, dupilumab is also FDA approved for use in nasal polyps and atopic dermatitis. Omalizumab is also FDA approved for use in chronic urticaria. ‡Nasal polyps predict an enhanced response to these T2 biologics when targeting asthma. The efficacy of each biologic for nasal polyps may differ. FDA, U.S. Food and Drug Administration; FeNO, fraction of exhaled nitric oxide; FVC, forced vital capacity; IgE, immunoglobulin E; OCS, oral corticosteroid.

rare instances, to dual therapies. Recommended management algorithms on the basis of response to biologic therapy are depicted in Figure 62.6.

Bronchial Thermoplasty

One alternative nonpharmacologic treatment goal for asthma is the mechanical reduction of airway smooth muscle mass to improve physiologic function. Bronchial thermoplasty is the application of controlled thermal energy via a radiofrequency catheter to reduce smooth muscle mass. In a clinical trial of thermoplasty or sham thermoplasty in patients with moderately severe asthma, thermoplasty reduced airway responsiveness to an inhaled constrictor, improved lung function, and improved asthma symptoms and quality of life; however, concurrent improvements were also seen in those receiving the sham procedure.[207,208] In addition, treatment requires a series of three bronchoscopies, exposing patients to the concomitant procedural risk, and requires providers have advanced procedural training. Long-term 5-year data demonstrate sustained improvements in asthma control, reduced exacerbations, decreased medication use, and a lack of evidence of long-term adverse effects.[209] Despite this, in 2014, the ERS/ATS severe asthma guidelines recommended against the widespread use of bronchial thermoplasty and suggested that this procedure should be recommended only in the context of a clinical trial or in a large academic center coupled with

a registry aimed at identifying predictors of response.[84] As for other expensive asthma therapies, it is imperative to identify responders and target this therapy to those who are most likely to benefit from the procedure.

ADDITIONAL MANAGEMENT STRATEGIES

Medication Adjustment Based on Asthma Control

All patients should be reassessed for control regardless of the therapy. Recent studies support the importance of focusing on asthma control as a means of reducing exacerbations and morbidity.[210] Depending on the extent of control, a more or less aggressive approach to symptom management may be necessary, such as dose adjustment or use of alternative medication class. Published guidelines provide a framework for medication choices when "stepping up" therapy to improve asthma control and "stepping down" therapy when control has been achieved (see Fig. 62.3).

Uncontrolled asthma is defined by the International ERS/ATS Guidelines for Severe Asthma[84] as presence of any of the following four criteria:

1. Poor symptom control, defined as an Asthma Control Questionnaire score consistently 1.5 or greater or Asthma Control Test score of 19 or less (or "not well controlled" by National Asthma Education and Prevention Program or GINA guidelines over the 3 months of evaluation)

Management Based on Response

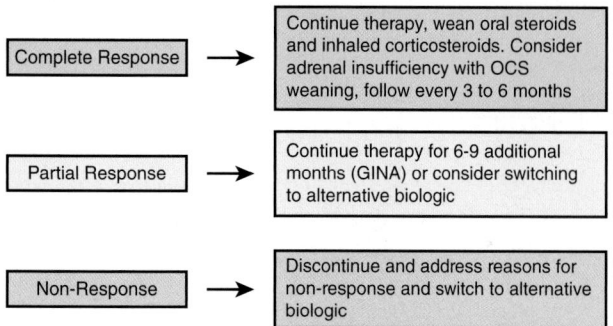

Consistently assess and document response markers: Asthma control, medication use, exacerbations, and biomarkers in all patients.

Fig. 62.6 Assessing response to biologic therapy. Before initiating biologic therapy, choose markers of response that will be monitored (e.g., exacerbations, oral corticosteroid use, asthma control, lung function, rescue bronchodilator use, patient comfort, and satisfaction). Most patients will experience at least a partial response to biologic therapy, 10–15% will have no response, and a small proportion will have a complete response. Assess response continuously and adjust asthma medications and/or biologics based on response. GINA, Global Initiative for Asthma; OCS, oral corticosteroids.

2. Frequent severe exacerbations, defined as two or more bursts of systemic corticosteroids (≥3 days each) in the previous year
3. Serious exacerbations, defined as at least one hospitalization, intensive care unit stay, or mechanical ventilation in the previous year
4. Airflow limitation, defined as FEV_1 less than 80% predicted (in the presence of reduced FEV_1/FVC defined as less than the lower limit of normal) following a withhold of both short- and long-acting bronchodilators

For patients with mild, intermittent asthma, with symptoms that return to baseline between episodes, as-needed use of a short-acting bronchodilator is usually sufficient to achieve relief of symptoms and is recommended per EPR guidelines. In contrast, in the most recent GINA guidelines, SABA-only treatment (without ICSs) is not recommended, even for patients with mild intermittent asthma. Because even patients with mild asthma show chronic airway inflammation, GINA guidelines suggest that all patients with mild asthma should receive a low-dose inhaled steroid, for use either as needed with SABA or in combination with a LABA (as budesonide/formoterol), or daily, to prevent risk of exacerbations. For all patients with persistent asthma (symptoms >2 times/week, nocturnal symptoms, or symptoms that affect activity), the addition of a controller medication is necessary and an ICS is the initial agent of choice.[133,211,212] As mentioned previously, when used properly, ICSs can ameliorate all asthma symptoms, improve airway physiology, and reduce hospitalizations and asthma mortality. Failure to respond to an ICS suggests either nonadherence to medications, uncontrolled trigger exposures and/or comorbidities, or a steroid-nonresponsive phenotype. Approximately 30–50% of asthmatics fall into the latter category and demonstrate noneosinophilic inflammation and associated decreased response to conventional asthma therapy with ICSs,[83,139] unlike patients with eosinophilic inflammation who demonstrate significant

response to a low dose of ICS.[213,214] LTMs are an alternative for patients who do not tolerate or respond to ICS and may provide additional symptom relief for patients with concomitant allergic rhinitis.[157,158]

Guidelines offer several different options for stepping up therapy. Some guidelines recommend the addition of a LABA to low-dose ICS (usually in a combination inhaler) based on a large amount of efficacy data.[108,215–217] Increasing the ICS dose is an alternative approach, and the preferred approach for pediatric patients. Recommendations regarding up-titration of inhaled steroids have typically focused on doubling the dose of ICSs in patients not well controlled on a low-dose ICS. However, there is increased recognition that doubling the dose is not consistently efficacious at improving asthma control or lung function measurements.[218] Furthermore, glucocorticoid resistance has been described in obese asthmatics.[219–221]

Once symptoms are controlled for a protracted period of time, therapy can be stepped down. Strategies for de-escalation of therapy are determined by a patient's controller regimen but may also be influenced by patient-specific factors. Patients on an ICS alone can be considered for a decrease in dose or dosing interval. Some data suggest that conversion to as-needed combined ICS/SABA may be effective with a lower total steroid dose.[144,222] However, an as-needed regimen is not yet part of NHLBI-EPR guidelines; it is, however, recommended by GINA. For patients on a combined ICS/LABA or ICS/LTM regimen, clinicians may focus first on reducing the ICS component for patients with steroid phobia or for whom steroid side effects are noted; alternatively, withdrawal of the nonsteroid agent may be appropriate for patients with high exhaled NO levels.[8] During down-titration of medications, care should be taken that patients not transition to LABA monotherapy, which is associated with worse outcomes.[108]

Difficult-to-Treat and Severe Asthma

Patients whose asthma symptoms are not controlled despite use of high-dose ICS and additional controller therapy (LABA or long-acting muscarinic antagonist), or whose symptoms require high-dose ICS to maintain control, are considered to have difficult-to-treat asthma.[8] Chronic use of systemic corticosteroids to control asthma is included in this definition. For many of these patients, modification of factors such as exposure to triggers, comorbid conditions (Table 62.5), incorrect inhaler technique, medication nonadherence, and adverse environmental exposures (tobacco smoke, particulates) may help to gain control of asthma and reduce medication requirements. Alternative diagnoses should also be considered, including bronchiectasis, COPD, vocal cord dysfunction, cardiac conditions, vasculitis, bronchomalacia, and lung masses. Those for whom asthma remains difficult to treat despite adequate control of these modifiable factors are considered to have *severe asthma*.[223]

Control of Triggers

Because treatment of comorbidities often improves the control of asthma, all difficult-to-treat patients with asthma should be evaluated for these underlying conditions.[224–229] Environmental factors and individual comorbid conditions have been shown to contribute to the pathogenesis and manifestations of asthma at all levels of severity

Table 62.5 Factors That Contribute to Worsening Asthma Control and Coexisting Conditions

Contributing Factor	Proposed Intervention
Tobacco use	Encourage tobacco cessation and assist with both nonpharmacologic and pharmacologic methods to help patients quit smoking; discuss avoidance of secondhand smoke
GERD	Consider empiric therapy for symptomatic GERD Barium swallow or pH probe study to diagnose GERD Impedance study if nonacid reflux is suspected Referral to gastroenterology for evaluation and treatment Consider surgical management for refractory cases
Atopy and allergic rhinitis	Consider empiric therapy with nasal steroids, nasal and oral antihistamines, leukotriene antagonists Consider skin prick testing or specific IgE testing to guide allergen identification and avoidance Referral to allergist or otolaryngologist for evaluation Consider allergen immunotherapy
Nasal polyps and chronic sinusitis	Refer to otolaryngologist for evaluation and treatment Possible surgical intervention for refractory cases Consider aspirin desensitization for patients with nasal polyps and aspirin sensitivity
Vocal cord dysfunction*	Laryngoscopy to diagnose vocal cord dysfunction Referral to speech pathologist for evaluation and treatment
Obesity*	Encourage weight loss Consider bariatric surgery
Obstructive sleep apnea*	Referral for sleep study and initiate therapy for sleep apnea Referral to sleep specialist for complex cases
Psychological factors*	Evaluate for anxiety and depression

*May coexist with asthma with overlapping symptoms (see also Chapter 61).
GERD, gastroesophageal reflux disease; Ig, immunoglobulin.

and therefore should be addressed as appropriate for each patient (Table 62.5). Cigarette smoking decreases asthma control and reduces the efficacy of corticosteroids.[230] All patients with asthma who smoke cigarettes should be strongly encouraged to quit.[231] Exposure to secondhand smoke should be avoided. Obesity complicates asthma through multiple mechanisms including reducing steroid efficacy and compounding symptoms and is reviewed thoroughly in Chapter 61.

Reduction of allergen exposure and provision of allergen-specific subcutaneous immunotherapy are common strategies for treating asthma. Allergic asthmatics benefit from allergen avoidance, but environmental control in the home or workplace is often difficult to achieve.[232] The most common allergens triggering asthma include molds, dust mites, and cat dander. Although overall data are mixed, several studies have shown clinical benefits from dust mite control measures (e.g., impermeable mattress covers, frequent vacuuming, cockroach control).[233–235] For patients with an allergic asthma phenotype, allergen-specific subcutaneous

immunotherapy may reduce asthma symptoms and improve bronchial hyperreactivity.[236,237] However, subcutaneous immunotherapy must take place under careful conditions owing to the risk of anaphylaxis, and the optimal duration of treatment is not completely clear. As an alternative, sublingual immunotherapy specific for dust mite allergen showed potential for reducing asthma exacerbations, is well tolerated, and is commercially available.[238]

Assessment and Management of Concomitant Diagnoses

Vocal Cord Dysfunction. *Vocal cord dysfunction* (VCD), also referred to as paroxysmal vocal fold motion, was first described as a separate clinical entity in 1983 and is one of the great mimics of asthma (see also Chapter 70). VCD presents more often in women than in men and is more common in persons 20 to 40 years old.[239,240] It is characterized by intermittent abnormal paradoxical adduction of the true vocal cords during breathing. Patients with VCD often experience shortness of breath, neck/chest tightness, stridor, wheezing, hoarseness, frequent throat clearing, and cough. VCD patients can have normal head and neck and lung examinations or abnormal examinations with upper airway noise or stridor. Although many causes of VCD have been identified, most patients experience one of three subtypes: psychogenic VCD, exercise-induced VCD, or irritant-associated VCD.

Psychogenic VCD is most often identified in those previously diagnosed with a psychiatric illness such as depression, anxiety, or factitious or somatoform disorder.[241] For these patients, the vocal cords are their "stress organ" and learning how to manage stress is key to treating their disease. Exercise-induced VCD is often described as episodic dyspnea or shortness of breath that manifests within the first 5 minutes of exercise and resolves abruptly. These patients are frequently misdiagnosed with exercise-induced bronchospasm but fail to respond to bronchodilator therapy or steroids.[242] Irritant-associated VCD is linked to chronic irritation of the throat resulting in vocal cord hypersensitivity. The irritants are categorized as either intrinsic (gastroesophageal reflux, laryngopharyngeal reflux, allergic rhinitis) or extrinsic (chemical or sensory irritants).

The diagnosis of VCD can be challenging because symptoms are frequently intermittent, and patients need to be symptomatic during testing. Difficulty in making the diagnosis is further complicated by the fact that up to 75% of asthmatics have coexistent VCD.[239,243] Pulmonary function studies can reveal normal spirometry (without bronchodilator responsiveness) or an abnormal truncated inspiratory flow volume loop. Methacholine challenge has been used as a provocative measure to recreate symptoms and induce paradoxical closure of the vocal cords. Flow volume loops before and after methacholine challenge in patients with VCD often demonstrate flattening of the inspiratory curve after methacholine challenge.[244] Flexible laryngoscopy and videolaryngostroboscopy are the gold standards for diagnosing VCD. Direct visualization of the cords classically demonstrates abnormal adduction of the anterior two-thirds of the true vocal cords with inspiration and "chinking" of the posterior cords; the chink describes the small triangular opening that remains patent at the posterior segment of the vocal cords.[245] The vocal cords can be seen in adduction during inspiration or during both inspiration and expiration.

Beyond treating the underlying disorder (gastroesophageal reflux disease, rhinitis, and depression), there is no specific medication that treats VCD. Acute severe VCD, manifesting as laryngospasm, can be managed with heliox to reduce airway resistance rapidly[246] or with anxiolytics. Long term, patients are often referred to speech therapy for initiation of relaxed throat breathing exercises and diaphragmatic breathing exercises. Although these exercises have been reported to be effective in case reports, randomized clinical trials to validate effectiveness are needed.

MANAGEMENT OF ACUTE ASTHMA

Asthma is a common cause of emergency department visits and hospital admissions. The treatment of acute asthma is based on the cornerstones of chronic asthma therapy but typically requires greater attention to patient monitoring and an escalation in the aggressiveness of asthma care.

Asthma exacerbations are characterized by increased shortness of breath, coughing, and/or chest tightness, and airflow limitation (as measured by decreased peak flow or FEV_1). Increased symptoms typically precede a detectable decrease in airflow,[247,248] although a subset of patients is at high risk of exacerbations due to poor perception of airflow limitation. In the outpatient setting, an increased requirement for rescue inhalers, especially in a patient previously on a stable regimen, suggests an asthma exacerbation. There is increased recognition that the pathophysiologic mechanisms underlying asthma exacerbations are as heterogenous as the underlying disease itself. Although we currently treat all exacerbations similarly, some data suggest that targeted therapies for asthma exacerbations and the management of triggers may be warranted and have the potential to reduce the morbidity associated with our current therapies.[249] Exacerbations have a significant impact on asthma morbidity and mortality, and therefore it is imperative to decrease the rate of asthma exacerbations whenever possible.[250] Research studies focused on asthma exacerbations have used a variety of definitions, which makes it particularly challenging to compare studies. Given the recognition that standardization was needed, the NIH convened a task force that defined an exacerbation as "a worsening of asthma requiring the use of systemic corticosteroids (or for patients on a stable maintenance dose, an increase in the use of systemic corticosteroids) to prevent a serious outcome."[251] Exacerbations are caused by a variety of triggers, including infection, environmental exposures, and allergens, as well as nonadherence with prescribed asthma medications.

Patients with asthma exacerbations require prompt evaluation and treatment to limit morbidity and mortality. Goals include relief of airflow obstruction and amelioration of respiratory symptoms. Patients with milder symptoms (with peak flow decrease by <20%) may be evaluated in an outpatient setting but should be referred to an acute care facility if they fail to respond promptly to aggressive treatment with bronchodilators and systemic glucocorticoids.[1] Conversely, certain patients are at high risk of asthma-related death and should be evaluated in the emergency department as soon as possible when their symptoms worsen. This includes patients with a history of recent exacerbation or previous near-fatal asthma, overutilization of SABAs or underutilization of ICS, recent oral glucocorticoid use, poor compliance with asthma action plans, or concomitant psychiatric disease.[247]

In the acute care setting, the severity of an asthma exacerbation should be assessed by physical examination, oximetry, and measurement of PEF. Use of accessory muscles, ability to complete sentences, and arterial oxygen saturation should all be evaluated. Patients require close monitoring during the early stages of treatment because it may take several hours for symptoms to resolve. Chest radiography is useful if pneumothorax is suspected but does not usually provide clues as to the etiology of an exacerbation. Arterial blood gas measurement typically reflects mild hypoxemia and respiratory alkalosis; the normalization of arterial P_{CO_2} in the absence of significant symptomatic improvement suggests impending respiratory failure. pH and P_{CO_2} on venous blood gases can also be used to monitor asthma in the critically ill[252,253]; anion gap metabolic acidosis may also be present, which is usually due to elevated lactate levels. Patients who fail to respond to albuterol administration within 30 to 60 minutes, with persistent dyspnea and peak flow less than 70% of baseline, require hospital admission.[1]

Key pharmacologic components of treatment include repeated or continuous short-acting bronchodilator administration (via nebulizer or metered-dose inhaler with a spacer) and systemic glucocorticoids.[254,255] The combination of SABAs and ipratropium at the initiation of treatment is associated with physiologic improvements and a reduced rate of hospitalization, but the benefits do not persist after hospitalization.[256] Systemic corticosteroids are unequivocally associated with a more rapid return to baseline function and are considered the first-line therapy for acute asthma exacerbations. More importantly, the early administration of steroids is important in reducing the need for hospitalization and improving asthma symptoms.[257,258] The initial dosing range for adult patients is from 1.5 to 2 mg/kg of intravenous methylprednisolone or the equivalent.[259] Oral steroids have been shown to have similar efficacy to intravenous preparations in the treatment of acute asthma exacerbations and therefore are an acceptable alternative in patients without life-threatening asthma.[260] ICSs are typically not used acutely, although data suggest that the addition of inhaled budesonide to systemic corticosteroids following an emergency department visit leads to improved symptoms and a decreased relapse rate.[261–263] Intravenous magnesium sulfate, usually given as a 2-g bolus or 40 mg/kg of body weight for children up to a maximal dose of 2 g, may act as a smooth muscle relaxant and has been shown to reduce hospital admission rates.[264] Supplemental oxygen to keep saturations above 90% helps maintain oxygen delivery to peripheral tissues and minimizes hypoxic pulmonary vasoconstriction.

Severe exacerbations of asthma are characterized by persistent reductions in PEF to less than 40% predicted with a poor response to initial treatment. These patients may demonstrate progressive hypercapnia, fatigue, altered sensorium, and dysrhythmias and are at high risk for respiratory arrest. Low-level noninvasive positive-pressure ventilation without positive end-expiratory pressure has been shown to reduce the rate of hospitalization and may be considered in alert, cooperative patients who are not in immediate need of intubation.[265] Heliox increases flow at the same pressure and may be a useful adjunct in patients with severe exacerbations that do not respond to initial emergency treatment.[266–268] Inhaled volatile anesthetics, such as halothane and isoflurane, are potent bronchodilators and have also been used for decades to treat refractory asthma.[269]

Intubation and mechanical ventilation are mandatory for patients in respiratory arrest or impending respiratory arrest. Mechanical ventilation in patients with severe asthma exacerbations may be complicated by immediate postintubation worsening of gas exchange and hemodynamic instability due to increased airway and intrathoracic pressures from dynamic lung hyperinflation. Provided that the patient is adequately oxygenated, briefly decreasing the mandatory respiratory rate to allow an extended expiratory phase is often successful in reducing intrathoracic pressure. Initial ventilator settings should be focused on minimizing dynamic hyperinflation by using a relatively low minute ventilation (with respiratory rate between 12 and 14/min and tidal volumes in the 6 to 8 mL/kg range), a high inspiratory flow rate, and minimal to no positive end-expiratory pressure.[270] With these low settings of rate and volume, the arterial P_{CO_2} may rise; this strategy of "permissive hypercapnia" is a sensible approach to avoiding barotrauma in severely obstructed patients (see Chapter 132). Aggressive sedation should be given to improve comfort and patient-ventilator synchrony. Short-term paralysis may be necessary in patients for whom ventilator synchrony cannot be achieved with sedation alone. Bronchodilator administration should be continued until airway resistance decreases.

CLINICIAN-PATIENT PARTNERSHIP

For chronic asthma, treatment should balance the best symptom control with the lowest possible dosage of medication.[1] Effective management requires that patients form a partnership with health care providers to ensure an appropriate flow of information, with the patients assuming a major role in the assessment and treatment of their disease. Through collaborative effort, a guided self-management plan can be developed, allowing patients to titrate their own treatment on the basis of changes in symptoms with some degree of independence. The use of such guided self-management reduces asthma morbidity in different patient populations and patient care settings.[271] Interestingly, patient-guided use of asthma medications based on symptoms was superior to physician and biomarker-based adjustments to asthma therapies as reported by the Asthma Clinical Research Network,[102] further highlighting the importance of actively involving patients in decisions regarding management of their asthma.

Crucial components of self-management plans include education, self-monitoring with symptoms and/or peak flow, regular review, and patient-directed self-management using a written action plan. Effective patient education is central to this approach. Better communication by health care providers translates into measurably better outcomes with no additional physician time commitment. Even for patients unable to engage in guided self-management, regular follow-up and medication review is beneficial because approximately 50% of patients on long-term therapy fail to take medications as directed at least some of the time.[272]

Key Points

- The approach to the diagnosis, assessment, and treatment of asthma has changed with the recognition that asthma is a heterogeneous disease encompassing many phenotypes with variable responses to therapy.
- Currently, the two main phenotypes appear to be *type 2* (T2)-high and T2-low asthma.
- T2-high asthma is characterized by increases in sputum and/or blood eosinophils and/or FeNO; in T2-low asthma, these biomarkers are not increased.
- Inhaled corticosteroids are the mainstay of asthma therapy; however, only 50% of patients have eosinophilic inflammation that predicts response to inhaled corticosteroids.
- Several biomarkers, including blood immunoglobulin E levels, blood eosinophils, and fraction of exhaled nitric oxide, can be used to diagnose mild to moderate asthma in patients and guide therapy toward biologics in patients with severe asthma.
- Multiple biologic therapies targeting T2 inflammatory pathways are available as add-on therapy for moderate to severe asthma.
- Assessment and management of asthma comorbidities, triggers, and medication nonadherence will help achieve asthma control, particularly for patients with moderate to severe asthma.
- Asthma education and collaboration between physicians and patients are essential in improving asthma-related outcomes.
- Future approaches to managing asthma will require better phenotyping of patients and better therapies for asthmatics with noneosinophilic inflammation.

Key Readings

Anderson SD. Indirect challenge test: airway hyperresponsiveness in asthma: its measurement and clinical significance. *Chest.* 2010;138:25S–30S.

Bleecker ER, FitzGerald JM, Chanez P, et al. Efficacy and safety of benralizumab for patients with severe asthma uncontrolled with high-dosage inhaled corticosteroids and long-acting beta2-agonists (SIROCCO): a randomised, multicentre, placebo-controlled phase 3 trial. *Lancet.* 2016;388(10056):2115–2127.

Carr TF, Kraft M. Management of severe asthma before referral to the severe asthma specialist. *J Allergy Clin Immunol Pract.* 2017;5(4):877–886.

Castro M, Corren J, Pavord ID, et al. Dupilumab efficacy and safety in moderate-to-severe uncontrolled asthma. *N Engl J Med.* 2018;378(26):2486–2496.

Global Initiative for Asthma. *Global Strategy for Asthma Management and Prevention;* 2019. www.ginasthma.org.

Lazarus SC, Krishnan JA, King TS, et al. Mometasone or tiotropium in mild asthma with a low sputum eosinophil level. *N Engl J Med.* 2019;380(21):2009–2019.

National Asthma Education and Prevention Program. *Expert Panel Report III: Guidelines for the Diagnosis and Management of Asthma (EPR-3);* 2017. https://www.nhlbi.nih.gov/health-topics/guidelines-for-diagnosis-management-of-asthma/.

Wang Z, Pianosi P, Keogh K, et al. In: *The Clinical Utility of Fractional Exhaled Nitric Oxide (FeNO) in Asthma Management.* Rockville: MD; 2017.

Wenzel SE. Asthma phenotypes: the evolution from clinical to molecular approaches. *Nat Med.* 2012;18(5):716–725.

Complete reference list available at ExpertConsult.com.

63 COPD: PATHOGENESIS AND NATURAL HISTORY

JEFFREY L. CURTIS, MD • MICHAEL H. CHO, MD, MPH •
NADIA N. HANSEL, MD, MPH

INTRODUCTION

COPD is a heterogeneous and variably progressive spectrum of lung pathologies primarily induced by injury and repair following prolonged oxidative inhalational exposures.[1,2] Most COPD in high-income nations results from direct *cigarette smoke* (CS) exposure but, worldwide, indoor and outdoor air pollution may be equally or more common risks.[3] COPD is highly prevalent. In many countries, it is the only leading non-communicable cause of death increasing in frequency.[4,5] COPD develops with a long latency, can progress despite removal of inciting factors,[6] and is greatly underdiagnosed.[7,8] Only some exposed individuals develop COPD, which is not explained solely by their premature death from other smoking-related diseases. The biologic basis for this restricted susceptibility is incompletely understood, but genetic predispositions are increasingly being identified.

The diagnosis of COPD currently requires incompletely reversible airflow obstruction (i.e., reduced expiratory airflow) during forced exhalation, as assessed by postbronchodilator spirometry.[9,10] In individual COPD patients, reduced maximum expiratory flow results from varying degrees of increased resistance in conducting airways and increased lung compliance from loss of lung elastic recoil. Both diagnosing COPD and classifying its severity currently depend on measuring *forced expiratory volume in one second* (FEV_1) and its ratio to *forced vital capacity* (FVC). Whether an abnormal FEV_1/FVC ratio, which defines airflow obstruction, should be based on a fixed ratio of 0.7 versus age-specific lower limits of normal remains controversial.[11] COPD was formerly attributed solely to accelerated loss of lung function relative to normal aging.[12] However, defective lung growth before adulthood, even without subsequent accelerated decline, was recently identified as an alternative pathway to COPD[13,14] (Fig. 63.1).

The validity of defining COPD by spirometry alone has been questioned based in part on results of two ongoing observational cohort studies, the *Genetic Epidemiology of COPD* (COPDGene)[15] and the *Subpopulations and Intermediate Outcomes in COPD Study* (SPIROMICS).[16] Both studies showed that some symptomatic ever smokers not meeting spirometric criteria used to diagnose COPD nevertheless exhibit characteristics of established COPD, including having acute respiratory events.[17,18] The Subpopulations and Intermediate Outcomes in COPD Study found that ever smokers with normal FEV_1 but FEV_1/FVC between 0.70 and the lower limits of normal had radiographic evidence of smoking-induced lung damage.[19] COPD also has significant systemic components that contribute greatly to functional impairment.[20] Collectively, these findings and those of other recent studies[21-23] suggest that spirometric criteria incompletely capture the range of pathologies induced by inhalational oxidative stress. Despite a recent proposal for a new approach,[24] no alternative classification has as yet gained international acceptance.

PATHOLOGIC CHANGES IN ESTABLISHED COPD

Clinical COPD phenotypes are heterogeneous[25,26] because inhalational stressors induce four key pathologic processes: small airway disease, mucus hypersecretion, emphysema,

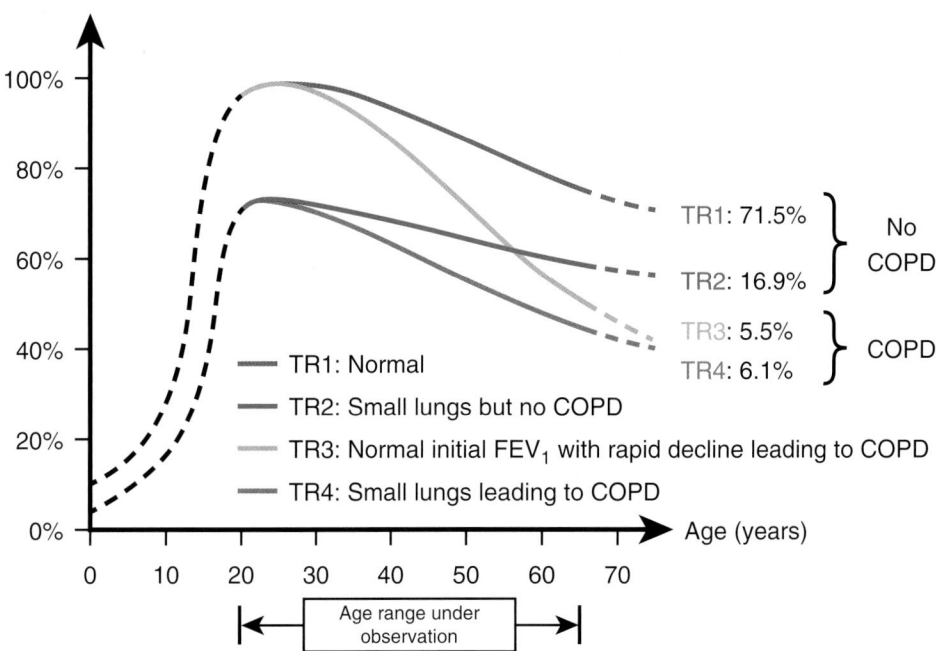

FEV$_1$ in percent of predicted maximally attained value

TR1: Normal
TR2: Small lungs but no COPD
TR3: Normal initial FEV$_1$ with rapid decline leading to COPD
TR4: Small lungs leading to COPD

TR1: 71.5% } No
TR2: 16.9% } COPD

TR3: 5.5%   } COPD
TR4: 6.1%

Age (years)

Age range under observation

Figure 63.1 **Both accelerated loss of lung function and defective lung growth contribute to development of COPD.** Distributions (indicated as percentages) of participants of the Framingham Offspring Cohort and the Copenhagen City Heart Study (N = 2864) into the four *trajectories* (TRs) defined according to baseline level of *forced expiratory volume in 1 second* (FEV$_1$) (below or above 80% of predicted value) and presence or absence of Global Initiative for Obstructive Lung Diseases grade >2 COPD at each study's final examination. The *solid lines* represent the schematic natural history of FEV$_1$ for the age range of this study; the *dashed lines* represent hypothetical trajectories. TR3 represents the classic pathway to COPD, whereas TR4 represents an alternate pathway to COPD. (From Lange P, Celli B, Agusti A, et al. Lung-function trajectories leading to chronic obstructive pulmonary disease. *N Engl J Med.* 2015;373:111–122.)

and vascular dysfunction. Recent correlations between lung histology and novel imaging modalities have accelerated understanding of the relationships among these processes.

SMALL AIRWAY DISEASE

Small airways are defined as those with an internal diameter less than 2 mm. In health, they contribute minimally to airflow resistance.[27] Because even a 50% loss of small airways only doubles airflow resistance, they have been termed the lung's "quiet zone."[28] However, in COPD, small airways become the principle site of obstruction.[29–31] *Small airway disease* (SAD) results from remodeling, obstruction by mucus, and disappearance of terminal and transitional bronchioles, the last airways before the gas exchanging region of the lung. SAD is an early pathologic lesion in susceptible smokers who develop COPD.[32] By the time that FEV$_1$/FVC ratios are abnormal, small airway loss is already considerable.[33,34] SAD leads to air trapping and dynamic hyperinflation, which can limit exercise capacity even in spirometrically mild disease.[35]

SAD cannot be visualized directly by conventional *computed tomography* (CT) in living humans, but it can be inferred from air trapping on expiratory CT scans as functional SAD.[36] A refinement, termed *parametric response mapping* (PRM), uses dynamic image registration to quantify changes in voxel density between inspiration and expiration. The PRM technique[37] permits phenotyping of COPD patients by identifying both functional SAD and emphysema. This approach has been validated in severe COPD by comparison to histologic SAD detected by micro-CT analysis of inflated frozen lung sections.[38] Importantly, serial PRM analysis indicates that SAD precedes emphysema[39] (Figs. 63.2 and 63.3). In mild-to-moderate COPD, where one finds the greatest rates of spirometric decline, SAD contributes more than emphysema does to FEV$_1$ decline; in advanced COPD, each contributes.[40]

CHRONIC BRONCHITIS AND MUCUS HYPERSECRETION

Chronic bronchitis (CB) is a common COPD phenotype, but it can also exist without airflow obstruction. CB is significantly associated with many occupational exposures.[41] CB is most commonly defined clinically as chronic cough with sputum production for 3 months in 1 year for 2 consecutive years.[41] CB is associated histologically and radiographically with airway wall thickening.[42] Findings from three observational cohorts indicate that CB independently contributes to multiple adverse respiratory outcomes in ever smokers.[43,44] Interestingly, the National Heart Lung and Blood Institute Pooled Cohort study recently confirmed increased risk of attributable hospitalizations and death in both smokers and nonsmokers with nonobstructive CB, but only smokers lost lung function over time.[45]

CB is increasingly viewed as a manifestation of hypersecretion and altered physical properties of airway mucus.[46,47] The healthy airway surface liquid consists of an aqueous periciliary layer[48] and an upper mucus layer containing secreted mucins. Mucins are large glycoproteins characterized by repeated threonine-rich domains modified by a range of complex O-linked polysaccharides. Airways express two types of mucins: tethered mucins, including MUC1, MUC4, MUC13, MUC16, which contribute to maintaining hydration of the periciliary layer; and secreted mucins, products of the *MUC5AC* and *MUC5B* genes. Both large and small airways are now known to secrete MUC5B and lesser amounts of MUC5AC in the physiologic state.

Oxidative stress adversely impacts mucus clearance by altering both airway surface liquid components. It induces mucus hyperconcentration,[49] in part due to smoking-induced disruption of the cystic fibrosis transmembrane conductance regulator.[50,51] It also causes hypersecretion of

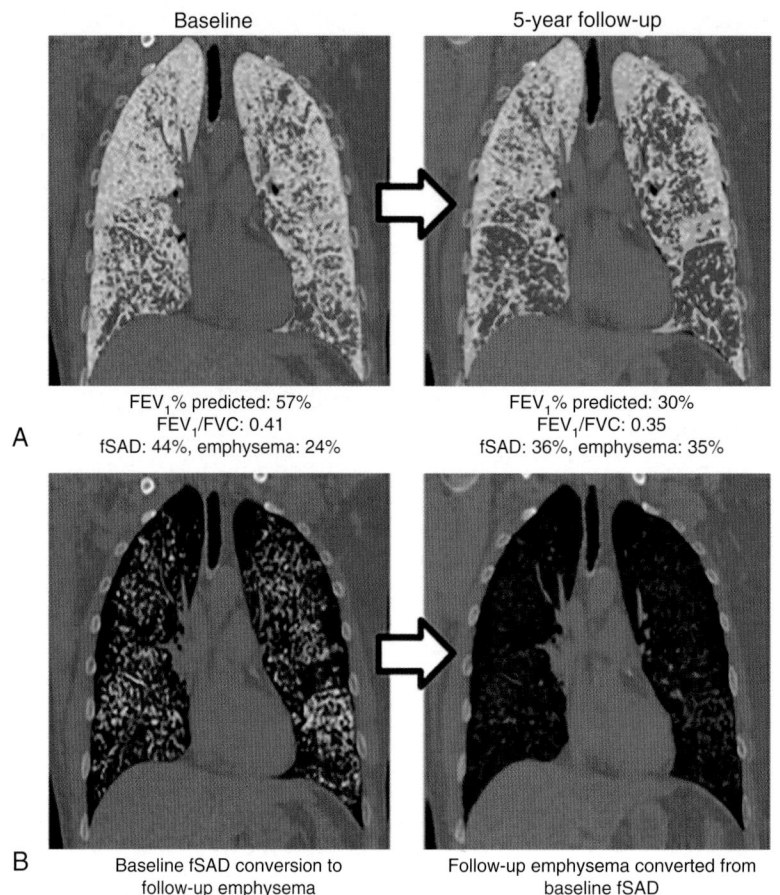

Baseline   5-year follow-up

A

FEV$_1$% predicted: 57%
FEV$_1$/FVC: 0.41
fSAD: 44%, emphysema: 24%

FEV$_1$% predicted: 30%
FEV$_1$/FVC: 0.35
fSAD: 36%, emphysema: 35%

B

Baseline fSAD conversion to
follow-up emphysema

Follow-up emphysema converted from
baseline fSAD

Figure 63.2 *Small airway disease* (SAD) **precedes emphysema in** *parametric response mapping* **(PRM) metrics in a representative male COPD patient.** Representative coronal computed tomographic sections of the same individual at baseline (*left*) and after 5-year follow-up (*right*). (A) All PRM metric values are depicted as normal lung parenchyma (*green*), functional small airway disease (fSAD; *yellow*) and emphysema (emph; *red*). (B) Only individual voxels classified as fSAD at baseline (*yellow*) that became emphysema 5 years later in this same subject (red) are shown. FEV$_1$, forced expiratory volume in 1 second; FVC, forced vital capacity. (From Labaki WW, Gu T, Murray S, et al. Voxel-wise longitudinal parametric response mapping analysis of chest computed tomography in smokers. *Acad Radiol.* 2019;26:217–223.)

MUC5AC, which has traditionally been considered to be the central abnormality in mucus clearance in COPD. However, in some patients, markedly decreased MUC5B may be more important.[52] By occluding terminal bronchi, mucus hypersecretion can contribute to SAD. However, not all COPD patients develop the symptomatic CB phenotype. Conversely, CB does not invariably lead to airflow obstruction,[53] although it appears to mark a group at increased risk.[54]

EMPHYSEMA

Emphysema is defined as permanent enlargement of airspaces distal to the terminal bronchioles due to alveolar wall destruction.[1] Three types of emphysema are recognized histologically and by CT: *centrilobular* (CLE), *panlobular* (PLE), and *paraseptal* (PSE) (see Fig. 20.24).[55] CLE (Fig. 63.4A and C) is common; among the three emphysema types, it is most closely associated with smoking history.[56] CLE is a frequent manifestation of spirometrically advanced COPD, but it can also be present with minimal or no airflow obstruction.[22] CLE begins with destruction of respiratory bronchioles within a single acinus and progresses by coalescence of such primary lesions.[57,58] Further progression can lead to confluent CLE, which extends across several secondary pulmonary lobules without generalized architectural

distortion, and to advanced destructive emphysema, with distortion from hyperinflation.[55]

By contrast, PLE affects all acini equally (see Fig. 63.4B and D). PLE is characteristic of homozygous *alpha$_1$-antitrypsin* (AAT) deficiency but has also been described in another genetic disease[59] and in users of intravenous methylphenidate.[60]

The third type of emphysema, PSE, forms by rupture of distal acini adjacent to the pleura.[61] PSE can develop along the chest wall, particularly in the upper and middle lobes, but is often prominent along the mediastinum, intralobar fissures, and bronchovascular bundles.[55] PSE is the type of emphysema most closely associated with bulla formation and spontaneous pneumothorax and, when adjacent to the trachea, with central airway expiratory collapse.[62] However, PSE is more commonly asymptomatic, least associated with impairment of lung function,[56] and even found to a minimal degree in healthy never smokers.[63,64] PSE in smokers is a highly inflammatory lesion associated with a greater lung density than is seen in CLE patients.[65]

Since the earliest modern descriptions of emphysema, there have been two major hypotheses about the initial mechanisms and anatomic sites of injury,[57,58,66] termed the Canadian and Denver schools, based on their recent proponents.[67] The Canadian school, which emphasized the role of

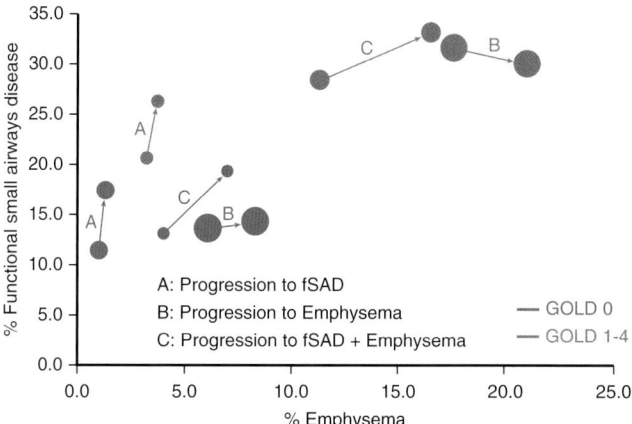

Figure 63.3 Evidence suggesting that emphysema evolves from *small airway disease* (SAD). Representation of the changes over 5 years in *parametric response mapping* (PRM) metrics among COPDGene participants initially without (*Global Initiative for Obstructive Lung Diseases* [GOLD] grade 0) vs. with COPD (GOLD grade 1–4). Data are from 725 high-resolution computed tomographic scans that showed interval progression. The center of each circle represents the mean coordinates (% emphysema and % functional SAD on PRM) for each type of progression (to functional SAD [fSAD; *A*], emphysema [*B*], or both [*C*]) at baseline and follow-up visits (identified by the direction of the arrows). The area of each circle is proportional to the number of subjects with a given type of progression (A, B, or C) within their GOLD grade (0 or 1–4). (From Labaki WW, Gu T, Murray S, et al. Voxel-wise longitudinal parametric response mapping analysis of chest computed tomography in smokers. *Acad Radiol.* 2019;26:217–223.)

SAD, has considerable support from analysis of human pathologic tissue[32–34,38,68] and, more recently, from imaging.[69,70] Because advanced stages of both CLE and PLE are associated with loss of terminal bronchioles,[33] SAD might contribute to development of either type of emphysema depending on genetic background. The Denver hypothesis, which focused on vascular endothelial cell apoptosis, originally derived from experimental results.[71–73] Recent support for this mechanism came from the Multi-Ethnic Study of Atherosclerosis COPD Study, which assessed pulmonary microvascular blood flow using dynamic contrast-enhanced MRI. Results showed 30% reductions in pulmonary microvascular blood flow even in mild COPD; correlations were strongest with emphysema and were independent of measures of SAD.[74]

Importantly, these two pathogenic mechanisms need not be mutually exclusive. Instead, varying degrees of epithelial damage, vascular injury, and *extracellular matrix* (ECM) degeneration[75,76] might contribute to emphysema development at specific disease stages or in different individuals. An additional seminal insight is that by transmitting mechanical stress to adjacent areas of normal lung, emphysema can become self-perpetuating.[77]

PULMONARY AND SYSTEMIC VASCULAR DYSFUNCTION

The healthy pulmonary circulation provides low resistance to blood flow, even during exercise (see also Chapter 85). It can do so in part by recruiting blood vessels, particularly in the upper lobes, not perfused at rest. An equally important contributor to low resistance is endothelial-dependent vascular relaxation, which results from the balance between the vasodilators, endothelial-derived nitric oxide and prostacyclin, and vasoconstrictors of the endothelin and serotonin pathways.[78]

In COPD, even in spirometrically mild stages, endothelial-derived nitric oxide production by *pulmonary artery* (PA) tissue is reduced in vitro, relative to PA tissue from never smokers or smokers without airflow obstruction.[79,80] Some pathology in COPD, especially the "vascular COPD phenotype,"[81] might represent pulmonary circulatory aspects of a generalized vascular response to inhaled insults. With worsening spirometric severity, mild to moderate elevations in PA pressures frequently develop, especially during exercise,[82,83] due to an abnormal increase in PA pressure relative to the rise in cardiac output. Mild *pulmonary hypertension* (pHTN) (20 mm Hg < PA pressure ≤ 35 mm Hg) is detectable in up to 90% of COPD patient with severe airflow obstruction[84] (Fig. 63.5).

Acute exacerbations of COPD (AE-COPD) are also accompanied by PA pressure elevations in groups including but not consisting entirely of those with left heart failure.[85] A ratio of PA to aortic diameters greater than 1.0 on CT scans was a strong independent predictor of AE-COPD in a study from two large cohorts.[86] In severe COPD, PA to aortic diameter ratio was significantly associated with resting pHTN in the absence of left heart failure and outperformed transthoracic echocardiogram as a predictor of pHTN.[87] Elevated PA to aortic diameter ratio detected right heart remodeling in mild-to-moderate COPD with preserved left ventricular function, independently of diastolic dysfunction.[88]

Severe pHTN (PA pressure > 35 mm Hg) is uncommon in COPD in the absence of sustained severe hypoxemia or of alternative causes including untreated sleep apnea, occult thromboembolic disease, or left-sided heart failure.[89–92] Although such severe pHTN can be accompanied by right heart failure (classical cor pulmonale), more common findings in COPD are pruning of pulmonary arteries with right ventricular enlargement[93] or even diminished right ventricular size (cor pulmonale parvus), which has been attributed to compression by lung hyperinflation.[94] Criteria have been proposed to distinguish classes of pHTN in COPD patients.[81,95,96]

COPD patients also exhibit systemic circulatory dysfunction. These findings, seen prominently in the renal circulation[97] and associated with microalbuminuria,[98,99] but also present elsewhere,[100] might partially explain some extrapulmonary manifestations of COPD.

EPIDEMIOLOGY

COPD AS A WORLDWIDE DISEASE

COPD is a global health problem and a leading cause of mortality throughout the world. The Global Burden of Disease Study reported a worldwide prevalence of 251 million COPD cases in 2016 and estimated that the disease caused 3.2 million deaths in 2015 (5% of all deaths globally in that year).[101] More than 90% of COPD deaths take place in low- and middle-income countries,[101] highlighting its significant worldwide public health impact. Further, COPD is likely to increase in developing countries due to aging and more widespread smoking.

COPD is also associated with significant economic burden. In the European Union, annual costs of health care and lost productivity due to COPD are estimated as

Centrilobular
Emphysema

Panlobular
Emphysema

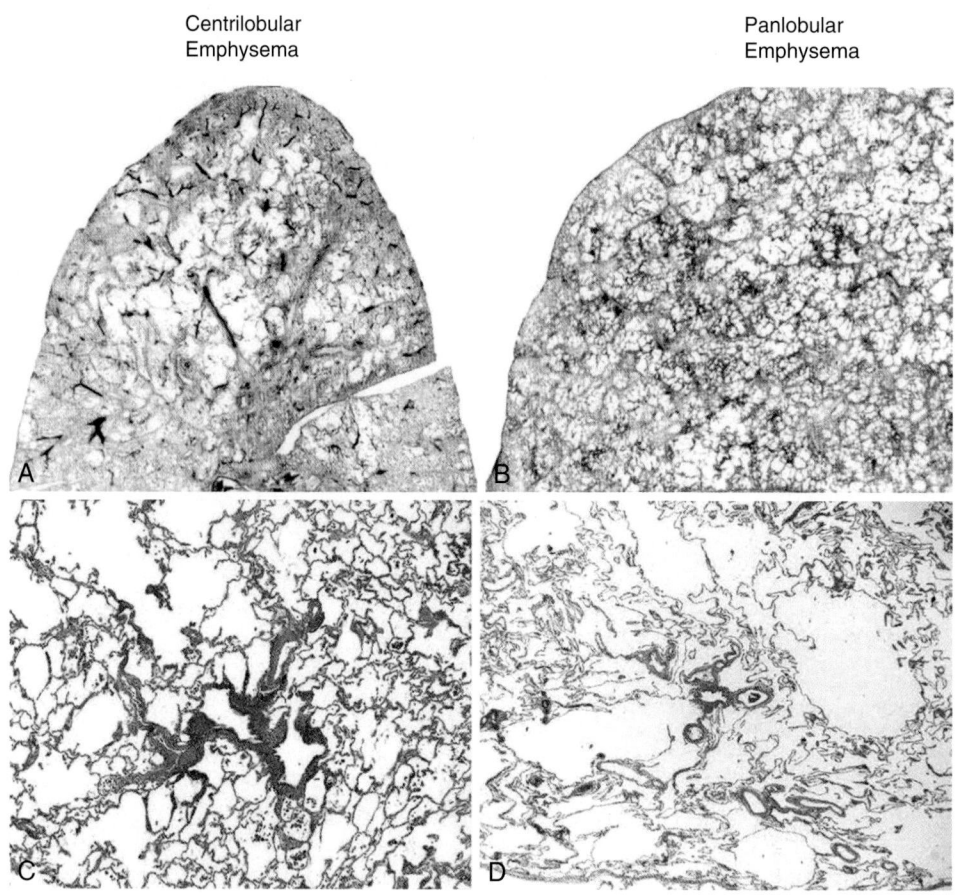

Figure 63.4 **Gross and histologic appearance of** *centrilobular emphysema* **(CLE) and** *panlobular emphysema* **(PLE).** (A–B) Paper-thin Gough-Wentworth sections prepared from whole lungs. (A) CLE in a smoker. (B) PLE in alpha$_1$-antitrypsin deficiency. The type and severity of emphysema may be difficult or impossible to determine on histopathologic grounds. (C–D) Hematoxylin and eosin–stained histologic sections. C, CLE with dilation of the air spaces surrounding the bronchiole. (D) PLE featuring a more diffuse air space dilation. (A–B, Original Gough sections prepared by T.V. Colby and the Charles B. Carrington Memorial Lung Pathology Library. C–D, From Leslie KO, Wick MR. *Practical Pulmonary Pathology: A Diagnostic Approach*, 2nd ed. Philadelphia: Saunders; 2011.)

€48 billion.[102] In the United States, the Centers for Disease Control and Prevention estimated the total medical cost attributable to COPD in 2010 at $32 billion, with the projected rise to $49 billion by 2020.[103] The greatest proportion of these costs comes from AE-COPD, especially from hospitalizations, which increase rapidly as COPD severity increases. Indirect costs are difficult to assess in COPD; however, in the United States an estimated 16.4 million days of work are lost due to COPD annually. The economic impact of COPD on workplace and home productivity, particularly in developing countries, may exceed the direct costs of disease management.

PREVALENCE AND INCIDENCE

The Global Burden of Disease Study reported a prevalence of 251 million cases of COPD globally in 2016, but estimates of COPD prevalence continue to vary by geographic location and also by differences in survey methods and diagnostic criteria.[103] The widespread under-recognition and under-diagnosis of COPD means that self-report surveys may underestimate its true prevalence.[104] In studies using spirometry, prevalence depends on the diagnostic criteria. Using the criteria suggested by the *Global Initiative for Obstructive Lung Diseases* (GOLD) will lead to higher prevalence in older individuals than using the lower limits of normal for the FEV$_1$/FVC ratio.[105] Partly due to global population growth, smoking prevalence, and aging, worldwide COPD prevalence increased by 44% between 1990

and 2015.[106] However, in the United States, the prevalence of COPD decreased from 7.2% in 2008 to 2009 to 6.4% in 2014 to 2015.[107] COPD prevalence is higher among adults with lower income, public insurance, and a history of smoking and varies by geographic location, ranging from 3.4% in Hawaii to 13.8% in West Virginia.[108] Existing data on COPD prevalence are limited or totally lacking in many regions of Europe; recently, however, by using inverse distance-weighted interpolation mapping, the mean prevalence in Europe was estimated to be as high as 12.4%, with significant variation across different areas.[109] Thus, standardized data on COPD prevalence across the globe remain lacking and incidence data are even fewer.

SMOKING AND OTHER ENVIRONMENTAL FACTORS

The primary cause of COPD in developed countries is exposure to tobacco smoke (either active smoking or secondhand smoke) (see also Chapter 65). Although tobacco smoking is a major risk factor, not all smokers develop COPD for several reasons, including differences in smoking behavior and in susceptibility to smoking. A dose-effect relationship between smoking and COPD risk has long been recognized. Recently, in the COPDGene cohort of current and former smokers, investigators found that, though smoking intensity is important, smoking duration is more strongly associated with estimates of COPD risk than is the number of cigarettes

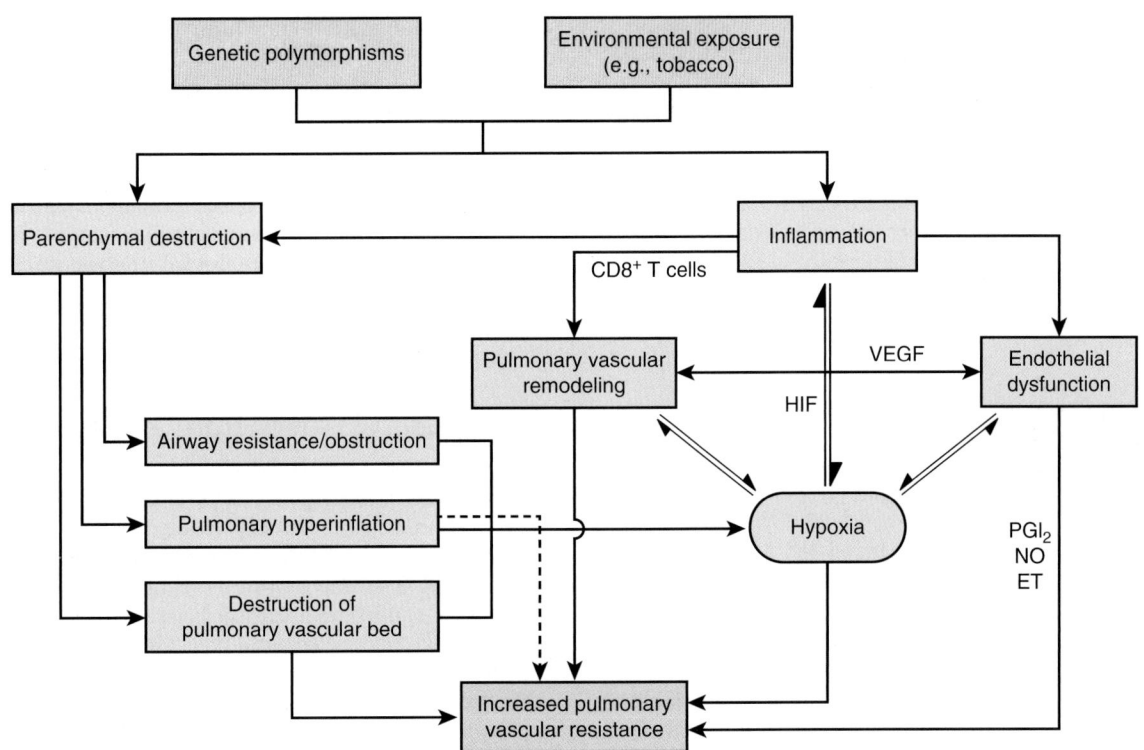

Figure 63.5 Cardiac, lung, and pulmonary vascular factors contributing to the development of pulmonary hypertension in COPD. The complex pathogenic interactions underlying increased *pulmonary vascular resistance* (PVR) in COPD. Genetic and environmental exposures contribute to parenchymal destruction and inflammation. Parenchymal destruction alters respiratory mechanics and causes destruction of the pulmonary vascular bed, which increases PVR and also leads to hypoxia. Inflammation is likely involved in pulmonary vascular remodeling and endothelial dysfunction, which also increases PVR and leads to hypoxia. The schema highlights the central role of hypoxia but also indicates that hypoxia is not essential to the development of an increased PVR in COPD. VEGF, vascular endothelial growth factor; HIF, hypoxia-inducible factors; PGI2, prostacyclin; NO, nitric oxide; ET, endothelin. (From Wrobel JP, Thompson BR, Williams TJ. Mechanisms of pulmonary hypertension in chronic obstructive pulmonary disease: a pathophysiologic review. *J Heart Lung Transplant.* 2012;31[6]:557-564.)

smoked per day or the composite index of pack-years.[110] It was hypothesized that a longer duration of smoking may be associated with accumulation of genetic and epigenetic changes or with sustained alterations in the lung microbiome contributing to disease progression. Further, accelerated decline in lung function persists even among those who smoke less than five cigarettes per day, reinforcing the view that there is no safe level of tobacco smoke exposure and that smoking cessation remains the primary intervention to modify disease risk.[111] Worldwide, however, it is estimated that 2–45% of patients with COPD never smoked,[3] and that non–tobacco-related exposures contribute substantially.

Indoor air pollution from biomass exposure has emerged as an important risk factor worldwide. In a recent meta-analysis including 35 studies with more than 70,000 participants, exposure to solid biomass fuel increased risk of COPD by 2.7 (95% confidence interval, 2.1 to 3.3) times compared to those without biomass fuel exposure.[112] Almost 3 billion people worldwide use biomass and coal as their main source of energy for cooking, heating, and other household needs; thus, in these communities, household air pollution is responsible for a large fraction of COPD risk.[101] Fewer studies have investigated the effect of indoor pollution in high-income countries, where indoor environmental exposure levels may be significantly lower than in low-income countries or in biomass-using homes. Still, research suggests that even low particulate levels may have adverse effects on the respiratory tract and are linked to

worse COPD outcomes.[113,114] This low level of indoor particulates may have tobacco and non-tobacco contributions, but there have also been consistent studies linking both cumulative home and workplace *secondhand smoke* exposure to COPD development.[115] Among those with COPD, evidence suggests that secondhand smoke exposure contributes to worse disease morbidity, including worse quality of life, dyspnea, and heightened risk for COPD exacerbation, even among those who are actively smoking.[116–119] (See also Chapter 102.)

Workplace exposures contribute to the burden of COPD, and estimates suggest that they may be the cause of 15–21% of COPD.[120–122] After accounting for smoking, occupational exposures to vapors, dust, and gases are associated not only with COPD risk but also with a higher degree of emphysema and with more disease of small and large airways.[123] For those with established COPD, occupational exposures are associated with greater morbidity, including shorter walk distance, greater breathlessness, worse quality of life, and increased exacerbation risk.[124]

Outdoor air pollution has long-term effects on lung function, with higher pollution exposure leading to more rapid lung function decline,[125–127] which may contribute to COPD development. Results from recent large cohort-based studies further strengthen the evidence supporting a link between ambient pollution exposure and COPD. Analysis of the UK Biobank data on more than 300,000 individuals aged 40 to 69 years associated air pollution with lower lung function and higher COPD prevalence.[128] In a cohort study conducted between

2000 and 2018 in six U.S. metropolitan regions, long-term exposure to ambient air pollutants, especially ozone, was significantly associated with increasing emphysema, assessed quantitatively using CT imaging, and with worsening lung function.[129] A large body of literature supports the contribution of ambient pollution exposure to several measures of COPD morbidity, including increased respiratory symptoms, risk of exacerbations, and higher mortality.[114] For example, exposure to ozone caused an additional 254,000 (95% confidence interval, 97,000 to 422,000) deaths and a loss of 4.1 million (range, 1.6 to 6.8 million) disability-adjusted life years from COPD in 2015.[130] (See also Chapter 102.)

EARLY CHILDHOOD FACTORS, ASTHMA AND BRONCHIAL HYPERREACTIVITY, AND NUTRITIONAL STATUS AS PREDISPOSITIONS TO COPD

There are additional risk factors for COPD, and it is becoming increasingly clear that respiratory health in adult life is influenced by factors affecting lung growth in early life. In particular, frequent childhood lower respiratory infections, asthma, and premature birth have been linked to increased COPD risk. As early as the 1970s, respiratory ailments during childhood were linked to adult respiratory disease and ventilatory limitation.[131] Subsequently, several studies have supported this hypothesis. For instance, recurrent childhood lower respiratory infections have been associated with COPD development.[132] In the COPDGene Study, reported childhood pneumonia was associated with 40% increased odds of COPD as well as increased COPD exacerbations and lower lung function. Having both pneumonia and asthma in childhood further increased the risk of developing COPD.[133]

Asthma is a chronic inflammatory respiratory disease with variable and reversible airway obstruction; however, persistent airway obstruction and an accelerated decline in lung function may develop, particularly in those with severe disease or frequent exacerbations.[134] Results from the European Community Respiratory Health Survey showed that subjects with a history of childhood asthma had a 10-fold increased risk of developing COPD.[135] Further, the combination of asthma and smoking can have a synergistic effect on lung function decline.[136] Increased *airway responsiveness*, a hallmark feature of asthma, has also been associated with lung function decline and COPD.[132,137] Airway responsiveness is also a common feature of COPD; results from the Lung Health Study demonstrated that baseline airway responsiveness is a strong predictor of future lung function decline among those with mild to moderate COPD[138] and that increased airway responsiveness is also associated with a higher risk of mortality from COPD.[139]

In addition to early respiratory conditions, nutritional status has been associated with lung health, and several studies have linked micronutrient and general nutritional status with lung function and COPD severity.[140,141] Hence, poor nutritional status may contribute to disease burden worldwide, particularly in low- and middle-income countries. Among COPD patients, nutritional status has been linked to worse morbidity. Polyunsaturated fatty acids have emerged as a dietary component capable of modifying inflammation; higher omega-3 and omega-6 intake

was associated with lower and higher COPD morbidity, respectively.[142]

Prematurity is often associated with low birth weight, recurrent respiratory infections, poor early lung function, and nutritional problems. Given that preterm birth appears to be increasing in most countries, it is becoming a rising concern for its potential contribution to the global COPD burden.[143,144] Thus, it is becoming increasingly important to recognize and reduce both environmental and nonenvironmental risk factors to COPD burden.

GENETICS OF COPD

METHODS OF DETERMINING SUSCEPTIBILITY

Studies in severe early-onset COPD[145] and in twins[146] confirmed that COPD has a genetic component. Notably, evidence for genetics persists even after controlling for CS exposure and excluding the most important known genetic risk factor, deficiency of AAT due to mutations of the *SERPINA1* gene. The clinical syndrome resulting from *AAT deficiency* (AATD) is considered later in this chapter. Heritability, the genetic contribution to disease susceptibility, for COPD has been estimated at 35–60%, depending on the study design and population.[146,147] Identifying the actual genetic sequences responsible for COPD heritability has been challenging. Studies using linkage and candidate gene approaches have proven hard to replicate. The most successful method of identifying susceptibility loci in the past decade has been *genome-wide association studies* (GWASs). Predicated on the existence of common variants (those present in at least 5% of the population) with weak effect sizes, the GWAS design requires very large cohorts.[148] Nonetheless, GWASs have identified dozens of replicated COPD risk loci.[149]

GWASs have several limitations. First, they are not optimal to identify the impact of rare variants. Studies attempting to identify rare variants have had variable results and produced no loci as convincingly replicated as AATD.[150–155] Second, GWASs usually identify a region, not the causal variant. Due to linkage disequilibrium, the "top" association is usually highly correlated with other genetic variants in the region. Third, the causal variant may act indirectly by affecting regulatory circuitry of genes millions of base pairs away. To define the function of a disease-associated locus, fine mapping, high-throughput variant screening,[156] and integrative omics that exploit intermediate phenotypes (such as gene expression or methylation)[157] have all been used.

Another key factor in genetic association is identifying the specific phenotype. To date, most COPD genetic association studies have been based on the GOLD definition, and hence on spirometric evidence of airflow limitation. GWASs of FEV_1 and FEV_1/FVC ratio in the general population have found similar associations to COPD studies, even though the former included those with and without obstructive prebronchodilator spirometry, and both smokers and nonsmokers.[158,159] Intriguingly, sensitivity analyses of population-based studies have not found substantial differences using pre- versus postbronchodilator spirometry or, for most loci, an effect in smokers versus nonsmokers. Gene-by-environment studies in COPD or lung function have largely not identified significant evidence of interaction,[160] which might be an issue of statistical power.[161]

For most GWASs, power is among the most important concerns. Thus, the analysis in large cohorts of lung function as a quantitative trait, rather than the binary trait of COPD versus healthy, has generally been more powerful. Such studies have identified hundreds of associations with FEV_1, FVC, and FEV_1/FVC ratio, most of which also show an association with COPD.[149,162]

COPD is heterogeneous, so analysis of specific phenotypes may yield additional insight into pathogenesis and hence the potential for targeted therapies. One study of severe COPD (GOLD stages 3 to 4) demonstrated associations not found in moderate COPD and also strengthened associations with previously identified loci.[163] Studies of phenotypes defined by imaging, such as emphysema and airway abnormalities, also discovered novel associations.[163–165] Notably, these studies identified significant associations of heterozygous *SERPINA1* Z alleles (e.g., MZ) with severe COPD and emphysema, a result not seen in milder COPD or in lung function studies. Although most studies of COPD-related phenotypes have suffered from smaller sample sizes,[166,167] large studies of cigarette smoking behavior have identified several regions of genetic susceptibility.[168]

However, GWASs have not disclosed associations in many important phenotypes, chief among them accelerated lung function decline. Although this trait is heritable,[169] to date GWASs have found interesting but not well-replicated results.[170,171] This failure for a longitudinal outcome, in contrast to successes using cross-sectional data, may be due to the smaller sample size, inadequate follow-up time, measurement error or random noise, or a lower overall contribution of genetic variants to this phenotype. Similar limitations may apply to studies of COPD exacerbations, for which the heritability has not been well studied. Surprisingly, most loci found in GWASs based on cross-sectional data do not appear to be associated with lung function decline.[172] Thus, while one of the main interests in COPD genetic association is to identify loci impacting ongoing inflammatory and destructive processes, these studies may have mostly identified developmental or early life processes that reduce attainment of maximal lung function by young adulthood,[172] thus increasing susceptibility to COPD via the alternative pathway (see Fig. 63.1).

CONFIRMED GENETIC RISK FACTORS

Despite these limitations, the discovery of dozens to hundreds of associated genetic loci holds great promise for elucidating COPD pathobiology. Only a few loci have been followed up by functional studies, though novel insights have already resulted (Table 63.1). The first GWAS-identified locus for COPD[173] is located at 15q25, which contains the nicotinic receptor genes *CHRNA3* and *CHRNA5*, and the iron-responsive element binding protein 2, which has a key role in iron homeostasis. Although this locus is clearly associated with smoking behavior, effects independent of smoking have been seen in some, but not all, genetic analyses.[162,174,175] Contemporaneous with identification of this locus by GWASs, the region was also linked to COPD via gene expression of iron-responsive element binding protein 2.[176] Iron homeostasis has intriguing connections to COPD; mice with reduced dietary iron intake or lacking the murine analog (iron regulatory protein 2) were less susceptible to CS-induced air space enlargement and lung injury, whereas increased iron loading increased severity of CS-induced airway phenotypes.[177]

This initial GWAS also identified an association with lung function and COPD at the 4q31 locus.[173,178] Functional studies including *expression quantitative trait loci* analysis and chromosomal conformation capture identified *hedgehog interacting protein* (HHIP) as the likely causal gene.[179] HHIP binds ligands of the hedgehog pathway, which regulates both embryonic body segmentation and adult stem cell maintenance. Subsequent studies identified influences of HHIP on noncanonical pathways, including those related to ECM.[179] The haploinsufficient *HHIP* mouse shows increased sensitivity to CS- and age-related emphysema, possibly related to increased oxidative stress.[180] Although *HHIP* variants have to date not been associated with lung function decline in humans, these data suggest that genes identified by GWAS could still have an effect later in life.

The 4q24 region harbors several susceptibility loci. The first is near the *family with sequence similarity, member 13 (FAM13A)* gene,[181] and additional studies support the likelihood that *FAM13A* is the effector gene at this locus.[182] Recent work identified *FAM13A* as a negative regulator of the β-catenin/Wnt pathway; *Fam13a$^{-/-}$* mice have increased levels of β-catenin and resistance to CS-induced emphysema.[183] A second locus in the 4q24 region is near *GSTCD, INTS12,* and *NPNT*. These genes are expressed by several airway cell types and appear to be at least partially coregulated.[184,185]

Though several other regions identified by genetic association have not been subject to functional study, other evidence implicates specific genes or pathways. The most significant signal in the *AGER* region is a nonsynonymous variant associated with lung function, COPD, soluble receptor for advanced glycation end product levels, and emphysema.[186] A nonsynonymous variant in *surfactant protein D (SFTPD)* was also previously identified in a candidate gene study.[187] Rare variant studies have found associations in small COPD cohorts by examining phenotype association and variant function in specific telomerase-related genes (*TERT* and *NAF1*).[152,188] A putative functional variant was identified in the *TGFB2* region, and genetic signals near *TGFBR3, ACVR1B, ITGA2, ITGAV, MFAP2, GDF5,* and *SMAD3*[149,162,189,190] lend strong support for the importance of the *transforming growth factor-β* (TGF-β) pathway in COPD pathogenesis. Associations near *KIAA0753, CEP72,* and *LRCC45*, as well as rare variant studies, all support a role for cilia-related genes.[149,162,191,192] Similarly, an association near *PTCH1* lends further support for the role of the hedgehog pathway.[193]

Importantly, the ability to identify a likely causal gene (and variant, and cell type) appears to be locus dependent. For example, an association near *desmoplakin (DSP)* colocalizes (is highly statistically likely to be due to the same variant) with expression of *DSP* in the lung.[158] However, other loci illustrate the complexities of identifying a causal gene. The *HTR4* locus was first identified as associating with lung function, and later with COPD.[158,175,193,194] Gene expression studies and murine knockouts support its role in pulmonary function[195,196]; however, gene expression of *HTR4* in the lung is low relative to other tissues, and newer gene expression and colocalization suggest a role for other genes

Table 63.1 Selected Putative Genes Identified from COPD Genetic Association Studies

Gene	Putative Function	Supportive Evidence (see text)	References
ADAM19	A disintegrin and metallopeptidase domain 19; member of a family of proteins involved in cell-cell and cell-matrix interactions through integrin binding, expressed in airway epithelium, smooth muscle, and inflammatory cells	Gene expression	158, 557
AGER	Receptor for advanced glycan end products; binds to molecules implicated in inflammation; soluble form (sRAGE) is a biomarker for emphysema	Nonsynonymous variant	186
CHRNA5	Neuronal acetylcholine receptor subunit alpha-5; affects cigarette smoking behavior	Coding variants	555
DSP	Desmoplakin, component of desmosomes required for epidermal integrity	Colocalized gene expression	158
FAM13A	Family with sequence similarity 13, member A; induces β-catenin degradation; increases fatty acid oxidation and reactive oxygen species	Reporter assay (variant), murine model	182, 183, 556
FBXO38	F-box protein 38; orphan F-box protein, may act by coactivating KLF family genes to affect airway remodeling	Colocalized splicing	197
HHIP	Hedgehog interacting protein; deficiency leads defects in branching morphogenesis, increased lymphoid aggregates, and increased oxidative stress	Chromosomal conformation capture (variant), murine model	179, 180
HTR4	5-hydroxytryptamine receptor 4; expressed in developing lung, murine model with increased airways resistance	Murine models	196, 558
IREB2	Iron responsive element binding protein 2; increases mitochondrial iron loading and mitochondrial dysfunction	Gene expression, murine model	176, 177
NPNT	Nephronectin; extracellular matrix protein located in the basement membrane, known role in kidney development, but also expressed in lung	Gene and protein expression	162
SFTPD	Surfactant protein D; component of pulmonary surfactant, and responsible for immune and inflammatory regulation (see below)	Nonsynonymous variant	187
TGFB2	Transforming growth factor β2; member of the TGFB family, with roles in wound healing, development, and fibrosis	Colocalized expression, functional assay	149, 189

in the region, particularly *FBXO38*.[197] An analysis of coding variation associated a nonsynonymous variant in *IL27* with COPD.[197] However, this variant is correlated with several other regulatory variants and with an inversion polymorphism that affects the expression of multiple genes, including *TUFM*, whose product interacts with *NLRX1*, a gene implicated in cytokine response, virus-induced autophagy, and COPD.[197] Thus, putative genetic association of specific genes and pathways with COPD susceptibility must always be considered in view of all available evidence.

Bioinformatic tools can help support specific gene sets, pathways, and cell types. Such approaches have implicated *IL17RD*, *CHIA*, genes in the integrin family including *ITGAV*, and genes involved in cell-matrix interactions like *ADAMTSL3*.[149,162] Consistently, tests of overall enrichment identify a strong signal related to lung development, based on (1) gene set enrichment and (2) overlap of associations with regulatory regions in fetal lung.[149,162] These studies also support a role for smooth muscle, and some additional support also exists for endothelial cells, alveolar epithelial type 2 cells, basal-like cells, and fibroblasts.[149,159,162]

PATHOGENESIS

MECHANISMS OF OXIDANT INJURY AND ANTIOXIDANTS

Oxidant stress and injury resulting from *reactive oxygen species* (ROS) is the ultimate trigger for the four major

pathologic changes (SAD, mucus abnormalities, emphysema, and pulmonary microvascular changes) culminating in distinct COPD clinical phenotypes. The principal ROS are superoxide anion, hydrogen peroxide, and the hydroxyl radical, the most damaging ROS.[198,199] ROS arise either exogenously, from CS and air pollution, or endogenously. Mainstream CS contains high concentrations of oxidants (1014 molecules/puff) and 3000 ppm nitric oxide/puff, and over 4700 chemical compounds.[200] ROS in CS range from short-lived oxidants, such as the superoxide radical and nitric oxide, to long-lived organic radicals, such as semiquinones.[199]

Aerosols from vaping and heat-not-burn tobacco products have much lower free radical levels than CS[201] but do emit volatile carbonyls, furans, and toxic metals, including chromium, lead, and nickel. Inhalational exposure to e-cigarette vapor causes adverse respiratory outcomes in animal models.[202–206] One study of e-cigarette users showed elevated lung concentrations of *neutrophil elastase* (NE) and the *matrix metalloproteinases* (MMPs)-2 and -9 with no change in antiprotease concentrations.[207] Insights have come from the public use data files for the Population Assessment of Tobacco and Health, which collected nationally representative, population-based, longitudinal data three times from 2013 to 2016. Results imply that use of e-cigarettes is a risk factor for respiratory disease, independent of combustible tobacco smoking, and that dual use, the most common pattern, is riskier than using either alone.[208] These devices were also recently associated with a syndrome of acute lung injury in humans[209] (see also Chapter 65).

Table 63.2   Categories of Lung Damage Due to Reactive Oxygen Species

Mediator	Target	Reaction	Result
Aldehydes	Proteins	Protein adduct formation	Altered protein function, indirect effect on gene expression via HDAC-2
Multiple reactive oxygen species	DNA	Double-strand breaks, ring-opened and rearranged guanine products	Apoptosis; accelerated senescence; DDR activation, leading to proinflammatory cytokine production; mutagenesis
Peroxide	Lipids	Peroxidation	Cell membrane damage, formation of reactive aldehydes
Peroxynitrite	Proteins	Tyrosine nitration	Altered protein function, MMP-9 activation, indirect effect on gene expression via HDAC-2
Reactive carbonyl species	Proteins and carbohydrates	Carbonylation	Potentially antigenic self-proteins

DDR, DNA damage response; HDAC-2, histone deacetylase 2; MMP-9, matrix metalloproteinase 9.

Smoking and other oxidative inhalational stressors induce endogenous ROS production by lung epithelial cells, *alveolar macrophages* (AMø), and other phagocytes. Reduced nicotinamide adenine dinucleotide phosphate oxidase is the principal intracellular ROS source, but mitochondrial respiration and the xanthine/xanthine oxidase system also participate.[199] The impact of oxidant stress is amplified in smokers due to the increased levels of iron in their lungs,[210] which, by redox cycling of Fe^{++} and Fe^{+++} (via the Fenton and Haber-Weiss reactions), can produce the highly toxic hydroxyl radical. Phagocytes also produce two very damaging oxidants, hypochlorous acid and hypobromous acid, via cell-type specific enzymes that include myeloperoxidase and eosinophil peroxidase. During severe AE-COPD, oxidant stress in the lungs increases markedly in parallel with neutrophil recruitment.[211] Oxidative stress can be measured by a host of biomarkers.[212]

Excessive ROS damage cells in multiple ways (Table 63.2).[198] Lipid peroxidation of polyunsaturated fatty acids causes them to reorient out of the membrane plane, making them targets for scavenger receptors.[213] Because the reaction of a radical with a nonradical always produces another free radical, lipid peroxidation can proceed as a chain reaction. One stable product of lipid peroxidation, 8-isoprostane, potently stimulates airway smooth muscle contraction via the thromboxane A_2 receptor.[214] ROS produce diffusible reactive aldehydes, including acrolein, that create protein adducts by targeting cysteine, histidine, and lysine residues. Such adducts impair the function of matrix components and of enzymes crucial to regulating gene expression, such as histone deacetylase 2, which is important for inactivation of proinflammatory genes.[215] The reaction of ROS with nitric oxide forms peroxynitrite, which causes tyrosine nitration, particularly of histone deacetylase 2,[216] perpetuating inflammatory mediator production.[217] Carbonylation describes two distinct kinds of damaging results of oxidants, both the direct non-enzymatic, irreversible oxidation of amino acid side chains, and non-oxidative covalent adduction of reactive carbonyl species generated by the oxidation of lipids or carbohydrates.[218] Multiple pathways lead to reactive carbonyl species, particularly by metal-catalyzed oxidation of lysine, arginine, proline, and threonine residues.[219] Carbonylation may be important in late stages of COPD because it renders proteins potentially antigenic.[220] Finally, ROS can damage DNA directly, particularly at guanine residues.[221]

Besides direct damage, excessive ROS subvert physiologic gene expression, which may be more consequential for COPD development. During homeostasis, controlled intracellular ROS production is a crucial component of signal transduction pathways central to cell proliferation, differentiation, migration, senescence, and apoptosis. ROS targeting of redox-reactive cysteine residues creates disulfide bonds, changing protein structure and hence function.[222] The most important ROS for such intracellular communication functions is hydrogen peroxide, a relatively weak oxidizer.[223] These changes are mostly reversible via thioredoxin and peroxiredoxin, which are themselves targets of redox cysteine regulation. Excessive intracellular ROS activate the *phosphoinositide 3'-kinase* (PI3K) pathway, which is coupled with multiple receptor tyrosine kinases that recognize growth factors, including *epidermal growth factor receptor* (EGFR), platelet-derived growth factor receptor, and *vascular endothelial growth factor* (VEGF) receptor. Thus, inappropriate ROS-induced PI3K activation can drive proliferation of multiple lung cell types.

Excessive ROS can also exaggerate the activation of several of the four major *mitogen-activated protein kinase* (MAPK) signaling cascades: extracellular signal-related kinases, c-Jun N-terminal kinases, p38 kinase, and the big MAP kinase 1. The MAPK cascades comprise triads of linked kinases that sequentially phosphorylate their downstream target. Like PI3K, MAPKs transduce signals from multiple cell-surface growth receptors,[224] so excessive ROS can bypass their physiologic control. One ROS target is apoptosis signal-regulated kinase 1, an upstream MAPK that regulates the c-Jun N-terminal kinases and p38 kinase MAPK pathways, ultimately triggering apoptosis in response to various cellular stressors.[222] ROS can also directly inhibit multiple phosphatases, some irreversibly, via formation of sulfinic and sulfonic acid adducts.[222] The net result is deranged signal transduction leading to dysplasia or cell death.

Finally, excessive ROS can subvert a key physiologic function of ROS, the cotranslational redox regulation of transcription factors such as p53, activator protein 1, cyclic adenosine monophosphate response element binding protein, early growth response protein-1, hypoxia inducible factor 1,

Table 63.3 Antioxidant Defenses of the Lungs[199,226]

NON-ENZYMATIC ANTIOXIDANTS

Glutathione, ascorbic acid (vitamin C)*

Uric acid, alpha-tocopherol (vitamin E), albumin†

ENZYMATIC ANTIOXIDANTS

Cu,Zn-SOD, EC-SOD, Mn-SOD, catalase, thioredoxin, glutathione peroxidase, heme oxygenase-1, glutathione-S-transferase

EC, extracellular; SOD, superoxide dismutase.
*These have higher concentrations in the airway lining fluid relative to plasma.
†These have lower concentrations in airway lining fluid than in plasma.

nuclear factor kappa B (NF-κB), and paired box containing proteins. This action is normally accomplished via the activity of the multifunctional DNA repair enzyme apurinic/apyrimidinic endodeoxyribonuclease 1 (Gene ID 328), better known in this role as redox factor-1.[225] By maintaining cysteine residues in the reduced state, redox factor-1 controls the DNA binding activity of these transcription factors. Unchecked intracellular ROS antagonizes this activity by directly oxidizing crucial cysteine residues, including in redox factor-1 itself. Redox factor-1 also targets the transcription factor commonly known as Nrf2 (nuclear factor, erythroid 2 like; Gene ID 4780). Nrf2 counters oxidative stress by activating genes whose promoters contain antioxidant response elements.[222] Thus, oxidative stress may contribute centrally to COPD development by inducing sustained adverse changes in gene expression, especially if there are changes in self-replicating committed progenitor cell types.

The lungs are defended against ROS by non-enzymatic and enzymatic antioxidants (Table 63.3). Non-enzymatic antioxidants include glutathione, ascorbic acid (vitamin C), and uric acid, and by alpha-tocopherol (vitamin E).[226] Glutathione and ascorbic acid are co-secreted by alveolar epithelial type 2 cells, whose loss in emphysema may thus accelerate deterioration of antioxidant defenses. Even in those without airflow obstruction, active smoking reduces lung concentrations of ascorbate, alpha-tocopherol, and especially glutathione.[198] In COPD, regardless of smoking status, glutathione concentrations are particularly decreased and fall further during severe AE-COPD.[211] There are also multiple enzymatic antioxidants, all altered in COPD.[199] These include three types of superoxide dismutase (Cu,Zn- extracellular [EC], expressed around airways and blood vessels[227]; and Mn), as well as catalase, thioredoxin, glutathione peroxidase, heme oxygenase-1, and glutathione-S-transferase.

SMOKING-INDUCED EPIGENETIC REPROGRAMMING OF THE AIRWAY EPITHELIUM

Epigenetic changes triggered by oxidative inhalational stress lead to SAD and chronic mucus hypersecretion, which collectively form the basis for the multiple clinical phenotypes seen in mild COPD. For small airways, efficient mucus clearance and local self-defense depend on the integrity of a normal pseudostratified epithelium composed of diverse cell types.[228] All these cell types derive from multipotent stem cells within the heterogeneous *basal cell* (BC) population (Fig. 63.6A).[229,230] BCs also give rise to two rare airway cell types, pulmonary neuroendocrine cells[231–233] and pulmonary

ionocytes, which are rich in cystic fibrosis transmembrane conductance regulator expression.[234] In human airways, only the respiratory bronchioles lack BCs, making that anatomic locus uniquely susceptible to inhalational damage,[235] and the initial site of CLE development. Unlike the predominance of ciliated cells (60–80%) in proximal airways, the most common small airway cell type is secretory cells, which produce CC-16 (secretoglobin family 1A member 1 [SCGB1A1]; Gene ID 7356) and other innate immune molecules (Table 63.4), including cathelicidin LL37, H-ficolin, lactoferrin, *secretory immunoglobin A* (sIgA), and surfactant proteins A and D. Most of these innate immune molecules have been shown to have altered expression in COPD.[236–247]

Smoking causes BC epigenetic reprogramming, inducing changes that include hyperplasia of BCs and mucus-producing goblet cells, squamous metaplasia, dropout of ciliated cells and secretory cells, and damage to remaining cilia (Fig. 63.6B).[248] These changes arise in all smokers and precede inflammatory cell inflammation,[249] implying that they are necessary but insufficient for progression to COPD. However, it is also possible that BC exhaustion could contribute to SAD and emphysema.[250]

Altered community structure of small airway epithelial cells results in part from an imbalance between signal transduction via Notch family members, which induce physiological secretory cell and neuroendocrine cell differentiation,[251,252] and EGFR, a receptor tyrosine kinase of the ErbB family. Oxidative stress induces EGF production by ciliated cells, and additionally, by increasing epithelial permeability, overcomes the normal sequestration of EGFR from its ligands on opposite sides of the polarized epithelium.[253,254] EGFR activation induces an alternative EGFR ligand, amphiregulin. By promoting its own expression, amphiregulin can drive epithelial hyperplasia even after oxidative stress is removed. Amphiregulin causes hyperplasia of BCs and mucus cells, which along with other smoking-induced alterations, culminates in an airway epithelium susceptible to bacterial invasion.[255]

Such bacterial invasion is facilitated by yet another result of BC epigenetic reprogramming, impairment of defensive systems reliant on small airway secretory cells (see Table 63.4). One defensive system is CC16/SCGB1A1, the most abundant protein in normal distal airway secretions, which blocks production of proinflammatory cytokines and lipid mediators by antagonizing NF-kB activation and by inhibiting phospholipase A₂. Loss of CC16/SCGB1A1 appears to contribute to SAD.[256] However, best characterized and potentially most important of these systems is immune exclusion of microbes by sIgA.[67] In normal small airways, sIgA is translocated into the airway lumen by the polymeric immunoglobulin receptor (see Fig. 63.4C). This requirement does not apply to more proximal airways, where sIgA can gain access to the lumen via submucosal glands. In lung tissue ranging from healthy never smokers to severe COPD, focal loss of the polymeric immunoglobulin receptor and luminal sIgA correlated tightly with small airway damage (see Fig. 63.4D).[257]

Loss of translocation of sIgA into the lumen of small airways permits bacteria to invade epithelial cells, which induces focal NF-κB activation.[257] The identity of these bacteria is so far unreported but plausibly includes *nontypeable*

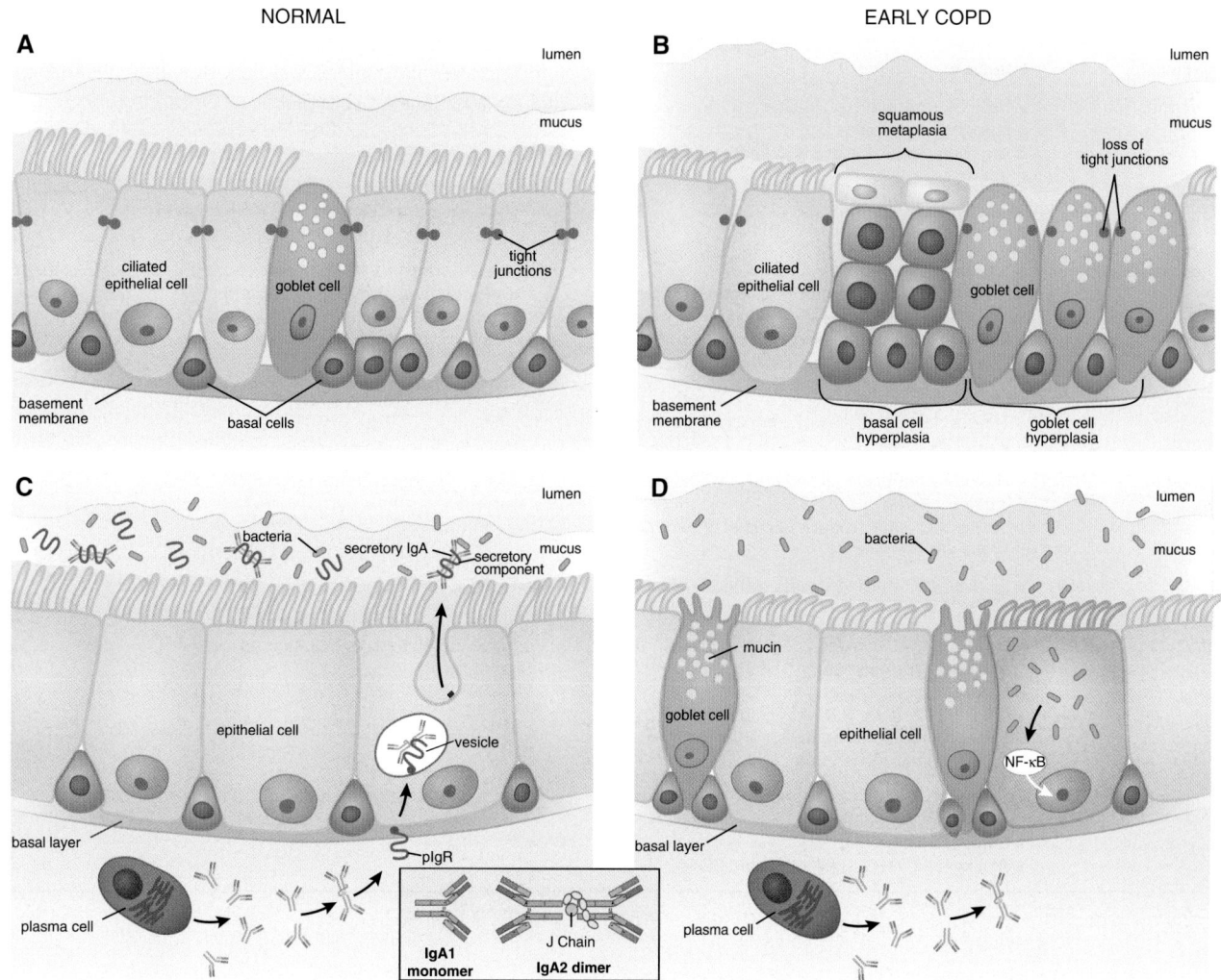

NORMAL

EARLY COPD

Figure 63.6 Epigenetic changes induced by smoking lead to progressive small airway damage and inflammation in early COPD. (A and C) Normal small airways. (B and D) Small airways in early COPD. (A–B) Cellular constituents. (A) Normal distal epithelium contains self-renewing basal cells, which differentiate into ciliated, mucus-producing goblet, and secretory (club) cells (not depicted), joined by tight junctions that form an impermeable barrier. Mucus is separated from the epithelial surface by a robust aqueous periciliary layer. (B) Smoking induces hyperplasia of basal and goblet cells, squamous metaplasia, loss of ciliated and club cells, a decrease in the periciliary layer and ciliary damage and crowding, and junctional barrier loss. (C–D) Role of secretory immunoglobulin A (IgA) in physiology and early COPD. (C) In normal small airways, dimeric IgA (*inset*) is transcytosed by the polymeric immunoglobulin receptor (pIgR) into the mucosal lumen. pIgR cleavage at the luminal surface liberates secretory IgA, which prevents bacterial invasion. (D) Smoking reduces pIgR expression, leading to localized secretory IgA deficiency in small airways, allowing bacteria to invade and induce sustained airway inflammation. NF-κB, nuclear factor-κB. (From Martinez FJ, Han MK, Allinson JP, et al. At the root: defining and halting progression of early chronic obstructive pulmonary disease. *Am J Respir Crit Care Med.* 2018;197:1540-1551. Illustration by Patricia Ferrer Beals.)

Haemophilus influenzae and *Streptococcus pneumoniae*, which both have this ability. Such invasion is facilitated due to the up-regulation by airway epithelial cells of both smokers and COPD patients of adhesion molecules that pathogens exploit: intercellular adhesion molecule 1, also known as CD54, by nontypeable *H. influenzae* and rhinovirus[258] and platelet activating factor by pneumococcus.[259] In advanced COPD, epithelial barrier integrity appears to be lost.[260]

Thus, the earliest stages of COPD pathology appear to result from impaired innate immune defenses. Active smoking may also prevent appropriate regulation by the adaptive immune system via the immunosuppressive properties of nicotine,[261] which reduces lymphocyte proliferation and impairs T cell polarization both directly[262,263] and indirectly via actions on *dendritic cells* (DCs).[264]

SMALL AIRWAY REMODELING AND MATRIX DAMAGE

The earliest overt lesion of COPD is small airway remodeling, which is the deposition of excess connective tissue in the subepithelial and adventitial compartments of the airway wall.[32,68] Remodeling is one component of SAD (along with obstruction by mucus and disappearance of terminal and transitional bronchioles). In later stages, these changes are accompanied by inflammatory cell infiltration, considered below.

The healthy lung ECM consists of the basement membrane to which cells attach plus the interstitial matrix. ECM is formed by collagen and elastin fibers interwoven by proteoglycans, fibronectin, and laminin.[75] Most abundant of

Table 63.4 Lung Host Defense and Homeostatic Soluble Mediators

Molecule	Function	Effect of Smoking and COPD	Reference
β-Defensins	▪ Have direct antimicrobial effects via membrane lysis ▪ Block bacterial toxins ▪ Are chemotactic for DCs and T cells via CCR6	Increased in sputum in COPD	236, 237
CC-16/SCGB1A1	▪ Reduces IL-8 production by epithelial cells ▪ Suppresses phospholipase A$_2$ and NF-κB	Airway levels lower in smokers and in COPD. Reduced serum concentrations independently associated with accelerated decline in FEV$_1$	238, 239, 256
Cathelicidin LL37	▪ Has direct antimicrobial effects ▪ Is chemotactic for neutrophils, monocytes, and T cells via FPRL-1 ▪ Reduces Mø responses to LPS ▪ Can damage epithelial cells at high concentrations	Elevated in sputum in COPD; reduced plasma levels independently associated with longitudinal loss of lung function in ever smokers	236, 240, 241
H-ficolin (ficolin 3)	▪ Opsonizes bacteria ▪ Triggers lectin pathway of complement activation ▪ Binds LPS	Not yet reported to play a role in smoking and COPD	242
Lactoferrin	▪ Has direct antibacterial and antiviral effects due to cationic charge ▪ Sequesters iron to reduce bacterial growth and biofilm formation	Reduced iron-to-lactoferrin ratios in BAL of smokers	243, 244
sIgA	▪ Binds to bacteria and viruses without activating complement	Reduced in BAL in COPD	245–247
Surfactant protein A	▪ Opsonizes bacteria and apoptotic cells without activating complement ▪ Binds LPS ▪ Blocks TLR2, TLR3, TLR4, MD2, and CD14 ▪ Enhances multiple negative regulators of AMø proinflammatory function	Reduced in BAL both by smoking and in COPD	242
Surfactant protein D	▪ Opsonizes bacteria and apoptotic cells without activating complement ▪ Binds LPS ▪ Blocks TLR2, TLR3, TLR4, MD2, and CD14	Reduced in BAL both by smoking and in COPD	242

AMø, alveolar macrophages; BAL, bronchoalveolar lavage; DC, dendritic cell; FEV$_1$, forced expiratory volume in 1 second; FPRL-1, formyl peptide receptor-like 1; IL, interleukin; LPS, lipopolysaccharide; Mø, macrophage; NF-κB, nuclear factor kappa B; SCGB1A1, secretoglobin family 1A member 1; TLR, toll-like receptor.

these are collagens, which can be divided into the interstitial type I and type III fibrillar collagens and the nonfibrillar type IV, which forms basement membranes. Elastin is chiefly responsible for lung elastic recoil and hence airflow velocity during exhalation. Elastin is particularly consequential because it is not typically replaced during adult life.[265] Proteoglycans consist of core proteins decorated by glycosaminoglycan(s) that sequester water and ions and regulate cellular migration. Rather than contributing to lung mechanical strength, fibronectin and laminin are important for promoting cell migration and survival and for storing growth factors that can be released during matrix damage. ECM also contains latent TGF-β, cytokines, proteases, and other enzymes essential for its continuous physiologic remodeling and for the participation of immune effectors in COPD pathogenesis.[266,267]

Smoking and development of COPD alter lung concentrations of these ECM constituents in a complex fashion. Elastin is increased in smokers without airflow obstruction, relative to both never smokers and COPD patients.[75] Despite up-regulation of elastin gene expression, advanced COPD is associated with reduced elastin content, including in small and large airways[75] but not in alveolar walls, where it is increased.[268] Genetic defects in elastin have been identified as a cause of severe emphysema.[269,270] Expression of tenascin C and its binding partner, fibronectin, is also increased

in COPD.[75,271,272] Tenascin and fibronectin may enhance COPD pathology by inducing MMP expression and activity and via tenascin's adverse effect on endothelial cell survival,[273] an example of how SAD could contribute to early pulmonary vascular disease. Collagen content of the alveolar walls appears to be increased in emphysema but is considerably disorganized.[274,275]

Remodeling is associated with up-regulation of the zinc finger transcription factor *Krüppel-like factor 5* (KLF5) in lung fibroblasts. KLF5 drives myofibroblast survival and differentiation; controls release of collagen and MMPs[276]; and regulates expression of platelet derived growth factor-α, fibroblast growth factor, VEGF, and TGF-β.[277] KLF5 is induced by the Ras-MAPK pathway downstream of multiple growth factors, and also by Wnt signaling, angiotensin II, and early growth response protein-1. Hence, KLF5 production may be one result of oxidant-induced aberrant gene regulation. Remodeled small airways also express multiple members of the TGF-β superfamily,[278] which have potentially profibrotic properties. One member, activin-A, is increased in COPD in parallel with decreases in its endogenous inhibitor, follistatin.[279] Activin-A has some potentially beneficial properties in smokers (e.g., stimulating development of *regulatory T cells* [T$_{reg}$][280]) but its profibrotic properties likely contribute to airway remodeling.

Tissue degradation around small airways in COPD has been shown by global gene analysis to predominate over repair.[281] This finding suggests that small airway narrowing due to remodeling may be only one feature of a process that simultaneously increases lung compliance even before the advent of overt emphysema. Such tissue degradation results from actions of proteases that destroy ECM faster than it can be replaced.

PROTEASES/ANTIPROTEASES

Since the initial recognition of the strong association between AATD and emphysema, an imbalance between proteases and antiproteases has been postulated to drive emphysema development.[282] As originally formulated, the most important contributor to this imbalance was believed to be NE,[283,284] but MMPs, especially macrophage-derived MMP-12,[285] are now considered more crucial for overall emphysema development.[266,286,287] A promoter variant in MMP12 has been associated with COPD onset and severity, though not all studies have replicated this finding.[163,288]

Nevertheless, neutrophil proteases are also crucial for lung destruction in COPD. Neutrophils are a major source of MMP-9, which, through the serial action of another neutrophil serine protease, prolyl endopeptidase, degrades collagen to release *N-acetyl-Pro-Gly-Pro* (Ac-PGP), a tri-peptide that is a potent neutrophil chemoattractant.[289,290] Ac-PGP shares sequence and structural homology with a domain of CXC chemokines containing a glutamic acid-leucine-arginine motif. Such acid-leucine-arginine+ CXC chemokines, particularly *interleukin* (IL)-8, have traditionally been considered the major drivers of neutrophil recruitment in COPD. However, Ac-PGP is a specific agonist for the chemokine receptors CXCR1 and CXCR2, which are required for its neutrophil chemoattractant activity.[291] Hence, in the process of damaging collagen, neutrophils induce a self-perpetuating loop for their own recruitment to the lungs.[292] This loop is normally broken when Ac-PGP is degraded by the aminopeptidase activity of leukotriene A_4 hydrolase, a proinflammatory enzyme that also generates a lipid neutrophil chemoattractant, leukotriene B_4. However, CS inhibits the aminopeptidase activity of leukotriene A_4 hydrolase,[293] thus amplifying neutrophil recruitment via the Ac-PGP loop.

Proteolytic damage initiated by SAD can spread into the surrounding tissues.[294] By eliminating tethering of small airways through destruction of bronchiolar-alveolar attachments,[295–297] proteolysis accelerates airflow obstruction and triggers the earliest damage leading to CLE.[34,298,299] These findings suggest that, although distinct *endotypes* (i.e., subtypes of a clinical disorder defined by a distinct pathophysiological mechanism[300]) likely contribute to the heterogeneity of COPD phenotypes,[25,301,302] there may also be a core pathologic pathway that evolves from airway epithelial epigenetic reprogramming to SAD and finally to CLE adjacent to individual airways. To date, the existence of this pathway is an extrapolation from cross-sectional histologic results, but it is supported by longitudinal imaging data[39] that, in advanced COPD, correlate to histology.[34,38,297] Hence, understanding the cell types contributing to proteolytic damage is key to developing novel therapies to arrest COPD progression.

INNATE CELLULAR RESPONSES

Lung *macrophages* (Mø) serve crucial immunoregulatory functions that minimize lung inflammation[303,304] but are also key sources of proteolytic enzymes that contribute to emphysema development[266,285–287] (see also Chapter 15). Mø are broadly distributed in the lungs, as in every other organ, and they appear to be essential for organogenesis[305] and for resistance to cellular stress.[306] The adult lung contains at least three types of Mø. *Alveolar Mø* (AMø) arise from a distinct progenitor during embryogenesis[307] and are maintained during health by low-level in situ proliferation.[308,309] Relative to DCs, AMø are poor antigen-presenting cells but can generate T_{reg}.[310] AMø from a subset of COPD patients exhibited impaired immune responses to TLR4 stimulation in vitro by respiratory pathogens or by molecules derived from them, which correlated with increased risk of future exacerbations.[311] Interstitial Mø, by contrast, are a minor population that express phenotypic markers suggesting that they derive from bone marrow via maturation of monocytes.[308,312–315] Interstitial lung Mø have been difficult to study but appear to segregate into several subsets with distinct anatomic localizations[315,316] and to be capable of immunoregulatory functions.[313,315,317] Finally, blood monocytes, which, in health, migrate through the lungs without differentiation,[312,318] can differentiate during acute inflammation into mature phagocytes with properties spanning the spectrum from those of Mø to DCs.[319]

Lung Mø numbers increase soon after initiation of smoking[320,321] and further increase during COPD progression.[68] The molecular basis for this expansion is incompletely defined, but evidence favors oxidant-induced resistance to apoptosis as the predominant factor.[322–324] Smoking and, to a greater extent, the progression of COPD itself are associated with defective AMø phagocytosis of bacteria and of apoptotic cells.[325,326] Defects in the latter process, also known as *efferocytosis*, are believed to foster lung inflammation.[327] AMø from COPD patients show a reduced ability to kill bacteria,[328] in part related to deficient Nrf2 activation.[329] Smoking additionally decreases the capacity of AMø to provide anti-inflammatory mediators to lung epithelial cells via extracellular vesicles.[330] Collectively, these changes, plus increased Mø production of proinflammatory cytokines in COPD,[331] likely exacerbate the focal immunocompromise resulting from small airway epithelial reprogramming.

DCs are essential in the regulation of both innate immunity, because they can prime *natural killer* (NK) cells for cytotoxicity, and adaptive immunity, because they are the preeminent antigen-presenting cell that activates and polarizes naive T cells.[332,333] The lungs contain three types of DCs, each with a specialized function[334]: *type 1 and type 2 conventional DCs* (cDC1 and cDC2, respectively) and plasmacytoid DCs. cDC1s reside in airway mucosa and vascular walls, cross-present antigens derived from apoptotic cells, and are essential to generate T_{reg} and thus to maintain self-tolerance at mucosal surfaces. On maturation in response to danger signals, cDC1s can elicit *type 1 T helper* (Th1) cells and cytotoxic T cell responses, which are essential for antiviral defenses but are also linked to COPD pathology. cDC2s, which are more numerous, reside primarily in the airway lamina propria and are the major producers of proinflammatory chemokines. cDC2s are also responsible for polarization of T cells to the

Th2 and Th17 phenotypes. Plasmacytoid DCs are widely distributed throughout the lung, including airways and alveolar septa. Their rapid ability to elaborate large amounts of type 1 interferons is essential for antiviral responses. Progression of COPD has been associated with increased numbers and activation state of all three lung DC subsets within lung parenchyma in some,[335–337] but not all, studies.[338,339]

Neutrophils have traditionally been considered to be crucial to COPD pathogenesis, primarily for their secretions of proteases,[340] but are also increasingly recognized to serve immunoregulatory functions that include mediator elaboration, activation of γδ T cells, and antigen presentation[341] (though the last action has been contested[333]). Constitutive migration of neutrophils through the lungs, following a circadian rhythm, appears important for IL-22–dependent production of antimicrobial peptides.[342] Neutrophils store preformed mediators, including *B-cell activating factor* (BAFF), and *a proliferation-inducing ligand/tumor necrosis factor ligand superfamily member 13* (APRIL) (which are B cell trophic factors), *TNF-related apoptosis-inducing ligand* (TRAIL), CXCL8, CCL20, and IL-1R antagonist. Neutrophil secretion of extracellular vesicles can profoundly influence their surroundings and sustain lung inflammation.[343,344]

Eosinophils are increased in the sputum of a sizeable percentage of patients with stable COPD, relative to healthy never smokers, with the exact frequency depending on the threshold considered abnormal.[345–350] Eosinophils are also elevated in bronchoalveolar lavage and lung tissue of some COPD patients,[347,351] even in the absence of peripheral blood eosinophilia,[352] and are associated with reticular basement membrane thickening.[351] Eosinophils potently produce chemokines and T2 cytokines. They can express class II major histocompatibility antigens and, in murine models, localize to the same areas of mediastinal lymph nodes as the DCs,[353] supporting the ability of eosinophils to polarize T cells to a Th2 phenotype. Eosinophils are also associated with a specific subtype of exacerbation risk, discussed below.

NK cells, by far the most numerous type of *innate lymphoid cell* (ILC), are common in healthy lungs. NK cells mediate rapid lysis of damaged cells, but require initial priming by cDCs,[354,355] which is increased in COPD.[356] Most lung NK cells display the differentiated (CD56^{dim}) phenotype associated with cytotoxicity, regardless of smoking status or COPD,[357,358] in contrast to other organs and within tumors, where cytokine-secreting CD56^{bright} NK cells predominate. Evidence supports a contribution of NK cell killing of airway epithelial cells to the development of SAD and the progression to emphysema,[356,358,359] although their role relative to that of CD3$^+$, CD8$^+$ cytotoxic lymphocytes remains to be defined.[360] The involvement of the other, far less common ILC subsets,[361] especially ILC2 and ILC3, in the development of specific COPD endotypes is highly plausible but as yet undefined.

MEDIATORS OF INFLAMMATION AND OF ITS RESOLUTION

In the stable state, COPD is characterized by increased expression of multiple proinflammatory cytokines (notably IL-1α, IL-1β, tumor necrosis factor-α, and IL-6) and chemokines (especially CXCL8).[361–363] However, no single mediator can account for the four key pathologies characterizing lung damage in COPD and, to date, the specific therapeutic blockade of individual mediators has had mixed results in arresting progression or reducing exacerbation frequency.[364] The anti-IL-1β *monoclonal antibody* canakinumab was ineffective (ClinicalTrials.gov NCT00581945). Infliximab, an anti–tumor necrosis factor-α monoclonal antibody, showed no benefit and was associated with increased cancers and other adverse events.[365] A monoclonal antibody against CXCL8 was ineffective,[366] and trials inhibiting its receptor, CXCR2, were equivocal, showing some promise but also potential for toxicity.[367,368]

Nevertheless, recent progress in identifying key roles for several of these soluble mediators suggests the possible existence of COPD endotypes that could be targeted selectively.[302] Mutually exclusive subsets of COPD patients with predominately Th2-high versus Th17-high inflammation appear to exist and to denote steroid-responsive versus unresponsive disease, respectively.[369,370] Hence, the future of targeted cytokine blockade will likely involve more precise selection of COPD patients based on specific types of inflammation. Attractive targets for this approach include more upstream cytokines produced by and near the epithelium, such as thymic stromal lymphopoietin (Gene ID: 85480)[371] and IL-33 (or its receptor, ST2),[372] which define the tissue niche for ILC2 cells.[373]

Rather than resulting passively from dilution of inflammatory mediators, resolution of inflammation is an active process. Resolution depends crucially on specific lipid mediators derived from essential polyunsaturated fatty acids, which fall into four families: lipoxins, resolvins, protectins, and maresins (the last short for *ma*crophage mediators in *res*olving *in*flammation).[374] Collectively, these lipids are termed *specialized pro-resolving mediators* (SPMs); they act via stereospecific G-protein–coupled receptors. SPM biosynthesis is tightly controlled spatially and temporally because individual cell types can both class-switch their lipid mediator production[375] and may lack enzymes needed for the initial or the final steps of production, necessitating transcellular biosynthesis.[376] Specific SPMs reduce leukocyte cytokine production and adhesion, arrest neutrophil migration and favor their apoptosis, enhance efferocytosis, and reduce antigen presentation and IL-12 production by DCs. SPMs appear to be reduced in COPD.[377] Because they favor resolution without being broadly immunosuppressive, SPMs are promising therapeutic agents.[378]

PULMONARY MICROVASCULAR CHANGES INDUCED BY OXIDANT INJURY

Oxidative stress causes endothelial cell death,[379–381] a process linked to atherogenesis in the systemic circulation. Potential contributors to endothelial cell death include apoptosis by p53 due to DNA damage[380] or ROS-induced activation of the MAPK family member apoptosis signal-related kinase,[222] and decreased Notch signaling.[382] The pulmonary microvasculature maintains distal lung architecture, as demonstrated both in human pathologic samples[72,383–385] and in animal models. Death of pulmonary microvascular endothelial cells can lead to irreversible destruction of entire secondary pulmonary lobules, as seen in severe confluent CLE and PLE. The peripheral blood of COPD patients contains elevated levels of circulating endothelial microparticles, an indicator of endothelial cell damage.[386-388] Microparticle concentrations fall following smoking cessation in those without airflow obstruction but not in those with COPD,[389] suggesting that endothelial cell death might be causally linked to loss of lung function.

Death of pulmonary microvascular endothelial cells could become self-sustaining via *endothelial monocyte activating protein 2* (EMAP-2), which causes endothelial cell apoptosis.[390,391] EMAP-2 (also known as p43; Gene ID 9255) is a noncatalytic component of the multi-aminoacyl-tRNA synthetase complex that also functions as a multifunctional proinflammatory cytokine when released by stressors such as hypoxia, lipopolysaccharide, viral infections, or CS.[392] Neutralizing antibodies against EMAP-2 block emphysema development in a murine CS exposure model.[393]

Additionally, as in other organs, the activation states and responses to injury of pulmonary microvascular endothelial cells is governed by tissue-resident parenchymal and stem cells by production of angiogenic factors such as VEGF-A, fibroblast growth factor-2, CXCL12, thrombospondin-1, and angiopoietins.[394] VEGF concentrations and endothelial expression of VEGF receptor are reduced in COPD.[72] Hence, damage to pericytes or airway mesenchymal cells, which could result from changes in their surrounding ECM, could be another reason for loss of pulmonary microvasculature in COPD.

It is known that prenatal lung development depends on reciprocal, mutually supportive signals between endothelial and epithelial cells. These reciprocal relationships are also likely necessary to sustain adult physiology. In the experimental model of compensatory lung hypertrophy following left pneumonectomy, propagation of alveolar epithelial type 2 cells requires endothelial expression of cell-bound MMP-14. Following activation by platelet-derived CXCL12, endothelial cells up-regulate MMP-14, which activates EGFR on alveolar epithelial progenitor cells.[395] This mechanism also sustains airway BCs,[395] further support that the epithelial and endothelial theories of emphysema origin are not mutually exclusive.

COPD AS A DISEASE OF ACCELERATED AGING

Age is one of the strongest risk factors for COPD development[396]; conversely, COPD is proposed to be a disease of accelerated aging.[397-400] Evidence supporting this hypothesis fits the framework of nine proposed hallmarks of normal aging,[401] which segregate into three categories (Fig. 63.7):

1. *Primary hallmarks*: genomic instability, telomere attrition, epigenetic alterations, and loss of proteostasis, all of which are intrinsically negative;
2. *Antagonistic hallmarks*: deregulated nutrient sensing, mitochondrial dysfunction, and cellular senescence, which are initially beneficial responses to the primary hallmarks but become detrimental when intense and sustained;
3. *Integrative hallmarks*: stem cell exhaustion and altered intercellular communication, including "inflamm-aging."[306]

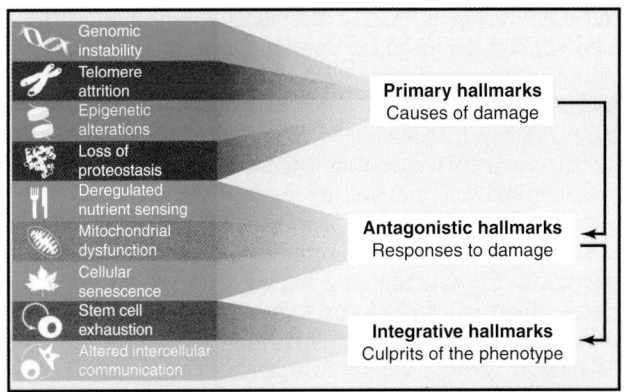

Figure 63.7 Functional interconnections between the hallmarks of aging. The proposed nine hallmarks of aging are grouped into three categories. *Top,* Those considered to be the primary causes of cellular damage. *Middle,* Those considered to be part of compensatory or antagonistic responses to the damage. These responses initially mitigate the damage but eventually, if chronic or exacerbated, become deleterious themselves. *Bottom,* Integrative hallmarks that are the end result of the previous two groups and that are ultimately responsible for the functional decline associated with aging. (From Lopez-Otin C, Blasco MA, Partridge L, Serrano M, Kroemer G. The hallmarks of aging. *Cell.* 2013;153:1194–1217.)

Primary Hallmarks

Genomic instability due to oxidant-induced DNA damage is found in smokers regardless of COPD status, but the oxidant-induced damage is greater in COPD, and increased DNA repair is restricted to those without airflow obstruction.[402,403] Ineffective DNA repair in COPD may result from selective reduction of Ku86, a component of the complex that repairs double-stranded DNA breaks.[402]

Telomeres support chromosome stability, but their maintenance requires telomerase because conventional DNA polymerases cannot completely replicate the ends of linear DNA stands. Telomerase is absent from most somatic cell types so that, with repeated cell division, telomere lengths fall, leading to replicative senescence or apoptosis. Pulmonary endothelial cell telomere length is reduced in COPD.[404] Shorter leukocyte telomere length associates with lower adult lung function and higher COPD prevalence.[405-407] Lower spirometry at a mean age of 50 years was predicted by faster leukocyte telomere length attrition between mean ages of 30 to 40 years (but not by leukocyte telomere length at baseline or follow-up). Because lung function was measured only once in that study, whether leukocyte telomere length reduction is causally related to spirometric decline remains unproven[408]; however, genetic defects in telomere maintenance have been identified in emphysema.[152,188]

Epigenetic alterations could contribute to COPD pathogenesis by perpetuating lung damage even after removal of the initiating stimulus. Epigenetic alteration is a composite term for processes that collectively regulate gene transcription. Types of epigenetic alteration include DNA methylation (which induces transcriptional repression), chromatin remodeling, reversible post-translational modifications of histones (including methylation, acetylation, phosphorylation, ubiquitination, SUMOylation, and adenosine diphosphate ribosylation), and alterations in transcription of noncoding RNAs.[409] Histone modifications either disrupt chromatin organization or provide new binding surfaces to recruit DNA-binding proteins to specific chromosomal regions, while noncoding RNA alterations can have broad-reaching effects on translation of multiple genes. Besides the changes in histone deacetylase 2 cited above, extensive changes in other enzymes mediating post-translational modifications are induced by smoking, both in epithelial cells in vitro and in CS-exposed mice.[410] The net effect of altered histone post-translational modifications is heterochromatin decay, which has been linked to cellular senescence. Smoking also induces AMø to down-regulate many, but not all, microRNAs (hence increasing expression of their target genes) via dysfunction of the cytosolic RNA endonuclease DICER.[411,412]

Proteostasis refers to the combination of maintenance of correct protein synthesis and folding, and the quality control mechanisms that rely on the ubiquitin-proteasome and autophagy-lysosomal pathways. Defective proteostasis can activate the unfolded protein response, which contributes to cell death in some variants of AATD.[413,414] In smokers, ROS-induced damage, especially carbonylation (see Table 63.3), greatly challenges protein quality control[219] and leads to rapid compensatory up-regulation of the unfolded protein response.[415] Proteasome function is defective in COPD, perhaps because it is overwhelmed. CS activates autophagy, which might initially play a protective role in lung epithelial cells. Indeed, autophagy is globally elevated in the lungs of COPD patients,[416] but multiple aspects of selective autophagy are impaired, contributing to ciliary dysfunction, which may reflect failure to complete autophagy ("incomplete autophagic flux").[417]

Antagonistic Hallmarks

Deregulated nutrient sensing degrades cellular homeostasis. The primary mediator of normal regulation is the intracellular signaling pathway shared by insulin and insulin-like growth factor-1 (IGF-1), termed insulin and IGF-1 signaling, the most evolutionarily conserved of any aging control mechanism. Levels of IGF-1 decline during normal aging,[418] which has been interpreted to indicate a down-modulation of the insulin and IGF-1 signaling pathway as a defensive strategy to minimize cell growth in the context of cellular damage.[401] Regulation of nutrients also involves (1) the PI3K-AKT–mammalian target of rapamycin pathway, which senses high amino acid levels, is partially controlled by the insulin and IGF-1 signaling pathway, and accelerates aging; (2) 5'-AMP-activated protein kinase (AMPK), which detects low energy states and inhibits mammalian target of rapamycin; and (3) sirtuins, which reciprocally regulate and are regulated by AMPK and that, by activating peroxisome proliferator activated receptor-γ coactivator 1α, suppress aging via mitochondriogenesis, enhanced antioxidant defenses, and improved fatty acid oxidation. COPD is characterized by abnormalities in all three pathways,[419–429] arguing that they may be therapeutic targets to combat progression both of COPD and of its comorbidities.[400,430]

Mitochondrial dysfunction, affected by multiple pathways that promote aging,[431] is also described in COPD.[432–435] In cultured murine alveolar epithelial cells, CS extract at nontoxic doses induced excessive fusion of mitochondria, an initially adaptive but ultimately potentially harmful response.[436]

Cellular senescence, a stable block on proliferation, results from DNA damage or telomerase attrition.[430] Senescence is of evolutionary benefit by blocking tumorigenesis, albeit at the cost of shortening lifespan. Senescence is triggered either by pathways distal to p53, Arf, and Rb tumor suppressor or by the DNA damage response, which is orchestrated by the ATR (gene ID: 472) and ATM (gene ID: 545) serine/threonine kinases.[437–439] Senescence is maintained by heterochromatin formation.[440] Senescent cells up-regulate NF-κB and CCAAT enhancer binding protein beta. By inducing a positive feedback loop via CXCR2 and its ligands,[441] these transcription factors reinforce growth arrest but also sustain local and systemic inflammation through the senescence-associated secretory phenotype (SASP).[442,443] The known secretome of SASP-affected cells, dominated by IL-6 and IL-1α/β, closely matches cytokines recognized to be central to COPD pathogenesis. However, invoking SASP as the sole mediator of COPD progression would be overly simplistic. The SASP secretome is heavily pro-angiogenic and lacks the angiostatic factors[442] believed to contribute to development of emphysema.

Integrative Hallmarks

Stem cell exhaustion leading to loss of regenerative capacity is one of the most obvious features of aging. It likely contributes to COPD progression, especially via reduction of bone marrow–derived endothelial progenitor cells, which are essential to maintain pulmonary microvascular integrity. Endothelial progenitor cell numbers are decreased in COPD in parallel with spirometrically defined disease severity.[388,444–448] Thus, failure of the bone marrow to supply sufficient endothelial progenitor cells might contribute to emphysema in some individuals.

Altered intercellular communication during aging compounds the previously mentioned hallmarks of aging, which are all cell-autonomous defects. Examples of altered intercellular communication include dysregulation of the renin-angiotensin and adrenergic systems, which collectively impair homeostatic responses to stress and fail to restrain inflammation. A key subset of altered intercellular communication is "inflamm-aging," a progressive increase in the proinflammatory state with greater chronological age. Inflamm-aging is the net result of the inflammatory cytokines produced by SASP and exhaustion of specific immune components, especially T cell function, which leads to reduced clearance of pathogens and damaged cells. The damage that incites SAD and the toxic state of the ECM in COPD provide nonresolvable triggers for the classic stimuli for inflamm-aging, namely ongoing inflammation, and for interference with counterinflammatory regulatory mechanisms.[449] Inflamm-aging also accelerates many cardiovascular and metabolic comorbidities of COPD.

ADAPTIVE IMMUNE INFLAMMATION AND AUTOIMMUNITY

Several lines of evidence support involvement of adaptive immune mechanisms in COPD pathogenesis (see also Chapter 16). More severe COPD stages, defined spirometrically, exhibit lymphocytic infiltration of lung parenchyma not seen in milder COPD, with eventual development of organized tertiary lymphoid tissue, known as lung lymphoid follicles.[68,450] The cytokine B-cell activating factor is a key trigger to this process.[451,452] Lung lymphoid follicles contain germinal centers, indicating class switching of B cells to produce high-affinity antibodies, which might contribute to host defense, but might also accelerate lung pathology. B cells have been strongly associated with emphysema in integrative genomic analyses[453,454] and experimental models.[455–457] Tissue-specific autoantibodies can be detected in advanced COPD,[458–465] potentially driven by smoking-induced modification of self-proteins.[220,466] These findings suggest that early damage triggered by innate immune mechanisms can lead to a break in self-tolerance accelerating lung destruction.

Simultaneously, components of protective physiologic adaptive immunity appear to be reduced in established COPD. CD8+ T cells have a deficient ability to protect against respiratory viruses in COPD, due to up-regulated expression of programmed cell death protein 1.[467] Because viral infections themselves can induce programmed cell death protein 1,[468] there is risk of a positive feedforward loop favoring recurrent virally induced exacerbations. In many COPD patients, lung CD4+ T cells display markedly reduced mRNA transcripts for the transcription factors controlling Th1, Th2, Th17, and *forkhead box P3* (FOXP3)+ T_{reg} subsets and their signature cytokines; these patients' lung CD4+ T cells produce little to no inflammatory cytokines following in vitro stimulation.[469] Therefore, defective T cell function may compound the already deficient immune defense of the distal airways in COPD.

One potential cause of adaptive immune involvement in COPD is loss of the physiologic restraint on inflammation provided by T_{reg}, which are increased in the distal lung parenchyma of smokers without airflow obstruction relative to never smokers, but markedly decreased in COPD.[459,469–472] T_{reg} typically control effector T cell populations such as Th1, Th2, and Th17 cells, and also NK cells,[473–477] all of which could contribute to specific lung damage. The mechanism of lung T_{reg} decrease in COPD is unknown but might involve their local conversion into Th17 cells.[478]

PHENOTYPIC HETEROGENEITY AND NATURAL HISTORY

SEX AS A FACTOR IN COPD HETEROGENEITY

COPD has historically been considered a disease of older men, but its prevalence among women has been increasing. This change is due to the narrowing gap in gender disparities in smoking prevalence in high-income countries and greater likelihood of biomass exposure among women in low-income nations. Thus, COPD now affects men and women almost equally.[479] However, female smokers who visit a physician are less likely than male smokers to be diagnosed with COPD, to receive spirometry testing, or to be referred to a pulmonologist.[480,481] Sex differences in lung size are present throughout childhood and adolescence and persist into adulthood.[482] On CT imaging, female smokers exhibit higher wall area percentage compared with male smokers, but lower luminal area, internal diameter, and airway thickness.[483] This sex difference in airway dimensions may explain differing susceptibility

to disease and phenotypic presentation. Women appear to be more susceptible to tobacco because they have more severe disease despite lower cumulative tobacco consumption, earlier onset of COPD, and faster decline in lung function.[480,484] Female sex hormones may increase metabolism of CS to generate oxidative stress and thus may contribute to greater airway injury[485]; however, postmenopausal women may have faster rates of lung function decline.[486] The role of estrogen and progesterone is unclear, and hormone replacement therapy has not been consistently associated with COPD risk.[487] Further, in terms of phenotypic presentation, women with COPD suffer disproportionately from higher levels of anxiety, depression, and worse dyspnea and symptom-related quality of life for the same degree of lung function impairment.[488] Yet, they may report lower prevalence of other symptoms, such as cough and sputum production. There are differences between the sexes in prevalence of related comorbidities that can affect health outcomes, including higher rates of chronic heart failure and osteoporosis in women but lower rates of ischemic heart disease and alcoholism.[488,489] Gender-linked disparities are also seen in patient perceptions, expectations of the health care system, and access to health care.[489] These differences suggest that varying approaches to individual treatment may be necessary to optimize care. Given the growing burden of COPD among women, understanding sex differences in disease diagnosis, presentation, and management is increasingly important.

AAT DEFICIENCY

AAT, a serine protease inhibitor (serpin) derived principally from hepatocytes, is the most prevalent anti-protease in peripheral blood. Normal AAT serum concentrations are 120 to 200 mg/dL. AAT concentrations are higher in children and, as an acute phase reactant, increase during infection and pregnancy. Although originally named for its ability to block trypsin activity in vitro, AAT provides 95% of the inhibition of NE. AAT binds NE in equimolar concentrations and inactivates it. Importantly, CS damages AAT by converting the active site Met[358] to methionine sulfoxide, reducing its association constant for NE 2000-fold.[490] AAT also blocks the neutrophil enzymes cathepsin G, proteinase 3 (as does alpha-2 macroglobulin but not secretory leukoprotease inhibitor), mast cell–derived tryptase and chymase,[491] and possibly other proteases.[491] AAT does not inhibit MMPs, except ADAM-17,[492] although it blocks Mø release of MMP-12 in response to CS.[493] Conversely, MMPs can degrade AAT, leading to a neutrophil chemoattractant moiety.[494]

The most common form of AATD causing lung disease in adults results from homozygous expression of the Z allele (PI*ZZ). The AAT in PI*ZZ individuals forms an insoluble protein whose egress from hepatocytes is reduced by 85%, has slower kinetics of NE inactivation,[490] and tends to polymerize, producing a proinflammatory molecule.[495,496] Serum AAT concentration in PI*ZZ individuals is typically less than 50 mg/dL (11 μM). Prevalence of PI*ZZ AATD is estimated at 1:2500 to 1:5000 individuals in North America and Europe.[497,498] Worldwide, heterozygosity of the S allele, an E264V mutation that also produces a misfolded protein, with the Z allele is even more common.[499] The overwhelming majority (estimated up to 95%) of those with AATD are undiagnosed. Unexpectedly, some individuals with PI*ZZ AATD can have normal lung function throughout their lives, even despite significant smoking.[500,501]

Multiple groups, including the World Health Organization, recommend testing for AATD in all patients with COPD or unexplained bronchiectasis, regardless of race, ethnicity, or age.[502] Those with confirmed concentrations at or below the low normal range should undergo genotyping for at least the Z and S alleles.[502] Augmentation therapy significantly slows the rate of decline in lung density in PI*ZZ cases as assessed by quantitative CT scanning, a surrogate measure for emphysema progression.[503] Augmentation therapy is not currently recommended for PI*ZZ individuals who continue to smoke.[502]

AATD is classically associated with early development of PLE with lower lobe predominance, but some individuals exhibit upper zone predominance.[504] Other pulmonary manifestations of AATD are chronic productive cough (in 40%), bronchiectasis (in 27%), asthma (in 35%), and partial reversibility of airway obstruction (in 61%).[505-507] AATD is associated with more frequent and more lethal anti–proteinase 3 vasculitis, hypothyroidism, and inflammatory bowel disease, particularly ulcerative colitis.[508] AATD is also associated with liver disease with manifestations that vary from cholestasis presenting in infancy and liver failure requiring transplantation in childhood to late-onset cirrhosis and hepatocellular carcinoma, which are significant causes of death in PI*ZZ never smokers older than 50 years.[509] Surprisingly, cirrhosis develops in only a minority of affected individuals, mostly men.[510]

AATD also provides insights into the pathogenesis of COPD in those without genetic deficiency due to its many immunomodulatory properties.[491,511] During inflammation, AAT is also produced by innate immune cells and has biphasic immunoregulatory properties; AAT initially induces IL-1β but later causes release of IL-1 receptor antagonist.[512,513] AAT regulates neutrophil chemotaxis in response to IL-8[492] and reduces release of neutrophil secondary and tertiary granules, both spontaneously and in response to tumor necrosis factor-α.[514] AAT shifts the balance of cytokine production from pro- to anti-inflammatory, particularly via multifactorial regulation of tumor necrosis factor-α release. AAT also favors development of T_{reg} over polarized T effector cell subsets.[491,511] Finally, AAT has antibacterial and antiviral properties.[491] Hence, immunomodulatory actions of AAT are important to all COPD patients.

PRESERVED RATIO IMPAIRED SPIROMETRY

Although current criteria for a diagnosis of COPD are based on rigid dichotomies between "normal" and "abnormal," as defined by spirometry, the distribution of lung function as plotted by FEV_1% predicted versus FEV_1/FVC ratios among ever smokers, and indeed in the general population, is a continuum that does not separate into distinct populations. A subset of ever smokers was identified in the COPDGene cohort with reduced FEV_1 but normal FEV_1/FVC; this group had greater dyspnea and radiographic abnormalities and worse exercise capacity relative to ever smokers with normal spirometry.[515,516] This subset is termed *preserved ratio impaired spirometry*

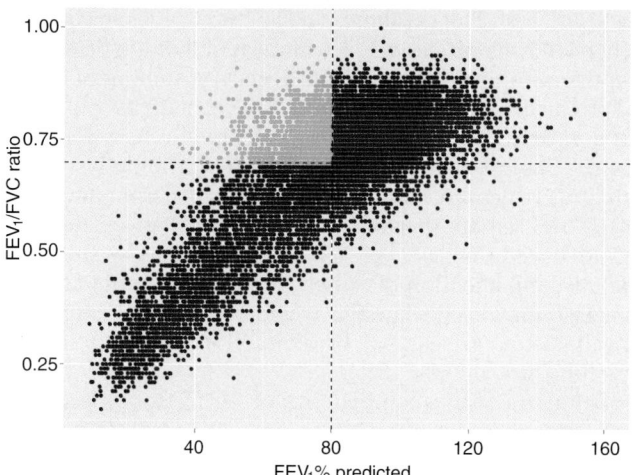

Figure 63.8 Distribution of spirometry in the Genetic Epidemiology of COPD cohort, which led to description of the *preserved ratio impaired spirometry* (PRISm) phenotype. *Forced expiratory volume in 1 second* (FEV₁) *% predicted is plotted on the x-axis while FEV₁/forced vital capacity* (FVC) *ratio is plotted on the y-axis. Dashed lines* represent fixed threshold criteria used to delineate PRISm subjects (highlighted in blue, upper left quadrant), control (upper right quadrant), and COPD (lower left quadrant) subjects. (From Wan ES, Castaldi PJ, Cho MH, et al. Epidemiology, genetics, and subtyping of preserved ratio impaired spirometry [PRISm] in COPDGene. *Respir Res.* 2014;15:89.)

(PRISm) (Fig. 63.8). Longitudinally, PRISm subjects show increased mortality, particularly due to cardiovascular causes; some develop overt COPD.[517,518]

PROGRESSION AND MORTALITY

Consistent with the observation that abnormal adult spirometry can result from failure to attain predicted lung size, and not simply from subsequent accelerated lung function decline (see Fig. 63.1), progression of COPD is variable among individuals. Both individuals with initially reduced FEV_1% predicted and those with increased lung function decline (mean loss ≥40 mL/yr, normal loss ≈20 mL/yr[486]) have the greatest risk of progression to overt COPD.[13,519] COPD resulting from biomass fuel exposure alone may have slower progression than disease resulting from tobacco smoking.[520,521] Evidence on whether the two exposures cause additive damage is conflicting.[522-524]

AE-COPD accelerates loss of lung function,[525,526] especially in those with spirometrically mild disease, but whether that is the case in ex-smokers has been questioned.[527] Interestingly, similar respiratory events did not increase the rate of spirometric decline in those without airflow obstruction or in PRISm subjects.[526] Recovery from exacerbations is variable and may be incomplete at 3 months in 7% of events.[528]

Eosinophilic COPD[351] has been suggested to be a subset of COPD patients distinct from the asthma-COPD overlap syndrome.[529] This concept arose from demonstration of eosinophilic lung inflammation in nonatopic individuals without history of asthma or marked bronchoreversibility.[347,351,352] It is supported by findings in longitudinal cohorts,[350,530] in randomized controlled trials,[348,531,532] and in the general population[533] that peripheral blood eosinophils identified patients at increased risk of exacerbations, often frequently. Such exacerbations are characterized by increased blood and sputum eosinophilia and are independent of those related to bacteria or viruses.[534–536] The most recent report of the GOLD Scientific Committee recommended measuring blood eosinophil absolute numbers (with thresholds of <100 and >300 eosinophils/μL) to aid in deciding which COPD patients should receive therapies containing inhaled corticosteroids.[537]

Due to the high burden of comorbidities associated with COPD,[400,538,539] the causes of mortality vary between individuals and are strongly affected by spirometric severity and smoking status.[540,541] Cardiovascular death and lung cancer predominate in less severe COPD stages, whereas the proportion of respiratory deaths rises considerably in advanced COPD.[542] Prognosis can vary greatly even among those with identical lung function. Relative to $FEV_1\%$ predicted alone, prediction of mortality is improved by multidimensional indices such as BODE (body mass index, airflow obstruction [$FEV_1\%$ predicted], dyspnea, and exercise capacity),[543] ADO (age, dyspnea, and airway obstruction [$FEV_1\%$ predicted]),[544] and DOSE (dyspnea, airway obstruction [$FEV_1\%$ predicted], smoking status, and exacerbation frequency),[545] although even these tools are limited.[546] pHTN of even moderate severity has a strong adverse impact on survival in COPD.[92,547–549] Prognostic indices incorporating imaging variables will likely improve future mortality predictions.[24,93]

No currently available pharmacologic intervention alters COPD progression or mortality. Lung volume reduction surgery is associated with decreased mortality in those with upper zone–predominant emphysema and low exercise capacity after pulmonary rehabilitation.[550] Supplemental oxygen reduces mortality in COPD patients with severe resting hypoxemia but not in those with only intermittent or moderate desaturation.[551–554]

Key Points

- Airflow obstruction in adults that meets the spirometric definition of COPD can result either from accelerated loss of initially normal lung function or from defective lung growth before adulthood.
- Most COPD in high-income nations results from direct cigarette smoke exposure, but workplace exposures and indoor and outdoor air pollution are also important and may be equal or greater risks worldwide.

- Clinical COPD phenotypes are heterogeneous because inhalational stressors induce four key pathologic processes: small airway disease, mucus hypersecretion, emphysema, and vascular dysfunction.
- Both mucus hypersecretion and the reduced defenses against bacterial invasion that lead to small airway disease are initiated by smoking-induced epigenetic reprogramming of airway basal progenitor cells. The subsequent progression of those two processes into phenotypic manifestations in individuals who develop COPD is highly variable for reasons that remain incompletely understood.
- Three types of emphysema are recognized histologically and are identifiable by computed tomographic scanning: centrilobular, panlobular, and paraseptal.
- COPD can be considered a disease of accelerated aging. Nine hallmarks of aging have been proposed, in the categories of damage, responses to damage, and integrative failure.
- Multiple groups, including the World Health Organization, recommend testing for alpha$_1$-antitrypsin disease in all patients with COPD or unexplained bronchiectasis, regardless of race, ethnicity, or age.[502] Those with confirmed concentrations at or below the low normal range should undergo genotyping.[502]

Key Readings

Agustí A, Hogg JC. Update on the pathogenesis of chronic obstructive pulmonary disease. *N Engl J Med.* 2019;381:1248–1256.

Barnes PJ, Baker J, Donnelly LE. Cellular senescence as a mechanism and target in chronic lung disease. *Am J Respir Crit Care Med.* 2019;200:556–564.

Celli BR, Wedzicha JA. Update on clinical aspects of chronic obstructive pulmonary disease. *N Engl J Med.* 2019;381:1257–1266.

Han MK, Agusti A, Calverley PM, et al. Chronic obstructive pulmonary disease phenotypes: the future of COPD. *Am J Respir Crit Care Med.* 2010;182:598–604.

Martinez FJ, Han MK, Allinson JP, et al. At the root: defining and halting progression of early chronic obstructive pulmonary disease. *Am J Respir Crit Care Med.* 2018;197:1540–1551.

Whitsett JA, Alenghat T. Respiratory epithelial cells orchestrate pulmonary innate immunity. *Nat Immunol.* 2015;16:27–35.

Complete reference list available at ExpertConsult.com.

64 COPD: DIAGNOSIS AND MANAGEMENT

MEILAN K. HAN, MD, MS • STEPHEN C. LAZARUS, MD, FCCP, FERS

INTRODUCTION AND HISTORY

Chronic obstructive pulmonary disease (COPD), as it is currently defined, is a spectrum of lung abnormalities characterized physiologically by persistent airflow obstruction. The histologic abnormalities seen most commonly are lung tissue destruction, or emphysema, and airway disease, recognized clinically as chronic bronchitis. From a historical perspective, emphysema was recognized first. Dating back to the 17th and 18th centuries, clinicians recognized what were termed abnormally "voluminous" lungs.[1] In 1789 Baillie published a series of illustrations demonstrating the classic pathologic features of emphysema. A bit later chronic bronchitis was described, best documented by the clinician, pathologist, and inventor of the stethoscope, Laennec. In his 1821 "A Treatise on the Diseases of the Chest," Laennec describes lungs that are hyperinflated and do not empty well.[2] But, upon pathologic inspection, he also noted the "bronchus of the trachea are often…filled with mucous fluid." At that time smoking was not common, and Laennec attributed the principal causes of this disease to environmental and genetic factors. However, it is important to note that Laennec identified both of the characteristic features of COPD: emphysema and chronic bronchitis.

By the 1940s, master clinicians were becoming familiar with an entity characterized by dyspnea on exertion in patients with physical signs of emphysema along with chronic bronchitis and asthma.[3] However, the ability to diagnose this entity reliably was not possible until the invention of spirometry. In 1846, John Hutchinson invented the spirometer, which was capable of measuring vital capacity, but 100 years later, it was Tiffeneau who introduced the concept of a timed vital capacity as a measure of airflow that allowed the spirometer to become a diagnostic instrument for airflow obstruction.[4] By the 1950s, clinicians recognized that specific spirometric and flow volume patterns indicated the presence of emphysema.[5] In fact, the first edition of Hinshaw and Garland's *Diseases of the Chest*, in 1956, depicted spirograms indicating airflow obstruction in emphysema.[6]

Groundwork for the modern definition of COPD was established at two major scientific conferences, the CIBA Guest Symposium[7] in 1959 and the *American Thoracic Society* (ATS) Committee on Diagnostic Standards[8] in 1962. The ATS committee defined chronic bronchitis clinically as chronic productive cough lasting at least 3 months, with bouts recurring over at least 2 years; emphysema was defined histologically as enlarged alveolar spaces; asthma was defined as airway hyperresponsiveness.[9] It was then that Dr. William Briscoe, at the ninth Aspen Emphysema Conference in 1965, first introduced the term COPD. Several years later Drs. Charles Fletcher and Richard Peto provided support for the link between smoking and the development of COPD in their 1976 landmark book documenting that continued smoking accelerates the loss of lung function, a process ameliorated by smoking cessation.[10]

The modern definition of COPD, as put forth by the ATS and *European Respiratory Society* (ERS), describes it as "a preventable and treatable disease state characterized by airflow limitation that is not fully reversible. The airflow

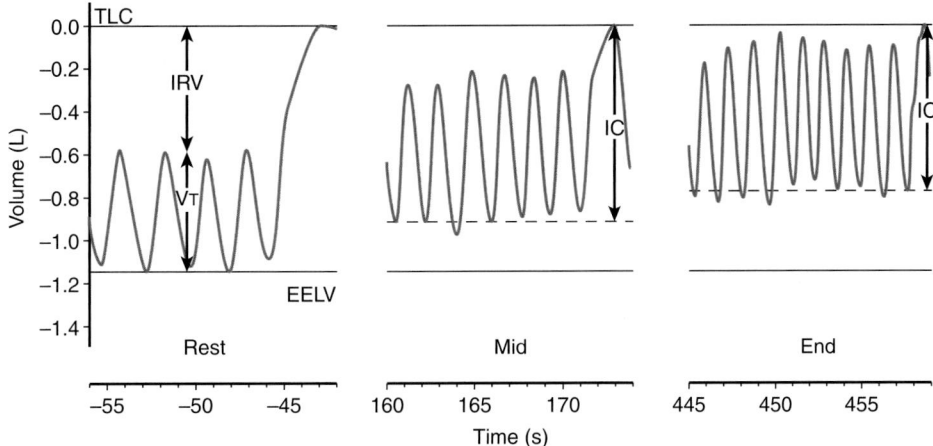

Figure 64.1 Dynamic hyperinflation. Volume tracing from a patient with severe COPD who demonstrated ventilatory-dependent dynamic hyperinflation. Inspiratory capacity (IC) decreases and end-expiratory lung volume (EELV) increases as ventilation increases during exercise. IRV, inspiratory reserve volume; TLC, total lung capacity; VT, tidal volume. (From Dolmage TE, Evans RA, Goldstein RS. Defining hyperinflation as "dynamic": moving toward the slope. *Respir Med.* 2013;107[7]:953–958.)

limitation is usually progressive and is associated with an abnormal inflammatory response of the lungs to noxious particles or gases, primarily caused by cigarette smoking. Although COPD affects the lungs, it also produces significant systemic consequences."[9] Although this definition describes a physiologic abnormality associated with exposure to noxious stimuli, the challenge that remains for both clinician and researcher is understanding the significant heterogeneity in disease presentation and progression that still exists within this umbrella definition.

CLINICAL FEATURES

SYMPTOMS

Individuals with early COPD are often asymptomatic. However, as the disease progresses, dyspnea, cough, and sputum production typically become more prominent. Any of these features should trigger an evaluation including spirometry both for diagnosis, if not already established, and for disease staging. Early in the disease course, dyspnea may be experienced only with exertion, and patients may attribute these symptoms to other factors and not seek treatment. Patients may also modify their activities to avoid dyspnea, and so the progression of pulmonary limitation may therefore be rather insidious. In fact, patients' activity may be severely limited even when they believe their disease process is still mild.[11] Eventually, however, as the disease progresses, dyspnea may ultimately be present with activities of daily living. Whereas the mechanism for dyspnea in COPD is likely multifactorial, exercise-induced air trapping, otherwise known as "dynamic hyperinflation," likely plays a significant role (Fig. 64.1).

As with dyspnea, cough may be attributed to other factors, such as smoking, and therefore patients may not complain about this symptom unless prompted. In general, sputum production is more common in current smokers, although, paradoxically, it may increase transiently after smoking cessation.[12] Although the presence of cough and sputum production in COPD is often more variable than the presence of dyspnea, it can significantly impact quality of life.[11]

Sputum, when present, tends to be mucoid, clear to white in appearance, and more purulent with exacerbations. Chronic bronchitis is also clinically significant because it is associated with more frequent exacerbations[13] and has specific therapeutic implications (see "Treatment").[14,15] Excessive sputum production (>2–3 tablespoons daily) may indicate the presence of bronchiectasis, which has been reported to range in prevalence from 29–52% in moderate to severe COPD and has been associated with increased mortality.[16] Hemoptysis may be seen with both chronic bronchitis and bronchiectasis, particularly during COPD exacerbations. However, the presence of hemoptysis in a patient with COPD should raise concern for other possible causes, including lung cancer, given the increased risk for lung cancer in this patient population.[17]

Several instruments have been developed to assess health status in COPD, most notably the *St. George's Respiratory Questionnaire*[18] (SGRQ) and the *COPD Assessment Test*[19] (CAT) (eFig. 64.1). Both are multidimensional instruments encompassing symptoms such as dyspnea, cough, and sputum production, as well as activity limitation. Both the SGRQ and CAT demonstrate rough but imperfect correlations with *forced expiratory volume in 1 second* (FEV_1) but, more important, demonstrate changes after interventions[20,21] and with exacerbations.[22,23] Although the SGRQ is longer and used primarily in the research setting, the CAT consists of only eight questions and is practical for use within the clinical setting. The *Modified Medical Research Council* (mMRC) scale is a 5-point dyspnea scale[24] that, although not developed specifically for COPD, is relevant because the measure is associated with mortality in COPD, either when used alone[25] or when used as part of the BODE (body mass index, obstruction, dyspnea, exercise capacity) composite index[26] (Tables 64.1 and 64.2).

PHYSICAL EXAMINATION

Early in the course of the disease, no specific abnormalities may be noted on physical examination. Wheezing may or may not be present and does not necessarily relate to the severity of airflow obstruction. Prolonged expiratory time

Table 64.1   The BODE Index: Four Variables Predictive of Survival in Patients with COPD

Variable	POINTS ON THE BODE INDEX			
	0	1	2	3
B: Body mass index (kg/m^2)*	>21	≤21	—	—
O: FEV$_1$ (% of predicted)†	≥65	50–64	36–49	≤35
D: Distance walked in 6 min (m)	≥350	250–349	150–249	≤149
E: mMRC dyspnea scale (score)	0–1	2	3	4

Values (0-3) are assigned to each variable and summed, providing a score from 0 to 10.
*Values for body mass index are 0 or 1 owing to the inflection point in the inverse relationship between survival and body mass index at a value of 21 kg/m^2.
†FEV$_1$ categories are based upon stages identified by the American Thoracic Society.
FEV$_1$, forced expiratory volume in 1 second; mMRC, modified Medical Research Council.
From Celli B, Goldstein R, Jardim J, Knobil K. Future perspectives in COPD. *Respir Med.* 2005;99:S41–S48.

is a more consistent finding in COPD, particularly as the disease progresses. A forced expiratory time of more than 6 seconds corresponds to an FEV$_1$/*forced vital capacity* (FVC) ratio of less than 50–60%.[27,28] In very severe disease, patients develop physical signs indicative of hyperinflation, including a barrel-shaped chest, decreased breath sounds, distant heart sounds, and increased resonance to percussion. Patients may breathe in a "tripod" position in which the individual leans forward and supports his or her upper body with extended arms. This maneuver takes advantage of the accessory muscles of the neck and upper chest to increase air movement. Patients with severe disease may also use pursed-lip breathing, which involves exhaling through tightly pressed, pursed lips. This technique creates back-pressure and is thought to reduce dynamic hyperinflation, although it may also work by reducing bronchoconstriction via neurally mediated mechanisms.[29]

In patients with severe disease, other systemic manifestations may include signs of right-sided heart failure, leading to lower extremity edema. An accentuated pulmonic component of the second heart sound (P2) may also be appreciated. Tar stains on the fingers from cigarette smoking may be present. Clubbing is not a typical feature of COPD, even when hypoxemia is present, and should suggest evaluation for other comorbidities, including lung cancer.

Two commonly recognized COPD subtypes are the "pink puffers" and "blue bloaters." Pink puffers, typically associated with significant emphysema, compensate by hyperventilation and often manifest muscle wasting and weight loss. Compared with blue bloaters, pink puffers are less hypoxemic and therefore appear "pink." Blue bloaters typically have chronic bronchitis and tend to have decreased ventilation and greater ventilation-perfusion mismatch than pink puffers, leading to hypoxemia and hence cyanosis and to right heart dysfunction with edema or "bloating."

PULMONARY FUNCTION TESTING AND DIAGNOSIS

Spirometry

Pulmonary function testing (PFT) (see Chapters 31 and 32) and, in particular, spirometry is essential to establish a diagnosis of COPD. Although symptoms suggest a diagnosis, unfortunately their predictive value for a diagnosis of COPD is poor.[30] Several screening tools have been developed, including questionnaires[31] used in conjunction with peak expiratory flow.[32] Several studies suggest that, among the various risk factors, older age and smoking history are the two most important risk factors for development of COPD.[30,31,33] Spirometry can be performed in the physician's office and should be done for any patient with symptoms (e.g., cough, sputum, dyspnea) and risk factors. When performing spirometry (see Chapter 31), a subject exhales forcefully, and the FEV$_1$ is compared against the total air exhaled, which is the FVC. COPD is defined by a reduction in the FEV$_1$/FVC ratio. The degree of FEV$_1$ reduction defines the severity of airflow obstruction. The flow-volume loop in COPD typically has a concave appearance that may be apparent before the FEV$_1$ and FEV$_1$/FVC ratio decrease significantly, and the volume-time curve demonstrates a prolonged expiratory time (Fig. 64.2).

The ATS and the *Global Initiative for Chronic Obstructive Lung Disease* (GOLD) recommend that postbronchodilator values be used to help distinguish COPD from asthma. GOLD recommends an FEV$_1$/FVC less than 0.70 as the threshold for presence of airflow obstruction.[34] Rather than using the fixed ratio, the ATS/ERS recommends using the fifth percentile for the lower limit of normal.[9] In general, the fixed ratio approach leads to overdiagnosis in older subjects because the FEV$_1$/FVC ratio declines with age, even in healthy individuals.[35] However, the fixed ratio approach carries the advantage of simplicity.

Although COPD severity has typically been graded based on FEV$_1$% predicted, which is part of the GOLD (see Fig. 64.7) and ATS/ERS recommendations, updates to the GOLD[34] recommendations now incorporate symptoms and exacerbation history as part of disease staging. Two or more exacerbations in the prior year or one severe (hospitalized) exacerbation are the thresholds used by GOLD to identify individuals at risk for future events. Finally, it should be noted that, although airflow obstruction as quantified by spirometry is the internationally accepted definition for COPD, more recent data demonstrate the prognostic significance both of symptoms and of significant radiographic abnormality among at-risk smokers who do not meet spirometric criteria for airflow obstruction.[36] However, for this population at the moment, there is no evidence to support specific management strategies other than smoking cessation, although at least one *National Heart, Lung, and Blood Institute* (NHLBI)-supported study is currently underway.[37]

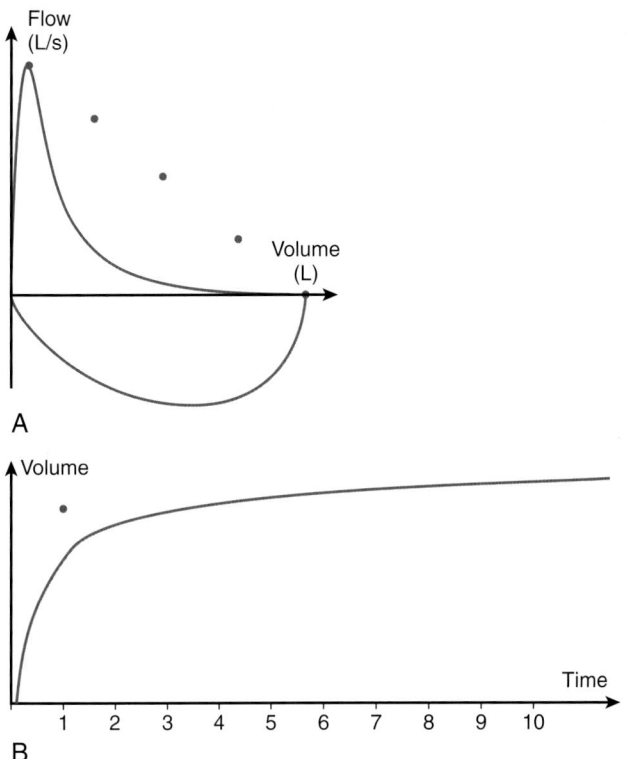

Figure 64.2 Flow volume loop in COPD. (A) The tracing shows a concave flow volume loop with reduction of flow at all lung volumes. The *dots* indicate the expected flow at various lung volumes. (B) The volume-time curve shows a prolonged expiratory time. The *dot* demonstrates the predicted forced expiratory volume in 1 second.

Table 64.2 Estimates of Mortality Based on BODE Index

	MORTALITY RATE (%)		
BODE Index Score	12 Months	24 Months	52 Months
0–2	2	6	19
3–4	2	8	32
5–6	2	14	40
7–10	5	31	80

Index score is used to predict mortality at different times.
Data from Celli BR, Cote CG, Marin JM, et al. The body-mass index, airflow obstruction, dyspnea, and exercise capacity index in chronic obstructive pulmonary disease. *N Engl J Med.* 2004;350(10):1005–1012.

Lung Volumes

Other lung volumes, including *total lung capacity* (TLC) and *residual volume* (RV), must be measured via plethysmography, not by dilution of a test gas, because of the heterogeneity of air flow and underestimation of volumes. Such tests are typically performed in a pulmonary function laboratory. TLC is increased in COPD, particularly in the presence of emphysema, where there is significant loss of elastic recoil resulting in lung hyperinflation. Increases in RV and functional residual capacity may also be seen. RV tends to increase to a greater extent than TLC, leading to an increase in the RV/TLC ratio. Vital capacity in COPD is also typically decreased because of hyperinflation.

Diffusing Capacity

Diffusing capacity for carbon monoxide (DL_{CO}) reflects the alveolar capillary blood volume and consequently is decreased in the presence of emphysema but may also be reduced in the presence of other abnormalities that affect the alveolar capillary bed, including pulmonary fibrosis and pulmonary vascular disease. Near-normal spirometry and lung volumes in the setting of severely reduced diffusing capacity and radiographic evidence of emphysema should suggest a possible diagnosis of combined pulmonary fibrosis and emphysema syndrome.[38]

Exercise Testing

The *6-minute walk test* (6MWT) is probably the most frequently used exercise test in COPD. The distance that a patient can walk in 6 minutes is termed the *6-minute walk distance* (6MWD).[39] Measuring distance walked during a defined time period was first described in the early 1960s.[40] An advantage of the 6MWT is that it requires little training to administer and no specialized equipment. Although a 6MWT is not required to make a diagnosis of COPD, it allows the clinician to measure oxygenation during ambulation and assess the potential need for supplemental oxygen. 6MWD is also frequently used during lung transplant evaluation to gauge functional status and prognosis. 6MWD relates to mortality in COPD and is a component of the BODE mortality index (Tables 64.1 and 64.2).[26] Although there is good correlation between 6MWD and peak oxygen uptake in end-stage lung disease,[41,42] the 6MWT should be considered complementary to cardiopulmonary exercise testing (see later). Most patients do not achieve maximal exercise capacity during the 6MWT, and consequently the 6MWD may better reflect functional exercise capacity.[43] The 6MWD also correlates better with quality-of-life measures; therapeutic interventions resulting in changes in 6MWD also correlate with improvements in dyspnea.[44–46] Some form of exercise testing is typically used before and after pulmonary rehabilitation to assess improvement.

Compared to the 6MWT, *cardiopulmonary exercise testing* (CPET) can provide diagnostic information regarding specific causes for dyspnea and exercise limitation. CPET can be performed with either a treadmill or cycle ergometer.[47] A large number of parameters can be measured or derived during a CPET, including *maximal oxygen uptake* ($\dot{V}O_2$), *carbon dioxide output* ($\dot{V}CO_2$), maximal work rate, and anaerobic threshold. CPET is also a necessary part of evaluation for *lung volume reduction surgery* (LVRS), because a low work rate after pulmonary rehabilitation predicts a survival benefit from LVRS (see Chapter 33).[48]

IMAGING

Chest radiography and *computed tomography* (CT) are the two imaging modalities most commonly used in COPD. Although not required to diagnose COPD, imaging can be helpful to rule out concomitant processes. Chest radiographs are frequently obtained to investigate dyspnea or hemoptysis or to look for pneumonia, heart failure, lung cancer, or pneumothorax. Chest radiography is not particularly sensitive or specific for the diagnosis of COPD. There are certain features, however, that are often seen in COPD. Radiolucency, diaphragmatic flattening, and increased

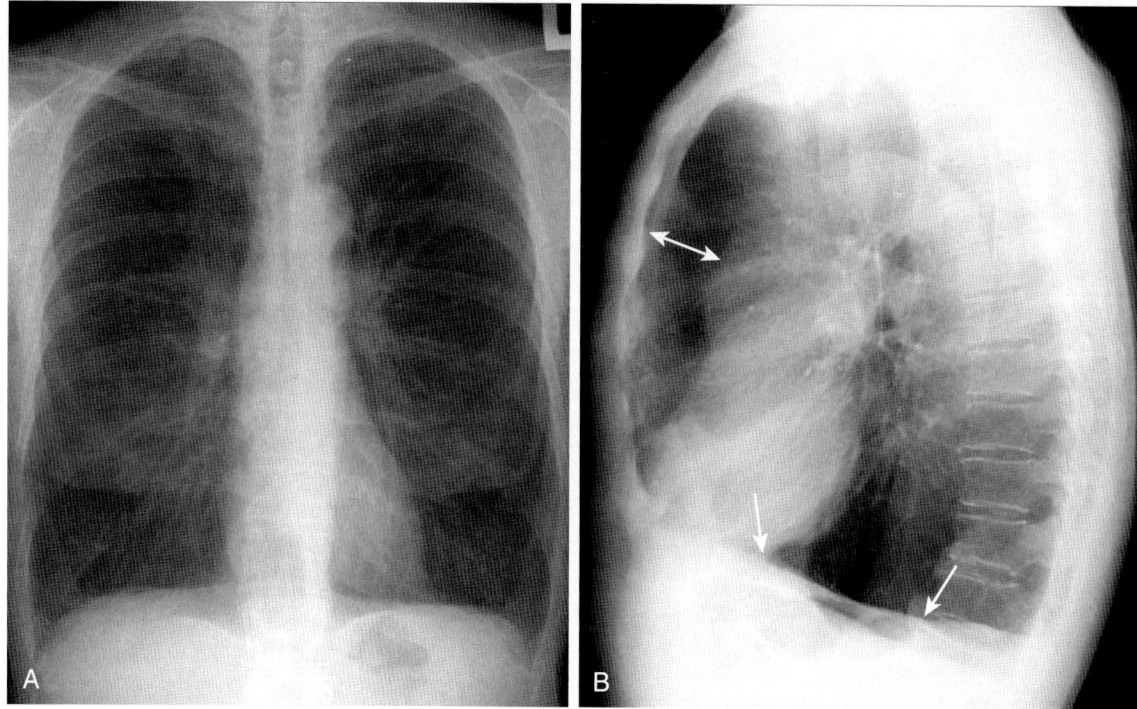

Figure 64.3 Centriacinar emphysema. Frontal (A) and lateral (B) chest radiograph in a 54-year-old female smoker with centriacinar emphysema. Note the very large lung volumes, with hyperlucency primarily seen in the upper lobes, consistent with a centriacinar emphysema pattern. Flattening of the diaphragms *(arrows)*, a prominent retrosternal clear space on the lateral radiograph *(double arrow)*, and a small-appearing heart on the frontal radiograph are findings consistent with abnormally increased lung volumes and are typical of advanced emphysema. The upper lobe lucency, typical of centriacinar emphysema, contrasts with the lower lobe predominant lucency seen in patients with panacinar emphysema. See Video 64.1 for computed tomography video of this patient.

retrosternal airspace on the lateral radiograph may be seen when hyperinflation is present (Fig. 64.3 and Video 64.1). On occasion, large bullae may manifest as radiolucent areas.

Chest CT allows better detection and quantification of emphysema than does traditional chest radiography. Areas of low attenuation are a marker of emphysema; thickened airways indicative of bronchial thickening may also be seen (Fig. 64.4). If expiratory views are obtained, areas of air trapping indicative of small airway obstruction and emphysema may also be seen. CT is not indicated in the routine diagnosis or evaluation of COPD but can be helpful when evaluating individuals with very severe COPD. CT imaging is required to quantify emphysema extent and distribution for the purposes of LVRS.[48] Individuals with very severe COPD undergoing transplant evaluation typically require a chest CT to rule out lung cancer and aid with surgical planning. CT imaging is also helpful when the clinician is concerned about a concomitant process such as interstitial lung disease, which may be suggested on PFT (see "Pulmonary Function Testing and Diagnosis"), or when hemoptysis or other unexplained changes in symptoms develop. Bronchiectasis, which may be reflected by copious sputum production and cough and has been associated with increased mortality,[16] is also best assessed on CT.

Although CT is not required for routine practice, the potential clinical importance of CT imaging is becoming better appreciated. Several studies demonstrate a strong relationship between emphysema and both lung function decline[49,50] and mortality.[51–53] Advances in CT technology allowing higher resolution at lower radiation dose, have

provided valuable information in research studies and offer potential for early diagnosis.[54] CT-defined small airway abnormality has also been associated with lung function decline and exacerbations.[55,56] Bronchial thickening as assessed by CT also appears to have a strong relationship with symptoms as measured by the SGRQ.[57]

The COPD patient population is at increased risk for lung cancer, and the mortality benefit of screening CTs in smokers has now been established in large US and European studies.[58–60] Therefore a low-dose screening CT for lung cancer in individuals age 55 to 74 years with at least a 30 pack-year smoking history, including those who quit in the preceding 15 years, may be appropriate, assuming the patient would be an eligible candidate for lung cancer treatment (see Chapters 20 and 75).

LABORATORY TESTING

Arterial Blood Gases

Arterial blood gases (ABGs) are not indicated as part of the routine evaluation for patients with mild to moderate COPD. For many patients, pulse oximetry will suffice to provide an estimate of oxygen saturation. However, ABGs can be helpful to assess hypoxemia and to provide information regarding hypercapnia, particularly in individuals with more severe disease or during an acute exacerbation. ABG abnormalities also tend to worsen during exercise[61] and sleep.[62] Early in the disease course, mild to moderate hypoxemia without hypercapnia is typically seen. Later in the disease course, hypercapnia may develop, particularly in individuals with FEV_1 less than 1 L.

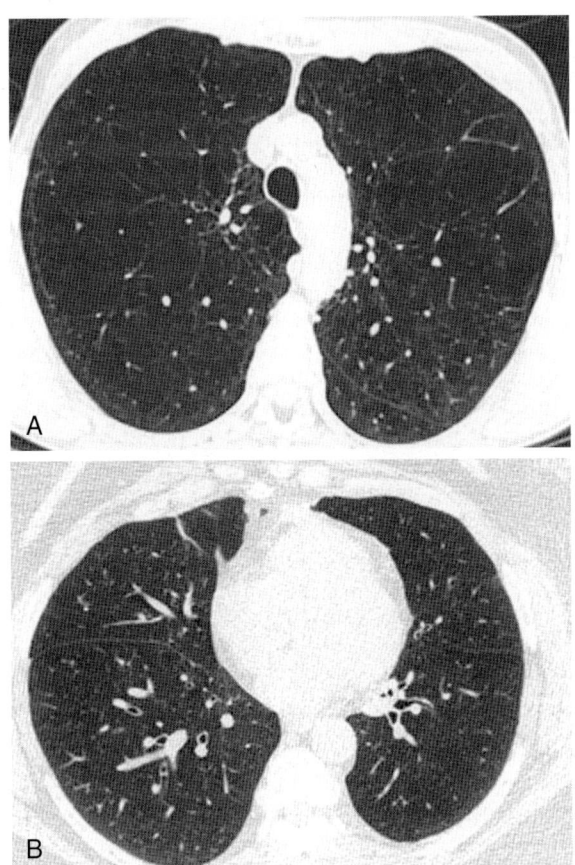

Figure 64.4 Two radiologic phenotypes of COPD. Computed tomography of two patients with COPD demonstrating the significant difference in the type of disease that may be present. Two patients with moderately severe disease are shown. (A) This patient demonstrates predominantly emphysema, whereas the second patient (B) demonstrates predominantly airway thickening. (From Han MK, Kazerooni EA, Lynch DA, et al. Chronic obstructive pulmonary disease exacerbations in the COPDGene study: associated radiologic phenotypes. *Radiology.* 2011;261:274–282.)

Erythrocytosis

Elevated hemoglobin may be seen in COPD, particularly in the presence of chronic hypoxemia. A hemoglobin value is also helpful in the evaluation of dyspnea because anemia is a common cause of dyspnea that should be excluded. In addition, DL_{CO} is most accurate when adjusted for hemoglobin.

Serum Bicarbonate

An elevated serum bicarbonate suggests chronic hypercapnia; in the setting of hypercapnia, serum bicarbonate is increased due to compensatory metabolic alkalosis (see Chapter 45).

Alpha₁-Antitrypsin Serum Levels

The ATS guidelines recommend testing for *alpha₁-antitrypsin* (A1AT) deficiency for all individuals with persistent airflow obstruction.[63] A1AT is a protease that inactivates neutrophil elastase. Clinical features suggestive of A1AT deficiency include emphysema at a young age, emphysema in an individual with minimal or no smoking history, lower lobe predominant emphysema, and a family history of emphysema. However, A1AT deficiency can also be present in patients with more typical COPD presentations. In individuals with established COPD, diagnostic testing is recommended. Concern for the diagnosis is raised based on A1AT serum levels below 11 micromol/L (≈50

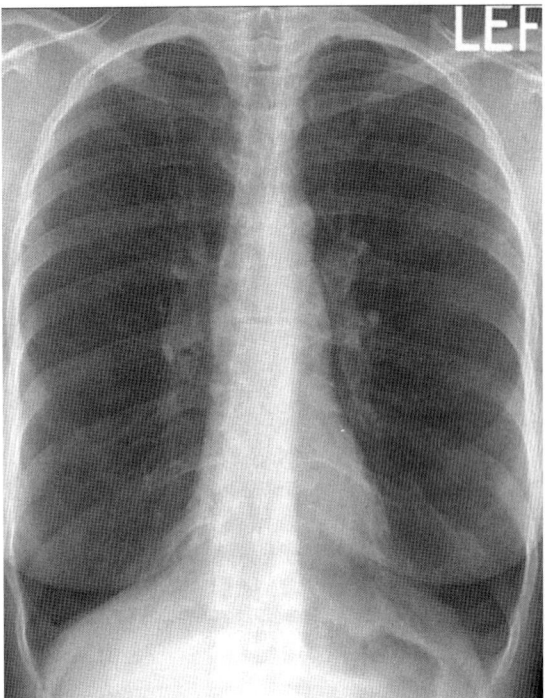

Figure 64.5 Panacinar emphysema. Frontal chest radiograph in a 51-year-old woman with alpha₁-antitrypsin deficiency presenting for lung transplant evaluation. Note the very large lung volumes with hyperlucency primarily seen in the bases, consistent with panacinar emphysema, as well as flattening of the diaphragms. Contrast the lower lobe lucency in this radiograph with Fig. 64.3, which shows upper lobe hyperlucency in a patient with centriacinar emphysema. See Video 64.2 for computed tomography video of this patient.

mg/dL using nephelometry [i.e., immunoturbidimetry] and 80 mg/dL by radial immunodiffusion) but should be confirmed with genotyping (high-risk genotypes include S, Z, and null alleles, with null as the most deficient). On occasion, the serum level and genotyping are discordant; in this situation, protein phenotype analysis via electrophoresis can identify alleles with abnormal protein migration patterns. The chest radiograph and CT show the predominantly lower lobe distribution of emphysema, consistent with a panacinar pattern (Fig. 64.5 and Video 64.2) and different from the more common centriacinar pattern (see Fig. 64.3 and Video 64.1).

Blood Eosinophils

Recent studies have demonstrated a relationship between blood eosinophil levels and response to *inhaled corticosteroids* (ICSs).[64,65] When eosinophil counts are less than 100 cells/µL, ICSs are less likely to be of benefit; in patients with blood eosinophils greater than or equal to 300 cells/µL, ICSs are more likely to reduce exacerbations.[66] Although conceptually sputum eosinophils would seem relevant in this regard and are associated with increased frequency of exacerbations,[67] because they are more difficult to collect, we do not have data from large therapeutic trials regarding the utility of sputum eosinophils to identify patients more likely to be responsive to ICSs.

Sputum

Sputum evaluation is not indicated in the routine diagnosis and care of the COPD patient. In patients with stable disease, sputum examination typically reveals a predominance of macrophages and few bacteria. During exacerbations, the number of organisms on Gram stain typically increases. The most common pathogens identified on sputum culture include *Haemophilus influenzae*, *Moraxella catarrhalis*, and *Streptococcus pneumoniae*.[68] Less frequently identified organisms include *Staphylococcus aureus*, *Pseudomonas aeruginosa*, and other gram-negative rods. However, the relationship between identification of organisms in sputum and their pathogenic contribution to acute exacerbations has been questioned because longitudinal studies have suggested that the incidence of bacterial isolation from sputum during an acute exacerbation of COPD was no different from that of the stable state,[69,70] although bacteria identified in sputum during stable COPD have been associated with a greater exacerbation frequency[71] and lung function decline.[72] In general, exacerbations typically respond to empirical treatment.

COMPLICATIONS

PNEUMOTHORAX

Pneumothoraces may develop spontaneously in patients with COPD. Depending on the degree of respiratory impairment, a pneumothorax may result in significant dyspnea and even acute respiratory failure. Pneumothoraces are treated similarly in COPD as in other conditions, although patients with severe emphysema are at increased risk for persistent air leaks, which may be difficult to treat (see also Chapter 110).

GIANT BULLAE

Emphysema may present with large bullae that can occupy a good portion of the hemithorax. Surgical treatment can be considered if compression of adjacent lung tissue is significant and surgical intervention is expected to improve pulmonary mechanics (see "Surgical Treatment of Emphysema").[60] Bullae may also become infected. An increased frequency of lung cancer has been reported in association with large bullae, seen either as a mass within the bulla or a thickening of the wall.[61,62]

PNEUMONIA

Pneumonia is not uncommon in patients with COPD and should be in the differential diagnosis for any patient with COPD presenting with increased dyspnea, cough, sputum production, and/or fever, which can make it difficult to distinguish from an acute exacerbation of COPD without a chest radiograph. Although COPD is believed to increase the risk for pneumonia, epidemiologic data are limited.[76,77] ICS, which are frequently used in the treatment of COPD because they reduce the frequency of COPD exacerbations, have been associated with an increased risk for pneumonia, particularly in older patients with COPD.[78] All patients with COPD should be immunized against *Pneumococcus*.[79]

RIGHT VENTRICULAR DYSFUNCTION

The *right ventricle* (RV) alters its structure and function due to the *pulmonary hypertension* (PH) associated with chronic lung disease (see Chapter 85). The prevalence of RV dysfunction in COPD is not known with certainty, but reported prevalence ranges from 1% to greater than 70%, depending on the patient population examined and the methodology used for defining PH.[79] When PH develops in the setting of COPD, the severity tends to be modest; severe resting PH due to COPD is relatively uncommon (see Fig. 85.2). Signs and symptoms of RV dysfunction include an increase in dyspnea, chest pain, and syncope. RV failure often presents with an increase in lower extremity edema, which should prompt further investigation. Other physical examination findings include RV heave, prominent pulmonic component to the second heart sound, tricuspid regurgitation murmur, and a right-sided S4. Electrocardiographic findings may include right axis deviation, evidence of RV hypertrophy, and right bundle-branch block (see Fig. 85.5), but overall these findings are rather insensitive for the diagnosis of PH. Echocardiography can be diagnostically helpful (see Fig. 83.3), although not infrequently, images are limited in patients with parenchymal lung disease and hyperinflation. In addition, the correlation between echocardiogram and right heart catheterization is imperfect; sensitivity tends to be better than specificity, suggesting that normal results on echocardiogram can help exclude significant RV dysfunction. Right heart catheterization remains the gold standard for diagnosis (see Fig. 83.7). PH in COPD is associated with worse outcomes, including increased risk for hospitalization[80] and worse survival.[81,82] There are few data to support the use of vasodilators for treatment of PH in COPD. Oxygen is the only therapy for PH in COPD and it improves mortality in appropriately selected patients (see Chapter 85).[83]

SLEEP DISORDERS

As many as 40% of COPD patients report sleep difficulties, such as poor sleep quality or difficulties initiating or maintaining sleep.[84] The combination of COPD and *obstructive sleep apnea* (OSA) is commonly referred to as "COPD-OSA overlap syndrome." The frequency of COPD-OSA overlap syndrome in the COPD patient population has been estimated to be approximately 16%,[85] which is roughly similar to that of the general population, although the consequences of OSA in patients with COPD are more significant. Compared to patients with OSA alone or with COPD alone, patients with COPD-OSA overlap syndrome tend to have more severe nocturnal hypercapnia, hypoxemia, and increased risk for PH.[86] OSA in COPD is also associated with poorer quality of life, frequent exacerbations, and increased mortality.[87,88] Diagnosis of OSA in COPD is important because *continuous positive airway pressure* (CPAP) therapy for patients with COPD-OSA overlap syndrome has been associated with both decreased risk of death and decreased incidence of severe exacerbations[88] (see Chapters 119 and 120).

SYSTEMIC MANIFESTATIONS AND COMORBIDITIES

Cardiovascular Disease

Ischemic cardiovascular disease is a leading cause of death in COPD.[89] Tobacco use is a shared risk factor that contributes to this association, but epidemiologic data suggest impaired lung function is an independent risk factor for increased cardiovascular mortality even when adjusted for smoking status.[90] Among those with COPD, an abnormal FEV_1 also predicts the presence of atherosclerosis[91] and cardiovascular mortality.[92,93] Patients with COPD are also at increased risk for hospitalization due to cardiovascular events.[94] Atherosclerosis is a disease of systemic inflammation,[95] which may help explain the link to COPD. Elevated C-reactive protein levels correlate not only with the presence of COPD but also with the presence of exacerbations, severity of lung function, and risk for hospitalization and death.[80] Although clinicians need to be aware of the increased risk for the presence of both disorders, no therapeutic strategies have yet been demonstrated to benefit this subgroup of patients specifically. Cardioselective β-blocker medications frequently used in patients with cardiovascular disease have traditionally raised safety concerns in patients with COPD. Indeed, a recent prospective randomized trial of 532 patients with moderate-severe exacerbation-prone COPD, but no established indication for β-blocker use, found that the risk of a COPD exacerbation was similar in the metoprolol and placebo groups but that hospitalization for exacerbation was more common in patients treated with metoprolol.[96]

Osteoporosis

A clear association between osteoporosis and COPD has been established, with studies suggesting a twofold to fivefold increase in prevalence of osteoporosis in patients with COPD compared with age-matched control subjects.[97,98] Multiple shared risk factors between COPD and osteoporosis likely influence this association, including oral and ICS use, smoking, and low body mass index. However, these factors do not completely explain the association because lower bone mineral density in patients with COPD has been documented even in the absence of systemic corticosteroids.[99] Clinicians must be mindful of this association in both their male and female patients with COPD. Pulmonary rehabilitation improves the functional status of patients with COPD and may diminish fracture risk by decreasing the risk of falls.[100]

Diabetes

Diabetes is another comorbidity with increased prevalence in COPD. Decreased lung function has been associated with the coexistence of metabolic syndrome and the development of insulin resistance and diabetes.[101–103] The cause for this association is not known with certainty. ICS may be a contributing factor. Some data suggest a dose-dependent association between ICS use and diabetes control or new-onset diabetes,[104] although a retrospective analysis of 8 COPD trials and 26 asthma trials found no association between ICS use and new-onset diabetes or hyperglycemia.[105]

Gastroesophageal Reflux Disease

The prevalence of *gastroesophageal reflux disease* (GERD) in COPD also appears to be increased.[106,107] Possible contributions to the development of GERD in COPD include respiratory medications that may lower esophageal sphincter tone and lung hyperinflation that may also compromise the antireflux barrier. More important, GERD in the setting of COPD has specific clinical implications. GERD in COPD is associated with poorer quality of life[108] and more frequent exacerbations.[107,109] GERD may also be more common in COPD patients with chronic bronchitis.[110] A clear cause for the association between GERD and COPD has not been identified. Unfortunately, only limited data suggest that treatment for GERD may reduce the risk of exacerbations.[111]

Depression and Anxiety

Coexistent depression and anxiety are prevalent in COPD,[112,113] with conservative estimates suggesting that in COPD the prevalence of anxiety ranges from 7–50%, and depression ranges from 10–57%.[114] Patients with severe COPD are among those most impacted by anxiety and depression.[115] Risk factors for depression in COPD also include limited mobility, need for supplemental oxygen therapy, comorbid conditions, and female gender.[116,117] Patients with COPD and comorbid depression and anxiety experience poorer clinical outcomes. Patients with anxiety are at increased risk for COPD exacerbations and higher mortality.[118] Depressive symptoms are also associated with increased risk of death.[119,120] Specific therapies for anxiety and depression have not been demonstrated to improve COPD outcomes, although pulmonary rehabilitation has been shown to improve not only anxiety and depression but also other outcomes in patients with COPD, including quality of life and functional capacity.[121]

DIFFERENTIAL DIAGNOSIS

Several disorders may mimic aspects of COPD, and certainly many conditions may be associated with dyspnea. However, there are a handful of disorders that are particularly challenging because they may be associated with cough, sputum production, airflow obstruction, or emphysema-like radiographic changes. Careful clinical assessment can help differentiate these disorders from COPD, although, in some instances these disorders may be present in addition to COPD.

CHRONIC OBSTRUCTIVE ASTHMA

Chronic asthma may be associated with the development of persistent airflow obstruction that is not completely reversible (i.e., due to "remodeling"). Hence a clear distinction from COPD may not be possible; chronic asthma may also coexist with COPD (asthma-COPD overlap).[122] However, several clinical features tend to be more likely associated with each of the two disorders. In general, the age of onset for asthma tends to be earlier. Asthmatic patients may have a history of atopy and a family history of asthma. Airflow obstruction abnormalities are usually less severe with asthma, with greater prevalence and magnitude of reversibility. Sputum production is less common in asthma. These patients also tend to have less of a smoking history and greater corticosteroid responsiveness than patients with COPD. Chronic asthma is also not associated with emphysema; the DL_{CO} is normal or increased in chronic asthma, whereas it is decreased in emphysema.

CHRONIC BRONCHITIS WITHOUT AIRFLOW OBSTRUCTION

Chronic cough and sputum production may be present in the absence of airflow obstruction. The accepted definition for chronic bronchitis is a productive cough lasting for 3 months, recurring over at least 2 successive years.[123] Diagnostically, this is often mistaken for COPD because chronic bronchitis, even in the absence of airflow obstruction, is often associated with smoking. Chronic exposure to poor air quality or industrial dusts/fumes also increase risk for this disorder. Although no specific therapies have been developed for chronic bronchitis without airflow obstruction, the morbidity and mortality associated with this disorder should not be ignored. Such patients still experience poorer quality of life and increased risk of death as opposed to healthy control subjects.[124–126] On a related note, the *Subpopulations and Intermediate Outcomes in COPD Study* (SPIROMICS) identified at-risk smokers with respiratory symptoms as defined by CAT score greater than or equal to 10 and with normal spirometry, and it demonstrated that these patients had increased frequency of exacerbations and thickened airway walls as measured by CT imaging.[127] Further analyses of sputum demonstrated increased mucin concentrations even among non-obstructed patients with either chronic bronchitis symptoms or elevated CAT scores.[128] It is not known with certainty which of these patients will ultimately develop airflow obstruction, although evidence suggests that the presence of chronic bronchitis is a risk factor for more rapid lung function decline.[129] Whether or not these patients ultimately develop spirometric airflow obstruction, their symptoms and morbidity suggest the need for specific therapies.

BRONCHIECTASIS

Bronchiectasis is characterized by dyspnea and, in particular, copious mucopurulent sputum that tends to be greater than in typical COPD. The diagnosis can be established with the aid of high-resolution CT scan wherein bronchial wall thickening and luminal dilation is seen. Bronchiectasis in COPD is associated with increased mortality.[16] Whereas mild bronchiectasis is commonly seen in both COPD and asthma, moderate to severe bronchiectasis should raise a clinician's concern for immunodeficiency, cystic fibrosis, rheumatic disorders, ciliary motility disorders, alpha$_1$-antitrypsin deficiency, allergic bronchopulmonary aspergillosis, mycobacterial infection, and recurrent aspiration. (See Chapter 69.)

BRONCHIOLITIS OBLITERANS

Bronchiolitis obliterans (BO) is also known as constrictive bronchiolitis. This disorder is characterized by submucosal fibrosis, resulting in narrowing of the bronchiolar lumen. BO is a known complication of lung, heart, and bone marrow transplants but also may be seen in association with connective tissue diseases and inflammatory bowel disease. Inhalation of dusts or toxins, infection, and drug reactions are less frequent causes of BO. In some cases no clear etiology is identified. As opposed to those with COPD, patients with BO may have no significant smoking history and typically do not have significant emphysema on CT, which may show only hyperinflation and air trapping. Mosaic attenuation indicative of localized air trapping is common. Bronchial wall thickening may also be present. PFT demonstrates severe, progressive, and irreversible airflow obstruction but is not typically associated with severe $D_{L_{CO}}$ impairment. Unfortunately, BO responds poorly to therapy. (See Chapter 72.)

DIFFUSE PANBRONCHIOLITIS

Diffuse panbronchiolitis is a rare form of bronchiolitis involving the upper and lower respiratory tracts seen primarily in Japan and only rarely outside the Far East.[130,131] Genetic factors, specifically human leukocyte antigen haplotypes, are thought to contribute to the pathogenesis and geographic distribution of this disease. Such patients typically present with chronic sinusitis, cough productive of copious sputum, dyspnea, wheezing, and weight loss. Airflow obstruction is a common feature, and high resolution CT may show diffusely thickened and dilated bronchi or tree-in-bud opacities corresponding to bronchiolitis. Confirming this diagnosis is important because diffuse panbronchiolitis often improves with macrolide antibiotics.

LYMPHANGIOLEIOMYOMATOSIS

Lymphangioleiomyomatosis is a rare disorder affecting women almost exclusively.[132] It is caused by a mutation in the tuberous sclerosis-1 or sclerosis-2 gene, either sporadically or in the setting of tuberous sclerosis, resulting in the proliferation of interstitial smooth muscle cells and pulmonary cyst formation. Other clinical characteristics include renal angiomyolipomas and chylous effusions. Lymphangioleiomyomatosis is also characterized by airflow obstruction and spontaneous pneumothoraces. Therefore it is not infrequently mistaken for emphysema. However, an expert radiologist should be able to distinguish pulmonary cystic changes from emphysematous holes. The presence of other characteristic clinical features can be helpful in the diagnosis. (See Chapter 97.)

TREATMENT

Until recently, treatment of COPD was focused entirely on relief of symptoms because treatment options were few and were believed to be largely ineffective. In fact, the literature reported that the only interventions that changed the natural history of COPD were smoking cessation[133,134] and oxygen in patients with hypoxemia.[135,136] More recently, however, clinical trials have demonstrated that pharmacologic treatments can prevent or attenuate acute exacerbations of COPD, and the data suggest that some can slow the inexorable loss of lung function over time, which is the hallmark of COPD.[137–139] These observations have appropriately shifted the focus to a more proactive approach, aiming to identify patients earlier in the course of their disease and to implement treatment regimens that would not only relieve symptoms but also prevent exacerbations, prevent disease progression, improve exercise tolerance, and improve quality of life.

GENERAL PRINCIPLES OF TREATMENT

Goals of treatment of COPD are to *reduce risk* by preventing and treating exacerbations, preventing disease progression, and reducing mortality; to *reduce symptoms*, which include relief of dyspnea, improved exercise tolerance, and improved health status; and, at the same time, to *minimize the adverse effects* of medications.

Reduction of Risk Factors

In the case of COPD, risk reduction refers to interventions that may decrease the likelihood of developing the disease, slow disease progression, decrease exacerbations, and reduce mortality. Although our knowledge of the factors that contribute to each of these is limited, there are substantial data on some factors that contribute to each of these.

Smoking Cessation. Throughout the developed world, cigarette smoking is the most important risk factor for the development of COPD. Public health and educational programs aimed at discouraging people from smoking ("primary prevention") and efforts to help active smokers stop are probably the most important interventions for COPD. In their landmark publication in 1977,[134] Fletcher and Peto showed that, in patients with COPD who stopped smoking, the accelerated loss of lung function slowed until it more closely paralleled the annual decrement seen in nonsmokers (Fig. 64.6). Nearly 2 decades later, the National Institutes of Health–sponsored Lung Health Study demonstrated that, in smokers with COPD, smoking cessation reduced the rate of decline in lung function, whereas inhaled bronchodilator therapy did not.[133] In a 14.5-year follow-up to the Lung Health Study, Anthonisen and colleagues[140,141] reported that the lung-function benefit continued for persistent quitters; there was also a mortality (all-cause) benefit for those who maintained abstinence. Perhaps more important, even those whose smoking cessation was intermittent experienced a benefit compared with continued smokers. Smoking cessation education and support should be offered to every patient with COPD at every visit. (For more details on smoking hazards and cessation, see Chapters 65 and 66).

Biomass Fuel. In the developing world, cigarette smoke is less of an issue than is exposure to smoke from biomass fuel, used for cooking and heating. The exposure is particularly great for women and their young children, who may spend the greater part of each day indoors with an unvented fire, fueled by wood, dung, or kerosene. Such exposure has been associated with chronic bronchitis and COPD.[142–145] Guarnieri and colleagues[146] showed that something as simple as a vented stove can decrease gene expression for markers of inflammation in sputum. (For more information, see Chapter 102.)

Environmental Controls. In addition to active and secondary smoke exposure, allergens and air pollutants may have an impact on COPD. Catastrophic air pollution events in the Meuse Valley, Belgium; Donora, Pennsylvania; and London, England[147–149] speak to the potential for air quality

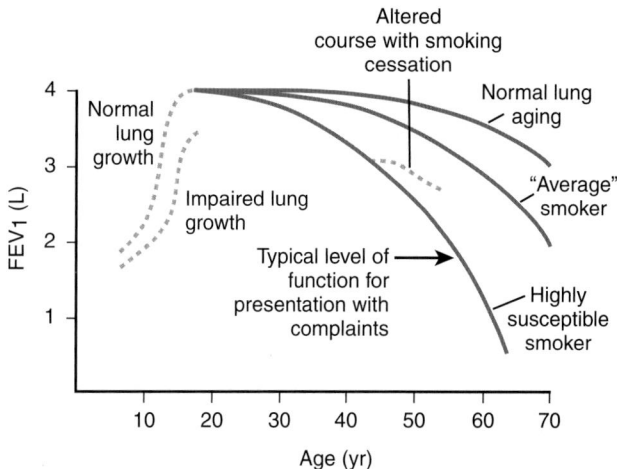

Figure 64.6 Fletcher-Peto curve of the natural history of COPD. Lung function increases with growth in childhood and adolescence. Fetal and childhood events can affect lung growth and development, resulting in reduced maximally attained lung function, for convenience shown here as a forced expiratory volume in 1 second (FEV_1) of 4 L. Actual predicted values depend on height and gender. After growth is completed, lung function remains constant for some time, the "plateau phase," after which lung function declines at an accelerating rate with age. Smoking reduces the duration of the plateau phase and accelerates the rate of lung function loss. Smoking cessation early in the course of the disease can reduce the rate of lung function loss to that of a nonsmoker. Patients typically present with symptoms when lung function declines below 50% of that in young adulthood but may have limitation much earlier.

to impact people with lung disease. In addition, a growing body of evidence suggests that long-term exposure to even low levels of air pollution increases the risk for COPD.[150] Also, people with COPD who also have allergic disease have higher levels of respiratory symptoms and are at higher risk for COPD exacerbations.[151] As a consequence, people with COPD should avoid noxious exposures, heed air quality warnings, and be cautious of ongoing occupational exposures.

Prevention of Respiratory Infections. A significant proportion of COPD exacerbations are triggered by respiratory infections. Although there are data to suggest that patients with COPD are more susceptible to respiratory infections because of impaired mucociliary clearance, a more important issue is that those with COPD are more susceptible to the *consequences* of respiratory tract infections. As a general rule, every patient with COPD should be immunized annually against influenza, which is effective at reducing the incidence of influenza, regardless of the severity of COPD,[152] and has been demonstrated to reduce mortality in older adults.[153,154] In addition, all should be vaccinated against *S. pneumoniae*. Despite a belief that older patients with COPD might not respond well to immunization, pneumococcal vaccines have been shown to be effective in this population.[155,156] Chronic antibiotics for prophylaxis are not a part of standard care for COPD because early trials showed they were not useful.[157–160] However, more recent trials with erythromycin and moxifloxacin have demonstrated a reduction in exacerbations.[161,162] There has been a particular interest in macrolide antibiotics because of their demonstrated value in diffuse panbronchiolitis and in cystic fibrosis and because they may have anti-inflammatory and antimicrobial properties. In a prospective, randomized, double-blind trial of 1142 patients with exacerbation-prone COPD, the NHLBI's COPD Clinical Research Network found that daily azithromycin for 1 year decreased the frequency of exacerbations by 27% and improved quality of life.[163] Enthusiasm for this approach has been tempered by the small risk of ototoxicity and by the potential for QTc prolongation by macrolides. Data suggest that screening subjects for history of cardiac disease and obtaining electrocardiograms before starting macrolides virtually eliminates the risk of cardiac rhythm disturbance.[164] Thus, in selected patients who neither have cardiac disease nor take concomitant medications that affect the QTc interval, and who experience frequent exacerbations with the attendant morbidity and mortality, the use of azithromycin is probably warranted.

Prevention of Exacerbations. Exacerbations of COPD are sentinel events and are closely associated with disease progression. Increasing severity of COPD is associated with increased exacerbations and need for hospitalization, but, for every stage of severity, severe exacerbations are associated with increases in short-term and long-term all-cause mortality.[165] Exacerbations are independently associated with prognosis, and mortality increases with the frequency of hospitalizations. In one study of 305 men with COPD, only 20–30% of patients who were readmitted for exacerbation after an initial hospitalized exacerbation survived 5 years.[166] Although supporting data are lacking, the hope is that, by preventing exacerbations, lung function may be preserved and deterioration prevented. ICSs, long-acting β-agonists, long-acting muscarinic antagonists, and macrolide antibiotics have all been shown to reduce exacerbations. Unfortunately, even patients taking these medications may still experience as many as 1.4 exacerbations per year.[167]

PHARMACOTHERAPY

The goals of treatment include dyspnea relief and exacerbation prevention with the aim to preserve functional status and quality of life. Most medications for COPD are administered by inhalation. Standard therapy consists of inhaled bronchodilators, either β-agonists or muscarinic antagonists (antimuscarinics or anticholinergics), and inhaled corticosteroids. The latter have been demonstrated to be most effective in patients at increased risk for exacerbations and who demonstrate increased peripheral blood eosinophils. Oral agents include phosphodiesterase-4 inhibitors (e.g., roflumilast) and, less commonly, methylxanthines (e.g., theophylline).

The choice of medications should be based on an assessment of the severity of airflow obstruction, symptoms, frequency and severity of exacerbations, the patient's functional limitation, and the availability and local cost of medications. Formerly, medication decisions were based primarily on severity of airflow obstruction; guidelines now, as exemplified by GOLD,[34] emphasize a metric that includes obstruction (GOLD grade), based on the FEV$_1$% predicted; symptoms, based on either the mMRC dyspnea scale[168] or the CAT[19]; and risk of exacerbations, based on

events documented in the prior year as a marker of future risk. Using this tool, patients can be categorized into class A, B, C, or D (Fig. 64.7), and GOLD provides specific treatment recommendations for each category at initial diagnosis (Table 64.3). Patients' level of symptoms and exacerbations should be further reviewed periodically and medications adjusted as outlined in Figure 64.8.

Bronchodilators

Bronchodilators are recommended for all patients with COPD. Pharmaceutical classes of bronchodilators include β-agonists, muscarinic antagonists (antimuscarinics or anticholinergics), and methylxanthines. Unlike asthma, where bronchodilator reversibility is part of the definition, airflow obstruction in COPD is often thought of as "irreversible." This is not, however, completely true. Although the diagnosis of COPD requires airflow obstruction that persists after bronchodilators, most patients with COPD demonstrate some improvement in spirometry. This response can vary from day to day.[169] In one study of 1552 patients with COPD who were tested with albuterol, ipratropium, or the combination on four occasions over 3 months, only 37–56% had 15% or better improvement in FEV$_1$ on all four test dates, but 90% or more had greater than or equal to 15% reversal on at least one occasion.[170] Therefore even patients who do not respond to bronchodilator testing in the pulmonary function laboratory should be given a clinical trial of bronchodilators. Although the increase in FEV$_1$ may be modest, it may be sufficient to improve lung emptying and, by this mechanism, reduce dynamic hyperinflation.[171–173] In multiple studies, bronchodilators have been shown to reduce dyspnea and increase exercise tolerance in patients with chronic stable COPD.[174,175]

β-Adrenergic Agonists

These medications bind directly to β-receptors located on airway smooth muscle and dilate the airway. Less prominent effects include increased ciliary beat frequency that promotes mucus transport along the mucociliary escalator[176] and improved respiratory muscle endurance.[177] β-Agonists are available in both short-acting and long-acting preparations and can be administered by inhalation, orally, subcutaneously, or intravenously. For treatment of COPD, β-agonists should only be given by inhalation because the other routes are associated with an unacceptably high risk of systemic adverse effects.

Short-acting β-agonists (SABAs) include albuterol (salbutamol), levalbuterol, terbutaline, and fenoterol. Albuterol is a racemic mixture of both (R)- and (S)-enantiomers of albuterol; levalbuterol is the (R)-enantiomer alone. The (R)-enantiomer is thought to be responsible for bronchodilation, whereas the (S)-enantiomer is believed to cause tremor, tachycardia, and perhaps airway inflammation. Thus levalbuterol would be expected to be better tolerated than albuterol. In fact, for most patients with stable COPD who use their SABA for symptom management, the added advantage of levalbuterol over albuterol[178] is probably not significant.[179] Albuterol is also available in combination with ipratropium (a muscarinic antagonist). Terbutaline inhalers are no longer sold in the United States; fenoterol is available in many parts of the world but not in the United States.

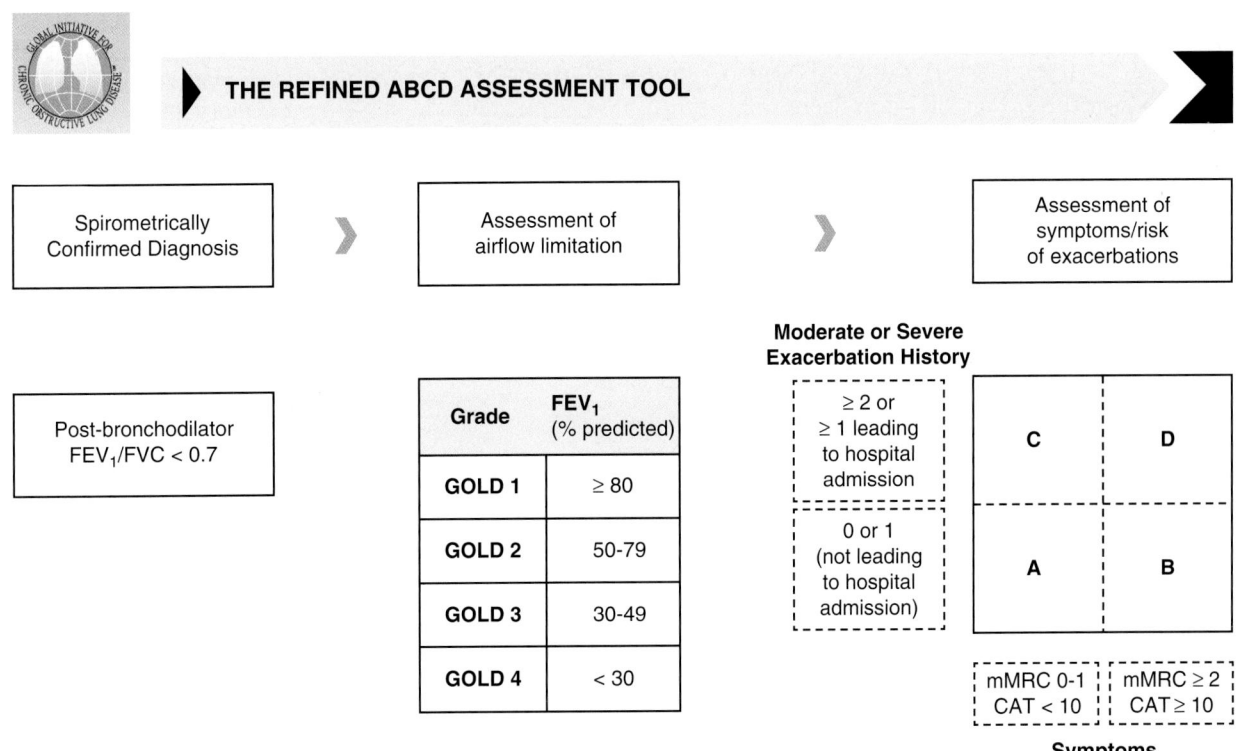

THE REFINED ABCD ASSESSMENT TOOL

Figure 64.7 *Global Initiative for Chronic Obstructive Lung Disease* **(GOLD) classification system.**[34] When assessing risk, two or more moderate exacerbations or one severe (hospitalized) exacerbation history places patients into the high-risk category. When assessing symptoms, Modified Medical Research Council (mMRC) dyspnea scale score of 2 or greater or COPD Assessment Test Score of 10 or greater places patients into the "high symptoms" category. CAT, COPD Assessment Test; FEV_1, forced expiratory volume in 1 second; FVC, forced vital capacity. (From Global Initiative for Chronic Obstructive Lung Disease. Global Strategy for the Diagnosis, Management, and Prevention of Chronic Obstructive Pulmonary Disease, 2019. http://www.goldcopd.org/.)

Table 64.3 Initial Pharmacologic Management of COPD

Patient Group	Initial Pharmacologic Treatment
A	Bronchodilator
B	Long-acting bronchodilator (LAMA *or* LABA)
C	LAMA
D	LAMA *or* LAMA + LABA* *or* ICS + LABA†

*Consider if highly symptomatic (e.g., CAT ≥ 20).
†Consider if eosinophil count is ≥ 300.
LABA, long-acting β-agonist; LAMA, long-acting muscarinic antagonists; ICS, inhaled corticosteroids.
From Global Initiative for Chronic Obstructive Lung Disease. Global Strategy for the Diagnosis, Management, and Prevention of Chronic Obstructive Pulmonary Disease, 2019. http://www.goldcopd.org/.

SABAs for inhalation are available in solution for administration by a nebulizer, metered-dose inhaler, and *dry powder inhaler* (DPI). The combination of albuterol and ipratropium is available in a soft mist inhaler. Many studies have shown that metered-dose inhalers, DPIs, and soft mist inhalers are as effective as nebulizers in patients who are able to use the devices properly. Unfortunately, the proper technique for using different devices is not the same, and patients need detailed instructions and periodic assessment of their technique. In addition, DPIs require a much higher inspiratory flow to inhale the proper dose than do metered-dose inhalers, and some patients with moderate to severe COPD may not be able to generate adequate flows. For these individuals and for those whose medical or mental status makes coordinated breathing efforts difficult, nebulized β-agonists may be preferable.[180]

The major advantage of SABAs is their rapid onset of action, within 5 to 15 minutes after inhalation. Their effects last for 2 to 6 hours. As noted earlier, most patients with COPD demonstrate a modest improvement in FEV_1, and many studies and meta-analyses support their use for COPD.[181] The combination of albuterol and ipratropium results in greater and more sustained improvement in lung function than either drug alone.[182–184] When used at the recommended doses, inhaled SABAs are thought to be safe. The major adverse effects include tremor, anxiety, tachycardia, and hypokalemia. In a retrospective case-control cohort study of more than 70,000 patients with COPD, initiation of short- or long-acting β-agonists was associated with increased risk for arrhythmias,[185] but the study did not account for multiple potential confounders. Adverse effects are dose dependent and are less common with inhaled compared with systemic dosing and with optimized inhaler technique. Fortunately, tachyphylaxis to the systemic side effects of β-agonists is greater than tachyphylaxis to the bronchodilator effect.

Long-acting β-agonists (LABAs) typically produce bronchodilation that lasts for 12 hours or more. Salmeterol was the first LABA to be studied extensively. Its onset of action is much slower than that of albuterol, on the order of 20 to 30 minutes. Formoterol has a similar duration of action to salmeterol but an onset of action nearly identical

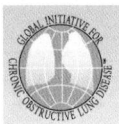

▶ **FOLLOW-UP PHARMACOLOGICAL TREATMENT**

1. IF RESPONSE TO INITIAL TREATMENT IS APPROPRIATE, MAINTAIN IT.
2. IF NOT:

✓ Consider the predominant treatable trait to target (dyspnea or exacerbations)
   -Use exacerbation pathway if both exacerbations and dyspnea need to be targeted

✓ Place patient in box corresponding to current treatment & follow indications

✓ Assess response, adjust and review

✓ These recommendations do not depend on the ABCD assessment at diagnosis

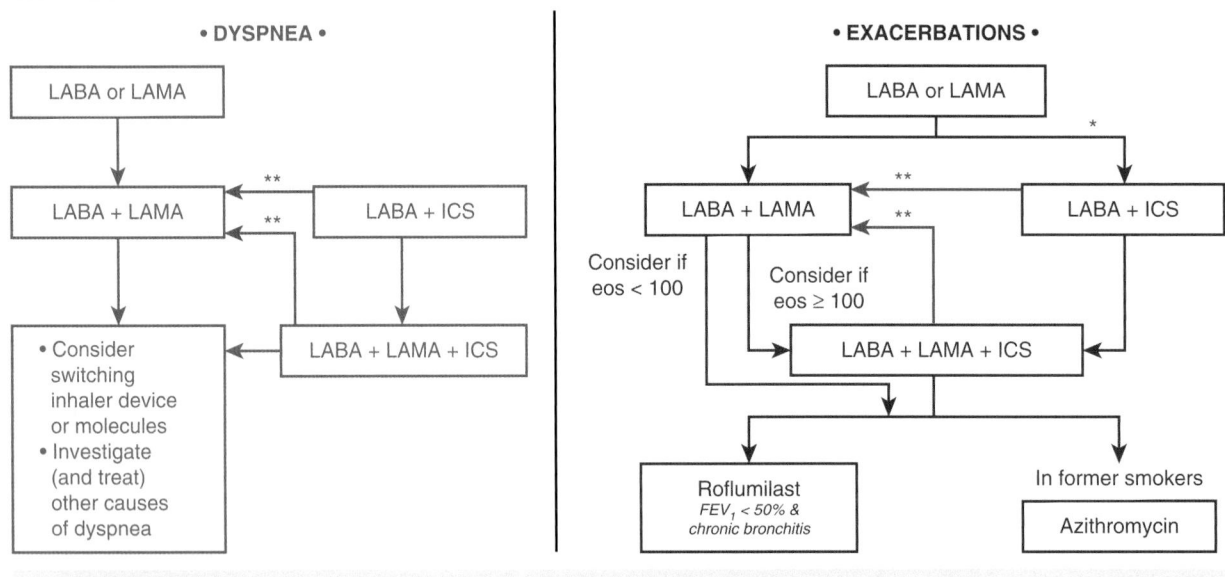

eos = blood eosinophil count (cells/μL)
*Consider if eos ≥ 300 or eos ≥ 100 AND ≥ 2 moderate exacerbations/1 hospitalization
**Consider de-escalation of ICS or switch if pneumonia, inappropriate original indication or lack of response to ICS

Figure 64.8 Follow-up pharmacologic treatment, _Global Initiative for Chronic Obstructive Lung Disease_ (GOLD). If response to initial treatment is appropriate, maintain it. If not, consider the predominant treatable trait to target (dyspnea or exacerbations), use exacerbation pathway if both exacerbations and dyspnea need to be targeted. FEV₁, forced expiratory volume in 1 second; ICS, inhaled corticosteroids; LABA, long-acting β-agonist; _LAMA_, long-acting muscarinic antagonists. (From Global Initiative for Chronic Obstructive Lung Disease. Global Strategy for the Diagnosis, Management, and Prevention of Chronic Obstructive Pulmonary Disease, 2019. http://www.goldcopd.org/.)

to albuterol. Both salmeterol and formoterol must be taken twice daily. Arformoterol is the (R)-enantiomer of formoterol. Indicaterol has a rapid onset and a duration of action of nearly 24 hours and thus requires only once-daily dosing. The bronchodilator effect of indicaterol is greater than that of salmeterol or formoterol. Vilanterol is another LABA with a rapid onset of action and a duration of action of approximately 24 hours. It is not used as monotherapy but has recently been approved in the United States and in Europe for use in combination with the ICS fluticasone or the long-acting muscarinic antagonist, umeclidinium.

Many studies have demonstrated a benefit of LABAs in patients with stable COPD.[78,186–193] Salmeterol and formoterol significantly improve lung function, dyspnea, and quality of life, and decrease the rate of exacerbations.[78,194–198] Salmeterol has been shown to reduce hospitalizations.[78] Indicaterol improves dyspnea and health status and reduces exacerbations.[199–202] The adverse effects reported with LABAs are similar to those described for SABAs. Of note, the association of LABA use with deaths that raised concern in the asthma community (see Chapter

62) has not been seen for COPD, and monotherapy with a LABA appears to be both safe and efficacious for COPD.

LABAs are frequently combined with an ICS in the same inhaler, and currently available preparations include fluticasone-salmeterol, budesonide-formoterol, mometasone-formoterol, and fluticasone-vilanterol. Many studies have shown that combination therapy is often more effective than either agent alone, and various guidelines provide recommendations for how and when to escalate treatment beyond short-acting bronchodilators. In general, ICS are reserved for patients who are prone to exacerbations.

Muscarinic Antagonists

Muscarinic antagonists, also known as anticholinergics or antimuscarinics, block the effects of acetylcholine on the M3 muscarinic receptors on airway smooth muscle. The M3 receptor is the predominant subtype of receptor mediating parasympathetic control of smooth muscle. Anticholinergics were used historically, long before β-agonists, in the form of stramonium and belladonna alkaloids,[203,204] then atropine. The newer quaternary amines, such as ipratropium and glycopyrrolate, as well as tiotropium and aclidinium, are better tolerated because they do not cross the blood-brain barrier. In addition, tiotropium, aclidinium, glycopyrrolate, and umeclidinium have pharmacokinetic selectivity for the M3 receptor and dissociate more rapidly from M2 receptors, which are found on cholinergic nerve terminals and inhibit acetylcholine release.[205] Thus the relative lack of M2 binding by these muscarinic antagonists may allow acetylcholine to bind to M2 receptors, thereby inhibiting further acetylcholine release and reducing bronchoconstriction.[206]

Short-acting muscarinic antagonists (SAMAs) include ipratropium and oxitropium. They increase FEV_1 with an onset of action of 10 to 15 minutes and a duration of action of 4 to 6 hours. Ipratropium improves lung function, increases exercise capacity, decreases dyspnea, and decreases cough.[207] Ipratropium monotherapy is more effective than SABAs at improving lung function, health status, and need for systemic corticosteroids,[208] but, when used in combination, their effects are additive and the duration is longer.[182-184]

Long-acting muscarinic antagonists (LAMAs) include tiotropium, aclidinium, umeclidinium, glycopyrrolate, and revefenacin. Most are slower in onset than ipratropium but last longer, with bronchodilation lasting at least 12 hours after aclidinium[209] and glycopyrrolate and more than 24 hours after tiotropium, umeclidinium, and revefenacin.[210-212] Tiotropium decreases symptoms, improves health status, and reduces exacerbations by 20–25%[213,214] and reduces hospitalizations.[211] It appears to improve the effectiveness of pulmonary rehabilitation, perhaps by decreasing dynamic hyperinflation.[215] When compared head-to-head with salmeterol, tiotropium increased time to first exacerbation and reduced the annual rate of exacerbations more than did salmeterol.[216] Although less data are available for the newer LAMAs, their effects on lung function and on dyspnea and exacerbations appear to be similar.[209]

In general, both SAMAs and LAMAs have good safety profiles. The most common side effects are dry mouth and urinary retention. Medication that contacts the eye, either by hand contact or by aerosolization, can cause blurred vision and can precipitate glaucoma. A retrospective database review[217] and a meta-analysis of ipratropium and tiotropium in COPD[218] suggested that anticholinergic therapy was associated with an increased risk of cardiovascular death, myocardial infarction, and stroke. However, a prospective study of almost 6000 patients with COPD who were treated with tiotropium or placebo found no increased risk of cardiovascular events or mortality.[219,220] A long-term study of more than 17,000 patients with COPD, designed specifically to examine safety of a soft mist Respimat device, concluded that tiotropium administered by the Respimat device had a safety profile similar to tiotropium delivered by the DPI HandiHaler device in patients with COPD and was not associated with an increased risk of death.[221]

Methylxanthines

Methylxanthines are nonselective inhibitors of phosphodiesterase and, by this mechanism, have a modest bronchodilator effect.[197,222,223] Theophylline is the most commonly used methylxanthine and, in stable COPD, its effect is greater than that of placebo but less than that of LABAs or LAMAs.

In addition to its bronchodilator effect, theophylline is reported to improve inspiratory muscle function[224-226] and to have anti-inflammatory effects.[227] Its effect on reducing symptoms is greater than its effect on airway function, suggesting that these alternative mechanisms may be important. However, a recent placebo-controlled, double-blinded study of low-dose theophylline (200 mg once or twice daily) as add-on therapy to inhaled corticosteroids found no difference in the rate of exacerbations[228] Further, because theophylline is a nonselective phosphodiesterase inhibitor, its actions are not all beneficial. The major adverse effects are insomnia, nausea, vomiting, cardiac arrhythmias, and seizures. These toxicities are dose dependent, but the onset of severe adverse events (e.g., ventricular arrhythmias, seizures) may not be heralded by warning symptoms, such as nausea or insomnia. In addition, blood levels are affected by age, liver disease, congestive heart failure, and many drug interactions. To minimize toxicity, current guidelines recommend targeting blood levels of 5 to 10 µg/mL rather than 15 to 20 µg/mL as was done previously. Because of its narrow therapeutic index and modest benefits, theophylline is not recommended as a first-line drug but can serve as an alternative for patients intolerant of LABAs and LAMAs or in settings where these drugs are too expensive.

Phosphodiesterase-4 Inhibitors

Phosphodiesterase-4 (PDE-4) inhibitors act by blocking the breakdown of cyclic adenosine monophosphate. By this mechanism, they decrease airway inflammation; they have no direct bronchodilator activity. Roflumilast is an oral PDE-4 inhibitor that has been approved for patients with chronic bronchitis and a history of exacerbations.[14] In a meta-analysis of 23 randomized trials of two different PDE-4 inhibitors (roflumilast and cilomilast), the PDE-4 inhibitors reduced exacerbations (odds ratio, 0.78; 95% confidence interval, 0.72–0.85) and produced a modest increase in FEV_1 (50 mL; 95% confidence interval, 39–52).[229] When roflumilast was added to salmeterol or tiotropium, the prebronchodilator FEV_1 increased.[14,15] Roflumilast appears to have greatest effect in patients with two or more exacerbations in the prior year or a hospitalized exacerbation[230] and high blood eosinophils.[231] Because its effect on exacerbations is much greater than its effect on airway function, guidelines recommend that roflumilast be used in combination with a long-acting bronchodilator.[34] Use of PDE-4 inhibitors has been limited by side effects. The most common are nausea, anorexia, abdominal pain, diarrhea, weight loss, sleep disturbances, and headache.[14,15,232] Monitoring weight during treatment is warranted.[34]

Corticosteroids

Inhaled Corticosteroids. Airway and systemic inflammation are critical components of the pathogenesis of COPD.[233-235] Therefore corticosteroids, with their anti-inflammatory effects, are an appealing intervention. ICS offer the additional advantage of minimizing systemic exposure. Early studies were not able to show that ICS altered the natural history of COPD. However, ICS have been shown to improve symptoms, lung function, and quality of life and to reduce the frequency of COPD exacerbations, especially in patients with an FEV_1 less than or equal to 60% of predicted. The improvement in FEV_1 achieved with ICS

(50–100 mL) is typically less than that observed with bronchodilators.[137,138] The reduction of exacerbations by ICS is more significant and is comparable to that observed with LABAs or LAMAs ($\approx$20–25%).[236–238] Guidelines recommend that ICS be used in combination with a long-acting bronchodilator in subjects who are prone to exacerbations but that they not be used as monotherapy.[34] Four large trials in which patients with COPD were treated with ICS for 3 to 5 years failed to demonstrate a reduction in loss of lung function over time.[137,138,239,240] However, in a post hoc analysis of the *Towards a Revolution in COPD Health* (TORCH) trial, in which 6112 subjects with moderate to severe COPD were randomly treated for 3 years with placebo, fluticasone, salmeterol, or the fluticasone-salmeterol combination, Celli and colleagues[241] reported that each active treatment arm reduced the rate of decline in FEV_1. Whether this benefit reflects the reduction in exacerbations or a more direct effect on the airway, perhaps by decreasing inflammation, is not known.

Most recently, ICS has been studied as part of "triple" combination therapy along with LABA and LAMA. The IMPACT study recently demonstrated among on-treatment subjects a reduction in all-cause mortality in the two ICS-containing arms (ICS/LABA/LAMA and ICS/LABA) compared to the non–ICS-containing arm (LABA/LAMA) of the study.[242] These are the strongest data to date demonstrating a role for ICS in reducing mortality in COPD. It should be noted, however, that the *InforMing the Pathway of COPD Treatment* (IMPACT) trial patient population had fairly severe COPD. The mean FEV_1% predicted was 45% and mean CAT score approximately 20. Nearly half the patient population experienced a moderate exacerbation in the prior year, and roughly one-quarter had experienced a hospitalized exacerbation in the prior year. Hence the results with respect to mortality reduction should be judged within the context of the patient population studied.

ICS are relatively safe, especially compared to systemic corticosteroids. The most common adverse effects are oral candidiasis (thrush) and dysphonia, both of which can be minimized by careful inhalation technique, followed by rinsing the mouth and gargling.[137,138] Increased skin bruising is probably a manifestation of steroid-induced capillary fragility. Reduced bone density has been reported after long-term treatment with triamcinolone,[243] but studies with budesonide and fluticasone have not found similar results, perhaps because these patients with COPD had a high prevalence of osteoporosis at baseline.[244,245] However, although ICS clearly reduce the frequency of exacerbations in COPD, they have been associated with an increased incidence of pneumonia.[78]

Systemic Corticosteroids. With rare exceptions, the use of systemic corticosteroids should be reserved for the treatment of exacerbations; in patients with stable disease, even when severe, the risk of adverse effects is probably greater than the likelihood of benefit. Chronic use of systemic corticosteroids is associated with increased mortality,[246,247] which may reflect corticosteroid effects or the underlying severity of the COPD. On occasion, in exacerbation-prone patients who require frequent courses of high-dose systemic corticosteroids, a very low daily dose of corticosteroids may protect against exacerbations and thereby reduce the total annual steroid exposure. If this unusual approach is followed, the lowest possible dose of corticosteroids should be used. If patients are reluctant to reduce their dose, they may be reassured by spirometry demonstrating a stability of FEV_1.

Combination Therapy

Patients who remain symptomatic after a period of treatment with a single long-acting bronchodilator (either LAMA or LABA) may benefit from addition of a second drug. Choices include either an ICS or a second long-acting bronchodilator from the other pharmacologic class. Accumulating data suggest that patients with significant dyspnea experience even greater benefit with dual bronchodilator therapy.[248] Increasing evidence also suggests that patients with elevated levels of blood eosinophils experience greater benefit with inhaled corticosteroids.[66,249] Although no threshold perfectly identifies ICS responders, an eosinophil count may be useful. Data suggest that ICS have little effect on exacerbation reduction at a blood eosinophil count less than 100 cells/μL, whereas greater than 300 cells/μL identifies patients with greatest likelihood to respond.

In two large trials, combination therapy improved outcomes significantly compared to each of the other treatment arms alone (placebo, LABA, ICS, LAMA). In the TORCH trial of 6112 patients with moderate to severe COPD, the combination of fluticasone-salmeterol improved lung function, health status, and exacerbations more than either agent alone[78] and was cost-effective.[250] In the *Investigating New Standards for Prophylaxis in Reduction of Exacerbations* (INSPIRE) trial, 1323 patients with severe COPD were randomly treated with fluticasone-salmeterol or tiotropium for 2 years.[251] There was no difference in exacerbations, but mortality was less in the fluticasone-salmeterol group, and health status was better, despite the finding that pneumonia was more frequent in the fluticasone-salmeterol group. Combinations of budesonide-formoterol, mometasone-formoterol, and fluticasone-vilanterol have also been shown to improve some clinical outcomes.

Several more recent studies have compared ICS/LABA to LABA/LAMA. The FLAME study compared fluticasone-salmeterol to indacaterol-glycopyrrolate for exacerbation reduction. The annual rate of moderate or severe exacerbations was higher in the fluticasone-salmeterol group compared to the indacaterol-glycopyrrolate group (1.19 vs. 0.98; rate ratio).[252] However, the IMPACT study also compared ICS/LABA to LABA/LAMA, specifically examining fluticasone-vilanterol versus umeclidinium-vilanterol, and found the annual rate of exacerbations to be *lower* with fluticasone-vilanterol than with umeclidinium-vilanterol (1.25 vs. 1.40).[242] It is not completely clear why these two studies produced different results, although several key study design aspects lend some insights. The IMPACT patient population had to have CAT greater than or equal to 10 and at least one moderate or severe exacerbation in the prior year if FEV_1 was less than 50% predicted and at least two exacerbations or one hospitalized exacerbation in the prior year if FEV_1 was greater than 50% predicted. There was also no medication "run-in" for IMPACT. Patients were transferred directly from maintenance medication to study medication. The FLAME study enrolled patients with at least one exacerbation in the prior year and also required a one-month run-in on tiotropium. Hence patients in IMPACT may have been sicker than those in FLAME.

Of interest, the IMPACT patient population also demonstrated increased ICS response with higher eosinophils that was not seen in the FLAME population,[253] again suggesting different types of patients. The SUNSET study compared patients on indacaterol-glycopyrrolate to those on fluticasone-tiotropium-salmeterol, where the fluticasone was withdrawn.[254] Here ICS withdrawal was associated with an increase in exacerbations for those with greater than or equal to 300 eosinophils/µL. The totality of the data would suggest that there are patients more likely to respond to ICS than others and that elevated eosinophils may be of assistance in identifying those patients. GOLD now identifies the threshold of 300 eosinophils/µL as those with greater likelihood to benefit from ICS, less than 100 eosinophils/µL as lower likelihood of benefit, and the range of 100 to 300 eosinophils/µL as an intermediate zone where ICS may be tried and response assessed.

Finally, guidelines suggest "triple inhaler therapy" for subjects whose symptoms or exacerbations are not controlled by any of the combinations already described.[34] Several recent studies support this recommendation, demonstrating greater lung function and symptom improvement and exacerbation reduction for ICS/LABA/LAMA compared to either ICS/LABA or LABA/LAMA.[242,255–258] The majority of these studies examined patients with significant symptoms as measured by CAT of 10 or greater and at least one exacerbation in the prior year, supporting triple therapy as a treatment option for patients with either persistent symptoms or exacerbations despite dual therapy.

Stepwise Pharmacologic Management

Enormous progress has been made from the time, not long ago, when few drugs for COPD were available in the therapeutic armamentarium. Now, many pharmaceutical categories have been shown to improve outcomes in COPD. Often there are many choices within each drug class and a variety of ways to progress through a therapeutic algorithm. The GOLD recommendations provide a framework for making these decisions.

In the past, recommendations for pharmacologic treatment were based primarily on spirometry. Recognizing that FEV_1 alone is a poor descriptor of disease status, the GOLD committee revised the approach to focus on symptoms and exacerbation history (see Fig. 64.7). Based on these variables, patients are assigned to groups A, B, C, or D, and recommendations for initial management are provided for each group (see Table 64.3).

After implementation of initial treatment, patients should be reassessed periodically to see if they are achieving goals of treatment. Common barriers to success include failure to adhere to prescribed regimen, poor inhaler technique, inappropriate choice of initial treatment, and comorbid conditions. For patients with good control, de-escalation should be considered. GOLD provides a second algorithm for follow-up management, where escalation and de-escalation or change in medications are based on dyspnea, exacerbations, and the presence or absence of peripheral blood eosinophilia (see Fig. 64.8).

Antioxidants and Mucolytics

Increased mucus production by hypertrophied and hyperplastic airway submucosal glands and goblet cells, together with impaired mucociliary clearance and cough, are frequent in patients with COPD. Although mucolytics have been evaluated in a number of long-term studies in COPD, the results are mixed and, in those studies demonstrating benefit (often those using higher doses), the effect is modest.[259–263] *N-acetylcysteine* (NAC) is a mucolytic and antioxidant that has been tested for its ability to slow the decline in lung function and prevent exacerbations. In the *Bronchitis Randomized on NAC Cost-Utility Study* (BRONCUS) trial, 523 patients at 50 centers were randomly assigned to 600 mg NAC or placebo daily. Patients were followed for 3 years. Neither the yearly rate of decline in FEV_1 nor the number of exacerbations per year differed between the NAC and the placebo group. However, subgroup analysis of those subjects who were not treated with an ICS suggested that NAC reduced exacerbations and hyperinflation.[264] A Cochrane review of 30 trials that included more than 7000 patients treated with NAC or other mucolytics concluded that there was a small effect on exacerbations but no effect on quality of life.[265] In its 2019 revision, the GOLD panel suggested that mucolytics may be useful in selected populations.[34]

Leukotriene Modifiers

Although the 5-lipoxygenase inhibitor zileuton and the cysteinyl leukotriene antagonists montelukast and zafirlukast are sometimes used for COPD, no data support their use, and guidelines do not recommend their use.[34]

NONPHARMACOLOGIC TREATMENT

Mucus Clearance

In patients with mucus hypersecretion and airflow obstruction, it may be very difficult to mobilize secretions. Maneuvers such as controlled cough[266] and the huff cough[267] can be helpful. In the former, patients take a deep breath, hold their breath for a few seconds, then cough two or three times with their mouth open and without taking another breath. The sequence is then repeated several times. Huff coughing involves one or two forced expirations starting at mid–lung volume and performed with the glottis open. Mucus clearance can also be facilitated by having patients breathe or cough through a device that generates high-amplitude oscillations[268] or with an external percussive device. These maneuvers are considered safe, but data supporting their use are limited.[269–272]

Oxygen

Two landmark studies conducted more than 30 years ago demonstrated the value of long-term oxygen therapy in patients with COPD and hypoxemia. The National Institute of Health's *Nocturnal Oxygen Therapy Trial* (NOTT) randomized 203 patients with COPD and hypoxemia to receive oxygen either for 12 hours overnight or for 24 hours/day for at least 12 months.[135] Overall mortality in the nocturnal oxygen group was 1.94 times that in the continuous oxygen group ($P = 0.01$). Almost simultaneously, the British mMRC compared the effect of oxygen administered for 15 hours/day with no oxygen (control) in 87 patients with

COPD, hypoxemia, carbon dioxide retention, and heart failure. Forty-five percent of the oxygen-treated patients died during the 5-year follow-up period compared with 67% of the control group.[136] In addition to this survival benefit, several studies have confirmed that administration of oxygen for at least 15 hours/day improves quality of life and neuropsychiatric metrics, reduces erythrocytosis, and improves pulmonary hemodynamics in patients with COPD and hypoxemia.[135,273,274]

Since then the National Institutes of Health sponsored the *Long-Term Oxygen Treatment Trial* (LOTT), which examined the benefits of supplemental oxygen therapy to patients with moderately low levels of oxygen[275] saturation. Specifically, patients with a blood oxygen saturation (peripheral capillary oxygen saturation, or SpO_2) from 89–93% at rest (moderate resting hypoxemia), or an SpO_2 below 90% during a 6MWT were randomized to 24-hour oxygen if their resting SpO_2 was 89–93% and oxygen only during sleep and exercise, if they had desaturation only during exercise. The primary outcome measure was time to first hospitalization or death. No significant difference in the primary outcome was seen between groups. Further, no differences were seen in quality of life, lung function, or 6MWD at the end of the study. Hence, although the NOTT and mMRC studies suggest mortality benefit of supplemental oxygen treatment with more severe hypoxemia, the LOTT study does not show clear benefit for treatment of individuals with more mild to moderate hypoxemia.

Indications for Oxygen.
Based on these data, guidelines recommend long-term administration of oxygen (>15 h/day) to patients with COPD with resting hypoxemia. Criteria include arterial *partial pressure of oxygen* (PO_2) less than 55 mm Hg, or arterial SpO_2 less than 88% while breathing room air at rest. For those whose resting arterial PO_2 is between 56 and 59 mm Hg, long-term oxygen treatment is indicated if they demonstrate erythrocytosis (hematocrit ≥ 55%) or right heart dysfunction. After an exacerbation or another acute respiratory event, patients often have hypoxemia that resolves slowly over 1 to 2 months. For this reason, patients given oxygen as they are recovering should be reevaluated after approximately 1 month to determine if they continue to meet criteria for long-term oxygen treatment.

Oxygen During Exercise.
Patients whose arterial PO_2 or SpO_2 are borderline at rest may develop worsening hypoxemia with exercise. This is especially true for patients with emphysema and a low diffusing capacity. Supplementary oxygen improves exercise endurance,[276,277] and even patients without hypoxemia may improve their exercise capacity with supplementary oxygen.[278] Although the LOTT study did not demonstrate benefit of oxygen therapy in this group of patients, it is still possible that supplemental oxygen during exertion is beneficial in some patients with mild hypoxemia at rest or exercise-related desaturation. Hence, although routine oxygen use in this group of patients is not recommended, individual patient factors may warrant a trial of oxygen.

If oxygen is prescribed, one of the goals of oxygen therapy is to permit patients to remain active. Ambulatory oxygen systems are intended to provide a lightweight, portable source of oxygen that can be carried as the patient pursues activities of daily living. Unfortunately, patients are often provided with "portable" systems that are not really conducive to ambulation. The standard E-cylinder, for example, weighs 22 pounds and must be pulled along on a bulky wheeled cart. Various lightweight oxygen reservoirs do exist, weighing as little as 4 pounds; portable oxygen concentrators weighing less than 3 pounds are another lightweight option. Health care providers must specify to oxygen vendors which ambulatory system they want for their patients.

Oxygen During Sleep.
Just as they do with exercise, patients with COPD may experience a significant drop in arterial oxygen tension during sleep, due to a combination of increases in ventilation-perfusion mismatch and a change in ventilatory pattern[279] (see also Chapter 117). In patients who are not hypoxemic at rest, the long-term consequences of these episodes of nocturnal hypoxemia are unknown, as are the benefits of long-term oxygen.[280–282] Although many clinicians prescribe nocturnal oxygen for these patients, there is no evidence to support this approach. The International Nocturnal Oxygen Trial, a 4-year, multicenter, randomized, placebo-controlled trial of nocturnal oxygen in COPD patients without resting hypoxemia or OSA, was completed in 2019, and results will be available soon.[283]

Oxygen for Air Travel.
When flying at altitudes higher than 12,000 feet, aircraft are pressurized to protect passengers and crew from hypoxemia, barotrauma, and other manifestations of altitude (see Chapter 106). The Federal Aviation Administration mandates that the cabin pressure must not drop below that of an altitude of 8000 feet (equivalent to 564 mm Hg). Although this pressurization is sufficient to prevent most barotrauma and altitude sickness, it does not eliminate the possibility of hypoxemia. Arterial PO_2 will drop and, in patients who are hypoxemic at rest at sea level or those who are borderline, the arterial PO_2 may fall to dangerous levels at altitude. Patients whose resting arterial PO_2 at sea level is greater than 70 mm Hg are likely to be safe to fly without supplementary oxygen.[284,285] When there is uncertainty about a patient's potential oxygen requirement at altitude, an altitude simulation test can be performed, using 16% oxygen to simulate the partial pressure of oxygen at 8000 feet.[286]

For patients who require in-flight oxygen, arrangements must be made with the airline in advance. In general, patients may not bring their own oxygen supply, and airlines usually charge for the oxygen they provide. Lightweight portable oxygen concentrators have become available, and these are approved by the Federal Aviation Administration for commercial air travel. Some airlines allow passengers to travel with their own concentrators (see Chapter 106).

Technical Issues for Oxygen Use.
Most patients receive oxygen via a nasal cannula. Flow rates should be adjusted to achieve an SpO_2 greater than 90% (arterial PO_2 > 60 mm Hg). In general, patients who use oxygen 24 hours/day should increase the oxygen flow by 1 L/min during sleep and exercise, to prevent drops in arterial PO_2 during these periods. Oxygen-conserving devices that improve the efficiency of oxygen delivery increase the time that a

given volume of portable oxygen will last, allowing patients greater mobility. These include nasal cannulae with reservoirs that store oxygen during exhalation for delivery during inhalation, as well as breath-activated regulators that deliver an oxygen pulse only during inspiration. For use in the home, electric-powered oxygen concentrators are the most convenient, for they do not require replacement or refilling as is the case with gas cylinders or liquid oxygen. It is important that patients who depend on a concentrator have back-up cylinders on hand, in case of a power failure. Ambulatory systems include E-cylinders on wheeled carts, lightweight aluminum cylinders, liquid oxygen reservoirs, and portable concentrators. Many of these ambulatory systems weigh as little as 3 to 4 pounds and provide oxygen for 4 to 6 hours at a flow of 2 L/min.

Noninvasive Ventilation

For patients with acute exacerbations of COPD with hypercapnia and acidosis, bilevel positive airway pressure decreases mortality, need for intubation, and hospital length of stay.[287] For patients with stable COPD, the use of nocturnal noninvasive ventilation has been proposed to prevent desaturations during sleep and to improve both nocturnal and daytime respiratory function by "resting" respiratory muscles. Unfortunately, studies have provided conflicting results, with several trials each demonstrating prolonged time to readmission or death,[288,289] improved survival that was not sustained beyond 36 months,[290] or no benefit.[291,292] Some experts suggest a trial of high-pressure or high-intensity nocturnal noninvasive ventilation in hypercapneic patients with COPD who desaturate during sleep despite supplementary oxygen, but this recommendation is not included in COPD management guidelines.

PULMONARY REHABILITATION

Pulmonary rehabilitation is a comprehensive program that combines exercise training, smoking cessation, nutrition counseling, and education, in an attempt to improve the functional capacity and quality of life of patients with COPD. Formal rehabilitation programs have been shown to improve exercise capacity and quality of life and to decrease dyspnea and health care utilization.[293–296] In addition, a Cochrane review has suggested that pulmonary rehabilitation decreases mortality.[297] Pulmonary rehabilitation should be offered to all patients with COPD who are symptomatic (see Chapter 139).

SURGICAL TREATMENT OF EMPHYSEMA

More than 50 years ago, anecdotal reports of symptomatic improvement in patients with emphysema who underwent resection of concomitant lung cancers or bullae led physiologists to consider LVRS to improve the mechanical efficiency of respiratory muscles. Because of hyperinflation, respiratory muscles are forced to operate on the disadvantageous part of the length-tension curve; reducing hyperinflation was predicted to improve force generation by respiratory muscles, to improve lung elastic recoil, and to improve expiratory flow rates. Unfortunately, early procedures were associated with an unacceptably high mortality rate. In 1995 Cooper and colleagues[298] reported on

their experience with 20 patients who underwent bilateral LVRS. By using a linear stapling device and strips of bovine pericardium to minimize air leak through the staple holes, they were able to eliminate this major cause of early mortality and reported very impressive improvements in FEV_1, arterial PO_2, 6MWD, dyspnea, and quality of life. This was followed by the *National Emphysema Treatment Trial* (NETT), a precedent-setting collaborative effort of the Centers for Medicare and Medicaid Services, the NHLBI, and the Agency for Healthcare Research and Quality. NETT enrolled 1218 patients with severe emphysema and compared LVRS to maximal medical treatment.[48] In patients with upper lobe–predominant emphysema and a low postrehabilitation exercise capacity, LVRS improved survival and quality of life.[299] In those patients with FEV_1 of 20% or less predicted and either homogeneous distribution of emphysema or DL_{CO} of 20% or less predicted, mortality was greater with LVRS compared to medical management.[300] These criteria are currently used to select patients for LVRS.

TREATMENT OF EMPHYSEMA WITH ENDOBRONCHIAL VALVES

Nonsurgical methods for reducing hyperinflation in severe emphysema have also been explored. In particular, endobronchial valves leading to lobar deflation mimic the mechanism of lung volume reduction surgery. The evidence basis for efficacy of this procedure is growing.[301–303] The LIBERATE study randomized 190 subjects to Zephyr endobronchial valve versus standard of care.[302] Patients with hyperinflation, greater than 50% emphysema in the target lobe, and at least 15% greater emphysema in the target versus ipsilateral lobes were enrolled. Patients also had to have no evidence of collateral ventilation between target and adjacent lobes. Endobronchial valve placement was studied in patients with both heterogeneous and homogenous emphysema. Patients receiving the valve demonstrated improvements in FEV_1, 6MWD, and SGRQ score. However, pneumothorax developed in 26.6% of valve-treated subjects. After the 45-day postprocedural period, patients treated with endobronchial valves trended toward lower numbers of exacerbations. This therapy is now clinically available and approved for treatment in many countries, including the United States. A second endobronchial valve, the Spiration valve, was also approved by the U.S. Food and Drug Administration in December 2018[303] (see Chapter 28).

ACUTE EXACERBATIONS

Definition

Perhaps surprisingly, it has not been easy to define an acute exacerbation of COPD. GOLD[34] states, "An exacerbation of COPD is an acute event characterized by a worsening of the patient's respiratory symptoms that is beyond normal day-to-day variations and leads to a change in medication."[304–306] This works sufficiently well that it allows classification of events in various studies and for comparisons across trials.

Triggers

Exacerbations of COPD are precipitated most often by respiratory tract infections. These may be viral or bacterial. A key event, even in individuals whose airways are chronically colonized by bacteria, may be the acquisition of bacterial strains that are new to that patient.[307] Many patients are sensitive to air pollutants and experience an exacerbation when ambient levels increase.[308-310] In perhaps 30% of patients with COPD, no cause for exacerbations can be identified. Of interest, some patients have an exacerbation whenever one of these events takes place; others rarely do. Those who experience two or more exacerbations per year are often defined as "frequent exacerbators" and pose a unique challenge for management.

Treatment

The goal of treatment is to minimize the impact of the current exacerbation, to minimize loss of lung function, and to prevent the development of subsequent exacerbations. The vast majority of exacerbations can be managed without hospitalization. Indications for hospitalization include severe dyspnea or respiratory insufficiency, severe underlying COPD, serious comorbidities, frequent exacerbator phenotype, older age, and insufficient support at home. Supplemental oxygen should be administered if necessary to achieve an SpO_2 greater than 88%. After 30 to 60 minutes, arterial blood gases should be assessed for evidence of carbon dioxide retention.

Bronchodilators. During an acute exacerbation, SABAs should be used aggressively, alone or in combination with muscarinic antagonists. Although metered-dose inhalers, when used correctly, can be as effective as nebulizers,[311] it can be difficult for severely dyspneic patients to coordinate their efforts to use a metered-dose inhaler or to generate sufficient inspiratory flow required for some devices. Therefore nebulizers are a reasonable approach for delivering bronchodilator therapy in the setting of an acute exacerbation.

Corticosteroids. Substantial data support the use of systemic corticosteroids for treatment of exacerbations of COPD. Their use is associated with a more rapid recovery, improvement in lung function and hypoxemia, and a reduced risk of relapse.[312-315] Guidelines recommend 40 to 60 mg prednisone per day for 2 weeks, but a more recent prospective trial of more than 300 patients found that 5 days of prednisone was not inferior to 14 days for preventing reexacerbation within 6 months and was associated with a significantly lower total corticosteroid exposure.[316] A retrospective study of more than 17,000 patients admitted to intensive care units with acute exacerbations found that those treated with more than 240 mg/day of methylprednisolone equivalents or 300 mg/day prednisone equivalents had greater mortality, length of stay, ventilator days, complications, and costs.[317]

Antibiotics. The use of antibiotics for exacerbations of COPD is somewhat controversial, largely because of the paucity of data documenting bacterial colonization or infection. Studies have suggested that nearly 50% of acute exacerbations are associated with *H. influenzae, S. pneumoniae,* and *M. catarrhalis.*[318] Even when patients are chronically colonized, changes in strain may be associated with exacerbations.[307] Sputum cultures are of limited utility because they do not distinguish between colonization and infection and because of the time required for results. Most guidelines recommend empirical treatment when infection seems likely, based on what are sometimes called the "Anthonisen criteria": increased dyspnea, sputum volume, and sputum purulence,[319] with greater weight given to meeting all three criteria. The recommended length of antibiotic treatment is 5 to 10 days.

DEVELOPMENT OF NEW TREATMENTS

Despite advances in recent years, treatment options for COPD are woefully inadequate. Other than smoking cessation and supplementary oxygen in patients who are hypoxemic, there are no treatments that clearly and consistently reduce mortality. Several factors have contributed to the lack of progress. COPD is highly heterogeneous: In some patients, emphysema predominates; in others, bronchitis predominates; and still others may have both. COPD is a systemic disease and, as a consequence, comorbid extrapulmonary conditions are common. Because treatment effects are small, very large studies are required to test potential new interventions. For all of these reasons, investigators are beginning to explore individual patient subtypes, looking for subpopulations that might benefit from unique therapeutic regimens, and for intermediate outcomes measures that might increase the efficiency of clinical trials. To this end, the NHLBI has funded the SPIROMICS,[320] a prospective observational study of COPD subjects and control subjects. Complementary studies, such as *Evaluation of COPD Longitudinally to Identify Predictive Surrogate Endpoints* (ECLIPSE)[321] and COPDGene,[322] will hopefully add to the explosion of knowledge in the next few years, aiming at improving treatment for patients with COPD.

> ### Key Points
>
> - COPD is a highly prevalent disease and a leading cause of mortality. COPD is significantly underdiagnosed.
> - COPD is characterized by airflow obstruction that is not fully reversible. Spirometry is required for diagnosis.
> - Older age and a history of smoking are the two most important risk factors for COPD.
> - Emphysema at a young age or in an individual with minimal or no smoking history should suggest alpha$_1$-antitrypsin deficiency.
> - Smoking cessation is the only intervention demonstrated to alter the course of lung function decline. Smoking cessation also conveys a long-term mortality benefit.
> - Pharmacotherapy is no longer for symptom relief only. Short- and long-acting muscarinic antagonists, long-acting β-agonists, and inhaled corticosteroids have been shown to improve exercise capacity, improve quality of life, and reduce exacerbations.
> - Choice of medications is based in part on the availability of medication and the patient's response. The Global Initiative for Chronic Obstructive Lung Disease has proposed a stepwise treatment algorithm, based on symptoms, and exacerbation history.
> - In patients with persistent hypoxemia, continuous oxygen treatment for at least 15 hours/day improves survival, quality of life, and a number of other measures.

- Patients with arterial PO_2 less than 55 mm Hg or SpO_2 less than 88% while breathing room air at rest or patients with arterial PO_2 56 to 59 mm Hg and erythrocytosis or right heart dysfunction should be offered continuous oxygen treatment.
- Pulmonary rehabilitation improves exercise capacity and quality of life and decreases dyspnea and health care utilization, as well as hospitalizations and mortality. Pulmonary rehabilitation should be offered to any patient who develops shortness of breath while walking.
- Lung volume reduction surgery may be beneficial for the small subgroup of patients with upper lobe–predominant emphysema and a low postrehabilitation exercise capacity. Endobronchial valve therapy may also benefit patients with emphysema.

Key Readings

Anthonisen NR, Skeans MA, Wise RA, et al. The effects of a smoking cessation intervention on 14.5-year mortality: a randomized clinical trial. *Ann Intern Med.* 2005;142:233–239.

Bafadhel M, Peterson S, De Blas MA, et al. Predictors of exacerbation risk and response to budesonide in patients with chronic obstructive pulmonary disease: a post-hoc analysis of three randomized trials. *Lancet Respir Med.* 2018;6:117–126.

Calverley PM, Anderson JA, Celli B, et al. Salmeterol and fluticasone propionate and survival in chronic obstructive pulmonary disease. *N Engl J Med.* 2007;356:775–789.

Celli BR, Cote CG, Marin JM, et al. The body-mass index, airflow obstruction, dyspnea, and exercise capacity index in chronic obstructive pulmonary disease. *N Engl J Med.* 2004;350:1005–1012.

Celli BR, Thomas NE, Anderson JA, et al. Effect of pharmacotherapy on rate of decline of lung function in chronic obstructive pulmonary disease: results from the TORCH study. *Am J Respir Crit Care Med.* 2008;178:332–338.

Continuous or nocturnal oxygen therapy in hypoxemic chronic obstructive lung disease: a clinical trial. Nocturnal Oxygen Therapy Trial Group. *Ann Intern Med,* 1980;93(3):391–398.

Cooper JA, Criner GJ, Diaz P, Fuhlbrigge AL, et al. A randomized trial of long-term oxygen for COPD with moderate desaturation. *N Engl J Med.* 2016;375:1617–1627.

Fishman A, Martinez F, Naunheim K, et al. A randomized trial comparing lung volume reduction surgery with medical therapy for severe emphysema. *N Engl J Med.* 2003;348(21):2059–2073.

Fletcher C, Peto R. The natural history of chronic airflow obstruction. *Br Med J.* 1977;1:1645–1648.

Global Initiative for Chronic Obstructive Lung Disease. *Global Strategy for the Diagnosis, Management, and Prevention of Chronic Obstructive Pulmonary Disease;* 2019. https://goldcopd.org/wp-content/uploads/2017/11/GOLD-2018-v6.0-FINAL-revised-20-Nov_WMS.pdf.

Leung JM, Sin DA. Asthma-COPD overlap syndrome: pathogenesis, clinical features, and therapeutic targets. *BMJ.* 2017;358:3772–3785.

Long term domiciliary oxygen therapy in chronic hypoxic cor pulmonale complicating chronic bronchitis and emphysema. Report of the Medical Research Council Working Party. *Lancet,* 1981;1(8222):681–686.

Mannino DM, Buist AS. Global burden of COPD: risk factors, prevalence, and future trends. *Lancet.* 2007;370(9589):765–773.

Tashkin DP, Celli B, Senn S, et al. A 4-year trial of tiotropium in chronic obstructive pulmonary disease. *N Engl J Med.* 2008;359:1543–1554.

Vestbo J, Edwards LD, Scanlon PD, et al. Changes in forced expiratory volume in 1 second over time in COPD. *N Engl J Med.* 2011;365:1184–1192.

Woodruff PG, Barr RG, Bleecker E, et al. Clinical significance of symptoms in smokers with preserved pulmonary function. *N Engl J Med.* 2016;374:1811–1821.

Complete reference list available at ExpertConsult.com.

65 SMOKING HAZARDS: CIGARETTES, VAPING, MARIJUANA

JEFFREY E. GOTTS, MD, PHD • NEAL L. BENOWITZ, MD

INTRODUCTION

From cigarette smoking to cocaine, this chapter covers the greatest preventable cause of lung disease and of other preventable smoking hazards. Despite significant public health efforts to control its use, cigarette smoking remains the leading global risk factor for disability-adjusted years of life lost.[1–4] Secondhand smoke causes tens of thousands of cardiovascular deaths and several thousand lung cancer deaths annually. *Electronic cigarettes* (e-cigarettes), which deliver nicotine in an aerosol of propylene glycol, vegetable glycerin, and flavorings, have jumped in prominence over the last 15 years, even as the health risks and the potential benefits for smoking cessation remain controversial. *E-cigarette/vaping–associated lung injury* (EVALI) is a newly described syndrome of acute respiratory distress syndrome of unclear mechanism associated with vaping *delta-9-tetrahydrocannabinol* (THC) obtained from the black market. Cannabis, now legalized in many states in the United States, has not been shown to cause COPD or cancer but is associated with upper airway irritation, wheezing, chronic cough, sputum production, and barotrauma. Finally, cocaine and methamphetamine have acute cardiovascular toxicity and are associated with pulmonary edema, alveolar hemorrhage, emphysema, and pulmonary hypertension. The important related topic of smoking cessation is covered in Chapter 66.

CIGARETTE SMOKING

EPIDEMIOLOGY OF CIGARETTE SMOKING

Currently, about 41 million individuals (19% of the adult population) in the United States are smokers of cigarettes or other combustible tobacco products, including cigars and cigarillos, pipes, and water pipes.[5] Heavy smoking (≥20 cigarettes/day) has declined substantially over the past 30 years, and in the United States, about 25% of smokers do not smoke every day. People who are less well educated and/or have unskilled occupations are more likely to smoke. For example, 37% of people with a high school education are smokers compared to 7.1% of those with a college degree. High rates are seen in those living below the federal poverty level (28%) and in those working in construction and extraction industries (30%).[6]

There are more than 1 billion smokers worldwide, the majority of whom live in low- and middle-income countries.[7] Tobacco use remains the leading global risk factor for disability-adjusted life years lost. The World Health Organization Framework Convention on Tobacco Control aims to reduce both the demand and the supply of tobacco around the world through educational, political, and legislative means.[8]

TOXICOLOGY OF CIGARETTE SMOKE

Tobacco smoke is an aerosol of droplets (particulates) containing water, nicotine and other alkaloids, and tar suspended in a gaseous phase. Tobacco smoke contains several thousand different chemicals, many of which may contribute to human disease.[9] The *particulate* phase contains major toxic chemicals, such as nicotine, benzo(a)pyrene and other polycyclic hydrocarbons, 4-(methylnitrosamino)-1-(3-pyridyl)-1-butanone, N'-nitrosonornicotine, β-naphthylamine, polonium-210, nickel, cadmium, arsenic, and lead. The *gaseous* phase contains carbon monoxide, acetaldehyde, acetone, methanol, nitrogen oxides, hydrogen cyanide, acrolein, ammonia, benzene, formaldehyde, nitrosamines, and vinyl chloride. Tobacco smoke contains a high concentration of free radicals and other oxidizing chemicals, as well as fine particulates, which contribute to disease. Tobacco smoke may produce illness by way of systemic absorption of toxins and/or cause local pulmonary injury by oxidants and other chemicals.

SMOKING-RELATED DISEASES

Tobacco use is a major cause of death from cancer, cardiovascular disease, and pulmonary disease (Table 65.1). Smoking is also a major risk factor for osteoporosis, reproductive disorders, and fire- and trauma-related injuries.

TABLE 65.1 Health Hazards of Tobacco Use (Risks Increased by Smoking)

CANCER (SEE TABLE 65.2)

CARDIOVASCULAR DISEASE

Sudden death
Acute myocardial infarction
Unstable angina
Stroke
Peripheral arterial occlusive disease (including thromboangiitis obliterans)
Abdominal aortic aneurysm

PULMONARY DISEASE

Lung cancer
Chronic bronchitis
Emphysema
Asthma
Increased susceptibility to/severity of pneumonia, influenza, and pulmonary tuberculosis
Increased susceptibility to desquamative interstitial pneumonia, respiratory bronchiolitis–interstitial lung disease, pulmonary Langerhans cell histiocytosis
Increased morbidity from viral respiratory infection

GASTROINTESTINAL DISEASE

Peptic ulcer
Esophageal reflux

REPRODUCTIVE DISTURBANCES

Reduced fertility in women
Erectile dysfunction
Premature birth
Lower birth weight
Ectopic pregnancy
Spontaneous abortion
Abruptio placentae
Orofacial clefts
Increased perinatal mortality (including sudden infant death syndrome)

ORAL DISEASE (SMOKELESS TOBACCO)

Oropharyngeal cancer
Leukoplakia
Dental caries
Periodontitis
Tooth staining

OTHER

Non–insulin-dependent diabetes mellitus
Earlier menopause
Osteoporosis
Hip fracture
Cataract
Age-related macular degeneration
Rheumatoid arthritis
Poor wound healing
Premature skin wrinkling
Aggravation of hypothyroidism
Altered drug metabolism or effects

TABLE 65.2 Cigarette Smoking and Cancer Risk

Cancer Site	Average Relative Risk
Lung	15.0–30.0
Urinary tract	3.0
Oral cavity	4.0–5.0
Oropharynx and hypopharynx	4.0–5.0*
Esophagus	1.5–5.0*
Larynx	10.0*
Pancreas	2.0–4.0
Nasal cavity, sinuses, nasopharynx	1.5–2.5
Stomach	1.5–2.0
Liver	1.5–2.5
Kidney	1.5–2.0
Uterine cervix	1.5–2.5
Acute myeloid leukemia	1.5–2.0

*Synergistic interaction with alcohol use.
Modified from Vineis P, Alavanja M, Buffler P, et al. Tobacco and cancer: recent epidemiological evidence. *J Natl Cancer Inst.* 2004;96(2):99–106; International Council for Research on Cancer. Tobacco smoking and involuntary smoking. IARC monographs on the evaluation of carcinogenic risks to humans. *IARC Sci Publ.* 2004;83.

associated with squamous cell carcinomas of the lung, head, and neck.[11] Lung cancer is the leading cause of cancer deaths in the United States and is predominantly attributable to cigarette smoking.[4] The risk of lung and other cancers is proportional to the number of cigarettes smoked per day and, even more strongly, to the duration of smoking.[12]

Workplace exposure to asbestos or α-radiation, the latter in uranium miners, synergistically increases the risk of lung cancer in cigarette smokers.[13] Alcohol use interacts synergistically with tobacco in causing oral, laryngeal, and esophageal cancer[14]; the mechanism of interaction may involve alcohol solubilizing tobacco carcinogens and/or alcohol-related induction of liver or gastrointestinal enzymes that metabolize and activate tobacco carcinogens. Smoking is associated with 15% of leukemia cases in adults and 20% of colorectal cancers.[15,16]

A detailed description of the epidemiology and the pathogenesis of smoking-induced lung cancer is presented in Chapters 73 and 74.

Chronic Lung Disease

Greater than 80% of COPD in the United States is attributable to cigarette smoking. Cigarette smoking also increases the risk for respiratory infection, including pneumonia, and results in greater disability from viral respiratory tract infections.[17,18] Pulmonary disease from smoking includes the overlapping syndromes of chronic bronchitis (cough and mucus secretion), emphysema, and airway obstruction.[19] Whereas the diagnosis of COPD is based on evidence of airflow obstruction on spirometry, smokers with normal spirometry can also have chronic respiratory symptoms, reduced exercise tolerance, and evidence of emphysema or bronchiolitis on imaging.[20]

Cancer

Smoking, the largest preventable cause of cancer (Table 65.2), is responsible for about 30% of cancer deaths.[10] Many chemicals in tobacco smoke may contribute to carcinogenesis as tumor initiators, cocarcinogens, tumor promoters, or complete carcinogens.[9] Complexes of tobacco smoke carcinogens with DNA are thought to be a crucial step in cancer induction. Cigarette smoking induces specific patterns of *p53* gene mutations

---

The pathologic changes in the lung produced by cigarette smoking include loss of cilia, mucous gland hyperplasia, increased number of goblet cells in the central airways, inflammation, goblet cell metaplasia, squamous metaplasia, mucus plugging of small airways, destruction of alveoli, and pruning of the distal small (<5 mm^2) pulmonary arteries[21,22] (see also Chapter 63). The mechanisms of injury are complex and include both innate and adaptive immune inflammatory pathways,[23] as well as direct injury by oxidant chemicals, increased elastase activity (a protein that breaks down elastin and other connective tissue), and decreased antiprotease activity.[24] A genetic deficiency of α_1-antiprotease (α_1-antitrypsin) activity produces a similar imbalance between pulmonary protease and antiprotease activity and is a risk factor for early and severe smoking-induced pulmonary disease.[25] Epigenetic changes related to cigarette smoking are associated with decreased lung function and may contribute to the pathogenesis of COPD.[26]

In addition to cigarette smoke–induced injury, the delivery of carbon monoxide from cigarette smoke serves to worsen the level of functioning in smokers who have significant COPD. Carbon monoxide avidly binds to hemoglobin, reduces the capacity of hemoglobin to carry oxygen, and impairs oxygen release at the tissues. Thus carbon monoxide exposure produces a functional anemia. Carboxyhemoglobin levels are typically 5–10% in smokers compared to 1% or less in nonsmokers. In a normal person, carbon monoxide from cigarette smoke causes few symptoms, but, in patients with pulmonary disease, carbon monoxide has the potential to cause significant impairment. Exposure to carbon monoxide at levels even less than that derived from cigarette smoking has been shown to reduce exercise tolerance in patients with COPD.

Cigarette smoking may contribute to the development of asthma, although this potential link could be confounded by the increased rate of pulmonary infections observed in smokers. A longitudinal study of 5800 individuals taking part in a national British cohort study suggested that regular smoking was associated with asthma in people between 17 and 33 years of age (*odds ratio* [OR], 4.4).[27] More recently, a longitudinal study of more than 46,000 women revealed increased adult-onset asthma in former smokers (*hazard ratio* [HR], 1.4; 95% *confidence interval* [CI], 1.1 to 1.7) and active smokers (HR, 1.4; CI, 1.2 to 1.8).[28] Current smokers, compared to never and ex-smokers, demonstrate higher asthma severity scores, more frequent asthma symptoms, and more frequent asthma attacks (OR, 2.4).[29] Silverman and coworkers[30] evaluated 1847 emergency department patients presenting with acute asthma and found that 35% of patients were current smokers. Half of these smoking asthmatic patients reported that cigarette use worsened their asthma symptoms.

The link between secondhand smoke and asthma would support the hypothesis that tobacco exposure worsens bronchial hyperresponsiveness. Several studies have reported increased prevalence of airflow obstruction and asthma in children exposed in utero to maternal smoking.[31,32] In addition, a study evaluating infants exposed to smoking mothers in their first year of life demonstrated they were 2.1 times more likely to develop asthma than were children of nonsmoking mothers.[33] Likewise, the Swiss Study on Air Pollution and Lung Disease in Adults suggested that secondhand smoke was associated with an increased risk for asthma (OR, 1.4) or reactive airway disease in nonsmoking adults.[34]

There are other links between smoking and both acute and chronic inflammatory lung conditions. In a small cohort of healthy nonasthmatic smokers, bronchoalveolar lavage fluid documented altered macrophage cytokine release, increased cellularity, and depressed levels of interleukin-6.[35] The risk of acute respiratory distress syndrome is increased in smokers[36] and, in experimental studies, smokers exposed to nebulized endotoxin had increased markers of lung injury and inflammatory cytokines in bronchoalveolar lavage.[37]

Cigarette smoking has been associated with multiple nonneoplastic pulmonary disorders other than emphysema and chronic bronchitis. These include respiratory bronchiolitis–associated interstitial lung disease, desquamative interstitial pneumonitis, pulmonary Langerhans cell histiocytosis, and cryptogenic interstitial fibrosing alveolitis.[38] Ninety percent of patients with pulmonary Langerhans cell histiocytosis are smokers. Respiratory bronchiolitis–associated interstitial lung disease and desquamative interstitial pneumonitis have similar histopathologic features and are characterized by the accumulation of pigmented macrophages within the alveoli. Respiratory bronchiolitis ("smoker's bronchiolitis") refers to the presence of pigmented macrophages, in the absence of respiratory symptoms or significant fibrosis.[39,40] Desquamative interstitial pneumonitis often affects individuals in their fourth or fifth decade of life, and the symptoms are more frequent in smokers.[41] Smoking may also have an association with idiopathic pulmonary fibrosis.[42] Smoking is over-represented in patients with idiopathic pulmonary fibrosis compared to the general population, and the overall OR for smoking as a risk factor for idiopathic pulmonary fibrosis has been reported to be 1.6.[43]

Infection

Cigarette smoking is a major risk factor for respiratory tract and other systemic infections. Both active and passive cigarette smoke exposure increase the risk for infection.[44,45] The mechanisms by which smoking increases risk are multifactorial and include structural and immunologic alterations. As mentioned previously, cigarette smoking causes structural changes in the respiratory tract. These changes include peribronchiolar inflammation and fibrosis, increased mucosal permeability, impairment of mucociliary clearance, changes in pathogen adherence, and disruption of the respiratory epithelium. A number of components of cigarette smoke, including acrolein, acetaldehyde, formaldehyde, free radicals produced from chemical reactions within the cigarette smoke, and nitric oxide, may contribute to the observed structural alterations in airway epithelial cells.

Immunologic mechanisms include alterations in cellular and humoral immune system function. These include a decreased level of circulating immunoglobulins, a depression of antibody response to certain antigens, a decrease in CD4$^+$ lymphocyte counts, an increase in CD8$^+$ lymphocyte counts, depressed phagocyte activity, and decreased release of proinflammatory cytokines. Many of the immunologic disturbances in smokers resolve within 6 weeks after smoking cessation, supporting the idea that smoking cessation

TABLE 65.3 Cigarette Smoking and Risk of Infection

	Odds Ratio (95% CI)
Tuberculosis	4.5 (4.0–5.0)
Legionnaires' disease	3.5 (2.1–5.8)
HIV infection	3.4 (1.6–7.5)
Periodontal disease	2.8 (1.9–4.1)
Pneumococcal pneumonia	2.6 (1.9–3.5)
Meningococcal disease	2.4 (0.9–6.6)
Influenza	2.4 (1.5–3.8)
Helicobacter pylori	2.2 (1.2–4.0)
Common cold	1.5 (1.1–1.8)

CI, confidence interval; HIV, human immunodeficiency virus.

is highly effective in a relatively short period of time in the prevention of infection.[44]

Cigarette smoking is associated with an increased risk for bacterial and viral infections (Table 65.3). Cigarette smoking is a substantial risk factor for pneumococcal pneumonia, especially in patients with COPD. Smoking is strongly associated with invasive pneumococcal disease in otherwise healthy adults.[18] A population-based case-control study showed smoking was the strongest independent risk factor for invasive pneumococcal disease among immunocompetent adults. The OR was 4.1 (95% CI, 2.4 to 7.3) for active smoking and 2.5 (95% CI, 1.2 to 5.1) for passive smoke exposure in nonsmokers compared to nonexposed nonsmokers. The attributable risk in this population was 51% for cigarette smoking and 17% for passive smoking, with a strong dose response. The risk for pneumococcal disease declined to nonsmoker levels 10 years after cessation. Cigarette smoking has also been shown to be associated with a nearly twofold increased risk for community-acquired pneumonia, with 32% of the risk attributable to cigarette smoking.[46]

Cigarette smoking increases both the incidence and severity of viral infections, including the common cold, influenza, and varicella. Influenza infections are more severe, with more cough, acute and chronic phlegm production, breathlessness, and wheezing in smokers.[17] Influenza infections produce more lost workdays in smokers compared to nonsmokers. Influenza vaccination is effective in preventing the disease in smokers, and smoking should be considered a high-priority indication for influenza vaccination. The development of varicella pneumonitis in adults is reported to be substantially greater in smokers compared to nonsmokers.[47] Of interest are early epidemiology studies of smoking and COVID-19 (SARS-CoV-2) infection. These studies suggest that smokers are less likely to become infected and less likely to be hospitalized but, once hospitalized, are more likely to progress in severity and more likely to die than never or former smokers.[48,49]

Tuberculosis is perhaps the most important smoking-associated infection. Cigarette smoking is a risk factor for tuberculin skin test reactivity, skin test conversion, and the development of active tuberculosis. A large case-control study from India examined smoking and tuberculosis in

men between 35 and 69 years of age. The tuberculosis prevalence *relative risk* (RR) was 2.9 (95% CI, 2.6 to 3.3) with ever smokers compared to never smokers, and the prevalence was higher with a higher level of cigarette consumption.[50] The mortality from tuberculosis among men 25 to 69 years old showed an RR of 4.5 (95% CI, 4.0 to 5.0) and 4.2 (95% CI, 3.7 to 4.8) for urban and rural residents, respectively. The authors found that the proportion of deaths from tuberculosis attributable to smoking was 61% greater than the proportion of deaths from vascular disease or cancer attributable to smoking. Thus, it is likely that smoking contributes substantially to the worldwide disease burden of tuberculosis.[51]

Of historical interest is the relationship between tuberculosis and the risk for cigarette smoking in the early 20th century. Before that time, chewing tobacco was the preferred type of tobacco. Public fear that users of chewing tobacco who spit in public places might be spreading tuberculosis is one of the factors that led to the increase in cigarette sales in the United States. This is nicely described by Kluger[52] as follows:

"Chewing tobacco was no longer merely messy but socially disagreeable in more crowded urban America, and its inevitable byproduct, spitting, was now identified as a spreader of tuberculosis and other contagions, and thus an official health menace. The leisurely pipe all at once seemed a remnant of a slower-tempo age, and cigar fumes were newly offensive amid thronged city life. The cigarette by contrast, could be quickly consumed and easily snuffed out on the job as well as to and from work."

Cardiovascular Disease

Although not the focus of this text, cardiovascular disease is common in patients with respiratory disease and often complicates management of respiratory illness. This relates to the fact that both diseases are common and both increase with age, and that smoking is a major risk factor for both respiratory disease and cardiovascular disease.

Cigarette smoking accounts for about 20% of cardiovascular deaths in the United States. Risks are increased for coronary artery disease, sudden death, cerebrovascular disease, and peripheral vascular disease, including abdominal aortic aneurysm.[9,53] Cigarette smoking accelerates atherosclerosis and promotes acute ischemic events. The mechanisms of the effects of cigarette smoking include (1) hemodynamic stress (nicotine increases the heart rate, transiently increases blood pressure, and increases myocardial work), (2) endothelial injury and dysfunction (nitric oxide release and resultant vasodilation are impaired), (3) development of an atherogenic lipid profile (smokers have on average higher low-density lipoprotein, more oxidized low-density lipoprotein, and lower high-density lipoprotein cholesterol than nonsmokers do), (4) enhanced coagulability, (5) arrhythmogenesis, and (6) relative hypoxemia from the effects of carbon monoxide.[54] As a compensation for the reduced oxygen-carrying capacity, polycythemia often develops in smokers, with hematocrit values of 50% or more. The polycythemia and the increased fibrinogen levels found in cigarette smokers also increase blood viscosity, which adds to the risk of thrombotic events. Cigarette smoking also produces insulin resistance, increases the risk of non–insulin-dependent diabetes, and induces a chronic inflammatory state, as evidenced by increased neutrophil count and increased levels of fibrinogen and C-reactive protein in the blood of smokers. Insulin resistance and chronic inflammation are thought to contribute to accelerated atherogenesis.

Cigarette smoking acts synergistically with other cardiac risk factors to increase the risk of ischemic heart disease. Although the risk of cardiovascular disease is roughly proportional to cigarette consumption, the risk persists even at low levels of smoking, that is, at one to two cigarettes per day.[55] Cigarette smoking reduces exercise tolerance in patients with angina pectoris and intermittent claudication. Vasospastic angina is more common, and the response to vasodilator medication is impaired in patients who smoke. The number of episodes and total duration of ischemic episodes, as assessed by ambulatory electrocardiographic monitoring in patients with coronary heart disease, are substantially increased by cigarette smoking.[56] The increase in relative risk of coronary heart disease because of cigarette smoking is greatest in young adults who, in the absence of cigarette smoking, would have a relatively low risk.[53] Women who use oral contraceptives and smoke cigarettes have a synergistically increased risk of both myocardial infarction and stroke. Data suggest that implementing smoking bans at the community level has an appreciable impact on lowering hospital admission rates for coronary artery disease.[57,58]

After acute myocardial infarction, the risk of recurrent myocardial infarction is higher, and survival is half over the next 12 years in persistent smokers as compared with quitters.[59] Smoking also interferes with revascularization therapy for acute myocardial infarction. After thrombolysis, the reocclusion rate is fourfold higher in smokers who continue than in those who quit.[60] The risk of reocclusion of a coronary artery after angioplasty or of occlusion of a bypass graft is increased in smokers.[61] Cigarette smoking is not a risk factor for hypertension per se but does increase the risk of complications, including the development of nephrosclerosis and progression to malignant hypertension.[62] Cigarette smoking has been shown to be a substantial contributor to morbidity and mortality in patients with left ventricular dysfunction. The mortality benefit of stopping smoking in such patients is equal to or greater than the benefit of therapy with angiotensin-converting enzyme inhibitors, β-blockers, or spironolactone.[63]

Wound Healing/Postoperative Complications

Cigarette smoking is a major cause of adverse postoperative events and delayed wound healing.[64,65] The mechanisms include cutaneous vasoconstriction (reducing skin blood flow), local thrombosis, and reduced oxygen-carrying capacity, all of which can delay tissue repair. Impaired clearance of secretions, altered immune function, altered collagen synthesis, and the influence of underlying tobacco-related diseases (e.g., COPD and altered cardiovascular function) also contribute to postoperative complications.

A meta-analysis of 107 studies found that smoking within 30 days of operation significantly increased complications as follows: general morbidity (RR, 1.5), wound complications (RR, 2.2), infections (RR, 1.5), pulmonary complications (RR, 1.7), neurologic complications (RR, 1.4), and admission to an intensive care unit (RR, 1.6).[64] A study of 489 adult patients undergoing ambulatory surgery demonstrated a significantly higher rate of respiratory complications (32.8% in smokers vs. 25.9% in nonsmokers) and wound infections (3.6% in smokers vs. 0.6% in nonsmokers).[66] Causes of major pulmonary events after pneumonectomy were sought in a retrospective analysis of 261 patients.[67] Patients who continued to smoke within 1 month of operation were determined to be at an increased risk of pulmonary events, which was associated with increased postoperative mortality. Cigarette smoking is associated with an increased risk of hepatic artery thrombosis after liver transplantation, and cessation 2 years before transplantation was associated with a decreased risk.[68] Similar data exist regarding renal transplantation and allograft survival in smokers compared to nonsmokers.[69] Recent studies describe substantially increased risk of postoperative complications in elective plastic surgery procedures, of wound complications after coronary bypass surgery, and of marginal ulcers after Roux-en-Y gastric bypass.[70-72]

Smoking cessation substantially reduces postoperative complications. Moller and colleagues[73] published the results of a randomized, controlled trial of smokers awaiting elective hip or knee surgery at three hospitals in Copenhagen. They compared 56 patients in a smoking cessation intervention arm (83% stopped or reduced smoking) versus 62 patients in a usual care arm. The overall complication rate was 18% in the intervention arm and 52% in the control group, a highly significant difference. The greatest differences were seen in wound complication rates (5% vs. 31%, respectively) and cardiovascular complications (0% vs. 2%, respectively).

The optimal window for smoking cessation intervention may be at 8 weeks before elective surgery, as suggested by data demonstrating that patients who had stopped smoking at least 2 months preoperatively had nearly maximal reduction in postoperative respiratory complications.[74] A meta-analysis of six trials of smoking cessation found that cessation reduced postoperative complications by 41% and that each week of cessation increased the magnitude of benefit by 19%.[75] An important issue related to elective surgery is that patients are often highly motivated to quit smoking just before surgery and can benefit from cessation counseling before surgery, as well as from in-hospital cessation counseling and medication in the postoperative setting. Specific issues related to smoking cessation are discussed in Chapter 66.

Other Complications of Cigarette Smoking

Cigarette smoking increases the risk of duodenal and gastric ulcers, delays the rate of ulcer healing, and increases the risk of relapse after ulcer treatment.[76] Smoking is also associated with esophageal reflux symptoms. Smoking produces ulcer disease by several proposed mechanisms: increasing acid secretion, reducing pancreatic bicarbonate secretion, impairing the gastric mucosal barrier (related to decreased gastric mucosal blood flow and/or inhibition of prostaglandin synthesis), reducing pyloric sphincter tone, and increasing the risk of *Helicobacter pylori* infection.[77]

Cigarette smoking is a risk factor for osteoporosis in that it reduces the peak bone mass attained in early adulthood and increases the rate of bone loss in later adulthood. Smoking antagonizes the protective effect of estrogen replacement therapy on the risk of osteoporosis in postmenopausal women.[78] Hip fractures are more common in women who smoke cigarettes. Cigarette smoking is a major cause of reproductive problems, including fetal growth restriction, preeclampsia, stillbirth, perinatal mortality, and sudden infant death syndrome.[79] Growth retardation from cigarette smoking has been termed *fetal tobacco syndrome*.[80] Cigarette smoking causes reproductive complications by causing placental ischemia mediated by the hypoxic effects of chronic carbon monoxide exposure, endothelial dysfunction, and the general increase in coagulability produced by oxidant chemicals in cigarette smoke.[81]

Other adverse effects of cigarette smoking include premature facial wrinkling, an increased risk of cataracts, age-related macular degeneration, olfactory dysfunction, and fire-related injuries. The last effect contributes significantly to the economic costs of tobacco use. Smoking reduces the secretion of thyroid hormone in women with subclinical hypothyroidism and increases the severity of clinical symptoms of hypothyroidism in women with subclinical or overt hypothyroidism, the latter effect reflecting antagonism of thyroid hormone action.[82] Cigarette smoking also potentially interacts with a variety of drugs by accelerating drug metabolism or by the pharmacologic interactions that nicotine and/or other constituents of tobacco have with other drugs (see Chapter 66).

Health Hazards of Secondhand Smoke

Considerable evidence indicates that exposure to secondhand smoke is harmful to the health of nonsmokers (Table 65.4).[83] The U.S. Environmental Protection Agency classifies secondhand smoke as a class A carcinogen, which means that it has been shown to cause cancer in humans.[84]

Secondhand smoke consists both of *sidestream* smoke generated while the cigarette is smoldering and of *mainstream* smoke exhaled by the smoker. Of the total combustion product from a cigarette, 75% or more enters the air. The constituents of secondhand tobacco smoke are qualitatively similar to those of mainstream smoke. However, some toxins, such as ammonia, formaldehyde, and nitrosamines, are present in much higher concentrations in secondhand tobacco smoke than in mainstream smoke. The Environmental Protection Agency has estimated that secondhand smoke is responsible for approximately 3000 lung cancer deaths annually in nonsmokers in the United States, is causally associated with 150,000 to 300,000 cases of lower respiratory tract infection in infants and young children up to 18 months of age, and is causally associated with the aggravation of asthma in 200,000 to 1 million children.[84] Secondhand smoke exposure promotes atherosclerosis and thrombosis by multiple mechanisms[85] and is estimated to be responsible for 40,000 cardiovascular deaths.[86] An appreciation of the hazards of secondhand tobacco smoke is important to the physician because it provides a basis for advising parents not to smoke when children are in the home,[87] insisting that child care facilities be smoke free, and recommending smoking restrictions in work sites and other public places.

TABLE 65.4 Health Hazards of Secondhand Tobacco Smoke in Nonsmokers

Children	Adults
Hospitalization for respiratory tract infection in first year of life	Lung cancer
Chronic respiratory symptoms	Myocardial infarction
Middle ear disease	Stroke
Asthma	Reduced pulmonary function
Reduced birth weight (maternal exposure)	Irritation of eyes, nasal congestion, headache
Sudden infant death syndrome	Cough

ELECTRONIC CIGARETTES

E-cigarettes, or electronic nicotine delivery devices, heat a nicotine solution to generate an aerosol that is inhaled without the combustion of tobacco and its toxic constituents. *Vaping* refers to the act of using of an e-cigarette. These devices have evolved substantially over the last decade but have in common (1) a reservoir that contains an e-liquid (propylene glycol, vegetable glycerin, nicotine, and flavorings), (2) a resistance metal coil (nickel, chromium, stainless steel, or a related alloy) that heats the e-liquid, (3) a wick (typically made of silica or cotton) that conducts the e-liquid to the coil, and (4) a battery that supplies electric current to the coil in response to airflow or a button push initiated by the user, generating a plume of small droplets (aerosol) (Table 65.5). E-cigarettes have been marketed with claims of health benefit compared with smoking cigarettes; they are marketed for use in reducing and quitting smoking, for use when a person is forbidden to smoke cigarettes, and for avoiding generating smelly and irritating secondhand smoke. The use of e-cigarettes in the United States has increased substantially since they were first marketed in 2006, with 2.8% (6.9 million) current e-cigarette users in 2017.[5] A concerning trend has been the explosive increase in e-cigarette use by young people, with 28% of high school students and 11% of middle school students reporting current e-cigarette use in 2019.[88]

As of 2020, there are thousands of e-cigarette devices on the U.S. market, and they vary with respect to size, power, coil architecture and metal type, and cartridge design. Some look like cigarettes and are disposable; others look like pens or cigars and have refillable tanks. E-cigarette liquids are sold over the Internet or in vape shops, in which the user can select the liquid, including the vehicle (varying proportions of propylene glycol and vegetable glycerin), nicotine concentration, and flavor. Over the last 3 years, pod-based devices with USB-compatible batteries, such as JUUL, have captured the majority of market share, in part because of overwhelming popularity with younger users.[88,89] Nicotine aerosolization depends on coil temperature (power), airflow, and the concentration of nicotine in the e-liquid, which ranges from 3 mg/mL or less for high-power devices to 60 mg/mL or higher for low-power devices, such as JUUL. More recently, vaping devices have been developed to aerosolize more viscous substances, such as *tetrahydrocannabinol* (THC) and cannabidiol-containing oils derived from cannabis. Vaping of THC-containing liquids has recently been implicated in an outbreak of severe acute respiratory disease (see "Cannabis" section).

TABLE 65.5   E-Cigarette Designs, Descriptions, and Brand Names*

Product	Description	Sample Brands†
Disposable e-cigarette	Cigarette-shaped device consisting of a battery and a cartridge containing an atomizer to heat a solution (with or without nicotine). Not rechargeable or refillable and is intended to be discarded after product stops producing vapor.	NJOY, Blu, Green Smoke
Rechargeable e-cigarette	Cigarette-shaped device consisting of a battery that connects to an atomizer used to heat a solution typically containing nicotine. Often contains an element that regulates puff duration and/or how many puffs may be taken consecutively.	V2 Cigs, Halo G6, MarkTen
Pen-style, medium-sized rechargeable e-cigarette	Larger than a cigarette, often with a higher-capacity battery, may contain a prefilled cartridge or a refillable cartridge (often called a clearomizer). These devices often come with a manual switch allowing the smoker to regulate length and frequency of puffs.	eGo, Kanger EVOD, Halo Triton
Tank-style, large-sized rechargeable e-cigarette	Much larger than a cigarette with a higher-capacity battery and typically contains a large, refillable cartridge. Often contains manual switches and a battery casing for customizing battery capacity. Can be easily modified.	Kanger Aerotank, Innokin iClear, Aspire Nautilus
Pod-style e-cigarette	Low-power devices, typically USB-rechargeable; e-liquid pods typically contain a high concentration of nicotine. Some pods are refillable.	JUUL, SMOK, Aspire AVP

*E-cigarettes come in various sizes and designs. All contain a cartridge, a heating element, and a battery and provide an aerosol containing nicotine.
†Some brands may have been discontinued.
Modified from Grana R, Benowitz N, Glantz SA. Background paper on e-cigarettes (electronic nicotine delivery systems). Prepared for the 7th Meeting of the WHO Study Group on Tobacco Product Regulation. San Francisco: University of California; 2013.

PULMONARY TOXICITY

Given the relatively recent introduction of e-cigarettes, it is not surprising that their health effects are controversial and poorly characterized. Indeed, it took many decades for the toxicity of combustible cigarettes to be fully appreciated. The simpler chemical nature of e-cigarette aerosol, lacking many of the harmful components of cigarette smoke, would seem to predict less short- and long-term pulmonary toxicity, but few rigorous studies have been performed.

Population-based studies of e-cigarette users have revealed increased reports of chronic cough, sputum production,[90–92] asthma diagnoses,[93,94] and dyspnea,[94] although limitations of all of these studies include a reliance on self-reporting and frequent dual use of e-cigarettes with combustible cigarettes. Chronic smokers who are able to switch from cigarettes to e-cigarettes typically report improvements in respiratory symptoms,[95,96] but most of these studies have not rigorously compared e-cigarette use to quitting smoking without the use of e-cigarettes. A recent study from the United Kingdom randomized 886 smokers interested in cessation, using e-cigarettes or nicotine-replacement therapies as choices. The primary outcome, 1-year abstinence from cigarettes, was more frequent in the e-cigarette group (18.0% vs. 9.9%, RR, 1.8 [CI, 1.3 to 2.6], respectively). Those randomized to e-cigarettes also had significant reductions in self-reported cough and wheeze, effects not fully accounted for by the increase in abstinence from smoking.[97]

Acutely, e-cigarette aerosol has variably been shown to cause obstructive physiology,[98–100] but whether long-term use results in persistent changes in spirometry is not yet clear. Bronchoscopic studies of healthy e-cigarette users have revealed erythematous mucosa with increased levels of inflammatory mucin proteins and damaging enzymes, including elastase, although many or most of the participants were former smokers.[101,102] Of note, the toxicity of e-cigarette aerosol is likely to be greater under high coil temperature conditions, which increase the production of toxic aldehydes and other oxidizing chemicals. A recent study in healthy young occasional cigarette smokers demonstrated impaired gas exchange after 15 minutes vaping an aerosol from a high-wattage (60-watt) device.[103] Case reports have identified several patterns of e-cigarette–associated respiratory disease, including organizing pneumonia, lipoid pneumonia, barotrauma, and hypersensitivity pneumonitis, although the incidence of these diseases and attributable risk from e-cigarettes at the population level remains unclear.[104] Experiments exposing mice to several months of e-cigarette aerosol have demonstrated major changes in surfactant and lipid metabolism, including oil-filled macrophages that stain with oil red O.[105]

E-CIGARETTES AND SMOKING CESSATION

There is currently considerable debate in the public health community about the safety and benefit of e-cigarettes. Most agree that e-cigarettes could be a health benefit if people would use e-cigarettes and stop smoking cigarettes entirely. A recent clinical trial demonstrated that e-cigarettes enhance smoking cessation with a substantially greater benefit than nicotine medication, although 80% of those who quit smoking with e-cigarettes continued to vape at 1 year.[97] Epidemiology studies in the United States find that regular use of e-cigarettes is associated with higher rates of quitting smoking, whereas other studies find that dual use of cigarettes and e-cigarettes may be associated with lower quit rates.[106,107] Many e-cigarette users report smoking fewer cigarettes per day while using e-cigarettes, but the health benefits of such reductions are not clear.

OTHER POTENTIAL TOXICITIES OF E-CIGARETTES

In addition to pulmonary toxicity, which was discussed earlier, there are concerns that e-cigarette use may cause cardiovascular toxicity, reproductive toxicity, and possibly impair brain development in adolescents. Whereas products of combustion are thought to be the main mediators of smoking-induced cardiovascular disease, constituents of concern with e-cigarettes include oxidant chemicals, nicotine, particulates, and possibly metals.[108]

The manner in which an e-cigarette is puffed depends on the concentration of nicotine in the e-liquid,[109] the power of the device,[110] and prior cigarette use,[111] among other factors. Similarly, aerosols generated by e-cigarettes vary based on the device, power setting, e-liquid composition, and characteristics of the puff, with longer puffs resulting in higher coil temperatures and greater carbonyl production.[112] Broadly speaking, e-cigarettes produce much lower levels of oxidants than cigarettes while delivering similar levels of nicotine and particulates. The particulates in e-cigarette aerosol are similar in number and size distribution to those in cigarette smoke but are primarily liquid, rather than carbonaceous, and their toxicity is unknown. Nicotine causes sympathetic neural activation, which has some potentially deleterious effects on cardiovascular hemodynamics (increased heart rate, blood pressure, and myocardial contractility) and may impair endothelial function and promote insulin resistance; however, its effects are certainly much less than those of the combustion products in cigarette smoke. Acutely, e-cigarette use produces endothelial dysfunction similar to cigarette smoking, but when smokers switch from cigarettes to e-cigarettes, endothelial function substantially improves.[113] E-cigarette use can enhance platelet aggregation, an effect not related to nicotine, but long-term effects on coagulation are unknown.[114,115] Nicotine has neuroteratogenic effects in the fetus, but e-cigarettes are likely less toxic than smoking, which exposes the fetus not just to nicotine but also to myriad other reproductive toxins.[116] In adolescent rodents, nicotine impairs brain maturation, which has been a concern in light of the large number of young people now using e-cigarettes, but whether nicotine will impair brain maturation in people has been difficult to assess due to many social and environmental confounders.[117]

The *U.S. Food and Drug Administration* (FDA) has the authority to regulate e-cigarettes but has only very recently begun to promulgate regulations.[118] FDA regulation will be particularly useful to ensure the safety of these products, limit marketing and access to youth, and restrict use in situations where smoking is banned—both to minimize environmental pollution with e-cigarette vapor and to mitigate the renormalization of smoking behavior. Some clinicians recommend and/or support e-cigarette use in patients who have been unable to quit smoking using traditional counseling and medications, although the use of e-cigarettes in such a role is not approved by the FDA.

CANNABIS

During the past decade, many U.S. states have legalized cannabis for medical or recreational use and, although federal laws remain on the books, enforcement has declined, with nearly 9.8% of the U.S. population 12 years of age and older reporting use during the past month in 2017–18 compared to 6.4% in 2008–09.[119] Use frequency varies widely, with approximately 4 million U.S. residents estimated to have *cannabis use disorder* in 2016.[120] Furthermore, with the growth of the marketplace for cannabis and its psychoactive constituent, THC, the last several years has seen the extraordinary growth of new methods of consumption. These include the extraction of THC using butane and other solvents into waxes and oils, which are then heated and inhaled, and the development of new vape pens designed to aerosolize viscous liquids, including oils.[121] These novel methods of use have the potential to deliver concentrations of THC that exceed the use of combustible cannabis by an order of magnitude, with unknown consequences for addiction and health.[122]

PULMONARY TOXICITY

In contrast to cigarette smoke, comparatively little is known about cannabis-related pulmonary toxicity, and what is known nearly exclusively concerns traditional combustible cannabis use. Not surprisingly, cannabis smoke contains many of the same carcinogens and toxicants as cigarette smoke; perhaps surprisingly, cannabis smoking has been associated with greater increases in carboxyhemoglobin and inhaled tar per "cigarette" than cigarette smoking.[123] Typically, cannabis smoke is inhaled less frequently, but more deeply, and includes a long breath-holding time.[123] Coughing at near-total lung capacity likely explains the association of cannabis smoking with barotrauma, including pneumothorax and pneumomediastinum.[124] Most studies of chronic cannabis smoking have reported increased symptoms of upper airway irritation, including laryngitis, wheezing, and chronic cough and sputum production.[125,126]

Few high-quality studies of pulmonary function have been performed, with some showing reductions in forced expiratory volume in 1 second/forced vital capacity and reduced diffusing capacity but others showing no differences compared to control subjects.[126] Of note, two studies using high-resolution computed tomography scans have not found evidence that cannabis smoking causes emphysema.[127,128] Bronchoalveolar lavage studies have revealed increased neutrophils and alveolar macrophages,[129] with impaired responses to bacterial challenge.[130] Of importance, pulmonary fungal infections have been reported in cannabis smokers who are immunocompromised by diabetes mellitus, leukemia, and chronic steroid use.[131] Despite containing many of the same carcinogens as tobacco smoke, cannabis smoke has not been clearly linked to lung cancer.[132] Most likely this is because cannabis smoking is generally much less frequent than cigarette smoking.

In the summer of 2019, a new syndrome of severe acute hypoxemic respiratory failure/acute respiratory distress syndrome was described, notable for the development of diffuse ground-glass opacities on computed tomography scan (frequently with subpleural sparing) in the context of gastrointestinal and constitutional symptoms.[133] Termed EVALI, this syndrome has been linked to the use of mostly illicitly produced THC-containing vape pens. At the time of this writing the etiology remains unclear, but high levels of vitamin E acetate have been found in many of the implicated devices and nearly all of the bronchoalveolar lavage samples of EVALI patients, suggesting that the toxicity may be due to vitamin E acetate.[134] Vitamin E acetate is used as a cutting agent for THC oil for resale or in the THC oil extraction process due to its similar viscosity and aerosol appearance. The Centers for Disease Control and Prevention have published recommendations for evaluating and caring for EVALI patients.[135]

CARDIOVASCULAR TOXICITY

The use of cannabis products containing THC has been associated with acute cardiovascular events, including myocardial infarction, stroke, arrhythmias, and sudden death.[136–138] The cardiovascular toxicity of marijuana smoking can be viewed as a result of one or more of these mechanisms: inhalation of combustion products (with a similar toxicity to cigarette smoking); direct sympathomimetic and other cardiovascular effects of THC; and indirect effects of THC related to extreme anxiety, hallucinations, and/or psychosis.[136] THC use acutely increases heart rate (20–100%), which can be associated with supine hypertension and increased myocardial work. Systemic catecholamine release can constrict coronary arteries and/or activate platelets. The net result can be markedly increased myocardial work and oxygen demand combined with an inadequate compensatory increase in coronary blood flow, resulting in myocardial ischemia or infarction. THC can also produce orthostatic hypotension, which poses a risk in the elderly. The cardiovascular impact of THC depends on the product (marijuana leaf vs. THC oil vs. edibles), dose consumed, route of administration, pattern of use, and degree of tolerance. Cardiovascular toxicity is likely to be greater in people with underlying cardiovascular disease.

COCAINE AND METHAMPHETAMINE

Cocaine and methamphetamine are sympathomimetic drugs that produce vasoconstriction, tachycardia, and hypertension. Cocaine hydrochloride may be inhaled nasally or injected; its free base form ("crack") can be smoked by a pipe or mixed with other substances, such as tobacco or cannabis, and smoked or vaped in an e-cigarette. Co-use of other substances with cocaine has made it challenging to discern its unique pulmonary toxicities. Smoking crack cocaine can result in hemorrhagic alveolitis and

diffuse alveolar damage with a prominent eosinophilic inflammatory component.[139] Pulmonary edema may be increased due to elevated left ventricular end-diastolic pressures related to cocaine's acute vasoconstricting and hypertensive effects. Other patterns of disease reported with cocaine include acute eosinophilic pneumonia,[140] barotrauma,[141] emphysema,[142] and pulmonary hypertension.[143] Excipients (i.e., inactive materials used as the vehicle for a drug), including talc and cotton, have been associated with foreign body granulomatosis,[144] and adulterants, including levamisole, have caused systemic illness, including vasculitis[145] (see Chapter 99).

Like cocaine, methamphetamine can be taken intravenously or smoked. Its use has been associated with many of the same pulmonary diseases as cocaine, including cardiogenic pulmonary edema and diffuse alveolar damage.[146] One important difference is that methamphetamine is more frequently associated with a progressive form of pulmonary hypertension that carries a dismal prognosis.[147] Both cocaine and methamphetamine can cause acute cardiovascular injury, including myocardial infarction, stroke, and dissecting aortic aneurysm, as well as aggravate ischemia in users with underlying cardiovascular disease. For patients suffering from pulmonary toxicity from cocaine and methamphetamine, the cornerstones of management are cessation counseling and supportive care. In addition, acute eosinophilic lung disease and organizing pneumonia may respond to corticosteroid therapy.[140]

Key Points

- Tobacco use remains the leading global risk factor for disability-adjusted years of life lost.
- In addition to causing cancer and COPD, smoking increases the risk for other pulmonary diseases, including respiratory infection (including pneumococcal pneumonia and tuberculosis), asthma, interstitial lung disease, and acute respiratory distress syndrome; it also increases the incidence of cardiopulmonary complications after surgery and in critically ill patients.
- Smoking causes 20% of cardiovascular deaths and increases the risk of peptic ulcer disease, diabetes mellitus, and osteoporosis.
- Secondhand smoke causes tens of thousands of cardiovascular deaths and several thousand lung cancer deaths annually.
- Electronic cigarettes deliver nicotine in an aerosol of propylene glycol, vegetable glycerin, and flavorings, and use has increased over the last 15 years, markedly so among young people, with 28% of high school students reporting current use in a 2019 survey.
- The health risks of electronic cigarettes and potential benefits in smokers remain controversial.
- Electronic cigarette/vaping–associated lung injury is a newly described syndrome of acute respiratory distress syndrome of unclear mechanism associated with vaping THC obtained from the black market.
- Cocaine and methamphetamine have acute cardiovascular toxicity and are associated with pulmonary edema, alveolar hemorrhage, emphysema, and pulmonary hypertension.

Key Readings

Agusti A, Hogg JC. Update on the pathogenesis of chronic obstructive pulmonary disease. *N Engl J Med.* 2019;381:1248–1256.

Barraza LF, Weidenaar KE, Cook LT, Logue AR, Halpern MT. Regulations and policies regarding e-cigarettes. *Cancer.* 2017;123(16):3007–3014.

DiGiacomo SI, Jazayeri M-A, Barua RS, Ambrose JA. Environmental tobacco smoke and cardiovascular disease. *Int J Environ Res Public Health.* 2018;16(1).

Gotts JE, Jordt S-E, McConnell R, Tarran R. What are the respiratory effects of e-cigarettes? *BMJ.* 2019;366:l5275.

Gronkjaer M, Eliasen M, Skov-Ettrup LS, et al. Preoperative smoking status and postoperative complications: a systematic review and meta-analysis. *Ann Surg.* 2014;259(1):52–71.

Hajek P, Phillips-Waller A, Przulj D, et al. A randomized trial of e-cigarettes versus nicotine-replacement therapy. *N Engl J Med.* 2019;380(7):629–637.

Huttunen R, Heikkinen T, Syrjänen J. Smoking and the outcome of infection. *J Intern Med.* 2011;269:258–269.

Jha P, Ramasundarahettige C, Landsman V, et al. 21st-century hazards of smoking and benefits of cessation in the United States. *N Engl J Med.* 2013;368:341–350.

Margaritopoulos GA, Vasarmidi E, Jacob J, Wells AU, Antoniou KM. Smoking and interstitial lung diseases. *Eur Respir Rev.* 2015;24(137):428–435.

Mills E, Eyawo O, Lockhart I, et al. Smoking cessation reduces postoperative complications: a systematic review and meta-analysis. *Am J Med.* 2011;124:144–154.

Morris MA, Jacobson SR, Kinney GL, et al. Marijuana use associations with pulmonary symptoms and function in tobacco smokers enrolled in the subpopulations and intermediate outcome measures in COPD Study (SPIROMICS). *Chronic Obstr Pulm Dis.* 2018;5(1):46–56.

Oh CK, Murray LA, Molfino NA. Smoking and idiopathic pulmonary fibrosis. *Pulm Med.* 2012;2012:808260.

Vanker A, Gie RP, Zar HJ. The association between environmental tobacco smoke exposure and childhood respiratory disease: a review. *Expert Rev Respir Med.* 2017;11(8):661–673.

Woodruff PG, Barr RG, Bleecker E, et al. Clinical significance of symptoms in smokers with preserved pulmonary function. *N Engl J Med.* 2016;374(19):1811–1821.

Complete reference list available at ExpertConsult.com.

66 *SMOKING CESSATION*

PAUL G. BRUNETTA, MD • LISA KROON, PHARMD

INTRODUCTION

Pulmonologists have a highly experienced view of the burden of tobacco-related diseases, which are reviewed in Chapter 65. Unfortunately, pulmonary specialists may have little understanding of the neuropsychiatric impact of nicotine addiction and the psychological underpinning of chronic tobacco use. Consequently, many providers may not be comfortable prescribing smoking cessation medications and thus may not provide optimal tobacco cessation support. The U.S. Public Health Service Guidelines recommend that all health care providers practice the "5 A's" as the primary approach for smoking cessation: (1) ask about tobacco use, (2) advise to quit, (3) assess readiness to quit, (4) assist in connecting to tobacco treatment, and (5) arrange follow-up to review progress toward quitting.[1] Despite the clarity of this approach, only 20.9% of smokers in the United States are provided counseling, and only 7.6% receive cessation medications.[2,3] Even in the setting in which a smoker develops cancer, a 2009 survey of National Cancer Institute–designated cancer centers revealed that only 21% of patients were offered cessation treatment services, and only 62% routinely received tobacco-education materials. This core gap is now being addressed by the National Cancer Institute Moonshot program, which has launched a national Cancer Center Cessation Initiative, providing support and grants to 20 centers in the United States.[4] The Department of Health and Human Services devoted the U.S. Surgeon General's 2020 report entirely to smoking cessation, underscoring the importance of preventing tobacco-related disease.[5] With this recent background in mind, this chapter is designed to familiarize health care practitioners with currently available support options, counseling, smoking cessation medications, and trends in their use.

Medications are a key component to increase the chance a smoker will quit successfully. Spontaneous cessation with the "cold turkey" approach (without medications or counseling) yields only a 2–5% cessation rate at 1 year.[2,3] Many smokers try unsuccessfully on multiple occasions to quit with an unsupported approach before a health care provider may start to discuss tobacco use. The combination of medications and counseling/behavioral support will provide patients with the best chance of quitting successfully. The availability of *nicotine replacement therapy* (NRT) *over the counter* (OTC) is important for some patients who may not interact with a health care provider during their quit attempt.[6]

NICOTINE ADDICTION

Tobacco use is motivated primarily by the desire for nicotine. Drug addiction is defined as the compulsive use of a psychoactive substance in which the consequences are detrimental to the individual or society. Understanding addiction is useful in providing effective smoking cessation therapy.[7] Nicotine is absorbed rapidly from tobacco smoke or e-cigarette vapor into the pulmonary circulation. It then moves quickly to the brain, where it acts on nicotinic cholinergic receptors to produce its gratifying effects within 10 to 15 seconds after a puff. Chronic exposure to high levels of nicotine will cause an increased concentration of nicotinic receptors in different regions of the brain, accounting for the development of tolerance and intense withdrawal symptoms. Nicotine has a half-life of approximately 2 hours. Nicotine from smokeless tobacco is absorbed more slowly and results in less intense acute pharmacologic effects. With long-term use of tobacco, physical dependence develops, associated with an increased number of nicotinic cholinergic receptors in the brain[8,9] (Fig. 66.1). When nicotine is unavailable, even for only a few hours, withdrawal symptoms begin, including anxiety, irritability, difficulty concentrating, restlessness, hunger, craving for tobacco, disturbed sleep and, in some people, depression.

Addiction to nicotine is multifactorial, including a desire for the direct pharmacologic actions of nicotine, relief of withdrawal symptoms, and learned associations. Smokers report a variety of reasons for smoking, including pleasure, arousal, enhanced vigilance, improved performance, relief of anxiety or depression, reduced hunger, and control of body weight. Environmental cues, such as after eating a meal, drinking coffee or an alcoholic beverage, talking on the phone, or being around friends who smoke, often trigger an urge to smoke. Compared to the general population

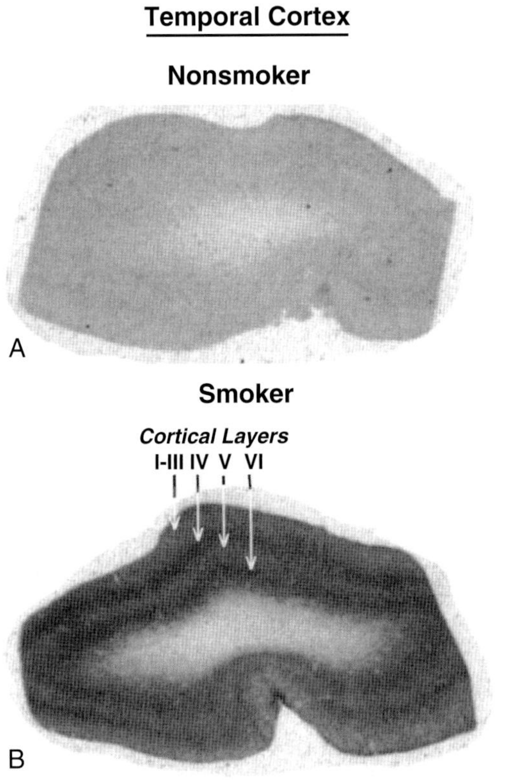

Temporal Cortex

Nonsmoker

A

Smoker

Cortical Layers
I-III IV V VI

B

Figure 66.1 Increased nicotinic receptors in the brains of smokers. A representative autoradiographic image of radiolabeled ligand binding to nicotinic receptors in comparable sections of autopsy-derived human temporal cerebral cortex from a nonsmoker (A) and a smoker (B). In the smoker, nicotinic receptors are clearly increased throughout multiple cortical layers. (From Perry DC, Dávila-García MI, Stockmeier CA, Kellar KJ. Increased nicotinic receptors in brains from smokers: membrane binding and autoradiography studies. *J Pharmacol Exp Ther.* 1999;289:1545–1552.)

in the United States, United Kingdom, and Australia, smoking is two to three times more prevalent among people with mental illness. It is particularly high among patients with schizophrenia, bipolar disorder, posttraumatic stress disorder, and alcohol or illicit drug use disorders.[10] Smoking and depression are strongly linked. Smokers are more likely to have a history of major depression than are nonsmokers. Smokers with a history of depression are also likely to be more highly dependent on nicotine and have a lower likelihood of quitting.[11] When they do quit, depression is more apt to be a prominent withdrawal symptom.

Often tobacco use begins in childhood or adolescence.[12] Risk factors for youth smoking include peer and parental influences; behavioral problems (e.g., poor school performance); personality characteristics, such as rebelliousness or risk taking, depression, and anxiety; and genetic influences. The adolescent's desire to appear older and more sophisticated, such as by emulating more mature role models, can be another strong motivator. Environmental influences, such as advertising and smoking in movies, also contribute. Smoking rates among adults have been declining in economically advanced countries. Similarly, initiation rates for youth have gradually declined over the past 3 decades, although this is counterbalanced by the rapid increase of e-cigarette use by youth over the past 5 years. Approaches to preventing tobacco use and addiction in youth include educational activities in schools,

aggressive antitobacco media campaigns, taxation of tobacco products, increasing the age for purchase from 18 to 21 years, changing the social and environmental norms (e.g., restricting indoor smoking and educating parents not to smoke around children), and deglamorizing smoking. Unfortunately, the current e-cigarette epidemic has intensified nicotine addiction in youth, and new data validate that e-cigarette use has increased cigarette use.[13]

NEUROBIOLOGIC MECHANISMS OF ADDICTION

(S)-Nicotine binds stereoselectively to *nicotinic cholinergic receptors* (nAChRs) in the brain, as well as in the autonomic ganglia, the adrenal medulla, and neuromuscular junctions. Most relevant to nicotine addiction are the receptors found throughout the brain, with the greatest number in the cortex, thalamus, and interpeduncular nucleus. There is also substantial binding in the amygdala, septum, brainstem motor nuclei, and locus coeruleus. The nAChR is a ligand-gated ion channel composed of five subunits. Most brain nAChRs are composed of α- and β-subunits. Usually, there are two α- and three β-subunits, with the α-subunits responsible for ligand binding and the β-subunits mediating other aspects of receptor function.[14] Nicotinic receptors in the brain have different chemical conductances for sodium and calcium and sensitivity to nicotinic agonists. Brain imaging studies in smokers have confirmed that smoking causes the upregulation of high-affinity nAChRs, which is maintained for up to 4 weeks after cessation of nicotine exposure.[15–17]

The various nicotinic receptors are believed to mediate different pharmacologic actions of nicotine, perhaps corresponding to the multiple effects of nicotine experienced by human smokers.[18] Adolescent nicotine exposure also appears to alter *gamma-aminobutyric acid* (GABA) signaling in the developing brain but not in the adult brain. GABA receptors are now known to alter the nicotine reward effect, which may have an impact on enhancing alcohol self-administration.[19]

Nicotinic receptor activation facilitates the release of neurotransmitters, including acetylcholine, norepinephrine, dopamine, serotonin, β-endorphin, GABA, and others.[20] Pharmacologically, nicotine is a stimulant. It enhances fast excitatory synaptic transmission, which may contribute to learning and memory.[21,22] Nicotine also releases growth hormone, prolactin, vasopressin, and adrenocorticotropic hormone. Behavioral rewards from nicotine and nicotine addiction appear to be linked largely to dopamine release[23] with an impact from GABA receptors as well.

Nicotine metabolism can vary significantly among individuals. *Cytochrome P-450* (CYP) isoenzymes impact the speed of metabolism and are categorized as poor, extensive, or ultrarapid.[24] These differences can have an impact on smoking behavior and the metabolism of nicotine replacement therapies. In addition, exposure to tobacco smoke has a wide-ranging impact on the metabolism of many drugs. Polycyclic aromatic hydrocarbons, products of combustion in cigarette smoke, upregulate certain CYP enzymes, primarily CYP1A2, and accelerate the metabolism of drugs that go through the CYP1A2 pathway. Several drugs have important pharmacokinetic interactions with smoking.

Table 66.1 Interaction Between Cigarette Smoking and Drugs

DRUGS		Interaction (Effects Compared With Nonsmokers)	Significance
Caffeine	Imipramine	Accelerated metabolism	May require higher doses in smokers, reduced doses after quitting
Chlorpromazine	Lidocaine		
Clozapine	Olanzapine		
Desmethyldiazepam	Oxazepam		
Estradiol	Pentazocine		
Estrone	Phenacetin		
Flecainide	Phenylbutazone		
Fluvoxamine	Propranolol		
Haloperidol	Theophylline		
Combined hormonal contraceptives		Enhanced thrombosis, increased risk of stroke and myocardial infarction	Do not prescribe to smokers, especially if ≥35 years old and smoke ≥15 cigarettes daily
Cimetidine and other H_2-blockers		Lower rate of ulcer healing, higher ulcer recurrence rates	Consider using mucosal protective agents
Propranolol		Less antihypertensive effect, less antianginal efficacy; more effective in reducing mortality after myocardial infarction	Consider the use of cardioselective β-blockers
Nifedipine (and probably other calcium blockers)		Less antianginal effect	May require higher doses and/or multiple-drug antianginal therapy
Diazepam, chlordiazepoxide (and possibly other sedative-hypnotics)		Less sedation	Smokers may need higher doses
Chlorpromazine (and possibly other neuroleptics)		Less sedation, possibly reduced efficacy	Smokers may need higher doses
Propoxyphene		Reduced analgesia	Smokers may need higher doses

Caffeine clearance is increased by more than 50% when a person smokes. Therefore, upon smoking cessation, it is advised that patients cut their caffeine intake by half. Nicotine in tobacco smoke also has pharmacodynamic interactions with certain drugs through antagonistic pharmacologic actions. (See Table 66.1 for pharmacokinetic and pharmacodynamic interactions with smoking.)

Nicotine causes an increase in the firing of ventral tegmental area neurons, resulting in release of dopamine in the nucleus accumbens.[23] Dopamine release is potentiated and sustained by nicotine-mediated release of glutamate.[25] Rapid dopamine release in the outer shell of the nucleus accumbens is characteristic of the effects of many addicting drugs (e.g., heroin, cocaine, and alcohol) and is thought to be an important site for drug-mediated reinforcement.[26] The addiction potential for inhaled nicotine is extremely high, in part due to the rapid attainment of the maximal concentration for nicotine achieved from an inhaled cigarette. NRT (e.g., patch, gum, and lozenge) has significantly slower and lower maximal concentration attainment and therefore has minimal addiction potential.

Acute exposure to nicotine produces stimulation of the release of dopamine from neurons in mesolimbic pathways, whereas chronic exposure to nicotine and other drugs of abuse produces other changes in mesolimbic function. Chronic nicotine exposure results in neuroadaptation, or the development of tolerance, and the absence of nicotine results in subnormal release of dopamine and other neurotransmitters. Thus, nicotine withdrawal may result in a state of deficient dopamine responses to novel stimuli in general and to a state of malaise and inability to experience pleasure. This has been termed *hedonic dysregulation* by Koob.[27] Hedonic dysregulation may explain craving, and

sensitivity to drug effects may explain why even a single slip might easily result in a return to compulsive drug use.

The release of various neurotransmitters discussed previously results in behavioral arousal, sympathetic neural activation, and a number of other effects believed to be rewarding.[28,29] The release of certain neurotransmitters has been linked to the reported reinforcing effects of nicotine. For example, enhanced release of dopamine and norepinephrine may be associated with pleasure and appetite suppression, the latter of which may contribute to lower body weight. Release of acetylcholine may be associated with improved performance on behavioral tasks and improvement of memory. Release of β-endorphin may be associated with reduction of anxiety and tension. Although smokers give different explanations for their smoking, most agree that smoking produces arousal, particularly with the first cigarettes of the day, and relaxation, particularly in stressful situations, which may in part be due to the relief of nicotine withdrawal throughout the day (Fig. 66.2).

SMOKING CESSATION

Among current cigarette smokers, approximately 70% would like to quit, and about half try to quit each year.[30,31] Spontaneous quit rates (i.e., without support) are about 1% per year. Simple physician advice to quit increases the quit rate to 3%. Minimal intervention programs increase quit rates to 5–10%, whereas more intensive treatments, including smoking cessation clinics, can yield quit rates of 25–30%.[32]

The main strategies for cessation are behavioral counseling, pharmacologic intervention, or a combination of the two, which is strongly recommended. Assessing triggers such as stress and exposure to family members or roommates who smoke is an important part of history taking before a therapeutic intervention is undertaken.

GUIDELINES

Evidence-based guidelines for the treatment of tobacco addiction emphasize identifying all tobacco users in a

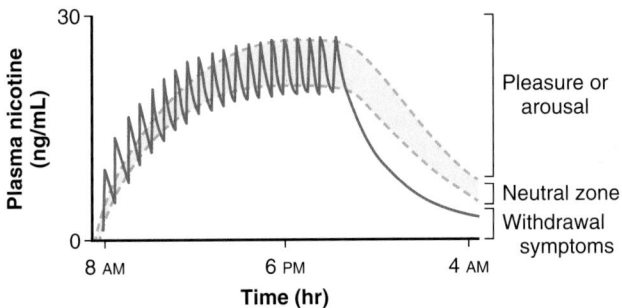

Figure 66.2 Nicotine levels in a person who smokes cigarettes. The peaks and troughs of nicotine concentrations throughout the day in a person smoking 20 cigarettes. Levels are low in the morning and drop rapidly with sleep. Smokers begin to experience withdrawal symptoms as the nicotine concentration drops below the shaded area, prompting another cigarette. The shaded area (neutral zone) represents the zone of nicotine concentrations in which the smoker is comfortable without pleasure/arousal or withdrawal symptoms. Note that the threshold levels for pleasure/arousal and withdrawal symptoms rise progressively during smoking due to development of tolerance. The magnitude of pleasure/arousal is greatest with the first cigarette of the day but becomes less intense with subsequent cigarettes. (From Benowitz NL. Cigarette smoking and nicotine addiction. *Med Clin North Am.* 1992;76:415–437.)

clinical practice setting and ascertaining each patient's intent with respect to quitting smoking (Fig. 66.3).[1,5,33,34] Identification of tobacco use is facilitated by the implementation of an office-based system so that patients are queried about tobacco use at every visit. Tobacco use should be treated as a vital sign, with reminders placed in the electronic medical record to screen patients. The practice of routinely recording a patient's tobacco use status increases the *odds ratio* (OR) for quitting by twofold.

Brief strategies to help a patient quit, which can be implemented in as little as 3 minutes, increase cessation rates significantly. In a meta-analysis of 31 trials, brief physician advice increased quit rates by 70%.[32] Intensive behavioral treatment of tobacco dependence produces higher success rates than does brief advice (the 5 A's) and is cost-effective. However, these intensive programs are less widely available and can be challenging to provide for busy clinicians. Nevertheless, clinicians with training in intensive smoking cessation therapy should be identified as a referral source and champion for smokers who are interested.

The 2008 Public Health Service guidelines and other international guidelines recommend that all smokers trying to quit should be offered pharmacotherapy (Table 66.2).[1,34] Three types of medications have been approved by the *U.S. Food and Drug Administration* (FDA) for smoking cessation: bupropion, which was originally marketed as an antidepressant drug, NRT, and varenicline (Table 66.3). Unfortunately, smoking cessation medications are underutilized by patients and providers. It is estimated that only approximately one-third of patients use medications when

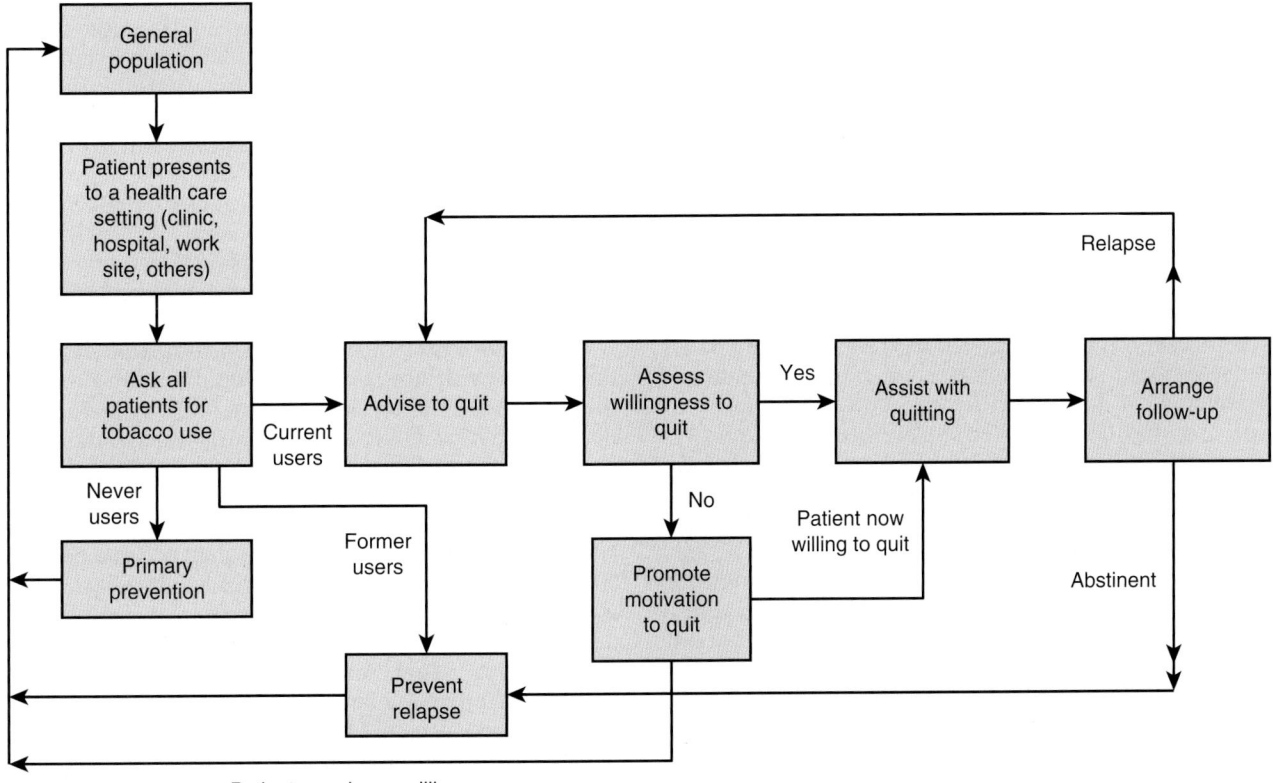

Figure 66.3 An algorithm for treating tobacco use. (From Clinical Practice Guideline Treating Tobacco Use and Dependence 2008 Update Panel, Liaisons, and Staff. A clinical practice guideline for treating tobacco use and dependence: 2008 update. A U.S. Public Health Service report. *Am J Prev Med.* 2008;35[2]:158–176.)

Table 66.2 General Clinical Guidelines for Prescribing Pharmacotherapy for Smoking Cessation

- In general, all smokers trying to quit smoking should be offered pharmacotherapy.

- There are seven first-line smoking cessation medications—five types of *nicotine replacement therapy* (NRT), sustained-release bupropion, and varenicline. Varenicline or the combination of nicotine patch plus ad libitum short-acting nicotine products appear to be most effective. However, the choice of first-line therapy should be governed by patient preference, familiarity of the clinician with the medication, contraindications for specific patients, and prior experience of the patient with specific pharmacotherapies.

- Second-line therapies include clonidine and nortriptyline. These should be reserved for individuals with contraindications to or failure of response to first-line medications.

- Bupropion and NRT may delay but not prevent weight gain after smoking cessation. It is recommended that patients start or increase physical activity, but strict dieting is discouraged because this appears to increase the likelihood of relapse to smoking. Patients should be reassured that weight gain after quitting is self-limited and poses much less of a risk to health than smoking.

- All first-line therapies appear to be safe for patients with chronic cardiovascular disease. The over-the-counter NRT therapies (gum, lozenge, and patch) contain precautions for use if the following exist: recent (≤2 weeks) myocardial infarction, serious or underlying arrhythmias, or serious or worsening angina pectoris. This labeling is for over-the-counter use only. Bupropion and varenicline are likely to be safer than smoking in the presence of cardiovascular disease.

- In individuals with prolonged withdrawal symptoms or those who are unable to abstain in the absence of medication, extended use or long-term therapy with NRT, bupropion, or varenicline appears to be safe and effective therapy.

Modified from 2008 PHS Guideline Update Panel, Liaisons, and Staff. Treating tobacco use and dependence: 2008 update U.S. Public Health Service Clinical Practice Guideline executive summary. *Respir Care.* 2008;53:1217–1222.

trying to quit.[31] Other drugs such as nortriptyline and clonidine have been shown in clinical trials to be effective in smoking cessation but have not yet been approved by the FDA for this purpose.

SMOKING CESSATION COUNSELING

Counseling smokers about the benefits of quitting and the health consequences of tobacco should be incorporated into routine medical practice and has been shown to be an effective method to improve cessation rates. Motivational interviewing, a patient-centered values-based form of counseling, has demonstrated a clear benefit in smoking cessation.[35,36] Based on a review of 188 randomized trials, personal advice and encouragement to stop smoking provided by a physician during a routine office visit resulted in an estimated 2% of all smokers stopping and not relapsing over 1 year.[37] Although this percentage seems low, it is both cost-effective and important when considering the large population and the risk for disease. Specific patient populations may have better results: 8% of pregnant smokers, 21% of healthy men at risk for cardiovascular disease, and 36% of survivors of *myocardial infarction* (MI) will stop smoking when receiving advice and encouragement. This high success rate likely reflects the patient's inherent motivation once challenged by a condition that has been caused by or may be aggravated by cigarette smoking.

Group counseling is less cost-effective than brief advice but is a highly effective option for smokers who are not successful with less intensive therapy. A review of 16 studies comparing group counseling found increased rates of cessation compared to self-help programs (16 studies; OR, 2.0) or no intervention (six studies; OR, 2.2).[32] There is no evidence that group counseling is more effective than a similar intensity of one-on-one counseling with a clinician.[38]

Telephone counseling is also effective in promoting cessation. In a large *randomized controlled trial* (RCT) of 1973 intensively counseled callers versus 1309 control subjects, telephone counseling through a quitline nearly doubled abstinence rates.[39] The 12-month self-reported cessation rates for those who made one or more cessation attempts was 23.3% in the treatment group and 18.4% in the control group. Telephone quitlines are available at no cost in most of the United States. Thus, when clinicians are unable to provide counseling due to lack of time, they can easily refer patients to a quitline, such as 800-QUIT-NOW in the United States, for cessation counseling and support.

Counseling for smokers during hospitalization has been found to be effective for patients admitted with cardiovascular disease; this is not well studied in other populations. Molyneux[40] evaluated 274 patients in an RCT and found that NRT given with brief counseling is more effective than counseling alone or usual care. Counseling alone was not more effective than usual care, and differences between all groups disappeared at 12 months. Counseling for hospitalized patients appears to be most effective when it includes at least 1 month of supportive contact after discharge.[41]

MOTIVATING SMOKERS TO QUIT

The well-known association between cigarette use and morbidities, such as lung cancer, MI, stroke, and COPD, is often insufficient to motivate many cigarette smokers to quit. This is likely due to the significant addiction to nicotine. A telephone-based survey conducted in 1999 found that only 29% of smokers felt that they were at greater risk of MI, and only 40% felt they were at greater risk for development of cancer compared to nonsmokers.[42] This clearly indicates denial of risk and may explain why many smokers only become motivated to quit when they develop a medical condition later in life.

As described previously, many smokers depend on nicotine to cope with stressors encountered in daily life because they perceive smoking as having a stress-reducing effect. Becoming a nonsmoker requires a profound change of self-image and a discovery of personal coping skills that may have not been used previously.

Health care providers' role in the motivation process can be substantial. The message to the smoker must be consistent and inspirational (Table 66.4). Patients respect advice from their provider, and hopelessness can be allayed by describing the many options available for cessation medications and counseling. Smoking cessation is the most important health initiative many patients will ever undertake and is highly cost-effective for the health care system. It is difficult to address smoking with patients when three or four medical issues are being managed in addition to smoking cessation. For this reason, a separate planned visit focused solely on smoking cessation is recommended.

Table 66.3   First- and Second-Line Smoking Cessation Medications

Pharmacotherapy	Precautions/ Contraindications	Adverse Effects	Dosage	Duration	Availability
FIRST-LINE					
Bupropion sustained release (SR)	Current or history of seizure Current or history of eating disorders	Insomnia, dry mouth, neuropsychiatric symptoms (rare)	150 mg every morning for 3 days then 150 mg twice daily (begin treatment 1–2 wk before quit date) Allow at least 8 hr between doses Avoid bedtime dosing	7–12 wk maintenance, up to 6 mo	Prescription
Varenicline	Renal impairment	Severe nausea, trouble sleeping, abnormal or vivid/strange dreams, neuropsychiatric symptoms (rare)	0.5 mg/day for 3 days 0.5 mg twice/day for next 4 days, then 1 mg twice/day Begin treatment 1 wk before quit date	3–6 mo	Prescription
Nicotine gum	Temporomandibular joint disorder	Mouth and throat irritation, dyspepsia, hiccups	First cigarette ≥30 min after waking: 2 mg First cigarette ≤30 min after waking: 4 mg Up to 24 pieces/day	3 mo	OTC
Nicotine lozenge		Mouth and throat irritation, dyspepsia, hiccups	First cigarette ≥30 min after waking: 2 mg First cigarette ≤30 min after waking: 4 mg Up to 20 pieces/day	3 mo	OTC
Nicotine inhaler	Bronchospastic disease	Mouth and/or throat irritation	6–16 cartridges/day	3–6 mo	Prescription
Nicotine nasal spray	Chronic nasal disorders, including rhinitis, polyps, and sinusitis Severe reactive airway disease	Nasal and/or throat irritation, ocular irritation/tearing, sneezing	1 dose = 1 spray in each nostril 8–40 doses/day Maximum of 5 doses/hr or 40 doses/day	3 mo	Prescription
Nicotine patch	Skin diseases, such as atopic or eczematous dermatitis	Local skin reactions, insomnia	>10 cigarettes daily: 21 mg 14 mg 7 mg ≤10 cigarettes daily: 14 mg 7 mg	 4 wk then 2 wk then 2 wk 6 wk then 2 wk	Prescription and OTC
SECOND-LINE					
Clonidine	Rebound hypertension	Dry mouth, drowsiness, dizziness, sedation	0.15–0.75 mg/day	3–10 wk	Prescription only (oral formulation, patch)
Nortriptyline	Risk of arrhythmias	Sedation, dry mouth	75–100 mg/day	3 mo	Prescription only

Note: Tapering will vary across different medications; information is available in the package insert and the regulatory approval label.
OTC, over the counter.
Modified from 2008 PHS Guideline Update Panel, Liaisons, and Staff. Treating tobacco use and dependence: 2008 update. US Public Health Service Clinical Practice Guideline executive summary. *Respir Care*. 2008;53:1217–1222.

Motivating patients to quit needs to be more than steering them away from the health consequences of tobacco-related disease but also steering them toward greater self-control, self-expression, independence, and positive role modeling. Table 66.4 provides a few simple framing do's and don'ts to keep in mind when talking with cigarette and e-cigarette users.

Exercise during trials of smoking cessation may reduce anxiety, tension, and stress but was not found to be an independent predictor of success in a RCT.[43] Walking on a regular basis is a reasonable initial step and, in many cases, improves self-esteem and investment in health.

Other interventions for smoking cessation, such as acupuncture and hypnotherapy, are available. In many cases the interventions are either incompletely studied or have poor study methodologic quality to render a solid recommendation. Both acupuncture and hypnotherapy have significant variability in the practice of the intervention. A recent systematic review of acupuncture suggested a short-term benefit, with greater benefit when used in

Table 66.4   Key Points When Counseling Smokers

DO'S

- Determine where the person is on the spectrum of smoking cessation (precontemplation, contemplation, action, maintenance, relapse). Your focus is to move them stepwise toward action, and after cessation keep them in maintenance.

- Dose adjust nicotine replacement therapy to the maximally effective dose based on the person's cigarette use, response to medications and frequency of urges.

- Ask "Have you used any tobacco or nicotine products in the past 30 days"?

DON'TS

- Ask "Do you smoke?" People with regular tobacco use may not identify as a regular smoker and answer *no* to this question.

- Call it a habit. Cigarette smoking and nicotine addiction is an acknowledged disease with significant withdrawal symptoms.

- Do not think that talking about a tobacco-related disease like lung cancer or COPD leads to an increased motivational level. Fear can reduce energy level and lead to discouragement. Frame the benefit of cessation in a positive manner (improved breathing, greater freedom, greater control of health).

combination with counseling.[44] Hypnotherapy was systematically reviewed across 14 studies of 1926 participants. The authors concluded there was insufficient evidence to determine if hypnotherapy was more effective than other forms of behavioral support or unassisted quitting.[45] Mobile phone texting and app-based smoking cessation interventions have been studied in multiple settings. A comprehensive review of 26 studies and 33,849 participants updated in 2018 concluded that there is moderate-certainty evidence that text-based interventions result in greater quit rates than minimal support.[45a] The evidence evaluating the benefit of smartphone apps was of low certainty, clearly suggesting the need for RCTs in this area.[45a,46]

PHARMACOTHERAPY FOR SMOKING CESSATION

All types of smoking cessation medications, if used properly, double to triple smoking cessation rates compared with placebo treatments.[33]

NICOTINE REPLACEMENT THERAPY

NRT is typically started on the person's designated quit date and includes nicotine gum, transdermal nicotine patches, nicotine nasal spray, nicotine inhaler, and nicotine lozenges. Patch, gum, and lozenge formulations are available over the counter, and the nicotine nasal spray and oral inhaler are by prescription only. All have comparable efficacy when used as monotherapy. In a randomized study, adherence was greatest for the patch, lower for gum, and very low for the spray and the inhaler.[47] The use of combination therapy (nicotine patch plus a short-acting NRT used as needed for cravings) appears to be more effective.[48]

Both the nicotine gum and lozenge are available in two doses: 2 mg and 4 mg. Their dose is based on when a patient

has the first cigarette upon waking. If it is within the first 30 minutes, the 4-mg dose is used; if a person waits more than 30 minutes after waking up, the 2 mg-dose is used. A person will use one piece every 1 to 2 hours while awake for the first 6 weeks, then taper over the next 6 weeks with instructions not to taper too quickly if experiencing significant urges. Optimal use of nicotine gum includes providing instructions on how to chew properly (i.e., use the chew-park-chew-park method) and to park in different areas of the mouth. A piece of gum will last about 30 minutes. Optimal use of nicotine lozenge[49] includes placing in the mouth and allowing to dissolve (it should not be chewed or swallowed) and to rotate to different areas of the mouth. A lozenge will dissolve over 20 to 30 minutes. Nicotine is absorbed across the buccal mucosa for both products. Patients should not eat or drink 15 minutes before or while using the gum or lozenge. Side effects of the gum and lozenge are primarily local and include mouth and throat irritation, upset stomach, and hiccups. The gum can also cause jaw muscle soreness.

Transdermal nicotine patches come in three strengths: 21 mg, 14 mg, and 7 mg; all deliver nicotine over a 24-hour period. A patch is applied in the morning and removed the next morning. If a patient experiences intrusive or disturbing dreams, the patch should be removed at bedtime. If a patient smokes more than 10 cigarettes a day (more than half a pack), then the 21 mg strength should be started; if a patient smokes less, then the 14-mg strength should be started (see Table 66.3 for full dosing information). It is important to rotate the sites where the patch is applied and to not use the same site for at least 1 week. The patch is generally applied to the upper body or upper outer part of the arm and to clean, dry skin (as hairless as possible) to ensure good adhesion. Although the patch provides a steady level of nicotine, the challenge becomes how to manage acute cravings; in this situation, combination NRT can be very effective, in which a short-acting NRT is used per its usual directions but on an as-needed basis.

Nicotine nasal spray is dosed one spray into each nostril and should be dosed one to two doses per hour. A patient should use at least eight doses per day for the first 6 to 8 weeks and then slowly taper over an additional 4 to 6 weeks as tolerated. It has unique side effects from the local irritation of the nasal mucosa (e.g., burning, sneezing, and watery eyes); with regular use, patients develop tolerance to these effects.

The nicotine inhaler delivers nicotine vapor across the mucosa of the mouth to the back of the throat. The nicotine is contained in a cartridge inserted into a plastic mouthpiece. A patient should use one cartridge every 1 to 2 hours, inhaling into the back of the throat or puffing in short breaths. The cartridge is depleted after 20 minutes of active puffing. Patients should not eat or drink 15 minutes before or while using the inhaler. Side effects of the inhaler are primarily local and include mouth and throat irritation, upset stomach, and hiccups. Although the labeling includes bronchospastic disease as a precaution, smoking cigarettes is likely a much greater trigger for irritation than the nicotine vapor from the inhaler.

All nicotine medications appear to be safe in patients with cardiovascular disease and can be offered to cardiovascular patients.[50–52] Although smoking cessation medications are recommended by the manufacturer for relatively short-term use (generally 3–6 months), the use of these medications for 6 months or longer (i.e., extended use) is safe and may be helpful in smokers who fear relapse without medications.[53]

In pregnancy, the two recommended interventions are counseling and the use of NRT. The safety of other medications, such as bupropion and varenicline, has not yet been adequately studied to support a clear recommendation for use in pregnancy. Potential fetal side effects are of paramount concern, and the opportunity to quit smoking still exists in the postpartum period. Pregnancy and the parent's concerns about immediate fetal health and postpartum secondhand smoke exposure to the infant can create a highly motivated focus to stop smoking and should receive extra support and attention.[54–56] Additional high-quality research is needed to determine optimal and safe non-NRT interventions or optimal combinations of therapies.

BUPROPION

Bupropion sustained release (Wellbutrin SR, formerly available as Zyban) is a dopamine-norepinephrine reuptake inhibitor originally marketed and still widely used as an antidepressant. Bupropion was found to aid smoking cessation independent of whether a smoker was depressed.[57] In this study, Hurt demonstrated that, with a 300 mg SR dose, 44% of patients quit at 7 weeks versus 19% of control subjects. This difference was sustained at 12 months (23% vs. 12%). This study also indicated that, when smokers quit, they gained less weight while taking bupropion compared to placebo.[38] An additional randomized, placebo-controlled trial demonstrated that the combination of bupropion with nicotine patch is safe and that bupropion alone or in combination was as effective or more effective than the patch alone.[58] The combination of bupropion and nicotine patch has been approved by the FDA for smoking cessation. Bupropion used for 1 year for relapse prevention was demonstrated to be safe and effective and significantly better at promoting cessation (55%) than placebo (42%).[59] Given its antidepressant properties, bupropion is a logical choice for smokers with depression but, as mentioned previously, has clear efficacy in smokers without depression as well.

Bupropion SR is by prescription only and is dosed at 150 mg daily for 3 days, then 150 mg twice a day for 12 weeks. Bupropion should be started 1 to 2 weeks before the quit date to ensure that therapeutic levels are attained because it has a long half-life (21 hours). Dose tapering is not needed at the end of 12 weeks. Bupropion in higher doses can cause seizures and should not be used in an individual with (or a history) of seizures or with eating disorders (bulemia or anorexia). Common side effects are dry mouth and insomnia.

VARENICLINE

Varenicline (Chantix), available by prescription only, is a nicotinic receptor partial agonist that selectively binds to α4β2 nicotinic cholinergic receptors in the brain. This receptor mediates dopamine release and is thought to be the major receptor involved in nicotine addiction. A partial agonist means that the drug activates the receptor but at a lower-level agonist activity (about 50% of that of nicotine)

and also blocks the effects of other agonists (e.g., nicotine) on the receptor. It primarily works to help alleviate nicotine withdrawal symptoms. In the case of a relapse, if a person smokes, the effects of the nicotine are likely blocked by varenicline.

Varenicline is initiated in a dose of 0.5 mg daily for 3 days, then 0.5 mg twice daily for 4 days, followed by a maintenance dose of 1 mg twice daily. Varenicline generally should be started 1 week before the quit date to ensure therapeutic levels are attained because it has a long half-life (24 hours). A flexible (quit within a month) or gradual (quit within 12 weeks) quit approach can also be used after starting varenicline. Lower doses may be used if nausea is a problem at higher doses. Because varenicline is eliminated by the kidneys, dose reduction is required in the presence of severe renal disease. The treatment duration is 3 months, and an additional 3 months is possible in selected patients who have significant urges and are at high risk of relapse.

In clinical trials, varenicline treatment for 12 weeks has been shown to be more effective than bupropion SR 300 mg or placebo. Continuous abstinence rates after study medication discontinuation out to 52 weeks were 29%, 21%, and 11% for varenicline, bupropion, and placebo, respectively.[60,61] Varenicline has also been shown to be effective in preventing relapse over 6 months. In a network meta-analysis, varenicline was associated with an increased odds of quitting, with an OR of 2.9 (2.4–3.5) compared to placebo, and varenicline monotherapy was comparable to dual NRT use (OR of 2.7 vs. placebo).[48] The common side effects of varenicline are nausea and insomnia; it is important to take it with food and a full glass of water.

Both bupropion and varenicline have been associated with a variety of neuropsychiatric symptoms described in the warnings and precautions sections of their respective FDA labels. A boxed warning for severe neuropsychiatric symptoms from varenicline was removed in December 2019 as a result of the *Evaluating Adverse Events in a Global Smoking Cessation Study* (EAGLES),[62] which demonstrated that varenicline and bupropion were not associated with an increased risk of neuropsychiatric symptoms compared with NRT or placebo. The American Thoracic Society released an official clinical practice guideline on initiating cessation treatment in tobacco-dependent adults in May 2020.[63] Five "strong" recommendations (based on National Academy of Medicine criteria) were developed from an analysis of the most recent published data and included (1) using varenicline rather than a nicotine patch, (2) using varenicline rather than bupropion, (3) using varenicline rather than a nicotine patch in adults with a comorbid psychiatric condition, (4) initiating varenicline in adults even if they are unready to quit, and (5) using controller therapy (varenicline, bupropion or nicotine patch) for an extended treatment duration more than 12 weeks. Patients should be monitored for neuropsychiatric events during treatment and instructed to discontinue bupropion or varenicline and contact a health care provider if they experience adverse events.

COMBINATION THERAPY

An important consideration in smoking cessation medication strategy is the use of combination therapies. Combined medications for smoking cessation can be more effective than individual therapies, particularly when combining long-acting medications such as nicotine patch or bupropion with short-acting NRT used at times of intense urges or cravings to smoke. Only bupropion and transdermal nicotine in combination have been approved by the FDA. However, a number of studies have looked at various combinations of medications.[63–67] Combination NRT (patch plus quick-acting NRT) is more effective than monotherapy and therefore is generally recommended over monotherapy.[48]

Combination therapies can also give people more flexibility in their plan, particularly if they start with one therapy and feel it is not fully effective and want to add a second therapy. Because there is significant individual variability in the metabolism of nicotine, some patients who rapidly metabolize nicotine may require higher doses of replacement therapy.[66] Experiencing breakthrough urges could suggest that some people are significantly underdosed by one form of NRT and that a second form or higher doses could be more effective. One prospective study found that the combination of bupropion and varenicline was more effective than varenicline alone in a specific subset of patients with a high level of dependency.[67] Published guidelines[1] have not kept pace with emerging combination data in the literature, and multiple publications have demonstrated that combinations of smoking cessation medications can be more effective than monotherapy. The safety of unapproved combination therapies is unclear and must be considered to enable an appropriate benefit versus risk assessment for an individual patient.

ELECTRONIC NICOTINE DELIVERY SYSTEMS AND E-CIGARETTES

The toxicity and side effects associated with e-cigarettes are emerging and are reviewed in Chapter 65. Several studies have begun to evaluate the use of e-cigarettes as a smoking cessation modality. However, the main concern is that this constitutes a switch from one highly addictive form of inhaled nicotine (cigarettes) to another highly addictive form of inhaled nicotine (e-cigarettes) without the intention to end nicotine addiction. The e-cigarette industry is not regulated, and there is no formal FDA-supported safety database providing accurate safety information. For these reasons, the use of e-cigarettes will remain controversial in clinical practice because their safety is unclear in comparison to health authority–approved cessation medications. Some studies have started to evaluate the use of e-cigarettes as a cessation aid. A systematic review in 2015 of the potential efficacy of e-cigarettes versus other cessation therapies revealed six RCTs and nine cohort studies of 7551 participants. Among 1242 smokers in the RCTs, 18% reported smoking cessation after using nicotine-containing e-cigarettes for a minimum duration of 6 months.[68] A separate retrospective study of 25- to 44-year-olds in the National Health Interview Survey database conducted by the Centers for Disease Control and Prevention[69] demonstrated that e-cigarette use was associated with higher quit attempts and greater smoking cessation (adjusted OR, 1.6; $P = 0.001$) in recent years compared to 2006 data. This could suggest that the new technology and media messaging associated with e-cigarettes provides an incentive to attempt quitting compared to other modalities. In contrast, a prospective cohort study from 2015–16[70] performed a random probability sample of 1284 U.S. adult smokers evaluated over 1 year. In this sample, the adjusted odds of quitting smoking were lower for those using e-cigarettes at baseline compared to those who did not use e-cigarettes (adjusted OR, 0.30). In summary, individual studies may suggest evidence for or against the potential benefit of e-cigarettes for smoking cessation but, in aggregate, in a systematic review,[71] there does not appear to be a place for their use, particularly when compared to approved smoking cessation medications.

Perhaps the most important recent trial[72] was an open-label RCT of 886 participants in the United Kingdom randomly assigned NRT (alone or combination) for 3 months versus an e-cigarette and refillable bottle of nicotine e-liquid (18 mg/mL), with all participants receiving 4 weeks of behavioral support. The 1-year abstinence from smoking was 18.0% in the e-cigarette group versus 9.9% in the NRT group (relative risk, 1.8; $P < 0.001$). Eighty percent of the participants in the e-cigarette group were using e-cigarettes at 12 months versus 9% in the NRT group. This important trial warrants significant analysis and context. Although the cessation rate was higher in the e-cigarette group at 1 year, the trial was not blinded, and the e-cigarette cessation rate was similar to rates seen with medications such as bupropion (≈20% at 1 year), varenicline (≈30% at 1 year), and a common combination of bupropion and patch (28% at 1 year[73,74]). The cessation rate of 9.9% with the convenience (multiple option) NRT treatment approach is significantly lower than a recent meta-analysis review of NRT, which yielded a 1-year point estimate of 19.8%. Of importance, as mentioned, 80% of participants in the e-cigarette group continued their use at 1 year, raising the concern about long-term safety and providing a contrast to NRT and other medications that have an intended use of approximately 3 months.

Because the health effects of e-cigarettes are only beginning to be understood, clinicians should recommend medications with a proven benefit and safety profile before considering new options. There may be a role for e-cigarettes in smokers who have a strong desire to quit smoking but refuse other cessation medications or have tried other interventions and found them to be unsuccessful. Even in this case, it is reasonable to recommend that e-cigarettes for smoking cessation should be used short term (3–6 months) because the medical goal is to end nicotine addiction.[75] Clinicians should educate patients about lung disease and other health risks that are emerging from vaping.

A recent cross-sectional analysis in the U.S. Population Assessment evaluated the risk of MI in cigarette users compared to e-cigarette users and to those with dual use. These data demonstrated that e-cigarette use and cigarette use conferred a similar risk of MI and demonstrated that dual use had an OR of 6.6 for an MI compared to never-cigarette or e-cigarette users.[76] The Forum of International Respiratory Societies has actively called for the regulation of e-cigarettes and the American College of Cardiology/American Heart Association Guidelines on the Prevention of Cardiovascular Disease (2019) recommend against the use of e-cigarettes for smoking cessation.[77] In light of the newly recognized epidemic of vaping-associated severe lung disease and associated deaths, it appears reasonable for all physicians to discourage e-cigarette use until both the short- and long-term dangers associated with their use are understood.[78]

BENEFITS OF QUITTING

The benefits of quitting smoking are substantial for smokers of any age. A person who quits smoking before age 50 years has half the risk of dying in the next 15 years compared with a continuing smoker.[79] Smoking cessation reduces the risks of developing lung cancer, with the risk falling to half that of a continuing smoker by 10 years and one-sixth that of a smoker after 15 years' cessation. Quitting smoking in middle age substantially reduces lung cancer risk, with a 50% reduction in risk if a lifelong smoker quits at age 55 years compared with age 75 years.[80] The risk of acute MI falls rapidly after quitting smoking and approaches non-smoking levels within 1 year of abstinence. Cigarette smoking produces a progressive loss of airway function over time characterized by an accelerated loss of *forced expiratory volume in 1 second* (FEV_1) with increasing age. Loss of FEV_1 due to cigarette smoking cannot be regained by cessation, but the rate of decline slows after smoking cessation and returns to that of nonsmokers[81] (see Fig. 64.6). Women who stop smoking during the first 3 to 4 months of pregnancy reduce the risk of having a low-birthweight infant to that of a woman who has never smoked.

After quitting, smokers gain an average of 10 pounds, which is often perceived by some smokers as undesirable and may be a barrier to quitting. Smokers tend to be thinner because nicotine increases energy expenditure and suppresses a compensatory increase in food consumption. Upon quitting, ex-smokers tend to reach the weight expected had they never smoked. Of course, the benefits of quitting far outweigh the risks associated with weight gain, and patients should be counseled accordingly.

RESOURCES FOR HEALTH CARE PROVIDERS

Most hospitals have smoking cessation services available that will enable referral of smokers if deemed necessary. Most states have free quitlines that can be accessed through a national network at 800-QUIT-NOW (800-784-8669) that provides smoking cessation information and counseling and has been shown to be effective. The American Lung Association (www.lung.org/quit-smoking) has a wealth of information and an online program called "Seven Steps to a Smoke-free Life" to which patients can be referred. The Centers for Disease Control and Prevention has information that can be downloaded for adults, youth, and Spanish-speaking patients (www.cdc.gov/tobacco/). Other web-based counseling resources include www.smokefree.gov and www.becomeanex.org. If patients do not have their own computer, the public library is a smoke-free environment where they can access computers. Patients suspected of having underlying depression, anxiety, or other substance abuse disorders may benefit from psychiatric referral to evaluate these conditions known to reduce the likelihood of smoking cessation. Finally, the Rx for Change:

Clinician-Assisted Tobacco Cessation training program is available; it equips practicing clinicians and health professional students with evidence-based knowledge and skills for how to assist patients with quitting. Lectures (with downloadable PowerPoint slides) and other educational materials have been created by pharmacists and experts in smoking cessation for the medical community as a free educational and clinical resource (http://rxforchange.ucsf.edu).

Acknowledgment

Many thanks to Dr. Neal Benowitz, who as a prior contributing author to this chapter provided much of the nicotine neurobiology information still featured.

> ### Key Points
>
> - Nicotine is an intensely addictive chemical that causes the upregulation of nicotinic cholinergic receptors in the brain.
> - Nicotine has a short half-life, and withdrawal symptoms can be severe.
> - Cigarette smoking is the most important preventable cause of respiratory disease.
> - Most smokers would like to quit smoking but have difficulty doing so because of nicotine addiction.
> - Smoking cessation counseling and medications are extremely underutilized in the United States and many countries around the world.
> - Smoking cessation medications come in two broad categories: nicotine replacement therapies and the oral medications bupropion and varenicline. Both individual therapies and combinations are effective.
> - E-cigarettes represent a new and addictive technology.
> - The efficacy of e-cigarettes for smoking cessation continues to be evaluated, but long-term data on safety are unknown. E-cigarettes are not recommended for smoking cessation by major medical societies.

Key Readings

Babb S, Malarcher A, Schauer G, Asman K, Jamal A. Quitting smoking among adults—United States, 2000–2015. *MMWR Morb Mortal Wkly Rep.* 2017;65:1457–1464.

Benowitz NL. Nicotine addiction. *N Engl J Med.* 2010;362(24):2295–2303.

Cahill K, Stevens S, Lancaster T. Pharmacological treatments for smoking cessation. *JAMA.* 2014;311(2):193–194.

Centers for Disease Control and Prevention. Surgeon General's Report on Smoking Cessation 2020. https://www.cdc.gov/tobacco/data_statistics/sgr/index.htm.

Croyle RT, Morgan GD, Fiore MC. Addressing a core gap in cancer care: the NCI Moonshot Program to help oncology patients stop smoking. *N Engl J Med.* 2019;380(6):512–515.

Fiore MC, Jaén CR, Baker TB, et al. *Treating Tobacco Use and Dependence: 2008 Update. Clinical Practice Guideline.* Rockville, MD: US Department of Health and Human Services. Public Health Service; 2008.

Gesthalter YB, Wiener RS, Kathuria H. A call to formalize training in tobacco dependence treatment for pulmonologists. *Ann Am Thorac Soc.* 2016;13(4):460–461.

Jha P, Ramasundarahettige C, Landsman V, et al. 21st-century hazards of smoking and benefits of cessation in the United States. *N Engl J Med.* 2013;368(4):341–350.

Leone FT, Zhang Y, Evers-Casey S, et al. Initiating pharmacologic treatment in tobacco-dependent adults. An official American Thoracic Society clinical practice guideline. *Am J Respir Crit Care Med.* 2020;202(2):e5–e31.

Complete reference list available at ExpertConsult.com.

67

CYSTIC FIBROSIS: PATHOGENESIS AND EPIDEMIOLOGY

STEVEN M. ROWE, MD, MSPH • GEORGE M. SOLOMON, MD •
ERIC J. SORSCHER, MD

INTRODUCTION

Cystic fibrosis (CF) is a multisystem genetic disease that affects children and young adults. CF is the most common monogenetic disease in white populations. The disease is caused by mutations in the *CF transmembrane conductance regulator* (CFTR) protein, an anion channel expressed on the epithelial surface. CF is typified by the presence of chronic upper and lower respiratory tract infection leading to bronchiectasis and end-stage lung disease. Manifestations in the pancreas, gastrointestinal tract, skin, and male reproductive tract are also prominent.

Understanding the biology and treatment strategies in CF is important for several reasons. First, CF is the most common cause of both chronic respiratory failure and pancreatic exocrine dysfunction in children and young adults. Second, it is a major cause of bronchiectasis and pansinusitis, among other sinopulmonary conditions in this age group, and therefore represents an essential consideration in the differential diagnosis of numerous clinical syndromes. Third, the pathobiology has substantial commonalities with other mucociliary disorders, thus representing common principles. Finally, advances in CF research have provided a roadmap for understanding the pathophysiology and treatment for other severe airway diseases, including COPD, asthma, and non-CF bronchiectasis. This chapter highlights the current understanding of CF pathobiology, with particular emphasis on the role of CFTR in disease pathogenesis.

HISTORICAL PERSPECTIVE

The first comprehensive description of CF as a distinct clinical entity was published in 1938 by Anderson, who named the disease "cystic fibrosis of the exocrine pancreas."[1] In 1945, Farber described the condition as a generalized *mucoviscidosis* resulting in obstruction of exocrine glands.[2,3] Also in the 1940s, clinical descriptions first linked mucoviscidosis to severe and recurrent lung infections. With the development of effective antimicrobials, new treatments to address severe pulmonary infection were applied to CF for the first time.

An extreme heat wave in the northeastern United States in the summer of 1948 led di Sant'Agnese[4] to describe high salt concentrations in the sweat of infants with CF and introduce the concept of abnormal ion transport as contributing to the disease. End-organ dysfunction in the sweat gland was among the first characteristics recognized for the disorder. Di Sant'Agnese demonstrated elevated levels of sweat sodium and chloride in greater than 98% of subjects with CF, a finding that remains a cornerstone for diagnosis today. A traditional Irish folk saying, "if your baby tastes of salt, he is not long for this world," may have presaged these fundamental scientific discoveries regarding sweat hypersalinity in CF.

Before identification of the *CFTR* gene and protein in 1989,[5–7] early observations led investigators to postulate an ion transport abnormality as a proximate cause of CF. To measure this phenomenon, Gibson and Cooke[8] developed the modern pilocarpine method of sweat chloride testing. Later, Quinton[9,10] demonstrated that sweat gland ducts in CF patients are impermeant to chloride. At the same time, a number of contributions regarding the physiology of ion transport within nasal epithelium by Knowles and colleagues[11,12] and subsequent membrane patch-clamp analysis of airway epithelial cells by Welsh and Liedtke[13] and Frizzell[14] provided conclusive evidence for defective chloride transport within plasma membranes of epithelial cells in the upper and lower respiratory tract of patients with CF, in addition to associated abnormalities of sodium uptake.[11,12] Transformational chromosome mapping technology applied by Collins, Riordan, and Tsui[6,15,16] identified the causative gene, which they named the *cystic fibrosis transmembrane conductance regulator*. This finding set the stage for molecular cloning of the gene; independent verification that *CFTR* encoded a chloride channel protein; elucidation of the most common mutation, F508del; and definition of myriad other disease-associated variants. These studies comprise the basis for current understanding of CF pathogenesis and new therapeutics directed toward the fundamental molecular defect.[17,18]

EPIDEMIOLOGY

CF is the most common monogenetic lethal disease in white populations, found in 1 in 2500 to 3500 live births in the United States, with lower frequencies among African Americans (1:17,000). There is a varied incidence in particular ethnic groups, ranging from 1:569 in an isolated Ohio Amish population to 1:90,000 in Asian populations.[19]

CFTR mutations are most prevalent among persons descended from central and northern European populations. Non-European white populations demonstrate intermediate rates of *CFTR* mutation, and Native Americans, Asian populations, and Black Africans demonstrate the lowest rates. Proposed reasons for the selectivity of *CFTR* mutations in these populations include a heterozygote advantage in epidemic illnesses, such as cholera, tuberculosis, or plague. Cholera is of particular interest because the absence of CFTR-dependent chloride transport could confer an advantage on *cyclic 3′,5′-adenosine monophosphate* (cAMP) activation by cholera toxin.[20] Conversely, selectively lower rates of *CFTR* mutations in populations living in tropical or semitropical environments could be due to propensity for excess salt loss conferred by heterozygosity. In white populations, approximately 1 in 25 is a carrier for a *CFTR* gene mutation,[21] resulting in a carrier rate of 2–5%. CF carriers do not exhibit manifestations of CF illness, although carrier status has been proposed to increase the propensity for a wide variety of respiratory and non-respiratory disorders.[22]

GENETIC BASIS

CF is an autosomal recessive condition caused by mutations of *CFTR*, a gene located on the long arm of chromosome 7.[6,15,16] CFTR encodes a protein in the *adenosine triphosphate* (ATP) *binding cassette* (ABC) transporter family, sharing primary and secondary structural elements with many other proteins in this group. The approximately 190-kB CFTR encodes 27 exons and a full-length protein consisting of two *membrane-spanning domains* (MSDs), two *nucleotide binding domains* (NBDs), and a single *regulatory domain* (R domain). A schematic of CFTR is shown in Figure 67.1; the protein crystal structure has been solved using cryoelectron microscopy, opening the door for structural-based drug design.[23,24]

A very large number of *CFTR* mutations have been linked to clinical disease, including a current estimate of more

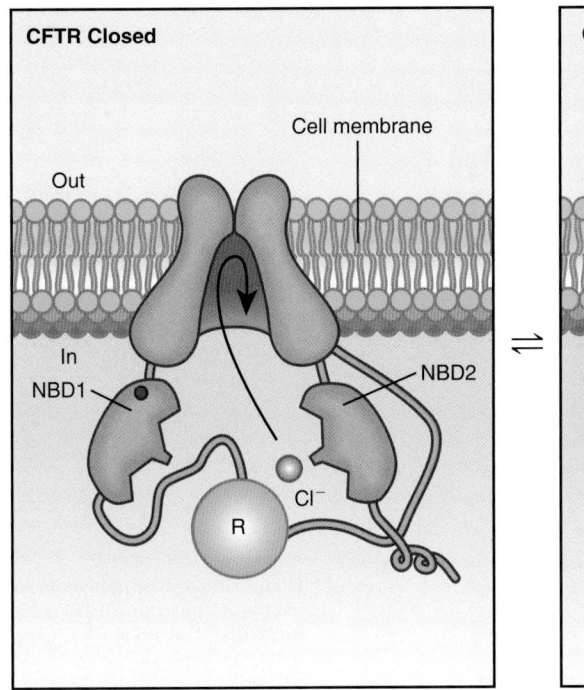
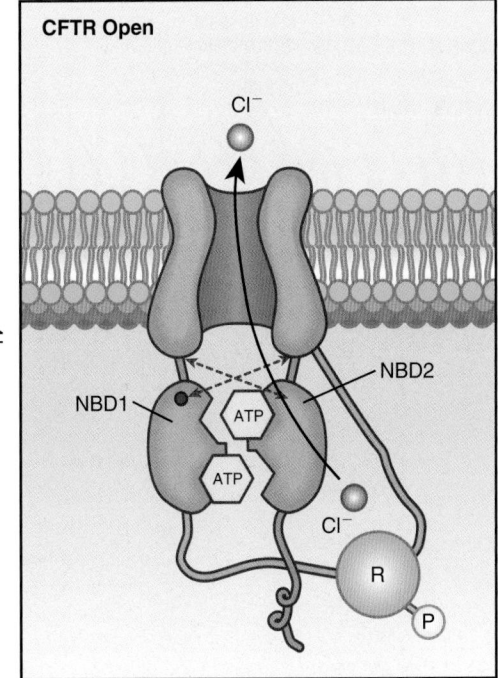

Figure 67.1 CFTR structure and domain assembly. Schematic representing the proposed structure of the *cystic fibrosis transmembrane conductance regulator* (CFTR) in its closed (*left*) and open (*right*) configurations. The two transmembrane spanning domains consist of six α-helices each and together form the channel pore. Gating of the channel is controlled by the two intracytoplasmic nucleotide binding domains (NBD1 and NBD2) as they bind and hydrolyze *adenosine triphosphate* (ATP) (*hexagons*) and a regulatory domain (R), which contains numerous sites of phosphorylation. Normal activation of the protein requires phosphorylation (P) of the regulatory domain. The NBDs bind and hydrolyze ATP, inducing channel gating by conferring opening of the pore through interfaces with the transmembrane domains via their extracellular loops (*dashed lines*), which also function to stabilize the overall protein structure. The location of the F508del mutation (*red dot*) is on the surface of NBD1, compromising its stability and interrupting interactions with the transmembrane domains.

than 1900 disease-associated variants, of which more than 350 are confirmed to cause disease.[19] That being said, a much smaller number of mutations account for the majority of disease in the CF patient population (eTable 67.1). For example, the most frequent 159 mutations account for 96% of defective CF alleles. As already stated, the most prevalent variant is F508del (c.1521_1523delCTT), which causes a three–base-pair nucleotide deletion and omission of phenylalanine at CFTR position 508. This mutation accounts for approximately 75% of CF-causing alleles, although distribution of the abnormality is heterogeneous among particular ethnic populations and as high as 86% in northern European white populations.[19]

F508del CFTR exhibits severe protein misfolding and leads to endoplasmic reticulum–associated retention and destruction of CFTR by the proteasome. The F508del defect represents a severe form of the prototypic class II variant (i.e., abnormalities resulting in premature degradation or incomplete maturation). Other less common CFTR variants fall into various mutation classes on the basis of molecular mechanism (Fig. 67.2). Additional classes include defects that confer incomplete CFTR synthesis due to premature termination codons (class I); disordered regulation and gating, causing diminished ATP binding and hydrolysis (class III), seen with the G551D mutation; defective chloride conductance (class IV); a reduced number of CFTR transcripts, such as due to a promoter or splicing abnormality (class V); and reduced protein stability at the cell surface, first reported as a defect in terminal CFTR variants that lack sequences anchoring the protein to the cell membrane (class VI). Ultimately, molecular classes reduce channel number, inhibit its function, or exhibit a combination of these effects, and the severity of these effects influences

clinical outcome. Mutations in class I, II, and III tend to cause severe CFTR functional abnormalities, whereas class IV, V, and VI variants may exhibit residual function, reducing their severity (i.e., mild/variable activity) and CF phenotype. It is notable that many variants exhibit features of more than one molecular category; thus, the system is imperfect but a useful construct that has guided drug discovery efforts. For example, whereas the F508del mutation principally reduces channel number through its class II defect in processing and trafficking, it also exhibits abnormal gating (class III) and class VI (reduced channel stability) properties.[25] Understanding the molecular abnormality in each mutational class is important for addressing the defect with pharmacologic interventions such as CFTR modulators, discussed in Chapter 68.

Despite extensive knowledge concerning various mutations in CFTR, only approximately 90% of CF patients have both of their disease-causing alleles identified, although this number is increasing with more frequent use of full-length CFTR sequence analysis. Moreover, the pathogenic role of many mutations remains unknown, and knowledge in this area has dramatically improved through the CFTR2 project, which critically evaluates CFTR variants in the context of clinical phenotype on a global scale (www.CFTR2.org).[26] It has been estimated that more than 1000 CFTR variants are present, causing disease in fewer than five CF patients each.[18] Common nucleotide transversions, such as M470V, are designated as simple polymorphisms rather than disease-causing alleles, despite a potential (secondary) role of M470V impacting expression and/or function of F508del CFTR.[19] Other polymorphisms, such as the poly-T sequence located within intron 8, can modify CFTR expression, thus acting as important covariates of disease.[27]

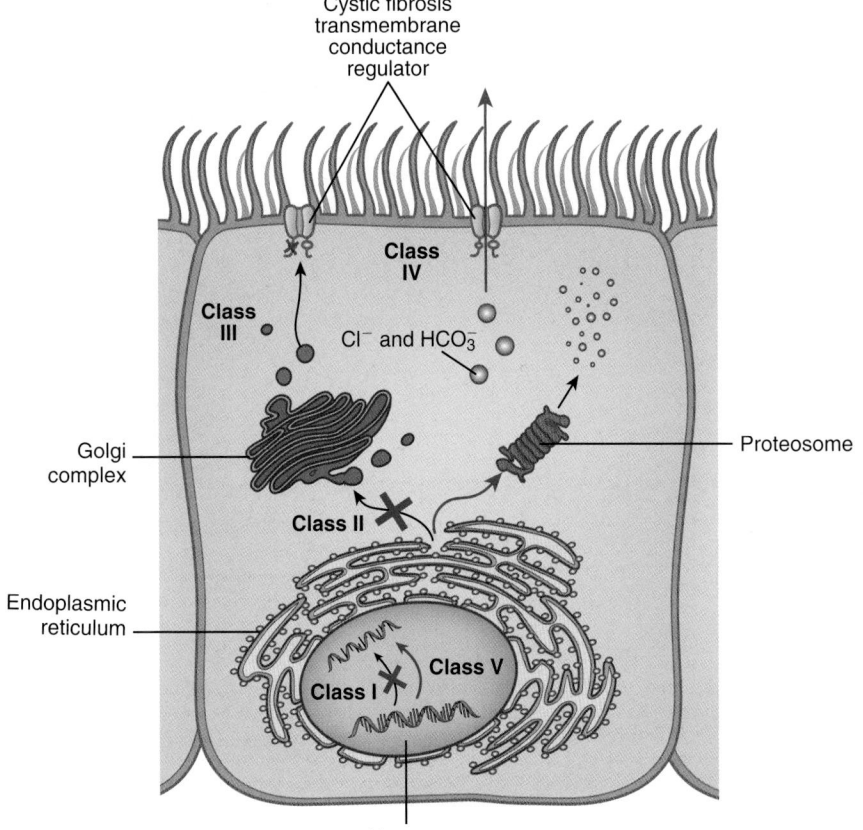

Figure 67.2 *Cystic fibrosis transmembrane conductance regulator (CFTR) gene mutations and molecular consequences.* Classes of defects in the CFTR gene product include the absence of synthesis (class I); defective protein maturation and premature degradation (class II); disordered regulation, such as diminished adenosine triphosphate binding and hydrolysis (class III); defective chloride conductance or channel gating (class IV); and a reduced number of CFTR transcripts due to a promoter or splicing abnormality (class V). Another class of defect has reduced protein stability at the cell surface (class VI, not shown).

The functional basis underlying specific *CFTR* mutations allows the correlation of genotype to phenotype, noting that other genetic modifiers and the environment also play prominent roles in disease expression. For example, when two severe (e.g., class I, II, or III) mutations are present, pancreatic insufficiency typically results, especially in patients homozygous for F508del. The finding of two severe mutations also confers risk for clinical manifestations, such as meconium ileus or hepatobiliary disease. On the other hand, presence of one or more mild/variable mutations may allow sufficient residual CFTR activity to diminish disease severity. CF patients with mild mutations often exhibit intermediate sweat chloride values, which correlate with pancreatic sufficiency.[19,28] When two mild/variable mutations are present, atypical forms of CF are more frequently observed, such as congenital absence of the vas deferens, "idiopathic" pancreatitis, or late-onset respiratory disease without other characteristic features of a complete CF phenotype.[27,29-31] Disease severity and expression can also be affected by non-*CFTR* genetic modifiers, which have been extensively studied. *Transforming growth factor* (TGF)-β has been shown to modify lung disease severity, specifically among subjects homozygous for F508del *CFTR*.[32,33] Other modifier loci on chromosome regions 4q35, 8p23, 11q25, and 19q13 confer increased risk of meconium ileus,[34,35] and various additional genes have been associated with acquisition of *Pseudomonas aeruginosa* infection.[36,37] Effect sizes for findings such as these have not been sufficient for routine use in the clinic, and a significant component of missing heritability may contribute to pulmonary decline in CF patients with two copies of F508del.

PATHOPHYSIOLOGY

CFTR AS AN ABC GENE

As described earlier, *CFTR* is a member of the ABC transporter or the traffic ATPase family of genes.[17,38,39] Proteins in this group are ancient and include hundreds of prokaryotic and eukaryotic polypeptides that transport nutrients, metabolites, toxins, and other small molecules across cellular membranes. All ABC proteins are characterized by two NBDs encoding canonical Walker A and B motifs (polypeptide sequences within the protein capable of binding and hydrolyzing ATP). CFTR gating, induced by ATP binding, hydrolysis, and release, confers conformational changes that allow pore opening and closing. Like other ABC proteins, CFTR encodes for two membrane-spanning domains with multiple α-helices that form highly selective passageways across lipid bilayers. Among ABC proteins, CFTR is atypical by virtue of a regulatory domain with numerous sites for *protein kinase A* (PKA)/cAMP-dependent phosphorylation, and a regulatory insertion in NBD1 shown to play an important role during channel gating[17,40,41] (see Fig. 67.1). Lasso helical structures near the CFTR amino-terminal region represent additional distinctive features of CFTR.[23,24]

STRUCTURE/ACTIVITY AND CFTR GATING MECHANISM

The CF gene product is composed of approximately 1500 amino acids and functions as a transporter of chloride ion

(Cl^-) and bicarbonate ion (HCO_3^-) in numerous epithelial tissues. Site-directed mutagenesis indicates that gating is enabled by PKA/cAMP-dependent phosphorylation of the R domain. The phosphorylation step has been shown to elicit a conformational change in the regulatory insertion, leading to NBD1/NBD2 heterodimerization and structural realignments of MSD1 and MSD2, which permit opening of the ion conductive pore.[42] Key interactions between intracellular loops of the transmembrane domains and NBDs are integral to CFTR stability and interdomain assembly, as well as to transmission of forces required for channel gating (see Fig. 67.1).[43-45] NBD dimerization is greatly augmented when two ATP binding sites (at the NBD1/2 interface) are occupied; closing of CFTR is attributable to ATP hydrolysis.[46,47] It should be noted that ATP binding is not absolutely required for ion transport by CFTR; so-called ATP-independent channels can also open, for example, based on the tendency of NBDs to realign spontaneously in the open or outward-facing channel conformation.[47] Transepithelial anion flow through CFTR is governed by the electrochemical driving force, and a CFTR bioelectric signature (using membrane patch-clamp analysis or planar lipid bilayer reconstitution) describes PKA/cAMP or PKA-dependent currents through an approximately 8-picosiemen channel with linear current/voltage relationship and characteristic opening bursts. CFTR therefore uses ATP binding to enable passive ion transport, rather than subserving a function more typical of the ABC gene family (i.e., pumping of larger metabolites with stoichiometric dependence on ATP hydrolysis).

BIOGENESIS AND PROCESSING OF NATIVE CFTR

Wild-type CFTR matures and reaches the cell surface by conventional pathways that include cotranslational insertion in the *endoplasmic reticulum* (ER) membrane and post-translational modifications, such as N-linked glycosylation (Fig. 67.3). Subdomain folding (e.g., within NBDs) and achievement of final tertiary structure requires complex domain-binding interactions—and represents a topic of intense interest—because CFTR misfolding is a crucial mediator of clinical disease.[43,44,48-51] Wild-type CFTR processing may not be completely efficient and, in most experimental expression systems that express too much CFTR, a portion of wild-type CFTR becomes targeted for hydrolysis by *ER-associated degradation* (ERAD) and can stimulate ER stress. For CFTR advancing from the ER to the Golgi apparatus, complex glycosylation takes place at two asparagine residues. CFTR reaching the Golgi apparatus is transported to the cell surface by vesicular traffic with subsequent recycling through sorting and recycling endosomes and reinsertion in the plasma membrane or routing to the lysosome (or other cellular compartments). The cell surface apparatus governing CFTR peripheral stability (i.e., at the plasma membrane) has been well characterized and includes ubiquitin conjugation to regulate internalization.[52]

CELLULAR DEFECTS ATTRIBUTABLE TO F508del CFTR

The vast majority of F508del CFTR is retained in the ER, heavily ubiquitinated, and routed to the proteasome by ERAD.[53]

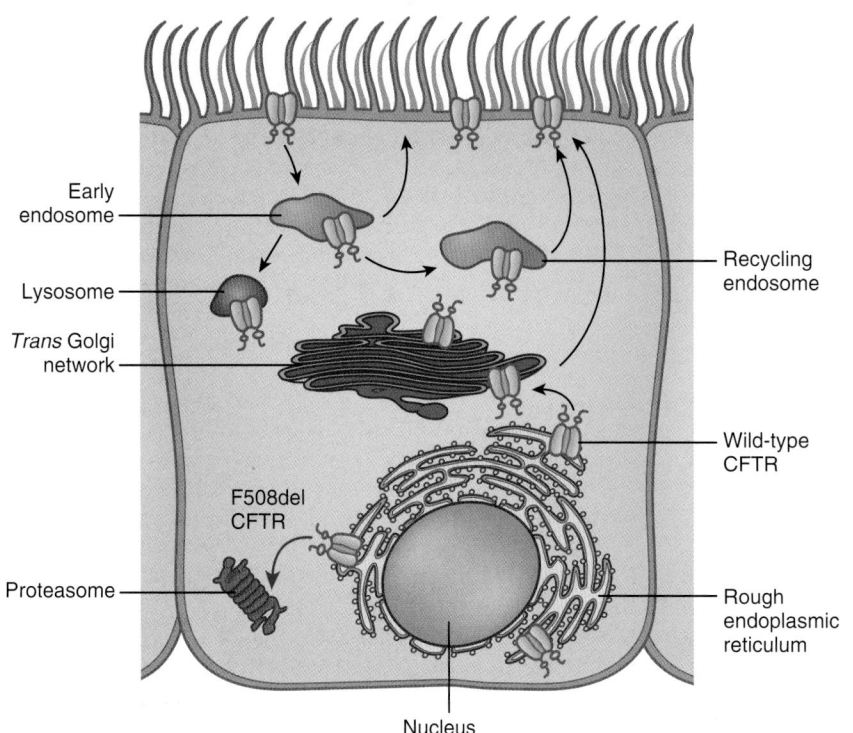

Figure 67.3 **Scheme of *cystic fibrosis transmembrane conductance regulator* (CFTR) biogenesis.** Biogenesis of CFTR in normal epithelial cell (*black arrows*) and F508del CF-affected epithelial cell (*red arrow*). In the normal epithelial cell, CFTR is synthesized in the rough endoplasmic reticulum, glycosylated and folded in the Golgi apparatus, and chaperoned to the cell surface. In the F508del-affected epithelial cells, the CFTR polypeptide is misfolded and tagged for premature degradation via endoplasmic reticulum–associated degradation (*red arrow*) before reaching the cell surface (class II mutation). (Modified from Ameen N, Silvis M, Bradbury NA. Endocytic trafficking of CFTR in health and disease. *J Cyst Fibros* 2007;6:1–14.)

As a consequence, F508del CFTR visualized by polyacrylamide gel electrophoresis is predominantly an ER-localized, approximately 150-kDa core glycosylated (band B) form. This is in contrast to a substantial portion of the post-ER wild-type protein, which migrates more slowly on polyacrylamide gel electrophoresis due to complex glycosylation (≈180-kDa band C). The F508del trafficking defect is temperature sensitive, and growth of epithelium at 27°C leads to measurable levels of F508del band C CFTR, with partial restoration of cell surface activity. Although likely not relevant in vivo, except perhaps at the nasal surface, this improvement in function at low temperature provided an early indication that pharmacologic intervention could diminish the cellular recognition machinery necessary for protein degradation.

Maturational processing abnormalities attributable to F508del arise from at least two distinct features.[43,44,54] Omission of F508, which is located on an externally exposed peptide loop of the first nucleotide binding domain, leads to pronounced loss of NBD1 stability as judged by thermal and isothermal calorimetry, protein aggregation, and protein yield measurements after recombinant overexpression.[43,44] In addition, F508 facilitates binding of NBD1 to a cytosolic loop from MSD2, and disruption of the NBD1/MSD2 interface (independent of NBD1 stability) leads to further impairment of F508del maturation. F508del CFTR molecules that do reach the cell surface, as shown through in vitro techniques, such as pharmacologic therapy or, alternatively, low temperature correction of cellular processing, display intrinsic channel gating abnormalities, diminished plasma membrane stability, and pronounced thermal unfolding with loss of function.[55,56] The observation of multiple distinct CFTR defects attributable to F508del presents a challenge to identifying single agents capable of restoring mutant CFTR to therapeutically relevant levels. Of note, intramolecular suppressor mutations

that specifically ameliorate F508del NBD1 instability or the defective NBD1/MSD1 interface have been well characterized.[43,44] CFTR constructs encoding these suppressors provide a means to improve F508del corrective strategies and have enabled compound library screening tailored to specific CFTR folding defects (see also later).

OVERVIEW OF LUNG PATHOPHYSIOLOGY

An improved understanding of CF pathogenesis has led to better diagnostic strategies, understanding of features leading to the onset and progression of respiratory decline, and therapeutic approaches to target the underlying disease. An overview is provided in Figure 67.4 and described in further detail later. Absent or dysfunctional CFTR results in diminished protein activity, leading to deficient chloride and bicarbonate transport across airway epithelium. Several key aspects of CF pathophysiology include delayed mucociliary clearance resulting from depletion of the periciliary compartment of the *airway surface liquid* (ASL), defects involving the rheologic properties of CF mucus that contribute to mucus stasis and adhesion to the epithelial surface, predisposition to early infection because of abnormal mucosal defense, and pronounced and/or dysregulated inflammation. These processes initiate and perpetuate a cycle of destruction that ultimately results in irreversible lung injury, bronchiectasis, and respiratory failure.[17,57]

In the respiratory tract, CF manifests with infected mucus that compromises the airway lumen and contributes to obstructive pulmonary disease and reduced FEV_1 (Fig. 67.5). Respiratory damage is thought to begin in the small airways, resulting in airflow obstruction detected by spirometry midflows (i.e., $FEF_{25\%-75\%}$). Submucosal gland hyperplasia and inspissated mucus secretions emanating from the glands are also prominent in early CF

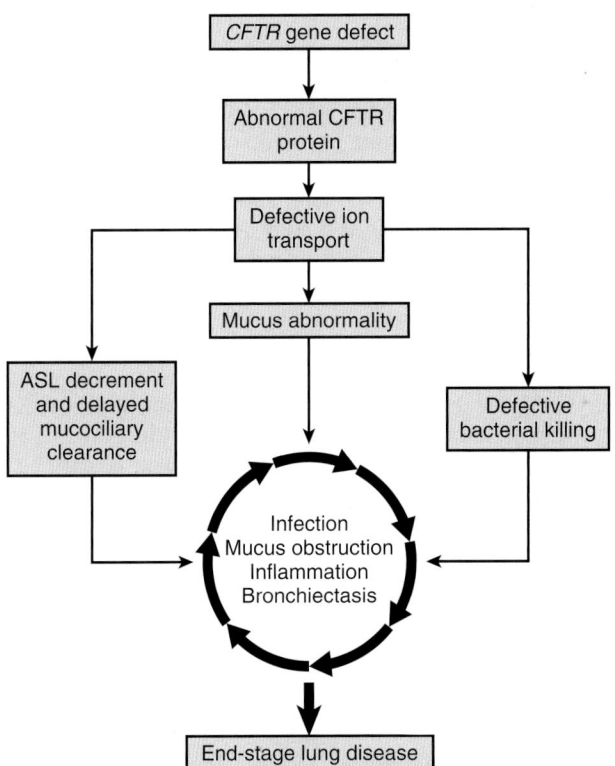

Figure 67.4 *Cystic fibrosis* **(CF) pathophysiology.** CF lung disease results from consequences of genetic mutations in the cystic fibrosis transmembrane conductance regulator gene (*CFTR*). Major operative pathways include reduced mucociliary clearance due to depleted airway surface liquid (ASL) hydration, abnormal mucus adhesion and viscosity, and defective bacterial killing, which each contribute to the cycle of destruction.

lungs. Radiographic changes consistent with small airway obstruction (e.g., tree-in-bud opacities) followed by bronchiectasis become apparent over time. Development of bronchiectasis leads to irreversible changes that predispose to worsening infection and accelerate disease pathogenesis.

CELLULAR FUNCTIONS OF THE *CFTR* GENE PRODUCT

The *CFTR* gene is hundreds of millions of years old on an evolutionary basis and used by diverse species, including fish, amphibians, fowl, and mammals.[58] Although best described as a chloride and bicarbonate transporter, the protein appears to regulate numerous cellular processes in addition to anion secretion (see also earlier). CFTR is situated within membrane complexes by virtue of its C-terminal anchoring sequence via a PDZ-type binding motif. CFTR is configured in close proximity to a number of integral membrane proteins, including other ion channels. By establishing electrochemical gradients, CFTR also exerts a regulatory influence on other apical ion transporters, including the *epithelial sodium channel* (ENaC), alternative chloride transporters, and bicarbonate/chloride exchangers.[59] Proteomic and transcriptome analyses demonstrate hundreds of cellular gene products that may directly bind or are impacted by CFTR.[60]

With the advent of single-cell sequencing came the surprising observation that CFTR is predominantly expressed in the airways in a minority cell type termed the *ionocyte*. The identification of the ionocyte as a major site of CFTR signaling has important implications for pathogenesis and gene therapy.[61,62] It is unknown whether the ionocyte regulates

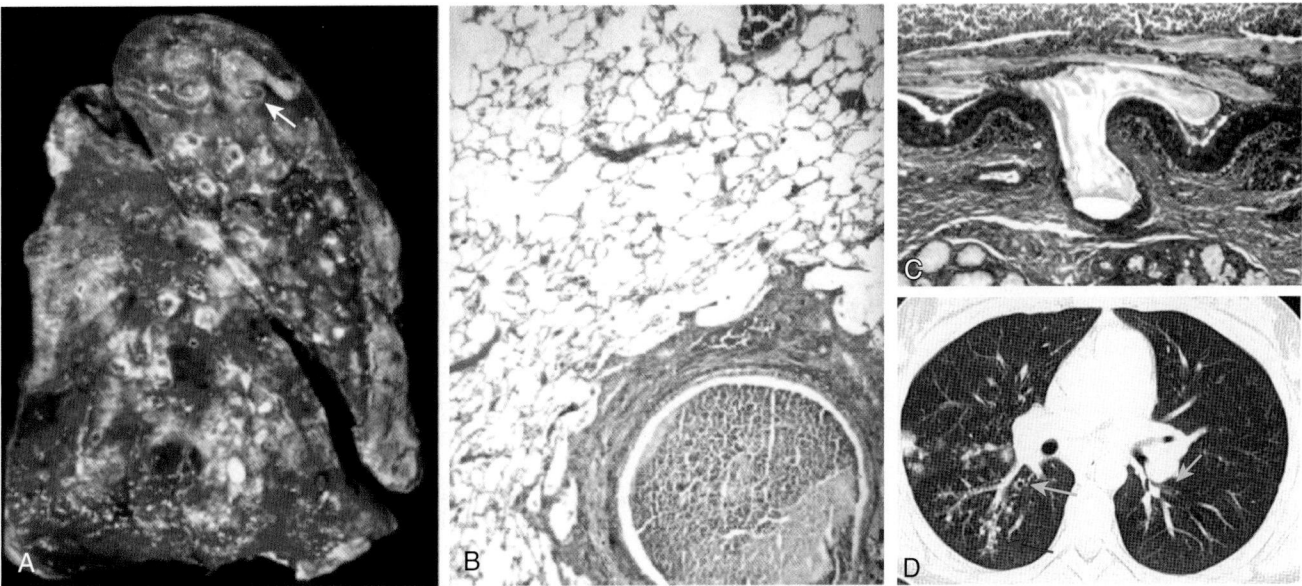

Figure 67.5 *Cystic fibrosis* **(CF) pathologic and radiologic correlation.** (A) Gross pathologic specimen of explanted CF lung from a patient with advanced CF. This specimen (sagittal section) shows heavy lungs characterized by ectatic bronchi (e.g., *arrow*) and numerous mucopurulent plugs. (B) Large airway pathology of CF. A large mucus plug filled with inflammatory infiltrate is seen, in addition to remodeling of the medium-size airway (hematoxylin-eosin stain). (C) Representative photomicrograph from a CF patient with end-stage lung disease is depicted. Note the thickening of the lamina propria (higher Reid index), the prominent arborized mucus plug extruding from the submucosal gland onto the airway lumen, and the hypertrophic surface epithelium (periodic acid–Schiff stain). (D) Axial high-resolution computed tomography image from a 16-year-old male patient with CF demonstrating mild to moderate multilobar bronchiectasis (*blue arrows*) and tree-in-bud opacities representing small airway mucus plugs (*red arrow*). (A–C, Courtesy Dr. David Kelly, University of Alabama, Birmingham.)

the ion transport environment of the epithelia by establishing electromotive forces or serves other unique functions yet to be discerned. This has notable implications for attempts to repair CFTR through gene therapy because it is not yet known if ionocyte repair will be a prerequisite for efficacy. In the lung, CFTR is also expressed in low numbers in surface epithelial cells and glandular epithelia, where it functions to regulate the formation and maturation of mucus.

REGULATION OF SWEAT CHLORIDE BY CFTR

The concentration of chloride in human sweat is determined by the balance of secretion and reabsorption of sodium and chloride in the sweat gland and duct. Chloride is secreted by two parallel pathways. One involves CFTR; the other uses a CFTR-independent, calcium-activated chloride channel. Because CFTR is not the only pathway by which chloride exits the apical membrane, chloride is secreted into sweat even in the absence of functional CFTR. Normally, sodium is reabsorbed along the sweat gland duct by ENaC in the apical membranes of ductular cells. Chloride follows sodium into the cell through CFTR. In CF, absent or defective CFTR significantly reduces chloride reabsorption, and the chloride content of sweat is therefore abnormally high, providing a convenient indicator of CFTR function. With differences in CFTR function either due to genetic variation or to drug therapy, sweat chloride is a dynamic and sensitive indicator of the modulation of CFTR activity.

REGULATION OF AIRWAY SURFACE LIQUID HOMEOSTASIS

The absence of apical CFTR leads to failure of chloride and bicarbonate secretion.[17,63] Because release of water into the periciliary region is driven in part by a CFTR-dependent osmotic gradient, CFTR deficiency leads to failure of mucus hydration, particularly when combined with excess mucus expression and secretion. Persistent airway fluid absorption through ENaC, which can be augmented by free nucleotides and other inflammatory stimuli, further exacerbates airway desiccation.[64–66] Hyperconcentrated mucus contributes to its elevated viscosity and correlates with disease severity across the spectrum of mucociliary diseases.[67] Osmotic forces induced by entangled mucus in the overlying mucus layer draw fluid from the periciliary layer, which normally provides the environment for appropriate ciliary function and mucus transport (Fig. 67.6). The harm caused by ASL dehydration is underscored by the therapeutic improvement among patients treated with hypertonic saline aerosols and dry powder mannitol to augment mucociliary clearance in CF lung disease by providing airway hydration, although their influence on the electrostatic environment of gel forming mucins has also been postulated.[67]

Through bicarbonate transport, CFTR serves to regulate airway pH. In people with CF and in CF pigs, the absence of the chloride bicarbonate exchanger ATP12a, present in mice, prevents compensation for airway pH abnormalities,[68] leading to an acidic airway surface. The acidic pH environment is postulated to have several effects, including a defect in bacterial killing through pH-sensitive defensins; this may be a crucial early event that initiates CF infections, particularly early in life when aspiration events are common and where fast-acting bacterial killing is highly relevant.[69] The absence of bicarbonate transport and the acidic pH environment also has consequences to the formation of mucus and its rheologic properties, as detailed later.

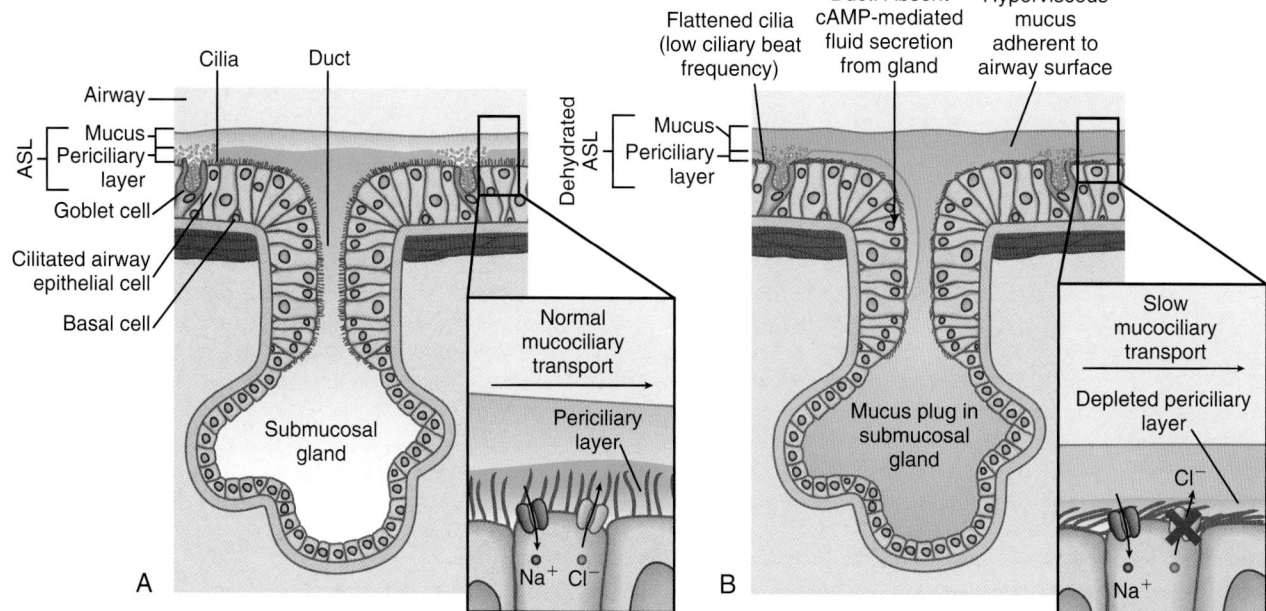

Figure 67.6 Schematic of the mucociliary transport defect in *cystic fibrosis* (CF). (A) In the healthy state, adequate airway surface homeostasis ensures effective transport of mucus extruding from airway surface goblet cells and the submucosal glands. The airway surface liquid (ASL) is maintained by fluid secretion via the cystic fibrosis transmembrane conductance regulator (CFTR) and fluid absorption via the epithelial sodium channel (ENaC) (*inset at right*) (CFTR, surface receptor in *blue*; ENaC, surface receptor in *red*). (B) In CF, the ASL is depleted through the absence of CFTR-mediated fluid secretion, accompanied by tonic fluid absorption via the ENaC. CFTR-dependent liquid dehydration decreases the depth of the ASL, including the periciliary layer, causing abnormal clearance of mucus from the epithelial cell surface in the airways. cAMP, cyclic monophosphate.

MUCUS BIOGENESIS, ADHESION, AND TRANSPORT

Hyperviscous respiratory secretions obstruct small- and medium-size airways in CF, leading to profound failure of mucociliary clearance that can be verified macroscopically by radioligand imaging[70] and direct visualization of the mucociliary transport apparatus in human nasal airways.[71] Quantitative analyses have indicated this is multifactorial, with airway dehydration and hyperviscous acidic mucus each contributing independently.[71,72] Even early in disease, before robust infection, insoluble mucus plaques (also called "flakes") can be observed in the bronchoalveolar lavage fluid of affected infants.[73] As mucus obstruction ensues, proinflammatory cytokines, such as interleukin-1β, are released, perpetuating mucus expression and exacerbating the consequences of CFTR deficiency.[73]

Specific mucins expressed in respiratory secretions include the gel-forming mucins MUC5B and MUC5AC, in addition to a complex array of extracellular proteins that participate in host defense.[74] Evidence for a primary biochemical defect in mucus composition includes the adhesion of large MUC5B strands in CF porcine airways or in those deficient in both bicarbonate and chloride transport[75] and the role of enzymatic release of mucus in the intestine.[76] Defective bicarbonate transport, in part through its effects on airway pH, contributes to mucus hyperviscosity through electrostatic forces.[77] Exocrine mucins (highly negative in charge) are produced intracellularly as compacted forms assisted by bound calcium, which shields the negative repulsive force between sulfates and other anionic groups on constituent mucins.[2] Under normal circumstances, bicarbonate secretion via CFTR, likely coordinated with mucus secretion, chelates the calcium and permits mucin expansion and a viscoelastic state compatible with physiologic clearance.[78] Failure of bicarbonate secretion results in defective mucin expansion, leading to hyperviscous secretion with abnormally adherent properties (i.e., mucus that is tightly bound to the respiratory surface and difficult to mobilize). Therapeutics in development to alter electrostatic interactions can ameliorate abnormal mucus rheology.[79] Excessive mucus adhesion that can be reversed by bicarbonate has been observed in the intestine of CF mice,[80,81] but this bicarbonate-mediated effect on mucus may not be sufficient to reverse airway mucus obstruction because CF mucus also becomes oxidized, a secondary phenomenon that also serves to increase its viscosity and may be less readily reversed. DNA strands released from dying bacteria, injured epithelial and inflammatory cells, and inflammatory secretions, such as *neutrophil extracellular trap* (NET)osis from polymorphonuclear leukocytes, represent important contributors to excess mucus viscosity and provide a rationale for the use of recombinant DNAse as an aerosolized mucolytic.

CYSTIC FIBROSIS EXOCRINE GLANDULAR EPITHELIUM

Submucosal glandular ducts filled with inspissated mucus are observed early in the course of CF pulmonary involvement. CFTR is highly expressed within epithelial cells of submucosal glands, where it functions to activate fluid and electrolyte secretion and promote release of mucus onto the airway surface.[3,82] The relative contributions of submucosal glands to overall CF respiratory pathophysiology are an area of considerable interest. Illustrating this notion, in CF rats, mucus stasis is only apparent with the development of glands as they age, even though both pH and airway dehydration are evident early in life, and is augmented by stimulation of mucus secretion.[83] Adhesive mucus at the outlet of gland ducts may further contribute to airway obstruction and provide a nidus for infection.

HOST DEFENSE AND INFECTION

CF lungs are characterized by intense neutrophilic inflammation with polymorphonuclear cells densely infiltrating airway secretions. Whether robust lung inflammation is mediated directly by CFTR, as opposed to a consequence of polymicrobial infection, is a topic of considerable debate. Sterile mucus obstruction plays an important role in experimental animals,[84] and interleukin-1β can serve as a positive feedback loop that furthers mucus stasis.[85] Neutrophil chemoattractants, such as interleukin-8, tumor necrosis factor-α, and a collagen fragment, proline-glycine-proline, are present at high levels in airway secretions, and abnormalities of CFTR-dependent macrophage function have also been implicated. Although anti-inflammatory therapies can improve lung function and slow the rate of CF respiratory decline, immune blockade also can predispose individuals to worsening lung infection, and the proper clinical balance has been difficult to achieve.[86]

Bacteria typically colonize the CF respiratory tract during infancy or early childhood. Longitudinal analysis of *P. aeruginosa* indicates sentinel infection due to a single genotype of the organism often persisting throughout the life of an individual patient.[87] The factors that lead to early colonization are not well understood. Studies have implicated acidic pH within the ASL, attributable to absent CFTR bicarbonate release, as a likely cause of the increased susceptibility to bacteria.[69] Findings such as these may, in some cases, be most relevant to early colonization events.[3]

Virulent respiratory pathogens such as *P. aeruginosa* evolve in a stereotypic fashion during the lifespan of individuals with CF and are characterized by rapid phenotypic change and hypermutability.[88] After several years of pulmonary infection, *P. aeruginosa* typically develops a mucoid phenotype in which considerable metabolic reserves are expended to synthesize and release the polyanionic protein, alginate. The appearance of mucoid *P. aeruginosa* in CF is a negative prognostic indicator. The selective advantage of alginate release has been attributed to the immunomodulating role of this exoproduct.[89,90] Studies have demonstrated the complexity of the CF microbiome, which can be altered during exacerbations by the presence of a dominant pathogen.[91] Further, co-culture studies provide evidence of synergistic interactions between bacteria that perpetuate and accelerate chronic infections.[92]

Animal Models of Cystic Fibrosis

Mouse models of CF have provided an important base of knowledge regarding the CF ion transport abnormality. A key strength of CF mice has been the ability to perform tissue-specific expression models, allowing the role of CFTR to be explored in various tissues[93]; humanized versions of mice have also informed therapeutic evaluation. Nevertheless, CF mice have proved more limited in elucidating features of lung disease pathogenesis, unless hyperexpression of ENaC is implemented, which provides a model of airway dehydration but not other characteristic features of CF lung disease.[94] Filling the gap, porcine, ferret, and rat models of CF pulmonary disease have proved highly informative. Mice are likely protected from CF lung disease due to several features, including important differences in cell types that populate the airway, the absence of airway glands that serve as reservoirs for mucus production (see Chapter 1 for background differences between mouse and human lungs), and expression of the aforementioned ATP12a exchanger that protects mice from pH abnormalities, in addition to high expression of alternative chloride channels such as TMEM12a.[68,95] Rats, ferrets, and pigs each provide increasingly more faithful disease modeling of the airway defects and have been crucial to insights regarding lung disease pathogenesis, particularly regarding mechanisms of mucociliary clearance and CF defects in host defense. Each species exhibits elements of airway disease due to mucus obstruction and host defense abnormalities; ferrets and pigs exhibit spontaneous and progressive lung disease, whereas infection must be experimentally initiated in CF rats. These species provide informative models to assess pathophysiology, although cost, experimental complexity, and reagent availability serve as limitations that counterbalance how well they each replicate CF lung disease.

When combined with the evaluation of very young CF patients by newborn screening, animal models have provided particularly important means to clarify relationships existing among initial bacterial colonization, chronic infection, and inflammation in CF lungs. Longitudinal monitoring of CF respiratory infection in humans and transgenic animals will also facilitate a more sophisticated understanding of the complex CF microbiome and could provide new therapeutic opportunities in the future, particularly as robust models of chronic infection evolve. As gene therapy advances, animal models will also be essential to assess issues of gene delivery, tissue and cellular level expression, and correction of physiology.[96]

CFTR AND PULMONARY REMODELING

Measurements in the CF porcine model indicate a change in tracheal diameter and density of submucosal glands before the advent of hyperviscous mucus obstruction. Similar findings have been reported in human CF lungs and in CF rats (i.e., preceding the appearance of other pulmonary manifestations).[97] For tissues such as porcine and human pancreas, fibrotic damage and fatty replacement can be profound, with extensive parenchymal scarring.[98] Myofibroblast proliferation has been implicated as mediating some of these effects, and TGF-β signal transduction, which engenders myofibroblast transformation, is markedly increased throughout the CF lung.[99] TGF-β is also a well-established genetic modifier of F508del homozygous CF lung disease,[32,100] and

these findings suggest that changes in TGF-β–dependent profibrotic pathways contribute to lung tissue remodeling, in addition to inflammatory responsiveness elicited by the cytokine.

Key Points

- *Cystic fibrosis* (CF) is the most common monogenic lethal disease in white populations and results from mutations in the *CF transmembrane conductance regulator (CFTR)* gene.
- *CFTR* genetic variants can be classified according to their molecular consequences to cell biology, which has implications for disease phenotype and for possible response to pharmacologic intervention.
- The most common *CFTR* mutation is F508del, one of more than 2000 variants, of which 350 have been confirmed to cause disease. Nearly 90% of CF individuals have one or more F508del alleles.
- CFTR is a tightly regulated anion channel of chloride and bicarbonate in the ABC transporter family. CFTR is expressed on epithelial cells and recently found on a novel cell, the ionocyte, and serves to regulate membrane potential and to influence the function of other channels.
- Absent CFTR causes delayed mucociliary clearance, abnormalities in mucus biogenesis and rheology, and host immunologic defects, which lead to chronic, progressive sinopulmonary infections and a cycle of lung destruction, bronchiectasis, and end-organ failure.
- Extrapulmonary manifestations are observed in numerous tissues that express CFTR, including the endocrine and exocrine pancreas, gastrointestinal tract, skin, bone, and male reproductive tract.

Key Readings

Boucher RC. Muco-obstructive lung diseases. *N Engl J Med.* 2019;380 (20):1941–1953.

Chen G, Sun L, Kato T, et al. IL-1β dominates the promucin secretory cytokine profile in cystic fibrosis. *J Clin Invest.* 2019;129(10):4433–4450.

Hoegger MJ, Fischer AJ, McMenimen JD, et al. Cystic fibrosis. Impaired mucus detachment disrupts mucociliary transport in a piglet model of cystic fibrosis. *Science.* 2014;345(6198):818–822.

Leung HM, Birket SE, Hyun C, et al. Intranasal micro-optical coherence tomography imaging for cystic fibrosis studies. *Sci Transl Med.* 2019;11(504):eaav3505.

Liu F, Zhang Z, Csanady L, Gadsby DC, Chen J. Molecular structure of the human CFTR ion channel. *Cell.* 2017;169(1):85–95 e88.

Montoro DT, Haber AL, Biton M, et al. A revised airway epithelial hierarchy includes CFTR-expressing ionocytes. *Nature.* 2018;560(7718):319–324.

Pezzulo AA, Tang XX, Hoegger MJ, et al. Reduced airway surface pH impairs bacterial killing in the porcine cystic fibrosis lung. *Nature.* 2012;487(7405):109–113.

Ratjen F, Bell SC, Rowe SM, Goss CH, Quittner AL, Bush A. Cystic fibrosis. *Nat Rev Dis Primers.* 2015;1:15010.

Stoltz DA, Meyerholz DK, Welsh MJ. Origins of cystic fibrosis lung disease. *N Engl J Med.* 2015;372(16):1574–1575.

Complete reference list available at ExpertConsult.com.

68 CYSTIC FIBROSIS: DIAGNOSIS AND MANAGEMENT

GEORGE M. SOLOMON, MD • WYNTON HOOVER, MD •
ERIC J. SORSCHER, MD • STEVEN M. ROWE, MD, MSPH

INTRODUCTION

Cystic fibrosis (CF) care has benefited from an increased understanding of CF pathobiology and from the partnership of academic and pharmaceutical research enterprises with a multinational team of care centers and the Cystic Fibrosis Foundation and other committed research entities. As a result, CF care constitutes a model for advancing treatment of chronic, life-threatening diseases through evidence-based quality improvement initiatives and comprehensive multidisciplinary care directed at multiple deleterious manifestations. It also provides a seminal example of the potential for translational medicine to deliver scientific discoveries that have transformed a universally fatal condition with targeted therapeutics addressing the underlying defect in the function of the *cystic fibrosis transmembrane conductance regulator* (CFTR). Future advances will capitalize on even more personalized therapies directed at the underlying cause of the condition and will address the potential for a genetic-based cure.

This chapter extends upon the concepts demonstrated by CF molecular pathobiology detailed in Chapter 67 to focus upon its diagnosis, prognosis, and natural history. CF therapeutics are also described, including the development of new therapies that target the basic defect.

DIAGNOSIS

OVERVIEW

The diagnosis of CF is predicated on clinical suspicion for the disease, as indicated by clinical manifestations or family history, or alternatively through newborn screening programs. Early detection through newborn screening is leading to recognition of illness before clinical findings become apparent. The first organized CF newborn screening programs were developed in the 1980s and implemented in Colorado (1987) and Australia and Europe (1980s)[1]

after retrospective studies demonstrated improved clinical outcomes and decreased mortality as a result of early disease detection.[2] The number of such programs in the United States and abroad has grown in the past decade, and all states in the United States implemented newborn screening programs after a U.S. Centers for Disease Control and Prevention/Cystic Fibrosis Foundation Consensus Statement in 2004 recommended this practice.[3] The report invoked emerging prospective data that screening and early interventions in CF infants led to improved nutritional, gastrointestinal, respiratory, and cognitive functioning.[4-7]

In North America, newborns are screened using a heel prick blood test for immunoreactive trypsinogen, a byproduct of prenatal pancreatic inflammation. In most U.S. states, this test is paired with a DNA probe panel for common *CFTR* mutations. Immunoreactive trypsinogen is not a highly specific measurement due to elevated levels observed in prematurity, traumatic delivery, and other neonatal gastrointestinal disorders.[8] Because of declining immunoreactive trypsinogen levels in the first few months after birth in CF and non-CF infants,[9] this test is only useful for screening during the first few weeks postnatally. Family history or clinical suspicion based on clinical findings becomes the main impetus for diagnostic evaluation once the neonatal period has passed.

If the immunoreactive trypsinogen is elevated or in situations where CF is suspected for other reasons, a diagnosis should be confirmed by sweat chloride testing per the algorithm at a certified sweat testing lab once the newborn reaches an age where this testing may be performed accurately (usually after 10 days of age). Sweat chloride measurements are available in many clinical laboratories and have been standardized to ensure accuracy. Because of high sensitivity, sweat chloride testing has a central role in establishing the diagnosis in both the Cystic Fibrosis Foundation and European algorithms, once a positive newborn screen or compatible clinical characteristics are established.

Diagnostic Algorithms

The diagnosis of CF is based on a positive newborn screening test in newborns or CF clinical characteristics (Table 68.1). In 2017, the Cystic Fibrosis Foundation published comprehensive diagnostic guidelines for infants and adults

with suspected CF[10] (Fig. 68.1) that emphasized a similar algorithmic approach for newborns, children, and adults. Similar European guidelines primarily differed only in the timing of *CFTR* mutation analysis and sweat chloride normative values.[11] There is good concordance when comparing the U.S. and European framework in terms of diagnostic accuracy.[12]

In the new approach, a low sweat chloride concentration (≤29 mmol/L) effectively rules out CF, whereas a high sweat chloride concentration (≥60 mmol/L) definitively establishes the diagnosis. In the case of clinical suspicion with an intermediate sweat chloride concentration (30 to 59 mmol/L), guidelines recommend performing *CFTR* sequencing or high-sensitivity DNA probe testing to establish the presence of *CFTR* mutations, usually coordinated through specialized commercial laboratories or via coordination and referral to a CF center for evaluation. Genetic confirmation by commercial *CFTR* sequencing in certified laboratories is recommended to confirm the diagnosis and to guide mutation-specific treatments, independent of the diagnostic yield of sweat chloride testing. Worldwide catalogs of CF phenotypic information by genotype are housed in the CFTR-2 repository (www.cftr2.org) and can help provide guidance about expected severity based on sequence information.

If two *CFTR* mutations are found, the diagnosis of CF is established. If one or zero mutations are present, then repeat sweat chloride testing is recommended. It should be noted that standard genetic panels (i.e., panels that test fewer than 40 mutations) are not sufficient in patients with elevated sweat chloride and atypical manifestations, because rare, partial function mutations are common in these cases and may not be detected by limited panels;

Table 68.1   Diagnostic Criteria for CF by Clinical Phenotypic and CFTR Functional Abnormalities

DIAGNOSIS OF CF CONFIRMED BY THE PRESENCE OF APPROPRIATE PHENOTYPIC CLINICAL FEATURES (ANY OF):

Chronic sinopulmonary disease
- Chronic cough and sputum production
- Persistent infection with characteristic pathogens (*Staphylococcus aureus, Pseudomonas aeruginosa,* other gram-negative organisms)
- Airflow obstruction
- Chronic chest radiographic abnormalities
- Sinus disease; nasal polyposis

Gastrointestinal and nutritional abnormalities
- Exocrine pancreatic insufficiency
- Recurrent pancreatitis
- Fat-soluble vitamin deficiency
- Meconium ileus; DIOS

Obstructive azoospermia in males

PLUS LABORATORY EVIDENCE OF CFTR ABNORMALITY (ONE OR MORE OF FOLLOWING):

Elevated sweat chloride

Disease-causing mutation in *CFTR* gene in both alleles

Characteristic bioelectric abnormalities (potential difference) in nasal epithelium

Abnormal ex vivo intestinal short-circuit current measurement

---

CF, cystic fibrosis; CFTR, cystic fibrosis transmembrane conductance regulator; DIOS, distal intestinal obstruction syndrome.

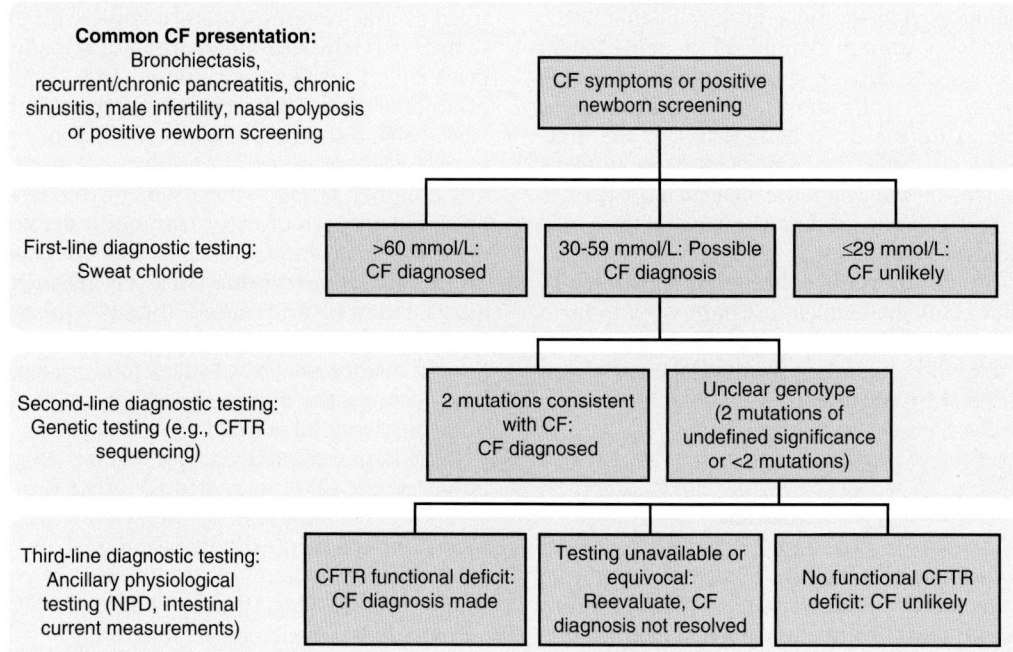

Figure 68.1 Diagnostic algorithm for *cystic fibrosis* (CF). Schematic depiction of algorithm for the diagnosis of CF in newborns through adults emphasizing sweat chloride as the cornerstone for diagnosis. Genetic testing for intermediate probability cases should trigger *cystic fibrosis transmembrane conductance regulator* (CFTR) sequencing because analysis for only a limited number of mutations can result in false-negative evaluations in this disease category. NPD, nasal potential difference. (Modified from Farrell PM, White TB, Ren CL, et al. Diagnosis of cystic fibrosis: Consensus guidelines from the Cystic Fibrosis Foundation. *J Pediatr.* 2017;181S:S4-S15.e1.)

they are also biased towards mutations prevalent in those of Caucasian descent. Some patients exhibit CF-like disease even in the absence of *CFTR* mutations, a finding that might be caused by changes in genes encoding other proteins that can mimic mutations in *CFTR* (i.e., mutations in the epithelial sodium channel) or in other noncoding regions of the *CFTR* gene itself.[13]

If clinical suspicion remains and sweat chloride is in the intermediate range, there are several alternatives to confirm CFTR functional deficits. *Nasal potential difference* (NPD) testing, available at many CF research centers, can be an acceptable alternative in cases of inconclusive sweat chloride or inadequate genetic analysis. Alternatively, intestinal current measurements to estimate CFTR activity require a biopsy of rectal mucosa but the test is only available at a few centers worldwide.[14,15] Other measures of pancreatic function, such as fecal elastase, may also help support a diagnosis in this setting.

It is increasingly recognized that CFTR-related disorders represent a spectrum of disease, with pancreatic-insufficient CF as the most severe form and borderline CF-like syndromes representing the other extreme (Fig. 68.2). It is notable that functional assessments of CFTR reflect this diversity, although the relationship between genotype and CFTR functional decrements can vary on an individual level and on the tissues affected.

Functional CFTR assays can help distinguish between mild and severe phenotypes by measuring the decrement in CFTR function along this continuum and can be informative beyond genotype information alone.[16] These tests are done at specialized centers throughout North America and usually are coordinated through CF referral centers. Cell-based assays are increasingly used to help resolve the functional implications of cryptic or ultra-rare mutations.

With widespread acceptance of newborn screening programs in the United States, it is now typical to diagnose CF before the onset of respiratory disease. A high index of suspicion must be maintained to ensure correct diagnosis in the event of screening failure or among individuals born before the initiation of newborn screening programs. Screening programs have led to the detection of CFTR-related dysfunction, as demonstrated by indeterminate range sweat chloride values in subjects without phenotypic CF. These individuals should be designated as having CFTR-related metabolic syndrome or, synonymously, a CF screen–positive inconclusive diagnosis. Current recommendations are that these individuals be followed annually by experienced CF providers because many have been reported to develop phenotypic CF later in life.[17] A significant number of CF patients may therefore present in adulthood because symptoms are unusual, subtle, or even absent early in life,

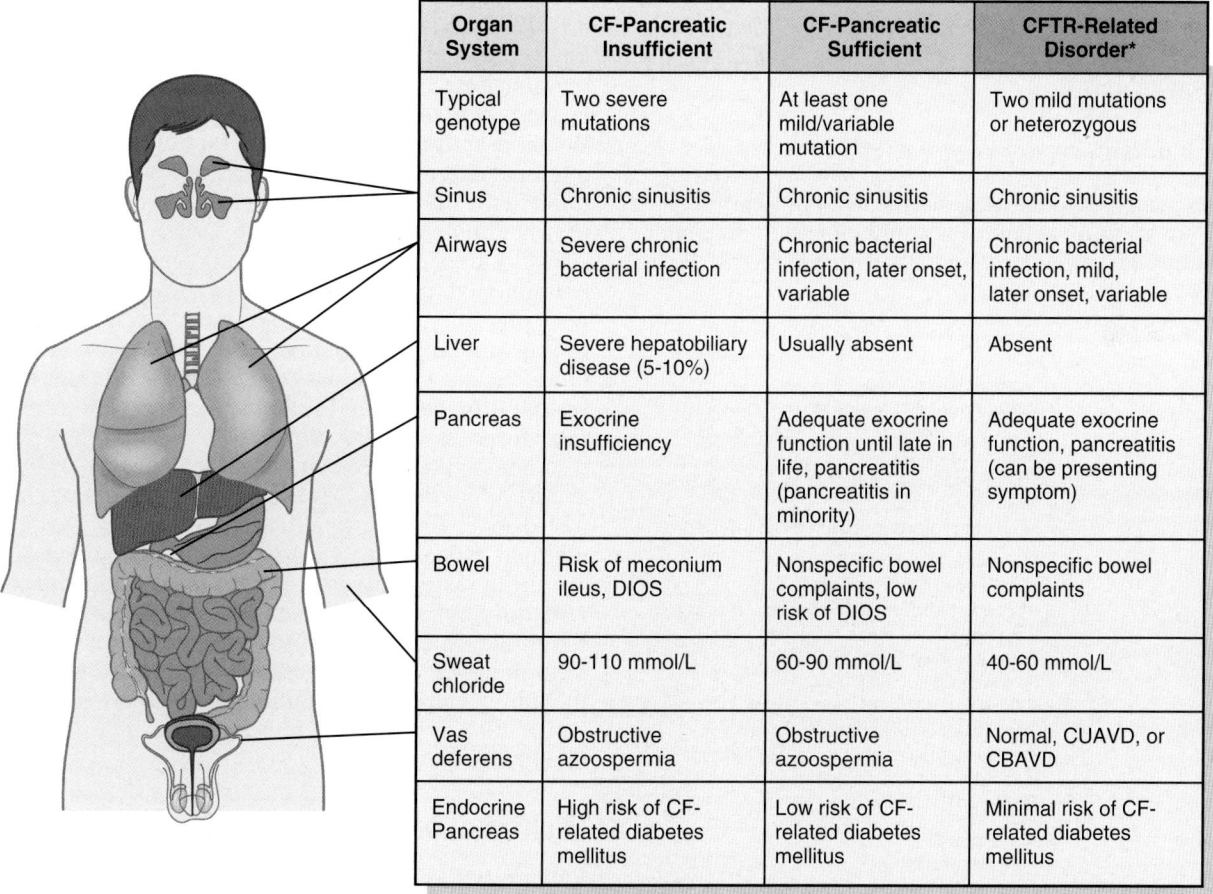

Organ System	CF-Pancreatic Insufficient	CF-Pancreatic Sufficient	CFTR-Related Disorder*
Typical genotype	Two severe mutations	At least one mild/variable mutation	Two mild mutations or heterozygous
Sinus	Chronic sinusitis	Chronic sinusitis	Chronic sinusitis
Airways	Severe chronic bacterial infection	Chronic bacterial infection, later onset, variable	Chronic bacterial infection, mild, later onset, variable
Liver	Severe hepatobiliary disease (5-10%)	Usually absent	Absent
Pancreas	Exocrine insufficiency	Adequate exocrine function until late in life, pancreatitis (pancreatitis in minority)	Adequate exocrine function, pancreatitis (can be presenting symptom)
Bowel	Risk of meconium ileus, DIOS	Nonspecific bowel complaints, low risk of DIOS	Nonspecific bowel complaints
Sweat chloride	90-110 mmol/L	60-90 mmol/L	40-60 mmol/L
Vas deferens	Obstructive azoospermia	Obstructive azoospermia	Normal, CUAVD, or CBAVD
Endocrine Pancreas	High risk of CF-related diabetes mellitus	Low risk of CF-related diabetes mellitus	Minimal risk of CF-related diabetes mellitus

Figure 68.2 Spectrum of cystic fibrosis disorders. A comparison between findings in severe *cystic fibrosis* (CF) and milder forms of the disease is shown. Although manifestations are variable, severity in each organ system is generally consistent with degree of *cystic fibrosis transmembrane conductance regulator* (CFTR) dysfunction conferred by genotype. CBAVD, congenital bilateral absence of the vas deferens; CUAVD, congenital unilateral absence of the vas deferens; DIOS, distal intestinal obstruction syndrome. *Refers to CFTR-related metabolic syndrome or CFTR-related disorders.

resulting in a delayed presentation. Oftentimes these CFTR-related metabolic syndrome–associated presentations are due to partially active *CFTR* alleles or other ameliorating mutations or factors resulting in milder CFTR functional defects (e.g., sweat chloride in the 30 to 59 mmol/L range or NPD in the intermediate severity range).[18] Recognition of the variable manifestations of CF is required to detect CF after early childhood.

Finally, the diagnosis of CFTR-related syndrome is usually made in older children and adults presenting with single-organ CF involvement (e.g., isolated bronchiectasis, sinusitis, pancreatitis, or congenital absence of the vas deferens) with inconclusive CFTR functional testing and genotype. The complexity of inconclusive diagnostic scenarios is outlined in eTable 68.1.

CLINICAL MANIFESTATIONS

CF has historically presented with protean manifestations and symptoms that may mimic or resemble other diseases. Usual presentations include early onset of respiratory tract findings, particularly persistent cough and recurrent or refractory chest radiographic changes. Gastrointestinal presentations are also prominent and include meconium ileus (in approximately 15% of patients) and failure to thrive with steatorrhea due to pancreatic insufficiency. A list of unusual presentations is compiled in Table 68.2. Clinical severity can vary widely; less severe disease states can be initially misdiagnosed as other more common respiratory conditions.

LOWER RESPIRATORY TRACT DISEASE

Progressive obstructive lung disease leading to bronchiectasis and respiratory failure accounts for the vast majority of mortality among individuals with the disease. Even

Table 68.2	Atypical Presentations of Cystic Fibrosis*
Respiratory	■ Bronchiolitis/asthma ■ ***Pseudomonas aeruginosa* or *Staphylococcus aureus* colonization of the respiratory tract** ■ Staphylococcal pneumonia ■ **Nasal polyposis** ■ **Nontuberculous mycobacterial infection**
Gastrointestinal	■ Meconium plug syndrome ■ Rectal prolapse ■ **Recurrent abdominal pain and/or right lower quadrant mass** ■ Hypoproteinemic edema ■ Prolonged neonatal jaundice ■ **Biliary cirrhosis with portal hypertension** ■ Vitamin deficiency states (A, D, E, K) ■ *Acrodermatitis enteropathica*–like eruption with fatty acid and zinc deficiency ■ **Recurrent pancreatitis**
Genitourinary	■ **Male infertility** ■ **Female infertility**
Other	■ Hypochloremic, hyponatremic alkalosis ■ **Mother of a child with cystic fibrosis**

*__Bold__ type signifies possible presentation in adolescents or adults with cystic fibrosis.

seemingly healthy infants with CF often have significant subclinical lung findings, including inflammation often disproportionate to the degree of infection.[19,20] The most common manifestation of lung disease is cough in association with bronchitis. Early in life, symptoms are often intermittent and exacerbated by episodes of acute respiratory tract infection that tend to exhibit a protracted course. With time, cough becomes a daily event. It is often more pronounced at night and on rising in the morning. With progression or during exacerbations of lung disease, cough typically becomes productive with tenacious, mucopurulent sputum secondary to chronic bacterial infection and neutrophilic inflammation, especially after the onset of chronic infection.

Hyperinflation of the lungs is common and often observed early in the progression of CF lung disease.[21] Asthmatic or bronchiolitic-type wheezing is often observed during the first 2 years of life but may be encountered at any age. Wheezing is noted in up to one-third of infants and may be present with or without evidence of atopy.[22] Early in life, CF can mimic the clinical manifestations of asthma and/or coexist with asthma, leading to delayed recognition if newborn screening is not definitive for a diagnosis.

Lung sounds are typically unremarkable at presentation; the first detectable abnormalities may be subtle retractions, diminished intensity of breath sounds, or prolongation of the expiratory phase. Once CF lung disease becomes clinically apparent, adventitious lung sounds are usually first noted in the upper lobes. CF patients may have only mild bronchitic findings for long periods during the time lung homeostasis is maintained but still manifest exacerbation of symptoms such as increased cough intensity and sputum production. Respiratory exacerbations often present as tachypnea, shortness of breath, malaise, anorexia, and weight loss. Viral respiratory tract infection is a frequent trigger, as are other infectious agents, cigarette smoke,[23] pollutants,[24] allergens, and respiratory irritants that have been implicated as disturbing lower airway physiology. Initiation of broad-spectrum antibiotic therapy and aggressive maneuvers to facilitate clearance of mucus are usually required to improve symptoms and restore lung function. Pulmonary exacerbations are now recognized as a major driver of overall disease progression, and aggressive attempts to recognize and treat these events before the advent of irreversible injury have become a priority.[25] As CF lung disease progresses, exacerbations characteristically become more frequent and severe, often requiring extended courses of intravenous antibiotics and hospitalization. End-stage lung damage associated with impairment of daily activities heralds a sequence of terminal events in the absence of lung transplantation, including hypoxemia, pulmonary hypertension, right ventricular dysfunction, hypercapnic respiratory failure, and death.

MICROBIOLOGY

Patients with CF demonstrate bacterial colonization of the airways early in life. Chronic infection of the lower airways, once established, is difficult to eradicate. *Staphylococcus aureus* and *Haemophilus influenzae* are usually the first organisms detected in CF lungs (Fig. 68.3) and often present with a comparatively benign clinical picture.[26] Historically, acquisition of *Pseudomonas aeruginosa* or *Burkholderia cepacia* was regarded as a particularly ominous clinical finding because these infections are associated with accelerated decline in lung function and increased mortality.[27] With the increased prevalence of microbiologic screening and more aggressive antimicrobial treatment regimens, a more broad and diversified group of respiratory pathogens has emerged.[28] These pathogens include *methicillin-resistant S. aureus* (MRSA), multidrug-resistant gram-negative rod bacteria, nontuberculous mycobacteria, and fungal organisms.[29] When present, these new opportunistic infections may be associated[30] with declining lung function. Often the clinical significance and complex factors contributing to the presence of these organisms in sputum culture are multifactorial and thus require careful clinical consideration to determine the appropriate timing and intensity of treatment. This is particularly true because certain organisms, such as nontuberculous mycobacterial and fungal organisms, may represent benign colonizers of CF lower airways.

The prevalence of *P. aeruginosa* increases with age, infecting more than two-thirds of patients by the third decade of life. The frequency of detection earlier in life has increased in the era of newborn screening and may be as high as 20% in children younger than 2 years; detection in infants at the time of diagnosis is common. Acquisition of *P. aeruginosa* increases longitudinally (see Fig. 68.3) and may be associated with genotype severity—individuals homozygous for F508del demonstrate a higher prevalence of chronic infection.[31] The effect of CFTR modulators on the eradication of bacteria appears promising at the population level based on the effect of ivacaftor in patients with gating mutations but continues to emerge for more common CFTR mutations[32,33] and for microbiome analyses.[34,35]

Nosocomial acquisition of new infections and transmission of multidrug-resistant organisms is a substantial concern in CF care.[36] Because eradication of sentinel infection has become an increasing priority, identification and earlier treatment of initial infection (e.g., due to *P. aeruginosa*) based on frequent sputum monitoring is recommended for those not previously colonized.[37–39] Sputum bacteriology correlates reasonably well with specimens obtained directly from the lower respiratory tract, although microbial sequencing is lending new insights into the validity of this conclusion.

Oropharyngeal swab cultures that yield *S. aureus* or *P. aeruginosa* are modestly predictive of results from bronchoscopic specimens, but negative pharyngeal cultures do not rule out growth of these organisms in lower airways.[40] Nevertheless, recent studies supporting sputum or oropharyngeal swab culture surveillance and subsequent treatment with intent to eradicate infection have demonstrated similar efficacy to more invasive detection regimens.[41] Other, more sensitive means to detect *P. aeruginosa*, such as polymerase chain reaction or circulating markers, may further improve sensitivity of noninvasive techniques. Quantitative bacteriology may be particularly useful for determining the relative contributions of isolated organisms in this setting.

As lung disease progresses, *P. aeruginosa* often becomes the predominant organism recovered from sputum and may be present in multiple strains with distinct antibiotic sensitivity patterns. The emergence of a mucoid phenotype due to elaboration of large amounts of *alginate*, an exopolysaccharide that protects the bacteria from adversity in its surroundings and also enhances adhesion to solid surfaces, is associated with worsened clinical outcome.[42] Mucoid organisms are found as microcolonies of pseudomonads embedded and growing in biofilms of alginate.[43] Biofilms inhibit phagocytosis and enhance bacterial adherence while limiting exposure to antibiotics and reactive intermediates produced by leukocytes.[44–47] Although the presence of a mucoid phenotype is clearly associated with colonization, new mucoid *Pseudomonas* infection or conversion to a mucoid phenotype may also be amenable to aggressive eradication strategies.[48,49] Isolation of *P. aeruginosa* from the lower respiratory tract of a child or young adult with chronic lung symptoms is highly suggestive of CF but has been reported in patients with primary ciliary dyskinesia, bronchiectasis, or other severe obstructive lung diseases.[50]

Although *P. aeruginosa* has remained the dominant pathogen in adult CF lung disease, MRSA has emerged as a significant contributor to disease progression and mortality.[51] In contrast, methicillin-susceptible strains are associated with improved outcomes.[52] Two studies using the U.S. CF registry have demonstrated an association between MRSA and worsened lung function, and another has shown MRSA infection to be an independent risk factor for mortality.[53,54] Considerable interest has emerged in the epidemiology and biologic significance of the staphylococcal chromosomal

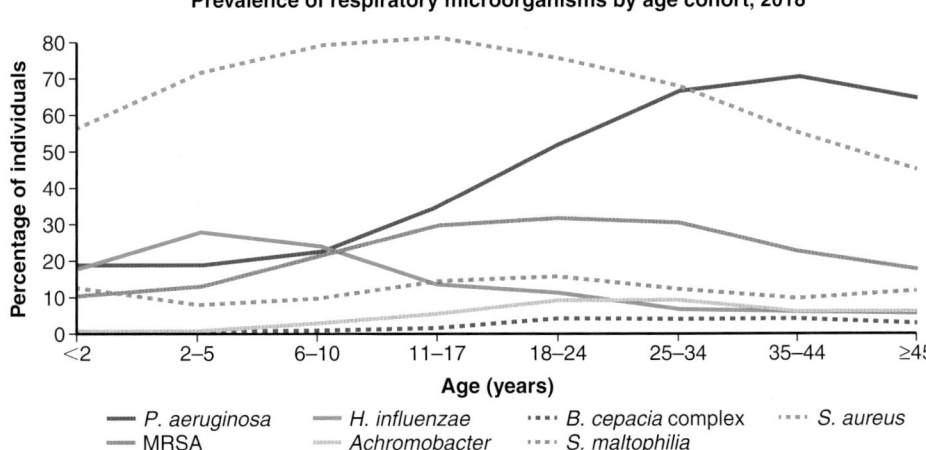

Prevalence of respiratory microorganisms by age cohort, 2018

Legend:
- P. aeruginosa
- MRSA
- H. influenzae
- Achromobacter
- B. cepacia complex
- S. maltophilia
- S. aureus

Figure 68.3 Alterations in sputum microbiology with age. Chronic infection with *Pseudomonas aeruginosa* and *methicillin-resistant Staphylococcus aureus* (MRSA) changes as a function of advancing age, based on data from cystic fibrosis care centers in the National CF Patient Registry. This is in contrast to a higher prevalence of *Haemophilus influenzae* and methicillin-sensitive *S. aureus* in childhood and adolescence among patients with cystic fibrosis. (Data from the Cystic Fibrosis Foundation, Patient Registry; Bethesda, MD; 2018.)

cassette containing the methicillin resistance gene and the Panton-Valentine leukocidin expressing strains, both of which have an effect on their virulence and impact disease severity.[29] Although the clinical significance of MRSA infection and colonization must be recognized, evidence is not sufficient to support aggressive eradication strategies in individuals with MRSA who are clinically stable.[55] Small-colony staphylococcus variants may also represent a distinct entity highly resistant to traditional therapy.[56] In addition, there is increasing recognition that MRSA exhibits biofilm-forming behavior in chronic infection.[57]

Numerous gram-negative pathogens in addition to *P. aeruginosa* have demonstrated a significant clinical impact on respiratory health, lending support to the notion that CF lung infection represents a significantly more complex microbiome than previously realized.[58] Of these, *B. cepacia* has remained the most ominous, due to its inherent multi-drug antibiotic resistance and association with rapid decline in CF pulmonary reserve.[59] Infection from *B. cepacia* can spread from patient to patient, requiring stringent infection control measures within CF care settings.[60,61] Infection has been linked to the rapid clinical deterioration and death of a small percentage of patients with what has been referred to as *cepacia* syndrome.[62] Molecular analyses have shown that *B. cepacia* complex is composed of at least nine phenotypically indistinguishable but genetically distinct species (genomovars).[38,63,64] Genomovars II (*Burkholderia multivorans*) and III (*Burkholderia cenocepacia*) have been associated with *cepacia* syndrome, and genomovar III includes a highly transmissible strain that may be linked to expression of the cable pilus, which enhances infectivity and virulence.[64–66] Other gram-negative rods present in CF sputum include mucoid *Escherichia coli*, *Stenotrophomonas maltophilia*, *Achromobacter xylosoxidans*, *Klebsiella*, and *Proteus*. Of these, *S. maltophilia* and *A. xylosoxidans* appear to have the strongest association with poor respiratory outcomes, but their clinical significance warrants further evaluation. Additional gram-negative organisms such as *Pandoraea* and *Ralstonia* sp have been isolated from CF sputum samples, but further clinical investigation will be necessary to determine their pathogenic significance. Obligate anaerobes have also been identified from CF lung tissue. These are typically undetected by standard clinical laboratory microbiologic analyses and may be found in large abscess cavities on rare occasions.[67,68]

Infection with *nontuberculous mycobacteria* (NTM) is increasingly observed in the CF population, presumably due to concomitant antibacterial therapy resulting in a favorable ecologic niche, host susceptibility, improved detection, and environmental prevalence.[69–74] Up to 20% of adult patients in some clinics are colonized by NTM, and its incidence has been increasing in recent years. Although culture positivity is sometimes transient, the deleterious clinical impact of these organisms once established is increasingly appreciated.[75] *Mycobacterium avium* complex infection is of variable clinical significance, whereas rapidly growing organisms such as *Mycobacterium abscessus* can exhibit a virulent course, prompting aggressive and prolonged treatment regimens.[72] In contrast, *Mycobacterium tuberculosis* infection has only been seen in sporadic cases. Studies to standardize treatment for these emerging pathogens in CF are underway.[76] (See also Chapter 55 for a detailed discussion of NTM infections in CF patients.)

Nearly 40% of individuals with CF will grow *Aspergillus fumigatus* in the sputum during their lifetime; patients who have severe lung disease appear to have an even higher incidence of sputum positivity.[77] The pathogenic nature of *Aspergillus* in an otherwise immunocompetent CF host is not well established, although it may contribute to the burden of excess mucus production. However, *Aspergillus* is clearly associated with *allergic bronchopulmonary aspergillosis* (ABPA). ABPA is present in approximately 2% of CF patients and adds a considerable burden of care.[78,79] ABPA is described later and in Chapters 69 and 96.

IMAGING

The earliest radiographic finding in CF lung disease is typically hyperinflation of the lungs, reflecting obstruction of small airways. Central airway thickening and linear opacities produce a "tram track" appearance representing bronchiectasis (eFig. 68.1) and often progress with age (Fig. 68.4, eFig. 68.2). Frequently, these findings are most

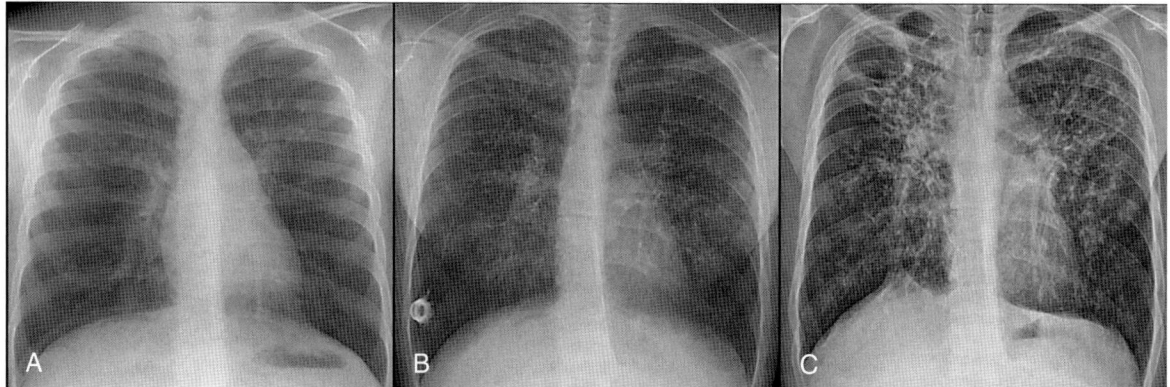

Figure 68.4 Cystic fibrosis: chest radiographic findings over 2 decades. (A) Frontal chest radiograph in a 9-year-old boy shows mid and upper lung predominant bronchovascular thickening, consistent with the bronchial wall thickening and bronchiectasis typical of cystic fibrosis. (B) Frontal chest radiograph performed in the same patient at age 19 years shows progression in the upper lobe predominant vascular thickening, now with a slightly more cystic appearance in the right upper lobe. (C) Frontal chest radiograph performed in the same patient at age 29 years, after the patient had become oxygen dependent, shows further worseninng of bronchial wall thickening and bronchiectasis, particularly in the right suprahilar region, now with hilar retraction suggesting upper lobe scarring. Bullae formation at the right apex is also now apparent. Note that the chest radiographic technique for this image used edge enhancement. (Courtesy Michael B. Gotway, MD.)

readily appreciated in the right upper lobe (eFig. 68.3) because this region is often involved before other areas. The appearance of bronchiectasis by *computed tomography* (CT) of the chest is highly characteristic of CF pulmonary involvement (see eFigs. 68.1B–E and 68.2B–E and Chapter 69). Although chest radiography is appealing due to accessibility and relatively low-dose radiation exposure, sensitivity for detecting acute or subtle chronic changes during a period of acute exacerbation remains limited.[80] Nonetheless, chest radiographs remain a standard first-line imaging test for surveillance and during acute exacerbations, for episodes of hemoptysis (eFig. 68.4), or to identify complications such as pneumothorax[81] (eFig. 68.5). Use of CF monitoring by chest CT is recommended biannually in stable CF patients.[82]

Chest CT, with its high-resolution cross-sectional imaging, is clearly superior for detecting mild disease and quantifying the extent and pattern of bronchiectasis (see eFigs. 68.1B–E and 68.2B–E).[83,84] Mosaic perfusion, manifesting as areas of inhomogeneous lung opacity resulting from air trapping and disordered parenchymal blood flow, is a common CT finding in patients with CF (eFig. 68.6). Small nodules due to bronchial and bronchiolar impaction are commonly observed (eFig. 68.7). CT studies have also demonstrated significant changes in young children, before obvious symptomatic disease, supporting the notion that CF lung disease begins early in life and disease detection is limited by the sensitivity of routine clinical procedures including spirometry.[83] Regardless of the imaging modality used, the degree of hyperinflation generally increases over time. As endobronchial infection and reactive inflammation emerge, peribronchial cuffing becomes increasingly apparent. Manifestations of bronchiectasis, including enlarged ring shadows or airway dilation and cysts, are common even early in life (see eFig. 68.1); upwards of 50% of CF patients demonstrate bronchiectasis by 3 to 5 years of age.[84]

During acute pulmonary exacerbation, a variety of radiographic findings may be noted. These include peripheral round densities and mucoid impaction seen radiographically as branching opacities. Such findings may be transient and resolve during therapy or be replaced by emergence of frank bronchiectatic or cystic changes. Additional findings, including subpleural blebs, often become evident during the second decade of life and are most prominent along the mediastinal border.[85]

The clinical justification for CT scanning in place of routine chest radiography is not well established. Clear indications may include management of a patient with focal disease being considered for lobectomy or of a patient experiencing acute deterioration—as a means to detect complications or evidence of new infection. Magnetic resonance imaging, which avoids radiation associated with CT, can define lung morphology, particularly as techniques have improved, although relative sensitivity and specificity of magnetic resonance techniques in CF have not yet been firmly established.[86] Recent imaging studies using hyperpolarized gas magnetic resonance imaging have begun to uncover early ventilation defects in young pediatric patients before obstruction is detected by spirometry. These findings correlate with the severity of obstruction; they mirror early defects of ventilation measured on more sensitive testing such as multiple breath washout and confirm that early imaging abnormalities are present in patients with preserved lung function.[87]

LUNG FUNCTION

Lung function in CF is believed to be normal at birth, although recent studies have demonstrated that, within weeks to months of delivery, the cycle of inflammation and infection has begun, and reduced cartilage size very early in life may predispose to airway obstruction.[88] Infants with CF can exhibit increased airway resistance, gas trapping, and diminished flow rates.[89–91] A few centers use infant pulmonary function testing to detect early evidence of airway obstruction and guide institution of therapeutic strategies before permanent lung injury has been established. *Lung clearance index*, a test performed by measuring the time for clearance of an inert gas through the multiple breath washout technique and a test not confounded by patient effort, has emerged as an important research tool used to detect early evidence of ventilation abnormality.[92–94] Reliable and consistent spirometry can be obtained routinely at 5 to 6 years of age, when children are able to cooperate.[95,96]

The earliest evidence of airway obstruction is typically limited to the small airways and thus is often first detectable by reduced forced mid-expiratory flow rates, reduced flows at low lung volumes, and gas trapping (i.e., elevated residual volume to total lung capacity ratio). Although infrequently applied during clinical management, abnormalities such as increased alveolar-arterial oxygen tension difference, frequency dependence of dynamic compliance, reduced response of flows to a helium-oxygen mixture, elevated slope of phase 3 of the single-breath nitrogen washout, and an elevated physiologic dead space are often present.[97] Spirometry is the most clinically useful test to follow the course of respiratory disease progression and is typically measured at each clinic visit. Equally important is assessment of the flow volume loop, which may demonstrate obstruction by concavity, with low flows especially in the terminal portion of the curve, earlier than either the *forced expiratory volume in 1 second* (FEV_1) or mean forced expiratory flow from 25–75% of the forced vital capacity. As discussed earlier, early ventilatory defects can be uncovered using imaging techniques in the research setting.

Over time, patients with active CF lung disease typically experience progressive deterioration of lung function. The annualized rate of decline in FEV_1 is approximately 2–3% of predicted FEV_1.[98] Despite recent advances, this progressive loss of pulmonary reserve often accelerates in young adulthood.[99] As respiratory disease progresses, peripheral airway obstruction yields to more generalized blockage and air trapping as increasingly damaged airways cease to contribute to gas exchange, mimicking a restrictive pattern by spirometry.[100]

The chronic cycle of inflammation and infection contributes to CF lung disease, and patients typically exhibit progressive decrements of arterial P_{O_2}. Oxygenation declines slowly throughout life but may not become symptomatically limiting until late in the disease course. Patients who are able to sustain adequate oxygenation usually function well despite the presence of obstructive impairment.

When arterial P_{O_2} values are chronically below 55 mm Hg, patients are at high risk for development of pulmonary hypertension.[101,102] Clinically significant hypoxemia most commonly presents during sleep, particularly during rapid eye movement–associated hypoventilation, and it is a significant factor leading to pulmonary hypertension.[103] Desaturation at rest or with exertion as measured during a 6-minute walk test is a negative prognostic indicator and associated with increased risk of CF mortality.[104] Elevation of arterial P_{CO_2} and FEV_1 less than 30% define end-stage CF lung disease. Patients with FEV_1 less than 30% of predicted, arterial P_{CO_2} greater than 50 mm Hg, or arterial P_{O_2} less than 55 mm Hg have a predicted 2-year mortality of 50% and should be considered for lung transplantation.[105] Other prediction tools can facilitate appropriate patient selection for referral and outperform reliance on any single criterion.[106]

Bronchial hyperresponsiveness is a consistent finding in asthma, but its presence and clinical significance in CF remains controversial.[107,108] Bronchial hyperresponsiveness in CF has been demonstrated during exercise testing, during bronchoprovocation testing, or by the response to bronchodilators, with two-thirds of CF patients demonstrating decreased forced expiratory flows after a bronchoconstrictive challenge. In contrast to cross-sectional studies, repeated tests every 1 to 3 months for a year have demonstrated bronchodilator responsiveness at least once in 95% of subjects.[109] Despite its frequency, the pathogenesis of bronchial hyperresponsiveness in CF is unclear. The finding is unrelated to the severity of pulmonary disease or indices of atopy but appears to be more prevalent during winter months. Hyperresponsiveness diminishes during acute exacerbations of CF lung disease, but often returns as lung function improves following 2 weeks of intensive antibiotic therapy. Patients with CF may also have a lack of response to bronchodilators that may be related to diminished tone in bronchiectatic airways.

Exercise tolerance in CF is related to the severity of airway obstruction.[110] Nearly 50% of patients with moderate to severe airway obstruction may experience oxygen desaturation to below 90% during peak exercise.[111] Persons with CF have higher than expected ventilatory muscle endurance, and this endurance can be further improved with inspiratory muscle training. However, improved inspiratory muscle strength and endurance do not augment exercise performance, suggesting that this is not the limiting factor in exercise.

Exercise therapy in CF has many physiologic and biologic benefits although it does not improve standard spirometry. Nevertheless, standardized aerobic and resistive exercise does improve cardiorespiratory fitness and *quality of life* (QOL) and has been associated with a reduced risk of hospitalization.[112] Maximum oxygen consumption during exercise has been suggested as a better predictor of survival than routine pulmonary function testing, although the test is time-consuming and not available in all clinical settings.[113] Several more clinically efficient measures of physical fitness show strong correlation with maximum oxygen consumption and CF disease prognosis, further reinforcing the notion that improved physical health through exercise may benefit overall clinical status.[114]

UPPER RESPIRATORY TRACT DISEASE

Chronic rhinosinusitis is present in virtually all patients with CF. CF sinus disease manifests as chronic, relapsing symptoms of increased upper airway secretions, moderate airflow obstruction, and widening of the nasal bridge.[115] This can be noted during imaging (eFig. 68.8) as opacification of the paranasal sinuses and has been reported in more than 90% of patients during the first year of life. Nasal polyps are seen in an additional 15–20% of individuals with CF.[116] Nasal polyps usually present towards the end of the first or during the second decade of life and may be the clinical finding that triggers diagnostic evaluation.[117] The presence of acute and chronic nasal obstruction can diminish olfactory function and contribute to diminished dietary intake with subsequent nutritional decline.[118] Despite the presence of pronounced radiographic abnormalities, nasal symptoms can be surprisingly well tolerated. Complaints related to acute or chronic sinusitis manifest in less than 10% of children and approximately 24% of adults.[119,120] Nevertheless, colonization of the upper airway may contribute to lower airway disease (e.g., as a reservoir for CF pathogens), although more recent pediatric literature suggests that there may be discordance between upper and lower airway tract flora.[121] In symptomatic patients, sinus débridement remains a mainstay of therapy for those who have not responded to medical treatments, but there is inconclusive evidence for the role of endoscopic sinus surgical treatment in management of symptoms of lower respiratory tract disease.[122]

COMPLICATIONS OF RESPIRATORY TRACT DISEASE

Atelectasis is present in approximately 5% of CF patients during the first 5 years of life and diminishes in frequency with advanced age.[123] Atelectasis can be lobar or subsegmental, with the right lung most commonly affected, and may develop concurrently with pulmonary exacerbations or in the absence of clinical symptoms. Occasionally, atelectasis results from endobronchial aspergillosis presenting as mucoid impaction and volume loss.[124] In most instances, however, a discrete mucous plug is not evident on bronchoscopy.

Pneumothorax (see eFig. 68.5) is a well-recognized CF complication caused by air trapping and subsequent rupture of subpleural blebs. Although the finding is equal among sexes and fairly rare (about 1% per year), incidence increases sharply with age and disease severity. Up to 20% of adults with CF experience at least one pneumothorax during their lifetime,[125] and recurrence is common. Typical presentations include acute onset of chest pain, dyspnea, respiratory distress, or hemoptysis.[126] Simultaneous bilateral pneumothoraces have been described and may constitute a medical emergency. Tension pneumothorax, which is more common in CF than in other obstructive lung diseases, may be life-threatening. Small asymptomatic pneumothoraces may be discovered in patients on routine surveillance chest radiography.

Hemoptysis is a relatively common event in CF (see eFig. 68.4) and is believed to result from mucosal erosions and bronchial artery hypertrophy, which are a consequence of chronic inflammation.[127] The presence of hemoptysis correlates with disease severity and is more common in the setting of chronic MRSA infection.[126] Blood streaking in the sputum is a frequent finding and may be intermittent and chronic. Massive hemoptysis (>240 mL blood in 24 hours) presents in approximately 5% of patients during their lifetime.[128] Due to the strong correlation between new-onset hemoptysis and exacerbation of lung infection, initial treatment should include antibiotic therapy, with omission of chest physiotherapy. Typically, aerosol treatments are temporarily held, and measures to promote clot stabilization are considered. There are anecdotal reports describing use of the antifibrinolytic agent tranexamic acid in this setting.[129] Beta-blockade has also been reported to provide benefit during acute and chronic hemoptysis, presumably by reducing blood pressure and blunting the sympathetic response to coughing.[130] Although bronchoscopy can help localize the site of bleeding, emergent bronchoscopy or radiographic imaging are of limited clinical utility and are not currently recommended in the emergent evaluation of hemoptysis. Instead, rapid assessment for emergent bronchial artery embolization (see eFig. 68.4F–G) is preferred. Advances in invasive vascular intervention and improved clinical management strategies have resulted in significantly reduced mortality, which was historically as high as 10% following massive hemoptysis.[131](See also Chapter 40.)

ABPA has a lifetime incidence of 2–8% among CF patients, although a few small cohort studies have reported incidence as high as 20%.[132,133] *Aspergillus* is a common environmental mold and is frequently recovered in sputum culture. Although up to 50% of patients with CF may demonstrate precipitating antibodies to *A. fumigatus* in their serum, an immunoglobulin E (IgE)-mediated allergic hypersensitization must develop to manifest symptoms of ABPA infection.[134] Clinical features include increased cough, dyspnea, wheezing, and expectoration of rusty-brown plugs with eosinophilic infiltrates by microscopy. Radiographic findings can be present, including a characteristic finger-in-glove pattern (see Fig. 96.7). Atelectasis and volume loss may also result from hyphae-laden mucoid impaction in segmental bronchi. A diagnosis of ABPA is made by fulfilling major and minor criteria that include characteristic clinical findings plus skin test hypersensitivity, elevated total IgE, and increased levels of IgG and IgE antibodies against *A. fumigatus* or other fungi.[78] (For full details on diagnosis, see Chapter 96.)

Staphylococcal and pseudomonal empyemas have been described in patients with CF, but respiratory tract infections typically spare the pleural space, making complications such as pleural effusion and empyema uncommon. Nonetheless, pulmonary exacerbations commonly present with pleuritic-type pain.[135]

Digital clubbing, which is caused by hyperplasia and hypertrophy of connective tissue and increased vascularity of the distal phalanges, appears in virtually all patients with advanced CF and is often present early in individuals with active lung disease (see Fig. 18.3). The cause of clubbing is unknown, and the finding may resolve following lung transplantation.[136] Severity generally correlates with extent of lung disease.[137] Hypertrophic pulmonary osteoarthropathy is a common clinical entity presenting with advanced CF lung disease in up to 15% of older adolescents

and adults.[102] Radiographic evidence for periostitis may be present in up to 8% of subjects (see eFig. 18.1). Distal aspects of the tibia, fibula, radius, and ulna are most commonly affected. Symptoms can include pain, bone tenderness, swelling, and warmth over the involved areas. Pain with ambulation or following strenuous physical exercise is common.[138] Hypertrophic pulmonary osteoarthropathy is worsened during periods of poorer respiratory health and exacerbation and tends to subside with resolution of pulmonary exacerbation. During end-stage lung disease, persistent joint symptoms may require chronic analgesic therapy. Rare instances of cutaneous vasculitis causing self-limited, painless, palpable purpura, typically involving the lower extremities, have also been reported in CF.[139–141]

Respiratory failure is the greatest contributor to mortality and is the cause of death in more than 90% of CF patients. In early CF, hypoxemia is observed during exertion or sleep and progresses in concert with lung disease.[103,142] Hypercapnia is a late finding reflecting advanced pulmonary decline, which often worsens during clinical exacerbation. Pulmonary hypertension and right ventricular dysfunction may develop late in the disease process, resulting in hepatic congestion and peripheral edema.[143] The role of pulmonary hypertension in CF is an area of considerable interest, particularly with regard to determining optimal treatment regimens.[144] Hypoxemia, if not recognized or adequately treated, contributes to worsening pulmonary hypertension and cardiac failure. Pneumothorax, hemoptysis, and infections such as respiratory syncytial virus or influenza can cause acute respiratory failure that is reversible with aggressive treatment.[145,146]

GASTROINTESTINAL MANIFESTATIONS

Meconium ileus is observed in approximately 15% of newborns with CF and is highly specific for the diagnosis of CF in the neonatal period. Failure to pass thick inspissated meconium during the first 48 hours of life is associated with abdominal distention and rapidly advances to bilious emesis. Affected infants are at risk for intestinal perforation and peritonitis accompanied by shock. Radiographic features are typical of high-grade bowel obstruction and reveal multiple dilated loops of intestine and air-fluid levels (eFig. 68.9). A granular appearance of the lower abdomen may be noted due to accumulated meconium containing small air bubbles. The colon is characteristically small when visualized with contrast imaging (eFig. 68.10). Scrotal and peritoneal calcification may be observed if the ileum has perforated in utero. Meconium obstruction of the colon can also interfere with passage of stool, but it presents a distinct clinical scenario that has been termed the meconium plug syndrome and is much less specific for CF.[147]

Beyond the newborn period, approximately 20% of CF patients develop the distal intestinal obstruction syndrome annually. This relatively common sequela is characterized by obstruction in the cecum, proximal colon, or terminal ileum associated with voluminous, viscous, and incompletely digested intestinal contents and is otherwise similar to meconium ileus (eFig. 68.11). Partial obstruction may manifest as a chronic or recurrent condition with intermittent crampy abdominal pain as the only symptom. Fulminant, complete obstruction is associated with failure to pass stool, resulting in abdominal distention and vomiting that may be bilious or fecal if allowed to progress. A mobile right lower quadrant mass may be palpable. Risk factors for distal intestinal obstruction syndrome include previous episodes, dehydration, change of diet, immobilization, bacterial overgrowth, hospitalization for pulmonary exacerbations, treatment with antibiotics, and constipating medications. Other causes of acute abdominal pain with obstruction should also be considered, including intussusception, intestinal adhesions from previous abdominal surgery, and appendicitis, which may be clinically less evident due to concurrent antibiotic therapy.[148] Appendicitis is thought to be uncommon in CF, with a 2% lifetime risk compared with 7–8% risk in the general population.[149] Nonfilling of the appendix with contrast enema has been observed in patients with CF. Radiographic and histologic findings of a dilated, mucus-filled appendix are typical features,[150,151] although the uninflamed appendix is also frequently enlarged on CT in the absence of appendicitis (eFig. 68.12). Inadequate pancreatic and bowel secretion of bicarbonate in CF may also contribute to duodenal irritation and recurrent epigastric pain by failing to buffer gastric acid.[152]

Gastroesophageal reflux is prevalent in CF, in part due to increased abdominal pressure associated with obstructive lung disease resulting in decreased lower esophageal sphincter tone. In addition, a direct effect of gastric acidification due to CFTR protein dysfunction resulting in decreased buffering capacity in the stomach may contribute.[153] Consideration of gastroesophageal reflux is important because the condition can impair nutritional status and may contribute to microaspiration, accelerating respiratory decline. The presence of gastroesophageal reflux has been associated with worsened outcome after lung transplantation, and patients with CF considered for transplant should be evaluated thoroughly in this regard. Certain transplant centers recommend surgical therapy for ongoing reflux during the peritransplant period.[154]

Rectal prolapse develops in nearly 20% of children with CF but is an infrequent event for adults.[155] Rectal prolapse in a child should raise suspicion for an underlying CF diagnosis, even if this is the only clinical finding. The clinical diagnosis of prolapse is often precipitated by the presence of bulky, sticky stools that adhere to rectal mucosa, associated poor nutritional status, and loss of perirectal fat that normally supports the rectum, as well as presence of high intra-abdominal pressure due to frequent paroxysmal coughing.

Colorectal carcinoma in adults with CF is up to 10 times more frequent than in the general population, probably as a consequence of chronic inflammation. Colorectal carcinoma is up to 30 times more frequent in CF patients after organ transplantation, probably due to the additional risk associated with immunosuppression.[156] Current recommendations include colonoscopy screening at age 40 years with 5-year rescreening and 3-year surveillance intervals (unless a shorter interval is indicated by individual findings) and a CF-specific intensive bowel preparation.[156] Organ transplant recipients with CF should initiate colorectal screening at age 30 years within 2 years of the transplantation because of their additional risk.

PANCREATIC DISEASE

Exocrine pancreatic insufficiency, due to intraductal obstruction by thickened, dehydrated secretions, is present from birth in approximately 85% of patients with CF.[157,158] Adequate exocrine pancreatic secretion is present in up to 15% of patients and has been associated with certain (residual function) CFTR genotypes. Insufficient release of pancreatic enzymes into the gut impairs fat and protein digestion and reduces absorption by the small bowel. Pancreatic insufficiency results in frequent bulky, greasy, foul-smelling stools and protuberance of the abdomen due to increased intraluminal bacterial gas production. Assessment of pancreatic function by enzyme-linked immunosorbent assay measurement of stool fecal elastase-1 is diagnostic in the clinical assessment of pancreatic insufficiency.[159] Complete fatty replacement of the pancreas is common, as judged by CT (eFig. 68.13), and pancreatic lipomatosis and fibrosis are characteristic of pediatric CF. Pancreatic ductal dilation and calcifications are also observed in CF patients. Rarely, there may be cystic replacement of the pancreas, referred to as pancreatic cystosis.

Untreated malabsorption due to exocrine pancreatic insufficiency results in nutritional failure and impaired linear growth, which has been linked to worsened clinical outcomes.[160] Patients with CF often grow slowly because of factors other than poor nutritional intake and intestinal malabsorption. For example, increased expenditure of energy to accomplish the work of breathing may be an important contributor, and systemic inflammation may also play a role.[158] Fat-soluble vitamin deficiency due to nutritional failure was historically common in young children with CF but is much less common in the era of early diagnosis via newborn screening with early vitamin and pancreatic enzyme replacement.

Symptomatic pancreatitis with paroxysmal pain develops in less than 1% of adolescent or adult CF patients, usually in those who maintain at least some residual exocrine pancreatic function.[161] Recurrent painful pancreatitis can be the presenting feature of CTFR-related disorders.[162,163]

HEPATOBILIARY DISEASE

Diagnosis of cystic fibrosis liver disease[164] is formally made by the presence of two or more of the following: hepatomegaly and/or splenomegaly, confirmed by ultrasonography; abnormalities of alanine aminotransferase, aspartate aminotransferase, and γ-glutamyltransferase greater than 1.5 to 2 times the upper limits of normal for more than 6 months after excluding other causes of liver disease; ultrasonographic evidence of coarseness, nodularity, increased echogenicity, or portal hypertension; or, liver biopsy showing focal biliary cirrhosis or multilobular cirrhosis. Histologically, CF liver damage manifests as focal biliary cirrhosis and has produced clinically significant liver pathology in greater numbers of CF patients as they live longer. One description of clinically significant disease includes the constellation of an abnormal physical exam, characteristic liver function testing, and radiographic findings.[165] Liver disease may present as hepatosplenomegaly or most commonly as persistent elevation of hepatic enzymes (aspartate aminotransferase/alanine aminotransferase and/or bilirubin and γ-glutamyltransferase). Current guidelines recommend a comprehensive evaluation for CF liver disease when enzymes are greater than 3 times the upper limit of normal or remain 1.5- to 2-fold increased for a period of 3 months. Patients with CF-associated liver disease rarely develop acute fulminant hepatic failure but may progress to advanced cirrhosis, portal hypertension, and clinically significant esophageal varices.[166] Steatosis is a common clinical finding and has been associated with malnutrition, essential fatty acid deficiency, and/or oxidative stress in the setting of CF hepatobiliary dysfunction.[165] Ultrasound is generally used to monitor severity of CF liver injury, including in longitudinal studies.

Biliary tract disease is common in CF. Cholelithiasis develops in approximately 10% of patients but causes significant clinical symptoms in less than 4% of cases.[167] The risk of stone formation is increased due to abnormal ion transport within the gallbladder, which may result in biliary colic or symptomatic cholelithiasis. A small or microgallbladder, seen in 20–30% of CF patients, is of unknown clinical significance.[168]

GENITOURINARY TRACT ABNORMALITIES

The vas deferens is absent in almost all adult men with CF.[169] Semen analysis can be used to identify the 1% of male CF patients who remain fertile. Volume of ejaculate in men with the disease is usually one-third to one-half of normal and exhibits complete absence of spermatozoa in addition to a number of chemical abnormalities that reflect aberrant secretions from the seminal vesicles.[170] Male infertility is increasingly overcome via sperm harvest paired with in vitro fertilization methods, which have become more widespread and effective. The patient and family may consider prenatal genetic testing of partners or spouses and early preimplantation genetic testing if in vitro fertilization methods are used. An increased incidence of inguinal hernia and hydrocele has also been reported.

Although significantly less common than vas deferens atresia, female infertility in CF may be as high as 20%.[171] Many women with CF and advanced lung disease and/or malnutrition are anovulatory. Another obstacle to conception is the presence of thick tenacious cervical mucus and increased endocervicitis. Dehydrated cervical mucus is characterized by abnormal electrolyte and other compositions, preventing the physiologic ferning of midcycle. As a result, CF abnormal mucus is thought to impede normal sperm migration.[171]

Pregnancy in women with CF appears to be increasing as clinical outcomes have improved. A longitudinal study of 325 pregnant women with CF demonstrated 258 live births (79%).[172] Pregnancy in women in a large observational study did not contribute to pulmonary decline or mortality over 2 years.[173] Successful pregnancy and delivery are possible and can be carried out safely, but it is essential that women with CF consider implications to their health as they embark on family planning.[174] CFTR modulators may increase fertility due to effects on cervical mucus; however, recommendations on their use during pregnancy are still emerging. Successful breastfeeding has also been reported among women with the disease.[175]

Urinary incontinence can be seen beginning in adolescence and does not clearly correlate with CF disease severity; rather, incontinence probably reflects chronic cough and increased abdominal pressure due to airflow obstruction.[176]

SWEAT GLAND DYSFUNCTION

Sweat sodium chloride is elevated in most CF patients due to abnormal reabsorption of chloride from the sweat duct lumen in the absence of CFTR (see also earlier). This may predispose individuals with CF to excessive salt loss in certain settings. Young children are especially susceptible to salt depletion, especially when exposed to warm, arid climates or when there is additional salt loss due to vomiting or diarrhea. Children in this circumstance typically present with lethargy, anorexia, and hypochloremic alkalosis and/or hyponatremia.[177]

TREATMENT

OVERVIEW

A concerted effort to address the pulmonary manifestations in a comprehensive fashion has led to improved CF outcomes.[178] Therapies including mucolytics,[179] hydrators of the airway surface,[180,181] inhaled antimicrobials,[182–184] systemic anti-inflammatory treatments,[185–187] and nutritional support are traditional mainstays of CF treatment (Table 68.3). These supportive therapies, in addition to comprehensive care undertaken at organized CF clinical centers, are partly responsible for a steadily improving life expectancy observed over the past 3 decades

Table 68.3 Supportive Cystic Fibrosis Therapeutics by Category

Agent	Predominant Mechanism of Action
RESTORATION OF AIRWAY SURFACE HYDRATION	
Hypertonic saline*	Osmotic increase of airway hydration; expectorant
Mannitol†	Osmotic increase of airway hydration; expectorant
MUCOLYTICS	
Dornase alfa	Cleavage of DNA polymers
ANTI-INFLAMMATORY	
Ibuprofen	Reduction of airway inflammation
ANTI-INFECTIVES	
Inhaled tobramycin	Chronic treatment of *Pseudomonas aeruginosa*
Inhaled aztreonam	Chronic treatment of *P. aeruginosa*
Dry powder tobramycin	Chronic treatment of *P. aeruginosa*
Azithromycin	Anti-inflammatory/anti-infective for chronic *P. aeruginosa* infection
NUTRITIONAL THERAPIES	
AquADEKs	Restoration of fat-soluble vitamin levels
Pancrelipase	Restoration of pancreatic enzyme levels

*Therapy commonly used but not approved by the U.S. Food and Drug Administration.
†Therapy approved in the United States, Europe, Australia, and New Zealand; other approvals under consideration.

in the United States (Fig. 68.5), resulting in a median life expectancy of 41 years in 2012 increasing to 47 years in 2018.[188] Similar improvements have been observed in other developed countries. More recently, treatments that address the basic defect by restoring CFTR function have emerged, resulting in marked clinical improvement for the majority of individuals with CF, promising to transform the disease.[189] Other therapies that address rare *CFTR* alleles not yet impacted by CFTR modulators, including genetic-based treatments, are in various stages of development (Fig. 68.6).

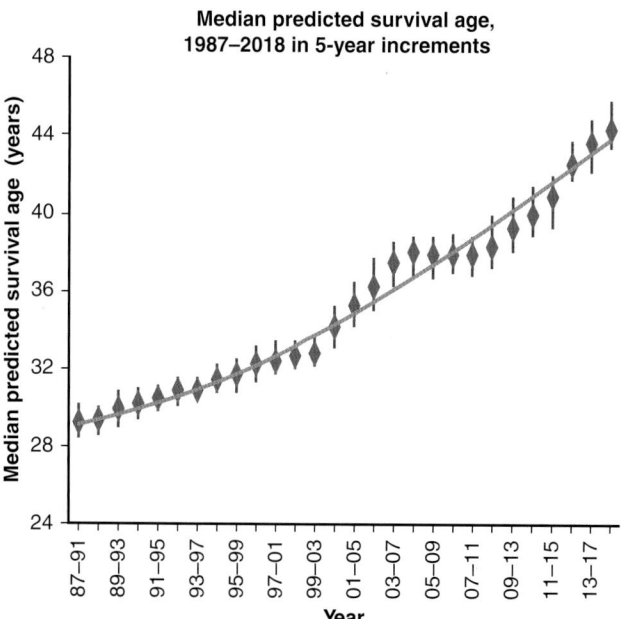

Figure 68.5 Median predicted survival in cystic fibrosis. Median predicted survival for *cystic fibrosis* (CF) patients in U.S. CF centers in the CF registry is depicted as the median for each 5-year time span from 1987 to 2018. Since the mid-1980s, predicted survival has increased from about 27 years of age to older than 40 years for the most recent 5-year time span. (Data from the Cystic Fibrosis Foundation Patient Registry, Bethesda, MD; 2018.)

MONITORING AND AGGRESSIVE APPROACH

Aggressive monitoring and treatment of pulmonary infections and other common CF complications have contributed significantly to improved clinical status in the disease.[99,190,191] Substantial attention has focused on efforts to delay or prevent chronic colonization with *P. aeruginosa*, with a number of studies evaluating various regimens to achieve sustained bacterial clearance. Coincident with this approach is increased attention to infection control as a means to forestall acquisition of virulent organisms, particularly in health care settings where risk from these pathogens is significant. Segregation of clinics by *Pseudomonas* status can reduce spread of highly prevalent organisms (i.e., standard infection control procedures alone may not be sufficient).[192,193] Observations of this type have led to rigorous guidelines for patient isolation and prevention against comingling and consequent infection.[194] Once established, *P. aeruginosa* is challenging to eradicate with antimicrobial therapy alone,[195–199] although this can be accomplished in certain patients,[49] including a subset of individuals initiating CFTR modulator therapy (see later). Chronic colonization with *Pseudomonas* is associated with a more rapid decline in respiratory status.[27,42,200] Virulent organisms such as *B. cepacia*[201,202] confer an even worse prognosis and have been associated with outbreaks due to nosocomial spread. Despite advances in lung function and inhibition of *Pseudomonas* growth, delaying progression of CF disease during adolescence remains a challenge. However, early aggressive care, particularly prior to substantial respiratory decline, is thought to forestall permanent loss of lung function.[203] As with chronic pulmonary infection, early and aggressive nutritional therapy, particularly among young children with CF, has been crucial to achieving improved outcomes.

CF centers have embarked on a rigorous quality improvement program to facilitate best practices in CF care. Outcomes are compared between centers and made publicly available to encourage continuous improvement.[204] A culture of cooperation among centers, patients, families, and the Cystic Fibrosis Foundation has led to evidence-based

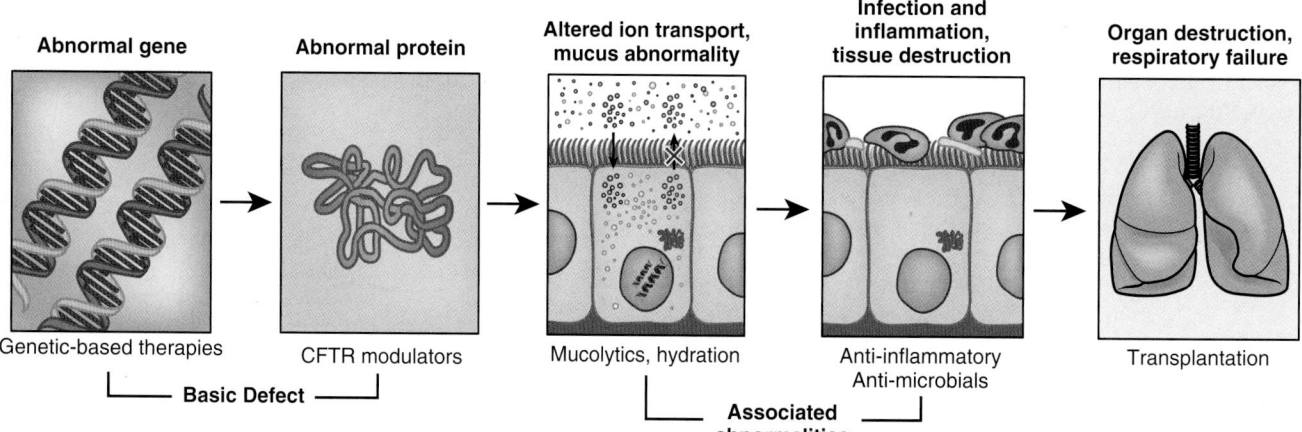

Figure 68.6 *Cystic fibrosis* (CF) therapeutics by category. This figure depicts the mechanisms and possible therapeutics for CF airway pathology. CF therapeutics attempt to address defective *cystic fibrosis transmembrane conductance regulator* (CFTR) function by genetic-based therapy or modulation of CFTR expression or function; to address the diminished airway surface liquid, abnormally viscous mucus, and disrupted mucociliary clearance; and, finally, to treat chronic airway infection and inflammation. When respiratory failure develops, lung transplantation is the remaining option.

guidelines, protocol-driven therapies, and rapid dissemination of results to facilitate advances in health care delivery.[205]

Cystic Fibrosis Transmembrane Conductance Regulator Potentiators, Correctors, and Other Treatments for the Basic Defect

On the basis of functional consequences of various *CFTR* mutations, specific therapeutic strategies to restore deficient or defective protein activity have been developed by altering CFTR expression or function (Fig. 68.7 and Table 68.4). Following ambitious high-throughput drug screening efforts to bolster their discovery,[206–210] benefits of these new CFTR modulators have rapidly come to fruition and expanded beyond initial indications. Rescue of CFTR protein function to sufficient levels, now termed "highly effective," as first established by the archetype CFTR modulator ivacaftor, is associated with marked improvement in the clinical outcome that is dramatically more efficacious than previous therapies.[189,211,212] *CFTR potentiators* activate CFTR channels located at the cell surface by potentiating cyclic adenosine monophosphate–mediated channel

gating.[206,213–215] Ivacaftor, a potentiator-type modulator that improves CFTR gating, was the first to be approved and was initially demonstrated in CF patients with the G551D gating mutation, an allele represented in approximately 4% of those with the disease. Subsequently, ivacaftor was also shown to activate 23 additional CFTR alleles as a monotherapy, based on clinical and in vitro data that justified[216,217] expansion of its indications. The highly efficacious treatment benefit observed with ivacaftor therapy led to strong interest in recapitulating the effect among other, more common *CFTR* alleles.[218] This includes correctors of F508del CFTR misfolding, termed CFTR correctors. *CFTR correctors* restore normal CFTR processing of the most common *CFTR* mutation, F508del, and of other alleles with class II properties, and are used in one or two corrector combinations with CFTR potentiators to restore CFTR function. Agents that induce translational readthrough (or suppression) of premature termination codons (class I) to induce expression of full-length CFTR are also under development.[219–222] *CFTR amplifiers* augment translation efficiency and thus increase protein levels, which could augment function for various CFTR genotypes. Approaches beyond these small molecule

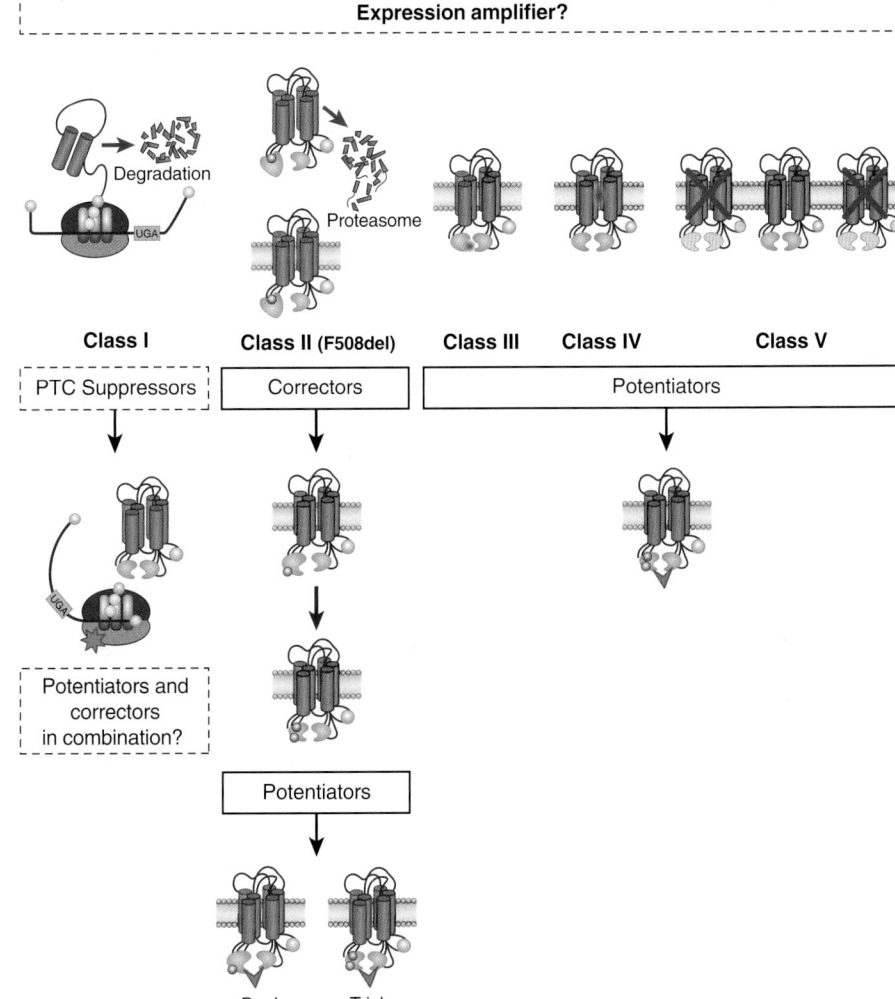

Figure 68.7 **Schematic of approach to *cystic fibrosis transmembrane conductance regulator* (CFTR) restoration with small molecules, by mutation class.** Therapeutic approaches with definitive studies are shown in solid boxes; those under investigation are noted by dashed boxes. CFTR mutations can be addressed pharmacologically based on their underlying molecular defect (see Chapter 67). CFTR expression amplifiers increase CFTR transcription and/or translation efficiency and would be expected to have broad-ranging effects across mutation classes. Nonsense mutations (a form of class I mutation) have the potential to be restored by *premature termination codon* (PTC)-suppressing drugs that induce full-length functional CFTR protein. Because some protein forms generated by translational readthrough are dysfunctional, the addition of correctors and potentiators may also be needed. Misfolded mutations (class II), including F508del, require multiagent therapy to restore processing and trafficking with a CFTR corrector and then to augment ion channel function with CFTR potentiators. CFTR proteins that are localized to the cell surface but are dysfunctional, or reduced in number, as in class III, IV, and/or V mutations (in addition to class VI, not shown), can be addressed by CFTR potentiators alone. *Green star,* PTC suppressor; *green circles,* correctors; *green chevrons,* potentiators. (Data from Mall MA, Mayer-Hamblett N, Rowe SM. Cystic fibrosis: Emergence of highly effective targeted therapeutics and potential clinical implications. *Am J Respir Crit Care Med.* 2019; and Bell SC, Mall MA, Gutierrez H, et al. The future of cystic fibrosis care: a global perspective. *Lancet Respir Med.* 2020;8[1]:65–124.)

Table 68.4 Approved Therapeutics Targeting Each CFTR Mutational Class

CFTR Modulator Class	Molecule	CFTR Mutations Affected	CFTR Mutation Class Affected
Potentiator	Ivacaftor	G551D/S	II
		Non-G551D gating mutations	III
		Surface localized CFTR Alleles	IV
		F508del*	V
Correctors	Lumacaftor (VX-809) (in combination with ivacaftor)	F508del (homozygous)	II
	Tezacaftor (VX-659) (in combination with ivacaftor)	F508del (homozygous) F508del heterozygous (with residual function mutation)	II
	Elexacaftor (VX-445) (in combination with tezacaftor and ivacaftor)	F508del (homozygous or heterozygous)	II

*Investigational.
CFTR, cystic fibrosis transmembrane conductance regulator.

CFTR modulators are also being advanced. For example, gene replacement by viral and nonviral gene therapy remains an approach under active investigation,[223] as well as newer strategies that attempt to express CFTR through translation of delivered mRNA alone.[224,225] Because many CF patients (≈40%) are complex heterozygotes and encode more than one *CFTR* mutation,[226] combination therapeutics addressing more than one *CFTR* variant or use of multidrug therapy will likely dictate a need for individualized therapeutics optimized for particular patients in the future.[218]

Cystic Fibrosis Transmembrane Conductance Regulator Potentiators. *CFTR potentiators* activate mutant CFTR localized to the cell surface by potentiating channel gating stimulated by physiologic activation of cyclic adenosine monophosphate.[206,210,227–229] The impetus for development included the anticipated need to activate F508del CFTR once localized to the cell surface, in addition to the need to activate other mutant channels residing at the plasma membrane but dysfunctional due to aberrant gating, impaired conductance, or a reduced number of channels due to mild processing mutations or splice variants. Early attempts at potentiation included use of genistein, a natural flavonoid molecule that demonstrates strong activation of CFTR but is poorly absorbed and exhibits other undesirable physiologic properties.[228,230,231] Subsequently, ivacaftor and other investigational CFTR potentiators were discovered via high-throughput screening approaches that identified small-molecule potentiators optimized for druglike qualities through traditional medicinal chemistry approaches.[206,210,228–230] Ivacaftor induced about 50% CFTR activity in G551D/F508del CFTR-expressing primary epithelial cells, a benchmark for preclinical development of CFTR modulators.[206]

In a landmark trial conducted in older children and adults (age 12 years and older) with CF and with at least one copy of the G551D-*CFTR* gating mutation, ivacaftor caused a roughly 10% absolute improvement in FEV_1% predicted at 24 weeks, an effect durable through 48 weeks of testing, providing confirmation of positive prior phase II testing results.[189] In addition, multiple secondary clinical end points showed meaningful and statistically significant improvements, including a 55% reduction in the probability of experiencing a pulmonary exacerbation, improved weight gain, and an improvement in respiratory symptoms. Posttreatment sweat chloride testing also exhibited marked improvements (mean of sweat chloride was about 55 mEq/L, a value below the traditional diagnostic threshold). In a smaller study that enrolled pediatric G551D CF patients 6 to 12 years old,[212] benefit was also documented by lung clearance index measurements in CF patients with minimal detectable lung function abnormality by spirometry, likely reflecting improved function of the small airways.[232] The degree of improvement in spirometry among participants of the phase III trial of ivacaftor compares favorably with that of commonly used therapies for chronic CF care. In clinical studies to date, ivacaftor appeared safe and well tolerated, although monitoring of liver function tests is recommended.[233]

These findings formed the basis of clinical approval for ivacaftor in CF patients with the G551D mutations, and this treatment has rapidly been deployed to children and adults with closely related mutations. Registry-based comparisons demonstrated a reduced rate of decline in FEV_1 in individuals treated with ivacaftor,[234] and multiple studies have demonstrated reduced rates of exacerbation coupled with an approximately 30% reduction in *Pseudomonas* infection rates (depending on the population) that have been durable over time.[32,33,235] Mechanistic evaluations have shown improved airway pH,[236] mucus clearance,[235] mucus plugging,[237,238] and radiographic parameters of mucosal thickening by CT imaging,[239] attributable to the improved CFTR function. More detailed microbiome analyses have shown the potential for rebound of bacterial counts in those that do not eradicate *Pseudomonas*,[35] and measures of airway inflammation have been conflicting. Long-term use has reduced the risk of bacterial acquisition, but initial attempts to augment bacterial eradication with ivacaftor use have not demonstrated efficacy, although further research into this concept is warranted given continued improvements in CFTR modulator efficacy and antimicrobial strategies.[240] The relatively large magnitude of weight gain observed with ivacaftor in CF patients with G551D-*CFTR* has been attributed to its beneficial effect on intestinal pH via bicarbonate secretion that improves enzyme function and raises the possibility that mucosal integrity might also be improved throughout the gut.[235,241] Other potential avenues for exploration include the effect of CFTR modulation on other manifestations of CF, such as glucose metabolism, innate immunity and leukocyte function, osteopenia, pancreatic insufficiency, and gastrointestinal absorption, many of which may be directly tied to CFTR activity.[242] As ivacaftor approval has extended to younger and younger children with CF, presently age 1 year and older, evidence has emerged that preservation of pancreatic function may be possible[243] and suggests the potential for the rescue of other organs if instituted early in life, as demonstrated in a G551D ferret model.[244]

Ivacaftor also increased CFTR activity in other class III mutations beyond G551D in vitro,[245] and the beneficial effects of ivacaftor were also observed in patients with other non-G551D gating mutations. Patients observed a large increase in FEV_1 and a similar decrease in sweat chloride compared with that seen in patients with G551D, indicating a class effect.[246] Ivacaftor also activates other groups of CFTR mutations that allow low levels of partially active CFTR channels to reach the cell surface; such mutations include conductance mutations, mild processing mutations, or noncanonical splice variants (meaning abnormal splicing does not take place with absolute fidelity, as with canonical splice mutations, leaving some channels with the wild-type sequence).[247] The beneficial effect of ivacaftor on partially active missense mutations from these CFTR classes is generally proportionate to basal CFTR function, reflecting the ability of increased gating to compensate in part for reduced surface expression or conductance.[217] In contrast, ivacaftor monotherapy had no meaningful effect in CF patients homozygous for F508del CFTR, establishing that CFTR potentiation alone is not effective without concomitant administration of a corrector molecule to bring F508del CFTR to the cell surface.[248] In sum, CFTR potentiator monotherapy can benefit approximately 10–15% of the CF population, noting this is often supplanted by dual corrector-potentiator therapy when a patient also expresses F508del.

Cystic Fibrosis Transmembrane Conductance Regulator Correctors. Significant efforts toward the goal of correcting the folding of F508del CFTR, thus restoring ion channel activity to the misfolded protein, have come to fruition, potentially transforming outcomes and rivaling the benchmark set by ivacaftor in G551D patients. With the use of multiagent corrector potentiator therapy, rescue of F508del CFTR function can be achieved efficiently, making highly effective CFTR corrector therapy applicable to nearly 90% of the population, as defined by genetics.[249] Early attempts included 4-phenyl butyrate to alter protein processing chaperones,[250,251] curcumin, and 8-cyclopentyl-1, 3-dipropylxanthine, which did not successfully translate from in vitro studies to clinical results.[252–254] More recent efforts have resulted from high-throughput library screens for chloride channel function following incubation of test compounds with F508del-expressing cells.[208,210,255] Pharmacologic activity of correctors includes improved processing and trafficking of CFTR and may also affect F508del CFTR half-life in the plasma membrane through altered surface recycling attributed to features of the cellular processing

machinery or reduced endocytic trafficking, depending on their underlying mechanism.[256] The correctors now in clinical use, lumacaftor and tezacaftor, have been shown to interact with CFTR directly and may offer greater specificity than agents that alter general aspects of cell folding or cellular quality control.[257,258] Success toward correction of F508del CFTR in patients was first seen during initial phase II testing of lumacaftor (formerly VX-809).[259] Although results established that improved function of F508del CFTR in patients was achievable by a systemically delivered small molecule, the degree of CFTR rescue was insufficient to confer clinical improvement. Because F508del CFTR also exhibits abnormal channel gating, in addition to aberrant cellular processing, an approach to address insufficient activity is to coadminister a CFTR potentiator with a CFTR corrector.[257] Following successful phase II testing,[260] lumacaftor-ivacaftor therapy was shown to be efficacious in individuals homozygous for F508del in two large randomized controlled studies; however, the magnitude of benefit was modest ($\approx$3% improvement in FEV_1 and $\approx$30% reduction in exacerbations) compared with prior experience with ivacaftor.[261] Long-term studies showed that the improved rates of exacerbation were sustained, and the reduced rate of lung function[262] decline and efficacy has been duplicated in younger patients.[263] Lumacaftor-ivacaftor was also associated with chest tightness upon initiation, a finding more common in individuals with severe pulmonary dysfunction, and lumacaftor induced drug-drug interactions involving CYP metabolism, including the induction of ivacaftor metabolism.[264] An alternative corrector, tezacaftor (formerly VX-661), which has a similar cellular mechanism as lumacaftor but more advantageous pharmacologic properties, resulted in similar efficacy as lumacaftor-ivacaftor (4% FEV_1 improvement), but did not induce chest tightness or induce the drug metabolism of ivacaftor.[265] Further, tezacaftor-ivacaftor was efficacious in people with CF who are complex heterozygotes for F508del CFTR and an array of CFTR mutations that are partially functional and responsive to ivacaftor in vitro; in these individuals, the magnitude of benefit was approximately 7% predicted FEV_1, reflective of both correction of the F508del mutation and potentiation of the residual functional allele.[217] Neither lumacaftor-ivacaftor nor tezacaftor-ivacaftor benefited CF patients heterozygous for F508del CFTR and a minimal function allele that does not respond to ivacaftor, providing evidence of a gene-dose effect but also illustrating the need to address this sizable population.[266]

Despite the success of corrector-potentiator therapy, the activity of correctors is inherently less efficient than potentiators for CFTR gating mutations, likely because F508del and trafficking is a multistep process, limiting the potential of any single pharmacologic intervention. Additive or synergistic rescue of F508del CFTR using more than one corrector with distinct mechanisms of action on the cellular level could potentially overcome this limitation, leading to efforts to advance multiagent corrector therapy, to be combined with CFTR potentiators.[267] The next-generation correctors, elexacaftor and other related agents, were discovered via high-throughput screening programs conducted in the presence of tezacaftor.[268,269] When used in combination, elexacaftor-tezacaftor-ivacaftor delivered pronounced efficacy in vitro, meeting or exceeding levels observed with ivacaftor in gating mutations, including in cells derived from individuals with only a single responsive F508del allele. Initial clinical results matched this pronounced benefit in patients heterozygous for F508del and a minimal function allele in comparison to placebo and in patients homozygous for F508del in comparison to tezacaftor-ivacaftor.[268] In confirmatory testing, results were recapitulated, with patients heterozygous for F508del and a minimal function allele exhibiting an approximately 14% improvement in FEV_1, a 50% reduction in exacerbations, and sweat chloride changes that were greater than 50 mmol/L.[270] Patients homozygous for F508del experienced a 10% additional improvement in FEV_1 over tezacaftor-ivacaftor comparator therapy.[271] Overall, prior experience guided by ivacaftor use in patients with gating mutations suggests highly effective CFTR modulator therapy is likely to be transformative and could substantially alter the progression of disease if initiated prior to substantial lung dysfunction. Longer-term evaluation studies are in progress, as are efforts to examine efficacy in patients younger than 12 years.

Presently, multiple other corrector-potentiator regimens are also in development with potentially unique pharmacologic features that could be advantageous. Successful further development could set the stage for comparator studies in the future or attempts to optimize CFTR modulator therapy at the individual level using cell-based assays or other techniques. There are also pronounced efforts to understand how highly effective CFTR modulator therapy could be brought to bear on rare mutations that may be susceptible to improved activity with various correctors and potentiators. Given that exceedingly rare mutations make up a disproportionately large number of patients in whom CFTR modulator therapy is not yet proven, alternative approaches beyond routine clinical trials will be needed to foster availability of effective modulator therapy to this group of patients.[272]

Translational Readthrough. Readthrough of *premature termination codons* (PTCs) represents a potential approach to address CF caused by nonsense mutations, which could also be applicable to many other genetic diseases. The approach was identified when certain aminoglycoside antibiotics were found to interact with the eukaryotic rRNA within the ribosomal subunits.[273] Through this interaction, the fidelity of eukaryotic translation can be altered by interrupting the normal proofreading function of the ribosome.[274-280] Insertion of a near cognate amino acid at a PTC allows protein translation to continue normally.[275] Specificity is conferred by greater termination codon fidelity at the authentic (3′) end of mRNA and has been established in vitro by demonstrating that there is no detectable elongation beyond native termination codons.[281-284] This has subsequently been investigated as a potential approach to a number of relatively common genetic diseases aside from CF in which premature termination codons are relatively prevalent, including Duchenne muscular dystrophy,[285-287] Hurler syndrome,[1,288,289] ceroid lipofuscinosis,[290] nephropathic cystinosis,[291] and expression of mutated p53.[292] Proof of concept experiments with aminoglycosides established that PTCs within *CFTR* in human subjects can be suppressed, resulting in the synthesis of full-length, functional CFTR protein.[281-284,293] The approach has

also demonstrated success in mouse models of CF.[294,295] Following two small pilot trials indicating restoration of chloride secretion in CF subjects harboring PTCs,[284,284] a double-blind, placebo-controlled trial showed correction of nasal ion transport specifically in subjects with nonsense mutations following topical administration of gentamicin and, as expected, not in CF controls homozygous for F508del.[283] A trial examining systemic gentamicin in seven French subjects with Y122X *CFTR*, a mutation highly susceptible to readthrough therapy, also indicated rescue of CFTR activity in the airway and sweat duct.[181] Not all aminoglycoside trials in CF have demonstrated success, suggesting variable levels of protein correction.[296] Regardless, due to the known toxicity and poor bioavailability of aminoglycosides, more efficacious agents that avoid undesirable properties of aminoglycosides will be needed for the long-term genetic treatment of CF. One promising approach uses medicinal chemistry optimization to identify the antimicrobial, toxic, and readthrough effects of aminoglycoside scaffolds, a strategy demonstrating initial success using in vitro reporters of efficacy and toxicity,[297] and cell- and animal-based models of CFTR rescue.[298] Addition of CFTR correctors and potentiators have the potential to augment function further by activating the processing and function of CFTR readthrough products, which include missense mutations from near-cognate amino acid insertion.[299,300]

Other attempts to address nonsense mutations include novel compounds without the disadvantages of aminoglycosides, and efforts remain ongoing in this regard. One such molecule, ataluren (formerly PTC124), induced translational readthrough in experimental systems.[301,302] Although the agent is available for the treatment of Duchenne muscular dystrophy, clinical development ultimately failed for people with CF[303] after mixed results in preceding clinical trials[220,293,304,305] that raised questions about insufficient efficacy.[306,307] The effects of readthrough agents are likely substantially affected by low levels of steady-state *CFTR* mRNA due to nonsense-mediated decay. The level of nonsense-mediated decay has been associated with readthrough efficacy and may need to be addressed to achieve effective CFTR rescue.[220,308] Given new knowledge regarding the best models to identify and optimize CFTR drug candidates that has emerged since the identification of ataluren, it is possible that identification of new chemicals using alternate readthrough assays that incorporate the influence of nonsense-mediated decay might yield more efficacious compounds. Other strategies such as pseudouridinylation of the mRNA encoding nonsense mutations or gene editing the PTC sequence are in early development.[309]

Gene Therapy

Within years after discovery of the *CFTR* gene, initial enthusiasm for gene therapy was robust, but variable efficiency of vectors coupled with heterogeneous transgene expression and adverse effects from inflammation impeded progress in this area. Using NPD as an outcome, viral vectors demonstrated transgene delivery using adenovirus[310,311] and adeno-associated adenovirus,[312] but positive results have not been observed by all groups conducting studies of this type.[313] Improvements in Cl^- transport using lipid-based gene transfer vectors were initially limited to modest changes,[314-316] improvements in specific subgroups,[315-319] or inconsistent CFTR expression[320–322] and therefore were not convincing. Depletion of immunogenic CpG motifs for plasmid delivery used during a large, long-term clinical trial by the UK Gene Therapy Consortium demonstrated safety and provided a roadmap for trials of this sort, but efficacy was again not convincing.[323] With the success of gene therapy in immune-privileged organs such as the eye, research into CF gene therapy has experienced renewed vigor, with the goal of a "one-time cure," especially for those not helped by CFTR modulator treatment. Use of the latest adeno-associated and hybrid lentiviral-based gene transfer is a major emphasis, but limitations including cargo size (noting CFTR is a large gene), durability of gene integration, and possible off-target effects remain challenging. Alternative approaches such as gene editing with CRISPR-Cas9 are also engendering considerable interest, although the efficiency of homology-directed repair of the target has been challenging thus far. All gene therapy approaches must navigate past the mucociliary barrier and must target specific cell types, such as basal progenitors, to induce sustained expression, unless repeat administration is envisioned.[324,325]

mRNA Replacement and Other Nucleotide Repair Strategies

Splicing mutation represents a relatively common minority of CFTR alleles seen in patients with CF. For example, one CF mutation is 3849+10kb C→T, which leads to inclusion of an 84-base pair cryptic exon in the mature mRNA.[326] This cryptic exon contains an in-frame nonsense codon, which leads to production of truncated nonfunctional proteins. Splicing machinery is heterogeneous both among patients and also among tissues within an individual, resulting in relatively heterogeneous expression of the disease. This forms the basis of examining usefulness of a CFTR potentiator in patients with relatively preserved CFTR expression due to alternatively spliced forms of CFTR and partially retained expression, and ivacaftor is now approved in the United States for the treatment of several noncanonical splice variants. The variation in splicing efficiency can also be exploited using antisense oligonucleotides to induce normal splicing by masking mutant splice sites.[309] Although this would require specific antisense oligonucleotides to be developed for each CFTR splice mutation, use of such technology has shown therapeutic efficacy in Duchenne muscular dystrophy.[327] Full-length RNA transduction is also being pursued for the treatment of genetic diseases and is being exploited in CF, with sequences optimized for translation efficiency. As with gene therapy, similar challenges with delivery of nucleotides and dependence on cell type will need to be addressed with these therapeutic strategies. To that end, editing the RNA sequence with nasal delivery showed promise using NPD as an outcome,[328] but it did not improve lung function following inhalation.[329]

RESPIRATORY THERAPIES

Physical Airway Clearance

The combination of cough augmented with chest vibration or percussion to loosen mucus represents a cornerstone of the daily care of CF to reduce airway obstruction and prevent CF exacerbations.[330] Daily clearance maneuvers, including chest physiotherapy by vibropercussion,

hand-administered therapy, or the chest physiotherapy vest clearance systems, are considered standard of care.[331,332] Alternative airway clearance techniques include positive expiratory pressure, huff coughing, and the use of vibratory flutter valves.[332]

Exercise therapy can provide additional improvement in mucus clearance in concert with physical maneuvers.[333] Standardized, aerobic exercise programs targeting 70–85% of maximal heart rate have demonstrated benefits with regard to exercise tolerance but do not improve lung function. Similar results have been obtained in isometric exercise programs.[334] Supervised pulmonary rehabilitation in severe CF lung disease can be an important supportive modality (see also Chapter 139).

Airway Rehydration Therapy

Rehydration of the airway surface liquid to augment mucociliary clearance can be achieved with nebulized *hypertonic saline* (HTS), which causes a durable increase in mucociliary clearance in CF subjects.[181] A multicenter, randomized, placebo-controlled trial of HTS showed a modest improvement in pulmonary function and a 56% reduction in frequency of CF pulmonary exacerbation despite relatively poor compliance.[180] Evidence suggests that the effects of HTS are additive to rhDNase.[180,335,336] In infants too young for reliable spirometry, HTS improved infant pulmonary function tests ($FEV_{0.5}$) and lung clearance index, an effort-independent measure of pulmonary obstruction through inert gas washout, although it did not alter an already low rate of pulmonary exacerbations.[337] Confirmatory studies have established that lung clearance index improvements are reproducible and associated with other indicators of clinical benefit, such as weight gain.[82,338,339]

Because a minority of subjects develop bronchospasm following administration of HTS, inhaled β_2-agonist is generally recommended before HTS dosing; moreover, HTS should be used cautiously in those with severe pulmonary obstruction. Many patients exhibit excessive cough following HTS administration (a feature that limits use), although this will often decrease with repeated HTS use.[180] Lower concentrations (3%) can sometimes be used when excess cough or bronchospasm is a problem with the standard HTS (7%).

Airway treatments with the nonabsorbable sugar mannitol to hydrate the mucosal surface by generating an osmotic gradient represent an alternative to HTS. Following success in early-phase trials,[340] two large-scale clinical trials demonstrated reduced exacerbations and a small increase in lung function.[341,342] On the basis of this success, inhaled mannitol therapy is approved for use in some countries (including the United States in 2019), though intolerance of dry powder inhalation has been a barrier to substantial uptake. Other strategies to circumvent CFTR by inducing non–CFTR-dependent fluid secretion or inhibiting epithelial sodium channel–mediated fluid resorption remain an active area of research and clinical development.[343]

Dornase Alfa

Use of inhaled recombinant human dornase alfa, a pharmacologic treatment to improve the physical properties of mucus, has been shown beneficial in randomized, placebo-controlled trials among CF subjects and was among the first

CF-specific medicines to be approved for respiratory disease. Dornase alfa causes dissolution of excess DNA debris that accumulates due to bacterial infection, mucus stasis, and the large influx of neutrophils into the CF airway lumen. The drug augments pulmonary function, diminishes frequency of pulmonary exacerbation, and enhances QOL.[179] Trials examining dornase alfa therapy in individuals with severe CF pulmonary disease (forced vital capacity < 40% predicted) also show benefit.[344] With regard to milder lung disease, dornase alfa stabilized inflammatory markers in bronchoalveolar lavage fluid of young children[345] and improved radiographic measures of gas trapping,[346] suggesting the potential to benefit even when mucus production is not clearly evident. The treatment also improved ventilation inhomogeneity as determined by the lung clearance index in pediatric patients with minimal decrements in spirometry.[347] Thus, dornase alfa therapy is recommended for CF patients in all ranges of disease severity.[348]

Inhaled Antibiotics

Refractory infection is a sine qua non of bronchiectasis, and aggressive antimicrobial therapy is a mainstay of chronic CF care. The inhaled route provides higher doses of antibiotics directly to the mucopurulent airways, and several treatment strategies have been shown to improve CF lung function and reduce pulmonary exacerbations. Intermittent use of chronic inhalational antibiotics is intended to target the airways while avoiding systemic toxicity and to limit emergence of bacterial resistance through continuous selection pressure. The first drug to be approved for this purpose was inhaled tobramycin, which has been shown to improve pulmonary function, reduce exacerbation rate, and increase weight gain compared with placebo when administered twice daily during alternate 4-week periods.[82,349] Concerns about daily burden of therapy and patient nonadherence have led to the development of a dry powder formulation, which was shown to be noninferior to conventional nebulized tobramycin and improved patient satisfaction when tolerated.[182]

The inhaled monobactam aztreonam has also been developed for chronic use in CF. Initial studies demonstrated improved QOL and a prolonged gap between exacerbations.[350,351] In a large 6-month trial involving CF patients older than 6 years who previously used inhaled tobramycin, improved FEV_1 and reduced exacerbations were observed with inhaled aztreonam given every other month[352] compared with inhaled tobramycin every other month. A similar study in subjects with milder lung function abnormalities demonstrated more modest improvements in FEV_1 and QOL.[353] Inhaled colistin is often used as an alternative antipseudomonal agent in subjects with resistant strains, although it is not approved by the U.S. Food and Drug Administration for this purpose and is associated with side effects such as bronchospasm.[82,354,355]

It is not yet clear which antimicrobial agent is best for individual patients, and the choice of agent is generally driven by the dominant pathogen, antimicrobial resistance patterns, and patient preference. Nevertheless, antimicrobial resistance profiles do not predict clinical response effectively. The difficulty in predicting response is probably due to intrinsic resistance conferred by biofilms and intermicrobial interactions that alter susceptibility in the lung but are not modeled in routine clinical bacterial culture methods, a limitation that poses substantial clinical challenges in antibiotic selection.[356] Continuous alternating 28-day cycles of inhaled tobramycin and aztreonam for individuals who experience increased infection or symptoms during off-cycle are frequently used and may be beneficial.[357] A number of other inhaled therapies are in development, and treatments that target dissolution of biofilms are of particular interest.

Bacterial Eradication

The primary morbidity and mortality in CF are attributable to obstructive respiratory disease associated with chronic endobronchial infection by opportunistic bacteria. *P. aeruginosa* infection is clearly associated with decline in respiratory function, and early acquisition of *Pseudomonas* is associated with increased morbidity and mortality.[27,358–363] Consequently, infection and eradication via treatment with anti-pseudomonal antibiotics has been sought as a means to sustain lung function and delay mortality.[44,364] Early bacterial isolates from CF lungs are present at lower density, are generally nonmucoid, and display favorable microbial resistance profiles, reflecting a potential window of opportunity for treatment and eradication.[365,366] As noted earlier, *Pseudomonas* infection becomes more prevalent with increasing age; positive respiratory tract cultures are reported in up to 30% of infants, 30–40% of children aged 2 to 10 years, and 60–80% of adolescents and adults.[367] Newborn screening for CF allows earlier identification of *P. aeruginosa* infection in children prior to onset of significant lung disease that limits efficacy of treatment. Following detection of *P. aeruginosa* in asymptomatic children, standard of care includes clinical interventions to eradicate the organism. Antimicrobial regimens differ depending on the clinical setting but, for individuals detected by surveillance, 28-day treatment periods with inhaled antibiotics are sufficient to achieve reasonable eradication rates.[368] More aggressive strategies should be reserved for extenuating circumstances, such as with clinical deterioration or advanced disease. Although several studies have validated efficacy of various treatment regimens, no single approach has demonstrated clear superiority.[369] Suppression and eradication of *Staphylococcus* species, including MRSA, is possible and is possibly associated with clinical benefit.[370,371] Of note, prophylaxis for *S. aureus* has led to increased *Pseudomonas* infection, warranting caution.[372]

Macrolide Therapy. Although macrolide antibiotics do not exhibit significant antipseudomonal properties, the utility of these agents in diffuse panbronchiolitis, a rare disease that resembles CF (including chronic infection with *P. aeruginosa*), led to therapeutic trials in CF patients.[373–376] In a multicenter, randomized, placebo-controlled trial, alternating-day oral azithromycin demonstrated improved pulmonary function accompanied by a large reduction in pulmonary exacerbations.[377] Similar results were seen in a Canadian study using clarithromycin.[378] Beneficial effects of azithromycin have also been observed in CF patients not chronically infected with *Pseudomonas* (presumably due to less well-described anti-inflammatory effects), suggesting a contributory mechanism independent of antimicrobial properties. One large clinical trial demonstrated reduced rates of exacerbation,[379] although an FEV_1 benefit was not observed. On the basis of current evidence, present guidelines assign a lower priority for chronic azithromycin in noninfected patients.[185] However, the use of azithromycin in young children has become more common because several trials have demonstrated safety and efficacy in decreasing pulmonary exacerbations and improving health metrics such as nutritional health. The rising incidence of NTM infections raises concern about long-term use of azithromycin due to the potential for inducible macrolide resistance. Some data suggested increased risk of promoting infection by NTM mycobacteria,[82] although this has been refuted by epidemiologic studies.[380] Nevertheless, annual screening for NTM is recommended and is particularly important among azithromycin-treated patients. Azithromycin use may inhibit the efficacy of inhaled tobramycin, a finding under evaluation in prospective clinical studies.[381]

Anti-inflammatory Therapy

Intense neutrophilic inflammation is characteristic of CF and remains a therapeutic target that has not been fully exploited.[69,382–384] Early trials utilizing chronic, alternate-day systemic corticosteroids showed a beneficial effect of prednisone (1 mg/kg) on CF lung function, but use remains limited by steroid toxicities, and chronic corticosteroid therapy is not generally recommended.[385–387] Inhaled steroids have frequently been studied in small trials. In some studies, reduced airway reactivity has been observed, but sustained effects on lung function have not been shown.[388,389] Use of oral steroids in CF is generally limited to individuals with an asthmatic phenotype. Concerns include the potential for bone demineralization, adrenal suppression, and growth retardation in pediatric patients.

A number of other anti-inflammatory molecules have been studied in CF, although identifying an appropriate therapeutic window that allows blockade of excessive inflammation without causing increased susceptibility to infection has been difficult. High-dose ibuprofen, a nonsteroidal anti-inflammatory drug, has been shown to diminish the rate of pulmonary function decline, but beneficial effects appear greatest in young children.[390] Other studies have confirmed these findings.[187,391] Despite this evidence, nonsteroidal anti-inflammatory drug therapy is not widely utilized in the United States due to concerns of chronic toxicities, particularly in older individuals, and the need for pharmacokinetic monitoring to achieve adequate serum levels.[392] For example, inadequate levels have been associated with paradoxical proinflammatory effects, leading to increased neutrophil migration.[187,393]

Attempts to extend the observed benefits of anti-inflammatory therapy to other eicosanoid-active agents (e.g., leukotriene inhibitors) have indicated variable results, including studies showing increased pulmonary complications with a nonselective leukotriene B4 antagonist.[394,395] Synthetic cannabinoids and more specific leukotriene modifiers are presently in development to improve efficacy. Along similar lines, initial attempts to block protease activity with inhaled antitrypsin were not effective,[396] although other inhaled neutrophil elastase inhibitors are under consideration. Other agents such as 3-hydroxy-3-methylglutaryl coenzyme reductase inhibitors, hydroxychloroquine, and methotrexate have not demonstrated convincing benefit, illustrating the challenge of successfully targeting this mechanism, which may be suited to young patients with less-established disease and fewer activated inflammatory pathways. Development remains challenging given limitations in anti-inflammatory biomarkers to guide early advancement, and given the large number of subjects needed to demonstrate reductions in exacerbations compared to improvements in lung function.[397]

OTHER SUPPORTIVE CARE

Pulmonary Exacerbations

Exacerbations of CF pulmonary disease are characterized by increased cough and sputum production, respiratory distress, diminished exercise tolerance, weight loss, decreased spirometry, worsened hypoxemia, or development of a major pulmonary complication such as hemoptysis.[398–401] Treatment includes intensified airway clearance measures and systemic antimicrobial therapy generally directed against the most recently acquired pathogens. Both inpatient and outpatient treatment are utilized; factors important to consider during management include severity of disease, baseline lung function, microbial organisms and resistance pattern, presence of additional complications, and the ability to adhere to an outpatient regimen. Acute pulmonary exacerbation is the most common indication for hospitalization in CF and is warranted when episodes are severe, refractory to outpatient care, or not suited to home therapy for psychosocial reasons. Hospitalization facilitates controlled administration of intravenous antibiotics to address exacerbating infections and provides a setting conducive to sustained intensification of chest physiotherapy. Although the historical standard for pulmonary exacerbations is hospital-based treatment, outpatient management that includes use of parenteral antimicrobials and mucus clearance procedures may achieve equivalent outcomes in appropriately selected patients.[402] In general, the primary goal in this setting is to improve clinical symptoms and to return pulmonary function to baseline. In some patients, however, lung function does not return to previous levels despite clinical improvement and can decline further in the days to weeks following intervention.[403–405] A severe decrement in spirometry from baseline at the onset of pulmonary exacerbation is a major risk factor for sustained loss of lung function, suggesting the need for early and aggressive treatment.[404–406]

Antibiotic therapy should be broad based due to the polymicrobial nature of CF lung disease and is typically selected on the basis of respiratory tract culture and susceptibility results. Notwithstanding this recommendation, in vitro sensitivity profiles are poor predictors of clinical response, indicating significant limitations to the general strategy.[406] Treatment of Pseudomonas is the first consideration, and two mechanistically distinct antibiotics should be administered to maximize efficacy. In some clinical scenarios where oral therapy is used, fluoroquinolones as single agents are a mainstay but can be associated with the risk of promoting bacterial resistance.[407] Aminoglycosides have optimal antimicrobial activity as intravenous anti-*Pseudomonas* drugs but require careful monitoring to optimize therapy. Traditional dosing of aminoglycosides two to three times a day has shifted in favor of once-daily dosing.[408,409] Aminoglycoside schedules in the range of 8 to 12 mg/kg once daily achieve higher peak concentrations (20 to 30 µg/mL) that potentiate bactericidal effect and limit toxicity by extending the duration of low, near-trough drug concentrations, which approach undetectable levels in the setting of normal renal function.[100,410] Patients should be monitored during aminoglycoside therapy for emergence of nephrotoxicity and ototoxicity. Aminoglycosides are usually paired with a β-lactam to maximize efficacy. A third antibiotic may also be useful for controlling MRSA or other atypical organisms. Although there is no consensus regarding duration of therapy, a clinical response with respect to symptoms or pulmonary function is usually apparent 4 to 7 days after initiating treatment, depending on severity of the initial decrement and degree of underlying lung disease. Ten to 14 days appear adequate to achieve maximal improvement in lung function and sustained health in most cases.[411,412] With refractory infection, treatment for 3 weeks or more is sometimes warranted but may not be successful. Certain studies have demonstrated that the FEV_1 reaches a plateau following 10 days of inpatient treatment, raising a question concerning the benefit (and risk) of longer hospital and parenteral antibiotic courses.[413] Each treatment schedule therefore requires careful and somewhat individualized assessment by the clinician. Shorter treatments may improve QOL and compliance, limit drug-associated morbidities, and be less costly. However, prolonged regimens may be necessary to clear an infection, achieve sustained benefit, and preclude early recurrence of exacerbation. Prospective comparator studies evaluating treatment duration are currently underway.[414] Extended courses of antibiotic therapy should also include longitudinal respiratory tract cultures for bacterial and fungal organisms because antibiotic sensitivities can shift.[415] For patients requiring frequent or long-term home antibiotic therapy, subcutaneous central intravenous catheters can provide stable intravenous access to facilitate treatment. Chronic port access carries a risk of catheter-associated infections and thrombosis.[416] For this reason, exogenous estrogen should be avoided in female patients with central venous catheters if possible.

TREATMENT OF LUNG COMPLICATIONS

Treatments directed to control airway infection, limit inflammation, and optimize airway clearance represent the cornerstone of therapy in both early and advanced CF lung disease. Hypoxemic respiratory insufficiency should be recognized and treated with supplemental oxygen. Low-flow oxygen is effective at relieving nocturnal, exertional, and resting hypoxemia and does not usually cause significant hypercapnia.[417]

Pulmonary hypertension (PH) and increased mortality are strongly associated with the development of nocturnal or resting hypoxemia.[418] The development of PH is correlated with declining lung function and the development of respiratory failure; however, direct evidence that it increases the risk of mortality is lacking.[419] Treatment

for PH, including diuretics, inotropic agents, and theophylline, provides little to no benefit in CF and is rarely used; however, sildenafil is associated with improved exercise capacity.[420,421] Right ventricular dysfunction is an end-stage finding in advanced disease with few viable treatment options beyond those that stabilize lung disease and symptomatically treat pulmonary hypertension.[422] Thus, advancing PH is largely an indication for referral for lung transplantation (see also Chapter 85).

Acute respiratory failure due to reversible insults can be managed by either noninvasive measures or invasive ventilatory support.[145,423,424] Although mortality associated with mechanical ventilation in CF is high, the intervention can be beneficial. It has been reported, for example, that one-third of CF patients with advanced lung disease survive events requiring intubation and ventilatory support.[146] Mechanical ventilation and extracorporeal membrane oxygenation can also be used as a bridge to lung transplant at appropriate centers[146,424–426] (see also Chapter 138).

Atelectasis in CF is managed by escalating the intensity and frequency of airway clearance, together with other therapies directed towards addressing pulmonary exacerbations. Systemic or inhaled corticosteroids may be helpful in the presence of asthma, ABPA, or significant airway inflammation refractory to antimicrobial therapy. There is little evidence that bronchoscopy and lavage are effective in treating atelectasis. However, bronchoscopic evaluation of atelectasis and treatment of mucoid impaction in association with endobronchial aspergillosis and ABPA have been described.[427,428]

ABPA is a common complication of CF, seen in about 10% of the CF population annually. ABPA typically responds to standard doses of systemic corticosteroids (1 mg/kg).[124] Inhaled corticosteroids,[429] paired with suppressive oral antifungal therapy,[430] and more recently, omalizumab[431] (an anti-IgE monoclonal therapy), has been shown to limit the systemic steroid burden in cases of steroid refractoriness or steroid intolerance.

Pneumothorax, when small and minimally symptomatic, may be managed by observation with the expectation of spontaneous resolution. Pneumothoraces of greater volume (e.g., >20%) or that compromise ventilation or physiologic stability require chest tube re-expansion immediately.[432] Recurrent pneumothoraces are common in advanced lung disease and are associated with higher mortality. Patients with nonexpandable lung after pneumothorax who experience significant morbidity may benefit from video-assisted thoracic surgery to take down adhesions followed by chemical and/or mechanical pleurodesis.[433] Prior pleurodesis is not considered a contraindication to lung transplantation, although it increases surgical complexity.[433]

Major hemoptysis is treated with antibiotics, limitation of aggressive physiotherapy, and inhaled respiratory health medications, although reinstitution of postural drainage therapy has become increasingly accepted in this setting. Supplemental vitamin K should be given if the prothrombin time is prolonged due to malabsorption. Clot stabilization with intravenous or inhaled tranexamic acid and systemic blood pressure reduction with beta-blockade may have some clinical utility but are not indicated as first-line therapies.[129,434] Massive hemoptysis may resolve with conservative therapy, but bronchial artery embolization provides more definitive clinical control and should be considered in recurrent or refractory cases of submassive bleeding.[130] Recurrent submassive or massive hemoptysis episodes should prompt consideration for lung transplant referral.

Treatment of Gastrointestinal Complications

Meconium ileus often can be relieved with enemas refluxing water-soluble radiographic contrast into the terminal ileum under fluoroscopy.[131] If this is not successful, or there is concern for intestinal perforation due to severity of involvement, surgical consultation should be sought. The distal intestinal obstruction syndrome is typically treated with large volume-balanced electrolyte solutions containing osmotic laxatives (polyethylene glycol) and mucolytics (N-acetylcysteine).[435] Contrast enemas that reach the terminal ileum can complement this therapy. In the setting of significant abdominal distension or intractable emesis, bowel obstruction or bilious/fecal emesis may require surgical intervention.[436] Rectal prolapse can be voluntarily reduced in patients experienced with techniques involving the abdominal, perineal, and gluteal muscles. Young children often require manual reduction by gentle pressure in the knee-chest position.[436] Pancreatic enzyme replacement therapy, improved nutritional status, and control of lung disease usually prevent recurrence. Surgical stabilization of the rectum is required if prolapse is chronic and refractory to medical management.

Liver disease is thought to result from abnormal bile secretion due to CFTR dysfunction. Ursodeoxycholic acid (ursodiol) is used to treat primary biliary cirrhosis.[155] Although its impact on CF liver disease is unclear, several studies have demonstrated that ursodiol improves or stabilizes liver function tests. Long-term effect on CF hepatocellular injury, however, remains unknown.[437] Thresholds for initiating therapy and clinical outcomes are under investigation, although current guidelines recommend aggressive nutritional support and consideration of ursodiol treatment.[438] Bleeding esophageal varices that complicate cirrhosis can often be managed with banding or sclerotherapy. Portal hypertension and severe, refractory variceal bleeding have been treated successfully with portosystemic shunt procedures.[439] CF hepatic failure and ascites are treated in standard fashion. Liver transplantation is successful in CF, with survival rates at 1 and 5 years reported at greater than 80%.[440] CFTR modulator therapy may be associated with elevated hepatic enzymes, but this is also seen sporadically in CF, often in association with treatment for pulmonary exacerbations.[264]

Hyperglycemia can complicate CF at any age but is generally first encountered during the second and third decades of life.[441,442] Ketoacidosis is not typically a feature of CF-related diabetes mellitus. Treatment of elevated blood glucose in CF has become more aggressive as patient longevity has improved. This is in part due to appreciation of complications from diabetes among older adults with CF and increased recognition concerning the impact of CF-related diabetes mellitus on pulmonary disease progression and its association with declining lung function.[443] Vascular disease affecting the retina and kidneys has been documented in CF patients who have had prolonged hyperglycemia.[443,444] Intensive screening and management regimens have been recommended for control of blood sugar,

including annual oral glucose tolerance testing for previously unaffected patients.[442,445–447] Insulin therapy is the mainstay of treatment, and the anabolic effects of insulin may be beneficial in this setting.[442,446–448] Increasing use of continuous glucose monitoring improves glucose control and clinical outcomes[449] (see also Chapter 128).

Surgical Therapy

Endoscopic sinus surgery and nasal polypectomy to relieve obstruction are the most common surgical procedures conducted in the CF patient population.[448,450,451] Although most individuals with CF experience improvement postoperatively, recurrence is common and often requires repetitive procedures.[452] The incidence of nasal polyposis tends to wane in adulthood.[450] More aggressive sinus surgery to marsupialize the sinus cavity may also be beneficial.[453] Other frequently encountered procedures include cholecystectomy to treat symptomatic gallstones.[452] Pulmonary resection has historically been considered when severe focal lung disease leads to clinical instability and accelerated decline in lung function. Although surgical therapy has been reported to stabilize the clinical course and reduce exacerbation frequency, such treatment has become rare due to improved therapeutic strategies and overall health of individuals with CF.[167,454–457] Patients under consideration for partial pneumonectomy must be carefully selected because short-term loss of lung function postoperatively is expected.[458] Massive hemoptysis refractory to standard interventional therapy may require lobectomy.

Lung Transplantation

Sequential double-lung transplantation is an accepted therapy for respiratory failure secondary to CF.[459] More than 3000 lung transplants have been performed for CF around the world, and the rate is increasing. The 5-year survival is just above 50% and improving, which compares favorably to survival following pulmonary transplantation performed in other lung diseases.[460] Given the limited survival and complexity of treatments required, consideration of lung transplantation requires careful psychological and social evaluation. Patients should be referred when death is expected over the ensuing 2 to 3 years.[106] Recent consensus guidelines emphasize early patient discussion and referral, especially with complicating factors that include patient size and gender, CF medical complications, and psychosocial barriers.[461] Following successful transplantation, CF patients may experience dramatically improved respiratory status and QOL, but significant medical treatment burden remains (see also Chapter 140).

Nutrition

Improved nutritional status in patients with CF is associated with better long-term clinical outcomes.[456] Individuals with the disease have increased caloric requirements attributable to intestinal malabsorption, increased work of breathing, and factors associated with infection and/or inflammation. Dietary recommendations include high caloric intake (20–50% greater than standard), high-protein diet with a moderate amount of dietary fat (35–45% of caloric intake), and limited processed carbohydrates.[462] Patients with a body mass index below the 25th percentile are typically considered to be in nutritional failure and warrant aggressive dietary counseling and supplementation. If nutritional adjustments are unsuccessful, consideration of appetite stimulants, gastrostomy tube feedings, or other approaches may be warranted. This is in part because supplementation with elemental dietary preparations by mouth is unlikely to be sustained over an extended period of time.

Almost all patients with CF require pancreatic enzyme replacement therapy due to cystic destruction of the exocrine pancreas early in life. The enzymes are supplied as capsules containing acid-resistant enteric-coated granules, with doses of lipase from 3,000 to 40,000 units. The replacement therapy is typically administered based on patient weight and adjusted to ameliorate symptoms of malabsorption such as abdominal cramping, excessive flatulence, and fatty stools. Dose ranges should be limited to current guidelines (2500 lipase units/kg/meal; 10,000 lipase units/kg/day), because more intense drug schedules have been associated with fibrosing colonopathy.[463-466] Recombinant forms are in development, and enzyme replacement cartridges for nocturnal use can improve absorption of nocturnal feeding.[467] With earlier use of highly effective CFTR modulator therapy, pancreatic enzyme replacement may not be needed if pancreatic function can be preserved.[468]

A daily multivitamin is standard in CF care, and additional supplementation is dependent on clinical evaluation. Vitamins A and E are often adequately supplied by a standard (daily) multiple-vitamin preparation. Vitamin A deficiency is readily corrected by dietary supplementation. Symptomatic deficiency is rare and may result in increased intracranial pressure, xerophthalmia, and night blindness. Vitamin D deficiency presenting as rickets is rarely seen. That being said, patients with CF often have inadequate levels of vitamin D (<30 to 60 ng/mL) that can be refractory to high-dose supplementation. Bone demineralization is common, and association of inadequate vitamin D levels with poor health-related outcomes in other clinical scenarios has led to recommendations of aggressive supplementation. Vitamin E is deficient only in non-supplemented patients and rarely causes increased red blood cell destruction or neuroaxonal dystrophy.[469] Insufficient vitamin K may result in bleeding diathesis. Although clinically significant hemorrhagic problems manifest mostly in children, vitamin K deficiency in the setting of hemoptysis may present a significant challenge in older CF patients. Other vitamins and trace minerals, specifically zinc, may be deficient and require supplementation on an individualized patient basis.[470]

Psychosocial Factors

With the advent of newborn screening and with individuals with CF surviving into adulthood, psychosocial aspects of CF have broadened and continue to affect patients, families, and the community. Medical therapies offer significant benefit but can be limited by problems with psychosocial well-being, attitude, and ultimately adherence to treatment. Approaches to delivery of clinical care that promote a positive self-image and support the patient and/or family efforts to manage their own medical therapy while maximizing health-related QOL are likely to have substantial impact on outcomes. Partnering strategies between providers and patients to sustain daily care routines are recognized as a beneficial approach in CF.[471]

Providers with expertise in psychosocial support are invaluable to the CF care team.[463] Major depression and anxiety disorder is a common comorbidity as patients grow older and can interfere with good clinical outcomes. Aggressive monitoring and treatment of these aspects of CF are warranted and recommended annually for all patients with CF.[472] At present, no CF-specific medical treatments for major depression have been investigated.

Key Points

- Effective treatment and monitoring through a network of specialized *cystic fibrosis* (CF) care and research centers has led to improvement in morbidity and mortality among patients with CF.
- The diagnostic paradigms emphasize early detection by newborn screening and a high index of suspicion to recognize atypical cases later in life, which are generally caused by *cystic fibrosis transmembrane conductance regulator (CFTR)* alleles coding for partially active CFTR.
- Aggressive treatment of CF pulmonary exacerbations is required to delay progression and reduce complications of end-stage lung disease.
- Treatment strategies for chronic lung disease generally address downstream manifestations of CF pathophysiology. Such therapies include airway clearance techniques, hydration of airway surface liquid, mucolytics to enhance mucus clearance, antimicrobials, and chronic use of anti-inflammatory agents.
- The successful development and approval of ivacaftor for CF patients with the G551D *CFTR* mutation has provided a roadmap invigorating investigators working to develop novel modulators of CFTR function to correct the underlying defect caused by the most common *CFTR* alleles.
- Combination CFTR modulator therapy has been developed to treat lung disease in all patients with F508del CFTR (≈90% of the U.S. CF population as defined by genotypic prevalence). The most recent of these is a triple combination (elexacaftor/tezacaftor/ivacaftor).
- Ongoing efforts are aimed at various gene-based methods to cure all patients with CF.

Key Readings

Bell SC, Mall MA, Gutierrez H, et al. The future of cystic fibrosis care: a global perspective. *Lancet Respir Med.* 2020;8(1):65–124. Erratum: *Lancet Respir Med.* 2019;7(12):e40.

Farrell PM, White TB, Ren CL, et al. Diagnosis of cystic fibrosis: a consensus guideline from the cystic fibrosis foundation. *J Pediatr.* 2017;181S:S4–S15.e1.

Heijerman HGM, McKone EF, Downey DG, et al. VX17-445-103 trial group. Efficacy and safety of the elexacaftor plus tezacaftor plus ivacaftor combination regimen in people with cystic fibrosis homozygous for the F508del mutation: a double-blind, randomised, phase 3 trial. *Lancet.* 2019;394(10212):1940–1948.

Mall MA, Mayer-Hamblett N, Rowe SM. Cystic fibrosis: emergence of highly effective targeted therapeutics and potential clinical implications. *Am J Respir Crit Care Med.* 2019. Epub ahead of print.

Middleton PG, Mall MA, Dřevínek P, et al.; VX17–445–102 Study Group. Elexacaftor-tezacaftor-ivacaftor for cystic fibrosis with a single Phe508del allele. *N Engl J Med.* 2019;381(19):1809–1819.

Complete reference list available at ExpertConsult.com.

69 *BRONCHIECTASIS*

GEORGE M. SOLOMON, MD • EDWARD D. CHAN, MD

INTRODUCTION

Bronchiectasis is defined by dilation, or ectasia, of the large airways or bronchi. The primary clinical manifestations of bronchiectasis are recurrent, chronic, or refractory infections. Other significant sequelae include hemoptysis, chronic airflow obstruction, and progressive impairment of pulmonary function.

There are varied pathways that lead to the development of bronchiectasis (Table 69.1 and Fig. 69.1). Broadly, bronchiectasis may develop because of an incidental event or episode that does not necessarily reflect impairment of the patient's intrinsic host defenses. Such examples include a necrotizing pneumonia after aspiration or chronic infection distal to an obstructing bronchial mass or foreign body. Often, however, bronchiectasis evolves due to underlying genetic risk factors and/or recurrent exposures to environmental mycobacteria. Regardless of the underlying etiology of bronchiectasis, superimposed bacterial infection is common and frequently drives the progression and exacerbation of bronchiectasis.

A central issue in understanding the pathogenesis of bronchiectasis is whether infection is truly the proximate cause of bronchiectasis or whether infections develop because of an underlying predisposing condition. For example, a commonly held adage is that many cases of bronchiectasis in adults are associated with childhood bouts of pertussis, measles, or other infections, including adenovirus.[1,2]

It is important to emphasize that these findings provide, at most, only an associative link and not a causal link.[1] Although childhood infections can undoubtedly cause bronchiectasis, one might be skeptical of this simple construct, asking why formerly common childhood illnesses resulted in bronchiectasis in only a small proportion of patients. Recently emerging is the concept that neutrophils and other inflammatory cells release elastase and reactive oxygen intermediates in response to infection, and that this unresolved inflammatory response to infection may damage airways.[3,4]

CLASSIFICATION SCHEMA

Although there is considerable overlap and coexistence among the various forms of bronchiectasis, the radiographic patterns and distribution may provide clues to diagnosis, management, and prognosis.[5] Thus, characterizing the morphologic features and distribution of bronchiectasis is a useful exercise. Bronchiectasis is most accurately diagnosed by *high-resolution computed tomography* (HRCT). Radiographic correlates to HRCT findings are summarized in eFigs. 69.1 to 69.3.

Cylindrical bronchiectasis is described as failure of the involved airways to taper progressively in their distal course. Usually, in this condition, the bronchial walls are smooth or regular. *Varicoid* bronchiectasis is an allusion to varicose veins and is marked by irregular dilation, narrowing, and outpouching of the airways. *Saccular* bronchiectasis, also known as *cystic* bronchiectasis, includes focal or cystic distortion of the distal airways. These bronchiectatic forms are summarized in Figure 69.2. Cystic distortion may become confluent, producing the appearance of bronchiectatic consolidation and volume loss (eFig. 69.4).

A traditional "wet" versus "dry" bronchiectasis paradigm is now less commonly used because newer paradigms regarding phenotypes have emerged based on underlying diagnosis, type of infectious agent(s) causing or exacerbating the bronchiectasis,[6] and clinical phenotype.[7]

The most well-characterized, clinically relevant example is the *frequent exacerbator* phenotype.[8] Within this group, frequent exacerbations are the strongest predictor of future exacerbation frequency. Patients with frequent

941

Table 69.1   Conditions Associated With Bronchiectasis

POSTINFECTIOUS CONDITIONS
Childhood lower respiratory tract infections
Granulomatous infections
Necrotizing pneumonias in adults
Other respiratory infections

PRIMARY IMMUNE DISORDERS
Humoral defects
Cellular and/or mixed disorders
Neutrophil dysfunction
Other

CYSTIC FIBROSIS (CF)
Classic CF
Variants of CF
Young syndrome

ALPHA$_1$-ANTITRYPSIN ABNORMALITIES
Deficiencies
Anomalies

HERITABLE STRUCTURAL ABNORMALITIES
Primary ciliary dyskinesia
Williams-Campbell syndrome
Mounier-Kuhn syndrome
Marfan syndrome
Sequestration, agenesis, hypoplasia

IDIOPATHIC INFLAMMATORY DISORDERS
Sarcoidosis
Rheumatoid arthritis
Ankylosing spondylitis
Systemic lupus erythematosus
Sjögren syndrome
Inflammatory bowel disease
Relapsing polychondritis

INHALATION AND OBSTRUCTION
Gastroesophageal reflux/aspiration
Pneumonia
Toxic inhalation/thermal injury
Postobstruction accident
Foreign body
Tumors, benign and malignant
Extrinsic airway compression
Allergic bronchopulmonary aspergillosis/mycosis

MISCELLANEOUS
Human immunodeficiency virus infection
Yellow nail syndrome
Radiation injury

exacerbations have a poorer *quality of life* (QOL), are more likely to be hospitalized and, at up to 5 years of follow-up, have a higher mortality, proportional to the number of exacerbations per year.[8]

EPIDEMIOLOGY

Incidence and prevalence of bronchiectasis is difficult to estimate but likely varies in different regions of the world.[9] The prevalence of *non-cystic fibrosis* (non-CF) bronchiectasis, based on narrow case-finding criteria, is estimated to be 139 cases per 100,000 persons, to be higher among women versus men (180 vs. 95 per 100,000), and to increase substantially with age (from 7 per 100,000 for ages 18–34 years to 812 per 100,000 for ages ≥75 years); annual incidence is estimated to be 29 cases per 100,000 persons. Disease prevalence based on broad case-finding criteria is estimated to be 213 cases per 100,000 persons.[9]

This study suggested that, in the United States (in 2013), between 340,000 and 522,000 adults were receiving treatment for bronchiectasis and that 70,000 adults were newly diagnosed with bronchiectasis. More recent data indicate that bronchiectasis is much more common than previously reported, and the incidence has risen with an estimated annual growth rate of 8% since 2001.[10–12] Whether these rising rates reflect a true increase in incidence and/or enhanced detection due to more frequent use of *computed tomography* (CT) scans is not known. The observation that bronchiectasis was the *primary* diagnosis in only a minority (<20%) of all the bronchiectasis-associated hospitalizations supports the concept that greater incidental diagnosis is being made, at least in part, from more frequent use of CT scans.[13]

There are significant economic burdens of increased incidence and prevalence of bronchiectasis. The major drivers of annual health care costs appear related to hospitalizations, but total cost is currently unknown.[14]

In the United States and many parts of the world, there appear to be increasing numbers of bronchiectasis cases associated with *nontuberculous mycobacteria* (NTM) (see Chapter 55).[15–23] NTM appears capable of both initiating[24] and driving the evolution of bronchiectasis[25,26] through a chronic neutrophil-driven process in the airways, resulting in enhanced airway damage and initiation of the vicious cycle of inflammation.

PATHOPHYSIOLOGY

Various mechanisms operate to produce bronchiectasis. In the simplest terms, they may be thought of in terms of *traction, pulsion,* and *weakness* of the airways. In most cases, the pathogenesis becomes inextricably linked with and propelled by the destructive effects of chronic infection, as summarized in Figure 69.1.

Traction bronchiectasis implies that local retractile forces dilate the airways. As the lung undergoes fibrotic changes due to disorders such as sarcoidosis, interstitial lung disorders, or infections such as tuberculosis, those increased forces are transmitted to the airways. In contrast, in normal lungs, airways are held patent by a combination of negative intrapleural pressure, which maintains the lungs in an inflated state, and the cartilaginous rings of the trachea and the large and medium airways. The distending forces of the negative intrapleural pressure are transmitted to the airways by a diffuse system of interstitial tethering.

Pulsion bronchiectasis implies that intense inflammation originating in the lumen leads to permanent airway dilation. The prototype is *allergic bronchopulmonary aspergillosis* (ABPA). In ABPA, there are intense, immunologically mediated reactions to inhaled *Aspergillus* lodged in the airways. The proliferating fungi form large mucoid conglomerates that fill the central airways; a sequela of this airway inflammatory process and mucoid impaction is bronchiectasis (eFig. 69.5).

Weakness of the airways may take many forms. Classic postinfectious bronchiectasis presumably is mediated in part by damage to the walls of the airways, resulting in secondary loss of structural integrity.[27,28] This is

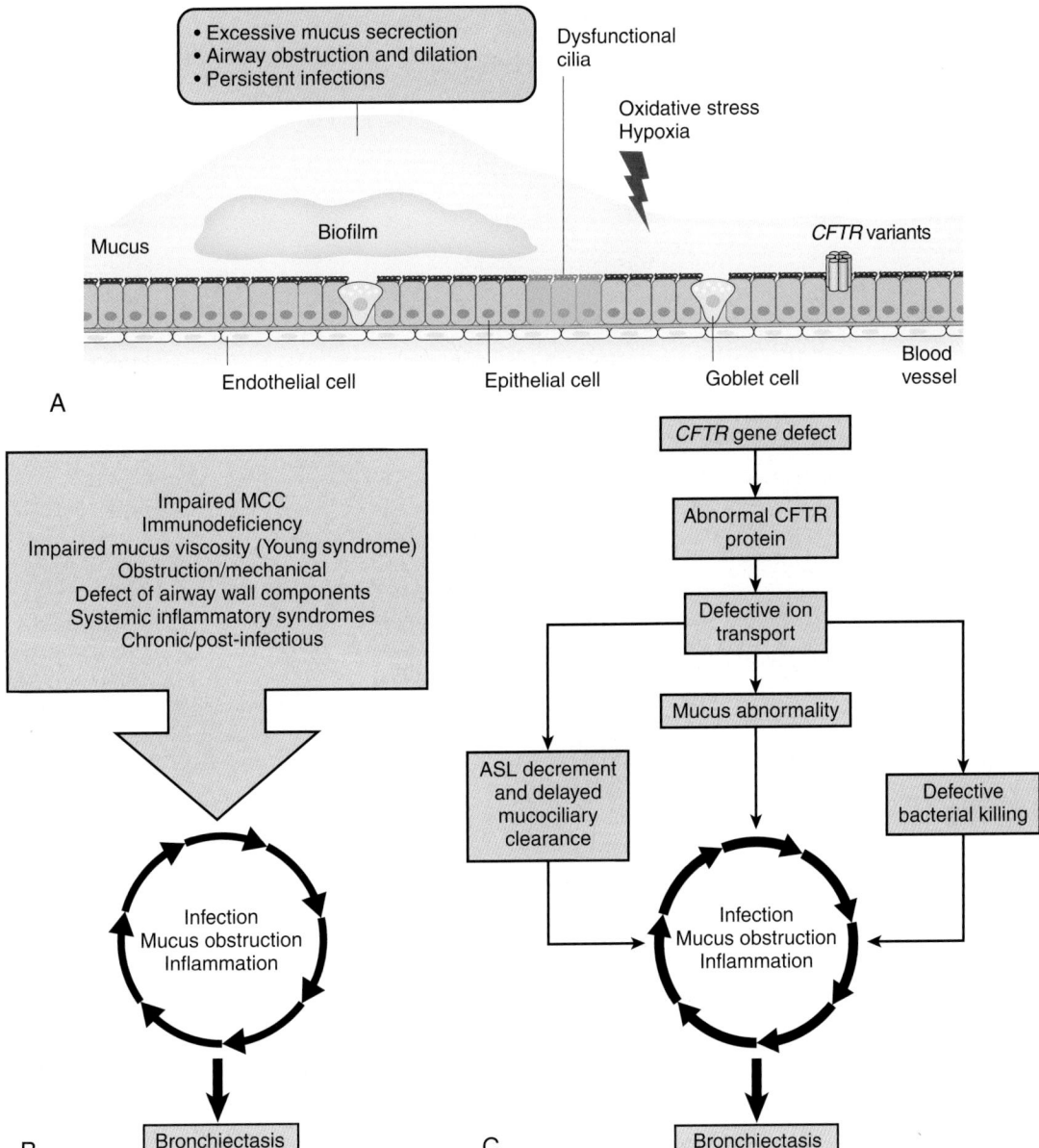

Figure 69.1 General pathophysiologic mechanisms for the development of bronchiectasis. (A) General pathophysiologic mechanisms in the airway epithelium leading to bronchiectasis. (B) Due to the underlying bronchiectatic defect (e.g., impaired *mucociliary clearance* [MCC]) and predisposition to infections (e.g., immunodeficiencies), there is biofilm formation and accumulation of mucus leading to chronic bacterial colonization. A vicious cycle ensues, wherein mucus accumulation predisposes to bacterial colonization and infection, which then incites more inflammation and bronchiectasis, leading back to greater impaired mucus clearance. (C) A prototypical example is cystic fibrosis, wherein a defect in the *cystic fibrosis transmembrane regulator* (*CFTR*) gene leads to a primary ion transport defect. These defects create abnormalities in *airway surface liquid* (ASL) and mucus clearance, inherent changes in airway mucus, and impaired bacterial killing resulting in the vicious cycle of bronchiectasis development in cystic fibrosis.

coupled with scarring and loss of volume of the local lung units, leading to regional increases in retractile forces. Examples of primary weakness of the airways contributing to bronchiectasis include Mounier-Kuhn syndrome (congenital tracheobronchomegaly due to atrophy of airway elastic fibers), Williams-Campbell syndrome (absence of cartilaginous rings in the segmental and subsegmental generations of bronchi), Marfan syndrome, and relapsing polychondritis.

Weakened airways and airway collapsibility impair the effectiveness of the cough mechanism. Coughing is an essential, primary element of lung defense. An effective cough sends columns of air rushing upward through the bronchial tree at peak speeds measured in the range of 600 mph.[29] To support these high flow rates, the cartilaginous rings must have the structural integrity to remain patent while the posterior membranous element invaginates into the lumen of the airway, thereby decreasing the cross-sectional diameter of the airway and accelerating airflow. Bronchoscopy of patients with bronchiectasis commonly reveals extraordinary collapsibility of the airways, virtually completely obstructing the bronchi with each cough. It seems likely that such amplified airway compressibility impedes the air-driven propulsion of secretions out of the

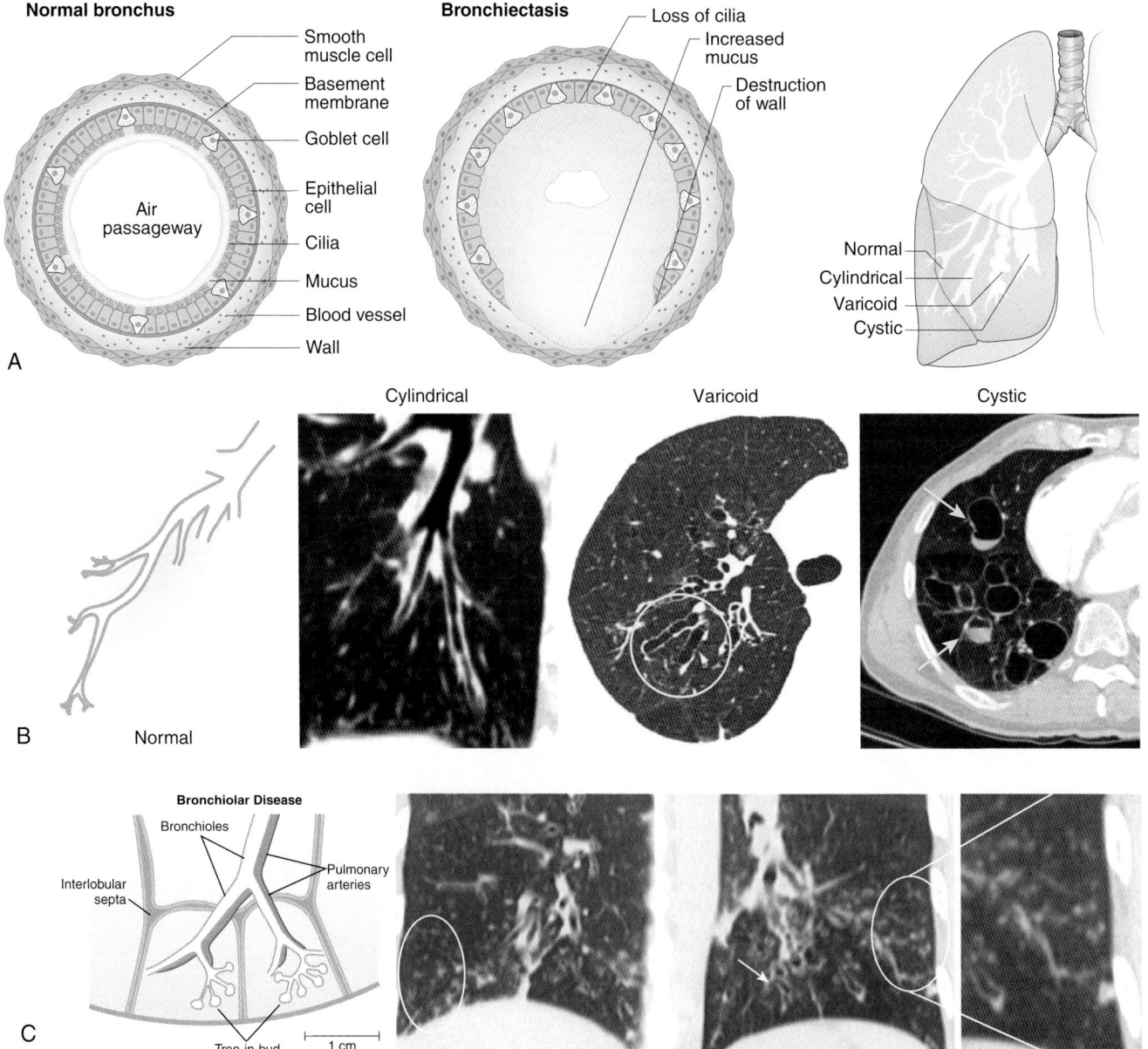

Figure 69.2 Radiographic examples of different forms of bronchiectasis. (A) The three top figures show a cross-section diagram of a normal airway, a bronchiectatic airway, and the three different forms of bronchiectasis on longitudinal view. (B) The middle panel shows a diagram of a normal bronchial tree demonstrating usual tapering as the airway branches distally (*far left*) and axial computed tomography images showing cylindrical bronchiectasis (*middle left*), varicoid bronchiectasis (*middle right, yellow circle*), and cystic bronchiectasis (*arrows, far right*). (C) The bottom panel shows a diagram of bronchiolitis (*left*) and a coronal computed tomography image (*right*) of inflammatory bronchiolitis manifested as tree-in-bud opacification (*white ovals*) (enlarged at *far right*) and bronchiectasis (*arrow*) in a patient with nontuberculous mycobacterial lung disease.

bronchial tree and helps perpetuate the chronic or recurring infections that mark most cases of bronchiectasis.

"VICIOUS CYCLE" AND MICROBIOLOGY

Because the lung is constantly exposed to the environment, resident or recruited lung phagocytes, such as macrophages, dendritic cells, and neutrophils, must play an important host defense role against inhaled or aspirated microbes. In addition, the host uses an array of other mechanisms to defend against microbial organisms that invade

the respiratory tract, including the cough reflex, mucociliary escalator, antimicrobial peptides (lysozymes, secretory leukocyte protease inhibitor, defensins, and cathelicidin), secretory *immunoglobulin* (Ig) A, and, with more sustained infection, recruited T-effector lymphocytes. Airway epithelial cells are also able to contribute to the lines of defense by secreting antimicrobial peptides.[30,31] (See Chapter 15.) Thus, in addition to the three aforementioned mechanisms by which physical forces or primary weakness of the airway walls may result in bronchiectasis, the other major element in the pathogenesis of bronchiectasis is the vicious cycle of recurrent or sustained infection and inflammation, as described by Cole.[32,33]

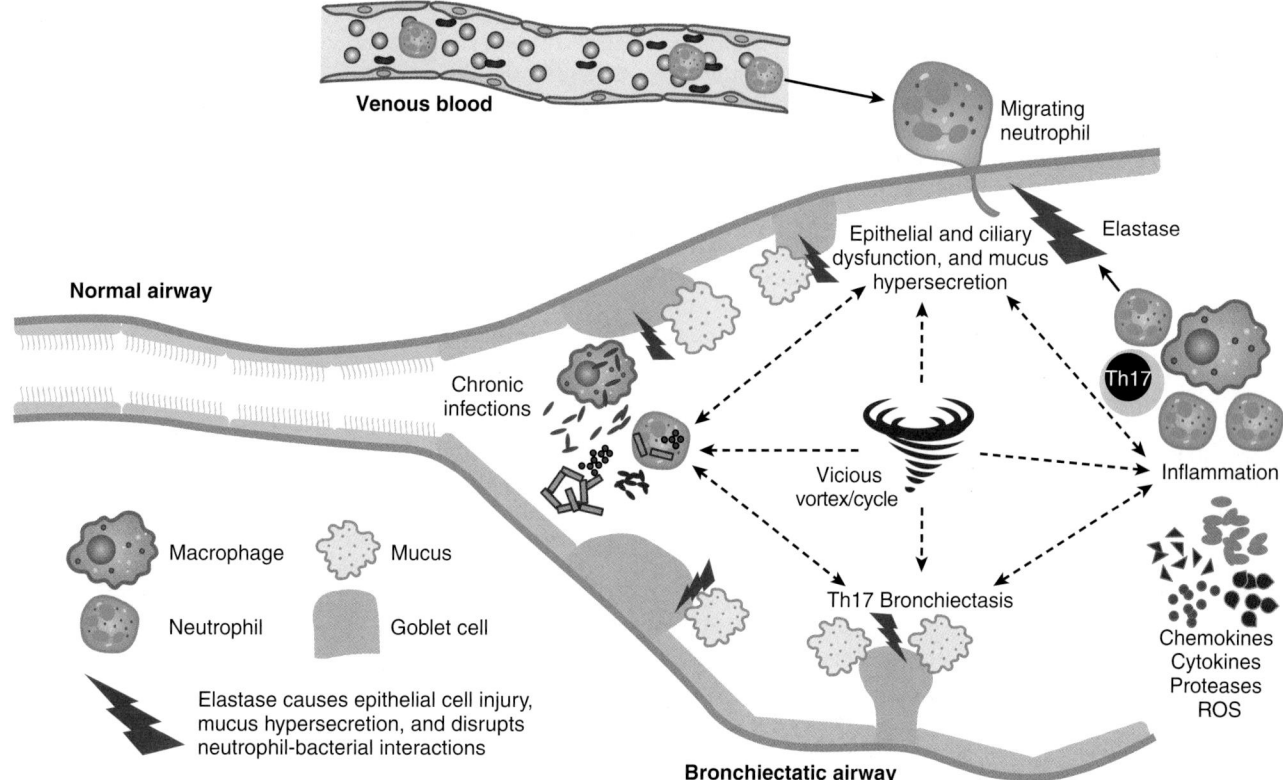

Figure 69.3 Cellular pathophysiologic mechanism of bronchiectasis. Cross-sectional view of the bronchiectatic airway demonstrating the components that play a role in the pathogenesis, including neutrophils, neutrophil elastase, goblet cells that produce mucus, and the chemokines and proinflammatory cytokines produced by macrophages and *T helper type 17 cells* (Th17). The epithelial and ciliary dysfunction, mucus hypersecretion, inflammation with unchecked protease (elastase) activity, chronic infection, and resultant bronchiectasis are intertwined and help perpetuate each other, creating the paradigm of the "vicious vortex/cycle" central to bronchiectasis pathogenesis. ROS, reactive oxygen species.

More recently, it has been proposed that a tetrad of events leads to bronchiectasis, the so-called "vicious vortex," a new term proposed because each of these factors may help perpetuate the other three (Fig. 69.3): (1) airway epithelial and ciliary dysfunction, and mucus hypersecretion; (2) chronic infections that induce further mucus hypersecretion; (3) inflammation, resulting in permanent airway injury and dilation; and (4) resultant bronchiectatic airways that are poor in mucociliary clearance, perpetuating the chronic infection, inflammation, and airway epithelial cell and ciliary dysfunction.[34] Transmural inflammation causes damage to the bronchi and bronchioles, which then become susceptible to chronic colonization by certain microorganisms, such as *Pseudomonas aeruginosa*, NTM, and *Aspergillus*, resulting in further injury and in less resistance to infection. Analysis of cellular and noncellular constituents in the bronchiectatic airways typically demonstrates intense infiltration by neutrophils, as well as by mononuclear cells and lymphocytes.[35] When the initial defenses are unable to contain the infection, an exuberant immune response ensues, orchestrated by airway epithelial cells and phagocytes through the release of inflammatory cytokines and chemokines that include macrophage inflammatory protein-2, *interleukin-8* (IL-8), and tumor necrosis factor-α. In consequence, airway infiltration by predominantly neutrophils, macrophages, and lymphocytes causes damage to the airway epithelium through the release of various proteolytic enzymes, such as neutrophil elastase and metalloproteinases, which results in erosion of mucosal barriers, creating

microabscesses that can harbor bacteria. For instance, neutrophil elastase has also been shown to cause ciliary dysfunction, mucous gland hyperplasia, and increased mucus secretion, thus further impairing clearance, summarized in Figure 69.3.[36–38]

Moreover, elastase and other proteases released by neutrophils can cleave Fcγ receptors and complement receptor 1 from neutrophil surfaces, as well as digest Ig and complement components from bacterial surfaces. These activities impair opsonization of bacteria and reduce recognition of bacteria by neutrophils, leading to decreased phagocytosis and bacterial killing (see Fig. 69.3).[39,40] Neutrophils undergo both necrotic and apoptotic forms of cell death. Necrotic neutrophils can incite more inflammation and the release of highly viscous DNA, which contributes to the volume and inspissated quality of bronchiectatic mucus. Although phagocytosis of apoptotic neutrophils—a process known as efferocytosis, which requires engagement of phosphatidylserine on apoptotic cells and phosphatidylserine receptor on macrophages—can limit inflammation, elastase can inhibit efferocytosis by cleavage of phosphatidylserine.[41] In summary, damaged airways are vulnerable to infection, begetting more damage.

Simple colonization and infection of the airways is not sufficient to produce true bronchiectasis. Sputum from patients with smoking-related chronic bronchitis typically yields organisms such as *Haemophilus influenzae*, *H. parainfluenzae*, *Streptococcus pneumoniae*, and *Moraxella catarrhalis*, a microbial spectrum similar to that seen with bronchiectasis.[42–45]

In addition, in this setting, there is heavy cellular traffic and the presence of a variety of inflammatory mediators. However, significant bronchiectasis is uncommon among patients with typical chronic bronchitis. Hence it is probable that systemic conditions or additional focal disturbances as described earlier are required for the development of classic bronchiectasis. Of note, however, the appearance in respiratory secretions of P. aeruginosa on a chronic or recurring basis does pose the risk for deleterious effects on ciliary function and other host defenses.[46] Pseudomonal infections may be of particular importance due to their role in the formation of biofilms (see later). Indeed, chronic P. aeruginosa infection or colonization plays a major role in the pathogenesis of bronchiectasis and poorer health outcomes, including increased exacerbations and hospital admissions and an approximately threefold increased risk of death.[47] In a longitudinal study of the microbiologic characteristics of 89 patients with bronchiectasis over a 5-year period, 47% were colonized with H. influenzae, 12% with P. aeruginosa, and 21% had no identifiable pathogen. After 5 years, there was a slight increase in the number of those colonized with P. aeruginosa. As expected, those with the mildest disease had no identifiable pathogens, whereas those with the worst disease were colonized with P. aeruginosa.[48]

Genetic techniques have been used to identify the bacterial flora in patients with bronchiectasis. Using 16S ribosomal RNA gene pyrosequencing of paired induced sputum and bronchoalveolar lavage samples, the bacterial flora of lower airway samples was analyzed in 41 adult patients with non-CF bronchiectasis.[49] A group of core bacterial species, defined as those frequently detected, was found to consist of commonly recognized pathogens (e.g., P. aeruginosa, H. influenzae, and S. pneumoniae) but also organisms not typically detected by routine cultures (e.g., Veillonella, Prevotella).[49] Studies genetically categorizing the lung microbiome in patients with bronchiectasis and determining its significance relative to clinical end points, such as exacerbations, continue to be advanced. Although a study showed that there was no significant difference in the overall microbial community diversity between patients with stable bronchiectasis and those with exacerbations, it was clear that Acinetobacter and Stenotrophomonas were seen primarily during exacerbations.[50] In an editorial that accompanied this report, the authors raised the critical question of whether analyzing the mountain of 16S ribosomal RNA–derived microbiota data ("the forest") masks the importance of individual microbes detected ("the trees").[51]

BIOFILMS

In 1984, Costerton[52] hypothesized that P. aeruginosa in human infections "attaches to solid or tissue surfaces and grows predominantly in biofilms." These natural and pathogenic biofilms are covered by an exopolysaccharide matrix (glycocalyx) that serves as a barrier against hostile factors, such as host immune cells and antibiotics.[52] Since this discovery, there has been clear evidence for the importance of biofilms in promoting chronic bacterial infection in the airways of CF patients,[53] and in promoting infections with NTM and methicillin-resistant Staphylococcus aureus.[54] In addition, biofilms have been identified in bronchoalveolar lavage of patients without overt signs of infection.[55] P. aeruginosa, among its various attributes, uses cilia-driven motility, which appears critically important in the aggregation phase of early biofilm formation.[56] Once biofilm formation commences, features of growth and gene activation that release virulence factors are influenced by a type of cell-cell communication called quorum sensing, in which the individual bacteria share genetic information in a paracrine fashion. Owing to a combination of physicochemical factors that protect the microbes from host defense cells and/or antibiotics, infection may persist despite aggressive treatment. In vitro testing indicates that bacteria embedded in biofilms can survive despite exposure to concentrations of antimicrobials that exceed the minimal inhibitory concentration by 1000-fold.[57] We may anticipate that future understanding and optimal management of patients with bronchiectasis will entail interventions to modify or interfere with biofilms.[56] Among potential treatments, macrolides inhibit quorum sensing,[58] and N-acetylcysteine disrupts biofilm formation and enhances bacterial killing in in vitro studies.[59]

ASSOCIATED DISEASE STATES AND ETIOLOGIC CONSIDERATIONS FOR BRONCHIECTASIS

APPROACH TO DIAGNOSIS OF BRONCHIECTASIS ETIOLOGY

A diverse set of medical conditions is strongly associated with or complicated by bronchiectasis. Given the increasing attention to developing treatments for these unique and diverse etiologies, a systematic approach to diagnosis is recommended (Fig. 69.4).[60–62] Of special importance is the recognition of CF because of the highly efficacious and more specific therapies available to these patients (see also Chapter 68).

In addition to this schema, determining the etiologic cause of bronchiectasis may be enhanced by understanding distribution patterns on HRCT imaging. The anatomic distribution of bronchiectasis associated with various etiologies is outlined in Figure 69.5 (also see eFig. 20.52).

LUNG INJURY DUE TO ACUTE INFECTION

In the modern era in industrialized nations, most adequately treated episodes of lower respiratory tract infection resolve without residual damage. However, among the older generations who were not protected by readily available antibiotics and vaccines, some individuals offer a convincing history of recurring, localized infections after a discrete episode of "pneumonia" in their childhood or early adult years that presumably produced irreversible damage leading to bronchiectasis.[1]

Specific pathogens believed to cause bronchiectasis include Bordetella pertussis, mucoid strains of S. pneumoniae, S. aureus, Klebsiella pneumoniae, adenoviruses, rubeola (measles), and influenza. Chronic granulomatous pathogens commonly related to bronchiectasis include Mycobacterium tuberculosis, Histoplasma capsulatum, and NTM such as Mycobacterium avium complex (MAC). In

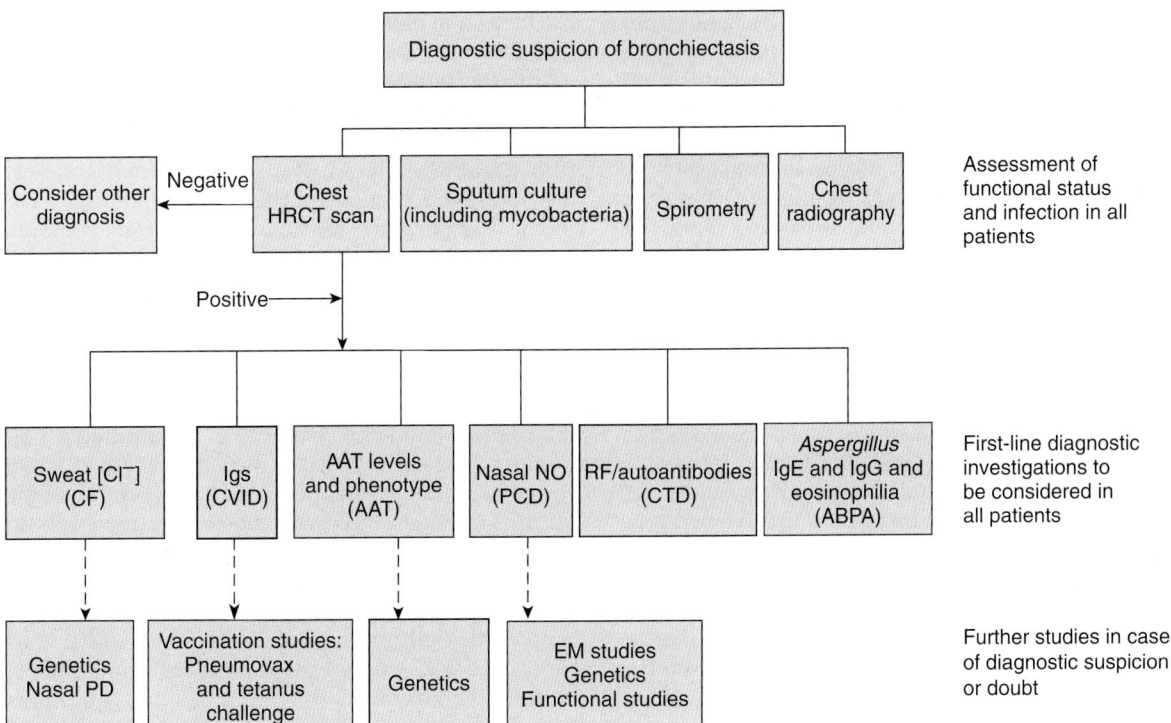

Figure 69.4 Diagnostic algorithm for the evaluation of suspected bronchiectasis. Although chest radiographs may suggest bronchiectasis, the diagnosis is confirmed by *high-resolution computed tomography* (HRCT). Sputum cultures and spirometry define the presence of infection and functional status. Subsequently, first-line laboratory and other ancillary tests are obtained to differentiate the more common causes of the bronchiectasis. Additional testing may be needed to diagnose less common causes if the initial evaluation is unrevealing. ABPA, allergic bronchopulmonary aspergillosis; AAT, alpha₁-antitrypsin; CF, cystic fibrosis; [Cl⁻], chloride concentration; CTD, connective tissue disease; CVID, common variable immunodeficiency; EM, electron microscopy; IgE, immunoglobulin E; IgG, immunoglobulin G; NO, nitric oxide; PCD, primary ciliary dyskinesia; PD, potential difference; RF, rheumatoid factor. (Modified from Drain M, Elborn S. Assessment and investigation of adults with bronchiectasis. *Eur Respir Monogr.* 2011;52:32–43.)

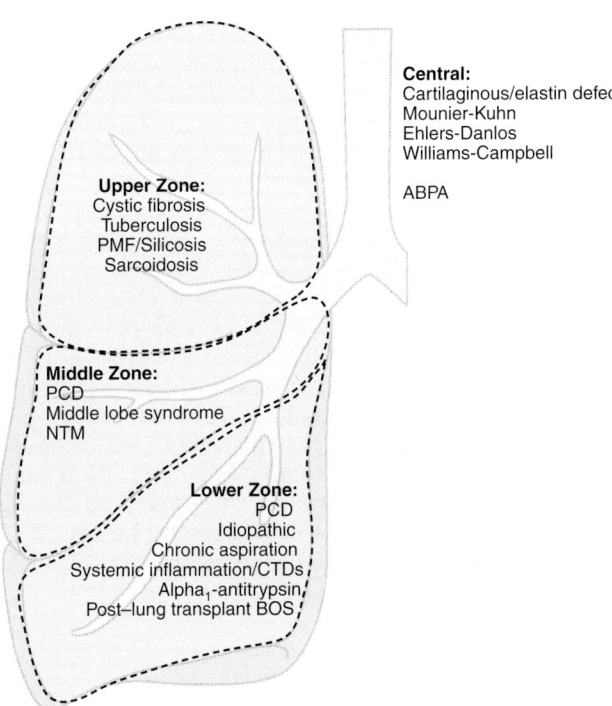

Figure 69.5 Anatomic clues to diagnosis of bronchiectasis. The causes of the bronchiectasis stratified by the predominant anatomic location of the lung abnormality; that is, upper, middle, or lower zone of the lungs and the central airway. ABPA, allergic bronchopulmonary aspergillosis; BOS, bronchiolitis obliterans syndrome; CTDs, connective tissue diseases; NTM, nontuberculous mycobacteria; PCD, primary ciliary dyskinesia; PMF, progressive massive fibrosis.

addition, mixed infection, including anaerobic mouth flora related to aspiration, may result in extensive damage to the parenchyma ("lung abscesses") with subsequent bronchiectasis.

BRONCHIECTASIS ASSOCIATED WITH NONTUBERCULOUS MYCOBACTERIA

NTM-associated bronchiectasis is discussed separately because the NTM may be a primary cause of bronchiectasis or a secondary infection complicating preexisting bronchiectasis. Chronic lung disease due to NTM is manifested by two main radiographic patterns, although both types may be found in a single patient: (1) an upper lobe fibrocavitary pattern seen mostly in persons with underlying lung disease, such as COPD, and (2) a nodular-bronchiectasis pattern with or without cavitary disease that often involves the right middle lobe, lingula, and/or right upper lobe seen in those with neither preexisting lung disease nor known genetic predisposition.[63,64] Although NTM can exacerbate preexisting bronchiectasis, such as that associated with CF,[65] *primary ciliary dyskinesia* (PCD),[66] prior tuberculosis,[67] and COPD,[68] it is also believed to cause bronchiectasis. Furthermore, there is increasing evidence that heterozygosity of the *cystic fibrosis transmembrane regulator* (CFTR) or *alpha₁-antitrypsin* (AAT) gene predisposes individuals to NTM infections resulting in secondary bronchiectasis.[69–71] Indeed, in the Bronchiectasis Research Registry for non-CF bronchiectasis, comparison of four different underlying causes for bronchiectasis—idiopathic, AAT deficiency, *common variable immunodeficiency* (CVID), and PCD—revealed that those with AAT deficiency were significantly more likely to have NTM isolated from their respiratory samples than those with the other three underlying conditions.[72]

In patients with NTM lung disease, a careful family history should be obtained for bronchiectasis. We recommend that patients with NTM lung disease be screened for CFTR abnormalities, AAT anomalies, CVID, and swallowing dysfunction and, in certain groups such as those with sinusitis, infertility, and lower lung zone bronchiectasis, for PCD. Individuals with NTM-associated bronchiectasis who have no known predisposing factors have been observed by clinicians to possess marfanoid physical features, such as constitutively slender body habitus, scoliosis, and pectus excavatum, more commonly than anticipated by chance alone.[71,73–77] Of interest, this phenotype in those with NTM lung disease seems disproportionately to involve predominantly slender white or Asian women,[78,79] although it is also seen in men.[80] We and others have postulated that these skeletal abnormalities may be a marker for an underlying and yet-to-be identified genetic predisposition speculated to be related to a minor variant of Marfan syndrome or ciliary dysfunction.[71,74–76,81–83] In those with the marfanoid body habitus, do the airways dilate because of an intrinsic structural defect? This hypothesis is plausible because fibrillin-1 is a component of the extracellular matrix, and a fibrillin mutation is the cause of Marfan syndrome. Is there an immune defect that increases the risks for infections that set in motion the coughing and inflammation that lead to bronchiectasis? This supposition is supported by the fact that the morphologic anomalies seen with Marfan syndrome have been associated with increased localized production of transforming growth factor-β, a cytokine that increases susceptibility to mycobacteria.[84–87]

More recently, it has been hypothesized, based on gene sequencing, that a combination of variants of ciliary, immune-related, connective tissue, and *CFTR* genes, in addition to other factors such as body weight, age, and environmental exposure, cooperate to increase vulnerability to NTM lung disease.[88,89]

Regardless of the presence or absence of an underlying predisposing condition for NTM lung disease, there is also increasing evidence and experience that aspiration from swallowing dysfunction or *gastroesophageal reflux* (GER) may predispose to NTM infection.[90–92]

CYSTIC FIBROSIS

CF and CF variants are arguably the most common causes of bronchiectasis in the United States and other industrialized nations of the Western Hemisphere today. Being the most common autosomal recessive disorder among whites (1 in 2000–2500 live births),[93] CF is increasingly prevalent as improved therapies allow those who are afflicted to live longer (see Chapter 67 for full details on the incidence and prevalence of CF).

In addition to "typical" cases in which CF is recognized early in life, variants may be present in the population that predispose to bronchiectasis in adults. Among a large series of adult patients with bronchiectasis associated with

NTM seen at National Jewish Health in Denver, 117 of 865 (13.5%) were found to have one or more abnormal alleles of the *CFTR* gene,[94] well in excess of the anticipated carrier rate of 6% in the general population. In 19 of these patients (2.2% overall), there were two abnormal alleles and, in the remaining 98 (11.3%), there was only one mutation. Of note, the mean age of these patients was 61 years. The clinical importance of these heterozygous mutations may be disputed; however, patients in this cohort had a high frequency of chronic airflow obstruction, sinusitis, difficulties with conception, and coinfection with pathogens typical of CF, including mucoid strains of *P. aeruginosa*, all features compatible with clinical CF.[94] Among another series of patients with bronchiectasis and/or NTM lung disease, 24 of 50 (48%) had one or more *CFTR* mutations.[95] Similarly, among a cohort of 63 patients with NTM lung disease studied at the National Institutes of Health, 36% had mutations in the *CFTR* gene.[96] Consistent with the assertion that these heterozygous mutations are clinically relevant is a series of 30 patients with clinical features of CF who were reported to have normal *CFTR* alleles on comprehensive gene sequencing.[97] The authors concluded that factors other than mutations in *CFTR* could result in a clinical condition consistent with CF. It is our contention that heterozygous anomalies in the CF gene act as a predisposing factor for NTM infections that lead to bronchiectasis.

Bronchiectasis has been described in a condition identified in the 1970s called Young syndrome. Although Young syndrome is not CF, it has a number of similar clinical features, such as bronchiectasis, sinusitis, and infertility.[98] However, unlike CF, the genetic basis for Young syndrome is not known and, because the definition includes azoospermia, it is seen only in men. Furthermore, whereas the azoospermia related to CF is due to congenital absence of the vas deferens, in Young syndrome it is due to obstruction in the distal epididymis (i.e., obstructive azoospermia).[99,100] In a comprehensive study of 15 patients with a clinical diagnosis of Young syndrome, the mean nasal mucociliary clearance was prolonged nearly threefold compared to nonsmoking control subjects, but the ciliary beat frequency and ultrastructural anatomy of the cilia were considered to be within normal limits.[100] Of interest, in one subject in whom a sample of epididymis was available, microtubular disarrangement, mostly missing or "displaced" microtubules, was seen in approximately 13% of the cilia examined.[100] Because the incidence of Young syndrome appears to be decreasing dramatically since it was originally reported in the 1970s, it has been hypothesized that Young syndrome may be due to poisoning from mercurous chloride (calomel), a compound contained in teething powder and antihelmintics, which has since been banned.[101,102] Furthermore, we posit that, with more comprehensive testing for the *CFTR* mutation, it is quite plausible that some cases diagnosed as Young syndrome were in fact CF.

DISORDERS OF IMMUNITY

The most common immunodeficiency associated with bronchiectasis is CVID. CVID is mostly sporadic but familial inheritance is seen in approximately 10% of cases.[103] CVID is best considered a syndrome comprised of a collection of diseases with different genetic defects and characterized by reduced or absent serum IgG, IgA, and/or IgM, as well as reduced or absent antibody production to specific antigen challenge after exclusion of defined causes of hypogammaglobulinemia.[104] Specific molecular defects have been described in 2–10% of CVID patients.[105,106] Several cellular defects have been described, with the most prominent one being failure of immature B cells to differentiate into memory B cells and plasma cells. However, an array of defects in other immune cell types are commonly seen in CVID, including impaired dendritic cell function and reduced number and function of CD4+ T-effector cells and T-regulatory cells.[103] Given the heterogenous clinical presentation, ranging from recurrent infections to autoimmune diseases, granulomatous inflammation, and lymphoid malignancies, CVID should not be viewed as a single disease entity.[103,107] It is believed that the recurrent infections with encapsulated bacteria, such as S. pneumoniae and H. influenzae, and subsequent uncontrolled inflammation underlie the pathogenesis of bronchiectasis in CVID, which aligns with the generally accepted hypothesis set forth by Cole,[34] that a vicious cycle of chronic infection and inflammation is a key driver of bronchiectasis. Thus, recurrent infections and resultant bronchiectasis should raise the suspicion for CVID and should prompt further evaluation for an underlying immune defect.

Deficiency of natural killer (NK) cells has also been linked to the development of bronchiectasis and, of interest, a deficiency of circulating NK-cell subsets has been described with CVID.[108] Other less common to rare primary antibody deficiencies that can result in bronchiectasis include IgG subclass deficiency (total IgG is normal, but there is decreased level of one or more IgG subclasses: IgG1, IgG2, IgG3, IgG4), selective IgA deficiency (seen in up to 10% of the population studied), and a specific antibody defect (normal IgG, IgG subclass, IgA, and IgM but impaired antibody response to polysaccharide antigens).[109–111] Although agammaglobulinemia and CVID may be the most common primary immunodeficiencies associated with bronchiectasis, several other genetic primary immunodeficiencies can manifest with bronchiectasis, including those associated with signal transducer and activator of transcription-3 (STAT-3) gain-of-function, phosphoinositol-3-kinase (PI3K) gain-of-function (activated PI3K delta syndrome or APDS), hyper-IgE syndrome (STAT-3 loss-of-function, DOCK8 and Tyk2 deficiency), cytotoxic T lymphocyte–associated protein 4 haploinsufficiency, and lipopolysaccharide-responsive beige-like anchor protein deficiency, among others.[112]

CVID in individuals older than 2 years is diagnosed by decreased serum levels of IgG and IgA of at least two standard deviations lower than normal for age and abnormal antibody responses to specific antigen challenge. For a specific diagnosis of CVID, the IgG level should be less than 4.5 g/L (normal: 7–18 g/L for adults), IgA should be absent or markedly reduced (normal: 0.7–3.5 g/L), and IgM should be normal or reduced (normal: 0.4–2.6 g/L). Rarely, IgM may be elevated due to a concomitant hyper-IgM syndrome or a class switch defect. An isolated reduction in IgG should prompt further analysis of IgG subclass deficiency (normal for adults in g/L: IgG1, 4.8–9.5; IgG2, 1.1–6.9; IgG3, 0.3–0.8; IgG4, 0.2–1.1).[103] In addition, it is important to exclude other causes of hypogammaglobulinemia, such as (1) nephrosis and other causes of Ig loss; (2) myriad drugs that can reduce Ig levels, including glucocorticoids, rituximab, alkylating agents, anticonvulsants (carbamazepine, valproic acid, phenytoin), and sulfasalazine; (3) underlying malignancy, such as chronic lymphocytic leukemia, lymphoma, and thymoma; and (4) various genetic abnormalities, such as X-linked agammaglobulinemia, Wiskott-Aldrich syndrome, ataxia telangiectasia, and severe combined immunodeficiency.[103,104,113] Of note, replacement with IgG does not always protect CVID patients from recurrent infections and bronchiectasis.[114] In patients with hypogammaglobulinemia on IgG replacement therapy, those able to secrete IgM (hyper-IgM syndrome) have a significantly lower risk of nontypeable H. influenzae carriage compared to those who lack IgM production (panhypogammaglobulinemia) despite equivalent trough levels of IgG.[115] Therefore, IgM probably plays a more prominent role in the protection against recurrent infection in CVID than previously thought, and patients should also be screened for low IgM because they might need prophylactic antibiotics in addition to IgG supplemention.[115]

Determining antibody responses to specific antigens (using commercially available vaccines) is most useful when there is a mild to moderate reduction in IgG.[103] Antibody responses to at least two protein-based vaccines (e.g., tetanus, diphtheria toxoid, or H. influenzae type b vaccine) should be assessed. A fourfold or greater increase in IgG level 4 weeks after immunization (or at least the presence of protective titers if less than a threefold increase from baseline) argues against CVID. The 23-valent pneumococcal vaccine (Pneumovax), which contains only polysaccharides, can be used to assess B cell responses independent of T cell help.[103] In contrast, the 13-valent pneumococcal vaccine (Prevnar) is used to assess B cell responses dependent on T cell help. In addition, in patients already receiving intravenous immunoglobulin, a Salmonella typhi polysaccharide vaccine may be used to assess the antigen response without discontinuing the therapy.[116] If testing for basal and stimulated immunoglobulins is suggestive of CVID, it is prudent to refer such patients to a clinical immunologist, because assessment of lymphocyte subset, B cell subsets, T cell function, and genetic testing for specific gene mutations are often warranted to prognosticate and formulate an optimal treatment regimen.

Among persons with acquired immunodeficiency syndrome, bronchiectasis has been identified in a significant proportion of those undergoing CT scans, including children.[117,118] Obviously this is skewed by the selection of those with respiratory problems for imaging. Presumably, the pathogenesis of the bronchiectasis involves severe, chronic, and recurrent infections with a variety of opportunistic pathogens.[119,120] An additional element that has not been fully addressed is the potential impact of oxidative damage associated with infection or other stressors on the AAT system.[121,122] Impairment of AAT function may contribute to the accelerated lung damage, including bronchiectasis, in persons with acquired immunodeficiency syndrome.[123,124]

Autosomal dominant hyper-IgE syndrome (AD-HIES) due to heterozygous STAT-3 mutation is a primary immunodeficiency characterized by eczema, elevated serum IgE, and connective tissue and skeletal findings, and recurrent infections of the skin (abscesses), joints, gums, sinuses, middle ear, airways, and lung parenchyma.[125] These infections include severe recurrent bronchopneumonia, especially due to *S. aureus*, which leads to bronchiectasis and pneumatoceles. In addition, bronchiectasis in AD-HIES can also result from impaired remodeling of lung tissue due to a STAT-3 defect.[126] Bronchiectasis in AD-HIES predisposes to opportunistic NTM infection and invasive fungal infection, which contribute significantly to mortality in AD-HIES.

Chronic granulomatous disease (CGD) is caused by a mutation in one of the components of the *reduced nicotinamide adenine dinucleotide phosphate* (NADPH)-oxidase complex, subsequently resulting in deficient NADPH-dependent reactive oxygen species production. Individuals with CGD are vulnerable to severe recurrent bronchopneumonia, particularly with *S. aureus* and fungal infections, which can result in structural lung damage.[127] Although patients are often identified in early childhood due to the typical and severe infections, mild forms of CGD may present in adulthood, and thus CGD could be a cause of unexplained bronchiectasis.[128]

ALPHA₁-ANTITRYPSIN ANOMALIES

AAT deficiency may be associated with bronchiectasis.[129–132] Parr and colleagues[130] examined 74 patients with the protease inhibitor ZZ genotype, the most common genotype that results in AAT deficiency, and found that 70 (95%) had bronchiectatic changes on CT scan involving an average of 3.7 lobes and 20 (27%) had "clinically significant bronchiectasis," defined as bronchiectasis affecting four or more lobes *and* "regular sputum production." In contrast, a study of more than 200 bronchiectasis patients found that the frequency of abnormal AAT genotypes was not significantly different from those without bronchiectasis.[133] Thus, based on these studies, it seems that AAT anomalies are uncommon in unselected patients with bronchiectasis, whereas bronchiectasis is common in patients with known AAT deficiency.[134] Because the "Z" isoform of AAT may polymerize in the lungs and act as a chemoattractant for neutrophils, which can then release inflammatory mediators and elastase that incite airway damage, this is a plausible mechanism by which an abnormal AAT protein may predispose to bronchiectasis.[135] However, caution must be exercised in ascribing bronchiectasis to AAT deficiency because one potential confounder is that COPD itself may be associated with bronchiectasis as discussed later.

COPD

Over the past decade, likely due to increasing use of HRCT scans, a relatively high prevalence of bronchiectasis has been reported in patients with moderate to severe COPD and the presence of bronchiectasis has been associated with increased morbidity and mortality.[136–140] Given the 30–60% prevalence of bronchiectasis found in COPD patients in these studies, it would be important to evaluate AAT phenotypes to determine whether the bronchiectasis is associated more closely with severe COPD itself, with associated AAT anomalies, or with both. In one study, COPD patients with bronchiectasis had higher levels of the neutrophil chemoattractant IL-8 in their sputa, increased bacterial colonization of their lower airways, and more severe exacerbations than those without bronchiectasis.[139] Whether bronchiectasis is a sequela in COPD patients with frequent exacerbations, identifies a subgroup of COPD patients with a different pathogenic mechanism, or both, remains to be determined.[141]

PRIMARY CILIARY DYSKINESIA

PCD is an uncommon inherited condition, with an estimated prevalence of 1:10,000. PCD is caused by mutations of various genes that encode for dynein proteins that are components of cilia or for cytoplasmic proteins responsible for cilia assembly.[142,143] Respiratory manifestations result from defective ciliary structure and function in the middle ear, nose, sinuses, and tracheobronchial tree, and include chronic oto-sinopulmonary disease.[142,144–146] Because ciliary function is critically important for proper organogenesis and laterality of organs during embryonic development, there may also be complex congenital heart disease and inversion of the normal anatomic locations for the organs of the thorax and abdomen, whether *situs inversus universalis* (Kartagener syndrome) or *partialis*[147] (eFig. 69.6). Reduced fertility is another hallmark feature among men and women with PCD due to abnormal ciliary function that results in impaired sperm motility or fallopian tube dysfunction, respectively.

Because of impaired function of ciliated respiratory epithelium, PCD patients typically have a history of recurrent otitis media, sinusitis, chronic rhinitis, bronchitis, and bronchiectasis. Newborns with PCD often experience respiratory distress shortly after birth despite term gestation, which is believed to be a consequence of defective ciliary function causing inefficient clearance of lung fluid. In contrast to CF, the bronchiectasis associated with PCD tends to be lower lung zone predominant and milder in severity.[66,148] Compared to those with other causes of non-CF bronchiectasis, those with PCD are generally younger, have lower lung function, and perhaps have more exacerbations/hospitalizations.[72] Although PCD-associated bronchiectasis may not manifest until the late teens or early adulthood, asymptomatic or symptomatic bronchiectasis may be seen by imaging in PCD-affected children of all ages, including those younger than 5 years.[147] *H. influenzae, S. aureus*, and smooth strains of *P. aeruginosa* are commonly found in children with PCD, but infection or colonization with mucoid strains of *P. aeruginosa* typically does not happen until adulthood.[66,149] Other historical and clinical features associated with PCD include parental consanguinity, nasal polyps, pectus excavatum, and scoliosis.[149,150]

In contrast to CF, PCD is a genetically heterogeneous disease with numerous implicated genes leading to various abnormalities in ciliary structure and function. As a consequence, diagnosing PCD is not a trivial process.[62,66,152–154] A complement of functional and genetic tests is of value to diagnose PCD, and multiple tests may be required to confirm the diagnosis.[153]

Behan and coworkers[155] formulated and validated a clinical scoring tool, the *Primary Ciliary Dyskinesia Rule* (PICADAR), to help clinicians diagnose PCD in patients with chronic productive cough, using seven clinical parameters: situs inversus (4 points), full-term gestation (2 points), neonatal chest symptoms (2 points), neonatal intensive care admittance (2 points), congenital cardiac defect (2 points), chronic rhinitis (1 point), and ear symptoms (1 point). This PICADAR tool demonstrated a sensitivity and specificity of 90% and 75% for PCD diagnosis with scores of 5 or more out of a possible 14 points. A modified PICADAR score was subsequently developed for PCD screening in adult bronchiectasis because gestational age is often not known and thus omitted from the scoring criteria; in addition, "neonatal chest symptoms" and "neonatal intensive care admittance" were combined to "neonatal respiratory distress."[156] Using a cutoff score of 2 or more points with the modified PICADAR score, the sensitivity and specificity for PCD were 100% and 89%, respectively.[156]

Nasal nitric oxide (nNO) is a noninvasive test that has emerged as a screening test due to its high sensitivity for PCD.[153] Although nNO testing is still often limited to a few centers, the development of electrochemical portable analyzers that are relatively easy to operate will likely increase the availability of PCD screening.[157] Affected individuals have nNO that is significantly lower (<77 nL/min) than the range seen in unaffected individuals. Hypothesized mechanisms for the low nNO in PCD include reduced NO synthesis by the abnormal airway epithelium, increased NO breakdown by denitrifying bacteria, reduced storage capacity of NO in the paranasal sinuses, and NO trapped in obstructed paranasal sinuses.[158] It should be noted that approximately one-third of patients with CF have nNO below the diagnostic threshold for PCD, which underscores the importance of eliminating CF as a potential cause in anyone suspected of having PCD.[66,153,154] nNO is measured by aspirating nasal air while instituting measures to prevent sampling air from the lower respiratory tract (exhaled NO), which typically has much lower NO levels than nNO. A meta-analysis of 12 studies (514 PCD patients and 830 non-PCD subjects) comparing nNO with either ultrastructural analysis by *transmission electron microscopy* (TEM) alone or TEM plus genetic testing found nNO had a sensitivity of 98% and specificity of 96%.[159] But it is important to emphasize that patients with low nNO may also have negative genetic testing or normal/nondiagnostic TEM analysis for PCD.[160] The specificity of low nNO for PCD may be further compromised if CF and patients with acute viral infections, chronic sinusitis, nasal polyposis, human immunodeficiency infection, cigarette smoking, and diffuse panbronchiolitis are not excluded, because these conditions may be associated with low nNO.[152,153]

Genetic testing for PCD is becoming more available with development of commercial testing panels. Currently, mutations of more than 40 genes have been identified to cause PCD. Because it is likely that not all genes associated with PCD have been identified, the sensitivity of genetic testing for PCD is estimated to be about 50–80% with the 26-gene panel, increasing to 94% with the 32-gene panel.[62,153,154] Biallelic autosomal mutations or hemizygous X-linked mutations in one of the approximately 40 PCD genes are present in greater than 70% of patients with PCD.[161] The majority

of these mutations are either deletion or nonsense mutations leading to a loss-of-function of ciliary proteins (e.g., DNAI1, DNAI2, or DNAH5) or cytoplasmic proteins involved in the preassembly of the cilia.[152] Mutation of any of the cytoplasmic proteins involved in cilia assembly results in loss of both outer and inner dynein arms, causing ciliary immotility or severe dysmotility, and mutation of genes that encode for dynein arm components results in partial or complete situs inversus. Complicating genetic diagnosis, several mutations implicated in PCD can be associated with normal ultrastructural findings (≈30% of cases) and may even demonstrate normal ciliary beat frequency and motility.[152,162]

The traditional gold standards for diagnosis of PCD are TEM of ciliated epithelium revealing ultrastructural defects of the cilia ultrastructure (e.g., absence of outer and/or inner dynein arms) and measurements of ciliary beat frequency or coordination via high-speed video microscopy. However, each has its own considerable limitations, as discussed later. Ultrastructural findings of abnormal cilia include complete or partial absence of outer or inner dynein arms, a lack of radial spokes, and transposition of one or more outer doublet microtubules into the central area of the cilia resulting in dyscoordinated and chaotic ciliary movement. These tests are limited by availability and expertise required, as well as the fact that, due to chronic sinopulmonary infection, the biopsied samples often contain inadequate or infection-induced damage to the ciliated epithelium, precluding accurate assessment.[152,163] Furthermore, based on clinical manifestations and genetic testing consistent with PCD, it is estimated that about 30% of PCD patients have normal or near-normal cilia ultrastructure, as exemplified by those with mutation of *DNAH11*.[152,154,164-166] Thus, absence of ultrastructural abnormalities does not rule out PCD.

Measurement of ciliary beat frequency and analysis of dysmotility, by high-speed video microscopy alone (120–500 frames/sec) or combined with ciliary wave form analysis (also known as ciliary beat pattern, which assesses ciliary coordination and the presence of a full sweep motion), require experienced investigators and specialized techniques. Despite optimal conditions, known limitations to assessing ciliary function include the presence of ciliary dysfunction due to infection, inflammation, and/or injury during sample collection, as well as the overlap of ciliary beat frequencies between PCD patients, disease controls, and even normal subjects.[152] Thus, an abnormal ciliary beat frequency or dysmotility does not definitively diagnose PCD and, conversely, a subset of genetically confirmed PCD patients have normal ciliary beat frequency. Hence, there was less enthusiasm for measurement of ciliary beat frequency in the 2018 guideline for diagnosing PCD.[153,154]

Among adult men, semen analysis may be useful to diagnose PCD. Dysmotile or immotile spermatozoa may be demonstrated using traditional light microscopy, using a slide prepared with a drop of nondiluted semen at 200× to 400× magnification. Abnormal motility is diagnosed if greater than 50% of sperm are immotile or nonprogressive, meaning that they move but do not make forward progression.[167] However, visualization of motile sperm does not rule out the possibility of PCD. Sperm tails may appear morphologically normal using light microscopy; therefore, ultrastructural analysis of the sperm flagella using TEM is needed to confirm the diagnosis. Sperm tails often, but not always, demonstrate the same inner and/or outer dynein arm defects present in the respiratory cilia.[168] Although infertility due to impaired or absent sperm motility is supportive of a diagnosis of PCD, fatherhood (or motherhood) of PCD subjects has been reported, and thus male (or female) fertility does not rule out a diagnosis of PCD.[169]

Given the complexities and uncertainties of the various tests available to confirm the diagnosis of PCD and the order they should be performed, a recently published American Thoracic Society guideline on PCD diagnosis generated an algorithm that aids clinicians in PCD assessment (eFig. 69.7).[153,154]

BRONCHIAL CARTILAGE OR ELASTIC FIBER DEFECTS

Mounier-Kuhn syndrome, or congenital tracheobronchomegaly, is a rare disorder associated with gross enlargement or dilation of the trachea and segmental bronchi[170] (eFig. 69.8). The underlying defect is atrophy and even absence of elastic fibers and smooth muscle tissues of the large airways.[171] Atrophy of the connective tissue between the rings may result in outpouchings (diverticulae) that can serve as reservoirs for recurrent infections. Clinically, Mounier-Kuhn patients may present in early childhood or as late as the fourth decade with recurring lower respiratory infections. The diagnosis is readily made by finding extraordinary dilation of the trachea and central bronchi on CT scans, especially in the presence of tracheal and/or bronchial diverticula (see eFig. 69.8); for men, transverse and sagittal tracheal diameter greater than 25 mm and greater than 27 mm, respectively, is considered abnormally enlarged, whereas in women, the respective values are greater than 21 mm and greater than 23 mm.[172] Special considerations in management include positive end-expiratory pressure support and silicone or metallic stenting. Lung transplantation is an option, although unique issues associated with Mounier-Kuhn syndrome include recurrent infections when tracheal diverticula are present and difficulty with bronchial anastomosis due to discrepancy in the airway diameters between the donor and the recipient lungs.

Williams-Campbell syndrome arises due to absence of cartilaginous rings in the fourth- to sixth-generation subsegmental bronchi in a symmetrical distribution, although more proximal bronchi may also be involved.[173] In addition to the subsegmental and segmental bronchiectasis, bronchomalacia of the more proximal airways may be seen[174] (eFig. 69.9). Familial cases have been reported in this condition, although the precise genetic defect is not known. Patients with Williams-Campbell syndrome are particularly predisposed to proximal bronchomalacia after transplantation due to the combined effects of cartilage deficiency in their mainstem bronchi in addition to the usual decrement of blood supply to the proximal airways due to loss of collateral circulation of the transplanted lung.[175]

CONNECTIVE TISSUE DISORDERS

Among the various formally described heritable disorders of the connective tissues, Marfan syndrome, caused by mutations of the *fibrillin 1 (FBN1)* gene, with more than 600 different mutations of *FBN1* identified, has been reported to be associated with bronchiectasis.[176–178] Other lung disorders associated with Marfan syndrome include distal acinar emphysema, cystic degeneration, spontaneous pneumothorax, bullae, apical fibrosis, and a congenital pulmonary malformation known as middle lobe hypoplasia.[178]

CONGENITAL AND DEVELOPMENTAL ANOMALIES

Conditions such as sequestration, agenesis, hypoplasia, and atresia may primarily cause bronchiectasis or may predispose to infections that secondarily cause bronchiectasis. Sequestrations presumably develop from accessory primordial lung buds, which may be invested within normal lung tissue (intralobar) or external to the normal lungs (extralobar). Sequestrations may or may not connect with the bronchial tree and often derive their blood supply directly from the aorta. Clinically, intralobar sequestration most commonly presents with recurrent and/or chronic lower respiratory tract infections beginning in the second or third decade of life, whereas extralobar sequestration is usually asymptomatic due to lack of communication with the airways. Radiographically, they usually appear as irregular, peculiar densities abutting the diaphragm in the posterior basal regions. Unilateral hyperlucent lung (Swyer-James-MacLeod syndrome) is characterized by unilateral bronchiolitis leading to hyperinflation. In some cases, bronchiectasis is present. The etiology and pathogenesis of this rare disorder are uncertain but may involve developmental or acquired disturbances of the bronchial tree.

IDIOPATHIC INFLAMMATORY DISORDERS

There is a wide array of idiopathic inflammatory conditions associated with bronchiectasis. They are all systemic illnesses that variably involve the lungs and may or may not result in bronchiectasis.

Sarcoidosis is by far the most common of these disorders (see Chapter 93). Broadly, sarcoidosis may involve the airways by several fundamental mechanisms: diffuse parenchymal scarring resulting in traction and airway distortion; endobronchial granulomatous inflammation, including stricture with poststenotic infection; or compression secondary to hypertrophic peribronchial lymphadenopathy.[179]

Rheumatoid arthritis (RA) may entail a variety of pulmonary manifestations. In two early series, bronchiectasis was seen in 3.2%[180] and 5.2%[181] of RA patients. More recently, bronchiectasis has been described in considerably higher percentages of RA patients undergoing HRCT scanning (20–35%)[182]; these studies were likely skewed by the selection of patients with respiratory problems. However, bronchiectasis was seen in 8% of RA patients without respiratory symptoms.[183] Of note, the majority of the patients in the previously discussed series did not have RA-associated interstitial lung disease as a presumed cause of the bronchiectasis. Potential causal mechanisms include increased propensity for infections, either intrinsic to RA or secondary to glucocorticoid or cytotoxic therapy. Clinically, the presence of bronchiectasis in RA patients was associated with an unfavorable prognosis in one series.[184]

Ankylosing spondylitis has been classically associated with upper lung zone fibrocystic degeneration and ankylotic fusion of the junctions of the ribs and vertebrae, resulting in restricted ventilation. However, in a large series from the Mayo Clinic, pulmonary involvement was described in only 1.2% of the patients.[185] Bronchiectasis independent of apical fibrocystic disease has been seen in a small series from the United Kingdom.[186]

Systemic lupus erythematosus may involve an assortment of pulmonary complications, including those intrinsic to the disorder itself, whereas others may be iatrogenic (see Chapter 92). Bronchiectasis was described in 21% of systemic lupus erythematosus patients studied with HRCT.[187] As with RA, the presence of Sjögren syndrome may be a comorbid element that predisposes to bronchiectasis.

Sjögren syndrome, keratoconjunctivitis sicca, and xerostomia (dry eyes and mouth) may exist in the primary form or in association with other collagen vascular diseases, such as RA or systemic lupus erythematosus. Pulmonary complications of Sjögren syndrome include lymphocytic interstitial pneumonia, lymphoma or pseudolymphoma, and/or pulmonary hypertension (see Chapter 92). Bronchiectasis has also been noted.[188–190] It is reasoned that lymphocytic inflammation results in impaired function of mucous glands, in turn resulting in decreased volumes and increased desiccation and viscosity of mucus. This leads to airway obstruction, poor clearance, and chronic infection. There have not been large CT scan surveys in patients with Sjögren syndrome to quantify the incidence of bronchiectasis.

Inflammatory bowel disease–associated bronchiectasis appears to be more common with ulcerative colitis than with Crohn disease.[191,192] In the majority of cases, the bowel disease antedates the lung manifestations, but the conditions may be temporally reversed. One unique observation of ulcerative colitis–associated bronchiectasis is that it may develop after therapeutic colectomy.[193] Proposed pathogenic relationships include a cryptogenic infection that incites both airway and intestinal inflammation, common epithelial targets of autoimmunity, or sensitizing agents that are inhaled and/or ingested, resulting in both lung and bowel disease.

Relapsing polychondritis is identified essentially as progressive inflammation, weakness, and deformity of cartilaginous structures, including the ears, nose, larynx, and tracheobronchial tree, typically associated with nonerosive polyarthritis. In addition, there may be inflammatory and/or functional disturbances of the eyes, auditory/vestibular components of the ears, and aorta (vasculitis with aneurysm). Respiratory involvement is characterized by tracheal and bronchial cartilage inflammation, resulting airway collapse, and airflow limitation (eFig. 69.10). Bronchiectasis in such patients may be due to primary bronchial damage and/or recurrent infection.[194]

ASPIRATION/INHALATION ACCIDENTS (See Also Chapter 43)

Spillage of foreign matter into the airways may result in bronchiectasis. There are two fairly distinct scenarios in which such matter might be aspirated into the lungs and cause sufficient damage to result in chronic deformity of the airways. One is the direct spillage of secretions from the oropharynx—infamous for containing a plethora of microorganisms, including microaerophilic and anaerobic bacteria—producing necrotizing pneumonia. The other is introduction of materials refluxed from the esophagus and/or stomach, which, in addition to the microorganisms noted earlier, contain food particles, hydrochloric acid, biliary or pancreatic secretions that contain various proteases, and microbes indigenous to the gut.[195]

Laryngeal protective functions are imperfect, and "microaspiration" is common. Thus, we might presume that aspiration leading to lower respiratory tract infections involves greater-than-usual volumes and/or more noxious contents. Also, it is reasonable to posit that once the airways have been damaged, a lesser inoculum may be adequate to incite the same damage, a variant of the "vicious cycle" theory.

Many factors influence the likelihood/frequency of aspiration. They include (1) depressed sensorium (trauma, alcohol or drug abuse, postictal confusion state, and general anesthesia), (2) altered brainstem function (cerebrovascular accident, polio, and primary neurologic diseases, such as multiple sclerosis, amyotrophic lateral sclerosis, or syringomyelia), (3) altered laryngeal structure/function (after surgery or irradiation), (4) esophageal disorders (dysmotility, obstruction by tumors or strictures, muscular dystrophy, achalasia, tracheoesophageal fistulas, or lower esophageal sphincter incompetence), and (5) gastric dysfunction (dysmotility or outlet obstruction).

Although all of these elements may contribute to the risk for infection (and bronchiectasis), it seems likely that GER is the most common factor. Among a cohort of bronchiectasis patients noted previously, approximately three-fourths of them had demonstrated abnormalities of esophageal morphologic features (dilation and thickening), function (dysmotility), anatomy (hiatal herniation), or competence (overt reflux).[196] Indeed, the frequency of esophageal disturbances was so high that one might question whether the esophageal findings were the cause of recurring infections/bronchiectasis or, in some cases, an effect. In the latter regard, among a series of patients with asthma and idiopathic pulmonary fibrosis, the incidence of esophageal dysfunction ranged from 80–95%.[197,198] It is plausible that labored breathing with wide disparities between intra-abdominal and intrathoracic pressure and/or chronic coughing, which stresses and dilates the diaphragmatic ring, might disrupt the lower esophageal sphincter and subject the esophagus to distending forces.[199] An additional factor that could contribute to GER disease is the medical therapy used for these lung disorders; anticholinergics, β_2-agonists, theophylline, and corticosteroids can impair lower esophageal sphincter function,[200] and broad-spectrum antibiotics alter gastroesophageal flora.

For those suspected of disordered swallowing, tailored hypopharyngography using contrast materials of varying consistency may identify unsuspected aspiration, even in the absence of awareness or coughing. A speech therapist can also instruct patients on safer techniques for eating, drinking, and swallowing.

Impaired esophageal motility may be suggested on CT scans of the lungs, manifesting as grossly dilated esophagus, excessive luminal air in the esophagus, and/or thickened esophageal walls. Impaired motility may often be demonstrated on a simple barium swallow. The extent of impaired contractility may be measured by esophageal manometry; this is essential if a reconstitution of the lower esophageal sphincter is contemplated. Demonstrating actual reflux may be challenging. If gross reflux is demonstrated on a routine study, it is sufficient for a presumptive diagnosis. However, if symptoms or other clinical features suggest GER disease, and the upper gastrointestinal series has negative results, an 18- to 24-hour pH probe with or without measurement of impedance may both identify and quantify reflux episodes.[197] Non-acid reflux may result in chronic cough and even lung injury.[201] Among the implications of these findings is that acid inhibition measures may not be sufficient to protect the airways. For individuals with evidence of recurrent aspiration, elevation of the head of the bed should be done routinely.

Toxic inhalation or thermal injury may also be associated with bronchiectasis. Acute and chronic inflammation of the tracheobronchial tree, bronchiolitis, bronchiolitis obliterans, and diffuse alveolar damage may be a consequence of exposure to toxic metal fumes (e.g., aluminum, cadmium, chromium, nickel) or toxic gases (e.g., ammonia, chlorine, phosgene, sulfur dioxide) (see Chapter 103). In severe cases, bronchiectasis may ensue because of infectious complications of the exposure, denuding of the ciliated epithelium, or progressive fibrosis. Similarly, chronic airway damage and bronchiectasis may evolve after thermal or smoke injury.

POSTOBSTRUCTIVE DISORDERS

Foreign bodies may be aspirated into the airways, especially in infants and children. Adults may aspirate with eating, trauma, or loss of consciousness. In some cases, the obstructing object may be radiopaque (teeth, bone, or metal objects) but, in most instances, the obstructing material (e.g., peanuts, vegetables) is not discernible by standard chest radiography. Tumors, benign or malignant, may also result in airway obstruction, poor drainage, recurrent/chronic infection, and bronchiectasis. The more common tumor types include bronchogenic carcinomas (particularly the squamous cell variety), carcinoid tumors, and papillomas. Extrinsic airway compression due most often to hypertrophic lymphadenitis from granulomatous diseases, such as sarcoidosis or infections and including tuberculosis or histoplasmosis, may severely narrow or even occlude large airways. In patients with "focal" bronchiectasis, particularly those with disease limited to only one region (eFig. 69.11), bronchoscopic examination to exclude an obstructing lesion should be performed early if other causes are not evident.

ALLERGIC BRONCHOPULMONARY ASPERGILLOSIS (See also Chapter 96)

ABPA is a relatively uncommon condition, estimated in approximately 2.5% of patients with asthma.[202] ABPA is a hypersensitivity reaction, usually to *Aspergillus fumigatus*, but other fungi, including *Candida albicans*, may also be a source of the antigenic stimulus (allergic bronchopulmonary mycoses). The exaggerated type 2 T helper cell response seen in ABPA is likely due to *human leukocyte antigen* (HLA)-DR2/5 polymorphism resulting in greater efficiency in presenting *Aspergillus* allergens to T cells.[203] As a result of type 2 T helper cell expansion and release of IL-4, IL-5, IL-9, IL-10, and IL-13, there is increased expansion and influx of eosinophils and mast cells, as well as isotype switching to IgG and IgE.[203]

ABPA may manifest with fever, wheezing, eosinophilia, and fixed or fleeting pulmonary opacification (often upper lobes). The opacifications range from subsegmental to lobar and are due to eosinophilic infiltration and/or lymphocytic interstitial pneumonia. Other radiographic findings include atelectasis due to mucus plugging, manifesting clinically as expectoration of thick, brown mucous plugs. The inflammation and distention from the plugs typically result in thin-walled bronchiectasis that is often multilobar and central (Fig. 69.6). The mucoid impaction may show high attenuation, reflecting the organism's ability to fix calcium salts, iron, and manganese (see eFig. 69.5D and F).

The diagnosis of ABPA should be considered in patients with asthma or CF who have frequent exacerbations requiring anti-inflammatory drugs to affect symptomatic relief. The diagnostic criteria for ABPA have evolved but include a number of clinical, radiographic, and laboratory features.[203] A more current diagnostic criterion was proposed by the International Society for Human and Animal Mycology, which allows a diagnosis of ABPA to be made in the absence of radiographic changes[202,204,205] (Table 69.2). However, many patients with ABPA do not have all the criteria, especially with early disease or if taking glucocorticoids. If patients fulfill all the criteria for ABPA except for bronchiectasis, they are diagnosed with seropositive ABPA, likely an early stage of disease.

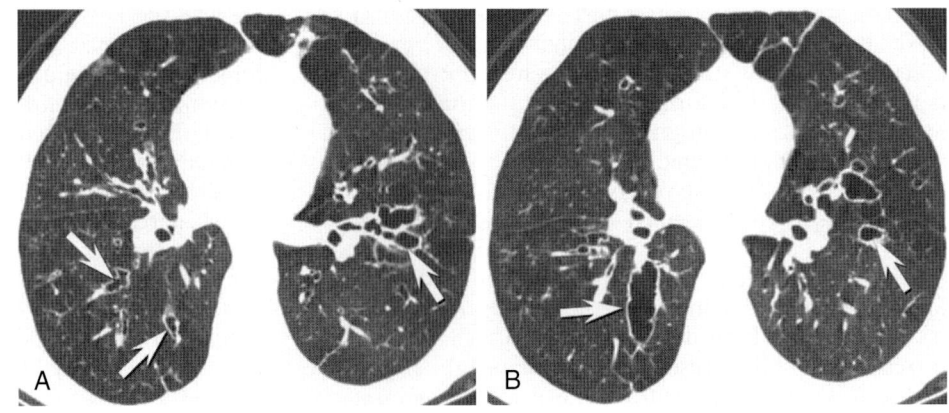

Figure 69.6 Bronchiectasis: allergic bronchopulmonary aspergillosis. (A–B) Axial chest computed tomography shows central bronchiectasis (*arrows*), typical of allergic bronchopulmonary aspergillosis. (Courtesy Michael B. Gotway, MD.)

Table 69.2 Diagnostic Criterial for Allergic Bronchopulmonary Aspergillosis

Predisposing condition: asthma or cystic fibrosis

ESSENTIAL CRITERIA

1. Type I immediate cutaneous hypersensitivity reaction (wheal and flare) to *Aspergillus fumigatus** or elevated serum IgE against *A. fumigatus* and

2. Elevated total IgE (>1000 IU/mL[†])

OTHER CRITERIA (≥2 OF 3 NEEDED)

1. Presence of serum precipitating or IgG against *A. fumigatus*

2. Radiographic pulmonary opacities consistent with ABPA (e.g., pulmonary opacification and/or bronchiectasis)

3. Total eosinophil count >500 cells/μL in patients not on recent corticosteroids

*Although cutaneous skin testing is nearly 100% sensitive and is a useful screening test for ABPA, it is not specific for ABPA.
[†]Total of IgE <1000 IU/mL may be acceptable if patient meets all other criteria.
ABPA, allergic bronchopulmonary aspergillosis; IgE, immunoglobulin E; IgG, immunoglobulin G.
From Agarwal R, Chakrabarti A, Shah A, et al; ABPA Complicating Asthma ISHAM Working Group. Allergic bronchopulmonary aspergillosis: review of literature and proposal of new diagnostic and classification criteria. *Clin Exp Allergy.* 2013;43:850–873.

Distinguishing ABPA from CF can be difficult, given the similarities between the two disorders, including the presence of bronchiectasis and positive serologic tests for *Aspergillus.* The CF Foundation has established diagnostic criteria for ABPA in CF patients: (1) clinical deterioration not attributable to another cause, (2) IgE greater than 1000 IU/mL, (3) skin test positivity to *Aspergillus*, (4) precipitating antibody or specific IgG to *Aspergillus*, and (5) abnormalities on chest imaging unresponsive to antibiotics or standard chest physiotherapy.[203]

IDIOPATHIC BRONCHIECTASIS

Depending on the extent of evaluation and perhaps referral bias, "idiopathic" bronchiectasis, for which no known predisposition is identified, is estimated to account for 25–50% of cases of bronchiectasis.[1,206,207] Although the diagnosis of idiopathic bronchiectasis can only be made after known causes of bronchiectasis are effectively excluded, it often has a characteristic phenotype of bilateral lower lobe bronchiectasis and chronic rhinosinusitis.[1] Genotyping studies of class I and class II major histocompatibility complex molecules indicate that allelic polymorphism for certain HLA subtypes are statistically associated.[208–211] NK cell activation may play a role. NK cells use their killer cell Ig-like receptors to recognize abnormal HLA-C molecules on the surfaces of infected cells, and genotypic analysis of HLA-C–killer cell Ig-like receptor combinations have supported a role for increased NK cell activation in the pathogenesis of idiopathic bronchiectasis.[208] However, to the best of our knowledge, functional studies to confirm excessive NK cell activity in patients with idiopathic bronchiectasis have not been done. Nevertheless, this hypothesis is supported by the presence of bronchiectasis in patients with the transporter-for-antigen-presentation deficiency

syndrome, a genetic disorder with impaired HLA class I expression and dysregulated NK, γδ cytotoxic T cell, and CD8[+] T cell function. In this disorder, the defective HLA class I expression results in increased NK and γδ T cell activities because HLA class I normally serves as an inhibitory ligand for these cell types.[212]

MISCELLANEOUS

There are numerous other causes of bronchiectasis, including such diverse entities as yellow nail syndrome and radiation therapy injury.

Yellow nail syndrome is an uncommon disorder marked by the triad of yellow, thick, dystrophic nails; chronic lymphedema of the face, hands, and lower extremities; and pleural effusions.[213] Women are more commonly affected than men; the median age of onset is 40 years, with cases ranging from infancy to the seventh decade. The most prominent pulmonary finding is bilateral exudative pleural effusions.[214] Recurrent sinusitis and lower respiratory tract infections are common, the latter resulting in bronchiectasis.[215] Contributing factors for bronchiectasis include abnormal lymphatic structure, increased vascular permeability, deficient immunoglobulin production, and/or ciliary dysfunction.

Radiation therapy, typically delivered for carcinoma of the breast or mediastinal tumors, including lymphomas, may result in profound damage to the central airways. This reaction is marked by focal damage to the cartilage and mucosa of the airways leading to distention and irregularities of the major bronchi in the field of irradiation. Bronchiectasis secondary to radiation therapy for neoplasms has become less common as radiation dosage and field used have become more refined. This condition may be recognized by lung parenchymal scarring in the field of irradiation (eFig. 69.12).

MANAGEMENT

The care of patients with bronchiectasis typically involves many layers, which may be partitioned into five broad components: airway hygiene, antimicrobial treatment, anti-inflammatory therapy, surgery, and miscellaneous. Although most patients with bronchiectasis require various elements of each of these components to enjoy optimal health, there is no standard formula for treating this disorder. The great majority of recurrently or chronically symptomatic patients benefit from a regular mucus-clearing regimen and periodic antibiotic therapy. For most patients, a pragmatic or trial-and-error approach is required to determine individual needs, preferences, and tolerances.

It is important to note that most elements described in this section have not been shown to be efficacious by randomized, controlled clinical trials. Thus, meta-analyses, such as those reported in the Cochrane Database of Systematic Reviews, generally cannot confirm the benefits or disutility of such approaches.[216–223] Perhaps because bronchiectasis is such a complex mix of varying conditions and has been an underappreciated "orphan" disease, a paucity of systematic research has been directed at this very troublesome disorder, although this is changing. The available evidence and assessment of the value of integrated therapies have been summarized in two guidelines by the British Thoracic Society[60] and the European Respiratory Society.[61]

AIRWAY HYGIENE AND HYPEROSMOTIC AGENTS

Airway hygiene consists of nonantibiotic therapies directed toward mobilizing and eliminating inflammatory secretions from the tracheobronchial tree and from the paranasal sinuses. Modern devices to facilitate airway clearance of secretions include the Flutter valve, Acapella valve, Aerobika valve, and high-frequency chest wall oscillation devices. See eFig. 69.13 for a summary of potential airway clearance therapies. Also included under this rubric are steps to prevent/limit aspiration of oropharyngeal or gastroesophageal contents into the airways.

Hypertonic saline, 3% or 7% two to four times daily, has been shown to accelerate mucus clearance, decrease exacerbations, and improve lung function in CF patients.[224] However, its role in non-CF bronchiectasis remains to be seen because studies show conflicting results. When hypertonic saline was used for mucus clearance as part of an algorithm in combination with protocolized chest physiotherapy, exacerbations were reduced.[225] Inhaled dry-powder mannitol, recently approved for adult CF patients,[226] appears promising in airway clearance in bronchiectatic patients,[227,228] although it may be difficult to tolerate.

The mucolytic drug N-acetylcysteine (600 mg twice daily) was found to be effective at reducing exacerbations when taken orally,[229] although studies to confirm this small sample size trial are needed. Other mucoactive drugs, such as recombinant human deoxyribonuclease, failed to reduce exacerbations and had a trend toward more frequent and severe exacerbations in patients with idiopathic bronchiectasis.[230]

ANTIMICROBIAL THERAPY

Antimicrobial therapy historically has been the centerpiece of bronchiectasis care. However, there is no clear consensus on the major questions in this area, including whether treatment should be given on a routine, periodic schedule (rotating) or an as-needed basis for clinical exacerbations. In a meta-analysis of the use of prolonged oral antibiotics for purulent bronchiectasis, sputum volume/purulence was shown to decrease, but there were no significant beneficial effects in regard to rates of exacerbations, lung function, or death.[231] There are also limited data on the empirical selection of an antimicrobial agent or treatment guided by species identification and in vitro susceptibility testing. For patients unresponsive to empirical antibiotics or who experience frequent exacerbations, it appears prudent to obtain comprehensive microbiologic cultures, including for NTM and fungal organisms, and to tailor antibiotics based on the type of organism identified and drug susceptibility profile.

Aerosolized antibiotics also appear promising in treating or preventing exacerbations. Given the role of chronic P. aeruginosa in the pathogenesis and prognosis of bronchiectasis, there is ongoing research to develop strategies for acute and chronic treatment of this infection.

The success of inhalational antibiotics targeted toward P. aeruginosa in CF lung disease has prompted extensive evaluation of this strategy in non-CF bronchiectasis. In the earliest studies, addition of inhaled tobramycin to oral ciprofloxacin for Pseudomonas-associated exacerbation of non-CF bronchiectasis showed improved microbiologic outcome; however, there was no additional clinical benefit over ciprofloxacin alone, perhaps due to approximately threefold greater incidence of bronchospasm in the tobramycin arm.[232] In patients with CF, inhaled tobramycin twice daily given in alternating months decreased the frequency of exacerbations due to P. aeruginosa.[233] Even in patients without CF, inhaled tobramycin was found to be efficacious.[234] In a randomized study of nebulized gentamicin (twice daily for 12 months) versus saline for 65 patients with non-CF bronchiectasis, the gentamicin-treated subjects had reduced microbial burden, airway neutrophils, and sputum purulence.[235] Improved exercise capacity, decreased exacerbation frequency, and better health-related QOL measure were also seen in the gentamicin arm, with the caveat that patients were not blinded to the treatment.[236] Compared to nebulized saline, nebulized gentamicin given prophylactically for 12 months also showed significant reduction in markers of inflammation in both the airways and circulation.[237]

Inhaled ciprofloxacin has been studied for its efficacy in preventing exacerbations from Pseudomonas and several other chronic infections associated with frequent exacerbations. In companion Phase III studies (RESPIRE 1 and 2), the effect of ciprofloxacin in varied on-off cycles was examined in reducing time to next exacerbation.[238,239] Given the inconsistent results on the primary end point, inhaled ciprofloxacin was not approved. In a separate trial of aerosolized liposomal ciprofloxacin (150 mg liposome encapsulated plus 60 mg of free ciprofloxacin) in 582 subjects, there was no significant difference in the time to first exacerbation between the ciprofloxacin and placebo arms, although the ciprofloxacin arm had a significant reduction in the annualized exacerbation frequency.[240]

Inhaled aztreonam was studied in two companion trials (AIR-BX1 and 2) for effects of improved QOL by the QOL-Bronchiectasis Questionnaire (QOL-B) in patients with chronic Pseudomonas infection. A total of 540 patients were randomized to receive on-off periods of 38 days of inhalational aztreonam versus placebo. There was no significant difference in the primary end point of improved QOL. Subsets of patients experienced reduced exacerbations and improved QOL, but inhaled aztreonam was not approved for use in this subset of bronchiectasis patients.[241]

Finally, inhaled colistin, at a dose of 1 million international units (aerosolized), was studied in a randomized trial versus saline in 144 subjects with P. aeruginosa in their sputum and who were randomized after a course of intravenous antipseudomonal antibiotics for an exacerbation. The median time to first exacerbation was not significantly different in the colistin subjects compared with the placebo subjects. The patients receiving colistin had improved QOL and reduced bacterial sputum density of Pseudomonas.[242]

In summary, the role of inhalational antibiotics is not supported by large-scale pivotal studies. However, in many of the studies, subsets of patients had improvements in QOL or bacterial density. Therefore, expert opinion advocates the use of these therapies in individualized therapeutic regimens for patients with chronic Pseudomonas or other gram-negative infections.

Due to the role of *Pseudomonas* in propagating pathology and accelerating clinical decline, attention has been paid recently to eradication of initial infections.[61] Several groups have evaluated eradication protocols predicated on a period of systemic antipseudomonal antibiotics followed by suppression with inhalational antibiotic therapies, with varied success at achieving long-term eradication.[243,244] Approaches to *P. aeruginosa* eradication are summarized in eFig. 69.14.

ANTI-INFLAMMATORY THERAPY

The rationale for using the anti-inflammatory agents in bronchiectasis is to dampen the inflammatory cascade, with the goals of reducing symptoms and limiting the progression of disease and decline in lung function. Anti-inflammatory agents that have been examined in bronchiectasis include the *nonsteroidal anti-inflammatory drugs* (NSAIDs) and inhaled corticosteroids. Intermittent macrolides have been studied for their antimicrobial activities as well as their anti-inflammatory and other nonmicrobicidal activities (see next section).[245]

Nonsteroidal Anti-inflammatory Drugs

Because prostaglandins may play a role in augmenting airway secretions, NSAIDs, by blocking the cyclooxygenase pathway, have been studied in bronchiectasis. In a double-blind, placebo-controlled study in patients with bronchorrhea due to chronic bronchitis, diffuse panbronchiolitis, and bronchiectasis, inhaled indomethacin significantly decreased both the amount of sputum and the perceived dyspnea.[246] Another mechanism by which indomethacin may help in bronchiectasis is via inhibition of both neutrophil chemotaxis and neutrophil degradation of fibronectin, thereby decreasing airway inflammation and purulence.[247] In a comprehensive Cochrane Database review of randomized trials of NSAIDs in CF patients, high-dose ibuprofen was shown to slow the progression of lung disease, especially in children.[248] In contrast, there have been no randomized, controlled trials on the use of NSAIDs in non-CF bronchiectatic patients.[249]

The anti-inflammatory properties of statins were studied in a Phase II trial demonstrating reduction in cough and improved QOL.[250] Although larger trials failed to replicate these findings, treatment was associated with improved cough and QOL, indicating that further exploration of statins is warranted.[251]

Inhaled Corticosteroids

Although some studies show improved symptoms and lung function in CF patients treated with *inhaled corticosteroids* (ICS),[252,253] others, including a review of clinical trials, have not found ICS to be beneficial.[254,255] In non-CF bronchiectasis, relatively small studies indicate that ICS provides symptomatic relief (e.g., reduction in dyspnea, cough, and sputum production).[256–259] High doses of ICS are typically tried in bronchiectasis because of the notion that neutrophils, dominant in bronchiectatic airways, are relatively resistant to the (apoptotic) effects of corticosteroids.[260] Although bronchiectatic patients are often treated with β_2-agonists and ICS based on extrapolation by clinicians of treatment for COPD and asthma, there is limited evidence of their efficacy with bronchiectasis. Martinez-Garcia and associates[260] performed a pilot study comparing high-dose budesonide 800 µg every 12 hours to budesonide 640 µg plus formoterol once daily and found that the combined treatment with the lower dose of ICS resulted in a greater improvement of dyspnea score, health-related QOL assessment, and reduced ICS-associated side effects, such as pharyngeal irritation and dysphonia. Because of the potential risk for pneumonia with ICS use, as has been documented with COPD,[261] it seems prudent to limit the duration of ICS whenever possible, while monitoring closely for worsening respiratory symptoms and function. It is clear that larger studies are needed to determine the benefits and risks of ICS, long-acting β_2-agonists, or the combination as maintenance treatment or rescue therapy for exacerbations.[262]

THERAPIES FOR TREATMENT OF FREQUENT EXACERBATIONS

Intermittent Macrolide Therapy

Independent of their antimicrobial properties, macrolide antibiotics hold promise in inhibiting disease activity in bronchiectasis because of their immunomodulatory effects.[263] Intermittent macrolide therapy may help in bronchiectasis by decreasing the chloride diffusion potential gradient across the airway mucosa (resulting in decreased sputum volume), reducing airway levels of the neutrophil chemokine IL-8, inhibiting both neutrophil and *Pseudomonas* migration, suppressing *Pseudomonas* quorum sensing, disrupting the established biofilm layer, and enhancing alveolar macrophage phagocytic ability.[264,265] Thus macrolide therapy is posited to antagonize several of the mechanisms of pulmonary exacerbation and pathogenesis of bronchiectasis.

Clinical trials have explored the benefits of macrolides. In older studies, clarithromycin, but not amoxicillin or cefaclor, was shown to reduce sputum production in patients with chronic bronchitis or bronchiectasis.[266] Beneficial effects plus improvement in lung function have been shown in various trials using intermittent azithromycin therapy in CF patients chronically infected with *P. aeruginosa* and also in younger CF patients before they have been colonized with *P. aeruginosa*.[267] In a double-blind, placebo-controlled trial of approximately 120 patients with non-CF bronchiectasis and a history of frequent pulmonary exacerbations, low-dose erythromycin (400 mg twice daily) for 12 months significantly reduced (1) the number of pulmonary exacerbations overall by roughly one-third, as well as in those with baseline *P. aeruginosa* airway infection, (2) sputum production, and (3) lung function decline as measured by *forced expiratory volume in 1 second* (FEV$_1$).[268] However, erythromycin prophylaxis was associated with increased frequency of macrolide-resistant oropharyngeal streptococci.[268] Two double-blind, placebo-controlled trials of azithromycin (250 mg daily for 12 months or 500 mg thrice weekly for 6 months) resulted in significantly lower rates of exacerbations compared to placebo.[269,270] In an individual patient data meta-analysis that comprised three studies totaling 341 subjects with bronchiectasis, long-term macrolide antibiotics significantly reduced the frequency of exacerbations, improved the time to first exacerbation, and enhanced the QOL, especially in those with *P. aeruginosa* infection, although there was no significant improvement in FEV$_1$.[271] Finally, in a recently published randomized, controlled trial of 90 patients with PCD, thrice weekly azithromycin therapy was found to reduce exacerbations compared to placebo patients.[272]

Azithromycin also carries risks. In one study there was a nearly threefold increase in macrolide resistance of bacteria in the azithromycin group and significantly higher incidence of abdominal pain and diarrhea, although these gastrointestinal symptoms did not prevent continuation of azithromycin.[273] In addition to the potential increase in antibiotic resistance in pyogenic bacteria, long-term azithromycin may predispose to drug-resistant NTM infections in patients with bronchiectasis.[273] Azithromycin was also shown to inhibit autophagy, a normal homeostatic cell recycling process increasingly recognized as important for the phagosomal killing of intracellular mycobacteria.[273] Other potential serious adverse effects of azithromycin include dysrhythmias and cardiac-related deaths, especially in those with underlying risk factors for cardiovascular disease.[274,275] In sum, at this time, because of their risk of harm, macrolides should probably be considered only in patients who would potentially benefit the most, for example, those with frequent exacerbations.

Inhibition of Neutrophil Elastase

Recurrent exacerbations in bronchiectasis are linked to neutrophilic influx into the airways. Subsequent elaboration of neutrophil serine proteases, including neutrophil elastase, may be at play in both chronic and acute inflammation. Thus, this pathway is postulated to drive recurrent cycles of inflammation and damage in the airways. Clinically, inhibition of these pathways is being explored to reduce the vicious cycle through inhibition of neutrophil elastase, which not only degrades elastin but also has other aforementioned deleterious effects. Recently, a large randomized control trial of a novel oral inhibitor of dipeptidyl peptidase I, a key enzyme in the activation of neutrophil elastase (INS1007, Insmed Corporation), has completed enrollment to demonstrate if this strategy reduces time to next exacerbation and frequency of exacerbation.[276] If successful, this strategy will add to the growing armamentarium for treatment of frequently exacerbating patients.

Recent expert guidelines suggest an integrated approach to treatment of frequent pulmonary exacerbations as outlined in eFig. 69.15.

SURGERY

The role of surgery in the management of bronchiectasis is uncertain. No formal systematic studies of the indications and efficacy of resectional surgery have been conducted among patients with bronchiectasis. Traditional indications for resectional surgery have included chronic disabling infection, recurrent infections of intolerable frequency, or irreversible lung damage distal to a foreign body or benign tumor. Hemoptysis that is life-threatening and/or recalcitrant to bronchial artery embolization may be an indication for surgery. A historical adage has been that surgery does not cure bronchiectasis. If true, it is likely due to our evolving understanding that most cases of bronchiectasis are due to innate risk factors that predispose to recurrence. However, surgery may be an appropriate palliative measure in selected cases, especially with severe localized disease, as not uncommonly seen in patients with NTM lung disease or in those with localized bronchiectasis and recalcitrant or recurrent superimposed infections.

Tracheal reconstruction surgeries, including tracheobronchoplasty or tracheal stenting, may confer symptomatic benefit for patients with Mournier-Kuhn.[277,278] Due to the rare nature of this disease, expert opinion from an experienced airway surgical team is vital for making this decision.

Bilateral lung transplantation has become increasingly recognized for patients who experience severe respiratory failure due to bronchiectasis. Due to the suppurative nature of bronchiectasis, single-lung transplantation is not recommended. Although limited evidence for long-term outcomes are available, single-center studies indicate that adults with bronchiectasis have similar long-term survival and recovery of lung function as other patient populations receiving bilateral lung transplant.[279] However, one study found that underlying immunodeficiency and pretransplantation diagnosis of chronic *Pseudomonas* infection may reduce posttransplantation outcomes.[280] The optimal timing is based on lung allocation scores. Although successful for some cases, there is limited evidence for optimal timing and tailoring of lung allocation scores for non-CF bronchiectasis, an area for future research.

MISCELLANEOUS

Additional measures, such as smoking cessation and vaccination against pneumococcal disease and influenza, are appropriate for all patients. Intuitively, these measures seem particularly important for those with bronchiectasis; however, no systematic information is available to confirm their usefulness in this setting. On the other hand, early recognition and remediation of exercise limitation and sleep-related hypoxia has demonstrated substantial benefits in regard to morbidity and mortality. As with all individuals, it seems sensible to ensure that patients with bronchiectasis have repleted vitamin D levels because this hormone has been shown to induce cathelicidin, an antimicrobial peptide.[281] Recently, it was reported that bronchiectasis patients with vitamin D deficiency have more frequent bacterial colonization (especially *P. aeruginosa*), worse airflow, more frequent exacerbations, higher levels of inflammatory markers in sputa, and more rapid decline in lung function over a 3-year follow-up than those with higher vitamin D levels.[282]

OVERALL APPROACH TO MANAGEMENT

Due to increasing complexity of bronchiectasis management, a thoughtful approach to management is necessary. Recent expert guidelines suggest several approaches. One strategy involves step-up therapy based on patient symptoms and severity of lung function and frequency of exacerbations.[283] In addition, a treatment strategy targeted toward aspects of pathophysiology with frequent reassessment of therapeutic response is a reasonable approach. Individualization of therapeutic approach is necessary and may vary by patient preference. We recommend the strategy outlined in Figure 69.7.

PROGNOSIS

All patients with bronchiectasis are affected by a poorer prognosis than age- and gender-matched healthy control subjects. Recent estimates demonstrate an approximately twofold increase in mortality in those with bronchiectasis compared to healthy normal subjects.[284] Recently published analyses have identified a host of factors predictive of excessive mortality.[285] Prospective evaluation of these analyses has aided in the development of two propensity scoring systems that assess long-term prognosis in non-CF bronchiectasis: the *FEV$_1$, Age, Chronic Colonization, Extension, Dyspnea* (FACED) Score[286] and the *Bronchiectasis Severity Index* (BSI).[287] Both identified increased risk of mortality and hospitalization on the basis of worsening lung function, age, presence of *P. aeruginosa*, degree of dyspnea, and extent of radiographic bronchiectasis. Both systems result in similar prediction of outcomes when validated head to head.[288] In addition, the BSI scoring system emphasizes the role of prior hospitalization and frequency of exacerbation in the prediction of risk of subsequent hospitalizations.

In addition to excess mortality attributed to bronchiectasis, many patients experience increased morbidity due to pulmonary and sleep-related complications.[289] Patients also have increased risk of nonpulmonary medical issues, including cardiovascular disease, GER disease, malignancy, and cerebrovascular diseases than age-matched healthy control subjects.[290]

Recent developments of QOL instruments, including the QOL-B, focused on bronchiectasis and have aided the assessment of patients and have served as key clinical trial end points.[291]

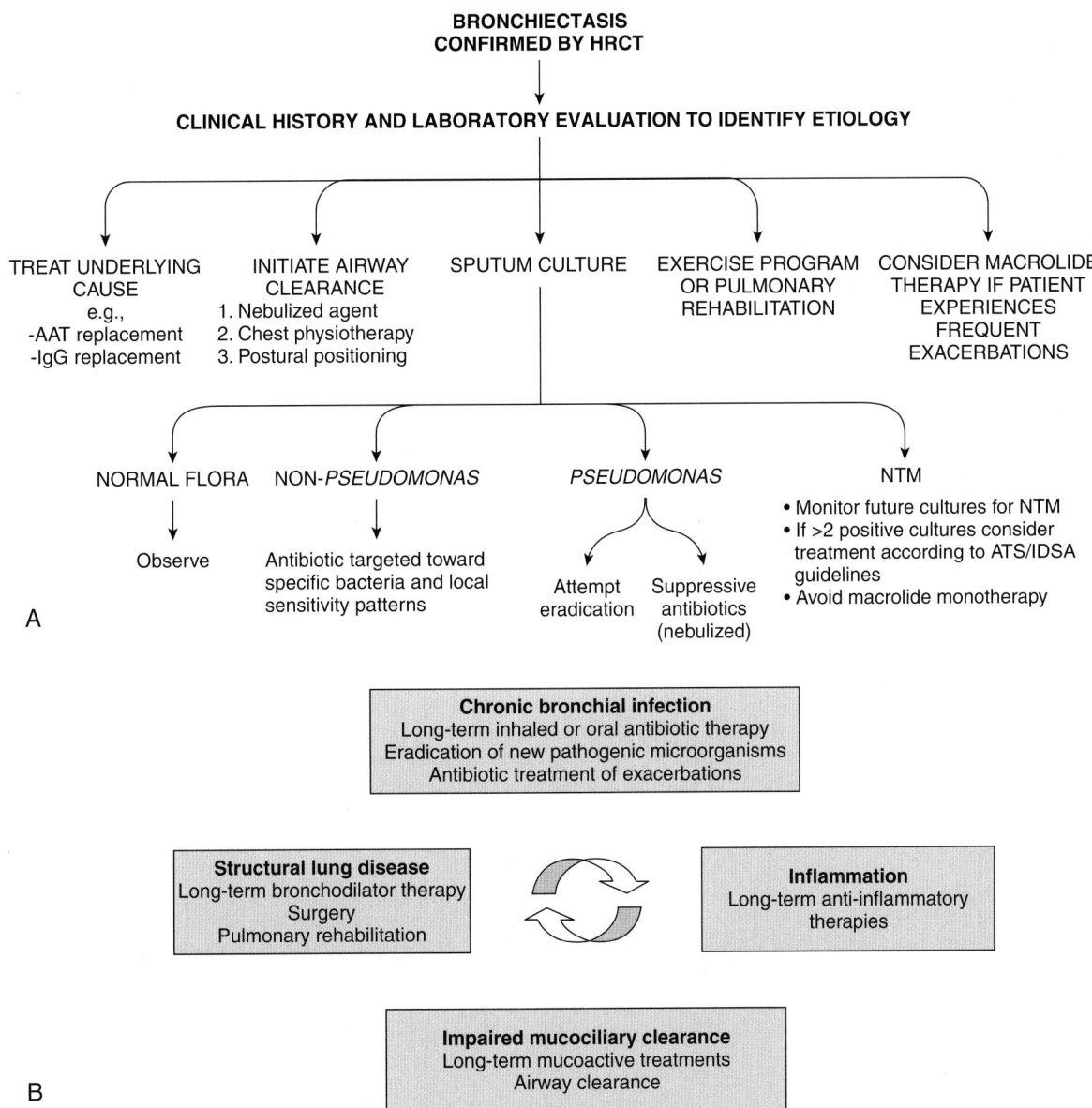

Figure 69.7 Comprehensive management of bronchiectasis. (A) Treatment includes measures that are common to all types and underlying causes of bronchiectasis, such as airway clearance, sputum microbial analysis, and pulmonary rehabilitation. More specific treatments are tailored to the underlying cause, such as *alpha$_1$-antitrypsin* (AAT) augmentation therapy for those with frank AAT deficiency or cystic fibrosis transmembrane regulator modifiers for those with cystic fibrosis. Antimicrobial therapy is based on whether it is for acute treatment or chronic suppressive therapy, and whether the goals are eradication or reducing the bacterial load to limit the symptoms. (B) Treatment strategies shown in the context of the vicious cycle hypothesis of bronchiectasis pathogenesis. ATS, American Thoracic Society; HRCT, high-resolution computed tomography; IDSA, Infectious Diseases Society of America; IgG, immunoglobulin G; NTM, nontuberulous mycobacteria. (A, Modified from McShane PJ, Naureckas ET, Tino G, Strek ME. Non-cystic fibrosis bronchiectasis. *Am J Respir Crit Care Med.* 2013;188(6):647–656; B, modified from Polverino E, Goeminne PC, McDonnell MJ, et al. European Respiratory Society guidelines for the management of adult bronchiectasis. *Eur Respir J.* 2017;50:1700629.)

Key Points

- Bronchiectasis is defined by the presence of permanent dilation of the medium to large bronchi. The main clinical significance of bronchiectasis is recurrent airway infections by bacterial and fungal organisms, resulting in chronic cough, sputum, weight loss, and respiratory compromise.

- Most bronchiectasis is due to a combination of host susceptibility factors, which may be overt or covert, recurrent infections, and the largely neutrophilic, inflammatory response. These factors lead to a vicious cycle of airway inflammation, infection, and mucus obstruction that may result in end-stage lung disease.

- Localized bronchiectasis is most often due to suboptimally treated bacterial infections, although bronchiectasis due to nontuberculous mycobacteria appears increasingly prevalent. Bronchiectasis due to nontuberculous mycobacteria is typically seen in postmenopausal women with lingular and right middle lobe involvement, although other lobes may be affected, and can also be seen in men, especially those with underlying COPD.

- Diffuse bronchiectasis is generally due to an underlying host disorder, such as cystic fibrosis, disorders of immunity, alpha$_1$-antitrypsin anomalies, COPD, primary ciliary dyskinesia, Mounier-Kuhn and Williams-Campbell syndromes, common variable immune deficiency, allergic bronchopulmonary aspergillosis, and chronic inflammatory states.

- Bronchiectasis has been associated with extrapulmonary disorders, such as ulcerative colitis and collagen vascular diseases. Severe fibrotic lung diseases from any cause may also result in a form of bronchiectasis known as traction bronchiectasis.

- The keys to management of bronchiectasis are the timely institution of empirical antimicrobials to treat the most likely pathogens and diligent airway clearance measures to improve symptoms. For patients unresponsive to empirical antibiotics or those with frequent exacerbations, sputum cultures should be obtained, drug susceptibility determined, and treatment tailored to more objective data. Surgical lung resection should also be considered for patients with severe localized disease recalcitrant to medical treatment; bilateral lung transplantation may be necessary for diffuse disease in appropriate patients.

- New approaches to the treatment of initial and chronic *Pseudomonas aeruginosa* infection are important in the consideration of infectious management.

- Prognostic guidelines and understandings of disease severity, including the frequent exacerbator phenotype, have helped to guide new research endeavors targeting appropriate populations.

- Strategies aimed at the vicious cycle of inflammation and infection show promise for improving quality of life and reduction of exacerbations. Anti-inflammatory agents, such as nonsteroidal anti-inflammatory drugs, inhaled corticosteroids, and low-dose intermittent macrolides, show promise in alleviating symptoms and reducing the rate of disease progression, but definitive recommendations for their use remain to be defined. Recent guidelines integrate these therapies for the treatment of patients with frequent exacerbations.

Key Readings

Chalmers JD, Aliberti S, Filonenko A, et al. Characterization of the "frequent exacerbator phenotype" in bronchiectasis. *Am J Respir Crit Care Med.* 2018;197(11):1410–1420.

Chalmers JD, Anne B, Chang AB, Chotirmall SH, et al. Bronchiectasis. *Nat Rev Dis Primer.* 2018;4(1):45.

Chalmers JD, Goeminne P, Aliberti S, et al. The bronchiectasis severity index. An international derivation and validation study. *Am J Respir Crit Care Med.* 2014;189(5):576–585.

Chang-Macchiu P, Traversi L, Polverino E. Bronchiectasis phenotypes. *Curr Opin Pulm Med.* 2019;25(3):281–288.

Hill AT, Sullivan AL, Chalmers JD, et al. British Thoracic Society guideline for bronchiectasis in adults. *Thorax.* 2019;74(suppl 1):1–69.

Polverino E, Goeminne PC, McDonnell MJ, et al. European Respiratory Society guidelines for the management of adult bronchiectasis. *Eur Respir J.* 2017;50:1700629.

Shapiro AJ, Davis SD, Polineni D, et al. American Thoracic Society Assembly on Pediatrics. Diagnosis of primary ciliary dyskinesia. An official American Thoracic Society clinical practice guideline. *Am J Respir Crit Care Med.* 2018;197:e24–e39.

Complete reference list available at ExpertConsult.com.

70 UPPER AIRWAY DISORDERS

CLARK A. ROSEN, MD • STEVEN D. PLETCHER, MD

INTRODUCTION

The upper airways extend from the nares to the subglottis and include diverse anatomic structures with a wide variety of functions. Along with assisting in breathing, the structures of the upper airway contain the nerves for the sensory functions of taste and smell, create a functionally safe swallow by separating the process of swallowing from that of breathing, and allow communication through the generation of voice and speech. The nasal cavity has a defined role in filtering and humidifying air for presentation to the lower airway.[1–3] The larynx protects the airway to prevent aspiration and regulates airflow and vocalization. The pharynx and oral cavity assist in these functions by controlling and shaping substances to be swallowed and modulating voiced sounds from the larynx into words and speech. The upper airway is controlled by both voluntary and involuntary mechanisms. Therefore, respiratory function can be affected through uncoordinated or inefficient muscular activity, centrally mediated neurologic reflex activity, and/or humoral or immunologic responses. The exact function of some areas within the upper airway, such as the paranasal sinuses, is unclear.

Pathologic changes in the upper airways are often associated with lower airway disease. Swallowing disorders may result in aspiration, leading to inflammatory and infectious complications in the lungs. Chronic inflammation of the paranasal sinuses is frequently associated with asthma and appears to be driven by similar inflammatory pathways, which has been called the *unified airway theory*.[4–7] This theory posits that the upper and lower airways can be considered one organ, sharing both the mechanisms of injury and the benefits from treatment. Long-standing infection in the sinuses has been implicated as a possible reservoir for recurrent pulmonary infection.[8–10] Laryngeal dysfunction may create symptoms similar to, and mistaken for, asthma. Finally, stenosis of the subglottis or cervical trachea is often misdiagnosed as asthma. This chapter discusses the anatomy and clinical conditions of the upper airway and their influence on lower airway function.

THE NOSE

ANATOMY, HISTOLOGY, AND PHYSIOLOGY

The nose is the initial site of air entry for the majority of breaths. The external nose has important structural components that, when compromised, may inhibit nasal airflow. The nasal dorsum is made up of three structurally distinct subunits (Fig. 70.1). The upper third of the nasal dorsum is supported by the nasal bones. At their distal end, the nasal bones articulate with the upper lateral cartilages in a region known as the keystone area. The upper lateral cartilages define the middle third of the nose. The structure of the lower third, or nasal tip, is defined primarily by the lower lateral cartilages. The nasal septum divides the right and left sides of the nose and provides additional structural support to the lower two-thirds of the nose. The quadrangular cartilage forms the anterior septum. The bone of the vomer, the perpendicular plate of the ethmoid, and the maxillary crest form the posterior and inferior aspects of the septum.

Airflow through the nose may be limited by the cross-sectional area of the external and internal nasal valves (Fig. 70.2). The external nasal valve area is determined by the relationship between the lower lateral cartilage, the septum, and the inferior turbinate. The internal nasal valve is determined by the angle between the upper lateral cartilage and septum. Facial musculature attaching to the upper and lower cartilages of the nose can widen these principal areas of resistance and enhance nasal breathing.[11,12] Patients with narrowing or structural weakness in these regions may suffer from nasal obstruction. The external and internal nasal valves are frequently the target of nasoseptal reconstructive surgery.

Another common area implicated in narrowing of the nasal cavity and subsequent nasal obstruction is the nasal

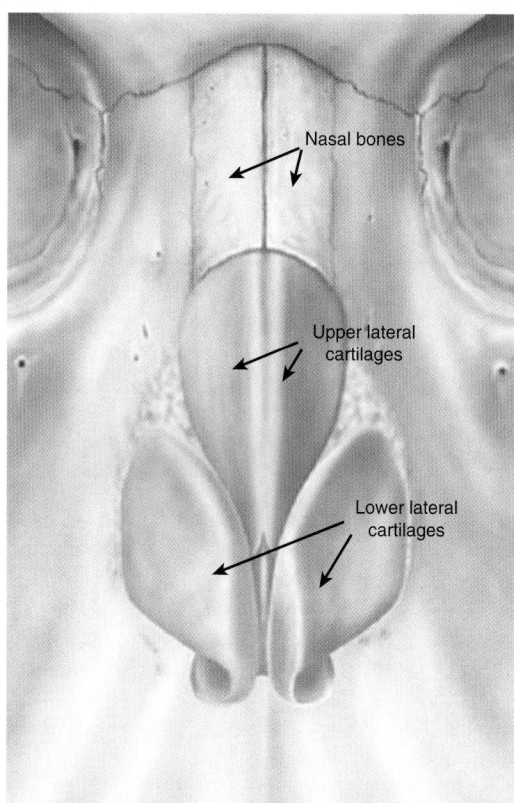

Figure 70.1 Vertical thirds of the nose. The upper, middle, and lower third of the nose are structurally supported by the nasal bones, the upper lateral cartilages, and the lower lateral cartilages, respectively. (From Hafezi F, Naghibzadeh B, Nouhi AH. Applied anatomy of the nasal lower lateral cartilage: a new finding. *Aesthetic Plast Surg.* 2010;342:244–248.)

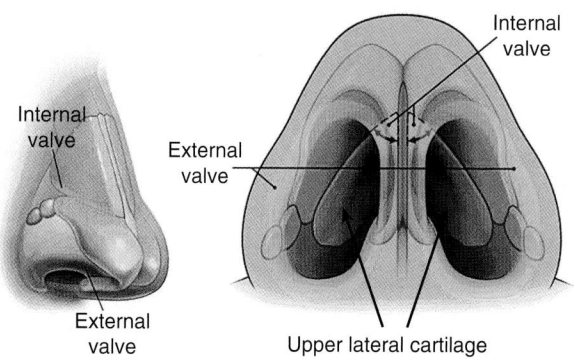

Figure 70.2 The internal and external nasal valves. The external nasal valve exists at the level of the inner nostril and is formed by the caudal edge of the lateral crus of the lower lateral cartilage, the soft tissue alae, the membranous septum, and the sill (the anterior nares) of the nostril. The internal nasal valve accounts for approximately half of the total airway resistance and is bordered medially by the septum, inferiorly by the nasal floor, laterally by the inferior turbinate, and superiorly by the caudal border of the upper lateral cartilage. (From Howard BK, Rohrich RJ. Understanding the nasal airway: principles and practice. *Plast Reconstr Surg.* 2002;109:1128–1146.)

septum. Deviation of the septum diminishes the cross-sectional area of the affected nasal passage and can significantly impact nasal airflow. Most patients have some degree of septal deviation, so anatomic changes in this area must be correlated with clinical findings when determining if a patient would benefit from treatment of a septal deviation. Nasal trauma may lead to septal deviations and

spurs; many patients will relate a history of trauma to the nose. Developmental variations are perhaps a more common cause of deviation and of spurs of the nasal septum than is trauma. Overgrowth of the quadrangular cartilage may result in bowing of the cartilage or in forming spurs at the junction of the cartilage and bones that make up the nasal septum. Nasal obstruction related to septal deviation may respond either to surgical or to medical treatment. In patients with concomitant turbinate hypertrophy or chronic rhinitis, treatment with intranasal corticosteroids may diminish mucosal swelling and provide an adequate airway despite the septal deviation. Surgery to straighten the septum has few risks and complications and is an effective method for improving the nasal airway in patients with narrowing secondary to septal deviation. Although implicated as a cause for acute or chronic rhinosinusitis, septal deviation is a very rare cause for inflammatory sinus disease. While a septoplasty may be indicated to improve nasal breathing or enhance surgical access for endoscopic sinus surgery, in the majority of cases, surgical correction of the septal deviation is unlikely to influence the disease course of acute or chronic rhinosinusitis.

Air that enters the nasal sill (or anterior nares) and passes through the internal nasal valve accelerates as it passes through this area of narrowing. There is also a change in direction of airflow because inspired air shifts from a vertical to a horizontal trajectory at this site. This combination of acceleration and change in flow vector causes the majority of airborne particles to be deposited in the anterior nasal cavity.[13,14] Airflow through the nose slows as the nasal passages widen beyond the internal nasal valve.

Upon entry into the nasal cavity the stratified squamous epithelium of the nasal sill quickly transitions to a respiratory epithelium. Located along the lateral nasal wall, the turbinates (or conchae) serve to warm and humidify air passing through the nasal cavity. Rich vasculature, including venous sinusoids, allows the turbinates to enlarge and shrink in response to various stimuli.[15–17] Fenestrated subepithelial capillaries facilitate heat and gas exchange, enhancing humidification during nasal inhalation.[17] Engorgement of the turbinates increases the surface area and mucosal contact with inspired air. The slowing of airflow beyond the internal nasal valve provides prolonged mucosal contact during nasal inspiration and allows efficient humidification and filtration of inspired air so that, even at extremes of ambient temperature and humidity, air that reaches the trachea is very close to body temperature and is at 98% humidity.

The respiratory mucosa of the turbinates contains both goblet cells and seromucous glands. These structures combine to produce a mucus blanket mobilized by coordinated beating of this ciliated epithelium. Nasal irritants, microbes, and other particles are swept through the nasal cavity by this mucociliary clearance mechanism to be swallowed, preventing exposure of the lower airways. The lower airways are further protected by immune function within the nasal mucosa. Both the innate and humoral immune arms of the immune system function within the nasal mucosa, resulting in the secretion of immunoglobulins (primarily immunoglobulin A)[18,19] and microbial toxins, such as lysozyme and lactoferrin.[20,21] Emerging evidence suggests that commensal microbes inhabiting the mucosal surface or mucus layer of the nasal cavity contribute to the host defense mechanisms within the nasal cavity through competitive colonization and immune regulation.[22,23]

The turbinates are dynamic structures that swell and shrink in response to multiple stimuli. Gravity, nasal irritants, allergic response, and autonomic neural input all regulate the blood supply and venous drainage of the submucosal tissue of the inferior turbinate, resulting in marked fluctuations in turbinate size.[17,24] The size of the inferior turbinate fluctuates throughout the day, with the left and right sides alternately swelling and shrinking in a phenomenon known as the nasal cycle.[24] Pathologic enlargement of the inferior turbinate is one of the most common causes of nasal congestion and nasal obstruction.[25,26]

The tubular structure of the turbinates contributes to a laminar airflow pattern through the nasal cavity.[27,28] Aggressive resection of the turbinates enlarges the cross-sectional area of the nasal cavity but risks paradoxical worsening of nasal obstruction by altering the flow pattern from laminar to turbulent. The humidification function of the turbinates can also be lost with resection, resulting in possible dryness and crusting. This constellation of symptoms after turbinate resection has been referred to as *empty nose syndrome*.[29] A conservative surgical approach to nasal obstruction with turbinate hypertrophy is therefore recommended in patients who do not receive adequate relief from medical therapy.

The superior aspects of the nasal septum, middle turbinate, and superior turbinate are lined with olfactory epithelium. Successful olfaction requires that airborne or mucus-soluble particles reach this epithelium. Odorant-specific receptors of the olfactory epithelium send projections intracranially through the bone of the cribriform plate. Axons from the olfactory epithelium synapse within the olfactory bulb, and these signals are then routed for central processing. Smell disorders may arise from mucosal inflammation and edema that prevent odorant exposure to the olfactory epithelium. This is frequently a reversible condition. Direct viral injury of the olfactory epithelium has also been postulated as a cause for smell loss, which may result in long-term dysfunction.[30,31] Acute smell loss has been identified as a key screening symptom for COVID-19 disease.[32–34] In a prospective tracking study of more than 2.5 million individuals in the United Kingdom and United States, including more than 18,000 who underwent polymerase chain reaction testing for severe acute respiratory syndrome coronavirus-2 infection, loss of smell was the symptom most strongly associated with a positive COVID-19 test, with an odds ratio of 6.4 in the UK cohort and 10.0 in the U.S. cohort. The odds ratio for skipped meals, fatigue, and fever were all less than 3 in both cohorts.[32]

Sneezing is a nonspecific, involuntary response to nasal irritation. Allergens, microbes, and other nasal irritants may precipitate this reaction when they contact the nasal mucosa and trigger histamine release. The trigeminal nucleus coordinates the sneeze reflex, which involves muscles of the pharynx, larynx, oral cavity, and chest wall. The pressure generated from a sneeze may expel irritants and can contribute to spread of infections. In susceptible individuals, sudden exposure to bright light may trigger the sneeze reflex. This photic sneeze reflex is an autosomal dominant trait impacting approximately one-fourth of the human population.[35]

PATHOLOGIC CONDITIONS OF THE NASAL CAVITY

Rhinitis

Rhinitis, or inflammation of the nasal cavity, may result from multiple causes. Rhinitis may be classified by duration (acute vs. chronic) and by cause (allergic vs. nonallergic). Acute rhinitis is a self-limited inflammation, most commonly secondary to viral infection. Many of the clinical features of acute rhinitis may result from the immune response to viral pathogens. Release of inflammatory cytokines and chemokines, including *interleukin* (IL)-6, tumor necrosis factor-α, and interferon-γ, results in tissue edema, increased mucus production, and vascular dilation.[36] The clinical manifestations of these changes are well known as symptoms of the common cold: nasal congestion and obstruction, increased nasal drainage, and diminished sense of smell. Nasal irritants, including perfumes, smoke, and cleaning products, can cause a similar constellation of symptoms, although typically of shorter duration.

Allergic Rhinitis

Epidemiology. *Allergic rhinitis* (AR) is a common disorder estimated to be the sixth most common chronic illness in the United States.[37] The prevalence of AR is 10–20% in the United States and Europe.[38] An estimated 18 million adults in the United States suffer from AR, resulting in significant health care expenditures.[39] A diagnosis of allergic rhinitis adds approximately $1500 per patient per year in direct health care costs.[39] A similar prevalence of AR is evident in children, and AR in this population is associated with a significant decrease in both physical and emotional health, as well as sleep disturbance.[40] Thirteen million Americans in the workforce suffer from AR, and it is estimated that 3.5 million workdays and 2 million school days are lost each year due to this condition.[41,42] Overall, annual direct and indirect costs of AR in the United States have been estimated at $5 to $8 billion and $11 billion, respectively.[43]

The incidence of allergic rhinitis has been rising over the past 3 decades. One explanation for this is the *hygiene hypothesis*, which proposes that early exposure to antigens allows for proper immune system development and a reduced risk for AR and other atopic disease.[44] With improved hygiene and a reduction in exposure to antigens, children may develop an exaggerated immune response, as demonstrated by AR. Early microbial exposure may be particularly important in the prevention not only of atopic but also of autoimmune disease.[45–48]

Diagnosis. AR symptoms may be seasonal or perennial, depending upon the specific allergen. Pollens from trees and grasses are the most common triggers for seasonal symptoms, whereas dust mites and pet dander represent common triggers for perennial disease. Offending allergens may be identified through a variety of approaches. Skin reaction to allergens may be measured through either prick testing or intradermal injection using serial end point dilution techniques. Both approaches carry a rare but important risk for anaphylaxis.[49] Testing centers must have personnel and equipment to deal with such emergencies. Immunoassays for allergen-specific *immunoglobulin* (Ig) E, such as ImmunoCAP (Phadia AB/ThermoFisher), have largely replaced radioallergosorbent tests as an alternative to intradermal skin testing. Immunoassays demonstrate a similar sensitivity as skin testing. The efficacy of both dermal testing and immunoassays depends on proper antigen selection. Knowledge of local flora is particularly important in patients with seasonal AR. This knowledge is also essential in identifying clinically significant allergens. Identification of offending allergens allows counseling of allergen avoidance and may be used to initiate immunomodulatory therapy.

Pathophysiology. After an initial allergen exposure, inhaled antigens provoke both early and late-phase reactions in the nasal cavity. The early phase is initiated by the recognition of a specific allergen by IgE subunits on the surface of mast cells and basophils. IgE activation results in antibody cross-linking, which, through a series of downstream mediators, causes degranulation of mast cells and basophils with release of preformed mediators, primarily histamine. Tryptase release and de novo formation of leukotrienes may also contribute to nasal inflammation and symptoms. Exposure to inflammatory mediators results in marked tissue edema and mucus secretion, which manifest clinically as rhinorrhea, nasal congestion, and obstruction, frequently in association with sneezing. These symptoms develop within minutes of allergen exposure.

The late phase of AR typically arises 4 to 8 hours after allergen exposure. Nasal congestion is typically the dominant symptom. Chemoattractants and adhesion molecules released in response to the initial inflammatory mediators promote infiltration of leukocytes, eosinophils, basophils, CD4+ lymphocytes, and monocytes. Activation of these cells results in the release of a second wave of inflammatory mediators.[50] The early and late-phase reactions in AR mimic those of allergic asthma.

Priming of the immune response may be important in the pathophysiology of AR. Repeated allergen exposure results in amplification of mucosal hyperresponsiveness. In patients with seasonal AR, the severity of allergic response depends not only on the current pollen count and allergen exposure but also upon the cumulative exposure for a given allergy season. Because of this phenomenon, severe symptoms of AR may persist late in the allergy season despite a waning pollen count. This increased allergen sensitivity may be secondary to both a neural hyperresponsiveness and amplification of the immune response through recruitment of mast cells and basophils. Immune system priming is not an allergen-specific phenomenon; patients also report increased sensitivity to nonspecific nasal irritants, including smoke and perfume.[51,52]

Association With Asthma. AR and asthma are linked through both pathophysiology and epidemiology.[50,52,53] Eighty percent of patients with allergic asthma also suffer from AR. The presence of AR is a risk factor for the future development of asthma. Guidelines suggest screening patients with persistent AR for asthma and evaluating asthmatic patients for rhinitis.[52,53]

The *unified airway theory* suggests that inflammatory cells from an inflamed area within the airway may impact distant airway locations. In patients with AR and asthma, segmental bronchial allergen challenge results in an inflammatory response not only in bronchi, but also in the nasal cavity.[54] When treated with intranasal corticosteroids, these same patients demonstrate a decrease in both nasal and bronchial hyperreactivity.[55,56]

Treatment. There are three primary modalities of treatment for AR: allergen avoidance, pharmacotherapy, and immunomodulatory treatments. Consensus panels suggest evaluating the severity and frequency of AR symptoms to guide treatment. Severity of symptoms is categorized as mild or moderate to severe as determined by the level of impact on daily activities and sleep disturbance. Symptoms are classified as *intermittent* if the duration is less than 4 days per week or for fewer than 4 weeks or as *persistent* if the duration satisfies both of these criteria.[53] Fig. 70.3 depicts a consensus management strategy for AR.[57] The vast majority of patients are effectively treated with pharmacotherapy and allergen avoidance. Saline irrigation results in modest symptomatic improvement and may reduce the need for medications with more significant side-effect profiles. Evidence-based AR treatment recommendations for allergen avoidance, individual medications, and immunotherapy were revised in 2010[58] and again in 2017[59] to incorporate considerations for combination pharmacotherapy options. Recommendations for allergen avoidance strategies for patients with AR are similar to those for patients with allergic asthma and require identification of offending allergens. After identification of clinically significant allergens, environmental precautions may be instituted.

Immunotherapy

Although pharmacologic treatment of AR may be quite effective in managing symptoms, immunotherapy offers the only approach known to impact the natural history of the disease. *Subcutaneous immunotherapy* (SCIT) regimens involve once- or twice-weekly subcutaneous antigen injections with gradual escalation of the antigen dose. This is the most well-studied and commonly used approach in the United States. More recently, *sublingual immunotherapy* (SLIT) has emerged as an option that avoids injection and may be administered at home. The *U.S. Food and Drug Administration* (FDA) has approved four SLIT treatments in the United States: Grastek (ALK-Abelló) for treatment of timothy grass or cross-reactive grass pollens, Oralair (Stallergenes SA) for treatment of five different grass pollens, Odactra (ALK-Abelló) for dust mites, and Ragwitek (ALK-Abelló) for short ragweed pollen.[60] Additional SLIT allergen extracts are approved in Europe and have been used off-label in the United States. The overall treatment course for SCIT or SLIT is 2 to 3 years.

With repeated allergen exposure, a shift in allergen-specific T cells to a regulatory phenotype results in suppression of type 2 T-helper inflammatory cytokines and enhanced production of IL-10 and antigen-specific IgG4. This results in suppression of allergen-specific IgE and mast cells and appears to inhibit antigen capture and presentation to T cells.[61] This immune modulation may also

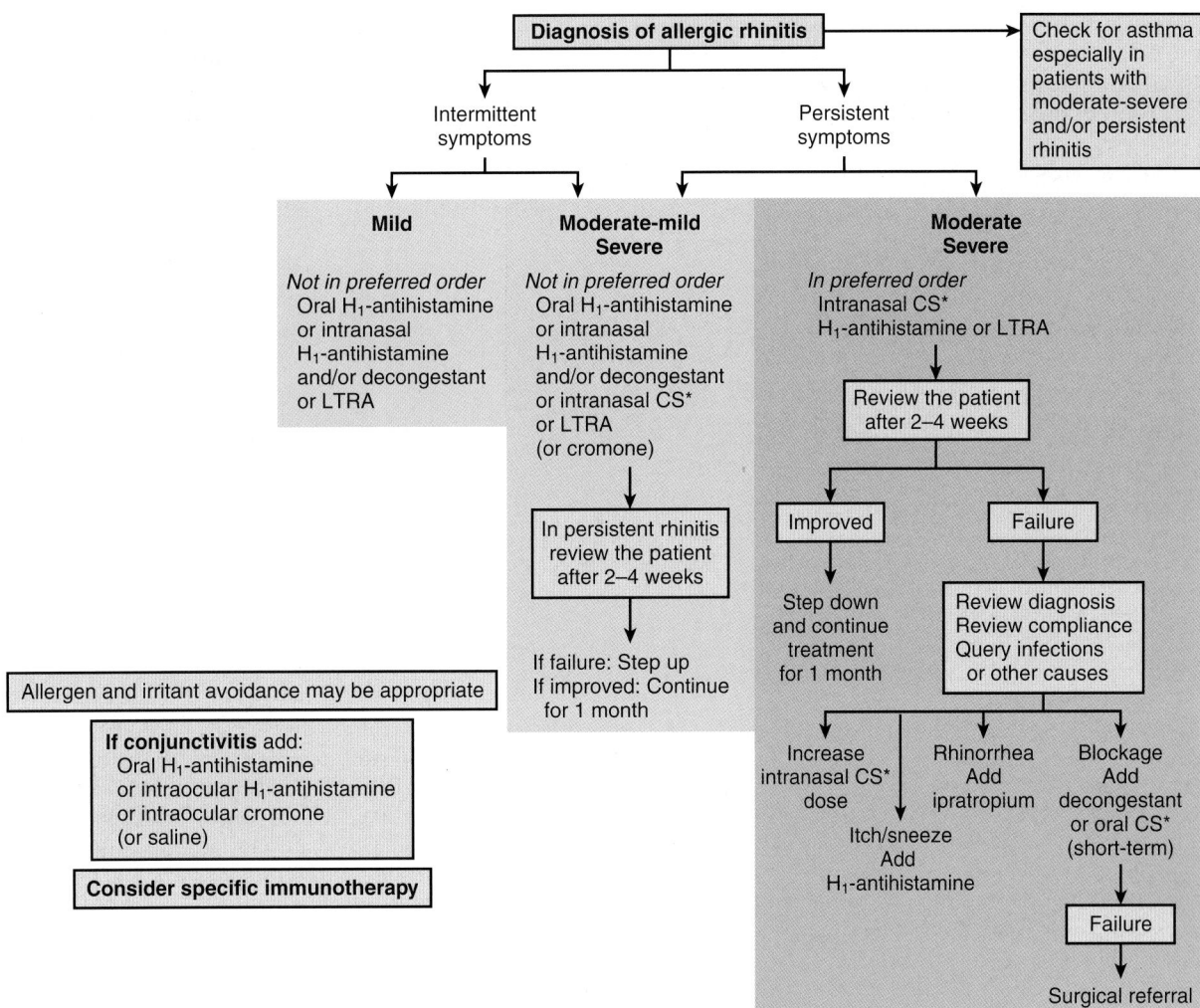

Figure 70.3 Algorithm for the management of allergic rhinitis. CS, corticosteroid; LTRA, leukotriene-receptor antagonist. *Total dose of topical CS should be considered if inhaled steroids are used for concomitant asthma. (From Bousquet J, Schünemann HJ, Samolinski B, et al. Allergic rhinitis and its impact on asthma (ARIA): achievements in 10 years and future needs. *J Allergy Clin Immunol.* 2012;130:1049–1062.)

diminish the onset of additional atopic disorders, such as asthma in patients with AR.

Systemic responses to immunotherapy are rare and typically mild. Nevertheless, deaths have been reported from anaphylactic response during immunotherapy, and vigilance is required. SCIT has a higher, although still very low, incidence of systemic response than SLIT; SLIT has a high rate of mild local (mucosal) side effects that rarely impact the treatment regimen.[62] Practitioners who administer allergy shots require appropriate training and access to emergency equipment to address the rare systemic response. With sublingual administration, patients often self-administer the allergen, and proper patient selection and education are critically important. Multiple trials demonstrate efficacy of both SCIT and SLIT; they appear to have similar efficacy, but head-to-head trials are lacking.[63–65] The determinants of SCIT versus SLIT use are evolving as additional sublingual options receive FDA approval and clinical experience in the United States increases.[66]

Nonallergic Chronic Rhinitis

Overall, nonallergic rhinitis is poorly characterized. *Vasomotor rhinitis* may happen in a subgroup of nonallergic patients thought to have aberrant parasympathetic innervation in the nose. Patients frequently note rhinorrhea in association with eating or a change in the weather. This disorder is more common in elderly patients and may respond well to ipratropium nasal spray. Additional noninflammatory disorders of the nasal cavity, including nonallergic rhinitis with eosinophilia, may improve with nasal steroid treatment. Symptomatic treatment with saline irrigation is another popular treatment for nonallergic rhinitis.

THE PARANASAL SINUSES

ANATOMY, HISTOLOGY, AND PHYSIOLOGY

The paranasal sinuses are aerated cavities within the skull that connect to the nasal cavity. There are four sets of paired sinuses: the maxillary, ethmoid, frontal, and sphenoid. The sinuses are lined with a pseudostratified, ciliated epithelium. Goblet cells within the epithelium produce mucus, and the coordinated action of the cilia moves this mucus through the sinus cavities and into the nose. Once thought to be sterile, it is now known that bacterial communities inhabit the

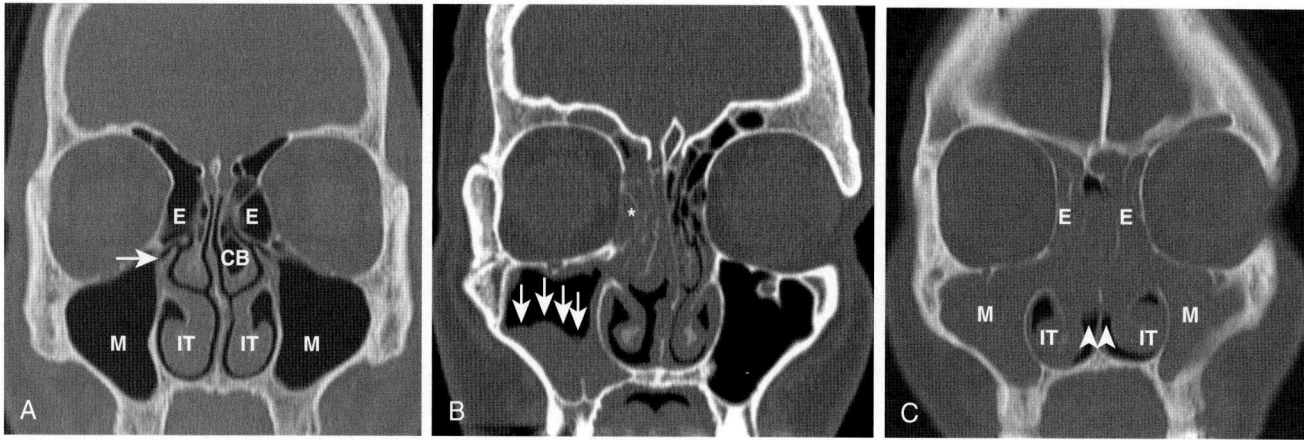

Figure 70.4 Coronal *computed tomography* (CT) imaging of the paranasal sinuses. (A) Normal anatomy, including well-aerated maxillary (M) and ethmoid (E) sinuses bilaterally, patency of the osteomeatal complex (*arrow*), and normal appearance of the inferior turbinates (IT). Incidentally noted is a left concha bullosa (CB), a normal variant involving aeration of the middle turbinate, which arises in approximately 30% of patients. (B) CT findings consistent with acute sinusitis. There is unilateral opacification of the ethmoid sinuses (*asterisk*) and a fluid level within the right maxillary sinus (*arrows*). Acute sinusitis may present with unilateral or bilateral disease, and routine CT imaging is not recommended. (C) Bilateral chronic sinusitis with nasal polyposis. There is complete opacification of the maxillary (M) and ethmoid (E) sinuses bilaterally. *Arrowheads* demonstrate bilateral nasal polyps, a soft tissue density within the nasal cavity and adjacent to the inferior turbinates (IT).

mucosal surfaces of the paranasal sinuses in both health and disease.[22,67,68]

The function of the sinuses has not been clearly established. They may serve a protective role in force dissipation with blunt trauma to the head or face. The paranasal sinuses can impact vocal resonance, which may have aided their evolution. The sinuses may allow for enhanced facial aesthetics. They may play a role in mucus production and immune surveillance in the nasal cavity.

The four paired sinuses are named after the bones they aerate. The maxillary and ethmoid sinuses are the first to develop and are present at birth. The frontal and sphenoid sinuses develop later. A visible frontal sinus is often not present until age 4 or 5 years, and continued aeration and development persist throughout the teenage years.[69] Asymmetric aeration of the sinuses is common, particularly in the later-developing frontal and sphenoid sinuses. The frontal sinus may be absent in up to 10% of normal patients.[70,71] An increased incidence of frontal sinus aplasia and diminished overall paranasal sinus aeration is seen in patients with congenital disorders that impact the sinuses, such as cystic fibrosis.[72]

Mucus produced in the sinuses is propelled into the nasal cavity by coordinated ciliary motion. The maxillary (Fig. 70.4) and sphenoid sinuses are connected to the nasal cavity by discrete ostia, which often have a diameter of no more than 4 mm. The ethmoid sinuses are made up of a labyrinth of small air cells located between the orbit and the nasal septum. The ethmoid sinus typically drains through clefts between air cells rather than through discrete ostia. Collectively, the anterior ethmoid air cells drain through the middle *meatus* located between the middle turbinate and the lateral nasal wall. Whereas the posterior ethmoid air cells drain through the superior meatus, which is located between the superior turbinate and lateral nasal wall, the frontal sinus drainage tract is determined by the variable anatomy of the underlying anterior ethmoid air cells and eventually leads to the middle meatus.

Blood supply to the paranasal sinuses is provided through both the internal and external carotid systems. The *sphenopalatine artery* (SPA) is the terminal branch of the internal maxillary artery, which originates from the external carotid artery. The SPA enters the nasal cavity through the sphenopalatine foramen just behind the posterior wall of the maxillary sinus. The majority of the blood supply to the nasal cavity is provided by the SPA. The blood supply to the superior nasal cavity and to much of the ethmoid system arises from the anterior and posterior ethmoid arteries. These vessels are branches from the ophthalmic artery of the internal carotid system and typically run within the skull base along the roof of the ethmoid sinuses. All of these vessels may contribute to refractory or "posterior" nosebleeds. Epistaxis originating from the SPA is amenable to embolization or surgical ligation of the SPA. The anterior and posterior ethmoid arteries are not amenable to embolization due to their origin from the ophthalmic artery and the associated risk for blindness. In cases of refractory epistaxis, these vessels are amenable to surgical ligation.[73]

PARANASAL SINUS DISEASE

Overall, inflammatory disease of the paranasal sinuses is poorly understood. Sinusitis represents a wide variety of pathologic conditions that may cause either acute or chronic inflammation. Paranasal sinus inflammation is almost inevitably accompanied by inflammation of the nasal cavity, or rhinitis. Thus, the term *rhinosinusitis* is commonly used to describe this condition.

Although the diagnosis of acute rhinosinusitis may be made with clinical symptoms and time course alone, objective evidence of sinus inflammation is required for a diagnosis of chronic rhinosinusitis.[74–76] Table 70.1 demonstrates the diagnostic criteria for acute, chronic, and recurrent acute rhinosinusitis. The duration of symptoms is the primary factor used to differentiate between acute and chronic rhinosinusitis. Acute sinusitis lasts up to 4 weeks. Patients

Table 70.1 Diagnostic Criteria for Rhinosinusitis

Term	Definition
ACUTE	
Acute rhinosinusitis	Up to 4 weeks of purulent nasal drainage (anterior, posterior, or both) accompanied by nasal obstruction, facial pain-pressure-fullness, or both: ■ *Purulent nasal discharge* is cloudy or colored, in contrast to the clear secretions that typically accompany viral upper respiratory infection and may be reported by the patient or observed on physical examination. ■ *Nasal obstruction* may be reported by the patient as nasal obstruction, congestion, blockage, or stuffiness, or may be diagnosed by physical examination. ■ *Facial pain-pressure-fullness* may involve the anterior face, periorbital region, or manifest with headache that is localized or diffuse.
Viral rhinosinusitis (VRS)	Acute rhinosinusitis caused by, or presumed to be caused by, viral infection. A clinician should diagnose VRS when symptoms or signs of acute rhinosinusitis are present for fewer than 10 days and the symptoms are not worsening.
Acute bacterial rhinosinusitis (ABRS)	Acute rhinosinusitis caused by, or presumed to be caused by, bacterial infection. A clinician should diagnose ABRS when: ■ Symptoms or signs of acute rhinosinusitis are present 10 days or more beyond the onset of upper respiratory symptoms, *or* ■ Symptoms or signs of acute rhinosinusitis worsen within 10 days after an initial improvement (double worsening).
CHRONIC AND RECURRENT	
Chronic rhinosinusitis	Twelve weeks or longer of two or more of the following signs and symptoms: ■ Mucopurulent drainage (anterior, posterior, or both) ■ Nasal obstruction (congestion) ■ Facial pain-pressure-fullness *or* ■ Decreased sense of smell *and* ■ Inflammation is documented by one or more of the following findings: 　■ Purulent (not clear) mucus or edema in the middle meatus or ethmoid region 　■ Polyps in nasal cavity or the middle meatus, *and/or* 　■ Radiographic imaging showing inflammation of the paranasal sinuses.
Recurrent acute rhinosinusitis	Four or more episodes per year of ABRS without signs or symptoms of rhinosinusitis between episodes. Each episode of ABRS should meet diagnostic criteria.

From Rosenfeld RM, Piccirillo JF, Chandrasekhar SS, et al. Clinical practice guideline (update): adult sinusitis. *Otolaryngol Head Neck Surg.* 2015;152(suppl 2):S1–S39; and Rosenfeld RM. Clinical practice guideline on adult sinusitis. *Otolaryngol Head Neck Surg.* 2007;137(3):365–377.

with signs and symptoms for 12 weeks or longer are diagnosed with chronic sinusitis. Patients with symptoms lasting from 4 to 12 weeks are deemed to have subacute sinusitis, and clinical judgment is recommended in determining whether to manage based on acute or chronic rhinosinusitis guidelines. Whereas the duration of symptoms is used to distinguish between acute and chronic disease, the pathophysiologic features, symptoms, and treatment of these entities are different. *Acute bacterial rhinosinusitis* is an acute infectious disorder, and patients present with fever and facial pain as characteristic symptoms. *Chronic rhinosinusitis* (CRS) is primarily an inflammatory disorder in which the role of microbes is not well established. Patients with CRS typically note nasal congestion, thick nasal drainage, and facial pressure, but fever[77] and pain are uncommon in the absence of acute exacerbations.

Objective findings of rhinosinusitis may be present on routine physical examination during evaluation of the anterior nasal cavity or anterior rhinoscopy. Acute rhinosinusitis may be diagnosed by history and anterior rhinoscopy alone; imaging studies are not recommended for uncomplicated acute sinusitis.[74–76,78] Objective evidence of inflammation in patients with chronic sinusitis is often difficult to establish on anterior rhinoscopy, so nasal endoscopy or imaging of the sinuses is often required to establish the diagnosis. With a nasal endoscope, the middle and superior meatus can be closely examined. Polyps or significant edema in these regions satisfies the objective criteria for

inflammation required for a CRS diagnosis. Thick mucus can be sampled under endoscopic guidance to guide antimicrobial therapy. *Computed tomography* (CT) (see Fig. 70.4) is the preferred method of imaging for the paranasal sinuses; radiographs of the paranasal sinuses lack sufficient specificity and sensitivity and have little clinical utility.[78] *Magnetic resonance imaging* (MRI) is not indicated for routine inflammatory sinus disease. MRI, however, is quite useful in the assessment of sinonasal tumors, intracranial complications of sinusitis, and encephaloceles, and in the diagnosis and treatment planning for invasive fungal sinusitis.

ACUTE RHINOSINUSITIS

Epidemiology

Acute rhinosinusitis is extremely common and typically of viral etiology. It is estimated that adults suffer two to five episodes of viral rhinosinusitis (i.e., the common cold) annually. School-age children may suffer 7 to 10 colds per year.[74] In the United States, upper respiratory tract infection is the third most common reason for a primary care provider consultation, with approximately one-third of these attributed to acute rhinosinusitis.[79] Gwaltney and colleagues[80] demonstrated that 60% of viral upper respiratory infections demonstrate radiologic evidence of inflammation within the ethmoid and maxillary sinuses on CT imaging. This study also highlights the futility of CT imaging for distinguishing between acute viral and acute bacterial rhinosinusitis.

From 0.5–2% of viral rhinosinusitis episodes will progress to *acute bacterial rhinosinusitis* (ABRS).[74] The proposed pathophysiology is that virally mediated mucosal inflammation and edema result in ciliary dysfunction and obstruction of the sinus ostia. This disruption of mucociliary clearance results in mucus stasis and a vulnerability to bacterial superinfection. The most common organisms seen in ABRS are noted in Table 70.2.

Treatment

Distinguishing the self-limited, viral-induced inflammation of the common cold from ABRS is a challenge often faced by primary care physicians. Clinical guidelines suggest that a detailed history is somewhat effective in making this distinction. Patients who do not demonstrate significant clinical improvement after 10 days or experience a worsening of symptoms after 5 days of the onset of symptoms, also referred to as double sickening, are more likely to have ABRS.[75,76,78] In addition, facial pain beyond what is expected from a viral upper respiratory infection or evidence of extrasinus extension of infection, such as periorbital edema, may be used to diagnose ABRS. Although patients who meet these clinical criteria demonstrate decreased duration and severity of symptoms when treated with antibiotics, the magnitude of improvement is relatively small.[75] Watchful waiting and antibiotic therapy are both reasonable options for patients with ABRS. A shared decision-making approach with patients is recommended, and updated guidelines provide patient education materials to help with this decision.[76] Patients who opt for watchful waiting should have access to medical professionals so that they may be treated with antibiotics if their symptoms worsen or fail to improve after 1 week. Patients with suspected complications of ABRS should be treated with antibiotics and referred to an otolaryngologist for urgent evaluation. Amoxicillin with or without clavulanate is recommended as a first-line treatment for uncomplicated ABRS, with trimethoprim-sulfamethoxazole encouraged for penicillin-allergic patients.[76,78] Alternatives for penicillin-allergic patients include doxycycline or a respiratory fluoroquinolone.[76,78,81] Diagnostic imaging, including both radiographs and CT images of the sinuses, do not adequately distinguish between ABRS and acute viral rhinosinusitis and are not recommended unless extrasinus spread of infection is suspected.[76,78]

Table 70.2 Microbiology of Acute Bacterial Rhinosinusitis in Adults

Organism	Range of Prevalence (%)
Streptococcus pneumoniae	20–43
Haemophilus influenzae	22–35
Streptococcus spp	3–9
Anaerobes	0–9
Moraxella catarrhalis	2–10
Staphylococcus aureus	0–8
Other	4

Recurrent acute rhinosinusitis, defined as four or more episodes of ABRS per year, may arise in the context of predisposing anatomic variations, exacerbations of CRS, immune compromise, or without identifiable predisposing factors.[75] Surgical intervention with widening of sinus ostia and removal of ethmoid septations may decrease the frequency and severity of symptoms.[82,83] Balloon sinus dilation, either in the clinic or in the operating room, may also be considered for treatment of recurrent acute rhinosinusitis. Whereas ABRS may be diagnosed without objective (endoscopic or CT) findings of inflammation, CT imaging demonstrating inflammation and elucidating patient anatomy is required before traditional endoscopic surgery or balloon sinus dilation for recurrent acute rhinosinusitis.[84] Although uncommon, complications arising from rhinosinusitis are seen more frequently in acute than in chronic rhinosinusitis. Infection may spread to the orbit or intracranial cavity, a complication more common in children.[85,86] Suppurative complications of acute rhinosinusitis frequently arise from infections of odontogenic origin, particularly from the *Streptococcus milleri* group. Urgent evaluation and treatment, often including surgical drainage of affected sinuses and associated abscesses, is required to minimize the risk for visual loss, seizures, meningitis, and even death.

Invasive fungal sinusitis is a life-threatening condition developing in patients with significant immune compromise. Diabetics with poorly controlled blood glucose levels and patients undergoing bone marrow transplantation are at highest risk. The diagnosis is suspected in this patient population with the development of facial pain, swelling, cranial neuropathies, or unexplained fevers. Imaging studies (CT and MRI) (Fig. 70.5) are helpful in raising suspicion for the diagnosis, particularly if there is loss of contrast enhancement on MRI.[87,88] The diagnosis is established by biopsy demonstrating fungal invasion into the sinus tissues. Frozen section of diseased tissue demonstrates good sensitivity and expedites this analysis.[89,90] Cultures may be helpful to guide antifungal treatment; the morphologic features of fungal elements seen on pathologic evaluation may also assist in identifying the offending fungi. Extrasinus invasion is most common with mucormycosis. Treatment involves surgical débridement, systemic antifungal medications and, when possible, reversal of the underlying immune dysfunction. Even with appropriate medical care, mortality for this condition approaches 50%.[91] Aggressive surgical débridement must therefore be considered in the context of the patient's goals of care.

A slowly progressive, indolent form of invasive fungal sinusitis is seen in patients with less severe immune compromise. Solid-organ transplant recipients and patients with chronic corticosteroid use are at risk for this disorder. *Aspergillus* is the most common pathogen. The treatment principles are the same as for patients with acute invasive fungal sinusitis.

CHRONIC RHINOSINUSITIS

Epidemiology

CRS has an uncertain incidence because the diagnosis often requires both subjective symptoms and nasal endoscopy or CT evaluation. Surveys, which rely only on patient symptom reports, suggest that more than 15% of

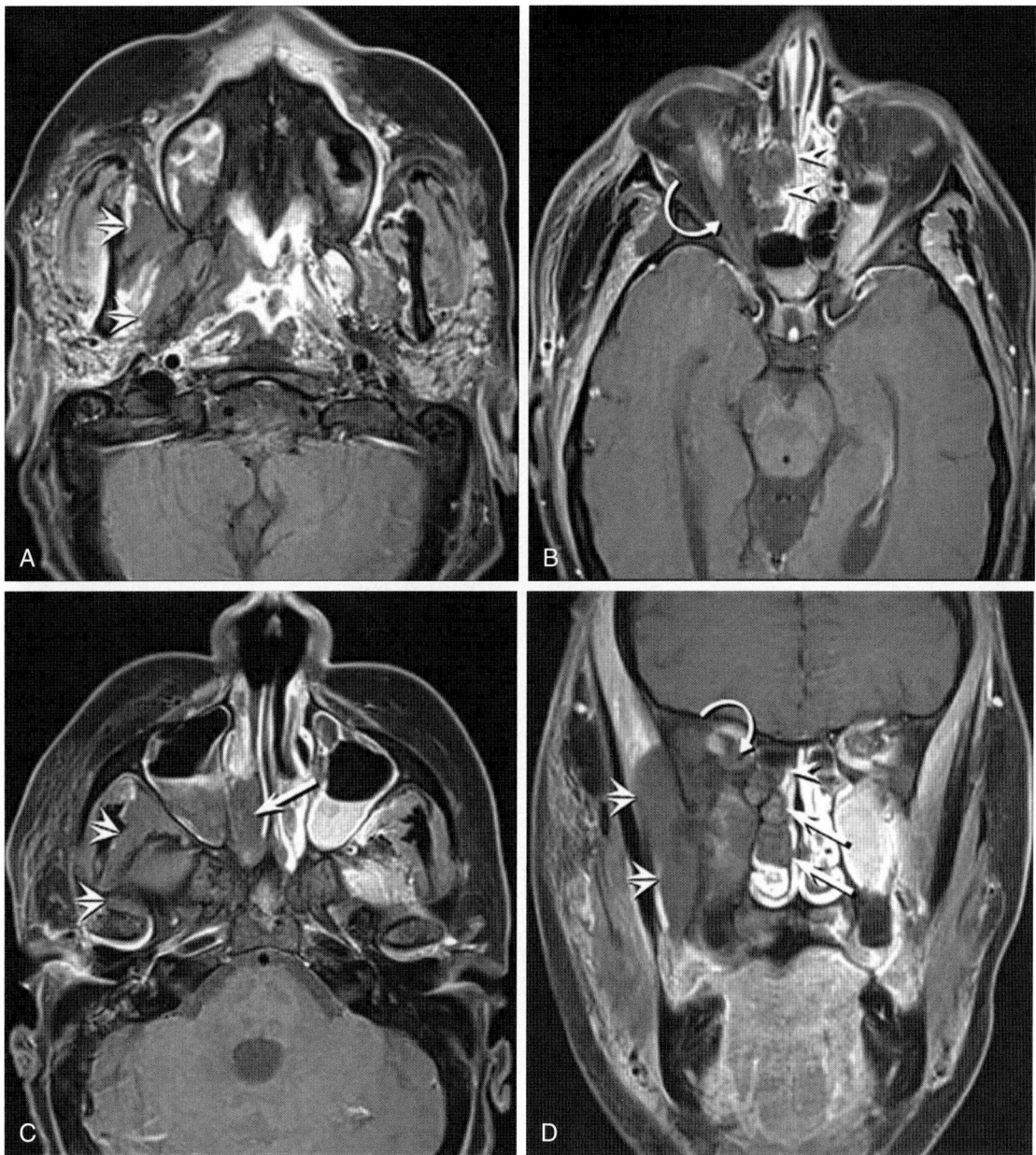

Figure 70.5 Angioinvasive fungal sinusitis. (A–C) Axial and (D) coronal contrast-enhanced fat saturation T1-weighted magnetic resonance images show necrotic tissue with loss of contrast enhancement. The abnormality extends from the right middle/superior turbinates (*arrows*) and posterior right ethmoid region (*arrowheads*) laterally as far as the right infratemporal fossa (*double arrowheads*). Note involvement of the posteroinferior right orbit, particularly the right inferior rectus muscle (*curved arrows*). (Courtesy Joseph M. Hoxworth, MD, Consultant and Associate Professor of Radiology, Department of Radiology, Mayo Clinic College of Medicine.)

the U.S. population suffers from CRS,[92,93] likely a significant overestimation of the true incidence.[74] The prevalence of physician-diagnosed CRS using diagnostic coding reporting in a limited geographic area was closer to 2%.[94] Nonetheless, the impact of CRS on overall quality of life is estimated to be similar to that of COPD and congestive heart failure.[95] In the United States, the overall cost burden for chronic sinusitis is estimated at $8.6 billion per year.[96]

Pathophysiology

CRS is characterized by persistent mucosal inflammation of the paranasal sinuses. The cause of this inflammation is variable and often poorly understood. Numerous theories have been proposed for mechanisms that drive the

inflammation in CRS, including systemic immune dysfunction,[97–99] staphylococcal superantigens,[100] pathologic bacterial biofilms,[101–103] aberrant immune response to fungus,[104] and microbial dysbiosis (e.g., imbalance of the resident microbial population).[22,105–108] Several subtypes of CRS have been well established.

The bacteriology of CRS differs from that of acute sinusitis. *Staphylococcus aureus, Pseudomonas aeruginosa,* and anaerobic bacteria are more commonly cultured from patients with chronic disease than with acute disease. Recent studies using culture-independent bacterial identification demonstrate that healthy sinuses contain diverse bacterial communities, which may serve a protective role in the sinuses. Chronically inflamed sinuses are characterized by a loss of bacterial diversity with overgrowth of a pathologic species[22,105–108] (see also Chapter 17).

Association With Allergy and Asthma

The role of allergy and atopy in CRS is unclear. Studies suggest a higher rate of positive skin tests in patients with CRS[109] but may be confounded by selection bias. Although a causal role for allergy in patients with CRS has not been demonstrated, in atopic patients with CRS, treatment of allergy improves patient outcomes.[110]

CRS with nasal polyps (CRSwNP) demonstrates a more clear association with asthma. Nearly 30–40% of patients with polyps describe wheezing and respiratory discomfort. In addition, 26% of patients with polyps report a diagnosis of asthma compared to 6% of control patients.[111] Patients with asthma also demonstrate a high incidence of sinus mucosal thickening on CT imaging.[112,113] Asthmatic patients also demonstrate a high incidence of nasal polyps; of note, nonatopic asthma is more strongly associated (13%) with nasal polyps than is atopic asthma (5%).[114] As additional evidence of the association of asthma and CRSwNP, asthmatic patients who undergo endoscopic sinus surgery for CRSwNP demonstrate clinical improvement in both upper and lower airway disease.[115–117]

CHRONIC RHINOSINUSITIS WITH NASAL POLYPOSIS

CRS patients are frequently categorized based upon the presence or absence of nasal polyps. A more detailed analysis of the pathophysiology of these patient populations demonstrates that both CRS with and without nasal polyps represents a heterogeneous group of disorders with distinct pathogenic mechanisms. Furthermore, the endotype (i.e., the CRS subtype associated with a pathobiologic mechanism) appears to predict the efficacy of various treatment approaches.[118] Many CRSwNP patients are characterized by type 2 inflammation: inflammatory pathways involving IL-4, IL-5, IL-13, and IgE, which strongly associate with tissue eosinophilia, asthma comorbidity, and severity of sinus disease (see Fig. 70.4C).[119] These patients typically respond well to systemic steroid treatment, which blunts type 2 inflammation, and they are good candidates for biologic therapy targeting IL-4, IL-13, IgE, and IL-5 (see "Treatment" section later).

Conversely, patients with a predominately IL-17–mediated response and neutrophilic inflammation may develop polyps but are generally refractory to corticosteroid treatment.[120] Long-term macrolide therapy has been proposed as an important treatment adjunct for CRSwNP patients with predominately neutrophilic inflammation.[118,121,122]

Although nasal polyps may be visible on anterior rhinoscopy and may even extend to or beyond the nasal vestibule, more frequently nasal endoscopy is required to visualize nasal polyps. Patients typically present with nasal congestion, obstruction, thick nasal drainage, and anosmia. Facial pressure is common. Severe pain, headache, and fever are unusual in the absence of acute exacerbations of chronic disease. Fatigue and difficulty sleeping are also common symptoms.

Patients with asthma and nasal polyps should be queried regarding sensitivity to aspirin and *nonsteroidal anti-inflammatory drugs* (NSAIDs). *Aspirin-exacerbated respiratory disease* (AERD) is found in a subset of CRSwNP patients and is characterized by nasal polyps, asthma, and NSAID sensitivity. Patients with AERD demonstrate abnormalities in arachidonic acid metabolism, characterized by increased production of proinflammatory products of the 5-lipoxygenase pathway after exposure to cyclooxygenase-1 inhibitors, such as aspirin and NSAIDs, which results in shunting through the lipoxygenase pathway and in upper and lower airway inflammation. Patients often develop persistent rhinitis in their late teenage years, with asthma and sinusitis developing over the next several years. Aspirin and NSAID sensitivity may develop at any point along the course of the disease.[123] AERD represents a significant proportion of patients with asthma (9%)[124] and CRSwNP (13%).[114] These patients demonstrate a more refractory clinical course in the treatment of their sinus disease. Aspirin desensitization improves both asthma and sinus disease in this patient population.[125–128]

Patients with unilateral nasal polyps should be evaluated for sinonasal neoplasms with imaging and consideration of biopsy. Before performing a biopsy of a sinonasal mass, the clinician should evaluate the relationship of the mass to the skull base to rule out an encephalocele. Assessment of surrounding vasculature is also critically important because both aneurysms of the carotid artery and juvenile nasal angiofibromas may present as a nasal mass. Biopsy of these entities may lead to severe hemorrhagic complications.

Allergic fungal rhinosinusitis (AFRS) is a distinct category of chronic sinusitis. Unlike the majority of chronic inflammatory sinus disease, AFRS is often unilateral. This diagnosis is established by the presence of nasal polyps, eosinophilic mucus with Charcot-Leyden crystals, and skin or blood testing demonstrating allergy to fungus.[129] The incidence of AFRS is higher in African American patients, and the disorder is more common in humid regions, including the southern United States.[130,131] Bone expansion and erosion may result in initial difficulty distinguishing AFRS from sinonasal neoplasms. In such cases MRI findings are also helpful in the diagnosis of AFRS (Fig. 70.6).

Congenital disorders resulting in impairment of mucociliary clearance have a high incidence of CRS. Because nasal polyps are unusual in pediatric patients, their presence should trigger evaluation for cystic fibrosis and ciliary dyskinesia. Pathologic evaluation of polyps in these patients is likely to demonstrate a neutrophilic infiltrate and a predominately type 1 T–helper cell–mediated inflammatory process.[132,133]

Treatment

Treatment of CRSwNP is challenging. Most patients receive only temporary, if any, benefit from antibiotic therapy.[76,78,134,135] Topical steroid sprays and saline irrigations often provide improvement[135,136] but rarely provide adequate symptomatic relief for patients with a significant polyp burden. Systemic steroid therapy frequently provides significant symptomatic improvement.[76,78,137] Unfortunately, systemic side effects limit long-term use of this medication, and symptoms often recur quickly after

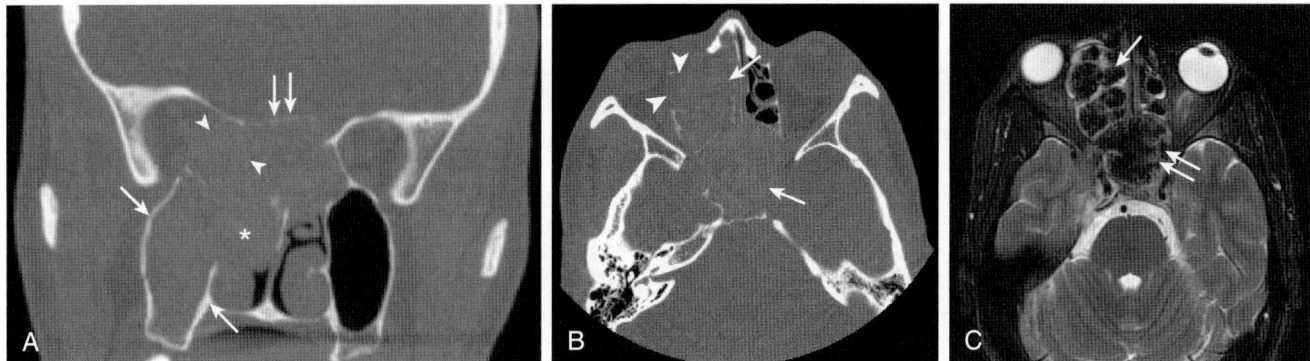

Figure 70.6 Allergic fungal rhinosinusitis. Coronal (A) and axial (B) computed tomography images demonstrate allergic fungal rhinosinusitis. The sinus contents are increased in density and expansile in nature with associated bone remodeling and erosion involving the medial right maxillary sinus (*single arrows*, A), sphenoid sinus walls and ethmoid partitions (*arrows*, B), and anterior skull base (*double arrows*, A). The right lamina papyracea (the medial wall of the orbit) has also been eroded (*arrowheads*, A–B), with the ethmoid contents bowing laterally into the medial right orbit. Lobulated opacity in the right nasal cavity (*asterisk*, A) is consistent with sinonasal polyposis, one of the diagnostic criteria for allergic fungal rhinosinusitis. Axial T2-weighted magnetic resonance imaging (C) demonstrates a loss of signal within the affected sinuses (*arrow*, right ethmoid sinuses; *double arrows*, sphenoid sinuses), which is characteristic of allergic fungal rhinosinusitis. (Courtesy Michael B. Gotway, MD.)

cessation of exogenous glucocorticoids. Initial enthusiasm for antifungal irrigations has waned with the publication of trials that demonstrate not only a lack of efficacy, but worsened symptoms when compared to placebo saline irrigation.[134,138] Current guidelines recommend against use of antifungal irrigations for patients with CRS.[78,139] Endoscopic sinus surgery with removal of polyps and cleaning of mucus and debris from within the sinuses results in significant symptomatic improvement.[140] Systemic corticosteroids are frequently initiated before surgery for CRSwNP to decrease mucosal inflammation, which improves hemostasis and endoscopic visualization during surgery. Corticosteroids also enhance control of asthma during endotracheal anesthesia and the postoperative period. Even in the setting of appropriately performed endoscopic sinus surgery, recurrence of polyps is common. Combining medical and surgical interventions is essential in this patient population. Surgery enhances postoperative access to the sinuses, allowing enhanced penetration of topical steroid irrigations. Steroid-impregnated implantable materials have also been used to extend the duration of symptomatic improvement after surgery.[141–143]

New biologic treatments hold promise for the treatment of CRS. Dupilumab (anti–IL-4 with anti–IL-13 activity) has been approved by the FDA for treatment of CRS with nasal polyps.[144,145] Studies evaluating this treatment focused on patients with severe disease burden and often with concomitant asthma, likely selecting for patients with type 2 inflammation. Concerns related to cost and requirement for continued therapy may limit the clinical utility of this medication. Omalizumab, an anti-IgE monoclonal antibody, has been used to treat refractory asthma and appears also to benefit patients with CRSwNP. Data on the efficacy of omalizumab as a treatment for CRSwNP have been submitted to the FDA with the goal of approval as a treatment for this disorder.[135,146] IL-5 is an important driver of eosinophil differentiation and survival, and anti–IL-5 antibodies (mepolizumab, benralizumab, reslizumab) have been FDA approved for treatment of eosinophilic asthma. Studies targeting patients with asthma have demonstrated some efficacy for CRS.[147,148]

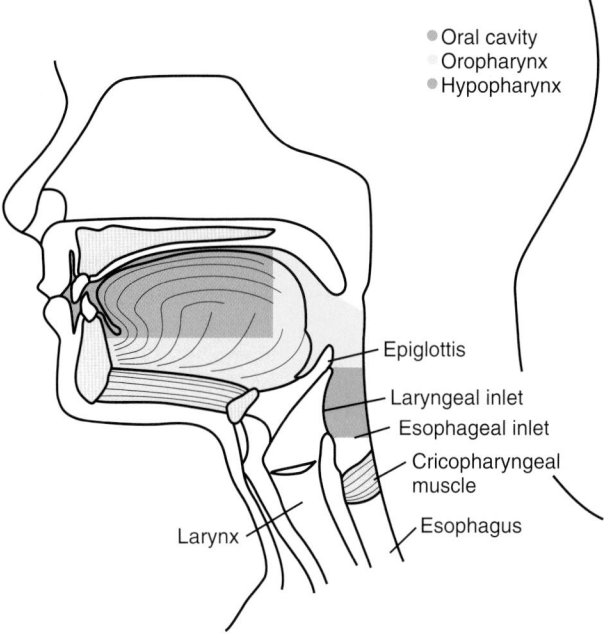

Figure 70.7 Schematic of the oral cavity (*green*), oropharynx (*yellow*), and hypopharynx (*blue*) along with the esophageal inlet and cricopharyngeal muscle.

THE ORAL CAVITY, OROPHARYNX, HYPOPHARYNX, AND LARYNX

ANATOMY, HISTOLOGY, AND PHYSIOLOGY

Oral Cavity

The *oral cavity* is defined as the space from the lips to the end of the hard palate. It contains the teeth, the buccal and gingival mucosa, the mandible and hard palate, the floor of the mouth, and the tongue anterior to the circumvallate papilla (Fig. 70.7). The oral cavity structures are mostly under voluntary control. The oral cavity functions to control the ingestion of food substances. The structures control the food during mastication and preparation of a bolus suitable for presentation to the oropharynx for reflexive swallowing. Mastication and preparation involve the muscles of mastication for opening and closing of the jaws and the muscles in the lips and cheeks to control the size of the cavity and the muscles of the tongue to move the food particles around the mouth and shape them into the required bolus. In addition to controlling the intake of substances, the structures in the oral cavity are responsible for voluntary modulation of air exhaled from the lungs. This voluntary control is used to control the rate of the air exhaled and to shape the noises created by airflow into speech and song.

Oropharynx

The *oropharynx* is defined as the space from the end of the hard palate to a plane parallel to the top of the epiglottis (see Fig. 70.7). This space includes the structures of the lateral pharyngeal walls, made up by the middle constrictors, the palatoglossus and the palatopharyngeus, the palatine tonsils, the soft palate and uvula, the vallecula, and the base of the tongue. Although these muscles and structures are under voluntary control for assistance in the rate of exhaled air from the lungs and shaping sounds released from the vocal tract, they are under reflexive control for swallowing. Once the sensory nerves are triggered by the exposure to a bolus of solids or liquids, the central nervous system sends a reflexive response to swallow. This reflex leads to an orderly contraction of the tongue base, soft palate, and lateral pharyngeal walls to propel the bolus posteriorly, seal off the nasopharynx, and propel the bolus to the hypopharynx, respectively.

Hypopharynx

The *hypopharynx* is defined as the space from a plane perpendicular to the tip of the epiglottis beyond the superior and lateral aspect of the larynx down to the esophageal inlet (see Fig. 70.7). This includes the structure of the lateral pharyngeal walls, including the inferior constrictors and mucosal membranes, as well as the bilateral pyriform sinuses. As for the oropharynx, the skeletal muscles that make up these structures are under voluntary control for assisting in regulation of airflow out of the lungs and shaping the airflow into speech and as reflexive central nervous system control for swallowing. The distal end of the hypopharynx culminates in the upper esophageal sphincter. This is a region of the pharynx that controls opening of the proximal esophagus to allow passage of food into the alimentary tract and to prevent the inadvertent regurgitation of food or secretions back into the pharynx and upper airway. Although the upper esophageal sphincter is several centimeters in length, the primary portion is made up of the cricopharyngeal muscle (see Fig. 70.7). This circumferential, sling-like skeletal muscle is maintained in a tonic contracted and closed state. The act of swallowing initiates reflexive inhibition of the neural input, resulting in muscular relaxation. As the larynx and pharynx are pulled upward and forward by the actions of other muscles, the relaxed upper esophageal sphincter is stretched open. This allows the passage of the food bolus. The bolus can fail to pass either because of failure of relaxation of the cricopharyngeal muscle segment or failure to stretch the area open through pull of coordinated muscles on the relaxed upper esophageal sphincter segment. Either will result in the retention of foods and secretions, which can then spill into the upper airway.

Larynx

The *larynx* is made of the bone, cartilage, and muscular and mucosal structures from the epiglottis to the bottom of the cricoid ring. It is divided into three regions based on the lymphatic drainage patterns. These regions include (1) the supraglottis from the tip of the epiglottis to the top of the vocal folds (also known as the vocal cords), including the upper part of the arytenoid; (2) the glottis, which includes the tissue from the top of the vocal folds to 1 cm below the top of the vocal folds; and (3) the subglottis, which is below the vocal folds to the first ring of trachea (Fig. 70.8).

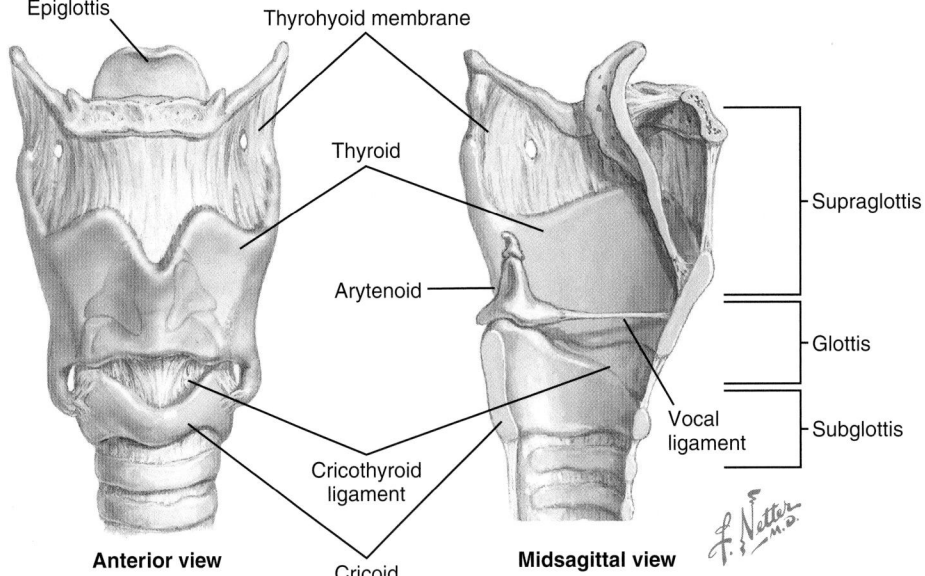

Figure 70.8 Schematic view of the larynx with the cartilage and ligamentous structures. The supraglottis, glottis, and subglottic subdivisions are marked. (Modified from Netter FH. *Atlas of Human Anatomy.* ed 5. Philadelphia: Elsevier; 2010. Netter illustration from www.netterimages.com, ID: 1495. Copyright Elsevier Inc. All rights reserved.)

Epiglottis   Thyrohyoid membrane   Thyroid   Arytenoid   Cricothyroid ligament   Cricoid   Vocal ligament   Supraglottis   Glottis   Subglottis   **Anterior view**   **Midsagittal view**

Bone and Cartilage. The structural bone and cartilages of the larynx include the hyoid bone, paired thyroid lamina, and cricoid ring. These structures have ligamentous and cartilaginous attachments to each other to allow them to function as one organ. Specifically, the hyoid is attached to the thyroid cartilage by the thyrohyoid ligament. The thyroid laminae are attached to the cricoid laterally by the fibrous cricothyroid joint and anteriorly by the cricothyroid ligament and membrane. The hyoid bone is attached to the skull base by the styloglossus muscle, to the mandible by the geniohyoid muscle, and to the tongue base by the hyoglossus muscle. The laryngeal cartilage is attached to the pharyngeal wall through the inferior pharyngeal constrictor muscle and to the cricoid ring by the cricothyroid joint, membrane, ligament, and muscle. The cricoid is attached to the trachea through fibrous attachments. These connections support the airway. Other cartilaginous structures within the larynx include the arytenoid complex cartilages known as cuneiform, corniculate, and arytenoid cartilages and the epiglottic cartilage. The mucosal and muscular structures of the larynx include the aryepiglottic folds connecting the arytenoid complex to the epiglottis; the false vocal folds, running from the body of the arytenoid to the base of the epiglottis; and the true vocal folds, running from the arytenoid to the thyroid cartilage (Fig. 70.9). The laryngeal ventricle is a cleft between the true and false vocal folds. It contains mucus-producing cells and minor salivary glands that lubricate the tissue of the larynx during breathing and speaking. In addition, the shape of the ventricle probably creates turbulence in airflow that is significant for vocal fold vibration during speaking[149] but of relatively little significance for airflow during breathing.

Arytenoid Complex. The arytenoid cartilage is attached to the cricoid ring through a series of anterior and posterior ligaments that form the capsule of the synovial cricoarytenoid joint. The corniculate and cuneiform cartilages have fibrous attachments to the arytenoids and are located on top of and anterior to the arytenoid cartilage, respectively.

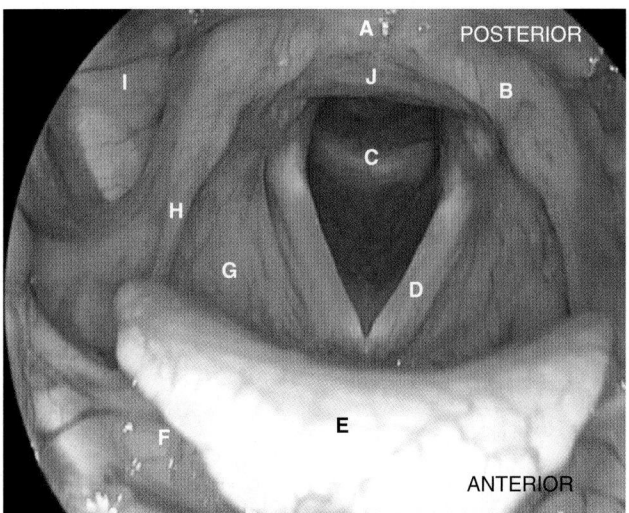

Figure 70.9 Upper airway anatomy: endoscopic view. *A,* Esophageal inlet; *B,* arytenoid; *C,* trachea; *D,* true vocal folds; *E,* epiglottis; *F,* vallecula; *G,* false vocal folds; *H,* aryepiglottic folds; *I,* pyriform sinus; *J,* interarytenoid region.

The true function of these structures is unknown, but they are thought to increase and stiffen the aryepiglottic fold and may therefore aid in prevention of aspiration during swallowing and prevent supraglottic collapse of the airway during breathing. The cricoarytenoid joint allows movement of the arytenoid on the cricoid ring for vocal fold abduction and adduction, which is controlled by the action of the intrinsic laryngeal musculature on the arytenoid. Specifically, the lateral cricoarytenoid muscle attaches from the lateral aspect of the cricoid to the muscular process on the posterolateral aspect of the arytenoid. Contraction of the lateral cricoarytenoid muscle creates inward rotation of the arytenoid on the cricoid and closes the laryngeal airway during swallowing, speaking, and exhalation. This activity is supplemented by the action of the interarytenoid muscle, which runs between the upper bodies of the arytenoids and pulls the arytenoids together. The interarytenoid muscle is probably more important during voice production than during breathing. The posterior cricoarytenoid muscle attaches from the posterior aspect of the cricoid ring also to the muscular process on the posterolateral aspect of the arytenoid. Contraction of the posterior cricoarytenoid muscle creates outward rotation of the arytenoid on the cricoid and opens the airway during inspiration.

Epiglottis. The epiglottis has ligamentous attachments to the hyoid bone (hyoepiglottic ligament) and thyroid cartilage (thyroepiglottic ligament) and fibromuscular attachments to the arytenoid complex (aryepiglottic fold). As the names of these attachments imply (origin to insertion), the epiglottis moves in relation to these supportive structures during breathing and swallowing. This movement is passive. As the tongue base and pharyngeal walls contract and the hyoid and attaching laryngeal supporting framework are pulled upward, the epiglottis tilts posteriorly (passive inversion) to cover the top of the airway and divert the bolus to be swallowed to the outside of the larynx (pyriform sinuses). The epiglottis does not completely cover the airway, but rather steers the bolus through the pyriform sinus and outside of the laryngeal airway. Patients who lose the epiglottis secondary to cancer treatment can be taught to swallow again by strongly contracting the tongue base to pull the larynx forward, thereby partially covering the laryngeal airway. Usually this results in a small amount of residue deposited on the top portion of the larynx and/or vocal folds that then must be cleared out of the larynx into the hypopharynx with a throat clear or cough and swallowed a second time. This is known as a "supraglottic swallowing technique" and is useful in preventing aspiration in cases of epiglottic loss or malfunction.

Mucosal and Fibromuscular Structures. The mucosal and fibromuscular structures include the aryepiglottic folds, false vocal folds, and true folds. As stated previously, the aryepiglottic folds run from the arytenoid complex to the epiglottis. They separate the pyriform sinus of the hypopharynx from the supraglottic larynx and form a sling of tissue around the vocal folds to prevent aspiration during swallowing. They consist of fibrofatty tissue and contain minor salivary glands and mucus-producing cells. If a significant portion of the aryepiglottic fold is removed during surgery, the liquid or food bolus can fall into the larynx and increase the risk for aspiration. At the inferior portion of the aryepiglottic fold is the false vocal fold. This is a fibrofatty collection of tissue also covered with epithelium containing minor salivary glands and mucus-producing cells. The true function of the false vocal folds is unknown, but they most likely affect the resonance characteristics of the voice rather than the process of breathing or swallowing. The aryepiglottic folds and false vocal folds are part of the supraglottis and can be covered with either respiratory epithelium or squamous epithelium.[150]

The true vocal folds are composed of the *thyroarytenoid* (TA) and *lateral cricoarytenoid* (LCA) muscle covered with mucosa. The mucosa is a stratified squamous epithelium supported by a specialized submucosa or lamina propria differentiated into three layers. This differentiation is likely secondary to use of the vocal folds for phonation, which causes the supporting fibroblasts to produce and secrete proteins and carbohydrates.[151] These extracellular particles are then layered in a particular order, with dense collagen as the deepest layer, an elastin-rich middle layer, and glycosaminoglycans and glycoproteins forming a spongy superficial layer. The middle and deep layer form a transition zone known as the vocal ligament, which runs from the anterior aspect of the thyroid cartilage to the vocal process of the arytenoid. This ligament allows the superficial layers to separate from the deeper layers as the vocal folds vibrate to produce voice and is probably responsible for the relatively wide vocal pitch range that humans are able to produce. The TA-LCA muscle runs from the anterior aspect of the thyroid cartilage and attaches along the body of the arytenoid cartilage. As the TA contracts, it adducts, tenses, shortens, and thickens the vocal fold. This is important because, as the TA-LCA muscle changes tension and shape, it has an indirect effect on the vocal fold mucosa, which is involved in vocal fold vibration. The vibration frequency of an object is related to the driving force for vibration and the tension and mass of the object. Therefore, as we adjust the tension in the vocal fold, through voluntary contraction of the intrinsic skeletal muscle of the larynx, we affect the frequency of vocal fold vibration, which is perceived as the pitch of the voice. In the case of vocal fold tension and mass, the most important muscles are the TA-LCA along with the cricothyroid muscle. As the cricothyroid muscle, which originates on the cricoid ring anteriorly and inserts on the thyroid cartilage, contracts, the thyroid cartilage is subluxed on the cricoid ring. This results in stretching the vocal fold and increasing the tension, which drives up the frequency of vibration and the pitch of the voice.

Pathophysiology. The pharynx and larynx have prominent and complex functions in the upper airway to separate the alimentary tract from the respiratory tract for human survival. For swallowing and breathing, the pharynx and larynx must work in a coordinated manner. If these systems fail to function properly, the airway can be obstructed or pharyngeal contents can be aspirated, leading to lung disease.

DISORDERS OF SWALLOWING

Epidemiology

Disorders of swallowing caused by either neurologic or muscular diseases interrupting the normal sequences of upper airway and pharyngeal activity can lead to the aspiration of pharyngeal contents either directly, during the swallowing act, or indirectly, from refluxed gastric contents. Aspiration of large quantities of liquid material or of large solid substances can lead to airway obstruction with asphyxiation and death. Acute aspiration of small amounts of substances has been shown to produce acute pulmonary inflammation.[152] Aspiration of acidic materials appears to be more inflammatory than aspiration of less acidic materials.[153] If the aspiration is an isolated single event, the inflammation resolves with little consequence.[152] However, repeated aspiration can damage the alveolar lining of cells and capillaries and lead to bacterial invasion, mucosal desquamation, and mononuclear cell inflammation.[153] In lung transplant patients, chronic aspiration of refluxed gastric contents has been associated with increased failure rates of grafts through the development of bronchiolitis obliterans syndrome.[154] Although the exact mechanism is unknown, it appears to be related to fibrosis developing as a response to chronic repeated inflammation. This response may be reduced through the use of agents that reduce inflammation[155] (see also Chapters 43 and 72).

Disorders of swallowing, commonly called dysphagia, affect 2–11% of the general population.[156] The etiology is varied. Dysphagia may arise in response to normal aging due to weakening of the pharyngeal musculature. Dysphagia may also arise from neurologic disease (e.g., stroke), motor neuron disease, or Parkinson disease, due to mistiming of the swallow with poor coordination or to weakness or spasticity of the pharyngeal musculature. Finally, dysphagia often results from medical intervention for the treatment of head and neck disease or after intubation for respiratory failure.

Dysphagia is reported to develop in 40–50% of patients intubated for more than 48 hours.[157–159] Furthermore, the incidence of postextubation dysphagia rises by 14% for each additional day of intubation and is significantly more common in older patients.[158,160] The cause of dysphagia due to prolonged intubation is not completely understood. However, because the incidence is remarkably high, all patients intubated for prolonged periods should be evaluated with at least a bedside swallow examination before the initiation of oral feeding after extubation.[157] Clinical studies have also revealed that aspiration after extubation from prolonged intubation may be silent due to changes in laryngeal and pharyngeal sensation; therefore, some authors recommend more aggressive intervention with *flexible endoscopic examination of swallowing* (FEES) to document aspiration.[160] Silent aspiration can be identified by FEES, but the procedure has no impact on outcomes. Although dysphagia with aspiration does not always lead to pneumonia,[160] dysphagia alone is correlated with prolonged hospital stays.[159] The incidence of postintubation dysphagia can be reduced by using smaller endotracheal tubes and by careful monitoring to prevent excessive endotracheal tube cuff pressure.[161,162]

Symptoms of Disorders of Swallowing

The most common symptoms in patients with disordered swallowing are chronic coughing, weight loss, and repeated episodes of pneumonia. On questioning, patients report that they cough during meals. In general, a greater difficulty with swallowing liquids is indicative of neurologic dysfunction or muscular weakness, and a greater difficulty with solids is more indicative of obstruction. The examiner should inquire about what substances cause the most difficulty, the timing of the cough in relation to eating, the length of time required to finish a moderate-sized meal, and where food appears to create the greatest difficulty during the swallow.

Coughing early during the act of swallowing indicates poor oral motor control of the bolus. Patients with neurologic disorders may notice that they cannot control the food within the oral cavity so that the food prematurely spills into the oropharynx or hypopharynx before the patient is ready to swallow. Patients find that substances that break apart easily or consist of both liquids and solids are most difficult because portions of the bolus can escape. Coughing during or after the swallow is most indicative of pharyngeal dysfunction due to either disordered reflex timing of the pharyngeal contraction or muscular weakness that prevents the bolus from moving through the pharynx as required.

Prolongation of mealtimes often leads to malnutrition and weight loss. Patients with an intact swallow mechanism can usually finish a complete meal in 15 minutes. Longer mealtimes are suggestive of dysphagia. When patients go beyond 30 minutes for a meal, they typically begin to lose interest in eating. In most cases, this prolongation is socially unacceptable, and dining companions begin to leave the table, forcing the patient to stop eating.

Dysphagia can be roughly divided into pharyngeal phase dysphagia and esophageal phase dysphagia. Patients with pharyngeal phase problems will complain of substances sticking in the back of their "throat" and coughing because of aspiration of retained substances, whereas patients with esophageal phase disorders will complain of food lodging in the chest that needs to be regurgitated or "washed down" with liquids. Cough may also be stimulated at the distal esophagus, but this is after the swallow and is generally nonproductive and not associated with the development of pneumonia.

Evaluation of Dysphagia

Evaluation is best done by a team of physicians and speech-language pathologists interested in disorders of swallowing. After a careful history, the patient can be given a sip of water during palpation of the laryngeal complex. As the patient swallows, the larynx should elevate briskly about 2 cm. In addition, the patient should not cough and should then be able to speak without a wet-sounding voice. If the patient passes this initial screening, then he or she should be asked to take multiple sips to see if the swallowing reflex breaks down. Next, complete head and neck evaluation and indirect endoscopy of the hypopharynx and larynx is undertaken to assess lip and tongue mobility and strength and for patterns of retained secretions or food particles. Patients with normal tongue function should be able to protrude the tongue and move it side to side without associated movement of the mandible. Retention of food particles within the oral cavity or inability to move the tongue freely is indicative of weakness or restricted motion. Indirect endoscopy identifying pooling at the base of the tongue within the vallecula is suggestive of weakness of the tongue base, pooling of secretions within the pyriform sinuses is indicative

of pharyngeal weakness, and pooling of secretions in the esophageal inlet is indicative of failure of cricopharyngeal opening or obstruction of the esophagus.

To confirm these patterns of weakness, FEES[163] or modified barium swallowing examination can be performed. These tests are usually performed by a qualified speech-language pathologist. Rather than just being a screening test for aspiration, these examinations should be used to identify which deficits within the swallowing act are responsible for the dysphagia. In addition, during FEES or a modified barium swallow, various adaptive/compensatory swallowing adjustments can be tried. These diagnostic evaluations result in essential treatment approaches and can direct treatment strategies.

Treatment

Treatment for disorders of swallowing involves precise identification of the region and type of the swallowing deficits. If muscular weakness is identified, patients can be given a series of exercises targeting specific areas either of the tongue base[164,165] or of the lateral pharyngeal walls.[166] If neurologic deficits are identified, resulting in reflex timing issues or if the muscular deficits are insurmountable, patients can be taught compensatory strategies to improve the safety of the swallow. These strategies include repositioning of the patient during the swallow so that the bolus is less likely to fall into the airway, chin tuck to keep the bolus in the mouth during mastication, or head turning to close off the weakened side of the pharynx during the swallow act. Finally, if none of these techniques is beneficial and the patient and the family are interested, a feeding tube can be inserted to prevent weight loss and lessen the burden of needing to ingest a sufficient amount of calories orally to maintain weight. If repeated aspiration persists, laryngotracheal separation or narrow field laryngectomy, a less invasive procedure for laryngeal diversion, should be considered.

GASTROESOPHAGEAL AND LARYNGOPHARYNGEAL REFLUX DISEASE

Association with Asthma and COPD

The relationship between reflux disease, asthma, and COPD is complex. Although the association between reflux and severe asthma is well accepted, the empirical evidence for causation of one by the other is lacking. Lung disease may be related to reflux disease by different mechanisms. First, direct microaspiration of contents refluxed into the lungs on a chronic basis may lead to pulmonary remodeling. The extent of injury is related to the amount and characteristics of the aspirate, the frequency of aspiration, and the effectiveness of protective lung-clearance mechanisms. This is one proposed mechanism for the development of bronchiolitis obliterans syndrome in transplant patients. Second, reflux or reduced clearance of food from esophageal dysmotility may cause vagally induced bronchospasm. Vagally induced bronchospasm is associated with increased acidification of the lower esophagus and may be ameliorated by deacidification of the gastric contents in patients with difficult-to-control asthma.[167] Treatment with a *proton pump inhibitor* (PPI) improves asthma control in individuals with symptomatic *gastroesophageal reflux disease* (GERD) but not in those without symptoms.[168,169]

However, as previously stated, the association between reflux disease and lung disease does not prove causation. Medications for the treatment of asthma may increase reflux, as may changes from chronic lung disease. Albuterol is known to lower the resting pressure of the lower esophageal sphincter and decrease esophageal contraction amplitude. These changes may increase the incidence of reflux.[170] Prednisone, which is often prescribed in patients with difficult to control asthma, has been shown to increase esophageal acid exposure times.[171] COPD can lead to hyperinflation with flattening of the diaphragm. The diaphragm, specifically the crura around the esophageal hiatus, forms a critical part of the lower esophageal sphincter, and flattening of the diaphragm decreases the protective reflux barrier of the diaphragm. An increased transdiaphragmatic pressure gradient, as seen in patients with COPD, predisposes to the movement of gastric contents into the esophagus.

Evaluation of Gastroesophageal Reflux Disease and Laryngopharyngeal Reflux Disease

There are no universally accepted physical findings in the upper aerodigestive tract pathognomonic for extraesophageal reflux disease.[172] *Extraesophageal reflux disease* refers to the manifestations of reflux such as laryngitis, dysphonia, cough, and bronchospasm, which are separate from the classic esophageal reflux symptoms such as heartburn. Although attempts have been undertaken to develop a reflux finding score for physical changes in the larynx in patients with presumed extraesophageal reflux,[173] attempts at validation of these findings through correlation with pH studies have been unsuccessful. Therefore, the various laryngeal examination findings previously ascribed to *laryngopharyngeal reflux disease* (LPRD) are nonspecific and must be taken into context of a larger evaluation process.

After a careful history for symptoms of both classic GERD and extraesophageal reflux disease has been completed, most patients will be placed on an empirical trial of antireflux medications in combination with behavioral modification instructions. If the trial results in amelioration of the symptoms, the symptoms are commonly believed to be secondary to reflux disease. This method of evaluation for reflux with an empirical trial of medications is problematic because there may be a considerable placebo effect. Meta-analysis of randomized controlled clinical trials has shown that the effect of medications in alleviating symptoms is not significantly different from the effect of placebo.[174] However, most of these trials did not rely on objective testing for LPRD as entrance criteria. Some clinicians proceed to 24-hour pH monitoring and/or impedance testing. The latter, when combined with pH testing, allows detection of both acid and non-acid reflux. Although 24-hour pH analysis is considered the gold standard for esophageal reflux, pH testing over shorter time periods is often very helpful. Testing of pH within the hypopharynx to assess extraesophageal spillage of gastric contents is an area in its infancy, and there is significant debate as to what constitutes an abnormal finding.[175]

Treatment of Gastroesophageal Reflux Disease

Treatment of GERD or extraesophageal reflux disease causing pulmonary problems is best started with dietary modifications and twice-daily PPI medications. The rationale for these aggressive management strategies is that the pharynx, larynx, and trachea have few, if any, natural protective mechanisms for the neutralization of aspirated gastric contents.[176,177]

If there is strong suspicion of GERD or extraesophageal reflux causing pulmonary disease, consideration can be given to surgical therapies, such as Nissen fundoplication. Studies evaluating the true response of symptoms from extraesophageal reflux disease to surgical intervention show conflicting results. This is due in part to the significant difficulty in diagnosing extraesophageal reflux accurately and in understanding the role extraesophageal reflux may play in the pulmonary disease process.[178] The best results are obtained when classic GERD is identified and surgery, such as Nissen fundoplication, is performed for significant reflux within the lower esophagus.[179–181]

PARADOXICAL VOCAL FOLD MOTION DISORDER AND LARYNGOSPASM

Definition and Diagnosis

Also known as vocal cord dysfunction or inducible laryngeal obstruction, *paradoxical vocal fold motion disorder* (PVFMD) is a descriptive term for inappropriate adduction of the vocal folds during breathing. The mistimed vocal fold closure creates difficulty breathing and is often misdiagnosed as asthma. The diagnosis of PVFMD is made on the basis of history, followed by spirometry and laryngeal examination. Patients present with a constellation of symptoms, including difficulty breathing; a sensation of a foreign body or lump in their throat; a dry, nonproductive cough; and possibly chest tightness. These symptoms can manifest at rest, after talking, or after physical exertion. A distinct subset of this condition is associated with physical exertion and exercise. This has been called exercise-related PVMD or, more recently, exercise-induced laryngeal obstruction. Often the symptoms are exacerbated as the patient increases the intensity of the precipitating behavior. The disease is commonly misdiagnosed as asthma; however, the symptoms are refractory to standard asthma management protocols. In patients with PVFMD, spirometry performed during an episode may reveal flattening of the inspiratory limb of the flow-volume curve, indicative of a variable extrathoracic obstruction[182–184] (see Fig. 32.2, right panel). Flexible laryngoscopy, considered by some to be the gold standard for diagnosis,[182,185,186] may reveal paradoxical closure of the vocal folds during breathing. Typically, paradoxical closure is observed during active inhalation through either the mouth or the nose but is considered pathognomonic by some when seen at the end of a speech utterance.[183] Provocation testing through increased exercise challenge, odor exposure, or even methacholine challenge may increase the sensitivity of laryngoscopy in the identification of paradoxical closure. However, even with these challenges, the sensitivity of endoscopy is still only 60% in patients with symptoms.[187] Therefore, a presumptive diagnosis and empirical treatment may be warranted in all patients with symptoms who do not respond well to medical management for asthma.

Laryngospasm, closing of the vocal folds preventing inhalation, is a physiologic protective reflex to prevent aspiration when foreign particles or liquid (e.g., drowning) stimulate the vocal folds or supraglottic structures. Laryngospasm is most commonly encountered during extubation from general anesthesia. It is managed with positive-pressure ventilation and small doses of paralytic agents to weaken vocal fold closure. Severe episodes are complicated by post-obstructive pulmonary edema, which can require management in the intensive care unit. In the absence of a known stimulus, recurrent episodes of laryngospasm can develop in patients with progressive neurologic disease[188,189] or can be associated with severe forms of PVFMD. These often lead to recurrent trips to the emergency department and can be misdiagnosed as bilateral vocal fold paralysis. Patients with recurrent episodic laryngospasm should undergo a complete neurologic examination to rule out a neurologic disorder. In the absence of neurologic disease, laryngospasm will often respond to the same management strategies used for patients with PVFMD.

Etiology

The etiology of PVFMD is unclear. PVFMD is associated with asthma and GERD.[190] High levels of stress, chronic postnasal drip, and environmental exposure to inhaled or aspirated irritants, allergies, or GERD may lead to laryngeal hyperresponsiveness, which in turn triggers paradoxical laryngeal closure. In one study,[190] when patients with PVFMD were compared with normative data on the Minnesota Multiphasic Personality Inventory, 40% of the patients with PVFMD demonstrated elevation on the hypochondriasis and hysteria scales and minor elevation on the depression scale, in a pattern consistent with conversion disorder. An additional 29% of these patients had significant differences in these scales but did not fit the classic conversion disorder pattern, whereas only 24% of patients had scores suggestive of no psychopathologic conditions.

The association of PVFMD with asthma, GERD, and environmental exposure to irritants raises the possibility of an organic cause in some patients with the disease. Some authors have suggested that, when an organic cause is suspected, the term *irritable larynx* should be used to describe the disorder.[184] In one study of patients with asthma, 19% had coexistent PVFMD, whereas only 5% of asymptomatic control subjects had any evidence of paradoxical vocal fold closure.[191] It is best to consider inappropriate adduction of the vocal fold during breathing as an abnormal physical examination finding with a wide range of etiologies: stress reactivity, GERD/LPRD, environmental exposure, peripheral neuropathy (sensory), or unable to be determined.

Treatment

The first step in the treatment of PVFMD is recognition of the disease. The clinical presentation is often confusing because patients may have coexistent asthma or GERD and may be resistant to the idea that behavioral change could result in any significant reduction in their symptom severity. One study estimated that the association with asthma and GERD is as high as 65% and 51%, respectively.[185] This association, along with a desire to use medication to treat the problems, usually leads to attempted medical trials for asthma management and therapy for GERD. With these strategies, the symptoms may be reduced modestly, but the acute attacks of intermittent dyspnea, cough, and chest tightness can still be difficult to control. Therefore, referral to an otolaryngologist to perform laryngeal endoscopy may be required. If the true coexistence of asthma is questionable because there is little, if any, response to bronchodilator therapy, repeat pulmonary function testing

before and after bronchodilator therapy, and possibly with methacholine challenge, is indicated. If test results are positive, management of the reactive airway disease should be maximized. If test results are negative, all medical therapy should be stopped because the asthma medications may be exacerbating the disease by irritating the laryngeal mucosa, increasing patient anxiety, or increasing the risk for gastroesophageal reflux. If symptoms lead to a suspicion that GERD or LPRD is a contributing factor, it is reasonable to treat the patient with dietary modifications and PPI therapy. Dietary modifications include eating small meals, avoiding foods known to cause reflux, and avoiding reclining after eating. Therapy with PPIs should be initiated on a twice-daily basis 30 to 60 minutes before the first and last meal of the day. Reflux that reaches the hypopharynx most frequently happens after meals. Therefore, PPIs should be given before the meal so that a therapeutic serum level can be achieved before the stimulation of acid production by the ingested food. If symptoms have not improved by 2 to 3 months after the initiation of therapy, formal pH impedance testing should be considered. It is also reasonable to consider that acid reflux may not be playing a significant role in the pathogenesis of the patient's disease.

After careful history and endoscopy to rule out other causes of airway obstruction, the treatment of acute episodes of PVFMD includes reassurance, breathing instruction, and possibly the use of a helium and oxygen mixture (heliox) to reduce the turbulence of airflow past an obstruction and thus reduce the pressure needed to generate airflow[192,193] (see also Chapter 39). Often, acute exacerbations will precipitate visits to an emergency department. The patient presents with dyspnea, a rapid respiratory rate, and stridor. Rather than immobile vocal folds or an obstructing mass lesion, endoscopy usually reveals that the vocal folds are held in a paramedian position through inspiration and expiration. If patients are asked to cough or clear their throat, the vocal folds will usually abduct. Vocal fold abduction can be further stimulated by reassuring the patient and attempting to provide a calm, relaxed environment. Inhaling through the nose and exhaling through the nose or pursed lips (metered breathing) may also be beneficial. Alternatively, the patient can be asked to breathe through a straw. Introducing a restriction in the airway with the nose and lips or with a straw facilitates the patient's ability to control his or her breath and promotes laryngeal relaxation with appropriate laryngeal activity. Respiratory control or metered breathing reduces the laryngeal hypersensitivity by reducing either the respiratory rate or breath volume or both. This type of respiratory retraining is the key to management of patients with PVFMD.[194,195]

Difficulties in establishing diagnostic criteria for PVFMD are even greater than for asthma. With asthma, objective pulmonary function measures can document reversible airflow obstruction, or methacholine bronchoprovocation can demonstrate bronchial hyperreactivity. Patients with PVFMD may show flattening of the inspiratory limb of the flow-volume curve, as is seen in patients with variable extrathoracic airway obstruction, but these changes can be transient or mimicked by submaximal inspiratory effort. Therefore, there are no objective measures of the disease, and establishing objective diagnostic criteria is not possible. Treatment may involve placebo effects from medications for other disorders, such as GERD or asthma, or active respiratory retraining to engage the patient in regaining control of his or her breathing, as described earlier. Due to the difficulty in establishing diagnostic criteria, there have been few randomized controlled trials of respiratory retraining in patients with PVFMD. Limited evidence from case series has shown a reduction in the severity of patient symptoms and improvements in quality of life, which can be maintained through periodic long-term follow-up.[196]

VOCAL FOLD PARALYSIS

Unilateral

Unilateral vocal fold paralysis rarely produces symptoms of airway obstruction other than dyspnea with phonation. Although changes in pulmonary function can be measured during both quiet and active breathing, these are rarely clinically significant.[197] When obstruction is present, the proposed mechanism is either (1) the action of inspiratory airflow producing a Bernoulli effect on the flaccid vocal fold (e.g., pulling the cord inward due to low pressure and thereby increasing obstruction) or (2) inappropriate reinnervation of the paralyzed vocal fold with active signals for adduction during inspiration (e.g., synkinesis).[198] The findings can be corrected through surgery to stabilize the flaccid vocal fold complex, botulinum toxin injections to reduce the effects of the inappropriate reinnervation, or surgery to reduce the nerve supply to the synkinetic vocal fold.[199] It is rare that any of the treatments are required for unilateral vocal fold paralysis.

Bilateral

Bilateral vocal fold paralysis most commonly develops secondary to surgery in the anterior compartment of the neck for thyroid disease.[200] The recurrent laryngeal nerves are either crushed or cut during the intervention, and vocal fold abduction for inspiration and adduction for phonation are lost. Immediately after the onset of the injury, some patients are able to tolerate the loss of vocal fold abduction because the vocal folds are flaccid and immobile in a lateral position. The voice is weak and breathy. However, the recurrent laryngeal nerve contains all axons for abduction and adduction in a single fascicle. As axons regrow, the vocal fold muscles may regain tone without active adduction or abduction. Because of the increased mass of the adductor muscles compared to the abductor muscle, the vocal folds adopt a more medial position. Vocal fold tone recovers in the majority of patients who sustain an injury to the recurrent laryngeal nerve.[201] This process of neural regeneration takes 3 to 9 months and leads to slowly progressive improvement in voice but progressive airway compromise. Patients often adapt to this progressive airway compromise by decreasing their level of activity.

A small percentage of patients develop bilateral vocal fold paralysis secondary to a Chiari malformation with increased intracranial pressure and compression of cranial nerve X in the foramen magnum by the base of the brain as it herniates through the foramen. This condition can be extremely difficult to diagnose. Finally, a small percentage of patients will have an idiopathic etiology. In these instances, the paralysis can develop bilaterally simultaneously or unilaterally, separated by years.[202]

Patients with bilateral vocal fold paralysis typically report minimal voice changes and note marked dyspnea on exertion. Careful history usually reveals the cause as prior surgical intervention,[200] and general examination reveals prolongation of inspiration with mild to moderate inspiratory stridor. Endoscopic examination reveals bilateral vocal fold immobility with possible elongation of the vocal folds on inhalation.[200] Pulmonary function testing demonstrates a classic pattern of variable extrathoracic obstruction with flattening of the inspiratory limb of the flow-volume curve and little change in the expiratory limb (see Fig. 32.2, right panel). When maximal inspiratory flow falls below 1.5 L/sec, most patients are markedly symptomatic, and intervention is warranted. If inspiratory flow is maintained around 2 L/sec, most patients can perform modest activity, such as climbing one flight of stairs or walking on level surfaces.

The treatment of bilateral vocal fold paralysis is aimed at enlarging the airway or bypassing the glottis with a tracheotomy. If patients choose the latter, consideration should be given to the creation of a skin-lined tracheostomy tract. This will reduce the risk for granulation tissue growth at the stoma, provide a safe stable stoma for patients to manage by themselves on a long-term basis, and allow patients to use an appliance that will hold a one-way valve so that digital occlusion is not required for phonation.[203] Bilateral vocal fold paralysis can also be treated by injecting botulinum toxin into the muscles of adduction. This reduces the adductor force and allows improved function of the abductor muscles. The voice is fairly well preserved because the patient can usually override some of the effects of the botulinum toxin. The disadvantage of this treatment option is that it requires repeat injections.[204] Transverse cordotomy or partial arytenoidectomy are also surgical options for treatment designed to remove the posterior portion of the vocal fold or a portion of the arytenoid cartilage, respectively. This enlarges the cartilaginous portion of the laryngeal airway by 1 to 2 mm without interfering too greatly with the anterior vibratory function of the vocal folds. However, because the posterior portion of the airway is enlarged on a static basis, air will leak out during phonation, and the voice will be reduced in volume and be breathy in quality. This is referred to as "the great compromise" because the larger the airway for breathing and activity tolerance, the worse the voice. The patient and surgeon must decide on a balance.[205] In addition, one or both of the vocal folds can be sutured in a lateral position through myriad different techniques referred to as suture lateralization. Some of these techniques are potentially reversible and can be used in patients in whom recovery of function is possible to improve their airway during this period.[206] Finally, experimental surgical strategies for management with electrical stimulation of the abductor muscles (laryngeal pacemaker) to open the glottis are being conducted.[207] Initial results indicate that abduction for breathing can be achieved without compromise of vocal fold closure for voice production. An alternative experimental approach involves surgical reinnervation of the posterior cricoarytenoid muscle to achieve vocal fold abduction. This approach sounds attractive but to date has not achieved consistent results.

LARYNGEAL STENOSIS

Scarring of the larynx, usually in the posterior portion, referred to as *posterior glottis stenosis* (PGS), most commonly develops secondary to endotracheal tube–related injury. In fact, when patients present with bilateral vocal fold immobility after prolonged intubation, 95% of the time the immobility is secondary to scar formation in and around the cricoarytenoid joints.[200] This is a decidedly different process from bilateral vocal fold paralysis, but clinically and endoscopically it can be difficult to distinguish the two because visual inspection reveals the vocal folds to be immobile in both situations. Helpful clinical clues to diagnosis are the events and timing around the onset of symptoms. The most common events associated with onset are prolonged intubation, multiple intubations, and/or intubation with an excessively large endotracheal tube. As the endotracheal tube rubs against the mucosa of the posterior larynx, the mucosa is eroded and inflammation develops. Reflux may play a role in adding to inflammation or mucosal erosion.[208] Secondary infection of the mucosal ulceration may also play a role in adding to inflammation. After the endotracheal tube is removed, the mucosa heals by secondary intention over a 6-week period. Thus, the patient notices deterioration of breathing more rapidly after a mucosal injury than after a neurologic injury; after a neurologic injury, as described earlier, the difficulty with breathing develops over a 3- to 6-month period as the nerve recovers partial tone.

Examination also reveals subtle differences in patients with PGS from those with bilateral vocal fold paralysis. Careful endoscopic evaluation usually reveals scar tissue over and around the cricoarytenoid joint. This can be subtle, with a relatively normal appearance and only slight reduction in the normal size and shape of the posterior portion of the larynx, or obvious, with overt scar tissue built up in the posterior portion of the glottis.[209] Finally, pulmonary function testing usually reveals a fixed extrathoracic pattern with flattening of both the inspiratory and expiratory limbs of the flow-volume loop.

Distinguishing between PGS and bilateral vocal fold paralysis is clinically significant because treatment options and outcomes are different. Both PGS and bilateral vocal fold paralysis can be treated with tracheotomy. In PGS, the initial surgical treatment should be aimed at release of the scar tissue holding the joint in the fixed position. If this is not possible due to loss or remodeling of the cartilaginous joint structure, portions of the cartilage or vocal fold can be removed. If possible, mucosal advancement flaps should be designed to cover the site of surgical excision. Because the tissue of the posterior glottis is scarred, a simple incision through prior scar tissue is less likely to provide sustained significant release and more likely to heal with recurrent scar. Injudicious surgery can make the problem worse. The majority of patients with either PGS or bilateral vocal fold paralysis can have successful endolaryngeal surgery that will enlarge the airway to prevent a lifetime of tracheotomy dependence.

UPPER AERODIGESTIVE TRACT MALIGNANCIES

Malignancies of the upper aerodigestive tract are a significant cause of morbidity and mortality. Cancers of the upper aerodigestive tract constitute approximately 4% of all malignancies.[210] *Squamous cell carcinoma* (SCC) is the predominant cancer in this location, and smoking and alcohol use are the traditional risk factors. Surgery, radiation, and chemotherapy all play an important role in the treatment of this disease; a thorough discussion of this topic is beyond the scope of this chapter.

In the oropharynx, recent evidence has identified *human papillomavirus* (HPV) as an emerging, and now dominant, cause of malignancies. In all, 80–90% of newly diagnosed SCC of the tonsils or base of the tongue are HPV induced. HPV-associated oropharyngeal SCC represents a distinct clinical entity with a significantly better prognosis than non–HPV-associated oropharyngeal SCC. National Cancer Center Network guidelines now recommend HPV testing for all oropharyngeal malignancies. HPV-16 is identified as the most common HPV subtype associated with oropharyngeal malignancy.[211] In SCC of the oral cavity, oral tongue, and larynx, HPV is less commonly found; in this region, tobacco and alcohol use remain the primary risk factors. Whereas the incidence of these non–oropharyngeal SCCs is declining likely secondary to a decrease in tobacco use, the incidence of oropharyngeal carcinoma is rising, likely due to HPV.

Laryngeal cancers usually present early with voice changes. However, if the cancer arises in the supraglottic area, the subglottis, or pyriform sinus, or if the patient ignores the changes in voice and the diagnosis is otherwise delayed, airway obstruction can be one of the presenting symptoms. In these instances, the diagnosis is made through endoscopic evaluation, and the airway should be managed with endoscopic debulking of the tumor before definitive therapy is undertaken.[212]

SUBGLOTTIS AND CERVICAL TRACHEA

ANATOMY, HISTOLOGY, AND PHYSIOLOGY

The subglottis is the area within the cricoid ring from the bottom of the vocal folds to the top of the first tracheal ring. The latter is the only complete ring in the airway and structurally functions to support the larynx and suspend the trachea. The subglottis is lined with a respiratory mucosa with goblet cells for mucus production and minor salivary glands as well. Mucus and saliva travel upward because of the actions of the ciliated epithelium and airflow and help humidify the airway and lubricate the vocal fold mucosa. In the adult human, the subglottis is the narrowest portion of the airway and ranges from 15 to 18 mm in diameter. It is roughly a round or slightly oval tubular space that is narrowest just below the vocal folds and widens out at the bottom at the transition into the cervical trachea. The space extends for 1 to 2 cm in vertical dimension from the bottom of the vocal folds to the first tracheal ring. The shape of the subglottis is probably important for establishing laminar flow through the glottis. This is important for both the clearance of secretions and generating flow that will efficiently drive vocal fold vibration. Irregularities in the subglottic mucosa often lead to turbulent airflow with crust formation, which can further compromise the airway. Below the subglottis lies the cervical trachea, consisting of the first four or five tracheal rings.

SUBGLOTTIC AND CERVICAL TRACHEAL STENOSIS

Pathophysiology

Because the subglottis is surrounded by a firm cartilaginous structure, and the mucosa lies over the surface with only a normal submucosa for support of the epithelium, the area is particularly prone to injury from surgical manipulation or intubation, reflux disease, and autoimmune disease. Injury to the mucosa by any one of the prior processes can lead to exposure of the perichondrium, which then responds with inflammation and scar tissue formation. The scar tissue impedes airflow and mucus clearance, which can create a fixed extrathoracic airway obstruction.

The cervical trachea is most commonly injured through intervention from prolonged intubation (eFig. 70.1) or tracheotomy. Again, sloughing of mucosa from traumatic manipulation due to a movement of an endotracheal tube or repetitive deep suctioning can lead to exposure of the cartilage with inflammation and secondary collapse. Neoplasia of the minor salivary glands or squamous mucosa can also lead to obstruction.

Diagnosis

The diagnosis of subglottic or cervical tracheal stenosis is made on the basis of the patient's medical history, surgical history, and symptoms. The symptoms are primarily dyspnea on exertion and stridor heard on inspiration and on expiration. If the patient has had a prior intubation or tracheotomy, the possibility of physical obstruction due to scarring should be considered. If a patient has known granulomatosis with polyangiitis, consideration should be given to involvement of the subglottic mucosa with inflammation, vasculitis, and granuloma formation (eFig. 70.2). In the case of idiopathic subglottic stenosis, patients are often treated for reactive airways disease without success.[213] These patients will benefit from early endoscopy/visualization of the subglottic region rather than weeks to months of ineffective treatment. As the name implies, there is no known cause for idiopathic subglottic stenosis. It has been presumed to be autoimmune, and the relationship with extraesophageal reflux disease is established, but the causal nature is unknown.[208,214] Because idiopathic subglottic stenosis is found almost exclusively in women, some authors have proposed a hormonal cause.

High-resolution CT imaging (see eFigs. 70.1 and 70.2) and/or three-dimensional reconstruction of the CT images may help in diagnosis and characterization of the stenotic airway segment. But these imaging modalities are not always available and, even if available, they may miss a short area of obstruction. Pulmonary function tests will demonstrate a characteristic plateau on the flow-volume curve (see Fig. 32.2, right panel), and the measured maximal flow can provide an estimate of the functional diameter of the flow-limiting segment (see eFig 32.3).

The diagnosis of stenosis is confirmed with endoscopic visualization of the area. Endoscopy of the subglottis and cervical trachea for confirmation of stenosis is easily accomplished with a transnasal scope in the office setting using local anesthesia. Lidocaine (4%) can be applied topically to the nose and can also be sprayed onto the vocal fold from above with a curved cannula or from below by injecting it percutaneously into the subglottis and asking the patient to cough. Then the flexible scope can be passed through the vocal folds and the area evaluated.

Treatment

Surgery is the primary mode of treatment of subglottic and cervical tracheal stenosis. The type of surgery, either endoscopic or open, and the use of adjuvant agents, such as steroid injections, or fibroblast activity inhibitors, such as mitomycin C, depend in part on the cause and characteristics of the stenosis. Usually treatment begins with an endoscopic approach. Rigid endoscopy allows palpation of the area to determine the nature of the scar tissue and the length of the segment of the airway that is involved. If the segment is relatively short (<1.5 cm in length), occludes less than 50% of the airway diameter, and is primarily soft tissue in nature, it will likely respond to endoscopic incision and dilation and/or balloon dilation performed in a nontraumatic manner.[215] The incisions, which can be made with either cold steel or a laser, control the area of injury and allow the surgeon to identify the nature of the stenosis without further injury of the cartilaginous airway support. If the laser is used injudiciously, however, the surgeon can create more injury and damage to the cartilage. New-generation lasers have a very short pulse structure, resulting in minimal heat dissipation into the tissue beyond what is seen. Once the extent of the stenosis is identified, the surgeon can use that information to decide on the amount of dilation that the area will accept. The area is then dilated with a balloon to the appropriate size.

For very short stenotic segments or webs, any technique, such as dilation alone, to break up the web usually works after one or two procedures. When performed with the appropriate technique, the area of stenosis should remain dilated after the procedure during visual inspection. If the area collapses immediately after the dilation, it is unlikely that the procedure will have lasting benefits. In addition to endoscopic incision and dilation, short and relatively discrete segments of cartilage collapse, such as may be seen at a tracheotomy site, can be resected endoscopically. Care should be exercised so that no more than 90 to 120 degrees of trachea are treated at one time. This may necessitate staging of the procedures with two or three attempts to resect the area.[216] The primary goal of endoscopy is to characterize the stenotic segment. If the segment is too long, involves too much cartilage, or collapses immediately after completion of the procedure, it is probably wise to proceed to open resection of the segment.

Acknowledgment

We thank Dr. Mark Courey for his contributions to this chapter in a previous edition of this textbook.

Key Points

- The upper airway contains diverse anatomic structures with a variety of functions that contribute to breathing, vocalization, smell, and taste.
- New-onset anosmia is the most specific early symptom of severe acute respiratory syndrome coronavirus-2 (SARS-CoV-2; COVID-19) infection.
- Asthma and chronic rhinosinusitis with nasal polyps are heterogeneous disorders. Subgroups of each disorder are driven by type 2 inflammation and respond to new biologic therapies.
- Allergic rhinitis and asthma are linked in both pathophysiologic and epidemiologic characteristics. Patients with persistent allergic rhinitis should be screened for asthma, and patients with asthma should be evaluated for allergic rhinitis.
- Although multiple medical therapies demonstrate efficacy in the treatment of allergic rhinitis, immunotherapy is the only approach known to alter the natural history of the disease.
- Asthmatic patients with comorbid chronic sinusitis often experience improvement in both upper and lower airway disease after both medical and surgical treatment of chronic rhinosinusitis.
- In swallowing, the oral cavity creates a bolus of the ingested substance and presents this, in an orderly fashion, to the oropharynx and hypopharynx, where the reflexive portion of swallowing takes place. This requires structural and functional integrity and is under control of the central nervous system.
- The larynx is divided into the supraglottis, glottis, and subglottis and functions to regulate inspiratory and expiratory airflow. During swallowing, the larynx is pulled up and forward, to allow the upper esophageal sphincter to open. The bolus passes through the pyriform sinus and into the esophagus.
- During breathing, the vocal folds normally open for inspiration and then close slightly during exhalation to control the rate of air egress. In paradoxical vocal fold motion disease, it is believed that these actions are reversed. The mechanism for this reversal is unknown. However, behavioral interventions designed to retrain breathing are often beneficial in patients demonstrating this finding.
- Paradoxical vocal fold motion disease can often be confused with asthma, but it is typically unresponsive to medical management.
- The contribution of gastroesophageal reflux disease and extraesophageal reflux disease to respiratory disorders is incompletely understood. Most of the evidence supporting an association is derived from studies that measure patient response to empirical therapy.
- Bilateral vocal fold paralysis, posterior glottic stenosis, and subglottic stenosis can often cause airway obstruction that may be misdiagnosed as asthma. Diagnosis requires suspicion based on events in the patient history and endoscopic evaluation. Treatment is usually surgical and is designed to enlarge the airway.

Key Readings

Abreu NA, et al. Sinus microbiome diversity depletion and *Corynebacterium tuberculostearicum* enrichment mediates rhinosinusitis. *Sci Transl Med.* 2012;4:151ra124.

Bousquet J, et al. Allergic rhinitis and its impact on asthma (ARIA): achievements in 10 years and future needs. *J Allergy Clin Immunol.* 2012;130:1049–1062.

Cao PP, et al. Pathophysiologic mechanisms of chronic rhinosinusitis and their roles in emerging disease endotypes. *Ann Allergy Asthma Immunol.* 2019;122(1):33–40.

Cope EK, et al. Compositionally and functionally distinct sinus microbiota in chronic rhinosinusitis patients have immunological and clinically divergent consequences. *Microbiome.* 2017;5(1):53.

Fokkens WJ, et al. European position paper on rhinosinusitis and nasal polyps 2012. *Rhinol Suppl.* 2012;1–298.

Forrest LA, Husein T, Husein O. Paradoxical vocal cord motion: classification and treatment. *Laryngoscope.* 2012;122:844–853.

Krouse JH, et al. Executive summary: asthma and the unified airway. *Otolaryngol Head Neck Surg.* 2007;136:699–706.

Langmore SE, Schatz K, Olsen N. Fiberoptic endoscopic examination of swallowing safety: a new procedure. *Dysphagia.* 1988;2:216–219.

Murry T, Cukier-Blaj S, Kelleher A, Malki KH. Laryngeal and respiratory patterns in patients with paradoxical vocal fold motion. *Respir Med.* 2011;105:1891–1895.

Orlandi RR, et al. International consensus statement on allergy and rhinology: rhinosinusitis. *Int Forum Allergy Rhinol.* 2016;6(suppl 1):S22–S209.

Rosenfeld RM, et al. Clinical practice guideline (update): adult sinusitis. *Otolaryngol Head Neck Surg.* 2015;152(suppl 2):S1–S39.

Shaker R, Kern M, Bardan E, et al. Augmentation of deglutitive upper esophageal sphincter opening in the elderly by exercise. *Am J Physiol.* 1997;272(6 Pt 1):G1518–G1522.

Complete reference list available at ExpertConsult.com.

71 LARGE AIRWAY DISORDERS

LAKSHMI MUDAMBI, MBBS • MESHELL JOHNSON, MD • SUIL KIM, MD, PHD

INTRODUCTION

The large intrapulmonary airways are the trachea, mainstem bronchi, and right bronchus intermedius. The trachea is a semirigid tube serving as a conduit for the entire tidal volume with each breath. It begins just below the larynx and extends approximately 10 to 16 cm to the main carina. The trachea is closely associated with the esophagus, which travels toward the gastroesophageal junction along the left posterior tracheal border; the thyroid gland, which sits anterolateral to the proximal cervical trachea; major blood vessels (e.g., aortic arch, innominate artery, superior vena cava, azygos vein); and mediastinal lymph nodes.

Like the trachea, the large bronchi are surrounded by smooth muscle, contain cartilage, and do not participate in gas exchange. The tracheobronchial mucosa consists of a ciliated pseudostratified columnar epithelium containing mucus-producing goblet cells, submucosal gland duct openings, and cough receptors and is one of the initial sites of innate defensive responses against inhaled invaders.

The subglottic, proximal one-third of the trachea is extrathoracic, whereas the distal two-thirds of the trachea is intrathoracic. The trachea contains 16 to 22 C-shaped cartilage rings anteriorly and laterally, which stiffen the trachea and are connected posteriorly by a membranous wall. The trachealis muscle runs longitudinally along the posterior membrane and is innervated by muscarinic output via the vagus nerve. The posterior membrane is somewhat flexible and moves inward during exhalation.

During cough, the flexible tracheal posterior membrane facilitates dynamic compression of the intrathoracic trachea, reducing tracheal cross-sectional area and increasing cough velocity (see Chapter 37). For example, a 50% decrease in tracheal diameter increases mean linear cough velocity fourfold,[1] improving mucus clearance.

Because the large airways contribute to innate airway host defense via cough and mucociliary clearance, are the site of most of the airflow resistance in airways, and are surrounded by critical mediastinal organs, it is no surprise that the manifestations of large airway disorders are protean and can be serious. Unlike the small airways, which are a "silent zone," the large airways are a common source of symptoms and can be evaluated via pulmonary function testing, imaging, and direct visualization (i.e., flexible bronchoscopy).

Large airway disorders can be classified into two general categories: those that are intrinsic, or within the airway or airway wall, and those that are extrinsic, or outside the airway. In intrinsic disorders, the large airways can become narrowed, fibrotic, thickened, or malacic; in extrinsic disorders, they can be compressed or invaded by benign or malignant lesions of surrounding organs, lymph nodes, or vasculature. The roles of the tracheobronchial airways in innate immune host defense are described in Chapter 15. This chapter focuses on the diagnosis and management of intrinsic and extrinsic large airway disorders.

CLINICAL FEATURES

For tracheal disorders, the most serious signs and symptoms are the acute onset of stridor or wheeze (see Videos 18.12 and 18.6) and respiratory distress suggesting possible life-threatening tracheal obstruction. Although the tracheal lumen diameter is often decreased by greater than 75% (to <5 mm) in patients with stridor or dyspnea at rest, these symptoms also depend on patient-specific factors, such as comorbid cardiac and pulmonary disease, functional status, and activity levels.[2] In a patient at risk of tracheal obstruction (e.g., lung cancer, prolonged intubation), these symptoms should prompt immediate evaluation and treatment, with the primary goal of maintaining a patent airway.

For the large airways, the most common symptoms are cough, sputum production, dyspnea, hemoptysis, and wheeze. Because these symptoms are nonspecific and are also found in patients with inflammatory and infectious

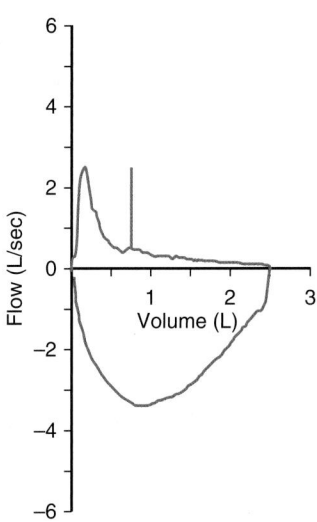

Figure 71.1 Flow-volume loop showing a characteristic rapid decrease in peak expiratory flow due to excessive tracheal collapse. Note that maximal expiratory flow (peak flow) is also reduced. (Courtesy Suil Kim, MD, PhD.)

lower airway diseases (e.g., asthma, COPD, bronchiectasis, pneumonia), large airway disease is often overlooked or misdiagnosed. The key to diagnosing a large airway disorder is having a high index of suspicion. For example, recurrent aspiration, recurrent pneumonia, or cough triggered by eating or drinking should suggest tracheoesophageal fistula in patients with risk factors such as esophageal cancer, tracheal cancer, prolonged intubation, or tracheostomy. In patients with respiratory symptoms suggestive of an obstructive airway disease or infection, the absence of a clinical response to bronchodilators or antibiotics should raise suspicion of a large airway disorder and trigger diagnostic testing rather than additional ineffective treatment.

DIAGNOSTIC APPROACH

The diagnostic approach to a suspected large airway disorder includes spirometry with flow-volume loops, chest imaging, and flexible bronchoscopy.

SPIROMETRY AND FLOW-VOLUME LOOPS

In stable patients, the first step in evaluating a suspected large airway disorder is to obtain spirometry with flow-volume loops, which may reveal plateaus of maximal inspiratory or expiratory airflow that help to localize obstruction (see Chapters 31, 32, and 39). For example, an inspiratory plateau suggests variable extrathoracic obstruction involving the proximal extrathoracic trachea (see Fig. 39.4). An expiratory plateau suggests variable intrathoracic obstruction involving the intrathoracic large airways, as can be seen in tracheobronchomalacia. Plateaus of both inspiratory and expiratory flows suggest fixed tracheal obstruction, as can be seen in tracheal stenosis. Certain features of the flow-volume loop, such as a sudden drop in expiratory flow (Fig. 71.1), plateauing of both inspiratory and expiratory flows, notching of expiratory flow, and oscillations

of expiratory flow (see Fig. 39.3), are highly suggestive of large airway disorders.

The classic curves showing the relationship between driving pressure and airflow through a series of critical orifices (see eFig. 32.3) indicate that the diameter of the tracheal lumen must be reduced to less than 8 mm to produce an abnormal flow-volume loop.[2] The FEV_1 is less sensitive than the flow-volume loop in detecting tracheal obstruction, remaining greater than 90% predicted until the orifice diameter is reduced to 6 mm.[3] Of note, in tracheobronchomalacia, airflow limitation on flow-volume loops does not correlate well with *computed tomography* (CT) evidence of tracheal collapse.[4] In clinical practice, the corollary also applies: CT and airway inspection can suggest near total collapse, while the airflow on flow-volume loops is essentially normal. Spirometry and flow-volume loops should be relied upon to determine if tracheal narrowing is physiologically significant.

CHEST IMAGING

After spirometry and flow-volume loops, chest imaging is the next step in evaluating suspected large airway disorders. Chest radiographs can reveal tracheal dilation (i.e., tracheomegaly or Mounier-Kuhn syndrome) or tracheal narrowing (i.e., saber-sheath trachea) but are rarely diagnostic. CT is the imaging test of choice to evaluate the trachea and large bronchi. An axial CT chest scan without contrast is often adequate to localize tracheobronchial pathology and determine if it is focal or diffuse and intrinsic or extrinsic. Contrast is recommended if there is suspicion for mediastinal tissue impinging on the trachea or bronchi, as in fibrosing mediastinitis, or if there is concern for abnormal venous collateral vessels, as in tracheal varices. Multiplanar or three-dimensional reconstructions can create a more complete visualization of tracheal lesions. Magnetic resonance imaging may provide added benefit in characterizing lesions compressing or invading the trachea, such as mediastinal masses or vascular anomalies.[5] If the history, examination, or flow-volume loops suggest tracheobronchial obstruction or collapse, inspiratory, end-expiratory, and/or dynamic CT images should be obtained to evaluate the tracheal lumen at different parts of the respiratory cycle, which is important in diagnosing *tracheobronchomalacia* (TBM) and *excessive dynamic airway collapse* (EDAC).

BRONCHOSCOPY

The definitive procedure for the diagnosis of large airway disorders is visualization of the airways using a flexible bronchoscope. Many large airways disorders cause characteristic mucosal and structural abnormalities that can be identified on white light (standard) bronchoscopy and diagnosed with endobronchial biopsies. Narrow band imaging, which makes blood vessels appear very dark, may be slightly more sensitive than white light bronchoscopy in detecting dysplasia but has not been routinely incorporated into airway inspections.[6]

Radial probe endobronchial ultrasound can be used to evaluate cartilage integrity and wall thickness in tracheobronchomalacia and to determine if malignancies of adjacent structures, such as the esophagus, are invading the trachea or left mainstem bronchus[7–9] (see Chapter 27). Flexible bronchoscopy can also be used to evaluate the shape and cross-sectional area of the lumen during quiet tidal breathing, forced breathing maneuvers, and cough (a technique termed dynamic bronchoscopy) in patients suspected of having TBM and/or EDAC.[10] For severely obstructed airways, thin and ultrathin bronchoscopes may be able to pass the obstruction safely and allow visualization of the airways distal to the lesion, providing valuable information for planning endobronchial therapy (see Chapter 27). In clinical practice, visual inspection remains the most common method of estimating luminal area and degree of obstruction.[11] Specialized airway sizing tools can be used to measure airway diameter before stent placement.

MANAGEMENT

The decision to treat large airway disease is based on the cause, symptoms, degree of obstruction, and the severity of potential complications. Infections and inflammatory diseases are managed medically unless there is compromise of the airway resulting in respiratory insufficiency. In asymptomatic patients with large airway disorders, regular surveillance is usually indicated. However, significant obstruction, disease progression, and concern for serious complications, such as hemoptysis, should prompt intervention even in patients without symptoms.

Management should be coordinated with a careful strategy to maintain airway patency. Flexible bronchoscopy through a benign or malignant tracheal stenosis can result in complete obstruction and respiratory failure due to edema or bleeding caused by scope trauma or biopsies. Rigid bronchoscopy can minimize these risks by allowing rapid dilation of benign stenosis and coring of malignant obstruction without interruption to ventilation. Endobronchial therapies include laser, microdébrider, electrocautery, airway stents, cryotherapy, and balloon dilation (see Chapter 28). There is growing evidence that endobronchial interventions for simple, benign strictures can produce long-lasting results.[12–15] In patients with life-threatening symptoms, such as massive hemoptysis and respiratory failure due to malignant large airway obstruction, endobronchial therapies can be used to palliate symptoms before definitive surgical resection for early-stage lung cancer or radiation therapy for unresectable disease.

Surgical resection is the definitive treatment for many tracheal diseases such as benign stenosis and localized tracheal tumors. The likelihood of a good surgical outcome depends on the cause of the large airway lesion, the natural history of the disease, whether the surgery is a reoperation, whether there was a previous tracheal appliance, and the location and length of resection (tracheal resections exceeding 4 cm in length are associated with increased anastomotic complications).[16,17]

STENOSIS AND MALACIA

Many large airway disorders decrease the cross-sectional area of the airway lumen, increasing resistance and reducing airflow if driving pressure remains constant.

The term *central airway obstruction* refers to airflow obstruction in the large airways, whereas the terms *tracheobronchial stenosis* and *tracheobronchial malacia* refer to relatively fixed narrowing of the large airways and weakness of the cartilaginous large airway walls, respectively.

STENOSIS

Large airway stenoses can be benign or malignant. They can be intrinsic and caused by exophytic growth into the airways, focal strictures (usually benign), granulation tissue, and airway wall thickening. They can also be extrinsic and caused by compression from structures outside the airways, or they can be both intrinsic and extrinsic (e.g., a combination of exophytic growth and compression). Multiple classification systems for tracheal stenosis based on the degree of obstruction,[18] the location of stenosis,[19] and symptoms, such as dyspnea, change in voice, and dysphagia,[20] or a combination of these features,[21–23] have been developed to facilitate evaluation and treatment of stenosis.

In stenosis, quantifying luminal obstruction is essential for planning interventions, making comparisons over time, and communicating among managing specialists. Numeric visual estimation by bronchoscopy is the most common method for measuring luminal obstruction. CT-based measurements of luminal cross-sectional area reduce interobserver variability and are more reproducible than visual estimates. New machine learning software also improves precision and accuracy of the measurements, but these technologies are not widely available.[11] Because luminal area can vary with the phases of respiration and along the length of the stenosis, it is difficult to measure stenoses reproducibly.

MALACIA

Malacia of the large airways leads to excessive airway collapse, narrowing the airway lumen and reducing airflow. Cartilage weakness causes malacia of the anterolateral cartilaginous walls, whereas laxity of the muscular posterior membrane results in excessive collapse of the posterior wall. Unlike stenosis, malacia of the intrathoracic large airways limits airflow only during expiration. Because standard CT scans are obtained at end-inspiration, and because symptoms of large airway obstruction are nonspecific and can be mistaken for more common obstructive airway diseases such as asthma and COPD, malacia tends to be missed. Suspicion for malacia is often raised by a narrowed tracheal lumen on expiratory CT or by abnormalities in the expiratory flow-volume loop mentioned above (see Figs. 71.1 and 39.3).

Similar to stenosis, the amount of airway collapse due to malacia is measured by CT and visual inspection. Several classification systems have been devised to assist clinicians in diagnosing malacia.[10] However, there may be poor concordance between the degree of collapse, airflow, and symptoms.[24] Thus, malacia can be overlooked in symptomatic patients with airflow limitation and overdiagnosed in patients without these features.

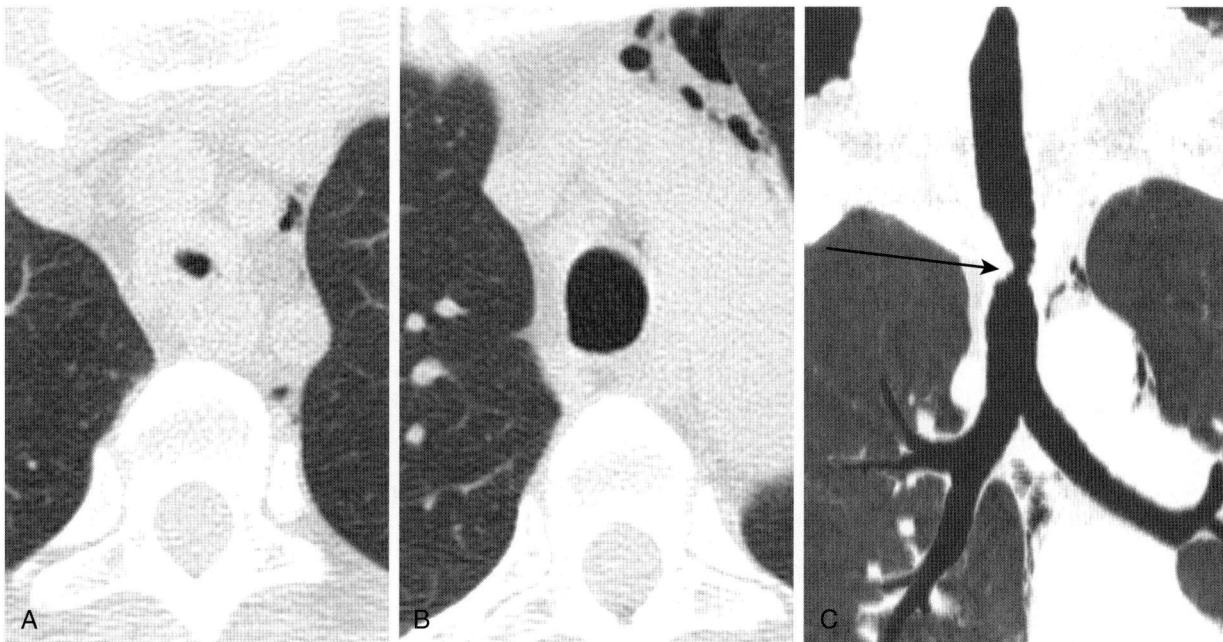

Figure 71.2 Tracheal stenosis. (A) Severe focal narrowing is present in the upper trachea in a patient with postintubation stricture. (B) The tracheal diameter is normal distal to the stricture. (C) Coronal reformatted minimum intensity projection image demonstrates the focal region of narrowing (*arrow*) in the upper trachea. (Courtesy Brett Elicker, MD, Department of Radiology, University of California San Francisco.)

INTRINSIC DISORDERS

For the intrinsic disorders, those primarily causing stenosis or obstruction are discussed before those primarily causing malacia.

BENIGN TRACHEAL STENOSIS

Benign tracheal stenosis is caused by a variety of disorders. Idiopathic laryngotracheal stenosis is characterized by mucosal and submucosal hypertrophy, sparing the cartilage. It is almost exclusively seen in women.[25] Causes of acquired tracheal stenosis include prolonged intubation, tracheostomy, infection, sarcoidosis, and autoimmune disease (e.g., *granulomatosis with polyangiitis* [GPA], ulcerative colitis).

Postintubation tracheal stenosis can result when endotracheal tube cuff pressure exceeds mucosal capillary pressure ($\approx$30 cm H_2O), resulting in mucosal ischemia. If ischemia is prolonged, the mucosa dies via necrosis and becomes fibrotic, causing tracheal stenosis (Fig. 71.2). Risk factors include female sex, obesity, diabetes mellitus, hypertension, and cardiovascular disease.[15]

Posttracheostomy tracheal stenosis results from damage to the tracheal cartilage during tracheostomy placement or from subsequent mucosal injury caused by the tracheostomy tube or cuff. Although the incidence of postintubation tracheal stenosis has decreased with the introduction of low-pressure endotracheal tube cuffs, the incidence of proximal tracheal stenosis has increased as greater numbers of percutaneous tracheostomies are performed.[26] Risk factors include the use of a percutaneous technique, the insertion of a tracheostomy tube size greater than 6, and obesity.[27]

Postinfectious tracheal stenosis is most commonly caused worldwide by tuberculosis. It is estimated that 10–37% of patients with pulmonary tuberculosis develop endobronchial disease at risk of progressing to airway stenosis.[28] Similarly, granulomatous infections with fungus and bacteria such as *Klebsiella rhinoscleromatis*[29] can lead to tracheal stenosis. Infections with human papillomavirus can cause tracheobronchial stenosis as a complication of recurrent respiratory papillomatosis (see later).

Large airway stenosis can be caused by GPA, sarcoidosis, amyloidosis, and inflammatory bowel diseases. The airways are involved in approximately 10–33% of patients with GPA.[30–32] Treatment of stenosis caused by immune or inflammatory disease consists of immune suppression and endobronchial interventions. Surgery can be considered in refractory cases.

When tracheal stenosis is caused by diseases not easily treated medically, the approach depends on several features. First, symptoms such as dyspnea, dysphagia, and dysphonia should be considered as indications for treatment, while asymptomatic patients can often be serially monitored with CT and airway inspection.[19–21] Second, spirometry and flow-volume loops may suggest critical stenosis requiring intervention. Third, CT can define the location and severity of stenosis, which is essential for procedural planning. Finally, flexible bronchoscopy remains the gold standard for characterizing the stenosis and directing therapy.[23]

A decision tool to treat benign tracheal stenosis is shown in Figure 71.3. Simple stenotic lesions (i.e., short-segment concentric stenosis, <1 cm in length, without malacia) can be treated with endobronchial interventions without surgery.[9–12] The optimal treatment for complex stenotic lesions (i.e., many shapes, long segments, >1 cm, with associated malacia) is surgical resection with reconstruction unless the stenosis is located high in the subglottis or is greater than 4 to 6 cm in length.[22] Dilation with or without

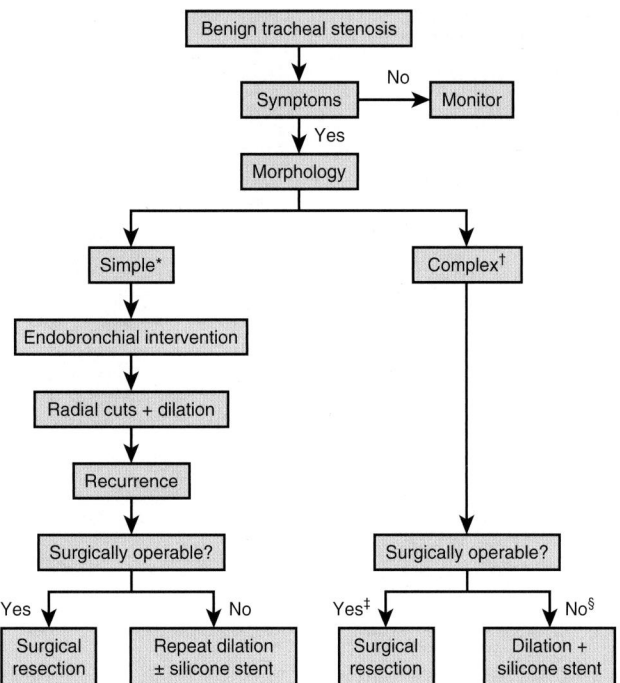

Figure 71.3 Decision tool for benign tracheal stenosis. Management is based on the presence of symptoms, the morphology of the stenosis, and the surgical operability of both the stenotic lesion and the patient. *Simple stenosis: concentric, <1 cm in length, without malacia. †Complex stenosis: many shapes, >1 cm in length, with malacia. ‡1–4 cm in length, not high subglottic, and operable candidate. §>4–6 cm in length, high subglottic, or inoperable candidate.

silicone stent placement may be the only option for patients who are ineligible for or awaiting surgery.

MALIGNANT LARGE AIRWAY DISEASE

Primary tracheal tumors (see Fig. 20.29) are rare, responsible for less than 0.2% of airway neoplasms,[33] and are usually malignant. Squamous cell carcinoma and adenoid cystic carcinoma account for approximately two-thirds of tracheal tumors.[34] Less common primary tracheal tumors include mucoepidermoid carcinoma and pleomorphic adenoma, indolent tumors that can invade locally and metastasize. Pulmonary carcinoid tumors most often arise in major bronchi but can rarely be found in the trachea.[35]

Squamous cell carcinomas generally affect men in their 60s. Adenoid cystic carcinomas show no gender predilection and present in a younger population (≈40s). Of interest, although smoking is associated with the development of squamous cell carcinoma of the trachea, it is not a risk factor for adenoid cystic carcinoma. Patients may be asymptomatic, with the lesion detected incidentally, or have symptoms such as chronic cough unresponsive to standard therapy, sputum production, wheezing, dyspnea, hemoptysis, and obstructive pneumonia. Squamous cell carcinoma of the large airways can invade surrounding structures and cause fistulas.

The approach to large airway tumors has two parts. First, complications such as massive hemoptysis or critical tracheobronchial obstruction should be urgently addressed to stabilize the patient.[36] Second, once the patient is stable, staging with *positron emission tomography*

(PET)-CT and invasive lymph node sampling should be expedited to determine optimal treatment. Surgical resection for localized malignant tracheal tumors yields 5- and 10-year survival rates of 39–79% and 18–51%, respectively.[37] For squamous cell carcinoma with nodal involvement, definitive chemotherapy plus radiation is an option. Palliative radiation alone can sometimes relieve symptoms of malignant central airway obstruction. For adenoid cystic carcinoma, the optimal management strategy is not clear, although the cancer is radiosensitive and radiation therapy is used to treat unresectable disease and residual disease after resection. For adenoid cystic carcinoma, complete surgical resection is a more important prognostic factor than nodal staging.[38]

TRACHEOBRONCHOPATHIA OSTEOCHONDROPLASTICA

Tracheobronchopathia osteochondroplastica (TPO) is a benign disorder of the trachea and mainstem bronchi. It is characterized by submucosal cartilaginous or bony nodules that connect to airway cartilage and protrude into the lumen of the large airways, sparing the posterior wall. The exact prevalence is unknown because it rarely causes symptoms and is often detected incidentally on imaging or bronchoscopy performed for other reasons. The etiology remains unknown, although associations with chronic inflammation, atrophic rhinitis, mycobacterial disease, and immunoglobulin A deficiency have been reported.[39-42] When present, symptoms include cough, dyspnea, wheeze, and recurrent airway infections, which may be mistaken for asthma or chronic bronchitis.[43] Large nodules can cause hemoptysis, lobar obstruction, and postobstructive pneumonia.[44] If located in the subglottis, nodules can lead to hoarseness and sore throat.

CT images show calcified nodules arising from cartilage rings in the anterolateral walls of the large airways (Fig. 71.4A). The posterior tracheal wall is spared, a key feature that distinguishes TPO from other causes of tracheal nodules, such as amyloidosis, sarcoidosis, fibromas, and carcinomas. TPO is diagnosed by recognizing submucosal nodules along the cartilaginous tracheal wall during airway inspection (see Fig. 71.4B). Biopsy is not required for diagnosis and is often unsuccessful because the nodules are heavily calcified. If biopsied, nodules reveal cartilaginous and osseous metaplasia.

The goal of treatment is to ameliorate symptoms. In rare cases of severe tracheobronchial obstruction (see Fig. 71.4C), therapeutic options include forceps removal, laser extraction, cryotherapy, external beam radiation, stent placement and, if endobronchial therapies are unsuccessful, surgical resection.[45,46] Tracheostomy has also been performed as a last resort when endobronchial interventions have failed.

TRACHEOBRONCHIAL AMYLOIDOSIS

Amyloidosis is characterized by the extracellular deposition of fibrillar protein in insoluble β-pleated sheets. Causes include chronic inflammation, plasma cell dyscrasias, heritable mutations that promote fibrillogenesis, and senescence

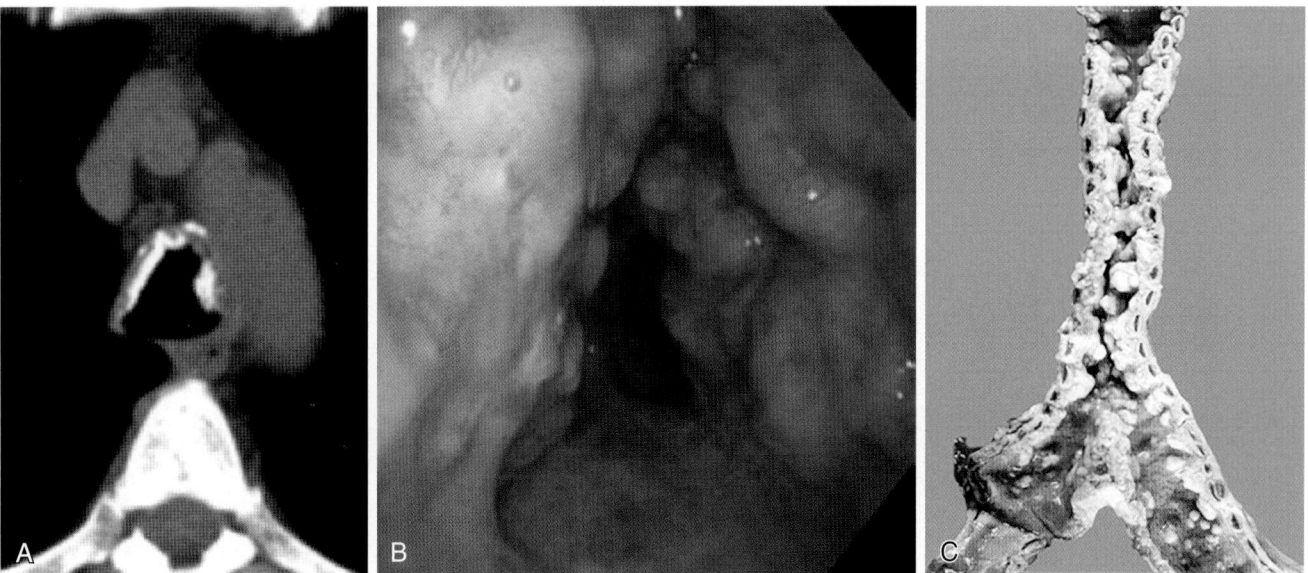

Figure 71.4 Tracheobronchopathia osteochondroplastica. (A) Axial computed tomography displayed in soft tissue windows shows partially calcified nodules involving only the anterior two-thirds of the trachea. (B) Airway inspection in the same patient shows submucosal nodules arising from the anterior tracheal wall and sparing the posterior wall. (C) Gross tracheal specimen from autopsy performed on a different patient shows extensive calcified and ossified nodules throughout the tracheal wall. (A–B, Courtesy Russell Miller, MD, Pulmonary Department, Naval Medical Center, San Diego. C, Courtesy Martha Warnock, MD, Department of Pathology, University of California San Francisco.)

(in senile systemic amyloidosis). Amyloidosis can be systemic or localized to a particular organ.[47] There are few data in the literature to determine the incidence or prevalence of systemic amyloidosis. A small Mayo Clinic study from Olmsted County, Minnesota, cited a yearly incidence of 5.1 to 12.8 per million person-years,[48,49] whereas a study from the United Kingdom estimated the incidence there at just more than 8.0 per million inhabitants per year.[50] Numbers for localized disease are more difficult to acquire.

Amyloid involvement of the respiratory tract is uncommon. Pulmonary amyloidosis can present as one of five subtypes: tracheobronchial, nodular (solitary or multiple), senile pulmonary, mediastinal-hilar, or diffuse interstitial.[51] *Tracheobronchial amyloidosis* (TBA) is a rare idiopathic disorder not typically associated with systemic or lung parenchymal amyloidosis.[52] As such, there is typically no association with other disease entities, such as plasma cell dyscrasias for primary or immunoglobulin light-chain amyloidosis, or inflammatory conditions, such as rheumatoid arthritis for secondary or serum amyloid protein A amyloidosis. Similarly, it is not known if there are any precipitants of this form of amyloid. TBA is estimated to account for only 1.1% of all amyloidoses.[53] The peak age of onset is 50 to 60 years of age, and it is equally prevalent in men and women.[51,54] Symptoms of TBA often go unnoticed because they are nonspecific and can include cough, dyspnea, hoarseness, or hemoptysis, leading to delays in diagnosis. Patients are often treated for recurrent pneumonia, asthma, or tracheobronchitis before the correct diagnosis is made.[47]

Amyloid is deposited in the submucosal tissue plane of the large airway circumferentially and can be associated with calcifications. CT images show diffuse circumferential wall thickening and nodularity of the trachea and mainstem bronchi (Fig. 71.5A).[55] The differential diagnosis includes infectious laryngotracheitis, radiation injury, submucosal tumor spread, and TPO. Flexible bronchoscopy

reveals diffuse mucosal edema and hyperemia, friable mucosa, or small nodules or masses occluding the trachea and mainstem bronchi (see Fig. 71.5B).[54] TBA lesions can be sessile, nodular, or polypoid. Sessile lesions are hard, yellow plaques that can cause airway stenosis if distributed diffusely. Nodular or polypoid lesions are firm and nonmobile with overlying hypervascular mucosa, which is friable and is often mistaken for malignancy. Endobronchial biopsy of amyloid lesions reveals amorphous hyaline material, positive Congo red staining, and yellow-green birefringence under polarized light.[52,56]

The goal of TBA treatment is maintaining a patent airway. Endobronchial interventions, such as *neodymium-doped yttrium aluminum garnet* (Nd:YAG) laser, argon plasma coagulation, stent placement, freezing, and resection, can be used singly or in combination to keep the large airways patent (see Chapter 28). Radiation therapy has been shown to slow the progression of TBA and is now considered a first-line therapy in patients with bulky or distal disease not amenable to endobronchial intervention.[56,57] The efficacy of various systemic therapies (e.g., corticosteroids, colchicine, autologous hematopoietic stem cell transplantation) is unclear.[53] Surgical resection should be considered for localized TBA if endobronchial or radiation therapy interventions have failed.

INFECTIONS

Infections can cause large airway obstruction and stenosis as a sequela of acute inflammation and scarring.[58] During the acute phase of infection, edema and necrosis can lead to airway obstruction with thickening of the airway walls and irregular luminal narrowing. Subsequent healing of these infections can result in fibrosis and stenosis. Although numerous agents cause infections in the respiratory tract, few have been linked to the development of tracheal stenosis.

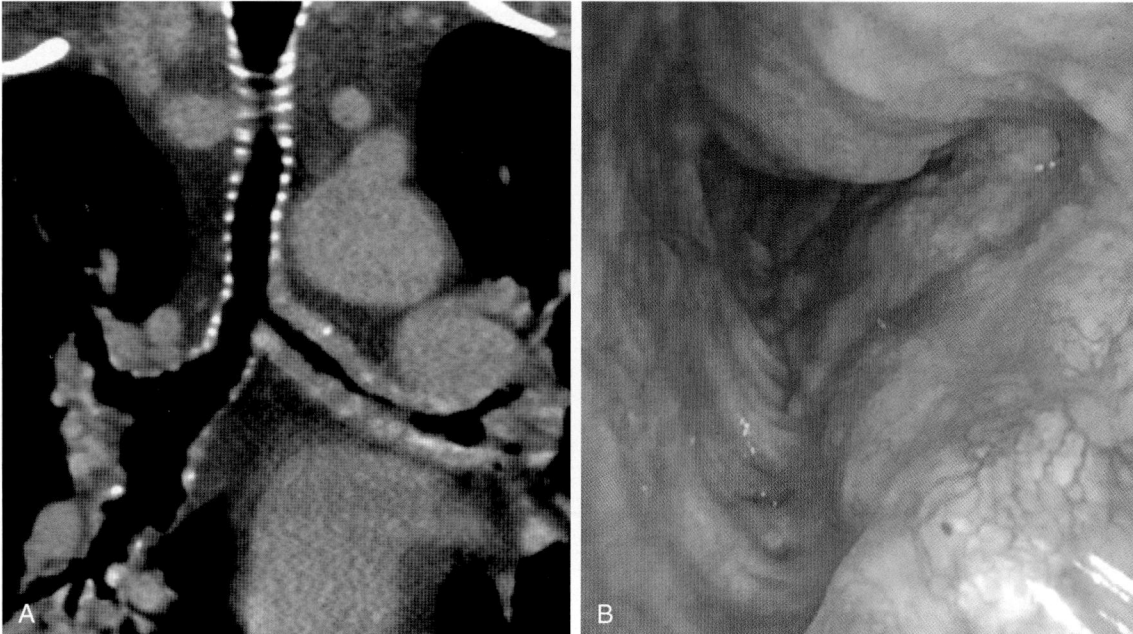

Figure 71.5 Tracheobronchial amyloidosis. (A) Coronal computed tomography displayed in soft-tissue windows shows diffuse circumferential thickening and irregularity of the left mainstem bronchus. (B) Airway inspection in the same patient shows hyperemic and thickened mucosa circumferentially with small nodules and sessile, yellow plaques narrowing the bronchial lumen. (Courtesy Lakshmi Mudambi, MD.)

Tuberculosis

Endobronchial tuberculosis is common,[59] and tracheobronchial stenosis has been reported in up to 90% of patients with endobronchial tuberculosis despite adequate treatment. In rare cases, airway stenosis can be the sole manifestation of infection. The most common symptom of tracheal tuberculosis is intractable cough.[59] CT images show circumferential tracheal thickening, deformation of the tracheal rings, and tracheal stenosis.[60] The presence of mediastinitis suggests active tuberculosis. Airway inspection reveals mucosal ulcers, surrounding erythema and edema, and hyperplastic inflammatory polyps.[61]

Fungal Infections

Fungal infections in immunosuppressed patients also cause large airway stenosis but are difficult to diagnose. *Aspergillus fumigatus* and, to a lesser extent, mucormycosis have been found to cause tracheobronchial infection[58,62] in patients at high risk for fungal infections, such as solid-organ transplant recipients or those with hematologic malignancies or neutropenia, or on immunosuppressive medication.[63] CT images may show parenchymal involvement in addition to irregular tracheal thickening. Flexible bronchoscopy can reveal white plaques, hyperemic mucosa, "sticky" secretions suggestive of fungal disease, and evidence of airway necrosis given the angioinvasive nature of these organisms.[64] White material may represent calcium deposited by the *Aspergillus* (see Fig. 26.3B). Biopsy of the plaques can be diagnostic[65] in the correct clinical setting of a severely immunocompromised patient with respiratory complaints in the absence of other pathogens. If the lesion fails to respond to appropriate antifungals, the resulting stenosis can be treated endobronchially using tracheal balloon dilation,[66] laser therapy, cryotherapy, stent placement, and surgical resection (see Chapter 28).

Bacterial Infections

Bacterial infections localized to the large airways are often overlooked because most instances of tracheitis or tracheobronchitis also involve concomitant infection of the lower respiratory tract. One organism associated with tracheal infections leading to obstruction and stenosis is *Klebsiella rhinoscleromatis*. *K. rhinoscleromatis* primarily infects the nares and paranasal sinuses but can also cause infection in the upper airway and trachea. The diagnosis is made by identifying the pathognomonic Mikulicz cells in the nodules of rhinoscleroma; these cells are round or oval macrophages with small nuclei that contain the causative bacterium, *K. rhinoscleromatis*.[67] This indolent infection is endemic in Africa, South America, and other developing countries and is quite rare in the developed world. Tracheal infection with *K. rhinoscleromatis* can ultimately lead to a chronic granulomatous infection resulting in diffuse tracheal stenosis.[29,68] Treatment may require surgical intervention for obstructing lesions and long-term antimicrobial therapy.

Respiratory Papillomatosis

Recurrent respiratory papillomatosis presents in a juvenile or an adult form (see Chapter 78). The juvenile form is caused by perinatal infection with *human papillomavirus* (HPV) and presents in childhood.[69] It is characterized by multiple benign airway papillomas and recurs frequently. HPV subtypes 6 and 11 cause greater than 90% of cases, whereas infection with subtypes 16 and 18 increases risk of malignant transformation to squamous cell carcinoma (see eFig. 78.25).[70] The adult form is more common in men and in smokers and is caused by HPV transmitted via oral sex.[71] In the adult-onset form, papillomas tend to be solitary or multilobulated and rarely recur after resection (see Fig. 26.3C).

Symptoms are nonspecific and include cough, dyspnea, wheeze and, if the larynx is involved, hoarseness. Rarely, respiratory papillomatosis can lead to critical tracheal obstruction. Endobronchial resection (see Chapter 28) and adjuvant medical therapy are the mainstays of treatment. Intralesional cidofovir, an antiviral nucleotide analogue, and bevacizumab, a vascular endothelial growth factor inhibitor, have shown promise in the treatment of recurrent, severe, or obstructive tracheobronchial papillomas.[72–74]

INFLAMMATORY

Granulomatous inflammatory diseases, such as sarcoidosis, inflammatory bowel disease, and GPA, and autoimmune conditions, such as relapsing polychondritis, can target the tracheobronchial tree. Scarring often results from the edema and necrosis seen with inflammation, causing stenosis. Chronic airway inflammation can also weaken cartilage, leading to tracheobronchial malacia.

Relapsing Polychondritis

Relapsing polychondritis is a rare autoimmune disorder characterized by inflammation of cartilage in the ears, nose, joints, and large airways. The airways are involved in about 50% of cases and account for about 10% of deaths.[55] The larynx and trachea are the most common sites of airway involvement. Repeated episodes of tracheal chondritis can lead to tracheal obstruction due to tracheomalacia and/ or tracheal stenosis. When smaller bronchi are involved, the respiratory phenotype is less severe than with tracheal disease.[75]

Spirometry and flow-volume loops may reveal plateaus of maximal airflow suggestive of tracheal obstruction (see "Diagnostic Approach" earlier), especially when cartilage fibrosis leads to tracheal stenosis. Of note, relapsing polychondritis does not cause a diffusion defect. CT images (see Fig. 20.30) reveal thickened cartilage in the cartilaginous tracheal wall with sparing of the posterior membrane (see Fig. 92.6). The parenchyma is also spared. PET scans may reveal high activity in tracheal cartilage, helping to distinguish between active and fibrotic lesions. Flexible bronchoscopy can delineate the degree of stenosis or malacia.

The mainstay of treatment is immunosuppression with systemic corticosteroids. Biologics have been studied, but the numbers of treated patients are small and the results inconsistent[76] (see Chapter 92). Stepwise treatment with positive pressure ventilation, tracheal stenting, and tracheostomy should be considered if tracheal obstruction due to relapsing polychondritis worsens despite maximal medical treatment.

Sarcoidosis

Sarcoidosis is characterized by the formation of noncaseating granulomas in one or more organs. The lung is involved in greater than 90% of sarcoidosis patients, with endobronchial involvement approaching 70%. In contrast, tracheal involvement is uncommon, seen in only 1–3% of all pulmonary cases.[28,77] In the trachea, sarcoidosis can present as intrinsic granulomatous infiltration or extrinsic compression from enlarged mediastinal lymph nodes. The proximal one-third of the trachea is more commonly affected than the distal trachea or lower airways.[28] Symptoms are nonspecific and include cough, dyspnea,

and wheeze. Bronchoscopic findings include cobblestone mucosa and whitish granulomatous material in areas of stenosis (see Fig. 26.2C). Like other forms of sarcoid, tracheal sarcoid is treated with systemic steroids. If there is evidence of reversible airway obstruction on spirometry, inhaled corticosteroids or bronchodilators may be considered[78] (see Chapter 93).

Granulomatosis with Polyangiitis

GPA is a necrotizing granulomatous vasculitis affecting small blood vessels in the upper and lower airways and kidneys (see Chapter 87). GPA has been reported to involve the tracheobronchial tree in 12–23% of patients.[30,31] Of interest, although GPA affects women and men equally, greater than 90% of patients with GPA-related tracheal stenosis are women.[79] The reason for this female predominance is unknown. GPA should also be considered in patients with unexplained hemoptysis (see Chapter 40).

CT images in patients with tracheal GPA show circumferential, smooth, or nodular mucosal thickening (see eFig. 70.2), irregular borders, and ulceration.[80] Although not commonly involved, the cartilage rings can be narrowed and deformed. Flexible bronchoscopy may reveal subglottic stenosis, tracheal stenosis, tracheal ulcers, and inflammatory pseudopolyps. Transbronchial biopsy is insensitive, revealing histopathologic features diagnostic of GPA in less than 20% of specimens.[30,81] In some patients, a presumptive diagnosis of an *antineutrophil cytoplasmic autoantibody*–associated vasculitis, such as GPA, can be made if the clinical picture and positive antineutrophil cytoplasmic antibody argue against an alternative etiology. Treatment depends on the seriousness of the disease. Severe tracheobronchial disease often responds to systemic treatment with the combination of corticosteroids together with either cyclophosphamide or rituximab. If tracheobronchial stenosis persists or recurs despite prolonged immunosuppressive therapy, endobronchial therapies, including tracheal dilation, conservative laser surgery, and stenting, should be considered.[82]

Inflammatory Bowel Disease

Pulmonary manifestations of inflammatory bowel disease are uncommon, and tracheal involvement is even rarer, reportedly as low as 0.2% for ulcerative colitis and 0.4% for Crohn disease.[83] Ulcerative colitis can manifest as a tracheobronchitis, producing dyspnea and hoarseness. CT scanning shows tracheobronchial wall thickening, and flexible bronchoscopy reveals tracheobronchial ulcers in the mucosa, severe luminal narrowing, and cobblestoning. If biopsied, the ulcers show necrosis with submucosal inflammation characterized by lymphoplasmacytic infiltration within the epithelium and lamina propria without granuloma formation.[84] Infection must be excluded. Exacerbations of the gastrointestinal and pulmonary systems often happen simultaneously, quite possibly due to their common embryologic tissue origin.[84] Crohn disease results in extraintestinal manifestations more often than ulcerative colitis but, similarly, pulmonary involvement is rare and can present as tracheitis, tracheobronchitis, or tracheal stenosis.[85] Treatment with high-dose corticosteroids is often successful.

BRONCHOLITHIASIS

Broncholithiasis is characterized by calcified material eroding into the tracheobronchial lumen, leading to inflammation and obstruction of the airway.[86] Most often, the calcified material is a calcified lymph node, often the result of earlier granulomatous infection, endemic fungal diseases such as *Histoplasma capsulatum*, or the result of silicosis.[87,88] Alternatively, broncholiths can originate from aspirated foreign material that has calcified within the tracheobronchial lumen, calcified endobronchial hamartomas, carcinoid tumors, or calcified tracheal cartilage rings that protrude into the lumen.[89] Clinically, broncholithiasis can range from being asymptomatic to causing cough, lithoptysis (expectoration of calcified material), postobstructive pneumonia, and hemoptysis. In severe cases, erosion of the broncholith into the tracheobronchial lumen can lead to a bronchoesophageal fistula.[90] Although chest radiographs may show calcifications within clusters of lymph nodes, diagnosis is most often made by CT scan (see eFig. 56.4). Bronchoscopy can sometimes miss the lesion if the broncholith only partially erodes into the airway.

Treatment is conservative if the patient is asymptomatic or has minimal symptoms, such as an infrequent cough. This involves cough suppression and treatment of any pneumonias. If the symptoms escalate, more definitive therapy is warranted, which can include bronchoscopy to evaluate the broncholith and facilitate its removal. If removal by forceps is not possible, bronchoscopy with Nd:YAG lasers (bronchoscopic lithotripsy) may be effective. If these methods are unsuccessful, surgery can be considered but should be reserved for those who are symptomatic and have not responded to endobronchial therapy.[87,91]

VASCULAR MALFORMATIONS

Tracheal varices are rare but are important to recognize because they are potential sources of massive hemoptysis if biopsied. They can be caused by obstruction of the pulmonary veins or of the superior vena cava due to pulmonary venous hypertension, portal hypertension, congenital cardiac diseases, or mediastinal masses.[92,93] In addition to hemoptysis, patients may present with symptoms of the underlying cause of the varices (e.g., superior vena cava syndrome). Diagnosis is made by bronchoscopy in the setting of hemoptysis or incidentally during bronchoscopy performed for another reason. Airway inspection reveals tracheal varices that appear as polypoid tracheal nodules along with dilated mucosal vessels. Tracheal varices should be suspected in patients with hemoptysis, tracheal nodules, and mediastinal collateral vessels on CT, a feature that distinguishes tracheal varices from other causes of tracheal nodules, such as amyloidosis and sarcoidosis. As mentioned, magnetic resonance imaging may be useful for identifying and mapping vascular abnormalities.

TRACHEOBRONCHOMALACIA AND EXCESSIVE DYNAMIC AIRWAY COLLAPSE

Tracheobronchomalacia (TBM) refers to weakness of the cartilaginous anterolateral walls of the trachea and mainstem bronchi. It is caused by cartilage breakdown that results in loss of structural rigidity and excessive collapse of the trachea and large bronchi during exhalation. In contrast, *excessive dynamic airway collapse* (EDAC) refers to exaggerated bulging of the posterior tracheal membrane into the airway lumen during exhalation. Both TBM and EDAC can cause severe, symptomatic upper airway obstruction and may present individually or together in the same patient.

In adults, TBM is most often acquired. Causes include chronic airway inflammation due to chronic bronchitis,[94] cystic fibrosis,[95] and gastroesophageal reflux[96]; cartilage inflammation due to relapsing polychondritis[97]; chronic extrinsic compression by adjacent structures, such as thyroid goiters[98] or tumors; cartilage necrosis induced by endotracheal and tracheostomy tubes[99]; and radiation. Tracheobronchomegaly (Mounier-Kuhn syndrome) can also cause TBM. In contrast, EDAC, which is mainly found in patients with chronic obstructive airway diseases, is thought to be caused by an increased transmural pressure gradient during exhalation[10] and by weakening of the muscular posterior membrane.[100]

Because symptoms due to TBM and EDAC are nonspecific (e.g., cough, dyspnea, recurrent airway infections), diagnosis requires a high index of suspicion and focused testing. As mentioned, flow-volume loops may show a rapid decline of expiratory flow after a sharp peak suggestive of large airway collapse (see Fig. 71.1) or signs of notching or oscillations of the expiratory flow (Fig. 39.3) to suggest the diagnosis; however, they are not by themselves diagnostic.[101,102] Traditionally, TBM and EDAC have been diagnosed when the cross-sectional tracheal area measured by bronchoscopy or dynamic CT (Figs. 71.6A–B) decreases by greater than 50% during forced exhalation as a result of exaggerated cartilaginous collapse (TBM; see Fig. 71.6C), posterior bulging into the lumen (EDAC; see Fig. 71.6D), or an overlap of both TBM and EDAC.[103–105] However, in many healthy control subjects without these conditions, their trachea collapses posteriorly by 50% or more on forced exhalation,[24] indicating that this threshold is inadequate to define abnormal collapse. Instead, tracheal collapse requiring treatment usually approaches 95–100% during forced exhalation[10,106,107] (see Fig. 39.3). Thus, reduced maximal expiratory flow rates and the appearance of the flow-volume curve, although not diagnostic, may be better indicators of clinically significant collapse than visual assessment.

The decision to treat TBM or EDAC should be based on the presence of symptoms due to excessive tracheal collapse. In an asymptomatic patient, treatment is generally not indicated. In a symptomatic patient, treatment of the underlying cause (e.g., bronchodilators and airway hygiene for COPD, steroids for relapsing polychondritis) may ameliorate symptoms. If medical management is ineffective, continuous positive airway pressure can pneumatically stent the airway open, reducing dynamic airway collapse and facilitating mucus clearance.[108,109] Airway stents[110,111] and surgery,[107] including tracheobronchoplasty (splinting of the posterior membrane with a polypropylene mesh or acellular dermis[113]) or tracheobronchial resection and reconstruction, can be considered in very symptomatic patients who do not respond to noninvasive treatment and have focal tracheobronchial disease. A successful stent trial helps identify patients who will benefit from surgical airway stabilization via tracheoplasty.[107] Successful endoscopic therapy

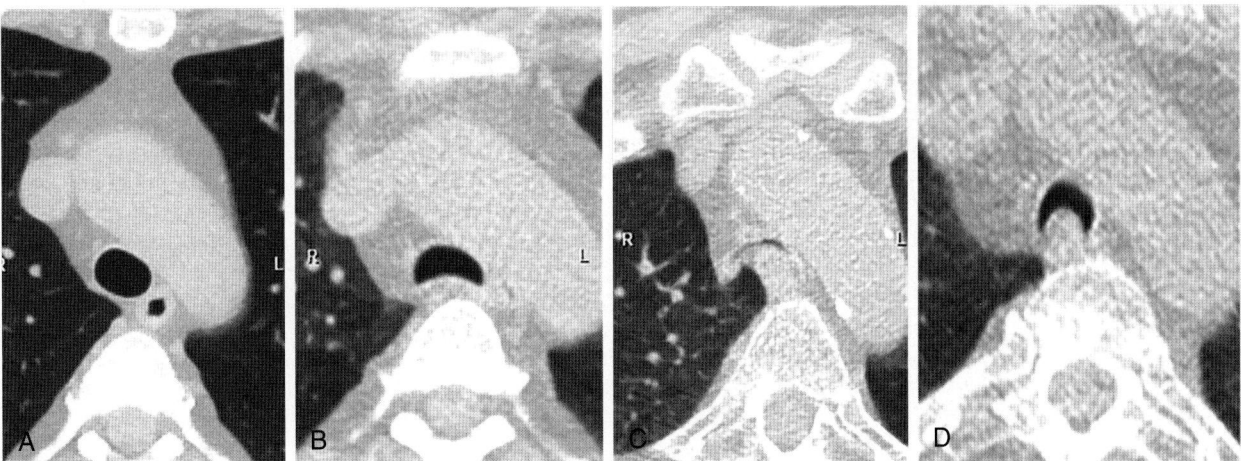

Figure 71.6 Tracheomalacia and *excessive dynamic airway collapse* (EDAC). (A–B) Normal, paired *computed tomography* (CT) images through the midtrachea at the level of the aortic arch show a normal trachea at full inspiration (A) and end-exhalation (B). The posterior tracheal membrane normally bows inward slightly at end-exhalation. (C) Tracheomalacia. The CT image shows excessive flattening of the anterolateral cartilaginous walls at end-exhalation. (D) EDAC. The CT image shows excessive bulging of the posterior membrane into the lumen at end-exhalation. (Courtesy Michael B. Gotway, MD.)

to tighten the posterior membrane with laser has also been reported but requires further study.[114]

EXTRINSIC DISORDERS

FIBROSING MEDIASTINITIS

Fibrosing mediastinitis, also termed sclerosing mediastinitis or mediastinal fibrosis, is a rare disease causing external tracheal compression. It is the result of an exaggerated granulomatous response in mediastinal lymph nodes to a variety of pathogens leading to fibrosis, compression, and invasion of adjacent structures, including the trachea, esophagus, and blood vessels (see Chapter 116). Common triggers include *Histoplasma capsulatum* and, to a lesser extent, *Mycobacterium tuberculosis*.[115] *Aspergillus flavus*, sarcoidosis, and immunoglobulin G4-related disease have also been reported to cause fibrosing mediastinitis.[116,117]

In addition to tracheal compression, the most serious complication of fibrosing mediastinitis is pulmonary arterial and venous obstruction (see Fig. 116.5). Most patients with fibrosing mediastinitis have unilateral disease and can remain undiagnosed for years because symptoms are nonspecific. Chest radiographs can reveal a widened mediastinum due to mediastinal adenopathy and fibrosis, but CT with contrast is indicated to assess the degree of mediastinal involvement along with the extent of airway narrowing and vascular compromise. Bronchoscopy can reveal narrowing of the tracheal lumen and massive tracheal variceal formation along the posterior tracheal wall if superior vena cava syndrome is present. There are no standard treatment options, but therapy focuses predominantly on symptomatic management, including stenting of arteries and veins.

FISTULAS

Tracheoesophageal fistulas (TEFs) are abnormal congenital or acquired connections between the trachea and esophagus. This section focuses on the acquired form, which is most often caused by esophageal or lung cancer. From 5–15% of patients with esophageal cancer and 1% of patients with lung cancer develop TEFs.[118–120] Less common, TEFs are caused by benign

conditions, such as prolonged intubation, tracheostomy, surgery, and radiation. Symptoms include cough with eating or drinking, recurrent pneumonia, recurrent aspiration, dysphagia, and malnutrition. In TEF due to cancer, survival has been reported to be a few weeks to months.[121–123]

Airway inspection is indicated in patients when symptoms, barium esophagram, or CT imaging suggest TEF. The fistula may be visible with heaped, irregular margins and secretions from the esophagus escaping into the trachea (Fig. 71.7A) and can be associated with significant tracheal stenosis. Small fistulas may be difficult to identify due to local erythema and edema. In such cases, orally administered methylene blue before bronchoscopy can help identify them.[124]

The goal of treatment is blocking the seepage of esophageal and stomach contents into the airways to prevent aspiration-related airway injury and pneumonia and to improve nutrition. This can be attempted by stenting or surgery. In benign TEF, surgical repair with curative intent is the preferred approach because it can produce good long-term results and because stents, while occasionally placed as a bridge to surgery, cannot be placed indefinitely.[125–127] In malignant TEF or in inoperable benign TEF, stenting of the trachea and/or esophagus can ameliorate symptoms and prolong survival.[7,118,121,122] Surgical repair is normally not attempted in malignant TEF because the underlying condition is incurable and because resection does not yield satisfactory results.[120]

To treat TEF, stents can be placed in the trachea, esophagus, or both. An esophageal stent is indicated in patients with esophageal stenosis and no tracheal obstruction. Side effects of esophageal stent placement include gastroesophageal reflux disease and dietary changes needed to maintain stent patency. On occasion, airway obstruction develops after placement of an esophageal stent, requiring removal or revision with or without placement of a tracheal stent.

Tracheal stenting is performed first if the patient has tracheal obstruction, if there is clinical concern for the development of tracheal obstruction after placement of an esophageal stent, or if the esophageal tumor is not causing stenosis (see Fig. 71.7B–E). Tracheal stents are usually well tolerated but may

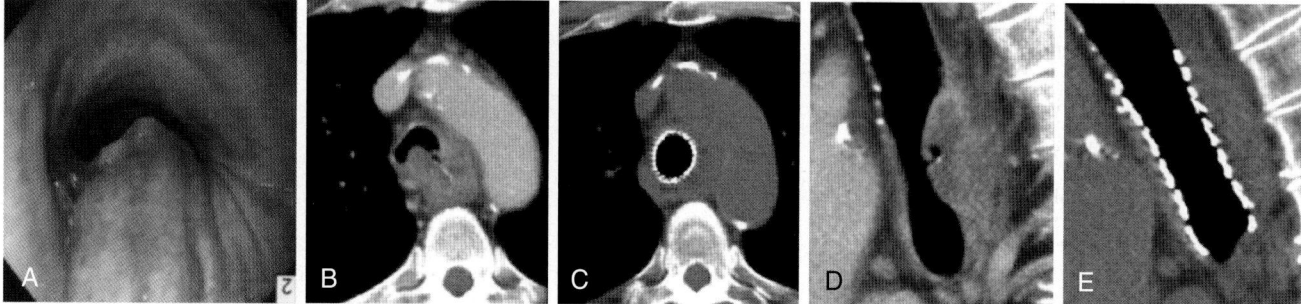

Figure 71.7 Tracheoesophageal fistula. (A) Airway inspection shows a mixed obstruction of the mid-trachea with necrosis and secretions, suggesting a fistula. (B–C) Paired axial computed tomography images show an esophageal mass invading the posterior trachea before (B) and after (C) placement of a covered self-expanding metal stent. (D–E) Paired sagittal computed tomography images clearly show a fistula (D) before stent placement (E). (Courtesy Lakshmi Mudambi, MD.)

produce an intractable cough. Patency is maintained with daily nebulization of bronchodilators and saline solutions.

Double stenting (i.e., placement of a tracheal and esophageal stent) can be considered if the patient has tracheal obstruction and a stenotic esophageal tumor causing dysphagia, a very large fistula not completely occluded by either a tracheal or esophageal stent, or tracheal obstruction that develops after placement of an esophageal stent.[7,128,129] Double stenting can increase the size of the fistula and prevent healing. It should be avoided in patients with potential for cure, surgical correction, or long-term survival.

EMERGING THERAPIES

THREE-DIMENSIONAL PRINTED AIRWAY STENTS

Airway stents are used to maintain tracheal patency and to block fistulous tracts in the trachea (see Chapter 28). In some patients, a deformed trachea can result in poor fit of commercially available stents, leading to complications such as migration, impaired mucus clearance, granulation tissue, and perforation. Three-dimensional printed airway stents address this issue by precisely fitting the patient's trachea. They have recently been approved by the U.S. Food and Drug Administration. The stents are made by injecting medical-grade silicone into a three-dimensional printed mold engineered from three-dimensional CT reconstructions of the patient's trachea.[130] The literature on three-dimensional printed stents is currently limited to case reports, but early results are promising.[131,132]

TRACHEAL REPLACEMENT

Primary tracheal resection with direct end-to-end anastomosis is the definitive treatment for various focal tracheal disorders. The principal limitation is involvement of more than 4 cm of trachea, which significantly increases the risk of anastomotic failure likely due to increased tension on the anastomosis.[16] In patients requiring long tracheal resections, several methods of tracheal replacement (e.g., synthetic prosthetics, allografts, autologous tissue, and tracheal transplantation) have been used to restore function. Currently, none of these methods meets the criteria of an ideal tracheal replacement. Such criteria would include lateral rigidity and stiffness, longitudinal flexibility, air-tightness, support of a functional ciliated respiratory epithelium, biocompatibility, and absence of need for immunosuppression.

Tracheal replacement with synthetic stents,[133,134] aortic allografts reinforced with tracheal stents,[135,136] and cadaveric tracheal allografts[137] has been associated with significant morbidity and mortality. Tracheal allotransplants have been used to reconstruct tracheas in benign tracheal disease.[138,139] This approach is limited by the need for immunosuppression (making it unsuitable for malignant disease), a compromised blood supply (risking necrosis of the transplanted trachea), and the lack of published data on long-term outcomes.[140] In malignant tracheal disease, autologous transplants constructed from fasciocutaneous, omental, or muscle flaps reinforced with strips of cartilage or mesh to simulate cartilage rings have been used in tracheal reconstruction.[141] Artificial tracheas made from biocompatible three-dimensional printed tubular scaffolds and the subject's own pluripotent stem cells have shown promise as tracheal substitutes and are an area of active research.[142]

Key Points

- Because symptoms due to large airway disorders are nonspecific and often mimic those of more common conditions, such as asthma or COPD, the diagnosis of large airway disorders requires a high index of suspicion.
- Spirometry with flow-volume loops, computed tomographic imaging, and flexible bronchoscopy provide complementary information required to evaluate large airway disorders.
- Of the diagnostic tests, flexible bronchoscopy is the gold standard test for the assessment of large airway disorders.
- Surgical resection is the definitive treatment of focal tracheal disease and should be considered in symptomatic patients.
- Endobronchial interventions are first-line therapies for several large airway disorders and can palliate symptoms in nonsurgical disease.
- Intervention for symptomatic tracheal collapse is usually not indicated until collapse approaches 95–100% of cross-sectional area of the trachea during forced exhalation and is supported by finding abnormal expiratory flows on spirometry or flow-volume loop.
- Novel therapeutic approaches, such as three-dimensional printing of tracheal stents and tissue-engineered tracheal replacements, show promise.

Key Readings

Boiselle PM, O'Donnell CR, Bankier AA, et al. Tracheal collapsibility in healthy volunteers during forced expiration: assessment with multidetector CT. *Radiology.* 2009;252:255–262.

Chung JH, Kanne JP, Gilman MD. CT of diffuse tracheal diseases. *AJR Am J Roentgenol.* 2011;196:W240–W246.

Dalar L, Karasulu L, Abul Y, et al. Bronchoscopic treatment in the management of benign tracheal stenosis: choices for simple and complex tracheal stenosis. *Ann Thorac Surg.* 2016;101:1310–1317.

Herth FJ, Peter S, Baty F, Eberhardt R, Leuppi JD, Chhajed PN. Combined airway and oesophageal stenting in malignant airway-oesophageal fistulas: a prospective study. *Eur Respir J.* 2010;36:1370–1374.

Kim SS, Khalpey Z, Hsu C, Little AG. Changes in tracheostomy- and intubation-related tracheal stenosis: implications for surgery. *Ann Thorac Surg.* 2017;104:964–970.

Majid A, Guerrero J, Gangadharan S, et al. Tracheobronchoplasty for severe tracheobronchomalacia: a prospective outcome analysis. *Chest.* 2008;134:801–807.

Miller RD, Hyatt RE. Obstructing lesions of the larynx and trachea: clinical and physiologic characteristics. *Mayo Clin Proc.* 1969;44:145–161.

Mudambi L, Miller R, Eapen GA. Malignant central airway obstruction. *J Thorac Dis.* 2017;9:S1087–S1110.

Murgu S, Colt H. Tracheobronchomalacia and excessive dynamic airway collapse. *Clin Chest Med.* 2013;34:527–555.

Murgu SD, Egressy K, Laxmanan B, Doblare G, Ortiz-Comino R, Hogarth DK. Central airway obstruction: benign strictures, tracheobronchomalacia, and malignancy-related obstruction. *Chest.* 2016;150:426–441.

Prince JS, Duhamel DR, Levin DL, Harrell JH, Friedman PJ. Nonneoplastic lesions of the tracheobronchial wall: radiologic findings with bronchoscopic correlation. *Radiographics.* 2002;22(Spec No):S215–S230.

Wright CD, Grillo HC, Wain JC, et al. Anastomotic complications after tracheal resection: prognostic factors and management. *J Thorac Cardiovasc Surg.* 2004;128:731–739.

Complete reference list available at ExpertConsult.com.

72 BRONCHIOLITIS

JOHN R. GREENLAND, MD, PHD • KIRK D. JONES, MD •
JONATHAN P. SINGER, MD, MS

INTRODUCTION

Although other chapters focus on the major diseases primarily affecting the large intrathoracic airways, including asthma, bronchitis, cystic fibrosis, and bronchiectasis, a constellation of entities primarily affect *peripheral* airways. Early diagnosis of these small airway diseases remains difficult, however. Early in the disease course, the large cross-sectional area and reduced airflow of peripheral airways protect patients from symptoms of dyspnea and limit detection of flow abnormalities on functional testing. Diseases affecting the peripheral airways may nonetheless have profound effects on lung function. Because pathologic narrowing of peripheral airways is difficult to detect, these airways may be considered a silent zone of the lung. Although tests to identify peripheral airway obstruction have suffered from a lack of sensitivity, heightened recognition of the entities affecting peripheral airways and diagnostic advances have increased the frequency of diagnosis. Nevertheless, the epidemiology of disorders of the peripheral airways remains largely unknown.[1] This chapter takes into account the heightened clinical recognition and evolving efforts at classification as our understanding of these entities advances. The chapter first reviews the anatomy of the peripheral airways. The predominantly inflammatory and fibrotic bronchiolitis entities are then addressed, with the recognition that there may be substantial overlap in clinical and histologic features.

ANATOMIC AND PHYSIOLOGIC FEATURES

Among other roles, the intrathoracic airways serve as a conduit between the outside environment and alveolar units. Moving distally from the trachea, the bronchi transition to bronchioles and ultimately to the terminal respiratory units. These transitions are defined by changes in the constellation of cell types and by architectural features.

Bronchi range in size from 10 down to 1 mm in diameter and are characterized by incomplete cartilaginous rings, ciliated epithelium, goblet cells, submucosal glands, and smooth muscle innervated by muscarinic output via the vagus nerve. Bronchioles are defined by their lack of cartilage; their sparse population of ciliated, simple, columnar epithelium and secretory club cells; and their lack of goblet cells and glands. Bronchiolar smooth muscle is not innervated by the vagus nerve, and the diameter of bronchioles typically ranges from 2 down to 0.5 mm. As bronchioles branch, they go from lobular to terminal and then respiratory segments. Terminal bronchioles are the last divisions of conducting airways, whereas alveoli bud from respiratory bronchioles (Table 1.2; see also Chapter 1).

Because of their relatively small total cross-sectional area, bronchi are responsible for most airflow resistance in the lung. In contrast, bronchioles contribute little to total airflow resistance at high and normal lung volumes. This limited contribution is attributable to dichotomous branching that arranges vast numbers of bronchioles in parallel. Within the conducting region of the lung, bronchioles branch into terminal bronchioles, whereas in the respiratory zone, where gas exchange takes place, respiratory bronchioles branch into alveoli. This branching translates into a much larger total cross-sectional area for bronchioles relative to bronchi. At low lung volumes, the relative contribution of bronchioles to total airflow resistance increases because, as residual volume is approached, the flexible, thin-walled bronchioles, supported only by connective tissue, may collapse. Despite significant disease of the bronchioles, however, *pulmonary function test* (PFT) results may be normal. In advanced disease, PFTs may demonstrate upward concavity (curvilinearity) of the flow-volume curve, especially at low lung volumes, an increased slope of phase III (the alveolar plateau) of the single-breath nitrogen washout test, and air trapping. Although mid–*forced expiratory lung flow* ($FEF_{25\%-75\%}$) had been proposed as an early criterion for post–lung transplantation bronchiolitis, subsequent studies have challenged its predictive utility.[2]

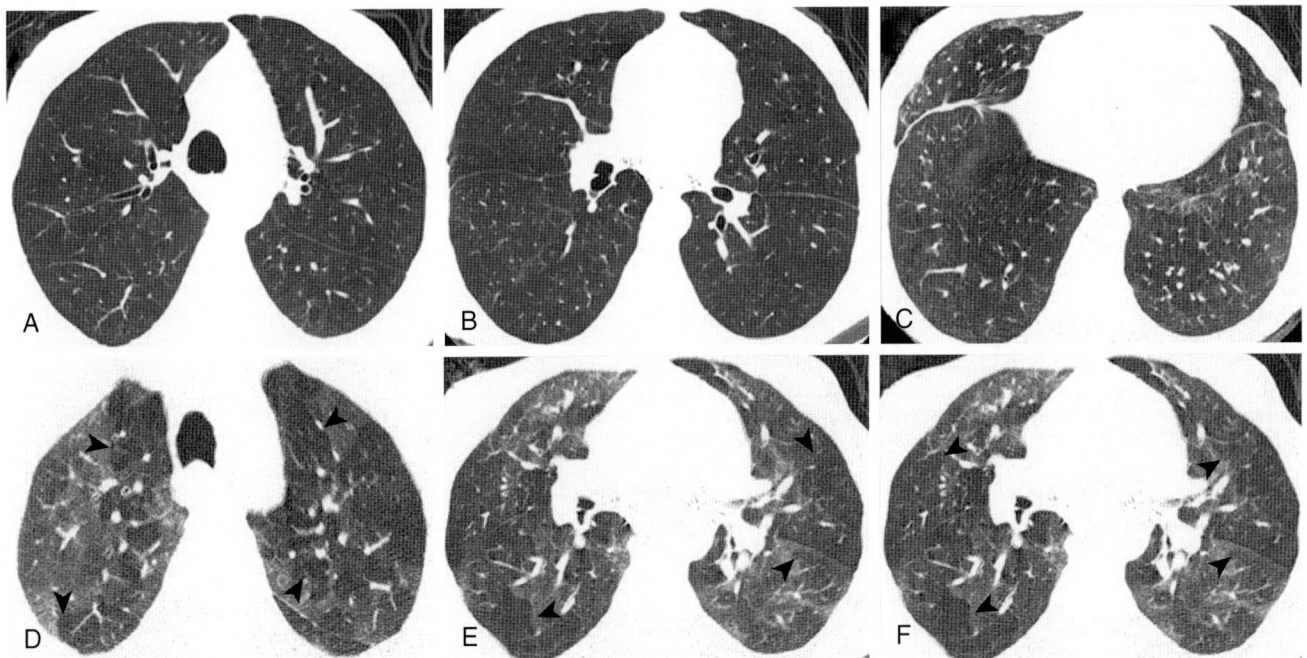

Figure 72.1 **High-resolution *computed tomography* (CT) scan demonstrating air trapping during expiration.** (A–C) Axial chest CT images performed through the upper (A), mid (B), and lower (C) lungs obtained during inspiration (see Video 140.2) in a bilateral lung transplant recipient show only minimal inhomogeneous lung opacity. Expiratory chest CT images performed through the upper (D), middle (E), and lower (F) lungs show extensive accentuation of the bilateral inhomogeneous opacity (see Video 140.3). The areas of increased attenuation represent normal collapsing lung during exhalation. The areas of relatively decreased attenuation (*arrowheads*) represent air trapping due to constrictive bronchiolitis as a result of chronic rejection.

Computed tomography (CT) scans or magnetic resonance imaging with hyperpolarized gases, similarly, may demonstrate inhomogeneity of ventilation and air trapping (Fig. 72.1, see Video 140.3); see also Chapter 10).

DEFINING BRONCHIOLITIS

Bronchiolitis refers to a nonspecific cellular and mesenchymal reaction of the bronchioles. Developing a straightforward classification, however, is difficult. Perhaps most important, bronchiolitis is a catchall term subsuming several unique clinical syndromes and a histopathologically diverse set of lesions identifiable in many diseases. Next, there are many diseases that, in addition to causing bronchiolitis, also cause disease proximal (e.g., bronchiectasis) or distal (e.g., organizing pneumonia) to the bronchioles. As a result, some avoid defining the precise site of involvement, instead referring to peripheral airways (<2 mm diameter) as small airways. Lastly, clinical bronchiolitis syndromes may demonstrate more than one histologic pattern temporally and spatially. These factors complicate defining a mutually exclusive classification system. Therefore, definitive diagnosis of a specific bronchiolitis entity requires clinical, diagnostic (imaging, PFTs), and frequently histopathologic evaluation. Definitive diagnosis depends on excluding bronchial and alveolar involvement seen in alternative diagnoses. A hybrid classification schema based on both histopathologic findings and clinical syndromes is presented in Fig. 72.2. The early branch points in this schema are driven by histopathologic findings, whereas later branch points are driven by clinical syndromes and exposures.

INFLAMMATORY AND INFECTIOUS BRONCHIOLITIS

This group of bronchiolitis syndromes involve inflammation or infection and are characterized by a predominantly cellular infiltration of the bronchioles. Cellular infiltration can be localized to the wall (mural) or lie within or around the bronchiole (Fig. 72.2).

INFLAMMATORY BRONCHIOLITIS

Infectious Bronchiolitis

Although relatively rare in adults, acute *infectious bronchiolitis* is common in infants and young children. Indeed, within the pediatric population, this entity is referred to simply as bronchiolitis. *Respiratory syncytial virus* infection is the cause of 70% of infectious bronchiolitis, although rhinovirus, metapneumovirus, influenza virus, and other viral and bacterial infections can also cause this syndrome.[3] Infection damages bronchiolar epithelial cells. Edema, epithelial sloughing, ciliary dysfunction, and mucus secretion result in small airway obstruction and atelectasis. In severe cases, there may be peribronchiolar lymphocytic infiltration and even mural necrosis (Fig. 72.3A, see Fig. 72.2 [classified under the category inflammatory bronchiolitis]). Bronchiolitis within the first few years of life can result in protracted wheezing and asthma development, particularly through the first decade and possibly into adulthood. Long-term sequelae appear to be modified by genetic and environmental factors, including environmental tobacco smoke exposure.[4]

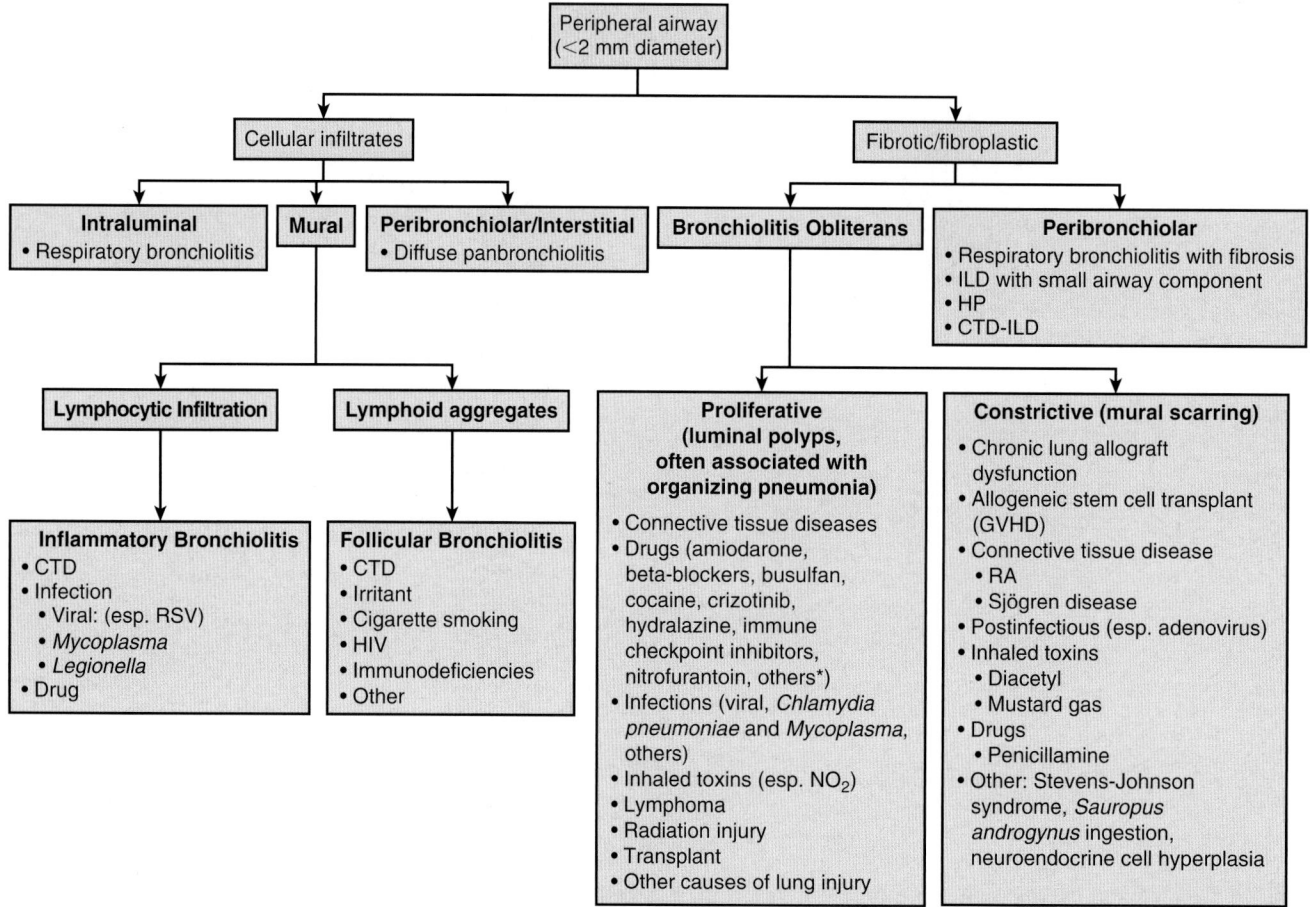

Figure 72.2 Classification schema for bronchiolitis. Traditionally, bronchiolitis has been defined by clinical syndromes and histopathologic lesions, making classification difficult. In this schema, early classification branch points are defined by histopathologic findings (e.g., cellular infiltrates in the small airways vs. fibrosis). Later branch points are defined by specific clinical entities. *See http://pneumotox.com/ for a complete list. CTD, connective tissue disease; esp., especially; GVHD, graft-versus-host disease; HIV, human immunodeficiency virus; HP, hypersensitivity pneumonitis; ILD, interstitial lung disease; NO$_2$, nitrogen dioxide; RA, rheumatoid arthritis; RSV, respiratory syncytial virus.

Typically affecting children younger than 2 years, bronchiolitis begins as an acute upper respiratory tract infection with rhinorrhea, nasal congestion, and/or cough. Within days the cough worsens, and dyspnea and fever develop. Although wheezing, chest wall retractions, and cyanosis may be seen, respiratory failure is uncommon. Examination typically demonstrates mildly depressed oxygen saturation, tachypnea, mild chest wall retractions, expiratory wheezing, and crackles. In more severe cases, nasal flaring, grunting, pronounced chest wall retractions, prolonged expiratory phase, and cyanosis may be seen. Epithelial sloughing with bronchiolar obstruction may cause hyperinflation and gas exchange abnormalities.[5] In general, infectious bronchiolitis is diagnosed based on clinical signs and symptoms. When obtained, radiographs may be normal or have evidence of pneumonia or bronchitis, whereas focal consolidation may be indicative of bacterial coinfection.[6,7] Outpatient supportive therapy with nasal bulb suctioning and hydration is usually sufficient, but some patients require hospitalization for fluid administration and/or respiratory support. This self-limiting infection typically resolves within weeks. A number of studies have investigated additional therapies and shown no clear evidence of benefit for bronchodilators,

corticosteroids, antibiotics, chest physiotherapy, or leukotriene inhibitors.[8,9] Of note, respiratory syncytial virus–specific monoclonal antibody therapies have not proven efficacious for acute management but are recommended as prophylaxis for selected high-risk infants.[8,10]

RESPIRATORY BRONCHIOLITIS

Respiratory bronchiolitis (RB) is a pathologic entity characterized by pigmented alveolar macrophage accumulation in respiratory bronchioles and adjacent alveoli. Peribronchiolar inflammation or fibrosis and epithelial metaplasia extending into adjacent alveoli (i.e., lambertosis) may be present (see Fig. 72.3B). Although nearly universally seen in cigarette smokers, it may also be seen after particulate exposures.[11–13] RB rarely causes symptoms or physiologic abnormalities per se. It is most commonly diagnosed incidentally by imaging (see Fig. 72.2 [classified under the intraluminal category]). In some cases, more extensive fibrosis extends into the alveolar septa and is associated with clinical and radiographic evidence of interstitial pneumonia. In these cases, the term *RB-associated interstitial lung disease* (RB-ILD) is applied (see Chapter 90).[11,12] In

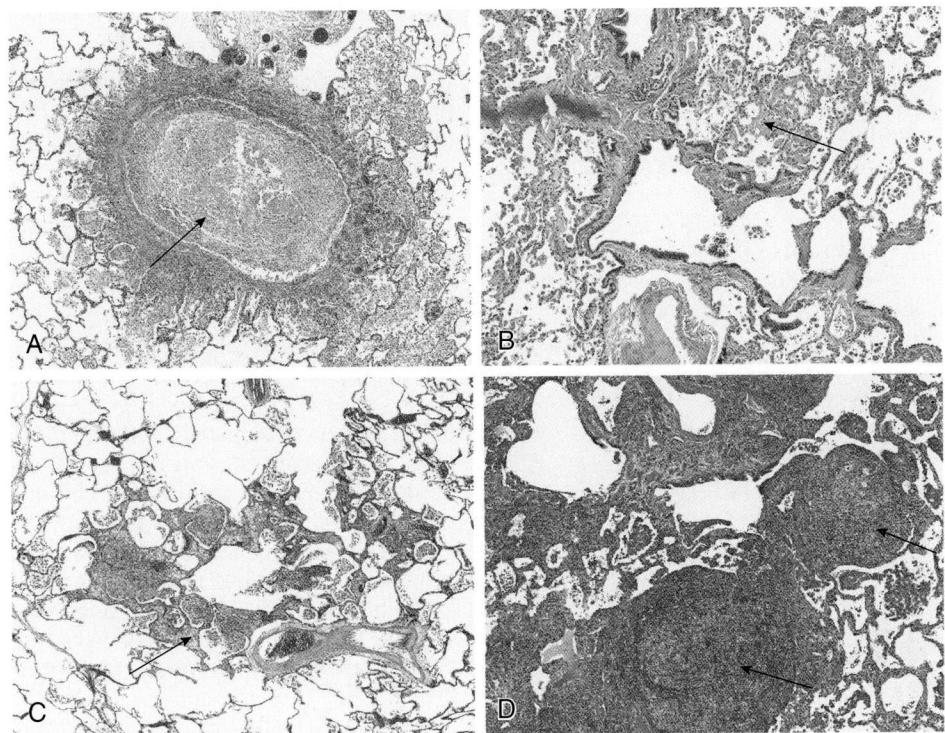

Figure 72.3 Pathologic patterns of bronchiolitis. (A) Infectious bronchiolitis. The bronchiolar wall shows marked acute inflammation with neutrophils and apoptotic debris (*arrow*) extending from the sloughed epithelial surface transmurally to the adjacent alveolar spaces. (B) Respiratory bronchiolitis. The terminal bronchiole and peribronchiolar alveolar spaces show consolidation by lightly pigmented "smoker's" alveolar macrophages (*arrow*). Mild peribronchiolar fibrosis is present. (C) Diffuse panbronchiolitis. The terminal bronchiole shows mural lymphoid inflammation, luminal inflammation and organization, and peribronchiolar interstitial expansion by foamy macrophages (*arrow*). (D) Follicular bronchiolitis. Prominent lymphoid aggregates with well-formed germinal centers (*arrow*) are noted adjacent to bronchioles.

RB-ILD, patients present with subacute cough, dyspnea, and crackles, as well as restriction and reduced diffusing capacity on PFTs.[14] *High-resolution computed tomography* (HRCT) imaging shows a distinctive pattern of bronchial wall thickening, centrilobular nodules, reticulation, and diffuse or patchy ground-glass opacities.[15,16] Smoking cessation leads to resolution or stabilization of disease in most patients, and the risk of progression to respiratory failure and death appears less than is observed with the related smoking-associated ILD—desquamative interstitial pneumonia.[17] Subjective and objective improvements after corticosteroid treatment have been described but not studied prospectively.[17]

DIFFUSE PANBRONCHIOLITIS

Diffuse panbronchiolitis (DPB) is an unusual inflammatory disease of the respiratory bronchioles. Formally described in 1969, a 1982 survey in Japan estimated a prevalence of 11 cases per 100,000 people.[18,19] Although reported outside of East Asia, this entity is predominantly observed among those with Japanese ancestry, which may reflect an increased prevalence of genetic risk factors.[20,21] On histologic examination, DPB is characterized by the triad of bronchiolocentric inflammation, lymphoid hyperplasia, and accumulation of interstitial foam cells (see Fig. 72.2 [classified under the category peribronchiolar/interstitial] and Fig. 72.3C).[22–24] Of note, similar findings are also seen in bronchiectasis, underscoring the importance

of developing a diagnostic approach to bronchiolitis that considers clinical, functional, radiographic, and histopathologic findings.

Given the rarity of DPB, epidemiologic data are limited. Clinically, DPB has a slight male predilection, and symptoms manifest in early to mid-adulthood.[19,20,24] Chronic sinusitis is exceedingly common and frequently precedes pulmonary symptoms. Before diagnosis, patients report years of nasal discharge or congestion, cough, dyspnea, and sputum production that exceeds 50 mL/day.[25] Radiographs demonstrate hyperinflation, diffuse small nodular opacities and, in advanced disease, ring shadows and "tram track" opacities consistent with bronchiectasis. In early disease, HRCT findings may include centrilobular nodules, sometimes termed a tree-in-bud pattern, and air trapping on expiratory images. Mosaic perfusion is atypical. In advanced disease, bronchiolar wall thickening, dilation, and cysts are seen.[26,27] PFTs demonstrate a progressive airflow obstruction with reduced diffusing capacity. Less commonly, a mixed obstructive-restrictive pattern may be observed.[21] Although clinical diagnostic criteria have been proposed for Japan, surgical lung biopsy is required in countries and populations in which the disease is rare.[20] If untreated, DPB leads to bronchiectasis, pulmonary hypertension, respiratory failure, and ultimately death. Although the etiology of DPB remains obscure, both genetic and environmental factors are believed to be important.[28–31] *Human leukocyte antigen* (HLA)-Bw54 is associated with a 13-fold increase in risk for diffuse panbronchiolitis.[29] Polymorphisms of the genes for *interleukin* (IL)-8[30] and mucins[31,32] have been associated with diffuse panbronchiolitis.

Macrolides are the cornerstone of treatment.[33] As with macrolide therapy for other forms of bronchiolitis, their salutary effects likely involve a variety of immunomodulatory mechanisms rather than antimicrobial properties.[34,35] More than 40 studies have described these immunomodulatory effects across a variety of disease states. Within diffuse panbronchiolitis, the most consistently reported effect of macrolides is suppression of neutrophilic airway inflammation, with associated decreases in neutrophil chemoattractants and other proinflammatory cytokines.[36] Of note, 14- and 15-membered lactone ring macrolides (e.g., erythromycin, clarithromycin, azithromycin) are effective in treating DPB, whereas 16-membered lactone ring macrolides (e.g., tylosin, spiramycin) are not. Macrolide therapy is generally continued for at least 6 months.[33] For severe cases, lung transplantation has been performed, although the disease may recur in the allograft.[37]

Originally DPB was a highly fatal disease. In the 1980s, 5- and 10-year survivals were approximately 62% and 33%, respectively. With macrolide therapy, increased disease diagnosis, and early, aggressive treatment of bacterial infections, 10-year survival now exceeds 90%.[34] Recurrent respiratory infections are common, and *Pseudomonas* infection, often arising late in the disease, is associated with markedly increased mortality.[20]

FOLLICULAR BRONCHIOLITIS

Follicular bronchiolitis (lymphoid hyperplasia) is characterized by peribronchiolar hyperplastic lymphoid follicles with germinal centers (see Fig. 72.3D).[38,39] These follicles, which have high endothelial venules, lymphatics, and defined zones with T cells and B cells with follicular dendritic cells, resemble Peyer patches in the gut and are termed *bronchus-associated lymphoid tissue* (BALT).[39] BALT is commonly observed in transbronchial biopsies from lung transplant recipients and is not generally thought to be pathologic in this context. Indeed, in mouse lung transplant models, BALT regulatory T cells were necessary for protection against antibody-mediated rejection.[40]

BALT hyperplasia is pathognomonic for follicular bronchiolitis. Although idiopathic primary pulmonary lymphoid hyperplasia has been described, follicular bronchiolitis commonly indicates pulmonary involvement of a systemic immunologic condition, such as rheumatoid arthritis, Sjögren syndrome, lupus, *coatomer-associated protein subunit alpha syndrome* (COPA), human immunodeficiency virus, Evans syndrome, bronchiectasis, and other infections or immunodeficiencies. It can also be seen in association with smoking or other irritants and other airway or interstitial lung disease states[39,41] (see Fig. 72.2 [classified under the lymphoid aggregates category]).

Clinical symptoms of follicular bronchiolitis are often mild, with cough and dyspnea being most consistently reported.[42,43] PFT findings may show restrictive, obstructive, or mixed patterns. HRCT findings include small (<3 mm) centrilobular or peribronchial nodules and ground-glass opacities.[44] Treatment is directed at the underlying disease.

BRONCHIOLITIS OBLITERANS

Bronchiolitis obliterans can be stratified into constrictive and proliferative bronchiolitis. Although there is some overlap between these entities, this stratification is largely supported by histopathologic and clinical evidence. Unique entities featuring bronchiolitis obliterans are listed in Fig. 72.2; more common entities are discussed in greater detail later.

Histologically, constrictive bronchiolitis defines a submucosal and peribronchiolar fibrotic process that circumferentially and externally compresses the bronchiolar lumen (Fig. 72.4A). Patchy and focal in distribution, progressive fibrosis observed in constrictive bronchiolitis ultimately results in slit-like or completely obliterated bronchiolar lumens. Clinically, patients describe progressive dyspnea and nonproductive cough. Auscultation demonstrates early inspiratory crackles and occasional squeaks. PFTs performed late in the course of disease demonstrate obstruction and air trapping. Radiographs may have normal findings or show hyperinflation. HRCT can demonstrate ground-glass nodules, air trapping and, in advanced disease, bronchiectasis. Currently, the most common presentation of constrictive bronchiolitis is in the context of *chronic lung allograft dysfunction* (CLAD) after lung transplantation.[45]

Histologically, proliferative bronchiolitis is defined by the proliferation of transluminal polypoid organizing fibroblastic tissue, also known as a Masson body (see Fig. 72.4B).[46] Isolated proliferative bronchiolitis is rare, observed only in specific inhalational (e.g., nitrogen gas) exposures or localized injuries. Much more commonly, fibroblastic tissue extends from the bronchioles into adjacent alveoli. The term organizing pneumonia defines this organizing fibroblastic tissue in alveoli. Given the relatively common coexistence of proliferative bronchiolitis and organizing pneumonia, the term *bronchiolitis obliterans with organizing pneumonia* (BOOP) had been used. There is little overlap, however, between the clinical entities featuring constrictive bronchiolitis and those featuring BOOP. Furthermore, BOOP presents as a restrictive pattern on PFTs compared with the obstructive pattern seen in constrictive bronchiolitis. For these reasons, this nomenclature caused confusion and, in response to this confusion, in 2002 the American Thoracic Society and European Respiratory Society jointly recommended abandoning the term BOOP in favor of organizing pneumonia with appropriate qualifiers. When idiopathic, the term cryptogenic organizing pneumonia is used[47] (see Chapter 90). In rare situations, acute injury causing proliferative bronchiolitis may progress into constrictive bronchiolitis.

Despite this evolution in nomenclature, "bronchiolitis obliterans" continues to be used imprecisely in clinical practice and in the biomedical literature. The terms BOOP, bronchiolitis obliterans with intraluminal polyps, and bronchiolitis obliterans applied to both bronchiolitis obliterans and organizing pneumonia persist. Of importance, organizing pneumonia tends to be responsive to corticosteroid treatment, whereas constrictive bronchiolitis is typically resistant. This absence of a precise nomenclature makes studies of the epidemiology, clinical features, and treatment responsiveness of "bronchiolitis obliterans" difficult to interpret. Given the substantial differences in both etiology

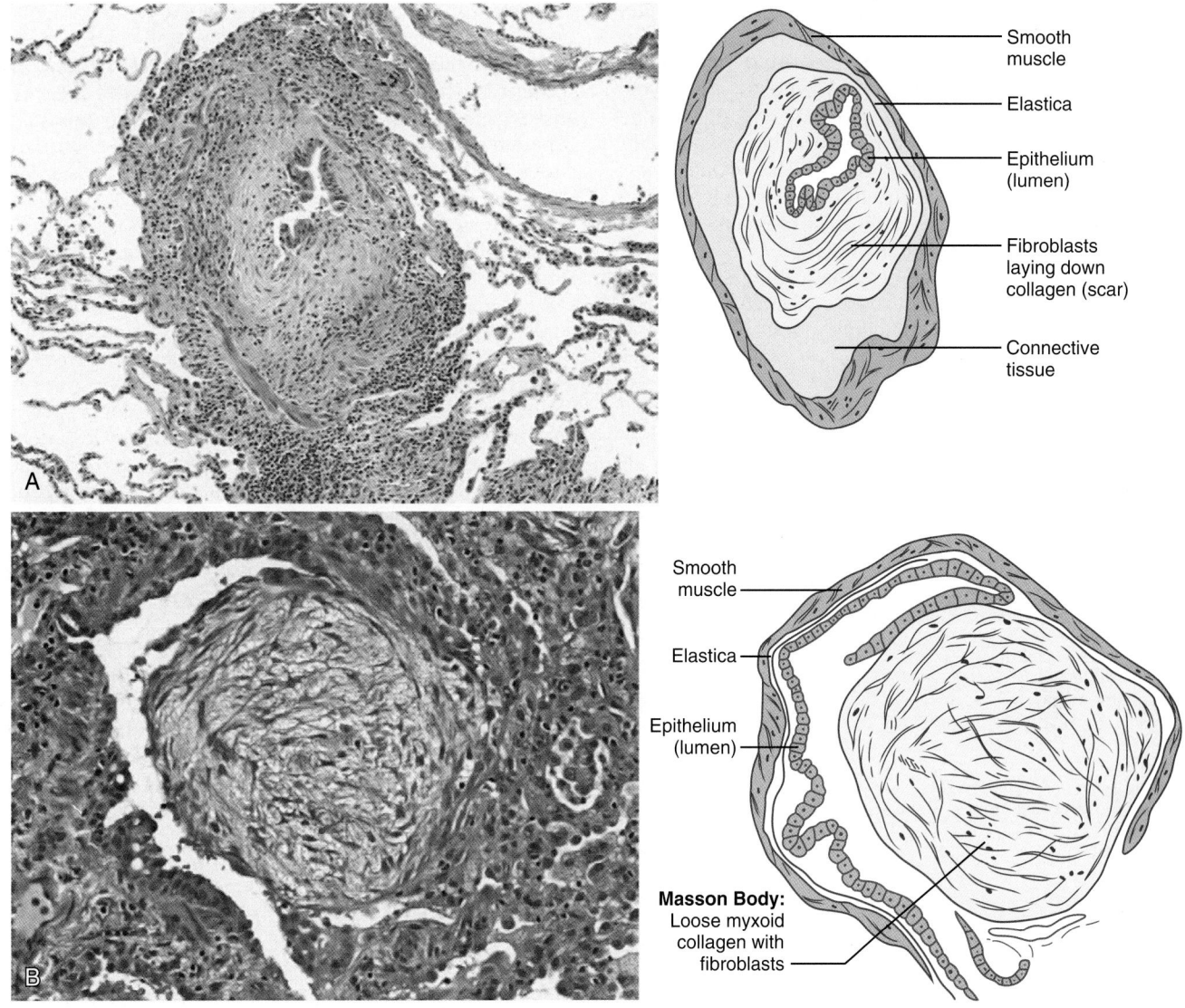

Figure 72.4 Pathologic patterns of bronchiolitis obliterans. (A) Constrictive bronchiolitis. Circumferential subepithelial intramural fibrosis is present. This fibrosis separates the normally approximated epithelium and elastica (the elastin-rich layer of the lamina propria). This scarring results in luminal constriction and narrowing, often with irreversible complete obstruction. (B) Proliferative bronchiolitis. Although the diameter of the airway remains unchanged, the functional area of the lumen is reduced by a rounded intraluminal polypoid plug of granulation tissue, extending from the subepithelium and filling the airway lumen (also known as a Masson body).

and prognosis, we favor using the terms *constrictive* and *proliferative* to define these bronchiolitis subtypes more clearly.

Although these categories are defined histopathologically, in practice, there is a lot of overlap. We will discuss the following entities, which are mostly constrictive but may exhibit proliferative features as well.

CONSTRICTIVE BRONCHIOLITIS AFTER LUNG TRANSPLANTATION (See Chapter 140)

Chronic Lung Allograft Dysfunction

Since the late 1980s, there have been steady increases in the rates of lung transplantation performed, with more than 4500 procedures worldwide in 2016. Although survival rates are improved compared with the pre-2008 era, the median posttransplantation survival is only 6.5 years.[48] The most common cause of death after the first year posttransplantation is *chronic lung allograft dysfunction* (CLAD).[49] CLAD is a clinical syndrome of obstructive or restrictive defects defined by a persistent, greater than 20% decline in *forced expiratory volume in 1 second* (FEV$_1$) from posttransplantation baseline, with baseline defined as the average of the two best posttransplantation FEV$_1$ measurements taken more than 3 weeks apart (see Table 72.1). Constrictive bronchiolitis is the most common pathologic feature in CLAD and is thought to be the main cause of decline in FEV$_1$, particularly for the predominantly obstructive form of CLAD, known as *bronchiolitis obliterans syndrome* (BOS). Registry data show the majority of lung transplant recipients die or develop CLAD within 4 years.[45] The presence of a total lung capacity decline of 10% or more and persistent chest CT opacifications define the restrictive allograft syndrome subtype of CLAD, for which pleural and/ or parenchymal fibrotic pathology are also associated.[50]

Adding to the confusion, this terminology has changed over time. Until 2014, BOS was defined as any decline in FEV_1, without regard to *forced vital capacity* (FVC), similar to what is currently called CLAD.[51,52] From 2014 to 2019, CLAD was defined by a decline in FEV_1 *or* FVC.[53] Since 2019, BOS has been considered only the obstructive subtype of CLAD, and CLAD is diagnosed only based on FEV_1.[49] Nonetheless, even in patients meeting criteria for restrictive allograft syndrome, explant tissue typically demonstrates concomitant constrictive bronchiolitis.

Various factors can cause persistent FEV_1 loss in lung transplant recipients, thought to be unrelated to CLAD or constrictive bronchiolitis, including chest wall disease, pleural effusions, pulmonary edema, airway stenosis, obesity, aging, diaphragmatic dysfunction, native lung hyperinflation, or scarring from focal infections. For these, the consensus definition recommends a resetting of the FEV_1 baseline once such factors have been stable for 6 months.[49] Whether or not this FEV_1 baseline is reset in practice, patients with incipient CLAD should undergo an evaluation for these potential confounders, including CT scans and bronchoscopy. Chest CT can also be useful in evaluating for restrictive versus obstructive CLAD, which would be associated with fibrotic changes or air trapping, respectively[54,55] (see Fig. 72.1 and Video 140.3). Transbronchial biopsy can be used to evaluate for acute rejection pathology but only rarely demonstrates histopathologic evidence of constrictive bronchiolitis.

The onset of CLAD is variable based on donor, recipient, and environmental factors (discussed later). Patients report progressive dyspnea and, occasionally, dry cough. In advanced disease with bronchiectasis, the cough is productive. Pulmonary function tests demonstrate irreversible airflow obstruction with reduced diffusing capacity. As CLAD progresses, findings consistent with bronchiectasis may be seen.

Table 72.1 Chronic Lung Allograft Dysfunction Classification System

CLAD 0	$FEV_1 > 80\%$ of baseline*
CLAD 1	$FEV_1 > 65–80\%$ of baseline
CLAD 2	$FEV_1 > 50–65\%$ of baseline
CLAD 3	$FEV_1 > 35–50\%$ of baseline
CLAD 4	$FEV_1 \le 35\%$ of baseline

*Baseline is the average of the two best *forced expiratory volume in 1 second* (FEV_1) measurements that are more than 3 weeks apart but can be adjusted in the case of 6 months of stability for certain non–*chronic lung allograft dysfunction* (CLAD) causes.
Modified from Verleden GM, Glanville AR, Lease ED, et al. Chronic lung allograft dysfunction: definition, diagnostic criteria, and approaches to treatment—a consensus report from the Pulmonary Council of the ISHLT. *J Heart Lung Transplant*. 2019;38:493–503.

Chronic Lung Allograft Dysfunction Pathogenesis. Constrictive bronchiolitis is likely a final histologic lesion resulting from a failure in epithelial cell regeneration in the context of chronic, predominantly alloimmune injury (Fig. 72.5). Emerging evidence suggests that epithelial integrity requires active signaling to prevent proliferation of the adjacent mesenchyme so that when damage to the epithelium

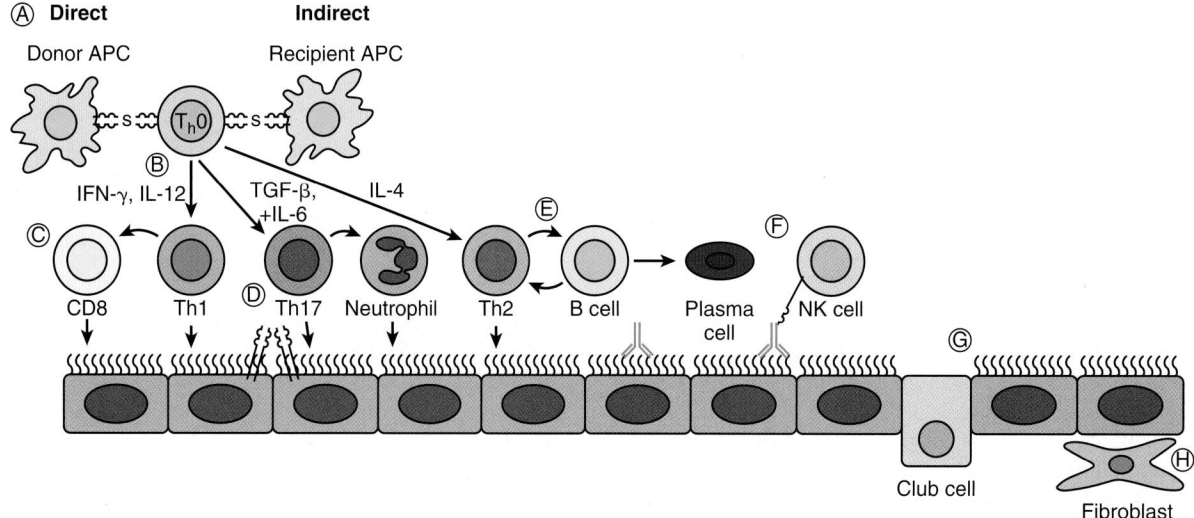

Figure 72.5 Overview of chronic lung allograft dysfunction pathogenesis. (A) Donor antigens are presented on donor *major histocompatibility complex* (MHC) (directly) or on recipient MHC (indirectly) to T cells. (B) T cells differentiate based on the local cytokine milieu into *T helper* (Th)1, Th2, or Th17 subtypes of CD4 cells and activated CD8 cells. (C) These cell types cause direct cytotoxicity in areas of vascular endothelium, manifest as A-grade rejection, and airway epithelium, termed B-grade rejection. (D) Airway injury drives epithelial cell damage responses, such as up-regulation of MHC leading to further amplification of alloimmune responses. (E) B cells interact with T cells and *antigen-presenting cells* (APCs), generating antibodies and differentiating into long-lived antibody-secreting plasma cells. (F) Antibodies also contribute to epithelial cell damage through complement fixation, direct cytotoxicity, or in concert with natural killer (NK) cells via antibody-dependent cell-mediated cytotoxicity. (G) Club cells and other cells responsible for protecting and regenerating the epithelium may initially compensate for the increased epithelial cell turnover but are eventually exhausted, particularly in the setting of compromised vasculature associated with transplantation. (H) Fibroproliferative cells may then replace denuded airway and commit the epithelium to fibrotic replacement via autocrine signaling. Of note, these steps (A–F) of chronic lung allograft dysfunction pathogenesis may not happen in this order or at all in cases. IFN-γ, interferon-γ; IL, interleukin; TGF-β, transforming growth factor-β.

exceeds its capacity for repair, profibrotic cells are activated to patch the denuded airway.[56] This biology may explain why a deficiency of club cells, cells that both protect and repopulate bronchiolar epithelium, is associated with constrictive bronchiolitis.[57,58] Other factors limiting epithelial cell regeneration, such as microvascular injury or telomere dysfunction, are also linked to CLAD risk.[59,60] Similarly, processes that result in airway injury have been linked to CLAD, including primary graft dysfunction[61]; infection with *Pseudomonas*,[62] *Aspergillus*,[63] cytomegalovirus,[64] and other viruses[65,66]; air pollution[67]; and gastroesophageal reflux.[68] Bronchioles might be particularly susceptible to potentiating effects of air pollution because the increase in cross-sectional area related to branching in the bronchiolar region results in a slowing of airflow and a preferential accumulation of airborne particles in this region.[69] Once shunted toward a fibrotic pathway, mesenchymal cells can then become self-perpetuating, further hampering restoration of normal physiology.[70]

Cellular Immune Responses. Among injury responses, alloimmune injury appears most important to CLAD pathogenesis. CLAD risk is linked to acute cellular rejection episodes.[71] Acute cellular rejection of the lung allograft is diagnosed on transbronchial biopsy specimens as perivascular lymphocytosis or lymphocytic bronchiolitis, classified as A-grade and B-grade rejection, respectively, based on *International Society of Heart and Lung Transplantation* (ISHLT) nomenclature (see Chapter 140).[72] Lymphocytic bronchitis (in the large airways) has also been associated with CLAD risk.[73,74] Severity of acute rejection appears important because untreated "minimal" or A1-grade acute cellular rejection does not appear to increase CLAD risk.[74-76]

Enhanced expression of donor *major histocompatibility complex* (MHC) antigens has also been found in bronchiolar and alveolar epithelium of lung transplant recipients with acute rejection and CLAD, likely secondary to type 1 lymphocytic inflammation.[77,78] Donor MHC antigens presenting donor self-antigen are then recognized by the recipient immune system, further propagating alloimmune responses.[79] An increasing burden of donor-recipient HLA mismatches has also been shown to be a CLAD risk factor.[80] In addition to this direct pathway of allorejection, there is also indirect antigen presentation, where recipient antigen-presenting cells present phagocytosed donor antigens.[81] Calcineurin inhibitor–based immunosuppression targets this type 1 immune response. Indeed, the clinical success of lung transplantation is coincident with the advent of calcineurin inhibitors. Of interest, although variability in tacrolimus-based immunosuppression levels has been associated with CLAD, suggesting a detrimental effect of transient lack of immunosuppression,[82] supratherapeutic immunosuppression levels are associated with increased infection risk but no change in rates of acute rejection.[83] Thus, although type 1 immune responses are potentially a potent driver of CLAD, this pathway is effectively inhibited by current immunosuppression strategies, suggesting that other pathways could be responsible for CLAD in practice.

Type 17 and, to a lesser extent, type 2 alloreactive T cell responses are also associated with CLAD and appear to be relatively resistant to calcineurin inhibitors.[84] In particular, type 17 inflammation can recruit neutrophils, and neutrophilic inflammation has been linked to early development of CLAD. A syndrome of greater than 15% neutrophils in bronchoalveolar lavage, combined with a 10% or greater decline in FEV_1, is often reversible with azithromycin treatment, at which point it is termed *neutrophilic reversible allograft dysfunction* (NRAD).[85] Clinical features of NRAD overlap with lymphocytic airway inflammation, which is associated with IL-17 and can reverse after azithromycin treatment.[86] Mechanistically, tacrolimus paradoxically increases the IL-17–dependent production of the neutrophil chemoattractant chemokine IL-8 by airway smooth muscle cells, and this effect can be reversed by azithromycin.[87]

Humoral Immune Responses. Lung transplant recipients may develop antibodies to donor HLA antigens. The de novo development of *donor-specific antibodies* (DSAs), in particular to HLA-DQ, has been linked to more rapid onset of CLAD.[88] A syndrome of *antibody-mediated rejection* (AMR) can manifest as obstructive or restrictive pulmonary function defects; histopathologic features of neutrophil margination, capillaritis, and/or arteritis; complement component 4d deposition on alveolar capillaries; and serologic evidence of DSA. Although some patients present with indisputable AMR, diagnostic uncertainty is common. Thus the ISHLT definition of AMR groups patients into "definite," "probable," and "possible" categories based on the presence of allograft dysfunction and four, three, or two of the following features, respectively: DSA, complement component 4d staining on lung biopsy, compatible lung histology, and exclusion of other causes.[89] Even within this definition, there is disagreement on the criteria for the component features.

Lung transplant recipients with severe AMR have substantial morbidity. Thus, some lung transplantation centers have treated de novo DSA and AMR with combination therapy that includes some or all of the following: corticosteroids, intravenous immunoglobulin, plasmapheresis, monoclonal antibodies to the B cell antigen CD20, proteasome inhibitors, and complement inhibitors.[90] However, there are no randomized controlled trial data to guide therapy. Although clearance of DSA with therapy is associated with freedom from BOS,[91] it is not clear that interventions that result in DSA clearance improve outcomes.[92,93] Crosstalk between alloreactive type 2 and follicular helper T cells and B cells via cytokines and costimulatory molecules results in B cell activation and differentiation into plasma cells. Thus, persistence of DSA may also be a biomarker for alloimmune responses more broadly.

Other Immune Responses. Autoimmune responses may also contribute to the development of CLAD. Lung injury may expose self-antigens that would otherwise be masked from the immune system. Type V collagen and K-α1 tubulin, in particular, are expressed in small airway epithelial cells and exposed during rejection and lung remodeling. Autoantibodies to these proteins are risk factors for CLAD in humans.[94] In rodent models, these autoantibodies can be induced by anti-MHC antibodies, and induction of tolerance to type V collagen can protect from allograft rejection in rodent models.[95]

Finally, innate immune responses play key roles in potentiating adaptive immune responses in the context of lung transplantation. Single nucleotide polymorphisms in innate immune genes, such as *toll-like receptor 4* (TLR4), have been linked to CLAD.[96] Natural killer cells are postulated to play important roles in both amplifying and dampening alloimmune responses, in primary graft dysfunction, in AMR, and in responses to infections.[97]

BRONCHIOLITIS OBLITERANS SYNDROME AFTER ALLOGENEIC STEM CELL TRANSPLANTATION

Although a mismatch between lung and immune system MHC antigens is present in both lung transplantation and allogeneic stem cell transplantation, constrictive bronchiolitis appears less frequent after the latter. In the context of allogeneic stem cell transplantation, the clinical syndrome of constrictive bronchiolitis is termed BOS, and the distinction between restrictive and obstructive forms of chronic lung dysfunction is not generally addressed. The comparison between these two contexts of BOS is complicated by differences in definitions, however. Pulmonary *graft-versus-host disease* (GVHD) resembles constrictive bronchiolitis histologically after lung transplantation. However, surgical lung biopsies are rarely performed to confirm the diagnosis, given the potential surgical risk. Thus, pulmonary GVHD is generally diagnosed as the clinical syndrome termed BOS.

BOS was defined in a 2014 consensus statement by the presence of all four of the following criteria: (1) an obstructive FEV_1/slow vital capacity ratio, (2) FEV_1 less than 75% of predicted with a 10% or greater decline over 2 years, (3) absence of infection, and (4) either evidence of extrapulmonary GVHD or evidence of air trapping by CT or spirometry.[98] With this definition, one study estimated the prevalence of GVHD at about 10% at 36 months after transplantation.[99] Other studies suggest a prevalence of as low as 2–3% at a similar time point after transplantation.[100] More liberal pulmonary GVHD diagnostic criteria have been proposed. For example, post–stem cell transplantation airflow obstruction, defined as greater than 5% per year decline in FEV_1 and minimum FEV_1/FVC of less than 0.8, has a reported prevalence of 26%.[101]

BOS is usually preceded or accompanied by typical findings of GVHD: mucositis, esophagitis, and/or skin rash.[102] Four to 6 months after the onset of GVHD, patients may develop dyspnea and a nonproductive cough that may be severe and rapidly progressive. Physical examination may reveal scattered wheezing and frequently bibasilar crackles. Hypoxemia is common.[100] Spirometry and radiographic findings are similar to those observed in BOS in lung transplantation.

Extrapulmonary GVHD, including skin, gastrointestinal, or hepatic inflammation, is the most significant risk factor for BOS. Other risk factors include a busulfan-containing preparative regimen, stem cells from the peripheral blood, viral infections, lung disease pre–stem cell or post–stem cell transplantation, and ABO blood type incompatibility.[103] Its rarity after autologous stem cell transplantation implies an association with alloimmune responses, but the pathogenesis remains incompletely understood. Quarterly spirometry for at least 1 to 2 years after allogenic stem cell transplantation and with new manifestations of GVHD can aid in early identification of BOS.[103] Mild declines in FEV_1 can be treated with inhaled corticosteroids with or without an inhaled β_2-agonist. With the diagnosis of BOS, treatment with a tapered steroid burst and initiation of fluticasone, azithromycin, and montelukast ("FAM") treatment are recommended.[104] Calcineurin inhibitors, lymphocyte proliferation inhibitors (e.g., mycophenolic acid), or sirolimus for systemic GVHD are generally continued. Additional therapies, including extracorporeal photopheresis and etanercept, have been added in cases of continued progression, without clear evidence of efficacy.[103] A trial of azithromycin for the prevention of post–stem cell transplantation GVHD was stopped early because of increased mortality attributed to the risk of hematologic relapse, so prophylactic azithromycin is generally not recommended.[105]

BRONCHIOLITIS OBLITERANS AND CONNECTIVE TISSUE DISEASES

Constrictive bronchiolitis may present uncommonly with connective tissue or collagen vascular diseases, in particular, rheumatoid arthritis.[106] It predominantly affects women who are at least 10 years out from a rheumatoid arthritis diagnosis. Patients present with rapid onset of progressive dyspnea, nonproductive cough, and spirometric evidence of airflow obstruction. In a case series, all-cause mortality was 27% over a median follow-up of 5 years, with FEV_1 stabilization achieved in the context of (although not necessarily because of) steroids, macrolide antibiotics, and other immunosuppression therapies.[107] Cases of constrictive bronchiolitis have also been reported with Sjögren syndrome.[108] Older literature linking bronchiolitis obliterans and other connective tissue diseases frequently refers to BOOP which, as discussed earlier, is a distinct pathobiology.

BRONCHIOLITIS OBLITERANS AFTER INFECTION

Although acute infectious bronchiolitis is common in children, postinfectious bronchiolitis obliterans is quite rare. The syndrome is defined by persistent airway obstruction, as assessed by symptoms, imaging, and spirometry, subsequent to a lower respiratory tract infection and unresponsive to at least 2 weeks of steroids and bronchodilators.[109] Despite similarity in the names, this disease entity appears distinct from acute bronchiolitis. Postinfectious bronchiolitis obliterans is most common in South America and linked to adenovirus infection, rather than respiratory syncytial virus infection. This epidemiologic difference has been linked to more potent T helper type 1 immune responses associated with adenoviral infection.[110] There are no well-controlled studies to guide management of these patients. Although lung function generally improves in pediatric patients, defects may persist.[111]

BRONCHIOLITIS FROM INHALED OR INGESTED TOXINS

A generalized inflammatory response of the peripheral airways may follow inhalation of toxicants in gases, vapors, fumes, or aerosols (see Chapter 103). The location of damage is determined in part by the toxicant solubility. Highly soluble irritants, such as sulfur dioxide and ammonia, dissolve in the lining fluid of the upper airway, causing damage primarily there. Less soluble gases, such as oxides of nitrogen, are able to pass into and therefore damage the peripheral airways.[112] Such exposures continue to represent significant industrial and environmental hazards.[113] Nitrogen dioxide for example, may be found in silo gas (silo filler's disease), jet and missile fuel, metal pickling fumes, and certain fires. Exposure results in an acute respiratory distress syndrome that evolves to proliferative bronchiolitis.[114] Acutely, patients may develop cough, dyspnea, cyanosis, hemoptysis, hypoxemia, and loss of consciousness. These symptoms and signs may last hours to weeks before resolving. Corticosteroid therapy is frequently used in the initial management, based on limited evidence.[113] Although most patients recover, some may die from respiratory failure. Finally, some patients develop irreversible obstructive abnormalities 2 to 8 weeks after exposure. Persistent obstruction may even be seen in patients who had no initial illness. Rather, these patients typically have a gradual onset of dyspnea and nonproductive cough that may progress to respiratory failure and death.[115]

Diacetyl and other alpha-diketones used in flavoring food have been linked to proliferative and constrictive bronchiolitis (see Fig. 72.2). These fumes are a particular risk in occupational settings where these chemicals are heated or powdered. In popcorn manufacturing, diacetyl-related constrictive bronchiolitis is termed popcorn lung.[116] Exposed workers are at increased risk for obstructive lung disease that may present with cough, wheeze, or dyspnea.[117] Diacetyl may directly activate fibroproliferative pathways in airway epithelial cells[118] or initiate autoimmune responses through hapten formation.[119] Diacetyl is found in many consumer products, including electronic cigarettes, although constrictive bronchiolitis from exposures outside of industrial settings appears extremely unusual.[116] Minimizing exposure and spirometric screening are reasonable prevention strategies.

Constrictive bronchiolitis has been reported through military exposures. A cohort of Iranian soldiers exposed to mustard gas during the Iran-Iraq war were found to have an increased frequency of chronic respiratory symptoms; a subset of these were diagnosed with constrictive bronchiolitis based on HRCT and, in some cases, lung biopsy. Minimal progression of obstruction was observed on spirometry, with a regimen including inhaled corticosteroid and long-acting β-agonist, azithromycin, and N-acetylcysteine.[120] A cohort of soldiers from the United States with otherwise unexplained dyspnea had a high prevalence of constrictive bronchiolitis based on surgical lung biopsy,[121] but subsequent studies have not confirmed this association.[122]

A number of other inhaled and ingested toxins have been linked to constrictive bronchiolitis. Treatment with penicillamine and gold have been linked to constrictive bronchiolitis, although in some cases it may be difficult to distinguish between medication effect and underlying disease.[123] *Sauropus androgynus*, a leafy vegetable popular in Asia and ingested for its slimming properties, has been linked to hundreds of cases of constrictive bronchiolitis.[124] Inhalational exposure during preparation of fiberglass with polymer resin and methylethyl ketone peroxide catalyst has been attributed as the cause of constrictive bronchiolitis among boat workers.[125]

TREATMENT OF CONSTRICTIVE AND PROLIFERATIVE BRONCHIOLITIS

Therapies to reverse the small airway remodeling observed in constrictive bronchiolitis have been largely ineffective. However, therapies to prevent progression of injuries preceding constrictive bronchiolitis have met with some success. In the case of exposure to toxic fumes, for example, corticosteroid therapy for organizing pneumonia or fibroproliferative bronchiolitis appears helpful.[126] In other contexts outside of lung transplantation, a trial of corticosteroids should be considered when there is evidence of these inflammatory bronchiolitis pathologies. If a response is identified, the corticosteroid should be continued for at least 2 to 3 months, then reduced slowly, to minimize the likelihood of relapse. In some cases it may be necessary to continue low-dose or alternate-day therapy for months or years.[127]

In the case of CLAD, azithromycin therapy has demonstrated efficacy in preventing progression and reversing acute airflow obstruction in a randomized trial.[128] This is thought to be particularly true for the subset of patients with NRAD; however, reversal of airway neutrophilia is not consistently linked to efficacy. Separately, prophylactic treatment with azithromycin started at the time of discharge from the initial transplantation was shown to be protective against CLAD development.[129] However, another trial of prophylactic azithromycin did not find evidence of protection from CLAD.[130] Together, these data suggest that macrolide therapy can be important for a subset of lung transplant recipients, but its efficacy for CLAD is modest when compared with its efficacy for diffuse panbronchiolitis.

Substantial attention is paid to identifying and treating other patient-specific risk factors for CLAD. Examples include surveillance bronchoscopy for acute rejection,[131] cytomegalovirus-specific antiviral prophylaxis,[132] reducing aspiration through lifestyle modifications and gastric fundoplication,[133] and treatment of certain community-acquired respiratory viral infections.[134-136]

Intensified corticosteroids do not improve outcomes for lung transplant recipients with CLAD. Of 30 lung transplant recipients randomized to the leukotriene inhibitor montelukast for CLAD, there was no overall benefit. Additional studies will be needed to determine whether certain subsets, such as those with milder airway dysfunction, might be more likely to benefit.[137] Extracorporeal photopheresis has been used to treat patients with CLAD but without high-quality evidence, and this therapy is the subject of an ongoing clinical trial.[138] Hydroxymethylglutaryl coenzyme A reductase inhibitors have been investigated for CLAD with mixed results.[139] Although there is little evidence that smooth muscle contraction plays a significant role, β-adrenergic agonists are frequently attempted to provide symptomatic relief. Lung transplantation is an option for some patients with CLAD and other forms of constrictive bronchiolitis.[140] After retransplantation, median CLAD-free survival is about 1 year less than after primary transplantation, based on registry data.[141]

Bronchopulmonary dysplasia, which has some features of bronchiolitis, is discussed at ExpertConsult.com.

Key Points

- Because of the large cross-sectional area of the peripheral airways, symptoms and physiologic changes of diseases involving the peripheral airways develop late in disease and can be silent.
- Bronchiolitis can be broadly categorized into inflammatory, proliferative, or constrictive subtypes.
- Inflammatory and proliferative bronchiolitis are more likely than constrictive bronchiolitis to be reversible or respond to immunosuppression. Certain bronchiolitis subtypes respond to macrolide antibiotics, especially diffuse panbronchiolitis and neutrophilic reversible allograft dysfunction.
- Constrictive bronchiolitis is the dominant pathology in chronic lung allograft dysfunction. Chronic lung allograft dysfunction is the major long-term limitation to survival after lung transplantation and appears to reflect multiple immune and nonimmune pathobiologies.
- Bronchiolitis obliterans after allogeneic stem cell transplantation results from chronic graft-versus-host disease.

Key Readings

Barker AF, Bergeron A, Rom WN, Hertz MI. Obliterative bronchiolitis. *N Engl J Med.* 2014;370(19):1820–1828.

Levine DJ, Glanville AR, Aboyoun C, et al. Antibody-mediated rejection of the lung: a consensus report of the International Society for Heart and Lung Transplantation. *J Heart Lung Transplant.* 2016;35(4):397–406.

Poletti V, Casoni G, Chilosi M, Zompatori M. Diffuse panbronchiolitis. *Eur Respir J.* 2006;28(4):862–871.

Verleden GM, Glanville AR, Lease ED, et al. Chronic lung allograft dysfunction: definition, diagnostic criteria, and approaches to treatment—a consensus report from the Pulmonary Council of the ISHLT. *J Heart Lung Transplant.* 2019;38(5):493–503.

Williams KM. How I treat bronchiolitis obliterans syndrome after hematopoietic stem cell transplantation. *Blood.* 2017;129(4):448–455.

Complete reference list available at ExpertConsult.com.

Index

Note: Page numbers followed by "f" indicate figures, "t" indicate tables, and "e" online-only material. Volume 1, pp 1-1004; Volume 2, pp 1005-1994.